12/25/05

To Mr. Paul Gordon —

Partner in neuro-archeology —
Digging for the roots of PLS —

All best wishes —
Buds Rosenzweig

MYOLOGY

NOTICE

Medicine is an ever-changing science. As new research and clinical experience broaden our knowledge, changes in treatment and drug therapy are required. The authors and the publisher of this work have checked with sources believed to be reliable in their efforts to provide information that is complete and generally in accord with the standards accepted at the time of publication. However, in view of the possibility of human error or changes in medical sciences, neither the authors nor the publisher nor any other party who has been involved in the preparation or publication of this work warrants that the information contained herein is in every respect accurate or complete, and they disclaim all responsibility for any errors or omissions or for the results obtained from use of the information contained in this work. Readers are encouraged to confirm the information contained herein with other sources. For example and in particular, readers are advised to check the product infomation sheet included in the package of each drug they plan to administer to be certain that the information contained in this work is accurate and that changes have not been made in the recommended dose or in the contraindications for administration. This recommendation is of particular importance in connection with new or infrequently used drugs.

MYOLOGY

BASIC AND CLINICAL

THIRD EDITION

VOLUME 1

EDITORS

Andrew G. Engel, M.D.
William L. McKnight Professor of Neuroscience
Mayo Clinic College of Medicine
Director, Neuromuscular Disease Research Laboratory
Consultant, Department of Neurology
Mayo Clinic
Rochester, Minnesota

Clara Franzini-Armstrong, Laurea
Professor, Department of Cell
and Developmental Biology
University of Pennsylvania School of Medicine
Philadelphia, Pennsylvania

McGraw-Hill
Medical Publishing Division

New York   Chicago   San Francisco   Lisbon   London   Madrid   Mexico City
Milan   New Delhi   San Juan   Seoul   Singapore   Sydney   Toronto

The **McGraw·Hill** Companies

Myology, Third Edition

Copyright © 2004, 1994, 1986 by The **McGraw-Hill** Companies, Inc. All rights reserved. Printed in the United States of America. Except as permitted under the United States copyright Act of 1976, no part of this publication may be reproduced or distributed in any form or by any means, or stored in a data base or retrieval system, without the prior written permission of the publisher.

1234567890 KGP KGP 0987654

   Set: ISBN 0-07-137180-X
Volume 1: ISBN 0-07-137181-8
Volume 2: IBBN 0-07-137182-6

This book was set in Palatino by PV&M Publishing Solutions.
The editors were Isabel Nogueira and Karen Davis.
The production supervisor was Catherine H. Saggese.
The cover designer was Janice Bielawa.
The index was prepared by Alexandra Nickerson.
Quebecor World/Kingsport was printer and binder.

This book is printed on acid-free paper.

Library of Congress Cataloging-in-Publication Data

Myology / Andrew G. Engel, Clara Franzini-Armstrong, [editors].—3rd ed.
   p. ; cm.
   Includes bibliographical references and index.
   ISBN 0-07-137180-X
   1. Muscles—Diseases.   2. Neuromuscular diseases.   3. Muscles—Physiology.
I. Engel, Andrew.   II. Franzini-Armstrong, Clara.
   [DNLM: 1. Muscles—anatomy & histology.   2. Muscles—physiology.
3. Neuromuscular Diseases.   WE 500 M997 2003]
RC925.M96 2003
616.7′4—dc21

2002043191

To Our Families, Students, and Coworkers
for their support, advice, and encouragement

CONTENTS

Contributors xiii
Preface xxi

VOLUME 1

PART 1 SCIENTIFIC BASIS

Section 1 DEVELOPMENT, DIFFERENTIATION, AND DIVERSITY

1 Embryonic Origins of Skeletal Muscles 3
  Charles P. Emerson, Jr.
  Stephen D. Hauschka

2 Assembly of the Skeletal Muscle Cell 45
  Joseph W. Sanger
  Jean M. Sanger
  Clara Franzini-Armstrong

3 Satellite and Stem Cells in Muscle Regeneration 66
  Richard Bischoff
  Clara Franzini-Armstrong

4 The Diversity of Muscle Fiber Types and Its Origin During Development 87
  Neal A. Rubinstein
  Alan M. Kelly

5 The Structure and Function of Motor Units 104
  Robert E. Burke

6 Extraocular Muscles 119
  Menachem Sadeh

Section 2 MUSCLE CONRACTION

7 Molecular Structure of the Sarcomere 129
  Roger W. Craig
  Raúl Padrón

8 Mammalian Muscle Myosin 167
  H. Lee Sweeney
  Anne Houdusse

9 Molecular Physiology of the Cross-Bridge Cycle 187
  Yale E. Goldman
  Earl Homsher

Section 3 THE CONTROL OF MUSCLE FIBER ACTIVITY

10 Ion Channels and Electrical Properties of Skeletal Muscle 203
   Karin Jurkat-Rott
   Frank Lehmann-Horn

11 The Membrane Systems of Muscle Cells 232
    Clara Franzini-Armstrong

12 Excitation-Contraction Coupling in Skeletal Muscle 257
    Kurt G. Beam
    Paul Horowicz

13 Activation of the Contractile Mechanism by Calcium 281
    Samuel Victor Perry

14 The Proteins of the Sarcotubular System 307
    Kimby N. Barton
    David H. MacLennan

Section 4 NEUROMUSCULAR TRANSMISSION

15 The Neuromuscular Junction 325
    Andrew G. Engel

16 Neuromuscular Transmission 373
    Karl L. Magleby

17 Nicotinic Acetylcholine Receptors: Structure, Function, and Antigenicity 397
    Jon M. Lindstrom

18 Function and Molecular Structure of Acetylcholinesterase 423
    Richard L. Rotundo

Section 5 MUSCLE AS A TISSUE

19a The Cytoskeleton: Maintenance of Muscle Fiber Integrity 443
     Clara Franzini-Armstrong
     Alan R. Horwitz

19b The Muscle Fiber Cytoskeleton: The Dystrophin System 455
     Eijiro Ozawa

20 The Extracellular Matrix 471
    Joshua R. Sanes

21 The Muscle Spindle 489
    Robert W. Banks
    David Barker

22 Microcirculation in Muscle 511
    O. Hudlicka
    M.D. Brown
    S. Egginton

23 Protein and Amino Acid Metabolism in Muscle 535
    R. Thomas Jagoe
    Nicholas E. Tawa, Jr.
    Alfred L. Goldberg

24 Lysosomal Metabolism and Its Relevance to Skeletal Muscle 565
    Joseph Alroy
    Edward H. Kolodny

PART 2 GENERAL APPROACHES TO NEUROMUSCULAR DISEASES

25 The Clinical Examination   599
Brenda L. Banwell
Manuel R. Gomez

26 Electrodiagnosis of Muscle Disorders   619
Jasper R. Daube
Devon I. Rubin

27 Muscle Imaging   655
Marianne de Visser
Carl D. Reimers

28 Functional Evaluation of Metabolic Myopathies   665
Ronald G. Haller
John Vissing

29 The Muscle Biopsy   681
Andrew G. Engel

30 Basic Reactions of Muscle   691
Betty Q. Banker
Andrew G. Engel

31 Ultrastructural Changes in Diseased Muscle   749
Andrew G. Engel
Betty Q. Banker

32 Immune Mechanisms in Muscle Diseases   889
Reinhard Hohlfeld

33 The Tools of Molecular Genetics and Their Application to the Study of Muscle Diseases   915
Eric A. Schon

COLOR PLATES
Color Plates 1–15 appear between pages 510 and 511.

Index   I-1–I-46

VOLUME 2

PART 3 DISEASES OF MUSCLE

Section 1 MUSCULAR DYSTROPHIES

34 Dystrophinopathies   961
Andrew G. Engel
Eijiro Ozawa

35 Emery-Dreifuss Muscular Dystrophy   1027
Nadir M. Maraldi
Luciano Merlini

36 Myotonic Dystrophy   1039
Peter S. Harper
Darren G. Monckton

37 The Limb-Girdle Muscular Dystrophies   1077
Carsten G. Bönnemann
Kate Bushby

38 Facioscapulohumeral Muscular Dystrophy and Scapuloperoneal Disorders   1123
Kevin M. Flanigan

39 Bethlem Myopathy   1135
Marianne de Visser
Anneke J. van der Kooi
G. Joost Jöbsis

40 Oculopharyngeal Muscular Dystrophy   1147
Bernard Brais
Fernando M. S. Tomé

41 X-Linked Vacuolar Myopathies   1163
Brenda L. Banwell

42 Distal Myopathies   1169
Bjarne Udd
Robert C. Griggs

43 Myofibrillar Myopathies   1187
Duygu Selcen
Andrew G. Engel

44 The Congenital Muscular Dystrophies   1203
Thomas Voit
Fernando M. S. Tomé

45 Cardiomyopathies Associated with Muscular Dystrophies   1239
Giovanni Nigro
Lucia I. Comi
Luisa Politano
Gerardo Nigro

Section 2   ALTERED EXCITABILITY OF THE CELL MEMBRANE

46 Nondystrophic Myotonias and Periodic Paralyses   1257
Frank Lehmann-Horn
Reinhardt Rüdel
Karin Jurkat-Rott

47 Generalized Peripheral Nerve Hyperexcitability (Neuromyotonia)   1301
Ian K. Hart
John Newsom-Davis

Section 3   HEREDITARY INCLUSION BODY MYOPATHIES

48 Hereditary Inclusion Body Myopathies   1311
Zohar Argov

Section 4 INFLAMMATORY MYOPATHIES

49 The Polymyositis and Dermatomyositis Syndromes   1321
Andrew G. Engel
Reinhard Hohlfeld

50 Inclusion Body Myositis   1367
Jacqueline Mikol
Andrew G. Engel

51 Virus-Related Muscle Diseases   1389
Marinos C. Dalakas

52 Parasitic Myositis   1419
Betty Q. Banker

53 Other Inflammatory Myopathies   1445
Betty Q. Banker
Andrew G. Engel

Section 5 CONGENITAL MYOPATHIES

54 Congenital Myopathies   1473
Kathryn North

Section 6 METABOLIC DISORDERS AFFECTING MUSCLE

55 Nonlysosomal Glycogenoses   1535
Salvatore DiMauro
Arthur P. Hayes
Seiichi Tsujino

56 Acid Maltase Deficiency   1559
Andrew G. Engel
Rochelle Hirschhorn
Maryann L. Huie

57 Disorders of Lipid Metabolism   1587
Stefano Di Donato
Franco Taroni

58 Mitochondrial Encephalomyopathies   1623
Salvatore DiMauro
Eduardo Bonilla

59 Malignant Hyperthermia   1663
Denise J. Wedel
David H. MacLennan

60 Myoglobinura   1677
Joern P. Sieb
Audrey S. Penn

61 Myopathies Due to Drugs, Toxins, and Nutritional Deficiency   1693
Joern P. Sieb

62 Endocrine Myopathies   1713
Eroboghene E. Ubogu
Robert L. Ruff
Henry J. Kaminski

63 Muscle Pain, Cramps, and Fatigue   1739
C. Michel Harper

Section 7   DISTURBANCES OF NEUROMUSCULAR TRANSMISSION

64 Acquired Autoimmune Myasthenia Gravis   1755
Andrew G. Engel
Reinhard Hohlfeld

65 The Lambert-Eaton Myasthenic Syndrome   1791
John Newsom-Davis

66 Congenital Myasthenic Syndromes   1801
Andrew G. Engel
Kinji Ohno
Steven Sine

Section 8   NEURAL DISEASES

67 Spinal Muscular Atrophies   1845
Sabine Rudnik-Schöneborn
Marianne de Visser
Klaus Zerres

68 Adult and Juvenile Amyotrophic Lateral Sclerosis and Related Motor Neuron Diseases   1865
Robert H. Brown, Jr.

69 Disease of Peripheral Nerves   1889
Peter James Dyck
Christopher Jon Klein

70 Congenital Deformities   1931
Betty Q. Banker

COLOR PLATES
Color Plates 1–15 appear between pages 1410 and 1411.

Index   I-1–I-46

CONTRIBUTORS

Joseph Alroy, D.V.M. [24]*
Associate Professor of Pathology
Tufts University Schools of Medicine
  and Veterinary Medicine
Boston, Massachussetts

Zohar Argov, M.D. [48]
Professor of Neurology
Department of Neurology
Hadassah University Hospital and Hebrew
University–Hadassah Medical School
Jerusalem, Israel

Betty Q. Banker, M.D. [30, 31, 52, 53, 70]
Emeritus Professor of Pathology
Dartmouth Medical College
Hanover, New Hampshire

Robert W. Banks, B.Sc., Ph.D., D.Sc. [21]
Lecturer
School of Biological and Biomedical Sciences
University of Durham
Durham, United Kingdom

Brenda L. Banwell, M.D., F.R.C.P.C. [25, 41]
Assistant Professor of Pediatric (Neurology)
Hospital for Sick Children
Toronto, Canada

David Barker, M.A., D.Phil., D.Sci. [21]
Emeritus Professor of Zoology
Department of Biological Sciences
University of Durham
Durham, United Kingdom

Kimby N. Barton, M.Sc. [14]
Associate Editor
Geriatrics & Aging Marketed Pharmaceuticals
  Division
Marketed Health Products Directorate
Ottawa, Canada

Kurt G. Beam, Ph.D. [12]
Professor of Anatomy and Neurobiology
Department of Anatomy/Neurobiology
Colorado State University
Fort Collins, Colorado

Richard Bischoff, Ph.D. [3]
Professor Emeritus
Department of Anatomy and Neurobiology
Washington University School of Medicine
St. Louis, Missouri

Eduardo Bonilla, M.D. [58]
Professor of Clinical Neurology
  and Clinical Pathology
Departments of Neurology and Pathology
Columbia University College of Physicians
  and Surgeons
New York, New York

Carsten G. Bönnemann, M.D. [37]
Assistant Professor of Neurology and Pediatrics
Departments of Neurology and Pediatrics
The Children's Hospital of Philadelphia
Pennsylvania Muscle Institute, University of
  Pennsylvania School of Medicine
Philadelphia, Pennsylvania

Bernard Brais, M.D., M.Phil., Ph.D. [40]
Associate Professor
Department of Medicine
Faculté de Médecine de l'Université de Montréal
Montreal, Canada

M. D. Brown, Ph.D. [22]
School of Sport and Exercise Sciences
University of Birmingham
Birmingham, United Kingdom

Robert H. Brown, Jr., D.Phil., M.D. [68]
Professor of Neurology
Harvard Medical School
Professor of Neurology
Massachusetts General Hospital
Boston, Massachusetts

*The number(s) in brackets following the contributor name refer to chapter(s) authored or co-authored by the contributor.

Robert E. Burke, M.D. [5]
Laboratory of Neural Control
National Institute of Neurological Disorders
  and Stroke
National Institutes of Health
Bethesda, Maryland

Kate Bushby, M.D., F.R.C.P. [37]
Professor of Neuromuscular Genetics
Institute of Human Genetics
School of Clinical Medical Sciences
University of Newcastle upon Tyne
Newcastle, United Kingdom

Lucia I. Comi, M.D. [45]
Associate Professor of Cardiology
Department of Clinical and Experimental Medicine
  and Surgery
2nd Naples University
Naples, Italy

Roger W. Craig, Ph.D. [7]
Professor of Biology
University of Massachusetts Medical School
Worcester, Massachusetts

Marinos C. Dalakas, M.D. [51]
Chief, Neuromuscular Diseases Section
National Institute of Neurological Disorders
  and Stroke
National Institutes of Health
Bethesda, Maryland

Jasper R. Daube, M.D. [26]
Professor of Neurology
Department of Neurology
Mayo Clinic College of Medicine
Rochester, Minnesota

Marianne de Visser, M.D., Ph.D. [27, 39, 67]
Professor of Neuromuscular Diseases
Department of Neurology
Academic Medical Center
Amsterdam, The Netherlands

Stefano Di Donato, M.D. [57]
Director, Department of Research and Diagnostic
Director, Division of Biochemistry and Genetics
Istituto Nazionale Neurologico C. Besta
Milan, Italy

Salvatore DiMauro, M.D. [55, 58]
Lucy G. Moses Professor of Neurology
Department of Neurology
Columbia University College of Physicians
  and Surgeons
New York, New York

Peter James Dyck, M.D. [69]
Professor of Neurology and Roy E.
  and Merle Meyer Professor of Neuroscience
Peripheral Neuropathy Research Laboratory
Mayo Clinic College of Medicine
Rochester, Minnesota

S. Egginton, Ph.D. [22]
Department of Physiology
University of Birmingham Medical School
Birmingham, United Kingdom

Charles P. Emerson, Jr., Ph.D. [1]
Director, Boston Biomedical Research Institute
Watertown, Massachusetts

Andrew G. Engel, M.D. [15, 29, 30, 31, 34, 43, 49, 50, 53, 56, 64, 66]
William L. McKnight Professor of Neuroscience
Mayo Clinic College of Medicine
Director, Neuromuscular Disease Research Laboratory
Mayo Clinic
Rochester, Minnesota

Kevin M. Flanigan, M.D. [38]
Associate Professor
Departments of Neurology, Human Genetics,
Pathology, and Pediatrics
University of Utah School of Medicine
Salt Lake City, Utah

**Clara Franzini-Armstrong, Laurea,
  member N.A.S., F.R.S.** [2, 3, 11, 19a]
Professor of Cell and Developmental Biology
University of Pennsylvania
  School of Medicine
Philadelphia, Pennsylvania

Alfred L. Goldberg, Ph.D. [23]
Professor of Cell Biology
Harvard Medical School
Boston, Massachussetts

Contributors

Yale E. Goldman, M.D., Ph.D. [9]
Professor of Physiology and Director Pennsylvania
  Muscle Institute
Department of Physiology
University of Pennsylvania School of Medicine
Philadelphia, Pennsylvania

Manuel R. Gomez, M.D. [25]
Emeritus Professor of Pediatric Neurology
Department of Neurology
Mayo Clinic College of Medicine
Rochester, Minnesota

Robert C. Griggs, M.D. [42]
Professor and Chair of Neurology
University of Rochester School of Medicine
  and Dentistry
Rochester, New York

Ronald G. Haller, M.D. [28]
Professor of Neurology
Neuromuscular Center
Institute for Exercise and Environmental Medicine
  of Presbyterian Hospital
Departments of Neurology and Internal Medicine
University of Texas Southwestern Medical School
  and Veterans Affairs Medical Center
Dallas, Texas

C. Michel Harper, M.D. [63]
Professor of Neurology
Department of Neurology
Mayo Clinic College of Medicine
Rochester, Minnesota

Peter S. Harper M.D. [36]
Professor
Institute of Medical Genetics
University of Wales College of Medicine
Cardiff, Wales, United Kingdom

Ian K. Hart, Ph.D., F.R.C.P. [47]
Senior Lecturer in Neurology
University Department of Neurological Science
Walton Center for Neurology and Neurosurgery
Liverpool, United Kingdom

Stephen D. Hauschka, Ph.D. [1]
Professor
Department of Biochemistry
University of Washington School of Medicine
Seattle, Washington

Arthur P. Hays, M.D. [55]
Associate Professor of Clinical Neuropathology
Department of Pathology
Columbia University College of Physicians
  and Surgeons
New York, New York

Rochelle Hirschhorn M.D., F.A.C.M.G. [56]
Professor of Medicine, Cell Biology and Pediatrics
New York University School of Medicine
Department of Medicine/Division
  of Medical Genetics
New York, New York

Reinhard Hohlfeld, M.D. [32, 49, 64]
Professor of Neurology
Institute for Clinical Neuroimmunology
Ludwig Maximilians University of Munich
Munich, Germany

Earl Homsher, Ph.D. [8]
Professor of Physiology
Center for Health Science
University of California at Los Angeles
Los Angeles, California

Paul Horowicz, Ph.D.[†] [12]
Former Professor of Physiology and Chair
Department of Physiology
University of Rochester School of Medicine
Rochester, New York

Alan R. Horwitz, Ph.D. [19a]
Department of Cell Biology
University of Virginia
Health Sciences Center
Charlottesville Virginia

Anne Houdusse, Ph.D. [8]
Équipe Motilité Structurale
Centre National de la Recherche Scientifique
Institute Curie
Paris, France

[†]Deceased.

O. Hudlicka, M.D., Ph.D. [22]
Professor
Department of Physiology
University of Birmingham Medical School
Birmingham, United Kingdom

Maryann L. Huie, Ph.D. [56]
Research Associate Scientist
Department of Medicine
Division of Medical Genetics
New York University School of Medicine
New York, New York

R. Thomas Jagoe, M.B., B.S., Ph.D., M.R.C.P. [23]
Senior Lecturer
Department of Medicine
University of Liverpool
Liverpool, United Kingdom

G. Joost Jöbsis, M.D., Ph.D. [39]
Department of Neurology
Slotervaart Hospital
Amsterdam, The Netherlands

Karin Jurkat-Rott, M.D., Ph.D. [10, 46]
Assistant Professor
Department of Applied Physiology
Ulm University
Ulm, Germany

Henry J. Kaminski, M.D. [62]
Professor of Neurology and Neurosciences
Case Western Reserve University and Cleveland
 Veterans Administration Center
Cleveland, Ohio

Alan M. Kelly, Ph.D., B.V.S.c, M.R.V.V.S. [4]
Dean Veterinary School
Professor of Pathology and Pathobiology
Member Pennsylvania Muscle Institute
University of Pennsylvania Veterinary School
Philadelphia, Pennsylvania

Christopher J. Klein, M.D. [69]
Assistant Professor of Neurology
Department of Neurology
Mayo Clinic College of Medicine
Rochester, Minnesota

Edwin H. Kolodny, M.D. [24]
Bernard A. and Charlotte Marden
 Professor and Chair
Department of Neurology
New York University School of Medicine
New York, New York

Frank Lehmann-Horn, M.D., Ph.D. [10, 46]
Professor and Chair
Department of Applied Physiology
Ulm University
Ulm, Germany

Jon M. Lindstrom, Ph.D. [17]
Trustee Professor of Neuroscience and Professor
 of Pharmacology
Medical School of the University of Pennsylvania
Philadelphia, Pennsylvania

David H. MacLennan, Ph.D., D.Sc., F.R.S.C., F.R.S.
[14, 59]
J. W. Billes Professor of Medical Research
 and University
Charles H. Best Institute
University of Toronto,
Toronto, Canada

Karl L. Magleby, Ph.D. [16]
Professor and Chair
Department of Physiology and Biophysics
University of Miami School of Medicine,
Miami, Florida

Nadir M. Maraldi, Ph.D. [35]
Professor of Histology and Chair, Department
 of Anatomical Science
University of Bologna
Director of Research
Laboratory of Cell Biology
National Research Council and Institute
 for Organ Transplants and Immunocytology
Rizzoli Orthopedic Institute
Bologna, Italy

Luciano Merlini, M.D. [35]
Neuromuscular Unit
Rizzoli Orthopedic Institute
Bologna, Italy

Contributors

Jacqueline Mikol, M.D. [50]
Professor of Pathology
Denis Diderot University
Neuropathologist
Hopital Lariboisiere
Paris, France

Darren G. Monckton, Ph.D. [36]
Reader in Genetics
Institute of Biomedical and Life Sciences
University of Glasgow
Glasgow, United Kingdom

John Newsom-Davis, M.D. [47, 65]
Professor Emeritus
Department of Clinical Neurology
University of Oxford
Oxford, United Kingdom

Gerardo Nigro, M.D. [45]
Assistant Professor
Department of Cardiology
2nd Naples University
Naples, Italy

Giovanni Nigro, M.D. [45]
Professor and Chair of Internal Medicine
Gaetano Conte Academy
Naples, Italy

Kathryn North M.D., M.B.B.S., B.Sc (Med), F.R.A.C.P. [54]
Professor of Paediatrics and Child Health
Faculty of Medicine
University of Sydney
Head, Neurogenetics Research Unit
The Children's Hospital at Westmead
Sydney, Australia

Kinji Ohno, M.D., Ph.D. [66]
Assistant Professor
Department of Neurology
Mayo Clinic College of Medicine
Rochester, Minnesota

Eijiro Ozawa, M.D., Ph.D. [19b, 34]
Emeritus Director General National Institute of Neuroscience
National Center of Neurology and Psychiatry
Kodaira, Tokyo, Japan

Raúl Padrón, Ph.D. [7]
Senior Investigator
Department of Structural Biology
Venezuelan Institute for Scientific Research
Caracas, Venezuela

Audrey S. Penn, M.D. [60]
Emeritus Professor of Neurology
Department of Neurology
Columbia University College of Physicians and Surgeons
New York, New York
Deputy Director
National Institute of Neurological Disorders and Stroke
National Institute of Health
Bethesda, Maryland

Samuel Victor Perry, Ph.D. [13]
Professor Emeritus
University of Birmingham School of Medicine
Department of Physiology
Birmingham, United Kingdom

Luisa Politano, M.D. [45]
Associate Professor of Medical Genetics
Department of Clinical and Experimental Medicine and Surgery
2nd Naples University
Naples, Italy

Carl D. Reimers, M.D. [27]
Department of Neurology
Saechsisches Krankenhaus
Arnsdorf, Germany

Richard L. Rotundo, Ph.D. [18]
Professor of Cell Biology and Anatomy
Department of Cell Biology and Anatomy
University of Miami School of Medicine
Miami, Florida

Devon I. Rubin, M.D. [26]
Assistant Professor
Department of Neurology
Mayo Clinic College of Medicine
Mayo Clinic
Jacksonville, Florida

Neil A. Rubinstein, M.D., Ph.D. [4]
Associate Professor of Cell
  and Developmental Biology
Department of Cell and Developmental Biology
University of Pennsylvania School of Medicine
Philadelphia, Pennsylvania

Reinhardt Rüdel, M.D. [46]
Professor and Chair
Department of General Physiology
University of Ulm
Ulm, Germany

Sabine Rudnik-Schöneborn, M.D. [67]
Consultant Clinical Geneticist
Institute of Human Genetics
Aachen University of Technology
Aachen, Germany

Robert L. Ruff, M.D., Ph.D. [62]
Professor and Vice Chair
Department of Neurology and Neurosciences
Case Western Reserve University
Veterans Administration Medical Center
Cleveland, Ohio

Menachem Sadeh, M.D. [6]
Associate Professor of Clinical Neurology
Department of Neurology
Wolfson Medical Center
Holon, Israel
Sackler School of Medicine
Tel Aviv University
Tel Aviv, Israel

Joshua R. Sanes, Ph.D. [20]
Alumni Endowed Professor of Neurobiology
Department of Anatomy and Neurobiology
Washington University School of Medicine
St. Louis, Missouri

Jean M. Sanger, Ph.D. [2]
Research Professor of Cell
  and Developmental Biology
Department of Cell and Developmental Biology
University of Pennsylvania School of Medicine
Philadelphia, Pennsylvania

Joseph W. Sanger, Ph.D. [2]
Professor and Interim Chair of Cell
  and Developmental Biology
Department of Cell and Developmental Biology
University of Pennsylvania School of Medicine
Philadelphia, Pennsylvania

Eric A. Schon, Ph.D. [33]
Professor of Genetics and Development
  (in Neurology)
Department of Neurology
Columbia University College of Physicians
  and Surgeons
New York, New York

Duygu Selcen, M.D. [43]
Assistant Professor of Neurology
Department of Neurology
Mayo Clinic College of Medicine
Rochester, Minnesota

Joern P. Sieb, M.D. [60, 61]
Privat Dozent
Department of Neurology
University of Bonn, Bonn, Germany
Chair, Department of Neurology
Stralsund General Hospital
Stralsund, Germany

Steven M. Sine, Ph.D. [66]
Professor of Physiology and Biophysics
Department of Physiology
  and Biomedical Engineering
Mayo Clinic College of Medicine
Rochester, Minnesota

H. Lee Sweeney, Ph.D. [8]
William Maul Measy Professor
  and Chair of Physiology
Department of Physiology
University of Pennsylvania School of Medicine
Philadelphia, Pennsylvania

Franco Taroni, M.D. [57]
Associate Neurologist and Senior Research Scientist
Division of Biochemistry and Genetics
Istituto Nazionale Neurologico C. Besta
Milan, Italy

Nicholas E. Tawa, Jr. M.D., Ph.D. [23]
Assistant Professor of Surgery (Cell Biology)
Department of Surgery
Beth Israel Deaconess Medical Center
Harvard Medical School
Boston, Massachusetts

Fernando M.S. Tomé, M.D., Ph.D. [40, 44,]
Professor "Agregado" (Neurology)
University of Lisbon
Former Director of Research
INSERM
Paris, France

Seiichi Tsujino, M.D. [55]
Section Chief, Department of Inherited Metabolic Disease, National Institute of Neuroscience
National Center of Neurology and Psychiatry
Tokyo, Japan

Eroboghene E. Ubogu, M.D. [62]
Instructor
Department of Neurology
Case Western Reserve University
Cleveland Veterans Administration Center
Cleveland, Ohio

Bjarne Udd, M.D., Ph.D. [42]
Associate Professor
Folkhalsan Genetic Institute, Biomedicum
University of Helsinki
Department of Neurology
University Hospital of Tampere
Neuromuscular Unit
Vasa Central Hospital
Finland

Anneke J. van der Kooi, M.D., Ph.D. [39]
Department of Neurology
Academic Medical Center
University of Amsterdam
Amsterdam, The Netherlands

John Vissing, M.D., Ph.D. [28]
Associate Professor
Department of Neurology
University of Copenhagen
Director
Neuromuscular Clinic
Rigshospitalit
Copenhagen, Denmark

Thomas Voit, M.D. [44]
Professor and Chair of Pediatrics
 and Pediatric Neurology
Managing Director
Center of Pediatric and Adolescent Medicine
University Hospital and University of Essen
Essen, Germany

Denise J. Wedel, M.D. [59]
Professor
Department of Anesthesiology
Mayo Clinic College of Medicine
Rochester, Minnesota

Klaus Zerres, M.D. [67]
Professor and Department Chair
Institute of Human Genetics
Aachen University of Technology
Aachen, Germany

PREFACE

A swell of enormous advances swept across the field of myology since the second edition of *Myology* was published in 1994. In the basic sciences, the molecular aspects of the development, organization, and function of muscle have been greatly extended. Myriad components have been added to the list of proteins that constitute the contractile, metabolic, and regulatory machinery of skeletal muscle. At the same time, the clinical significance of some of the heretofore unknown molecules was revealed by pathologic effects of their mutant alleles in both previously identified and newly recognized diseases.

Building on the pioneer discoveries of the past, recent research on muscle differentiation has painted a complete picture of the regulatory genes, signaling networks, and cellular mechanisms that control the embryonic origins of muscle progenitors and their subsequent differentiation to form mature muscle fibers (Chapter 1). That precise coordination and appropriate timing of developmental events are essential for the normal development of muscle and other tissues is now well recognized (Chapter 2). A disruption or inappropriate activation of this stereotyped developmental program in muscle and other tissues is a recurrent theme in the congenital muscular dystrophies and in the myofibrillar and congenital myopathies (Chapters 42, 43, and 54). The recent discovery of stem cells (other than satellite cells) in muscle and other tissues has raised hopes that stem cells derived from muscle or bone marrow could be used for therapeutic intervention; however, the therapeutic potential of stem cells remains unrealized (Chapters 3 and 34).

Intrinsic and environmental (including hormonal) factors shape the destiny of the muscle fibers, so that they become tuned to their varied roles in motor activity. Awareness of these developmental strategies provides a framework for understanding the reactions and adaptations of muscle in disease (Chapters 4 and 5).

The extraocular muscles harbor subcategories of muscle fibers highly specialized for extremely fast as well as slow, tonic movements. These muscles are either preferentially involved or spared in a variety of neuromuscular diseases. Their vulnerability in neuromuscular junction diseases and mitochondrial myopathies, and in oculopharyngeal dystrophy is well known, yet they are spared in most other muscle diseases (Chapter 6).

The building blocks of the muscle fiber—myofibrils, the accompanying membrane systems, and the cytoskeletal network that binds them together—have revealed unexpected complexities of composition and structure. The recent additions to the muscle protein catalogue reveal that appropriate muscle function depends directly on functional integration of all major and minor components of the muscle fiber (Chapter 7). For example, 12 mutations of major structural and regulatory myofibrillar components result in hypertrophic cardiomyopathy; and myosin heavy-chain isoforms are implicated in a form of inclusion body myopathy and hyaline body myopathy (Chapters 8, 48, and 54). A variety of myopathies stem from mutations of structural proteins less directly involved in the contractile functions: limb-girdle muscular dystrophy type 2G (telethonin), limb-girdle muscular dystrophy type 1A (myotilin), desminopathy, and nemaline myopathy (see below) (Chapters 37, 43, and 54).

Knowledge of the number, functional properties, and molecular aspects of plasmalemmal ion channels and pumps has greatly expanded in recent times. Chapter 10 reviews the classical channels responsible for excitatory activity and the equally important channels that contribute to the resting membrane potential, volume regulation, and signal transduction. Understanding the functional role of these channels sets the stage for grasping the complexities of the myotonias, periodic paralyses, and neuromyotonias (Chapters 36, 46, and 47). Muscle activation and the control of muscle fiber activity require a complex machinery based on specialized membrane systems that may occupy a third or more of the fiber volume (Chapters 11–14). Advances in this area have revealed how calcium channels in plasmalemma (the dihydropyridine receptors) and in the sarcoplasmic reticulum (the ryanodine receptors) cross talk and thus influence each other's ctivity. This close functional interaction may well explain that mutations in either channel can cause malignant hyperthermia (Chapter 59). Phospholamban (PLN) is an accessory protein that regulates the activity of the sarcoplasmic reticulum (SR) Ca^{2+} pump (SERCA) in slow skeletal and cardiac muscle. By decreasing the affinity of SERCA 2a for Ca^{2+}, PLN has dramatic beneficial effects on cardiac function. Thus modifying PLN/SERCA 2a interaction sites may be a promising therapeutic approach to heart failure (Chapter 14).

The mechanism of a protein's action is best understood after its architecture is deciphered at the atomic level. This is dramatically illustrated in Color Plates 1–5. In 1994, understanding of mechanochemical transduction by myosin cross-bridge action had just been revolutionized by the first crystal structures of the myosin molecule. Since then, the structure of other sarcomeric proteins in various functional states has been resolved (Chapters 7–9 and 13, and Color Plates 1–3). The first atomic models of large intramembrane proteins—the SR Ca^{2+} pump, voltage gated ion channels, and the extracellular part of the acetylcholine receptor—are now also available (Chapters 10, 14, 17, and 66, and Color Plates 4–6). The selectivity filter of the potassium channel, seen in its fine detail (Color Plate 5), is a marvel worthy of the 2003 Nobel prize; and the conformational changes in the SR Ca^{2+} pump that accompany the active transport of two Ca^{2+} ions involve impressively large to-and-fro movements in cytoplasmic domains of an innately flexible molecule (Color Plate 4).

Understanding the cytoskeletal network of muscle has been revolutionized by the realization that several macromolecular complexes initially thought to act independently are closely intertwined. Thus, the internal desmin scaffolding and its association with the plasmalemma are intimately linked to dystrophin- utrophin- and spectrin-based networks as these connect through the plasmalemma to the extracellular matrix (Chapters 19a and 19b). This has reinforced the notion that maintenance of sarcolemmal integrity is not limited to dystrophin and dystrophin-associated proteins but involves other components of the subplasmalemmal cytoskeleton and associated integral membrane proteins (Chapters 34 and 37).

The extracellular matrix plays a complex role as an "insoluble" network of proteins that traps bioactive molecules, contributes to fiber differentiation, and dictates specializations at the neuromuscular and myotendinous junction (Chapter 20). An exciting development of the past decade has been that defects in the extracellular matrix have pathogenic effects. Thus, mutations in laminin α2 (Chapter 44) and collagen VI (Chapters 39 and 44) cause muscular dystrophies; perlecan defects underlie the Schwartz-Jampel syndrome (Chapter 63); and mutations in ColQ result in a congenital myasthenic syndrome (Chapter 66).

An increased understanding of the structure and function of the neuromuscular junction (Chapters 15–18) proved to be a stepping stone to unraveling the complexities of the autoimmune and genetic disorders of neuromuscular transmission (Chapters 64–66).

The immense advances in the basic sciences were paralleled by a corresponding expansion of the horizons of clinical myology. The identification of disease genes and mutations has become increasingly important for accurate diagnosis, genetic counseling, and disease prevention. In the *dystrophinopathies*, better understanding of the structure and functional domains of dystrophin has provided new insights into pathogenic effects of dystrophin mutations and clues for designing constructs for possible gene therapy. Improved methods for detecting small DNA rearrangement of the dystrophin gene and for identifying carriers have been devised. The potentials of gene therapy with viral vectors has been explored in animal models but targeting the entire striated musculature, efficient delivery to the host's myofiber nuclei, and long-term expression of the transduced gene are yet to be realized. However, at least some frameshifting dystrophin mutations may be amenable to antisense-induced skipping of the mutant exon, aminoglycosides may suppress some stop codon mutations, and myostatin blockade may mitigate the course of the disease (Chapter 34).

The *classic form of myotonic dystrophy* (DM1) caused by a CTG_n expansion in the 3' untranslated region of the *DMPK* gene is now matched by *myotonic dystrophy type 2* [DM2, or proximal myotonic myopathy (PROMM)] caused by a $CCTG_n$ expansion in the *ZNF9* gene. The multisystem effects of both disorders have been traced to repressed expression of other genes by the expanded mRNAs. In DM1, this effect has now been attributed to sequestration of nuclear transcription factors of selected genes by the abnormal DM1 mRNAs (Chapter 36).

The mechanism by which deletion of an integral number of repeats in the telomeric region of chromosome 4 causes *facioscapulohumeral dystrophy* (FSHD) has been debated over the past decade. Current evidence, based on detailed microarray studies, indicates FSHD-specific alterations in at least 27 genes. Several of these genes are targets of MyoD, suggesting a defect of myogenic differentiation; others are involved in response to oxidative stress (Chapter 38).

Oculopharyngeal muscular dystrophy is now known to be caused by short (GCG_{8-13}) expansions of alanine codons in the first exon of the *PABP1* that encodes the nuclear polyadenylate-binding protein. Polymerization of the polyalanine domains results in formation of characteristic intranuclear filaments that may trap mRNA (Chapter 40).

The number of genetically defined *limb-girdle dystrophies* has increased from one dominant and three recessive forms in 1994 to six dominant and 10 recessive forms in 2004 (Chapter 37).

During the same period, the number of genetically distinct *congenital muscular dystrophies* grew from three to 10 and, with the exception of integrin α7-deficient muscular dystrophy, they all involve the muscle fiber basement membrane. Aberrant O-glycosylation of α-dystroglycan has been identified in five congenital muscular dystrophies, highlighting the crucial role of α-dystroglycan in maintaining basement membrane function in different organs, and especially in muscle and brain (Chapter 44). Both the autosomal dominant *Bethlem myopathy* and the autosomal recessive *Ulrich's congenital muscular dystrophy* were traced to mutations in collagen type VI (Chapters 39 and 44).

Different types of *X-linked vacuolar myopathies*, one with excessive autophagy and one with cardiomyopathy and mental retardation (Danon disease), are now recognized. Danon disease results from defects in the lysosome-associated membrane protein 2 (LAMP2), and is reproduced in mice by targeted disruption of *lamp2* (Chapter 41).

Among the *distal myopathies*, the genetic basis of tibial muscular dystrophy has been traced to mutations in titin. The chromosomal loci of the distal myopathies named after Welander and after Laing have been identified but the disease genes and their mutations are not yet known (Chapter 42).

The term *myofibrillar myopathy* (MFM) has been applied to disorders associated with characteristic changes in trichromatically stained frozen sections, ectopic accumulation of multiple proteins in abnormal fiber regions, disintegration of myofibrils that begins at the Z-disk and, frequently, distal as well as proximal weakness, cardiomyopathy, and peripheral neuropathy. A small proportion of MFM patients carry disease-associated mutations in desmin, αB-crystallin, or myotilin. In most patients, however, the molecular basis of the disease awaits discovery (Chapter 43).

In the *congenital myopathies* the genetic basis of nemaline myopathy has been traced to mutations in thin-filament associated proteins (nebulin, α-actin, α- and β-tropomyosin, and slow-troponin-T). The typical form of multiminicore disease is caused by mutations in selenoprotein N, which is also implicated in a form of the rigid spine syndrome; and the cause of hyaline body disease resides in the slow β cardiac myosin heavy-chain (Chapter 54).

Two eloquent messages emerge from these chapters: First, a decade ago only defects in dystrophin, α-sarcoglycan, and laminin α2 were recognized as proteins associated with muscular dystrophy. Today, an array of other proteins—in the plasmalemma, the internal and external cytoskeleton, the sarcomere as well as a chaperone protein, enzymes, and defects in RNA metabolism—are implicated. Second, the molecular and the phenotypic distinctions between congenital dystrophies, limb-girdle dystrophies, and some congenital myopathies are becoming blurred.

At least two genetically distinct forms of *hereditary inclusion body myopathies* have emerged: A dominant form caused by mutations in heavy myosin chain IIA is associated with early contractures, ophthalmoplegia and proximal weakness; and a recessive form caused by mutations in UDP-N-acetylglucosamine 2-epimerase/N-acetylmannosamine kinase, encoded by *GNE*, a bifunctional key enzyme in sialic acid synthesis. Interestingly, *GNE* mutations spare the quadriceps muscle in middle-eastern Jews but not in Japanese patients (Chapter 48).

The immunopathogenesis of T-cell-mediated *inflammatory myopathies* is now investigated by laser-assisted dissection of single inflammatory cells combined with single-cell PCR amplification of the sequences of the T-cell receptor. However, the antigen(s) recognized by the autoaggressive T cells remain unidentified (Chapter 49). The etiology of sporadic *inclusion body myositis* remains elusive despite numerous tantalizing clues that relate it to Alzheimer disease, and the observation that expression of the small-heat shock protein, αB-crystallin, is upregulated in numerous nonvacuolated fibers.

Novel *glycogenoses* caused by defects in aldolase A and in β-enolase were discovered, branching enzyme deficiency is turning out to be more heterogeneous than was thought, and the pathogenesis of Lafora disease (polyglucosan storage disease) is becoming clarified (Chapter 55). In acid maltase deficiency, no fewer than 70 mutations have been identified over the past decade, and enzyme replacement therapy of infantile patients is off to a promising start (Chapter 56). The concept of *mitochondrial encephalomyopathies* has also expanded. Mitochondrial DNA (mtDNA) is now known to harbor more than 150 mutations (compared to about 30 in 1994), and a number of nuclear mutations instigating defects in the respiratory chain or in intergenomic communication have been identified. The basis of mtDNA depletion and of multiple mtDNA deletions has been related to alterations of the nucleotide pool (Chapter 58).

In *myasthenia gravis* (MG), the muscle specific protein kinase (MUSK) has emerged as a novel autoantigen, but an animal model based on immunization with MUSK or detailed analysis of end plate pathology and physiology in a series of MUSK-antibody-positive MG patients is unavailable (Chapter 65). The *congenital myasthenic syndromes* (CMSs) are now known to arise from defects in five end-plate-associated proteins (choline acetyltransferase, the acetylcholine receptor, acetylcholinesterase, rapsyn, and the skeletal muscle sodium channel $Na_v1.4$) that harbor no fewer than 144 mutations. Clinical, morphologic, and electrophysiology clues now allow rational therapy for most CMSs (Chapter 66).

Among the *motor neuron diseases*, it is now realized that mutations in the telomeric form of the *SMN1* gene underlie all three forms of spinal muscular atrophy, and that the number of centromeric *SMN2* copies modulate disease severity (Chapter 67). And now, the serendipitous observation that SMN2 protein level is upregulated by valproic acid has raised hopes that juvenile and adult cases of spinal muscular atrophy may become therapeutically accessible. Mutations in three proteins—superoxide dismutase 1, alsin, and dynactin—have been implicated in familial forms of amyotrophic lateral sclerosis (ALS). Analysis of the deleterious effects of the mutant alleles may eventually provide clues to the cause, pathogenesis, and treatment of sporadic ALS. Of further interest, one-half of ALS patients have detectable reverse transcriptase in serum, pointing to a possible retroviral instigator (Chapter 68).

The clinical spectrum and molecular diversity of hereditary motor and sensory as well autonomic neuropathies have also expanded over the past decade. New methods have been devised to assess sensory and autonomic dysfunction and loss, and specific prevention and therapy have become available for a number of metabolic and immune neuropathies.

But the miraculous progress of the past decade has also challenged the traditional classification and categorization of neuromuscular diseases. Mutations in diverse genes can have converging functional and pathologic effects and, conversely, different mutations in a given gene can produce divergent clinical phenotypes. As examples, consider mutations in dysferlin, myotilin, or caveolin causing limb-girdle dystrophy or distal myopathy; mutations in lamin A/C resulting in Emery-Dreifuss dystrophy, cardiac conduction defect, lipodystrophy, axonal neuropathy, mandibuloacral dysplasia, or progeria; mutations in $Na_v1.4$ causing different forms of periodic paralysis, myotonia, or a CMS; and mutations in either $Na_v1.4$ or $Ca_v1.1$ causing hypokalemic periodic paralysis. Thus neither the traditional classification of diseases by their clinical or morphologic phenotype, nor their categorization by the mutated gene, the altered protein and, still less, by an ever increasing number of alphanumeric labels, is entirely satisfactory.

The third edition of *Myology* is organized in two volumes, comprising three parts. Part 1 (Chapters 1–24) deals with the development, differentiation and diversity of skeletal muscles, muscle contraction, the control of muscle fiber activity, neuromuscular transmission, and muscle as a tissue. Part 2 (Chapters 25–33) focuses on the general approaches to neuromuscular diseases. Part 3 (Chapters 34–70) presents the various disorders of muscle. Here the traditional phenotype-based classification of muscle diseases is retained, because phenotypic features of a given patient are the starting point for further studies and the subsequent molecular diagnosis. The biochemical aspects of glycogen, lipid, and mitochondrial metabolism, presented as separate chapters in Part 1 in the second edition, are now presented in the context of the corresponding clinical chapters in Part 3. Most chapters were thoroughly revised or written de novo, and eight new chapters were added. The new titles are: Extraocular Muscles (Part 1), Immune Mechanisms in Muscle Diseases (Part 2), Bethlem Myopathy, X-Linked Vacuolar Myopathies, Myofibrillar Myopathies, Cardiomyopathies Associated with Muscular Dystrophies, Generalized Peripheral Nerve Hyperexcitability, and Hereditary Inclusion Body Myopathies (Part 3).

We are grateful to the 97 contributing authors whose hard work has brought the third edition of *Myology* to life. Cleo Schaefer provided secretarial assistance. The Muscular Dystrophy Association and the National Institutes of Health were generous in their support of our laboratories during the period that this book was written. We also thank the staff at McGraw-Hill—Karen Davis, Muza Navrozov, and Isabel Nogueira—for their expert and devoted assistance in editing and producing this book.

Andrew G. Engel, M.D.

Clara Franzini-Armstrong, Laurea

MYOLOGY

1
Scientific Basis

SECTION 1

Development, Differentiation, and Diversity

Chapter 1
Embryonic Origins of Skeletal Muscles*

CHARLES P. EMERSON, JR.
STEPHEN D. HAUSCHKA

Specification of Mesoderm and Skeletal Muscle
  Progenitors
  FORMATION OF MESODERM AND PARAXIAL MESODERM IN
    VERTEBRATE EMBRYOS
  SPECIFICATION AND SEGMENTATION OF PARAXIAL MESODERM
  PARAXIAL MESODERM ORIGINS OF BODY AND HEAD MUSCLE
    PROGENITORS
  REGULATORS OF MYOGENESIS IN INVERTEBRATE EMBRYOS
Molecular Control of Muscle Differentiation
  MYOBLAST PROLIFERATION
  MYOCYTE DIFFERENTIATION
  EXERCISE-MEDIATED SKELETAL MUSCLE REGULATION
  FAST AND SLOW MUSCLE ENHANCERS AND CONTROL ELEMENTS
  ALTERNATIVE RNA SPLICING REGULATION OF MUSCLE PROTEIN
    EXPRESSION
  MUSCLE REGULATORY ELEMENTS AND THERAPEUTIC
    APPLICATIONS
Building Muscle Anatomy
  MIGRATION OF MUSCLE PROGENITORS TO ANATOMIC SITES
  SPECIFICATION OF ANATOMIC MUSCLES
  MYOCYTE FUSION AND MUSCLE FIBER FORMATION
  FORMATION OF THE MYOTOME
  COORDINATION OF MYOTOME AND TENDON DIFFERENTIATION

Skeletal muscle is specialized for mechanical force generation and motor activity in multicellular animals. A complexity of evolutionarily conserved proteins and regulatory mechanisms is now known to control muscle formation and function in invertebrate and vertebrate embryos, through the process of skeletal myogenesis. Skeletal muscle cells are highly specialized by virtue of the expression of a large set of muscle-specific contractile proteins that undergo an orderly assembly

*This chapter is dedicated to Howard Holtzer, Irwin R. Konigsberg, and David Yaffe, who were pioneers in the field of skeletal myogenesis. Their studies of myoblasts were the foundation for recent discoveries of regulatory genes and signaling networks that control muscle formation in embryos.

to form myofibrils, sarcoplasmic reticulum, and energy-generating machinery to regulate contraction in response to neural and mechanical signals. This chapter reviews current knowledge of skeletal myogenesis, including regulatory mechanisms that control the formation and differentiation of muscle progenitors in embryos and form functionally specialized muscles in adults.

Recent progress in the field of myogenesis has been facilitated by knowledge of the biochemistry and cytoarchitecture of contractile proteins. This has been one of the leading areas of structural biology over the past 60 years, beginning with the work of Albert Szent-Györgyi, and the discovery by Ross Harrison, 100 years ago, that muscle differentiation can be investigated in tissue culture explants of embryonic muscle. The biochemistry of muscle contractile proteins, together with morphologic and ultrastructural insights into the assembly and organization of muscle proteins within muscle fibers, have provided a rich resource of data that made possible the identification of contractile protein genes, leading to the discovery of the regulatory genes that control contractile protein gene expression during muscle progenitor differentiation. Utilization of tissue culture approaches to investigate the process of muscle differentiation led to the identification of embryonic muscle progenitors, "myoblasts," and opened the door to experimental investigations of the cellular and molecular mechanisms controlling the formation of myoblasts and their differentiation, including the important roles of cell proliferation, G1-specific cell cycle withdrawal, contractile protein gene expression, myofibril assembly, and cell-cell fusion in the formation of functional, multinucleated muscle fibers. These pioneering discoveries have been the basis for the current era of discovery of the genetic and cellular mechanisms that control the embryonic origins of muscle progenitors and their differentiation to form anatomic muscles.

Skeletal myogenesis in vertebrate and invertebrate embryos has been a major field of investigation over the past 20 years. These studies have led to the discovery of regulatory genes and signaling networks that control the embryonic origins and differentiation of muscle progenitors and coordinate muscle formation with the differentiation of tendons, bones, and vascular tissues to build functional muscle anatomy in the embryo. Muscle and skeletal anatomy is complex and richly varied among different groups of animals. Comparative studies of myogenesis are providing significant insights into the conserved and divergent mechanisms for skeletal myogenesis in embryos and the developmental mechanisms underlying evolutionary variations in muscle anatomy and function as a major adaptive force in animal evolution. Much of our current understanding of skeletal myogenesis has come from studies of avian and mouse embryos. However, important contributions are now coming from comparative studies of myogenesis in other vertebrates and invertebrates, including *Xenopus laevis*, zebrafish and protochordates, *Drosophila melanogaster*, and *Caenorhabditis elegans*. Finally, the discoveries in the genetic control of myogenesis continue to provide paradigms for a broader understanding of tissue and organ formation in animals and new experimental tools for the development of cell and gene therapies in the treatment of human muscle damage and disease.

Specification of Mesoderm and Skeletal Muscle Progenitors

FORMATION OF MESODERM AND PARAXIAL MESODERM IN VERTEBRATE EMBRYOS

Mesoderm Formation

Mesoderm forms during embryogenesis by the cell movements of gastrulation, a process that leads to the formation of the primary embryonic tissue layers of the embryo—the endoderm, mesoderm, and ectoderm—and establishes the anteroposterior (AP*) and dorsoventral (DV) axes of the embryo's body. The paraxial mesoderm, which is the part of the mesoderm that forms along the embryo's axis, is the source of progenitors that form skeletal muscles in the embryo. Following fertilization, the zygotic embryo undergoes a precisely regulated period of DNA replication, cytokinesis, and mitosis—referred to as *cleavage*—leading to the formation of a multicellular, blastula-stage embryo (Fig. 1-1). During cytokinesis and cleavage, the cytoplasm of the fertilized egg, including "maternal" RNAs and proteins, is distributed to specific embryonic blastomeres to establish the spatial patterning of key developmental regulators in the developing embryo. Maternal mRNAs are produced during oogenesis and prelocalized in the egg cytoplasm in a translationally inactive state. These mRNAs are translationally activated after distribution to specific blastomeres, producing transcription factor and signal transduction regulators that orchestrate the cellular movements of gastrulation and initiate specification of the primary tissue layers of the embryo. The three primary embryonic tissue layers of the embryo are produced by the directed cell movements of gastrulation. These primary tissues include the endoderm layer on the inside of the embryo, the ectoderm layer on the outside of the embryo, and the mesoderm layer between the ectoderm and endoderm. Each of these primary embryonic tissues gives rise to distinct lineages of progenitors that form the tissues and organs of the body.[1-3] The mesoderm is the source of all skeletal muscle progenitors in the head and body of the embryo as well as progenitors for a diversity of other tissues, including heart, skin, bones, tendons and vascular tissue, and blood.

*A list of abbreviations used in this chapter is given at the end of the chapter.

Paraxial Mesoderm Formation

Paraxial mesoderm lies on either side of the neural tube along the embryo's axis and is the source of muscle progenitors (Fig. 1-2). In amphibian embryos, paraxial mesoderm locates on either side of the blastopore lip, the site of the "primary organizer," which provides inductive signals to control the migration and specification of mesodermal progenitors.[4] During gastrulation, cells that converge and involute adjacent to the primary organizer undergo convergence-extension movements along the midline to the ventral pole of the embryo.[5,6] The paraxial mesoderm in the anterior embryo forms the presomitic mesoderm, which, in turn, gives rise to the muscle progenitors of the myotomal muscles of the tadpole tail, the first and primary muscles formed in the amphibian embryo. Paraxial mesoderm in avian and mammalian embryos also forms by convergence movements of embryonic cells to the primitive streak at the embryo midline, where these cells ingress into the region of the node at the posterior end of the primitive streak and then populate either side of the midline.[7] The signals and cell biological processes that orchestrate "convergent extension" movements of mesodermal cells during gastrulation are not well understood. Recent embryologic and genetic studies in zebrafish and *Xenopus* embryos suggest that these movements are controlled by noncanonical Wnt signaling through regulation of the cytoskeleton for cell motility.[3,8]

The cellular mechanics of gastrulation and paraxial mesoderm formation vary among vertebrates, reflecting evolutionary adaptations in egg structure and embryo environment. However, the inductive signals for paraxial mesoderm specification are significantly conserved in evolution. Localized inductive signaling centers—referred to as the primary organizer in amphibian embryos[4] and the node in bird and mammalian embryos[7]—produce signals that induce neighboring, migrating populations of embryonic cells to form the mesoderm and endoderm. Genetic and embryologic investigations have identified specific signaling ligands that mediate the organizer/node function. Among these are the transforming growth factor beta (TGF-β) ligand. *Nodal* and its downstream signal transduction effectors are key mediators of organizer functions in amphibian, zebrafish, and mouse and likely also chick embryos, as reviewed by Whitman.[2] *Nodal* is expressed in the organizer/node and has multiple developmental functions. In the mouse embryo prior to and during gastrulation, these functions include control of extraembryonic endoderm and ectoderm formation, AP axis orientation, mesoderm formation, and left-right embryo symmetry.[1] In fish and frog embryos, BMP4 and soluble BMP antagonists (Chordin, Noggin, and follistatin) are produced by the organizer, forming a gradient of BMP signaling activity in the region of paraxial mesoderm formation.[9] Experimental blockage of BMP signaling by implantation of Noggin-expressing cells into the axial region of chick embryos converts lateral plate mesoderm into paraxial mesoderm, whereas treatment of embryos with BMP4 converts paraxial mesoderm into lateral plate mesoderm.[10] Furthermore, zebrafish embryos with mutations that alter levels of BMP signal have patterning defects reflected in altered amounts of mesodermal tissues, including paraxial mesoderm,[11,12] indicating that BMPs form a morphogen

Chapter 1. Embryonic Origins of Skeletal Muscles

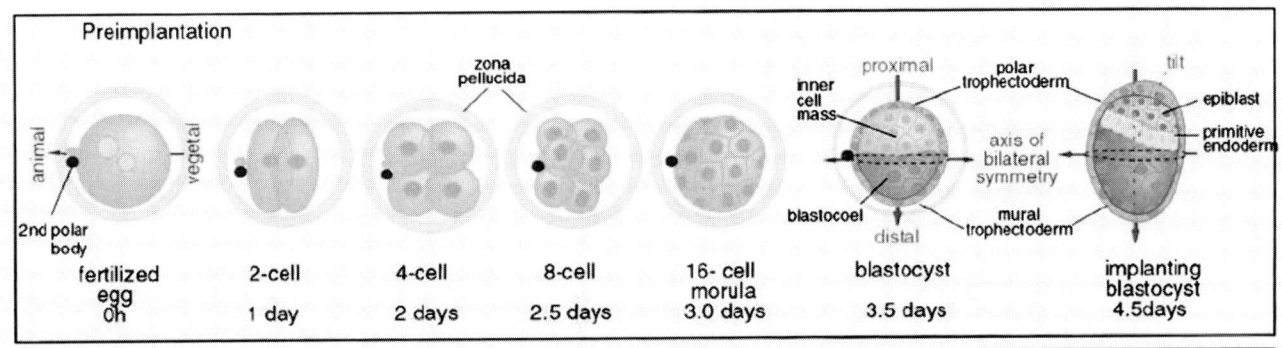

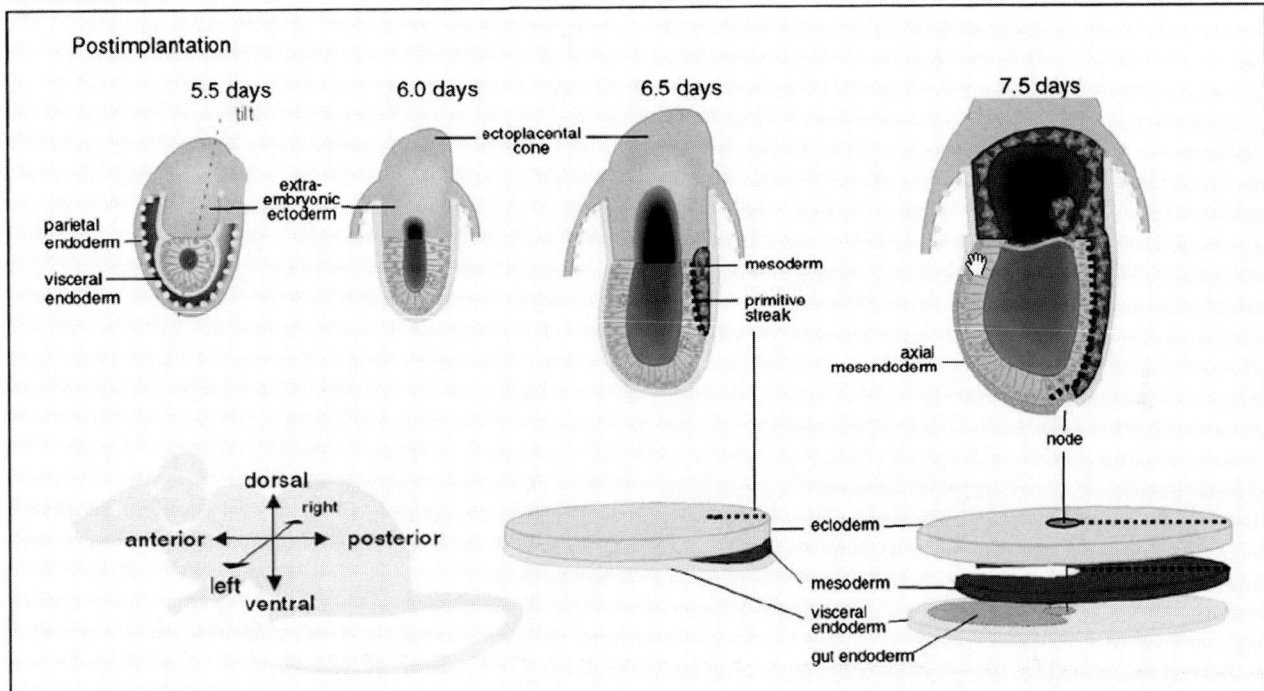

FIGURE 1-1. The first 7.5 days of mouse embryo development following fertilization. Preimplantation development is depicted on the top row with postimplantation development on the bottom (not drawn to scale). The germ layers of the 6.5- and 7.5-day embryos are also shown as flattened sheets for ease of comparison with other vertebrate and mammalian embryos. The major axes of the embryo are shown superimposed on the profile of an adult mouse (*From Beddington and Robertson.*[417] *Reproduced by permission.*)

gradient to pattern the specification of mesoderm and muscle progenitors along the dorsovental axis of the embryo.

SPECIFICATION AND SEGMENTATION OF PARAXIAL MESODERM

Signaling and Transcription Factor Regulation

Specification of paraxial mesoderm is controlled by distinct signals in the anterior and posterior regions of the embryo.[13] Mouse embryos mutant in PDGF do not form the anterior paraxial mesoderm from which cervical muscles derive.[14] Mutations in fibroblast growth factor (FGF), Wnt signal transduction components, and the T-box transcription factor genes *Brachyury* and *Tbx6* block formation of the posterior paraxial mesoderm, which forms the thoracic, limb, and tail muscles. FGF functions as a positive signal to promote paraxial mesoderm formation, as evidenced by the finding that FGFR-1 receptor (−/−) mutant cells fail to migrate through the primitive streak and to form paraxial mesoderm, but instead form a secondary neural tube, which normally is derived from the ectoderm.[15–17] Thus, in the absence of FGF signaling, cells fated to become mesoderm undergo a "default" regulatory response that allows them to respond to neural tube–inducing signals that activate the neural tube regulatory gene network. In support of this mechanism, frog embryos expressing dominant negative FGFR-1 mRNA are blocked in FGF signaling and fail to form trunk and tail mesoderm.[18] FGF8 is the likely ligand that mediates FGFR-1 function for paraxial mesoderm specification, as its expression is localized in midline cells of the primitive streak and FGF8 (−/−) embryos also are defective in paraxial mesoderm formation elevated.[19] Also, experimentally elevated FGF signaling in frog, fish, and chick embryos induces neural tube–fated cells to become paraxial mesoderm.[20,21]

Wnt3a ligand is an additional positive regulatory signal for paraxial mesoderm specification. Paraxial mesoderm does not form in Wnt3a (−/−) embryos, but becomes neural tissue.[22] Furthermore, genetic studies show that Lef1 and Tcf1, the transcription factor effectors of Wnt signal transduction, are required for paraxial mesoderm formation; in the absence of their function, mesoderm precursors also become neural tissue.[23]

The T-box transcription factor genes Brachyury and Tbx6 are the likely upstream regulators of FGF and Wnt signaling for paraxial mesoderm specification. Embryos mutant for each of these genes are deficient in mesoderm and form excess neural tube tissue.[24,25] pMesogenin, a basic helix-loop-helix (bHLH) transcription factor, is expressed in posterior paraxial mesoderm in an overlapping pattern with Tbx6 and Brachyury. pMesogenin (−/−) mutant embryos also fail to form posterior paraxial mesoderm, and its ectopic expression in Xenopus activates T-box gene expression,[26] suggesting that pMesogenin functions directly to control T-box regulatory genes and repress the regulatory network for neuroectoderm specification.

Segmentation and Somite Formation

As the AP axis of the embryo forms, the paraxial mesoderm undergoes a process of segmentation to establish the characteristic metameric body plan of vertebrates. In bird and mammalian embryos, segmentation is closely coupled with somite formation. Somites are epithelial clusters of about 1000 paraxial mesoderm cells that form by epithelialization of the paraxial mesoderm along either side of the neural tube (Fig. 1-3). Fish and frog embryos develop more rapidly than avian and mammalian embryos, forming free-swimming neonates within 24 to 48 h. Paraxial mesoderm in these embryos becomes segmented without epithelialization and somite formation.[27] As discussed further on, the processes of segmentation and somite formation are coupled to the gene regulat-ory program that initiates expression of regulatory genes for specification of muscle and other mesoderm progenitors.

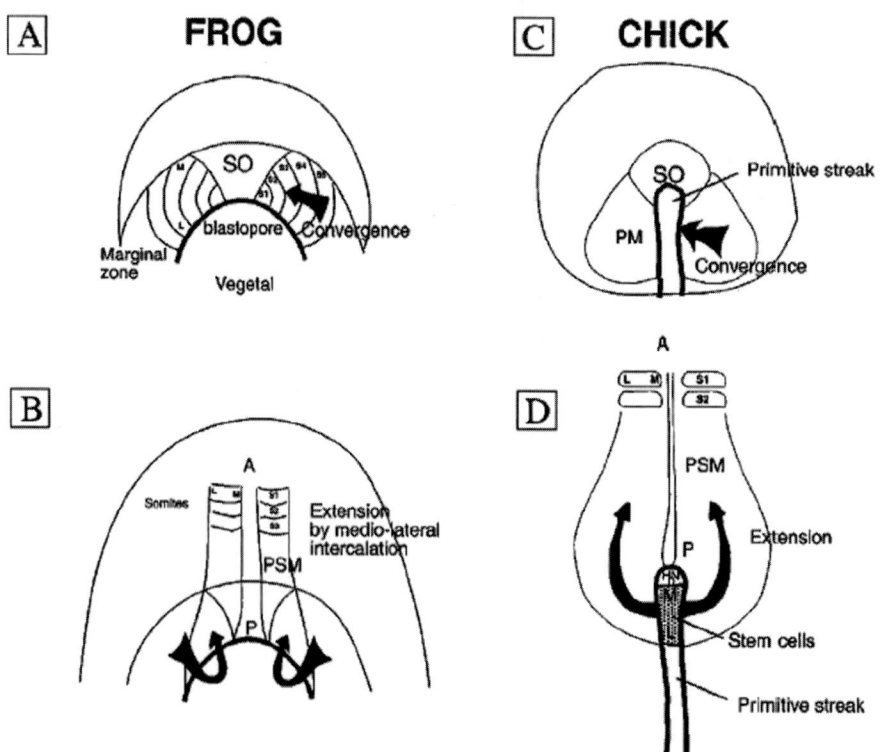

FIGURE 1-2. Gastrulation and the formation of the paraxial mesoderm in frogs (A, B) and chicks (C, D). A. Vegetal view of a Xenopus embryo at the beginning of gastrulation. The presumptive territory of the paraxial mesoderm lies on either side of the Spemann organizer (SO) in the marginal zone. Prospective somites are thought to be organized in a prepattern reflecting their future anteroposterior distribution along the axis (S1-Sn) (Keller 2000). During gastrulation, cells of the prospective paraxial mesoderm converge toward the blastopore (thick black line), where they involute. The black arrow shows the direction of the convergence movements. M–L: Future somatic mediolateral axis. B. Caudal view of a Xenopus embryo at the neurula stage. The anterior paraxial mesoderm has involuted and forms the presomitic mesoderm (PSM) by extension movements due to mediolateral intercalation of cells. Involution (black arrows) continues at the blastopore level (thick black line). C. Dorsal view of a gastrulating chick blastoderm. The presumptive territories of the paraxial mesoderm (PM) are found in the epiblast, lateral to the forming primitive streak (thick black line). Convergence movements of these territories will bring the cells to the streak, where they ingress to form the paraxial mesoderm. The Spemann organizer (SO) corresponds to the Hensen's node in chicks and is located at the rostral tip of the streak. D. Dorsal view of a chicken embryo at the neurula stage. The presumptive territories of the paraxial mesoderm have not ingressed into the primitive streak (thick black line) and are found resident as a stem cell population in the Hensen's node (HN) and the rostral primitive streak. This stem cell population will generate the PSM by extension movements (black arrows) over the entire length of the axis. A = Anterior; L = lateral; M = medial; P = posterior. (From Pourquie.[418] Reproduced by permission.)

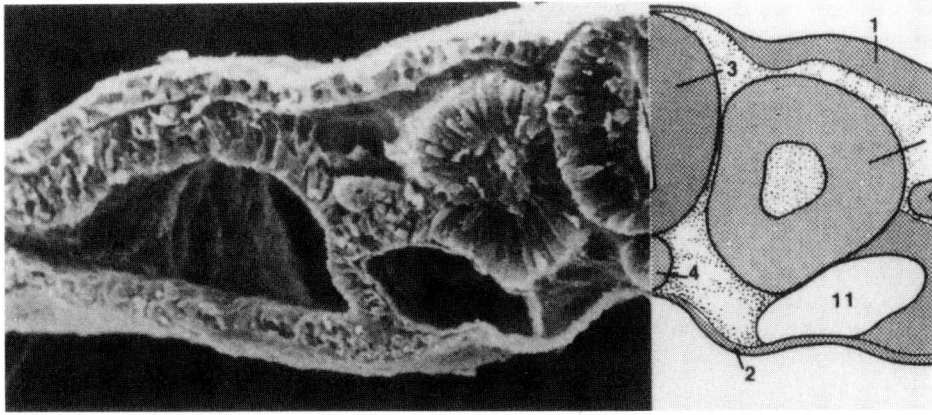

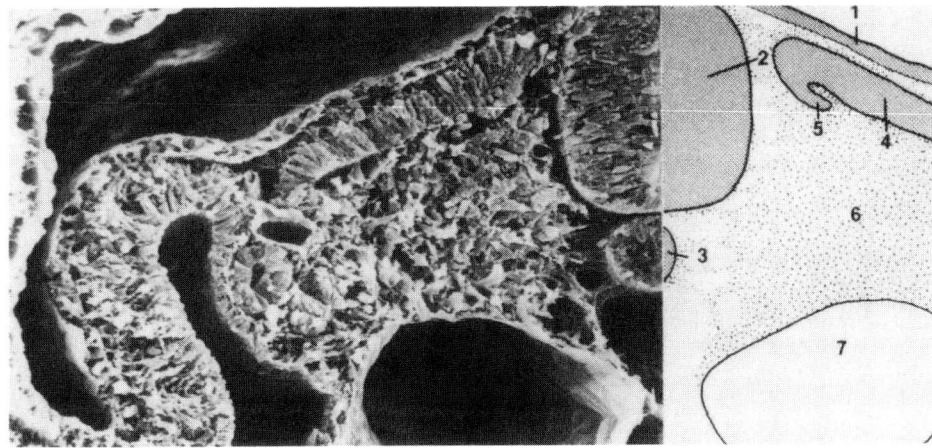

FIGURE 1-3. Scanning electron micrographs and diagrammatic representations of sections through the prospective wing bud regions of the chick embryo at about 45 h (panel A) and 55 h (panel B) of development. Panel A structures: 1 = ectoderm; 2 = endoderm; 3 = neural tube; 4 = notochord; 5 = somite; 6 = intermediate mesoderm; 7 = wolffian duct; 8 = somatopleure; 9 = splanchnopleure; 10 = body cavity coelom; 11 = aorta. Panel B structures: 1 = ectoderm; 2 = neural tube; 3 = notochord; 4 = dermatome; 5 = dorsomedial limp region of myotome formation; 6 = scleratome; 7 = aorta; 8 = pronephric duct; 9 = Wolffian duct; 10 = serous epithelium underlying region of wing bud somatopleure (mesenchyme + overlying ectoderm); 11 = body cavity coelom; 12 = lateral limiting sulcus. (*From Jacob and Christ.*[419] *Reproduced by permission.*)

Epithelial somites are organized as thick-walled vesicles of high columnar epithelial cells arranged radially around a small cavity of mesenchymal cells. Embryos of different vertebrate groups form variant numbers of somite pairs, reflecting evolutionary variations in cervical, thoracic, lumbar, and sacral anatomy.[28] Chick embryos have 45 somite pairs, formed at 90-min intervals, between days E2 and E4 of development. Mouse embryos form 60 somite pairs between 8.0 and 11.5 days postcoitum (dpc). Paraxial mesoderm segmentation and somite formation are tightly coordinated processes in bird and mouse embryos.

Segmentation is controlled by a segmentation clock that functions as a molecular oscillator, as evidenced by the cyclic expression of specific mRNAs that define the timing of segmentation and somite formation and define the posterior boundaries of newly formed segments (Fig. 1-4).[29–31] These cyclically expressed mRNAs are regulated by Notch developmental signaling ligand, including Hairy/E(spl) transcription factor, Lunatic fringe (Lfng), which encodes a glycosyltransferase-modifying enzyme of Notch ligand, and DeltaC, a related Notch ligand. The oscillatory expression of these cycling genes initiates when paraxial mesoderm cells populate the primitive streak. Interestingly, the cyclic expression of cycling genes is not blocked by protein synthesis inhibitors, indicating that segmentation is controlled by a posttranslational oscillator.[29] Mutations that disrupt expression of many Notch signaling pathway genes also disrupt somite boundary formation, indicating that Notch signaling either participates as a downstream output regulator of clock activity or is a component of the clock itself.[32,33] Lfng is an highly unstable, negative regulator of Notch signaling activity whose expression itself is controlled by Notch signaling. As such, Lfng can function as an oscillatory regulator of the clock through establishment of a negative feedback loop that drives the oscillation of Notch signaling (Fig. 1-5).[34]

FGF has an important role in establishing segment and somite boundaries in response to the segmentation clock by controlling the pattern of *Hox* gene expression in the paraxial mesoderm along the AP axis of the embryo.[35] *FGF8* expressed in the paraxial mesoderm generates a moving wavefront that defines a boundary of new somite formation, based on the finding that ectopic FGF expression in the paraxial mesoderm repositions somite boundaries and disrupts the AP expression of *Hox* genes. Somite epithelialization is controlled by β-Catenin-mediated Wnt signaling[36] and by *Paraxis*, a bHLH transcription factor gene that is expressed in paraxial mesoderm and in newly formed somites and is required for somite epithelialization.[37] *Paraxis* (−/−) mouse embryos do not form epithelial somites, but undergo segmentation, as evidenced by the segmental activation of muscle-specific reg-

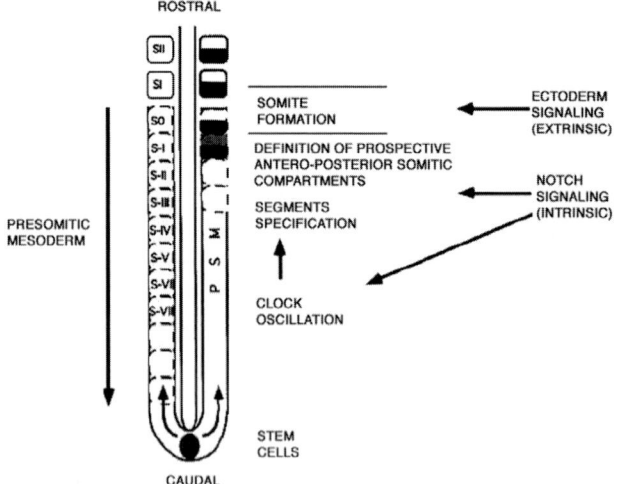

FIGURE 1-4. Major regulatory processes involved in formation of presomitic mesoderm (PSM) and somites (S) in the chick embryo. Somites are numbered according to the nomenclature defined by Ordahl.[420] Twelve presumptive somites are present in chick presomitic mesoderm. These presumptive somites are labeled with a negative sign, according to the somite nomenclature. S0 corresponds to the newest forming somite. (*From Pourquie.[418] Reproduced by permission.*)

ulatory genes, although the later patterning of somite tendon, bone, and vascular progenitors is disrupted. The epithelial somite appears to provide a structural scaffold for spatially patterning multiple lineages.[38] Consistent with this possibility, paraxial mesoderm in frog and fish embryos gives rise almost exclusively to segmented myotomal muscles along the body axis without undergoing somite epithelialization. Only a few cells in each segment form sclerotomal cartilage progenitors. This is in marked contrast to somites of birds and mammals, which produce large numbers of sclerotomal progenitors for vertebrae and ribs as well as progenitors for tendons, dermal tissues, and vascular tissues.

PARAXIAL MESODERM ORIGINS OF BODY AND HEAD MUSCLE PROGENITORS

Body Muscle Progenitors

Paraxial mesoderm in birds and mammals is the source of somite progenitors of muscles, vertebrae, and ribs as well as tendons, blood vessels, and dermis. The paraxial mesoderm origins of these progenitor lineages has been established using "lineage marking" and "cell-fate mapping" techniques. Individual or small clusters of cells in the early embryo are "marked" either by localized microinjection with visible dyes, by expression of "reporter" transgenes such as lacZ or GFP, or by engraftment of tissues from closely related species that are distinguishable by species-specific cell markers such as pigment,[4] cellular antigens,[39] and nucleolar morphology (Fig. 1-6).[40] Once marked, cell movements, mitotic divisions, and fates of individual or clusters of cells can be traced by microscopy in the living embryo or after fixation. Lineage tracing approaches continue to be a rich source of information on the origins and developmental histories of muscle and other progenitor lineages in embryos[41–43] as well as an important experimental tool for investigating the regulatory and signal networks controlling the origins and differentiation of muscle progenitors.[39,44–48] In embryos with small cell numbers, such as *C. elegans* or tunicates, the fates of every cell in the embryo, including muscle progenitors, have been traced directly using live cell and confocal microscopy.[49,50] Lineage tracing methods also have been used in combination with surgical grafting and clonal cell culture and explant studies as experimental tools to investigate the regulatory genes and signals that control the specification of muscle progenitors in embryos.

Cell fate specification is a genetic regulatory process that leads to the formation of the precursor lineages that form differentiated cell types. In the case of skeletal muscle, these precursors are referred to as *skeletal myobl*asts. Cell-fate specification is investigated using a combination of surgical grafting and lineage marking techniques to test the potentials of different embryonic tissues to form specific tissues and organs when transplanted to ectopic sites in embryos or into tissue culture. Such experiments determine whether explanted tissues can survive, proliferate, and differentiate at ectopic sites in the embryo or whether cells in these explants are induced to form different tissues characteristic of those formed at their site of engraftment. Using this experimental paradigm, embryologists have discovered that tissues in the early embryo are unspecified and plastic. These tissues have the potential to change their developmental fates in response to inductive signals when transplanted to

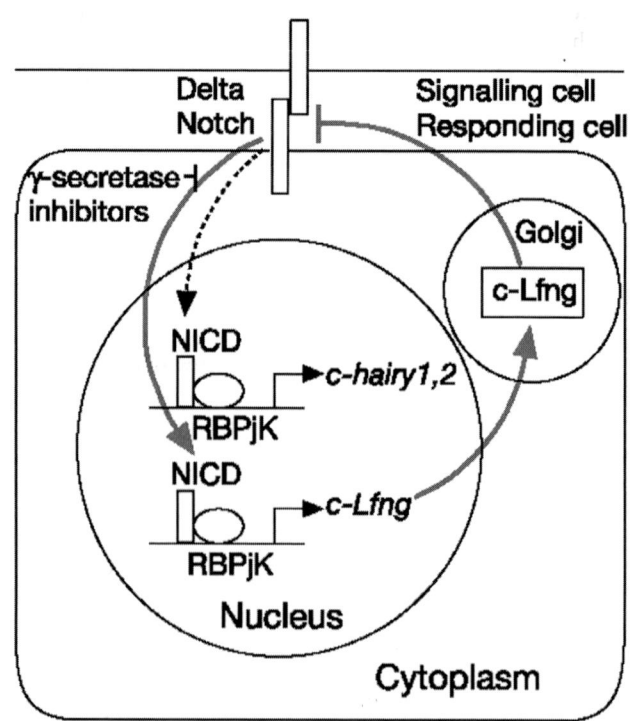

FIGURE 1-5. Model of a negative feedback oscillator mechanism for segmentation of paraxial mesoderm. Notch signaling activates cyclic gene transcription. Lfng then closes the loop by modifying Notch, thereby inhibiting Notch signaling. This negative effect is transient owing to the rapid turnover of Lfng. NICD, Notch$_{icd}$. (*From Dale et al.[34] Reproduced by permission.*)

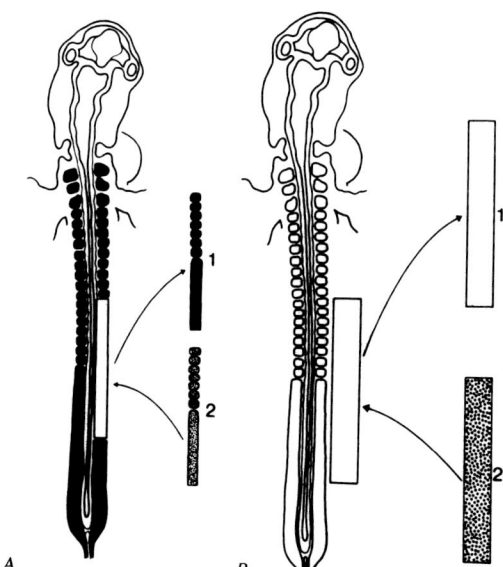

FIGURE 1-6. Chick-quail grafting experiments to determine the developmental fate maps of muscle precursor cells. *A.* Removal of wing-level brachial somatic mesoderm (somites + unsegmented plate) from stage 13 chick embryo and replacement with comparable region from a quail embryo donor. *B.* Removal of somatopleural tissue (mesoderm + overlying ectoderm) from wing-level stage 13 chick embryo and replacement with comparable region from a quail embryo. (*From Jacob et al.[421] Reproduced by permission.*)

different sites in the embryo. Their capacity for respecification, however, becomes progressively restricted as the embryo develops. Such findings have led to the idea that spatially distributed inductive signals are produced within the early embryo to specify the developmental fates of groups of embryonic cells, which will then produce progenitor lineages to form the differentiated tissues and organs of the body. Skeletal myoblasts arise from paraxial mesoderm in response to inductive signals that are now being discovered. By definition, myoblast progenitors that have become specified can proliferate, yet they stably inherit the potential to differentiate into skeletal muscle, even in the artificial environment of clonal cell culture.[51,52] Myoblasts are in a remarkably stable state, making it possible to establish immortalized skeletal myoblast cell lines with unlimited potential for proliferation and for muscle differentiation.[53,54] Such myoblast cell lines are widely utilized in molecular and cell biological studies of muscle differentiation.

Fate-mapping studies show that somites include multipotential progenitors that form all of the body musculature of vertebrate embryos as well as progenitors for vertebral cartilage and ribs, tendons, vascular tissue, and dermis.[44,45,55–57] These somite progenitor lineages arise from localized cell populations within the newly formed somite, as first evidenced by the patterned expression of different lineage-specific transcription factors immediately following somite formation to initiate the specification of somite-derived lineages (Fig. 1-7).[38] Epaxial muscle progenitors in the dorsal medial somite activate *Myf5* and *MyoD*, myogenic regulatory factor (MRF) genes that control the specification of epaxial muscles as well as all other myogenic lineages in the vertebrate embryo.

Ventral somite cells activate *Pax1* and *Pax9*, which define a domain of progenitors that form the sclerotome.[58]

Sclerotomal cells expressing *Pax1* undergo an epithelial-to-mesenchymal transformation and then migrate ventrally under the notochord and neural tube at the embryo midline to give rise to cartilage that forms vertebrae and ribs. Dorsal somite cells remain part of an epithelial sheet and flatten to form the dermamyotome, a columnar epithelium just below the surface of the dorsal ectoderm that gives rise to dermal progenitors.[59,60] Cells at the medial and lateral margins of the dermamyotome form a dorsomedial (DML) lip, which is the source of epaxial muscle progenitors, and a ventrolateral (VLL) lip, which is the source of hypaxial muscle progenitors (Fig. 1-7). Occipital and cervical somites, which are first to form during AP axis formation, form only a VLL, the source of progenitors for neck, tongue, and larynx skeletal muscles. In the thoracic and trunk regions, the DML is the source of epaxial muscle progenitors, which form the deep back and intercostal muscles.[61] Grafting and lineage tracing studies show that the DML also is a source of nonmyogenic dermatome progenitors.[62,63] The VLL of thoracic and trunk somites gives rise to three distinct muscle progenitor lineages: (1) myotomal progenitors that migrate ventromedially under the dermatome to form the ventral aspect of the myotome; (2) hypaxial progenitors that delaminate in small numbers from the newly formed VLL and migrate to sites of abdominal muscle formation; and (3) limb progenitors that delaminate from the lateral edge of fore- and hindlimb-level somites and migrate into the limb bud, where they localize in the dorsal and ventral muscle-forming regions. Mesenchymal cells in the central portion of the somite give rise to endothelial cells that vascularize surrounding axial tissues.[64,65] In the limb, endothelial cells arise from bipotential somite progenitors that also give rise to the limb muscle progenitors. The central "intercalated" region of the dermamyotome gives rise to a discrete population of muscle progenitors.[46,66] Tendon progenitors for axial muscles arise from a *Scleraxis*-expressing cell population localized at the margin between the VLL and the sclerotome.[57] Tendon progenitors for limb muscles arise from a distinct population of lateral plate mesoderm cells that migrate into the limb bud prior to somite-derived limb muscle progenitors.[67]

Head Muscle Progenitors

Skeletal muscles of the head derive from paraxial mesoderm on either side of the future brain (Fig. 1-8).[68] Current knowledge of the origins of head muscle progenitors comes largely from embryologic and surgical studies of avian embryos. Craniofacial muscles are anatomically complex, and their embryologic origins have been traced using techniques for cell transplantation and retroviral cell-fate mapping as well as gene expression studies.[69–71] Progenitors for branchial arch and extraocular muscles arise from unsegmented mesoderm in the head, in contrast to the progenitors of neck, tongue, and laryngeal muscles, which arise from the most anterior somites, the first to form in the embryo. Extraocular muscle progenitors arise from prechordal mesoderm adjacent to the anterior neural plate and from the paraxial mesoderm adjacent to the posterior midbrain; first branchial arch progenitors arise from mesoderm at the level of the mesocephalon and second and third arch progenitors from

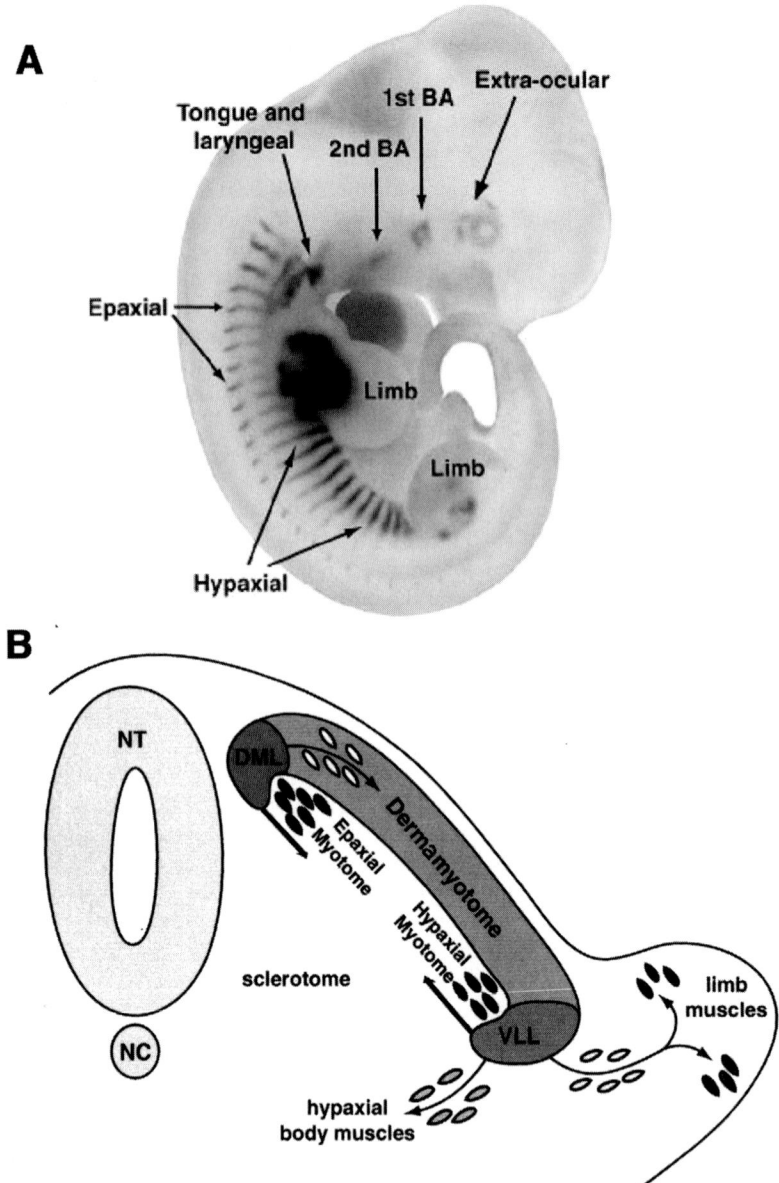

FIGURE 1-7. A. Myogenic progenitors in the mouse embryo 11.5 dpc, as visualized through expression of the *MyoD* Core Enhancer/*LacZ* reporter. *MyoD* transgene expression is localized to trunk somite progenitors at the sites of epaxial, hypaxial, and limb muscle differentiation, and the head mesoderm progenitors, including the first and second branchial arches (BA), the tongue and larynx, and the extraocular muscles. B. Somite origins of myogenic progenitors for epaxial, hypaxial, and limb muscles in bird and mouse embryos. Muscle progenitors originate in the dorsomedial and ventrolateral lips of the dermamyotome. Cells of the dorsomedial lip (DML) migrate ventrolaterally, differentiate, and form the myotomal muscles, which will give rise to epaxial deep back muscles. The ventrolateral lip (VLL) provides progenitors that migrate ventrally to form the ventral body wall muscles, migrate dorsolaterally to form the hypaxial myotome, and delaminate from the VLL to migrate to the dorsal and ventral muscle-forming regions of the limb, where they differentiate to form the limb musculature. (*From Pownall et al.[27] Reproduced by permission.*)

more posterior mesoderm near the hindbrain. Head and neck mesodermal progenitors migrate from the embryo's axis to specific sites of myogenesis and anatomic muscle formation (Fig. 1-9).

Developmental Signals for Specification of Body and Head Muscle Progenitors

Cell and tissue transplantation and lineage-marking experiments reveal that myogenic progenitors become specified for myogenesis in response to inductive signals from surrounding tissues.[38] Individual paraxial mesodermal cells in *Xenopus* embryos at the early gastrula stage are fated to become muscle, but they fail to do so when grafted to ectopic sites. During later gastrula stages, such single cells are competent to differentiate into muscle as single cells and therefore have become specified for myogenesis.[72] Significantly, in contrast to single cells, clusters of early gastrula paraxial mesodermal cells are competent for muscle differentiation, indicating that local "community effect" signaling between paraxial mesodermal cells mediates muscle specification.[73] An embryonic eFGF signaling ligand has been identified as the "community effect" signal for paraxial mesoderm specification,[74] likely through its function to activate MRF muscle specification genes, as discussed below.[75]

Paraxial mesoderm of avian embryos in the early gastrula stage is fated to become muscle but is also unspecified. Grafts of these cells do not form muscle when transplanted into Henson's node at the anterior midline. Instead, engrafted paraxial mesodermal cells form notochord, which is the normal fate of node cells.[41] Specification of muscle progenitors occurs later, following somite formation, as revealed by chick-quail somite grafting studies.[76,77] In these experiments, medial and lateral fragments of somites from the newest formed somites of stage 12 quail embryos were engrafted

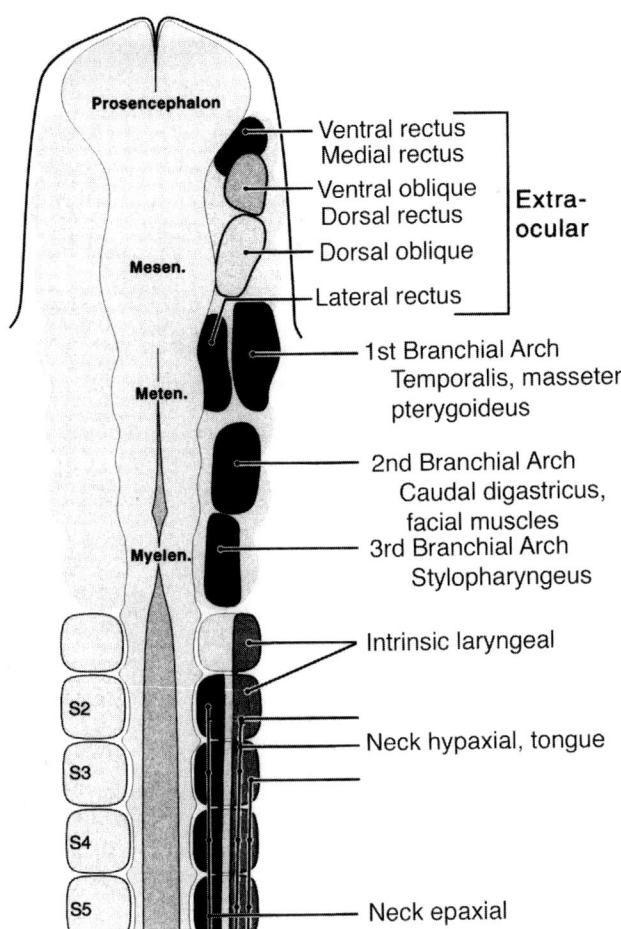

FIGURE 1-8. Paraxial mesoderm origins of the anatomic muscles of the head and neck of the chick embryo. S1–S5 are the first somites formed along the embryo AP axis. Mesen. = mesencephalon; Meten. = metencephalon; Myelen. = myelencephalon. (*From Noden.*[70] *Reproduced by permission.*)

into equivalent somites in chick embryos in normal and reversed dorsoventral and mediolateral orientations. The developmental fates of transplanted quail cells and host chick cells were monitored by histologic analysis using the species-specific quail nucleolar marker. Newly formed somites at this stage are at the level of the forelimb bud and give rise to epaxial myotomal muscles from DML progenitors of the medial somite and migratory limb muscle progenitors from the VLL of the lateral somite. Nomenclature identifies somite I as the most posterior, newest formed somite at any embryonic stage; more anterior somites have increasing numerals. When medial and lateral fragments of limb-level somites I to III were exchanged, medial (epaxial) and lateral (limb) muscle progenitor cells adopted fates dictated by their new positions relative to the embryo axis; however, somite fragments isolated anterior to somite III were no longer plastic in their capacity to contribute to epaxial and migratory limb progenitors, indicating that these more mature somite cells have become specified during a 4- to 5-h interval after somite formation. Interestingly, dye marking studies in the chick[41] and LacZ retrospective marking studies in the mouse[78] reveal that medial and lateral somite cells arise from separate populations of paraxial mesoderm progenitors, further establishing that the fates of medial and lateral cells in newly formed somites are unspecified at the time of somite formation. Similarly, reversal of the dorsoventral orientations of fragments of newly formed somites does not disrupt formation of normal sclerotome in the ventral somite and dermatome in the doral somite, showing that dorsal and ventral somite cells also are unspecified at the time of somite formation.[79] By this test, the fates of sclerotome progenitors in the ventral somite are specified later than epaxial myotomal progenitors in the dorsal somite, indicating that these specification processes are regulated by distinct control mechanisms.[46]

The developmental timing for specification of limb muscle progenitors is controversial. Somite progenitors that migrate into the limb bud are myogenic when engrafted to an ectopic site in the ventral somite, which normally forms the sclerotome, suggesting that migrating progenitors are specified to myogenesis.[47] However, somite-derived muscle progenitors also can form cartilage when dissociated from the limb mesenchyme and engrafted into the cartilage-forming region of the limb bud, suggesting that some limb muscle progenitors remain unspecified even after they become localized in muscle-forming sites in the limb bud.[80]

The plasticity of cells in newly formed somites for alternative fates provides evidence that somite specification is

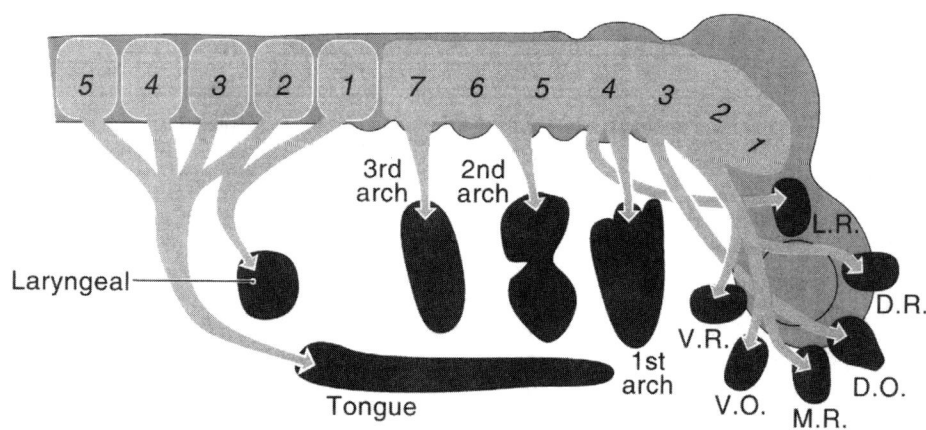

FIGURE 1-9. Movements of head muscle precursors in the chick embryo. VR=ventral rectus; MR, medial rectus; VO=ventral oblique; DR=dorsal rectus; DO=dorsal oblique; LR=lateral rectus. (*From Noden.*[70] *Reproduced by permission.*)

controlled by positional signals from tissues surrounding the somite. Direct evidence for such signaling came from surgical studies of the role of neural tube and notochord interactions in chick embryos.[81] Ablation of neural tube and notochord blocks the formation of epaxial myotomal muscles from DML progenitors but not the formation of hypaxial muscles and limb muscles derived from VLL progenitors on the lateral somite. These findings reveal that DML progenitors for epaxial myotome formation are controlled by neural tube/notochord signals and that the signals for epaxial and hypaxial myogenesis are distinct. Neural tube/notochord interactions for epaxial myotome differentiation are required only until just prior to the initiation of myotome differentiation in somite VIII in stage 12 chick embryos.[82] As discussed in more detail below, epaxial progenitor specification is now known to be controlled by multiple interacting developmental signals, including Sonic hedgehog (Shh), Wnts, and BMPs. The signaling interactions required for specification of head and somite body myogenic progenitors also are distinct. Somites engrafted into the head mesoderm and, similarly, head mesoderm engrafted into the body axis do not respond to axial neural tube/notochord signals for myogenesis.[83,84] Thus, distinct signaling mechanisms control the myogenic specification of head, epaxial, and hypaxial progenitors.

MRF Transcription Factors for Specification of Body and Head Muscle Progenitors

The myogenic regulatory factors (MRFs) are an evolutionarily conserved family of four bHLH transcription factors with regulatory functions in the specification and differentiation of muscle progenitors in vertebrate and invertebrate embryos. The MRFs were identified in molecular screens for regulatory genes with dominant regulatory activities to convert 10T1/2 cells into myogenic progenitors. 10T1/2 is a fibroblastic cell line established from mouse embryos that can be induced to form skeletal muscle, fat, and cartilage in response to brief treatment with 5′-azacytidine, a cystidine nucleotide analogue that inhibits DNA methylating enzymes.[85] 5′azacytidine also leads to high-frequency clonal conversions of 10T1/2 to form stable lineages of myoblasts, chondroblasts, and adipoblasts. These clonal lines can proliferate indefinitely and retain the potential to differentiate into muscle, cartilage, and fat in response to reduced levels of proliferation factors in the serum component of tissue culture medium. 10T1/2 cell, therefore, is a multipotential cell model for studies of the specification of muscle, cartilage, and fat progenitors.[86]

The high frequencies of 5′-azacytidine-induced 10T1/2 clonal conversion to myoblast lineages were the basis for a master regulatory gene model for myoblast specification and for an experimental strategy to test this model by DNA transfection and gene-transfer techniques.[86,87] 5′-azacytidine, through its known activity as an inhibitor of DNA methylation, was predicted to activate a dominantly acting muscle master regulatory gene by demethylating regulatory sequences controlling its expression. Evidence for dominant muscle regulatory genes was also provided by heterokaryon studies, which showed that myoblast nuclei could transactivate the expression of muscle-specific genes in nonmuscle nuclei.[88,89] This model also predicted that dominant regulatory genes for myogenesis could be identified using a DNA transfection approach.[86] DNA transfection studies revealed that genomic DNA from 5-azacytidine-derived myoblasts and recombinant human genomic DNA in cosmid libraries could convert 10T1/2 cells to stable myogenic progenitor lineages[87,90] at frequencies of single-gene transfer.[91] MyoD was the first MRF to be cloned, using cDNA transfection in the 10T1/2 myogenic conversion assay.[92] *MyoD* is a bHLH transcription factor consistent with its function as a muscle master regulator. Furthermore, MyoD expression, once activated, is maintained by autoregulation, providing a mechanism to stabilize the specification of myogenic progenitors.[93] Subsequent to the discovery of MyoD, three additional bHLH MRFs—*Myf5, Myogenin,* and *MRF4*—were identified, based on their sequence homology with MyoD and their activities to convert 10T1/2 cells to muscle in the 10T1/2 cDNA transfection assay.[94] Invertebrates, *C. elegans, Drosophila*, sea urchins, tunicates, and ancestral vertebrates have a single *MyoD*-related MRF gene that converts 10T1/2 cells to myogenic progenitors and is expressed and functions in skeletal myogenic lineages during embryogenesis, as discussed below.

MRF expression is highly restricted to skeletal muscles in vertebrate and invertebrate embryos.[27] *Myf5* and *MyoD* are expressed in proliferative myoblasts in cell culture and in head, epaxial, hypaxial, and limb body muscle progenitors in embryos, indicating their progenitor-specific functions (Figs. 1-7 and 1-10). *MyoD* expression persists in newly formed differentiated muscle fibers, whereas *Myf5* expression ceases during differentiation. *Myf5* transcripts also are transiently expressed at very low levels in the brain, neural tube, and paraxial mesoderm of avian and mouse embryos, although Myf5 protein has not been detected, suggesting that Myf5 mRNAs expressed in nonmyogenic cells are translationally regulated.[95,96] *Myogenin* and *MRF4* are activated during muscle differentiation, indicating their functions in muscle differentiation.

The timing of *Myf5* and *MyoD* activation in muscle progenitors is specific to the progenitor lineages that form different anatomic muscles in the head and body.[70] In avian embryos, *Myf5* and *MyoD* are coactivated in DML epaxial muscle progenitors in coordination with somite formation. In mouse embryos, *Myf5* is activated in DML epaxial progenitors in newly formed somites, but *MyoD* is not activated until 2.5 days later, well after myotome differentiation has initiated.[97] DML progenitors maintain MRF expression and are a source of myogenic progenitors that migrate from the DML ventrolaterally under the dermamyotome, where they initiate *Myogenin, MRF4,* and contractile protein gene expression and form the dorsal aspect of myotomal muscles.[98,99] Following dermamyotome formation, *Myf5* and *MyoD* are activated in the VVL, and these progenitors migrate ventromedially under the dermamyotome to form the ventral aspect of the myotome. Additionally, in the trunk region of the embryo, small numbers (50 to 100) of cells on the ventrolateral edge of the dermamyotome delaminate from the ventral aspect of the dermamyotome and migrate to sites of myogenesis in the limb and abdomen, where appendicular muscles are formed. These migratory myogenic cells do not activate *Myf5* and *MyoD* until they have completed their migration and are localized in the dorsal and ventral muscle-forming regions of the limb and in muscle-forming regions of the abdomen, where they proliferate to build skeletal muscles. Head mesodermal cells also migrate from head mesoderm along the neural tissue in the head to sites of facial and eye muscle differentiation, where they then activate *Myf5* or *MyoD*[69–70] (Fig. 1-10). The different developmental timing and patterning of cell migration and *Myf5* and *MyoD* activation in the embryo provides evidence that myogenesis is controlled by a complexity of local cell interactions and signals that differ at various anatomic sites.

Gene-targeting studies in the mouse embryo establish that MRFs have essential regulatory functions in both the specification and the differentiation of muscle progenitors. Mice with targeted mutations in *Myf5* (−/−) and *MyoD* (−/−) are viable and fertile,[100–103] whereas *Myf5* (−/−); *MyoD* (−/−) compound mutant embryos lack all muscle progenitors and skeletal muscles but form other anatomic tissues normally, including other somite-derived tissues. However, note that the original *Myf5* (−/−) allele produced by gene targeting has rib deficiencies, which are an artifact of the aberrant activity of a *neo* selectable marker gene cassette used in the gene targeting.[102] *Myf5* (−/−) mice with a deleted *neo* cassette form ribs and muscles normally and are viable and reproductive as adults.[104] *Myf5* (−/−); *MyoD* (−/−) compound mutant embryos do not express *Myogenin* and *MRF4* in muscle progenitors and are completely defective in muscle differentiation. Therefore *Myf5* and *MyoD* have redundant functions in the specification of muscle progenitors, whereas *Myogenin* and *MRF4* function in muscle differentiation. (However, also note that further studies are required to investigate myogenesis in compound *Myf5;MyoD* mutant embryos that have alleles cleanly deleted of their *neo* selection cassettes[103] in order to definitively test whether *MRF4* and *Myogenin* can function in earlier processes of progenitor specification in the absence of *Myf5* and *MyoD* function.) In adults, *MyoD* and likely *Myf5* have additional regulatory functions in fiber-type differentiation[104] and satellite cell recruitment for muscle regeneration.[105]

Lineage marking experiments in *Myf5* (−/−) and *MyoD* (−/−) mutant embryos provide important evidence that *Myf5* and *MyoD* are required for specification of muscle progenitors. The cell fates of epaxial muscle progenitors in *Myf5* (−/−) embryos have been traced by targeting *LacZ* transgene into the *Myf5* locus to both disrupt *Myf5* function and provide a lineage tracer. This approach was used to assay the cellular fates of homozygous heterozygous *Myf5* mutant somite cells in epaxial muscle progenitors, which are highly delayed in the activation of *MyoD*. A histoenzymatic β-glactosidase assay identifies *LacZ*-expressing progenitors.[106] As *MyoD* is not activated in epaxial muscle progenitors in the mouse, *Myf5* expression and function can be examined independent of *MyoD* in the epaxial muscle progenitors of embryos with *LacZ*-targeted *Myf5* mutations, independent of *MyoD*, which is not activated for 3 days following the time of normal *Myf5* activation. In these mice, the *LacZ* transgene is activated normally in *Myf5*-expressing epaxial lineages in heterozygous *Myf5* (−/+) and homozygous *Myf5* (−/−) mutant embryos; however, *LacZ*-expressing progenitors in *Myf5* (−/−) mutant embryos remain localized at the DML in relatively few numbers and are blocked in the initiation of myotone differentiation for 3 days until *MyoD* is activated. At that time, *LacZ*-expressing DML cells recover their activity

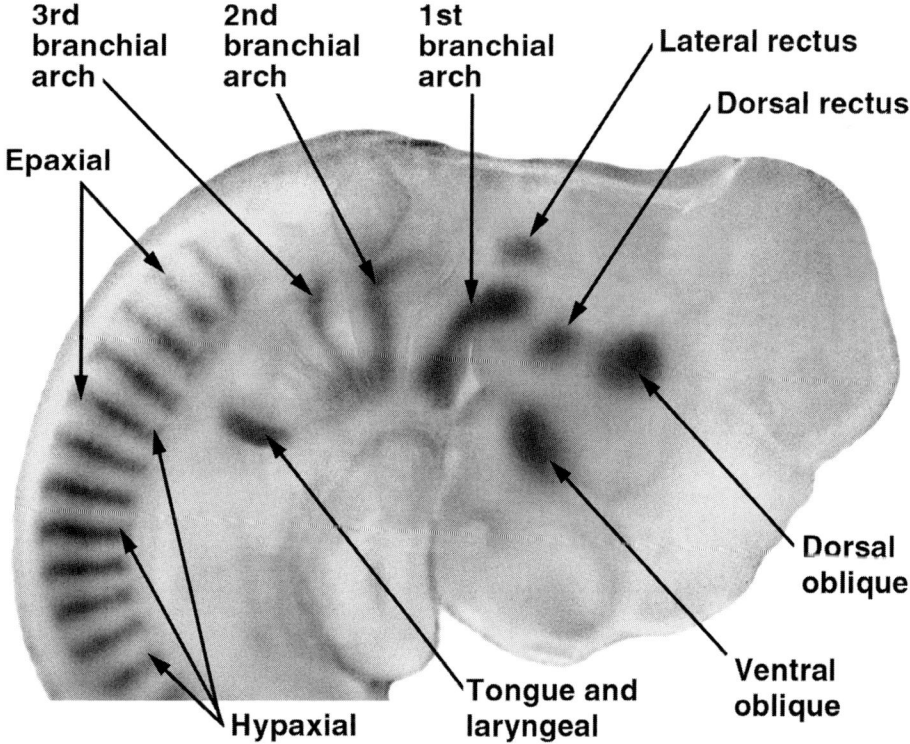

FIGURE 1-10. *Myf5* expression in head and body muscle progenitors of the chick embryo. In situ hybridization assay of *Myf5* expression in stage 19 chick embryos. (*From Noden.*[70] *Reproduced by permission.*)

to differentiate and form the myotone. These findings indicate, therefore, that *Myf5* is required for the proliferation, migration, and differentiation of myogenic progenitors, consistent with the results of cell culture studies of *Myf5* (−/−) and *MyoD* (−/−) mutant myoblasts.[219] Significantly, some *LacZ*-expressing *Myf5* (−/−) mutant progenitors were observed to migrate aberrantly into the dermatome and sclerotome, where they express sclerotome- and dermamyotome-specific marker genes. This important observation provides evidence that *Myf5* function is essential for epaxial progenitors to become specified to myogenesis. In the absence of *Myf5* function, DML cells remain multipotential, with the potential for specification to dermal and sclerotome lineages if they migrate to ectopic sites within the somite. Further evidence for the function of MRFs in muscle progenitor specification comes from cell-fate studies of limb muscle progenitors in *Myf5* (−/−); *MyoD* (−/−) double embryos, using *MyoD* core enhancer (CE)-*LacZ* transgene as a lineage tracer.[107] In *Myf5* (−/−) and *MyoD* (−/−) double embryos, somite progenitors migrate to the limb bud normally but then further migrate aberrantly and have cartilage cell morphology when they are found in ectopic sites of chondrogenesis. Both of these studies indicate *Myf5* and *MyoD* are regulators of genes that control the specification of multipotential somite cells as well as genes that are required for their local migration and proliferation. The specific genes controlled of *Myf5* and *MyoD* for muscle progenitor specification remain unknown.

MRFs function together with other mesodermal regulators, as revealed by the finding that MyoD fails to convert endodermally derived liver cells to myogenesis unless MyoD-expressing liver cells are combined as heterokaryons with mesodermally derived fibroblasts.[108] Furthermore, ectopic MyoD expression in nonmesodermal lineages in mouse embryos,[109] totipotential embryonic stem cells,[110] and *Xenopus* embryos[111] does not convert these cells to differentiated muscle, although ectopic MyoD expression does activate a partial program of myogenesis, including expression of chromosomal *MyoD* and a few muscle differentiation genes, including α-actin. Finally, MyoD mRNA and protein are abundantly expressed in paraxial mesoderm of early gastrula cells of *Xenopus* embryos, and yet these expressing cells remain unspecified, as shown by transplantation to ectopic sites in the embryo, where they fail as individual cells to undergo muscle differentiation.[72] These mesodermal MRF cooperating genes remain to be identified.

Signaling and Transcriptional Networks for Myf5 and MyoD Regulation

As *Myf5* and *MyoD* expressed in paraxial mesoderm control muscle progenitor specification, investigations have focused on understanding the molecular, genetic, and embryologic mechanisms controlling the activation of these key MRF regulators. Transgenic studies in the mouse reveal that *Myf5* is controlled by distinct transcription enhancers for activation in epaxial, hypaxial, limb, and head muscle progenitor lineages (Fig. 1-11).[63,112–117] Such modular *Myf5* transcriptional regulation provides evidence that distinct regulatory mechanisms control myogenesis at the different sites of anatomic muscle formation in the embryo. *Myf5* transcription enhancers controlling head and epaxial progenitor expression are localized in the intragenic region between *MRF4* and *Myf5*, in the *Myf5* gene itself for hypaxial progenitor expression, and in the 58-kb region upstream of the *MRF4-Myf5* locus for limb expression. The distal limb enhancer region also includes an enhancer for expression in differentiated myotomal muscle. *MRF4* regulatory elements are located in its promoter region distinct from these *Myf5* enhancers.[118–120] The physical proximity of *Myf5* and *MRF4* indicates the presence of specificity and/or boundary elements within the locus to direct the activities of their specific enhancers to their respective promoters. The linkage of the *MRF4* and *Myf5* is conserved in birds[121] and zebrafish.[122] *Myf5*

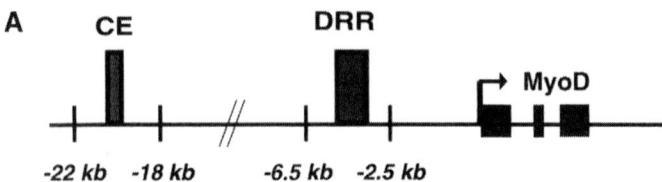

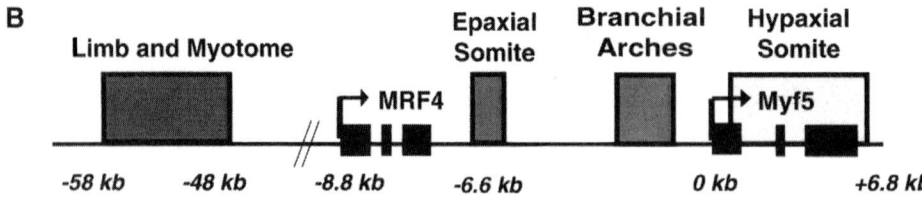

FIGURE 1-11. Multiple transcriptional control elements regulate *Myf5* and *MyoD* expression in muscle progenitors of the mouse embryo. A. *Myf5* is controlled by lineage-specific transcription enhancers in the *MRF4-Myf5* locus for expression in each of the muscle progenitor domains, including the epaxial (DML), hypaxial (VLL), limb, and branchial arches. There is also a transcription enhancer that controls expression in the differentiating myotome, located distally near the limb enhancer. B. *MyoD* is controlled by two transcription enhancers, the core enhancer (CE), which is activated in all muscle progenitor lineages, and the distal regulatory region (DRR), which is activated in all newly differentiated muscles. (*From Pownall et al.*[27] *Reproduced by permission.*)

transcriptional regulatory sequences have been identified in zebrafish[123] and Xenopus.[124]

In contrast to Myf5, MyoD activation in epaxial, hypaxial, branchial arch, and limb progenitors is controlled by a single core enhancer (CE)[125,126] and by a distal regulatory region (DRR), which maintains expression in differentiating muscle (Fig. 1-11).[127,128] The MyoD CE enhancer is activated in muscle progenitors in Myf5 (−/−); MyoD (−/−) mutant embryos under the control of currently unknown upstream regulators independent of cross regulation by Myf5.[107] By contrast, DRR activity requires Myf5 and MyoD, consistent with later activity in differentiating muscle.[129] Human and mouse CE element sequences are highly conserved, and linker scanning mutagenesis has identified CE sequences that are essential for its activity in muscle progenitors, indicating that the CE is under positive regulation.[130] An E-box bHLH transcription factor binding site controls CE activity specifically in DML and VLL but not limb and branchial arch progenitors. The bHLH regulator that interacts with this E-box site for DML- and VLL-specific MyoD transcription is unknown, as are the DRR transcription factor regulators. However, DRR (−/−) and compound mutant DRR (−/); Myf5 (−/−) embryos express chromosomal MyoD appropriately in the limb and branchial arches and in the DML and VLL progenitors,[131] indicating that the CE enhancer or another as yet unidentified enhancer is functionally redundant with the DRR. Avian MyoD is also controlled by multiple transcription enhancers, as identified by mouse transgenesis and myoblast transfection studies.[132,133] Interestingly, the sequence of the epaxial myotome-specific quail MyoD enhancer is very divergent from that of the mouse and human CE and DRR enhancers and therefore is a divergent regulatory element. This possibility is consistent with the observation that MyoD and Myf5 are coactivated in avian DML progenitors, whereas MyoD is activated several days after Myf5 in the mouse DML.[134]

Developmental signals control the transcriptional activation of Myf5 and MyoD in muscle progenitors (Fig. 1-12).[38] In avian embryos, MyoD and Myf5 are activated in epaxial progenitors of newly forming somites by neural tube and notochord signals,[81] which have distinct signaling functions.[82,135] In addition, the overlying surface ectoderm and the lateral plate mesoderm both also produce signals that function with notochord and dorsal neural tube signals to activate and localize MyoD and Myf5 expression in discrete populations of epaxial progenitors in the dorsomedial somite.[136] Sonic hedgehog is the notochord signal for Myf5 activation in epaxial progenitors. Explant and grafting studies in the avian embryo first identified notochord-produced Sonic hedgehog (Shh) as an inductive signal for Myf5 and

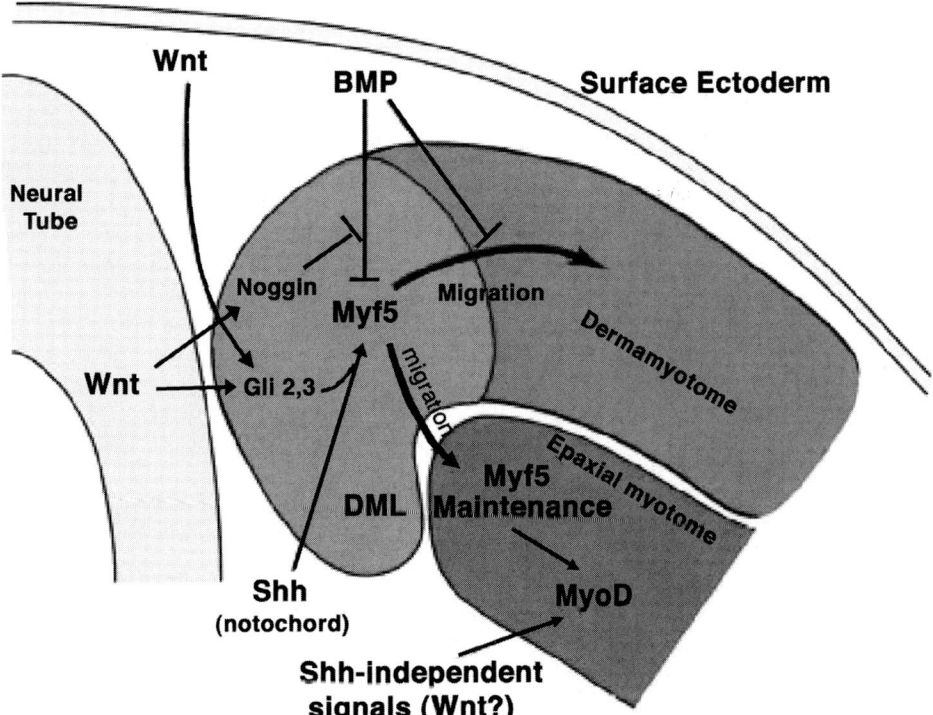

FIGURE 1-12. Model for Myf5 regulation for epaxial progenitor specification in bird and mouse embryos by cooperative Shh, Wnt, and BMP signaling. Glis are activated during somite formation in response to Wnt signaling from the surface ectoderm and dorsal neural tube to initiate Shh signaling in newly formed somites. Wnts also induce Noggin expression in the DML to create a localized domain of Shh signaling, protected from inhibitory BMPs. Long-distance Shh signaling from the notochord activates Myf5 through direct, positive regulation by Gli transcription factors, which bind to and activate the Myf5 epaxial enhancer. When Myf5-expressing cells migrate from the DML, they encounter a high BMP signal from the lateral somite that represses activity of the Myf5 epaxial enhancer. Dorsally migrating DML cells contribute to the growth of the dermamyotome. Ventrally migrating DML cells maintain Myf5 expression by an Shh-independent Myf5 myotome-specific enhancer and then initiate contractile protein expression and myotome differentiation under the control of differentiation-specific transcription factors Myogenin, MRF4, and Mef2c. (From Pownall et al.[27] Reproduced by permission.)

MyoD activation in epaxial progenitors.[82,137,138] Furthermore, *Shh* (−/−) mutant mouse embryos are blocked in *Myf5* activation specifically in epaxial progenitors but not in hypaxial, limb, or head muscle progenitors.[139] Occipital somites, which form first in the embryo, express low levels of *Myf5*, presumably under the control of a different signal.[63,140] Shh regulates *Myf5* activation in epaxial progenitors directly through Gli transcription factor effectors, which bind to an essential Gli binding site in the epaxial-specific *Myf5* transcription enhancer.[63] Shh also has an antiapoptotic activity,[141–144] but follows *Myf5* activation in the dorsal somite.[139] Hedgehog signaling in zebrafish embryos controls the specification of the "slow" adaxial and pioneer muscles but not myotomal muscles, indicating some divergence in hedgehog function.[145] *MyoD* and *Myf5* are activated in adaxial and pioneer muscle progenitors in response to multiple Hedgehog proteins, including *Sonic Hedgehog, Tiggywinkle Hedgehog*, and *Echidna Hedgehog*.[146] Adaxial progenitors initiate differentiation and the expression of "slow" myosin heavy chain and then migrate laterally through the somitic mesoderm to form "slow" adaxial muscles. Adaxial specification is mediated through Gli transcription factors,[122] as is also the case for Shh-mediated epaxial progenitor specification in the avian and mouse embryo. Shh induction of *Myf5* in epaxial progenitors is tightly coordinated with segmentation and somite formation during AP axis formation in avian and mouse embryos[138,147] and is mediated directly through an epaxial-specific Myf5 transcription enhancer, which has Gli binding site required for its activation (Fig. 1-13).[63] Paraxial mesoderm does not express Gli transcription factors, and during somite epithelialization, *Gli2* and *Gli3* are activated under the control of β-catenin-mediated Wnt signaling to initiate Shh signaling and the activation of MRF expression.[147] BMP4 produced by the lateral plate mesoderm provides an inhibitory signal that restricts expression of *Myf5* and *MyoD* to the medial somite.[148] Surgical ablation of the lateral plate mesoderm leads to ectopic expression of *MyoD* and *Myf5* throughout the medial and lateral aspects of the dermamyotome and, conversely, ectopic expression of BMP4 in the medial somite blocks *MyoD* and *Myf5* in medial epaxial progenitors. The patterning function of BMP4 is mediated through the localized expression of Noggin, a secreted BMP antagonist, in the DML, under the control of Wnt 11 signaling from the neural tube.[136,149,150] Noggin locally blocks the repressive activity of BMP4 signaling to restrict *MyoD* and *Myf5* expression to epaxial progenitors in the DML. The molecular mechanisms by which BMP signaling antagonizes Shh and Wnt signaling are currently unknown.

MyoD is coactivated with *Myf5* in epaxial progenitors in avian embryos under independent regulation by distinct developmental signals. Misexpression studies show that *MyoD* is activated in epaxial and limb progenitors, under positive control by Wnt signaling and negative control by Notch signaling.[151,152] Wnt signaling controls *MyoD* activation in epaxial progenitors through *QSulf1*, a Shh-regulated, extracellular N-acetyl glucosamine 6-0 sulfatase that controls Wnt signaling by localized populations of QSulf1-expressing cells.[153] Notch signaling negatively regulates *MyoD* but not *Myf5*. Progenitors with activated notch signaling migrate to form myotomes that, remarkably, do not express contractile proteins.[151] These observations provide support for the notion that *MyoD* is a differentiation initiator. In mouse embryos, *MyoD* is activated 2.5 days later, and its expression is predominant in the differentiating myotome and not epaxial progenitors, also indicating its downstream function in muscle differentiation.[128,134]

In *Xenopus* embryos, *XmyoD* and *Xmyf5* are activated in paraxial mesoderm of early gastrula-stage embryos, and their expression is spatially patterned and timed differently, indicating distinct modes of regulation. *Xmyf5* and *XmyoD* activation for myotome formation is controlled by interacting activating and inhibitory signals, as in birds and mammals, but there is apparent divergence in the specific signaling pathways utilized in different vertebrate embryos. In *Xenopus*, *XmyoD* is positively controlled and patterned in muscle progenitor formation in the dorsal mesoderm by FGF and Wnt signaling and by localized expression of Noggin and Chordin, which block the inhibitory signaling activity of BMP signals from the dorsal and ventral marginal zones of the embryo.[154,155] The antagonistic signaling from dorsal and ventral marginal zones in the embryo specifies the full range of mesodermal progenitors, including muscle progenitors, along the dorsoventral axis. eFGF, an embryonic FGF isoform,

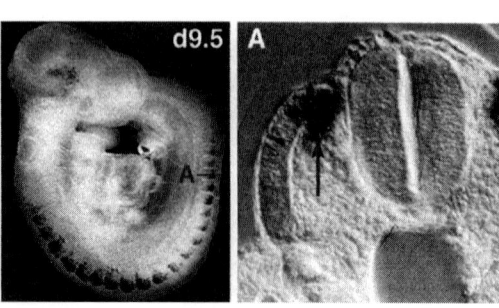
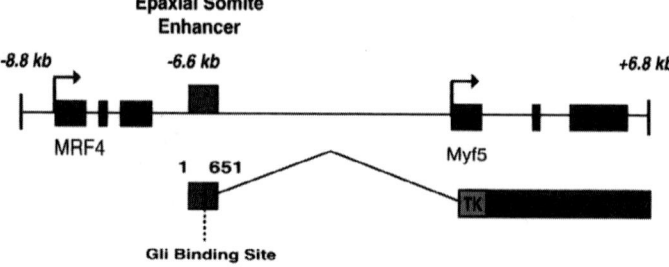
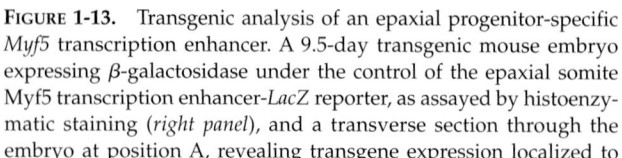

FIGURE 1-13. Transgenic analysis of an epaxial progenitor-specific *Myf5* transcription enhancer. A 9.5-day transgenic mouse embryo expressing β-galactosidase under the control of the epaxial somite Myf5 transcription enhancer-*LacZ* reporter, as assayed by histoenzymatic staining (*right panel*), and a transverse section through the embryo at position A, revealing transgene expression localized to somite DML (*left panel*). The schematic shows the position of the *Myf5* epaxial-specific enhancer, located 6.6 kb 5′ of the Myf5 promoter, immediately 3′ of the *MRF4* gene. Below is the 651-bp enhancer at its essential Gli binding site, as cloned into the *LacZ* transgene reporter. (*From Gustafsson et al.*[63] *Reproduced by permission.*)

induces *XmyoD* expression in ectoderm explants, and this induction is not blocked by cycloheximide inhibitors of protein synthesis, indicating that *XmyoD* is a primary target of FGF regulation.[75] XWnt8 functions cooperatively with eFGF to activate *XmyoD* at early gastrula stages.[156] BMP signaling controls the ventral expression of the Wnt antagonist, *Sizzled*, which in turn functions together with the dorsally expressed Wnt inhibitor *FrzB* to localize Wnt signaling for myogenesis to the lateral mesoderm, thus restricting *XmyoD* expression to muscle progenitors.[157] Wnt signaling though β-catenin has a direct role in the induction of *Xmyf5*, based on the finding that lithium can induce ectopic *Xmyf5* expression in dorsal and ventral mesoderm independent of protein synthesis. Lithium activates Wnt signaling by blocking the activity of GSK3-β, which inhibits the accumulation of β-catenin and the formation of transcription complexes for Wnt-mediated transcription. A role for Shh signaling in *Xmyf5* regulation has not been documented in *Xenopus*, although BMP signaling patterns *Xmyf5* expression to the dorsolateral mesoderm,[155,158] acting in coordination with dorsally localized Noggin and the other BMP antagonists, Chordin and Follastatin, to establish a dorsoventral BMP signaling gradient.[159]

Overall, significant progress has been made toward understanding the interacting signaling and transcriptional networks that control specification of epaxial myotomal muscle progenitors in vertebrate embryos through studies of *Myf5* and *MyoD* regulation. The signaling and transcriptional networks that control *Myf5* and *MyoD* regulation for hypaxial, limb, and head muscle progenitor specification are not yet established but should provide important insights into the evolution and developmental regulation of anatomic muscle formation.

REGULATORS OF MYOGENESIS IN INVERTEBRATE EMBRYOS

Global Myogenic Regulators

Muscle progenitors in invertebrate embryos also arise from the mesoderm following gastrulation, under the control of conserved and divergent gene regulatory pathways. In the nematode *C. elegans*, mesoderm formation has been investigated using combined genetic and cell biological approaches. *C. elegans* has a short 4-day life cycle, transparent embryos with small numbers of cells individually identifiable by confocal microscopy, and a complexity of differentiated tissues, including skeletal muscle. Adult *C. elegans* has 959 cells, including 95 striated body wall muscles and a variety of nonstriated (single sarcomere) muscles, including pharyngeal, intestinal, and reproductive muscles.[49] Cell lineages of *C. elegans* embryos are invariant, making it possible to catalogue precisely the developmental lineage history of all mesodermal and muscle progenitors as well as other progenitor lineages in the wild type and to trace the fates of specific lineages in mutant embryos. The four-cell *C. elegans* embryo has a single, multipotential mesendodermal EMS cell that gives rise to an E progenitor lineage to form the endoderm and to an M lineage to form the mesoderm. The mesoderm lineage gives rise to the two skeletal muscle lineages that form the body wall muscles and the sex myoblasts, as well as to a nonmuscle lineage of coelomocytes, which are blood cells, and SM lineages that form the reproductive uterine and vulval muscles. As in vertebrates, Wnt signaling has a major function in mesoderm specification for myogenesis through its control of the fates of the mitotic progeny of the single EMS cell, which gives rise to a mesodermal M progenitor and an endoderm E progenitor. Wnt signaling controls the expression of a downstream GATA transcription factor that controls specification of the endoderm E lineage. Mutations that disrupt Wnt signaling allow the EMS cell to proceed along a default regulatory pathway to form two cells with mesectodermal fates.[160] The gene regulatory pathway for endoderm formation in vertebrates is also controlled by Wnt signaling and GATA transcription factors, indicating conservation of this regulatory pathway.

In the fruit fly *Drosophila*, Twist, a bHLH transcription factor, is a key regulator for mesoderm specification during gastrulation. Later in development, Twist functions as a regulatory switch for specification of visceral and heart muscle progenitors.[161] Activated in mesodermal progenitors in the ventral mesodermal progenitors, *twist* is under the control of the transcription factor Dorsal. Dorsal is encoded by a maternally localized mRNA[162] in response to Dpp, a TGF-β ligand that has analogous functions to the TGF-β ligand Nodal, controlling dorsal ventral patterning in vertebrate embryos.[2,163] In the mouse and *C. elegans*, Twist is not expressed during mesoderm formation and therefore does not have an early function in mesoderm specification. However, as for *Drosophila*, Twist homologue lineages in *C. elegans* and mouse embryos have important functions in the mesoderm later in development. *Twist* (−/−) mutant mouse embryos have defects in mesodermal patterning.[164] In *C. elegans*, Twist homologue *hlh-8* is expressed in M-lineage cells, including smooth muscle (SM) and coelomocyte progenitors, and *hlh-8* misexpression and RNA inhibition disrupt the specification of a subset of nonskeletal muscle mesoderm lineages as well as expression of mesoderm-specific target genes that have consensus DNA binding sites in their promoters.[165] The DNA binding sites in *hlh-8* target genes are similar to those recognized by mammalian and *Drosophila* Twist, including *ceh-24*, an NK-class gene, and *egl-15*, an FGFR receptor gene. These genes are related to Twist targets in *Drosophila*, which include *tinman*, the NK-class homeobox gene, and *DFR1/heartless*, an FGFR receptor gene, both of which function in the specification of heart muscle mesodermal progenitors.[166,167] These observations indicate that the downstream transcriptional targets in the mesoderm specification process are conserved in evolution.[165]

Ascidians, which are protochordates, utilize a Gli- and Zic-related zinc finger transcription factor, Macho-1, as global regulator of myogenic lineage specification.[168] Macho-1 is differentially localized in the "myoplasm" of the egg and becomes distributed during cleavage to the myogenic progenitor lineage. Morpholino inhibition of Macho-1 function blocks tail myogenesis; when misexpressed, Macho-1 converts nonmuscle lineages into muscle, identifying Macho-1 as a muscle determinant and master regulator of muscle specification. The roles of Zic-related genes in vertebrate embryos remain to be investigated, although it is notable that Zic genes are expressed in somites[169] and are members of the Gli superfamily of transcription factors that mediate the Sonic hedgehog signaling for specification of epaxial muscle lineages.[170]

MyoD-Related Orthologues

The genomes of invertebrates have single MyoD-related *MRF* genes that are remarkably conserved in sequence and myogenic function with their vertebrate orthologues. The activities of invertebrate MRFs convert 10T1/2 cells to myogenesis,[171] and the activities of vertebrate MRFs rescue CeMyoD (*hlh1*) mutant phenotypes in *C. elegans*.[172] Invertebrate and vertebrate MRFs have a conserved HLH domain of 50 to 60 amino acids that forms two helices in the central region of these proteins separated by a loop region of random coil.[173] The HLH domain functions as a leucine zipper interaction domain to form homo- and heterodimers with related bHLH proteins, specifically E12/E47 bHLH transcription factors, which are widely expressed in many tissues. E proteins form heterodimers with MRFs to enhance their binding to E-box sites[174] and enhance the myogenic activity of XMyoD in ectopic expression assays in *Xenopus* embryos.[175] Alone, E proteins do not have myogenic activity.[176] Gene-targeting studies also show that E-protein genes are nonessential for myogenesis in mice[177] or *C. elegans*,[172] indicating either that other related bHLH proteins can substitute for E proteins as partners or that MRFs can function as homodimers.

Ascidians have a single MyoD-related orthologue that produces multiple MyoD isoforms through alternative splicing. This gene is expressed specifically in both primary and secondary muscle progenitors for tail myotomal muscle formation.[178] In contrast to ascidians and vertebrates, *Drosophila* and *C. elegans* MyoD orthologues are also expressed and function in only a subset of skeletal myogenic lineages.[179,180] *C. elegans* embryos with mutations of *hlh-1* form muscles that are functionally defective, indicating that *hlh-1* regulates muscle differentiation but not muscle progenitor specification.[181] However, mosaic analysis studies reveal that *hlh-1* is required for progenitor specification in adults, as *hlh-1* mutant adult muscle progenitors undergo cell-fate transformations to differentiate into other cell types[182] similar to the cell-fate transformations observed in *Myf5* (−/−) mutant epaxial progenitor cells in mouse embryos.[106] Therefore *hlh-1* has multiple myogenic functions that are different in the embryo and adult.

Drosophila embryos express the MyoD orthologue Nautilus in a small subset of larval muscles, and *nautilus* (*nau*) (−/−) mutants have differentiation defects in these muscles.[183] Although *nau* is not a global regulator of myogenic specification or differentiation, genetic studies have identified another class of global myogenic regulators in *Drosophila*. These include *twist* (*twi*), which encodes a bHLH transcription factor related to MRFs and is required during later development for muscle specification, as discussed above.[48] Twist, however, controls the expression of a downstream Zic finger transcription factor, *lame duck* (*lmd*), also known as *gleeful* (*gif1*), which is a global regulator of myogenesis in *Drosophila*.[184,185] lmb is essential for the specification of fusion-competent myoblasts, likely through its function as a direct transcriptional regulator of *Dmef2*,[186,187] which is a transcription factor regulator of contractile protein gene expression during muscle differentiation. Misexpression of lmb protein in *Drosophila* embryos converts neuronal lineages into muscle, establishing its function as a global regulator. lmb is a member of the Gli superfamily, suggesting that its myogenic regulatory function is related to that of Glis for epaxial myogenesis in vertebrate embryos.[63]

Molecular Control of Muscle Differentiaton

MYOBLAST PROLIFERATION

Myf5- and *MyoD*-expressing myoblasts are a renewable source of progenitors that proliferate at sites of anatomic muscle formation in the embryo. Their daughter cells undergo G1-specific cell-cycle withdrawal to initiate myocyte differentiation. Differentiation includes the activation of the muscle-specific transcription factor genes *Myogenin*, *MRF4*, and *MEF2C*, which coordinate the transcriptional activation of contractile and membrane protein genes. Differentiating myocytes also undergo cell-cell fusion to form multinucleated myotubes and muscle fibers. The cellular and molecular regulatory processes of myocyte differentiation have been elucidated through studies of myocyte differentiation in the simplified environment of cell culture. Recent investigations of muscle differentiation have focused on myogenesis in the embryo, providing an understanding of the genetic and cellular regulatory mechanisms that organize muscle differentiation with the embryo's body plan and in relation to blood vessels, tendons, and bones to form functional muscles.

G1-Specific Cell-Cycle Regulation

Myf5- and *MyoD*-expressing myoblasts proliferate in the embryo at sites of myogenesis and initiate differentiation in response to local signaling cues that are not well understood. Myoblasts explanted from embryonic muscle-forming regions can be maintained in their proliferative state by mitogens in serum, embryo extract, or specific growth factors. Single myoblasts also will proliferate as clones in which cells retain their potential to differentiate into muscle.[51] Myoblast proliferation and differentiation are tightly interlocked regulatory processes that can be manipulated by controlling the concentrations of mitogenic growth factors in culture medium. Mitogens in serum and embryo extract or growth factors such as FGF support myoblast proliferation,[188] while growth factor depletion leads to the rapid, G1-specific cessation of cell proliferation and the initiation of contractile protein gene expression (Fig. 1-14).[189] Myoblasts isolated from different muscle-forming regions of the embryo can grow as clones in cell culture but respond differentially to mitogens, indicating that myogenic progenitors from these different sites are adapted to respond to different proliferation and differentiation signals (Fig. 1-15).[190,191] Embryonic myoblasts in culture also require extracellular matrix substrate to support their proliferation and differentiation,[52] likely through integrin-mediated matrix interactions (see Chap. 19a).[192]

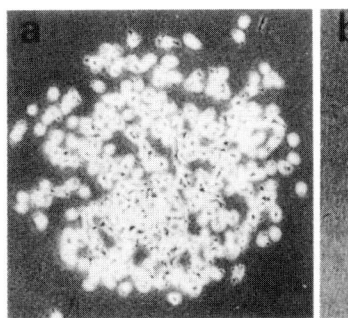 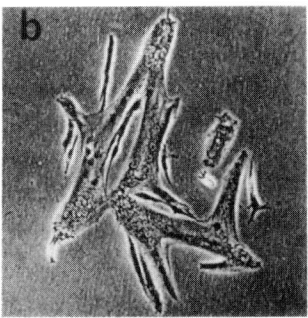

FIGURE 1-14. Illustration of MM14 mouse myoblast response to mitogen-rich and mitogen-depleted media. *a.* Typical MM14 clone 3 days after exponential growth in mitogen-rich medium. *b.* Typical MM14 clone 24 h after being cultured in mitogen-depleted medium. Cells are multinucleated, express contractile proteins, and are postmitotic. (*From Linkhart et al.[422] Reproduced by permission.*)

Myoblasts initiating differentiation undergo G1-specific cell-cycle withdrawal, as established by thymidine incorporation and cinematographic and immunostaining analyses.[193–195] Myoblast differentiation in culture can be monitored cytologically using myoblast fusion or antibodies to muscle-specific proteins such as myosin and creatine kinase.[196,197] Myoblast fusion is temporally coordinated with the process of differentiation, particularly during later stages of myogenesis in embryos.[198] However, in cell culture, G1-specific cell-cycle withdrawal and the initiation of differentiation, as assayed by activation of muscle protein synthesis, does not require myoblast fusion. This is shown experimentally by blocking fusion with low-calcium-containing medium and assaying contractile protein expression in postmitotic myocytes.[199] In the embryo, the epaxial progenitors that form the myotome become postmitotic and initiate contractile protein gene expression as mononucleated myocytes after they migrate locally from the DML under the dermatome to form the myotome. These myocytes later fuse to form the deep back and intercostal muscles.[200,201] At other sites of myogenesis in the embryo, such as the limb, cell-cycle withdrawal and fusion are temporally more closely coordinated.[198]

Nuclei in differentiated myocytes and muscle fibers remain postmitotic and do not undergo DNA replication except under exceptional circumstances such as viral infection.[202] Myocytes in the early stages of cell differentiation, however, can be stimulated to reenter the cell cycle in response to high levels of mitogens, indicating that activation of muscle protein gene expression does not irreversibly commit myocytes to a postmitotic program. Notably, however, skeletal myocytes stimulated to reenter the cell cycle shut down contractile protein expression antithetics.[203] In adults, satellite cells in the muscle sarcolemma can be activated to the cell cycle in response to unknown signals induced by muscle damage. These cells then provide a source of proliferative cells for muscle regeneration (see Chap. 3). Satellite cells most likely arise from somite progenitors during embryogenesis[204] and, in adults, lie in a mitotically dormant state under the sarcolemma of muscle fibers until they are recruited for muscle generation.[205] Multipotential stem cells also may contribute progenitors for muscle regeneration; the source of signals that control their proliferation and differentiation is unknown.[206]

Growth Factor Control of Proliferation

In cell culture and in the embryo, FGF2 is a key growth factor regulator of proliferation and of embryonic myoblasts and adult satellite cells and an inhibitor of differentiation in cell culture (see Chap. 3).[188,207] Retroviral studies in chick embryos provide evidence that FGF is a key signaling regulator of proliferation and differentiation of limb myoblasts.[208] Somite precursors infected with FGFR1-expressing retrovirus migrate normally to the limb bud but fail to differentiate, whereas somite precursors infected with retrovirus expressing dominant negative FGFR1 (ΔFGFR1) undergo premature muscle differentiation within the somite, prior to their migration to the limb.[208,209] These findings indicate that the proliferation of limb muscle progenitors is maintained by FGF signaling through the FGFR1 receptor during migration to the somite and that the initiation of differentiation is controlled by loss of FGFR1 receptor and FGF signaling once progenitors have migrated into the dorsal and ventral muscle-forming regions of the limb bud. The TGF-β ligand GDF-10

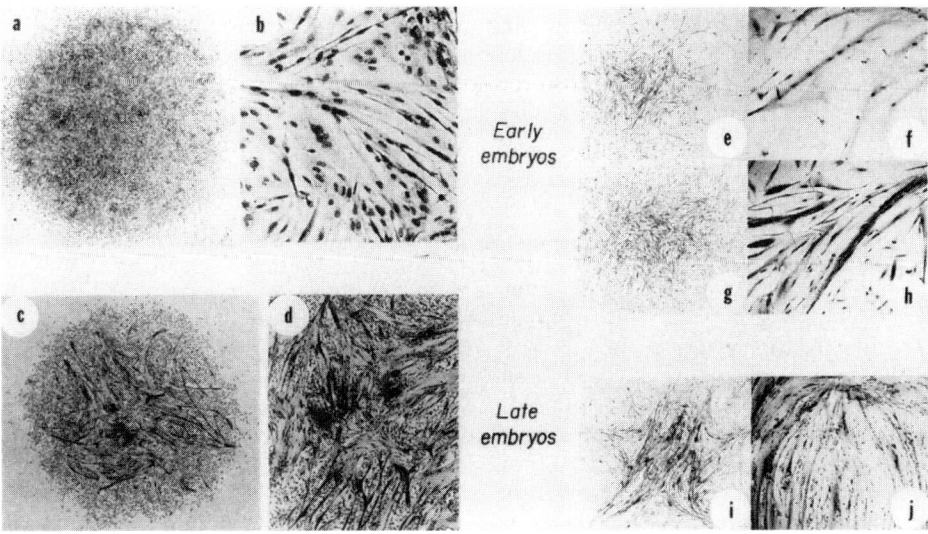

FIGURE 1-15. Photomicrographs depicting the typical clonal morphologies of early and late muscle colony-forming (MCF) cells obtained from human (*a* to *d*) and chick (*e* to *j*) leg muscle regions. Human early and late MCF clones from 36- and 127-day fetuses; chick early MCF clones from stage 22 and 23 embryos and late MCF clones from stage 29 embryo. (*From Bonner and Hauschka.[407,423] Reproduced by permission.*)

also has a role in the control of muscle differentiation in the embryo. Mice and cattle mutant for *GDF-10* have significantly increased muscle mass.[210,211] GDF-10 is expressed in the myotome of developing embryos, suggesting a role for its function in the control of myoblast proliferation and differentiation. Shh also controls muscle proliferation and differentiation in the limb. Retroviral misexpression of Shh in limb progenitors increases muscle growth, likely by promoting myoblast proliferation[212] to control the initiation of differentiation.[213] How Shh, GDF-10, and FGF signaling are coordinated to control myogenesis remains to be determined.

Insulin-like growth factors (IFG I and IGF II) have dual functions in the control of myoblast and satellite cell proliferation and differentiation (see Chap. 3).[214] Drug inhibitor studies reveal that the mitogenic activity of IGFs is mediated through Ras/Raf-1/MAP kinase pathways, whereas their differentiation-promoting activities are initiated through the PI3 kinase/P70 S6Kinase pathway.[215] The myogenic activities of IGF I and II are mediated through a type I igf-I receptor, as mouse embryos with targeted mutations of igf-I or the type I igf-I *receptor* are highly deficient in skeletal muscles and die at birth for lack of a diaphragm to breathe.[215,216] The muscle-deficient phenotypes in igf-I mutant embryos resemble the differentiation-deficient phenotypes of *Myogenin* (−/−) mice,[217,218] likely reflecting a role for IGF1 in *Myogenin* regulation, as discussed below.

Myf5 and MyoD Control of Proliferation and Differentiation

Myf5 and MyoD proteins have regulatory functions in the control of myoblast proliferation and differentiation. Myoblasts isolated from *MyoD* (−/−) and *Myf5* (−/−) mutant mouse embryos proliferate poorly and differentiate prematurely in culture.[219] The target genes regulated by Myf5 and MyoD for myogenic specification and cell-cycle regulation are not yet established, but this is an exciting area of current investigation, stimulated by the development of microchip expression array, chromatin immunoprecipitation, and subtractive cDNA cloning technologies. Some MyoD target genes involved in the myogenic conversion of 10T1/2 cells have been identified by microchip array analysis using estrogen-inducible MyoD expression vectors in combination with cycloheximide blockage to distinguish primary and secondary target genes.[220] These studies have identified a spectrum of cell-cycle and differentiation genes,[220] including progenitor-specific genes that are expressed in proliferative myoblasts prior to the initiation of differentiation.[221]

The growth factors that control myoblast proliferation and differentiation likely transduce their activities through posttranslational modifications of Myf5 and MyoD proteins and their associated partners and cofactors. MRFs are phosphoproteins.[222] Many mitogens, including bFGF, activate signal transduction pathways for protein phosphorylation,[223] providing a connection between growth factor control of myogenesis and MRF functions in myoblast differentiation. In vitro, protein kinase C (PKC)-mediated phosphorylation of the critical threonine residue in Myogenin inhibits its DNA binding activity.[224] In 10T1/2 cells, however, FGF can inhibit MRF4-induced myoblast differentiation independent of the phosphorylation status of this threonine residue or other phosphorylated serine residues in the basic DNA-binding domain, indicating that the mitogenic activity of FGF on myoblast proliferation is mediated indirectly, perhaps through control of the phosphorylation of MRF cofactors. Activated *Ras* oncogene proteins also transduce their signals to inhibit myoblast differentiation,[225,226] although this inhibition is not mediated directly by PKC, but through a currently unknown component of the Ras signaling pathway.[227] Cyclic AMP-mediated PKA phosphorylation also can block the transcription factor activity of MRFs.[228] Casein kinase II promotes myoblast differentiation, apparently through phosphorylation of E proteins, which may act by enhancing formation of E protein–MRF heterodimers.[229]

In proliferating myoblasts, Myf5 and MyoD levels are controlled by cell-cycle-specific turnover mechanisms that are modulated during cell-cycle withdrawal and the initiation of differentiation. MyoD turnover is controlled through cyclinD, cdk-dependent phosphorylation of Rb.[230–232] MyoD is a phosphoprotein, and its phosphorylation status influences its stability. MyoD turnover is controlled during G1/S by cyclin-dependent kinases (cdks), which phosphorylate MyoD at S200 for degradation through a ubiquitin-based proteosome mechanism.[233] During the initiation of myoblast differentiation in response to reduced mitogen activity, MyoD is stabilized by inhibition of cdk activity and its association with pRb, which allows myoblasts to exit from the cell cycle.[234–236] Myf5 is regulated through cell-cycle-regulated protein degradation during mitosis and transcriptional repression during differentiation.[237,238] The roles of IGF and FGF signaling in the cell-cycle control of MyoD and Myf5 turnover and transcriptional activity remain to be elucidated.

Myf5 and MyoD regulate the activation of *Myogenin*, *MRF4*, and *Mef2c* as direct transcriptional targets. Myogenin, MRF4, and Mef2c function as transcription factor regulators of muscle protein genes, as discussed below. Mouse transgenic studies have identified control sites (E boxes) for MyoD and Myf5 binding in their promoters and 5′ flanking regions and show that these sites are essential for their activation during myoblast differentiation.[118,120,239,240] The *Myogenin* and *MRF4* regulatory elements have both E-box and MEF2 binding sites. Mutational disruption of these sites leads to loss of expression of LacZ reporter transgenes in specific embryonic muscles, indicating that their expression is activated by MRFs, likely by *Myf5* and *MyoD* expressed in myoblasts, and then maintained in myocytes by MRF and Mef2 autoregulation.

MYOCYTE DIFFERENTIATION

Transcriptional Control of Contractile Protein Genes

G1-specific myoblast withdrawal from the cell cycle is closely coupled with activation of contractile, scaffolding, and control protein genes of the myofibril.[196] Contractile protein accumulation is controlled by the coordinated transcriptional activation of muscle genes, as established by kinetic studies of the accumulation of contractile proteins and their mRNAs during growth factor–mediated induction of myoblast differentiation[241,242] by nuclear runoff transcription assays of contractile protein genes in myoblasts and newly differentiating myocytes[243] and by molecular studies of differentiation-specific contractile protein gene enhancers.[244,245] The contractile protein genes activated during myoblast differentiation include isoforms for all of the functionally related muscle-specific myofibrillar proteins, including Myosin Heavy and Light Chains, α-Actin, Tropomyosin, and Troponins I, T, and C, as well as proteins involved in synapse formation and calcium signaling. Contractile protein genes first activated in embryonic muscle also include skeletal and cardiac isoforms of actin, troponin, and myosin, which are replaced later in development by skeletal isoforms. The temporally coordinated activation of contractile protein genes during myoblast differentiation provided a basis for the idea that myoblast differentiation is controlled by muscle-specific gene regulators that coordinate muscle gene activation, later identified as the MRFs and MEF2 transcription factors.

Contractile protein genes are activated during the initiation of myocyte differentiation by the muscle-specific transcription factors, Myogenin, MRF4, and Mef2, in combination with other muscle-restricted and general transcription factors, as discussed below. Myogenin and MRF4 share extensive sequence homology with Myf5 and MyoD and also convert 10T1/2 cells to myogenesis in cDNA transfection assays.[246–248] However, in contrast to Myf5 and MyoD, Myogenin and *mrf4* have later regulatory functions in the control of muscle differentiation. Mouse embryos with mutations in *Myogenin* (−/−)[217,218] and *mrf4* (−/−)[249] activate *Myf5* and *MyoD* and form muscle progenitors, but they have defects in muscle differentiation. Muscle differentiation defects in *mrf4* (−/−) embryos are more severe in *MyoD* (−/−); *mrf4* (−/−) compound mutant embryos, establishing that *MyoD* also has muscle differentiation functions.[250,251] In frog embryos, *XMyogenin* and *xmrf4* are differentially expressed in physiologically specialized fast and slow muscles, suggesting their additional specialized functions in fiber-type differentiation.[252,253] *xmrf4* is activated during muscle innervation as well as during muscle regeneration.

MEF2 proteins function cooperatively with MRFs in the control of contractile protein gene activation during muscle differentiation. Vertebrates have four *mef2* genes, *mef2a, b, c,* and *d*. These are members of the MADS domain family of transcription factors that function cooperatively with MRFs for the control of contractile protein genes.[254,255] *mef2* genes are expressed in skeletal, cardiac, and smooth muscle and in brain. *mef2c* is expressed in differentiating skeletal and cardiac muscles, and its expression is activated with Myogenin during the initiation of myoblast differentiation.[256] MEF2C protein functionally and physically interacts with bHLH MRFs through its MADS domain to enhance the transcriptional activities of MRFs and thus activate muscle transcription enhancers. The genetic requirements for *mef2c* function in vertebrate myogenesis have not yet been established; however, *Drosophila* has a single *mef2* gene, *Dmef2*, that is essential for the differentiation of skeletal and cardiac muscles.[186,187]

Muscle-Specific Promoters and Enhancers

Muscle-specific regulatory elements have been identified in the 5' and 3' of the coding regions of contractile protein genes as well as within their introns and promoters. All of the regulatory elements found in more distant locations from contractile protein genes exhibit the properties of tissue-specific enhancers, as do most of the regulatory elements found within introns when assayed for transcriptional activity using DNA transfection and transgene reporter gene assays. Tissue-specific enhancers are operationally defined as DNA sequences that confer elevated transcriptional activity to virtually any basal promoter and that exhibit about the same relative activity when placed at variable distances, orientations, and 5' versus 3' locations relative to the basal promoter. The tissue specificity of many contractile protein enhancers permits their function in skeletal as well as cardiac muscle, but usually not in smooth muscle. A common feature of muscle-specific enhancers as well as muscle-specific promoters is the presence of multiple muscle gene control elements located within several hundred base pairs of contiguous DNA sequence (see below). Now that the human and mouse genomic sequences are completed, it is possible to employ sophisticated database search algorithms to identify putative regulatory regions containing clusters of putative transcription factor binding sites.[257–259] Once identified, such putative regulatory sequences can be tested for transcription factor–binding and muscle-specific transcriptional activity using reporter gene expression assays. The functionality of specific regulatory sequences has been defined by gel shift and DNAase or chemical footprinting to map DNA-binding sites, in combination with site-directed mutagenesis and reporter gene assays to test transcriptional functions. Such studies have identified MRF (E box) and MEF2 binding sites in almost all muscle-specific regulatory elements and established the essentiality of these elements for muscle-specific transcription. Muscle-specific regulatory elements have sites for binding of more generally expressed transcription factors that function cooperatively with MRFs and Mef2, as discussed below.

As a rule, muscle-specific enhancers are highly conserved between different vertebrate species. They have been identified in cytoskeletal, postsynaptic membrane, myofibril, and metabolic muscle protein genes.[260] Data for chicken, quail, mouse, and rat enhancers are almost identical to the corresponding human enhancers. Among the best characterized are enhancers for acetycholine receptor subunits, troponins, myosin heavy and light chains, and desmin. Enhancers for muscle membrane proteins have not been characterized. Muscle protein gene enhancers are usually located in the 5' flanking regions of muscle genes, although some are located in introns and 3' flanking regions.[261,262]

The mouse *mck* enhancer and promoter regulatory elements are among the best-characterized muscle gene enhancers (Fig. 1-16).[263,264] The muscle-specific *mck* enhancer is defined by a 170-bp minimal sequence in which seven control elements reside; within this region, 60 bp contain no essential control elements. The *mck* enhancer can be further subdivided into a 110-bp fragment containing only two E boxes and an A/T-rich element, which also retains enhancer activity. Muscle enhancers are controlled by positive control elements and interacting transcription factors, including MRFs and Mef2C, such that mutation of E-box- and A/T-binding sites leads to loss of enhancer activity. The functional requirements of specific enhancers for activation of their chromosomal genes

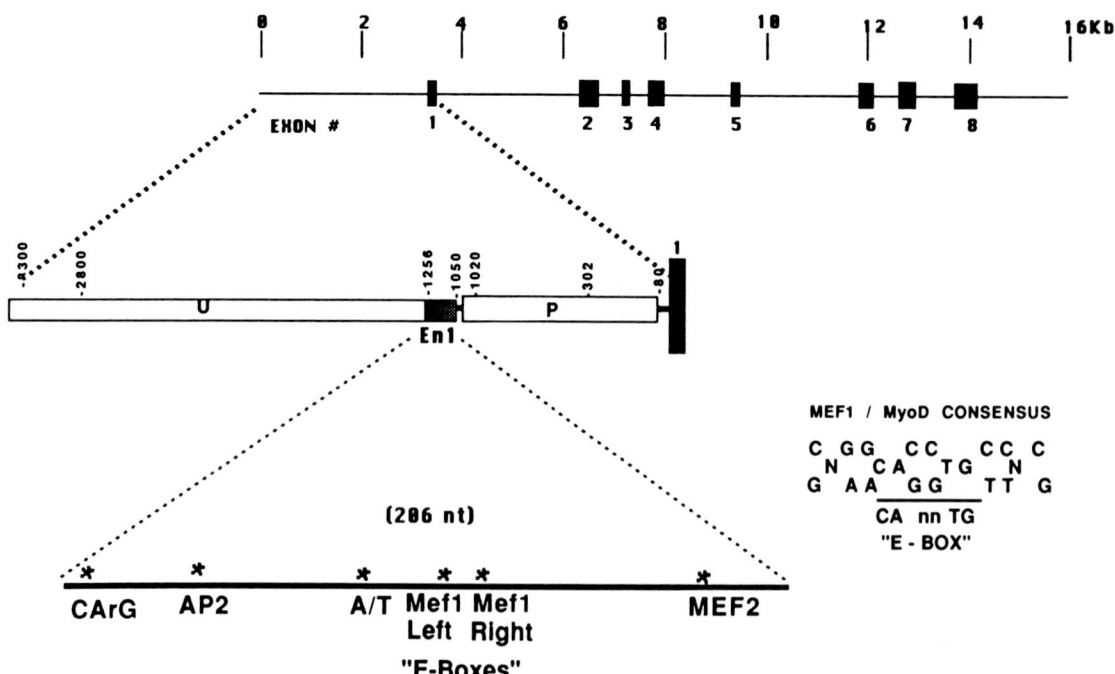

FIGURE 1-16. Diagrammatic representation of the mouse *mck* gene. Top diagram represents 16-kb genomic region of the *mck* gene, with 8 exons represented by solid rectangles. Middle diagram represents 5'-flanking region of *mck* gene from − 3300 bp to the first exon. U = (−3300 to −1257) upstream flanking region, which appears to contain regulatory elements important for MCK expression in slow muscle fibers as well as elements that increase overall expression in both skeletal and cardiac muscle; En1 = 206-bp enhancer (−1256 to −1050); P = promoter region, which contains elements that synergize with the enhancer to provide high expression in both skeletal and cardiac muscle in vivo; not shown is the intron-1 modulatory region, which provides high expression when combined with region P. Lower diagram represents the 206-bp enhancer with known control elements; sequence to the right indicates (MEF1/MyoD E-box consensus sequence. (*From Hauschka.*[264] *Reproduced by permission.*)

have not been investigated extensively using gene-targeting approaches to determine the degree of redundancy of muscle regulatory elements. Deletion of the *mlc1f/3f* enhancer in mouse embryos leads to precocious MLC expression in early mesoderm prior to its normal activation in myotomal muscles, indicating the presence of negative regulatory elements within the enhancer to restrict its activity to muscle.[265] Gene-targeting studies of other muscle enhancers could provide insights into the positive and negative regulatory elements required for the timing of activation and muscle specificity of muscle gene regulatory elements.

Many muscle genes with highly active enhancers also have muscle-specific promoters. Among the most extensively characterized promoters are those in human and avian α-*Cardiac Actin*; *Acetylcholine Receptor γ subunit* (*AChR-γ*); human, mouse, and rat *Aldolase*; and human muscle-specific subunit of *Phosphoglycerate Mutase* (*PGAM-M*). The mouse *mck* has a 350-bp promoter region that is active in both transient cell culture assays and transgenic mouse assays.[263] Muscle-specific enhancers may also be embedded in the promoters of muscle genes, as is the case for α-cardiac actin.[266] Muscle enhancers and promoters share a common set of sequence-specific DNA-binding sites. These elements are typically 6 to 9 bp in length and bind either muscle-specific or ubiquitous transcription factors, as determined by gel-shift and DNA footprinting assays. Contractile protein gene expression is dependent on an array of transcription factors, including skeletal muscle–specific factors such as the MRFs and MEF2C as well as more ubiquitous factors such as SRF, MCAT/TEF1, and MEF3/Trex, AP-2, and SP-1. The transcriptional activities of these factors depend on their relative concentrations, the concentrations of coactivators, and their interacting activating or repressing auxiliary factors, as well as their posttranslational modifications such as phosphorylation, acetylation, ubiquitinylation, and the physical state of chromatin encompassing individual enhancer/promoter regions. As a general rule, transcription factors have limited access to control elements in regions containing hypoacetylated histones and ready access in chromatin regions containing acetylated histones. Interestingly, repressed and activated chromatin states are regulated by histone deacetylases (HDACs) and histone acetylases (HATs), which can interact with many of the MRF and Mef2 muscle transcription factors; the latter are presumed to target HATs and HDACs to specific gene regions to facilitate subsequent local activation or repression of chromatin.[267–269] How transcription factors target HATs to chromatin regions that are repressed remains a mystery, but likely other chromatin remodeling factors such as swi/snf are involved. Such factors modify chromatin at more global levels, thereby permitting local rearrangements to provide transient access of transcription factors and associated HATs to control elements.

Control Elements for Muscle-Specific Promoters and Enhancers

Six major control elements have been identified in muscle-specific promoters and enhancers: MEF1/E-box, A/T-rich,

MEF2, CArG/SRE, MCAT/TEF1, and MEF3/Six4/Trex. Certain Sp-1-like sites also appear important in muscle gene promoter activity, but probably do not confer muscle specificity. AP-2 sites are also present in muscle enhancers and appear to be occupied in vivo, but their ubiquitous distribution in nonmuscle genes makes it unlikely that they confer muscle specificity.* Muscle enhancers and promoters typically contain multiple control elements for factor binding. For example, the 206-bp mouse *mck* enhancer contains at least six control elements [two E boxes and one each A/T-rich, CArG/SRE, MEF2, and Ap-2 site (Fig. 1-16)],[270] and the 173-bp *Mlc1/3* enhancer has at least six control elements (3 E boxes and one each CArG/SRE, MEF2, and AP-4 site).[271] The 5'-to-3' order, nearest neighbor relationships, and intervening nucleotides between control elements are variant within highly conserved mouse, rat, and human *MCK* enhancers. The two conserved E boxes are separated by slightly different numbers of base pairs, implying that these elements interact independently with DNA-binding proteins and that the two complexes need not be anchored on exactly the same faces of the DNA helix. An additional puzzle is that one or more of the elements may appear to be redundant or dispensable, even though they are conserved between species. An alternative possibility is that transfection and transgenic assays used to investigate the functionality of these elements lack the sensitivity and specificity to demonstrate all essential functions. Muscle elements are also variant in their core and flanking DNA sequences. For example, the core sequences of the *MCK* enhancer CArG/SRE element is CCATGTAAGG, and its transcriptional activity (based on the percent of total activity lost following mutation) is relatively "weak"; by contrast, the core sequence of the "strongest" CArG/SRE in the α-*skeletal actin* promoter is CCAAATATGG.[272] Given that the consensus CArG/SRE site is CC(A/T)$_6$GG, it may not be surprising that the *MCK* control element is not as transcriptionally active as the α-*skeletal actin* element. Such conserved, minor sequence variations in muscle control elements likely provide fine tuning control of the quantitative activities of muscle gene enhancers in response to different physiologic signals. Subtle sequence variations in control elements apparently can have significant quantitative effects on muscle enhancer activity, as shown in E-box replacement studies within the quail *TnI* enhancer, establishing the functional importance of both the core and the flanking sequences in muscle control elements.[273]

MRF/E box. The myogenic activities of MRFs are mediated through their basic domain on the N-terminal side of helix-1, which is responsible for sequence-specific binding of MRFs to E-box consensus binding sites on the muscle-specific regulatory elements of muscle genes and includes about 20 amino acids arranged in three clusters of basic residues. The N-terminal cluster appears partially dispensable, since the 12 amino acids within the two C-terminal clusters (located closest to helix 1) exhibit sequence-specific binding to generic E-box motifs. A basic amino acid domain on the N-terminal side of helix-1 is responsible for sequence-specific DNA binding of MRFs to E-box sites.[274] When the basic domains of either MyoD or Myogenin are replaced with the basic regions of E-12 or *Drosophila* Achaete Scute bHLH transcription factors, these chimeric proteins can dimerize with E proteins and bind E boxes in vitro, but they do not convert 10T1/2 cells to myogenesis or transactivate muscle enhancers on reporter genes.[176,274] This suggests that the basic amino acid domain of MRFs has specificities for muscle gene-regulatory elements. Sequence comparisons of basic regions of bHLH factors reveal that the MRFs have a conserved alanine-threonine dipeptide, located between these two essential basic amino acid clusters, that is absent from all other bHLH factors, including E proteins.[275] When the appropriate residues within the E-protein basic regions of the MyoD-E12 and myogenin-E12 chimeric proteins are mutated to alanine-threonine (so as to conform to the conserved MDF sequence at these positions), their myogenic transcriptional activities are restored.[274,276] The mechanisms by which this two–amino acid sequence confers myogenic transcriptional activity to MRFs remain unknown, although they probably involve site-specific phosphorylation.

Sequences of flanking control elements can determine transcriptional activity of enhancers. A particularly informative quantitative comparison has been carried out with the *MCK* enhancer Right E Box and an E box in the myosin light chain 1/3 enhancer, which has the identical core sequences but variant flanking sequences, as in the following:

CCCCAAC<u>ACCTG</u>CTGCCT (*MCK*) vs. ATTTTGC<u>ACCTG</u>GCTGC-TAT (*MyLC1/3*)

Fluorescence anisotropy reveals that MyoD/E12 and Myogenin/E12 heterodimers bind the *MCK* enhancer E box with approximately equal affinity and with much higher affinity than they bind the *MyLC1/3* E box. MyoD/MyoD homodimers bind the *MCK* E-box sequence with highest affinity, followed by E12/E12 and Myogenin/Myogenin. Interestingly, while both MRF homodimers bind the two E boxes with positive cooperativity, the E12 homodimers bind with negative cooperativity. Thus, the binding affinities of heterodimers are greater than those of homodimers. MyoD/MyoD and MyoD/E12 dimers have relatively weak but similar stability in solution without DNA, but they are less stable than E12/DNA. Therefore the thermodynamically preferred mechanism of heterodimer binding would be for E12 to bind as a monomer to the E box and then for an MRF to bind to the E12/DNA complex. In essence, the E-box

---

*The nomenclature of muscle control elements and their binding factors is confusing due to the historical contexts in which they were identified. For example, skeletal and cardiac α-*actin* CArG boxes and CArG binding factors are essentially identical to serum response factor (SRF) binding elements (SREs). CArG/SRE is thus used below to indicate these control elements, and SRF is used to specify CArG/SRE binding factors. Similarly, MCAT and MCAT binding factors are identical to TEF1 binding sites and the TEF1 transcription factor; MCAT/TEF1 is thus used below to indicate these control elements, and TEF1 is used to specify MCAT/TEF1 binding factors. The nomenclature for A/T-rich muscle control elements is problematic because the CArG/SRE and MEF2 control elements are also both A/T-rich (consensus sites CC(A/T)$_6$GG and YTA (A/T)$_4$TAR, respectively; Y = pyrimidine, R = purine). As a general rule, SRF does not bind to A/T-rich sites that do not contain the critical Cs and Gs flanking the core A/T portion of the CArMEF2 consensus sequence, but the more permissive planking nucleotides within the mef2 consensus permit MEF2 binding to some A/T-rich control elements. SRF and MEF2 also can form heterodimers, which likely influences their binding to specific sites. Oct-1 and Mhox are other transcription factors known to bind to A/T-rich elements.

DNA sequence would mediate the interaction of bound monomeric E12 with monomeric MRFs.[277] While it is certainly worth considering the implications of these thermodynamic considerations, such an order-of-binding hypothesis does not concur with studies of the *acetylcholine receptor α-subunit* enhancer, which binds myogenin/E12 as heterodimers.[278]

Although the 70 amino acids of the MyoD bHLH domain are sufficient to convert 10T1/2 cells to myogenesis in DNA transfection assays, the more divergent flanking N- and C-terminal domains of MyoD also have regulatory functions. The N-terminal and C-terminal portions of MRFs, when fused to the DNA-binding domain of the yeast GAL4 transcription factor, behave as general transcription activation domains in nonmuscle cells.[279,280] A cysteine-histidine (C-H) N-terminal domain is conserved in MyoD, Myf5, and Myogenin and can function in chromatin remodeling of target muscle protein differentiation genes, as revealed by chromatin nuclease hypersensitivity of transfected cells. This domain also is required for high-efficiency myogenic conversion of 10T1/2 cells.[281,282] An amphipathic helical C-terminal domain of MyoD is more efficient in the transactivation of muscle protein enhancer reporter genes in 10T1/2 cell transfection assays than is the C-terminal domain of Myogenin, which has functions as a general transcriptional activation domain. Together, these findings provide evidence for the functional diversity of MRFs. However, the relationship between differences in the domain functions of MyoD and Myogenin and their respective functions in progenitor specification and muscle differentiation are not yet understood. In addition to heterodimer formation with E proteins, MyoD also can form heterodimers with Id proteins. Id proteins lack a basic, DNA-binding domain, and overexpression also. Id-MyoD heterodimers do not bind to DNA target sequences. Id inhibits the myogenic acitivies of MyoD in transfection assays.[283] It is notable, however, that Id and MRFs are not coexpressed in embryonic tissues, so an in vivo myogenic regulatory function for Id proteins is unlikely.

CArG/SRF and its accessory factors. Serum response factor (SRF) is a MADS box–containing transcription factor that controls muscle gene expression in response to growth and differentiation signals. MADS boxes are 58 amino acid domains in which the C-terminal half functions in protein-protein dimerization between identical or other MADS box proteins, and the N-terminal half functions in DNA binding.[284] SRF homodimers bind the approximate palindromic consensus CArG/SRE sequence $CC(A/T)_6GG$, and induce extreme local DNA bending, as much as 72 degrees. Importantly, the binding interaction between SRF and the CArG/SRE site occurs within the DNA minor groove. SRF mRNA is detected in vertebrate embryos prior to neurulation, and while the gene is expressed ubiquitously thereafter, the SRF protein is most abundant in cardiac, smooth, and skeletal muscle tissues.[285] CArG/SRE elements function as key regulatory components of growth factor response genes such as cfos and are located in regulatory elements of a variety of muscle genes, raising the question of how generally expressed factors contribute to tissue specificity. Studies have attempted to answer this question by examining both the CArG/SRE DNA motifs within SRF-regulated genes, and by identifying and characterizing SRF accessory factors. Identification of the Elk-1/SRF and MAL-SRF complexes and delineation of how environmental signals modulate these interactions to affect the expression of different target genes is an instructive paradigm.[286] Myocardin, a cardiac and smooth muscle–specific transcription factor that associates with SRF, provides additional insight into how SRF exhibits transcriptional selectivity through recruitment of transcription factor complexes to DNA sites.[287]

SRF function can also be modified by the ubiquitous factor YY1, which possesses both SRF-enhancing and -inhibiting activities, depending on the ratios of active YY1 and SRF on the particular CArG/SRE sequence and on its position relative to the TATA box. YY1 is a 441–amino acid zinc finger transcription factor that binds the consensus site CGCCAT-NTT. Since the core YY1 binding motif is CCAT, YY1 can bind the flanking portions of some $CC(A/T)_6GG$ CArG/SRE sites, such as those in the *cfos* and *α-skeletal actin* promoter, even when many of the flanking nucleotides of the YY1 consensus binding sequence are not present. Recent studies suggest that changes in the actin cytoskeletal organization modify SRF binding to CArG/SRE motifs by modulating YY1-dependent inhibition[288] and by affecting interactions of SRF with a transcriptional coactivator MAL.[286] SRF transcriptional activity can also be modified by auxiliary factors that do not possess any DNA-binding domains. For example, the newly discovered 73–amino acid partial homeodomain protein HOP binds to SRF and inhibits its binding to the CArG/SRE control elements.[289,290] Interestingly, HOP also inhibits the myocardin-mediated transcriptional activation of muscle genes containing critical CArG/SRE control elements, presumably due to preventing productive association of SRF with myocardin at these regulatory sites.

MEF2. Muscle enhancer binding factor 2 (MEF2) transcription factors bind to MEF2 control sites within the MCK enhancer[291] and are identical to a family of four transcription factors called RSRF (related to serum response factor) (MEF2A, B, C, and D), three of which are alternatively spliced.[292] Each of the MEFs contains an N-terminal 58–amino acid MADS domain that functions in the formation of MEF2 homo- and heterodimers as well as for DNA binding to A/T-rich sequences. MEF2 MADS domains, however, do not permit MEF2 dimerization with other MADS proteins such as SRF. MEF2s also contain a conserved 28–amino acid MEF2 domain immediately C-terminal of the MADS domain and then one or more transactivation domains C-terminal of the MEF2 domain. Portions of the MEF2 domain are involved in DNA binding and other portions participate in interactions with auxiliary proteins.[293] Although MEF2 isoforms are ubiquitously expressed, significant developmental changes in *MEF2* expression patterns are observed. MEF2C mRNA is first detected in E7.5 mouse embryos within pre-cardiac mesoderm. MEF2A, MEF2C, and MEF2D transcripts are expressed in cardiac tissue by E8.5, and MEF2C mRNA is detected in somites by E9, about a day after *Myf5* activation and a few hours prior to *Myogenin*. MEF2A and MEF2D mRNAs are expressed by E9.5. MEF2 isoforms are expressed in limb buds at E11.5 and specifically in muscle tissue at later stages. MEF2D is expressed in proliferating myoblasts prior to differentiation, MEF2A is expressed as myoblasts commence differentiation, and MEF2C is expressed during later phases of differentiation. MEF2 also may activate *Myogenin* during early phases of skeletal muscle terminal differentiation.[256] Interestingly, while *Myogenin* expression occurs slightly prior to MEF2C expression in somites, the *Myogenin* promoter contains critical MEF2 control elements, indicating that its maintenance is under the control of MEF2.[240,294]

MEF2s bind the 10-bp consensus sequence $CTA(A/T)_4$ TAG, but MEF2B binds with lower affinity. Nucleotides flanking core MEF2 elements can also influence DNA binding affinity. Computer-based nucleotide frequency analysis of MEF2 sites in eight muscle genes identifies a weighted 12-bp MEF2 recognition sequence as $(G/t)CTA(T/A)(A/t)(A/t)ATA(G/a)(A/c)$. MEF2 interaction with its DNA control elements occurs primarily within the minor groove, with only one amino acid making major groove hydrogen bond interactions with two adjacent bases. MEF2 binding to DNA induces changes in the double helix conformation that differ from those induced by SRF-DNA interactions. Therefore MEF2-DNA interactions induce changes in DNA structure that facilitate its interactions with specific base pairs within the recognition motif. As these conformational changes involve parameters such as DNA bending and overwinding of DNA regions, these local physical changes would certainly propagate to surrounding DNA, causing secondary effects on transcription factor binding to neighboring control elements.

MEF2s interact with other regulatory proteins via their MADS and MEF2 domains, including MEF2 dimers' interactions with MRF/E12 heterodimers via the MEF2 MADS domain and the MRF bHLH regions. Significantly, this interaction does not require that each transcription factor be bound to its cognate control element.[293,295] These findings imply that MEF2-MRF complexes can assemble independently at either control element, and that more distant MEF2 and E-box control elements can be looped together via interactions between the MEF2 dimer bound to one element and the MyoD/E12 heterodimer bound to the other element. MEF2 also interacts with TEF1 and Vestigial-like factor 2; but the TEF-1 synergy requires binding of both MEF2 and TEF-1 to their respective control elements. The extent to which these multiple protein-protein interactions occur in vivo remains to be determined. A less understood parameter is the role of chromatin remodeling in controlling the access of MRFs, MEF2s, and TEF1 to their cognate binding sites.[296,297]

A/T-rich site binding factors. A/T-rich sites in muscle gene enhancers such as MCK are superficially similar to CArG/SRE and MEF2 sites, but they may not contain the stipulated non-A/T flanking base pairs. Factor interactions with these sites can be distinguished by competition and footprinting assays. An A/T-rich consensus sequence $T(A/T)ATAAT(A/T)A$ has been proposed based on the DNA-binding activity of MHox, a mesoderm-restricted homeodomain factor that may play critical roles in the expression of MRF genes as well as muscle structural genes.[298] Interestingly, the MCK enhancer A/T-rich control element binds Mhox, the ubiquitous transcription factor Oct1, and MEF2, even though the element is not a perfect binding site for any of these factors. However, when the site was mutated to create consensus Mhox-, Oct1-, or MEF2-binding sites, only the MEF2 site enhanced transcription, implying that MEF2 occupancy of this control element may be responsible for the element's transcriptional activity. Mhox or Oct1 occupancy of muscle gene A/T-rich sites to exclude MEF2 access also could provide an additional level of muscle gene regulation.

MCAT/TEF1. TEF1 factors are members of the TEA DNA-binding domain transcription factors. There are currently four known vertebrate TEF1 genes: NTEF-1, RTEF-1, DTEF-1, and ETEF-1. Their relative mRNA levels in skeletal and cardiac muscle are RTEF-1 > NTF-1 > DTEF-1, and RTEF-1 = DTEF-1 > NTEF-1, respectively.[299] There also is evidence for alternative splicing of TEF1 transcripts in and near the TEA domain, and these isoforms exhibit altered DNA binding specificities and transcriptional activities. Based on sequence analysis of nearly 20 different MCAT sites in 10 different muscle genes, CATTCCT has been established as the consensus muscle gene MCAT site. However, TEF1s also bind elements with variant sequences, including the GT-IIC element CATTCC and the SphI and SphII elements CATACT and CATGCT. Due to the low nucleotide binding constraints, putative TEF1 binding sites can very frequently be found in DNA sequence searches, which require that their identity be confirmed by mutational and DNA-binding studies.

TEF1 interacts with a variety of other regulatory factors via its TEA domain. It binds to SRF via the SRF MADS domain; when transcriptional synergy between the two factors was tested with the proximal *skeletal α-actin* promoter, binding of TEF1 and SRF to both of the adjacent control elements was required.[300] TEF1 also interacts with MEF2 via association with the MEF2 MADS and adjacent domains. When tested with the *myosin light chain* and *β-myosin heavy chain* promoters in transactivation assays, both promoters exhibited transcriptional synergy upon cotransfection with MEF2C and either RTEF-1 or DTEF-1, but not with NTEF-1. Gel mobility shift studies using a fragment of the myosin light chain promoter in which the MEF2 and MCAT control elements are separated by only 2 bp indicated that the factors interact when bound to DNA because competition with excess MEF2 oligonucleotides abolished both MEF2 and TEF1 binding. Finally, TEF1 interacts with the bHLH leucine zipper factor Max, which binds an E-box site in the *cardiac α-myosin heavy chain* promoter that overlaps an MCAT site, and both factors need to bind their corresponding DNA sites for transcriptional synergy to occur. The transcriptional readout from the SRF-TEF1, MEF2-TEF1, and Max TEF1 interactions thus differs from the proposed MEF2-MRF interaction (see above) in that synergy could be detected when only one of the factors is bound to its cognate DNA site.

An additional transcriptional link between TEF1 and MEF2 is Vestigial, a protein known to interact with the *Drosophila* TEF1 homologue Scalloped.[300] *Drosophila* Vestigial affects both wing and indirect flight muscle development. Among three mammalian vestigial homologues, Vgl-2 is expressed in differentiating somites and is skeletal muscle–specific in adult mice. Coexpression of Vgl-2 with MEF2 or MyoD in transactivation assays caused a marked increase in muscle gene expression levels. As with the studies described above, TEF1 and MEF2 must be bound to their respective control elements in order to exhibit transcriptional activation by the addition of Vgl-2. An additional

Vestigial-like factor "VITO-1" has recently been identified, which is also expressed primarily in the myogenic lineage.[301]

Six4/MEF3/Trex. The *MCK* Trex (transcriptional regulatory element X) control element was identified via mutagenesis of a highly conserved but novel sequence within the human, mouse, rat, and rabbit *mck* enhancers.[302] Portions of the sequence within the Trex region superficially resemble M-CAT/TEF1 and GATA elements, but extensive factor binding and site-directed mutagenesis disproved strong interactions with these factors. The Trex factor has recently been identified as Six4, a nuclear factor containing a Six domain and a homeodomain region that was originally discovered in the developing retina and subsequently identified as the *Myogenin* and muscle *aldolase* enhancer MEF3 control element binding factor.[303] Surprisingly, the *MCK* Trex/Six4 element sequence is sufficiently different from the *Myogenin* and *aldolase* MEF3 sites. Identification of the *MCK* enhancer Trex element as a Six4/MEF3 binding site will disclose a broader consensus sequence for Six4/MEF3/Trex control elements, thereby facilitating searches for these in other muscle gene enhancers and promoters. Mutagenesis and gel mobility shift studies of *MCK* enhancer regions immediately adjacent to the Trex element indicate that an additional unidentified factor binds to the conserved 3'-flanking region. Six4 transcriptional activity is potentiated by Eya, which is targeted to the nucleus via interaction with the conserved Six and homeodomains of Six4.[304] Six4 gene knockout studies have shown that the gene is not essential for mouse development and has no apparent muscle developmental defects. This is probably due to compensation by other Six proteins, most likely Six2 and/or Six5, since they share Six4's capacity for translocating Eya to the nucleus.[304] Studies of Six and Eya protein accumulation within the limb buds of 3- to 8-week human embryos and its correlation with MRF gene expression indicate that Six1, 4, and 5 and their potential coactivators Eya1 and Eya2 are not detected until after the appearance of *Myf5* and coincidentally with the detection of *Myogenin* transcription, indicating that Six and Eya proteins are not essential for the early aspects of MRF gene activation. Six4/MEF3/Trex factor and control elements may have additional roles in muscle fiber-type-specific gene expression.[303]

Myoblast-Specific Transcriptional Control Elements

The muscle control elements described above regulate contractile protein gene expression when replicating myoblasts initiate differentiation. There are distinct control elements that regulate a subset of muscle-specific genes expressed in proliferative myoblasts. These include MRFs, *Myf5* and *MyoD*, and also structural genes such as β-enolase and desmin.[305] In proliferative myoblasts, expression of these genes is controlled by distinct transcription enhancers that differ from those that regulate the contractile protein gene activation during muscle differentiation.[306] Further studies of the myoblast-specific control elements could provide an understanding of Myf5 and MyoD functions in proliferative myoblasts as well as lead to the development of therapeutic tools to manipulate muscle progenitors for repair of damaged muscles.

Transgenic Analysis of Skeletal Muscle Control Elements

Much of our current knowledge of muscle-specific regulatory promoters and enhancers and their interacting transcription factors comes from transient transfection studies of reporter genes in tissue culture cells as well as from DNA-binding studies with purified transcription factors. These approaches are productive but subject to limitations related to overexpression of reporter genes and to the more permissive regulatory state of tissue culture cells. Transgenic studies of skeletal muscle gene expression in embryos have provided a means to verify conclusions drawn from transfection transient assays and an opportunity to analyze the response of skeletal muscle gene regulatory elements to physiologic stimuli that cannot be accurately reproduced in cell culture. Transgenic studies are still in their infancy. The activity of transgenes is affected by their genomic integration and by potential cross-species incompatibilities between control elements and transcription factors. Lesser effects of this type could be anticipated in studies of human and rat muscle genes in transgenic mice; but even in these cases, it is possible that a single base pair change within a critical control element could alter the relative transcriptional activity of a transgene. That said, it is worth noting that mouse MCK transgenes are expressed at high levels in the skeletal muscles of transgenic Xenopus and zebrafish (Hauschka, unpublished).

Transgenic analysis has been used to identify regulatory elements for several muscle genes: chicken *Skeletal α-Actin*, human *Skeletal α-Actin, Acetylcholine Receptor*; human *Aldolase A*; *Desmin*; mouse *MCK*; human *Myoglobin*; quail *TnI-fast*, human *TnI slow*; *Myosin Heavy Chain*; and rat *Myosin Light Chain (MCK) 1/3*. These studies have delineated gene regulatory regions for skeletal and/or cardiac muscle and fast versus slow skeletal muscle fibers: *MCK*[263,307] and *MLC 1/3*[308] and AChR at the neuromuscular junction.[309]

Transgenic findings have both confirmed and challenged concepts of MCK gene regulation, based on cell culture transfection studies.[307] In concurrence with in vitro data, the 206-bp 5' enhancer (Figs. 1-11 and 1-12) is essential for high-level transgene expression; however, in contrast to the results of transfection studies, this enhancer activity is 100- to 1000-fold more active in combination with the entire 5'-promoter region (−1020 to +7) (Fig. 1-12) than with the 80-bp proximal MCK promoter region (Fig. 1-12). Similar synergy between the proximal promoter and enhancer is observed when the enhancer is combined with the highly conserved 350-bp proximal promoter region. Furthermore, the enhancer and entire promoter regions each exhibit similar low muscle-specific expression as transgenes, but the promoter has only about 2 percent of the enhancer's activity when tested in vitro.

A second unanticipated result of transgenic analysis concerns the transcriptional activities of individual enhancer control elements. In cell culture transfection studies, the MEF1/E box and A/T-rich elements are essential for enhancer activity. Mutations of the MEF2/E-box site cause a 90-fold decrease in activity of the enhancer alone and a 30-fold decrease in activity of the enhancer plus entire promoter; but in transgenic mice, mutations of the MEF2/E-box site have no disruptive effects. The paradoxical behavior of the

MEF1/E-box mutation remains to be explained. By contrast, in transfection assays, mutation of the A/T-rich element causes a 15-fold decrease in activity when tested in the enhancer alone and a 10-fold decrease when tested in the context of the enhancer plus entire promoter[271] and more than a 100-fold reduction in transgene expression in transgenic mice. The Trex control element also is functionally required in transgenic assays, as mutation of the Trex element reduced expression in slow soleus muscle, and to a lesser extent in fast EDL muscle. Studies involving viral-mediated transduction of similar mutant and wild-type muscle gene regulatory regions into adult mouse muscles may be informative with respect to determining the basis of these unanticipated differences.

EXERCISE-MEDIATED SKELETAL MUSCLE REGULATION

Advances are now being made toward an understanding of the transcriptional responses of muscle genes to exercise and hypertrophy.[310,311] Current studies include molecular analyses of humans subjected to various training or disuse paradigms as well as experimental studies of muscle activity and atrophy in experimental animals and muscle cell cultures. For example, endurance training under normal oxygen levels vs. hypoxic conditions reveals an 80 percent increase in hypoxia-inducible factor 1-α (HIF-1α) mRNA under both normal and hypoxic conditions, whereas myoglobin transcripts increase only during oxygen deprivation.[312] Animal studies reveal that strenuous muscle activity leads to a transient 10-fold increase in cFos, crystallin, and heat-shock protein 70 transcripts, while increases in myoglobin mRNA require much longer periods of intense muscle activity.[313] Attempts to identify critical control elements within muscle genes that respond to exercise and stretch-induced hypertrophy are in progress, focusing on regulatory elements controlling *MCK*,[314] *α-MyHC*,[315] and *Skeletal α-Actin*.[316] Animal and muscle cell culture studies are providing some conflicting results; for example, stretch-induced hypertrophy in young chickens is accompanied by increased expression of *Skeletal α-Actin* dependent upon intact SRF and TEF-1 elements within the proximal 100-bp promoter region, whereas cell culture studies indicate that mechanical stretching causes a repression in *Skeletal α-Actin* expression mediated via the TEF-1 binding site.[317] Comparative studies of human and rat *β-Myosin Heavy Chain* promoter function in transgenic mice subjected to decreased weight bearing of the slow soleus muscles, similar to that encountered in space flight and during chronic immobilization, identify an MCAT control element in the rat regulatory element that responds to non-weight-bearing conditions; however, a related MCAT element in the human *β-Myosin* promoter does not exhibit this activity,[318] indicating species-specific differences in physiologic response elements of muscle genes.

FAST AND SLOW MUSCLE ENHANCERS AND CONTROL ELEMENTS

Skeletal muscles have different relative proportions of fast and slow muscle fibers, which express different contractile protein isoforms and have different metabolic activities. Fast and slow muscle fibers are typically classified by their differential expression of specific myosin heavy-chain (MyHC) isoforms. Adult mouse hindlimb muscle fiber types are subdivided into fast types IIb (containing MyHC IIb), IIx/d (containing MyHC types IIx and IId), IIa (containing MyHC IIa), and slow type I (b-MyHC) (see Chap. 5). Muscle fibers containing each of these MyHC isoforms exhibit unique myosin ATPase activities and unloaded shortening velocities, and their overall energy metabolism exhibits corresponding differences. Slow-twitch muscles such as the soleus and back muscles, used for sustained locomotion and posture activities, contain mostly type I fibers and express relatively high levels of βMyHC and oxidative enzymes. Fast-twitch muscles, such as the EDL, used for strong-force rapid-response activities, contain mostly type II fibers and express relatively high levels of MyHC types IIx and IId and various proportions of oxidative and glycolytic enzymes. While contractile protein gene expression in these fiber types is developmentally programmed, this expression can be altered by muscle activity patterns and by disuse; the transcriptional mechanisms responsible for these activity-dependent gene regulatory process are being intensively studied.[319,320]

Recent attention has focused on muscle hypertrophy and the role of calcineurin in the regulation of NFAT and downstream transcription factors such as MEF2 and associated HATs and HDACs.[321] Transcriptional co-activator, peroxisome-proliferator-activated receptor-gamma coactivator-1 (PGC-1γ), previously implicated in mitochondrial biogenesis and oxidative metabolism, controls the formation of slow-twitch muscle fibers.[322] Overexpression of PGC-1α in fast muscle fibers via MCK-regulated PGC-1α transgene converts fast type II muscle fibers to a primarily slow type I phenotype. This process appears to involve calcineurin modifications of PGC-1α, followed by MEF2-mediated effects on muscle gene expression. These signals may well impinge on the fiber-type-specific clusters of control elements FIRE and SURE, or to other fiber-type-specific control elements identified in fast and slow muscle enhancers/promoters.[323,324]

SKELETAL AND CARDIAC TRANSCRIPTION ENHANCERS AND CONTROL ELEMENTS

Many skeletal muscle genes are expressed in cardiac muscle under the control of distinct regulatory elements. These elements probably have different relative functionality in one or the other striated muscle type, as illustrated by the skeletal and cardiac control elements in the MCK enhancer.[270] When tested in skeletal muscle cell cultures, MCK enhancers with MEF1/E-box site mutations have nearly 100-fold reduced activity, whereas these same mutations reduce activity less than sevenfold in cardiomyocyte cultures from newborn rats. As MRFs are not expressed in cardiomyocytes, unknown cardiomyocyte E-box-binding factors must utilize these control elements for regulating the MCK gene in cardiac muscle. Similarly, mutations of the MCK enhancer CArG/SRE site cause no more than a 2-fold reduction in activity in skeletal muscle cultures, whereas the same mutations reduce activity by 20-fold in heart muscle cultures. The 1-kb proximal promoter, which has a highly conserved 350-bp region adjacent to the TATA box, is essentially dispensable for activity of the MCK enhancer in skeletal muscle cultures, whereas expression in cardiac muscle cultures is reduced 10-fold following mutagenesis. Significantly, the promoter region is much more important for high-level expression in *both* striated muscle types when tested in transgenic mice, as discussed above.

Other transcription factors that provide relative cardiac selectivity to the expression of muscle genes include GATA-4/5/6, HF-1a, HF-1b, MEF2-D, NKX2.5, and TEF-1. A primary focus of current cardiac gene regulation studies is understanding the regulatory factors that control cardiac hypertrophy in response to injury, specifically the integration of physiologic signals such as Ca-regulated changes in CAM kinase and calcinurin with the modification of NFAT and MEF2 transcription factors and associated HATs and HDACs. These factors impinge on the expression of specific cardiac contractile protein and metabolic genes. Cardiac muscle gene control mechanisms have recently been reviewed.[325–327]

ALTERNATIVE RNA SPLICING REGULATION OF MUSCLE PROTEIN EXPRESSION

In addition to transcriptional control, alternative RNA splicing is an important mechanism controlling muscle gene expression during myocyte differentiation in vertebrate and invertebrate embryos.[328–331] Molecular studies have localized muscle-specific positive and negative regulatory sequences in the introns and splice junctions of alternatively spliced exons, providing evidence that these regulatory elements are sites of interaction with regulatory factors.[332–336] However, the nature and functions of specific RNA splicing factors have lagged behind.[337] Discovery of muscle-specific splicing factors and regulatory mechanisms controlling the alternative RNA splicing of contractile protein genes will be a significant advance toward understanding the fundamental processes of muscle differentiation and will provide opportunities for development of therapies in the treatment of muscular dystrophies, as discussed below.[338,339]

MUSCLE REGULATORY ELEMENTS AND THERAPEUTIC APPLICATIONS

Muscle Gene Regulatory Cassettes

The regulatory regions and control elements of muscle genes have applications to human gene therapy treatment of genetic neuromuscular disorders such as Duchenne muscular dystrophy (DMD). In addition, the possibility of using skeletal muscle as a bioreactor for synthesis and secretion of proteins such as growth hormone is being explored. For such applications, skeletal muscle gene regulatory components are valuable tools, as they confer muscle specificity to the expression of therapeutic proteins. When combined with viral vector-delivery therapies, muscle specificity of expression decreases the likelihood of deleterious effects due to high-level expression of inappropriate proteins in nonmuscle tissues. Stimulation of an immune response to the therapeutic protein may thus be limited.

DMD is among the most common neuromuscular diseases, occurring about 1 per 3500 male births (see Chap. 34). Dystrophin is the largest human gene yet mapped. The coding portion of the skeletal muscle isoform spans more than 2.4 million bp on the X chromosome and is composed of 79 multiply spliced exons. The *Dystrophin* gene contains seven promoters that regulate its expression in striated muscle, neuronal cells, and other nonmuscle cells.[340] A muscle promoter is located more than 200 kb 5' of the first translated exon, and its regulatory regions are poorly understood. Due to the Dystrophin gene's immense physical size, it is not presently feasible to design vector-mediated strategies for treating DMD with the native gene. Current therapeutic strategies thus envision miniaturizing the dystrophin protein and substituting alternative muscle-specific regulatory control regions so that these miniproteins can be packaged within viral vectors and expressed in skeletal muscles.

Most experimental studies of DMD gene therapy have utilized the *mdx* mouse model. *mdx* mice have a point mutation in exon 23, in which the glutamine CAA codon is changed to the TAA STOP codon. The N-terminal portion of Dystrophin that is synthesized does not localize to the sarcolemma and is rapidly degraded; this leads to the concomitant absence of most DGC components from the sarcolemma. The *mdx* mice exhibit a milder form of dystrophy than that observed in most DMD patients; however, pathology of the *mdx* diaphragm is severe,[341] and the threshold for contraction-induced injury is greatly reduced.[342] The severity of the *mdx* phenotype can be increased by the status of other genes; e.g., *mdx*, *MyoD*−/− mice exhibit poor muscle regeneration and much greater muscle pathology.[343] An X-linked canine dystrophin gene mutation (GRMD) is also available for gene therapy studies. This is an important model for human DMD treatment because the size of canine muscles provides a more equivalent load-bearing physiological comparison to human muscle than the tiny muscles of dystrophic mice. The GRMD allele is a point mutation in the consensus splice acceptor site in intron 6 of dystrophin. This leads to the skipping of exon 7, translation of out-of-frame codons in exon 8, and truncation of the nascent Dystrophin polypeptide due to a premature STOP codon. Affected male pups exhibit variable disease phenotypes and may die within days, months, or years of birth.[344]

Initial attempts to develop a gene therapy for DMD concentrated on expressing various Dystrophin cDNAs under the control of constitutive viral promoters. These studies were carried out in cell culture and succeeded in demonstrating that modified forms of the Dystrophin protein could be localized correctly in the cell membrane.[345,346] These studies encouraged use of similar techniques to express both full-length and truncated Dystrophin cDNAs in *mdx* mice. Truncated Dystrophin cDNAs are of therapeutic interest because the packaging size of viral vectors is considerably smaller than that of full-length dystrophin. The potential therapeutic value of a 6.3-kb human Dystrophin cDNA (approximately half the normal size, containing the N-and C-terminal domains and lacking most of the central rod domain) was suggested by the fact that a similar truncated protein causes a particularly mild Becker muscular dystrophy. Direct injection of fusion genes containing full-length or truncated human Dystrophin cDNAs into *mdx* muscle results in partial restoration of Dystrophin immunostaining and the occurrence of peripheral myonuclei in about 1 percent of the fibers in the injected regions.[347] Subsequent studies achieved higher levels of dystrophin expression via the injection of *mdx* muscles with either adenovirus[348] or retrovirus[349] constructs containing the human 6.3-kb Dystrophin cDNA. This latter study also achieved continual Dystrophin expression for at least 9 months as well as restoration of at least one of the Dystrophin-associated glycoproteins (DAGs). As greater knowledge of Dystrophin's structure-function has accumulated, it has now become feasible to construct even smaller functional Dystrophins.[350] These have been tested for function in transgenic *mdx* mice and for their ability to reverse or retard muscle degeneration following their intramuscular injection when packaged in adeno-associated virus (AAV), as described below.

Muscle-specific gene regulatory regions are now being used routinely for experimental studies of Dystrophin expression in *mdx* mice. The majority of these studies use either various portions of the MCK promoter and enhancer or the human skeletal muscle Actin promoter. Initial studies with MCK regulatory components used a 6.7-kb genomic fragment containing the well-defined enhancer and promoter regions plus 5' flanking and intron-1 regions known to contain additional regulatory elements ligated to the full-length mouse dystrophin cDNA (Fig. 1-13) to generate transgenic *mdx* mice. These mice exhibit complete restoration of normal cardiac and skeletal muscle phenotypes, including all of the DAGs, peripheral nuclei, lack of fiber degeneration, normal serum Creatine Kinase levels, and normal levels of muscle power and force generation.[351] Muscles of transgenic mice in which the Dystrophin cDNA was transcribed under the control of a different version of the mouse MCK gene also had extensive replacement of dystrophin and DAGs, but the fiber-to-fiber expression levels within individual muscles and between different mice varied widely.[352]

Although the initial attempts at DMD gene therapy in mice are promising, many technical modifications are necessary before this approach can be applied to humans. The size of the regulatory gene cassette-Dystrophin cDNAS construct needs to be reduced for more efficient gene transfer via the currently approved viral vectors. AAV is presently the viral vector of choice, primarily due to safety considerations. The challenge of building miniaturized regulatory cassette-Dystrophin cDNA constructs is great due to the very limited ~4.8-kb packaging size of AAV. Small MCK regulatory cassettes with high transcriptional activity contain a conserved proximal promoter region plus the MCK enhancer, with two purposeful mutations that were predicted to increase transcriptional activity. The most active cassette, "CK6," exhibits high transcriptional activity in skeletal muscle cultures and muscle tissue in vivo and exceedingly *low* activity in fibroblast and immune dendritic cell cultures and in muscle connective tissue and liver in vivo. CK6 activity is about fivefold greater in skeletal muscle cell culture assays than that of unmodified MCK promoter-enhancer cassettes. Expression level comparisons of CK6 to a standard high-activity CMV cassette indicates that it has about 8 percent of the activity of CMV. Adenoviral vectors containing CK6 exhibit strong tissue-specific expression in skeletal muscle fibers, no expression in muscle connective tissue, and virtually no expression in liver when injected intramuscularly or administered via the tail vein. Subsequent studies also showed that CK6-containing vectors exhibit 1000-fold lower expression in human immune system dendritic cells; and studies in *mdx* mice indicate that proteins expressed under the control of CK6 do not stimulate a substantial immune response. The CK6 regulatory cassette has also been used to express a ~4-kb microDystrophin cDNA in both transgenic *mdx* mice and AAV-injected *mdx* mouse muscle.[350] In transgenic mice, the presence of microdystrophin throughout development and adulthood provided substantially improved muscle strength compared to control *mdx* mice; and importantly, when the CK6-microDystrophin is incorporated into AAV vectors and injected into *mdx* muscle tissue, extensive muscle regions exhibiting intense immunostaining for microDystrophin are detected, and these persist for several months.

Compensatory Protein Strategies

The concept that Dystrophin deficiency might be compensated for by the upregulation or vector-mediated overexpression of one or more other proteins grew out of β-globinopathy studies in which vector-mediated overexpression or upregulation of the fetal isoform could partially compensate for mutations in the adult gene.

Utrophin. The analogy to globinopathy treatment strategies was immediately recognized when *Utrophin*, the autosomal homologue of Dystrophin, was discovered.[353] A particularly attractive attribute of compensatory protein overexpression strategies for DMD therapy is that patients would be unlikely to develop an immune response against compensatory proteins because their immune systems should recognize these proteins as "self." In contrast, DMD patients, especially those with large deletions of the dystrophin gene, may initiate an immune response against one or more "novel" epitopes present in micro-, mini-, or even full-length dystrophin proteins provided by standard gene therapy protocols.

Unlike Dystrophin, Utrophin is ubiquitously expressed. In developing and regenerating skeletal muscle, Utrophin is detected throughout the sarcolemma, but upon fiber maturation, Utrophin becomes localized to the neuromuscular and myotendinous junctions. Evidence for Utrophin's functional compensation for Dystrophin deficiency was obtained by overexpressing Utrophin in transgenic *mdx* mouse muscle.[354] Utrophin as well as the otherwise absent DGC components was observed throughout the sarcolemma. Subsequent to these studies, a large effort has been mounted by many investigators to identify gene response elements and signals capable of upregulating Utrophin expression in *mdx* mice. One particularly novel approach has been the attempt to design an artificial Zn-finger transcription factor whose regulated expression might potentially control levels of Utrophin expression in dystrophic muscle.[355] Other investigators have discovered that distinct regions in the 3' untranslated region of Utrophin transcripts are responsible for targeting and stabilizing Utrophin mRNAs in skeletal muscle cells.[356] Exploitation of these mRNA targeting motifs might provide the possibility of transporting "excess" Utrophin mRNA from neuromuscular junction and myotendinous regions of muscle fibers to regions lacking utrophin. Additional clues to natural mechanisms of Utrophin upregulation may come from studies of the extraocular eye muscles and distal toe muscles in DMD patients, where Utrophin expression has been found to be naturally high, thereby sparing these muscles from the dystrophic pathology.[357]

Muscle Integrin-cytoskeletal complex. Mechanical linkage between the skeletal muscle cytoplasm and extracellular matrix occurs via an Integrin-cytoskeletal complex as well as through the Dystrophin complex.[358] The physiologic importance of this linkage is demonstrated by the fact that mutations in the relatively muscle-specific α7-Integrin gene cause a congenital dystrophic myopathy.[359] The membrane-spanning Integrin α7β1 heterodimer binds to laminin-2 in the extracellular matrix, and it is linked to γ-actin cytoskeleton filaments via α-Actinin/Vinculin/Talin complexes. In mdx mice the dystrophin mechanical linkage between the cytoskeleton and extracellular matrix is abolished, but the Integrin linkage persists. Interestingly, overexpression of α7-Integrin transgenes driven by an MCK regulatory cassette in severely affected mdx/Utrophin −/− mice partially rescues the dystrophic phenotype, even though members of the DGC remain absent from the sarcolemma.[360] This important study suggests that contraction-mediated mechanical stress to the muscle membrane can be ameliorated by increasing the function or levels of the integrin-cytoskeletal complex and that this can occur independently of the DGC complex. Upregulation of α7-Integrin levels in DMD patients using vectors with muscle regulatory cassettes is thus an alternative therapeutic strategy that deserves further investigation.

GalNAc transferase. The compensatory properties of GalNAc transferase-2 in DMD were discovered via basic studies of neuromuscular junction (NMJ) glycoproteins. GalNAc transferase-2 is the enzyme responsible for carrying out the terminal linkage of βN-acetylglucosamine (GalNAc) to carbohydrate moieties on a number of glycoproteins found in the NMJ. Interestingly, when GalNAc transferase-2 is expressed extrasynaptically in transgenic mice, it can link the same GalNAc moiety to the DGC component α-dystroglycan. When GalNAc transferase-2 transgenes are overexpressed in mdx mice, the usual pathologic phenotype and creatine kinase leakage are markedly reduced, and the levels of utrophin and many of the DGC proteins increase.[361] However, a potential therapeutic complication is that GalNAc transferase-2 overexpression in normal mice severely reduced the number of synaptic secondary folds, and Schwann cell processes were observed in the synaptic cleft. These changes might lead to their own physiologic problems, but this was not noted in the mdx study.

Targeted Gene Correction and STOP Codon Skipping Strategies

Additional approaches for muscle gene therapy involve strategies designed to correct mutations in the patient's genomic DNA or within mRNA transcripts. Correction strategies for point mutations and small deletions in a variety of genetic diseases have involved strategies that directly target the mutation site and others that circumvent the mutation via the alteration of splicing signals. Attempts to correct Dystrophin point mutations in the mdx mouse and grmd dystrophic dog have involved the use of chimeric RNA/DNA oligonucleotides[362] and short-fragment homologous replacement.[363] Correction rates in the 1 to 10 percent range have been reported for the mdx mutation, depending on whether the correction frequency is based on the ratio of Dystrophin-positive to -negative fibers per se or on the number of Dystrophin-positive fibers per fiber that accumulated the labeled RNA/DNA oligonucleotide following intramuscular injection or following the treatment of cultured mdx satellite cells. These targeted correction frequencies are extremely impressive, but their potential shortcoming is that both the mdx mouse and grmd dog exhibit revertant muscle fibers. While this potential artifact has been addressed in the experimental designs and data interpretations, it remains possible that true correction frequencies are not as high as they seem. However, if the correction frequency were only 0.01 to 0.1 percent, the strategy would be well worth further development. Attempts to correct Dystrophin gene mutations at the mRNA level have employed antisense RNA to induce exon skipping during splicing reactions so as to avoid STOP codons caused by deletion mutations.[364] In cell culture studies, as many as 75 percent of the muscle fibers exhibited Dystrophin staining following this treatment. Other mRNA correction strategies have used aminoglycoside antibiotics to translate through STOP codons.[365] Due to the prevalence of STOP mutations among DMD patients, perfected versions of this strategy could be applicable to more than 10 percent of the patient pool.

Building Muscle Anatomy

Anatomic muscles form by the localized migration of populations of progenitors from somites along the AP axis of the embryo to the sites of muscle formation. Myf5 and MyoD are then activated in these localized somite progenitors to establish populations of muscle progenitors that differentiate and build anatomic muscles. The specification of muscle, bone, and tendon progenitors to build functional skeletal anatomy is controlled by shared developmental signals, including Hedgehogs, FGFs, BMPs, and Wnts, which spatially and temporally coordinate the formation of muscles with their functionally and anatomically related tendon, bone, and vascular tissues.[366] Recent studies have identified transcriptional and signaling regulators that control migration of muscle progenitors, myocyte fusion for fiber formation, and muscle patterning to build functional musculoskeletal anatomy.

MIGRATION OF MUSCLE PROGENITORS TO ANATOMIC SITES

Muscle progenitors that form head and appendicular body muscles of the body delaminate from lateral edges of epithelial dermomyotomes of somites located along the AP axis of the embryo. Once delaminated, these progenitors migrate directionally in cell clusters to sites of muscle formation.[367] Muscle precursors from individual somites undergo some intermingling with muscle precursors from adjacent somites, but the AP overlap within single muscles is typically limited to two to three somites to either side.[368] The migratory pathways of head and appendicular muscle progenitors have been mapped by lineage tracing techniques,[68,369] and genetic studies have identified transcription factor/signaling pathways that control the migration of somite progenitors to form abdominal and limb muscles in vertebrate embryos (Fig. 1-17).[370] Pax3, first identified as the Splotched mutation in mice, is a paired box transcription factor that is essential for the directed migration of somite progenitors to the anatomic sites of hypaxial and limb muscle formation.[371] Epaxial muscles form normally along the embryo axis in Pax3 (−/−) embryos, but migratory hypaxial and limb muscle progenitors fail to migrate and then undergo apoptosis.[372] However, Pax3 (−/−) mutant somite cells transplanted directly to the limb bud undergo muscle differentiation, establishing that Pax3 functions to regulate somite cell migration and not myogenesis.[371]

The migration of somite progenitors to abdominal and limb sites of myogenesis is controlled by the scatter factor/hepatocyte growth factor (SF/HGF) signaling. Pax3 regulates genes that control SF/HGF signaling for cell migration. Pax3 regulates c-met, which encodes a tyrosine kinase receptor for the SF/HGF ligand.[373] c-met is expressed by lateral dermomyotomal cells that fail to delaminate from the somite in c-met (−/−) and SF/HGF (−/−) embryos, which are completely blocked in the formation of all abdominal and limb muscles. The SF/HGF ligand is expressed specifically in developing limb buds and other sites along migratory pathways, under the control of morphogenic signals in the limb, including Shh and FGF.[370] Ectopic application of SF/HGF in chick embryos promotes delamination of lateral cells and generalized migration but is not sufficient for their directed migration to specific sites of myogenesis.[374] The signaling clues for directed migration of muscle progenitors are unknown. The Lbx1 transcription factor is expressed in migratory muscle progenitors, under the control of Pax3. Muscle progenitors in Lbx1 (−/−) mutant mice delaminate normally from the somite but then migrate aberrantly, leading to an absence of muscle progenitors in the limb and abdomen.[375,376] Lbx1 presumably controls the expression of target genes that mediate the receptiveness of muscle progenitors to guidance signals along their migration pathways. Significantly, Lbx1 is expressed in fin migratory progenitor muscles in zebrafish, indicating that the mechanisms for muscle progenitor migrations are conserved among vertebrates.[377]

SPECIFICATION OF ANATOMIC MUSCLES

An important question is whether the somites at different levels along the AP axis are prespecified to form the characteristic anatomic muscles and vertebrae at these locations or, alternatively, whether the anatomy of these muscles and bones is determined by extrinsic cues located along the embryo axis. Interestingly, grafting studies show that paraxial mesoderm and somites from different AP levels are prespecified for level-specific muscles and bones. Paraxial mesoderm transplanted from posterior to more anterior axial regions forms muscles and vertebrae with the anatomic characteristics of their more posterior origins, and vice versa. The AP specification of muscles and vertebral anatomy is reflective of the patterning of hox gene transcription in the paraxial mesoderm along the AP axis.[378] Hox expression, referred to as the HOX code, demarcates the cervical, thoracic, lumbar, and sacral anatomic domains of the vertebrate body plan and show species-specific variations, reflecting variations in somite numbers among vertebrates reflective of their variant cervical and thoracic bone and muscle anatomy.[28] Transgenic studies show that misexpression of hox genes along the AP axis of mouse embryos leads to anatomic transformations of vertebrae,[379,380] providing evidence for the functionality of HOX genes in patterning of AP anatomy. HOX genes likely function to determine bone and muscle morphology through their regulation of genes that control

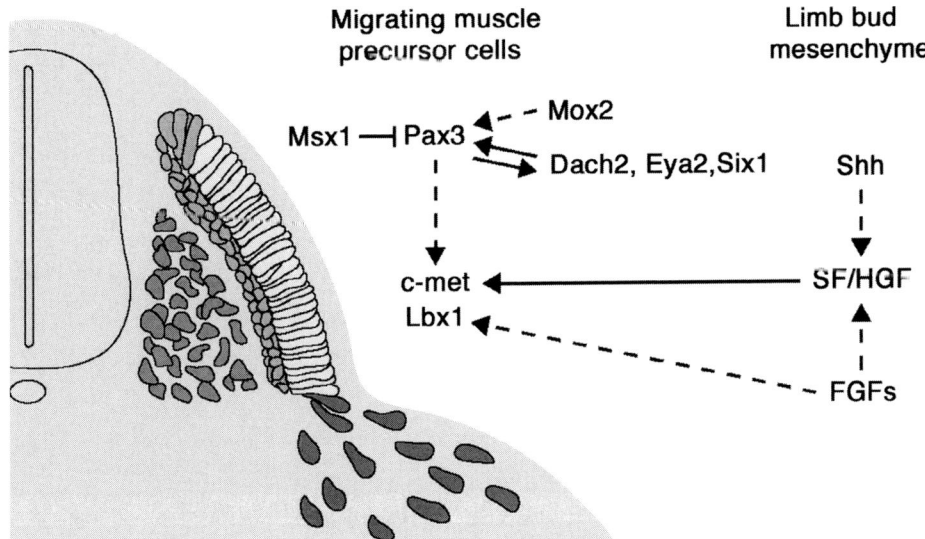

FIGURE 1-17. Schematic diagram of the genetic hierarchy that controls the development of migrating muscle precursor cells. Migrating muscle precursor cells and their dermomyotome progenitors express various genes encoding transcription factors, most notably Pax3. Pax3 controls, directly or indirectly, c-met and Lbx1 expression in migrating precursors. SF/HGF ligand produced in limb mesenchyme controls the activity of its c-met receptor. Genes that pattern the limb also control expression of SF/HGF and Lbx1. (From Birchmeier and Bromann.[370] Reproduced by permission.)

the differential proliferation and adhesion of somite progenitors at different levels along the AP axis.[381]

MYOCYTE FUSION AND MUSCLE FIBER FORMATION

Multinucleated muscle fibers are formed by cell-cell fusion of myocytes in most organisms.[196,382,383] Body wall muscles of some primitive organisms such as nematodes are mononucleated. Fusion and differentiation are not mechanistically coupled processes. Epaxial myotomal muscles formed from DML somite progenitors initially differentiate as mononucleated myocytes,[384] as do slow muscle progenitors in zebrafish embryos.[145] Myocytes fuse later to form larger multinucleated muscle fibers. Myocyte fusion requires calcium ions, suggesting that fusion is mediated by cadherin-based membrane interactions. Notably, blockage of myoblast fusion by reduction of calcium in the cell culture medium does not block myocyte differentiation and contractile protein activation. Extracellular matrix materials, including collagen, are essential for myoblast proliferation and differentiation in culture, and integrins are required for myocyte fusion.[385]

Genetic studies of muscle patterning in *Drosophila* have identified a pathway of genes that couple membrane events of myocyte fusion with intracellular, Rac-mediated signaling controlling cytoskeletal functions for cell morphology.[386,387] Somatic muscles in *Drosophila* are formed from two different myogenic lineages: founder cells and fusion-competent myoblasts (FCMs). These lineages arise from mesoderm expressing high levels of *Twist*. Founder cells are specified at defined anatomic sites of myogenesis in response to developmental signals that activate an array of transcription factor "muscle identity genes."[388] These founders act as cellular "seeds" that fuse with an invariant array of FCMs to establish the unique anatomic identity of muscles. In FCMs, *lmb* is expressed at high levels and is required for their specification and for activation in this lineage of the muscle differentiation gene MEF2;[389] *lmd* was also identified as *gleeful* (*gif1*) in a microarray screen to identify Twist target genes.[185] Each hemisegment of the larva has up to 30 different muscles with precisely defined fiber sizes, determined by fusion. These fibers range in size from 3 to 4 nuclei to 20 to 25 nuclei.[390] Muscle founder cells and FCMs are specified by independent signaling and transcriptional regulatory mechanism and then undergo fusion, although neither myoblast lineage fuses with itself. The extent of fusion and subsequent fiber size is determined by the muscle founder. Muscle identity genes in the founder exert their control of fusion in part by regulation of the timing of expression of fusion genes.

The genes that control cell-cell fusion have been identified in *Drosophila* genetic screens for mutations that disrupt myogenesis and fiber formation (Fig. 1-18). Such fusion genes include *myoblast city* (*mbc*), *Dmef2*, *blown fuse* (*blow*), and *Dtitin*, which are expressed in both founders and FCMs. Additional fusion genes include *dumbfounded* (*duf*) and *sticks and stones* (*sns*), which encode immunoglobulin superfamily members. These proteins are probably located on the cell surface based on their structural homology to known transmembrane or signaling proteins. Significantly, *duf* and *sns* are differentially expressed in founders and FCMs, respectively, and Duf functions as an attractant, providing a mechanism to explain the known asymmetry of fusion between founders and FCMs. Two cytoplasmic proteins required for fusion have also been identified: *antisocial* (*ants*) and *rolling pebbles* (*rols*), which have similar multiple protein interaction domains. Yeast two hybrid interaction screens show that Ants interacts with both Duf and Mbc. The latter is another cytoplasmic protein that interacts with the cytoskeleton and is likely to link the cytoskeletal rearrangement processes to the membrane changes that occur during fusion. Consistent with this finding, Ants and Rols are differentially expressed in founders, which express Duf, and not in FCMs, and Rols is not required for the initial fusion of founders with FCMs to form fibers with two to three nuclei, but is for later fusions to form larger fibers. Rols, therefore, has regulatory functions to control both fiber size and muscle identity. Two additional fusion genes encode extracellular proteins that

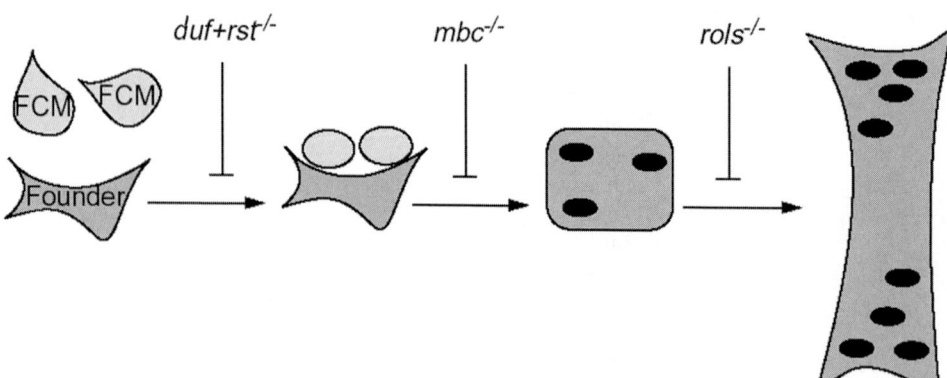

FIGURE 1-18. Genetic control of myoblast fusion. Myoblast fusion is a multistep process. First, fusion-competent myoblasts (FCMs) are attracted toward founder cells. In *duf+rst*, double mutant FCMs are not attracted and their filopodia extend in random orientations rather than toward the founders. Second, FCMs associate with the founders and then fuse to form bi- or trinucleate muscle precursors that are recruited to the founder's pattern of gene expression under the control of *mbc*. Last, in a process that requires *rols*, additional FCMs fuse with the muscle precursors to form multinucleate myotubes. (*From Taylor.*[386] *Reproduced by permission.*)

may function as myoblast attractants, suggesting their redundancy, although cellular expression and timing differ. An immunoglobulin superfamily protein, *roughest* (*rst*), is structurally related to Duf protein, which is expressed in both founders and FCMs, with different developmental timing; while *hebris* (*hbs*) is related structurally to Sns and human Nephrin and is expressed in FCMs but not founders, providing a basis to mediate asymmetrical fusion between these two myoblast lineages. The biochemical mechanisms by which adhesions between these cell surface molecules mediate appropriate cytoskeletal changes to promote membrane fusion remain to be discovered. Interestingly, many of the same proteins identified for myoblast fusion are also essential for fusion of visceral muscles to form the musculature of the gut lining of *Drosophila*. *Drosophila* fusion genes are evolutionarily conserved, raising the possibility that these or related genes control myoblast fusion in vertebrates.

FORMATION OF THE MYOTOME

Myotomal muscles are the first to form in vertebrate embryos and develop into the deep back and intercostal muscles of adults. The cellular processes leading to myotome differentiation and formation of anatomic muscles have been investigated in detail in the avian embryo (Fig. 1-19).[62,391,392] Myotomal muscle is formed from a renewable source of epaxial progenitors in the somite DML, which also gives rise to the growth of the dorsal dermatome. These progenitor cells undergo local, directed migration under the dermatome, become postmitotic, and initiate contractile protein expression. DML progenitors migrate in multiple waves, with individual cells following different migratory paths. Myocytes become organized in parallel arrays within the myotome, growing by the continued orderly migration of myocytes from DML progenitors. Myocytes then extend processes directly beneath the overlying dermamyotome toward the posterior edge of the somite. Cell elongation begins at the anterodorsomedial corner of the dermamyotome and progresses ventrolaterally along the entire anterior margin of the dermamyotome of each somite segment. As development progresses, these elongated myotomal cells eventually span the gap between adjacent vertebrae formed from sclerotomal progenitors. This is achieved by the formation of an intervertebral fissure that bisects each of the nascent vertebrae. The two halves then separate and fuse with the neighboring vertebral halves that abut their anterior and posterior borders by a process referred to as *resegmentation*. Each subset of myotomal cells is associated with the more ventral progenitors for tendon and bones that form the functional anatomic associations with the myotomal muscles. The anterior portions of each myotome become associated with tendons forming at the posterior portion of each vertebra when the vertebral halves move apart and undergo fusion. The myotomal midregion then spans the gap between vertebrae, and each myotomal caudal region becomes associated with the anterior portions of the more posterior vertebrae. At the end of this process, the myotomal cells form a set of primitive intervertebral muscles, linking adjacent vertebrae through interactions with tendons. Later in development, myocytes in the myotome fuse to form multinucleated fibers that become the epaxial, deep back, and intercostal muscles of the neonate.

COORDINATION OF MYOTOME AND TENDON DIFFERENTIATION

The myotomal muscle formation is tightly orchestrated with the formation of tendons and vertebral cartilage and ribs, to which these muscles will form attachments. Lineage marking studies reveal that the vertebrae and rib cartilage and tendons in the body derive from discrete populations of *Pax1*-expressing sclerotomal progenitors in the ventral aspect of the somite.[57,393] Sonic hedgehog signaling is required for the initial specification of both muscle progenitors at the DML and sclerotome progenitors in the ventral somite.[139,394] Tendons that form the attachments between vertebrae and myotomal muscles are derived from a localized population of *Scleraxis* (*Scx*)-expressing somite sclerotomal cells. These cells are intercalated between the bone-forming sclerotome progenitors of the more ventral somite progenitors and the myotomal muscles forming from DML and VLL progenitors migrating under the dermotome. *Scx*-expressing cells line the anterior border of one somite and posterior border of the next somite, in association with the developing vertebrae, which form by resegmentation of these two adjacent somites.[395] These *Scx*-expressing tendon progenitors, referred to as the *syndetome*, derive from the dorsolateral domain of the sclerotome in early somites (Fig. 1-20). They form between adjacent myotomes, dorsomedial and ventrolateral to the sclerotome, prefiguring the sites of muscle and bone attachments. Surgical grafting and misexpression studies reveal that *Scx* expression in the syndetome is controlled by FGF8 and FGF4 signals produced by the overlying myotomal primordia.[57] The same signals also control the waves of migration of DML myotomal progenitors to build the myotomal muscles.[396]

A continuous signaling dialogue also coordinates tendon and body muscle progenitor specification and differentiation in *Drosophila*. Body wall musculature of *Drosophila* comprises 600 individual muscles that are attached to the cuticle through epidermal-like tendon cells located at either end of the fiber beneath the cuticle. The identities of individual muscle groups and initial myogenesis are controlled by the muscle identify genes and fusion regulatory genes independent of tendon formation.[397] However, once multinucleated muscle fibers have formed, they then migrate directionally and are patterned under the cuticle in response to attractant signals produced by tendon progenitors. Attachment of the muscle fiber to tendon precursor cell at each end of the fiber leads to cessation of muscle fiber migration. Tendon precursors are specified independent of muscle, under the control of *Stripe*. This three–zinc finger transcription factor gene also controls production of the unknown muscle attractant, likely related to neural axon guidance factors. Once attached, muscle cells, in turn, produce Vein, a neuregulin-related signaling ligand, which promotes and maintains tendon survival and functional differentiation.

A role for neuregulin-like signaling in vertebrate tendon differentiation during muscle attachment is not yet known. However, as is the case in *Drosophila*, tissue ablation studies establish that tendon and muscles initially differentiate inde-

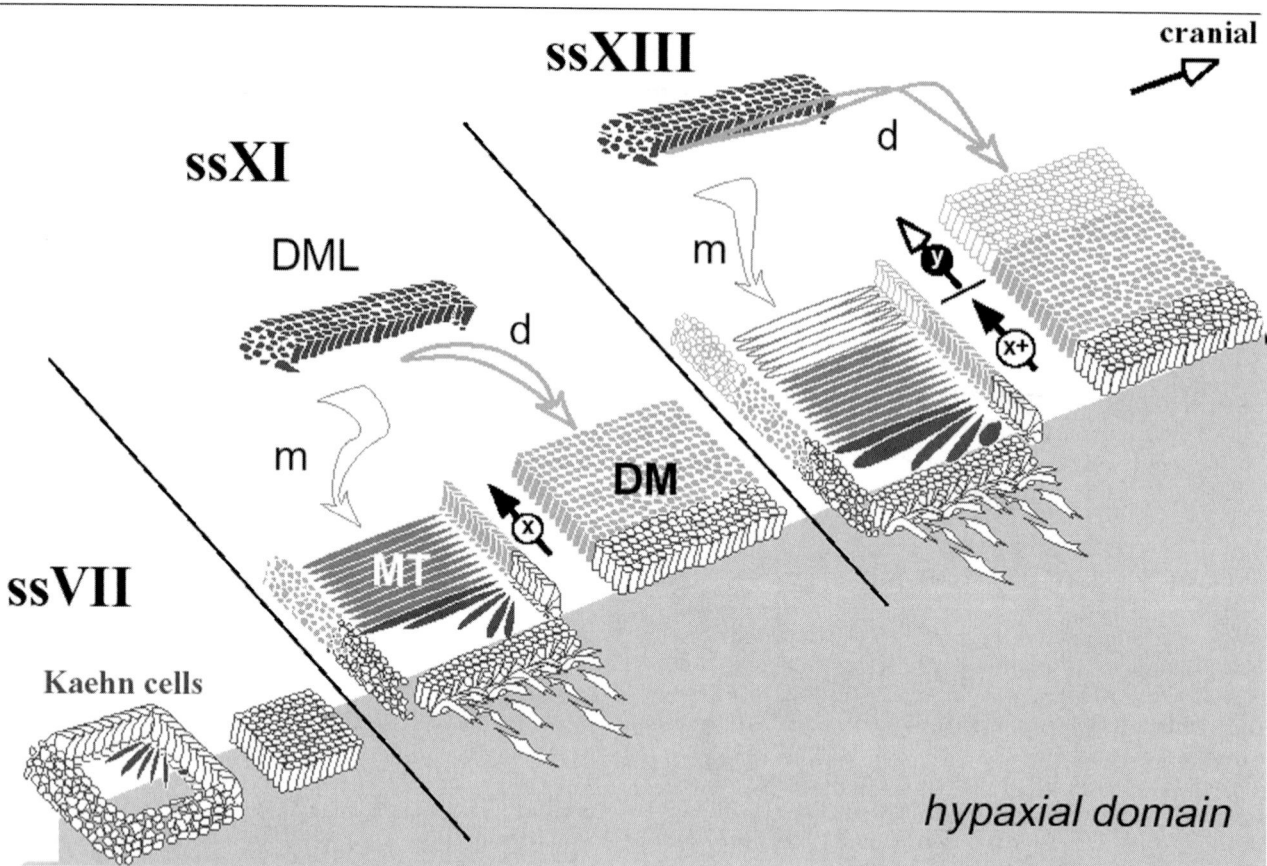

FIGURE 1-19. DML-directed growth and morphogenesis of the epaxial primary myotome and dermamyotome. At somite stage VII, new myotome and dermamyotome cells generated by the DML are displaced laterally as an intermingled stream of cells fated to enter either the myotome or dermamyotome. DML-dependent growth occurs through the asymmetric addition of new cells to the medial-most margin of the myotome (m) and dermamyotome (d), resulting in the medial displacement of the DML. The net growth increment of the somite between somite stages VII and XI is indicated by the arrow marked "x." Note that Kaehn cells (the oldest myotome cells in each segment) as well as some dermamyotome cells that were at the original site of birth of the Kaehn cells are progressively displaced laterally as the somite grows. During the interval between somite stages XI and XIII, that process continues (growth increment "y"), but maturing myocytes in the lateral region of the myotome undergo hypertrophy, thus further expanding the myotome and possibly (to an unknown extent) through secondary addition of new myocytes intercalated from the cranial or caudal dermamyotomal lips and/or other sources (x+). The dermamyotome continues to expand through hyperplasia. In forelimb-level somites, cells in the region of the dermamyotome migrate into the hypaxial domain, where they form blood vessels and limb muscles. (*From Ordahl et al.*[62] *Reproduced by permission.*)

pendently—for example, in the limb. Despite this initial independent formation, segregation of tendon primordia to form independent tendons requires association of tendon primordia with muscles, implicating a role for muscle signaling in the terminal steps of tendon differentiation.[67] Finally, differentiating tendon cells produce unique extracellular matrix and adhesion proteins for muscle and cuticle attachment. Novel transmembrane adhesion proteins adapted for muscle attachment and tensile strength have been identified in genetic screens for muscle attachment mutants (*mup* and *mua* genes) in *C. elegans*.[398–400] These proteins have modular domains related to matrilins, a recently discovered family of proteins found in connective tissues, including tendons. Matrilins associate with collagens and aggrecan to connect intermediate filaments with extracellular collagen matrix and thus provide tensile strength for contraction.

LIMB FORMATION AND MUSCLE PATTERNING

Limb Muscle Progenitors

Limb muscles are derived from somite progenitor cells delaminating from the lateral edges of those four to five somite pairs that are aligned along the AP axis with the regions of fore- and hindlimb bud formation. Lineage marking and grafting studies show that medial and lateral aspects of limb-level somites can give rise to migratory limb progenitors,[401] and cervical and interlimb somites flanking the limb level can also give rise to limb progenitors if engrafted in place of limb-level somites.[80,369,402] Thus, extrinsic factors produced by tissues lateral to somites at the limb-bud level control the migration of lateral somite cells into the limb bud. Lineage marking studies using replication-dependent

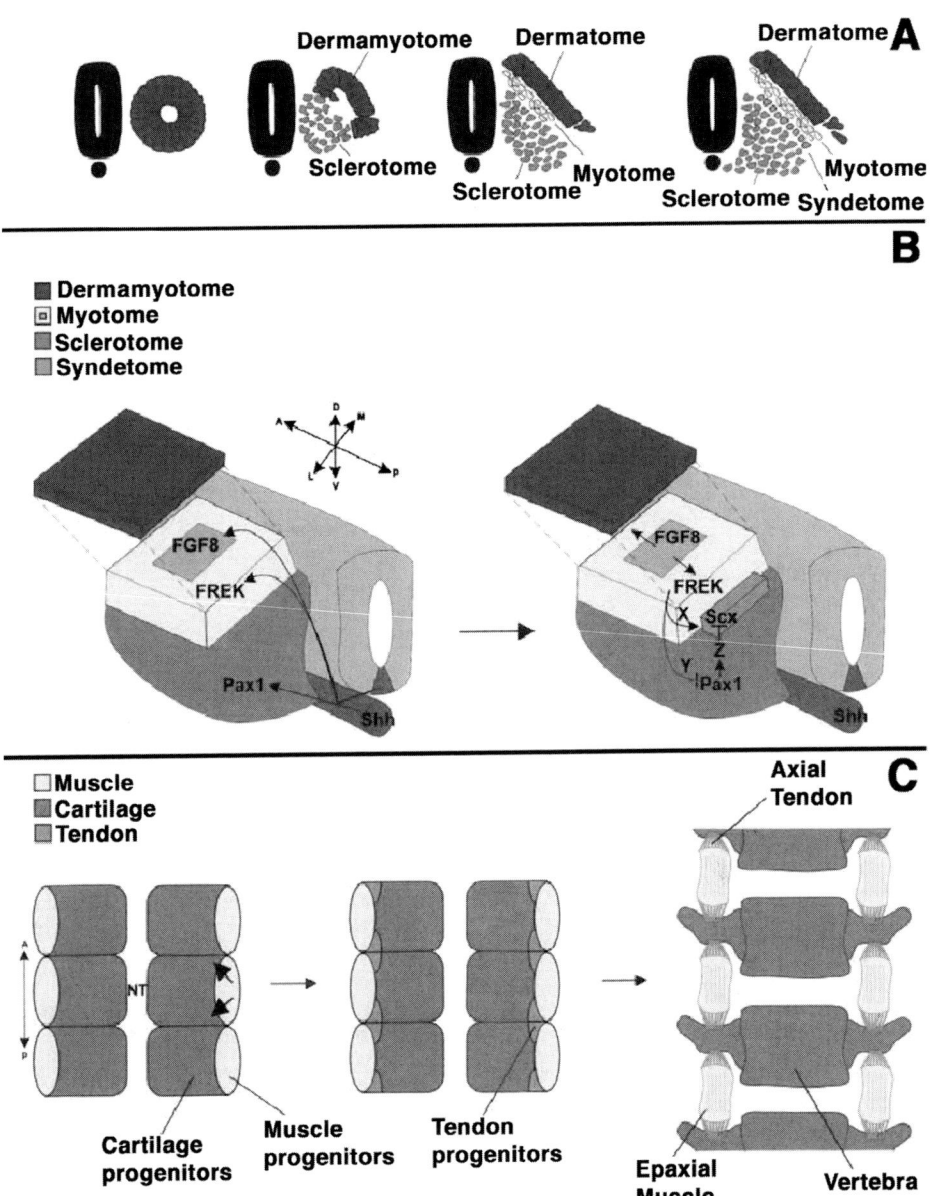

FIGURE 1-20. Model for syndetome tendon formation. A. Series of transverse sections depicting somite development from an epithelial (*left*) to a fully compartmentalized somite (*right*). In response to signals from surrounding tissues, the newly formed epithelial somite is divided into an epithelial dorsal dermamyotome and a mesenchymal ventral sclerotome. Slightly later, the dermamyotome is subdivided into the myotome and overlying dermatome, which remains dorsal. Finally, in response to myotomal signals, the sclerotome is subdivided into the ventral sclerotome and dorsal syndetome. The neural tube and notochord are indicated in black. B. Overview of signals involved in induction of *Scx* expression in the syndetome. During early somite development (*left*), Shh, secreted from the notochord and floorplate, induces both Pax1 in the ventral somite and the FGF/FREK signaling pathway of the myotome. During subsequent somite development (*right*), myotomal FGFs signal to FREK-expressing cells, which, in turn, activate Scx (via factor X) within the abutting sclerotome, giving rise to the syndetome. Sclerotomal Pax1 indirectly represses Scx (via factor Z), but this effect is counteracted by FGF8/FREK signaling (via factor Y). Arrows indicate anteroposterior (AP), dorsoventral (DV), and mediolateral (ML) axes. C. Schematic illustrating interactions between muscle (myotome) and cartilage (sclerotome) progenitors that function to place tendon progenitors (syndetome) at the junction of the other two. Six somites, three on either side of the neural tube (NT), and their derivatives, are depicted in frontal view. An inductive interaction between muscle and cartilage progenitors (*arrows, left*) leads to establishment of a tendon progenitor population between them; thus, the tendon primordials are, from inception, in the same relative spatial setting later required for their mature role as connectors of muscle to cartilage, as shown here in the attachment of epaxial muscle to vertebrae (*right*). (From Brent et al.[57] Reproduced by permission.)

retroviral marking techniques reveal that limb muscle progenitors migrating from limb-level somites are bipotential. These cells populate the dorsal and ventral regions around a central chondrogenic core and give rise to the primary muscles of the dorsal and ventral muscle masses and to the associated vasculature.[56,65] Lateral plate mesoderm progenitors migrate to the central region of the limb bud and differentiate into cartilage and tendons under the control of Indian Hedgehog, an Shh-related signaling ligand. This core of chondrogenic cells then gives rise to the complex bone and tendon anatomy of the limb and digits under the dorsoventral (DV), posterodistal (PD), and anteroposterior (AP) patterning control of interacting and spatially patterned developmental signaling ligands, Wnt, FGF, BMP, and Shh.[403,404]

Clonal cell culture studies and quail-chick somite grafting studies have provided evidence that individual somite progenitors are biased for fast and slow fiber formation.[405,406] However, recent cell lineage marking studies also reveal that somite precursors migrating to the limb give rise to both fast and slow muscle fibers and contribute to the formation of all the 45 morphologically and functionally distinct anatomic muscles of the limb.[56] These findings indicate that the mechanisms for fast and slow muscle specification are largely controlled by extrinsic signals within the limb bud itself.

Human Limb Morphogenesis

The major stages of human limb morphogenesis and myogenesis are illustrated in Fig. 1-21. Limb buds first appear at about the 28th day of development; within 5 to 7 days, they have acquired the morphology seen in Fig. 1-21B. At this stage there is no apparent organization within the limb mesoderm. The leg bud elongates considerably during the next 5 days, and regional densities become evident within portions of the central chondrogenic core (Fig. 1-21C), but the shape and unstructured appearance of cells within the peripheral myogenic regions remain unchanged from their appearance at day 35. During the next 3 days the embryo attains the overall appearance shown in Fig. 1-21A. This figure provides a good illustration of the slightly more advanced morphogenesis of digits in the arm bud compared to the leg bud. A longitudinal section through the leg bud at this stage (Fig. 1-21D) indicates distinct metachromatic staining within the central cartilaginous matrix of the developing femur as well as the initial segregation of muscles within the dorsal and ventral premuscle masses. At higher magnification, cells within the peripheral mesoderm have separated into loose tissue regions and more compact myogenic zones. Myogenic cells closest to the developing bones have elongated and become organized into parallel arrays. Although no multinucleated cells are observed at day 43, a few short myotubes are present by day 45. The cell shapes and alignments observed at this stage are essentially indistinguishable from the morphology of cells in myogenic regions of the chick wing bud at comparable stages of development. The rapidity with which the human leg bud acquires a superficially complete arrangement of muscles is striking (Fig. 1-21E). Within 5 days, all of the bone rudiments have formed and the major anatomic muscles have become segregated. However, the actual amount of differentiated muscle within what appear to be well-formed muscles is extremely small.

From the seventh week onward, muscle development continues at somewhat different rates within each muscle; even within individual muscles, myotube formation appears slightly more advanced in proximal regions. In a comparative sense, the histologic development of 62-day human leg muscle is virtually identical to that of 11-day chick embryo leg muscle. During the next 10 days of human development, muscle fibers in the proximal gastrocnemius become two to three times more numerous, but mononucleated cells still account for at least 50 percent of the cellular mass. Proliferation and accompanying myotube formation occur rapidly throughout the next 3 weeks of development. By day 95, less than 20 percent of the cell mass remains mononucleated. By the 20th week of development, only a few single cells persist within the muscle fiber interstices, and most of these are closely applied to the fiber surface. Fiber nuclei have elongated and are evenly distributed along the length of each fiber. By this stage, the fibers are strikingly cross-striated and

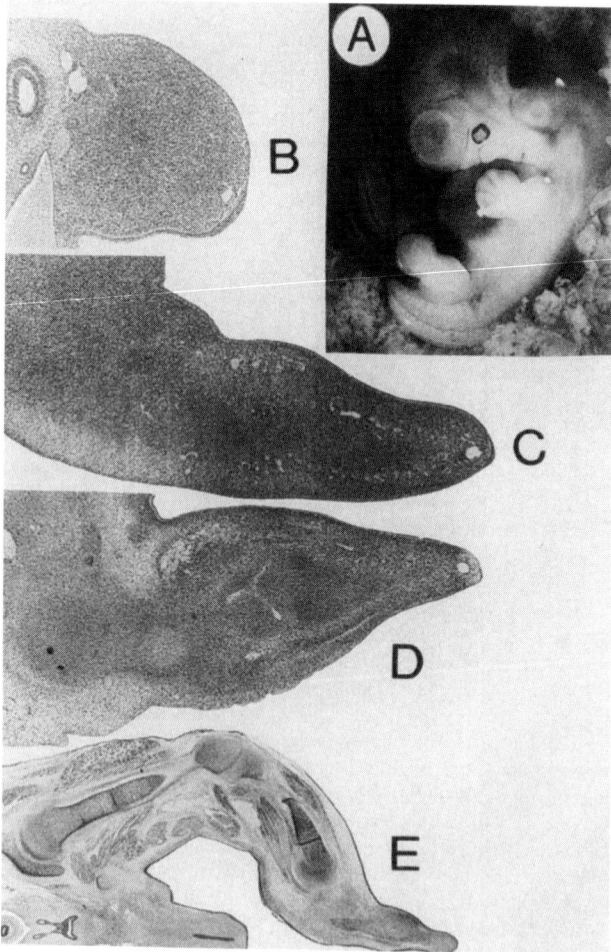

FIGURE 1-21. Photomicrographs depicting progressive stages in human limb muscle development. *A.* A 43-day fetus. *B.* A 35-day leg bud. *C.* A 40-day leg bud.; *D.* A 43-day leg bud. *E.* A 50-day leg bud. See text for more complete descriptions. (*From Hauschka.[407] Reproduced by permission.*)

are arranged in discrete fiber bundles. The overall appearance seen in the 21-week gastrocnemius muscle is actually achieved several weeks earlier, and this same general histologic appearance remains essentially unchanged throughout the remainder of human fetal development. During the interval between weeks 7 and 14, the most conspicuous histologic change is the rapid increase in myotubes; but concomitant with this activity, the mass of the leg as well as the number of single cells within the muscle regions, as determined by dissection and enzymatic dissociation, increase by about 100-fold.[407]

Limb Muscle and Tendon Patterning

Limb muscle precursors initially migrate and localize in discrete dorsal and ventral regions of the limb bud mesenchyme located above and below the chondrogenic core.[67] The newly formed muscle fibers align in orientations that precede and predict later compartments that will segregate into anatomically distinct muscles. The prospective segregation borders then become demarcated by furrows that gradually extend over the muscle mass surface. In E3 chick embryos, the prospective muscle regions are histologically indistinguishable from all of the other limb mesenchyme.[408] Their boundaries are delineated by the expression of *Myf5* and *MyoD*, which are activated as somite progenitors localized to these regions.[27] By E4, the prospective muscle masses become histologically distinguishable from the surrounding limb mesenchyme, but the future boundaries between the prospective limb muscles are not evident (Fig. 1-7). By E5, the ventral and then the lateral muscle masses start splitting into progressively larger numbers of longitudinal muscle bands, and by E7.5, the ventral mass has become partitioned into 11 anatomically distinct muscles[409] (Fig. 1-22). Similar descriptive studies of muscle cleavage within the lower leg region of the rat embryo indicate that the dorsal and ventral premuscle masses become segregated into all of their definitive muscles during the embryonic period spanning E14 to E17.[410]

The extrinsic factors and tissue interactions controlling morphogenesis and muscle patterning in limb are unknown. The patterning of dorsal and ventral muscles and bones is determined early by Wnt7a signaling from the dorsal surface ectoderm, mediated through the transcription factor Lmx1.[411] Later processes such as innervation, limb growth, and tendon morphogenesis are not required for the initiation of limb muscle patterning. For example, muscle patterning is normal in chick limbs that have been denervated as well as in limbs that are missing distal structures beyond the elbow region.[412,413] Aneural mouse limbs have most but not all aspects of normal muscle patterning, although some muscles fail to survive and some smaller muscles undergo initial cleavage or may fuse with neighboring muscles.[114] Tendon effects on muscle patterning initially are nonessential, as muscles and their tendinous insertions are patterned independently and then subsequently connect.[415] The orientation of fibers within developing muscles, the segregation of muscle masses into anatomically discrete muscles, and at least some of the subdivisions within individual muscles occur well before the muscles exhibit attachments to tendons and bones, although this does not exclude the possibility that

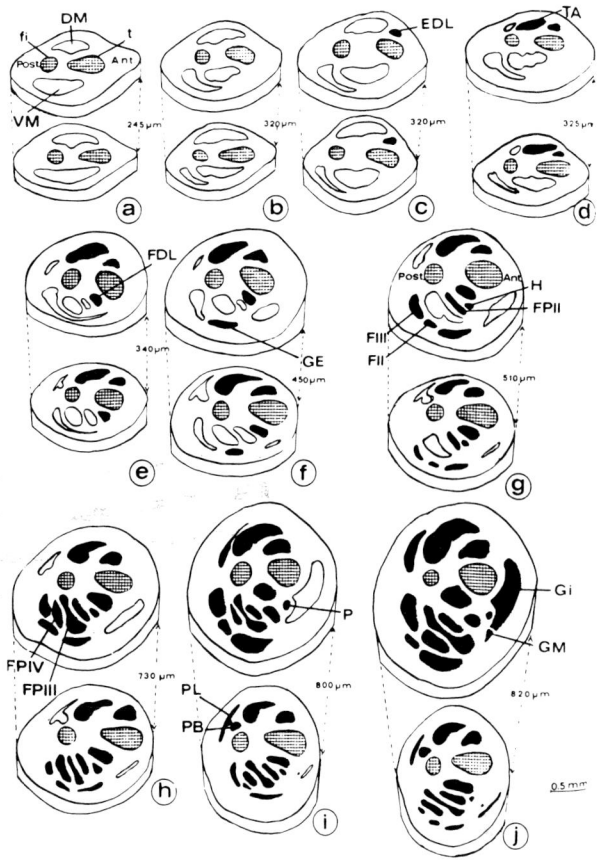

FIGURE 1-22. Diagrammatic representation of progressive compartmentalization of the anterior and posterior premuscle masses of chick embryos between days E5 and E7.5. Each time frame (a, b, c, etc.) is separated by about 6 h. The distance between the proximal and distal sections at each time frame is specified in microns on the dashed line to the right of each time frame. Skeletal elements are cross-hatched, fully partitioned anatomic muscles are shown in black, and muscle masses that have not yet become fully partitioned are shown in white. Muscle splitting occurs in an anterior-to-posterior direction along the limb. DM = dorsal premuscle mass; VM = ventral premuscle mass; fi = fibula; t = tibia; EDL = extensor digitorum longus; TA = tibialis anterior; FDL = flexor digitorum longus; GE, Gi, and GM = gastrocnemius pars externa, pars interna, and pars media; FII and FIII = flexor performans perforatus digiti II and III; FPII, FPIII, and FPIV = flexor perforatus digiti II, III, and IV; H = flexor hallucis longus; P = plantaris; PL = peroneus longus; PB = peroneus brevis. (*From Pautou et al.*[409] *Reproduced by permission.*)

muscles and tendons exchange signals, as discussed. The stage at which these attachments occur is unique for each muscle and appears to be independent of other aspects of muscle maturation. Myogenic cells themselves, however, have a role in maintaining partitions established between segregating muscle regions. Somites transplanted from *crooked neck dwarf* mutant chickens' embryos form premuscle masses within wild-type host limbs and initiate muscle splitting, but then re-fuse into a single mass.[416] As somites contribute only muscle progenitors to the limb, these findings establish that somite-derived muscle cells produce yet to be identified factors required to maintain muscle compartments once muscle splitting has occurred.

List of Abbreviations

AAV	adeno-associated virus	MyHC	myosin heavy chain
AP	anteroposterior	NMJ	neuromuscular junction
bHLH	basic helix-loop-helix	PD	posterodistal
DML	dorsomedial	PKC	protein kinase C
DV	dorsoventral	SF/HGF	scatter factor/hepatocyte growth factor
FCMs	fusion–competent myoblasts	Shh	Sonic hedgehog
FGF	fibroblast growth factor	TGF-β	transforming growth factor beta
IGF	insulin-like growth factor	VLL	ventrolateral
MRF	myogenic regulatory factor		

References

1. Beddington RS, Robertson EJ: Anterior patterning in mouse. *Trends Genet* 14:277, 1998.
2. Whitman M: Nodal signaling in early vertebrate embryos: Themes and variations. *Dev Cell* 1:605, 2001.
3. Kuhl M: Non-canonical Wnt signaling in *Xenopus*: Regulation of axis formation and gastrulation. *Semin Cell Dev Biol* 13:243, 2002.
4. Spemann H, Mangold H: Induction of embryonic primordia by implantation of organizers from different species, in Willier BH, Oppenheimer JM (eds): *Foundations of Experimental Embryology*. New York: Hafner; 1924, p 144.
5. Keller RE: The cellular basis of epiboly: An SEM study of deep-cell rearrangement during gastrulation in *Xenopus laevis*. *J Embryol Exp Morphol* 60:201, 1980.
6. Elul T, Koehl MA, Keller R: Cellular mechanism underlying neural convergent extension in *Xenopus laevis* embryos. *Dev Biol* 191:243, 1997.
7. Tam PP, Goldman D, Camus A, Schoenwolf GC: Early events of somitogenesis in higher vertebrates: Allocation of precursor cells during gastrulation and the organization of a meristic pattern in the paraxial mesoderm. *Curr Top Dev Biol* 47:1, 2000.
8. Topczewski J, Sepich DS, Myers DC, et al: The zebrafish glypican knypek controls cell polarity during gastrulation movements of convergent extension. *Dev Cell* 1:251, 2001.
9. Zimmerman LB, De Jesus-Escobar JM, Harland RM: The Spemann organizer signal noggin binds and inactivates bone morphogenetic protein 4. *Cell* 86:599, 1996.
10. Tonegawa A, Funayama N, Ueno N, Takahashi Y: Mesodermal subdivision along the mediolateral axis in chicken controlled by different concentrations of BMP-4. *Development* 124:1975, 1997.
11. Kishimoto Y, Lee KH, Zon L, et al: The molecular nature of zebrafish swirl: BMP2 function is essential during early dorsoventral patterning. *Development* 124:4457, 1997.
12. Nguyen VH, Schmid B, Trout J, et al: Ventral and lateral regions of the zebrafish gastrula, including the neural crest progenitors, are established by a bmp2b/swirl pathway of genes. *Dev Biol* 199:93, 1998.
13. Kimelman D, Griffin KJ: Vertebrate mesendoderm induction and patterning. *Curr Opin Genet Dev* 10:350, 2000.
14. Soriano P: The PDGFalpha receptor is required for neural crest cell development and for normal patterning of somites. *Development* 124:2691, 1997.
15. Ciruna B, Rossant J: FGF signaling regulates mesoderm cell fate specification and morphogenetic movement at the primitive streak. *Dev Cell* 1:37, 2001.
16. Chapman AE: Characterization of a 140-kd cell surface glycoprotein involved in myoblast adhesion. *J Cell Biochem* 25:109, 1984.
17. Yamaguchi TP, Takada S, Yoshikawa Y, et al: T (*Brachyury*) is a direct target of Wnt3a during paraxial mesoderm specification. *Genes Dev* 13:3185, 1999.
18. Amaya E, Musci TJ, Kirschner MW: Expression of a dominant negative mutant of the FGF receptor disrupts mesoderm formation in *Xenopus* embryos. *Cell* 66:257, 1991.
19. Sun X, Meyers EN, Lewandoski M, Martin GR: Targeted disruption of Fgf8 causes failure of cell migration in the gastrulating mouse embryo. *Genes Dev* 13:1834, 1999.
20. Burdsal CA, Flannery ML, Pedersen RA: FGF-2 alters the fate of mouse epiblast from ectoderm to mesoderm in vitro. *Dev Biol* 198:231, 1998.
21. Griffin KJ, Amacher SL, Kimmel CB, Kimelman D: Molecular identification of spadetail: Regulation of zebrafish trunk and tail mesoderm formation by T-box genes. *Development* 125:3379, 1998.
22. Yoshikawa Y, Fujimori T, McMahon AP, Takada S: Evidence that absence of Wnt-3a signaling promotes neuralization instead of paraxial mesoderm development in the mouse. *Dev Biol* 183:234, 1997.
23. Galceran J, Farinas I, Depew MJ, et al: Wnt3a−/−like phenotype and limb deficiency in Lef1(−/−)Tcf1(−/−) mice. *Genes Dev* 13:709, 1999.
24. Chapman DL, Agulnik I, Hancock S, et al: Tbx6, a mouse T-box gene implicated in paraxial mesoderm formation at gastrulation. *Dev Biol* 180:534, 1996.
25. Schulte-Merker S, Smith JC: Mesoderm formation in response to Brachyury requires FGF signalling. *Curr Biol* 5:62, 1995.
26. Yoon JK, Moon RT, Wold B: The bHLH class protein pMesogenin1 can specify paraxial mesoderm phenotypes. *Dev Biol* 222:376, 2000.
27. Pownall ME, Gustafsson MK, Emerson CP Jr: Myogenic regulatory factors and the specification of muscle progenitors in vertebrate embryos. *Annu Rev Cell Dev Biol* 18:747, 2002.
28. Burke AC: Hox genes and the global patterning of the somitic mesoderm. *Curr Top Dev Biol* 47:155, 2000.
29. Palmeirim I, Henrique D, Ish-Horowicz D, Pourquie O: Avian hairy gene expression identifies a molecular clock linked to vertebrate segmentation and somitogenesis. *Cell* 91:639, 1997.
30. McGrew MJ, Pourquie O: Somitogenesis: Segmenting a vertebrate. *Curr Opin Genet Dev* 8:487, 1998.
31. Evrard YA, Lun Y, Aulehla A, et al: Lunatic fringe is an essential mediator of somite segmentation and patterning. *Nature* 394:377, 1998.
32. Conlon RA, Reaume AG, Rossant J: Notch1 is required for the coordinate segmentation of somites. *Development* 121:1533, 1995.
33. Aulehla A, Johnson RL: Dynamic expression of lunatic fringe suggests a link between notch signaling and an autonomous cellular oscillator driving somite segmentation. *Dev Biol* 207:49, 1999.
34. Dale JK, Maroto M, Dequeant ML, et al: Periodic notch inhibition by lunatic fringe underlies the chick segmentation clock. *Nature* 421:275, 2003.
35. Dubrulle J, McGrew MJ, Pourquie O: FGF signaling controls somite boundary position and regulates segmentation clock control of spatiotemporal Hox gene activation. *Cell* 106:219, 2001.
36. Linask KK, Ludwig C, Han MD, et al: N-cadherin/catenin-mediated morphoregulation of somite formation. *Dev Biol* 202:85, 1998.
37. Burgess R, Rawls A, Brown D, et al: Requirement of the paraxis gene for somite formation and musculoskeletal patterning. *Nature* 384:570, 1996.
38. Borycki A-G, Emerson CP Jr: Multiple tissue interactions and signal transduction pathways control somite myogenesis, in Ordahl C (ed): *Somitogenesis*. Vols 47–48. San Diego, CA: Academic Press, 1999.
39. Williams BA, Ordahl CP: Fate restriction in limb muscle precursor cells precedes high-level expression of MyoD family member genes. *Development* 127:2523, 2000.
40. LeDouarin NM, Jotereau FV: Origin and renewal of lymphocytes in avian embryo thymuses studied in interspecific combinations. *Nat New Biol* 246:25, 1973.
41. Selleck MA, Stern CD: Fate mapping and cell lineage analysis of Hensen's node in the chick embryo. *Development* 112:615, 1991.
42. Stern CD, Hatada Y, Selleck MA, Storey KG: Relationships between mesoderm induction and the embryonic axes in chick and frog embryos. *Development*, Suppl 151, 1992.
43. Trainor PA, Tam PP: Cranial paraxial mesoderm and neural crest cells of the mouse embryo: Co-distribution in the craniofacial mesenchyme but distinct segregation in branchial arches. *Development* 121:2569, 1995.
44. Tajbakhsh S, Bober E, Babinet C, et al: Gene targeting the myf-5 locus with nlacZ reveals expression of this myogenic factor in mature skeletal muscle fibres as well as early embryonic muscle. *Dev Dyn* 206:291, 1996.
45. Eloy-Trinquet S, Mathis L, Nicolas JF: Retrospective tracing of the developmental lineage of the mouse myotome. *Curr Top Dev Biol* 47:33, 2000.
46. Dockter J, Ordahl CP: Dorsoventral axis determination in the somite: A re-examination. *Development* 127:2201, 2000.
47. Ordahl CP, Williams BA, Denetclaw W: Determination and morphogenesis in myogenic progenitor cells: An experimental embryological approach. *Curr Top Dev Biol* 48:319, 2000.
48. Baylies MK, Bate M, Ruiz Gomez M: Myogenesis: A view from *Drosophila*. *Cell* 93:921, 1998.
49. Sulston JE, Schierenberg E, White JG, Thomson JN: The embryonic cell lineage of the nematode *Caenorhabditis elegans*. *Dev Biol* 100:64, 1983.

50. Nishida H: Cell lineage analysis in ascidian embryos by intracellular injection of a tracer enzyme. III. Up to the tissue restricted stage. *Dev Biol* 121:526, 1987.
51. Konigsberg IR: Clonal analysis of myogenesis. *Science* 140:178, 1963.
52. Hauschka SD, Konigsberg IR: The influence of collagen on the development of muscle clones. *Proc Natl Acad Sci USA* 55:119, 1966.
53. Yaffe D: Retention of differentiation potentialities during prolonged cultivation of myogenic cells. *Proc Natl Acad Sci USA* 61:477, 1968.
54. Lim RW, Hauschka SD: EGF responsiveness and receptor regulation in normal and differentiation-defective mouse myoblasts. *Dev Biol* 105:48, 1984.
55. Christ B, Ordahl CP: Early stages of chick somite development. *Anat Embryol (Berl)* 191:381, 1995.
56. Kardon G, Campbell JK, Tabin CJ: Local extrinsic signals determine muscle and endothelial cell fate and patterning in the vertebrate limb. *Dev Cell* 3:533, 2002.
57. Brent AE, Schweitzer R, Tabin CJ: A somitic compartment of tendon progenitors. *Cell* 113:235, 2003.
58. Peters H, Wilm B, Sakai N, et al: Pax1 and Pax9 synergistically regulate vertebral column development. *Development* 126:5399, 1999.
59. Li L, Cserjesi P, Olson EN: Dermo-1: A novel twist-related bHLH protein expressed in the developing dermis. *Dev Biol* 172:280, 1995.
60. Olivera-Martinez I, Coltey M, Dhouailly D, Pourquie O: Mediolateral somitic origin of ribs and dermis determined by quail-chick chimeras. *Development* 127:4611, 2000.
61. Venters SJ, Ordahl CP: Persistent myogenic capacity of the dermomyotome dorsomedial lip and restriction of myogenic competence. *Development* 129:3873, 2002.
62. Ordahl CP, Berdougo E, Venters SJ, Denetclaw WFJ: The dermomyotome dorsomedial lip drives growth and morphogenesis of both the primary myotome and dermomyotome epithelium. *Development* 128:1731, 2001.
63. Gustafsson MK, Pan H, Pinney DF, et al: Myf5 is a direct target of long-range Shh signaling and Gli regulation for muscle specification. *Genes Dev* 16:114, 2002.
64. Wilting J, Brand-Saberi B, Huang R, et al: Angiogenic potential of the avian somite. *Dev Dyn* 202:165, 1995.
65. Ambler CA, Nowicki JL, Burke AC, Bautch VL: Assembly of trunk and limb blood vessels involves extensive migration and vasculogenesis of somite-derived angioblasts. *Dev Biol* 234:352, 2001.
66. Sporle R: Epaxial-adaxial-hypaxial regionalisation of the vertebrate somite: Evidence for a somitic organiser and a mirror-image duplication. *Dev Genes Evol* 211:198, 2001.
67. Kardon G: Muscle and tendon morphogenesis in the avian hind limb. *Development* 125:4019, 1998.
68. Noden DM: The embryonic origins of avian cephalic and cervical muscles and associated connective tissues. *Am J Anat* 168:257, 1983.
69. Noden DM: Patterning of avian craniofacial muscles. *Dev Biol* 116:347, 1986.
70. Noden DM, Marcucio R, Borycki AG, Emerson CP Jr: Differentiation of avian craniofacial muscles: I. Patterns of early regulatory gene expression and myosin heavy chain synthesis. *Dev Dyn* 216:96, 1999.
71. Hacker A, Guthrie S: A distinct developmental programme for the cranial paraxial mesoderm in the chick embryo. *Development* 125:3461, 1998.
72. Kato K, Gurdon JB: Single-cell transplantation determines the time when Xenopus muscle precursor cells acquire a capacity for autonomous differentiation. *Proc Natl Acad Sci USA* 90:1310, 1993.
73. Gurdon JB: A community effect in animal development. *Nature* 336:772, 1988.
74. Standley HJ, Zorn AM, Gurdon JB: eFGF and its mode of action in the community effect during Xenopus myogenesis. *Development* 128:1347, 2001.
75. Fisher ME, Isaacs HV, Pownall ME: eFGF is required for activation of XmyoD expression in the myogenic cell lineage of Xenopus laevis. *Development* 129:1307, 2002.
76. Ordahl CP, Le Douarin NM: Two myogenic lineages within the developing somite. *Development* 114:339, 1992.
77. Williams BA, Ordahl CP: Emergence of determined myotome precursor cells in the somite. *Development* 124:4983, 1997.
78. Eloy Trinquet S, Nicolas JF: Clonal separation and regionalisation during formation of the medial and lateral myotomes in the mouse embryo. *Development* 129:111, 2002.
79. Christ B, Brand-Saberi B, Grim M, Wilting J: Local signalling in dermomyotomal cell type specification. *Anat Embryol* 186:505, 1992.
80. Kieny M, Pautou MP, Chevallier A: On the stability of the myogenic cell line in avian limb bud development. *Arch Anat Microsc Morphol Exp* 70:81, 1981.
81. Rong PM, Teillet MA, Ziller C, Le Douarin NM: The neural tube/notochord complex is necessary for vertebral but not limb and body wall striated muscle differentiation. *Development* 115:657, 1992.
82. Pownall ME, Strunk KE, Emerson CP Jr: Notochord signals control the transcriptional cascade of myogenic bHLH genes in somites of quail embryos. *Development* 122:1475, 1996.
83. Noden DM: Interactions and fates of avian craniofacial mesenchyme. *Development* 103:121, 1988.
84. Mootoosamy RC, Dietrich S: Distinct regulatory cascades for head and trunk myogenesis. *Development* 129:573, 2002.
85. Taylor SM, Jones PA: Multiple new phenotypes induced in 10T1/2 and 3T3 cells treated with 5-azacytidine. *Cell* 17:771, 1979.
86. Konieczny SF, Emerson CP Jr: 5-Azacytidine induction of stable mesodermal stem cell lineages from 10T1/2 cells: Evidence for regulatory genes controlling determination. *Cell* 38:791, 1984.
87. Konieczny SF, Baldwin AS, Emerson CP Jr: Myogenic determination of 10T1/2 cell lineages: Evidence of a simple genetic regulatory system, in Emerson CP Jr, Fischman D, Nadal-Ginard B, Siddiqui M (eds): *Molecular Biology of Muscle*. Vol 29. New York: Liss; 1986, p 21.
88. Blau HM, Pavlath GK, Hardeman EC, et al: Plasticity of the differentiated state. *Science* 230:758, 1985.
89. Wright WE: Expression of differentiated functions in heterokaryons between skeletal myocytes, adrenal cells, fibroblasts and glial cells. *Exp Cell Res* 151:55, 1984.
90. Lassar AB, Paterson BM, Weintraub H: Transfection of a DNA locus that mediates the conversion of 10T1/2 fibroblasts to myoblasts. *Cell* 47:649, 1986.
91. Pinney DF, Pearson-White SH, Konieczny SF, et al: Myogenic lineage determination and differentiation: Evidence for a regulatory gene pathway. *Cell* 53:781, 1988.
92. Davis RL, Weintraub H, Lassar AB: Expression of a single transfected cDNA converts fibroblasts to myoblasts. *Cell* 51:987, 1987.
93. Thayer MJ, Tapscott SJ, Davis RL, et al: Positive autoregulation of the myogenic determination gene MyoD1. *Cell* 58:241, 1989.
94. Emerson CP: Myogenesis and developmental control genes. *Curr Opin Cell Biol* 2:1065, 1990.
95. Daubas P, Tajbakhsh S, Hadchouel J, et al: Myf5 is a novel early axonal marker in the mouse brain and is subjected to post-transcriptional regulation in neurons. *Development* 127:319, 2000.
96. Kiefer JC, Hauschka SD: Myf-5 is transiently expressed in nonmuscle mesoderm and exhibits dynamic regional changes within the presegmented mesoderm and somites I-IV. *Dev Biol* 232:77, 2001.
97. Buckingham M, Tajbakhsh S: Expression of myogenic factors in the mouse: Myf-5, the first member of the MyoD gene family to be transcribed during skeletal myogenesis. *Comptes Rendus Acad Sci, Serie Iii, Sci Vie* 316:1032, 1993.
98. Pownall ME, Emerson CP Jr: Sequential activation of three myogenic regulatory genes during somite morphogenesis in quail embryos. *Dev Biol* 151:67, 1992.
99. Hinterberger TJ, Sassoon DA, Rhodes SJ, Konieczny SF: Expression of the muscle regulatory factor MRF4 during somite and skeletal myofiber development. *Devel Biol* 147:144, 1991.
100. Rudnicki MA, Braun T, Hinuma S, Jaenisch R: Inactivation of MyoD in mice leads to up-regulation of the myogenic HLH gene Myf-5 and results in apparently normal muscle development. *Cell* 71:383, 1992.
101. Rudnicki MA, Schnegelsberg PN, Stead RH, et al: MyoD or Myf-5 is required for the formation of skeletal muscle. *Cell* 75:1351, 1993.
102. Braun T, Rudnicki MA, Arnold HH, Jaenisch R: Targeted inactivation of the muscle regulatory gene Myf-5 results in abnormal rib development and perinatal death. *Cell* 71:369, 1992.
103. Kaul A, Koster M, Neuhaus H, Braun T: Myf-5 revisited: Loss of early myotome formation does not lead to a rib phenotype in homozygous Myf-5 mutant mice. *Cell* 102:17, 2000.
104. Hughes SM, Taylor JM, Tapscott SJ, et al: Selective accumulation of MyoD and myogenin mRNAs in fast and slow adult skeletal muscle is controlled by innervation and hormones. *Development* 118:1137, 1993.
105. Cornelison DD, Olwin BB, Rudnicki MA, Wold BJ: MyoD(-/-) satellite cells in single-fiber culture are differentiation defective and MRF4 deficient. *Dev Biol* 224:122, 2000.
106. Tajbakhsh S, Rocancourt D, Buckingham M: Muscle progenitor cells failing to respond to positional cues adopt non-myogenic fates in myf5 null mice. *Nature* 384:266, 1996.
107. Kablar B, Krastel K, Ying C, et al: Myogenic determination occurs independently in somites and limb buds. *Dev Biol* 206:219, 1999.
108. Schafer BW, Blakely BT, Darlington GJ, Blau HM: Effect of cell history on response to helix-loop-helix family of myogenic regulators. *Nature* 344:454, 1990.
109. Faerman A, Pearson-White S, Emerson C, Shani M: Ectopic expression of MyoD1 in mice causes prenatal lethalities. *Dev Dyn* 196:165, 1993.
110. Dekel I, Magal Y, Pearson-White S, Emerson CP, Shani M: Conditional conversion of ES cells to skeletal muscle by an exogenous MyoD1 gene. *New Biol* 4:217, 1992.
111. Hopwood ND, Gurdon JB: Activation of muscle genes without myogenesis by ectopic expression of MyoD in frog embryo cells. *Nature* 347:197, 1990.
112. Carvajal JJ, Cox D, Summerbell D, Rigby PWJ: A BAC transgenic analysis of the Mrf5/Myf5 locus reveals interdigitated elements that control activation and maintenance of gene expression during muscle development. *Development* 128:1857, 2001.
113. Hadchouel J, Tajbakhsh S, Primig M, et al: Modular long-range regulation of myf5 reveals unexpected heterogeneity between skeletal muscles in the mouse embryo [In Process Citation]. *Development* 127:4455, 2000.
114. Patapoutian A, Miner JH, Lyons GE, Wold B: Isolated sequences from the linked Myf-5 and MRF4 genes drive distinct patterns of muscle-specific expression in transgenic mice. *Development* 118:61, 1993.

115. Summerbell D, Ashby PR, Coutelle O, et al: The expression of Myf5 in the developing mouse embryo is controlled by discrete and dispersed enhancers specific for particular populations of skeletal muscle precursors. *Development* 127:3745, 2000.
116. Zweigerdt R, Braun T, Arnold HH: Faithful expression of the Myf-5 gene during mouse myogenesis requires distant control regions: A transgene approach using yeast artificial chromosomes. *Dev Biol* 192:172, 1997.
117. Buchberger A, Nomokonova N, Arnold HH: Myf5 expression in somites and limb buds of mouse embryos is controlled by two distinct distal enhancer activities. *Development* 130:3297, 2003.
118. Black BL, Martin JF, Olson EN: The mouse MRF4 promoter is trans-activated directly and indirectly by muscle-specific transcription factors. *J Biol Chem* 270:2889, 1995.
119. Naidu PS, Ludolph DC, To RQ, et al: Myogenin and MEF2 function synergistically to activate the MRF4 promoter during myogenesis. *Mol Cell Biol* 15:2707, 1995.
120. Pin CL, Ludolph DC, Cooper ST, et al: Distal regulatory elements control MRF4 gene expression in early and late myogenic cell populations. *Dev Dyn* 208:299, 1997.
121. Saitoh O, Fujisawa-Sehara A, Nabeshima Y, Periasamy M: Expression of myogenic factors in denervated chicken breast muscle: Isolation of the chicken Myf5 gene. *Nucleic Acids Res* 21:2503, 1993.
122. Coutelle O, Blagden CS, Hampson R, et al: Hedgehog signalling is required for maintenance of myf5 and myoD expression and timely terminal differentiation in zebrafish adaxial myogenesis. *Dev Biol* 236:136, 2001.
123. Chen YH, Lee WC, Liu CF, Tsai HJ: Molecular structure, dynamic expression, and promoter analysis of zebrafish (*Danio rerio*) myf-5 gene. *Genesis* 29:22, 2001.
124. Polli M, Amaya E: A study of mesoderm patterning through the analysis of the regulation of Xmyf-5 expression. *Development* 129:2917, 2002.
125. Goldhamer DJ, Faerman A, Shani M, Emerson CP Jr: Regulatory elements that control the lineage-specific expression of myoD. *Science* 256:538, 1992.
126. Goldhamer DJ, Brunk BP, Faerman A, et al: Embryonic activation of the myoD gene is regulated by a highly conserved distal control element. *Development* 121:637, 1995.
127. Asakura A, Lyons GE, Tapscott SJ: The regulation of myoD gene-espression—conserved elements mediate expression in embryonic axial muscle. *Dev Biol* 171:386, 1995.
128. Chen JC, Love CM, Goldhamer DJ: Two upstream enhancers collaborate to regulate the spatial patterning and timing of MyoD transcription during mouse development. *Dev Dyn* 221:274, 2001.
129. Kablar B, Krastel K, Ying C, et al: MyoD and Myf-5 differentially regulate the development of limb versus trunk skeletal muscle. *Development* 124:4729, 1997.
130. Kucharczuk KL, Love CM, Dougherty NM, Goldhamer DJ: Fine-scale transgenic mapping of the MyoD core enhancer: MyoD is regulated by distinct but overlapping mechanisms in myotomal and non-myotomal muscle lineages. *Development* 126:1957, 1999.
131. Chen JC, Ramachandran R, Goldhamer DJ: Essential and redundant functions of the MyoD distal regulatory region revealed by targeted mutagenesis. *Dev Biol* 2002. In press.
132. Pinney DF, de la Brousse FC, Faerman A, et al.: Quail myoD is regulated by a complex array of cis-acting control sequences. *Dev Biol* 170:21, 1995.
133. Dechesne CA, Wei Q, Eldridge J, et al: E-box- and MEF-2-independent muscle-specific expression, positive autoregulation, and cross-activation of the chicken MyoD (CMD1) promoter reveal an indirect regulatory pathway. *Mol Cell Biol* 14:5474, 1994.
134. Tajbakhsh S, Rocancourt D, Cossu G, Buckingham M: Redefining the genetic hierarchies controlling skeletal myogenesis: Pax-3 and Myf-5 act upstream of MyoD. *Cell* 89:127, 1997.
135. Munsterberg AE, Lassar AB: Combinatorial signals from the neural tube, floor plate and notochord induce myogenic bHLH gene expression in the somite. *Development* 121:651, 1995.
136. Hirsinger E, Duprez D, Jouve C, et al: Noggin acts downstream of Wnt and sonic hedgehog to antagonize BMP4 in avian somite patterning. *Development* 124:4605, 1997.
137. Munsterberg AE, Kitajewski J, Bumcrot DA, et al: Combinatorial signaling by sonic hedgehog and wnt family members induces myogenic bHLH gene expression in the somite. *Genes Dev* 9:2911, 1995.
138. Borycki A-G, Mendham L, Emerson CP Jr: Control of somite patterning by sonic hedgehog and its downstream signal response genes. *Development* 125:777, 1998.
139. Borycki AG, Brunk B, Tajbakhsh S, et al: Sonic hedgehog controls epaxial muscle determination through Myf5 activation. *Development* 126:4053, 1999.
140. Zhang XM, Ramalho-Santos M, McMahon AP: Smoothened mutants reveal redundant roles for Shh and Ihh signaling including regulation of L/R asymmetry by the mouse node. *Cell* 105:781, 2001.
141. Asakura A, Tapscott SJ: Apoptosis of epaxial myotome in Danforth's short-tail (Sd) mice in somites that form following notochord degeneration. *Dev Biol* 203:276, 1998.
142. Cann GM, Lee JW, Stockdale FE: Sonic hedgehog enhances somite cell viability and formation of primary slow muscle fibers in avian segmented mesoderm. *Anat Embryol (Berl)* 200:239, 1999.
143. Kruger M, Mennerich D, Fees S, et al: Sonic hedgehog is a survival factor for hypaxial muscles during mouse development. *Development* 128:743, 2001.
144. Teillet M, Watanabe Y, Jeffs P, et al: Sonic hedgehog is required for survival of both myogenic and chondrogenic somitic lineages. *Development* 125:2019, 1998.
145. Blagden CS, Currie PD, Ingham PW, Hughes SM: Notochord induction of zebrafish slow muscle mediated by sonic hedgehog. *Genes Dev* 11:2163, 1997.
146. Lewis KE, Currie PD, Roy S, et al: Control of muscle cell-type specification in the zebrafish embryo by hedgehog signalling. *Dev Biol* 216:469, 1999.
147. Borycki A, Brown AM, Emerson CP Jr: Shh and Wnt signaling pathways converge to control Gli gene activation in avian somites. *Development* 127:2075, 2000.
148. Pourquie O, Coltey M, Breant C, Le Douarin NM: Control of somite patterning by signals from the lateral plate. *Proc Natl Acad Sci USA* 92:3219, 1995.
149. Marcelle C, Stark MR, Bronner-Fraser M: Coordinate actions of BMPs, Shh and Noggin mediate patterning of the dorsal somite. *Development* 124:3955, 1997.
150. Reshef R, Maroto M, Lassar AB: Regulation of dorsal somitic cell fates: BMPs and Noggin control the timing and pattern of myogenic regulator expression. *Genes Dev* 12:290, 1998.
151. Hirsinger E, Malapert P, Dubrulle J, et al: Notch signalling acts in postmitotic avian myogenic cells to control MyoD activation. *Development* 128:107, 2001.
152. Delfini M, Hirsinger E, Pourquie O, Duprez D: Delta 1-activated notch inhibits muscle differentiation without affecting Myf5 and Pax3 expression in chick limb myogenesis. *Development* 127:5213, 2000.
153. Dhoot GK, Gustafsson MK, Ai X, et al: Regulation of Wnt signaling and embryo patterning by an extracellular sulfatase. *Science* 293:1663, 2001.
154. Harland R, Gerhart J: Formation and function of Spemann's organizer. *Annu Rev Cell Dev Biol* 13:611, 1997.
155. Dosch R, Gawantka V, Delius H, et al: Bmp-4 acts as a morphogen in dorsoventral mesoderm patterning in *Xenopus*. *Development* 124:2325, 1997.
156. Christian JL, Moon RT: Interactions between Xwnt-8 and Spemann organizer signaling pathways generate dorsoventral pattern in the embryonic mesoderm of *Xenopus*. *Genes Dev* 7:13, 1993.
157. Marom K, Fainsod A, Steinbeisser H: Patterning of the mesoderm involves several threshold responses to BMP-4 and Xwnt-8. *Mech Dev* 87:33, 1999.
158. Suzuki A, Kaneko E, Maeda J, Ueno N: Mesoderm induction by BMP-4 and -7 heterodimers. *Biochem Biophys Res Commun* 232:153, 1997.
159. Re'em-Kalma Y, Lamb T, Frank D: Competition between noggin and bone morphogenetic protein 4 activities may regulate dorsalization during *Xenopus* development. *Proc Natl Acad Sci USA* 92:12141, 1995.
160. Maduro MF, Meneghini MD, Bowerman B, et al: Restriction of mesendoderm to a single blastomere by the combined action of SKN-1 and a GSK-3beta homolog is mediated by MED-1 and -2 in *C. elegans*. *Mol Cell* 7:475, 2001.
161. Baylies MK, Bate M: Twist: A myogenic switch in *Drosophila*. *Science* 272:1481, 1996.
162. Jiang J, Kosman D, Ip YT, Levine M: The dorsal morphogen gradient regulates the mesoderm determinant twist in early *Drosophila* embryos. *Genes Dev* 5:1881, 1991.
163. Harland RM: Developmental biology. A twist on embryonic signalling. *Nature* 410:423, 2001.
164. Chen ZF, Behringer RR: Twist is required in head mesenchyme for cranial neural tube morphogenesis. *Genes Dev* 9:686, 1995.
165. Harfe BD, Vaz Gomes A, Kenyon C, et al: Analysis of a *Caenorhabditis elegans*: Twist homolog identifies conserved and divergent aspects of mesodermal patterning. *Genes Dev* 12:2623, 1998.
166. Lee YM, Park T, Schulz RA, Kim Y: Twist-mediated activation of the NK-4 homeobox gene in the visceral mesoderm of *Drosophila* requires two distinct clusters of E-box regulatory elements. *J Biol Chem* 272:17531, 1997.
167. Beiman M, Shilo BZ, Volk T: Heartless, a *Drosophila* FGF receptor homolog, is essential for cell migration and establishment of several mesodermal lineages. *Genes Dev* 10:2993, 1996.
168. Nishida H, Sawada K: Macho-1 encodes a localized mRNA in ascidian eggs that specifies muscle fate during embryogenesis. *Nature* 409:724, 2001.
169. Nagai T, Aruga J, Takada S, et al: The expression of the mouse Zic1, Zic2, and Zic3 gene suggests an essential role for Zic genes in body pattern formation. *Dev Biol* 182:299, 1997.
170. Wallis DE, Muenke M: Molecular mechanisms of holoprosencephaly. *Mol Genet Metab* 68:126, 1999.
171. Venuti JM, Goldberg L, Chakraborty T, et al: A myogenic factor from sea urchin embryos capable of programming muscle differentiation in mammalian cells. *Proc Natl Acad Sci USA* 88:6219, 1991.
172. Zhang JM, Chen L, Krause M, et al: Evolutionary conservation of MyoD function and differential utilization of E proteins. *Dev Biol* 208:465, 1999.
173. Shirakata M, Friedman FK, Wei Q, Paterson BM: Dimerization specificity of myogenic helix-loop-helix DNA-binding factors directed by nonconserved hydrophilic residues. *Genes Dev* 7:2456, 1993.

174. Lassar AB, Davis RL, Wright WE, et al: Functional activity of myogenic HLH proteins requires hetero-oligomerization with E12/E47-like proteins in vivo. *Cell* 66:305, 1991.
175. Rashbass J, Taylor MV, Gurdon JB: The DNA-binding protein E12 cooperates with XMyoD in the activation of muscle-specific gene expression in *Xenopus* embryos. *EMBO J* 11:2981, 1992.
176. Davis RL, Cheng PF, Lassar AB, Weintraub H: The MyoD DNA binding domain contains a recognition code for muscle-specific gene activation. *Cell* 60:733, 1990.
177. Zhuang Y, Soriano P, Weintraub H: The helix-loop-helix gene E2A is required for B cell formation. *Cell* 79:875, 1994.
178. Meedel TH, Lee JJ, Whittaker JR: Muscle development and lineage-specific expression of CiMDF, the MyoD- family gene of *Ciona intestinalis*. *Dev Biol* 241:238, 2002.
179. Krause M, Fire A, Harrison SW, et al: CeMyoD accumulation defines the body wall muscle cell fate during *C. elegans* embryogenesis. *Cell* 63:907, 1990.
180. Michelson AM, Abmayr SM, Bate M, et al: Expression of a MyoD family member prefigures muscle pattern in *Drosophila* embryos. *Genes Dev* 4:2086, 1990.
181. Chen L, Krause M, Sepanski M, Fire A: The *Caenorhabditis elegans* MYOD homologue HLH-1 is essential for proper muscle function and complete morphogenesis. *Development* 120:1631, 1994.
182. Harfe BD, Branda CS, Krause M, et al: MyoD and the specification of muscle and non-muscle fates during postembryonic development of the C. elegans mesoderm. *Development* 125:2479, 1998.
183. Abmayr SM, Keller CA: *Drosophila* myogenesis and insights into the role of nautilus. *Curr Top Dev Biol* 38:35, 1998.
184. Duan H, Skeath JB, Nguyen HT: *Drosophila* Lame duck, a novel member of the Gli superfamily, acts as a key regulator of myogenesis by controlling fusion-competent myoblast development. *Development* 128:4489, 2001.
185. Furlong EE, Andersen EC, Null B, et al: Patterns of gene expression during *Drosophila* mesoderm development. *Science* 293:1629, 2001.
186. Bour BA, O'Brien MA, Lockwood WL, et al: *Drosophila* MEF2, a transcription factor that is essential for myogenesis. *Genes Dev* 9:730, 1995.
187. Lilly B, Zhao B, Ranganayakulu G, et al: Requirement of MADS domain transcription factor D-MEF2 for muscle formation in *Drosophila*. *Science* 267:688, 1995.
188. Clegg CH, Linkhart TA, Olwin BB, Hauschka SD: Growth factor control of skeletal muscle differentiation: Commitment to terminal differentiation occurs in G1 phase and is repressed by fibroblast growth factor. *J Cell Biol* 105:949, 1987.
189. Konigsberg IR: Diffusion-mediated control of myoblast fusion. *Dev Biol* 26:133, 1971.
190. Bonner PH: Clonal analysis of vertebrate myogenesis. V. Nerve-muscle interaction in chick limb bud chorio-allantoic membrane grafts. *Dev Biol* 47:222, 1975.
191. Miller JB, Stockdale FE: Developmental origins of skeletal muscle fibers: Clonal analysis of myogenic cell lineages based on expression of fast and slow myosin heavy chains. *Proc Natl Acad Sci USA* 83:3860, 1986.
192. Menko AS, Boettiger D: Occupation of the extracellular matrix receptor, integrin, is a control point for myogenic differentiation. *Cell* 51:51, 1987.
193. Bischoff R, Holtzer H: Mitosis and the processes of differentiation of myogenic cells in vitro. *J Cell Biol* 41:188, 1969.
194. Buckley PA, Konigsberg IR: Myogenic fusion and the duration of the post-mitotic gap (G1). *Dev Biol* 37:193, 1974.
195. Konigsberg IR, Sollmann PA, Mixter LO: The duration of the terminal G1 of fusing myoblasts. *Dev Biol* 63:11, 1978.
196. Okazaki K, Holtzer H: Myogenesis: Fusion, myosin synthesis, and the mitotic cycle. *Proc Natl Acad Sci USA* 56:1484, 1966.
197. Sutherland WM, Konigsberg IR: CPK accumulation in fusion-blocked quail myocytes. *Dev Biol* 99:287, 1983.
198. Buckley PA, Konigsberg IR: Do myoblasts in vivo withdraw from the cell cycle? A reexamination. *Proc Natl Acad Sci USA* 74:2031, 1977.
199. Emerson CP Jr, Beckner SK: Activation of myosin synthesis in fusing and mononucleated myoblasts. *J Mol Biol* 93:431, 1975.
200. Denetclaw WF, Ordahl CP: The growth of the dermomyotome and formation of early myotome lineages in thoracolumbar somites of chicken embryos. *Development* 127:893, 2000.
201. Kahane N, Cinnamon Y, Kalcheim C: The origin and fate of pioneer myotomal cells in the avian embryo. *Mech Dev* 74:59, 1998.
202. Iujvidin S, Fuchs O, Nudel U, Yaffe D: SV40 immortalizes myogenic cells: DNA synthesis and mitosis in differentiating myotubes. *Differentiation* 43:192, 1990.
203. Latham KE, Konigsberg IR: Mitogen stimulation affects contractile protein mRNA abundance and translation in embryonic quail myocytes. *Mol Cell Biol* 9:3203, 1989.
204. Armand O, Boutineau AM, Mauger A, et al: Origin of satellite cells in avian skeletal muscles. *Arch Anat Micros Morphol Exp* 72:163, 1983.
205. Beauchamp JR, Heslop L, Yu DS, et al: Expression of CD34 and Myf5 defines the majority of quiescent adult skeletal muscle satellite cells. *J Cell Biol* 151:1221, 2000.
206. Seale P, Asakura A, Rudnicki MA: The potential of muscle stem cells. *Dev Cell* 1:333, 2001.
207. Seed J, Hauschka SD: Clonal analysis of vertebrate myogenesis. VIII. Fibroblasts growth factor (FGF)-dependent and FGF-independent muscle colony types during chick wing development. *Dev Biol* 128:40, 1988.
208. Itoh N, Mima T, Mikawa T: Loss of fibroblast growth factor receptors is necessary for terminal differentiation of embryonic limb muscle. *Development* 122:291, 1996.
209. Flanagan-Steet H, Hannon K, McAvoy MJ, et al: Loss of FGF receptor 1 signaling reduces skeletal muscle mass and disrupts myofiber organization in the developing limb. *Dev Biol* 218:21, 2000.
210. McPherron AC, Lawler AM, Lee SJ: Regulation of skeletal muscle mass in mice by a new TGF-beta superfamily member. *Nature* 387:83, 1997.
211. McPherron AC, Lee SJ: Double muscling in cattle due to mutations in the myostatin gene. *Proc Natl Acad Sci USA* 94:12457, 1997.
212. Duprez D, Fournier-Thibault C, Le Douarin N: Sonic Hedgehog induces proliferation of committed skeletal muscle cells in the chick limb. *Development* 125:495, 1998.
213. Bren-Mattison Y, Olwin BB: Sonic hedgehog inhibits the terminal differentiation of limb myoblasts committed to the slow muscle lineage. *Dev Biol* 242:130, 2002.
214. Florini JR, Ewton DZ, Magri KA, Mangiacapra FJ: IGFs and muscle differentiation. *Adv Exp Med Biol* 343:319, 1993.
215. Coolican SA, Samuel DS, Ewton DZ, et al: The mitogenic and myogenic actions of insulin-like growth factors utilize distinct signaling pathways. *J Biol Chem* 272:6653, 1997.
216. Powell-Braxton L, Hollingshead P, Warburton C, et al: IGF-I is required for normal embryonic growth in mice. *Genes Dev* 7:2609, 1993.
217. Nabeshima Y, Hanaoka K, Hayasaka M, et al: Myogenin gene disruption results in perinatal lethality because of severe muscle defect (see comments). *Nature* 364:532, 1993.
218. Hasty P, Bradley A, Morris JH, et al: Muscle deficiency and neonatal death in mice with a targeted mutation in the myogenin gene. *Nature* 364:501, 1993.
219. Montarras D, Lindon C, Pinset C, Domeyne P: Cultured myf5 null and myoD null muscle precursor cells display distinct growth defects. *Biol Cell* 92:565, 2000.
220. Bergstrom DA, Penn BH, Strand A, et al: Promoter-specific regulation of MyoD binding and signal transduction cooperate to pattern gene expression. *Mol Cell* 9:587, 2002.
221. Wyzykowski JC, Winata TI, Mitin N, et al: Identification of novel MyoD gene targets in proliferating myogenic stem cells. *Mol Cell Biol* 22:6199, 2002.
222. Naya FS, Olson E: MEF2: A transcriptional target for signaling pathways controlling skeletal muscle growth and differentiation. *Curr Opin Cell Biol* 11:683, 1999.
223. Hunter T, Karin M: The regulation of transcription by phosphorylation. *Cell* 70:375, 1992.
224. Li L, Zhou J, James G, et al: FGF inactivates myogenic helix-loop-helix proteins through phosphorylation of a conserved protein kinase C site in their DNA-binding domains. *Cell* 71:1181, 1992.
225. Lassar AB, Thayer MJ, Overell RW, Weintraub H: Transformation by activated ras or fos prevents myogenesis by inhibiting expression of MyoD1. *Cell* 58:659, 1989.
226. Konieczny SF, Drobes BL, Menke SL, Taparowsky EJ: Inhibition of myogenic differentiation by the H-ras oncogene is associated with the down regulation of the MyoD1 gene. *Oncogene* 4:473, 1989.
227. Mitin N, Kudla AJ, Konieczny SF, Taparowsky EJ: Differential effects of Ras signaling through NFkappaB on skeletal myogenesis. *Oncogene* 20:1276, 2001.
228. Li L, Heller-Harrison R, Czech M, Olson EN: Cyclic AMP-dependent protein kinase inhibits the activity of myogenic helix-loop-helix proteins. *Mol Cell Biol* 12:4478, 1992.
229. Hardy S, Kong Y, Konieczny SF: Fibroblast growth factor inhibits MRF4 activity independently of the phosphorylation status of a conserved threonine residue within the DNA-binding domain. *Mol Cell Biol* 13:5943, 1993.
230. Skapek SX, Rhee J, Spicer DB, Lassar AB: Inhibition of myogenic differentiation in proliferating myoblasts by cyclin D1-dependent kinase. *Science* 267:1022, 1995.
231. Novitch BG, Mulligan GJ, Jacks T, Lassar AB: Skeletal muscle cells lacking the retinoblastoma protein display defects in muscle gene expression and accumulate in S and G2 phases of the cell cycle. *J Cell Biol* 135:441, 1996.
232. Novitch BG, Spicer DB, Kim PS, et al: pRb is required for MEF2-dependent gene expression as well as cell- cycle arrest during skeletal muscle differentiation. *Curr Biol* 9:449, 1999.
233. Song A, Wang Q, Goebl MG, Harrington MA: Phosphorylation of nuclear MyoD is required for its rapid degradation. *Mol Cell Biol* 18:4994, 1998.
234. Reynaud EG, Pelpel K, Guillier M, et al: p57(Kip2) stabilizes the MyoD protein by inhibiting cyclin E-Cdk2 kinase activity in growing myoblasts. *Mol Cell Biol* 19:7621, 1999.
235. Porrello A, Cerone MA, Coen S, et al: p53 regulates myogenesis by triggering the differentiation activity of pRb. *J Cell Biol* 151:1295, 2000.
236. Kitzmann M, Vandromme M, Schaeffer V, et al: cdk1- and cdk2-mediated phosphorylation of MyoD Ser200 in growing C2 myoblasts: Role in modulating MyoD half-life and myogenic activity. *Mol Cell Biol* 19:3167, 1999.

237. Lindon C, Montarras D, Pinset C: Cell cycle-regulated expression of the muscle determination factor Myf5 in proliferating myoblasts. *J Cell Biol* 140:111, 1998.
238. Lindon C, Albagli O, Domeyne P, et al: Constitutive instability of muscle regulatory factor Myf5 is distinct from its mitosis-specific disappearance, which requires a D-box-like motif overlapping the basic domain. *Mol Cell Biol* 20:8923, 2000.
239. Edmondson DG, Cheng TC, Cserjesi P, et al: Analysis of the myogenin promoter reveals an indirect pathway for positive autoregulation mediated by the muscle-specific enhancer factor MEF-2. *Mol Cell Biol* 12:3665, 1992.
240. Yee SP, Rigby PW: The regulation of myogenin gene expression during the embryonic development of the mouse. *Genes Dev* 7:1277, 1993.
241. Devlin RB, Emerson CP Jr: Coordinate accumulation of contractile protein mRNAs during myoblast differentiation. *Dev Biol* 69:202, 1979.
242. Devlin RB, Emerson CP Jr: Coordinate regulation of contractile protein synthesis during myoblast differentiation. *Cell* 13:599, 1978.
243. Bucher EA, Maisonpierre PC, Konieczny SF, Emerson CP Jr: Expression of the troponin complex genes: Transcriptional coactivation during myoblast differentiation and independent control in heart and skeletal muscles. *Mol Cell Biol* 8:4134, 1988.
244. Konieczny SF, Emerson CP Jr: Differentiation, not determination, regulates muscle gene activation: Transfection of troponin I genes into multipotential and muscle lineages of 10T1/2 cells. *Mol Cell Biol* 5:2423, 1985.
245. Jaynes JB, Chamberlain JS, Buskin JN, et al: Transcriptional regulation of the muscle creatine kinase gene and regulated expression in transfected mouse myoblasts. *Mol Cell Biol* 6:2855, 1986.
246. Wright WE, Sassoon DA, Lin VK: Myogenin, a factor regulating myogenesis, has a domain homologous to MyoD. *Cell* 56:607, 1989.
247. Edmondson DG, Olson EN: A gene with homology to the myc similarity region of MyoD1 is expressed during myogenesis and is sufficient to activate the muscle differentiation program. *Genes Dev* 3:628, 1989.
248. Rhodes SJ, Konieczny SF: Identification of MRF4: A new member of the muscle regulatory factor gene family. *Genes Dev* 3:2050, 1989.
249. Olson EN, Arnold HH, Rigby PW, Wold BJ: Know your neighbors: Three phenotypes in null mutants of the myogenic bHLH gene MRF4. *Cell* 85:1, 1996.
250. Rawls A, Valdez MR, Zhang W, et al: Overlapping functions of the myogenic bHLH genes MRF4 and MyoD revealed in double mutant mice. *Development* 125:2349, 1998.
251. Valdez MR, Richardson JA, Klein WH, Olson EN: Failure of Myf5 to support myogenic differentiation without myogenin, MyoD, and MRF4. *Dev Biol* 219:287, 2000.
252. Nicolas N, Gallien CL, Chanoine C: Expression of myogenic regulatory factors during muscle development of Xenopus: Myogenin mRNA accumulation is limited strictly to secondary myogenesis. *Dev Dyn* 213:309, 1998.
253. Charbonnier F, Gaspera BD, Armand AS, et al: Two myogenin-related genes are differentially expressed in Xenopus laevis myogenesis and differ in their ability to transactivate muscle structural genes. *J Biol Chem* 277:1139, 2002.
254. Molkentin JD, Olson EN: Combinatorial control of muscle development by basic helix-loop-helix and MADS-box transcription factors. *Proc Natl Acad Sci USA* 93:9366, 1996.
255. Naya FJ, Wu C, Richardson JA, et al: Transcriptional activity of MEF2 during mouse embryogenesis monitored with a MEF2-dependent transgene. *Development* 126:2045, 1999.
256. Edmondson DG, Lyons GE, Martin JF, Olson EN: Mef2 gene expression marks the cardiac and skeletal muscle lineages during mouse embryogenesis. *Development* 120:1251, 1994.
257. Konig S, Burkman J, Fitzgerald J, et al: Modular organization of phylogenetically conserved domains controlling developmental regulation of the human skeletal myosin heavy chain gene family. *J Biol Chem* 277:27593, 2002.
258. Wasserman WW, Palumbo M, Thompson W, et al: Human-mouse genome comparisons to locate regulatory sites. *Nat Genet* 26:225, 2000.
259. Pennacchio LA, Rubin EM: Genomic strategies to identify mammalian regulatory sequences. *Nat Rev Genet* 2:100, 2001.
260. Rosenthal N: Muscle cell differentiation. *Curr Opin Cell Biol* 1:1094, 1989.
261. Rosenthal N, Kornhauser JM, Donoghue M, et al: Myosin light chain enhancer activates muscle-specific, developmentally regulated gene expression in transgenic mice. *Proc Natl Acad Sci USA* 86:7780, 1989.
262. Konieczny SF, Emerson CP Jr: Complex regulation of the muscle-specific contractile protein (troponin I) gene. *Mol Cell Biol* 7:3065, 1987.
263. Shield MA, Haugen HS, Clegg CH, Hauschka SD: E-box sites and a proximal regulatory region of the muscle creatine kinase gene differentially regulate expression in diverse skeletal muscles and cardiac muscle of transgenic mice. *Mol Cell Biol* 16:5058, 1996.
264. Donoviel DB, Shield MA, Buskin JN, et al: Analysis of muscle creatine kinase gene regulatory elements in skeletal and cardiac muscles of transgenic mice. *Mol Cell Biol* 16:1649, 1996.
265. Jiang P, Song J, Gu G, et al: Targeted deletion of the MLC1f/3f downstream enhancer results in precocious MLC expression and mesoderm ablation. *Dev Biol* 243:281, 2002.
266. Latinkic BV, Cooper B, Towers N, et al: Distinct enhancers regulate skeletal and cardiac muscle-specific expression programs of the cardiac alpha-actin gene in Xenopus embryos. *Dev Biol* 245:57, 2002.
267. Puri PL, Iezzi S, Stiegler P, et al: Class I histone deacetylases sequentially interact with MyoD and pRb during skeletal myogenesis. *Mol Cell* 8:885, 2001.
268. Steinbac OC, Wolffe AP, Rupp RA: Histone deacetylase activity is required for the induction of the MyoD muscle cell lineage in Xenopus. *Biol Chem* 381:1013, 2000.
269. Zhang CL, McKinsey TA, Olson EN: Association of class II histone deacetylases with heterochromatin protein 1: Potential role for histone methylation in control of muscle differentiation. *Mol Cell Biol* 22:7302, 2002.
270. Amacher SL, Buskin JN, Hauschka SD: Multiple regulatory elements contribute differentially to muscle creatine kinase enhancer activity in skeletal and cardiac muscle. *Mol Cell Biol* 13:2753, 1993.
271. Ernst H, Walsh K, Harrison CA, Rosenthal N: The myosin light chain enhancer and the skeletal actin promoter share a binding site for factors involved in muscle-specific gene expression. *Mol Cell Biol* 11:3735, 1991.
272. Muscat GE, Gustafson TA, Kedes L: A common factor regulates skeletal and cardiac alpha-actin gene transcription in muscle. *Mol Cell Biol* 8:4120, 1988.
273. Yutzey KE, Konieczny SF: Different E-box regulatory sequences are functionally distinct when placed within the context of the troponin I enhancer. *Nucleic Acids Res* 20:5105, 1992.
274. Brennan TJ, Chakraborty T, Olson EN: Mutagenesis of the myogenin basic region identifies an ancient protein motif critical for activation of myogenesis. *Proc Natl Acad Sci USA* 88:5675, 1991.
275. Davis RL, Weintraub H: Acquisition of myogenic specificity by replacement of three amino acid residues from MyoD into E12. *Science* 256:1027, 1992.
276. Weintraub H, Dwarki VJ, Verma I, et al: Muscle-specific transcriptional activation by MyoD. *Genes Dev* 5:1377, 1991.
277. Maleki SJ, Royer CA, Hurlburt BK: Analysis of the DNA-binding properties of MyoD, myogenin, and E12 by fluorescence anisotropy. *Biochemistry* 41:10888, 2002.
278. Spinner DS, Liu S, Wang SW, Schmidt J: Interaction of the myogenic determination factor myogenin with E12 and a DNA target: Mechanism and kinetics. *J Mol Biol* 317:431, 2002.
279. Braun T, Winter B, Bober E, Arnold HH: Transcriptional activation domain of the muscle-specific gene-regulatory protein myf5. *Nature* 346:663, 1990.
280. Schwarz JJ, Chakraborty T, Martin J, et al: The basic region of myogenin cooperates with two transcription activation domains to induce muscle-specific transcription. *Mol Cell Biol* 12:266, 1992.
281. Gerber AN, Klesert TR, Bergstrom DA, Tapscott SJ: Two domains of MyoD mediate transcriptional activation of genes in repressive chromatin: A mechanism for lineage determination in myogenesis. *Genes Dev* 11:436, 1997.
282. Bergstrom DA, Tapscott SJ: Molecular distinction between specification and differentiation in the myogenic basic helix-loop-helix transcription factor family. *Mol Cell Biol* 21:2404, 2001.
283. Benezra R, Davis RL, Lockshon D, et al: The protein Id: a negative regulator of helix-loop-helix DNA binding proteins. *Cell* 61:49, 1990.
284. West AG, Shore P, Sharrocks AD: DNA binding by MADS-box transcription factors: A molecular mechanism for differential DNA bending. *Mol Cell Biol* 17:2876, 1997.
285. Croissant JD, Kim JH, Eichele G, et al: Avian serum response factor expression restricted primarily to muscle cell lineages is required for alpha-actin gene transcription. *Dev Biol* 177:250, 1996.
286. Miralles F, Posern G, Zaromytidou AI, Treisman R: Actin dynamics control SRF activity by regulation of its coactivator MAL. *Cell* 113:329, 2003.
287. Hauschka SD: Myocardin: A novel potentiator of SRF-mediated transcription in cardiac muscle. *Mol Cell* 8:1, 2001.
288. Ellis PD, Martin KM, Rickman C, et al: Increased actin polymerization reduces the inhibition of serum response factor activity by Yin Yang 1. *Biochem J* 364:547, 2002.
289. Chen F, Kook H, Milewski R, et al: Hop is an unusual homeobox gene that modulates cardiac development. *Cell* 110:713, 2002.
290. Shin CH, Liu ZP, Passier R, et al: Modulation of cardiac growth and development by HOP, an unusual homeodomain protein. *Cell* 110:725, 2002.
291. Gossett LA, Kelvin DJ, Sternberg EA, Olson EN: A new myocyte-specific enhancer-binding factor that recognizes a conserved element associated with multiple muscle-specific genes. *Mol Cell Biol* 9:5022, 1989.
292. Pollock R, Treisman R: Human SRF-related proteins: DNA-binding properties and potential regulatory targets. *Genes Dev* 5:2327, 1991.
293. Black BL, Olson EN: Transcriptional control of muscle development by myocyte enhancer factor-2 (MEF2) proteins. *Annu Rev Cell Dev Biol* 14:167, 1998.
294. Cheng TC, Wallace MC, Merlie JP, Olson EN: Separable regulatory elements governing myogenin transcription in mouse embryogenesis. *Science* 261:215, 1993.
295. Molkentin JD, Black BL, Martin JF, Olson EN: Cooperative activation of muscle gene expression by MEF2 and myogenic bHLH proteins. *Cell* 83:1125, 1995.

296. McKinsey TA, Zhang CL, Olson EN: Control of muscle development by dueling HATs and HDACs. *Curr Opin Genet Dev* 11:497, 2001.
297. Rupp RA, Singhal N, Veenstra GJ: When the embryonic genome flexes its muscles. *Eur J Biochem* 269:2294, 2002.
298. Cserjesi P, Lilly B, Bryson L, et al: MHox: A mesodermally restricted homeodomain protein that binds an essential site in the muscle creatine kinase enhancer. *Development* 115:1087, 1992.
299. Azakie A, Larkin SB, Farrance IK, et al: DTEF-1, a novel member of the transcription enhancer factor-1 (TEF-1) multigene family. *J Biol Chem* 271:8260, 1996.
300. Maeda T, Gupta MP, Stewart AF: TEF-1 and MEF2 transcription factors interact to regulate muscle-specific promoters. *Biochem Biophys Res Commun* 294:791, 2002.
301. Mielcarek M, Gunther S, Kruger M, Braun T: VITO-1, a novel vestigial related protein is predominantly expressed in the skeletal muscle lineage. *Gene Expr Patterns* 2:305, 2002.
302. Fabre-Suver C, Hauschka SD: A novel site in the muscle creatine kinase enhancer is required for expression in skeletal but not cardiac muscle. *J Biol Chem* 271:4646, 1996.
303. Spitz F, Demignon J, Porteu A, et al: Expression of myogenin during embryogenesis is controlled by Six/sine oculis homeoproteins through a conserved MEF3 binding site. *Proc Natl Acad Sci USA* 95:14220, 1998.
304. Ohto H, Kamada S, Tago K, et al: Cooperation of six and eya in activation of their target genes through nuclear translocation of Eya. *Mol Cell Biol* 19:6815, 1999.
305. Taylor JM, Davies JD, Peterson CA: Regulation of the myoblast-specific expression of the human beta-enolase gene. *J Biol Chem* 270:2535, 1995.
306. Lamande N, Brosset S, Lucas M, et al: Transcriptional up-regulation of the mouse gene for the muscle-specific subunit of enolase during terminal differentiation of myogenic cells. *Mol Reprod Dev* 41:306, 1995.
307. Nguyen QG, Buskin JN, Himeda CL, et al: Transgenic and tissue culture analyses of the muscle creatine kinase enhancer Trex control element in skeletal and cardiac muscle indicate differences in gene expression between muscle types. *Transgenic Res* 12:337, 2003.
308. Donoghue MJ, Alvarez JD, Merlie JP, Sanes JR: Fiber type- and position-dependent expression of a myosin light chain-CAT transgene detected with a novel histochemical stain for CAT. *J Cell Biol* 115:423, 1991.
309. Klarsfeld A, Bessereau JL, Salmon AM, et al: An acetylcholine receptor alpha-subunit promoter conferring preferential synaptic expression in muscle of transgenic mice. *EMBO J* 10:625, 1991.
310. Hamilton MT, Booth FW: Skeletal muscle adaptation to exercise: A century of progress. *J Appl Physiol* 88:327, 2000.
311. Baldwin KM, Haddad F: Effects of different activity and inactivity paradigms on myosin heavy chain gene expression in striated muscle. *J Appl Physiol* 90:345, 2001.
312. Vogt M, Puntschart A, Geiser J, et al: Molecular adaptations in human skeletal muscle to endurance training under simulated hypoxic conditions. *J Appl Physiol* 91:173, 2001.
313. Neufer PD, Ordway GA, Williams RS: Transient regulation of c-fos, alpha B-crystallin, and hsp70 in muscle during recovery from contractile activity. *Am J Physiol* 274:C341, 1998.
314. Tsika RW, Hauschka SD, Gao L: M-creatine kinase gene expression in mechanically overloaded skeletal muscle of transgenic mice. *Am J Physiol* 269:C665, 1995.
315. Vyas DR, McCarthy JJ, Tsika GL, Tsika RW: Multiprotein complex formation at the beta myosin heavy chain distal muscle CAT element correlates with slow muscle expression but not mechanical overload responsiveness. *J Biol Chem* 276:1173, 2001.
316. Carson JA, Schwartz RJ, Booth FW: SRF and TEF-1 control of chicken skeletal alpha-actin gene during slow-muscle hypertrophy. *Am J Physiol* 270:C1624, 1996.
317. Carson JA, Booth FW: Effect of serum and mechanical stretch on skeletal alpha-actin gene regulation in cultured primary muscle cells. *Am J Physiol* 275:C1438, 1998.
318. Tsika RW, McCarthy J, Karasseva N, et al: Divergence in species and regulatory role of beta-myosin heavy chain proximal promoter muscle-CAT elements. *Am J Physiol Cell Physiol* 283:C1761, 2002.
319. Hughes SM, Salinas PC: Control of muscle fibre and motoneuron diversification. *Curr Opin Neurobiol* 9:54, 1999.
320. Talmadge RJ: Myosin heavy chain isoform expression following reduced neuromuscular activity: Potential regulatory mechanisms. *Muscle Nerve* 23:661, 2000.
321. Crabtree GR, Olson EN: NFAT signaling: Choreographing the social lives of cells. *Cell* 109(suppl):S67, 2002.
322. Lin J, Wu H, Tarr PT, et al: Transcriptional co-activator PGC-1 alpha drives the formation of slow-twitch muscle fibres. *Nature* 418:797, 2002.
323. Calvo S, Venepally P, Cheng J, Buonanno A: Fiber-type-specific transcription of the troponin I slow gene is regulated by multiple elements. *Mol Cell Biol* 19:515, 1999.
324. Calvo S, Vullhorst D, Venepally P, et al: Molecular dissection of DNA sequences and factors involved in slow muscle-specific transcription. *Mol Cell Biol* 21:8490, 2001.
325. Chien KR: Genomic circuits and the integrative biology of cardiac diseases. *Nature* 407:227, 2000.
326. Frey N, Olson EN: Cardiac hypertrophy: The good, the bad, and the ugly. *Annu Rev Physiol* 65:45, 2003.
327. Nicol RL, Frey N, Olson EN: From the sarcomere to the nucleus: Role of genetics and signaling in structural heart disease. *Annu Rev Genomics Hum Genet* 1:179, 2000.
328. George EL, Ober MB, Emerson CP Jr: Functional domains of the *Drosophila melanogaster* muscle myosin heavy-chain gene are encoded by alternatively spliced exons [published erratum appears in Mol Cell Biol 1989;9(9):4118]. *Mol Cell Biol* 9:2957, 1989.
329. Perry SV: Vertebrate tropomyosin: Distribution, properties and function. *J Muscle Res Cell Motil* 22:5, 2001.
330. Bucher EA, Dhoot GK, Emerson MM, et al: Structure and evolution of the alternatively spliced fast troponin T isoform gene. *J Biol Chem* 274:17661, 1999.
331. Sironi M, Cagliani R, Pozzoli U, et al: The dystrophin gene is alternatively spliced throughout its coding sequence. *FEBS Lett* 517:163, 2002.
332. Ladd AN, Charlet N, Cooper TA: The CELF family of RNA binding proteins is implicated in cell-specific and developmentally regulated alternative splicing. *Mol Cell Biol* 21:1285, 2001.
333. Standiford DM, Sun WT, Davis MB, Emerson CP Jr: Positive and negative intronic regulatory elements control muscle-specific alternative exon splicing of Drosophila myosin heavy chain transcripts. *Genetics* 157:259, 2001.
334. Dye BT, Buvoli M, Mayer SA, et al: Enhancer elements activate the weak 3′ splice site of alpha-tropomyosin exon 2. *RNA* 4:1523, 1998.
335. Selvakumar M, Helfman DM: Exonic splicing enhancers contribute to the use of both 3′ and 5′ splice site usage of rat beta-tropomyosin pre-mRNA. *RNA* 5:378, 1999.
336. Duriez P, Lesimple M, Allo MR, Hardy S: Alternative splicing of *Xenopus* alphafast-tropomyosin pre-mRNA during development: Identification of determining sequences. *DNA Cell Biol* 19:365, 2000.
337. Ladd AN, Cooper TA: Finding signals that regulate alternative splicing in the post-genomic era. *Genome Biol* 3(rev 0008): 2002.
338. Philips AV, Cooper TA: RNA processing and human disease. *Cell Mol Life Sci* 57:235, 2000.
339. Mann CJ, Honeyman K, Cheng AJ, et al: Antisense-induced exon skipping and synthesis of dystrophin in the mdx mouse. *Proc Natl Acad Sci USA* 98:42, 2001.
340. Sadoulet-Puccio HM, Feener CA, et al: The genomic organization of human dystrobrevin. *Neurogenetics* 1:37, 1997.
341. Stedman HH, Sweeney HL, Shrager JB, et al: The mdx mouse diaphragm reproduces the degenerative changes of Duchenne muscular dystrophy. *Nature* 352:536, 1991.
342. Petrof BJ, Shrager JB, Stedman HH, et al: Dystrophin protects the sarcolemma from stresses developed during muscle contraction. *Proc Natl Acad Sci USA* 90:3710, 1993.
343. Megeney LA, Kablar B, Garrett K, et al: MyoD is required for myogenic stem cell function in adult skeletal muscle. *Genes Dev* 10:1173, 1996.
344. Bartlett RJ, Winand NJ, Secore SL, et al: Mutation segregation and rapid carrier detection of X-linked muscular dystrophy in dogs. *Am J Vet Res* 57:650, 1996.
345. Lee CC, Pearlman JA, Chamberlain JS, Caskey CT: Expression of recombinant dystrophin and its localization to the cell membrane. *Nature* 349:334, 1991.
346. Dickson G, Pizzey JA, Elsom VE, et al: Distinct dystrophin mRNA species are expressed in embryonic and adult mouse skeletal muscle. *FEBS Lett* 242:47, 1988.
347. Acsadi G, Dickson G, Love DR, et al: Human dystrophin expression in mdx mice after intramuscular injection of DNA constructs. *Nature* 352:815, 1991.
348. Ragot T, Vincent N, Chafey P, et al: Efficient adenovirus-mediated transfer of a human minidystrophin gene to skeletal muscle of mdx mice. *Nature* 361:647, 1993.
349. Dunckley MG, Love DR, Davies KE, et al: Retroviral-mediated transfer of a dystrophin minigene into mdx mouse myoblasts in vitro. *FEBS Lett* 296:128, 1992.
350. Harper SQ, Hauser MA, DelloRusso C, et al: Modular flexibility of dystrophin: Implications for gene therapy of Duchenne muscular dystrophy. *Nat Med* 8:253, 2002.
351. Cox GA, Cole NM, Matsumura K, et al: Overexpression of dystrophin in transgenic mdx mice eliminates dystrophic symptoms without toxicity. *Nature* 364:725, 1993.
352. Matsumura K, Lee CC, Caskey CT, Campbell KP: Restoration of dystrophin-associated proteins in skeletal muscle of mdx mice transgenic for dystrophin gene. *FEBS Lett* 320:276, 1993.
353. Perkins KJ, Davies KE: The role of utrophin in the potential therapy of Duchenne muscular dystrophy. *Neuromuscul Disord* 12(suppl 1):S78, 2002.
354. Tinsley JM, Potter AC, Phelps SR, et al: Amelioration of the dystrophic phenotype of mdx mice using a truncated utrophin transgene. *Nature* 384:349, 1996.
355. Corbi N, Libri V, Fanciulli M, et al: The artificial zinc finger coding gene "Jazz" binds the utrophin promoter and activates transcription. *Gene Ther* 7:1076, 2000.
356. Gramolini AO, Belanger G, Jasmin BJ: Distinct regions in the 3′ untranslated region are responsible for targeting and stabilizing utrophin transcripts in skeletal muscle cells. *J Cell Biol* 154:1173, 2001.

357. Dowling P, Culligan K, Ohlendieck K: Distal mdx muscle groups exhibiting up-regulation of utrophin and rescue of dystrophin-associated glycoproteins exemplify a protected phenotype in muscular dystrophy. *Naturwissenschaften* 89:75, 2002.
358. Burkin DJ, Kaufman SJ: The alpha7beta1 integrin in muscle development and disease. *Cell Tissue Res* 296:183, 1999.
359. Hayashi YK, Chou FL, Engvall E, et al: Mutations in the integrin alpha7 gene cause congenital myopathy. *Nat Genet* 19:94, 1998.
360. Burkin DJ, Wallace GQ, Nicol KJ, et al: Enhanced expression of the alpha 7 beta 1 integrin reduces muscular dystrophy and restores viability in dystrophic mice. *J Cell Biol* 152:1207, 2001.
361. Nguyen HH, Jayasinha V, Xia B, et al: Overexpression of the cytotoxic T cell GalNAc transferase in skeletal muscle inhibits muscular dystrophy in mdx mice. *Proc Natl Acad Sci USA* 99:5616, 2002.
362. Bertoni C, Lau C, Rando TA: Restoration of dystrophin expression in mdx muscle cells by chimeraplast-mediated exon skipping. *Hum Mol Genet* 12:1087, 2003.
363. Kapsa RM, Quigley AF, Vadolas J, et al: Targeted gene correction in the mdx mouse using short DNA fragments: Towards application with bone marrow–derived cells for autologous remodeling of dystrophic muscle. *Gene Ther* 9:695, 2002.
364. Aartsma-Rus A, Bremmer-Bout M, Janson AA, et al: Targeted exon skipping as a potential gene correction therapy for Duchenne muscular dystrophy. *Neuromuscul Disord* 12(suppl 1):S71, 2002.
365. Barton-Davis ER, Cordier L, Shoturma DI, et al: Aminoglycoside antibiotics restore dystrophin function to skeletal muscles of mdx mice. *J Clin Invest* 104:375, 1999.
366. Brent AE, Tabin CJ: Developmental regulation of somite derivatives: Muscle, cartilage and tendon. *Curr Opin Genet Dev* 12:548, 2002.
367. Bagnall KM, Higgins SJ, Sanders EJ: The contribution made by cells from a single somite to tissues within a body segment and assessment of their integration with similar cells from adjacent segments. *Development* 107:931, 1989.
368. Lance-Jones C: The somitic level of origin of embryonic chick hindlimb muscles. *Dev Biol* 126:394, 1988.
369. Chevallier A, Kieny M, Mauger A: Limb-somite relationship: Origin of the limb musculature. *J Embryol Exp Morphol* 41:245, 1977.
370. Birchmeier C, Brohmann H: Genes that control the development of migrating muscle precursor cells. *Curr Opin Cell Biol* 12:725, 2000.
371. Daston G, Lamar E, Olivier M, Goulding M: Pax3 is necessary for migration but not differentiation of limb muscle precursor in the mouse. *Development* 122:1017, 1996.
372. Borycki AG, Li J, Jin F, et al: Pax3 functions in cell survival and in *Pax7* regulation. *Development* 126:1665, 1999.
373. Epstein JA, Shapiro DN, Cheng J, et al: Pax3 modulates expression of the c-Met receptor during limb muscle development. *Proc Natl Acad Sci USA* 93:4213, 1996.
374. Brand-Saberi B, Muller TS, Wilting J, et al: Scatter factor/hepatocyte growth factor (SF/HGF) induces emigration of myogenic cells at interlimb level in vivo. *Dev Biol* 179:303, 1996.
375. Gross MK, Moran-Rivard L, Velasquez T, et al: Lbx1 is required for muscle precursor migration along a lateral pathway into the limb. *Development* 127:413, 2000.
376. Brohmann H, Jagla K, Birchmeier C: The role of Lbx1 in migration of muscle precursor cells. *Development* 127:437, 2000.
377. Neyt C, Jagla K, Thisse C, et al: Evolutionary origins of vertebrate appendicular muscle. *Nature* 408:82, 2000.
378. Nowicki JL, Burke AC: Hox genes and morphological identity: Axial versus lateral patterning in the vertebrate mesoderm. *Development* 127:4265, 2000.
379. Lufkin T, Mark M, Hart CP, et al: Homeotic transformation of the occipital bones of the skull by ectopic expression of a homeobox gene. *Nature* 359:835, 1992.
380. Kostic D, Capecchi MR: Targeted disruptions of the murine Hoxa-4 and Hoxa-6 genes result in homeotic transformations of components of the vertebral column. *Mech Dev* 46:231, 1994.
381. Salser SJ, Kenyon C: A *C. elegans* Hox gene switches on, off, on and off again to regulate proliferation, differentiation and morphogenesis. *Development* 122:1651, 1996.
382. Mintz B: Do cells fuse in vivo? *In Vitro* 5:40, 1970.
383. Lipton BH, Konigsberg IR: A fine-structural analysis of the fusion of myogenic cells. *J Cell Biol* 53:348, 1972.
384. Holtzer H, Marshall JH Jr, Finck H: An analysis of myogenesis by the use of fluorescent antimyosin. *J Biophys Biochem Cytol* 3:705, 1957.
385. Schwander M, Leu M, Stumm M, et al: Beta1 integrins regulate myoblast fusion and sarcomere assembly. *Dev Cell* 4:673, 2003.
386. Taylor MV: Muscle differentiation: How two cells become one. *Curr Biol* 12:R224, 2002.
387. Dworak HA, Sink H: Myoblast fusion in *Drosophila*. *Bioessays* 24:591, 2002.
388. Frasch M: Controls in patterning and diversification of somatic muscles during *Drosophila* embryogenesis. *Curr Opin Genet Dev* 9:522, 1999.
389. Duan H, Skeath JB, Nguyen HT: *Drosophila* lame duck, a novel member of the Gli superfamily, acts as a key regulator of myogenesis by controlling fusion-competent myoblast development. *Development* 128:4489, 2001.
390. Bate M, Rushton E: Myogenesis and muscle patterning in *Drosophila*. *Comptes Rendus Acad Sci, Ser Iii, Sci Vie* 316:1047, 1993.
391. Denetclaw WF Jr, Berdougo E, Venters SJ, Ordahl CP: Morphogenetic cell movements in the middle region of the dermomyotome dorsomedial lip associated with patterning and growth of the primary epaxial myotome. *Development* 128:1745, 2001.
392. Cinnamon Y, Kahane N, Bachelet I, Kalcheim C: The sub-lip domain—A distinct pathway for myotome precursors that demonstrate rostral-caudal migration. *Development* 128:341, 2001.
393. Huang R, Zhi Q, Schmidt C, et al: Sclerotomal origin of the ribs. *Development* 127:527, 2000.
394. Chiang C, Litingtung Y, Lee E, et al: Cyclopia and defective axial patterning in mice lacking sonic hedgehog gene function. *Nature* 383:407, 1996.
395. Brand-Saberi B, Christ B: Evolution and development of distinct cell lineages derived from somites. *Curr Top Dev Biol* 48:1, 2000.
396. Kahane N, Cinnamon Y, Bachelet I, Kalcheim C: The third wave of myotome colonization by mitotically competent progenitors: Regulating the balance between differentiation and proliferation during muscle development. *Development* 128:2187, 2001.
397. Volk T: Singling out *Drosophila* tendon cells: A dialogue between two distinct cell types. *Trends Genet* 15:448, 1999.
398. Hong L, Elbl T, Ward J, et al: MUP-4 is a novel transmembrane protein with functions in epithelial cell adhesion in *Caenorhabditis elegans*. *J Cell Biol* 154:403, 2001.
399. Bercher M, Wahl J, Vogel BE, et al: mua-3, a gene required for mechanical tissue integrity in *Caenorhabditis elegans*, encodes a novel transmembrane protein of epithelial attachment complexes. *J Cell Biol* 154:415, 2001.
400. Hahn BS, Labouesse M: Tissue integrity: Hemidesmosomes and resistance to stress. *Curr Biol* 11:R858, 2001.
401. Ordahl CP: Developmental regulation of sarcomeric gene expression. *Curr Topics Dev Biol* 26:145, 1992.
402. Mauger A, Kieny M, Chevallier A: Limb-somite relationship: Myogenic potentialities of somatopleural mesoderm. *Arch Anat Microsc Morphol Exp* 69:175, 1980.
403. Johnson RL, Tabin CJ: Molecular models for vertebrate limb development. *Cell* 90:979, 1997.
404. Niswander L: Interplay between the molecular signals that control vertebrate limb development. *Int J Dev Biol* 46:877, 2002.
405. Miller JB, Crow MT, Stockdale FE: Slow and fast myosin heavy chain content defines three types of myotubes in early muscle cell cultures. *J Cell Biol* 101:1643, 1985.
406. Nikovits W Jr, Cann GM, Huang R, et al: Patterning of fast and slow fibers within embryonic muscles is established independently of signals from the surrounding mesenchyme. *Development* 128:2537, 2001.
407. Hauschka SD: Clonal analysis of vertebrate myogenesis. 3. Developmental changes in the muscle-colony-forming cells of the human fetal limb. *Dev Biol* 37:345, 1974.
408. Hilfer SR, Searls RL, Fonte VG: An ultrastructural study of early myogenesis in the chick wing bud. *Dev Biol* 30:374, 1973.
409. Pautou MP, Hedayat I, Kieny M: The pattern of muscle development in the chick leg. *Arch Anat Microsc Morphol Exp* 71:193, 1982.
410. Condon K, Silberstein L, Blau HM, Thompson WJ: Development of muscle fiber types in the prenatal rat hindlimb. *Dev Biol* 138:256, 1990.
411. Riddle RD, Ensini M, Nelson C, et al: Induction of the LIM homeobox gene Lmx1 by WNT7a establishes dorsoventral pattern in the vertebrate limb. *Cell* 83:631, 1995.
412. Landmesser L, Morris DG: The development of functional innervation in the hind limb of the chick embryo. *J Physiol* 249:301, 1975.
413. Shellswell GB: The formation of discrete muscles from the chick wing dorsal and ventral muscle masses in the absence of nerves. *J Embryol Exp Morphol* 41:269, 1977.
414. Hughes DS, Ontell M: Morphometric analysis of the developing, murine aneural soleus muscle. *Dev Dyn* 193:175, 1992.
415. Kieny M, Chevallier A: Autonomy of tendon development in the embryonic chick wing. *J Embryol Exp Morphol* 49:153, 1979.
416. Kieny M, Mauger A, Hedayat I, Goetinck PF: Ontogeny of the leg muscle tissue in the crooked neck dwarf mutant (cn/cn) chick embryo. *Arch Anat Microsc Morphol Exp* 72:1, 1983.
417. Beddington RS, Robertson EJ: Axis development and early asymmetry in mammals. *Cell* 96:195, 1999.
418. Pourquie O: Vertebrate somitogenesis. *Annu Rev Cell Dev Biol* 17:311, 2001.
419. Jacob M, Christ B, Jacob HJ: On the migration of myogenic stem cells into the prospective wing region of chick embryos. A scanning and transmission electron microscope study. *Anat Embryol* 153:179, 1978.
420. Ordahl CP: Myogenic lineages within the developing somite, in *Molecular Basis of Morphogenesis*. New York: Liss; 1993, p 165.
421. Jacob M, Christ B, Jacob HJ: The migration of myogenic cells from the somites into the leg region of avian embryos. An ultrastructural study. *Anat Embryol* 157:291, 1979.
422. Linkhart TA, Hauschka SD: Clonal analysis of vertebrate myogenesis. VI. Acetylcholinesterase and acetylcholine receptor in myogenic and non-myogenic clones from chick embryo leg cells. *Dev Biol* 69:529, 1979.
423. Bonner PH, Hauschka SD: Clonal analysis of vertebrate myogenesis. I. Early developmental events in the chick limb. *Dev Biol* 37:317, 1974.

Chapter 2

Assembly of the Skeletal Muscle Cell

JOSEPH W. SANGER
JEAN M. SANGER
CLARA FRANZINI-ARMSTRONG

Myotubes to Muscle Fibers to Muscle Bundles
Fusion of Mononucleated Cells to Form Multinucleated Muscle Fibers
Myofibrillogenesis
    THE ASSEMBLY OF MYOFIBRILS
    MYOFIBRILS AND THE CYTOSKELETON
Developmental Changes in Microtubules and Intermediate Filaments
Renewal of Myofibrillar Proteins within Muscle Cells
Assembly and Organization of the Membrane System
    TRANSITION: ENDOPLASMIC RETICULUM TO SARCOPLASMIC RETICULUM
    ASSEMBLY OF CALCIUM RELEASE UNITS: TARGETING OF COMPONENTS TO JUNCTIONAL DOMAINS
    ASSEMBLY OF CALCIUM RELEASE UNITS: THEIR DOCKING AND MATURATION
    DEVELOPMENT OF T TUBULES AND MEMBRANE-TO-MYOFIBRILAR LINKAGE
Conclusions

Chapter 1 of this book discusses the formation of the precursors of skeletal muscle cells from an undifferentiated mass of cells in the mesoderm of the vertebrate embryo, and Chap. 4 defines the organization of diverse fiber types into muscles. This chapter covers biogenesis of the multinucleated adult muscle fiber with its cytoskeletal, membranous, and myofibrillar components (Fig. 2-1). The transmembrane and extracellular proteins necessary for the maintenance of myofibril alignment and for transmission of contractile force are defined in Chaps. 19 and 20.

Myotubes to Muscle Fibers to Muscle Bundles

Skeletal muscle fibers are multinucleated cells formed from the fusions of mononucleated myocytes (Figs. 2-2 and 2-3). Myocytes are the postmitotic daughters of myoblasts, the stem cells of developing muscle. Quiescent stem cells (i.e., satellite cells) are associated with muscle fibers. Exposure of vertebrate muscle fibers to tritiated thymidine led to the discovery that all the nuclei in an adult muscle fiber were postmitotic, and this was extended to myotubes in culture.[4–7] In response to injury or exercise, mononucleated satellite cells divide and either fuse with injured fibers or form entirely new myotubes (see Chap. 3).[8–10]

The multinucleated skeletal muscle cells that originate from myocyte fusions during embryogenesis are termed *myotubes*. Two (or three in larger animals) waves of mononucleated cell proliferation result in the formation of initial or primary myotubes and later secondary myotubes that share a common basal lamina and are coupled by gap junctions (see Chap. 4). These junctions are believed to be important during the critical transition between myotubes and muscle fibers (Fig. 2-4).[11–15]

During maturation of the myotube, the centrally positioned nuclei move to the periphery and the primary and secondary myotubes lose their interconnecting junctions. These myotubes gain their own basal lamina (endomysium) and become independent adult muscle fibers, each with its own innervation.[13–15] Neighboring muscle fibers aggregate to form muscle bundles or fascicles, with each bundle encased in a connective tissue called *perimysium*. The component muscle fibers rarely run the length of a muscle bundle, particularly if the muscle is very long.[16,17] In one study of feline sartorius muscle, only 7 of approximately 1000 cells ran the whole length of the bundle.[17] Appropriately placed tendons connect the muscle fibers to each other and to the bone.

Innervation and vascularization, other important aspects of myogenesis, are covered in Chaps. 15 and 22.

Fusion of Mononucleated Cells to Form Multinucleated Muscle Fibers

The fusion of myocytes to form myotubes proceeds through several different stages: cell differentiation, cell attachment, cell alignment, and finally membrane fusion.[8,9] The actual myoblast-to-myoblast and myoblast-to-myotube fusions are unpredictable and unsynchronized; they span a relatively long period in muscles of higher vertebrates. In the cross-striated muscles of the model organism *Drosophila*, however, the fusion process is more synchronized; it also takes place in only a few hours.[8,9] A number of mutations that interfere with the fusion of *Drosophila* myoblasts are in proteins that may enable myoblasts to attach and align with one another before fusion. Current work is focused on determining the function of these newly discovered proteins and on identifying their vertebrate homologues (see Chap. 1 for a detailed genetic analysis of myoblast formation and myocyte fusion).

The fusion process that leads to myotube formation in vertebrate muscles can be observed more clearly in movies of myocytes in tissue culture.[5,7,18] The mononucleated myocytes migrate in the culture dish and align in different arrays before fusion: Some fuse end-to-end and others side-to-side (Fig. 2-2). The myotubes derived from myoblast fusion, in turn, elongate by fusing with mononucleated myocytes at their elongating ends (Fig. 2-3A) or by fusion with other myotubes (Fig. 2-3B). These fusions result in myotubes that can reach several centimeters in length and

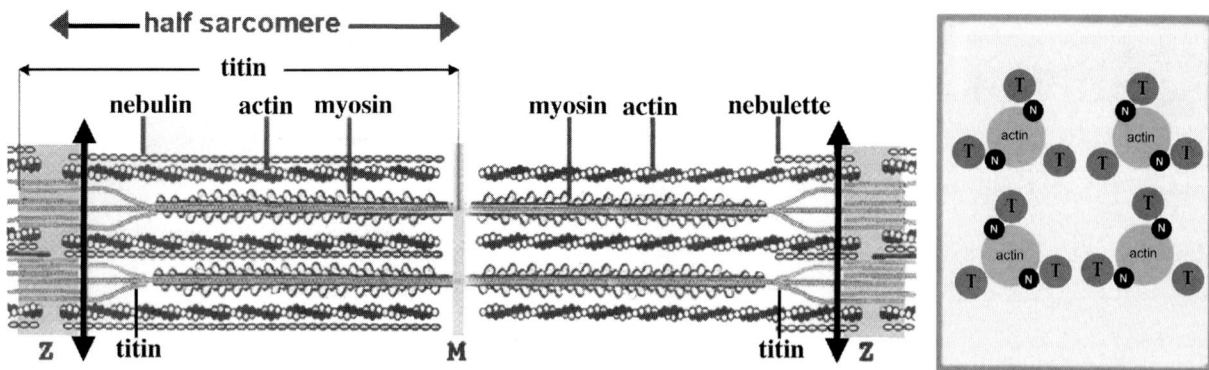

FIGURE 2-1. *A*. Diagram of a sarcomere structure. The left side illustrates the components of a skeletal muscle sarcomere. One of the two nebulin molecules that are embedded in the Z bands at the C-terminus and extend the entire length of each thin filament is shown. The right side illustrates a cardiac sarcomere: a smaller nebulin isoform, nebulette, begins within the Z band and extends a short distance along the thin filament. Both nebulin and nebulette are associated with the surface of thin filaments. Three of the six titins associated with each half thick filament are shown. Titins run on the surface of thick filaments; their C-termini meet at the M line and their N termini overlap within the Z band. The double arrow at either end of the sarcomere represents the position of a cross section that is viewed edge-on at a higher magnification in (*B*). *B*. Cross section of the actin, nebulin (dark profiles), and titin (T) filaments at the edge of the Z band to show the relative proportions of titin filaments to nebulin-actin filaments. It is not clear how the transition from the threefold symmetry of thick filaments and the twofold symmetry of actin filaments is accommodated at the Z lines. *(Modified from Sanger and Sanger[1] and Turnacioglu et al.[2] Reproduced by permission)*

contain several hundred centrally localized nuclei (Fig. 2-2). The uniform alignment of myotubes seen in vivo does not occur in tissue culture unless there is application of directional vectors of tension or deposition of aligned extracellular matrices.[19–21]

Migration of cells is important for the formation of large myotubes. Prevention of the migration of cultured mononucleated myoblasts and myocytes by a reagent such as cytochalasin, an inhibitor of actin polymerization, will inhibit fusion when the cells are at low density.[22,23] Myoblasts, prevented by cytochalasin from completing cytokinesis, an actin-dependent process, will form binucleated myocytes, which are not elongated. When the cytochalasin is removed, the ends of the binucleated myocytes become very motile and the cells elongate to from a small binucleated myotube. The ends of these myotubes will fuse with other binucleated myotubes to form an interconnecting contractile network that does not, however, reorganize to form long myotubes of large diameter.

Observation of myocytes in culture clearly shows that simple proximity is not enough to trigger fusion.[7] The cells may move alongside each other for fairly long periods of time

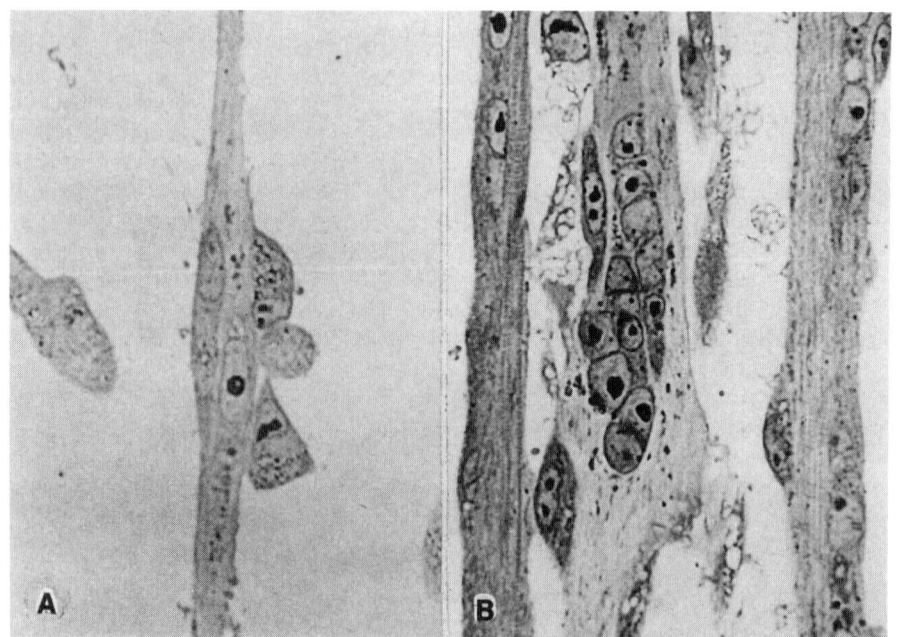

FIGURE 2-2. Light micrographs of embryonic chicken skeletal myocytes in culture. *A*. The elongated spindle-shaped cell in the middle of the field is a young myotube that has formed from the fusion of myoblasts after 72 h in tissue culture. Several mononucleated cells are associated with this myotube, and some may later fuse with it. *B*. A sister culture at 96 h shows three elongated myotubes with an increased number of nuclei and myofibrils (Myofibrils can be clearly seen in the leftmost myotube.) The width of each field in *A* and *B* is about 81 μm. *(From Fischman.[3] Reproduced by permission.)*

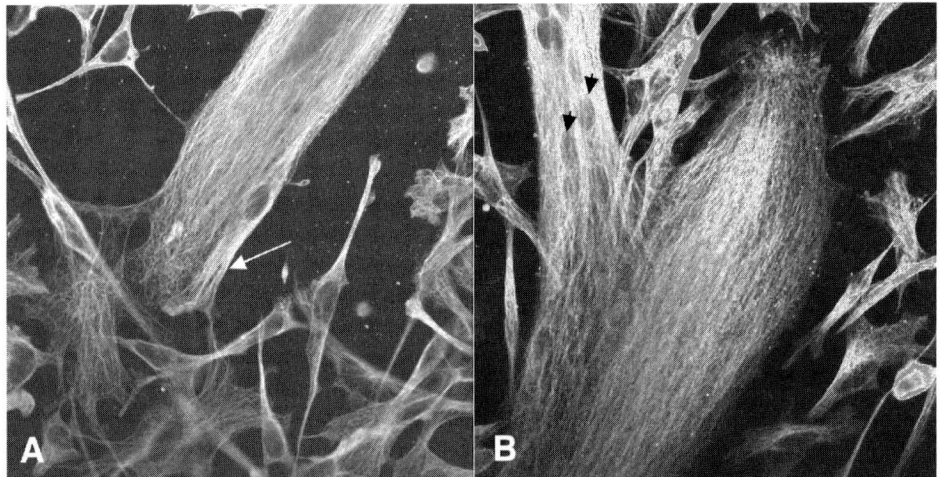

FIGURE 2-3. *A.* Four-day-old culture of quail skeletal muscle cells fixed and immunolabeled with antibodies against tubulin, showing abundant bundles of longitudinally oriented microtubules. An elongated mononucleated cell (arrow) is aligned with an elongated myotube. Note the variable orientation of other mononucleated cells near the myotube. *B.* Two elongated myotubes are closely associated. The nuclei (arrowheads) in one of the myotubes can be detected by their negative images.

before an unpredictable fusion event occurs. In vitro studies of muscle cultures have led to the identification of a number of molecules that are involved in fusion: cell adhesion molecules, metalloproteases, phospholipases, and calmodulin[24–31]; the general idea is that intimate adherence of the future partners is a prerequisite for fusion, but that other events must take place. For example, if the concentration of extracellular Ca^{2+} is lowered, fusion will be inhibited in a reversible manner,[25] presumably because Ca^{2+} is needed by N-cadherin molecules on adjacent cells to mediate the attachment that is important for fusion.[25] There is some evidence for an additional non-calcium-mediated attachment. Myocytes and myotubes express neural cell adhesion molecule (NCAM)* on their surfaces. If the level of NCAM expression rises, increased numbers of nuclei are detected in the myotubes.[26] Muscle cells also have surface-attached extracellular proteins that undergo modification via N-linked glycosylation. If this process is inhibited in muscle cultures, fusion is inhibited.[27]

It is assumed that cell fusion in myogenesis must be similar to other fusion processes that are more readily observable using electrophysiologic measurements and electron microscopic techniques such as rapid freeze and freeze-fracture (e.g., sperm-egg fusion, fusion of secretory vesicles with the cell surface, membrane fusion of enveloped viruses). In these nonmuscle systems, the initial fusion of the two different lipid layers requires the catalytic action of a protein, a fusigen, and goes through the initial formation of a very small pore. An initial small pore has been detected in conductance measurements of fusing muscle cells and judged to be 1 or 2 nm in diameter, increasing within milliseconds to establish a larger continuity between the two cells.[32] Thus, in addition to adhesion molecules allowing the cells to come to a close proximity (see above), a yet unidentified fusogenic protein may be necessary for myotube formation.

Satellite cells are nestled next to the adult fiber but retain their cellular identity. So at the developmental stage, when satellite cells are formed, fusogenic properties are lost. It is not known whether this is due to lack of adhesion proteins or of a fusigen. Injury to the muscle fiber leads to the mitotic stimulation of the satellite cells, to the recruitment of some myoblast precursors from the bone marrow to muscle, and

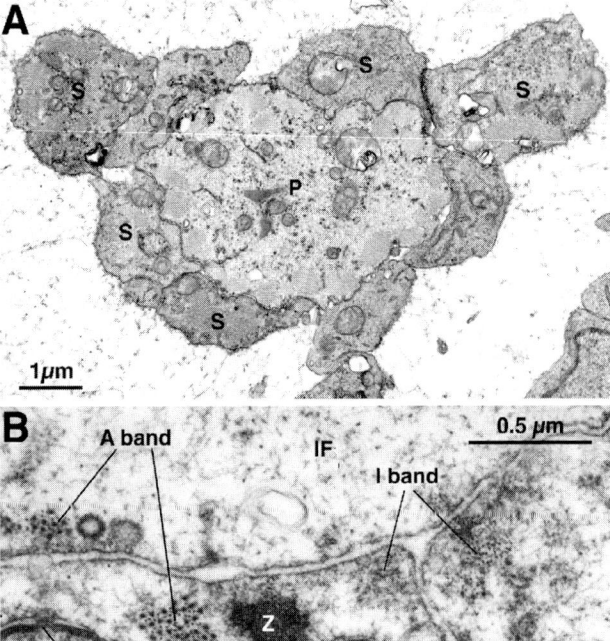

FIGURE 2-4. *A.* Electron micrograph of a cross section from the gastrocnemius of a chicken embryo at day 9 in ovo. The primary myotube (P) is surrounded by several closely adhering secondary myotubes (S). Gap junctions are present between the primary and secondary myotubes. Bar = 1 μm. (*From Takekura and Franzini-Armstrong.*[13] *Reproduced by permission.*) *B.* Cross section of a leg muscle from a 12-day in ovo chick. Note the association of developing myofibrils (A band, I band) with the cell surfaces in both primary and secondary myotube. Note also the cross sections of numerous intermediate filaments (IF) in the cytoplasm. (NP = nuclear pore.) (*From Fischman.*[12] *Reproduced by permission.*)

*A list of the abbreviations used in this chapter is given at the end of the chapter.

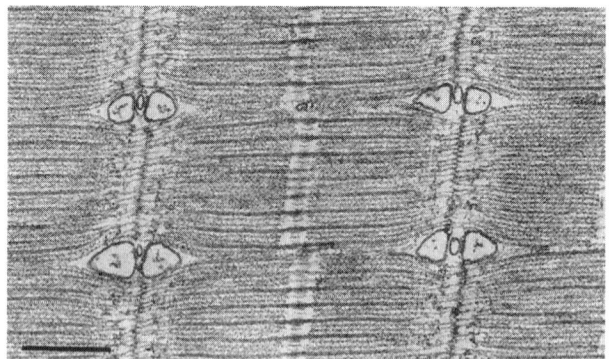

FIGURE 2-5. Longitudinal section of adult fish skeletal muscle. Myofibrils, T tubules, and sarcoplasmic reticulum (SR) form a highly ordered arrangement, with a precise disposition of SR–T-tubule triads at the Z lines. The uniform lengths of the thick and thin filaments are clearly observed in this image. Bar = 0.5 μm.

to fusion events.[10,33] This stimulation may be coupled to the enhanced expression of adhesion and/or fusigenic proteins.

An understanding of the fusion process is critical for the use of stem cell therapies designed to introduce compensatory molecules into muscle fibers, but it may also produce other advances.[34–36] It is often forgotten that adult muscle cells are not only contractile but also secretory cells: Plasma gelsolin, for example, is secreted by muscle fibers.[37] Since muscle cells can last the lifetime of the individual and are very large, they may conceivably be recruited as factories for the production of needed molecules that are not normally made.[34–36] An understanding of the fusion process should permit a more effective way of constructing these helpful "Trojan horse" cells.

An adult muscle fiber contains a highly stereotyped and muscle fiber type–specific disposition of cytoskeletal, cytoplasmic, and membrane-limited organelles. These are briefly introduced here. The myofibrils, responsible for contraction, occupy a large portion of the fiber volume. Their alternate brands are aligned across the fiber to form the cross striation; they are composed of contractile filaments and the associated cross-linking and scaffolding proteins that hold the filaments in a defined array and determine their length (Figs. 2-2 and 2-5; see also Chap. 7). The myofibrils are held within a cytoskeleton scaffolding that connects them transversely to each other and to the cell surface at periodic locations along their length (at the Z line and less strongly at the M line). A related scaffolding connects the myofibrils to the myotendinous junctions at their ends. Rib-like attachments between the Z bands of peripheral myofibrils and the cell surfaces are called *costameres* (Fig. 2-6). They appear electron-dense in ultrastructural images and contain vinculin. At the ends of myofibrils are focal adhesions that attach the myofibrils to the cell membrane (see also Chaps. 19a and b and 20). Along the entire periphery of the muscle cell is a subcortical cytoskeleton (see Chap. 19a and b). Intermediate filaments comprise a major fibrous polymer network that courses along the cell and across the muscle cell at the level of the Z bands (Fig. 2-7).[40] Direct short links between the Z line and the membrane systems is also present at the Z line (Fig. 2-8; see also "Assembly and Organization of the Membrane System," below). Microtubules constitute another polymer system that is distributed along the long axis of the muscle cell (Fig. 2-3). Microtubules are less abundant in adult than in developing skeletal muscle cells.[41] The membrane systems comprising transverse tubules and the sarcoplasmic reticulum responsible for calcium handling are precisely associated with the myofibrils (Figs. 2-8 and 2-9; see also Chap. 11). Mitochondria (see Chap. 60) represent a third membranous system within the muscle cell, often distributed in a sarcomeric pattern or just segregated to the sides of

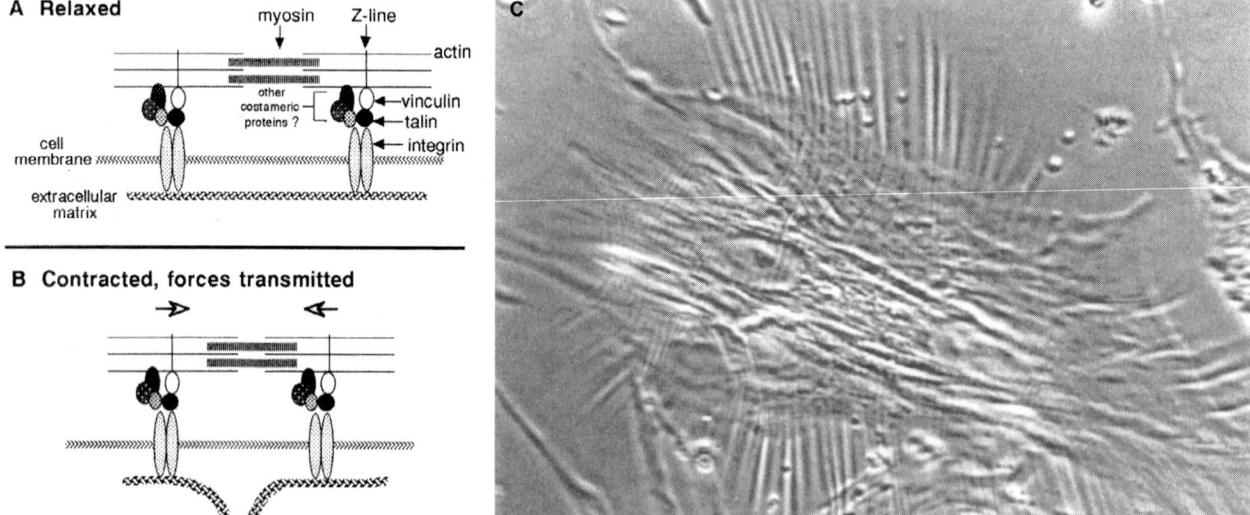

FIGURE 2-6. Costameres. A. Diagram summarizing the relationships between myofibrils, plasmalemma, and extracellular matrix at costameres. In a relaxed (extended) muscle, the plasmalemma is smooth. B. In a shortened, contracted state, the membrane between adjacent costameres is wrinkled. C. Adult rat cardiomyocyte in vitro contracting on a deformable surface. Accordion-like wrinkles form between the Z-bands. (*From Danowski et al.[38] Reproduced by permission.*)

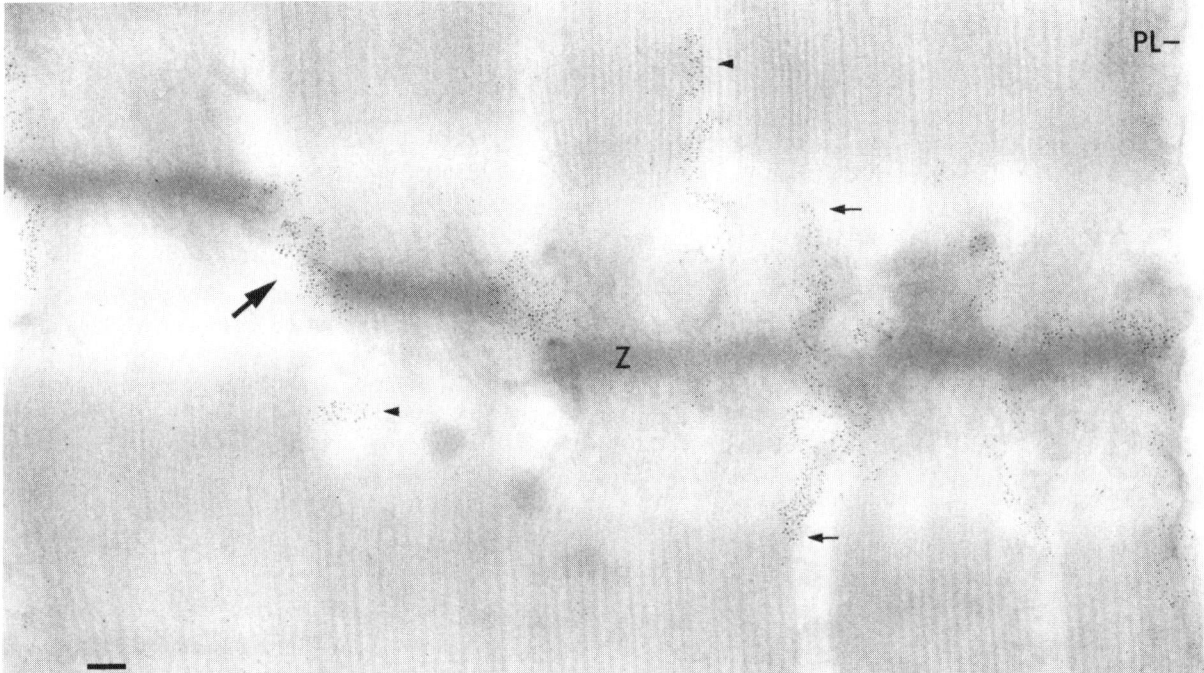

FIGURE 2-7. Immunoferritin labeling of desmin in an ultrathin cryosection of leg muscle from a 1-day-old chick. Most of the labeling is in the intermyofibrillar spaces at the level of the Z band (large arrows). The ferritin clusters indicate the positions of the desmin intermediate filaments that are part of the complex cytoskeletal network at the Z bands. Evidence of desmin filament labeling is also present in regions away from the Z bands (arrowheads and small arrows). In electron micrographs, desmin filaments are seen to course circumferentially aound the myofibrils at the Z line and to run parallel to the myofibrils in a longitudinal direction. Note the evidence for the desmin filaments extending from the Z band to the plasmalemma (PL). Bar = 0.1 μm. (*Courtesy of KT Tokuyasu.*)

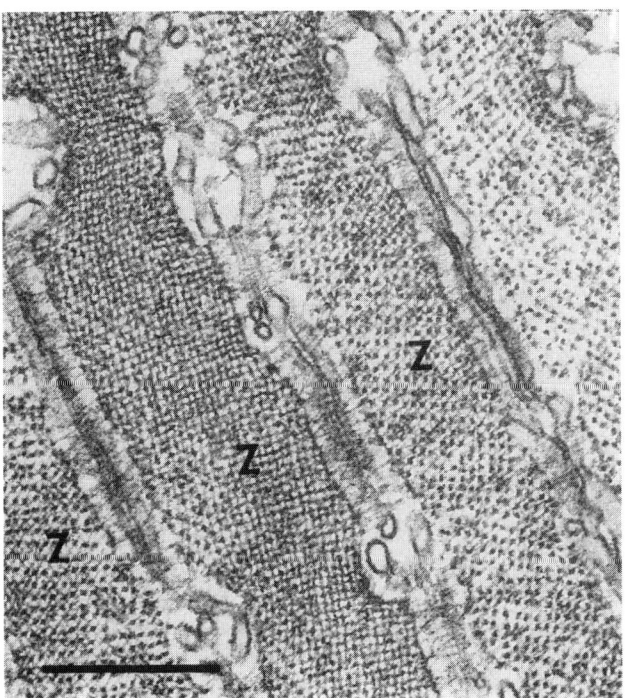

FIGURE 2-8. Electron micrograph from a thin cross section of fish muscle at the level of the Z band (Z). The spaces between the myofibrils are occupied by SR membrane profiles, which are connected by short filaments to the Z lines. The newly discovered protein obscurin may be a component of these filaments. Bar = 0.5 μm. (*From Nunzi and Franzini-Armstrong.*[39] Reproduced by permission.)

the muscle cells (Fig. 2-9). Intermediate filaments may be responsible for the close association between mitochondria and myofibrils.[42] Between the fibrous and membranous elements are a host of soluble proteins, many of them enzymes for glycogenolytic and glycolytic processes as well as lipids, carbohydrates, ribosomes, and other RNA molecules. Twenty percent of the proteins in muscle by weight are readily extractable by low-salt solutions and are termed *sarcoplasmic proteins*.[43,44] The glycogenolytic and glycolytic enzymes, as a group, are more abundant than either the actin or titin proteins in the muscle cells (see also Chap. 55). Several of these enzymes spend time bound to the fibrous elements of the sarcomere.[45]

Myofibrillogenesis

THE ASSEMBLY OF MYOFIBRILS

Coordinated expression of myofibrillar muscle-specific proteins (actin, myosin, tropomyosin, and α-actinin) is an early event in muscle differentiation.[46,47] This expression shift occurs before fusion, and indeed it is the beginning of the muscle-specific expression program that marks the transition from an undetermined myoblast to a determined myoblast (see Chap. 1). The newly synthesized proteins must come together in highly complex myofibrils, raising a

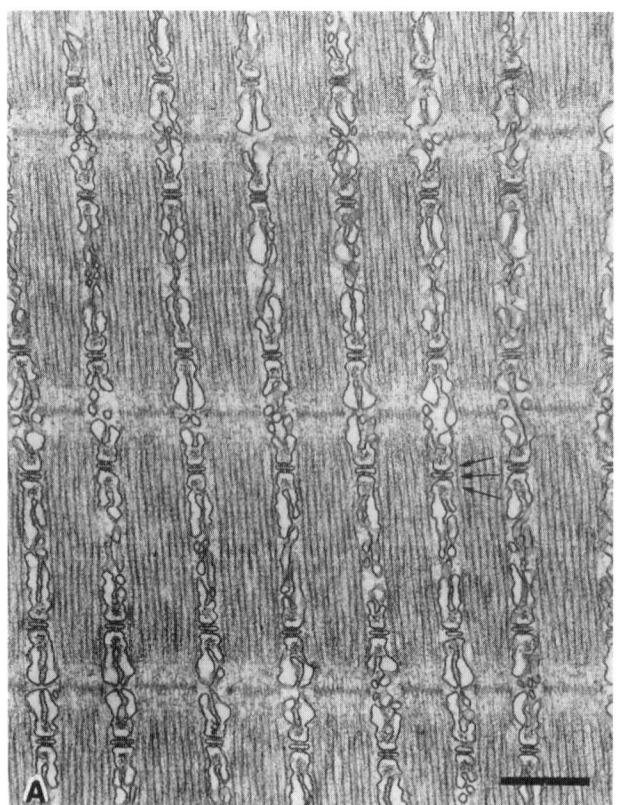 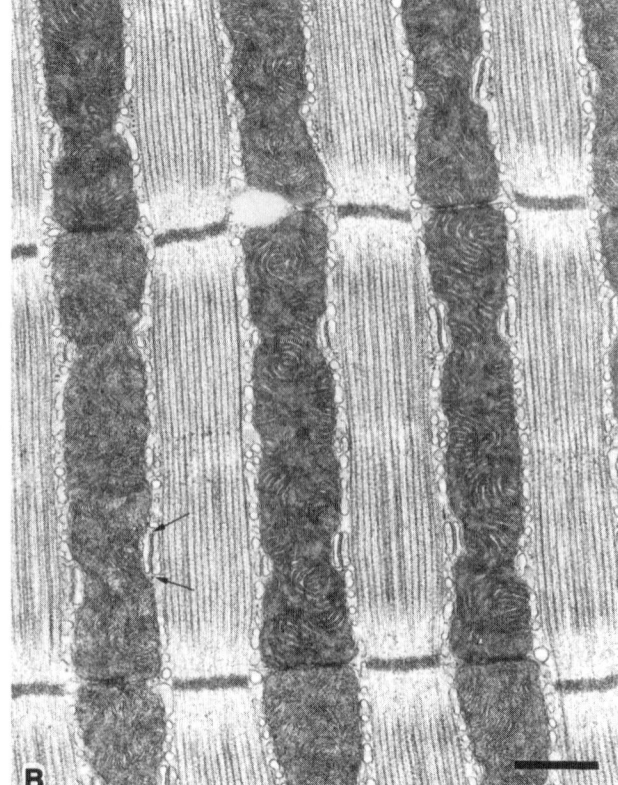

FIGURE 2-9. Longitudinal sections from two very fast muscles at the same magnification: (A) the swim bladder muscle in toadfish and (B) the flight muscle of the dragonfly. Mitochondria are between the myofibrils in the continuously active dragonfly muscle (B) but are segregated in the center and periphery of the fiber in toadfish muscle (not shown). The calcium release units are in the form of transversely oriented triads in toadfish (A; three arrows) and longitudinal dyads in dragonfly (B; two arrows). The thin and thick filaments are about 1.5 times longer in dragonfly muscle than in the toadfish. In marked contrast to the uniform length of A bands in vertebrate cross-striated muscles, invertebrate cross-striated muscles exhibit a wide variability in A-band lengths and sarcomeres that range from 1 to 25 μm. Bar = 0.5 μm.

number of questions. How are the myofibrils of a muscle cell formed? Is there a particular order in the assembly of different components of the myofibril? How do the myofibrils elongate as a muscle cell lengthens? Is the assembly process in developing muscles the same as that used for repair of muscle or in hypertrophy? How are proteins exchanged within a myofibril during the lifetime of the muscle cell?

The first clusters of thick and thin filaments, forming the nascent myofibrils, are positioned in close association with the peripheral cell membrane (Fig. 2-4). As shown by autoradiography, newly synthesized proteins continue to be incorporated at the cell periphery as the cells grow.[48] This indicates that as development progresses and the diameters of the cells increase, the cells fill themselves with myofibrils from the periphery inward. Indeed, the organization of nascent myofibrils gradually increases in order and complexity from periphery to center in a developing myotube (Fig. 2-10). Myofibril maturation involves an increase in the order of thin and thick filaments, more evident dense bodies, and the transition between dense bodies and Z lines (Fig. 2-10).[49]

Light microscopy—combined with standard histologic stains, immunolabeling, and specifically labeled proteins for dynamic in vivo studies—has played a major role in clarifying myofibrillogenesis.[50–52] Probes that are visible with light microscopy and specific for individual cytoskeletal proteins allow myofibril assembly to be studied in live cells in vitro, documenting whether a new myofibril is being formed or an existing one is being disassembled. To generated suitable probes, fluorescent dyes have been coupled to purified cytoskeletal proteins, followed by microinjection of trace amounts of the labeled proteins into live myocytes.[53–58] More recently, green fluorescent protein (GFP) technology has been applied to questions of myofibrillogenesis, allowing time-lapse observations over periods of many hours or days in a simple culture chamber on the microscope stage.[59] Expression of fragments of a sarcomeric protein linked to GFP can specify the region of the protein required for its proper localization in the myofibril. The development of brighter blue, yellow, or red fluorescent proteins along with the existence of GFP presents the future possibility of following two or three labeled proteins in the same muscle cell.

Early histologic observations of developing muscle showed that striations gradually appear from apparently "homogeneous" or unbanded fibers containing a high density of proteins.[50] However, microinjection of fluorescently labeled α-actinin, the major protein of Z bands, showed that this protein is localized in dense bodies, marking a striated pattern within narrow fibrils at very early stages of myogenesis (Fig. 2-11).[55,56] The spacings between these α-actinin bodies (Z bod-

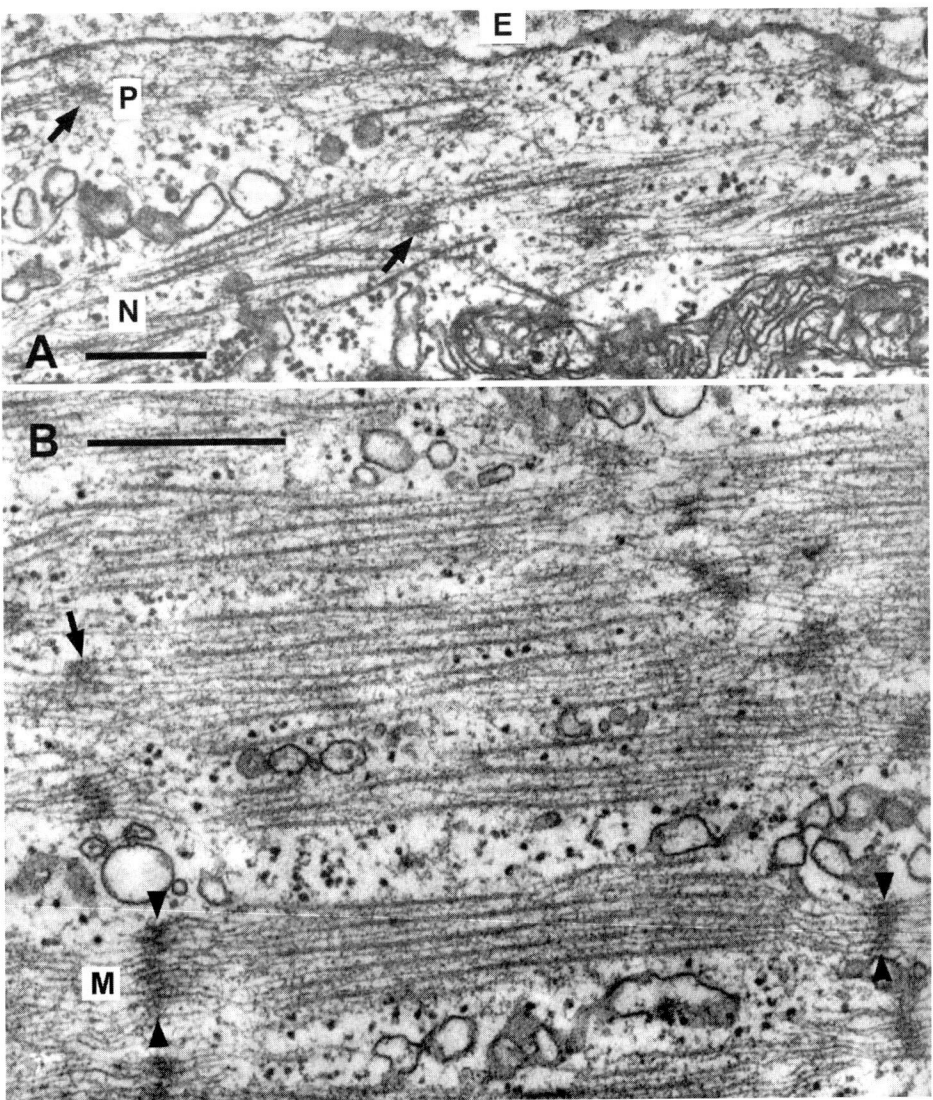

FIGURE 2-10. Developing myotubes from a limb bud of a larval newt. A. The extracellular material (E) is organized in a primitive basal lamina. A premyofibril (P), constituted of fairly disordered filaments and a small Z body (arrow), is associated with the cell surface. Deeper into the cell is a nascent myofibril (N) consisting of overlapping thick and thin filaments and a larger Z body (arrow). B. The thick filaments become better aligned and form distinct A and I bands as one progresses deeper into a myotube (from top to bottom). The Z bodies (arrow) fuse to form the Z bands (arrowheads) of mature myofibrils (M). (Modified from Kelly.[49] Reproduced by permission.)

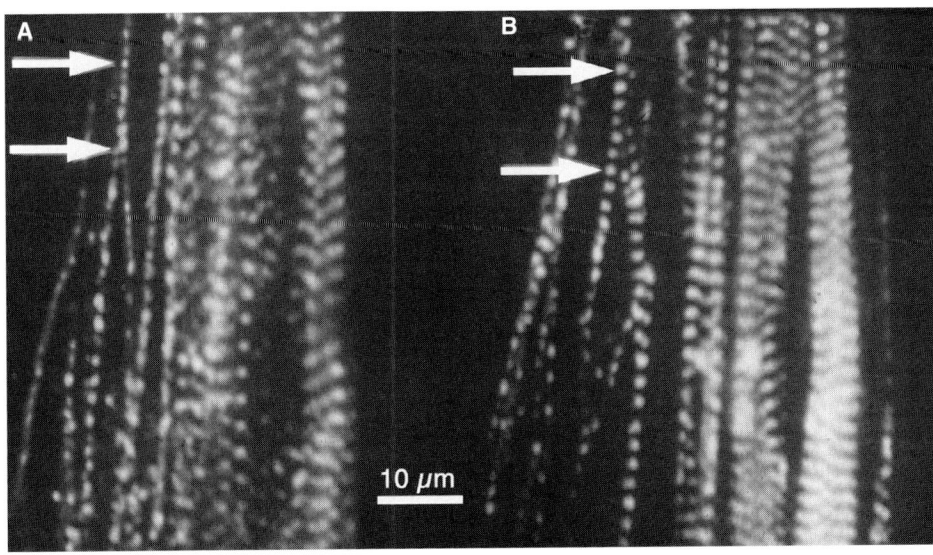

FIGURE 2-11. Images at two time points, separated by about 25 h, of a living embryonic chick myotube microinjected with fluorescently labeled α-actinin. The labeled α-actinin is in the Z bodies of the premyofibrils (between arrows in A) and in the Z bands of the mature myofibrils (between arrows in B). The region of the premyofibril marked in A has grown to form mature sarcomeres in B. Bar = 10 μm. (From Sanger et al.[55] Reproduced by permission.)

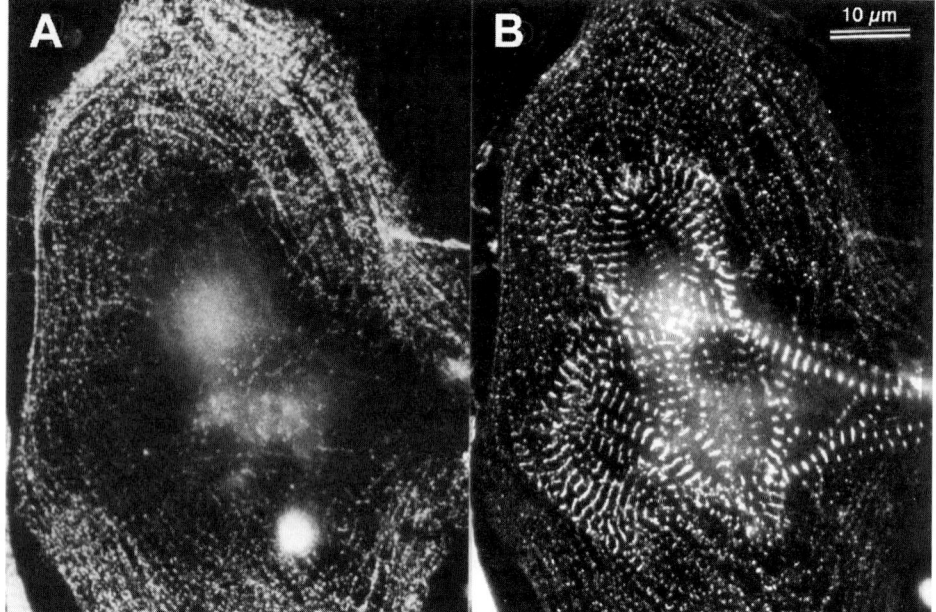

FIGURE 2-12. Spreading embryonic chick cardiomyocyte in culture, doubly labeled with antibodies against nonmuscle myosin IIB (A) and muscle-specific α-actinin (B). The nonmuscle myosin II is located exclusively at the periphery of the cell, where small periodically located beads of α-actinin mark the position of dense bodies belonging to premyofibrils. Nonmusclemyosin II is absent from the central region of the cell, where well-delineated bands of α-actinin show the presence of myofibrillar Z lines. Bar = 10 μm. (From Rhee et al.[60] Reproduced by permission.)

ies) ranged from 0.3 to 1.0 μm, much smaller than the 2.0- to 2.5-μm sarcomeric Z-band spacings of α-actinin in mature myofibrils.[55,56] The Z bodies mark the boundaries of minisarcomeres just as the Z bands in mature myofibrils mark the boundaries of sarcomeres. In contrast to α-actinin, actin initially is in an unbanded pattern, although in the same location as the banded α-actinin fibrils. Two isoforms of myosin II, nonmuscle and muscle-specific, are colocalized with unbanded actin and banded α-actinin fibrils.[60,64,65] At the earliest stages, nonmuscle myosin is present in bands that alternate with the Z bodies (Figs. 2-12 and 2-13).[55,58] These initial fibrils with their minisarcomeric pattern of α-actinin and nonmuscle myosin II, along with the overlapping thin filaments, have been termed *premyofibrils* (Fig. 2-14).[60] Muscle-specific isoforms of tropomyosin and troponin colocalize with actin in the premyofibrils as well.[58,62,63] Cap-Z and proteins that may influence actin filament length, tropomodulin and nebulin, appear early, but thin filament length is quite variable until later stages.[63–65] In later stages, muscle myosin appears first in an unstriated pattern, followed by clearly delineated A bands. Coincident with the appearance of muscle myosin, the sarcomeric spacings between the Z bodies increase in length,

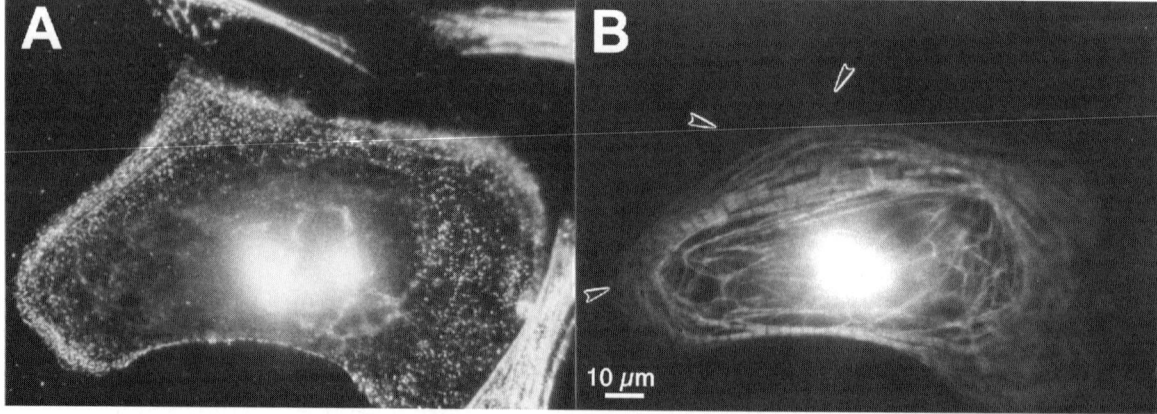

FIGURE 2-13. Embryonic chick cardiomyocyte stained with antibodies directed against nonmuscle myosin IIB (A) and muscle-specific myosin II (B). Arrowheads mark the margin of the cell. Nonmuscle myosin is present at the very edge of the cell and becomes less frequent as one moves inward. Muscle-specific myosin II, on the other hand, is absent from the premyofibrils along the cell periphery. Some regions, especially on the right side of the cell, contain both types of myosin in nascent myofibrils, but the area with clearly delineated A-bands of muscle myosin (mature myofibrils) is largely devoid of the nonmuscle myosin IIB. Bar = 10 μm. (From Rhee et al.[60] Reproduced by permission.)

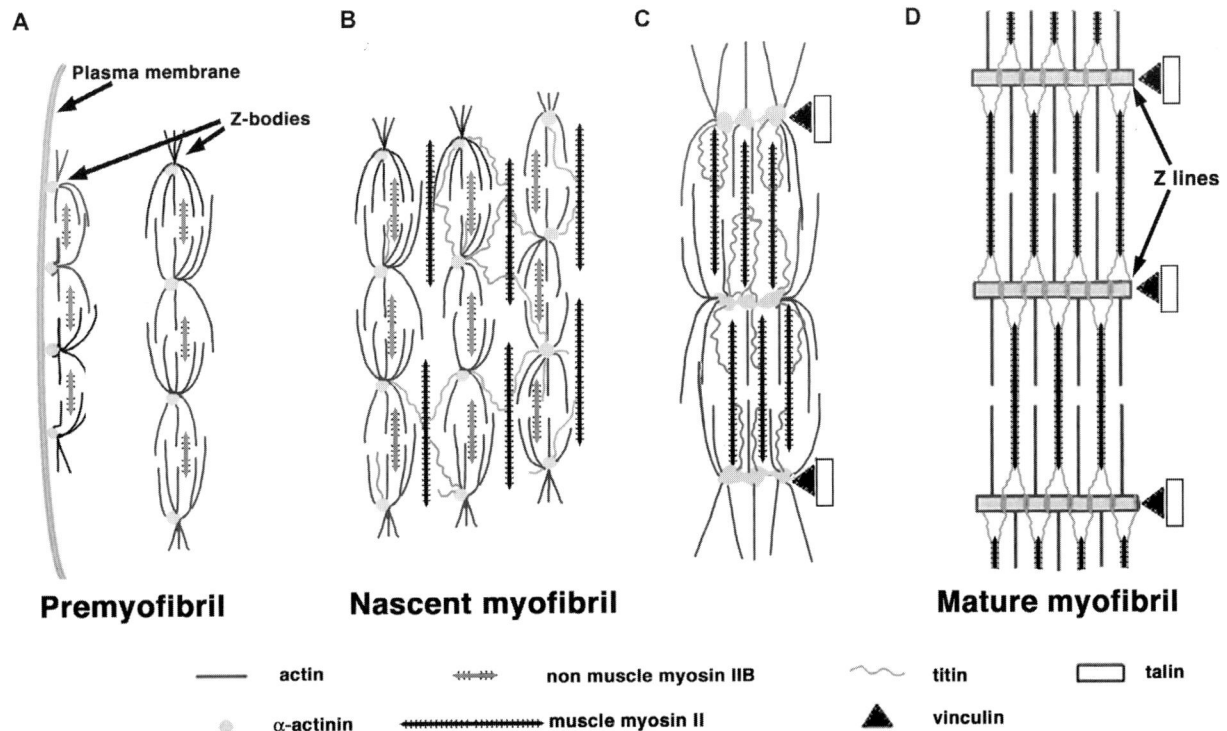

FIGURE 2-14. Model of myofibrillogenesis. A. The first fibrils (premyofibrils) form along the cell membrane where periodically disposed Z bodies composed of α-actinin and associated actin filaments are located. Myosin filaments composed of nonmuscle myosin II are located in bands between the Z bodies. Actin filaments from adjacent Z bodies overlap with each other, resulting in a continuous pattern of staining with phalloidin or actin antibody. B. Nascent myofibrils acquire thick filaments composed of muscle myosin presumably by the linking action of titin. Shorter nonmuscle myosin filaments coexist for a brief period of time with muscle myosin filaments. The muscle filaments overlap along the nascent myofibril, yielding a continuous staining pattern with muscle-specific myosin antibodies. C. The next step in the nascent myofibril is the lateral association of α-actinin-rich Z bodies, perhaps driven by the lateral pull of interactions between titin and thick filaments and between thick and thin filaments. The nonmuscle myosin II filaments are lost during this stage. Simultaneously, the spacing between Z bodies increases and an actin-free band (the H zone) appears as a result of the presence of the longer muscle myosin filaments and of the ordering action of titin. D. In mature myofibrils Z bodies have fused to form mature Z bands; nonmuscle myosin II is absent, and muscle myosin filaments are now aligned into A bands. The costameric proteins talin and vinculin first associate with mature myofibrils at the edge of the cell (C and D). (Modified from Dabiri et al.[66] Reproduced by permission.)

reaching 2.0 μm or more (Fig. 2-11). Comparable changes in patterns of α-actinin and myosins were also seen in developing myofibrils in cultures of precardiac mesoderm,[61,61a] and in embryonic cardiomyocytes.[60,66,67]

Fully formed myosin filaments composed of muscle-specific myosin are dispersed in the cytoplasm in proximity to assembling myofibrils, presumably to be incorporated later into the sarcomeres.[68] The giant protein titin appears to localize in developing myofibrils concurrently with muscle-specific myosin, leading to the idea that the N-terminus of titin associates with α-actinin in the forming Z bands and promotes myosin's insertion into the myofibrils when its C-terminus binds myosin filaments.[67–70] The myosin-associated proteins, C-protein and myomesin, appear later in the well-ordered A bands of mature myofibrils.[66,68]

There are currently three theories to explain the steps in the assembly of myofibrils.[61a,66] The premyofibril model proposes that the formation of mature myofibrils is preceded by two intermediary structures: premyofibrils and nascent myofibrils (Fig. 2-14).[60,67,70] Premyofibrils, characterized by banded patterns of sarcomeric α-actinin-rich Z bodies and nonmuscle myosin II, form at the edges of myocytes and develop into mature myofibrils. The Z bodies act as nucleating sites for the early polymerization of polarized actin filaments (Fig. 2-14A) and nonmuscle myosin associated with this actin. The actin filaments are of variable lengths and overlap each other in the fibers, so that labeling of actin does not show striation. During the transition from premyofibril to mature myofibril, it is postulated that nascent myofibrils form in which filaments of nonmuscle and muscle-specific myosin II coexist (Fig. 2-14B). Titin is thought to play a role in linking preformed muscle-specific myosin filaments to the nascent sarcomeres. In these early stages the myosin filaments have a disordered disposition, so that myosin appears to be nonstriated in the light microscope. Subsequently there is a loss of the nonmuscle myosin filaments, fusion of Z bodies into Z bands, and the alignment of the thick muscle myosin filaments into A bands (Figs. 2-14C and D). Since the muscle myosin filaments are

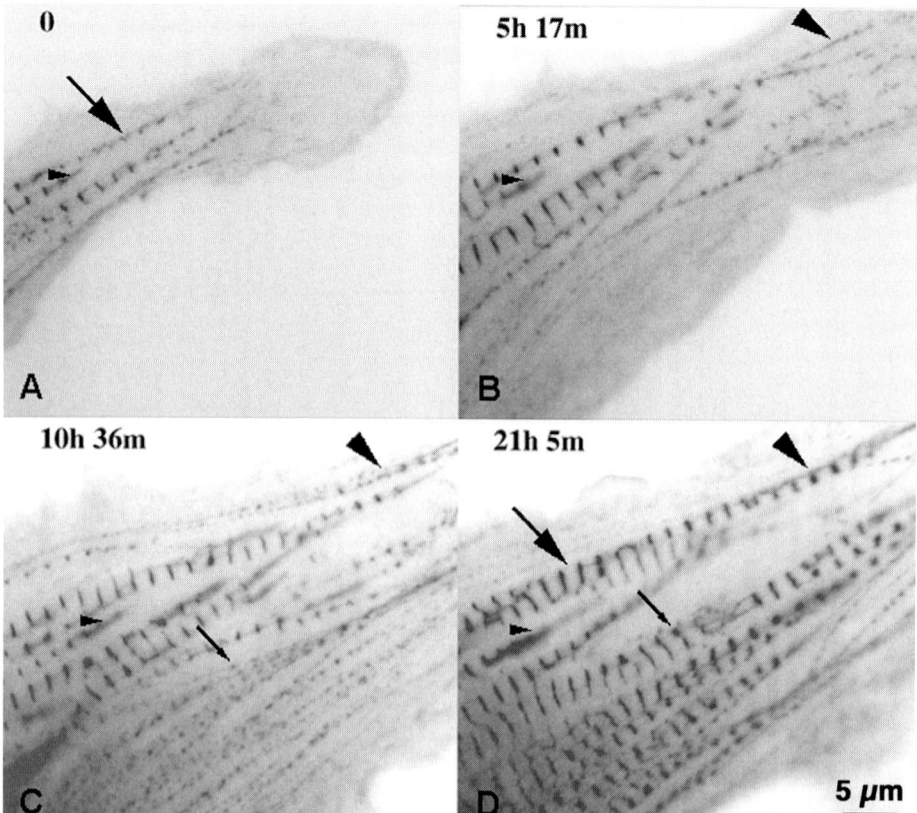

FIGURE 2-15. Four images from a time-lapse sequence of a spreading embryonic chick cardiomyocyte transfected with GFP–α-actinin. This cell was contracting as it spread in culture. The time of appearance of premyofibrils in the lower right spreading margin of cytoplasm is set to 0 (A), and at 21 h 5 m, myofibrils with solid Z bands had formed (D). The image is shown in reverse contrast to render the Z bands and Z bodies more visible. The same prominent adhesion plaque is marked in each section of the figure as a reference mark (A to D; small horizontal arrowhead). Note the amount of cell spreading with respect to this adhesion plaque. As the cell spreads toward the lower right of the image, punctate Z bodies appeared and assembled into linear arrays that fused laterally into Z bands of myofibrils. A myofibril indicated by a large arrow in (A) doubles in length over the next 21 h (D). This appears to happen by the lateral fusion of myofibrils (B to D; large oblique arrowheads). Scale = 5 μm. (From Dabiri et al.[66] Reproduced by permission.)

longer than the nonmuscle myosin filaments, this results in an elongation of the sarcomere. Mature myofibrils are the culmination of this changeover (Fig. 2-14D).[60,67]

This interpretation of myofibrillogenesis was supported by observations of live cardiomyocytes, previously transfected with GFP–α-actinin probe (Fig. 2-15).[66] Premyofibrils deposited at the edges of the spreading cell. The intensities of the Z bodies increased, indicating that additional molecules were adding to the recently formed premyofibrils. The spacings between the Z bodies gradually increased. Three to four premyofibrils fused together at the level of their aligned Z bodies to form nascent and mature myofibrils. Over the next few hours, the beaded Z bands of the mature myofibrils underwent a dramatic change to a fine line of the Z bands, typical of adult myofibrils.[66]

An earlier model for myofibrillogenesis postulated that the earliest fibrils are not muscle-specific premyofibrils but are simply equivalent to the stress fibers that are present in other cells, notably fibroblasts, and are composed of nonmuscle proteins.[71] These stress fiber–like structures were postulated to serve as temporary templates along which muscle-specific actin and myosin filaments and dense bodies lined up and formed mature myofibrils, followed by disassembly of the template fibril.[71] However, except for the nonmuscle myosin II, premyofibrils contain muscle-specific proteins (sarcomeric α-actinin, nebulin, tropomyosin, and troponin), and their response to inhibitors of polymerization (e.g., DNase I and vitamin D–binding protein) are not the same as shown by stress fibers.[72] Thus premyofibrils are distinct from stress fibers.

A third hypothesis for myofibrillogenesis proposes that spatially separate complexes of actin filaments, titin, and Z bodies (called I-Z-I brushes or I-Z-I bodies) and groups of muscle myosin thick filaments assemble independently of one another and become spliced together by titin filaments, which would grab the preformed myosin filaments and assemble them into A bands.[47,68] The fairly well aligned disposition of the I-Z-I brushes in this model would be determined by interactions with cytoskeleton rather than with myosin.[68] A major disagreement between this splicing model and the premyofibril model centers on whether nonmuscle myosin II is present in the earliest fibrils[60,73,74] or whether these fibrils are actually randomly oriented I-Z-I brushes unconnected by nonmuscle myosin.[75,76] The premyofibril and splicing models do agree on one aspect: There is a spatially distinct assembly of thick myosin filaments and Z bodies with associated actin filaments.[61a,66]

The premyofibril model was developed using cultured avian muscle cells. Is there support for this paradigm in other systems? Myoblasts isolated from the myotomes of Xenopus can be placed in tissue culture and in less than a day mature myofibrils are detected.[77] When filaments of nonmuscle myosin II were prevented from polymerizing, myofibrillogenesis was inhibited in these cells.[77] Removal of the inhibitor led to the assembly of myofibrils, supporting a role for nonmuscle myosin II in the assembly of myofibrils. Young myotubes that formed in cultures from a myogenic mouse cell line assembled fibrils with alternating bands of nonmuscle myosin II and α-actinin at their ends.[58] Mature myofibrils subsequently lost nonmuscle myosin and acquired muscle myosin.[58,78] These observations are consistent with a premyofibril model of myofibrillogenesis in mouse skeletal muscle cells.

How is the elongation of a myofibril coupled to the elongation of a muscle cell? Since the sarcomere length is approximately constant in a given muscle, elongation means addition of new sarcomeres, and this occurs at a very fast rate and in a manner dependent on the muscle.[79,80] In a mouse at birth, there are about 700 sarcomeres/myofibril in the soleus and 900 in the biceps brachii. The soleus muscle reaches the adult length at 6 weeks by adding sarcomeres at rates of 21 sarcomeres/myofibril per day for the first 2 weeks after birth, reaching a peak of 57 sarcomeres/myofibril per day for the next 2 1/2 weeks and decreasing to 19 sarcomeres/myofibril per day before reaching 2200 sarcomeres/myofibril at 6 weeks. The biceps brachii muscle assembles sarcomeres at a linear rate of 26 sarcomeres/myofibril per day, increasing its 900 sarcomeres to 1800 sarcomeres in 7 weeks.[79,80] The majority of studies in muscles from vertebrates suggest that individual sarcomeres are added to the ends of myofibrils[47,68,79,80] by unknown mechanisms through which scattered thin and thick filaments at the end of the elongating muscle cell interdigitate to assemble a sarcomere. A second mechanism, so far observed only in invertebrates, is based on the intercalation of a new Z line in the center of the A band of an existing sarcomere. The new Z lines would then nucleate new thin filaments on either side, and the thick filaments on either side of the split would regrow the missing half filaments.[81] Both models are based on images of fixed and stained cells examined with light and electron microscopy.[47,68,81]

In the only in vivo study of elongating myofibrils in vertebrated muscles, a different type of myofibril elongation was observed.[66] One myofibril was observed to double in length from 14 sarcomeres to 28 by fusing laterally with a newly formed adjacent myofibril (Fig. 2-15). The rate of new sarcomere addition for cells in the same culture (24 new sarcomeres/myofibril per day) (Fig. 2-15) is comparable to the in situ rates (see above), leaving the possibility that myofibril fusion may account for some of the in situ growth in fiber length.[79,80]

MYOFIBRILS AND THE CYTOSKELETON

Clusters of proteins that attach cytoskeletal filaments to the cell membrane have been studied extensively in nonmuscle cells, where they are referred to as *focal adhesions*.[82] Many of these proteins have also been found to be concentrated in regions of muscle cells where myofibrils contact the sarcolemma laterally and at their ends.[83,84] The membrane attachments at the ends of myofibrils are similar in structure and composition to focal adhesions of nonmuscle cells, with high concentrations of integrin, vinculin, α-actinin, and talin.[83–87] In a study of myofibrillogenesis in culture, α-actinin was the first protein detected at the terminal insertions of the forming myofibrils,[70] consistent with the fact that myofibrils always terminate at the Z line. Later, integrin, vinculin, and talin were also identified (Fig. 2-16).[83–88]

Costameres, the protein scaffolds that provide lateral attachments of the Z line of peripheral myofibril to the sarcolemma, are composed of some of the same proteins found in focal adhesions.[39,83,85–88] Evidence that Z bands adjacent to the sarcolemma might be coupled to the cell membrane came first from electron micrograph evidence of osmiophilic material between Z bands and membrane.[88] Subsequently, vinculin was shown to be localized in rib-like (hence costamere) staining patterns at peripheral Z bands of cardiac and skeletal muscles.[85,86] Vinculin and talin are initially associated only with the ends of the myofibrils (Figs. 2-14 and 2-16) and only later with the Z bands.[58,73,82,84,89] Not all muscle fibers have obvious costameres, since in some

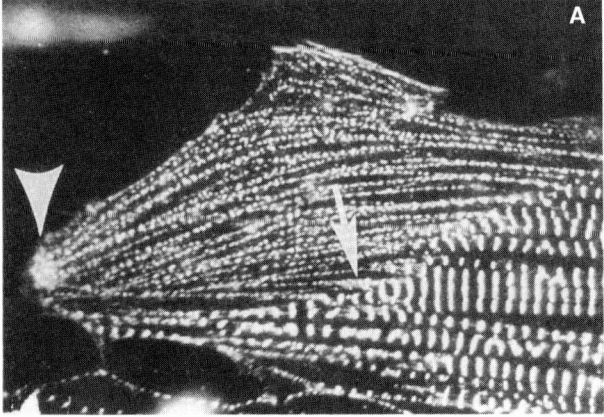 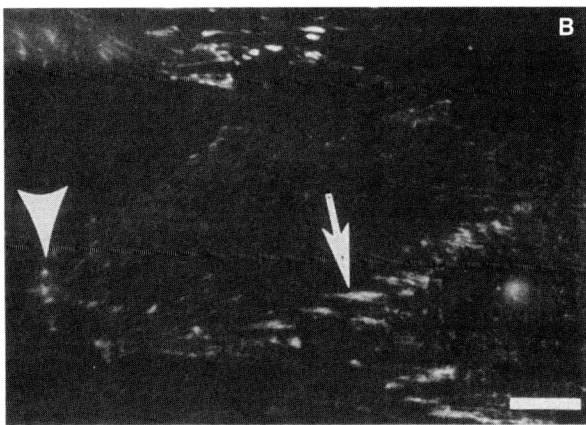

FIGURE 2-16. Cultured cardiomyocyte double-labeled with (A) muscle-specific α-actinin and (B) vinculin antibodies to show sites of adhesion of premyofibrils (arrowheads) and mature myofibrils (arrows) to the plasmalemma. Vinculin is detected at the ends of the premyofibrils and the mature myofibrils. While vinculin is detected at some Z bands of the mature myofibrils, no vinculin is detected associated with the Z bodies of the premyofibrils. Bar = 10 μm. *(From Schultheiss et al.[89] Reproduced by permission.)*

of them a wide band of cytoplasm separates the myofibrils from the plasmalemma. However, all fibers clearly have transverse networks that are responsible for transverse connections between myofibrils and plasmalemma and between adjacent myofibrils in the depth of the fiber. The term *costamere* has been extended to include these deeper connections.

The importance of vinculin for muscle attachment was demonstrated in the muscles of the nematode *Caenorhabditis elegans*. A mutation in the nematode vinculin gene leads to the detachment of muscle from the cell wall, disorganized arrays of muscle, and paralysis of the worms.[90] The disorder was reversed by injection of DNA encoding wild-type vinculin.[90] This insight into the important role of vinculin in muscle attachment has been extended to vertebrates, where antisense oligonucleotides directed against vinculin mRNA were added to cultures of mouse cardiomyocytes, decreasing the amount of vinculin by 43 to 48 percent and inducing the misalignment of the Z bands and of thin and thick filaments.[91] In parallel experiments, use of random oligonucleotides had no effect on vinculin synthesis or myofibril structure.[91]

Contraction of cardiac muscle cells on a deformable substrate provides direct evidence for myofibril-surface attachments at the sites of costameres (Fig. 2-6).[38] When muscle that had been microinjected with fluorescent vinculin contracted on an elastic substrate, accordion-like ripples formed in a pattern corresponding to the Z-band costameres.

Integrin is also located at the costameres of adult vertebrate skeletal muscle fibers. This location is acquired gradually: At 8 days of culture, embryonic vertebrate myotubes have integrin foci only at the ends of myofibrils,[87] but by 20 to 30 days in culture, integrin bands are found along the surface of many of the myotubes at the Z-band level.[83] In contrast to embryonic avian muscles, in developing cross-striated muscle of *Drosophila*, integrin is present at the earliest stages of development.[92] The absence of integrin in mutant flies leads to abnormal myofibrillogenesis.[93]

Developmental Changes in Microtubules and Intermediate Filaments

Microtubules are abundant in embryonic muscle cells (Fig. 2-3) but less frequent in adult fibers.[94] Depolymerization of microtubules both in vivo and in culture causes the formation of disorganized myofibrils.[95] Apparently, the organized longitudinal arrangement of microtubules, which is stabilized by microtubule-associated proteins (MAPs), is the important factor. Inhibiting the synthesis of a MAP by antisense RNA did not affect myoblast fusion but resulted in short myotubes with a rounded shape. Within the cells, microtubules were disorganized and myofibrils could not be detected.[96]

Further evidence for the importance of microtubule stability can be inferred from the posttranslational modifications of tubulin that occur prior to myofibrillogenesis. Microtubules are stabilized by the posttranslational detyrosination of tubulin in the myoblast prior to fusion and by acetylation, which occurs after the myocytes have fused.[97] A skeletal muscle ring-finger protein (MuRF) binds and stabilizes microtubules localized to the Z bands of the sarcomeres, suggesting that there may be an interaction between myofibrils and the stabilized arrays of microtubules.[98] Future work is needed to determine how these stabilized microtubules influence myofibrillogenesis other than by maintaining the elongated shape of the cells.

Intermediate filaments are a major component of skeletal muscle cells, both in developing cells (Fig. 2-17) and in adult fibers.[99–105] Many classes of intermediate filament proteins are present in skeletal muscle: desmin, vimentin, synemin, paranemin, nestin, syncoilin, desmuslin, and even cytokeratins.[40,102–106] Desmin, the most abundant, is one of the first muscle-specific proteins to appear in developing muscle cells.[69,102] The expression of vimentin and nestin, on the other hand, is downregulated in adult skeletal muscle cells.[102–104] Intermediate filaments are present at the Z-line level of the adult muscle as well as in longitudinal bands running parallel to the myofibrils, and their presence in the cytoskeleton may be important in integrating the mechanical properties of muscles.[105]

Desmin, however, is not essential for the assembly and alignment of myofibrils. Mice lacking desmin assemble myofibrils in both skeletal and cardiac muscle cells.[107] Desmin-null skeletal muscles are less susceptible to injuries compared to normal skeletal muscle cells,[108,109] perhaps because the absence of intermediate filaments allows the muscle to be more compliant, permitting the myofibrils to slide by one another. In slow-twitch fibers of desmin-null mice, mitochondria lose their alignment along the myofibrils and become concentrated at the fiber periphery.[42] Although it is not clear that desmin binds to mitochodndria, plectin, a desmin-binding protein, may mediate an inter-

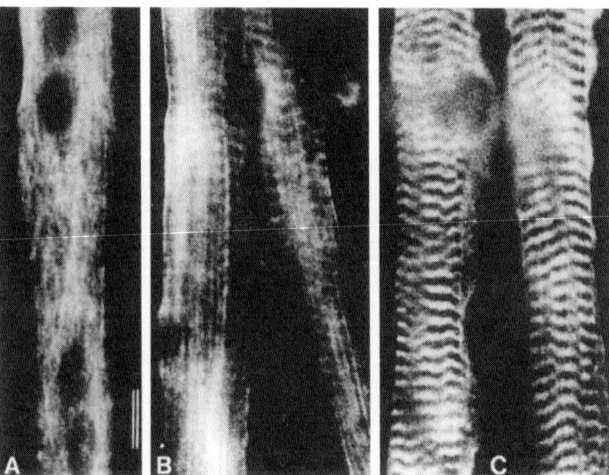

FIGURE 2-17. Localization of desmin by fluorescence immunolabeling in avian myotubes at three different stages of maturation in tissue culture. *A.* In a 2-day-old myotube, desmin is located in fibers that run along the whole length of the cell. *B.* By 6 days in culture, the myotube exhibits desmin at the Z bands and fibers along the long axis of the myotube. *C.* By 22 days in culture, most of the desmin is concentrated in the Z bands. Bar = 10 μm. (*From Bennett et al.*[100] *Reproduced by permission.*)

action with mitochondria.[110,111] Support for this view comes from the fact that mice lacking dystonin, a protein that cross-links intermediate filaments, also show mitochondrial misalignment.[112]

Renewal of Myofibrillar Proteins within Muscle Cells

Mature myofibrils appear at first sight to be very stable structures (Fig. 2-5). And yet it has been known for some time that the protein components of the sarcomeres have surprisingly short half-lives of 6 to 9 days (e.g., myosin heavy chain, 5.9 days; actin, 7.7 days; light chains, 9 days).[113] In a study of avian skeletal muscle cells in tissue culture, even titin, the largest protein in the body at a molecular weight of 3 million Da, was found to have a half-life of about 2.9 days.[114] These measurements indicate that within the same myofibril, individual components are replaced at different rates.

What is the import of these turnover numbers for the exchange of molecules within a sarcomere? With a 5.9-day half-life, myosin heavy chains are replaced at the rate of about 50 molecules per day in a thick filament that contains 600 myosin heavy chains. A 9-day half-life for myosin light chains indicates that 66 of these molecules are replaced every day. Since each myosin heavy chain binds two light chains, approximately half of the newly synthesized heavy chains will bind newly synthesized light chains and the other half will bind light chains present in the cytoplasmic pool (see below). The 3-day half-life of titin implies that 2 of the 12 titin filaments associated with a single thick filament must be replaced every day. Finally, the turnover rate for actin means that 23 of the 360 actin molecules in the 1-μm-long thin filament are replaced daily.

To determine if there were particular sites in myofibrils where newly synthesized myosin molecules became inserted into A bands, skeletal muscle cells were induced to synthesize a new myosin isoform.[115,116] The new isoform was detected along the whole length of the A bands of all myofibrils, with a higher concentration at the ends of the A bands.[115,116]

Such a high turnover rate indicates that the myofibrillar proteins can rapidly exchange with the cytoplasmic pool. Indeed, studies of cultured muscle cells—into which trace amounts of fluorescently labeled sarcomeric proteins, actin, α-actinin, myosin light chains, and tropomyosin, were injected—demonstrated that the proteins became incorporated into their appropriate sites in the myofibrils within 1 to 6 h of microinjection.[53,57,117–121] When the fluorescently labeled proteins were photobleached, they were replaced by unbleached fluorescent proteins at rates that varied for each protein[117,118] but that were much faster than the half-lives of sarcomeric proteins determined by radioisotopes. This suggests that the dynamic equilibrium between myofibrillar and cytoplasmic pools is independent of the synthesis of new protein molecules and that a cytoplasmic pool of molecules is always present, as shown for myosin light chains and actin.[122,123] However, when a new isoform is synthesized (e.g., in response to environmental or hormonal stimuli), the new protein readily gains access to the myofibrils. Mutated sarcomeric molecules might also exchange rapidly and thus lead to defective myofibrils.

Assembly and Organization of the Membrane System

The membrane systems responsible for the calcium cycle [the SR and the transverse (T) tubules (see Chap. 11)] are intimately associated with the contractile apparatus both structurally and functionally. Biogenesis of the membrane systems involves four series of events with partial temporal overlap. One event is the gradual transition of the ER in the differentiating myotube from the generic, housekeeping form to the specialized form to dedicated to calcium homeostasis. A second series of events is the segregation of proteins involved in the two main SR functions to distinct domains: the free and junctional SR (see Chap. 11). The free SR, constituting the majority of SR surface, is dedicated to calcium pumping; the junctional SR stores and releases calcium. A third event to be considered is the association of SR first with the plasmalemma and later with T tubules to form calcium release units (CRUs). The initial association of the SR with exterior membranes (plasmalemma and T tubules) requires a specific docking step, which precedes accrual of junctional SR-specific proteins to CRUs. A fourth developmental event is the linkage of the developing SR, the T tubules, and the CRUs to the myofibrils, resulting in a highly stereotyped, species- and fiber type–specific ultrastructural arrangement of the membrane systems.

A recent book covers aspects of SR differentiation in detail.[124]

TRANSITION: ENDOPLASMIC RETICULUM TO SARCOPLASMIC RETICULUM

Differentiation of the sarcoplasmic reticulum should be seen in the context of a set of functions common to the endoplasmic reticulum of all cells: the sequestering, storing, and releasing of Ca^{2+}. These tasks are achieved by actively pumping Ca^{2+} by means of a Ca^{2+}-activated ATPase (the SERCA, or sarco–endoplasmic reticulum calcium pump), which, in different varieties, is present in all cells (see Chap. 14); by storing the ions in the lumen with the aid of high-capacity, low-affinity calcium-binding proteins (calreticulin in a large variety of cells; calsequestrin in muscle and some neurons); and by releasing the calcium via two members of a unique family of calcium channels: the IP3 receptor and the ryanodine receptor (RyR). In nonmuscle cells, small membrane-limited organelles, the calciosomes, contain calcium-handling proteins.[125,126] Whether the calciosome should be considered as organelle that is structurally and functionally separate from the ER and whether all Ca^{2+}-handling organelles are calciosomes have been the subject of discussion.[127–129] In skeletal muscle, the great majority of the internal membranes are dedicated to Ca^{2+}

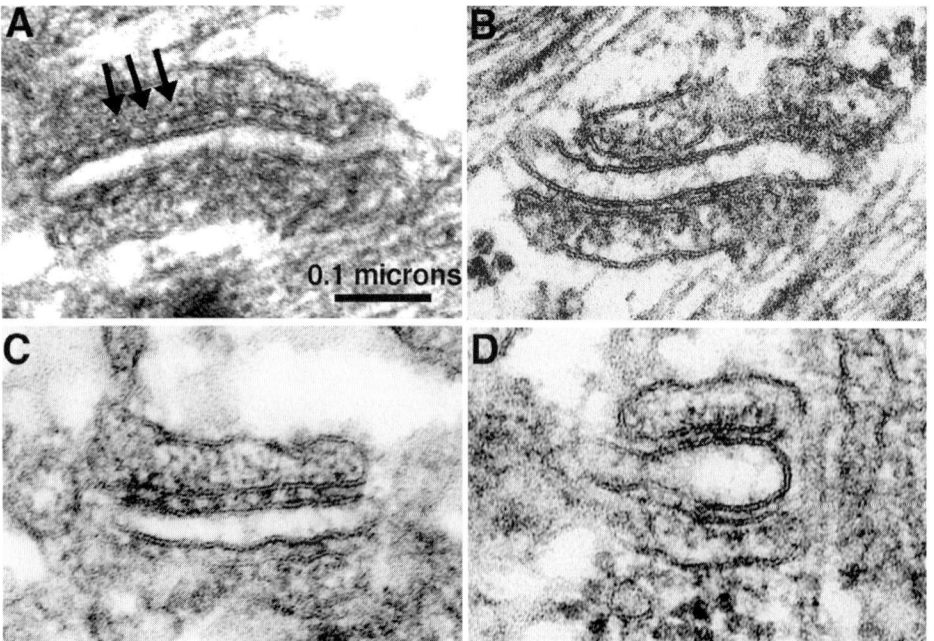

FIGURE 2-18. Examples of triads in diaphragm from wild type (*A*), dyspedic (*B*), dysgenic(*C*), and double mutant dysgenic/dyspedic (*D*) mice of perinatal age. Docking of SR to T tubules occurs normally despite the lack of either RyRs (*B*), DHPRs (*C*), or both. Note that arrangement of calsequestrin in the SR lumen is also unaffected by the lack of RyR or of the RyR/DHPR relationship, indicating that targeting of calsequestrin and triadin/junctin does not require the presence of RyR and that feet are appropriately targeted and disposed in the absence of DHPR (*C*). Not shown is evidence that DHPRs are appropriately targeted to sites of SR-surface docking in the absence of RyR. (See Refs. 168 and 169.)

handling, and thus in a sense the SR constitutes a giant "calciosome" which is continuous along and across the whole fiber. Skeletal and cardiac muscles contain specific forms of the various proteins dedicated to calcium handling, some unique to either muscle, some in common (see Chap. 14).

During skeletal muscle differentiation, the ER, identified through the luminal protein BiP, is transformed into the SR through a gradual but not complete replacement of generic ER proteins with SR-specific proteins functioning in the calcium cycle.[124,130–132] The major SR-specific proteins—calsequestrin,[133] SERCA,[132,134] and RyRs[135–137]—are upregulated at early stages of myogenesis and are detected in the SR in parallel with early myofibrillogenesis.[138–141] The two RyR isoforms present in skeletal muscle are regulated independently.[141] Dihydropyridine receptors (DHPRs), the channels of plasmalemma and T tubules that are part of CRUs, are also expressed during early myogenesis.[135] The SR proteins, like the contractile proteins, exhibit tissue specificity in their expression during muscle development, indicating that their induction is under the control of a common myogenic differentiation program.[137] The Ca^{2+} ATPase (SERCA) is by far the major protein in the SR. Accumulation of this protein in the nascent SR membrane is in parallel to the gradual structural transition of the SR into its mature form and probably drives an increase in surface area of the SR.[124,142] In the adult muscle cells a small complement of generic ER, RER, Golgi system, and accessory membranes remain associated with the perinuclear regions.

ASSEMBLY OF CALCIUM RELEASE UNITS: TARGETING OF COMPONENTS TO JUNCTIONAL DOMAINS

CRUs are composed of junctional SR (jSR) cisternae and junctional domains of plasmalemma/T tubules. The formation of CRUs requires the active segregation of transmembrane and luminal CRU proteins [e.g., ryanodine receptors, junctin, triadin, calsequestrin, and the RyR-associated proteins, calmodulin, FKBP12 (FK-binding protein 12), Homer, etc. (see Chaps. 11, 12, and 14) to the jSR cisternae, whereas the Ca^{2+} pump remains the major component of the free SR membrane by default. In the surface membrane, DHPRs, the calcium channels that act as voltage sensors of e-c coupling, become segregated into the junctional domains in parallel with the RyR, with which they become associated.[138,139,143–148] Segregation of the calcium storage and calcium release pro-

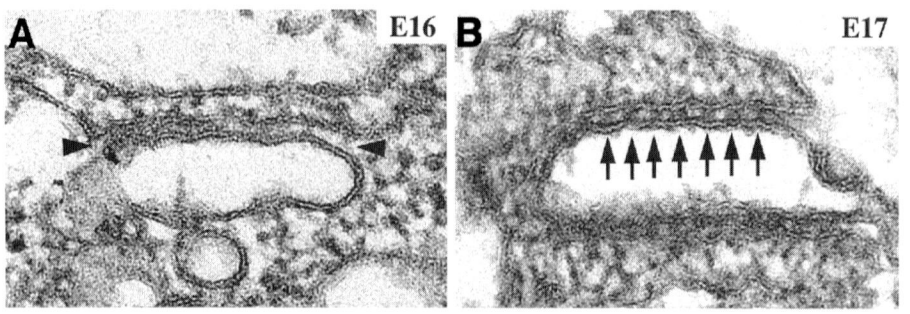

FIGURE 2-19. In the initial stage of CRU differentiation, the SR docks to the T tubules (*A*) and calsequestrin is present in its lumen. Maturation of the junction involves accrual of RyRs (feet; arrows in *B*); increase in the SR luminal content of calsequestrin; the clustering of calsequestrin at the junction, presumably due to junctin/triadin and the trapping of DHPR (not shown). (*From Takekura et al.*[166] *Reproduced by permission.*)

teins into junctional domains of the SR and clustering of DHPRs into junctional domains of the plasmalemma are early events during muscle differentiation.

The molecular basis for the targeting of various junctional SR components and of the surface membrane to CRUs is just beginning to be explored. Two null mutations—the dysgenic mutations resulting in lack of α1 subunit of DHPRs and the dyspedic mutations in which RyR1 is missing—indicate that RyR and DHPR reach the developing CRUs independently of one another and that they are not needed for targeting of other CRU components. Dysgenic CRUs contain RyRs and calsequestrin. Dyspedic CRUs have clusters of DHPRs and contain triadin and calsequestrin.[149–153] The various DHPR subunits, on the other hand, are interdependent for appropriate localization. The small subunits facilitate the incorporation of channels into the plasma membrane, forming a stable complex with the α1 subunit.[154] The association of β subunits with α1 is required for the targeting into triads.[155] Expression of α1 and its subsequent, independent location at CRUs is necessary for the proper targeting and distribution of α2.[156] The triad targeting signal for skeletal α1 is in the COOH terminus.[157]

Calsequestrin is one of the earliest CRU proteins to appear in the SR.[133] When it is overexpressed in skeletal or cardiac muscle, calsequestrin segregates into SR subdomains.[158–160] The synthetic pathway for this protein involves a passage through the Golgi for glycosylation.[161] However, glycosylation is not required for CRU targeting,[162] nor are the acidic carboxy terminal domain[163] and a number of phosphorylation sites.[164]

SR-plasmalemma junctions have been observed by electron microscopy in parallel with the differentiation of the first myofibrils.[143,145,165] SR-to-plasmalemma docking (see below) precedes delivery of most junctional proteins (except perhaps for calsequestrin) to junctional domains of the SR.[144,166] However, docking may not be necessary for the appropriate targeting of junctional proteins, since the junctional SR supramolecular complex can form in the absence of docking, at least in cardiac muscle (see Chap. 11). It is not known whether DHPR clustering into junctional domains is independent of SR docking, since the two events have never been detected separately.

ASSEMBLY OF CALCIUM RELEASE UNITS: THEIR DOCKING AND MATURATION

A major step in CRU formation is the docking of SR to plasmalemma/T tubules. Dysgenic (α1s DHPRs null) and dyspedic (RyR1 null) mutations and the double null obtained from mating of the two mutants have been very useful in unraveling the requirements for this step. Despite lack of either one or both of the two major interacting proteins and retarded or incomplete development of the myotubes, junctions between jSR and plasmalemma/T tubules are formed in dysgenic and dyspedic muscle fibers (Fig. 2-18).[149–152,167–169] A converse observation is that expression of RyR1 and DHPR in nonmuscle cells does not lead to the formation of CRUs, despite appropriate targeting of the two proteins to ER and plasmalemma, respectively.

These studies have led to the hypothesis that an initial docking step, independent of the RyR/DHPR interaction, is necessary for the formation of CRUs.[170] The challenge has been taken up by H. Takeshima, who has identified a probable candidate for the CRU docking protein in junctophilin, a protein of the SR that is thought to span the SR-plasmalemma gap and interact with the latter's lipids.[171]

The necessity for an initial docking step preceding accrual of CRU proteins is confirmed by ultrastructural observations of CRU differentiation during pre-and postnatal development of cardiac and skeletal muscle in vivo in which accumulation of proteins at the junction and their assembly are observed to follow gradually after an initial association of the SR with plasmalemma and/or T tubules (Fig. 2-19).[144,145]

Based on the above observations, the sequence of events illustrated in Fig. 2-20 has been proposed. First, SR docks,

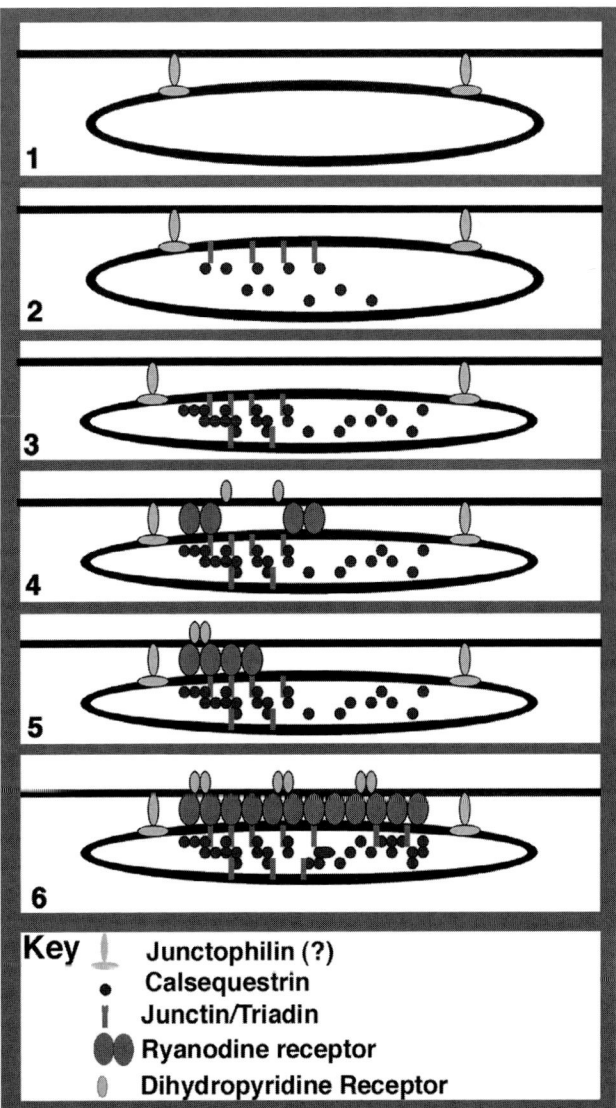

FIGURE 2-20. The sequence of CRU differentiation events involves (1) an initial docking due to junctophilin; (2) arrival of junctin/triadin and calsequestrin; (3) bundling of calsequestrin by triadin/junctin; (4) trapping of RyRs and DHPRs; (5) self-assembly of RyR into arrays and linking of DHPRs to RyR; and (6) maturation by the addition of more junctional protein.

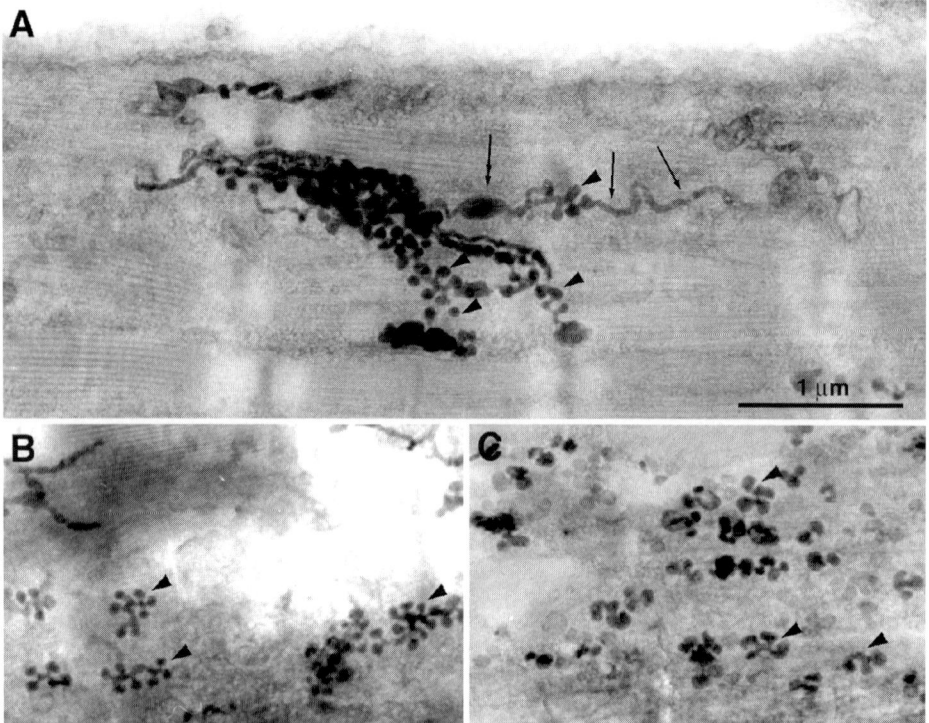

FIGURE 2-21. Mouse diaphragm at (A) embryonic day 16, (B) postnatal day 4, (C) day 14. A. Initial development of T tubules involves the formation of multiple clusters of caveolae (arrowheads), which are continuous with the nascent, mostly longitudinal T tubules (arrows). The frequency and clustering of caveolae at the fiber edge are higher at early (B) than at later stages of development (C). (See Franzini-Armstrong: Dev Biol 146:353, 1991.)

probably via junctophilin's action (step 1). An initial accumulation of calsequestrin, either simultaneously with the docking or even, in part, preceding it (step 2), is followed immediately by the condensation of calsequestrin due to the arrival of junctin/triadin (step 3). RyR and DHPR appear with a slight delay but simultaneously with each other (step 4). RyRs self-assemble into ordered arrays and induce formation of DHPR tetrads (step 5). Accrual of more proteins results in maturation of the junction (step 6). Normally, SR docking and the initial molecular differentiation of the junctional membrane domains occur concurrently or with minimal delay, suggestive of a hightly coordinated and possibly interdependent process.[166]

DEVELOPMENT OF T TUBULES AND MEMBRANE-TO-MYOFIBRILLAR LINKAGE

Development of T tubules is not a primary event in muscle differentiation. Early myofibrillogenesis, initial differentiation of the SR, and the formation of peripherally located CRUs at the surface of the myotube precede formation of T tubules by one to several days, depending on the species.[138,145,166,173] Interestingly, the control signal dictating the specific timing for T-tubule formation is lost during in vitro differentiation, in which SR and T tubules develop simultaneously.[139,164,167,174]

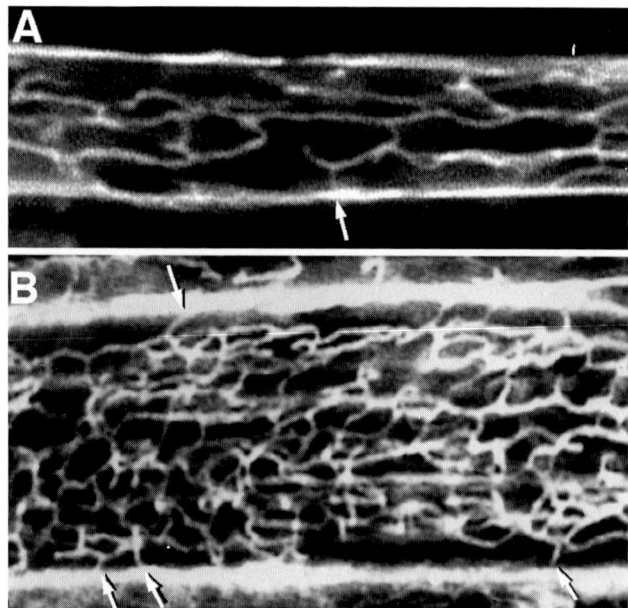

FIGURE 2-22. Labeling of T tubules by a fluorescent lipid-soluble marker in developing myotubes from chick embryos. A. T tubules initially invade the muscle fiber in longitudinal orientation, starting from widely spaced invagination sites (arrows). B. With further differentiation, the tubules become more frequent and acquire a transverse orientation. (See Refs. 145 and 166.)

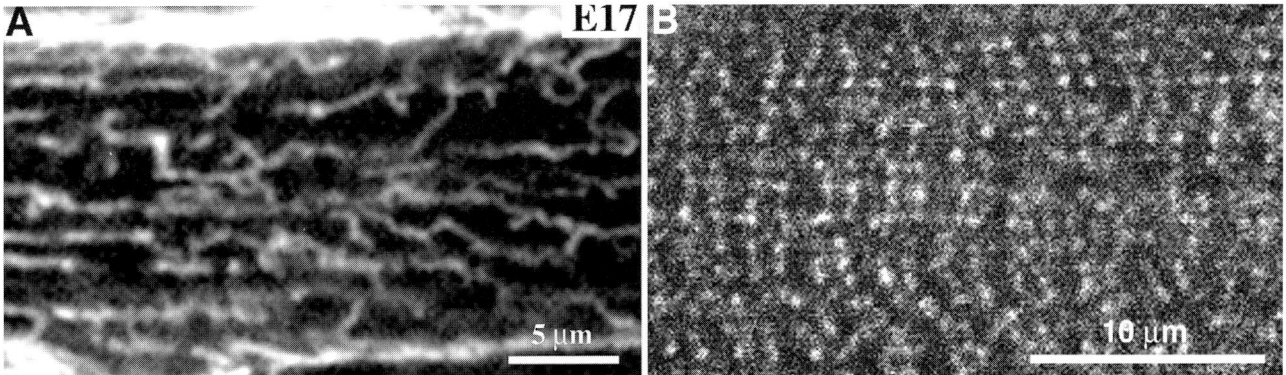

FIGURE 2-23. At embryonic day E17 in mouse diaphragm, T tubules are predominantly longitudinal (A), but triads (as evidenced by immunolabeled RyR foci) are already arranged in a sarcomere-related transverse arrangement (B). (See Ref. 166.)

Nascent T tubules are continuous with clusters of caveolae,[174] and caveolar invagination activity is very high during periods of initial T-tubule formation (Fig. 2-21). The abrupt change in membrane curvature that is necessary in order to form the T tubules is probably due to the recruitment of selected lipids by caveolin-3. Indeed, this protein is associated with nascent T tubules and the labyrinthine structures that accompany them in developing muscle.[175] A null mutation for caveolin-3 results in defective T tubules but, interestingly, not in complete loss of the tubules.[176] The immature T tubules are quite tortuous (Fig. 2-21) but become gradually more straight in time, presumably in parallel to the disappearance of caveolin from their surface.

The initial burst of T-tubule formation occurs at the time of myotube-to-myofiber transition (Fig. 2-22) and is accompanied by a marked increase in the frequency of CRUs and in a shift in the location of the units. Before T-tubule formation CRUs are at the fiber surface, but as soon as T tubules appear peripherally located CRUs disappear and internal CRUs, formed by SR–T tubule junctions, become numerous.[145,172] It is not known what determines the shift of CRU protein targeting from peripherally located to internal jSR.

The free SR is associated with the Z lines of the myofibrils as soon as the latter are formed.[177] A clue to the molecular basis for this association has come with the discovery of a novel large myofibrillar protein (obscurin) and its link to SR ankyrin.[181,182] Early T tubules, on the other hand, have a longitudinal orientation, not related to the bands of the sarcomere (Fig. 2-22).[138,143,165,166,172,177–180] The mature transverse arrangement of the tubules is achieved over a period that may be quite prolonged (up to about 3 weeks after birth in the mouse). The specific association of T-tubule networks with the bands of the myofibrils, either at the Z lines or at the A-I junctions, is apparently driven by the association of CRUs with the myofibrils, since the latter precedes the former during differentiation.[166] The mature position of triads relative to the bands of the sarcomere (e.g., at the edges of the A band for mouse skeletal muscle) is achieved early both in vitro and in vivo (Fig. 2-23) and is followed by a gradual shift from an initial longitudinal to a final transverse orientation (Fig. 2-24). Linkage of CRUs to myofibrils also precedes their rotation from a prevalently longitudinal to the mature transverse orientation.

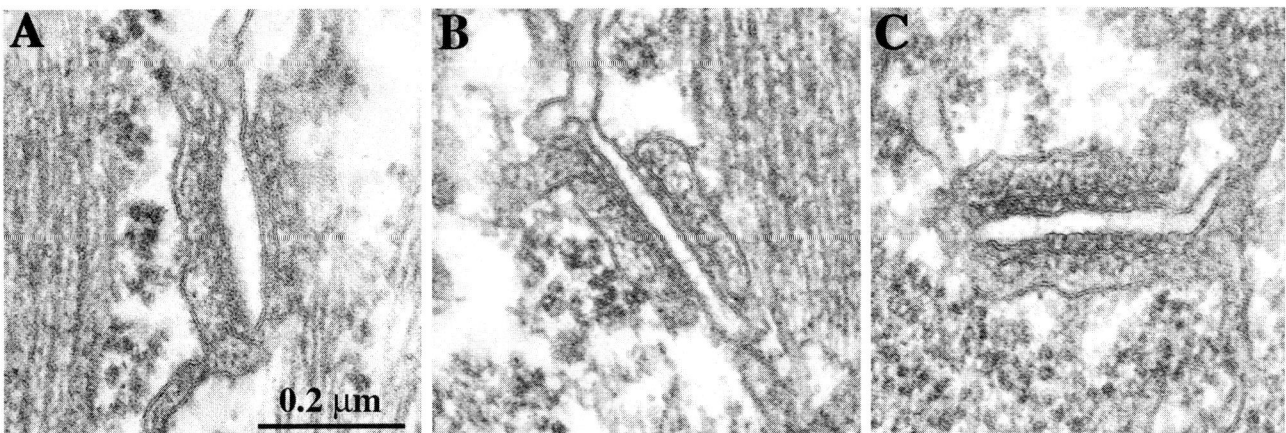

FIGURE 2-24. Triads in developing muscle have variable orientation, from transverse to oblique and longitudinal. In all images the long axis of the fiber is longitudinal. (See Ref. 166.)

Conclusions

Progress in understanding myofibrillogenesis was made in the past by the study of fixed cells using both light and electron microscopy. Now live-cell imaging of myofibrillogenesis and the assembly of membranes is increasing our knowledge. Nevertheless, all players are not yet in and we are very far from understanding the complex interplay of myofibrils, membranes, and cytoskeleton that determines how two such different muscle fibers as illustrated in Fig. 2-9 are assembled from similar types of molecules. This chapter focuses on vertebrate muscles. Model organisms, such as *Drosophila* and *C. elegans*, where genes are more easily manipulated will also continue to guide experiments in vertebrate systems.

List of Abbreviations

CRU	calcium release unit
DHPR	dihydropyridine receptor
ER	endoplasmic reticulum
FKBP12	FK-binding protein 12
GFP	green fluorescent protein
jSR	junctional sarcoplasmic reticulum
MAPs	microtubule-associated proteins
MuRF	muscle ring-finger protein
NCAM	neural cell adhesion molecule
RER	rough endoplasmic reticulum
RyR	ryanodine receptor
SERCA	sarco–endoplasmic reticulum calcium pump
SR	sarcoplasmic reticulum
T tubule	transverse tubule

References

1. Sanger JW, Saner JM: Fishing out proteins that bind to titin. *J Cell Biol* 154:21, 2001.
2. Turnacioglu KK, Mittal B, Dabiri G, et al: Zeugmatin is part of the Z-band targeting region of titin. *Cell Struct Funct* 22:73, 1997.
3. Fischman DA: The development of striated muscle, in Bourne G (ed): *The Structure and Function of Muscle*, 2d ed. Vol 1. New York: Academic Press; 1972; pp-75–148.
4. Stockdale FE, Holtzer H: DNA synthesis and myogenesis. *Exp Cell Res* 24:508, 1961.
5. Konigsberg IR: Clonal analysis of myogenesis. *Science* 140:1273, 1963.
6. Okazaki K, Holtzer H: Myogenesis, fusion, myosin synthesis and the mitotic cycle. *Proc Natl Acad Sci USA* 56:1484, 1966.
7. Capers CR: Multinucleation of skeletal muscle in vitro. *J Biophys Biochem Cytol* 7:559, 1960.
8. Taylor M: Muscle differentiation: How two cells become one. *Curr Biol* 22:R224, 2002.
9. Doberstein SK, Fetter RD, Mehta AY, Goodman CS: Genetic analysis of myoblast fusion: Blown fuse is required for progression beyond the prefusion complex. *J Cell Biol* 136:1249, 1997.
10. Labarge MA, Blau HM: Biological progression from adult bone marrow to mononucleate muscle stem cell to multinucleate muscle fiber in response to injury. *Cell* 111:589, 2002.
11. Kelly AM, Zacks SI: The histogenesis of rat intercostals muscle. *J Cell Biol* 42:135, 1969.
12. Fischman DA: An electron microscope study of myofibril formation in embryonic chick skeletal muscle. *J Cell Biol* 32:557, 1967.
13. Takekura H, Franzini-Armstrong C: Differentiation of membrane systems during development of slow and fast skeletal muscle fibres in chicken. *J Muscle Res Cell Motil* 14:633, 1993.
14. Yiping L, Appelt D, Kelly AM, Franzini-Armstrong C: Differences in the histogenesis of EDL and diaphragm in rat. *Dev Dynam* 193:359, 1992.
15. Rubinstein NA, Kelly AM: Development of muscle fiber specialization in the rat hind limb. *J Cell Biol* 90:128, 1981.
16. Lieber RL, Friden J: Functional and clinical significance of skeletal muscle. *Muscle Nerve* 23:1647, 2000.
17. Loeb GE, Pratt CA, Chanaud CM, Richmond FJ: Distribution and innervation of short interdigitated muscle fibers in parallel-fibered muscles of the cat hindlimb. *J Morphol* 191:1, 1987.
18. Dabiri GA, Ayoob JP, Turnacioglu KK, et al: Use of Green Fluorescent Proteins linked to cytoskeletal proteins to analyze myofibrillogenesis in living cells. *Methods Enzymol* 302:171, 1999.
19. Vanderburgh HH, Karlisch P, Farr L: Maintenance of highly contractile tissue-cultured avian skeletal myotubes in collagen gel. *In Vitro Cell Dev Biol* 24:166, 1988.
20. Vandenburgh HH, Hatfaludy S, Karlisch P, Shansky J: Mechanically induced alterations in cultured skeletal muscle growth. *J Biomech* 24:91, 1991.
21. Clark P, Dunn GA, Knibbs A, Peckham M: Alignment of myoblasts on ultrafine gratings inhibits fusion in vitro. *Int J Biochem Cell Biol* 34:816, 2002.
22. Sanger JW, Holtzer S, Holtzer H: Effects of cytochalasin-B on muscle cells in tissue culture. *Nature New Biol* 229:121, 1971.
23. Sanger JW: The use of cytochalasin-B to distinguish myoblasts from fibroblasts in cultures of developing chick striated muscle. *Proc Natl Acad Sci USA* 71:3621, 1974.
24. Wakelman MJO: The fusion of myoblasts. *Biochem J* 228:1, 1985.
25. Knudsen KA, Myers L, McElwee SA: A role for the Ca2+-dependent adhesion molecule N-cadheren in myoblast interaction during myogenesis. *Exp Cell Res* 188:175, 1990.
26. Dickson G, Peck D, Moore SE, et al: Enhanced myogenesis in NCAM transfected mouse myoblasts. *Nature* 344:348, 1990.
27. Wayne S, Jamieson JC, Spearman MA, Wright JA: Studies on the effect of ketaconazole on the fusion of L6 myoblasts. *Mol Cell Biochem* 92:137, 1990.
28. Knudsen KA, McElwee, Smith L: A role for the neural cell adhesion molecule, NCAM, in myoblast interaction during myogenesis. *Dev Biol* 138:159, 1990.
29. Rosen GD, Sanes JR, LaChance R, et al: Roles for the integrin VLA-4 and its counter receptor VCAM-1 in myogenesis. *Cell* 69:1107, 1992.
30. Yagami-Hiromasa T, Sato T, Kurisaki T, et al: A metalloprotease-disintegrin participating in myoblast fusion. *Nature* 377:652, 1995.
31. Wakelam MJO: Inositol phospholipid metabolism and myoblast fusion. *Biochem J* 214:77, 1983.
32. Rash JE, Fambrough D: Ultrastructural and physiological correlates of cell coupling and cytoplasmic fusion during myogenesis in vitro. *Dev Biol* 30:166, 1973.
33. Ferrari G, Cusella-De Angelis G, Coletta M, et al: Muscle regeneration by bone marrow-derived myogenic progenitors. *Science* 279:1528, 1997.
34. Blau HM, Dhawan J, Pavlath GK: Myoblasts in pattern formation and gene therapy. *Trends Genet* 9:269, 1993.
35. Ozawa CR, Springer ML, Blau HM: A novel means of drug delivery: Myoblast-mediated gene therapy and regulatable retroviral vectors. *Annu Rev Pharmacol Toxicol* 40:295, 2000.
36. Partridge T: The current status of myoblast transfer. *Neurol Sci* 21:S939, 2000.
37. Kwiatkowski DJ, Mehl R, Izumo S, et al: Muscle is the major source of plasma gelsolin. *J Biol Chem* 263:8239, 1988.
38. Danowski BA, Imanaka-Yoshida K, Sanger JM, Sanger JW: Costameres are sites of force transmission to the substratum in adult rat cardiomyocytes. *J Cell Biol* 118:1411, 1992.
39. Nunzi G, Franzini-Armstrong C: Trabecular network in adult skeletal muscle. *J Ultrastruct Res* 73:21, 1980.

40. Price M: Striated muscle endosarcomeric and exosarcomeric lattice. *Adv Struct Biol* 1:175, 1991.
41. Cartwright J, Goldstein MA: Microtubules in soleus muscles of the postnatal and adult rat. *J Ultrastruct Res* 79:74, 1982.
42. Milner DJ, Mavroidis M, Weisleder N, Capetanaki Y: Desmin cytoskeleton linked to muscle mitochondrial distribution and respiratory function. *J Cell Biol* 150:1283, 2000.
43. Scopes RK: Characterization and study of sarcoplasmic proteins, in *The Physiology and Biochemistry of Muscle as a Food*. Vol 2. Madison, WI: University of Wisconsin Press, 1970; pp 471–492.
44. Masters C: Interactions between glycolytic enzymes and components of the cytomatrix. *J Cell Biol* 99:222s–225s, 1984.
45. Chowrashi P, Mittal B, Sanger JM, Sanger JW: Amorphin is phosphorylase; phosphorylase is an alpha-actinin-binding protein. *Cell Motil Cytoskel* 53:125–135, 2002.
46. Devlin RB, Emerson CP: Coordinate regulation of contractile protein synthesis during myoblast differentiation. *Cell* 13:599, 1978.
47. Epstein HF, Fischman DA: Molecular analysis of protein assembly in muscle development. *Science* 251:1039, 1991.
48. Morkin E: Postnatal muscle fiber assembly: Localization of newly synthesized myofibrillar proteins. *Science* 167:1499, 1970.
49. Kelly DE: Myofibrillogenesis and Z-band differentiation. *Anat Rec* 163:403–426, 1969.
50. Boyd JD: Development of striated muscle, in Bourne GH (ed): *Structure and Function of Muscle*. Vol 1. New York: Academic Press; 1960, p63.
51. Engel WK, Horvath B: Myofibril formation in cultured skeletal muscle cells studied with antimyosin fluorescent antibody. *J Exp Zool* 144:209, 1960.
52. Wang SM, Greaser ML, Schultz E, et al: Studies on cardiac myofibrillogenesis with antibodies to titin, actin, tropomyosin, and myosin. *J Cell Biol* 107:1075, 1988.
53. Glacy SD: Pattern and time course of rhodamine-actin incorporation in cardiac myocytes. *J Cell Biol* 96:1164, 1983.
54. Sanger JW, Mittal B, Sanger JM: Analysis of myofibrillar structure and assembly using fluorescent labeled contractile proteins. *J Cell Biol* 98:825, 1984.
55. Sanger JM, Mittal B, Pochapin M, et al: Myofibrillogenesis in living cells microinjected with fluorescently labeled alpha-actinin. *J Cell Biol* 102:2053, 1986.
56. Sanger JM, Mittal B, Pochapin M, et al: Observations of microfilament bundles in living cells microinjected with fluorescently labeled contractile proteins. *J Cell Sci* (suppl 5):17, 1986.
57. Dome JS, Mittal B, Pochapin MB, et al: Incorporation of fluorescently labeled actin and tropomyosin into muscle cells. *Cell Diff* 23:37, 1988.
58. Sanger JW, Chowrashi P, Shaner NC, et al: Myofibrillogenesis in skeletal muscle cells. *Clin Orthop Rel Res* 403S:S153, 2002.
59. Sanger JW, Sanger JM: Green fluorescent proteins improve myofibril research. *Biophoton Int* 8:44, 2001.
60. Rhee D, Sanger JM, Sanger JW: The premyofibril: Evidence for its role in myofibrillogenesis. *Cell Motil Cytoskel* 28:1, 1994.
61. Imanaka-Yoshida K, Knudsen KA, Linask KK: N-Cadherin is required for the differentiation and initial myofibrillogenesis of chick cardiomyocytes. *Cell Motil Cytoskel* 39:52, 1998.
61a. Du A, Sanger JM, Linask KK, Sanger JW: Myfibrillogenesis in the first cardiomyocytes formed from isolated quail precardiac mesoderm. *Dev Biol* 57:382,2003.
62. Komiyama M, Zhou ZH, Maruyama K, Shimada Y: Spatial relationship of nebulin relative to other myofibrillar proteins during myogenesis in embryonic chick skeletal muscle cells in vitro. *J Musc Res Cell Motil* 13:48, 1992.
63. Moncman CL, Wang K: A 107 kD nebulin like protein in cardiac muscle. *Cell Motil Cytoskel* 32:205, 1995.
64. Schafer DA, Waddle JA, Cooper JA: Localization of CapZ during myofibrillogenesis in cultured chicken muscle. *Cell Motil Cytoskel* 25:317, 1993.
65. Almenar-Queralt A, Gregorio CC, Fowler VM: Tropomodulin assembles early in myofibrillogenesis in chick skeletal muscle: Evidence that thin filaments rearrange to form striated myofibrils. *J Cell Sci* 112:1111, 1999.
66. Dabiri GA, Turnacioglu KK, Sanger JM, et al: Myofibrillogenesis in living embryonic cardiomyocytes. *Proc Natl Acad Sci USA* 94:9493, 1997.
67. Sanger JW, Sanger JM: Myofibrillogenesis in cardiac muscle cells, in Dube D (ed): *Myofibrillogenesis*. New York: Springer-Verlag. 2001, pp; 3–20.
68. Holtzer H, Hijikata T, Lin ZX, et al: Independent assembly of 1.6 micron long bipolar MHC filaments and I-Z-I bodies. *Cell Struct Func* 22:83, 1997.
69. Hill CS, Duran S, Lin Z, et al: Titin and myosin, but not desmin, are linked during myofibrillogenesis in postmitotic multinucleated myoblasts. *J Cell Biol* 103:2185, 1986.
70. Sanger JW, Ayoob JC, Chowrashi P et al: Assembly of myofibrils in cardiac muscle cells. *Adv Exp Med Biol* 481: 89, 2000.
71. Dlugosz AA, Antin PB, Nachmias VT, et al: The relationship between stress fiber-like structures and nascent myofibrils in cultured cardiac myocytes. *J Cell Biol* 99:2268, 1984.
72. Sanger JM, Dabiri G, Mittal B, et al: Disruption of microfilament organization in living nonmuscle cells by microinjection of plasma vitamin D-binding protein or DNase I. *Proc Natl Acad Sci USA* 87:5474, 1990.
73. Fallon JR, Nachmias VT: Localization of cytoplasmic and skeletal myosins in developing muscle cells by double immunofluorescence. *J Cell Biol* 87:237, 1980.
74. Conrad AH, Jaffredo T, Conrad GWC: Differential localization of cytoplasmic myosin II isoforms A and B in avian interphase and dividing embryonic and immortalized cardiomyocytes and other cell types in vitro. *Cell Motil Cytoskel* 31:93, 1995.
75. Lu MH, DiLullo C, Schultheiss T, et al: The vinculin/sarcomeric-alpha-actinin/alpha-actin nexus in cultured cardiac myocytes. *J Cell Biol* 117:1007, 1992.
76. Ehler E, Rothen BM, Hammerle SP, et al: Myofibrillogenesis in the developing chicken heart assembly of Z-disk, M-line and the thick filaments. *J Cell Sci* 112:1529, 1999.
77. Ferrari MB, Ribbeck K, Hagler DJ, Spitzer NC: A calcium signaling cascade essential for myosin thick filament assembly in Xenopus myocytes. *J Cell Biol* 141:1349, 1998.
78. Morgan JE, Beauchamp JR, Pagel CN, et al: Myogenic cell lines derived from transgenic mice carrying a thermolabile T antigen: A model system for the derivation of tissue-specific and mutation-specific cell lines. *Dev Biol* 162:486, 1994.
79. Williams PE, Goldspink G: Longitudinal growth of striated muscle fibres. *J Cell Sci* 9:751, 1971
80. Williams PE, Goldspink G: Changes in sarcomere length and physiological properties in immobilized muscle. *J Anat* 127:459, 1978.
81. Jahromi SS, Charlton MP: Transverse sarcomere splitting. A possible means of longitudinal growth in crab muscles. *J Cell Biol* 80:736, 1979.
82. Jockusch BN, Bubeck P, Giehl P, et al: The molecular architecture of focal adhesions. *Annu Rev Cell Dev Biol* 11:379, 1995.
83. Mondello MR, Bramanti P, Cutroneo G, et al: Immunolocalization of the costameres in human skeletal muscle: Confocal scanning laser microscope investigations. *Anat Rec* 245:481–487, 1996.
84. Tidball JG, O'Halloran T, Burridge K: Talin at myotendinous junction. *J Cell Biol* 103:1465, 1986.
85. Craig SW, Pardo JV: Gamma actin, spectrin, and intermediate filament proteins colocalize with vinculin at costameres, myofibril-to-sarcolemma attachment sites. *Cell Motil* 3:449, 1983.
86. Pardo JV, Siliciano JD, Craig SW: A vinculin-containing cortical lattice in skeletal muscle: Transverse lattice elements ("costameres") mark sites of attachment between myofibrils and sarcolemma. *Proc Natl Acad Sci USA* 80:1008–1012.
87. Bozyczko D, Decker C, Muschler J, Horwitz AF: Integrin on developing and adult skeletal muscle. *Exp Cell Res* 183:72, 1989.
88. Pierobon-Bormoli S: Transverse sarcomere filamentous systems: "Z- and M-cables." *J Muscle Res Cell Motil* 2:401, 1981.
89. Schultheiss T, Lin ZX, Lu MH, et al: Differential distribution of subsets of myofibrillar proteins in cardiac nonstriated and striated myofibrils. *J Cell Biol* 110:1159, 1990.
90. Barstead RJ, Waterstone RH: Vinculin is essential for muscle function in the nematode. *J Cell Biol* 114:715, 1991.
91. Shiraishi I, Simpson DG, Carver W, et al: Vinculin is an essential component for normal myofibrillar arrangement in fetal mouse cardiac myocytes. *J Mol Cell Cardiol* 29:2041, 1997.
92. Volk T, Fessler LI, Fessler JH: A role for integrin in the formation of sarcomeric cytoarchitecture. *Cell* 63:525, 1990.
93. Fassler R, Rohwedel J, Maltsev V, et al: Differentiation and integrity of cardiac muscle cells are impaired in the absence of beta-1 integrin. *J Cell Sci* 109:2989, 1996.
94. Goldstein MA, Cartwright J: Microtubules in adult mammalian muscle, in Dowben RM, Shay JW (eds): *Cell and Muscle Motility*. New York: Plenum Press; 1982, pp 85–92.
95. Warren RH: Microtubular organization in elongating myogenic cells. *J Cell Biol* 63:550, 1968.
96. Mangan ME, Olmsted JB: A muscle-specific variant of microtubule-associated protein 4 (MAP4) is required in myogenesis. *Development* 122:771, 1996.
97. Gundersen GG, Khawaja S, Bulinski C: Generation of a stable posttranslationally modified microtubule array is an early event in myogenic differentiation. *J Cell Biol* 109:2275, 1989.
98. Spencer JA, Eliazer S, Ilaria RL, et al: Regulation of microtubule dynamics and myogenic differentiation by MURF, a striated muscle ring-finger protein. *J Cell Biol* 150:771, 2000.
99. Ishikawa H, Bischoff R, Holtzer H: Mitosis and intermediate-sized filaments in developing skeletal muscle. *J Cell Biol* 38:538, 1968.
100. Bennett GS, Fellini SA, Toyama Y, Holtzer H: Redistribution of intermediate filament subunits during skeletal myogenesis and maturation in vitro. *J Cell Biol* 82:577, 1979.
101. Saitoh O, Arai T, Obinata T: Distribution of microtubules and other cytoskeletal filaments during myotube elongation as revealed by fluorescence microscopy. *Cell Tissue Res* 252:263, 1988.
102. Gard D, Lazarides E: The synthesis and distribution of desmin and vimentin during myogenesis. *Cell* 19:263, 1980.
103. Small JV, Furst DO, Thornell LE: The cytoskeletal lattice of muscle cells. *Eur J Biochem* 208:559, 1992.
104. Boudriau S, Vincent M, Cote CH, Rogers PA: Cytoskeletal structure of skeletal muscle: Identification of an intricate exosarcomeric microtubule

lattice in slow-and-fast twitch muscle fibers. *J Histochem Cytochem* 41:1013, 1993.
105. Lazarides E: Intermediate filaments as mechanical integrators of cellular space. *Nature* 283:249, 1980.
106. O'Neill A, Williams MW, Resneck WG, et al: Sarcolemmal organization in skeletal muscle lacking desmin: Evidence for cytokeratins associated with the membrane skeleton at costameres. *Mol Biol Cell* 13:2347, 2002.
107. Shah SB, Peters D, Jordan KA, et al: Sarcomere number regulation maintained after immobilization in desmin-null mouse skeletal muscle. *J Exp Biol* 204:1703, 2001.
108. Sam M, Shah S, Friden J, et al: Desmin knockout muscles generate lower stress and are less vulnerable to injury compared with wild-type muscles. *Am J Physiol Cell Physiol* 279:C1116, 2000.
109. Shah SB, Su F-C, Jordan K, et al: Evidence for increased myofibrillar mobility in desmin-null mouse skeletal muscle. *J Exp Biol* 205:321, 2002.
110. Hijikata T, Murakami T, Imamura M, et al: Plectin is a linker of intermediate filaments to Z-discs in skeletal muscle. *J Cell Sci* 112:867, 1999.
111. Reipert S, Steinboeck F, Fischer I, et al: Association of mitochondria with plectin and desmin intermediate filaments in striated muscle. *Exp Cell Res* 252:479, 1999.
112. Dalpe G, Mathieu M, Comtois A, et al: Dystonin-deficient mice exhibit an intrinsic muscle weakness and an instability of skeletal muscle cytoarchitecture. *Dev Biol* 210:367, 1999.
113. Zak R, Martin AF, Prior G, Rabinowitz M: Comparison of turnover of several myofibrillar proteins and critical evaluation of double isotope method. *J Biol Chem* 252:3430–3435, 1977.
114. Isaacs WB, Kim IS, Fulton AB: Biosynthesis of titin in cultured skeletal muscle cells. *J Cell Biol* 109:2189–2195, 1989.
115. Franchi LL, Murdoch A, Brown WE, et al: Subcellular localization of newly incorporated myosin in rabbit fast skeletal muscle undergoing stimulation-induced transformation. *J Muscle Res Cell Motil* 11:227, 1990.
116. Wenderoth MP, Eisenberg BR: Incorporation of nascent myosin heavy chains into thick filaments of cardiac myocytes in thyroid-treated rabbits. *J Cell Biol* 108:2771, 1987.
117. McKenna NM, Meigs JB, Wang YL: Identical distribution of fluorescently labeled brain and muscle actins in living fibroblasts and myocytes. *J Cell Biol* 100:292, 1985.
118. McKenna NM, Meigs JB, Wang YL: Exchangeability of alpha-actinin in living cardiac fibroblasts and muscle cells. *J Cell Biol* 101:2223, 1985.
119. Mittal B, Sanger JM, Sanger JW: Visualization of myosin in living cells. *J Cell Biol* 105:1753–1760, 1987.
120. Mittal B, Sanger JM, Sanger JW: Binding and distribution of filamin in permeabilized and living non-muscle and muscle cells. *Cell Motil Cytoskeleton* 8:345–359,1987.
121. Imanaka-Yoshida K, Danowski BA, Sanger JM, Sanger JW: Contractile protein dynamics of myofibrils in paired adult rat cardiomyocytes. *Cell Motil Cytoskel* 26:301.1993.
122. Horvath BZ, Gaetjens E: Immunochemical studies on the light chain from skeletal muscle myosin. *Biochem Biophys Acta* 263:779, 1972.
123. Shimizu N, Obinata T: Actin concentration and monomer-polymer ratio in developing chicken skeletal muscle. *J Biochem (Tokyo)* 99:751, 1986.
124. Martonosi A: *The Development of Sarcoplasmic Reticulum*. Sydney, Australia: Harwood Academic Publishers; 2001.
125. Volpe P, Krause KH, Hashimoto S: "Calciosome," a cytoplasmic organelle: The inositol 1,4,5-trisphosphate-sensitive Ca^{2+} store of non muscle cells? *Proc Natl Acad Sci USA* 85:1091–1095, 1988.
126. Krause KH, Pittet D, Volpe P, et al: Calciosome, a sarcoplasmic reticulum-like organelle involved in intracellular Ca^{2+}-handling by non-muscle cells: Studies in human neutrophils and HL-60 cells. *Cell Calcium* 10:351–361, 1989.
127. Pozzan T, Volpe P, Zorzato F, et al: The Ins(1,4,5)P3-sensitive Ca^{2+} store of non-muscle cells: Endoplasmic reticulum or calciosomes? *J Exp Biol* 139:181–193, 1988.
128. Pozzan T, Rizzuto R, Volpe P, et al: Molecular and cellular physiology of intracellular calcium stores. *Physiol Rev* 74:595–636, 1994.
129. Rossier MF, Putney JW Jr: The identity of the calcium-storing, inositol 1,4,5-triphosphate-sensitive organelle in non-muscle cells: Calciosome, endoplasmic reticulum... or both? *Trends Neurosci* 14:310–314, 1991.
130. Villa A, Podini P, Nori A, et al: The endoplasmic reticulum-sarcoplasmic reticulum connection. II. Postnatal differentiation of the sarcoplasmic reticulum in skeletal muscle fibers. *Exp Cell Res* 209:140, 1993.
131. Volpe P, Villa A, Podini P, et al: The endoplasmic reticulum–sarcoplasmic reticulum connection: Distribution of endoplasmic reticulum markers in the sarcoplasmic reticulum of skeletal muscle fibers. *Proc Natl Acad Sci USA* 89:6142, 1992.
132. Kaprielian Z, Fambrough DM: Expression of fast and slow isoforms of the Ca^{2+} ATPase in developing chick skeletal muscle. *Dev Biol* 124:490, 1987.
133. Zubrzycka E, MacLennan DH: Assembly of the sarcoplasmic reticulum: Biosynthesis of calsequestrin in rat skeletal muscle cell culture. *J Biol Chem* 251:7733, 1976.
134. Holland PC, MacLennan DH: Assembly of the sarcoplasmic reticulum: Biosynthesis of the adenosine triphosphatase in rat skeletal muscle culture. *J Biol Chem* 251:2030, 1976.
135. Marks AR, Taubman MB, Saito A, et al: The ryanodine receptor/junctional channel complex is regulated by growth factors in a myogenic cell line. *J Cell Biol* 114:303, 1991.
136. Airey JA, Borisy MD, Sutko JL: Ryanodine receptor is expressed during differentiation in the muscle cell lines BC3H1 and C2c12. *Dev Biol* 148:365, 1991.
137. Arai M, Otsu K, MacLennan DH, et al: Regulation of sarcoplasmic reticulum gene expression during cardiac and skeletal muscle development. *Am J Physiol* 262:C614, 1992.
138. Flucher BE, Takekura H, Franzini-Armstrong C: Development of the excitation-contraction coupling apparatus in skeletal muscle: Association of sarcoplasmic reticulum and transverse tubules with myofibrils. *Dev Biol* 160:135–147, 1993.
139. Flucher BE, Andrews SB, Daniels MP: Molecular organization of transverse tubule/sarcoplasmic reticulum junctions during development of excitation-contraction coupling in skeletal muscle. *Mol Biol Cell* 5:1105, 1994.
140. Franzini-Armstrong C, Jorgensen AO: Structure and development of e-e coupling units in skeletal muscle. *Annu Rev Physiol* 56:509, 1994.
141. Sutko JO, Airey JA, Murakam K, et al: Foot protein isoforms are expressed at different times during embryonic chick skeletal muscle development. *J Cell Biol* 113:793, 1991.
142. Schiaffino S, Margreth A: Coordinated development of the sarcoplasmic reticulum and T system during postnatal differentiation of rat skeletal muscle. *J Cell Biol* 41:855, 1969.
143. Varga S, Marrtonosi A: Giant sarcoplasmic reticulum vesicles—A study of membrane morphogenesis. *J Muscle Res Cell Motil* 13:497, 1992.
144. Protasi F, Sun, X-H, Franzini-Armstrong C: Formation and maturation of calcium release units in developing and adult avian myocardium. *Dev Biol* 173:265, 1996.
145. Takekura H, Sun X-H, Franzini-Armstrong C: Development of the excitation-contraction coupling apparatus in skeletal muscle: Peripheral and internal calcium release units are formed sequentially. *J Muscle Res Cell Motil* 15:102, 1994.
146. Carl SL, Felix K, Caswell AH, et al: Immunolocalization of triadin, DHP receptors, and ryanodine receptors in adult and developing skeletal muscle of rats. *Muscle Nerve* 18:1232, 1995.
147. Yuan S, Arnold W, Jorgensen AO: Biogenesis of transverse tubules and triads: Immunolocalization of the 1,4-dihydropyridine receptor, TS28, and the ryanodine receptor in rabbit skeletal muscle developing in situ. *J Cell Biol* 112:289, 1991.
148. Jorgensen AO, Kalnins VI, Zubrzycka E, et al: Assembly of the sarcoplasmic reticulum: Localization by immuno fluorescence of sarcoplasmic reticulum proteins in differentiating rat skeletal muscle cell cultures. *J Cell Biol* 74:287, 1977.
149. Flucher BE, Andrews SB, Fleischer S et al: Triad formation: Organization and function of the sarcoplasmic reticulum calcium release channel and triadin in normal and dysgenic muscle in vitro. *J Cell Biol* 123:1161, 1993.
150. Powell JA, Petherbridge L, Flucher BE: Formation of triads without the dihydropyridine receptor alpha subunits in cell lines from dysgenic skeletal muscle. *J Cell Biol* 134:375, 1996.
151. Franzini-Armstrong C, Pincon-Raymond M, Rieger F: Muscle fibers from dysgenic mouse in vivo lack a surface component of peripheral couplings. *Dev Biol* 146:364, 1991.
152. Takekura H, Nishi M, Noda T, et al. Abnormal junctions between surface membrane and sarcoplasmic reticulum in skeletal muscle with a mutation targeted for the ryanodine receptor. *Proc Natl Acad Sci USA* 92:3381, 1995.
153. Takekura H, Franzini-Armstrong C: Correct targeting of dihydropyridine receptors and triadin in dyspedic mouse skeletal muscle in vivo. *Dev Dynam* 21:372, 1999.
154. Gerster U, Neuhuber B, Groschner K, et al: Current modulation and membrane targeting of the calcium channel alpha1C subunit are independent functions of the beta subunit. *J Physiol* 517:353, 1999.
155. Neuhuber B, Gerster U, Doring F, et al: Association of calcium channel alpha1S and beta1a subunits is required for the targeting of beta1a but not of alpha1S into skeletal muscle triads. *Proc Natl Acad Sci USA* 95:5015–5020, 1998.
156. Flucher BE, Phillips JL, Powell JA. Dihydropyridine receptor alpha subunits in normal and dysgenic muscle in vitro: Expression of alpha 1 is required for proper targeting and distribution of alpha 2. *J Cell Biol* 115:1345, 1991.
157. Flucher BE, Kasielke N, Grabner M: The triad targeting signal of the skeletal muscle calcium channel is localized in the COOH terminus of the alpha(1S) subunit. *J Cell Biol* 151:467, 2000.
158. Gatti G, Podini P, Meldolesi J: Overexpression of calsequestrin in L6 myoblasts: Formation of endoplasmic reticulum subdomains and their evolution into discrete vacuoles where aggregates of the protein are specifically accumulated. *Mol Biol Cell* 8:1789, 1997.

159. Sato Y, Ferguson DG, Sako H, et al: Cardiac-specific overexpression of mouse cardiac calsequestrin is associated with depressed cardiovascular function and hypertrophy in transgenic mice. *J Biol Chem* 273:28470, 1998.
160. Jones LR, Suzuki YJ, Wang W: Regulation of Ca2+ signaling in transgenic mouse cardiac myocytes overexpressing calsequestrin. *J Clin Invest* 101:1385, 1998.
161. Thomas K, Navarro J, Benson RJ, et al: Newly synthesized calsequestrin, destined for the sarcoplasmic reticulum, is contained in early/intermediate Golgi-derived clathrin-coated vesicles. *J Biol Chem* 264:3140, 1989.
162. Nori A, Valle G, Massimino ML, et al: Targeting of calsequestrin to the sarcoplasmic reticulum of skeletal muscle upon deletion of its glycosylation site. *Exp Cell Res* 265:104, 2001.
163. Nori A, Gola E, Tosato S, et al: Targeting of calsequestrin to sarcoplasmic reticulum after deletion of its carboxy terminus. *Am J Physiol* 277:C974, 1999.
164. Nori A, Furlan S, Patiri F, et al: Site-directed mutagenesis and deletion of three phosphorylation sites of calsequestrin of skeletal muscle sarcoplasmic reticulum. Effects on intracellular targeting. *Exp Cell Res* 260:40, 2000.
165. Kelly AM: Sarcoplasmic reticulum and t tubules in differentiating rat skeletal muscle. *J Cell Biol* 49:335, 1971.
166. Takekura H, Flucher B, Franzini-Armstrong C: Sequenstial docking, molecular differentiation and positioning of T-tubule/SR junctions in developing mouse skeletal muscle. *Dev Biol* 239:204, 2001.
167. Flucher BE, Phillips JL, Powell JA, et al: Coordinated development of myofibrils, sarcoplasmic reticulum and transverse tubules in normal and dysgenic mouse skeletal muscle in vivo and in vitro. *Dev Biol* 150:266, 1992.
168. Protasi F, Takekura H, Wang Y, et al: RYR1 and RYR3 have different roles in the assembly of calcium release units of skeletal muscle. *Biophys J* 79:2494, 2000.
169. Felder E, Allen PD, Protasi F, et al: SR-surface membrane docking in the absence of dihydropyridine receptors and ryanodine receptors. *Biophys J* 82:3144, 2002.
170. Flucher BE, Franzini-Armstrong C: Formation of junctions involved in excitation-contraction coupling in skeletal and cardiac muscle. *Proc Natl Acad Sci USA* 93:265, 1996.
171. Takeshima H, Komazaki S, Nishi M, et al: Junctophilins: A novel family of junctional membrane complex proteins. *Mol Cell* 6:11, 2000.
172. Yuan S, Arnold W, Jorgensen AO: Biogenesis of transverse tubules: Immunocytochemical localization of a transverse tubular protein (TS28) and a sarcolemmal protein (SL50) in rabbit skeletal musde in situ. *J Cell Biol* 110:1187, 1990.
173. Ishikawa H: Formation of elaborate networks of T-system tubules in cultured skeletal muscle with special reference to the T system formation. *J Cell Biol* 38:51, 1968.
174. Parton RG, Way M, Zorzi N, et al: Caveolin-3 associates with developing T-tubules during muscle differentiation. *J Cell Biol* 136:137, 1997.
175. Galbiati F, Engelman JA, Volonte D, et al: Caveolin-3 null mice show a loss of caveolae, changes in the microdomain distribution of the dystrophin-glycoprotein complex, and T-tubule abnormalities. *J Biol Chem* 276:21425, 2001.
176. Walker SM, Schrodt GR, Bingham M: Electron microscope study of the sarcoplasmic reticulum at the Z line level in skeletal muscle fibers of newborn rats. *J Cell Biol* 39:469, 1968.
177. Edge MB: Development of the apposed sarcoplasmic reticulum at the T system and sarcolemma and the change in orientation of triads in rat skeletal muscle. *Dev Biol* 2:634, 1970.
178. Schiaffino S, Cantini M, Sartore S: T-system formation in cultured rat skeletal tissue. *Tissue Cell* 9:437, 1977.
179. Veratti E: Investigations on the fine structure of striated muscle fiber. *J Biophys Biochem Cytol* 10(suppl):1, 1961.
180. Flucher BE: Structural analysis of muscle development: Transverse tubules, sarcoplasmic reticulum and the triad. *Dev Biol* 154:245, 1992.
181. Bagnato P, Barone V, Giacomello E, et al: Binding of an ankyrin-1 isoform to Obscurin suggests a molecular link between the sarcoplasmic reticulum and the myofibrils in striated muscles. *J Cell Biol* 160:245, 2003.
182. Kontrogianni-Konstantopoulos A, Jones EM, vanRossum DB: Obscurin is a ligand for small ankyrin in skeletal muscle. *Mol Biol Cell* 14:1138, 2003.

Chapter 3
Satellite and Stem Cells in Muscle Regeneration

RICHARD BISCHOFF
CLARA FRANZINI-ARMSTRONG

The Satellite Cell
    SATELLITE CELLS ARE UBIQUITOUS IN ADULT SKELETAL MUSCLE
    SATELLITE CELLS ARISE FROM MYOGENIC CELLS DURING EMBRYOGENESIS
    SATELLITE CELLS BECOME SPECIALIZED DURING DEVELOPMENT
    SATELLITE CELLS DIFFER FROM EMBRYONIC MYOGENIC CELLS

Satellite Cell Dynamics
    SATELLITE CELLS AS COMMITTED STEM CELLS

Other Myogenic Stem Cells
    SATELLITE CELLS CAN MIGRATE AND CROSS THE BASAL LAMINA
    SATELLITE CELLS IN CULTURE
    SATELLITE CELLS MODULATE THEIR CELL CYCLE IN RESPONSE TO GROWTH FACTORS

Regeneration of Muscle
    NEW MYONUCLEI ARISE FROM SATELLITE CELLS, BUT SURVIVING MYOFIBERS AID IN HEALING
    THE REGENERATING RESPONSE DEPENDS ON THE TYPE OF INJURY
    REMOVAL OF NECROTIC DEBRIS FACILITATES REGENERATION
    REGENERATION TAKES PLACE WITHIN EMPTY ENDOMYSIAL TUBES
    MUSCLE INJURY STIMULATES THE ACTIVATION AND PROLIFERATION OF SATELLITE CELLS

Contribution of Stem Cells Other Than Satellite Cells to Muscle Growth and Regeneration

The Influence of Innervation and Activity on Regeneration
    MOTOR NERVES INFLUENCE THE ACTIVITY OF SATELLITE CELLS
    MUSCLE OVERUSE PRODUCES SATELLITE CELL ACTIVATION

Progress in understanding the early events of skeletal muscle regeneration was accelerated by the discovery of satellite cells in 1961.[1,2] Prior to this time it was recognized that mononucleated myoblasts have a role in regeneration, but the origin of these cells was unknown. Satellite cells are the major source of myogenic cells in adult mammalian muscle; they proliferate following muscle trauma and form new myofibers through a process equivalent to embryonal myogenesis. In addition to satellite cells, a smaller number of mononucleated stem cells capable of proliferation and of differentiation into a variety of progenies populate the muscle. These constitute a dynamic and partially transient population. Proliferation of satellite cells is evoked not only by acute muscle injury but also by overuse. In fact, it seems likely that the extent of satellite cell activity, perhaps even as a part of normal muscle physiology, has been underestimated. Further interest in satellite cells arises from their potential use in transplant therapy for neuromuscular diseases.[3] The recent interest in stem cells other than satellite cells arises from their high proliferation potential and malleability, which is of importance in possible therapeutic strategies.

This chapter focuses on the properties and activities of satellite and other stem cells and their behavior during muscle regeneration. Several excellent and comprehensive reviews offer historical perspective and cover additional topics not stressed here.[4–14] The chronicle of satellite cells since their discovery is well documented in three symposium volumes sponsored by the Muscular Dystrophy Association.[3,15,16]

The Satellite Cell

SATELLITE CELLS ARE UBIQUITOUS IN ADULT SKELETAL MUSCLE

Definition and Structure

Satellite cells were first described in adult muscle, where they possess several distinctive features related to their normal state of quiescence. They are spindle-shaped cells with a central nucleus located very close to the outer surface of the muscle fibers (Fig. 3-1). The cells are located in a depression or groove, which may be very shallow or deeper, of the muscle fiber surface; they share a common basal lamina, so that the contour of the basal lamina covering both cells is continuous (Fig. 3-2). The gap between the plasmalemmae of the two cells is ~15 nm,[17,18] and this close apposition is maintained throughout the area of cell contact. The extracellular matrix closely binds the two cells together, so that when the muscle fiber shortens, the satellite cell also passively changes length (Fig. 3-3). However, there are no specialized junctional complexes between satellite cells of adult muscle and myofibers, and microelectrode recordings have failed to detect electrical coupling between them.[19] The cytoplasm of satellite cells is sparse and contains most of the common organelles, but in small numbers (Fig. 3-2).[17,18,20,21] Centrioles are commonly seen in satellite cells,[17,21,22] but they disappear after the cell fusion that occurs during myogenesis.[23]

The nucleus of the satellite cell is oval, often in line with adjacent myonuclei, and contains more heterochromatin than do the myonuclei. Although nuclei with large amounts of heterochromatin are considered to be inactive, the presence of some ribosomes, rough endoplasmic reticulum, and Golgi apparatus in the cytoplasm suggests that even mitotically dormant satellite cells have a modest synthetic program.

Satellite Cells Markers

In mammalian and avian muscle, myonuclei are at the cell periphery; even though the satellite cell nuclei are more heterochromatic than the myonuclei, distinction between the two is not reliable at the light microscope level. Various staining methods for light microscopy have been implemented for mammalian muscle[24–27] but have not been widely accepted. Identification at the electron microscope, based on the position under the basal lamina is reliable for the majority of the cells, but a few blood-derived cells may gain entry through the endomysial tube, particularly following myofiber damage (see "Regeneration of Muscle," below).[18,28] The cell from a denervated muscle illustrated in Fig. 3-4, for example, may be either a satellite cell that

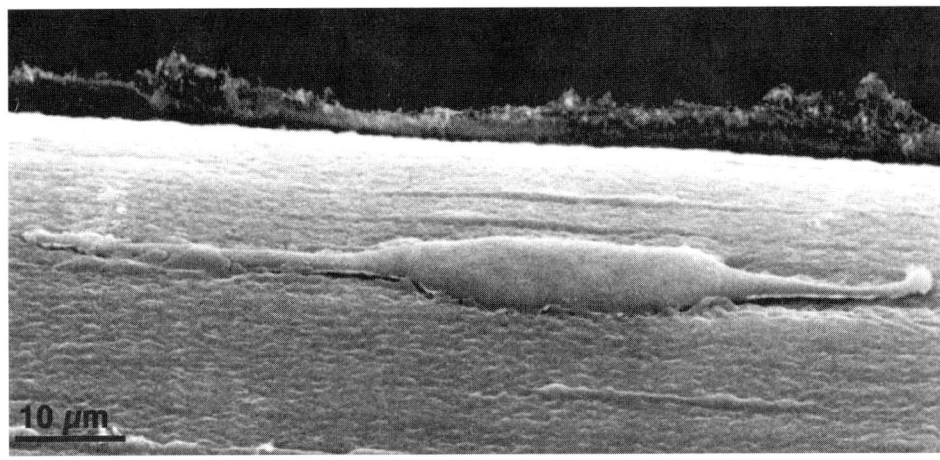

FIGURE 3-1. Scanning electron micrograph showing an elongated, spindle-shaped satellite cell on the surface of a frog muscle fiber. Basal and reticular laminae were eliminated by maceration after fixation. (*From Mazanet R et al: Dev. Biol. 93:22, 1982. Reproduced by permission.*)

has been activated or a cell of blood origin "invading" the endomysial tube.[18]

More promising is the relatively recent identification of satellite cell markers that can be used either for immunochemistry or cell sorting (Fig. 3-5).[29–31] The neural cell adhesion molecule (N-CAM)* is a large cell surface glycoprotein that exists in numerous isoforms.[32] Clear proof of the presence of N-CAM on satellite cells was obtained using a purified polyclonal antibody to chicken N-CAM, which binds to quiescent satellite cells identified ultrastructurally in adult rat muscle.[34] However, a monoclonal antibody against human N-CAM binds to proliferating satellite cells and myotubes in regenerating muscle but not to quiescent satellite cells.[33–36] Monoclonal antibody CD56 from a human leukemia cell immunogen[37,38] reacts with an isoform of N-CAM (CD34) that appears to be related to an antigen on natural killer T lymphocytes and to proliferating and quiescent human satellite cells and myotubes in vivo and in vitro.[37–42] CD34 is also present on the surface of "side population" cells in the interstitium.[43] Pax7 is a paired box transcription factor that was isolated as a gene specifically expressed in satellite cell–derived myoblasts and also in resident satellite cells.[44,45] Other markers of quiescent adult satellite cells are Myf5[40]; M-cadherin, located at the interface of satellite cells and muscle[30]; and syndecans, receptors for growth factors.[46] With the recent identification of other stem cells in muscle—i.e., the "side population" cells (see below)—criteria for satellite cell identification have become more stringent. For example, satellite cells are negative for Sca-1 and CD45, markers present on pluripotential and hematopoietic stem cells, respectively.[43]

Distribution and Frequency

Satellite cells are present in all vertebrates examined, but their frequency varies widely depending on location, muscle type, age, and species. Satellite cells constitute 3 to 10 percent of the subbasal lamina population of muscle nuclei (reviewed in Ref. 18).

*A list of the abbreviations used in this chapter is given at the end of the chapter.

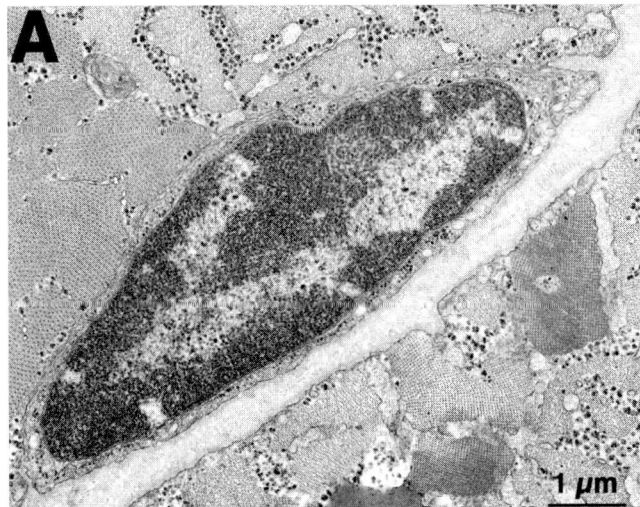 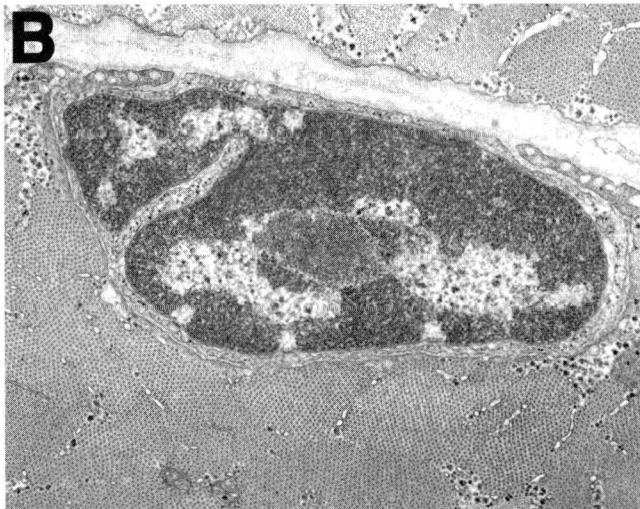

FIGURE 3-2. Profiles of satellite cells at the periphery of frog skeletal muscle fibers. The heterochromatic nucleus and scarce cytoplasm are typical of inactive cells. Cells in both images are covered by the muscle fiber's basal lamina, but the cell at right is in a deeper groove. (*From de Maruenda and Franzini-Armstrong.[18] Reproduced by permission.*)

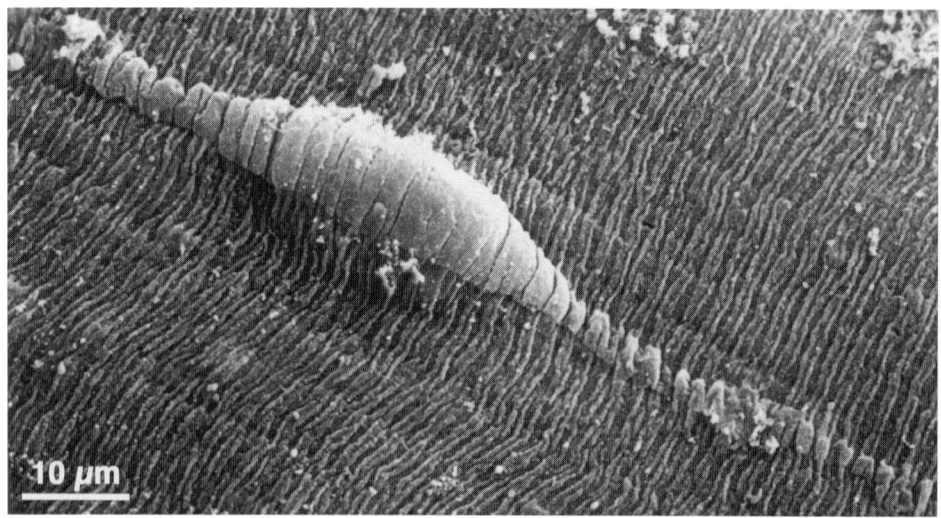

FIGURE 3-3. Detail of a satellite cell on the surface of a frog muscle fiber. The image is similar to Fig. 3-1, but in this case the muscle fiber greatly shortened before fixation, pulling the surface of the muscle cell into deep ridges and compressing the satellite cell along its length. (*From Mazanet et al: Dev Biol 93:22,1982.*)

Along the myofiber. The frequency of satellite cells is about 20-fold greater at the neuromuscular junction than at nonjunctional regions in both adult rat[47,48] and human[49] muscle. Schwann cells covering the nerve ending (see Chap. 15) and satellite cells occupy analogous compartments within the basal lamina of their respective fibers, but they are topologically separated from one another by the fusion of the muscle and nerve basal laminae at the edge of the myoneural junction (Fig. 3-6). Nevertheless, direct plasmalemmal contact between Schwann cell and satellite cell has been reported in developing rats.[49] There are no known functional relationships between satellite cells and the neuromuscular junction, although innervation of the myofiber has been reported to influence proliferation of associated satellite cells.

Muscle type. The frequency of satellite cells is different in fast and slow muscle fibers of the adult rat. In fast-twitch muscle, satellite cells make up 1 to 4 percent of nuclei within the basal lamina, while slow-twitch muscle contains three to four times as many.[50–52] The difference is even greater in terms of the number of satellite cells per unit muscle tissue, since the nucleus:cytoplasm ratio is lower in fast-twitch muscle.[50,51] For example, the adult soleus (slow) contains about 5000 satellite cells per cubic millimeter, while the tibialis (fast) contains about 900.[50] Factors that govern satellite cell frequency are not known, but they apparently are expressed during muscle maturation, since there is little difference at birth. The size of the myofiber per se is probably not important, nor are metabolic properties, since certain glycolytic myofibers (type IIB) have as many satellite cells as oxidative myofibers.[51] Similar findings have been reported for other species as well.[49,52–56]

Age. Satellite cells are most abundant during early development, when they contribute to muscle growth; thereafter, they decline in frequency in two stages. First, there is a sharp postnatal drop to the adult level, which is reached at about age 2 months in mice and 9 years in humans.[56–59] During this period in the mouse, satellite cells decline from about 32 percent of sublaminal nuclei at birth to less than 5 percent at 2 months. This decline mostly reflects the increase in myonuclei owing to fusion of satellite cell progeny during growth, but individual muscles vary in satellite cell population dynamics. In the rat extensor digitorum longus, for example, both the percentage and absolute number of satellite cells per muscle decline, but in the soleus the percentage declines while the absolute number remains constant.[52,60] Second, there is a smaller, gradual loss of satellite cells as senility approaches,[61,62] indicating limited proliferative potential.[63,64] Alternatively, there is evidence that some satellite cells may leave their sublaminal location during aging.[62]

SATELLITE CELLS ARISE FROM MYOGENIC CELLS DURING EMBRYOGENESIS

During myogenesis, muscle cells are grouped in clusters, consisting initially of primary myotubes and mononucleated myogenic cells and subsequently of a single primary

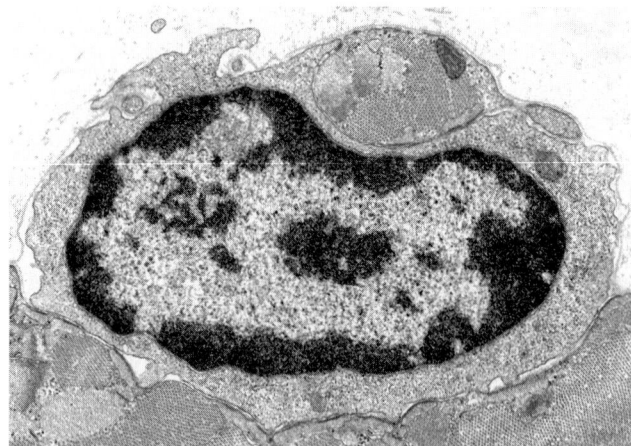

FIGURE 3-4. Cross section at the periphery of a frog muscle fiber that has been denervated. A mononucleated cell is caught in the process of crossing the basal lamina, but it is not clear in which direction it is moving. It is also not possible to tell whether this is a satellite cell or an invading blood-derived cell. (*From de Maruenda and Franzini-Armstrong.[18] Reproduced by permission.*)

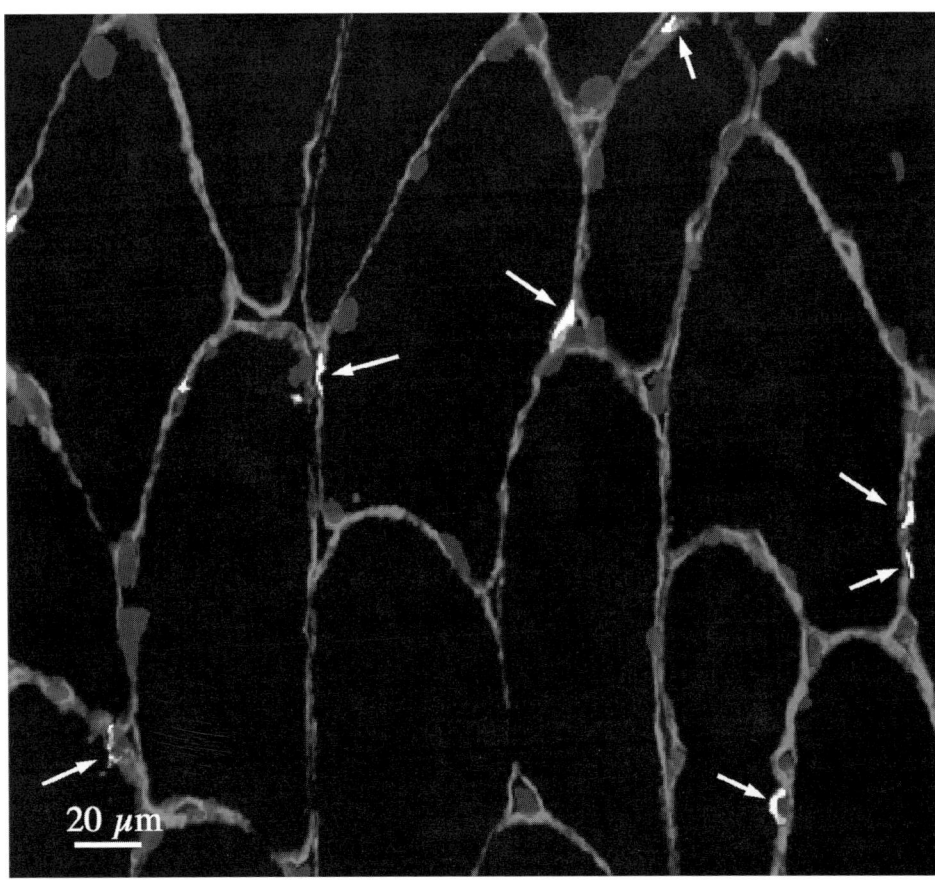

FIGURE 3-5. Cross section of the tibialis anterior from a rat, immunolabeled with antibodies against the satellite cell marker M-cadherin (*courtesy of A. Wernig*) and against dystrophin (*courtesy of L. Kunkel*). Brightly labeled satellite cells (arrows) are located in close proximity to the fiber surface delineated by a light gray line of labeled dystrophin. Nuclei, stained with DAPI, appear as dark gray shapes. (*Courtesy of D Fisher and TS Khurana.*)

myotube surrounded by secondary myotubes and mononucleated cells (see Chap. 4).[65] Eventually primary and secondary myotubes separate, but each bears adherent satellite cells under a common basal lamina. The two generations of myotubes form gap junctions briefly before separation.[66–68] Satellite cells proliferate during early development and later withdraw from the cell cycle and become quiescent. About 20 percent of rat satellite cells are labeled 1 h after a single injection of tritiated thymidine (^{3}H-TdR) at 2 weeks after birth.[69] Since generally DNA synthesis occupies about a third of the cell cycle, a labeling index of 20 percent indicates that most of the satellite cells are cycling at this time. By 3 weeks, however, the labeling index has dropped to around 5 percent[51,70] and satellite cells with heterochromatic nuclei (presumably quiescent) first become evident.[20] Satellite cell ontogeny in the chick presents a similar picture, but quiescent cells appear earlier in development.[71] Transplanted primary neonatal myoblasts can also give rise to functional satellite cells.[72] On the basis of the total lack of satellite cells in the Pax7 (–/–) mouse, it has been proposed that activation of this transcription factor is the step that separates satellite cells from other muscle-derived stem cells, restricting their future potential.[73] This would be consistent with the increased hematopoietic potential of mononucleated cells in the Pax7 (–/–) null muscle.

Satellite cells are often envisaged as becoming "trapped" beneath the basal lamina as it forms during development, implying that it is the basal lamina that binds the satellite cells to the myofiber surface. Instead, myogenic cells collect on the surface of myotubes even before a basal lamina forms, and it has been demonstrated that the cells have an adhesive affinity for myotubes that is maintained in the adult (see Fig. 3-3).[75] Furthermore, satellite cells appear able to migrate across the basal lamina in a variety of experimental conditions.[75–78] Clearly, the sublaminal position of satellite cells is elective, not compulsory.

SATELLITE CELLS BECOME SPECIALIZED DURING DEVELOPMENT

There is evidence of heterogeneity among myogenic cells during early development, and it is likely that this variation is transmitted to the satellite cells. Comprehensive

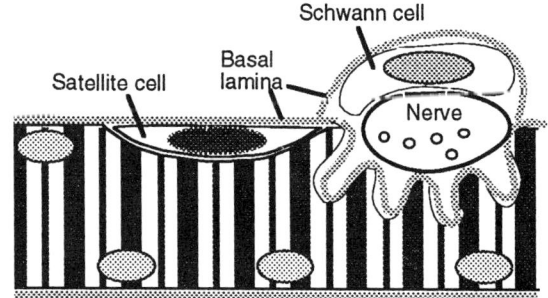

FIGURE 3-6. Diagram showing the position of satellite cells and Schwann cells in relation to the basal lamina at the myoneural junction.

studies of the requirements of myogenic cells for proliferation in low-density culture (clonal growth) have shown that there are at least three different classes of cells that arise in the chick embryo between days 3 and 12.[79–81] The appearance of one cell type requires functional innervation at about the period when myotubes first appear.[82,83] The expression of two muscle-specific antigens—H36, a cell surface glycoprotein, and desmin, a cytoskeletal protein—also differentiates early myogenic cell populations.[84] These early differences occur in presatellite cells, i.e., before the basal lamina forms, but they may be the basis of subsequent changes expressed in satellite cells. Another muscle-specific marker, B-enolase, is expressed in proliferating myogenic cells and alters its isoform type at about the time satellite cells first appear.[85]

SATELLITE CELLS DIFFER FROM EMBRYONIC MYOGENIC CELLS

Satellite cells and myogenic cells respond differently to certain phorbol esters that act as tumor promoters in vivo.[86–90] Myogenic cells resistant to phorbol ester first appear at about embryonic day 17 in the mouse,[88] which is about the same time the myofiber basal lamina forms.[91] Satellite cells from adult mouse cultured for 2 days express acetylcholine-activated membrane channels and bind alpha-bungarotoxin, while myogenic cells cultured under the same conditions are negative for both tests of acetylcholine receptors.[92,93] This difference, however, may simply reflect more rapid differentiation of satellite cells in vitro, since embryonal myoblasts do express receptors at 3 days in vitro.[92] Both the amount and type of acetylcholinesterase are different in myotubes derived from satellite cells compared with those from embryo-derived myogenic cells.[86,94]

Since the frequency and development of satellite cells varies depending on fiber type, it is possible that the cells carry information specified by fiber type and that this may be passed on to myotubes that differentiate in vitro (Fig. 3-7). This has been tested, with variable results (see also Chap. 4). In one study, satellite cells cultured from adult chicken fast or slow muscle form myotubes that express different myosin light chains but the same heavy chains.[95,96] However, monoclonal antibodies directed against myosin heavy chains showed that myotubes in high-density cultures from fast muscle contained only fast-type myosin, but myotubes from slow muscle made fast myosin (75 percent) and a combination of fast and slow myosins (25 percent).[97] Clonal growth showed that there are at least two different types of satellite cells in adult muscle. The commitment to make a particular type of myosin is not a stable property of the satellite cells, however, since prolonged proliferation in culture resulted in changes in the type of myosin expressed.[98] Since the antibodies used in these studies recognize only an epitope of the corresponding myosins, there is no assurance that the isoforms expressed in culture correspond to those expressed in vivo or that "fiber types" in vitro reflect those in vivo.[98] In addition, expression of differences in culture may be restricted to avian satellite cells, since rat satellite cells from fast or slow muscle make uniform myosin heavy and light chains as judged by biochemical and immunochemical analysis.[99] Still, these results taken together indicate clear dif-

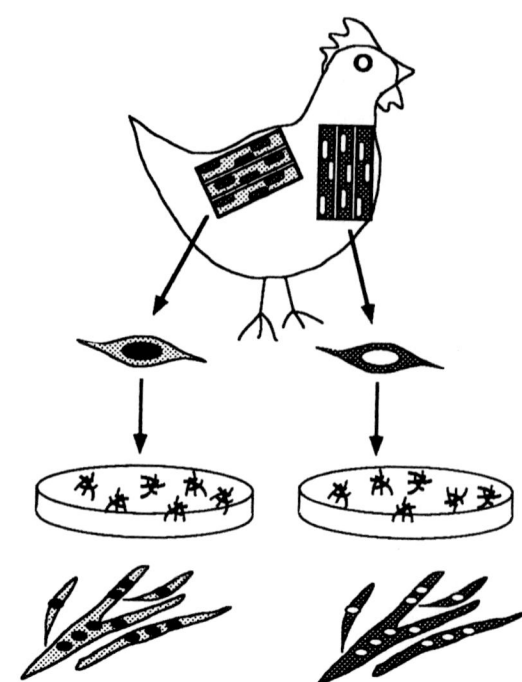

FIGURE 3-7. Diagram showing an experimental test for the specificity of satellite cells in different muscle types. Satellite cells are isolated by enzymatic digestion from either fast or slow muscle and grown in culture as single cells to form myogenic clones. The type of either myosin isoform or other fiber-specific marker made by myotubes in each clone is determined by immunocytochemistry. (*From Feldman and Stockdale.*[97] *Reproduced by permission.*)

ferences in satellite cells in the absence of external influences. The question arises whether satellite cells are so specialized as to preclude function as universal myogenic stem cells for all types of skeletal muscle.

Satellite Cell Dynamics

SATELLITE CELLS AS COMMITTED STEM CELLS

Stem cells in adults are generally considered to be associated with renewal tissues (e.g., gut, marrow, epidermis); but, in view of the regenerative ability of muscle, one may ask whether satellite cells are a class of reserve stem cells that are called into action under special circumstances. Stem cells, by definition, are capable of proliferation, production of specialized progeny, and self-maintenance.[100] Since it is clear that satellite cells proliferate and give rise to progeny that fuse and make muscle-specific proteins,[76,101] the critical point is self-maintenance, or the ability to maintain their numbers (Fig. 3-8). This property has been tested by asking whether the number of myogenic stem cells persists over an extended period of cell proliferation. During postnatal growth in the rat, the number of myonuclei increases more than fourfold,[102] indicating extensive proliferation of satellite cells, yet the absolute number of satellite cells per muscle has been found to remain constant during this period.[103,104]

Similarly, in adult muscle, many studies have demonstrated that regeneration and satellite cell frequency are undiminished after two or more rounds of muscle injury and regeneration.[102–109] A myotoxic anesthetic such as bupivacaine hydrochloride (Marcaine) kills most myofibers but not satellite cells and leaves the nerve and blood supply in place to facilitate rapid regeneration. Repeated injections of Marcaine have shown that muscle has a remarkable capacity for recurrent regeneration without exhausting the supply of myogenic stem cells.[110–112] For example, weekly intramuscular injection of Marcaine into the adult rat tibialis anterior for 6 months produces at least 20 cycles of regeneration and degeneration.[112] Since the frequency of satellite cells in this muscle is about 4 percent[48] and the original number of myonuclei is restored by a week after Marcaine injection,[112,113] each weekly cycle involves 4 to 5 satellite cell doublings or a total of at least 80 doublings for the 6-month period. Even though this is probably an overestimate, it is impressive that muscle is able to regenerate continuously for a quarter of the rat life span.[112] Within 24 h of isolating muscle fibers, 98 percent of satellite cells express MyoD, indicating activation of myogenesis.

Satellite cells can be liberated from adult muscle by enzymes that dissolve the basal lamina[114,115] and can be stimulated to proliferate in culture by a variety of growth factors.[76,116] The objective is to test whether cultured satellite cells continuously produce differentiation-competent progeny over a period within the limits of senescence of normal diploid cells, which is about 50 doublings for fetal cells and about half that for adult cells.[117,118] The best approach is clonal growth of isolated satellite cells followed by repeated subcloning until the cells exhibit senescence. Satellite cells isolated from adult human muscle can maintain themselves and still yield fusion-competent progeny through 25 to 30 doublings in vitro, while cells from fetuses can proliferate 60 to 70 times.[62,63,119] This is an enormous growth potential (27 doublings yield $>10^8$ cells) and represents one of the greatest in vitro proliferative capacities of any cell type.[118] Recent evidence indicates that subpopulations of satellite cells may actually have even higher capability of clonal expansion (reviewed in Ref. 4).

Several types of myopathies, including human Duchenne muscular dystrophy (DMD), are characterized by continuous degeneration-regeneration, which includes extensive satellite cell proliferation.[120,121] Cells cultured from dystrophic individuals have reduced numbers of doublings in vitro,[62,122,123] suggesting that progressive loss of muscle in DMD may result from proliferative senescence of satellite cells as well as from excessive formation of connective tissue (see Chap. 34).

Since satellite cells have an impressive capacity for growth and self-maintenance and have a myogenic function, they must be considered to be committed stem cells. It has been proposed that satellite cells can be induced to differentiate into other cells of their immediate lineage,[124] but this hypothesis has not been submitted to a full clonal test that would exclude contributions by other cells in the muscle.[4] Thus it is not clear at this time whether all satellite cells or at least a subpopulation of satellite cells have sufficient plasticity to be considered multipotent stem cells.

Other Myogenic Stem Cells

Two recent discoveries of direct relevance to muscle have focused interest on the questions of the origin, role and therapeutic potential for stem cells in muscle and other tissues.[4,72,125,126] One of the new findings is that stem cells derived from tissues other than muscle, particularly bone marrow, may have myogenic potential[127]; a second observation is that the interstitial connective tissue of muscle contains a population of precursor cells distinct from satellite cells and with a higher degree of plasticity—the so-called "side population" cells.[43] This population of cells is probably responsible for interconversions between the restricted lineage that includes myoblast, fibroblast, chondroblast, osteoblast, and adipocyte. Similar observations on precursor cells in other tissues have challenged the dogma that mononuclear cells derived from adult, postmitotic tissues can differentiate and contribute only to the tissue from which they originate.[126] The potential of these stem cells for extensive proliferation has stimulated testing of the small population of stem cells present in many tissues as possible agents for the delivery of normal genes into damaged or injured tissues, with some success.[128]

Some of the side population cells are probably circulating donor cells derived from the bone marrow, and a subpopulation of these is capable of myogenesis. It was shown, however, that this contribution occurs only in damaged muscle and that it is well detectable only after irradiation that impairs repair from the endogenous cells.[128–130] These cells share a common marker, CD34, with satellite cells. Immunohistochemical staining of mouse muscle for CD34 and laminin reveals numerous CD34-positive cells outside

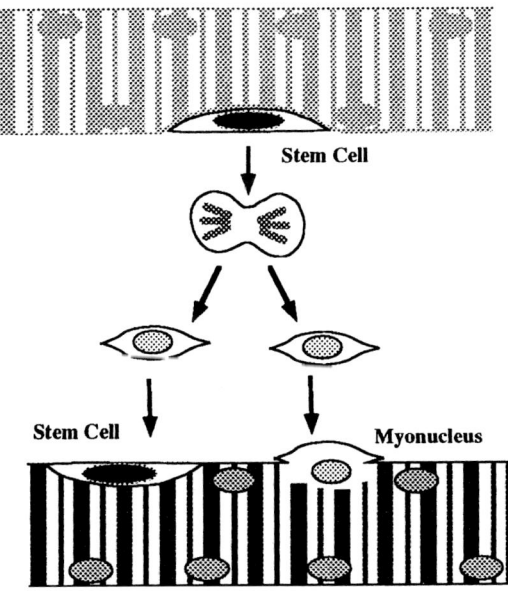

FIGURE 3-8. For satellite cells in adult muscle to function as stem cells, their mitotic divisions must yield, on average, one daughter that differentiates and one that remains as a stem cell, although not all divisions need be asymmetrical, as depicted here.

the basal lamina.[131] Two CD34-positive fractions, one positive for CD45 (a hematopoietic cell line marker) and one negative for it can be isolated by cell sorting. The CD45+ line, which is also Sca1+, is hematopoietic, while the CD45−Sca1+ line is myogenic.[132] It seems likely that the hematopoietic cells are part of a circulating set of stem cells that are rapidly sequestered into tissues.[4,132] It should be noted that side population cells and other possible stem cells in the muscle constitute a minute fraction of the monucleated cell population in an adult muscle, which is dominated by the satellite cells.

SATELLITE CELLS CAN MIGRATE AND CROSS THE BASAL LAMINA

Quiescent satellite cells become activated during injury-induced muscle regeneration and migrate considerable distances within the muscle. In a focal crush injury, satellite cells several millimeters from the site of injury are stimulated to proliferate and later migrate toward the crush, probably remaining within the basal lamina.[133] Free grafting of larger muscles, which involves separation of the muscle from tendon, blood vessels, and nerves, gives rise to a central area of ischemic necrosis from which satellite cells migrate beneath the basal lamina of degenerating myofibers toward the ends of the muscle.[134] Later, during subsequent revascularization, satellite cells from the periphery may migrate back toward the center, where they undergo myogenesis.[135] This was confirmed in longitudinally split autografts in which half of the muscle was freeze-killed: the necrotic half was repopulated by satellite cells migrating in from the viable half.[136]

Although the basal lamina is often viewed as a barrier to cell migration, there is evidence that activated satellite cells can move across the basal lamina in both directions. During a 2- to 3-week postnatal period in rat development, proliferating satellite cells marked in situ by infection with a retrovirus subsequently gave rise to progeny, some of which moved across the basal lamina and fused with neighboring myofibers.[77] Since the basal lamina thickens and strengthens with age,[137,138] the basal lamina of the adult may be a more effective barrier. Inward migration through the basal lamina was observed in juvenile rat and quail muscle that was injected with autologous satellite cells grown in tissue culture and labeled with ^{3}H-TdR.[74] Labeled myonuclei were found in apparently undamaged myofibers at some distance from the injection site, suggesting that the satellite cells were able to migrate through the tissue, penetrate the basal lamina, and fuse. This was the first evidence that satellite cell grafts could contribute nuclei to host myofibers, thus paving the way for subsequent trials of myoblast transfer therapy for muscle disease.[4,139,140]

The local application of myotoxic snake venom and other types of stress induce translaminar migration of satellite cells from undamaged myofibers.[141,142] However, it has been surprisingly difficult to catch satellite cells in the act of migrating and crossing the basal lamina in this and other types of injuries, although separation of the cells from the myofiber has been detected.[133,143–145] Thus, after a latent period for activation, the cells presumably move quite rapidly away from the fiber surface. In addition to migrating within a muscle, satellite cells are also capable of moving between adjacent muscles under certain conditions. In a series of experiments using genetic variants of metabolic enzymes to identify donor and host tissue in the adult mouse, it was shown that grafted regenerating muscle becomes invaded by myogenic cells from neighboring muscle.[146–152] However, experiments carried out in the adult rat failed,[153] and it was suggested that the thicker epimysium of rat muscle may block invasion.[110] Indeed, a damaged epimysium allowed transmuscle invasion.[154]

The behavior of satellite cells in vitro also showed two alternatives. In cultured myofibers mechanically dissected from adult rat, the satellite cells were segregated within the basal lamina and escaped only after the basal lamina was torn with a microneedle.[115,155] In a similar preparation from juvenile quail, however, about 20 percent of the myofibers showed spontaneous outgrowth of satellite cells.[156,157]

Taken together, these various reports indicate that satellite cells have extensive capacity for motility. In circumstances involving muscle injury or insult, satellite cells may move long distances beneath the basal lamina, leave the myofiber, and migrate throughout the muscle or even pass into adjacent muscles. It should not be inferred, however, that migration is commonplace. It is likely that in normal muscle, except for limited movement during development while the basal lamina is still fragile, most satellite cells remain in contact with the same myofiber for the life of the animal. Even during muscle regeneration following global injury, most new myofibers are surrounded by sleeves of old basal lamina, indicating that satellite cells remain within the basal lamina tubes to undergo myogenesis.

SATELLITE CELLS IN CULTURE

In the process of producing a primary muscle culture, satellite cells are released from adult muscle by mincing and with the aid of enzymes, such as trypsin or pronase, which dissolve the basal lamina.[114,115] The resulting suspensions of cells are contaminated with fibroblasts and other nonmyogenic cells, but some of these may be removed by selective attachment[158] or density gradient centrifugation.[159,160] Satellite cells obtained from adults undergo a lag period of about 24 h in culture before they begin to divide, while cells from neonates proliferate much sooner.[161] This difference probably reflects the fact that many of the neonatal cells are proliferating in vivo but become quiescent in the adult. The cultures are generally initiated in medium containing serum (and chick embryo extract in some cases) to begin growth and later may be switched to serum-free medium for testing various growth factors. Because serum and embryo extract contain a variety of hormones and unspecified growth factors, the specific conditions needed to activate proliferation of isolated satellite cells in vitro are unknown.

Satellite cells may also be placed in culture while still associated with the myofiber, and this preparation more closely reflects conditions in vivo. With appropriate enzyme preparations, myofibers isolated from adult rat flexor digitorum brevis retain normal morphologic specializations and each contains two to three satellite cells beneath the basal

Chapter 3. Satellite and Stem Cells in Muscle Regeneration

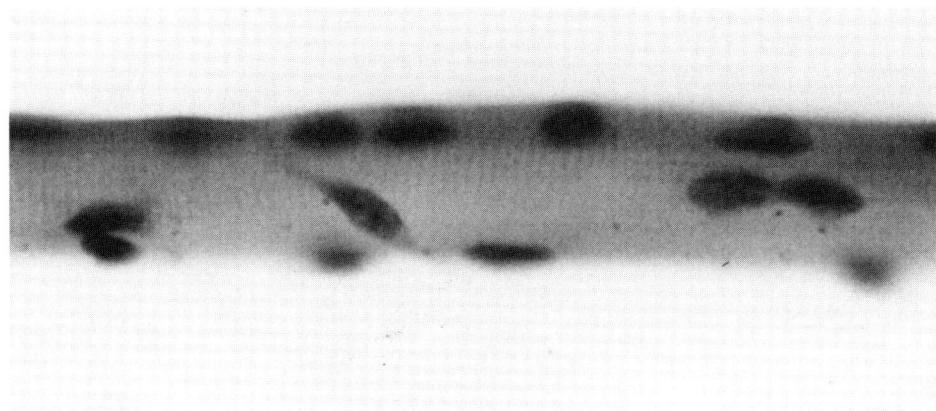

FIGURE 3-9. Light micrograph of part of a single myofiber after a few hours in culture, showing a spindle-shaped satellite cell with tabs of basophilic cytoplasm at either end and many myonuclei. Hematoxylin, ×1000.

lamina (Fig. 3-9).[75,100,162] Such preparations provide ideal material for testing factors that may initiate and maintain satellite cell proliferation and for studying satellite cell–myofiber interactions. When maintained in medium containing 10 percent serum, most of the satellite cells remain quiescent in the G_O phase of the cell cycle for at least several days. Given the appropriate growth factors, the satellite cells divide and their progeny fuse to form multinucleated myotubes. Myogenesis from satellite cells can occur in association with the viable myofiber (Fig. 3-10) or in the "empty" endomysial tube after the myofiber has been killed (Fig. 3-11).

SATELLITE CELLS MODULATE THEIR CELL CYCLE IN RESPONSE TO GROWTH FACTORS

Quiescent satellite cells reenter the cell cycle under a wide variety of conditions (injury, overwork, denervation, exercise, stretch), so it may be anticipated that the signal pathways involved are complex. To simplify analysis, potential growth factors have been tested using cultured cells of several types, each having advantages and drawbacks. The following discussion is drawn largely from studies of satellite cells from adult muscle. Reviews of growth-active substances for myogenic embryo cells and cell lines have been published.[163–166] Similar factors affect myoblasts during embryonal myogenesis (see Chap. 1).

Satellite cells in adult muscle are quiescent, or in the G_O phase of the cell cycle,[167,168] and are thought to be acted on by at least two different types of growth factors before commencing sustained proliferation. The cell must first be induced to enter the G_1 phase of the cell cycle by a competence factor and then stimulated to traverse the remainder of the cell cycle and undergo mitosis by a progression factor. Results from other cell types suggest that competence factors are needed only while the cell passes a critical point in G_1 (restriction point), while progression factors are needed

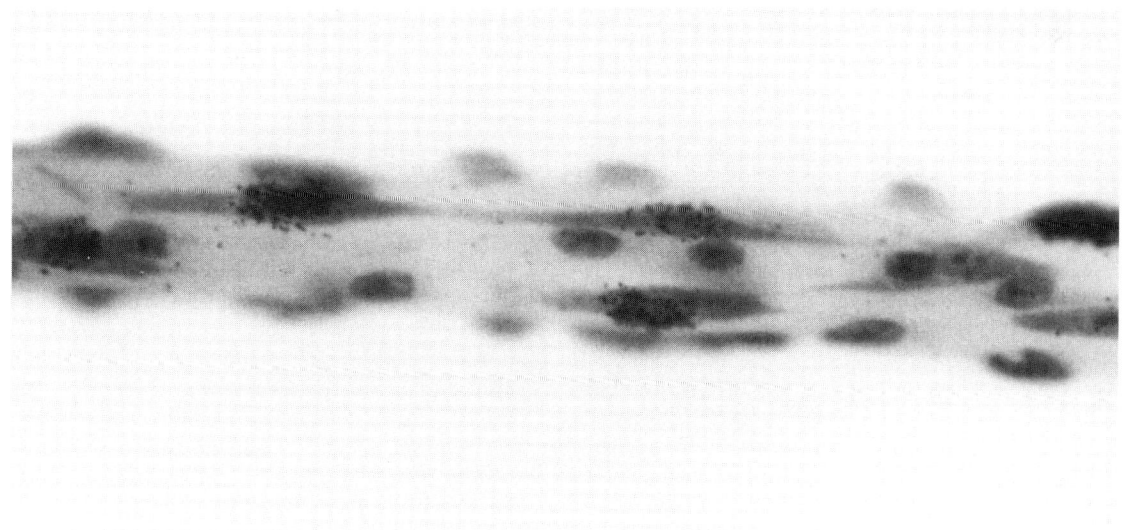

FIGURE 3-10. Radioautograph of a single, viable myofiber grown in vitro for 2 days in muscle growth factor and labeled with ³H-TdR. Most of the satellite cells have incorporated the nucleotide into their DNA and are overlain by silver grains in the emulsion. The satellite cells proliferate on the surface of the myofiber, beneath its basal lamina. All myonuclei are unlabeled. Hematoxylin, ×1100. (From Bischoff.[101] Reproduced by permission of the American College of Sports Medicine.)

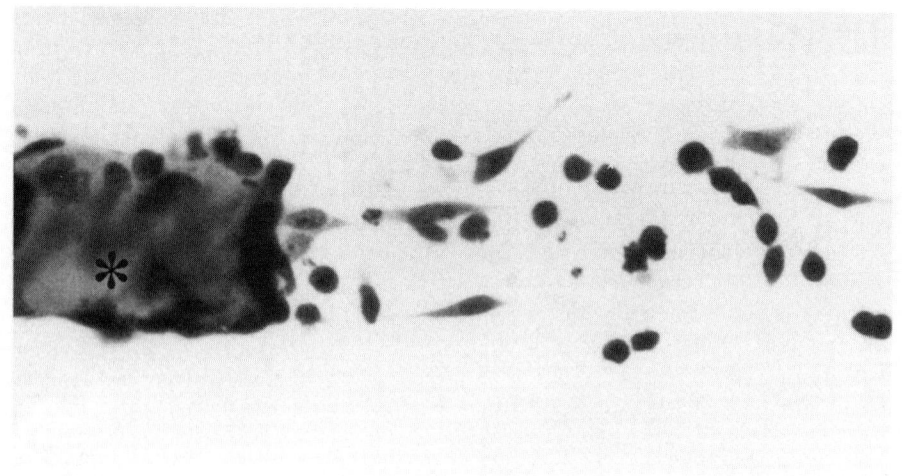

FIGURE 3-11. Light micrograph of single myofiber killed at 0 time with bupivacaine hydrochloride (Marcaine) and cultured in muscle growth factor for 2 days. Satellite cells are proliferating in association with the mass of necrotic myofibrils (asterisk) and also within the endomysial tube, not visible in this preparation. Hematoxylin, ×1100.

continuously to sustain proliferation.[169] Two growth factors, fibroblast growth factor (FGF) and insulin-like growth factor (IGF), have been extensively tested with satellite cells and found to be candidates for a competence factor (FGF) and a progression factor (IGF).

Fibroblast Growth Factors

FGFs are a group of structurally related, monomeric proteins (~150 amino acids) coded by at least six separate genes.[170] The proteins differ in isoelectric point, with acidic and basic classes; they also display extensive microheterogeneity, believed to result from partial degradation during extraction.[170] All stimulate the proliferation of fibroblasts and bind to heparin, a property widely used for their purification.[171] FGF was first isolated from brain and pituitary[172,173] and is also present in chick embryo extract,[174] which has been used for many years to stimulate the growth of myogenic cells. FGF stimulates the proliferation and inhibits differentiation of cultured satellite cells,[116,175–178] even in serum-free medium.[116,176,179] Since serum, or an alternate source of progression factors, such as IGF, is not needed for FGF-stimulated proliferation, it is unlikely that FGF functions for satellite cells as a competence factor in the sense originally proposed.[180] Autocrine secretion of IGFs in myogenic cell lines,[181] such as fetal rat myoblasts,[182] may explain the ability of FGF to stimulate the proliferation of satellite cells in serum-free medium. As a further complication, proliferating rat satellite cells have also been found to produce FGF in culture.[183,184] Receptors for FGF have been detected on mononucleated cells of several myogenic lines,[185,186] but satellite cells have apparently not been tested. There is evidence that FGF is bound to heparan sulfate proteoglycan components in the extracellular space,[187] and that its effects are reduced by addition of heparin or heparan sulfate proteoglycan to the culture medium.[188,189]

Interestingly, satellite cells on single isolated myofibers remain quiescent when grown in serum-containing medium, and FGF is the only defined substance found to induce their proliferation.[75] Since the satellite cells are enclosed in a basal lamina containing heparan sulfate proteoglycan,[190] it might be expected that the FGF response would be attenuated by its binding to the matrix; however, maximum stimulation occurs with as little as 1 ng/mL, comparable to the dose in other sensitive cells.[191,192]

The level of FGF in vivo varies with physiologic changes in the muscle. FGF has been found in the basal lamina of normal adult muscle, and the amount is elevated in mouse dystrophic muscle (mdx) and after muscle injury (see Chap. 20).[193–197] Following hypertrophy induced by synergist ablation, a condition known to involve satellite cell activation,[145] there is an increase in the content of a growth factor with the properties of FGF.[192] Finally, in electrically stimulated rabbit muscle, there is increased expression of FGF associated with both satellite cell proliferation and capillary growth.[198]

In summary, FGF is present in satellite cells and early myotubes and is stored in the basal lamina of mature muscle bound to proteoglycans. Injury may lead to the release of FGF either directly from the myofiber or indirectly via enzymatic degradation of the basal lamina. FGF is a multifunctional molecule which, besides stimulating satellite cell proliferation, could enhance revascularization,[187] fibroplasia,[199] and innervation.[196,200] Although this scheme is attractive, many details remain to be proven.

Insulin-like Growth Factors

The IGFs are single-chain proteins (~70 amino acids), highly conserved among species and related to insulin.[201] IGF-I is the mediator of growth hormone action, while IGF-II may function to stimulate cell proliferation during development.[198] Both IGFs are secreted by a variety of tissues and are carried in the circulation by specific binding proteins that compete with cellular IGF receptors and thus modulate growth factor activity.[202] The response of satellite cells to IGF is enhanced by dexamethasone,[203] a phenomenon that may be related to the observation that dexamethasone suppresses secretion of IGF-binding protein[204] and elevates IGF receptors[205] in myogenic cell lines. There is no information as yet on the autocrine secretion of IGFs by satellite cells in vitro, but cultured fetal rat myoblasts[182,206] and various myogenic cell lines[181,207] produce both types of IGF.

IGFs promote the differentiation of cultured satellite cells in serum-free medium; they enhance the uptake of amino acid and strongly stimulate protein synthesis[208,209]; in combination with FGF, they also stimulate proliferation.[116,179,198,208] The action of IGFs is mediated by cell surface receptors of two different types: the type I receptor is a multiunit complex closely related to the insulin receptor, while the type II receptor is a monomeric protein identical to the mannose-6-phosphate receptor.[210] In human,[209] avian[211] and rodent[212] satellite cell cultures, the effects of both IGF-I and -II are mediated by the type I receptor in both myoblasts and myotubes. Quiescent satellite cells on single myofibers in vitro do not proliferate in response to IGF or high concentrations of insulin, which stimulate the type I receptor.[75] Satellite cells activated by exposure to muscle growth factor or FGF are dependent on serum for continued proliferation, and the serum requirement can be replaced by IGF.[75,168]

In general, IGF stimulates satellite cell proliferation in vivo, but only if the cells are already in the cell cycle. Treatments that increase mRNA for IGF-I in muscle have no effect on the incidence of satellite cells in mature muscle but double the satellite cell frequency in young, growing rats.[213,214,217] Although aged rats have reduced levels of circulating IGF-I, restoring this to the value found in young animals by injection of growth hormone does not improve muscle regeneration.[215] Regeneration may be less dependent than embryonic growth on circulating IGF, because autocrine secretion of IGF is stimulated by injury. Messenger RNA for IGF-I is elevated in muscle within 24 h after injury, peaks at 3 days, and returns to normal values by 10 days—a time course that closely matches satellite cell proliferation in regenerating muscle.[216] The same pattern is found in hypophysectomized animals, showing that endogenous IGF synthesis during regeneration is independent of growth hormone.[217,218] Cytologic studies reveal IGF-I in satellite cells and early myotubes beginning 24 h after injury.[219] A splice variant of the IGF may directly control protein synthesis in response to muscle stretch.[220]

Other Growth Factors

Injured muscle itself appears to release an endogenous growth factor for satellite cells. A saline extract of crushed muscle contains a high-molecular-mass (~100 kDa) mitogen that is specific for both source and target tissue.[99,221,222] The factor binds heparin, as does FGF, but possesses different target cell specificity and produces additive effects with FGF; its activity is not suppressed by neutralizing antibodies to FGF. This muscle growth factor, which has not yet been purified, acts as a competence factor to commit quiescent satellite cells to enter the cell cycle and is required for only 10 h, after which the cells continue to proliferate for at least several days in the presence of serum.[153] Angiogenic activity has also been identified in crushed muscle extract,[223,224] and partially purified muscle growth factor is a potent chemoattractant for satellite cells.[225]

Although a small number of growth factors, such as FGF and IGF, exercise a decisive role in satellite cell proliferation, many other substances may modulate growth. Platelet-derived growth factor (PDGF) stimulates proliferation of many mesodermal cells, especially smooth muscle and fibroblasts, and is implicated in wound healing.[226,227] Skeletal myoblasts from embryos and myogenic cell lines respond to[228,229] and produce[230,231] PDGF. PDGF is also a chemoattractant for embryo myoblasts,[232] but neither rat serum nor pure PDGF stimulates proliferation of quiescent satellite cells on single fibers.[75] Growth of mouse satellite cells in vitro is weakly stimulated by PDGF, but interleukin-6, transforming growth factor alpha, and leukemia inhibitory factor are much more potent mitogens.[233]

Several factors that inhibit satellite cell proliferation have also been identified. These may play a role in maintaining quiescence of satellite cells in mature muscle in G_O and in suppressing further divisions after regeneration is complete. The best-studied negative growth factor is transforming growth factor beta (TGF-β), consisting of at least five closely related homodimeric proteins (~112 amino acids per chain) first purified from platelets but also present in a wide variety of cells and tissues.[234] The biological activities of TGF-β are diverse and depend on the cell type and state of differentiation. With rat satellite cells, low concentrations of TGF-β depress proliferation and totally block fusion in serum containing medium,[235] but substantial proliferation can occur at high concentrations of mitogen, especially FGF.[116]

In sum, the dominant role of TGF-β appears to be as an inhibitor of differentiation, while its effect on proliferation depends on cell type and species. In terms of satellite cell physiology, such a factor might act to suppress fusion during the early stages of muscle generation or regeneration. It may also play a role in preventing differentiation of satellite cells, while other factors promote withdrawal from the cell cycle and quiescence.

Another negative-acting growth factor, which appears to be mediated through cell contact, has been identified from studies of single myofibers and attached satellite cells. Response of quiescent satellite cells to mitogen is reduced by 30 to 40 percent when the cells are in contact with the plasmalemma of the myofiber but not when the myofiber is killed, leaving the cells in contact with only the basal lamina (Fig. 3-12).[236] Thus inhibition is exerted by the plasmalemma

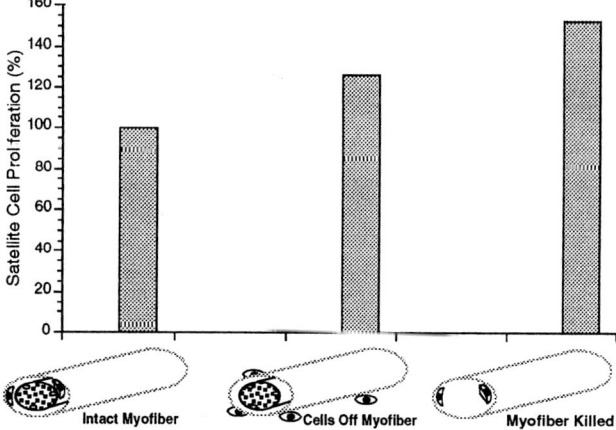

FIGURE 3-12. Experiments to test the effect of the viable myofiber and its basal lamina on proliferation of satellite cells in response to muscle growth factor. Proliferation of cells in contact with the myofiber and basal lamina (left) is enhanced if satellite cells are removed by centrifugation (center) or if the myofiber is killed (right), leaving the cells in the basal lamina tube. (From Bischoff.[236] Reproduced by permission.)

and not the basal lamina. The inhibition can also be removed by growing the myofibers in tetrodotoxin,[165] which blocks sodium channels. This suggests that electrical activity in the plasmalemma may regulate the response of satellite cells to growth factors.

In sum, many factors, each with pleiotropic effects, influence the growth and differentiation of satellite cells. The challenge is to understand their mechanism of action and determine which ones are physiologically relevant for satellite cells in the animal. Successful regeneration requires a number of processes such as cell proliferation, phagocytosis, revascularization, and reinnervation; it would be advantageous for a single multifunctional molecule, such as FGF, to regulate several of these events. There is evidence that growth factors are made by activated satellite cells themselves, and this may provide an autocatalytic mechanism for magnifying the effect of injury. Finally, microenvironmental factors—including contact between satellite cell and myofiber and position of the satellite cell on the myofiber in relation to site of injury and to the end plate—may modulate response to soluble growth factors.

Regeneration of Muscle

Some of the events involved in muscle regeneration following a crush injury are summarized in Fig. 3-13. The following sections focus on factors affecting the behavior of satellite cells during regeneration.

NEW MYONUCLEI ARISE FROM SATELLITE CELLS, BUT SURVIVING MYOFIBERS AID IN HEALING

Myonuclei lost as a result of injury are replaced mostly by the proliferation and fusion of satellite cells.[14] In cases where injured myofibers exhibit *partial* necrosis,[237,238] the surviving stump may undergo changes that facilitate regeneration, such as formation of sarcoplasmic outgrowths populated with migrating myonuclei.[239–241] These outgrowths provide a mechanism for the rapid establishment of functional continuity across a lesion as the outgrowths from opposite stumps meet and fuse.[242–244] This process has been termed *continuous regeneration*,[240] as opposed to *discontinuous regeneration* mediated by satellite cell activity. The role of continuous regeneration has been controversial, owing in part to the difficulty in distinguishing sarcoplasmic buds from early myotubes derived from satellite cells.[240,245–247] Recent experiments with single viable myofibers in culture have shed light on the morphologic plasticity of mature myofibers and their possible role in continuous regeneration.

Single myofibers isolated from adult rat muscle and deprived of all satellite cells remain viable and contractile for at least several weeks in culture.[75,248] After about 5 days in vitro, pseudopodial sprouts arise from the myotendinous junctions of the myofiber and rapidly elongate and branch as they extend over the substratum. Myonuclei from the original portion of the myofiber move into the sprouts, which now resemble embryonic myotubes. Remodeling of

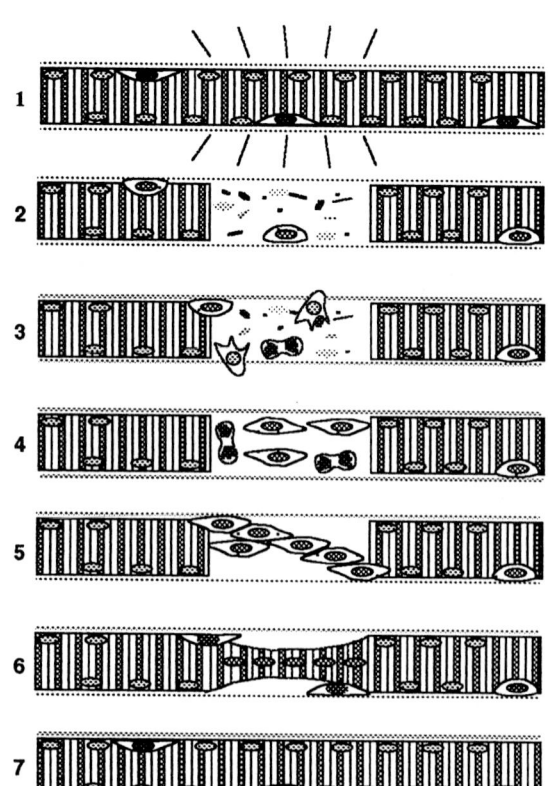

FIGURE 3-13. Muscle regeneration following a crush injury. (1) Mechanical trauma destroys the integrity of the myofiber plasmalemma, leading to ingress of extracellular calcium. (2) The myofiber undergoes necrosis and autodigestion by intrinsic proteases, but the endomysial tube and satellite cells remain. Segments of the myofiber adjacent to the injury may heal over and remain viable. (3) Macrophages, derived from blood monocytes, penetrate the endomysial tube and complete the removal of necrotic debris. Satellite cells become activated and enter the cell cycle. (4) The cells proliferate while attached to the inner surface of the basal lamina, forming a "basophilic cuff" of tissue. (5 and 6) Satellite cells begin to withdraw from the cell cycle and fuse to form multinucleated myotubes. These may subsequently fuse with the surviving stump myofibers, thus providing continuity across the injury. (7) The original myofiber and complement of satellite cells are restored. There are many variations on this basic scheme, depending on type and extent of injury, species, age, and other factors. This series of events presumably occurs continuously in dystrophic muscle.

the myofiber is accompanied by biochemical changes, such as the appearance of extrajunctional acetylcholine receptors and acetylcholinesterase activity[248] and a shift in creatine kinase isozyme profile from muscle type to brain type.[75] The remodeling of the myofiber is accelerated by the fusion of myoblasts[249] with the elongating sprouts.[75] Sprouting may also provide segment of the myofiber that has embryonic characteristics and is more conducive to reinnervation.

THE REGENERATING RESPONSE DEPENDS ON THE TYPE OF INJURY

The extent of muscle regeneration in space and time is influenced by the type of injury. Focal injury, as produced by micropuncture[238,250] or overwork,[251,252] involves the degeneration of one or a few myofibers; the resulting proliferation of satellite cells is limited to the necrotic myofibers. With more severe injuries, the regenerative signal spreads to adjacent nonnecrotic tissue, and the response is proportional to the amount of injury. Satellite cell proliferation occurs with greater magnitude and longer duration following a crush injury than after a cut.[253] The regenerative signal appears to travel both parallel and perpendicular to the principal myofiber axis, and the response includes activation, proliferation, and migration of satellite cells.[134–141]

Many types of injury do not create a uniform damage; in these cases the survival of undamaged myofibers within the injured area may complicate subsequent experimental analysis. Transient ischemia of an entire muscle, as is produced in free grafts, leads to degeneration of the central core of myofibers, but most of the peripheral myofibers survive.[254,255] Marcaine[113] kills most but not all myofibers,[256] leading to unexpected persistence of biochemical markers of mature muscle.[257,258]

The most dramatic display of the regenerative ability of muscle is that of minced muscle regeneration, in which a whole muscle is chopped into small fragments before grafting.[259,260] Although all myofibers are destroyed and neurovascular pathways are severely disrupted, the mince is capable of surprisingly good regeneration (~30 percent of original), albeit often accompanied by increased formation of connective tissue.[261] Mincing is the best preparation for quantitative biochemical studies, since there are no residual normal myofibers; but the adhesions to adjacent muscles that develop during healing, probably owing to the destruction of the epimysium, make it difficult to harvest the grafts cleanly.[258,260]

REMOVAL OF NECROTIC DEBRIS FACILITATES REGENERATION

The initial stages of myofibrillar breakdown have been described in vivo[250,262] and in single cultured myofibers.[75,155,248] Within minutes after injury, the myofibers undergo hypercontraction, probably as a result of the rapid influx of extracellular calcium,[238,250] and tear apart into a series of contraction clots composed of a dense irregular mass of myofilaments. The endomysial tube, composed of basal and reticular laminae, survives many types of injury and spans the region between contraction clots, leaving transparent chambers containing a few myonuclei, mitochondria, and membrane fragments (Fig. 3-14). These elements disappear from the cultured myofibers within 24 h, presumably owing to the action of endogenous proteases.[263–265] The clots of myofilaments persist for many days in vitro and are removed in vivo by the action of macrophages.

The onset and rate of phagocytosis in vivo is proportional to the preservation of the vascular supply, which carries macrophage precursor cells derived from the bone marrow to the site of injury; endogenous macrophages are rare in normal adult muscle.[266] Following Marcaine-induced muscle injury, which leaves the vascular supply intact, neutrophils appear early (peak = 12 h) and disappear, while macrophages

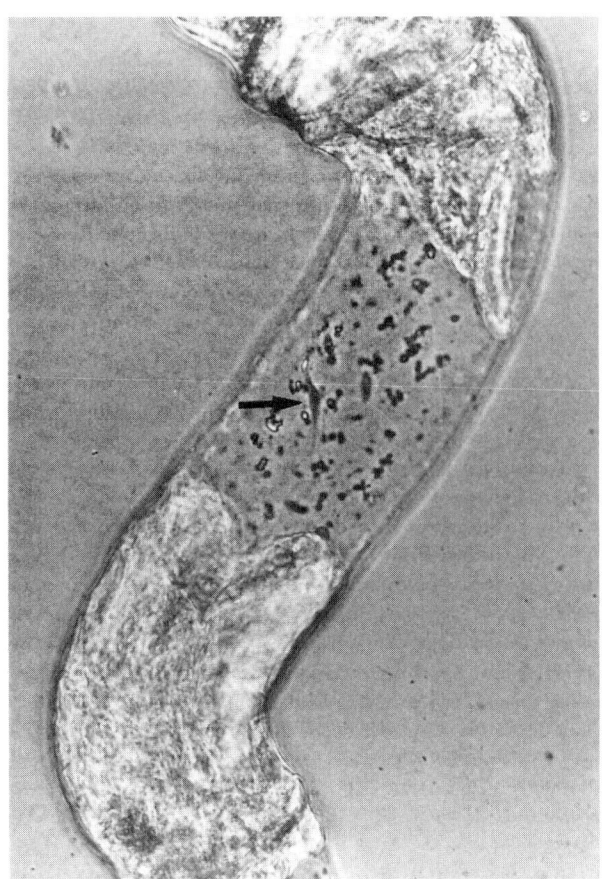

FIGURE 3-14. Micrograph of a necrotic myofiber a few minutes after its removal from adult rat muscle. The myofibrils have broken up in the center of this segment and retracted into contraction clots at either end, leaving a transparent chamber of endomysial tube. Several myonuclei and a satellite cell (arrow) are visible in the chamber, as well as other debris. Phase contrast, ×600. (From Bischoff.[155] Reproduced by permission of Wiley-Liss.)

arise later (peak = 2 days) and persist longer.[267] Ischemic injury produced by free grafting of small muscles is repaired in a centripetal gradient reflecting the ingrowth of new vessels, and macrophages do not reach the center of the graft until 5 days postinjury.[255,262]

Since intrinsic degeneration can remove only a small portion of necrotic tissue, it seems likely that macrophage activity is important for subsequent regeneration, if only for physical reasons. Indeed, destruction of macrophage stem cells by irradiation leads to persistence of necrotic myofibers in minced grafts and inhibition of muscle regeneration.[268] Reconstitution of the marrow restores regeneration,[268] and enhancement of phagocytic activity by adding extra macrophage stem cells to a muscle mince promotes regeneration and results in reduced fibrosis.[269] Besides removing degenerating myofibers, macrophages may stimulate regeneration by secreting effector molecules that act as mitogens, induce chemotaxis, and promote revascularization.[270] Although complete regeneration in vivo clearly requires the activities of macrophages, tissue culture studies have shown that the early stages of regeneration, including proliferation and fusion of satellite cells, can occur in their absence.[76,101,115]

REGENERATION TAKES PLACE WITHIN EMPTY ENDOMYSIAL TUBES

The endomysial tube, which completely encloses the myofiber and associated satellite cells, is not phagocytosed following injury and is, in fact, the only element of the original myofiber that persists. It appears to play several important roles in regeneration, including (1) sequestering of myogenic cells, (2) spatial orientation of nascent myotubes, (3) promoting growth and differentiation, and (4) furnishing essential cues for reinnervation.

The basal lamina is composed of several glycoproteins and collagens combined in a single integrated structure that extends from the plasmalemma to the reticular lamina (see Chap. 20) and connects transmembrane proteins (see Chap. 19). Some basal lamina components disappear during muscle necrosis[271,272] but others persist, and the complex appears, by electron microscopy, to be largely unaltered. Although satellite cells are able to cross the basal lamina under certain circumstances, most cells remain within the endomysial tubes during regeneration following most types of muscle injury.[273–278] In studies of single myofibers in culture, satellite cells do not cross the endomysial tube in mechanically dissected myofibers[117]; but following enzymatic dissociation, some satellite cells are able to migrate away from the myofibers,[76,101] probably owing to alteration of the basal lamina. Fusion of satellite cell progeny to form multinucleated myotubes occurs earlier where the cells are retained within the basal lamina.[115] Thus, the endomysial tube may facilitate regeneration by keeping most satellite cells within a confined space and separate from other non-muscle elements (except macrophages) to promote their interaction.

During regeneration, myotubes form within the old endomysial tubes, which thereby impose spatial orientation on the regenerate.[278] This initial orientation is later superseded by other forces within the tissue, such as tension and stress.[279–281] In minced regenerates, the new myotubes initially reflect the random position of the fragments; but by 7 days, all myotubes become oriented parallel to the axis of the muscle.[259,260]

The intimate contact that occurs between the basal lamina and satellite cells during regeneration suggests that the matrix may play a role in regulating growth and differentiation. Myogenic cell lines adhere preferentially to laminin[282] via a cell surface integrin (see Chap. 19a),[283] and this attachment stimulates their proliferation, mobility, and differentiation.[284,285] Satellite cells cultured on Matrigel, a mixture of basal lamina components, exhibit enhanced long-term survival and differentiation,[286,287] attributed to entactin, a minor basal lamina glycoprotein.[287] Certain components of the basal lamina, such as heparan sulfate proteoglycan, are able to bind growth factors that are somehow made available to satellite cells following injury.[183] Alternatively, the basal lamina may act as a barrier to limit access of satellite cells to growth factors. Finally, the original synaptic sites on the basal lamina instruct ingrowing nerves in the formation of new synapses and may be essential for the reinnervation of regenerating muscle (see Chap. 20).[288]

Despite the preservation of basal lamina following necrosis and the wealth of possibilities in modulating regeneration, there have been few direct experiments in vivo. A comparison of muscle injury induced by barium salt, which leaves the basal lamina intact, and trypsin, which dissolves the basal lamina, revealed equally good myotube orientation and regeneration.[289] Procedures for the preparation of empty segments of basal lamina[290] may be useful for further investigation of its role in regeneration.

MUSCLE INJURY STIMULATES THE ACTIVATION AND PROLIFERATION OF SATELLITE CELLS

The onset and duration of satellite cell proliferation is difficult to determine in vivo owing to the uncertainty of cell identification. Many nonmyogenic cells are present in injured muscle, and some may resemble satellite cells.[28] Several strategies have been used to overcome this problem. Schultz et al.[135] used isolated single myofiber segments from rats to identify labeled satellite cells in radioautographs following a crush injury and administration of ^{3}H-TdR at intervals. Satellite cells begin DNA synthesis about 15 h after injury at the crush site and several hours later in the adjacent undamaged tissue, suggesting a slow spread of the activation signal. Similar results were obtained for the onset of DNA synthesis (12 to 18 h) by labeling dividing cells with bromodeoxyuridine,[291] but proliferating macrophage precursors may have been included in this study, since all cells within the endomysial tubes were scored. Nevertheless, these values are in agreement with in vitro results; satellite cells on single myofibers first enter DNA synthesis at 16 h after mitogen stimulation.[168] Soluble factors from crushed muscle enhance regeneration of minced muscle.[222]

A different approach was used by McGeachie and Grounds[292,293] to study the timing of mouse muscle regeneration. Cycling cells were labeled with ^{3}H-TdR at intervals following injury and scored for labeling after they fused with myofibers. This avoids the problem of identifying satellite cells per se and permits determining the number of divisions before fusion by counting radioautographic silver grains above labeled myonuclei. These studies showed that satellite cells begin to synthesize DNA at 30 h after a cut or crush injury and a few hours later in minced or free muscle grafts.[253,294,295] Progeny begin to fuse and form multinucleated myotubes after only two divisions, but proliferation of satellite cells continues for up to 9 days, depending on the severity of injury.[292] There are also surprising differences between mouse strains in the onset, duration, and effectiveness of regeneration.[216,268,296]

Myoblast transplantation experiments have revealed that cultured myoblasts contain an undifferentiated population of cells that are capable of self-renewal and may be the major contributor to tissue regeneration after grafting.[297–299] Migration of myogenic cells occurs extensively during both the embryogenesis and regeneration of skeletal muscle. Hepatocyte growth factor (HGF) and TGRF-β exhibit significant chemotactic activity. The dose-response curves for both of these factors is bell-shaped, with maximum activity in the range of 1 to 10 ng/mL.[225]

Contribution of Stem Cells Other Than Satellite Cells to Muscle Growth and Regeneration

Two recent observations have raised the immediate question of how large is the contribution of stem cells other than satellite cells to muscle growth and regeneration and what is their potential for myogenesis. Cells derived from genetically marked bone marrow transplanted into immunodeficient mice migrate into areas of induced muscle degeneration, undergo myogenic differentiation, and participate in the regeneration of the damaged fiber.[126] In addition, stem cells other than satellite cells, the so-called side population cells, are present in the muscle interstitium. It has been proposed that progenitor cells in the interstitial spaces may be responsible for the apparently large increase in total number of fibers in the early postnatal growth of mouse muscle.[131] This hypothesis, however, fails to take into account several observations that point to satellite cells as major contributors to postnatal growth. One is the result of careful structural analysis showing that in fact all future muscle fibers are already present at birth,[300,301] so that postnatal growth does require new nuclei but does not produce new myofibers. The second observation is that satellite cells proliferate actively in the early postnatal period and also decline in frequency during that time and thus they are the most likely source of new myonuclei (see "Age-Related Satellite Cell Frequency,"). The third is that in the absence of satellite cells (in Pax7 null mutant mice), postnatal muscle growth is greatly reduced.[45]

The contribution of cells other than satellite cells to muscle regeneration in vivo is also likely not very large. One bit of evidence for this statement comes from the observation that in muscular dystrophy, regeneration begins to fail at the time when the proliferative potential of satellite cells begins to decline (see comment under "Satellite Cells as Committed Stem Cells, above").[302] Donor nuclei from bone transplant have been detected within muscle fibers after a period of 13 years in a patient with DMD, indicating long-term persistence. However, the nuclei were few and failed to correct the disease.[303] Kinetic analysis of proliferating myoblasts indicates that satellite cells alone can account for full regeneration.[304] A more precise estimate of a contribution to 3.5 percent of the fibers during regeneration after injury has been obtained using green fluorescent protein–tagged mononucleate muscle stem cell from adult bone marrow.[305] Interestingly, this work indicates a stepwise progress from marrow cells to satellite cells to regenerating myoblasts. In the mouse, it has also been reported that transplantation of a muscle-derived population of cells capable of multipotent differentiation improved the efficiency of muscle regeneration and dystrophin delivery to dystrophic muscle.[306] The kinetics of myoblast proliferation in the regenerating muscle indicate that satellite cells are sufficient for full regeneration.[304]

Pluripotent mesenchymal stem cells from the bone marrow can be engrafted into other tissues,[307] but it is not clear whether the bone marrow is the continuing source of these primitive stem cells in the muscle.

The Influence of Innervation and Activity on Regeneration

MOTOR NERVES INFLUENCE THE ACTIVITY OF SATELLITE CELLS

During muscle development, early proliferation and fusion of satellite cells to form primary myotubes is independent of nerves, but the formation of secondary myofibers from satellite cells requires innervation.[308,309] Perinatal denervation of muscles results in a decrease in the growth of satellite cells,[47,310] suggesting that nerves act by stimulating the proliferation of satellite cells. Since satellite cells are not directly innervated, the effect is probably mediated by the myofiber or brought about by the release of soluble substances from the nerves.

The effect of nerves on satellite cells in mature muscle is controversial. Early studies suggest that denervation prior to transplantation enhances subsequent regeneration.[311–314] Denervation produces in both the muscle and nerve a variety of changes that could facilitate early regeneration,[315–317] including an increase in the frequency of satellite cells. These were first interpreted as arising from sequestration of nuclei from the atrophying myofibers into mononucleated cells,[24,318,319] but later studies disproved this process and showed that denervation leads to activation and proliferation of pre-existing satellite cells.[26,320–323] There is little agreement on the timing and magnitude of the satellite cell response, but it probably depends on species, age, and muscle type. For example, satellite cells in the adult rat soleus double in frequency (= 4 to 8 percent) at 3 to 4 days postdenervation.[324,325] In adult mice, increased proliferation of satellite cells has been observed for as long as 4 weeks postdenervation.[326] The newly formed satellite cells may fuse with their associated myofibers,[326] migrate away from the myofibers and fuse to form new myotubes in the interstitum,[320,321] or form new myotubes in association with the degenerating myofibers.[327,328] The response of satellite cells to denervation may prepare the muscle for subsequent reinnervation but cannot ameliorate the severe atrophy that occurs in the absence of reinnervation. Despite extensive degenerative changes during long-term denervation (7 months), muscle still contains numerous satellite cells and is capable of substantial recovery on reinnervation[329] or stimulation[328,330]; however, in some conditions the satellite cells may be depleted.[327]

The stimulus for satellite cell proliferation in denervated muscle is unknown. One possibility is that satellite cell proliferation may result from release of the inhibition imposed by myofiber activity.[325] Also, since many fibroblasts and other nonmuscle cells proliferate in response to denervation,[329,331,332] the muscle or nerve may release nonspecific growth factors.

MUSCLE OVERUSE PRODUCES SATELLITE CELL ACTIVATION

Traditional views of the effect of exercise on muscle growth and fiber type transformation have emphasized the response of preexisting myofibers, but further studies established satellite cell–derived myogenesis as a major response to various types of exercise as well as experimental overwork paradigms such as synergist removal and stretch. This section focuses on satellite cell activity following muscle overwork.

Overuse of untrained muscle, especially exercise involving eccentric (lengthening) contractions, leads to damage. Physiologic mechanisms of exercise-induced muscle injury have been reviewed[333,334] and are not discussed here. The muscle damage is reflected in the release of creatine kinase and myofibrillar proteins into the plasma,[334,335] elevated autophagic elements,[337,338] disorganization of myofibrils,[339,340] and focal necrosis of myofibers.[252,341–345]

Satellite cell activity has been documented following various courses of exercise. A single running session of adult rats produces a threefold increase in satellite cell proliferation 24 h later,[251] and prolonged treadmill sessions leads to tripling of satellite cell frequency[344] and increased labeling with ^{3}H-TdR.[345] Weight lifting in cats results in focal necrosis, proliferation of satellite cells, and evidence of new myofiber formation based on histology and fiber counts.[343,346,347] Muscle overwork in humans also produces myofiber necrosis and regeneration.[342,348]

Another strategy for overwork is the tenotomy or removal of a synergist; this causes stretch and increased use of the remaining muscle and leads to a compensatory hypertrophy. Satellite cells promptly begin to proliferate and increase in frequency threefold in the soleus of adult rats at about a week postsurgery.[325,339] Comparable stimulation is found in other muscles.[144,323,349,350] Despite increased satellite cell proliferation, there is no evidence of a net increase in the number of myofibers (hyperplasia)[351,352]; it appears that satellite cell activity contributes solely to addition of myonuclei to preexisting myofibers and to replacement of necrotic myofibers.[145,353,354]

The most interesting overwork paradigm is wing weighting, in which growth of the tonic anterior latissimus dorsi (ALD) muscle results from stretch and overload induced by attaching weight to a bird's humerus. Initial report of substantial increase in total number of myofibers in chickens[355] was later confirmed in quail, which show a 50 percent increase in myofibers in the ALD after a month of weighting. The new myofibers appear not to arise from splitting or branching of preexisting myofibers[355, 356] and there is clear evidence of ^{3}H-TdR incorporation by satellite cells, which begins at 1 day and peaks by about a week.[357] It was observed that the frequency of satellite cells on mature myofibers does not change during this period, indicating that the satellite cell daughters fuse promptly with the myofibers.[358] However, the discovery of myotube formation in the interstitium around mature myofibers[76,359,360] suggests that, instead of fusing with their associated myofibers, some of the new satellite cells migrate away to undergo de novo myogenesis in the interfascicular connective tissue space. Although there is some disagreement about the amount of myofiber damage and necrosis,[359,360] which may depend on avian species and muscle region, it appears to be minimal as compared with other overwork paradigms.

In summary, many types of overwork produce activation and proliferation of satellite cells. It is not yet clear whether the satellite cell response is a primary result of overwork or a secondary consequence of induced myofiber injury. The additional satellite cells may contribute to (1) augmentation of nuclear number of existing myofibers, (2) repair or regeneration of damaged myofibers, or (3) formation of new myofibers. The degree of each response varies with type of overwork, species, and muscle, among other factors.

List of Abbreviations

ALD	anterior latissimus dorsi	mRNA	messenger ribonucleic acid
DMD	Duchenne muscular dystrophy	N-CAM	neural cell adhesion molecule
FGF	fibroblast growth factor	PDGF	platelet-derived growth factor
HGF	hepatocyte growth factor	RNA	ribonucleic acid
^{3}H-TdR	tritiated thymidine	TGF-β	transforming growth factor beta
IGF	insulin growth factor		

References

1. Mauro A: Satellite cells of skeletal muscle fibers. *J Biophys Biochem Cytol* 9:493, 1961.
2. Katz B: The terminations of the afferent nerve fibre in the muscle spindle of the frog. *Phil Trans R Soc Lond [Biol]* 243:221, 1961.
3. Griggs RC, Karpati G (eds): *Myoblast Transfer Therapy* New York: Plenum Press, 1990.
4. Grounds MD, White JD, Rosenthal N, et al: The role of stem cells in skeletal and cardiac muscle repair. *J Histochem Cytochem* 50:589, 2002.
5. Carlson BM, Faulkner JA: The regeneration of skeletal muscle fibers following injury: A review. *Med Sci Sports Exerc* 13:187, 1983.
6. Allbrook DB, Baker WD, Kirkaldy-Willis WH: Muscle regeneration in experimental animals and man. *J Bone Joint Surg* 48:153, 1966.
7. Campion DR: The muscle satellite cell: A review. *Int Rev Cytol* 87:255, 1984.
8. Cedars MG, Miller TA: A review of free muscle grafting. *Plast Reconstr Surg* 74:712, 1984.
9. Faulkner JA, Carlson BM: Skeletal muscle regeneration: A historical perspective. *Fed Proc* 45:1454, 1986.
10. Marechal G: Regeneration of mammalian striated muscle. *Biomed Biochim Acta* 45:S125, 1986.
11. Maxwell LC, Moody MR: Muscle fiber regeneration in grafted skeletal muscles. *J Reconstr Microsurg* 4:161, 1988.
12. Grounds MD: Towards understanding skeletal muscle regeneration. *Pathol Res Pract* 187:1, 1991.
13. Field EJ: Muscle regeneration and repair, in Bourne GH (ed): *Structure and Function of Muscle*. New York: Academic Press, 1960, p 139.
14. Plaghki L: Regeneration et myogenese du muscle strié. *J Physiol (Paris)* 80:51, 1985.
15. Mauro A (ed): *Muscle Regeneration*. New York: Raven Press, 1979.
16. Mauro A, Shafiq SA, Milhorat AT (eds): *Regeneration of Striated Muscle, and Myogenesis* Amsterdam: Excerpta Medica, 1970.

17. Ishikawa H: Electron microscopic observations of satellite cells with special reference to the development of mammalian skeletal muscles. *Zeitschr Anat Entwick* 125:43, 1966.
18. Castillo de Maruenda E, Franzini-Armstrong C: Satellite and invasive cells in frog sartorius muscle. *Tissue Cell* 10:749, 1978.
19. Bader CR, Bertrand D, Cooper E, Mauro A: Membrane currents of rat satellite cells attached to intact skeletal muscle fibers. *Neuron* 1:237, 1988.
20. Schultz E: Fine structure of satellite cells in growing skeletal muscle. *Am J Anat* 147:49, 1976.
21. Muir AR, Kanji AHM, Allbrook DB: The structure of satellite cells in skeletal muscle. *J Anat* 99:435, 1965.
22. Snow MH: Myogenic cell formation in regenerating rat skeletal muscle injured by mincing: 1. A fine structural study. *Anat Rec* 188:181, 1977.
23. Connolly JA, Kiosses BW, Kalnins VI: Centrioles are lost as embryonic myoblasts fuse into myotubes in vitro. *Eur J Cell Biol* 39:341, 1986.
24. Ontell M: Muscle satellite cells: A validated technique for light microscopic identification and a quantitative study of changes in their population following denervation. *Anat Rec* 178:211, 1974.
25. Cull-Candy SG, Miledi R, Nakaiima Y, Uchitel OD: Visualization of satellite cells in living muscle fibers of the frog. *Proc R Soc Lond (Biol)* 209:536, 1980.
26. Larocque AA, Politoff AL, Peters A: The visualization of myosatellite cells in normal and denervated muscle: A new light microscopic staining technique. *Anat Rec* 196:373, 1980.
27. Herrera AA, Banner LR: The use and effects of vital fluorescent dyes—Observation of motor-nerve terminals and satellite cells in living frog muscles. *J Neurocytol* 19:67, 1990.
28. Trupin GL, Hsu L, Hsieh Y-H: Satellite cell mimics in regenerating skeletal muscles, in Mauro A (ed): *Muscle Regeneration* New York: Raven Press, 1979, p 101.
29. Webster C, Pavlath GK, Parks DR, et al: Isolation of human myoblasts with the fluorescence-activated cell sorter. *Exp Cell Res* 174:252, 1988.
30. Grounds MD: Muscle regeneration: Molecular aspects and therapeutic implications. *Curr Opin Neurol* 12:535, 1999.
31. Walsh FS, Ritter MA: Surface antigen differentiation during human myogenesis in culture. *Nature* 289:60, 1981.
32. Hawke TJ, Garry DJ: Myogenic satellite cells: Physiology to molecular biology. *J Appl Physiol* 91:534, 2001.
33. Cunningham BA, Hemperly JJ, Murray EA, et al: Neural cell adhesion molecule: Structure, immumoglobulin-like domains, cell surface modulation, and alternative RNA splicing. *Science* 236:799, 1987.
34. Walsh FS, Dickinson G, Moore SE, Barton CH: Unmasking N-CAM. *Nature* 339:516, 1989.
35. Covault J, Sanes JR: Distribution of N-CAM in synaptic and extrasynaptic portions of developing and adult skeletal muscle. *J Cell Biol* 102:716, 1986.
36. Hurko O, Walsh FS: Human fetal muscle-specific antigen is restricted to regenerating myofibers in disease adult muscle. *Neurology* 33:737, 1983.
37. Wakshull E, Bayne EK, Chiquet M, Fambrough DM: Characterization of a plasma membrane glycoprotein common to myoblasts, skeletal muscle satellite cells, and glia. *Dev Biol* 100:464,1983.
38. Lanier LL, Le AM, Civin CL, et al: The relationship of CD16 (Leu-11) and Leu-19 antigen expression of human peripheral blood NK cells and cytotoxic T lymphocytes. *J Immunol* 136:4480, 1986.
39. Lanier LL, Testi R, Binal J, Phillips JH: Identity of Leu-19 (CD56) leukocyte differentiation antigen and neural cell adhesion molecule. *J Exp Med* 169:2233, 1989.
40. Schubert W, Zimmermann K, Cramer M, Starzinskipowitz A: Lymphocyte antigen leu19 as a molecular marker of regeneration in human skeletal-muscle. *Proc Natl Acad Sci USA* 86:307, 1989.
41. Beauchamp JR, Heslop DR. Yu S, et al:. Expression of CD34 and Myf5 defines the majority of quiescent adult skeletal muscle satellite cells. *J Cell Biol* 151:1221, 2000.
42. Alameddine H, Sharp N, Dehaupas M, et al: Lymphocyte Leu-19 antigens expression in regenerating canine muscles. *J Neurol Sci* 98S:296, 1990.
43. Mechtersheimer G, Staudter M, Moller P: Expression of the natural killer cell associated antigens CD56 and CD57 in human neural and striated muscle cells and in their tumors. *Can Res* 51:1300, 1991.
44. Asakura A, Seale P, Girgis-Gabardo A, et al: Myogenic specification of side population cells in skeletal muscle. *J Cell Biol* 159:123, 2002.
45. Seale P, Sabourin LA, Girgis-Gabardo A, et al: Pax7 is required for the specification of myogenic satellite cells. *Cell* 102:777, 2000.
46. Cornelison DD, Filla MS, Stanley HM: Syndecan-3 and syndecan-4 specifically mark skeletal muscle satellite cells and are implicated in satellite cell maintenance and muscle regeneration *Dev Biol* 239:79, 2001.
47. Kelly AM: Perisynaptic satellite cells in the developing and mature rat soleus muscle. *Anat Rec* 190:891, 1978.
48. Kelly AM: Variations in satellite cell distribution in developing and mature muscles of the rat, in Mauro A (ed): *Muscle Regeneration* New York: Raven Press, 1979, p 167.
49. Wokke JHJ, Vandenoord CJM, Leppink GJ, Jennekens FGI: Perisynaptic satellite cells in human external intercostal muscle—A quantitative and qualitative study. *Anat Rec* 223:174, 1989.
50. Schmalbruch H, Hellhammer U: The number of nuclei in adult rat muscles with special reference to satellite cells. *Anat Rec* 189:169, 1977.
51. Kelly AM: Satellite cells and myofiber growth in the rat soleus and extensor digitorum longus muscles. *Dev Biol* 65:1, 1978.
52. Gibson MC, Schultz E: The distribution of satellite cells and their relationship to specific fiber types in soleus and extensor digitorum longus muscles. *Anat Rec* 202:329, 1982.
53. Matthew CA, Moore MJ: Numbers of myonuclei and satellite cell nuclei in latissimus dorsi muscles of the chicken. *Cell Tissue Res* 248:235, 1987.
54. Sandset PM, Korneliussen H: Myosatellite cells associated with different muscle fiber types in the Atlantic hagfish. *Cell Tissue Res* 195:17, 1978.
55. Kryvi H, Eide A: Morphometric and autoradiographic studies on the growth of red and white axial muscle fibres in the shark *Etmopterus spinax*. *Anat Embryol (Berl)* 151:17, 1977.
56. Saito Y: Muscle fibre type differentiation and satellite cell population in Werdnig-Hoffmann disease. *J Neurol Sci* 68:75, 1985.
57. Allbrook DB, Han MF, Hellmuth AE: Population of muscle satellite cells in relation to age and mitotic activity. *Pathology* 3:233, 1971.
58. Cardasis CA, Cooper GW: An analysis of nuclear numbers in individual muscle fibers during differentiation and growth: A satellite cell-muscle fiber growth unit. *J Exp Zool* 191:347, 1975.
59. Cullen MJ, Watkins SC: The role of satellite cells in regeneration in diseased muscle. *Adv Physiol Sci* 24:341, 1981.
60. Schultz E: Satellite cell behavior during skeletal muscle growth and regeneration. *Med Sci Sports Exerc* 21:S181, 1989.
61. Schmalbruch H, Hellhammer U: The number of satellite cells in normal human muscle. *Anat Rec* 185:279, 1976.
62. Snow MH: The effects of aging on satellite cells in skeletal muscle of mice and rats. *Cell Tissue Res* 185:399, 1977.
63. Hauschka SD, Linkhart TA, Clegg C, Merrill G: Clonal studies of human and mouse muscle, in Mauro A (ed): *Muscle Regeneration* New York: Raven Press, 1979, p 311.
64. Blau HM, Webster C: Isolation and characterization of human muscle cells. *Proc Natl Acad Sci USA* 78:5623, 1981.
65. Kelly AM, Zacks SI: The histogenesis of rat intercostal muscle. *J Cell Biol* 42:135, 1969.
66. Rash JE, Staehelin LA: Freeze-cleave demonstration of gap junctions between skeletal myogenic cells. *Dev Biol* 36:455, 1974.
67. Schmalbruch H: Skeletal muscle fibers of newborn rats are coupled by gap junctions. *Dev Biol* 91:485, 1982.
68. Yiping L, Appelt D, Kelly AM, et al: Differences in the histogenesis of EDL and diaphragm in rat. *Dev Dynam* 193:359, 1992.
69. Moss FP, Leblond CP: Satellite cells as the source of nuclei in muscles of growing rats. *Anat Rec* 170:421, 1971.
70. Snow MH: Myogenic cell formation in regenerating rat skeletal muscle injured by mincing: II. An autoradiographic study. *Anat Rec* 188:210, 1977.
71. Armand O, Kieny M: Ontogeny of the myosatellite cell. *Arch Anat Microsc Morphol Exp* 73:75, 1984.
72. Heslop L, Beauchamp J, Tajbakhsh S, et al: Transplanted primary neonatal myoblasts can give rise to functional satellite cells as identified using the Myf5nlacZl+ mouse. *Gene Ther* 8:778, 2001
73. Seale P, Asakura A, Rudnicki MA: The potential of muscle stem cells *Dev Cell* 1:333, 2001.
74. Bischoff R, Lowe M: Cell surface components and the interaction of myogenic cells, in Milhorat AT (ed): *Exploratory Concepts in Muscular Dystrophy II*. Amsterdam: Excerpta Medica, 1974, p 17.
75. Lipton BH, Schultz E: Developmental fate of skeletal muscle satellite cells. *Science* 205:1292, 1979.
76. Bischoff R: Proliferation of muscle satellite cells on intact myofibers in culture. *Dev Biol* 115:129, 1986.
77. Kennedy JM, Eisenberg BR, Reid SK, et al: Nascent muscle fiber appearance in overloaded chicken slow-tonic muscle. *Am J Anat* 181:203, 1988.
78. Hughes SM, Blau HM: Migration of myoblasts across basal lamina during skeletal muscle development. *Nature* 345:350, 1990.
79. Bonner PH, Hauschka SD: Clonal analysis of vertebrate morphogenesis: I. Early developmental events in the chick limb. *Dev Biol* 37:317, 1974.
80. Hauschka SD: Clonal analysis of vertebrate myogenesis: II. Environmental influences upon human muscle differentiation. *Dev Biol* 37:329, 1974.
81. White NK, Bonner PH, Nelson DR, Hauschka SD: Clonal analysis of vertebrate myogenesis: IV. Medium-dependent classification of colony-forming cells. *Dev Biol* 44:346, 1975.
82. Bonner PH: Nerve-dependent changes in clonable myoblast populations. *Dev Biol* 66:207, 1978.
83. Bonner PH: Differentiation of chick embryo myoblasts is transiently sensitive to functional denervation. *Dev Biol* 76:79, 1980.
84. Kaufman SJ, George-Weinstein M, Foster RF: In vitro development of precursor cells in the myogenic lineage. *Dev Biol* 146:228, 1991.
85. Peterson CA, Cho M, Rastinejad F, Blau HM: Beta-enolase is a marker of human myoblast heterogeneity prior to differentiation. *Dev Biol* 151:626, 1992.

86. Cohen R, Pacifici M, Rubinstein N, et al: Effect of a tumour promoter on myogenesis. *Nature* 266:538, 1977.
87. Cossu G, Molinaro M, Pacifici M: TPA induced inhibition of the expression of differentiative traits in cultured myotubes: Dependence on protein synthesis. *Differentiation* 21:62, 1982.
88. Cossu G, Molinaro M, Pacifici M: Differential response of satellite cells and embryonic myoblasts to a tumor promoter. *Dev Biol* 98:520, 1983.
89. Cossu G, Cicinelli P, Fieri C, et al: Emergence of TPA-resistant "satellite" cells during muscle histogenesis of human limb. *Exp Cell Res* 160:403, 1985.
90. Cossu G, Ranaldi G, Senni MI, et al: "Early" mammalian myoblasts are resistant to phorbol ester-induced block of differentiation. *Development* 102:65, 1988.
91. Ontell M, Kozeka K: Organogenesis of the mouse extensor digitorum longus muscle: A quantitative study. *Am J Anat* 171:149, 1984.
92. Eusebi F Molinaro M: Acetylcholine sensitivity in replicating satellite cells. *Muscle Nerve* 7:488, 1984.
93. Cossu G, Eusebi F, Grassi F, Wanke E: Acetylcholine receptor channels are present in undifferentiated satellite cells but not in embryonic myoblasts in culture. *Dev Biol* 123:43, 1987.
94. Senni MI, Castrignano F, Poiana G, et al: Expression of adult fast pattern of acetylcholinesterase molecular forms by mouse satellite cells in culture. *Differentiation* 36:194, 1987.
95. Matsuda R, Spector DH, Strohman RC: Regenerating adult chicken skeletal muscle and satellite cell cultures express embryonic patterns of myosin and tropomyosin isoforms. *Dev Biol* 100:478, 1983.
96. Mouly V, Lemonnier M, Libri D, et al: Transformation and cloning of different types of myoblasts during avian development, in Pette D (ed): *The Dynamic State of Muscle Fibers*. Berlin: de Gruyter, 1990, p 651.
97. Feldman JL, Stockdale FE: Skeletal-muscle satellite cell diversity—Satellite cells form fibers of different types in cell culture. *Dev Biol* 143:320, 1991.
98. Stockdale FE: The myogenic lineage—Evidence for multiple cellular precursors during avian limb development. *Proc Soc Exp Biol Med* 194:71, 1990.
99. Dusterhoft S, Yablonka Reuveni Z, Pette D: Characterization of myosin isoforms in satellite cell cultures from adult-rat diaphragm, soleus and tibialis anterior muscles. *Differentiation* 45:185, 1990.
100. Potten CS, Loeffler M: Stem cells: Attributes, cycles, spirals, pitfalls and uncertainties. *Development* 110:1001, 1990.
101. Bischoff R: Analysis of muscle regeneration using single myofibers in culture. *Med Sci Sports Exerc* 21:S164, 1989.
102. Enesco M, Puddy D: Increase in the number of nuclei and weight in skeletal muscle of rats of various ages. *Am J Anat* 114:235, 1964.
103. Hellmuth AE, Allbrook D: Satellite cells as the stem cells of skeletal muscle, in Kakulas BA (ed): *Basic Research in Myology*. Amsterdam: Excerpta Medica, 1973, p 343.
104. Gibson MC, Schultz E: Age-related differences in absolute numbers of skeletal muscle satellite cells. *Muscle Nerve* 6:574, 1983.
105. Church JCT: Cell quantitation in regenerating bat web muscle, in Mauro A, Shafiq SA, Milhorat AT (eds): *Regeneration of Striated Muscle, and Myogenesis*. Amsterdam: Excerpta Medica, 1970, p 101.
106. Schultz E, Jaryszak DL: Effects of skeletal muscle regeneration on the proliferation potential of satellite cells. *Mech Ageing Dev* 30:63, 1985.
107. Gulati AK: Pattern of skeletal muscle regeneration after reautotransplantation of regenerated muscle. *J Embryol Exp Morphol* 92:1, 1986.
108. Morlet K, Grounds MD, McGeachie JK: Muscle precursor replication after repeated regeneration of skeletal-muscle in mice. *Anat Embryol* 180:471, 1989.
109. Mong FS: Satellite cells in the regenerated and regrafted skeletal muscles of rats. *Experientia* 44:601, 1988.
110. Bradley WG: Muscle fiber splitting, in Mauro A (ed): *Muscle Regeneration* New York: Raven Press, 1979, p 215.
111. Basson MD, Carlson BM: Myotoxicity of single and repeated injections of mepivacaine (Carbocaine) in the rat. *Anesth Analg* 59:275, 1980.
112. Sadeh M, Czyzewski K, Stern LZ: Chronic myopathy induced by repeated bupivacaine injections. *J Neurol Sci* 67:229, 1985.
113. Hall-Craggs ECB: Rapid degeneration and regeneration of a whole skeletal muscle following treatment with bupivacaine (Marcaine). *J Anat* 107:546, 1974.
114. Bischoff R: Enzymatic liberation of myogenic cells from adult rat muscle. *Anat Rec* 180:645, 1974.
115. Bischoff R: Tissue culture studies on the origin of myogenic cells during muscle regeneration in the rat, in Mauro A (ed): *Muscle Regeneration*. New York: Raven Press, 1979, p 13.
116. Allen RE, Boxhorn LK: Regulation of skeletal-muscle satellite cell-proliferation and differentiation by transforming growth factor-beta, insulin-like growth factor-I, and fibroblast growth-factor. *J Cell Physiol* 138:311, 1989.
117. Hayflick L: The limited in-vitro lifespan of human diploid cells strains. *Exp Cell Res* 37:614, 1965.
118. Stanulis-Praeger B: In-vitro studies of aging. *Clin Geriatr Med* 5:23, 1989.
119. Ham RG, St. Clair JA, Meyer SD: Improved media for rapid clonal growth of normal human skeletal muscle satellite cells. *Adv Exp Med Biol* 280:193, 1990.
120. Wakayama Y, Schotland DL, Bonilla D, Orecchio E: Quantitative ultrastructural study of muscle satellite cells in Duchenne dystrophy. *Neurology* 29:401, 1979.
121. Wakayama Y, Schotland DL: Muscle satellite cell populations in Duchenne dystrophy, in Mauro A (ed): *Muscle Regeneration*. New York: Raven Press, 1979, p 121.
122. Blau HM, Webster C, Pavlath GK: Defective myoblasts identified in Duchenne muscular dystrophy. *Proc Natl Acad Sci USA* 80:4856, 1983.
123. Wright WE: Myoblast senescence in muscular dystrophy. *Exp Cell Res* 157:343, 1985.
124. Asakura A Komaki M, Rudnicki M: Muscle satellite cells are multipotential stem cells that exhibit myogenic, osteogenic, and adipogenic differentiation *Differentiation* 68:245, 2001.
125. Blau HM, Brazelton TR, Weiman JM: The evolving concept of a stem cell: Entity or function? *Cell* 105:829, 2001
126. O'Brien K, Muskiewicz K, Gussoni E: Recent advances in and therapeutic potential of muscle-derived stem cells. *J Cell Biochem (Suppl)* 38:80, 2002.
127. Ferrari G, Cusella-De Angelis G, Coletta M, et al: Muscle regeneration by bone-marrow-derived myogenic progenitors *Science* 279:1528, 1998.
128. Gussoni E, Soneoka Y, Strickland CD, et al: Dystrophin expression in the mdx mouse restored by stem cell transplantation. *Nature* 401:390, 1999.
129. Bittner RE, Schofer C, Weipoltshammer K, et al: Recruitment of bone-marrow-derived cells by skeletal and cardiac muscle in adult dystrophic mdx mice. *Anat Embryol* 199:391, 1999.
130. Ferrari G, Stornaiuolo A, Sartori S, et al: Bone marrow transplantation as a source of myogenic progenitors: Differentiation of stem cells into muscle. *Cell Transplant* 8:195, 1999.
131. Tamaki T, Akatsuka A, Ando K, et al: Identification of myogenic-endothelial progenitor cells in the interstitial spaces of muscle. *J Cell Biol* 157:571, 2002.
132. McKinney-Freeman SL, Jackson KA, Camargo FD, et al: Muscle derived hematopoietic stem cells are hematopoietic in origin. *Proc Natl Acad Sci USA* 98:13699, 2001.
133. Schultz E, Jaryszak DL, Valliere CR: Response of satellite cells to focal skeletal muscle injury. *Muscle Nerve* 8:217, 1985.
134. Schultz E, Albright DJ, Jaryszak DL, et al: Survival of satellite cells in whole muscle transplants. *Anat Rec* 222:12, 1988.
135. Phillips GD, Lu D, Carlson BM: Survival of myogenic cells in freely grafted rectus femoris and extensor digitorum longus muscles. *Am J Anat* 180:365, 1987.
136. Phillips GD, Hoffman JR, Knighton DR: Migration of myogenic cells in the rat extensor digitorum longus muscle studied with a split autograft model. *Cell Tissue Res* 262:81, 1990.
137. Vracko R: Effects of aging and diabetes on basal lamina thickness of six cell types, in Kefalides NA (ed): *Biology and Chemistry of Basement Membranes*. New York: Academic Press, 1978, p 483.
138. Kovanen V, Suominen H, Risteli J, et al: Type IV collagen and laminin in slow and fast skeletal muscle in rats—Effects of age and life-time endurance training. *Coll Rel Res* 8:145, 1988.
139. Partridge TA: Invited review: Myoblast transfer—A possible therapy for inherited myopathies. *Muscle Nerve* 14:197, 1991.
140. Huard J, Bouchard JP, Roy R, et al: Human myoblast transplantation—Preliminary results of 4 cases. *Muscle Nerve* 15:550, 1992.
141. Klein-Ogus C, Harris JB: Preliminary observations of satellite cells in undamaged fibers of the rat soleus muscle assaulted by a snake-venom toxin. *Cell Tissue Res* 230:671, 1983.
142. Maltin CA, Harris JB, Cullen MJ: Regeneration of mammalian skeletal muscle following the injection of the snake-venom toxin, taipoxin. *Cell Tissue Res* 232:565, 1983.
143. Ontell M: Evidence for myoblastic potential of satellite cells in denervated muscle. *Cell Tissue Res* 160:345, 1975.
144. Salleo A, La Spada GF, Falzea G, et al: Response of satellite cells and muscle fibers to long-term compensatory hypertrophy. *J Submicrosc Cytol* 15:929, 1983.
145. Snow MH: Satellite cell response in rat soleus muscle undergoing hypertrophy due to surgical ablation of synergists. *Anat Rec* 227:437, 1990.
146. Partridge TA, Sloper JC: A host contribution to the regeneration of muscle grafts. *J Neurol Sci* 33:425, 1977.
147. Partridge TA, Grounds M, Sloper JC: Evidence of fusion between host and donor myoblasts in skeletal muscle grafts. *Nature* 273:306, 1978.
148. Grounds M, Partridge TA, Sloper JC: The contribution of exogenous cells to regenerating skeletal muscle: An isoenzyme study of muscle allografts in mice. *J Pathol* 132:325, 1980.
149. Watt DJ, Lambert K, Morgan JE, et al: Incorporation of donor muscle precursor cells into an area of muscle regeneration in the host mouse. *J Neurol Sci* 57:319, 1982.
150. Grounds MD, Partridge TA: Isoenzyme studies of whole muscle grafts and movement of muscle precursor cells. *Cell Tissue Res* 230:677, 1983.
151. Watt DJ, Morgan JE, Clifford MA, et al: The movement of muscle precursor cells between adjacent regenerating muscles in the mouse. *Anat Embryol (Berl)* 175:527, 1987.

152. Morgan JE, Coulton GR, Partridge TA: Muscle precursor cells invade and repopulate freeze-killed muscles. *J Muscle Res Cell Motil* 8:386, 1987.
153. Ghins E, Colson-Van SM, Marechal G: The origin of muscle stem cells m rat triceps surae regenerating after mincing. *J Muscle Res Cell Motil* 5:771, 1984.
154. Schultz E, Jaryszak DL, Gibson MC, et al: Absence of exogenous satellite cell contribution to regeneration of frozen skeletal muscle. *J Muscle Res Cell Motil* 7:361, 1986.
155. Bischoff R: Regeneration of single skeletal muscle fibers m vitro. *Anat Rec* 182:215, 1975.
156. Konigsberg UR, Lipton BH: The regenerative response of single mature muscle fibers isolated in vitro. *Dev Biol* 45:260, 1975.
157. Konigsberg IR: Regeneration of single muscle fibers in culture and in vivo, in Mauro A (ed): *Muscle Regeneration*. New York: Raven Press, 1979, p 41.
158. Richler C, Yaffe D: The in vitro cultivation and differentiation capacities of myogenic cell lines. *Dev Biol* 23:1, 1970.
159. Yablonka-Reuveni Z, Nameroff M: Skeletal muscle cell populations: Separation and partial characterization of fibroblast-like cells from embryonic tissue using density centrifugation. *Histochemistry* 87:27, 1987.
160. Morgan JE: Myogenicity in vitro and in vivo of mouse muscle cells separated on discontinuous Percoll gradients. *J Neurol Sci* 85:197, 1988.
161. McFarland DC, Pesall JE, Gilkerson KK, Ferrin NH: Comparison of the proliferation and differentiation of myogenic satellite cells and embryonic myoblasts derived from the turkey. *Comp Biochem Physiol (A)* 100:439, 1991.
162. Bekoff A, Berz W: Properties of isolated adult rat muscle fibers maintained in tissue culture. *J Physiol* 271:537, 1977.
163. Florini JR: Hormonal control of muscle growth. *Muscle Nerve* 10:577, 1987
164. Florini JR, Magri KA: Effects of growth factors on myogenic differentiation. *Am J Physiol* 256:C701, 1989.
165. Florini JR, Ewton DZ, Magri KA: Hormones, growth-factors, and myogenic differentiation. *Annu Rev Physiol* 53:201, 1991.
166. Dayton WR, Hathaway MR: Myogenic cell-proliferation and differentiation. *Poultry Sci* 70:1815, 1991.
167. Schultz E, Gibson MC, Champion T: Satellite cells are mitotically quiescent in mature mouse muscle: An EM and radioautographic study. *J Exp Zool* 206:451, 1978
168. Bischoff R: Cell cycle commitment of rat muscle satellite cells. *J Cell Biol* 111:201, 1990.
169. Pardee AB: G1 events and regulation of cell proliferation. *Science* 246:603, 1989.
170. Baird A, Bohlen P: Fibroblast growth factors, in Sporn MB, Roberts AB (eds): *Peptide Growth Factors and Their Receptors: 1*. New York: Springer-Verlag, 1991, p 369.
171. Klagsbrun M, Sullivan R, Smith S, et al: Purification of endothelial cell growth factors by heparin affinity chromatography. *Meth Enzymol* 147:95, 1987.
172. Gospodarowicz D, Weseman J, Moran J: Presence in brain of a mitogenic agent promoting proliferation of myoblasts in low density culture. *Nature* 256:216, 1975.
173. Gospodarowicz D: Purification of a fibroblast growth factor from bovine pituitary. *J Biol Chem* 250:2515, 1975.
174. Kimura I, Gotoh Y, Ozawa E: Further purification of a fibroblast growth factor-like factor from click embryo extract by heparin-affinity chromatography. *In Vitro Cell Dev Biol* 25:236, 1989.
175. Allen RE, Dodson MV, Luiten LS: Regulation of skeletal muscle satellite cell proliferation by bovine pituitary fibroblast growth factor. *Exp Cell Res* 152:154, 1984.
176. Allen RE, Dodson MV, Boxhorn LK, et al: Satellite cell proliferation in response to pituitary hormones. *J Anim Sci* 62:1596, 1986.
177. DiMario J, Strohman RC: Satellite cells from dystrophic (mdx) mouse muscle are stimulated by fibroblast growth-factor in vitro. *Differentiation* 39.42, 1988.
178. Greene EA, Allen RE: Growth-factor regulation of bovine satellite cell growth in vitro. *J Anim Sci* 69:146, 1991.
179. Allen RE, Rankin LL: Regulation of satellite cells during skeletal-muscle growth and development. *Proc Soc Exp Biol Med* 194:81, 1990.
180. Stiles CD, Capone GT, Antoniades HN, et al: Dual control of cell growth by somatomedins and platelet-derived growth factor. *Proc Natl Acad Sci USA* 76:1279, 1979.
181. Florini JR, Magri KA, Ewton DZ, et al: "Spontaneous" differentiation of skeletal myoblasts is dependent upon autocrine secretion of insulin-like growth factor-II. *J Biol Chem* 266:15917, 1991.
182. Hill DJ, Crace CJ, Nissley SP, et al: Fetal rat myoblasts release both rat somatomedin-C/insulin-like growth factor I and multiplication stimulating activity in vitro: Partial characterization and biological activity of myoblast-derived SM-C/IGF 1. *Endocrinology* 117:2061, 1985.
183. Alterio I, Courtois Y, Robelin J, et al: Acidic and basic fibroblast growth factor mRNAs are expressed by skeletal muscle satellite cells. *Biochem Biophys Res Commun* 166:1205, 1990.
184. Le Moigne A, Martelly I, Barlovatz-Meimon G, et al: Characterization of myogenesis from adult satellite cells cultured in vitro. *Int J Dev Biol* 34:171, 1990.

185. Olwin BB, Hauschka SD: Cell-surface fibroblast growth-factor and epidermal growth-factor receptors are permanently lost during skeletal muscle terminal differentiation in culture. *J Cell Biol* 107:761, 1988.
186. Moore JW, Dionne C, Jaye M, et al: The messenger RNAs encoding acidic FGF, basic FGF and FGF receptor are coordinately down-regulated during myogenic differentiation. *Development* 111:741, 1991.
187. Folkman J, Klagsbrun M, Sasse J, et al: A heparin-binding angiogenic protein-basic fibroblast growth factor is stored within basement membrane. *Am J Pathol* 130:393, 1988.
188. Kardami E, McClure S, Strohman RC: Heparin-like components may regulate skeletal muscle growth and differentiation, in Emerson, C, Fischman, D, Nadal-Ginard, B, Siddiqui, MAQ (eds): *Molecular Biology of Muscle Development*. New York: Liss, 1986, p 133.
189. Kardami E, Spector D, Strohman RC: Heparin inhibits skeletal muscle growth in vitro. *Dev Biol* 126:19, 1988.
190. Sanes JR, Schachner M, Covault J: Expression of several adhesive macromolecules (N-CAM, L1, J1, NILE, uvomorulin, laminin, fibronectin, and a heparan sulfate proteoglycan) in embryonic, adult, and denervated adult skeletal muscle. *J Cell Biol* 102:420, 1986.
191. Bischoff R: Control of satellite cell proliferation, in Griggs R, Karpati G (eds): *Myoblast Transfer Therapy*. New York: Plenum Press, 1990, p 147.
192. Rapraeger AC, Krufka A, Olwin BB: Requirement of heparan sulfate for bFGF-mediated fibroblast growth and myoblast differentiation. *Science* 252:1705, 1991.
193. DiMario J, Buffinger N, Yamada S, et al: Fibroblast growth factor in the extracellular matrix of dystrophic (MDX) mouse muscle. *Science* 244:688, 1989.
194. Yamada S, Buffinger N, Dimario J, et al: Fibroblast growth factor is stored in fiber extracellular matrix and plays a role in regulating muscle hypertrophy. *Med Sci Sports Exerc* 21:S173, 1989.
195. Anderson JE, Liu L, Kardami E: Distinctive patterns of basic fibroblast growth-factor (bFGF) distribution in degenerating and regenerating areas of dystrophic (mdx) striated muscles. *Dev Biol* 10:96, 1991.
196. Vaca K, Stewart SS, Appel SH: Identification of basic fibroblast growth-factor as a cholinergic growth-factor from human-muscle. *J Neurosci Res* 23:55, 1989.
197. Gurthridge M, Wilson M, Cowling J, et al: The role of basic fibroblast growth factor m skeletal muscle regeneration. *Growth Factors* 6:53, 1992.
198. Morrow NG, Kraus WE, Moore JW, et al: Increased expression of fibroblast growth factors in a rabbit skeletal muscle model of exercise conditioning. *J Clin Invest* 85:1816, 1990.
199. Davidson JM, Broadley KN: Manipulation of the wound-healing process with basic fibroblast growth factor. *Ann NY Acad Sci* 638:306, 1991.
200. Smith RG, Vaca K, McManaman J, et al: Selective effects of skeletal muscle extract fractions on motoneuron development in vitro. *J Neurosci* 6:439, 1986.
201. Rechler MM, Nissley SP: Insulin-like growth factors, in Sporn MB, Roberts, AB (eds): *Peptide Growth Factors and Their Receptors: 1*. New York: Springer-Verlag, 1991, p 263.
202. Hintz RL: Plasma forms of somatomedin and the binding protein phemonenon. *Clin Endocrinol Metab* 13:31, 1984.
203. Dodson MV, Allen RE, Hossner KL: Ovine somatomedin, multiplication-stimulating activity, and insulin promote skeletal muscle satellite cell proliferation in vitro. *Endocrinology* 177:2357, 1985.
204. McCusker RH, Clemmons DR: Insulin-like growth-factor binding-protein secretion by muscle-cells—Effect of cellular differentiation and proliferation. *J Cell Physiol* 137:505, 1998.
205. Whitson PA, Stuart CA, Huls MH, et al: Dexamethasone effects on creatine kinase activity and insulin-like growth factor receptors in cultured muscle cells. *J Cell Physiol* 140:8, 1989.
206. Hill DJ, Crace CJ, Fowler L, et al: Cultured fetal rat myoblasts release peptide growth factors which are immunologically and biologically similar to somatomedins. *J Cell Physiol* 119:349, 1984.
207. Tollefsen SE, Lajara R, McCusker RH, et al: Insulin-like growth-factors (IGF) in muscle development—Expression of IGF-I, the IGF-I receptor, and an IGF binding-protein during myoblast differentiation. *J Biol Chem* 264:13810, 1989.
208. Roe JA, Harper JMM, Buttery PJ: Protein-metabolism in ovine primary muscle cultures derived from satellite cells—Effects of selected peptide hormones and growth-factors. *J Endocrinol* 122:565, 1989.
209. Shimizu M, Webster C, Morgan DO, et al: Insulin and insulin-like growth factor receptors and responses in cultured human muscle cells. *Am J Physiol* 251:E611, 1986.
210. Herington AC: Insulin-like growth factors: Biochemistry and physiology. *Baillieres Clin Endocrinol Metab* 5:531, 1991.
211. Sun SS, McFarland DC, Ferrin NH, et al: Comparison of insulin-like growth-factor interaction with satellite cells and embryonic myoblasts derived from the turkey. *Comp Biochem Physiol [A]* 102:235, 1992.
212. Dodson MV, Allen RE: Interaction of multiplication stimulating activity/rat insulin-like growth factor II with skeletal muscle satellite cells during aging. *Mech Ageing Dev* 39:121, 1987.
213. McCusker RH, Campion DR: Effect of growth hormone-secreting tumors on skeletal muscle cellularity in the rat. *J Endocrinol* 111:279, 1986.

214. Beermann DH, Liboff M, Wilson DB, et al: Effects of exogenous thyroxine and growth hormone on satellite cell and myonuclei populations in rapidly growing rat skeletal muscle. *Growth* 47:426, 1983.
215. Ullmam M, Ullman A, Sommerland H, et al: Effects of growth hormone on muscle regeneration and IGF-I concentration in old rats. *Acta Physiol Scand* 140:521, 1990.
216. Grounds MD, McGeachie JK: A comparison of muscle precursor replication in crush-injured skeletal-muscle of Swiss and balbc mice. *Cell Tissue Res* 255:385, 1989.
217. Edwall D, Schalling M, Jennische E, et al: Induction of insulin like growth factor I messenger ribonucleic acid during regeneration of rat skeletal muscle. *Endocrinology* 124:820, 1989.
218. Sommerland H, Ullman M, Jennische E, et al: Muscle regeneration: The effect of hypophysectomy on cell proliferation and expression of insulin-like growth factor-1. *Acta Neuropathol (Berl)* 78:264, 1989.
219. Jennische E, Hansson HA: Regenerating skeletal muscle cells express insulin-like growth factor I. *Acta Physiol Scand* 130:327, 1987.
220. Goldspink G, Williams P, Simpson H: Gene expression in response to muscle stretch. *Clin Orthop Rel Res* 403:S146, 2002.
221. Bischoff R: A satellite cell mitogen from crushed adult muscle. *Dev Biol* 115:140, 1986.
222. Bischoff R, Heintz C: Enhancement of skeletal muscle regeneration *Dev Dynam* 201:41, 1994.
223. Phillips GD, Schilb LA, Fiegel VD, et al: An acid/ethanol extract from skeletal muscle stimulates angiogenesis in the rabbit cornea and monocyte and endothelial cell chemotaxis in vitro. *Proc Soc Exp Biol Med* 197:458, 1991.
224. Phillips GD, Knighton DR: Angiogenic activity in damaged skeletal muscle. *Proc Soc Exp Biol Med* 193:197, 1990.
225. Bischoff R: Chemotaxis of skeletal muscle satellite cells *Dev Dynam* 208:505, 1997.
226. Ross R, Glomset B, Karija B, et al: A platelet-derived serum factor that stimulates the proliferation of arterial smooth muscle cells in vitro. *Proc Natl Acad Sci USA* 71:1207, 1974.
227. Ross R, Raines EW, Bowen-Pope DF: The biology of platelet derived growth factor. *Cell* 46:156, 1986.
228. Yablonka-Reuveni Z, Balestreri TM, Bowen-Pope DF: Regulation of proliferation and differentiation of myoblasts derived from adult-mouse skeletal-muscle by specific isoforms of PDGF. *J Cell Biol* 111:1623, 1990.
229. Jin P, Sejersen T, Ringertz NR: Recombinant platelet-derived growth factor-BB stimulates growth and inhibits differentiation of rat L6 myoblasts. *J Biol Chem* 266:1245, 1991.
230. Sejersen T, Betsholtz C, Sjolund M, et al: Rat skeletal myoblasts and arterial smooth muscle cells express the gene for the A chain but not the gene for the B chain (c-sis) of platelet-derived growth factor (PDGF) and produce a PDGF-like protein. *Proc Natl Acad Sci USA* 83:6844, 1986.
231. Jin P, Rahm M, Claesson-Welsh L, et al: Expression of PDGF A-chain and B-receptor during rat myoblast differentiation. *J Cell Biol* 110:1665, 1990.
232. Venkatasubramanian K, Solursh M: Chemotactic behavior of myoblasts. *Dev Biol* 104:428, 1984.
233. Austin L, Burgess AW: Stimulation of myoblast proliferation in culture by leukemia inhibitory factor and other cytokines. *J Neurol Sci* 101:193, 1991.
234. Roberts AB, Sporn MB: The transforming growth factor-betas, in Sporn MB, Roberts AB (eds): *Peptide Growth Factors and Their Receptors: 1*. New York: Springer-Verlag, 1991, p 419.
235. Allen RE, Boxhorn LK Inhibition of skeletal muscle satellite cell differentiation by transforming growth factor-beta. *J Cell Physiol* 133:567, 1987.
236. Bischoff R: Interaction between satellite cells and skeletal-muscle fibers. *Development* 109:943, 1990.
237. Echeverria OM, Ninomiya JG, Vazquez-Nin P: Microscopical and electrophysiological studies on the healing-over of striated fibers of cremaster muscle of the guinea pig. *Acta Anat* 128:274, 1987.
238. Carpenter S, Karpati G: Segmental necrosis and its demarcation in experimental micropuncture injury of skeletal-muscle fibers. *J Neuropathol Exp Neurol* 48:154, 1989.
239. Shafiq SA, Gorycki MA: Regeneration in skeletal muscle of mouse: Some electron-microscope observations. *J Pathol Bacteriol* 90:123, 1965.
240. Hall-Craggs ECB: The regeneration of skeletal muscle fibers per continuum. *J Anat* 117:171, 1974.
241. Ali MA: Myotube formation in skeletal muscle regeneration. *J Anat* 128:553, 1979.
242. Gay AJ, Hunt TE: Reuniting of skeletal muscle fibers after transection. *Anat Rec* 120:853, 1954.
243. Webb P: The effect of innervation, denervation, and muscle type on the reunion of skeletal muscle. *Br J Surg* 60:180, 1973.
244. Stuart A, McComas AJ, Goldspink G, et al: Electrophysiological features of muscle regeneration. *Exp Neurol* 74:148, 1981.
245. Clark WEL, Blomfield LF: The efficiency of intramuscular anastomoses with observation on the regeneration of devascularized muscle. *J Anat* 79:15, 1945.
246. Clark WEL: An experimental study of the regeneration of mammalian striped muscle. *J Anat* 80:24, 1946.
247. Aloisi M, Mussini I: Number of satellite cells and muscle regeneration, in Freilinger G, Holle J, Carlson BM (eds): *Muscle Transplantation*. Vienna: Springer-Verlag, 1981, p 29.
248. Bischoff R: Plasticity of the myofiber-satellite cell complex in culture, in Pette D (ed): *Plasticity of Muscle*. Berlin: de Gruyter, 1980, pp 119–129.
249. Hinterberger TJ, Barald KF: Fusion between myoblasts and adult muscle fibers promotes remodeling of fibers into myotubes in vitro. *Development* 109:139, 1990.
250. Karpati G, Carpenter S: A new experimental model for the study of skeletal muscle cell damage, repair and regeneration in vivo, in Ebashi S (ed): *Muscular Dystrophy*. Tokyo: University of Tokyo Press, 1980, p 323.
251. Darr KC, Schultz E: Exercise-induced satellite cell activation in growing and mature skeletal muscle. *J Appl Physiol* 63:1816, 1987.
252. Irintchev A, Wernig A: Muscle damage and repair in voluntarily running mice: Strain and muscle differences. *Cell Tissue Res* 249:509, 1987.
253. McGeachie JK, Grounds MD: Initiation and duration of muscle precursor replication after mild and severe injury to skeletal muscle of mice: An autoradiographic study. *Cell Tissue Res* 248:125, 1987.
254. Carlson BM, Gutmann E: Contractile and histochemical properties of minced muscle grafts regenerating in normal and denervated rat limbs. *Exp Neurol* 50:319, 1976.
255. Carlson BM, Hansen-Smith FM, Magon DK: The life history of a free muscle graft, in Mauro A (ed): *Muscle Regeneration*. New York: Raven Press, 1979, p 493.
256. Carlson BM: A quantitative study of muscle fiber survival and regeneration in normal, predenervated and Marcaine-treated free muscle grafts m the rat. *Exp Neurol* 52:421, 1976.
257. Kelly AM, Rubenstein NA: Patterns of myosin synthesis in regenerating normal and denervated muscles of the rat, in Pette, D (ed): *Plasticity of Muscle*. Berlin: de Gruyter, 1980, p 161.
258. Mong FSF, Hays AP, Miranda AF: Creatine kinase isoenzyme transitions in muscle grafts of mice. *Cell Diff* 11:141, 1982.
259. Carlson BM: Regeneration of the completely excised gastrocnemius muscle in the frog and rat from minced muscle fragments. *J Morphol* 125:447, 1968.
260. Carlson BM: The regeneration of minced muscles, in Wolsky A (ed): *Monographs in Developmental Biology*. Basel: Karger, 1972, p 128.
261. Zacks SI, Sheff MF: Periosteal and metaplastic bone formation in mouse minced muscle regeneration. *Lab Invest* 46:405, 1982.
262. Hansen-Smith FM, Carlson BM: Cellular responses to free grafting of the extensor digitorum longus muscle of the rat. *J Neurol Sci* 41:149, 1979.
263. Pennington RJT: Proteinases of muscle, in Barrett AJ (ed): *Proteinases in Mammalian Cells and Tissues*. Amsterdam: North-Holland, 1977, p 516.
264. Mayer M: Regulation of myofibrillar protease, plasminogen activator and protein degradation in cultured myoblasts. *Prog Clin Biol Res* 180:543, 1985.
265. Zaidi SIM, Narahara HT: Degradation of skeletal-muscle plasma membrane proteins by calpain. *J Membr Biol* 110:209, 1989.
266. Abood EA, Jones MM: Macrophages in developing mammalian skeletal muscle: Evidence for muscle fibre death as a normal developmental event. *Acta Anat* 140:201, 1991.
267. Orimo S, Hiyamuta E, Arahata K, Sugita H: Analysis of inflammatory cells and complement C3 in bupivacaine-induced myonecrosis. *Muscle Nerve* 14:515, 1991.
268. Grounds MD: Phagocytosis of necrotic muscle in muscle isografts is influenced by the strain, age, and sex of host mice. *J Pathol* 153:71, 1987.
269. Meyer S, Kenan S, Yarom R: Enhancement of muscle regeneration by bone marrow cells in the monkey. *Experientia* 40:490, 1984.
270. Rappolee DA, Werb Z: Secretory products of phagocytes. *Curr Opin Immunol* 1:47, 1988.
271. Gulati AK: Basement membrane component changes in skeletal muscle transplants undergoing regeneration or rejection. *J Cell Biochem* 27:337, 1985.
272. Stauber WT, Fritz VK, Dahlmann B: Extracellular matrix changes following blunt trauma to rat skeletal muscles. *Exp Mol Pathol* 52:69, 1990.
273. Allbrook DB: An electron microscopic study of regenerating skeletal muscle. *J Anat* 96:137, 1962.
274. Church JCT: Satellite cells and myogenesis; a study in the fruit bat web. *J Anat* 105:419, 1969.
275. Schmalbruch H: The morphology of regeneration of skeletal muscles in the rat. *Tissue Cell* 8:673, 1976.
276. Schmalbruch H: Regeneration of soleus muscles of rat autografted in toto as studied by electron microscopy. *Cell Tissue Res* 177:159, 1977.
277. Jirmanova H, Thesleff S: Ultrastructural study of experimental muscle degeneration and regeneration in the adult rat. *Z Zellforsch* 131:71, 1970.
278. Vracko R, Benditt EP: Basal lamina: The scaffold for orderly cell replacement. Observations on regeneration of injured skeletal muscle fibers and capillaries. *J Cell Biol* 55:406, 1972.
279. Vandenburgh HH: Motion into mass: How does tension stimulate muscle growth? *Med Sci Sports Exerc* 19:S142, 1987.
280. Vandenburgh HH: Dynamic mechanical orientation of skeletal myofibers in vitro. *Dev Biol* 93:438, 1982.

281. Vandenburgh HH, Swasdison S, Karlisch P: Computer-aided mechanogenesis of skeletal-muscle organs from single cells in vitro. *FASEB J* 5:2860, 1991.
282. Kuhl U, Ocalan M, Timpl R, von der Mark K: Role of laminin and fibronectin in selecting myogenic versus fibrogenic cells from skeletal muscle cells in vitro. *Dev Biol* 117:628, 1986.
283. von der Mark H, Durr J, Sonnenberg A, et al: Skeletal myoblasts utilize a novel beta-1 series integrin and not alpha-6-beta-1 for binding to the e8 and t8 fragments of laminin. *J Biol Chem* 266:23593, 1991.
284. Ocalan M, Goodman SL, Kuhl U, et al: Laminin alters cell shape and stimulates motility and proliferation of murine skeletal myoblasts. *Dev Biol* 125:158, 1988.
285. von der Mark K, Ocalan M: Antagonistic effects of laminin and fibronectin on the expression of the myogenic phenotype. *Differentiation* 40:150, 1989.
286. Yablonka-Reuveni Z, Bowen-Pope DF, Hartley RS: Proliferation and differentiation of myoblasts: The role of platelet derived growth factor and the basement membrane, in Pette D (ed): *The Dynamic State of Muscle-Fibers*. Berlin: de Gruyter, 1990, p 693.
287. Funanage VL, Smith SM, Minnich MA: Entactin promotes adhesion and long-term maintenance of cultured regenerated skeletal myotubes. *J Cell Physiol* 150:251, 1992.
288. Bader D: Reinnervation of motor endplate-containing and motor endplate-less muscle grafts. *Dev Biol* 77:315, 1980.
289. Caldwell CJ, Mattey DL, Weller RO: Role of the basement-membrane in the regeneration of skeletal-muscle. *Neuropathol Appl Neurobiol* 16:225, 1990.
290. Carlson EC, Carlson BM: A method of preparing skeletal-muscle fiber basal laminae. *Anat Rec* 230:325,1991.
291. Hurme T, Kalimo H: Activation of myogenic precursor cells after muscle injury. *Med Sci Sports Exerc* 24:197, 1992.
292. Grounds MD, McGeachie JK: A model of myogenesis in vivo derived from detailed autoradiographic studies of regenerating skeletal muscle, challenges the concept of quantal mitosis. *Cell Tissue Res* 250:563, 1987.
293. McGeachie JK, Grounds MD: Applications of an autoradiographic model of skeletal muscle myogenesis in vivo, in Kakulas BA, Mastaglia FL (eds): *Pathogenesis and Therapy of Duchenne and Becker Muscular Dystrophy*. New York: Raven Press, 1990, p 151.
294. Roberts P, McGeachie JK, Grounds MD, Smith ER: Initiation and duration of myogenic precursor cell replication in transplants of intact skeletal-muscles—An autoradiographic study in mice. *Anat Rec* 224:1, 1989.
295. Grounds MD, McGeachie JK: Myogenic cell replication in minced skeletal-muscle isografts of Swiss and balbc mice. *Muscle Nerve* 13:305, 1990.
296. Mitchell CA, McGeachie JK, Grounds MD: Cellular differences in the regeneration of murine skeletal muscle: A quantitative histological study in SJL/J and BALB/c mice. *Cell Tissue Res* 269:159, 1992.
297. Baroffio AM, Hamann L, Bernheim M-L, et al: Identification of self-renewing myoblasts in the progeny of single human muscle satellite cells. *Differentiation* 60:47, 1996.
298. Beauchamp JR, Morgan JE, Pagel CN, et al: Dynamics of myoblast transplantation reveal a discrete minority of precursors with stem cell-like properties as the myogenic source. *J Cell Biol* 144:1113, 1999.
299. Yoshida NS, Yoshida K, Koishi K, et al: Cell heterogeneity upon myogenic differentiation: Down-regulation of MyoD and Myf-5 generates "reserve cells." *J Cell Sci* 111:769, 1998.
300. Ontell M, Kozeka K: The organogenesis of murine striated muscle: A cytoarchitectural study *Am J Anat* 171:133, 1984.
301. Ontell M, Hughes D, Bourke D: Morphometric analysis of the developing mouse soleus muscle. *Am J Anat* 181:279, 1988.
302. Ferrari G, Stornaiuolo A, Mavilio F: Failure to correct muscular dystrophy. *Nature* 411:1014, 2001.
303. Gussoni E, Bennett RR, Muskiewicz KR, et al: Long-term persistence of donor nuclei in a Duchenne muscular dystrophy patient receiving bone marrow transplantation.*J Clin Invest* 110:807, 2002.
304. Zammit PS, Heslop L, Hudon V, et al: Kinetics of myoblast proliferation show that resident satellite cells are competent to fully regenerate skeletal muscle fibers. *Exp Cell Res* 281:39, 2002.
305. LaBarge MA, Blau HM:Biological progression from adult bone marrow to mononuclear muscle stem cell to multinucleate muscle fiber in response to injury. *Cell* 111:589, 2002.
306. Qu-Petersen Z, Deasy B, Jankowski R, et al: Identification of a novel population of muscle stem cells in mice: Potential for muscle regeneration. *J Cell Biol* 157:851, 2002.
307. Flake AW: Human mesenchymal stem cells engraft and demonstrate site-specific differentiation after in utero transplantation in sheep. *Nat Med* 6:1282, 2000.
308. Harris AJ: Embryonic growth and innervation of rat skeletal muscles: 1. Neural regulation of muscle fibre numbers. *Philos Trans R Soc London (Biol)* 293:257, 1981.
309. Phillips WD, Bennett MR: Differentiation of fiber types in wing muscles during embryonic development: Effect of neural tube removal. *Dev Biol* 106:457, 1984.
310. Ross JJ, Duxson MJ, Harris AJ: Neural determination of muscle fibre numbers in embryonic rat lumbrical muscles. *Development* 100:395, 1987.
311. Studitsky AN: The neural factor in the development of transplanted muscle, in Milhorat AT (ed): *Exploratory Concepts in Muscular Dystrophy: 11*. Amsterdam: Excerpta Medica, 1974, p 351.
312. Carlson BM, Gutmann C: Regeneration in free grafts of normal and denervated muscles in the rat: Morphology and histochemistry. *Anat Rec* 183:47, 1975.
313. Carlson BM: The biology of muscle transplantation, in Freilinger G (ed): *Muscle Transplantation*. New York: Springer-Verlag, 1981, p 1.
314. Thompson N: Autogenous free grafts of skeletal muscle: A preliminary experimental and clinical study. *Plast Reconstr Surg* 48:11, 1971.
315. Thompson N: A review of autogenous skeletal muscle grafts and their clinical applications. *Clin Plast Surg* 1:349, 1974.
316. Carlson BM, Gutmann E: Regeneration in grafts of normal and denervated rat muscles: Contractile properties. *Pflugers Arch* 333:215, 1975.
317. Schiaffino S, Sjostrom M, Thornell LE, et al: The process of survival of denervated and freely autotransplanted skeletal muscle. *Experientia* 31:1328, 1975.
318. Lee JC: Electron microscopic observations on myogenic free cells of denervated skeletal muscle. *Exp Neurol* 12:123, 1965.
319. Hess A, Rosner S: The satellite cell bud and myoblast in denervated mammalian muscle fibers. *Am J Anat* 129:21, 1970.
320. Snow MH: A quantitative ultrastructural analysis of satellite cells in denervated fast and slow muscles of the mouse. *Anat Rec* 207:593, 1983.
321. Schultz E: Changes in the satellite cells of growing muscle following denervation. *Anat Rec* 190:299, 1978.
322. McGeachie J, Allbrook D: Cell proliferation in skeletal muscle following denervation or tenotomy. *Cell Tissue Res* 193:259, 1978.
323. Salleo A, LaSpada G, Falzea G, et al: "Activation" of satellite cells produced by compensatory hypertrophy, denervation and neostigmine treatment. *Adv Physiol Sci* 24:255, 1981.
324. Aloisi M, Mussini I, Schiaffino S: Activation of muscle nuclei in denervation and hypertrophy, in Kakulas B (ed): *Basic Research in Myology*. Amsterdam: Excerpta Medica, 1973, p 338.
325. Hanzlikova V, Mackova EV, Hnik P: Satellite cells of the rate soleus muscle in the process of compensatory hypertrophy combined with denervation. *Cell Tissue Res* 160:411 1975.
326. McGeachie JK: Sustained cell-proliferation in denervated skeletal muscle of mice. *Cell Tissue Res* 257.455, 1989.
327. Anzil AP, Wernig A: Muscle fibre loss and reinnervation after long-term denervation. *J Neurocytol* 18:833, 1989.
328. Schmalbruch H, Alamood WS, Lewis DM: Morphology of long-term denervated rat soleus muscle and the effect of chronic electrical stimulation. *J Physiol* 441:233, 1991.
329. Irintchev A, Draguhn A, Wernig A: Reinnervation and recovery of mouse soleus muscle after long-term denervation. *Neuroscience* 39:231, 1990.
330. Alamood WS, Lewis DM, Schmalbruch H: Effects of chronic electrical-stimulation on contractile properties of long-term denervated rat skeletal-muscle. *J Physiol* 441:243, 1991.
331. Murray MA, Robbins N: Cell proliferation in denervated muscle: Identity and origin of dividing cells. *Neuroscience* 7:1823, 1982.
332. Connor EA, McMahan UJ: Cell accumulation in the junctional region of denervated muscle. *J Cell Biol* 104:109, 1987.
333. Appell JH, Soares JMC, Duarte JAR: Exercise, muscle damage and fatigue. *Sports Med* 13:108, 1992.
334. Armstrong RB, Warren GL, Warren JA: Mechanisms of exercise induced muscle-fiber injury. *Sports Med* 12:184, 1991.
335. Clarkson PM, Dedrick ME: Exercise induced muscle damage, repair, and adaptation in old and young subjects. *J Gerontol* 43:M91, 1988.
336. Mair J, Koller A, Artner-Dworzak E, et al: Effects of exercise on plasma myosin heavy chain fragments and MRI of skeletal muscle. *J Appl Physiol* 72:656, 1992.
337. Salminen A, Vihko V: Autophagic response to strenuous exercise in mouse skeletal muscle fibers. *Virchows Arch (B)* 45:97, 1984.
338. Salminen A: Lysosomal changes in skeletal muscles during the repair of exercise injuries in muscle fibers. *Acta Physiol Scand (Suppl)* 539:1, 1985.
339. Newham DJ, McPhail G, Mills KR, et al: Ultrastructural changes after concentric and eccentric contractions of human muscle. *J Neurol Sci* 61:109, 1983.
340. Ogilvie RW, Armstrong RB, Baird DE, et al: Lesions in the rat soleus muscle following eccentrically biased exercise. *Am J Anat* 182:335, 1988.
341. Armstrong RB, Ogilvie RW, Schwane JA: Eccentric exercise-induced injury to rat skeletal muscle. *J Appl Physiol* 54:80, 1983.
342. Hikida RS, Staron RS, Hagerman FC: Muscle fiber necrosis associated with human marathon runners. *J Neurol Sci* 59:185, 1983.
343. Giddings CJ, Neaves WB, Gonyea WJ: Muscle fiber necrosis and regeneration induced by prolonged weight-lifting exercise in the cat. *Anat Rec* 211:133, 1985.

344. Umnova MM, Seene TP: The effect of increased functional load on the activation of satellite cells in the skeletal-muscle of adult rats. *Int J Sports Med* 12:501, 1991.
345. McCormick KM, Thomas DP: Exercise-induced satellite cell activation in senescent soleus muscle. *J Appl Physiol* 72:888, 1992.
346. Gonyea WJ, Sale DG, Gonyea FB, et al: Exercise induced increases in muscle fiber number. *Eur J Appl Physiol* 55:137, 1986.
347. Giddings CJ, Gonyea WJ: Morphological observations supporting muscle fiber hyperplasia following weight-lifting in cats. *Anat Rec* 233:178, 1992.
348. Appell HJ, Forsberg S, Hollmann W: Satellite cell activation in human skeletal-muscle after training—Evidence for muscle-fiber neoformation. *Int J Sports Med* 9:297, 1988.
349. Schiaffino S, Pierobon Bormioli S, Aloisi M: The fate of newly formed satellite cells during compensatory muscle hypertrophy. *Virchows Arch B Cell Pathol* 21:113, 1976.
350. Salleo A, Anastasi G, Laspada G, et al: New muscle fiber formation during compensatory hypertrophy. *Med Sci Sports Exerc* 12:268, 1980.
351. Snow MH, Chartkoff BS: Frequency of bifurcated muscle fibers in hypertrophic rat soleus muscle. *Muscle Nerve* 10:312, 1987.
352. Gollnick PD, Timson BF, Moore RL, et al: Muscular enlargement and number of fibers in skeletal muscles of rats. *J Appl Physiol* 50:936, 1981.
353. Salleo A, La Spada GF, Falzea G, et al: Response of satellite cells and muscle fibers to long-term compensatory hypertrophy. *J Submicrosc Cytol* 15:929, 1983.
354. James NT, Cabric M: Quantitative analyses of normal and hypertrophic extensor digitorum longus muscles in mice. *Exp Neurol* 76:284, 1982.
355. Sola OM, Christensen DL, Martin AW: Hypertrophy and hyperplasia of adult chicken anterior latissimus dorsi muscles following stretch with and without denervation. *Exp Neurol* 41:76, 1973.
356. Alway SE, Gonyea WJ, Davis ME: Muscle fiber formation and fiber hypertrophy during the onset of stretch-overload. *Am J Physiol* 259:C92, 1990.
357. Winchester PK, Davis ME, Alway SE, et al: Satellite cell activation in the stretch-enlarged anterior latissimus-dorsi muscle of the adult quail. *Am J Physiol* 260:C 206, 1991.
358. Winchester PK, Gonyea WJ: A quantitative study of satellite cells and myonuclei in stretched avian slow tonic muscle. *Anat Rec* 232:369, 1992.
359. Winchester PK, Gonyea WJ: Regional injury and the terminal differentiation of satellite cells in stretched avian slow tonic muscle. *Dev Biol* 151:459, 1992.
360. McCormick KM, Schultz E: Mechanisms of nascent fiber formation during avian skeletal-muscle hypertrophy. *Dev Biol* 150:319, 199

Chapter 4

The Diversity of Muscle Fiber Types and Its Origin during Development

NEAL A. RUBINSTEIN
ALAN M. KELLY

Recognition of Fiber-Type Diversity by Histochemistry
Recognition of Diversity by Myosin Heavy-Chain Isoforms
Recognition of Diversity by Physiologic Properties
Correlation of Fiber Types with Myosin Heavy-Chain Isoforms
Diversity as Demonstrated by Other Contractile Protein Isoforms
Fiber Types in Allotypical Muscles
Model for Contemplating Fiber-Type Diversity
Origins of Muscle Fiber Diversity
STEP I: DETERMINATION OF MYOGENIC CELLS
STEP II: SPECIFICATION OF FAST OR SLOW PROGRAMS
STEP III: SPECIFICATION OF A FAST SUBTYPE
STEP IV: MODULATION AND PLASTICITY
Four Stages of Muscle Specialization
THE RELATIONSHIP BETWEEN MUSCLE HISTOGENESIS AND THE EMERGENCE OF FIBER-TYPE DIVERSITY
THE ABILITY OF MOTOR NEURONS TO MODULATE FIBER TYPES
SYNAPTOGENESIS AND FIBER-TYPE DIVERSITY
SIGNAL TRANSDUCTION PATHWAYS AND EXPRESSION OF THE SLOW FIBER PHENOTYPE

Actively contracting striated muscle is the most energy-demanding tissue in the body. In this competitive world, therefore, efficiency of skeletal muscle contraction coupled with resistance to fatigue is crucial to survival. Skeletal muscles, however, are required to generate a wide range of forces and movements. Animals have adapted to these demands by developing specialized muscles and muscle fibers with a diverse range of properties. Scientists have long recognized that muscles differ both in their speed of contraction and in their color, some appearing red while others are white.[1] Speed of contraction and color, however, do not always coincide. While all the slowly contracting muscles are red, the fast-contracting muscles can be either red or white.[2]

Today, we understand that the speed of contraction of a muscle is directly related to its myosin adenosine triphosphatase (ATPase)* activity and is also correlated with the presence of specific isoforms of most of the myofibrillar

*A list of abbreviations used in this chapter is given at the end of the chapter.

contractile proteins as well as isoforms of the Ca^{2+}-sequestering enzymes of the sarcoplasmic reticulum.[3] Barany,[4] for example, demonstrated that fast- and slow-contracting muscles contained myosins that differed in their actin-activated and Ca^{2+}-dependent ATPase activities and that these ATPase activities correlated with the speed of contraction of the muscles. The dichotomy between the contractile protein isoforms of fast- and slow-contracting muscles was soon confirmed biochemically for the myosin heavy chains (MyHCs)[5,6]; the myosin light chains (MyLCs)[7]; troponins T, I, and C; the actinins; and C proteins.[8,9] Virtually every contractile protein exists in isoforms, which are discretely distributed between fast- and slow-contracting muscles.

The red color of a muscle is related to the concentration of the oxygen-sequestering molecule myoglobin and is also correlated with high concentrations of enzymes of aerobic metabolism and with the amount of vascularization. Pette and colleagues,[10] for example, demonstrated that muscles could be distinguished by the activities of enzymes involved in energy metabolism and that ratios of selected enzymes could be useful for distinguishing metabolic types of muscles. Resistance to fatigue is also correlated with the oxidative capacity of a muscle, since this metabolic pathway is efficient with respect to energy yield per mole of substrate[11]; muscles with high oxidative enzyme activity can maintain constant loads for long periods with comparatively small expenditures of energy (see Chap. 5).

Individual fibers of all these muscles can also be classified as fast or slow, red or white, by the same properties that distinguish whole muscles. Muscles, then, can be composed of a heterogeneous population of cells or fibers, so that they may tune their efficiency for the range of forces, velocities, and endurances they are required to generate. The initial attempts to distinguish among individual fibers depended on histochemical reactions, either for myofibrillar actomyosin ATPase activity or for aerobic or glycolytic enzyme activities. This approach usually identified a small number of fiber types.[12–14] As an increasing number of myofibrillar protein isoforms were discovered and it was discerned from biochemical studies that the oxidative enzymes could vary over a very wide range of activities in any of the described fiber types,[15] it became clear that the true number of distinctly defined muscle fibers superseded the number recognized by histochemistry alone. Moreover, patterns of contractile protein isoforms and enzyme activities in developing and pathologic muscles refused to correlate with standard, histochemically derived fiber types.[16,17] Hence, although the histochemical identification of fiber types is a clinically useful tool for pathologists, neurologists, and other physicians involved in diagnosing muscular or neuromuscular disorders, it is important to understand exactly what the technique does or does not reveal. Any attempt to create a more comprehensive and therefore a necessarily more complex system for describing muscle fiber types[18] may not find immediate clinical relevance; it may, however, contribute to our understanding of muscle as a dynamic tissue.

With these ideas in mind, we will now examine the extent of diversity of several contractile proteins and the difficulties of classifying fibers into distinct, nonoverlapping types of cells. We will also examine the development of fiber type specialization and the means of generating and maintaining fiber-type diversity. Several excellent recent reviews present more detailed analyses of contractile protein diversity and metabolic enzymes in skeletal muscles.[19,66]

Recognition of Fiber-Type Diversity by Histochemistry

The enormous diversity among mammalian muscle fibers can be recognized by physiologic, biochemical, or histochemical methods. Present histochemical techniques depend on differences either in the oxidative/glycolytic enzyme activity levels or in the myofibrillar ATPase activity of the distinct fiber types. As mentioned above, the speed of contraction of a muscle fiber is dependent on the ATPase activity of its myosin, and each myosin isoform has a distinct level of activity. Following the demonstration that myosins displayed different acid and alkaline labilities, Guth and Samaha[12] developed a histochemical staining method for the myofibrillar ATPase activity after either acid or alkali preincubation of the sections. In their method, the ATPase activity in fast fibers was alkali-stable and acid-labile; i.e., they showed high ATPase activity after alkaline preincubation and low ATPase activity after acid preincubation. Slow fibers showed just the opposite: alkaline lability and acid stability. Brooke and Kaiser[13] further refined the method with a range of pH preincubations, and they were able to distinguish three fiber types (Fig. 4-1). Type I fibers, the slow fibers, showed a stable, high ATPase activity after preincubation at either pH 4.3 or 4.6 but very low ATPase activity after preincubation at pH 10.4. Fast fibers, or type II fibers, could be subdivided into two types. Type IIa showed a strong reaction after preincubation at pH 10.4 but no reaction after preincubation at pH 4.3 or 4.6. A second type of fiber, type IIb, was also strongly reactive after preincubation at pH 10.4 and negative after preincubation at pH 4.3. After preincubation at pH 4.6, however, it showed moderate activity.

The underlying assumption of the ATPase technique is that each staining pattern corresponds to a distinct myosin isoform. Several limitations, however, must be recognized in interpreting the staining patterns. First, what happens when distinct myosin isoforms show almost identical staining patterns? For example, in 1988, a new fast fiber type was identified by the newly discovered MyHC it contained.[20] This fiber type, IIx (or IId), is difficult to distinguish from type IIb fibers using histochemistry.[21] Like the IIb fibers, it shows a strong reaction after preincubation at pH 10.3 and no reaction after preincubation at pH 4.3. After preincubation at pH 4.6, however, it shows a slightly darker reaction

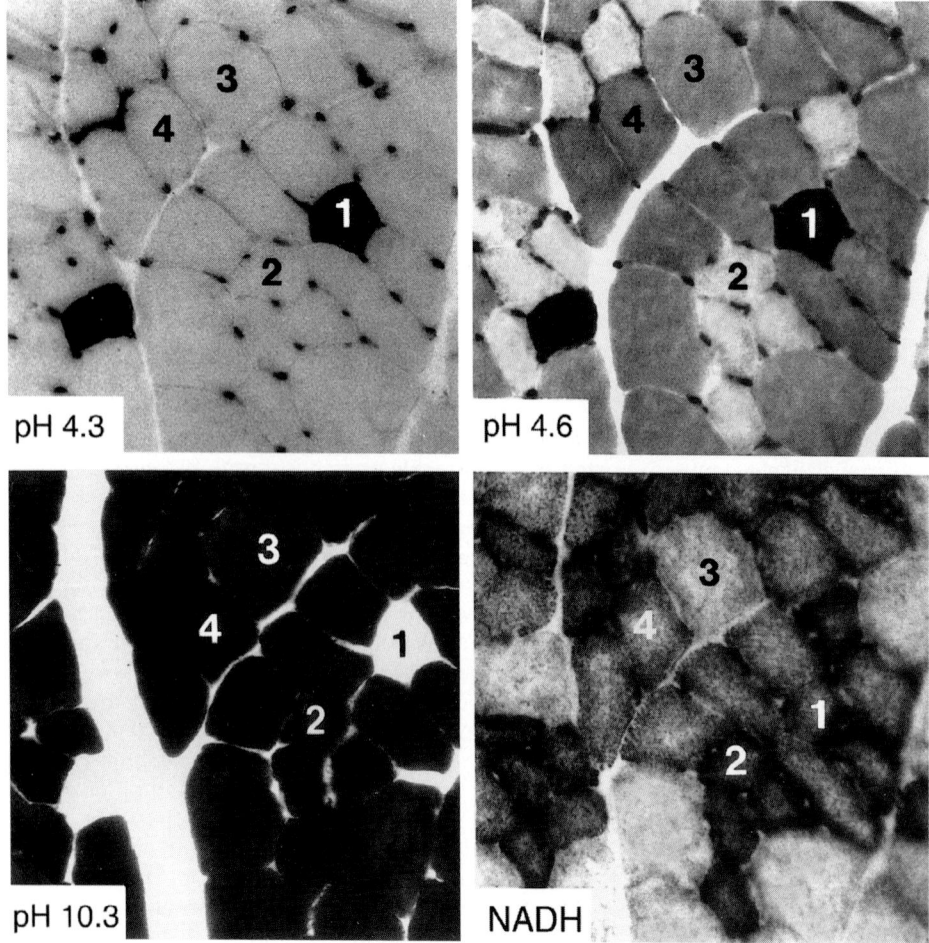

FIGURE 4-1. Serial cross sections of rat extensor digitorum muscles. Sections were stained for myofibrillar actomyosin ATPase activity after preincubation at pH values 4.3, 4.6, and 10.3 and for NADH tetrazolium reductase. Comparison of all four staining patterns allows four fiber types to be distinguished (the numbers designate single fibers whose MyHCs were analyzed) (see Fig. 4-2). Preincubation at pH 4.3 distinguished slow-twitch, type I fibers (fiber 1) from fast-twitch type II (fiber numbers 2, 3, and 4) fibers. Preincubation at pH 10.3 showed the inverse staining pattern. After preincubation at pH 4.6, the fast-twitch type II fibers could be divided into two distinct fiber types: those staining lightly (fiber 2, for example) and those staining with intermediate color (fibers 3 and 4). Fibers 3 and 4 could be further distinguished from each other by their reaction for NADH tetrazolium reductase. Fiber 4 shows more reaction than fiber 3. In these sections, then, fiber 1 is type I (slow-twitch), fiber 2 is IIa, fiber 3 is IIb, and fiber 4 is IIx (see Table 4-1). (*Figure courtesy of Dr. Dirk Pette.[30] With permission.*)

Table 4-1. HISTOCHEMICAL REACTIONS OF MAJOR ADULT FIBER TYPES[a]

Classification	pH 4.3	pH 4.6	pH 10.4	Metabolic Profile
I	++++	++++	0	High ox, low or moderate glycolytic
IIa	0	0	++++	Moderate ox
IIb	0	+	++++	Low to moderate ox, high glycolytic
IId	0	++	++++	Moderately high ox
IIm	+++	+++	++	Not available

[a]The left portion of this table indicates the histochemical myofibrillar ATPase reactions of mammalian muscle fibers after preincubation at the indicated pH. While the ATPase activity of all the last fiber types (type II fibers) shows alkali stability, they can be subdivided by their varying stability after acid preincubations. The right portion of the table indicates the metabolic profile, predominantly the oxidative capacity, of each fiber type. Both histochemical methods have biochemical correlates.

than does the IIb fiber (Table 4-1). But in a muscle that contains only one or the other fiber type, it is difficult to determine which fiber is present by histochemical means, and it is likely that the IIb fibers described in previous papers were actually a heterogeneous population of—at least—IIb and IIx fibers. In fact, although the human genome contains the IIb myosin gene,[22] no IIb myosin is expressed in human fibers, and the IIb fiber type identified in humans expresses the IIx—rather than the IIb—myosin isoform.[23] Also, while the IIb fiber is the predominant fast-twitch fiber type in rats, the IIx fiber is the predominant fast fiber type in rabbits.[23a] Prior to the discovery of the IIx, however, the IIx fiber in rabbits had been identified as a IIb fiber.

A second limitation is seen in fibers that do not show a typical staining pattern, stable at one pH, labile at another. We know today that fibers of this type represent a heterogeneous group. For example, a distinct fast-contracting fiber type, IIm, is found in the jaw-closing muscles of most carnivores and most primates except humans.[12,24,25] This fiber type is correlated with a very rapid contraction time and a distinct "superfast" myosin (see below). In the histochemical reaction, it shows moderate activity after preincubation at pH 10.3 and very strong reaction after preincubation at pH 4.3 or 4.6[24] (see Table 4-1).

When developing or regenerating fibers are examined, a continuum of staining patterns can be seen, from fibers that are stable at acid pH and moderately stable at alkaline pH (the so-called Ic fibers) to fibers which are stable at alkaline pH and moderately stable at acid pH (the IIc fibers). As Guth showed almost 20 years ago,[16] erroneous interpretations may result from the application of the myofibrillar ATPase histochemical method to developing muscles; similar confusion in staining patterns may arise in adult skeletal muscles undergoing regeneration after injury.

As discussed below, the Ic and IIc fiber types in adult animals appear to be promiscuous, synthesizing at least two different myosin isoforms in different ratios; but in chronically stimulated or developing muscles, the fibers identified as the c-type fibers additionally contain the developmental isoforms of the MyHC[26] (Table 4-2). Similarly, regenerating muscles and muscles undergoing any type of functional change (e.g., by denervation, cross-innervation, chronic stimulation) are also composed of fibers with a heterogeneous population of myosins.[27] Hence, the histochemical ATPase profiles of a muscle will reflect only an approximation of the number of fiber types within that muscle, since the ATPase profile of any individual fiber can reflect a heterogeneous population of distinct fiber types that cannot be distinguished by this histochemical method.

Another popular histochemical method for examining diversity is to stain for enzymes of the oxidative or tricarboxylic acid (TCA) pathway or the Embden-Meyerhof (glycolytic) pathway. Fibers that stain intensely for enzymes of the TCA or terminal oxidative process are considered *red fibers*, while those that show lower staining levels are *white fibers*.[28] Although these terms subsequently became synonymous with slow- and fast-contracting fibers as defined by the ATPase reaction or by physiologic methods, this correlation was not exact. While all slow-contracting fibers are red, fast-contracting fibers could be either red or white. Moreover, intermediately staining fibers were also identified histochemically[29] (see Chap. 5).

Table 4-2. CORRELATION OF MyHCS WITH HISTOCHEMICALLY DEFINED FIBER TYPES

Fiber Type	MyHC	Location
I	Cardiac β	Slow-twitch skeletal[38]
Extraocular	IIeom	EOM[36] and larynx[143]
IIm	IIm	Branchial arch muscles except humans[24,25]
IIa	IIa	Predominant fast fibers in leg and trunk
IIb	IIb	muscles and diaphragm (IIx not in
IIx(d)	IIx(d)	humans)[23]
Ic	I > IIa, emb, neo	May be transitional types in fibers
IIc	I < IIa, emb, neo	undergoing changes[29,31]
?	Embryonic	Early development and regeneration; also adult EOM[34,36]
?	Neonatal/perinatal	Perinatal period; adult EOM[36]
?	Slow tonic	EOM, tensor tympani, some intrafusal fibers[31,36]
?	Cardiac α	Some jaw muscles; adult EOM[36]

The two schemes for fiber classification (metabolic enzymes and myofibrillar ATPase activities), while each discerning three major groups of fibers, are not interchangeable. Guth and Yellin[18] described the dynamic nature of fiber types in mammalian muscles, referring to the demonstration that each of the three fiber types defined by the ATPase reaction showed a wide range of metabolic enzyme activities. Nemeth et al.[15] examined the myofibrillar ATPase activity as well as the SDH and phosphorylase activities of over 2500 fibers in the adult rat. They showed that each of the three fiber types identified by the ATPase method could contain widely varying and overlapping concentrations of the two metabolic enzymes, although the content of metabolic enzymes correlated with the fatigue index (see Chap. 5). Quantitative electron microscopy shows a similar variable and overlapping content of mitochondria within each ATPase-defined fiber (see Chap. 11).

It appears, then, that while histochemical methods for defining diversity among fibers are well accepted and frequently used, they pose difficulties that a more biochemical analysis of diversity would not: the latter would reduce subjective judgments, would allow us to interpret intermediate or changing fiber types and to quantitate small differences among fibers, and would distinguish among similarly staining but distinct fiber types.[19,30] A biochemical approach to fiber-type diversity might also allow us to concentrate on the dynamic nature of the muscle fiber and to abandon the histochemical nomenclature suggesting a small number of static fiber types. We must keep in mind, however, that the histochemical identification of fiber types can be a useful tool for clinical studies.

Recognition of Diversity by Myosin Heavy-Chain Isoforms

While early studies indicated the presence of only two MyHC isoforms, fast and slow, a variety of immunochemical, biochemical, and molecular biological methods have expanded the number of recognizable isoforms considerably. Today, in mammalian muscles, we can identify at least 12 MyHC isoforms whose expression can be identified at some time during development or in distinct muscles or muscle fibers (Table 4-2). These include one slow tonic isoform and two isoforms normally found in cardiac muscle. The slow tonic isoform is expressed in only a narrow range of muscles, including the extraocular and tensor tympani muscles and certain intrafusal fibers,[31] while the slow-twitch isoform found in most slow-twitch fibers is identical to the cardiac β isoform.[32] Recently, the second cardiac heavy chain, the α chain, has also been found expressed in jaw muscles and in extraocular muscles.[33–35]

Two isoforms, embryonic and neonatal, are considered developmental isoforms, since they are predominantly found in developing muscle fibers; however, they have recently been identified in adult extraocular muscles.[36] Finally, at least five distinct fast-twitch isoforms are seen. The type IIa, IIb, and IIx (IId) are the most widely expressed in muscles throughout the body; the IIeom[36] and IIm[24] are expressed in extraocular and branchial arch–derived muscles, respectively. In humans, however, the IIm MyHC may exist only as a pseudogene.[37]

The chromosomal localization and organization of the family of MyHC genes expressed in skeletal muscles has now been characterized. In *Drosophila*, there are two MyHC isoforms resulting from differential splicing from a single gene. In the mammalian systems, however, there is no evidence for differential splicing; rather, each MyHC isoform is the product of a distinct gene.[38] The two cardiac isoforms have been localized on chromosome 14 in the human.[39] The α and β genes are tandemly linked, separated by approximately 5 kb of intergenic DNA, in the order $5'\rightarrow\beta\rightarrow\alpha\rightarrow3'$.[40]

Most of the other sarcomeric MyHC genes known to be expressed in skeletal muscle are not linked to the cardiac genes; in the human, these are clustered on chromosome 17[41]; they are tandemly linked in the order $5'\rightarrow$embryonic$\rightarrow$IIa$\rightarrow$IIx$\rightarrow$IIb$\rightarrow$perinatal$\rightarrow$extraocular$\rightarrow3'$.[22] This is unlike the organization of the sarcomeric actin and the myosin light-chain gene families, which are dispersed throughout the genome.[42] Whether this organization in some way reflects the development or physiologic expression of these genes is a question for future investigators. However, in other gene families, the chromosomal order of members has been retained during evolution[42,43]; in the human β-like globin gene family, the order of the globin genes is important for correct developmental expression.[44] The importance of the organization of the skeletal MyHC gene locus, however, is suggested by its evolutionary conservation between humans and mice.[41] The physiologic or developmental requirement for this organization, however, has not been discerned. It should be noted that the expression of the cardiac α and β genes in skeletal muscle demonstrates that there is no obligatory physical linking of all MyHC genes expressed in any one skeletal muscle.

With the recent completion of the human genome project, investigators have identified several other sequences similar to skeletal MyHC gene sequences (Ref. 44a; R. Schachat, unpublished). Their expression patterns, however, have not yet been determined. None of these are linked to the cardiac or previously-identified skeletal MyHC loci. Of these, one localized on chromosome 7 is homologous to the IIm gene, but it may be a pseudogene (R. Schachat, unpublished). Another, on chromosome 19, shows 75 percent identity to a nonmuscle MyHC. Both chromosome 3 and chromosome 20 also contain MyHC sequences. Whether any of these MyHCs are found in skeletal muscle or whether they have any specific distribution among skeletal muscles or their fiber types is not yet known.

Recognition of Diversity by Physiologic Properties

Burke used physiologic properties to categorize the motor units of cat hindlimb muscles.[11] Using three specific properties—twitch contraction time, tetanus tension, and fatigue index—he separated motor units into three nonoverlapping types. These are the FF units (fast-twitch, fatigable), FR (fast-twitch, fatigue-resistant), and S (slow, fatigue-resistant). As all the fibers of a motor unit essentially have identical properties,[45] these definitions can also be used to categorize fiber types. A more detailed discussion of this definition of diversity by physiologic properties—including its correlation with other methods of fiber-type classification—can be found in Chap. 5. Other physiologic correlates of fiber types are discussed in the following section.

Correlation of Fiber Types with Myosin Heavy-Chain Isoforms

Clearly, the number of MyHC isoforms in any particular species does not correlate with the histochemically defined number of fiber types, and attempts have been made to correlate the two (Table 4-2). In a set of elegant experiments, Termin et al.[30] combined standard ATPase and metabolic enzyme histochemistry with microdissection and analyses of individual fibers. Figure 4-1 shows a set of serial cross sections of a rat extensor digitorum longus muscle stained for myofibrillar actomyosin ATPase after precincubation at different pH values and for NADH tetrazolium reductase. The MyHC isoforms of the numbered fibers are displayed on gradient polyacrylamide gels in Fig. 4-2. In these experiments, they determined that type I fibers contained the type I MyHC (labeled fiber 1 in Figs. 4-1 and 4-2), while type IIa and IIb fibers contained the IIa and IIb MyHCs, respectively (fibers 2 and 3, respectively, in Figs. 4-1 and 4-2). The IIx isoform could be found in fibers of the rat extensor digitorum longus (EDL), where they were shown to have a slightly different reactivity after acid preincubation than did the IIb fibers, and they had a higher NADH tetrazolium reductase activity (fiber 4 in Figs. 4-1 and 4-2). As mentioned above, fibers previously identified as IIb fibers in the human contain only IIx MyHC, as the IIb isoform is not expressed in humans.[23] Moreover, the majority of fast-twitch fibers in the rabbit, previously identified as IIb by histochemistry, contain only the IIx MyHC.

Hybrid fibers containing multiple MyHCs have also been detected in adult rat muscles. Type Ic fibers contained both I and IIa MyHCs with type I in excess; IIc fibers also contained I and IIa MyHCs with type IIa in excess. This, of course, raises the question of whether Ic and IIc fibers are stable fiber types or different stages of transition from one fiber type to another. While there is a relationship between shortening velocities and the MyHC content of individual fibers, there is considerable overlap in these measurements, and they cannot detect the specific contribution of individual isoforms to contractile properties. Stretch activation kinetics, on the other hand, can clearly distinguish between fibers containing a single isoform without any overlap in measurements; moreover, hybrid fibers such as the Ic and IIc fibers have stretch activation kinetics directly related to the ratio of isoforms within them.[46,47]

Diversity as Demonstrated by Other Contractile Protein Isoforms

The components of the calcium activation complex (troponins T, I, and C and tropomyosin) also exist in multiple isoforms. A four-member multigene family encodes the tropomyosins: α-TM, β-TM, TPM 3, and TPM 4.[48] Each of these genes generates a number of tissue and developmental stage–specific isoforms through multiple mechanisms: alternative exons, splicing, use of different promoters, and differential 3' end processing. Of these multiple genes, the α-TM, β-TM, and TPM 3 genes generate isoforms specific to skeletal muscle.[48,49] For example, although the α-tropomyosin gene can generate at least six messenger ribonucleic acids (mRNAs), only one is apparently used in skeletal muscle.[50,51] The α and β skeletal tropomyosins are not distributed to fast and slow fibers, respectively.[52] In fact, the tropomyosin isoforms are the only contractile proteins that break the fast-slow dichotomy—i.e., distinct isoforms for the fast- versus the slow-twitch fibers. In vivo, dimerization of tropomyosin subunits occurs, and α/α, α/β, and β/β dimers are found.

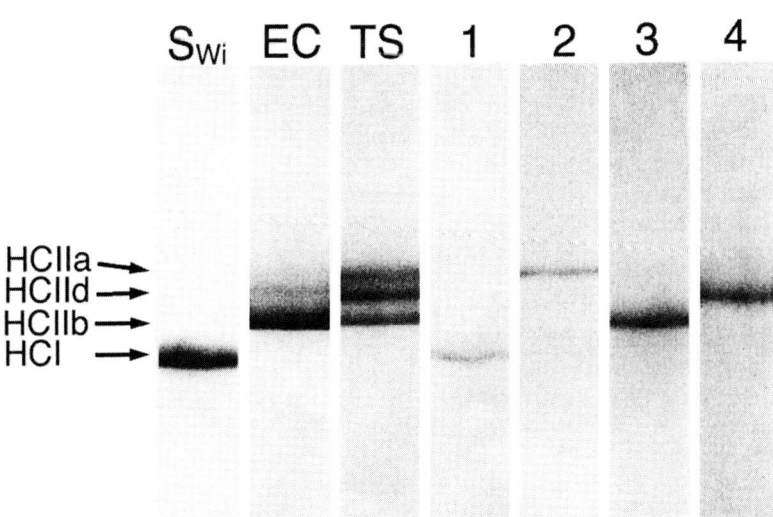

FIGURE 4-2. Gradient gel electrophoresis of microdissected fragments from histochemically classified single fibers. The numbered fibers in Fig. 4-1 were dissected and their MyHCs separated on 5 to 8% polyacrylamide gels. The numbers correspond to the same fibers as those in Fig. 4-1. Electrophoresis of whole muscle extracts are included for comparison. Swi, soleus, Wistar strain; EC, normal extensor digitorum longus; TS, 28-day stimulated tibialis anterior. (*Figure courtesy of Dr. Dirk Pette.[30] With permission.*)

In the human genome, eight striated muscle troponin genes can be identified: three for troponin I (TnI: slow skeletal, fast skeletal, and cardiac); three for troponin T (TnT: slow skeletal, fast skeletal, cardiac); and two for troponin C (TnC: fast skeletal and a cardiac/slow skeletal isoform). Mapping studies have shown that the genes for the TnI and TnT subunits are organized as pairs at three distinct chromosomal sites, each containing a TnT-TnI closely linked. Despite this suggestive organization, however, there is no obligatory linkage of expression of the members of each pair. For example, although the paired fast skeletal TnT/TnI genes are normally coexpressed, the other pairings (slow skeletal TnI/cardiac TnT and cardiac TnI/slow skeletal TnT) do not show obligatory coexpression.[53]

The troponin T (TnT) gene may offer the most complex range of contractile protein isoforms. Unlike the MyHC genes, the TnT isoforms are generated by differential splicing of the RNA transcript.[54] Nadal-Ginard and colleagues[55] have shown that differential splicing can account for as many as 64 distinct TnT fast isoforms, although considerably fewer than this number have been identified in rabbit fast muscles; three major fast isoforms of TnT account for most of the TnT expression in adult fast rabbit muscles.[56,57]

There is no one-to-one correlation of TnT isoforms and MyHC isoforms. However, there does appear to be a correlation among fast TnT isoforms and specific tropomyosin dimers and α-actinin isoforms. These combinations of TnT, tropomyosin, and actinin isoforms have been termed *canonical programs* by Schachat et al.[56]; the ratio of these contractile isoforms in any individual fiber can be represented by various combinations of canonical programs. Each of the canonical programs is named for a given TnT isoform. For example, the TnT-lf program contains TnT-lf, α/β dimers of tropomyosin, and α-actinin-lf/s. Likewise, TnT-2f, α/α tropomyosin dimers, and α-actinin-2f are coexpressed, as are TnT-3f, α/β or β/β dimers of tropomyosin and α-actinin-lf/s. In physiologic terms, the TnT-2f program is the most calcium-responsive, while the TnT-3f program provides the most graded response to calcium and perhaps should be found in fibers that are more like slow-twitch fibers in their responsiveness. The TnT-lf program bridges the gap between the two extremes.

With regard to the MyLCs, type IIb fibers appear to have a higher ratio of the MyLC 3f/MyLC 1f, while the type IIa fibers have a lower ratio.[58-60] Other proteins of the contractile apparatus, including C-protein,[61] titin,[62] nebulin,[63] and α-actinin[64] also exist in multiple isoforms distributed unevenly between fast- and slow-twitch muscles.

In rat muscle, there can be a correlation between the MyHC isoform and the TnT canonical program[65]: coexpression of TnT-2f with the IIb MyHC, TnT-3f with the IIa MyHC, and TnT-4f with the IIx MyHC isoform. In an excellent review of myofibrillar protein isoforms, Schiaffino and Reggiani[66] assembled all this data to provide a tentative scheme of isoform distribution along the various fast-fiber types of rat and rabbit skeletal muscles. In this scheme, at one end of the spectrum were type IIb fibers with the IIb MyHC, a higher MyLC 3f/1f ratio, TnT-2f, α/α tropomyosin dimers, and α-actinin-2f. These fibers would be expected to combine the fastest shortening velocity with the most rapid response to calcium. At the other extreme were type IIa fibers with the IIa MyHC, a lower MyLC 3f/1f ratio, TnT-3f, α/β or β/β tropomyosin dimers, and α-actinin 1f/s. These fibers would contract more slowly than the other fast-twitch fibers and show a graded calcium responsiveness.

Fiber Types in Allotypical Muscles

Vertebrate limb muscles have always been the paradigm for studies of myogenesis, including descriptions of fiber types and their development. Hoh and Hughes,[67] however, have pointed out that several other muscle groups have functional specializations and patterns of MyHC gene expression distinct from those seen in limb muscles. The patterns of gene expression in these muscle "allotypes" appear to be intrinsically controlled and probably arise from rules governing gene expression that are unique to each allotype. Allotypes of skeletal muscle would include the jaw closing muscles, the extraocular muscles (see Chap. 6), and the diaphragm. In this paradigm, then, each allotype is characterized by its potential to produce a specific set of fiber types. Exogenous factors such as innervation or hormones may modulate the muscle fiber characteristics of that muscle *within the range of options open to that allotype*; they are unable, however, to convert one allotype into another. For example, the jaw-closing muscles of the cat uniquely express the superfast-twitch IIm MyHC.[24] If these muscles are minced, reimplanted into the bed of a limb fast-twitch muscle, and innervated by a limb motor neuron, they make the superfast IIm MyHC unique to the jaw-closing muscles rather than the fast-twitch MyHCs normally found in that limb muscle.[67]

This concept suggests that the possible fates of satellite cells of jaw-closing muscles and those of limb muscles have already been determined by their previous developmental history, and hence are products of distinct lineages of myoblasts.

Model for Contemplating Fiber-Type Diversity

Previous models for fiber diversity have been either quantal or continuous.[56] As can be seen from the above discussion, any type of model could be proposed, depending on the particular properties on which the model is based; while continuous models may more closely approximate the true dynamic state of muscle fibers, they do not provide any relatively simple way to describe changes during pathologic or developmental situations. Quantal models, on the other hand, are less useful in describing the dynamic processes that occur during normal and abnormal situations but are more helpful in describing that state of a fiber at any point in time.

We have briefly discussed three properties of skeletal muscles that show divergence among fibers: MyHC isoforms, TnT isoforms, and metabolic enzymes. In general, the MyHC isoforms are discretely distributed among normal adult muscle fibers; normally, only one or predominantly one isoform is found per fiber. The TnT isoforms are distributed in a less discrete manner. Fast and slow isoforms are confined to fast- and slow-twitch fibers; but among the fast fibers, a myriad of TnT isoforms exist, often multiple isoforms in each cell. Yet, as mentioned above, there is some correlation with MyHCs; during chronic stimulation, there is a transition from IIb MyHC and the TnT-1f and TnT-2f isoforms to the IIa MyHC and the TnT-3f isoform.

Finally, the levels of oxidative enzymes do not strictly correlate with MyHC isoforms. While fibers containing the slow MyHC are normally high in oxidative enzymes, both fibers with IIa and IIb myosins can have widely varying levels of oxidative enzymes, particularly as an animal proceeds through adolescence to maturity.

It may be best to classify muscle fibers by their most discretely differentiated properties—which today are their MyHCs. As Fig. 4-3A shows, we can imagine the properties of a fiber type as filling a triangle. Properties are entered in the triangle at different levels, and the variability of that particular property in the fiber type is proportional to the width of the triangle at that level. At the top level of the triangle, then, are the properties that are most discretely distributed, such as the MyHCs. At lower levels of the triangle, we would place properties that show some restrictions (when correlated with the MyHC isoform) but not a strict one-to-one correlation. An example of this type of property would be the TnT isoforms. Finally, at the bottom of the triangle, we would place properties showing the most variability within fibers defined by that specific MyHC isoform. This would include the oxidative and glycolytic enzymes.

Moreover, relationships among fiber types could be seen by overlapping the various triangles (fiber types) where they have overlapping properties. As an example, the IIb and IIa fiber types in Fig. 4-3B would partially overlap at the TnT level, since they both express the TnT-1f isoform but not the TnT-2f and 3f isoforms; and they would overlap considerably at the bottom level, since both show a wide range of

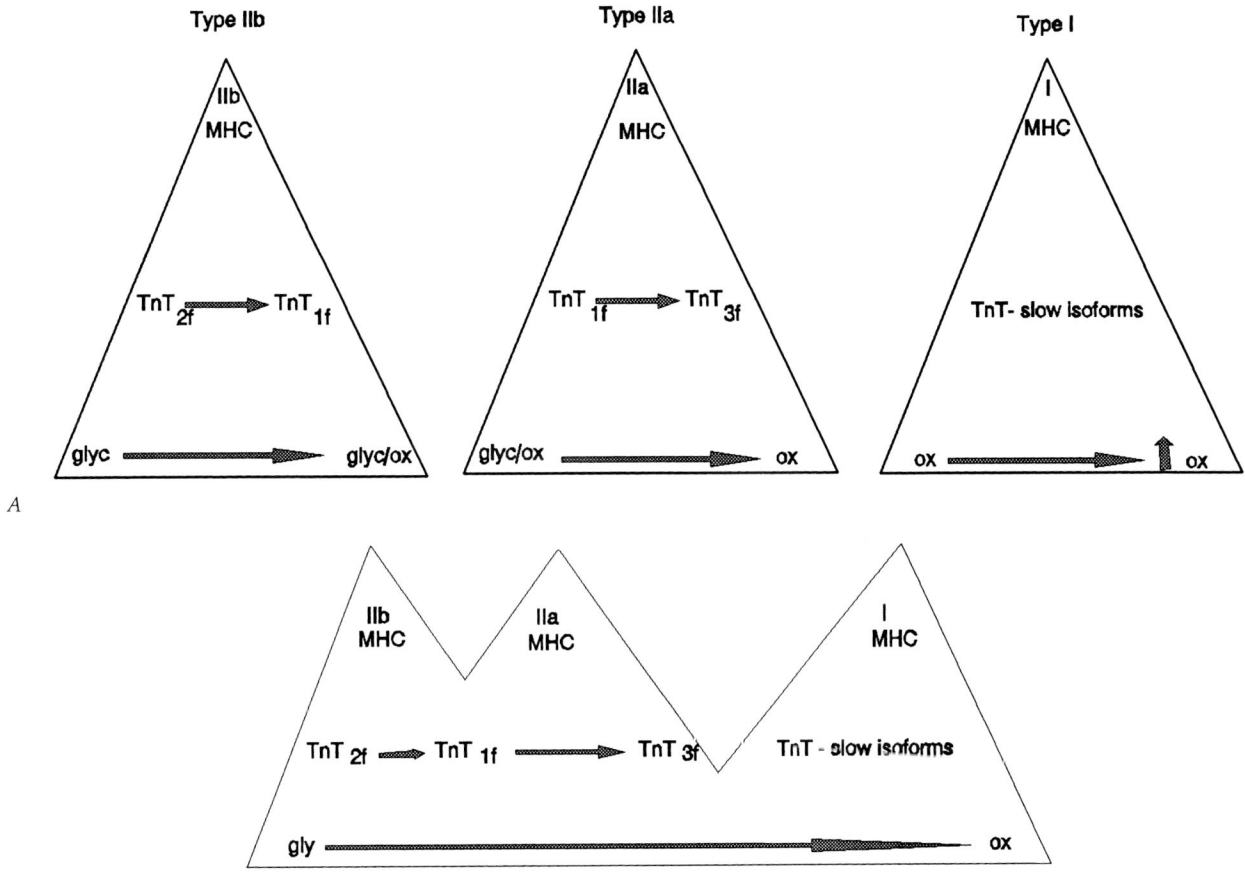

FIGURE 4-3. Representation of the properties of fiber types. A. In this scheme, fiber types are classified by their most discretely distributed property, the myosin heavy chain (MyHC). The totality of diversity within each fiber type is then represented by a triangle, with each property entered at a level whose width is proportional to the variability of the property in that fiber type (when compared to the MyHC). Hence, MyHCs, which are most discretely distributed among fibers, are found at the narrowest width of the triangle, while the more variable metabolic enzymes are found at the widest point. B. The relationship among fibers as well as their interconvertibility is demonstrated by overlapping the triangular representations of fiber types at the level of less discretely distributed properties. This demonstrates the continuum of some properties, such as the metabolic enzymes, among fibers, and the discontinuity of other properties, such as the MyHCs. The degree of overlap—i.e., the number of levels at which overlapping properties between two fibers can be seen—also represents the ease of conversion between those two fiber types. Properties at levels that are not overlapping, such as the MyHCs, are more difficult to switch.

metabolic enzyme concentrations. The type I fiber, however, would only overlap the IIa and IIb fiber types at the level of oxidative enzymes but not at considerably higher levels, since there is normally no sharing of fast or slow contractile protein isoforms by fibers of the opposite type. The degree of overlap of fiber triangles would suggest the ease with which the fibers are interconvertible. That the IIa and I fiber representations overlap only at the level of the oxidative enzymes is consistent with the usual dichotomy between fast and slow contractile protein isoforms.

In each muscle there may be preferential combinations of multiple properties, although there would be some fibers that would show more or less divergence from the preferential combinations. Moreover, the preferential combinations might differ among muscles and would certainly differ among allotypes. Concentration on the preferential combinations of properties would focus our attention on the quantal nature of fiber types and would certainly be a manageable way to classify fibers in a clinical setting. Attention to the divergent combinations would focus our attention on the dynamic nature of fiber types and would be more relevant to someone trying to understand the development and maintenance of dynamic fiber types.

Origins of Muscle Fiber Diversity

As we have now discussed, mature muscle is made up of fibers with a continuum of specialized properties. These properties, however, do not emerge simultaneously; rather, diversification appears to require that prospective muscle cells make a series of gradually more refined choices that will, in the end, limit the complement of properties expressed by each fiber. Each of these steps may prejudice the plasticity of fibers in the mature animal. When and how this diversity is choreographed in the embryo is a focus of research in developmental biology. Current work has begun to synthesize a model that encompasses both of the two very distinct types of developmental programs previously hypothesized. One program was dependent upon lineage directives that are inherited by differentiating muscle cells from their progenitors. Another program, independent of lineage directives, suggested that myoblasts were homogeneous and capable of giving rise to all of the different types of fibers in muscle. In these two situations, the role played by the environment is very different. If the population of precursor myoblasts has already acquired a predetermined, inherent fate, the environment will at most select which cells will survive and differentiate in a given location and which one of an already limited number of options the fiber will adopt. By contrast, if the precursor myoblasts are naive and capable of giving rise to multiple types of muscle cells, the local environment must play an instructive role in selecting specific phenotypes.

The concept that myoblasts were naive cells that followed one or another path of differentiation determined by exogenous cues after they were fused into a myotube or myofiber arose from the observation that plasticity is a hallmark of vertebrate skeletal muscle.[3,19] In response to a variety of hormonal perturbations, changes in neural activity, and a wide variety of exogenous cues, a muscle fiber can change from one type to another. Hence, the demonstration that chick myoblasts give rise to distinct families of myotubes in vitro and that the progeny of these myoblasts stably maintain that phenotype in culture through many generations came as a surprising and provocative finding.[68–70] From this work and work discussed below, one can conclude that myoblasts are a heterogeneous population of cells, are biased to specific phenotypes, and are capable of securely "remembering" these instructions through a series of cell divisions. These findings have prompted the interpretation that myofiber diversity is conceived by diverse lineages of myoblasts, fibers derived from each of these pedigrees being constrained to a subset of phenotypes that they may subsequently express. This strategy presumably requires that myoblasts committed to the same lineage must recognize and fuse with one another to initiate production of a specific fiber type. These data together suggest that the final generation of a diverse group of muscle fiber types is the result of multiple inductive influences imposed on cells that have already been restricted by their lineage.

Four Stages of Muscle Specialization

We have arbitrarily divided the generation of diversity into four steps, although the timing of each step and even the temporal overlapping of steps during development are not clear. These four steps do outline the minimum number of decisions that are necessary for generating a mature fiber type from an uncommitted mesenchymal cell.

STEP I: DETERMINATION OF MYOGENIC CELLS

Discovery of myoD, myogenin, myf-5, and MRF4 and their related helix-loop-helix gene family has provided significant insight into the events that regulate commitment of cells to the myogenic lineage[71] (see Chap. 1). This step confers stability and memory to myoblasts committed to the muscle lineage. Since these proteins can migrate back to the nucleus and activate their own and each others' transcription, they have the capacity to establish a stable, cell-autonomous pathway of differentiation in relative isolation from in vivo environmental influences. These factors may also have selective effects on determination and differentiation of muscle phenotypes, since they are expressed in a defined sequence during muscle development.[72–74] The role of these myogenic regulatory factors in determining the lineage of myogenic cells is discussed in Chap. 1 and is not discussed further here.

STEP II: SPECIFICATION OF FAST OR SLOW PROGRAMS

Although this decision occurs in individual, presumptive myoblasts, it becomes manifest only at the time myotubes express one phenotype versus another.[75] The dichotomy between fast and slow fibers involves MyHC genes on separate chromosomes[22] and may be tightly regulated, since fast-to-slow transformations are difficult to obtain under normal circumstances.

The generation of two distinct types of muscle fibers—fast and slow—may have been the earliest evolutionary solution to diversity. Clonal cell culture studies carried out with myoblasts obtained from chick and human embryos indicated the occurrence of distinct myoblast populations with distinct morphologies and differing dependence on innervation.[76] While it was initially suggested that each fiber type might be derived from one of these particular unique myoblast types, current data suggest no straightforward correlation between these myoblast types and the later muscle fiber phenotypes. However, clonal analyses of myogenic precursors in embryonic avian limbs did reveal that there are distinct populations in the limbs already committed to form fast or slow fibers after differentiation in vitro and in vivo.[69,77] This work suggests that at least initially, slow and fast muscle fibers form via a mechanism intrinsic to the cell (see Ref. 78 for review).

Work in zebrafish has shown that the binary decision between fast and slow myoblast lineages occurs at an even earlier stage of development—within precursor myogenic cells prior to somite formation—and depends on short-range interactions. Devoto et al.[79] have identified two distinct populations of myogenic precursor cells. The adaxial cells are large cells located adjacent to the notochord, while the lateral presomitic cells are smaller, more irregular cells distal to the adaxial cells. The adaxial cells eventually migrate through the length of the somite and form a monolayer of superficial cells that later generate the adult slow muscle cells. The presomitic cells assume a position deeper in the somite and eventually generate the fast fibers of the adult animal.

Commitment of the adaxial cells to the slow muscle lineage is dependent on the glycoprotein Sonic hedgehog (SHH) and its associated signal transduction pathways.[80,81] Supported by both in vivo and in vitro experiments,[82] the current hypothesis is that induction of the slow lineage requires a high concentration of SHH. Therefore, SHH secreted by the midline structures induces the slow lineage commitment only in the layer of cells closest to the notochord (the adaxial cells). Myoblasts distal to this layer (the presomitic cells) do not receive a threshold SHH signal and follow a default pathway: the fast muscle lineage. The percentage of cells committed to the slow lineage can be increased by addition of exogenous SHH; moreover, injection of SHH mRNA into individual presomitic cells induces the commitment to slow fibers in these cells, which would normally have generated the fast muscle lineage.[83]

Little work has been done with this paradigm outside of the zebrafish system. In avians, however, Stockdale and colleagues have demonstrated that the neural tube enhances the number of slow muscle fibers, an effect that can be mimicked by exogenous SHH.[84] Moreover, this commitment to the diverging destinies of myoblasts occurs within the somite, prior to migration into the limb.[85] and occurs independently of signals from the mesenchyme through which the myoblasts migrate from somite to limb bud.[86] This process has not yet been investigated in amniotes.

STEP III: SPECIFICATION OF A FAST SUBTYPE

In mammals, there may be only one slow-twitch subtype[87]; among the fast fibers, however, there are at least as many different subtypes as there are fast MyHC isoforms. It is interesting, then, that in humans the MyHC genes that define these subtypes are closely grouped at one locus on human chromosome 17.[22] The decision to generate diverse fast fiber types may represent a late event in evolution and apparently involves less restrictive programming than the original decision to become either fast or slow, since switching among fast subtypes can occur with less extensive reprogramming than transformations from fast to slow. This commitment is not neurally determined.

Expression of the MyHC isoforms that distinguish these subtypes occurs later in development than stage II specification, but this tells us nothing of when the decision to differentiate into IIa, IIx, or IIb fibers was made originally. For example, expression of the type IIb MyHC in IIb fibers occurs in response to the development of thyroid function[88,89]; but prior to this, prospective IIb fibers must have made the decision to respond in a selective way to systemic increases in the levels of thyroid hormone. It is not known, however, whether the division of fast fibers into IIa, IIb, or IIx fibers is a result of distinct myoblast lineages or merely a reflection of the plasticity of fiber phenotypes that is a hallmark of vertebrate skeletal muscle. It is probable, on the other hand, that the fast IIm fibers descend from myoblasts with a predetermined lineage,[67] since these cells can stably maintain the ability to generate type IIm fibers (see below).

Despite the extensive sequence homology among the fast MyHC genes and proteins, these isoforms cannot completely substitute for each other. In elegant knockout experiments, Leinwand and colleagues have demonstrated that the IIx null mutant has a severe phenotype that includes muscle weakness, aberrant kinetics of muscle contraction and relaxation, kyphosis, and growth inhibition.[90] The muscles of these mutants generate normal amounts of force but have altered kinetic properties. These defects occur even though the absence of the IIx isoform is compensated by an increase in the IIa isoform. In fact, the IIx null mice have normal amounts of MyHCs in their muscles because of this compensation. The IIb null mutants, however, show a much milder phenotype,[91] even though this isoform makes up more than 70 percent of the MyHCs in the mouse. The muscles of these animals, however, show a reduced generation of force. The mild phenotype of the IIb null mutant might not be surprising, since the human does not express this isoform at all,[23] which could be considered a pseudo-IIb null mutant itself.

The complexity of fiber specialization is further illustrated by studies of MyLC, tropomyosin, and troponin C and I and T gene expression in developing rats and humans. These studies show that during early myogenesis, the fast and slow isoforms of these contractile proteins are not coordinately regulated with the MyHCs.[92] Instead, each of these contractile protein genes appears to have its own determinants of mRNA accumulation. During the later stages of myogenesis, there is a surge of mRNA accumulation of the fast isoform genes of these contractile proteins, which leads to establishment of a coordinated "fast" phenotype as fibers progressively diversify. These findings suggest that fiber specialization is the product of multiple regulatory events.[92]

STEP IV: MODULATION AND PLASTICITY

As a result of the lineage decisions made under stages I, II, and III, myoblast pedigrees are established and a plan of diversity is introduced early in muscle histogenesis. As the animal matures, the fundamental diversity is modulated to produce the appropriate number and position of each fiber type. The array of mechanisms involved are probably distinct from those operating in steps I, II, or III. These mechanisms include, but are not limited to, temporal and positional factors, synaptogenesis, imposed neural activity (as the animal learns increasingly complex skills of locomotion), and activation of specific signal transduction pathways.

THE RELATIONSHIP BETWEEN MUSCLE HISTOGENESIS AND THE EMERGENCE OF FIBER-TYPE DIVERSITY

In addition to becoming restricted to a particular lineage, myoblasts must also become positionally restricted so that the correct fiber phenotypes are generated in their stereotypical locations within the muscle. In the rat hindlimb, for example, most slow fibers have an axial distribution surrounding the tibia and fibula, whereas fast IIb fibers are distributed more peripherally.[87,93,94] It is debated whether this pattern is preprogrammed into myoblasts prior to their migration into the limb or enter the limb naive to their future pattern and are instructed by the environment. Evidence exists for both arguments. For example, if embryonic chick trunk somitic mesoderm is transplanted to the position of the brachial somites, the normal complement of brachial muscles is generated,[95] and these muscles contain the same fiber type distributions as normal muscle. This suggests that the cells of trunk and brachial somites are capable of establishing equivalent fiber-type patterns and that nonequivalence must materialize in the environment into which the prospective myoblasts mature. Contradicting this is recent work suggesting that the pattern of fast and slow fibers within developing muscles is established independently of cues from the surrounding tissues and is somehow programmed within the myoblasts while still within the somite.[86] In this work, somites or lateral plate mesoderm were transplanted between chicken and quail embryos. The resulting pattern of fast and slow fibers in the limb was dependent only on the origin of the somite cells, not the lateral plate mesenchymal stroma through which the myoblasts migrated into the limb.

Whether the final pattern of fiber types arises from an environment-independent or -dependent mechanism, the temporal signals influencing specialization are tied in a general way to the pattern of muscle histogenesis. All muscle fibers do not form simultaneously. Rather, a series of generations of fibers occurs, with later generations forming along the walls of earlier generations. This appears to be a common system of instruction among vertebrates, since similar programs are seen in mammals,[94,96,97] including humans,[98,99] and in birds.[100] Muscle histogenesis is initiated by the differentiation of primary generations of myotubes[101–103] (Fig. 4-4A). In the primordia of most muscles, primary myotubes are linked by gap junctions[101] and function as an electrical syncytium.[104] As gap junctions break down, the primary cells move apart (Fig. 4-4B). As this occurs, new generations of myoblasts cluster around the primary cells and use their walls as a cellular scaffold to support the formation of secondary orders of myotubes (Fig. 4-4B). Gap junctions interconnect these primary and secondary orders of myotubes so that each cluster appears to function as an individual unit. At the

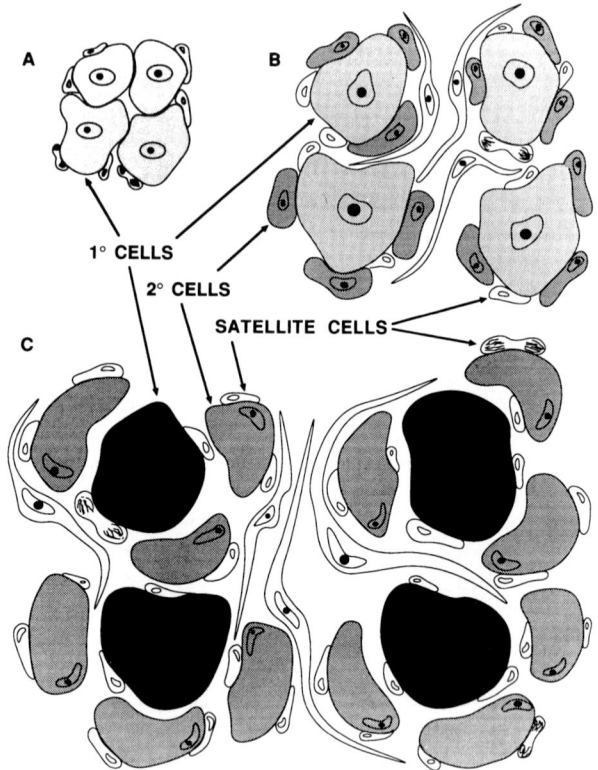

FIGURE 4-4. Model of the histogenesis and emergence of specialization in human fetal muscle. Cells are represented as in cross section; those with centrally drawn nuclei are myotubes. A. Fetal limb muscle, 9 to 10 weeks' gestation. The early muscle primordium is represented by four primary myotubes. At these stages, primary cells express embryonic and slow MyHCs. Plasma membranes of primary cells are closely apposed and probably interconnected by gap junctions. They are surrounded by replicating myoblasts. B. Progressive assembly of muscle, 13 to 18 weeks' gestation. Primary myotubes have enlarged and are separated from one another. Primary cells continue to express slow MyHC. They are ensheathed by myoblasts and by a secondary generation of myotubes that use the walls of the primary cell as a scaffold upon which to differentiate. Secondary myotubes express embryonic and perinatal but not slow MyHC and most will differentiate into fast fibers. C. Growth at 20 to 22 weeks' gestation. Primary and secondary fibers are now separated and new fiber formation is completed. Myoblasts remaining on the walls of fibers can fuse with primary or secondary fibers or become the satellite cells of adult muscle. As a result of the temporal pattern of histogenesis, primary and secondary fibers with differing phenotypes are intermingled in a mosaic.

same time, basal laminar material is deposited around each cluster, insulating one from another. Each of these primary/secondary cell clusters is initially innervated as a single unit by multiple axon sprouts [101] (Fig. 4-5B). With further growth, the gap junctions between primary and secondary cells break down and the cells segregate from one another (Fig. 4-4C), taking groups of axons with them (Fig. 4-5C). As this occurs, each fiber is individually wrapped by basal lamina so that it becomes an independent unit of contraction (Fig. 4-4C). Those myoblasts that do not participate in secondary fiber histogenesis persist on the walls of the now defined population of fibers and, through fusion, contribute to their growth[101] (Fig. 4-4C). A small proportion remain as the satellite cells of mature muscle.

A major developmental function of the primary myotubes is thought to be that of fiber alignment within each muscle. It may be advantageous to initially align only a small number of primary myotubes between their tendon attachment sites and then to utilize these as a scaffold for aligning the much larger number of secondary myotubes. Recent studies have shown that the primary and secondary myotube phases seen in small rodent muscles may be followed by tertiary and even higher-order phases of myotube formation in larger muscles of humans and sheep.[98,105,106] For example, the sheep tibialis cranialis (TC), which has as many as 30,000 fibers, presumably encounters a more complex morphogenesis problem with respect to fiber alignment than does a mouse EDL muscle of about 1100 total fibers. This potential problem may be overcome by adding additional developmental phases of myotube formation. Instead of requiring each of the approximately 440 primary myotubes in the TC muscle to control the alignment of 70 or so secondary myotubes, the addition of a third phase of myotube formation permits the several thousand primary and secondary fibers to serve as alignment guides for a relatively smaller number of tertiary myotubes.[106] These myotube types were not observed by earlier investigators because of the practical decision to focus attention toward small diameter rodent muscles containing relatively few total fibers; this was critical to the goal of examining the sequential histogenesis of entire muscles at the electron microscopic level.

The outcome of this step-by-step pattern of muscle assembly is that fibers with differing ancestry are intermingled in a mosaic reminiscent of the distribution of histochemically distinct fiber types in adult muscle. This similarity has attracted a number of studies, and it is now recognized that *the pattern of fiber specialization is linked to this plan of histogenesis*. Diversity emerges late in mammals, including rats[87] and humans,[98,101,107] coincident with the inception of secondary cell formation. Primary cells initially express embryonic MyHC followed shortly by slow MyHC[72,87] (Fig. 4-6). Primary myotubes located in specific regions of the muscle later lose this expression and go on to accumulate perinatal MyHC, followed by one of the adult fast MyHCs. Those that continue to express slow MyHC become the slow fibers of adult muscle. This relationship between muscle histogenesis and fiber type patterns must also take into consideration the preprogramming of the various—at least fast and slow—lineages. We can conclude, then, that myoblasts with identical lineage predetermination will fuse with each other as primary or as secondary generation fibers. This process is less

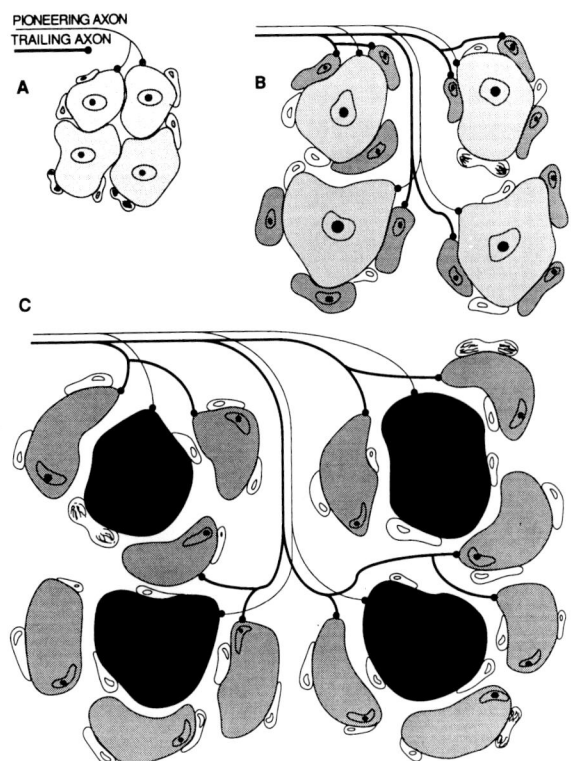

FIGURE 4-5. Theoretical scheme representing successive assembly of motor units during muscle histogenesis. *A.* A pioneering axon innervates four primary myotubes. A trailing axon from a later differentiating motor neuron has not yet found its target myotubes. *B.* Primary myotubes are separated from one another and are ensheathed by secondary generation cells. This organization suggests that at this stage, each primary/secondary cell cluster functions as a single unit. Each is innervated, polyneurally, by pioneering and trailing axons. *C.* Primary and secondary fibers intermingle in a mosaic. Polyneural innervation has been eliminated. Pioneering axons innervate primary slow fibers as one unit and trailing axons innervate secondary fibers as a larger, fast motor unit. By this model, the checkerboard intermingling of motor units is a consequence of the temporal patterns of muscle and nerve development.

clear in the chick where diversity arises early and is apparent among primary cells before secondary cells emerge.[68]

Despite the delay in emergence of fiber diversity in mammalian development, it is worth noting that even in the rat, the organization of primary cells varies from muscle to muscle very early in histogenesis[102,103] (Fig. 4-6). In the anlage of the diaphragm and soleus muscles, for example, primary myotubes are juxtaposed to one another through their entire length, and their membranes are extensively coupled by gap junctions. In the anlage of the EDL, by contrast, primary myotubes are coupled only at the myotendinous junctions but are detached and surrounded by mononucleated cells in the belly of the muscle. The significance of these variations in grouping and probably also in electrical coupling is not fully understood, yet they mark the identity of a muscle even in its primordium. Segregation of primary cells in the primordial EDL appears contrived to propagate the

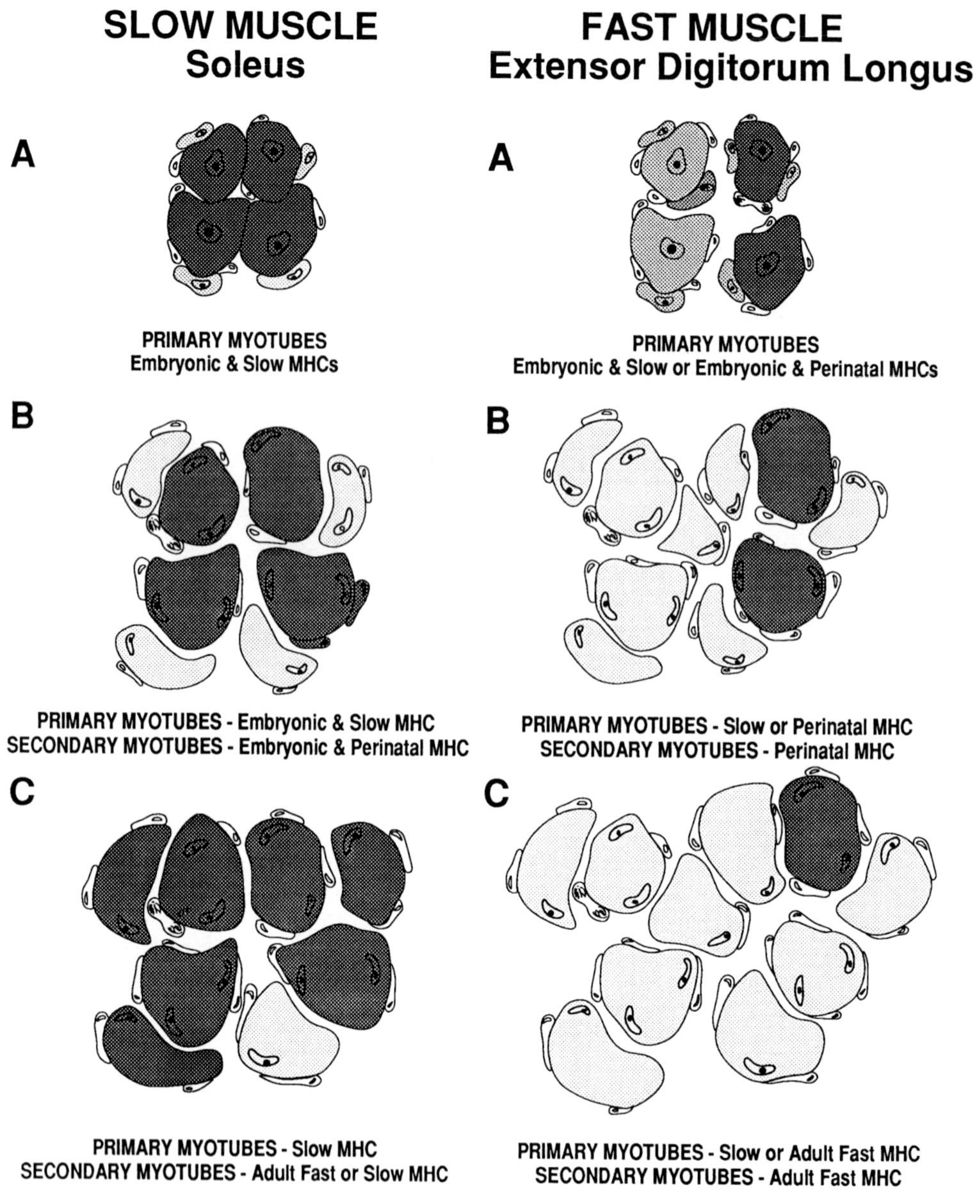

SLOW MUSCLE
Soleus

A

PRIMARY MYOTUBES
Embryonic & Slow MHCs

B

PRIMARY MYOTUBES - Embryonic & Slow MHC
SECONDARY MYOTUBES - Embryonic & Perinatal MHC

C

PRIMARY MYOTUBES - Slow MHC
SECONDARY MYOTUBES - Adult Fast or Slow MHC

FAST MUSCLE
Extensor Digitorum Longus

A

PRIMARY MYOTUBES
Embryonic & Slow or Embryonic & Perinatal MHCs

B

PRIMARY MYOTUBES - Slow or Perinatal MHC
SECONDARY MYOTUBES - Perinatal MHC

C

PRIMARY MYOTUBES - Slow or Adult Fast MHC
SECONDARY MYOTUBES - Adult Fast MHC

FIGURE 4-6. Accumulation of MyHCs in the soleus and extensor digitorum longus (EDL) muscles of the rat hindlimb during development. *A.* Development in the fetus. Primary myotubes of the soleus all express slow MyHC (dark stippling) and embryonic MyHC. In the EDL at this stage, primary myotubes form a heterogeneous population; some express embryonic and slow MyHCs whereas others express embryonic and perinatal MyHCs (intermediate stippling). At an earlier stage, all primary myotubes in the EDL express embryonic and slow MyHCs. Secondary myotubes begin to appear at this stage. They express embryonic and perinatal MyHCs. *B.* Development in the neonate. In the soleus, all primary fibers continue to express slow MYHC. They will become slow fibers in the adult. By contrast, secondary fibers in the soleus initially accumulate adult fast MyHCs (light stippling), principally fast IIa MyHC. In the EDL, many primary fibers and all secondary fibers express perinatal MyHC. They will mature into fast IIa, IIb, and probably IIx fibers in the adult. *C.* Adult phenotype. In the soleus, all primary cells continue to accumulate slow MyHC, but many secondary cells have now shifted from fast to slow MyHC accumulation. As a result, the soleus becomes increasingly specialized as a slow muscle. In the mature EDL, by contrast, many primary slow fibers switch to fast MyHC accumulation and the EDL is increasingly specialized as a fast muscle.

large numbers of secondary cells that characterize histogenesis in this future fast muscle (see Fig. 4-6).

With few exceptions, all secondary cells in fetal rat muscle initially express embryonic MyHC followed by perinatal MyHC and most differentiate into fast fibers[68,87,94,108] (Fig. 4-6). The decision to express neonatal MyHC as opposed to slow MyHC therefore introduces a strong bias toward fast patterns of differentiation.[108] This choice is made well before the adult MyHCs are expressed, meaning that muscle specialization is a progressive, incremental process.

In developing human muscle, primary generation fibers (Wolfart B fibers)[109] emerge between 8 and 10 weeks of gestation.[98,99,107] All fibers of this generation express slow MyHC. Secondary generation fibers (Wolfart A fibers) progressively form between 10 and 18 weeks of gestation and most mature to express fast-twitch MyHCs.[98,99]

THE ABILITY OF MOTOR NEURONS TO MODULATE FIBER TYPES

One consequence of the sequential ordering of fiber diversity is that primary and secondary cells commonly have differing programs of MyHC expression. This occurs despite junctional coupling and mutual innervation by groups of axons[101] (Fig. 4-5B). Hence, it is unlikely that the origins of diversity are induced by differential patterns of activity. Moreover, there is little evidence that motor neurons initially display differential patterns of activity capable of driving fiber-type specialization.[110] Other data support the concept that early fiber diversity is independent of innervation. In the absence of innervation in both the rat and the chick, a pattern of fast and slow fibers still appears.[111–116] Insightful results have also been obtained from studies involving transplantation of wing buds in the chick.[117] Wing buds were excised at a stage before they were penetrated by nerve and transplanted into the pelvic region of recipient chicks to produce supernumerary limbs. Though the wing became innervated by foreign axons from lumbar motor neurons, fiber specialization within the wrist muscles of the supernumerary limb was virtually identical to that of normally innervated wrist muscles. All of these studies show that although fetal muscle growth is dramatically affected, absence of nerve does not inhibit the emergence of a characteristic distribution of fiber types.

In the adult animal, however, the distinct properties within individual fast and slow fibers are partly the result of innervation by different types of motor neurons, since cross-innervation of fast and slow muscles causes a reciprocal transformation of the muscles' properties.[118,119] Eccles et al.[120] have demonstrated that fast and slow motor neurons have different frequencies of impulse activity; and in fact, the effect of cross-innervation of a fast muscle with a slow motor neuron can be mimicked by chronic stimulation of the fast muscle's own intact motor neurons at the low chronic frequencies characteristic of slow motor neurons (see Ref. 121 for review). Physiologic changes with chronic low-frequency electrical stimulation include slowing of the contraction and relaxation times and increased fatigue resistance. These functional changes reflect changes in gene expression, leading to a transformation from fast to slow fibers. Contractile proteins such as MyHCs and troponins, membrane-associated proteins involved in excitation-contraction coupling, and energy metabolism all show this fast-to-slow transformation. The changes in MyHCs are sequential, in the order IIb→IIx→IIa→I. A slow-to-fast transformation can be induced by denervation of the slow motor neuron.[122] Hence, in the adult animal, changes in impulse activity can lead to changes in fiber types.

The dichotomy between the results seen with aneural developing muscle versus those seen with denervated adult muscle experiments depicts an additional facet of muscle phenotypic control. Neural control is imposed on a prearranged plan of diversity, and regulation of slow MyHC synthesis—and therefore the slow fiber type—comes to be modulated by the nerve as the animal matures and learns antigravity postural movements. There is, then, a distinction between the nerve-independent *initiation* of the slow lineage seen in the zebrafish work and the nerve-dependent *maintenance* of the slow phenotype in adult animals.[122]

Even in the adult, however, the motor neuron does not interact with a naive cell; rather, the way in which an individual fiber will respond to these changes in impulse pattern appears to be influenced by its initial specification. In cross-innervation studies involving insertion of a fast nerve into a slow muscle, not all fibers are interconverted.[118,123] Similarly, from chronic stimulation studies, it is known that there are limitations in the capacity of fibers to adjust to incoming stimuli. Stimulated fast fibers of the rat EDL, for example, resist expression of slow myosin.[124] These boundaries appear to be rooted in the inaugural program and have been described as the "adaptive range" of fibers.[123,125] In some instances environmental cues may challenge and effectively override the original specification.[126]

There is also evidence to suggest that modulated fibers retain an inherent bias toward their original phenotype. The development of the rat soleus muscle and the cat jaw-closing muscles demonstrate these interactions.[67,122] The first fibers formed in the rat soleus (the primary generation fibers) become the slow fibers of the adult animal, whereas almost all secondary generation fibers initially differentiate as fast type IIa fibers[96] (Fig. 4-6). With maturity, as demands for posture and weight bearing increase, the secondary cells transform into slow type I fibers (Fig. 4-6 and Ref. 126). This is a neurally dependent process[126] that does not occur if the soleus is denervated at birth.[122] Moreover, the transition from type II to type I fiber appears to be reversible, since a population of fast fibers that are interpreted as secondary generation cells reemerges after denervation of the mature soleus.[126] Conversely, primary slow fibers of the EDL gradually transform to a fast IIa phenotype as the animal matures[87,127] (Fig. 4-5). But upon denervation, the number of slow fibers gradually increases; it is claimed that this proceeds to match the number of slow fibers present early in development.[122]

Finally, studies involving transplantation of myoblasts from jaw-closing muscles in the cat illustrate more of the interplay between intrinsic programs and the environment. As has been discussed, jaw-closing muscles uniquely express the superfast-twitch IIm MyHC in the cat.[24] When myoblasts from these muscles are transplanted to the bed of a limb muscle such as the EDL, they regenerate and express IIm MyHC and not limb fast MyHCs, regardless of whether they are innervated by the EDL nerve or not.[67] By contrast, when transplanted to the bed of the soleus and subsequently innervated, the soleus nerve has the capacity to override the program of IIm MyHC expression and switch fibers to slow MyHC expression. Hence, the slow motor neuron but not the fast motor neuron in the limb can override the IIm lineage of these jaw-closing fibers.

Taken together, these findings suggest that epigenetic modulations of muscle phenotype involve competitive interactions between an exogenous cue and an endogenous program and require continual reinforcement.

SYNAPTOGENESIS AND FIBER-TYPE DIVERSITY

Mechanisms of differentiation that are intrinsic to the muscle may play an active role in spatially sorting the distribution of terminal axons at the initiation of synaptogenesis. One possibility is that motor neuron differentiation is induced by target-derived molecules. Alternatively, the nerve may have the capacity to recognize appropriate myotube targets so that synaptogenesis occurs as a marriage between predetermined types of motor neurons and muscle fibers. Unfortunately, answers to this question are obscured by the presence of polyneural innervation during fiber formation. Unlike mature muscle, in which each fiber is innervated by just one motor neuron, muscles of fetal and newborn animals are innervated by several motor neurons.[128] Synapse elimination during the perinatal period reduces the number of innervating motor neurons to just one per fiber. Motor neurons rearrange themselves during this period, so that appropriate innervation is achieved. Most though not all studies indicate that the nervous system selectively innervates early muscle fibers and suggest that synapse elimination does not serve to significantly increase the precision of innervation[129–131] (but see Jones et al., 1987).[132] This fits with the concept that synaptogenesis in the peripheral nervous system is appropriate from the outset.[133]

We have proposed that the early specificity of innervation is biased by the relative timing of muscle assembly from primary and secondary cells and the concurrent growth of peripheral nerve from pioneering, followed by trailing, axons.[96] This scheme is outlined in Figs. 4-4 and 4-5. It provides a framework for thought but is probably an oversimplification. Additional explanation comes from studies of reinnervation of the neonatal rat soleus after nerve crush. Of 12 motor units in the reinnervated soleus, 10 were biased, either fast or slow, in their fiber-type composition.[129,134] This implies (1) that motor neurons recognize their muscle targets and (2) that differentiating fibers carry specific recognition markers. The process may entail competitive pursuit for molecules of differential adhesion.[135] However, expression of such markers must be transient during mammalian development, since reinnervation of muscle in mature animals is described as nonselective, proceeding on a first-come, first-served basis,[136] with the result that "type grouping" occurs. Type grouping does not occur in lower vertebrates or in invertebrates during reinnervation, prompting speculation that in these species reinnervating motor neurons either show preference for their original target or, alternatively, the process is as nonselective as in mammals but target muscle fibers lack plasticity.

The motor neuron may also regulate the number of primary and secondary generation cells in each muscle. Studies of fiber number in large and small breeds of swine indicate that the total fiber number of each muscle is under genetic control,[137] but experimental studies also suggest that fiber number can be modified by factors as complex as maternal nutrition[138] and by direct and indirect effects of innervation on primary and secondary myotube survival. Since neuronal development is also under genetic control, the overall mechanisms that regulate primary and secondary fiber number must involve the integration of genetic programs specifying myogenic and neuronal development with environmental signals.

While genetic mechanisms may specify the numbers of primary myotubes initially formed, the fraction of surviving primary myotubes is dependent on functional innervation.[113,115,139] Interestingly, the dependence of primary myotube survival on innervation varies between different muscles. For example, virtually all primary myotubes in the rat fourth lumbrical muscles depend on innervation,[140] while only about 20 percent of the primary myotubes in the rat soleus and EDL muscles are dependent on innervation for their survival.[111] Analysis of the dependence of secondary myotube formation upon innervation is even more complex due to the possibility of indirect effects via interactions between primary myotubes and secondary myoblasts/myotubes. Generalizations from one set of experiments to the next is also complicated by the possibility of species differences between the innervation dependence of secondary myotube formation within even the same muscle. For example, secondary myotube formation in mouse EDL muscles exhibits little innervation dependence,[115,139] while there appears to be a rather strict dependence in the rat EDL.[111] In contrast, mouse and rat soleus muscles exhibit 20 to 30 percent fewer muscle fibers, respectively, when they develop under aneural conditions.[111] During chicken muscle development, there appears to be an innervation dependence on primary myotube formation but no direct innervation effect on secondary myotube formation; however, the survival of secondary myotubes depends on the survival of the primary myotubes with which they are associated.[115]

SIGNAL TRANSDUCTION PATHWAYS AND EXPRESSION OF THE SLOW FIBER PHENOTYPE

At least two signal transduction pathways have been described that may contribute to the fiber-specific synthesis of slow muscle proteins. First, calcineurin, a cyclosporine-sensitive, calcium-regulated serine/threonine phosphatase, has been implicated in this process.[141] The myogenic cell line C2C12 was transfected with reported genes linked to the well-characterized slow muscle–specific promoters of the myoglobin and the troponin I slow (TnIs) genes. Cotransfection with calcineurin caused activation of these constructs but not constructs containing fast muscle–specific promoters. They additionally showed that cognate binding sites for NFATs (nuclear factor of activated T cells, the substrate for calcineurin phosphatase) were present on the slow promoters; excision of these binding sites disrupted their calcineurin-mediated activation. In the intact animal, cyclosporine induced a slow-to-fast transformation of fiber types, as would be expected if calcineurin were responsible for the maintenance of the slow phenotype.

Other work has suggested that Ras may be involved in the activity dependent regulation of slow muscle genes.[142] Regeneration of the slow soleus muscle in vivo, in the presence of the normal soleus motor neuron, resulted in slow fiber types, while regeneration after denervation prevented the appearance of the slow phenotype. Transfection of the regenerating, denervated cells in vivo with a constitutively active Ras construct resulted in both increased activity of MAPK and appearance of slow MyHC. A dominant negative Ras mutant blocked the appearance of the slow MyHC.

In a regenerating fast muscle, however, Ras did not induce significant slow MyHC.

Better insight into the fundamental mechanisms controlling the generation of diversity should be of importance to muscle pathologists, for an awareness of the strategies of development provides a framework for understanding the reactions and adaptations of muscle in disease.

List of Abbreviations

ATPase	adenosine triphosphatase	RNA	ribonucleic acid
EDL	extensor digitorum longus	SDH	succinic dehydrogenase
mRNA	messenger RNA	SHH	sonic hedgehog
MyHC	myosin heavy chain	TCA	tricarboxylic acid
MyLC	myosin light chain	TnT	troponin T
NFATs	nuclear factor of activated T cells	TnI	troponin I

References

1. Ranvier L: De quelques faits relatifs a l'histologie et a la physiologie des muscles stries. *Arch Physiol Nor Pathol* 1:5, 1874.
2. Paukal E: Die Zuckungsformen von Kaninchenmusckeln verschiedener Farge and Structur. *Arch Anat Physiol* 100, 1904.
3. Pette D: *Plasticity of Muscle*. Berlin: de Gruyter, 1979.
4. Barany M: ATPase activity of myosin correlated with speed of muscle shortening. *J Gen Physiol* 50(Suppl):197, 1967.
5. Arndt I, Pepe FA: Antigenic specificity of red and white muscle myosin. *J Histochem Cytochem* 23:159, 1975.
6. Nakamura A, Sreter F, Gergely J: Comparative studies of light meromyosin paracrystals derived from red, white, and cardiac muscle myosins. *J Cell Biol* 49:883, 1971.
7. Sarkar S, Sreter FA, Gergely J: Light chains of myosins from white, red, and cardiac muscles. *Proc Natl Acad Sci USA* 68:946, 1971.
8. Dhoot GK, Perry SV: Distribution of polymorphic forms of troponin components and tropomyosin in skeletal muscle. *Nature* 278:714, 1979.
9. Reinach FC, Masaki T, Shafiq S, et al: Isoforms of C-protein in adult chicken skeletal muscle: Detection with monoclonal antibodies. *J Cell Biol* 95:78, 1982.
10. Staudte HW, Pette D: Correlations between enzymes of energy-supplying metabolism as a basic pattern of organization in muscle. *Comp Biochem Physiol B* 41:533, 1972.
11. Burke RE, Levine DN, Tsairis P, Zajac FE III: Physiological types and histochemical profiles in motor units of the cat gastrocnemius. *J Physiol* 234:723, 1973.
12. Guth L, Samaha FJ: Qualitative differences between actomyosin ATPase of slow and fast mammalian muscle. *Exp Neurol* 25:138, 1969.
13. Brooke MH, Kaiser KK: Three "myosin adenosine triphosphatase" systems: The nature of their pH lability and sulfhydryl dependence. *J Histochem Cytochem* 18:670, 1970.
14. Brooke MH, Kaiser KK: Three human myosin ATPase systems and their importance in muscle pathology. *Neurology* 20:404, 1970.
15. Nemeth P, Hofer HW, Pette D: Metabolic heterogeneity of muscle fibers classified by myosin ATPase. *Histochemistry* 63:191, 1979.
16. Guth L, Samaha FJ: Erroneous interpretations which may result from application of the "myofibrillar ATPase" histochemical procedure to developing muscle. *Exp Neurol* 34:465, 1972.
17. Guth L: Fact and artifact in the histochemical procedure for myofibrillar ATPase. *Exp Neurol* 41:440, 1973.
18. Guth L, Yellin H: The dynamic nature of the so-called "fiber types" of mammalian skeletal muscle. *Exp Neurol* 31:227, 1971.
19. Pette D: The Dynamic State of Muscle Fibers. Berlin: de Gruyter, 1990.
20. Bar A, Pette D: Three fast myosin heavy chains in adult rat skeletal muscle. *FEBS Lett* 235:153, 1988.
21. Schiaffino S, Gorza L, Sartore S, et al: Three myosin heavy chain isoforms in type 2 skeletal muscle fibres. *J Muscle Res Cell Motil* 10:197, 1989.
22. Shrager JB, Desjardins PR, Burkman JM, et al: Human skeletal myosin heavy chain genes are tightly linked in the order embryonic-IIa-IId/x-IIb-perinatal-extraocular. *J Muscle Res Cell Motil* 21:345, 2000.
23. Smerdu V, Karsch-Mizrachi I, Campione M, et al: Type IIx myosin heavy chain transcripts are expressed in type IIb fibers of human skeletal muscle. *Am J Physiol* 267:C1723, 1994.
23a. Aigner S, Gohlsch B, Hamalainen N, et al: Fast myosin heavy chain diversity in skeletal muscles of the rabbit: Heavy chain IId, not IIb predominates. *Eur J Biochem* 211:367, 1993.
24. Rowlerson A, Pope P, Murray J: A novel myosin present in cat-jaw-closing muscles. *J Muscle Res Cell Motil* 4:443, 1981.
25. Rowlerson A, Mascarello F, Veggetti A, Carpene E: The fibre-type composition of the first branchial arch muscles in Carnivora and Primates. *J Muscle Res Cell Motil* 4:443, 1983.
26. Maier A, Gambke B, Pette D: Degeneration-regeneration as a mechanism contributing to the fast to slow conversion of chronically stimulated fast-twitch rabbit muscle. *Cell Tissue Res* 244:635, 1986.
27. Rubinstein N, Mabuchi K, Pepe F, et al: Use of type-specific antimyosins to demonstrate the transformation of individual fibers in chronically stimulated rabbit fast muscles. *J Cell Biol* 79:252, 1978.
28. Dubowitz V, Pearse A: A comparative histochemical study of oxidative enzyme and phosphorylase activity in skeletal muscle. *Histochemie* 2:105, 1960.
29. Gauthier GF, Padykula HA: Cytological studies of fiber types in skeletal muscle. A comparative study of the mammalian diaphragm. *J Cell Biol* 28:333, 1966.
30. Termin A, Staron RS, Pette D: Myosin heavy chain isoforms in histochemically defined fiber types of rat muscle. *Histochemistry* 92:453, 1989.
31. Mascarello F, Carpene E, Veggetti A, et al: The tensor tympani muscle of cat and dog contains IIM and slow-tonic fibres: An unusual combination of fibre types. *J Muscle Res Cell Motil* 3:363, 1982.
32. Lompre AM, Nadal-Ginard B, Mahdavi V: Expression of the cardiac ventricular alpha- and beta-myosin heavy chain genes is developmentally and hormonally regulated. *J Biol Chem* 259:6437, 1984.
33. d'Albis A, Janmont C, Mira J-C, Couteaux R: Characterization of a ventricular myosin isoform in rabbit masticatory muscles: Developmental and neural regulation. *Basic Appl Myol* 1:23, 1981.
34. Rubinstein NA, Hoh JFY: The distribution of myosin heavy chain isoforms among rat extraocular muscle fiber types. *Invest Ophthalmol Vis Sci* 41:3391, 2000.
35. Rushbrook JI, Weiss C, Ko K, et al: Identification of alpha-cardiac myosin heavy chain mRNA and protein in extraocular muscle of the adult rabbit. *J Muscle Res Cell Motil* 15:505, 1994.
36. Wieczorek DF, Periasamy M, Butler-Browne GS, et al: Co-expression of multiple myosin heavy chain genes, in addition to a tissue-specific one, in extraocular musculature. *J Cell Biol* 101:618, 1985.
37. Schachat F, Briggs M: Identification of two patterns of exon organization in the human striated muscle myosin heavy chain genes. *Mol Biol Cell* 10s:34a, 1999.
38. Emerson CP, Bernstein SI: Molecular genetics of myosin. *Annu Rev Biochem* 56:695, 1987.
39. Saez LJ, Gianola KM, McNally EM, et al: Human cardiac myosin heavy chain genes and their linkage in the genome. *Nucleic Acids Res* 15:5443, 1987.
40. Mahdavi V, Chambers AP, Nadal-Ginard B: Cardiac alpha- and beta-myosin heavy chain genes are organized in tandem. *Proc Natl Acad Sci USA* 81:2626, 1984.
41. Weiss A, McDonough D, Wertman B, et al: Organization of human and mouse skeletal myosin heavy chain gene clusters is highly conserved. *Proc Natl Acad Sci USA* 96:2958, 1999.
42. Robert B, Barton P, Minty A, et al: Investigation of genetic linkage between myosin and actin genes using an interspecific mouse back-cross. *Nature* 314:181, 1985.

43. Gaunt SJ, Singh PB: Homeogene expression patterns and chromosomal imprinting. *Trends Genet* 6:208, 1990.
44. Hanscombe O, Whyatt D, Fraser P, et al: Importance of globin gene order for correct developmental expression. *Genes Dev* 5:1387, 1991.
44a. Desjardins PR, Burkman JM, Shrager JB, et al: Evolutionary implications of three novel members of the human sarcomeric myosin heavy chain gene family. *Mol Biol Evol* 19:375, 2002.
45. Nemeth PM, Pette D, Vrbova G: Comparison of enzyme activities among single muscle fibres within defined motor units. *J Physiol* 311:489, 1981.
46. Hilber K, Galler S: Mechanical properties and myosin heavy chain isoform composition of skinned skeletal muscle fibres from a human biopsy sample. *Pflugers Arch* 434:551, 1997.
47. Hilber K, Galler S, Gohlsch B, Pette D: Kinetic properties of myosin heavy chain isoforms in single fibers from human skeletal muscle. *FEBS Lett* 455:267, 1999.
48. Lees-Miller J, Helfman D: The molecular basis for tropomyosin isoform diversity. *Bioessays* 13:429, 1991.
49. Gunning P, Gordon M, Wade R, et al: Differential control of tropomyosin mRNA levels during myogenesis suggests the existence of an isoform competition–autoregulatory compensation control mechanism. *Dev Biol* 138:443, 1990
50. Forry-Schaudies S, Hughes SH: The chicken tropomyosin 1 gene generates nine mRNAs by alternative splicing. *J Biol Chem* 266:13821, 1991.
51. Wieczorek DF, Smith CW, Nadal-Ginard B: The rat alpha-tropomyosin gene generates a minimum of six different mRNAs coding for striated, smooth, and nonmuscle isoforms by alternative splicing. *Mol Cell Biol* 8:679, 1988.
52. Bronson DD, Schachat FH: Heterogeneity of contractile proteins. Differences in tropomyosin in fast, mixed, and slow skeletal muscles of the rabbit. *J Biol Chem* 257:3937, 1982.
53. Barton PJ, Cullen ME, Townsend PJ, et al: Close physical linkage of human troponin genes: Organization, sequence, and expression of the locus encoding cardiac troponin I and slow skeletal troponin T. *Genomics* 57:102, 1999.
54. Breitbart RE, Nguyen HT, Medford RM, et al: Intricate combinatorial patterns of exon splicing generate multiple regulated troponin T isoforms from a single gene. *Cell* 41:67, 1985
55. Breitbart RE, Nadal-Ginard B: Developmentally induced, muscle-specific trans factors control the differential splicing of alternative and constitutive troponin T exons. *Cell* 49:793, 1987.
56. Schachat R, Briggs M, Williamson E, et al: Expression of fast thin filament proteins. Defining fiber archetypes in a molecular continuum, in Pette D (ed): *The Dynamic State of Muscle Fibers*. Berlin: de Gruyter, 1990.
57. Briggs MM, Lin JJ, Schachat FH: The extent of amino-terminal heterogeneity in rabbit fast skeletal muscle troponin T. *J Muscle Res Cell Motil* 8:1, 1987.
58. Greaser ML, Moss RL, Reiser PJ: Variations in contractile properties of rabbit single muscle fibres in relation to troponin T isoforms and myosin light chains. *J Physiol (Lond)* 496:85, 1988.
59. Bottinelli R, Betto R, Schiaffino S, Reggiani C: Unloaded shortening velocity and myosin heavy chain and alkali light chain isoform composition in rat skeletal muscle fibres. *J Physiol (Lond)* 481:663, 1994.
60. Wada M, Pette D: Relationships between alkali light-chain complement and myosin heavy-chain isoforms in single fast-twitch fibers of rat and rabbit. *Eur J Biochem* 214:157, 1993.
61. Yamamoto K, Moos C: The C-proteins of rabbit red, white, and cardiac muscles. *J Biol Chem* 258:8395, 1983.
62. Horowits R: Passive force generation and titin isoforms in mammalian skeletal muscle. *Biophys J* 61:392, 1992.
63. Labeit S, Kolmerer B: The complete primary structure of human nebulin and its correlation to muscle structure. *J Mol Biol* 248:308, 1995.
64. Schachat FH, Canine AC, Briggs MM, Reedy MC: The presence of two skeletal muscle alpha-actinins correlates with troponin-tropomyosin expression and Z-line width. *J Cell Biol* 101:1001, 1985.
65. Schmitt TL, Pette D. Corelations between troponin-T and myosin heavy chain isoforms in normal and transformed rabbit muscle fibers, in Pette D (ed): *The Dynamic State of Muscle Fibers*. Berlin: de Gruyter, 1990, p 293.
66. Schiaffino S, Reggiani C: Molecular diversity of myofibrillar proteins: Gene regulation and functional significance. *Physiol Rev* 76:371, 1996.
67. Hoh JFY, Hughes S: Myogenic and neurogenic regulation of myosin gene expression in cat jaw-closing muscles regenerating in fast and slow limb muscle beds. *J Muscle Res Cell Motil* 9:57, 1988.
68. Stockdale FE, Miller JB, Feldman JL, et al: Myogenic cell lineages. Commitment and modulation during differentiation of avian muscle, in Kedes L, Stockdale FE (eds): *Cellular and Molecular Biology of Muscle Development*. New York: Liss, 1989.
69. Miller JB, Stockdale FE: Developmental origins of skeletal muscle fibers: Clonal analysis of myogenic cell lineages based on expression of fast and slow myosin heavy chains. *Proc Natl Acad Sci USA* 83:3860, 1986.
70. Miller JB, Crow MT, Stockdale FE: Slow and fast myosin heavy chain content defines three types of myotubes in early muscle cell cultures. *J Cell Biol* 101:1643, 1985.
71. Olsen E: MyoD family. A paradigm for development. *Genes Dev* 4:1454, 1990.
72. Lyons GE, Ontell M, Cox R, et al: The expression of myosin genes in developing skeletal muscle in the mouse embryo. *J Cell Biol* 111:1465, 1990.
73. Hinterberger TJ, Sassoon DA, Rhodes SJ, Konieczny SF: Expression of the muscle regulatory factor MRF4 during somite and skeletal myofiber development. *Dev Biol* 147:144, 1991.
74. Bober E, Lyons GE, Braun T, et al: The muscle regulatory gene, Myf-6, has a biphasic pattern of expression during early mouse development. *J Cell Biol* 113:1255, 1991.
75. Hughes SM, Blau HM: Muscle fiber pattern is independent of cell lineage in postnatal rodent development. *Cell* 68:659, 1992.
76. Seed J, Hauschka SD: Temporal separation of the migration of distinct myogenic precursor populations into the developing chick wing bud. *Dev Biol* 106:389, 1984.
77. DiMario JX, Fernya SE, Stockdale FE: Myoblasts transferred to the limbs of embryos are committed to specific fibre fates. *Nature* 362:165, 1993.
78. Stockdale FE: Mechanisms of formation of muscle fiber types. *Cell Struct Funct* 22:37, 1997.
79. Devoto SH, Melancon E, Eisen JS, Westerfield M: Identification of separate slow and fast muscle precursor cells in vivo, prior to somite formation. *Development* 122:3371, 1996.
80. Barresi JJ, Stickney HL, Devoto SH: The zebrafish slow-muscle-omitted gene product is required for Hedgehog signal transduction and the development of slow muscle identity. *Development* 127:2188, 2000.
81. Currie PD, Ingham PW: Induction of a specific muscle cell type by a hedgehog-like protein in zebrafish. *Nature* 382:452, 1996.
82. Norris W, Neyt C, Ingham PW, Currie PD: Slow muscle induction by Hedgehog signalling in vitro. *J Cell Sci* 113:2695, 2000.
83. Blagden CS, Currie PD, Ingham PW, Hughes SM: Notochord induction of Zebrafish slow muscle is mediated by Sonic Hedgehog. *Genes Dev* 11:2163, 1997.
84. Cann GM, Lee JW, Stockdale FE: Sonic hedgehog enhances somite cell viability and formation of primary slow muscle fibers in avian segmented mesoderm. *Anat Embryol* 200:239, 1999.
85. Van Swearingen J, Lance-Jones C: Slow and fast muscle fibers are preferentially derived from myoblasts migrating into the chick limb bud at different developmental times. *Dev Biol* 170:321, 1995.
86. Nikovits W, Cann GM, Huang R, et al: Patterning of fast and slow fibers within embryonic muscles is established independently of signals from the surrounding mesenchyme. *Development* 128:2537, 2001.
87. Narusawa M, Fitzsimons RB, Izumo S, et al: Slow myosin in developing rat skeletal muscle. *J Cell Biol* 104:447, 1987.
88. Gambke B, Lyons GE, Haselgrove J, et al: Thyroidal and neural control of myosin transitions during development of rat fast and slow muscles. *FEBS Lett* 156:335, 1983.
89. Russell SD, Cambon N, Nadal-Ginard B, Whalen RG: Thyroid hormone induces a nerve-independent precocious expression of fast myosin heavy chain mRNA in rat hindlimb skeletal muscle. *J Biol Chem* 263:6370, 1988.
90. Sartorius CA, Lu BD, Acakpo-Satchivi L, et al: Myosin heavy chains IIa and IId are functionally distinct in the mouse. *J Cell Biol* 141:943, 1998.
91. Acakpo-Satchivi LJ, Edelmann W, et al: Growth and muscle defects in mice lacking adult myosin heavy chain genes. *J Cell Biol* 139:1219, 1997.
92. Sutherland CJ, Elsom VL, Gordon ML, et al: Coordination of skeletal muscle gene expression occurs late in mammalian development. *Dev Biol* 146:167, 1991.
93. Lyons GE, Haselgrove J, Kelly AM, Rubinstein NA: Myosin transitions in developing fast and slow muscles of the rat hindlimb. *Differentiation* 25:168, 1983.
94. Condon K, Silberstein L, Blau HM, Thompson WJ: Development of muscle fiber types in the prenatal rat hindlimb. *Dev Biol* 138:256, 1990.
95. Lance-Jones C: Motoneuron cell death in the developing lumbar spinal cord of the mouse. *Brain Res* 256:473, 1982.
96. Rubinstein NA, Kelly AM: Development of muscle fiber specialization in the rat hindlimb. *J Cell Biol* 90:128, 1981.
97. Kelly AM, Rubinstein NA: Development of neuromuscular specialization. *Med Sci Sports Exerc* 18:292, 1986.
98. Draeger A, Weeds AG, Fitzsimons RB: Primary, secondary and tertiary myotubes in developing skeletal muscle: a new approach to the analysis of human myogenesis. *J Neurol Sci* 81:19, 1987.
99. Butler-Browne GS, Barbet JP, Thornell LE: Myosin heavy and light chain expression during human skeletal muscle development and precocious muscle maturation induced by thyroid hormone. *Anat Embryol* 181:513, 1990.
100. McLennan IS: Neural dependence and independence of myotube production in chicken hindlimb muscles. *Dev Biol* 98:287, 1983.
101. Kelly AM, Zacks SI: The histogenesis of rat intercostal muscle. *J Cell Biol* 42:135, 1969.
102. Ontell M, Kozeka K: Organogenesis of the mouse extensor digitorum longus muscle: A quantitative study. *Am J Anat* 171:149, 1984.
103. Ontell M, Bourke D, Hughes D: Cytoarchitecture of the fetal murine soleus muscle. *Am J Anat* 181:267, 1988.
104. Dennis MJ, Ziskind-Conhaim L, Harris AJ: Development of neuromuscular junctions in rat embryos. *Dev Biol* 81:266, 1981.

105. Maier A, McEvawn JC, Dodds KG: Myosin heavy chain composition of single fibres and their origins and disribution in develoing fascicles of sheep tibialis cranialis muscles. *J Muscle Res Cell Motil* 13:551, 1992.
106. Wilson SJ, McEwarn JC, Sheard PW, Harris AJ: Early stages of myogenesis is a large mammal: Formation of successive generations of myotubes in sheep cranialis muscle. *J Muscle Res Cell Motil* 13:534, 1992.
107. Barbet JP, Thornell LE, Butler-Browne GS: Immunocytochemical characterisation of two generations of fibers during the development of the human quadriceps muscle. *Mech Dev* 35:3, 1991.
108. Whalen RG: Myosin isoenzymes as molecular markers for muscle physiology. *J Exp Biol* 115:43, 1985.
109. Wolfart G: Quantitativ-histologische Studien an der Skelettmuskulatur warend der Entwicklung und bei der Atropie nach Nervendruchshneidung. *A Mikr-Anat Forsch* 5:480, 1942.
110. Navarette R, Vrbova G: Changes of activity patterns in slow and fast muscles during post natal development. *Dev Brain Res* 81:11, 1983.
111. Wilson SJ. Harris AJ: Formation of myotubes in aneural rat muscles. *Dev Biol* 156:509, 1993.
112. Condon K, Silberstein L, Blau HM, Thompson WJ: Differentiation of fiber types in aneural musculature of the prenatal rat hindlimb. *Dev Biol* 138:275, 1990.
113. Fredette BJ, Landmesser LT: A reevaluation of the role of innervation in primary and secondary myogenesis in developing chick muscle. *Dev Biol* 143:19, 1991.
114. Phillips WD, Bennett MR: Differentiation of fiber types in wing muscles during embryonic development: Effect of neural tube removal. *Dev Biol* 106:457, 1984.
115. Ashby PR, Wilson SJ, Harris AJ: Formation of primary and secondary myotube in aneural muscles in the mouse mutant peroneal muscular atrophy. *Dev Biol* 156:519, 1993.
116. Condon K, Silberstein L, Blau H, Thompson W: Differentiation of fiber types in aneural musculature of the prenatal rat hindlimb. *Dev Biol* 138:275, 1990.
117. Laing NG, Lamb AH: The distribution of muscle fibre types in chick embryo wings transplanted to the pelvic region is normal. *J Embryol Exp Morphol* 78:67, 1983.
118. Buller AJ, Eccles JC, Eccles RM: Interactions between motoneromes and muscles in respect of the characteristic speeds of their responses. *J Physiol* 150:417–439, 1960.
119. Weeds AG, Trentham DR, Kean CJ, Buller AJ: Myosin from cross-reinnervated cat muscles. *Nature* 247:135, 1974.
120. Eccles J, Eccles R, Lundberg A: The action potential of alpha motoneurones supplying fast and slow muscles in rat. *J Physiol* 142:275, 1958
121. Pette D, Vrbova G: What does chronic electrical stimulation teach us about muscle plasticity? *Muscle Nerve* 22:666, 1999.
122. Rubinstein NA, Kelly AM: Myogenic and neurogenic contributions to the development of fast and slow twitch muscles in rat. *Dev Biol* 62:473, 1978.
123. Gundersen K, Leberer E, Lomo T, et al: Fibre types, calcium-sequestering proteins and metabolic enzymes in denervated and chronically stimulated muscles of the rat. *J Physiol* 398:177, 1988.
124. Kirschbaum BJ, Kucher HB, Termin A, et al: Antagonistic effects of chronic low frequency stimulation and thyroid hormone on myosin expression in rat fast-twitch muscle. *J Biol Chem* 265:13974, 1990.
125. Westgaard RH, Lomo T: Control of contractile properties within adaptive ranges by patterns of impulse activity in the rat. *J Neurosci* 8:4415, 1988.
126. Kugelberg E: Adaptive transformation of rat soleus motor units during growth. *J Neurol Sci* 27:269, 1976.
127. Whalen RG, Johnstone D, Bryers PS, et al: A developmentally regulated disappearance of slow myosin in fast-type muscles of the mouse. *FEBS Lett* 177:51, 1984.
128. Brown MC, Jensen JKS, Van Essen DC: Poly-neuronal innervation of skeletal muscle in new-born rats and its elimination during maturation. *J Physiol* 261:387, 1976.
129. Thompson WJ, Condon K, Astrow SH: The origin and selective innervation of early muscle fiber types in the rat. *J Neurobiol* 21:212, 1989.
130. Gordon H, Van Essen DC: Specific innervation of muscle fiber types in a developmentally polyinnervated muscle. *Dev Biol* 111:42, 1985.
131. Fladby T, Jansen JK: Selective innervation of neonatal fast and slow muscle fibres before net loss of synaptic terminals in the mouse soleus muscle. *Acta Physiol Scand* 134:561, 1988.
132. Jones SP, Ridge RM, Rowlerson A: The non-selective innervation of muscle fibres and mixed composition of motor units in a muscle of neonatal rat. *J Physiol* 386:377, 1987.
133. Purves D, Lichtman JW. *Principles of Neural Development.* Sunderland, MA: Sinauer, 1985.
134. Soileau LC, Silberstein L, Blau HM, Thompson WJ: Reinnervation of muscle fiber types in the newborn rat soleus. *J Neurosci* 7:4176, 1987.
135. Soha JM, Callaway EM, Van Essen DC: Lack of fiber type selectivity during reinnervation of neonatal rabbit soleus muscle. *Dev Biol* 131:401, 1989.
136. Kugelberg E, Edstrom L, Abbruzzese M: Mapping of motor units in experimentally reinnervated rat muscle. Interpretation of histochemical and atrophic fibre patterns in neurogenic lesions. *J Neurol Neurosurg Psychiatry* 33:319, 1970.
137. Strickland NC, Hande SE: The numbers and types of muscle fibres in large and small breeds of pigs. *J Anat* 147:181, 1986.
138. Wilson SJ, Ross JJ, Harris AJ: A critical period for formation of secondary myotubes defined by prenatal undernourishmen in rats. *Development* 102:815, 1988.
139. Ashby PR, Pincon-Raymond M, Harris AJ: Regulation of myogenesis in paralyzed muscles in the mouse mutants peroneal muscular atrophy and muscular dysgenesis. *Dev Biol* 156:529, 1993.
140. Ross JJ, Duxson MJ, Harris AJ: Neural determination of muscle fibre numbers in embryonic rat lumbrical muscles. *Development* 100:395, 1987.
141. Chin ER, Olson EN, Richardson JA, et al: A calcineurin-dependent transcriptional pathway controls skeletal muscle fiber type. *Genes Dev* 12: 2499, 1998.
142. Murgia M, Serrano AL, Calabria E, et al: Ras is involved in nerve-activity-dependent regulation of muscle genes. *Nat Cell Biol* 2:142, 2000.
143. Briggs MM, Scohachat F: Early specialization of the superfast myosin in extraocular and laryngeal muscles. *J Exp Biol* 203:2485, 2000.

Chapter 5
The Structure and Function of Motor Units

ROBERT E. BURKE

Definitions
Anatomy
   MOTOR NUCLEI
   MUSCLE ARCHITECTURE
   ANATOMY OF MUSCLE UNITS
Physiologic Properties of Motor Units
   IDENTIFICATION OF MOTOR UNIT TYPES
   MOTOR UNIT TYPES AND MUSCLE FIBER HISTOCHEMISTRY
   DEVELOPMENT OF MOTOR UNIT TYPES
   MUSCLE UNIT FORCE OUTPUT AND INNERVATION RATIOS
Motor Units in Human Muscle
Motor Units In Action
   INTERRELATIONS BETWEEN MOTOR NEURON AND MUSCLE UNIT PROPERTIES
   MECHANISMS THAT CONTROL MUSCLE OUTPUT
   RECRUITMENT CONTROL
   FORCE GRADATION BY MOTOR NEURON FIRING RATE
Synthesis

Definitions

Skeletal muscles are collections of striated muscle fibers, usually arranged in parallel bundles (fascicles) and enclosed by connective tissue. When examined in detail, many skeletal muscles exhibit complex internal architectures. From a functional point of view, muscles are simply collections of muscle units. A muscle unit is the set of muscle fibers that is innervated by a single motor neuron within the spinal cord or brainstem. The combination of motor neuron and muscle unit make up a motor unit, which is the indivisible quantal element of muscle action.[1] The mechanical actions exerted by collections of motor units may involve complex synergies within as well as between anatomic muscles, and the forces they deliver to the skeleton depend critically on the details of fiber arrangements within the muscle.[2]

Motor neurons belong to the small class of central nervous system (CNS)* neurons having axons that leave the CNS. They are the largest neurons in the CNS and are unique in that they innervate nonneuronal peripheral tissue (i.e., skeletal muscle fibers). There are three categories of motor neurons: (1) alpha, or skeletomotor, motor neurons, which innervate exclusively the large extrafusal skeletal muscle fibers; (2) gamma, or fusimotor, motor neurons, which innervate exclusively the small intrafusal muscle fibers within the muscle spindle stretch receptors; and (3) beta, or skeletofusimotor, motor neurons, which innervate both extra- and intrafusal muscle fibers.[3] This chapter focuses on the motor neurons that innervate extrafusal muscle units in limb and trunk muscles of mammals and humans. The limited available evidence suggests that alpha and beta motor neurons and their respective extrafusal muscle units are essentially similar,[3,4] and the following discussion does not distinguish between them.

A given motor neuron can innervate dozens to thousands of muscle fibers (the "innervation ratio"), but—in normal adult animals—each muscle fiber receives innervation from one and only one motor neuron. A motor unit represents a biological amplifier of dramatic proportions. Figure 5-1 illustrates the relative sizes of a motor neuron and part of a representative muscle unit. The volume of a motor axon 20 cm long (2 to 3×10^6 μm^3) is almost an order of magnitude larger than the cytoplasmic volume of a typical alpha motor neuron (3 to 5×10^5 μm^3). The volume of a *single* muscle fiber can be an order of magnitude larger than the motor neuron plus its axon. When multiplied by the dozens or hundreds of muscle fibers in the muscle, a single motor neuron thus controls the responses of muscle tissue that can be two to four orders of magnitude larger in volume. A more long-term aspect of this amplification is the "trophic" control of the properties of every fiber in the muscle unit by the innervating motor neuron (see Chap. 4). From both viewpoints, it is clear that a large volume of muscle tissue is controlled in multiple ways by a much smaller neuron.

For reasons of experimental methodology, current information about the physiology of motor units is most complete for certain muscles in experimental animals, particularly the cat and rat. However, evidence from other species, including humans, strongly suggests that the basic organization of motor unit populations is similar in all mammals. Points of similarity vastly outweigh differences. In this respect, information that has been developed from studies of motor unit populations in animals is clearly relevant to understanding the situation in normal and diseased human skeletal muscle.

Anatomy

MOTOR NUCLEI

Motor neurons are anatomically and functionally inseparable from the muscle units they innervate. The motor neurons that innervate units in a particular anatomic muscle are collected into longitudinal clusters within the ventral horn of the spinal cord.[5] Such nuclei are located within the ventral horn gray matter in predictable locations in both animal[6] and human spinal cords.[7] Although there is evidence for some topographic organization between the longitudinal position of motor neurons and the location of their muscle units within the muscle,[8] such subsets exhibit a great deal of overlap in position even in muscles that have definable compartments.[9]

By definition, the number of motor units in a given muscle equals the number of its motor neurons. In limb muscles, motor unit numbers vary from dozens to many hundreds, depending on muscle size and function as well as the overall size of the animal in question.[10] Paradoxically, the small

---

*A list of abbreviations used in this chapter is given at the end of the chapter.

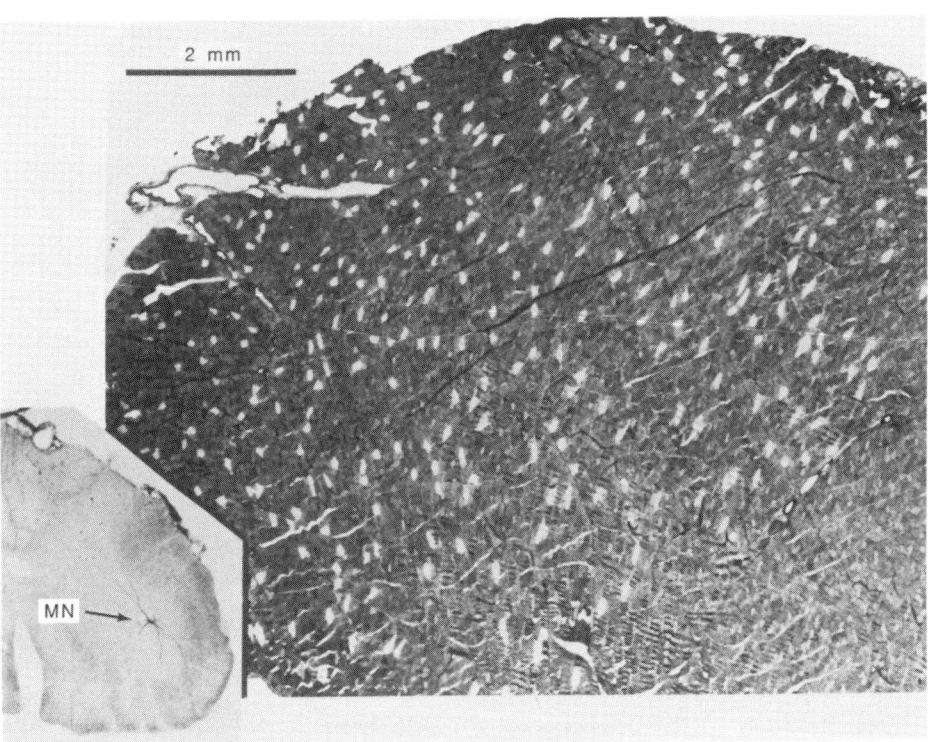

FIGURE 5-1. A motor unit depicted to scale. The large panel shows a representative cross section of a cat medial gastrocnemius muscle in which the muscle fibers of a single fast-twitch, fatigable (type FF) muscle unit had been depleted of glycogen during repetitive stimulation. (Preparation by Dr. Peter Tsairis from work reported in Ref. 32.) The depleted unit fibers are scattered among fibers with normal glycogen content. The inset photomicrograph shows a single type FF motor neuron (arrow, MN) stained by intracellular injection of a tracer substance, horseradish peroxidase, in a cross section of spinal cord. (Unpublished photomicrograph; see Ref. 88.) Note the large territory occupied by evenly scattered muscle unit fibers (see also Fig. 5-3) and the disparity between the sizes of the motor neuron and muscle unit.

extraocular muscles contain some of the largest numbers known (>1000 motor units; see Ref. 11). Estimates of motor unit numbers in human muscles, which are important in the evaluation of motor neuron disease and the effects of aging, can be obtained only indirectly.[12,13]

MUSCLE ARCHITECTURE

Somatic muscles exhibit a wide range of internal architectures that are clearly related to their evolution and function.[14] Muscle fibers are grouped into clusters, or fascicles, by connective tissue sheets that transmit forces to the robust aponeuroses and tendons that anchor the muscle to the skeleton. Fibers belonging to a given muscle unit are normally distributed to multiple such fascicles. Sometimes the aponeuroses are folded into complex sheets to create internal "compartments" that can produce different force vectors on the skeleton.[15] Some anatomically defined muscles have distinctly different heads (e.g., the human biceps brachii), while others have broad origins or insertions (e.g., the human deltoid), allowing muscle units in different parts of the muscle to act differentially during movement.

Although exceptions are numerous, it is fair to say that limb and trunk muscles exhibit two basic internal architectures. Both are governed in part by the fact that individual muscle fibers are usually considerably shorter than the length of the muscle belly in which they reside. Fiber lengths are constrained presumably because conduction of action potentials along muscle fibers is relatively slow (2 to 10 m/s), and action potentials generated by the centrally placed neuromuscular junctions (NMJs) must reach and activate the distal ends of fiber while the central region can still sustain force.[16]

One solution to this problem is to pack fascicles of short muscle fibers at an angle along the muscle axis, producing pinnate (feather-like) muscles (Fig. 5-2A). Pinnate muscles can generate large output forces because they pack a large cross-sectional area of muscle fibers into a relatively small volume. The price for this is that the working range over which pinnate muscles can effectively generate force (the force/length curve) is limited, although changes in fiber angulation during stretch mitigates this somewhat (Fig. 5-2A).

An alternative design is to arrange fascicles of short muscle fibers in serial compartments along the muscle axis, sometimes separated by tendinous inscriptions to transmit longitudinal force (Fig. 5-2B). This is found in the human rectus abdominus and cat semitendinosus.[17] Another alternative for parallel architecture is to arrange relatively short muscle fibers in fascicles that are staggered along the major axis of the muscle. The interdigitated fibers are usually tapered on both ends[18] and are somehow linked to an intramuscular connective tissue stroma that delivers output force to the skeletal attachments (Fig. 5-2C).[16] Muscles with serial compartments can work effectively over larger length excursions than pinnate muscles, but their maximum force output per unit weight is less because they have fewer sarcomeres in parallel.

ANATOMY OF MUSCLE UNITS

Obviously, the anatomy of muscle units must conform to variations in the internal architecture of the muscle in which they reside. As they approach their target muscle, each motor axon divides into a complex arborization such that each terminal branch ends in a neuromuscular junction (see Chap. 15) located roughly halfway along each of the fibers in its muscle unit. The distribution of fibers in an individual muscle unit can be revealed by stimulating its motor neuron or motor axon for periods of time long enough to deplete intrafiber glycogen[19] (see Fig. 5-1). Normally, muscle unit fibers are scattered within a territorial volume smaller than the volume of the muscle belly (Fig. 5-2).[20,21] They are intermingled with fibers belonging to many other muscle units, with few apposed fibers from the same unit (Figs. 5-1 and 5-3).[22] The average fiber density in the unipinnate cat gastrocnemius is 3 to 8 fibers per 100,[20] suggesting that the territory of one muscle unit may be shared by at least 15 to 30 others (see also Ref. 23). This estimate may be low, because overlapping muscle unit territories usually have different shapes. Rare glycogen-depletion observations of a motor unit in a patient with myokymia (Fig. 3.42 in Ref. 24) and electromyographic (EMG) data from human muscle units[12,25] indicate that the density and spatial dispersion of muscle unit fibers in humans are similarly arranged.

In compartmentalized pinnate muscles, muscle units usually occupy a single compartment,[9] so that their action is functionally uniform (Fig. 5-2A). This is also true for units in serially compartmentalized muscles (Fig. 5-2B).[17] Muscle

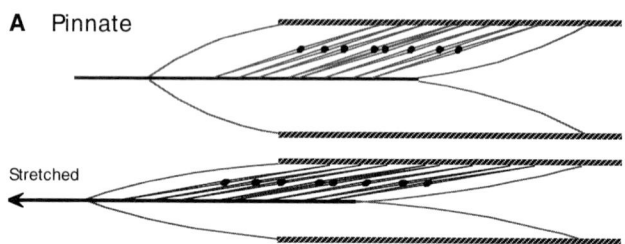

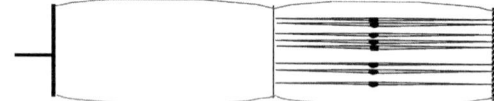

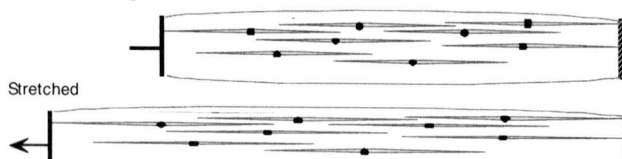

FIGURE 5-2. Diagrams to illustrate alternative patterns of intramuscular architecture. A. In the pinnate (feather-like) design, muscle fibers in muscle units are arranged at an angle to the axis of the muscle, running between fibrous aponeuroses of origin (cross-hatched) and insertion (solid lines). The neuromuscular junctions (NMJs; black dots) in a representative muscle unit are aligned along the muscle axis. Stretch elongates the fibers and decreases their angulation. B. In a muscle with serial compartments, fibers of muscle units are arranged in parallel to the muscle axis and NMJs are aligned in rows perpendicular to the axis. Individual muscle units are confined to one compartment. C. In a muscle with interdigitated muscle fibers, muscle unit fibers are arranged parallel with the muscle axis but staggered along its length, with many originating and ending on endomysial connective tissue stroma. Note that NMJs are scattered along the muscle axis.

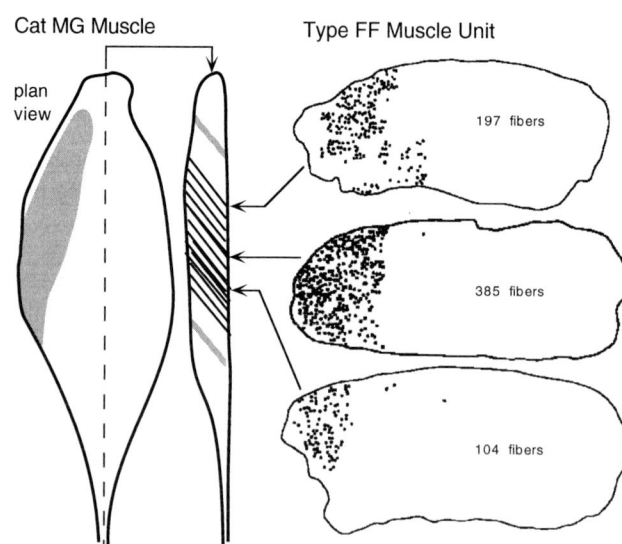

FIGURE 5-3. Mapping of muscle unit fibers in a cat medial gastrocnemius muscle. The diagrams on the left show a plan view and a longitudinal section of this flat unipinnate muscle. The projected muscle unit territory is indicated on the former by the shaded area. Approximate fiber angulation is shown on the latter. On the right are maps of glycogen-depleted fibers of a single type FF muscle unit, showing how their numbers change along the muscle axis because of fiber angulation. The middle map is from the section shown in Fig. 5-1. (*Adapted from Burke RE, Tsairis P: Anatomy and innervation ratios in motor units of cat gastrocnemius. J Physiol (Lond) 234:749–765, 1973. With permission.*)

units in serially interdigitated muscles like the cat tenuissimus and sartorius (Fig. 5-2C) are distributed throughout the entire length of these long, strap-like muscles, presumably within longitudinally interdigitated fascicles that are somehow mechanically linked.[16,26] The intermingling of muscle unit territories is the primary reason for the familiar difficulty in isolating the EMG discharges of individual motor units in normal muscles when even modest numbers are concurrently active.

The normal dispersion of muscle unit fibers, which arises during development, is disrupted when a cut muscle nerve grows to reinnervate the denervated muscle. Reinnervation of mature muscle after nerve injury or in motor neuron diseases is accompanied by local sprouting of motor axons that results in collections of contiguous fibers with the same histochemical type (called "type grouping")[27] many of these can be innervated by the same motor neuron.[28] This implies that the characteristics of many of the reinnervated muscle fibers change to match the innervating motor neuron.[29,30]

Physiologic Properties of Motor Units

Most muscles are made up of heterogeneous populations of motor units that display wide ranges in twitch contraction times and maximum force outputs.[31] These features are interrelated, such that the slowest-twitch units produce, on average, the smallest forces, whereas the fastest units produce the largest forces (Fig. 5-4, MG). In contrast, a few muscle, such as the soleus muscle of the cat, contain a relatively homogeneous population of slow-twitch units that exhibited a correspondingly limited range of individual force outputs (Fig. 5-4, SOL). Twitch contraction times and maximum force outputs exhibit continuous distributions, so that labels such as "large" or "small" and "fast" or "slow" are not very useful. Accordingly, several schemes have been developed for classifying motor units into distinct groups, or "types," based on additional physiologic properties of the muscle unit portion.[32,33]

IDENTIFICATION OF MOTOR UNIT TYPES

One such scheme is based on two such properties: (1) relative resistance to fatigue during a standard stimulation sequence (fatigue index, in which low values indicate marked fatigability) and (2) the presence or absence of decline in force output during low-frequency tetanization (the "sag" property) (see Fig 5-5).[32,34] These properties are correlated with contraction time and maximum force output, and allow identification of three main clusters of the cat gastrocnemius muscle units (Fig. 5-6). Units that exhibit sag in unfused tetani (open circles) are relatively fast contracting, while units without sag (stippled circles) contract more slowly. Fast-twitch units with fatigue index ≤ 0.25 are called "fast-twitch, fatigable" or type FF units, while fast-twitch units that are more resistant to fatigue (fatigue index ≥ 0.75) are

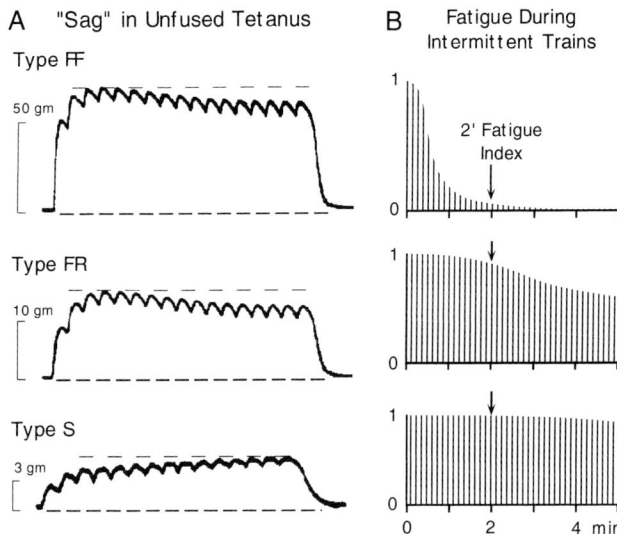

FIGURE 5-5. Two physiologic properties that separate motor units in cat muscles into three categories. *A.* During stimulus trains at intervals 25 percent longer than the twitch contraction time, fast-contracting units (types FF and FR) exhibit an early maximum in force output that later declines ("sags") to a lower plateau force. More slowly contracting units (type S) do not show this sag. *B.* Representative normalized force profiles during standardized sequences of repetitive stimulation, showing different degrees of fatigue sensitivity. When assessed after 2 min of stimulation (arrows; 2' fatigue index), force declines in some units to less than 25 percent of the initial value, while in others remains greater than 75 percent. When combined with the presence or absence of sag, this separates muscle units into three distinct categories called type FF (fast-twitch fatigable), type FR (fast-twitch, fatigue-resistant), and type S (slow twitch).

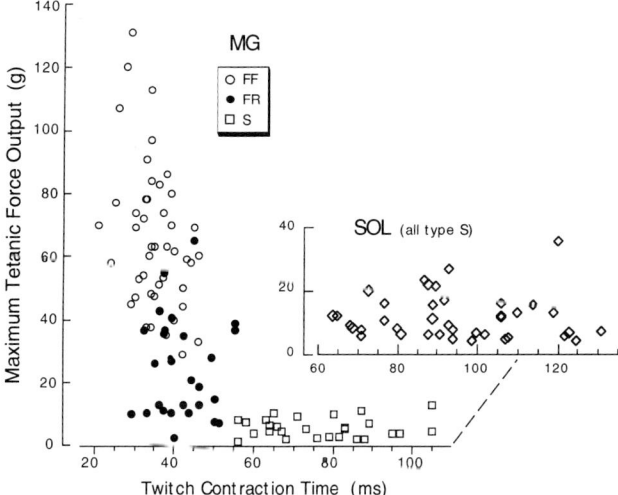

FIGURE 5-4. Superimposed scatter plots of twitch contraction time (abscissae) and maximum isometric force output (ordinates) of individual muscle units in cat medial gastrocnemius (MG; main graph) and soleus (SOL; inset graph). Rapidly contracting units in the MG sample exhibit a wide range of tetanic forces, while more slowly contracting MG units are uniformly small. Symbols denote motor unit types described in Fig. 5-6. SOL units are all type S but have, on average, slower contraction times and larger force outputs compared to type S units in MG. (*Adapted from Burke RE, Tsairis P: The correlation of physiological properties with histochemical characteristics in single muscle units. Ann NY Acad Sci 228:145–159, 1974. With permission.*)

called "fast-twitch, fatigue-resistant," or type FR units. Most type FF units produce larger force outputs than type FR units, while type S units have uniformly small force outputs (see also Fig. 5-7). Some fast-twitch units have fatigue indices intermediate between those of FF and FR units and are sometimes denoted type F(int).[35] The motor units in the homogeneous cat soleus (Fig. 5-4) are all type S. As discussed below, this scheme can also predict the histochemical fiber type of the muscle units.

In contrast, motor unit populations in small distal limb muscles, such as the cat lumbrical[36,37] or human forearm and hand (see below), either exhibit more continuous distributions of mechanical properties, with little indication of the clusters that suggest underlying "types," or more overlapping properties of units that can be only provisionally classified.[38] One study of lumbrical muscles in the rat suggests the presence of at least two distinct groups of units can be distinguished by the presence or absence of sag in unfused tetani, although other properties are distributed continuously and all units are fatigue-resistant.[39] In summary, it seems likely that motor unit populations in small, distal limb muscles are less readily distinguished by their mechanical properties as compared to those in larger, more proximal muscles. This argues that there is no universal system for motor unit classification, so that inferences about the functional roles of different unit types must be made with due care.

MOTOR UNIT TYPES AND MUSCLE FIBER HISTOCHEMISTRY

Modern histochemical and ultrastructural methods have confirmed the view of early histologists that most limb and trunk muscles of mammals are heterogeneous mixtures of different kinds of muscle fibers[40] (see also Chap. 4). Three or perhaps four histochemical categories are sufficient to classify the majority of fibers in normal limb and trunk muscles,[24,40] although there is a remarkable diversity of myosin isoforms within the categories.[41] In this chapter, the terminology suggested by Brooke and Kaiser[42] and based on myosin ATPase activity is used to denote histochemical fiber types (see Table 5-1). Type 1 fibers exhibit low intensities of staining for myofibrillar ATPase after preincubation at alkaline pH, while type 2 fibers have high staining intensities. Type 2A and 2B fibers can be distinguished by different ATPase staining after preincubation at less acidic pH. Type 1 and 2A fibers also show relatively high activity for oxidative enzymes, while type 2A fibers have markedly lower activities.

The technique of glycogen depletion[19] mentioned above made it possible to "label" the muscle fibers of an individual muscle unit with known physiologic properties. This permits matching the mechanical properties that identify motor unit type with the histochemical characteristics of the fibers within the same motor unit. In cat muscles, the muscle fibers of physiologic type FF units all exhibit the type 2B histochemical profile, type FR muscle units have the type

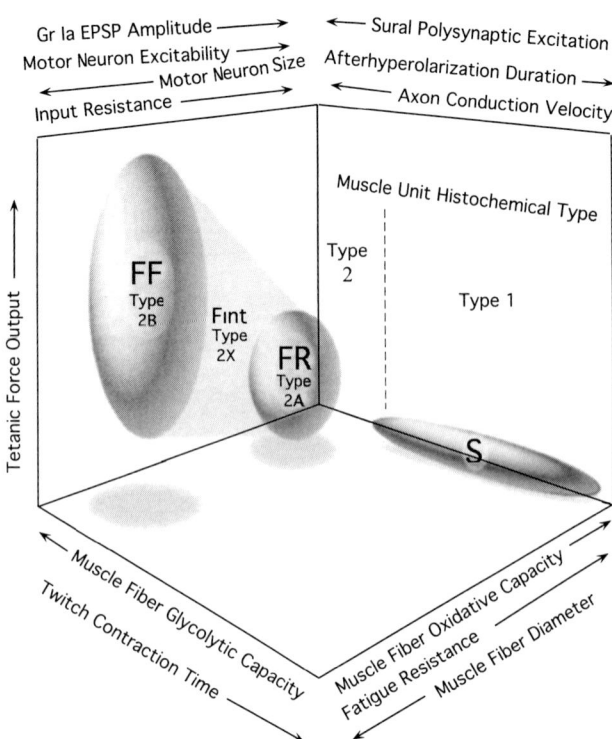

FIGURE 5-7. Schematic three-dimensional diagram patterned after Fig. 5-6 to illustrate the interrelations between physiologic motor unit properties and muscle fiber histochemistry (main panel and lower axes) as well as with intrinsic motor neuron properties and the characteristics of two synaptic input systems (upper axes). Further discussion and references are given in the text.

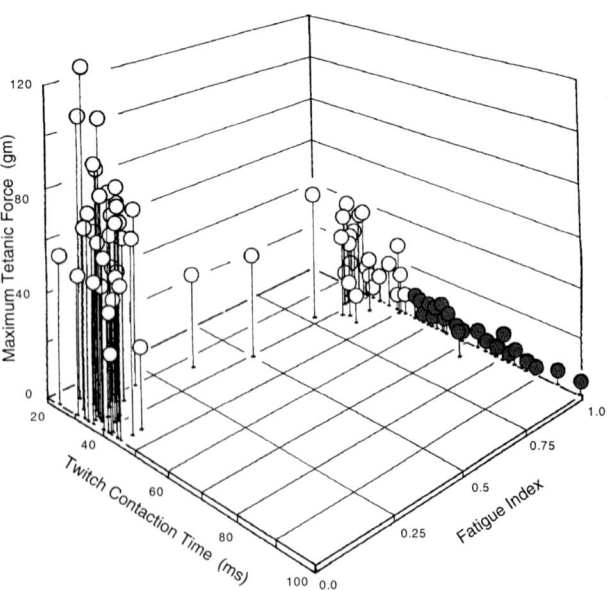

FIGURE 5-6. Three-dimensional display of four physiologic properties of muscle units in the cat gastrocnemius muscle. It expands the graph in Fig. 5-4 along a third axis to show the distribution of fatigability (Fatigue Index; Fig. 5-5B) and also denotes the presence or absence of sag in unfused tetani (Fig. 5-5A; open and stippled symbols, respectively). The three major clusters are the FF, FR, and S motor types, while the two fast-twitch units with fatigue indices between 0.25 and 0.75 are F (int) units. (*Adapted from Burke RE, Levine DN, Tsairis P, Zajac FE: Physiological types and histochemical profiles in motor units of the cat gastrocnemius. J Physiol (Lond) 234:723–748, 1973. With permission.*)

2A profile, and type S units all show type 1 histochemistry (Table 5-1).[32,35,43,44] Glycogen-depleted type F(int) units in cat muscles are less well characterized because of their infrequent occurrence. However, the few that have been studied by glycogen depletion have histochemical profiles that are either intermediate between the 2A and 2B characteristics (see Table 2, "unclassified" unit, in Ref. 32) or are simply type 2A.[45] On the other hand, Larsson and coworkers[46] have shown by glycogen depletion that rat motor units with the F(int) physiologic profile are made up of fibers with a distinct myosin subtype, called type 2X (see also Ref. 39).

In normal adult muscles, the fibers of an individual muscle unit all have the same histochemical type,[32] although there is somewhat more heterogeneity in self-reinnervated muscle units.[30] Studies of individual muscle fibers isolated from single glycogen-depleted muscle units show a quite remarkable degree of biochemical[47,48] as well as mechanical[49] uniformity. Although there is some debate about how much variation within the muscle unit is required for histochemical "uniformity,"[50] the bulk of available evidence is consistent with the notion that the motor neuron specifies the characteristics of its muscle unit in considerable although perhaps not complete detail.

There are obvious correlations between the physiologic and histochemical profiles of motor units (Table 5-1 and Fig. 5-7). In both rat and cat muscle, the intensity of myofibrillar ATPase staining after preincubation at alkaline pH is directly related to twitch contraction speed[32,48] and myosin heavy-chain composition.[51,52] This association fits with the widely held supposition that myofibrillar ATPase activity and myosin composition are important rate-limiting factors controlling contraction speed.[52] However, other steps in the excitation-contraction coupling sequence, particularly the influence of the sarcoplasmic reticulum and the intrafiber action of Ca^{2+}, are also clearly important (see Chap. 14 and Refs. 53 and 54).

Relative resistance to fatigue is also well correlated with the histochemically and biochemically demonstrable capacity of muscle fibers to metabolize substrates (fatty acids as well as glucose) by oxidative pathways associated with mitochondria (Table 5-1 and Refs 32, 48, and 55). The type 2B fibers charateristic of type FF motor units normally contain high concentrations of glycogen but relatively low concentrations of mitochondria and oxidative enzymes. They also exhibit low myoglobin content, large fiber diameter, and sparse capillary supply. These fibers apparently depend primarily on anaerobic glycolytic mechanisms using intrafiber glycogen stores to generate ATP, which accounts for their inability to produce effective force after glycogen depletion during prolonged activation.

In contrast, type 1 muscle fibers characteristic of type S muscle units have high concentrations of mitochondria, oxidative enzymes, and myoglobin but relatively low glycogen content.[56] They also exhibit relatively high local concentrations of capillaries.[57,58] When supplied with blood-borne metabolites and oxygen, type S muscle units resist fatigue for prolonged periods as long as intramuscular circulation is not compromised. The type FR units, with type 2A muscle fibers, represent a crossover category in that they contain both aerobic and anaerobic enzyme systems as well as considerable stored glycogen. Although not as resistant to fatigue as the type S, type FR units combine the advantages of relatively rapid contraction with considerable resistance to fatigue during sustained activation.

It should be noted that the oxidative capacities of all types of muscle fibers exhibit parallel increases and decreases with exercise training and detraining, respectively,[59] or prolonged electrical stimulation.[60] There is also considerable variation in metabolic enzymes within a given histochemical fiber type, if not within a given muscle unit.[40,48] It may be that such variations underlie the range of physiologic properties exhibited by individual motor units of a given type (e.g., Fig. 5-6; see also Ref. 61)

The definition of a relatively few histochemical types of muscle fibers provides a useful framework for discussion of muscle and motor unit heterogeneity. However, as noted above, neither the types as described nor the criteria for classification should be considered as universally applicable. Muscle unit physiologic properties vary with muscle and species, and it should be expected that typing criteria may differ accordingly. Indeed, some motor unit populations may not exhibit clearly separable categories. Although the available data do not negate the utility of motor unit classification, they do caution against using the notion of "types" in an overly rigid way.

DEVELOPMENT OF MOTOR UNIT TYPES

The early development of differentiated muscle fiber types is discussed in Chaps. 2 and 4. However, it is important here to note evidence suggesting that particular groups of motor neurons may innervate developing myotubes selectively before fiber-type differentiation. This implies a degree of genetic prespecification between motor neurons and their muscle units[62,62a] as well as their intended target muscles.[63] This could account for instances of topographic relation between the position of motor neurons within a motor nucleus and the location of their muscle units within the target muscle.[64] Furthermore, studies of muscle structure and function in human twins suggest that the composition of motor unit pools is under strong genetic control. The histochemical fiber type proportions in limb muscles of identical human twins exhibit a much higher concordance than is found in fraternal twins.[65] Although many open questions remain, the weight of existing evidence is compatible with

Table 5-1. GENERAL CHARACTERISTICS OF MOTOR UNITS IN CAT MUSCLES

	Muscle Unit Properties		
Motor unit types	FF	FR	S
Twitch contraction speed	Fast	Fast	Slow
Tetanic force output	Large	Modest	Small
Resistance to fatigue	Least	Fairly high	Very high
	Associated Muscle Fiber Characteristics		
Histochemical types	2B	2A	1
Alkaline ATPase	High	High	Low
Acidic ATPase	Moderate	Low	High
Oxidative enzymes	Low	Medium to high	High
Myoglobin	Low	High	High
Phosphorylase	High	High	Low
Glycogen	High	High	Low
Capillary supply	Sparse	Rich	Very rich
Average fiber diameter	Large	Moderate to large	Small

the notion that motor neurons and muscle fibers are in some way specified genetically to produce motor units with a range of properties matched to the functional demands placed on that motor unit population.

MUSCLE UNIT FORCE OUTPUT AND INNERVATION RATIOS

For any given muscle, the average number of muscle fibers per motor unit (the innervation ratio) is simply the number of muscle fibers divided by the number of innervating alpha motor neurons.[66] However, the large range (up to 100-fold) in maximum isometric forces found in many motor unit populations[31] (see also Fig. 5-6) is usually attributed to equivalent variations in innervation ratios around that average. Small force units generally have motor axons with relatively slow conduction velocities, leading to the inference that small-diameter axons branch less profusely than large axons.[67] A comprehensive study of this issue[68] indeed showed a direct exponential relation between axonal conduction velocity and tetanic force of type S and type FR motor units in many muscles of the cat hindlimb, although the largest force, type FF units, do not obey the same relation (Fig. 5-8).

Normal neuromuscular junctions are sufficiently powerful that all of the muscle unit fibers are activated by each motor neuron impulse (see Chap. 16). Accordingly, the maximum (tetanic) isometric force produced by an individual muscle unit is the product of three factors: (1) the number of fibers in the unit (the innervation ratio), (2) the average cross-sectional area of those fibers, and (3) the maximum force developed per unit of fiber area (called *specific force*). Despite significant technical problems, innervation ratios and average fiber areas are in principle directly measurable in glycogen-depleted muscle units, but specific force can only be inferred indirectly.

The relative importance of specific force output in regulating total unit force remains controversial.[34,69] Estimates of specific force that take account of the average tetanic force and relative proportion of each motor unit type, along with the average size and proportion of the associated muscle fiber type, suggest that specific force for type I fibers is considerably lower than that of type 2 fibers.[20,31] On the other hand, direct measurements of specific force in chemically skinned slow- and fast-twitch fibers indicate little difference.[70,71] Studies of this issue in glycogen-depleted muscle units have found that the range of tetanic force output of single units can be explained mainly by differences in inner-vation ratio, with small contributions from differences in average fiber area and calculated specific force.[45,72] There is no doubt that innervation ratio is a major determinant of muscle unit force output, but perhaps not the only one.

Motor Units in Human Muscle

Although there is a large literature on EMG studies of motor units in human muscle, information about the mechanical properties of human muscle units is much more limited. More than 50 years ago, Denny-Brown[73,74] recorded force changes produced by single motor units in human muscle in a case of motor neuron disease, but further progress had to await development of computer averaging techniques. These were used to educe the mechanical twitch responses of individual human motor units from total muscle force, the averages synchronized either to stimulation of intramuscular nerve branches[75] or to the EMG of a single motor unit during steady voluntary contractions ("spike-triggered averaging").[76] There are technical limitations inherent in both approaches. The mechanical responses educed during spike-triggered averaging are not really isolated twitches but rather components in unfused tetanic responses.[77,78] In addition, true tetanic responses of individual units cannot be obtained with this approach. Although these problems are partially overcome using electrical stimulation of individual motor axons,[79] both methods suffer from mechanical distortion due to variable compliance in the mechanical coupling between the active muscle unit and the force-measuring device.[80,81] Therefore some care is required in comparing results from human muscle with those from animal studies, which are more easily controlled.

Despite these methodologic limitations, the available evidence suggests that human muscle units display many of the same basic correlations found in animal muscle, discussed in preceding sections. For example, in a classic study using spike-triggered averaging, Milner-Brown and coworkers[82] found a three-fold range in twitch contraction times in the

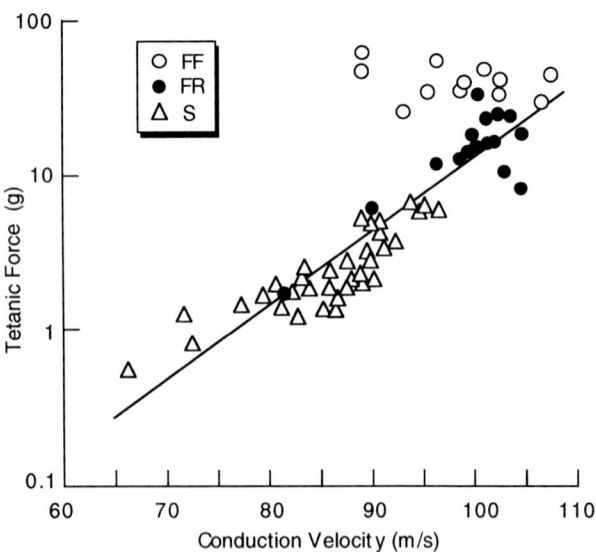

FIGURE 5-8. Scatter plot of the relation between motor axon conduction velocity (abscissa) and maximum tetanic force output (ordinate, note logarithmic axis) in a large sample of motor units from cat peroneus brevis obtained in a single animal. Data from type S (triangles) and type FR (filled circles) muscle units fit an exponential relationship (line), but those from FF units fall above the line. Note some overlap in force ranges between unit type clusters. (*Adapted from Emonet-Denand F, Hunt C, Petit J, et al: Proportion of fatigue-resistant motor units in hindlimb muscles of cat and their relation to axonal conduction velocity. J Physiol (Lond) 400:135–158, 1988. With permission.*)

human first dorsal interosseous (1DI) muscle (30 to 90 ms) and a 100-fold range in twitch force (approximately 0.1 to 10 g) (see Fig. 5-8). Twitch forces in 1DI units are also positively correlated with motor axon conduction velocities.[83] Studies of 1DI using intramuscular stimulation[84,85] showed that the largest force units were not only fast-contracting but also sensitive to fatigue, while the smallest force units were slowly contracting and uniformly resistant to fatigue (but compare Ref. 86). However, these properties are distributed continuously, without clear evidence of the type of clustering seen in cat MG units (Fig. 5-6). In this respect, the human work is similar to the results from small distal muscles in animals (see above).

For technical reasons, it is more difficult to obtain such data from larger, more proximal muscles. Nevertheless, Garnett and coworkers[87] used intramuscular electrical stimulation to demonstrate that motor units in the human medial gastrocnemius display correlated variations in force output, contraction time, and relative fatigability that resemble the patterns found in cat MG units. In summary, the patterns of motor unit properties in both large and small human muscles resemble those found in other mammals, suggesting that data from animals are relevant to human myology.

Motor Units in Action

The preceding material presented a static picture of motor unit anatomy and physiology. However, the business of motor units is to generate muscle force that either moves body segments or resists movement imposed by the environment (e.g., gravity). The following material deals with this aspect, starting with motor neurons and their synaptic inputs.

INTERRELATIONS BETWEEN MOTOR NEURON AND MUSCLE UNIT PROPERTIES

The variations in the properties of muscle units are matched by correlated variations in the characteristics of motor neurons and of the synaptic inputs to them. For example, the conduction velocities of motor axons are logarithmically related to muscle unit tetanic force as well as to motor unit types (Fig. 5-8). Additional interrelations are illustrated in the three-dimensional summary diagram in Fig. 5-7, which is based on Fig. 5-6. The ovals denote the clusters of data points that depend on muscle unit mechanical properties (lower axes labels) and associated histochemical fiber types. The axis labels above the diagram illustrate correlations with motor neuron properties—including cell size,[88] input resistance,[89] and excitability (measured as rheobase current, upper left axis)—while the trends in afterhyperpolarization (AHP) duration[90] and motor axon conduction velocity[68] are denoted along the upper right axis. Although these motor neuron properties exhibit essentially continuous distributions without the clusters found for muscle unit properties, Zengel and coworkers[90] found that the combination of motor neuron input resistance and rheobase successfully predicted muscle unit type in over 95 percent of a sample in cat gastrocnemius.

The correlations of motor unit type with AHP duration and motor neuron rheobase are particularly important. The AHP duration, which depends on a calcium-activated potassium conductance,[91] is the major factor that controls motor neuron firing rates, producing lower firing frequencies in type S units than in the fast-twitch types.[92,93] Rheobase (the electric current required to initiate an action potential) is an inverse measure of the motor neuron's intrinsic excitability, which varies in the sequence: FF < FR < S.[89,90] In addition, under certain conditions, motor neurons exhibit a nonlinear response to depolarization called *plateau potentials*.[94] Plateau potentials reflect activation of an all-or-none inward Ca^{2+} current that can produce sustained depolarization of the cell, with persistent firing, that can persist until it is gated off by an inhibitory hyperpolarization.[93] This mechanism can be modulated by serotonin and other neuromodulators.[95] There is some evidence that plateau potentials are more easily evoked in type S motor neurons,[96] which complements their innate excitability.

The synaptic inputs that drive motor neuron activity also exhibit systematic differences related to motor unit type.[31] For example, the direct (monosynaptic) excitatory postsynaptic potentials (EPSPs) produced by large-diameter group Ia afferents from muscle spindle stretch receptors are largest in motor neurons that innervate type S muscle units, somewhat smaller in type FR cells, and smallest in type FF cells (upper left axis in Fig. 5-7).[97,98] This fits with the fact that the small-force type S motor units are more readily activated in stretch reflexes than the fast-twitch types.[99,100] Several other synaptic input systems display similar gradations in efficacy.[101] On the other hand, some polysynaptic input systems, including pathways activated by some large-diameter cutaneous afferents that operate through one or more intermediate spinal interneurons (upper right axis in Fig. 5-7), produce excitation in motor neurons that is strongest among the fast-twitch unit types.[101,102] Such differences in synaptic organization are important to the ways in which the CNS controls the activity of different types of motor units.

MECHANISMS THAT CONTROL MUSCLE OUTPUT

Neural control of limb and trunk movement resides ultimately in the regulation of forces applied to the skeleton. This is accomplished by controlling the numbers and identities of motor units active at any moment, referred to as recruitment,[1] and by controlling the firing rate of the active motor neurons,[103] a process often referred to as *rate coding*. Recruitment and variation in motor neuron firing rates act together to govern the force output of muscle.[31,92,104] The relative importance of the two mechanisms can vary between different muscles. For example, the motor unit population of intrinsic muscle of the human hand is apparently completely recruited at about 50 percent of maximum voluntary contractile force (MVC),[76,105] while in larger muscles, like the biceps brachii, complete recruitment is attained only at larger MVC (about 70 to 80 percent).[105] Above these levels, further increases in output force must depend on increasing firing rates in already recruited units.

RECRUITMENT CONTROL

If all motor units were identical, recruitment would be a matter of addition and subtraction. However, data from human subjects as well as experimental animals clearly show that recruitment under many conditions is an ordered process, beginning with the smallest-force and slowest-contracting units and progressing to include units with larger and larger forces and faster contraction times as output demand increases.[31,100,106–109] An example of this from the human first dorsal interosseous pool is shown in Fig. 5-9, from the work of Milner-Brown and colleagues.[76,82]

This orderly sequencing, often referred to as the *size principle*[31,101,106] has been found during both voluntary and reflex muscle activation. Because force output and contraction speed are correlated with motor unit types (Fig. 5-6), the usual recruitment sequence begins with type S units, progresses to include type FR, and ends with type FF, as force demand increases.[110] It also seems likely that recruitment within a given motor unit type is also orderly.[100,107] Thus a general recruitment sequence of S to FR to FF can be thought of as a continuum, with probable overlaps between the groups, resulting from a continuous spectrum of functional motor neuron thresholds produced by a combination of intrinsic motor neuron properties and the characteristics of synaptic drive to them.

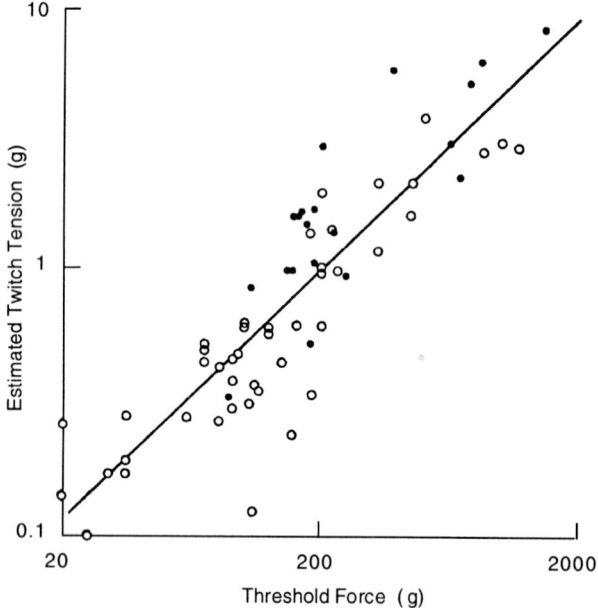

FIGURE 5-9. Scatter diagram of the relation between twitch force (ordinate) and the muscle force threshold at which each unit was recruited during slowly rising ramp contractions of first dorsal interosseus muscles in a normal human subject. Twitch tensions were educed from aggregate muscle force by the spike-triggered averaging method (see text). Filled circles denote a single experiment. Note that both scales are logarithmic, although the best-fitting equation to the data is linear with a slope of 0.005. (*Adapted from Milner-Brown HS, Stein RB, Yemm R: The orderly recruitment of human motor units during voluntary isometric contractions. J Physiol (Lond) 230:359–370, 1973. With permission.*)

There is some debate about the precision of size-ordered recruitment under special conditions. Although there is clear evidence for stochastic variability in the recruitment thresholds of individual motor units in relation to population discharge during stretch reflex activation,[111,112] such natural variability does not negate the idea of orderly recruitment. However, there are examples of apparent preferential recruitment of relatively high-threshold motor units under certain conditions (reviewed in Ref. 113). Most of these have been found in human subjects, in finger muscles during electrical stimulation of cutaneous afferents,[114] and in ankle extensor muscles during controlled lengthening.[115,116] It was recently shown that a large fraction of human extensor carpi radialis motor units exhibit different functional thresholds when activated reflexly or by transcranial magnetic stimulation.[117] It is difficult to demonstrate such selective recruitment and its functional importance has been questioned.[108,118] However, the existence of this phenomenon clearly demonstrates the importance of synaptic organization of synaptic drive to motor neuron control.

Instances of apparent selective recruitment among usually high-threshold motor units depends on the existence of synaptic inputs that preferentially excite motor units at the "large," or fast-twitch, end of the size spectrum.[101,102] Given the mechanical and metabolic advantages of size-ordered recruitment discussed below, one can ask what functional role such input systems could have. There are at least two possibilities. Rapidly alternating movements[119] or precise control of muscle force during active lengthening[115] might require the relatively fast relaxation found in fast-twitch muscle units. It also seems possible that synchronous activation of an entire motor unit pool, as occurs during very rapid ("ballistic") contractions (Fig. 5-10),[120] might be most efficiently generated by activating units at both ends of the size spectrum by differentially organized synaptic systems.[31,113] The observed general pattern of differential synaptic inputs can produce an increase in "recruitment gain," which may have utility in a wide range of movements.[121]

Functional Motor Unit Pools

The idea of recruitment order is inextricably bound to the notion of motor unit "pools" within which recruitment takes place. Historically, functional motor unit pools have been thought of as equivalent to motor nuclei—i.e., the group of motor neurons that innervate an anatomic muscle. However, motor neurons that innervate distinct compartments (see above) within a single "muscle" like the human biceps brachii can be selectively recruited during different movement tasks[122] and should probably be regarded as separate functional pools. More interesting are examples in which a single mechanical compartment contains motor units that exhibit clearly distinct recruitment patterns which depend on different synaptic drives. One such example is the anterior sartorius muscle of the cat, which is shared by two motor unit populations, one of which is active only during the flexion phase of walking while the other is active only in the extension phase.[123] The soleus muscle of the cat is a single-compartment model that also appears to have two functional populations of motor units that differ in their responses to certain synaptic inputs.[124]

On the other hand, natural movements usually involve coordinated actions by many muscles. This implies that the synaptic drives to motor units in different muscles must be appropriately linked during specific motor tasks. Functional motor unit pools thus may range from subsets within one intramuscular compartment up to collections of motor units in many different muscles. One would expect that recruitment orders occur in size/type-ordered sequences irrespective of whether the functional pools are large or small, although this has been difficult to demonstrate experimentally.[118]

FORCE GRADATION BY MOTOR NEURON FIRING RATE

In their pioneering study of the electrical activity of individual motor units, Adrian and Bronk[103] showed that motor neuron discharge frequency changes during voluntary contractions. In general, human motor units exhibit two types of firing behaviors, one during steady or slowly changing force output and the other during rapid, forceful contraction (Fig. 5-10). As motor neurons are recruited during slowly increasing force output, they begin to regular firing at frequencies between 5 and 10 Hz, often with a direct relation between minimum frequency and recruitment threshold. As force increases, so does firing rate, up to maximum steady rates of 20 to 40 Hz.[10] In some distal arm and hand muscles in humans, the majority of units exhibit similar minima and maxima;[80,104] in other samples from both proximal and distal human muscles, peak firing frequencies at a given submaximal contraction strength are higher for low threshold than for high-threshold units during isometric trapezoidal contractions.[125] Interestingly, low-threshold motor units in the human trapezius muscle, which has an important postural component, show much less rate modulation during slow contractions than the higher-threshold units.[126] Maximum firing rates depend in part on the duration of spike afterhyperpolarizations (AHPs).[92] AHPs are more prolonged in motor neurons of slow-twitch units than of fast in some muscles,[127] but this less apparent in others.[128] Such differences may account for some of the diversity of firing rate limits from human studies.

In contrast to slow or steady contractions, motor neuron firing rates during rapid movements can be quite high for brief periods (>50 Hz), representing "instantaneous frequencies" calculated from the intervals between successive action potentials (Fig. 5-10) (see also Refs. 120 and 129). Individual motor neurons recorded during free locomotion in normal cats also exhibit instantaneous firing rates up to 40 Hz.[130] The onset of sudden movements is sometimes associated with short-interval "doublet" firing of some human[131] and animal motor units.[130,132] The fact that such rapid firing is usually limited to a few intervals, mainly at the start of bursts, probably depends on the enhancement of the AHPs in motor neurons during later times in repetitive firing.[133]

Repetitive activation of muscle produces markedly nonlinear increases in force production (for review, see Ref. 134), and the same is true for individual muscle units (Fig. 5-11A).[135] Complete fusion of mechanical responses during repetitive motor neuron firing requires very high frequencies (>100 Hz) for slow- as well as fast-twitch muscle.[136] Although motor

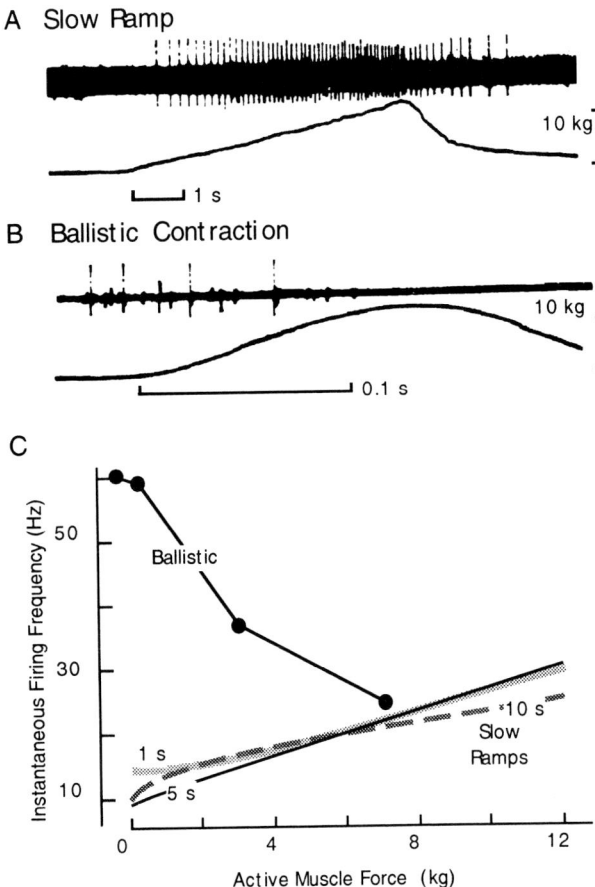

FIGURE 5-10. Recordings of discharge patterns in a motor unit in human tibialis anterior during voluntary contractions at different speeds. The upper records show EMG potentials from the same unit (large deflection; upper traces) and ankle dorsiflexion force (lower traces) during a slow ramp (A) and a very rapid, ballistic contraction (B); note different time scales. In (B), several addition units with smaller EMG signatures are evident. During the ballistic contraction, all units became active within about 20 ms of one another before output force showed an increase, and the entire burst lasted only about 100 ms. C. Graph of firing frequency of the same motor unit (ordinate) during three ramp contractions of 1, 5, and 10 s duration to the same final force (abscissa). The firing frequencies (shaded and dashed lines) followed essentially the same trajectory and showed approximately the same range despite the different slopes of slow force increase. In contrast, the unit's instantaneous frequency was much higher at the onset of the ballistic contraction (maximum 60 Hz) but rapidly declined thereafter. (*Adapted from Desmedt JE, Godaux E: Ballistic contractions in man: Characteristic recruitment pattern of single motor units of the tibialis anterior muscle. J Physiol (Lond) 264:673–694, 1977. With permission.*)

neurons never reach such high firing frequencies, a substantial fraction of the maximum isometric force (the P_t curve in Fig. 5-11C) can nevertheless be developed even during short bursts of motor neuron activity at more modest firing rates because of the nonlinear force/frequency response of muscle. The shape of the P_t curves as in Fig. 5-11C is essentially the same for both fast- and slow-twitch muscle units when the interval between activations (the reciprocal of pulse frequency)

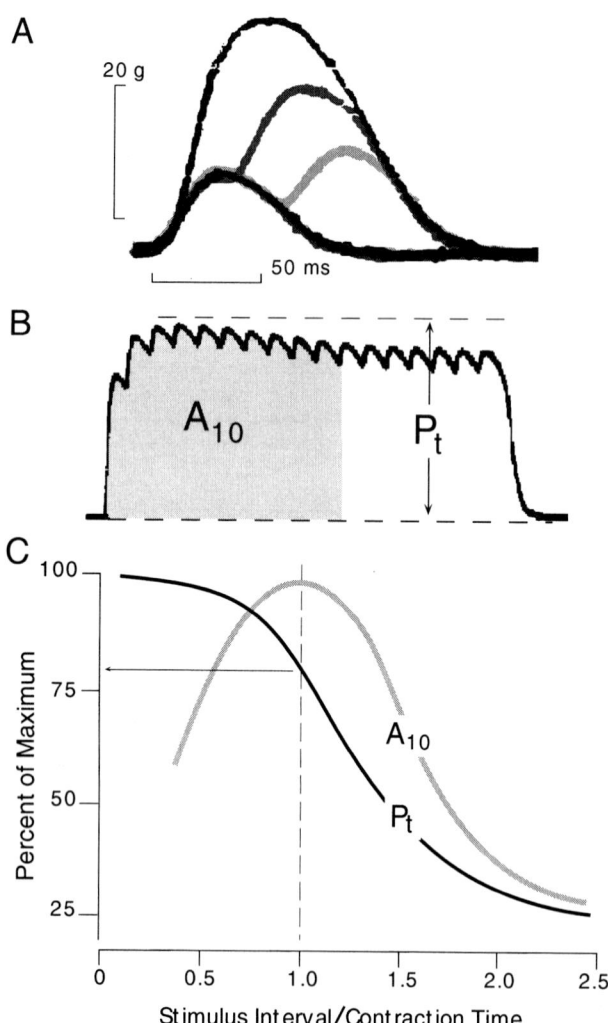

is scaled by the isometric twitch contraction time of the muscle unit in question.[135] The same seems to be true for human motor units.[137] Peak isometric forces developed during unfused tetani can reach 75 to 80 percent of the theoretical maximum at interstimulus intervals near the twitch contraction time, which translates into frequencies of about 33 Hz for a fast unit with contraction time of 30 ms and about 10 Hz for a slow unit with contraction time of 100 ms. If one integrates the force produced by the same number of sequential pulses in unfused tetani at different steady frequencies, the curve reaches a peak at interpulse intervals near the isometric twitch contraction (A_{10} in Fig. 5-11C) (see Ref. 135). This suggests that motor neuron firing at frequencies near the reciprocal of isometric twitch contraction times represents an optimum for both fast- and slow-twitch motor units.

Force output from muscle units is also very sensitive to the pattern of motor neuron firing intervals—i.e., to the time history of activation.[135] Insertion of a single extra activation at a short interval doublet, especially at the onset of much lower-frequency firing, can markedly enhance isometric force output that may persist for many seconds. An extreme example of this "catch" effect[138] in a type S motor unit is shown in Fig. 5-12. Human muscle units exhibit a similar phenomenon,[139] and introduction of an initial doublet reduces the effects of fatigue in human motor units.[140] Doublet firing occurs in human and animal motor units,[131,141] although the functional role of the resulting catch phenomenon remains unclear.[10] Figure 5-12 also illustrates the effects of increasing or decreasing later intervals in otherwise steady stimulus trains. Such irregularities in motor neuron firing intervals are the rule rather than the exception during actual movements, which suggests that firing pattern as well as frequency per se are both used by the nervous system to modulate muscle unit force output.

It should be noted that activation history shows also a more slowly decaying modulation of muscle unit force output

FIGURE 5-11. Examples of nonlinear dependence of force output on stimulation interval in individual muscle units. A. Nonlinear enhancement of isometric force and force-time integral with double pulse stimulation at three intervals (10, 40, and 65 ms) in a type FR muscle unit. Double responses are superimposed on a single twitch response. Note the large enhancement of peak force and force-time integral at the shorter intervals. B. Unfused tetanus in a different type FR unit showing sag from the maximum force (P_t) with constant interval stimulation. The force-time integral under 10 successive responses (A_{10}) is denoted by the shaded area. C. Generalized cartoon of the relations between P_t and A_{10} and stimulus intervals during tetanic stimulation when stimulation intervals are normalized by the twitch contraction time. Peak force output, P_t, increases monotonically as stimulation intervals decrease, reaching about 80 percent of maximum with intervals near the twitch contraction time (horizontal arrow). In contrast, A_{10} exhibits a maximum with stimulus intervals near the twitch contraction time and falls with longer and shorter intervals. The force-time integral provides an index of the work that a muscle unit could produce if the muscle were allowed to shorten. The same relations are found for both fast- and slow-twitch muscle units when scaled by their respective contraction times. (*From Burke RE, Rudomin P, Zajac FE: The effect of activation history on tension production by individual muscle units. Brain Res 109:515–529, 1976. With permission.*)

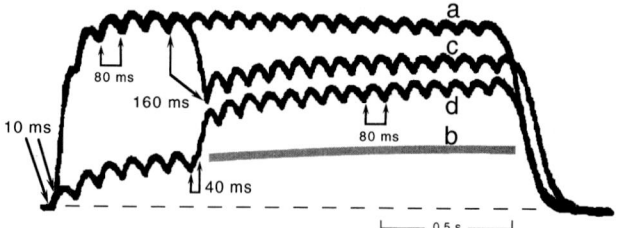

FIGURE 5-12. An example of the influence of stimulation pattern on force output during low-frequency (interval 80 ms) unfused tetani in a type S muscle unit. Introduction of a single extra pulse with interval of 10 ms (doublet) at the onset of the tetanus (response "a") produced a threefold increase in sustained force output ("catch" effect) for several seconds over the force that would have resulted without the extra impulse (shaded line "b"). Prolonging a single interval within a train with an initial doublet dropped the sustained force to an intermediate value (response "c"), while reducing a single interval in a train without an initial doublet increased the subsequent force (response "d"). This catch property is also found in fast-twitch muscle units but its time course is limited by the sag property. (*From Burke RE, Rudomin P, Zajac FE: The effect of activation history on tension production by individual muscle units. Brain Res 109:515–529, 1976. With permission.*)

called posttetanic potentiation (PTP), by which twitch and unfused tetanic forces are markedly enhanced for many seconds following a high-frequency tetanization.[134] In fact, such enhancements can follow in the wake of prolonged activation at any frequency, so that the phenomenon can be thought of simply as "postactivation" potentiation. Except for some special cases like type S units in the cat soleus, both fast- and slow-twitch motor units exhibit PTP.[31] Enhanced motor performance following warmup exercise undoubtedly depends, at least in part, on such effects.

Synthesis

An ideal goal for motor unit research would be to visualize the ebb and flow of activity among all of the motor units in a given motor pool—along with muscle lengths, tendon forces, and limb kinematics—during the performance of a normal behavior such as walking and running. Although this is unattainable at present, it has been possible to record simultaneously EMGs and tendon forces in the cat medial gastrocnemius (MG) and soleus muscles during treadmill walking and running (Fig. 5-13).[110] The cat MG motor unit pool has been intensively studied,[31] permitting inferences about which motor units may be active at different levels of MG force output. If we assume that recruitment is ordered strictly according to increasing force output of the individual muscle units,[100,142] the cumulative force produced by the MG motor unit population (Fig. 5-6) increases nonlinearly as recruitment progresses from the small force S units, through medium force FR units, and finally as it begins to activate the large force FF units (solid line in Fig. 5-13). The type S units, though making up about a quarter of the MG pool, produce in aggregate only about 5 percent (about 400 g) of the total MG force available (8 kg). However, this small output force is what the MG muscle generates during quiet standing in normal cats.

Type FR units make up the next quarter of the MG population. Since they produce larger individual forces than S units (Fig. 5-6), the slope of cumulative force versus recruitment increases more rapidly, to reach about 25 percent of maximum output force (about 2 kg) by the stage of complete FR unit recruitment. At this point, the MG pool is about 55 to 60 percent recruited and the active units are sufficient to generate the range of MG tendon forces that are observed during treadmill locomotion, from slow walk to rapid trot.[110] Only movements like gallop and vertical jumping required recruitment of the fatigue-sensitive type FF units, which make up the remaining 40 to 45 percent of the MG pool. These FF units generate three-quarters of the total theoretical MG force.

Figure 5-13 is essentially a thought experiment based on plausible assumptions,[110] but it serves as a useful frame of reference for thinking about how motor unit populations may be used to satisfy the wide range of mechanical demands placed on most mammalian muscles. There is sufficient force-generating capacity in the fatigue-resistant S and FR unit populations to produce the entire range needed from the MG population for postural maintenance as well as repetitive movements during a wide range of locomotion

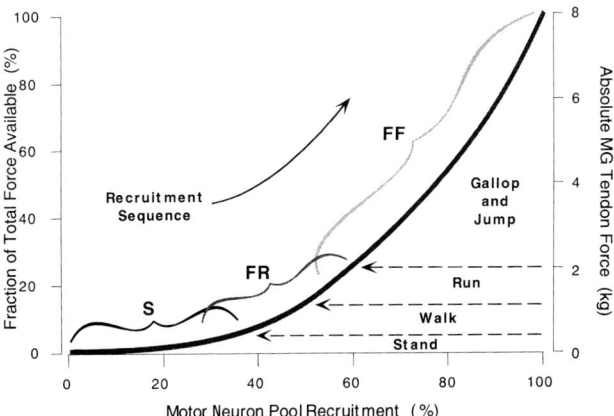

FIGURE 5-13. Graph showing the nonlinear increase in force (solid line, referred to the left ordinate) that would be produced by the motor unit population of the cat medial gastrocnemius muscle if units are recruited strictly according to their maximum force outputs (abscissa). Regions occupied by the different motor unit types are denoted by brackets. The absolute forces that would be produced by this recruitment sequence are shown in the right ordinate, along with the tendon force measured in freely moving cats during quiet standing, walking and running, and galloping and jumping. (*From Walmsley B, Hodgson JA, Burke RE: Forces produced by medial gastrocnemius and soleus muscles during locomotion in freely moving cats. J Neurophysiol 41:1203–1216, 1978. With permission.*)

speed. The large population of strong but fatigue-sensitive type FF units, which make up about 70 percent of the MG muscle bulk, are required only for infrequent movements that demand near-maximum force output. This organization appears precisely suited to the lifestyle demands of a sedentary predator like the cat. In contrast, the MG muscle in the skunk contains only type S and FR motor units, which is well matched to the requirement for great fatigue resistance in this wide-ranging scavenger with few natural enemies.[143] Human muscles appear to represent an intermediate design.

Muscles represent the major bulk of body tissue. Accordingly, they must be optimized not only to meet motor demands but also for metabolic efficiency. Human type 1 muscle fibers require much less energy, measured as the rate of ATP consumption, than type 2 fibers during isometric contraction, but this difference is reversed during shortening.[71] These characteristics apparently reflect the properties of the different myosin isoforms found in heterogeneous mammalian muscles. However, one cannot neglect the metabolic cost of muscles when they are inactive. Fatigue resistance is conferred by high oxidative capacity, which implies a relatively high cost of maintenance when inactive in the form of substrate utilization and oxygen extraction at rest.[144] The fatigue-sensitive type FF motor units probably have a lower maintenance cost than either S or FR units, so that their numbers can be sustained despite their relative bulk. There is evidence that the relative proportions of fiber types in human muscle are under strong genetic control.[65] Therefore the differences in motor unit populations between muscles and species appear to represent evolutionary specializations that match mechanical demands to metabolic costs.

List of Abbreviations

1DI	first dorsal interosseus		FR	fast-twitch, fatigue-resistant
AHP	afterhyperpolarization		MG	medial gastrocnemius
CNS	central nervous system		MVC	maximum voluntary contractile force
EMG	electromyogram		NMJ	neuromuscular junction
EPSP	excitatory postsynaptic potential		PTP	posttetanic potentiation
F(int)	fast-twitch, intermediate		S	slow-twitch, fatigue-resistant
FF	fast-twitch, fatigable			

References

1. Liddell EGT, Sherrington CS: Recruitment and some other factors of reflex inhibition. *Proc R Soc Ser B* 97:488–518, 1925.
2. Gans C: Fiber architecture and muscle function, in Terjung RJ (ed): *Exercise and Sport Sciences Reviews*. Philadelphia: The Franklin Institute, 1982; pp 160–207.
3. Laporte Y, Emonet-Denand F, Jami L: The skeletofusimotor or b-innervation of mammalian muscle spindles. *Trends Neurosci* 4:97–99, 1981.
4. Burke RE, Tsairis P: Histochemical and physiological profile of a skeletofusimotor (beta) unit in cat soleus muscle. *Brain Res* 129:341–345, 1977.
5. Burke RE, Strick PL, Kanda K, et al: Anatomy of medial gastrocnemius and soleus motor nuclei in cat spinal cord. *J Neurophysiol* 40:667–680, 1977.
6. Romanes GJ: The motor cell columns of the lumbo-sacral spinal cord of the cat. *J Comp Neurol* 94:313–363, 1951.
7. Sharrard WJW: The distribution of the permanent paralysis in the lower limb in poliomyelitis. *J Bone Joint Surg* 37:540–558, 1955.
8. Swett J, Eldred E, Buchwald JS: Somatotopic cord-to-muscle relations in efferent innervation of cat gastrocnemius. *Am J Physiol* 219:762–766, 1970.
9. English AW, Weeks OI: Compartmentalization of single muscle units in cat lateral gastrocnemius. *Exp Brain Res* 56:361–368, 1984.
10. Enoka RM, Fuglevand AJ: Motor unit physiology: Some unresolved issues. *Muscle Nerve* 24:4, 2001.
11. Goldberg SJ, Shall MS: Motor units of extraocular muscles: Recent findings, in Binder MD (ed): *Peripheral and Spinal Mechanisms in the Neural Control of Movement. Progress in Brain Research*. Vol 123. (Amsterdam: Elsevier, 1999; pp 221–232.
12. McComas AJ: Motor units: How many how large what kind? *J Electromyogr Kinesiol* 8:391–402, 1998.
13. Shefner JM: Motor unit number estimation in human neurological diseases and animal models. *Clin Neurophysiol* 112:955–964, 2001.
14. Lieber RL, Friden J: Functional and clinical significance of skeletal muscle architecture. *Muscle Nerve* 23:1647–1666, 2000.
15. Windhorst U, Hamm TM, Stuart DG: On the function of muscle and reflex partitioning. *Behav Brain Sci* 12:629–681, 1989.
16. Loeb GE, Pratt CA, Chanaud CM, et al: Distribution and innervation of short interdigitated muscle fibers in parallel-fibered muscles of the cat hindlimb. *J Morphol* 191:1–15, 1987.
17. Bodine SC, Roy RR, Meadows DA, et al: Architectural histochemical and contractile characteristics of a unique biarticular muscle: The cat semitendinosus. *J Neurophysiol* 48:192–201, 1982.
18. Chanaud CM, Pratt CA, Loeb GE: Functionally complex muscles of the cat hindlimb: 2. Mechanical and architectural heterogenity within the biceps-femoris. *Exp Brain Res* 85:257–270, 1991.
19. Edström L, Kugelberg E: Histochemical composition distribution of fibres and fatiguability of single motor units. Anterior tibial muscle of the rat. *J Neurol Neurosurg Psychiatry* 31:424–433, 1968.
20. Burke RE, Tsairis P: Anatomy and innervation ratios in motor units of cat gastrocnemius. *J Physiol (Lond)* 234:749–765, 1973.
21. Enoka RM: Morphological features and activation patterns of motor units. *J Clin Neurophysiol* 12:538–559, 1995.
22. Bodine S, Garfinkel A, Roy R, et al: Spatial distribution of motor unit fibers in the cat soleus and tibialis anterior muscles: Local interactions. *J Neurosci* 8:2142–2152, 1988.
23. Roy RR, Garfinkel A, Ounjian M, et al: Three-dimensional structure of cat tibialis anterior motor units. *Muscle Nerve* 18:1187–1195, 1995.
24. Dubowitz V, Brooke MJ: *Muscle Biopsy: A Modern Approach*. Philadelphia: Saunders, 1973.
25. Buchthal F, Schmalbruch H: Motor unit of mammalian muscle. *Physiol Rev* 60:90–142, 1980.
26. Lev-Tov A, Pratt CA, Burke RE: The motor unit population of the cat tenuissimus muscle. *Neurophysiol* 59:1129–1142, 1988.
27. Karpati G, Engel WK: "Type grouping" in skeletal muscles after experimental reinnervation. *Neurology* 18:447–455, 1968.
28. Kugelberg E, Edström L, Abbruzzese M: Mapping of motor units in experimentally reinnervated rat muscle. *J Neurol Neurosurg Psychiatry* 33:319–329, 1970.
29. Rafuse VF, Gordon T: Incomplete rematching of nerve and muscle properties in motor units after extensive nerve injuries in cat hindlimb muscle. *J Physiol (Lond)* 509:909–926, 1998.
30. Unguez GA, Roy RR, Pierotti DA, et al: Further evidence of incomplete neural control of muscle properties in cat tibialis anterior motor units. *Am J Physiol* 268:C527–C534, 1995.
31. Burke RE: Motor units: Anatomy physiology and functional organization, in Brooks VB (ed): *Handbook of Physiology: Sec. 1. The Nervous System*. Vol II. *Motor Control*. Part 1. Washington, DC: American Physiological Society, 1981; pp 345–422.
32. Burke RE, Levine DN, Tsairis P, et al: Physiological types and histochemical profiles in motor units of the cat gastrocnemius. *J Physiol (Lond)* 234: 723–748, 1973.
33. Burke R: Revisiting the notion of "motor unit types," in Binder M (ed): *Peripheral and Spinal Mechanisms in the Neural Control of Movement. Progress in Brain Research*. Vol. 123. Amsterdam: Elsevier, 1999; pp 167–175.
34. Burke RE: Motor unit types: Some history and unsettled issues, in Binder M, Mendell L (eds): *The Segmental Motor System*. New York: Oxford University Press, 1990; pp 207–221.
35. McDonagh JC, Binder MD, Reinking RM, et al: Tetrapartite classification of motor units of cat tibialis anterior. *J Neurophysiol* 44:696–712, 1980.
36. Appelberg B, Emonet-Denand F: Motor units of the first superficial lumbrical muscle of the cat. *J Neurophysiol* 30:154–160, 1967.
37. Kernell D, Ducati A, Sjöholm H: Properties of motor units in the first deep lumbrical muscle of the cat's foot. *Brain Res* 98:37–55, 1975.
38. Schieber MH, Chua M, Petit J, et al: Tension distribution of single motor units in multitendoned muscles: Comparison of a homologous digit muscle in cats and monkeys. *J Neurosci* 17:1734–1747, 1997.
39. Gates HJ, Ridge RMAP, Rowlerson A: Motor units of the fourth deep lumbrical muscle of the adult rat—Isometric contractions and fibre type compositions. *J Physiol (Lond)* 443:193–215, 1991.
40. Bottinelli R, Reggiani C: Human skeletal muscle fibres: Molecular and functional diversity. *Prog Biophys Mol Biol* 73:195–262, 2000.
41. Pette D, Staron RS: The molecular diversity of mammalian muscle fibers. *News Physiol Sci* 8:153–157, 1993.
42. Brooke MH, Kaiser KK: Muscle fibre types: How many and what kind? *Arch Neurol (Chicago)* 23:369–379, 1970.
43. Dum RP, Kennedy TT: Physiological and histochemical characteristics of motor units in cat tibialis anterior and extensor digitorum longus muscles. *J Neurophysiol* 43:1615–1630, 1980.
44. Dum RP, Burke RE, O'Donovan MJ, et al: Motor unit organization in the flexor digitorum longus muscle of the cat. *J Neurophysiol* 47:1108–1125, 1982.
45. Bodine S, Roy R, Eldred E, et al: Maximal force as a function of anatomical features of motor units in the cat tibialis anterior. *J Neurophysiol* 57: 1730–1745, 1987.
46. Larsson L, Edström L, Lindegren B, et al: MHC composition and enzyme-histochemical and physiological properties of a novel fast-twitch motor unit type. *Am J Physiol* 261:C93–C101, 1991.
47. Nemeth PM, Solanski L, Gordon DA, et al: Uniformity of metabolic enzymes within individual motor units. *J Neurosci* 6:892–898, 1986.
48. Nemeth PM: Metabolic fiber types and influences on their transformation, in Binder MD, Mendell LM (eds): *The Segmental Motor System*. New York: Oxford University Press, 1990; pp 258–277.
49. Nemeth PM, Rosser BWC, Wilkinson RS: Metabolic and contractile uniformity of isolated motor unit fibres of snake muscle. *J Physiol (Lond)* 434:41–55, 1991.
50. Larsson L: Is the motor unit uniform? *Acta Physiol Scand* 144:143–154, 1992.
51. Reiser PW, Moss RL, Gulian GG, et al: Shortening velocity in single fibers from adult rabbit soleus muscles is correlated with myosin heavy chain composition. *J Biol Chem* 260:9077–9080, 1985.

52. Bottinelli R, Canepari M, Pelligrino MA, et al: Force-velocity properties of human skeletal muscle fibres: Myosin heavy chain isoform and temperature dependence. *J Physiol (Lond)* 495:573–586, 1996.
53. Heilmann C, Pette D: Molecular transformations in sarcoplasmic reticulum of fast-twitch muscle by electro-stimulation. *Eur J Biochem* 93:437–446, 1979.
54. Bottinelli R, Canepari M, Reggiani C, et al: Myofibrillar ATPase activity during isometric contraction and isomyosin composition in rat single skinned muscle fibres. *J Physiol (Lond)* 481:663–675, 1994.
55. Kugelberg E, Lindegren B: Transmission and contraction fatigue of rat motor units in relation to succinate dehydrogenase activity of motor unit fibres. *J Physiol (Lond)* 288:285–300, 1979.
56. Peter JB, Barnard RJ, Edgerton VR, et al: Metabolic profiles of three fiber types of skeletal muscle in guinea pigs and rabbits. *Biochemistry* 11:2627–2633, 1972.
57. Reis DJ, Wooten GF: The relationship of blood flow capillary density and twitch characteristics in red and white skeletal muscle in cat. *J Physiol (Lond)* 210:121–135, 1970.
58. Romanul FCA: Capillary supply and metabolism of muscle fibers. *Arch Neurol* 12:497–509, 1965.
59. Booth FW, Thomason DB: Molecular and cellular adaptation of muscle in response to exercise—Perspectives of various models. *Physiol Rev* 71:541–585, 1991.
60. Pette D, Vrbova G: Adaptation of mammalian skeletal muscle fibers to chronic electrical stimulation. *Rev Physiol Biochem Pharmacol* 120:115–202, 1992.
61. Burke RE, Tsairis P: The correlation of physiological properties with histochemical characteristics in single muscle units. *Ann NY Acad Sci* 228:145–159, 1974.
62. Miller JB, Stockdale FE: What muscle cells know that nerves don't tell them. *Trends Neurosci* 10:325–329, 1987.
62a. Fladby T, Jansen JK: Development of homogeneous fast and slow motor units in the neonatal mouse soleus muscle. *Development* 109:723–732, 1990.
63. Milner LD, Rafuse VF, Landmesser LT: Selective fasciculation and divergent pathfinding decision of embryonic chick motor axons projecting to fast and slow muscle regions. *J Neurosci* 18:3297–3313, 1998.
64. Bennett M, Ho S: The formation of topographical maps in developing rat gastrocnemius muscle during synapse elimination. *J Physiol (Lond)* 396:471–496, 1989.
65. Komi PV, Viitasalo JHT, Havu M, et al: Skeletal muscle fibres and muscle enzyme activities in monozygotic and dizygotic twins of both sexes. *Acta Physiol Scand* 100:385–392, 1977.
66. Eccles JC, Sherrington CS: Numbers and contraction values of individual motor units examined in some muscles of the limbs. *Proc R Soc Lond B* 106:326–357, 1930.
67. Morgan DL, Proske U: On the branching of motoneurons. *Muscle Nerve* 24:372–379, 2001.
68. Emonet-Denand F, Hunt C, Petit J, et al: Proportion of fatigue-resistant motor units in hindlimb muscles of cat and their relation to axonal conduction velocity. *J Physiol (Lond)* 400:135–158, 1988.
69. Stein RB, Gordon T, Totosy De Zepetnek J: Mechanisms for respecifying muscle properties following reinnervation, in Binder MD, Mendell LM (eds): *The Segmental Motor System*. New York: Oxford University Press, 1990; pp 278–288.
70. Lucas SM, Ruff RL, Binder MD: Specific tension measurements in single soleus and medial gastrocnemius muscle fibers of the cat. *Exp Neurol* 95:142–154, 1987.
71. He Z-H, Bottinelli R, Pelligrino MA, et al: ATP consumption and efficiency of human single muscle fibers with different myosin isoform composition. *Biophys J* 79:945–961, 2000.
72. Chamberlain S, Lewis DM: Contractile chacteristics and innervation ratio of rat soleus motor units. *J Physiol (Lond)* 412:1–21, 1989.
73. Denny-Brown D, Pennybacker JB: Fibrillation and fasciculation in voluntary muscle. *Brain* 61:311–334, 1939.
74. Denny-Brown D: Interpretation of the electromyogram. *Arch Neurol Psychiatry* 61:99–128, 1949.
75. Buchthal F, Schmalbruch H: Contraction times and fibre types in intact human muscles. *Acta Physiol Scand* 79:435–452, 1970.
76. Milner-Brown HS, Stein RB, Yemm R: The contractile properties of human motor units during voluntary isometric contractions. *J Physiol (Lond)* 228:285–306, 1973.
77. Calancie B, Bawa P: Limitations of the spike triggered averaging technique. *Muscle Nerve* 9:78–83, 1986.
78. Romaiguère P, Vedel J-P, Pagni S, et al: Physiological properties of the motor units of the wrist extensor muscles in man. *Exp Brain Res* 78:51–61, 1989.
79. Taylor A, Stephens JA: Study of human motor unit contractions by controlled intramuscular microstimulation. *Brain Res* 117:331–335, 1976.
80. Monster AW, Chan H: Isometric force production by motor units of extensor digitorum communis muscle in man. *J Neurophysiol* 40:1432–1443, 1977.
81. Thomas C, Bigland-Ritchie B, Westling G, et al: A comparison of human thenar motor-unit properties studied by intraneural motor-axon stimulation and spike triggered averaging. *J Neurophysiol* 64:1347–1351, 1990.
82. Milner-Brown HS, Stein RB, Yemm R: The orderly recruitment of human motor units during voluntary isometric contractions. *J Physiol (Lond)* 230:359–370, 1973.
83. Dengler R, Stein R, Thomas C: Axonal conduction velocity and force of single human motor units. *Muscle Nerve* 11:136–145, 1988.
84. Stephens JA, Usherwood TP: The mechanical properties of human motor units with special reference to their fatiguability and recruitment threshold. *Brain Res*. 125:91–97, 1977.
85. Thomas CK, Johansson RS, Bigland-Ritchie B: Attempts to physiologically classify human thenar motor units. *J Neurophysiol* 65:1501–1508, 1991.
86. Fuglevand AJ, Macefield VG, Bigland-Ritchie B: Force-frequency and fatigue properties of motor units in muscles that control digits of the human hand. *J Neurophysiol* 81:1718–1729, 1999.
87. Garnett R, O'Donovan M, Stephens J, et al: Motor unit organization of human medial gastrocnemius. *J Physiol (Lond)* 287:33–43, 1979.
88. Burke RE, Dum RP, Fleshman JW, et al: An HRP study of the relation between cell size and motor unit type in cat ankle extensor motoneurons. *J Comp Neurol* 209:17–28, 1982.
89. Fleshman JW, Munson JB, Sypert GW, et al: Rheobase input resistance and motor-unit type in medial gastrocnemius motoneurons in the cat. *J Neurophysiol* 46:1326–1338, 1981.
90. Zengel JE, Reid SA, Sypert GW, et al: Membrane electrical properties and prediction of motor-unit type of cat medial gastrocnemius motoneurons in the cat. *J Neurophysiol* 53:1323–1344, 1985.
91. Safronov BV, Vogel W: Large conductance Ca^{2+}-activated K^+ channels in the soma of rat motoneurones. *J Membr Biol* 162:9–15, 1998.
92. Kernell D: Organized variability in the neuromuscular system—A survey of task-related adaptations. *Arch Ital Biol* 130:19–66, 1992.
93. Powers RK, Binder MD: Input-output functions of mammalian motoneurons. *Rev Physiol Biochem Pharmacol* 143:137–263, 2001.
94. Hultborn H: Plateau potentials and their role in regulating motoneuronal firing, in Binder MD (ed): *Peripheral and Spinal Mechanisms in the Neural Control of Movement. Progress in Brain Research*. Vol. 123. Amsterdam: Elsevier, 1999; pp 39–56.
95. Delgado-Lezama R, Hounsgaard J: Adapting motoneurons for motor behavior, in Binder MD (ed): *Peripheral and Spinal Mechanisms in the Neural Control of Movement. Progress in Brain Research*. Vol. 123. Amsterdam: Elsevier, 1999; pp 57–63.
96. Heckman CJ, Lee RH: Synaptic integration in bistable motoneurons, in Binder MD (ed): *Peripheral and Spinal Mechanisms in the Neural Control of Movement. Progress in Brain Research*. Vol. 123. Amsterdam: Elsevier, 1999; pp 49–56.
97. Burke RE, Rymer WZ, Walsh JV: Relative strength of synaptic input from short latency pathways to motor units of defined type in cat medial gastrocnemius. *J Neurophysiol* 39:447–458, 1976.
98. Fleshman JW, Munson JB, Sypert GW: Homonymous projection of individual group Ia-fibers to physiologically characterized medial gastrocnemius motoneurons in the cat. *J Neurophysiol* 46:1339–1348, 1981.
99. Burke RE: Firing patterns of gastrocnemius motor units in the decerebrate cat. *J Physiol (Lond)* 196:631–645, 1968.
100. Zajac FE: Coupling of recruitment order to the force produced by motor units: The "size principle hypothesis" revisited, in Binder M, Mendell L (ed): *The Segmental Motor System*. New York: Oxford University Press, 1990; pp 96–111.
101. Binder MD, Heckman CJ, Powers RK: The physiological control of motoneuron activity, in Rowell LB, Shepherd JT (eds): *Handbook of Physiology*: Sec. 12. *Exercise: Regulation and Integration of Multiple Systems*. New York: Oxford University Press, 1996, pp 3–53.
102. Burke RE, Jankowska E, ten Bruggencate G: A comparison of peripheral and rubrospinal synaptic input to slow and fast twitch motor units of triceps surae. *J Physiol (Lond)* 207:709–732, 1970.
103. Adrian ED, Bronk DW: The discharge of impulses in motor nerve fibres. Part II. The frequency of discharge in reflex and voluntary contractions. *J Physiol (Lond)* 67:119–151, 1929.
104. Milner-Brown HS, Stein RB, Yemm R: Changes in firing rate of human motor units during linearly changing voluntary contractions. *J Physiol (Lond)* 230:371–390, 1973.
105. Kukulka CG, Clamann PH: Comparison of the recruitment and discharge properties of motor units in human brachial biceps and adductor pollicis during isometric contraction. *Brain Res* 219:45–55, 1981.
106. Henneman E, Mendell LM: Functional organization of motoneuron pool and its inputs, in Brooks VB (ed): *Handbook of Physiology*: Sec. I. *The Nervous System*. Vol II. *Motor Control*. Part 1. Bethesda, MD: American Physiological Society, 1981; pp 423–507.
107. Cope TC, Clark BD: Motor-unit recruitment in the decerebrate cat: Several unit properties are equally good predictors of order. *J Neurophysiol* 66:1127–1138, 1991.
108. Cope TC, Pinter MJ: The size priniciple: Still working after all these years. *News Physiol Sci* 10:280–286, 1995.
109. Tansey KE, Botterman BR: Activation of type-identified motor units duing centrally evoked contractions in the cat medial gastrocnemius muscle: I. Motor-unit recruitment. *J Neurophysiol* 75:26–59, 1996.

110. Walmsley B, Hodgson JA, Burke RE: Forces produced by medial gastrocnemius and soleus muscles during locomotion in freely moving cats. *J Neurophysiol* 41:1203–1216, 1978.
111. Gossard J-P, Floeter MK, Kawai Y, et al: Fluctuations of excitability in the monosynaptic reflex pathway to lumbar motoneurons in the cat *J Neurophysiol* 72:1227–1239, 1994.
112. Rall W, Hunt CC: Analysis of reflex variability in terms of partially correlated excitability fluctuations in a population of motoneurons. *J Gen Physiol* 39:397–422, 1956.
113. Burke RE: Selective recruitment of motor units, in Humphrey DR, Freund H-J (eds): *Motor Control: Concepts and Issues*. Chichester, UK: Wiley, 1991; pp 5–21.
114. Garnett R, Stephens JA: Changes in the recruitment threshold of motor units produced by cutaneous stimulation in man. *J Physiol (Lond)* 311: 463–473, 1981.
115. Nardone A, Romano C, Schieppati M: Selective recruitment of high-threshold human motor units during voluntary isotonic lengthening of active muscles. *J Physiol (Lond)* 409:451–471, 1989.
116. Howell JN, Fugelvand AJ, Walsh ML, et al: Motor unit activity during isometric and concentric-eccentric contractions of the human first dorsal interosseus muscle. *J Neurophysiol* 74:901–904, 1995.
117. Morita H, Baumgarten J, Petersen N, et al: Recruitment of extensor-carpi-radialis motor units by transcranial magnetic stimulation and radial-nerve stimulation in human subjects. *Exp. Brain Res* 128:557–562, 1999.
118. Cope TC, Sokoloff AJ: Orderly recruitment tested across muscle boundaries, in Binder MD (ed): *Peripheral and Spinal Mechanisms in the Neural Control of Movement. Progress in Brain Research*. Vol 123. Amsterdam: Elsevier, 1999; pp 177–190.
119. Smith JL, Betts B, Edgerton VR, et al: Rapid ankle extension during paw shakes: Selective recruitment of fast ankle extensors. *J Neurophysiol* 43: 612–620, 1980.
120. Desmedt JE, Godaux E: Ballistic contractions in man: Characteristic recruitment pattern of single motor units of the tibialis anterior muscle. *J Physiol (Lond)* 264:673–694, 1977.
121. Kernell D, Hultborn H: Synaptic effects on recruitment gain: A mechanism of importance for the input-output relations of motoneurone pools? *Brain Res* 507:176–179, 1990.
122. Van Zuylen EJ, Gielen CCAM, Denier van der Gon JJ: Coordination and inhomogeneous activation of human arm muscles during isometric torques. *J Neurophysiol* 60:1523–1548, 1988.
123. Hoffer JA, Loeb GE, Sugano N, et al: Cat hindlimb motoneurons during locomotion: III. Functional segregation in sartorius. *J Neurophysiol* 57: 554–562, 1987.
124. Sokoloff AJ, Cope TC: Recruitment of triceps surae motor units in the decerebrate cat: II. Heterogeneity among soleus motor units. *J Neurophysiol* 75:2005–2016, 1996.
125. De Luca CJ, Foley PJ, Erim Z: Motor unit control properties in constant-force isometric contractions. *J Neurophysiol* 76:1503–1516, 1996.
126. Westgaard RH, De Luca CJ: Motor control of low-threshold motor units in the human trapezius muscle. *J Neurophysiol* 85:1777–1781, 2001.
127. Burke RE: Motor unit types of cat triceps surae muscle. *J Physiol (Lond)* 193:141–160, 1967.
128. Bakels R, Kernell D: Average but not continuous speed match between motoneurons and muscle units of rat tibialis anterior. *J Neurophysiol* 70:1300–1306, 1993.
129. Grimby L, Hannerz J: Firing rate and recruitment order of toe extensor motor units in different modes of voluntary contraction. *J Physiol (Lond)* 264:865–879, 1977.
130. Hoffer J, Sugano N, Loeb G, et al.: Cat hindlimb motoneurons during locomotion. II. Normal activity patterns. *J Neurophysiol* 57:530–553, 1987.
131. Denslow JS: Double discharges in human motor units. *J Neurophysiol* 11: 209–215, 1948.
132. Eken T: Spontaneous electromyographic activity in adult rat soleus muscle. *J Neurophysiol* 80:365–376, 1998.
133. Baldissera F, Gustafsson B, Parmiffiani F: Saturating summation of the afterhyperpolarization conductance in spinal motoneurones: A mechanism for secondary range repetitive firing. *Brain Res* 146:69–82, 1978.
134. Partridge LD, Benton LA: Muscle the motor, in Brooks BV (ed): *Handbook of Physiology*: Sec. I. *The Nervous System*. Vol II: Part 1. Bethesda, MD: American Physiological Society, 1981; pp 43–106.
135. Burke RE, Rudomin P, Zajac FE: The effect of activation history on tension production by individual muscle units. *Brain Res* 109:515–529, 1976.
136. Buller AJ, Lewis DM: The rate of tension development in isometric tetanic contractions of mammalian fast and slow skeletal muscle. *J Physiol (Lond)* 179:337–354, 1965.
137. Macefield VG, Fuglevand AJ, Bigland-Ritchie B: Contractile properties of single motor units in human toe extensors assessed by intraneural motor axons stimulation. *J Neurophysiol* 75:2509–2519, 1996.
138. Burke RE, Rudomin P, Zajac FE: Catch property in single mammalian motor units. *Science* 168:122–124, 1970.
139. Thomas CK, Johansson RS, Bigland-Ritchie B: Pattern of pulses that maximize force output from single human thenar motor units. *J Neurophysiol* 82:3188–3195, 1999.
140. Bigland-Ritchie B, Zijdewind I, Thomas CK: Muscle fatigue induced by stimulation with and without doublets. *Muscle Nerve* 23:1348–1355, 2000.
141. Gorassini M, Eken T, Bennett DJ, et al: Activity of hindlimb motor units during locomotion in the conscious rat. *J Neurophysiol* 83:2002–2011, 2000.
142. Zajac FE, Faden JS: Relationship among recruitment order axonal conduction velocity and muscle-unit properties of type-identified motor units in cat plantaris muscle. *J Neurophysiol* 53:1303–1322, 1985.
143. Van de Graaff KM, Frederick EC, Williamson RG, et al: Motor units and fiber types of primary ankle extensors of the skunk Mephitis mephitis. *J Neurophysiol* 40:1424–1431, 1977.
144. Ong T, Hayes D, Armstrong R: Distribution of microspheres in plantaris muscles of resting and exercising rats as a function of fiber type. *Am J Anat* 182:318–324, 1988.

Chapter 6
Extraocular Muscles

MENACHEM SADEH

Anatomy

Cellular Organization and Layers of Extraocular Muscles

The Innervation and Synapses of Extraocular Muscles

Physiologic Aspects of Extraocular Muscles

Structure-Function Correlations

Proprioception by Extraocular Muscles

Pathologic Reactions

Involvement in Diseases

Development

The main function of limb and axial muscles is to produce movement of the joints over which they pass. In contrast, the role of the extraocular muscles (EOMs)* is to subserve the function of a sensory organ—the eye. To accomplish clear and single vision of an object, its image must be positioned by the EOMs close to the center of the fovea and held there steadily. Furthermore, binocular vision requires that the image be held in corresponding parts of the retinas of both eyes. The systems of eye movements for gaze shifting and gaze holding are subdivided as vestibuloocular, visual fixation, optokinetic, smooth pursuit, saccadic, and vergence. These movements meet the need for controlling ocular motility during brief and sustained head motion, fixation, smooth tracking of a moving object, and shifting of gaze for looking at targets (for review, see Ref. 1). Thus, the EOMs can move the globe at a velocity as high as 500 degrees per second and yet keep fixation on a stationary object. Therefore it is not surprising that the EOMs differ morphologically, physiologically, and immunocytologically from other skeletal muscles. The chapter deals mostly with human EOMs.

Anatomy

The eyeball is embedded in orbital fat, to which it attaches by a thin membranous sac termed Tenon's capsule; this, in turn, attaches anteriorly to the conjunctiva and posteriorly to the orbital fat surrounding the optic nerve. This capsule is a cone-shaped envelope forming the socket in which the eye rotates. Its outer firm segment is penetrated by the four rectus muscles. These muscles as well as the superior oblique arise from a fibrous ring (the annulus of Zinn) at the orbital apex; the inferior oblique arises from the orbital surface of the maxilla.

*A list of abbreviations used in this chapter is given at the end of the chapter.

The four rectus muscles lie lateral, medial, superior, and inferior to the globe and insert to anterior to the equator of the globe. The superior oblique, placed at the superior and medial side of the orbit, first passes through a fibrocartilaginous ring (the trochlea), changes direction posterolaterally, and then inserts posterior to the equator. The inferior oblique inserts on the lateral part of the sclera behind the equator.

The EOMs rotate the eye about three axes, x (parasagittal), y (transverse), and z (vertical), which pass through the globe's center of rotation. The medial and lateral recti rotate the eye horizontally; since they lie symmetrically on the opposite sides of the globe, they have antagonistic action of adduction and abduction. The action of the other four EOMs is more complicated, because the orbit is aimed outward at approximately 23 degrees. Thus they have secondary and tertiary actions that depend on the globe's position in the orbit.

Proximally to its insertion, each rectus muscle traverses a ring or sleeve of collagen near the equator.[2] These fibrous pulleys are connected to the orbital wall by suspensor bands that contain elastic fibers and smooth muscle rich in autonomic innervation; they are influenced by catecholamines, acetylcholine, and nitric oxide.[3] The pulleys serve to prevent sliding of the rectus muscles during ocular movements, keeping the functional origin and fixing their direction even at extremes of gaze.[4]

Cellular Organization and Layers of Extraocular Muscles

Extraocular muscle fibers are smaller and more variable in size than limb muscle fibers. They are often round rather than polygonal and are separated by more abundant endomysial connective tissue enriched in capillaries. They differ ultrastructurally from limb muscles, having more mitochondria and abundant sarcoplasmic reticulum delineating the myofibrils (Fig. 6-1).

The rectus and oblique muscles are composed of two layers of fibers. An inner global layer extends from its origin to a long tendinous insertion on the globe. A peripheral orbital layer forms a C-shaped mantle around the global layer. Histologic studies of humans and monkeys reveal that the orbital layer of each rectus muscle inserts not on the globe but on its pulley through a short tendon; only the global layer inserts on the sclera (Fig. 6-2). MRI studies in vivo confirm this dual insertion.[5] Thus only the global layer of each rectus muscle rotates the globe; the orbital layer sets the position of the pulley and thereby alters the muscle's rotational axis.[5]

Generally, muscle fibers in the orbital layer have a smaller diameter, are richer in mitochondria, and are surrounded by more capillaries than those in the global layer. In human rectus muscles the global layer contains 8000 to 16,000 fibers, with little variability among the different recti. The orbital layer contains about three-fourths as many fibers as the global layer, with larger variability among the rectus muscles.[6] Recently, an additional marginal-zone layer has been described in human EOM.[7] This layer is peripheral to the

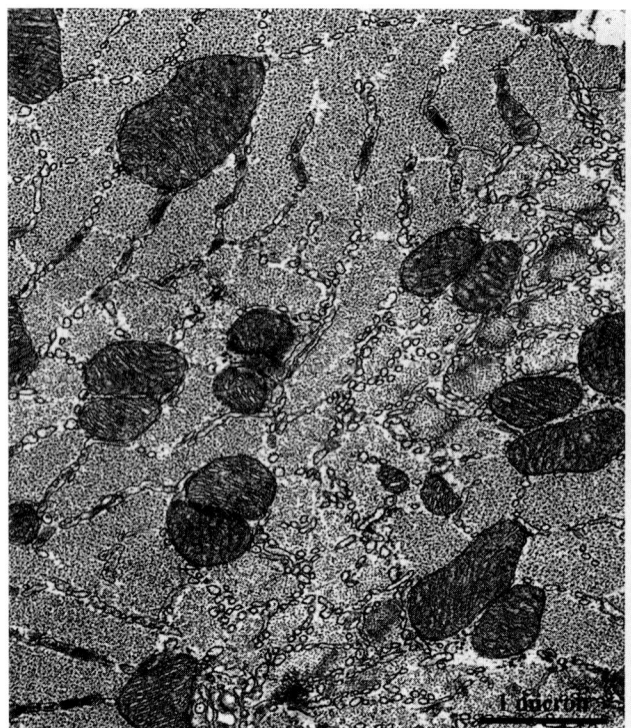 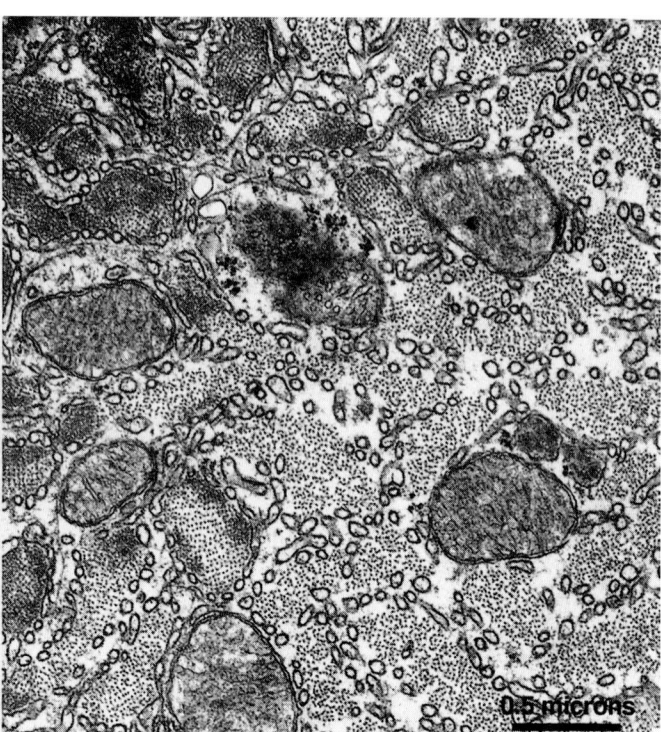

FIGURE 6-1. Transverse sections of a muscle from the mouse inferior rectus (probably a global, intermediate, singly-innervated fiber) showing relatively small myofibrils surrounded by well-developed sarcoplasmic reticulum. Mitochondria are large and abundant at all levels of the sarcomere. Bars: 1 μm (left), 0.5 μm (right).

orbital layer and contains larger fibers than the orbital layer. The levator palpebrae superioris (levator) and accessory extraocular muscles of nonhumans consist of one layer only.

Historically, EOM fibers were classified in many different ways. In 1949, Kruger[8] divided skeletal muscle fibers into two morphologic and functional types: *Fibrillenstruktur* (fibrillar structure) and *Felderstruktur* (plain structure). Dietert in 1965 applied this oversimplified classification to the EOMs.[9] In 1974, Durston,[10] studying baboon EOMs, termed the *Felderstruktur* fibers "coarse" and subdivided the *Fibrillenstruktur* fibers as "granular" and "fine" according to their morphology and intermyofibrillar network. This terminology was also applied to human EOMs.[11] In 1971, however, Mayr[12] recognized six types of EOM fibers in the rat according to their location, histochemical features, ultrastructural details, and pattern of innervation. Spencer and Porter[13] in 1988 compared different mammalian EOMs and proposed a classification based on six fiber types, and this work has been widely used.[14] An important component in the classification is the heavy-chain isoform of myosin, whose expression correlates well with the contractile characteristics and fatigue resistance of the muscle fibers.

1. Orbital singly-innervated fibers. These fibers, which correspond to Durston's coarse fibers, constitute 80 percent of the fibers in the orbital layer. They exhibit fast myofibrillar ATPase (i.e., they stain dark with ATPase reaction at pH 9.4 to 10.4) as well as high oxidative activity with numerous mitochondria in clusters. They express fast myosin isoform along their length, but co-express neonatal/embryonic (developmental) myosin in their proximal and distal segments.15 This fiber type is considered to be the most fatigue-resistant among mammalian skeletal muscle fibers.14

2. Orbital multiply-innervated fibers. These exhibit longitudinal structural and immunohistologic heterogeneity. The proximal and distal parts have fine structure (fitting Durston's fine fiber); they express slow myofibrillar ATPase (i.e., they stain dark with ATPase reaction after preincubation at pH 4.3) and developmental myosin isoform.[15] In their central segment, the fibers react for fast myofibrillar ATPase and express the fast isoform of the heavy-chain myosin, here resembling orbital singly-innervated fibers.

3. Global red singly-innervated fibers. These comprise about one-third of the global layer. Histochemically and ultrastructurally, they resemble orbital singly-innervated fibers but do not contain developmental myosin and show no longitudinal heterogeneity. They are considered to be fast-twitch and highly fatigue-resistant fibers.[14]

4. Global intermediate singly-innervated fibers. This fiber type comprises 25 percent of the global layer. The fibers have a granular appearance in the trichrome stain, contain type IIB myosin-like isoform, stain dark for ATPase at pH 9.4, have moderate oxidative and anaerobic enzyme activities, and have a high mitochondrial content, suggesting that they are fast-twitch and intermediate fatigue-resistant fibers.[14]

5. Global pale singly-innervated fibers. These fibers constitute one-third of the global layer, have a granular

appearance on the trichrome stain, and may correspond to Durston's granular fibers. They also contain a type IIB myosin-like isoform, have high anaerobic enzyme activity, and have a paucity of mitochondria, suggesting they are fast-twitch with low fatigue resistance.

6. Global multiply innervated fibers. These fibers account for the remaining 10 percent of the global layer. They exhibit end plates along their length, contain few and small mitochondria, have acid-stable ATPase activity, and harbor a slow-myosin isoform.[14]

The above classification was modified for human EOMs by Wasicky et al.[7] On the basis of a combination of histochemical and immunohistochemical techniques, these authors recognize three fiber types in the global layer—namely, granular singly-innervated (analogous to global pale singly-innervated fibers and global intermediate singly-innervated fibers), coarse singly-innervated (analogous to global red), and global multiply-innervated; and two fiber types in the orbital layer: orbital multiply-innervated and orbital singly-innervated fiber. In the newly described marginal zone, they detect one type of singly-innervated fiber, and low- and high-oxidative multiply-innervated fibers. They also note that the fibers in the marginal zone are larger than those in the orbital layer and that they coexpress both developmental and fast-myosin heavy-chain isoforms. Except for the marginal zone, this classification resembles the mammalian EOM classification. However, in nonhuman mammals the global multiply-innervated fiber shows low oxidative enzyme activity;[14] while in humans they react strongly for oxidative enzymes.[7] The last is consistent with the presence of numerous small mitochondria in human global multiply-innervated fibers.[16] Table 6-1 summarizes the properties of EOM fiber types.

The levator contains four types of uniformly distributed fibers: Three resemble those of singly-innervated global layer fibers and the fourth is a slow-twitch fiber type.[17]

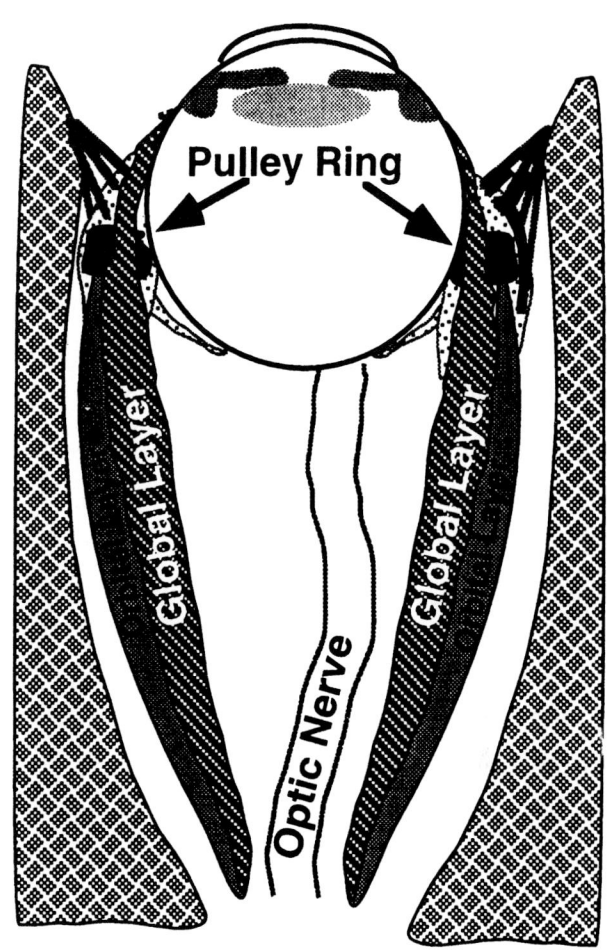

FIGURE 6-2. Schematic representation of orbital structures and their relation to rectus muscles layers. (*From Demer JL, Oh SY, Poukens V: Evidence for active control of rectus extraocular muscle pulleys. Invest Ophthalmol Vis Sci 41:1280–1290, 2000, with permission from the Association for Research in Vision and Ophthalmology.*)

Table 6-1. PROPERTIES OF FIBER TYPES

Fiber type	Orbital Layer		Global Layer			
	SIF	MIF	Red SIF	Intermediate SIF[a]	Pale SIF[a]	MIF
Percent	80%	20%	32.5%	25%	32.5%	10%
Network	Coarse	Fine	Coarse	Granular	Granular	Fine
ATPase 9.4	+	−	+	+	+	−
Myosin isoforms	Fast throughout; developmental at ends	Developmental at ends; fast in center	IIA-like	IIB-like	IIB-like	Slow
Oxidative activity	High	High	High	Moderate	Low	Animals, low; human, high
AChR expression	Fetal and adult	Fetal and adult	Mainly adult	Mainly adult	Mainly adult	Fetal and adult
Innervation	Single	Multiple at ends, singly at center	Single	Single	Single	Multiple
Function	Fast-twitch, fatigue-resistant	Slow at ends, fatigue-resistant at center	Fast-twitch, fatigue-resistant	Fast-twitch, intermediate fatigability	Fast-twitch, fatigable	Slow
Insertion	Pulley		Globe			

KEY: SIF = Singly-innervated fiber. MIF = Multiply-innervated fiber.
[a]Global intermediate and pale multiply-innervated fibers are considered as one type in humans.

The Innervation and Synapses of Extraocular Muscles

The EOMs are much more richly innervated than limb muscles. For example, in the cat EOM, a motor unit contains about 15 muscle fibers.[18] In humans, the abducens motor nucleus motor contains about 5000 neurons,[19] and the lateral rectus muscle comprises about 25,000 fibers.[6] Taking into account the fact that about half of the abducens motor neurons connect to the opposite medial rectus nucleus, this implies 10 muscle fibers per motor unit in the lateral rectus. By contrast, the biceps brachii muscle contains about 130 motor units and several hundred fibers per motor unit. There are two main types of motor innervation and end plates. About 80 to 85 percent of EOM nerve fibers are large and myelinated; they innervate a single end plate in the middle third of each muscle fiber. These end plates are wide, compact or lobulated, and plaque-like[19] (Fig. 6-3). The remaining 15 to 20 percent of nerve fibers are small and innervate numerous small end plates distributed along the length of muscle fiber in grape-like endings[20] (Figs. 6-4 and 6-5).

All orbital and global singly innervated fibers carry plaque-like end plates. Global multiply innervated fibers possess *en grappe* (grape-like) endings along their length, whereas orbital multiply innervated fibers have a single *en plaque* (plaque-like) synapse at the end plate zone and numerous *en grappe* endings along their proximal and distal segments.[15] Groups of small motor neurons identified just outside the main group of neurons of cranial nerve nuclei III, IV, and VI are thought to innervate the multiply innervated fibers.[21]

EOM end plates express both the adult epsilon and the fetal gamma subunit of the acetylcholine receptor (AChR). By contrast, adult skeletal muscle possesses only the adult α_2–β–ϵ–δ AChR. In the rat, all orbital layer and global layer *en grappe* endings (namely, all multiply innervated fibers) coexpress the adult and fetal AChR.[22] All *en plaque* endings of the orbital layer exhibit the gamma subunit. Thus, all orbital layer end plates on the multiply and singly innervated fibers coexpress fetal and adult AChR isoforms. The global layer *en plaque* end plates also express fetal AChR, but only at the periphery of the innervation zone.[22] The levator contains no multiply innervated fibers and no fetal AChR.[23]

Physiologic Aspects of Extraocular Muscles

The physiologic characteristics of multiply and singly innervated fibers differ considerably. The singly innervated fiber responds to a nerve stimulus with a unitary end plate potential that evokes a spreading action potential along the muscle fiber, which generates phasic tension. Thus, singly innervated fibers resemble nonocular muscle fibers in their electrophysiologic and contractile properties. By contrast, the global multiply innervated fibers respond to nerve stimuli with a compound end plate potential and a graded, voltage-dependent response or a slow peak potential,[24] producing sustained or tonic tension.[24,25] The membrane time constant and effective resistance of these fibers are very large;[24,25] hence, they resemble the amphibian slow tonic fibers.[26]

The orbital multiply innervated fibers show action potential responses around their plaque-like end plates; these do not propagate into the proximal and distal fiber segments,[27] which have tonic, nontwitch properties. The twitch and tonic functions of the orbital multiply innervated fibers coincide with the structural and immunohistochemical heterogeneity of these fibers.

The twitch motor units are classified into four types, according to contraction time, tetanic fusion frequency, and fatigue resistance: fast-fatigable, fast fatigue-resistant, slow-

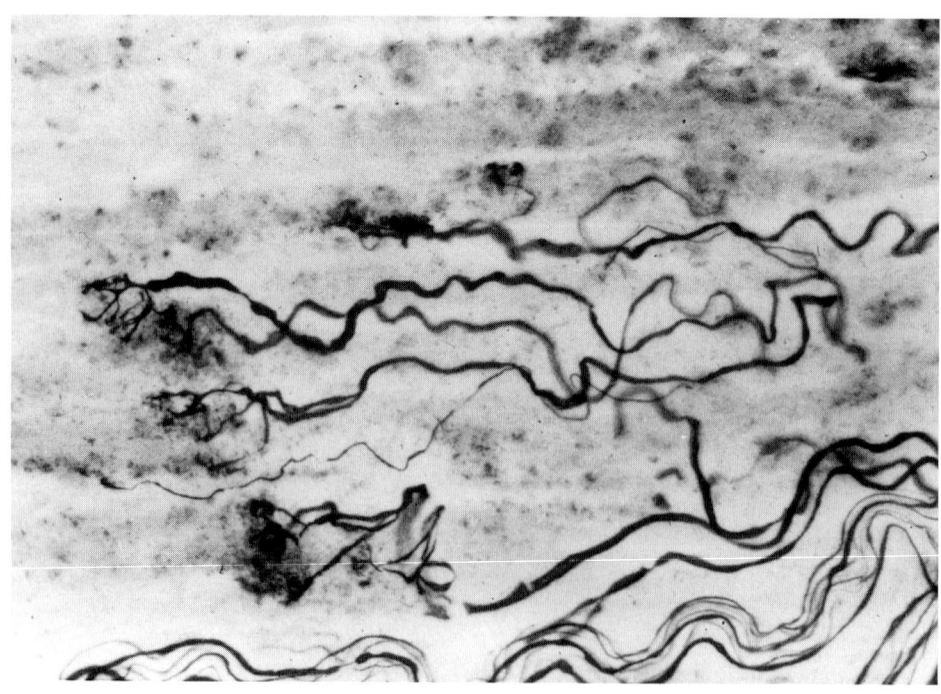

FIGURE 6-3. End plate band of orbital layer. Thick axons innervate large *en plaque* endings. (Bromoindoxyl acetate stain for cholinesterase and silver/gold impregnation for axons.)

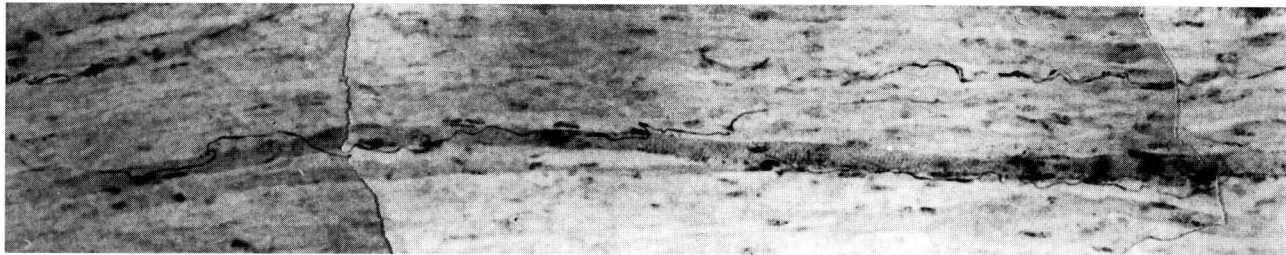

FIGURE 6-4. A thin axon travels along muscle fiber innervating multiple small *en grappe* synapses. (Bromoindoxyl acetate stain for cholinesterase and silver/gold impregnation for axons.)

fatigable, and slow fatigue-resistant,[17] fairly corresponding with the morphologic classification. Electromyographic (EMG) recording displays motor units that are confined either to the global layer or to the orbital layer as well as bilayer units whose fibers split between the two layers.[28] Most bilayer units are fast-fatigable.[28]

The maximum firing rate of ocular motor neurons is 600/s, compared with 125/s for spinal motor neurons. The EOMs never become slack and sustain tension even at rest. They produce tension much faster than limb muscles, with a time to peak tension of less than 5 ms. Initial reports suggested that the force output per unit cross-sectional area of EOMs is about half of that produced by limb muscles.[29,30] However, recent in situ measurements indicate that the tension output of EOMs does not differ from that of limb muscles.[31] The earlier findings are explained by the in vitro evaluations of contractility or by failure to recognize that orbital layer fibers insert on the pulley rather than the globe.

Structure-Function Correlations

A burst of neural activity in oculomotor nuclei, called a *pulse*, is required to produce a rapid movement, such as a saccade. To hold the eye in its new position, a steady neural activity, called a *step*, is required.[1] A neural network, termed a *neural integrator*,[1] synthesizes the velocity (pulse) and position (step) components of ocular movements.

According to Collins, initiation of saccades requires co-activation of both fiber layers.[32] However, orbital fibers discharge throughout the entire oculomotor range, with only step activity even during saccades, whereas global fibers display both pulse and step activity.[32] Collins proposed fixation as an important function of the orbital layer. He also indicated that the main load on an active agonist EOM is opposing the viscosity arising from the relaxing antagonist. On the basis of these observations, Demer et al.[5] proposed another role for the orbital layer. They pointed out that a phasic pulse of force is unnecessary to achieve a brisk motion of the pulley against the elasticity of the pulley suspension. Instead, they suggested that the orbital layer is continuously active against the elastic load of the pulley suspension, consistent with the fatigue-resistant nature of the orbital singly-innervated muscle fibers.

If the rule, valid for limb muscles, that all fibers of an individual motor unit are of the same type is applicable for EOMs, then bilayer motor units would consist of orbital singly-innervated fibers and global red singly-innervated fibers that share similar morphologic, histochemical, and contractile properties. These units may have a role in coordination of ocular rotation with pulley position.[6] The global fast-fatigable intermediate and pale singly-innervated fibers may function during saccade to generate the high transient force necessary for overcoming the viscous load of the relaxing antagonist.[5] These notions are further supported by the finding that botulinum-induced damage to orbital singly-innervated fibers resulted in an abnormal static alignment but normal saccade kinematics.[33]

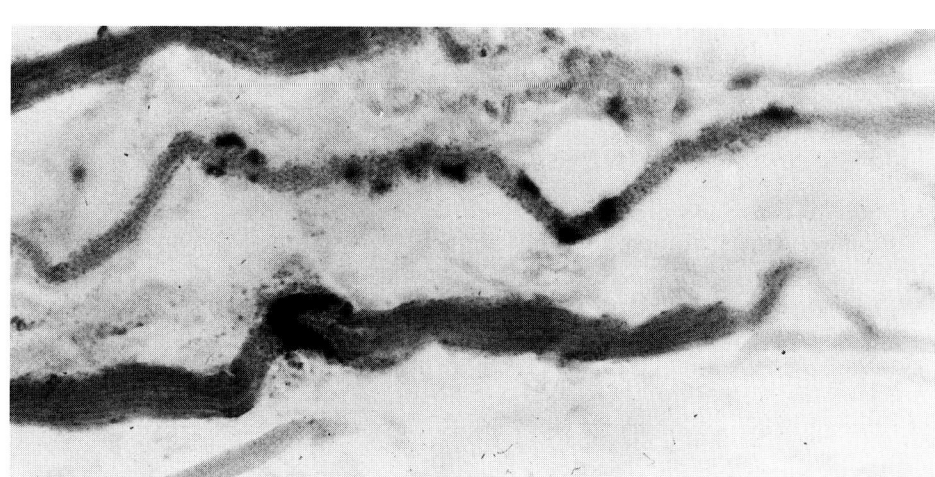

FIGURE 6-5. Two muscle fibers of the global layer. One possesses a single *en plaque* ending and the other multiple small *en grappe* endings. (Bromoindoxyl acetate stain for cholinesterase.)

However, there are a number of unresolved questions:

1. The bilayer motor units are reported to be physiologically fast-fatigable,[28] but all orbital singly-innervated fibers should be fast fatigue-resistant by histochemical criteria.[14] Moreover, all orbital singly-innervated fibers are histochemically similar and do not show the heterogeneity suggested by the physiologic studies. The same ocular motor neurons discharge for all type of ocular movements, and they discharge during pulse and step activity.[34] Moreover, EMG studies confirm that the same motor units are active during all classes of eye movements.[35] This leads to the conclusion that each muscle fiber contributes to all classes of eye movements.
2. The homogeneity of motor neurons versus the diversity of muscle fibers challenges the notion of fiber-type uniformity in a given motor unit or that the physiologic and anatomic properties of muscle fibers within a motor unit are dictated by the firing pattern of the innervating motor neuron. The order of motor-unit recruitment is not known. Is the size principle applicable to EOMs? Are there motor units that are recruited for small sacades and additional ones for larger saccades?
3. The role of the multiply-innervated fibers is obscure, although global multiply-innervated fibers may play a role in proprioception (as discussed below).

Proprioception by Extraocular Muscles

Vision provides the brain with continuous although somewhat late feedback on the precision of the outcome of gaze commands. A corollary discharge, or an efferent copy, by which information of the intended ocular movement is transmitted to higher centers, also plays a role in monitoring gaze. Considerable clinical and experimental evidence indicates that proprioception plays an important role in modifying alignment, and programming smooth pursuit and saccades (for reviews, see Refs. 36 and 37). There is general agreement that the feedback information from EOMs to the central nervous system (CNS) travels at first with cranial nerves III, IV, and VI and then crosses to the ophthalmic branch of the trigeminal nerve, being conveyed to the trigeminal ganglion and nuclei.[36,37] However, there is controversy regarding the sensory receptor within the EOM. The presence of muscle spindles varies among different species. Muscle spindles are found in human infants and the elderly in a similar number to that found in hand muscles.[38,39] Monkeys and cats, however, lack muscle spindles but still have stretch reflexes,[40] suggesting that receptors other than muscle spindles are important for proprioception. (However, in another study in monkeys, monosynaptic stretch reflex was absent.[41]) The proprioceptive properties of EOM spindles were questioned on the basis of structural considerations as well.[36] Thus the physiologic significance of EOM spindles remains unknown.

Golgi tendon organs are present in monkeys and sheep but not in humans.[42,43] Therefore the myotendinous cylinders (palisade endings), which are present in both humans and animals, are likely the main proprioceptive receptors in humans.[42–46] Myotendinous cylinders are encapsulated in junctions of single muscle fibers with tendons. Each cylinder is innervated by a small myelinated nerve that penetrates the capsule, loses its myelin sheath, and then ramifies, forming the palisade ending, and contacts both collagen fibrils and the sarcolemma through varicose terminals[41] (Fig. 6-6). In humans, the terminals at the myoneural contact were proven by AChR labeling and electron microscopy to be motor, whereas the terminals contacting collagen fibrils are presumably sensory.[42] Thus, these endings likely have combined proprioceptor and effector qualities. However, in the rabbit EOM, the myotendinous cylinders seem to possess only motor endings.[43] In contrast, according to another study, different axons approach the outer muscle surface and the collagen fibers.[44] Innervated myotendinous cylinders are associated with the global multiply-innervated fibers only. Since there have been no recordings from myotendinous

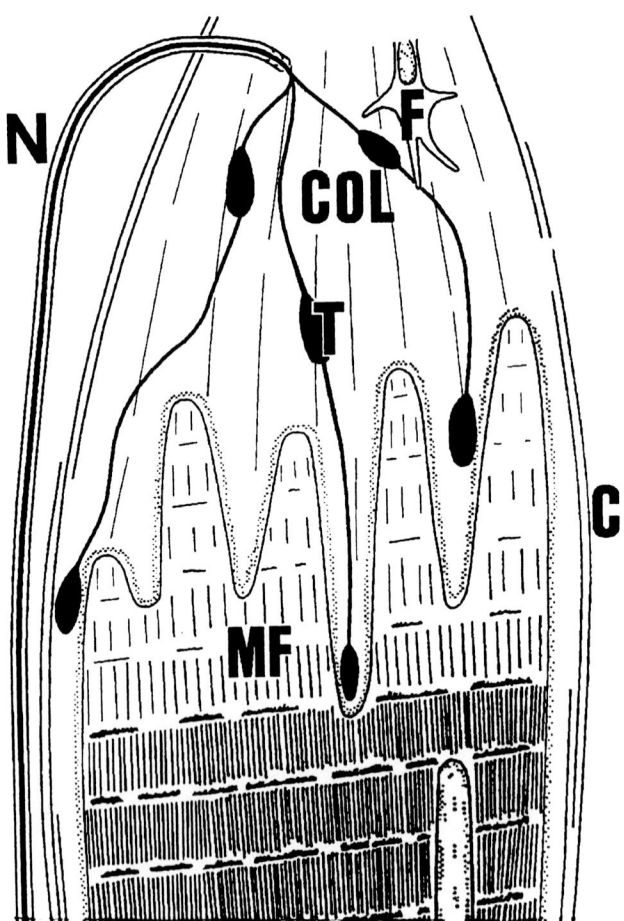

FIGURE 6-6. Schematic representation of an innervated myotendinous cylinder. Nerve fiber (N) enters an encapsulated (C) myotendinous ending and ramifies. Terminals (T) contact with collagenous fibrils (COL) and sarcolemma outside the muscle fiber (MF). F represents a fibrocyte. (*From Lukas JR, Blumer R, Denk M, et al: Innervated myotendinous cylinders in human extraocular muscles. Invest Ophthalmol Vis Sci 41:2422–2431, 2000, with permission from the Association for Research in Vision and Ophthalmology.*)

cylinder afferents, their role and the significance of their association with the global multiply-innervated fibers remains speculative. To conclude, the mechanisms of proprioception in EOMs, the function of palisade endings, and the significance of muscle spindles await clarification.

Pathologic Reactions

EOMs are also distinctive in their pathologic responses. Denervation by section of the oculomotor nerve causes mild atrophy and mild ultrastructural alterations.[47] Reinnervation is not followed by fiber-type grouping except for grouping of multiply-innervated fibers.[10] However, these experiments are not analogous to the chronic denervation-reinnervation process. There is no information about the pathologic changes in chronic denervation, as in amyotrophic lateral sclerosis, in which the EOMs are involved only at a very late stage of the disease. Interestingly, denervated multiply-innervated fibers acquire twitch properties and the ability to generate action potentials. After reinnervation, the slow peak potentials reappear.[48]

Conflicting results were reported concerning the effects of retrobulbar injection of local anesthetics. Carlson and Rainin[49] describe massive degeneration followed by regeneration, whereas Porter et al.[50] find a mild myopathic response largely restricted to the global singly-innervated fibers and no involvement of the multiply-innervated fibers. They suggested a mitigated myotoxicity of local anesthetics in EOMs. However, retrobulbar injection of EOMs by bupivacaine is not comparable with an intramuscular injection of limb muscles. Intramuscular injection into EOMs does produce large necrosis; therefore the degree of resistance of EOMs to local anesthetics is unclear.

Injection of botulinum toxin into skeletal muscle results in denervation atrophy, followed within a few months by complete recuperation due to nerve sprouting. Therefore treatment by botulinum toxin injection, widely used for various purposes, must be repeated. By contrast, a single injection of botulinum into EOMs results in permanent paralysis and can thus correct strabismus. Only the orbital singly-innervated fibers become permanently denervated, whereas other fiber types are preserved.[51] The levator responds to botulinum toxin as do the limb and facial muscles.[52]

Involvement in Diseases

EOMs are preferentially involved or spared in a variety of neuromuscular diseases. The vulnerability of EOMs in myasthenia gravis (MG) is well known, and often EOMs are exclusively affected (ocular MG). This was at first attributed to the exclusive presence of multiply-innervated fibers in EOMs, but sera from patients with ocular MG reacted with either both types of end plates or selectively with end plates on multiply- or singly-innervated fibers.[53] Later it was suggested that the γ subunit of AChR may serve as the antigenic target for the antibodies.[54] Indeed, antibodies against the γ subunit have been identified in myasthenic patients,[55] but their presence did not correlate with ocular symptoms. Moreover, in about 50 percent of ocular MG patients, no AChR antibodies are detected. Furthermore, neither multiply-innervated fibers nor fibers containing the fetal AChR occur in the levator, the most commonly affected EOM in MG. Muscle-specific kinase (MuSK) antibodies, recently demonstrated in 17 out of 24 patients with generalized MG but without anti-AChR antibodies, were not detected in ocular MG.[56] Therefore some as yet unidentified autoantibodies or antibody specificities may cause the ocular disease. Other explanations for the vulnerability of EOMs in MG have been suggested.[57]

EOMs are often spared in muscular dystrophies. The clinical and pathologic sparing of EOMs was investigated in Duchenne dystrophy.[58,59] Also, there is no significant pathologic involvement of the EOMs in experimental models of dystrophies, such as the mdx mouse,[60] or in gamma- or delta-sarcoglycan-[61] and α-2 laminin-deficient mice,[62] even though these mice lack sarcolemma-associated cytoskeletal or basal lamina proteins essential for sarcolemmal support. The levator and retractor bulbi of these animals do show central nuclei, presumably due to cycles of degeneration and regeneration.[61,63] Porter[64] extensively reviewed hypotheses for this selective sparing. The proposed protective mechanisms included: reduced sarcolemmal stress during contraction because of the smallness of the fibers,[63] better intracellular buffering of free calcium, enhanced antioxidant capacity, and an adaptive response related to overexpression of utrophin. Recently, McLoon and Wirtschafter[65] have demonstrated that satellite cells of adult uninjured EOMs continually divide and add new myonuclei to EOM fibers. This active rebuilding may allow EOMs to respond to muscle fiber injury associated with sarcolemmal protein deficiency.

Because of their high mitochondrial content and elevated oxidative enzyme activity, the EOMs are susceptible to mitochondrial cytopathies. EOMs are also preferentially affected in oculopharyngeal muscular dystrophy, Graves' ophthalmopathy, and congenital fibrosis of the EOM.

Development

Embryologically, EOMs develop from rostral condensations of mesoderm, called somitomeres,[66] rather than from the conventional somites from which limb and axial muscles grow. The connective tissue of the orbit arises from the neural crest.[67] Myoblast aggregates are contacted by oculomotor nerves and migrate to the developing orbit. There are two or three phases of myotube formation. The global multiply-innervated fibers are formed first and the orbital layer fibers last.[68] Like in the skeletal muscle system, there is overproduction of motor neurons and multiple axonal contacts with the same muscle fiber. After competitive elimination of extra nerve terminals and massive apoptotic death of motor neurons, only one axon innervates each singly-innervated fiber. The steps in synapse formation and innervation of multiply-innervated fibers is unknown.

Fiber categorization is established by the time of birth.[68] During infancy, EOMs mature with increase of their mitochondrial content (for a comprehensive review of EOM development, see Ref. 14).

Comparison of gene expression in rat EOM and limb muscle at the mRNA level reveals four new genes that are upregulated in EOM.[69] Their nature awaits clarification. Another interesting finding in this study was the upregulation in EOM of semaphorin A/V, a substance implicated in axonal guidance and synaptogenesis, that may play a role in the innervation of multiply–innervated fibers. Further advances in molecular genetics and proteonomics will likely shed more light on the development and functional significance of the different EOM fibers types.

List of Abbreviations

CNS   central nervous system
EMG   electromyogram
EOMs extraocular muscles
MG   myasthenia gravis
MuSK muscle-specific kinase

References

1. Leigh RJ, Zee DS: *The Neurology of Eye Movements*, 3rd ed. New York: Oxford University Press, 1999.
2. Demer JL, Miller JM, Poukens V, et al: evidence for fibromuscular pulleys of the recti extramuscular muscles. *Invest Ophthalmol Vis Sci* 36:1125–1136, 1995.
3. Demer JL, Poukens V, Miller JM, et al: Innervation of extraocular pulley smooth muscle in monkeys and humans. *Invest Ophthalmol Vis Sci* 38:1774–1785, 1997.
4. Clark RA, Miller JM, Demer JL: Location and stability of rectus muscles pulleys: Muscles paths as a function of gaze. *Invest Ophthalmol Vis Sci* 38:227–240, 1997.
5. Demer JL, Oh SY, Poukens V: Evidence for active control of rectus extraocular muscle pulleys. *Invest Ophthalmol Vis Sci* 41:1280–1290, 2000.
6. Oh SY, Poukens V, Demer JL: Quantitative analysis of rectus extraocular muscles layers in monkey and humans. *Invest Ophthalmol Vis Sci* 42:10–16, 2001.
7. Wasicky R, Ziya-Ghazvini F, Blumer R, et al: Muscle fibers types of human extraocular muscles: A histochemical and immunohistochemical study. *Invest Ophthalmol Vis Sci* 41:980–990, 2000.
8. Kruger P: Die Innervation der tetanischen und tonischen Fasern der quergestreiften Skeletmuskulatur der Wirbeltiere. *Anat Anz* 97:169–175, 1949.
9. Dietert SE: The demonstration of different types of muscle fibers in human extraocular muscle by electron microscopy and cholinesterase staining. *Invest Ophthalmol* 4:51–63, 1965.
10. Durston JHJ: Histochemistry of primate extraocular muscles and the change of denervation. *Br J Ophthalmol* 58:193–216, 1974.
11. Ringel SP, Wilson WB, Barsten MT, Kaiser KK: Histochemistry of human extraocular muscles. *Arch Ophthalmol* 96:1067–1072, 1978.
12. Mayr R: Structure and distribution of fiber types in the external eye muscles of the rat. *Tissue Cell* 3:433–462, 1971.
13. Spencer RF, Porter JD: Structural organization of the extraocular muscles, in Büttner-Enneyer JA (ed): *Reviews in Oculomotor Research*. Vol 2. Neuroanatomy of the Oculomotor System. New York: Elsevier, 1988; pp 33–73.
14. Porter JD, Backer RS, Ragusa RJ, Brueknek JK: Extraocular muscles: Basic and clinical aspects of structure and function. *Surv Ophthalmol* 39:451–484, 1995.
15. Jacoby J, Ko K, Weis C, Rushbrook JI: Systemic variation in myosin expression along extraocular muscle fibers of the adult rat. *J Musc Res Cell Motil* 11:25–40, 1989.
16. Carry MR, Ringel SP, Starcevich JM: Mitochondrial morphometrics of histochemically identified human extraocular muscle fibers. *Anat Rec* 214:8–16, 1986.
17. Porter JD, Burns LA, May PJ: Morphological substrate for eye lid movements: Innervation and structure of primate levator palpebrae superioris and orbicularis oculi muscles. *J Comp Neurol* 287:64–81, 1989.
18. Goldberg S, Shall MS: Motor units of extraocular muscles: Recent findings, in Binder MD (ed): *Progress in Brain Research*. Vol 123. New York: Elsevier, 1999; pp 221–232.
19. Vijayashankar N, Brody HJ: A study of aging in the human abducens nucleus. *J Comp Neurol* 173:433–438, 1977.
20. Kupfer C: Motor innervation of extraocular muscle. *J Physiol* 15:522–526, 1960.
21. Büttner-Enneyer JA, Horn AKE, Scherberger H-J, Henn V: The location of motor neurons innervating slow extraocular muscle fibers in monkey. *Soc Neurosci Abstr* 24:145, 1998.
22. Kaminsky HJ, Kusner LL, Block CH: Expression of acetylcholine receptor isoforms at extraocular muscle endplates. *Invest Ophthalmol Vis Sci* 37:345–351, 1996.
23. Kaminsky HJ, Kusner LL, Nash KV, Ruff RL: The γ-subunit of the acetylcholine receptor is not expressed in the levator palpebrae superioris. *Neurology* 45:516–518, 1995.
24. Chiarandini DJ, Stefani F: Electrophysiological identification of two types of fibres in rat extraocular muscles. *J Physiol* 290:453–465, 1979.
25. Bondy AY, Chiarandini DJ: Ionic basis for electrical properties of tonic fibres in rat extraocular muscles. *J Physiol* 295:473–481, 1979.
26. Stefani F, Steinbach AB: Resting potential and electrical properties of frog slow muscle fibres. *J Physiol* 203:383–401, 1979.
27. Jacoby J, Chiarandini DJ, Stefani E: Electrical properties and innervation of fibers in the orbital layer of rat extraocular muscles. *J Neurophysiol* 61:116–125, 1989.
28. Shall MS, Goldberg SJ: Lateral rectus EMG and contractile responses elicited by cat abducens motor neurons. *Muscle Nerve* 18:948–955, 1995.
29. Close RI, Luff AR: Dynamic properties of inferior rectus muscle of the rat. *J Physiol* 236:259–270, 1974.
30. Goldberg SJ, Wilson KE, Shall MS: Summation of extraocular motor unit tensions in the lateral rectus muscle of the rat. *Muscle Nerve* 20:1229–1235, 1997.
31. Frueh BR, Gregorevic P, Williams DA, Lynch GS: Specific force of the rat extraocular muscles, levator and superior rectus, measures in situ. *J Neurophysiol* 85:1027–1032, 2001.
32. Collins CC: The human oculomotor control system, in Lennerstrand G, Bach-y-Rita P (eds): *Basic Mechanisms of Ocular Motility and Their Clinical Implications*. New York: Pergamon, 1975; pp 145–180.
33. Stahl JS, Averbuch-Heller L, Remler BF, Leigh RJ: Clinical evidence of extraocular muscle fiber-type specificity of botulinum toxin. *Neurology* 51:1093–1099, 1998.
34. Robinson DA: Oculomotor unit behavior in the monkey. *J Neurophysiol* 33:393–404, 1970.
35. Scott AB, Collins CC: Division of labor in human extraocular muscles. *Arch Ophthalmol* 90:319–322, 1973.
36. Ruskell JL: Extraocular muscle proprioceptors and proprioception. *Prog Retin Eye Res* 18:269–291, 1999.
37. Weir CR, Knox PC, Dutton GN: Does extraocular muscle proprioception influence oculomotor control? *Br J Ophthalmol* 84:1071–1074, 2000.
38. Lukas JR, Aigner M, Blumer R, et al: Number and distribution of neuromuscular spindles in human extraocular muscles. *Invest Ophthalmol Vis Sci* 35:4317–4327, 1995.
39. Ruskell GL: The fine structure of human extraocular muscle spindles and their proprioceptive capacity. *J Anat* 167:199–214, 1989.
40. Cooper S, Fillenz M: Afferent discharges in response to stretch from the extraocular muscles of the cat and monkey and the innervation of these muscles. *J Physiol* 127:400–413, 1955.
41. Keller EL, Robinson DA: Absence of a stretch reflex in extraocular muscles of the monkey. *J Neurophysiol* 34:908–919, 1971.
42. Lukas JR, Blumer R, Denk M, et al: Innervated myotendinous cylinders in human extraocular muscles. *Invest Ophthalmol Vis Sci* 41:2422–2431, 2000.
43. Blumer R, Wasicky R, Hetzenecker M, Lukas JR: Innervated myotendinous cylinders in rabbit EOMs. *Exp Eye Res* 73:787–796, 2001.
44. Bruenech R, Ruskell GL: Myotendinous nerve endings in human infant and adult extraocular muscles. *Anat Rec* 260:132–140, 2000.
45. Richmond FJR, Johnston WSW, Baker RS, Steinbach MJ: Palisade endings in human extraocular muscles. *Invest Ophthalmol Vis Sci* 25:471–476, 1984.
46. Ruskell GL: The fine structure of innervated myotendinous cylinders in extraocular muscles of rhesus monkeys. *J Neurocytol* 7:693–708, 1978.

47. Porter JD, Burns LA, McMahon EJ: Denervation of primate extraocular muscle: A unique pattern of structural alterations. *Invest Ophthalmol Vis Sci* 30:1894–1908, 1989.
48. Bondi AY, Chiarandini DJ, Jacoby J: Induction of action potentials by denervation of tonic fibers in rat extraocular muscles. *J Physiol* 374:165–178, 1986.
49. Carlson BM, Rainin EA: Rat extraocular muscle regeneration: Repair of local anesthetic-induced damage. *Arch Ophthalmol* 103:1373–1377, 1985.
50. Porter JD, Edney DP, McMahon EJ, Burns LA: Extraocular myotoxicity of the retrobulbar anesthetic bupivacaine hydrochloride. *Invest Ophthalmol Vis Sci* 29:163–174, 1988.
51. Spencer RF, McNeer KW: Botulinum toxin paralysis of adult monkey extraocular muscle: Structural alteration in orbital singly innervated muscle fibers. *Arch Ophthalmol* 105:1703–1711, 1987.
52. Porter JD, Strebeck S, Capra NF: Botulinum-induced changes in monkey eyelid muscle: Comparison with changes seen in extraocular muscles. *Arch Ophthalmol* 109:396–404, 1991.
53. Oda K, Shibasaki H: Antigenic difference of acetylcholine receptor between single and multiple form endplates of human extraocular muscle. *Brain Res* 449:337–340, 1988.
54. Horton RM, Manfredi AA, Conti-Tronconi BM: The "embryonic" gamma subunit of the nicotinic acetylcholine receptor is expressed in adult extraocular muscle. *Neurology* 43:983–986, 1993.
55. Tzartos A, Seybold M, Lindstrom J: Specificities of antibodies to acetylcholine receptors in sera from myasthenia gravis patients measured by monoclonal antibodies. *Proc Natl Acad Sci USA* 79:188–192, 1982.
56. McConville J, Hoch W, Newsome-Davis J, Vincent A: Antibodies to the muscle specific kinase, MusK, in generalized and ocular myasthenia gravis seronegative for acetylcholine receptor antibodies (abstr). *J Neurol Sci* 187(suppl 1):s122–s123, 2001.
57. Kaminski HJ, Maas E, Spiegel P, Ruff RL: Why are eye muscles frequently involved in myasthenia gravis? *Neurology* 40:1663–1669, 1990.
58. Kaminski HJ, Al-Hakim M, Leigh RJ, et al: Extraocular are spared in advanced Duchenne dystrophy. *Ann Neurol* 32:586–588, 1992.
59. Khurana TS, Prendergast RA, Alameddine H, et al: Absence of extraocular muscle pathology in Duchenne muscular dystrophy: Role for calcium homeostasis in extraocular muscle sparing. *J Exp Med* 182:467–475, 1995.
60. Ragusa RJ, Porter JD: Extraocular muscle in the mdx mouse: Absence of pathology correlates with superoxide dismutase activity (abstr). *Mol Biol Cell* 5:26a, 1994.
61. Porter JD, Merriam AP, Hack AA, et al: Extraocular muscle is spared despite the absence of an intact sarcoglycan complex in gamma- or delta-sarcoglycan-deficent mice. *Neuromuscul Disord* 11:197–207, 2001.
62. Porter JD, Karathanasis P: Extraocular muscle in merosin-deficient muscular dystrophy: Cation homeostasis is maintained but is not mechanistic in muscle sparing. *Cell Tissue Res* 292:495–501, 1998.
63. Karpati G, Carpenter S: Small-caliber skeletal muscle fibers do not suffer deleterious consequences of dystrophic gene expression. *Am J Med Genet* 25:653–658, 1986.
64. Porter JD: Commentary: Extraocular muscle sparing in muscular dystrophy: A critical evaluation of potential protective mechanisms. *Neuromuscul Disord* 8:198–203, 1998.
65. McLoon LM, Wirtschafter JD: Continuous myonuclei addition to single extraocular myofibers in uninjured adult rabbits. *Muscle Nerve* 25:348–358, 2002.
66. Couly GF, Coltey PM, Le Dourain NM: The developmental fate of the cephalic mesoderm in quail-chick chimeras. *Development* 114:1–15, 1992.
67. Nodem DM: Cell movements and control of patterned tissue assembly during craniofacial development. *J Craniofac Genet Dev Biol* 4:192–213, 1991.
68. Porter JD, Baker RS: Prenatal morphogenesis of primate extraocular muscle: Neuromuscular junction formation and fiber type differentiation. *Invest Ophthalmol Vis Sci* 33:657–670, 1992.
69. Niemann CU, Krag TOB, Khurana TS: Identification of genes that are differentially expressed in extraocular and limb muscle. *J Neurol Sci* 179:76–84, 2000.

SECTION 2

Muscle Contraction

Chapter 7
Molecular Structure of the Sarcomere

ROGER W. CRAIG
RAÚL PADRÓN

Introduction
Structure and Function of Striated Muscle
   THE STRUCTURE OF THE VERTEBRATE STRIATED MUSCLE FIBER
   CONTRACTION OF MUSCLE: SLIDING FILAMENTS
The Thick Filament
   POLYMERIZATION OF MYOSIN TO FORM FILAMENTS
   STRUCTURE OF THE MYOSIN MOLECULE
   MOLECULAR ARRANGEMENT OF MYOSIN HEADS
   STRUCTURE OF THE THICK-FILAMENT BACKBONE
   MYOSIN-BINDING PROTEINS
The M Line
   STRUCTURE
   PROTEIN COMPONENTS AND INTERACTIONS
   MODEL
   FUNCTION
Titin Filaments
   MOLECULAR STRUCTURE, INTERACTIONS, AND ORGANIZATION
   FUNCTION IN MYOFIBRILLOGENESIS
   MECHANICAL FUNCTION
The Thin Filament
   POLYMERIZATION OF ACTIN TO FORM FILAMENTS
   REGULATORY PROTEINS OF THE THIN FILAMENT
   MOLECULAR MODEL OF THE THIN FILAMENT
   NEBULIN
   CAPPING PROTEINS
   "SOLUBLE" ENZYME BINDING TO THE THIN FILAMENT
The Z Line
   STRUCTURE
   COMPOSITION
   MODEL
Intermediate Filaments
Diseases of the Sarcomere

Introduction

Striated muscles are organs specialized for the rapid generation of movement and force in a specific direction. Their highly ordered structure, from the gross down to the molecular level, reflects this function. In this chapter we discuss the molecular organization of the elementary contractile unit of striated muscle, the sarcomere, a beautifully ordered multiprotein macromolecular machine, whose complex structure is based on the modular design of its protein components and their polymers.

The sarcomere possesses three crucial properties that are critical to its function: (1) its ability to shorten rapidly and efficiently, (2) its ability to switch on and off in milliseconds, and (3) its precision self-assembly and structural regularity. These properties can be understood in terms of the structures and interactions of its constituent proteins, which fall into three major functional classes: contractile, regulatory, and structural. Myosin and actin are the *contractile* proteins that assemble into polymeric filaments (the thick and thin filaments), which interact with each other to generate force and shortening. Troponin and tropomyosin are the major *regulatory* proteins of the sarcomere, binding to actin and regulating actin-myosin interaction and hence contraction in response to changes in Ca^{2+} concentration. The structure of the sarcomere is integrated, stabilized, and laid down during development, using an assortment of *structural* proteins that associate with the actin and myosin filaments. Myosin-binding proteins help to specify the structure of the myosin filament, contribute to the precise organization of its molecules during development, and also modulate contraction in cardiac muscle. Capping proteins, which attach to the ends of the thin filament, prevent polymerization or depolymerization of actin, thus helping to maintain precise filament length necessary for efficient contraction. Cross-linking proteins in the M and Z lines link the thick and thin filaments, respectively, into ordered, longitudinally registered three-dimensional (3D) lattices. Intermediate filaments attach to the Z and M lines, reinforcing sarcomeric structure and linking adjacent sarcomeres to each other both longitudinally and transversely. Finally, the giant proteins titin and nebulin specify the assembly of the thick and thin filaments in the sarcomere, and titin in addition plays a critical mechanical role in contraction.

Structure and Function of Striated Muscle

THE STRUCTURE OF THE VERTEBRATE STRIATED MUSCLE FIBER

Vertebrate striated muscle fibers are single, multinucleate, membrane-bounded cells, typically 10 to 100 μm in diameter and several centimeters long. Under the light microscope they show a regular pattern of transverse stripes (Fig. 7-1A). The fibers are packed with numerous myofibrils (Fig. 7-1B), about 1 to 3 μm in diameter, each enveloped by sarcoplasmic reticulum (SR*)[1] membrane (see Chap. 11) and running par-

*A list of abbreviations used in this chapter is given at the end of the chapter.

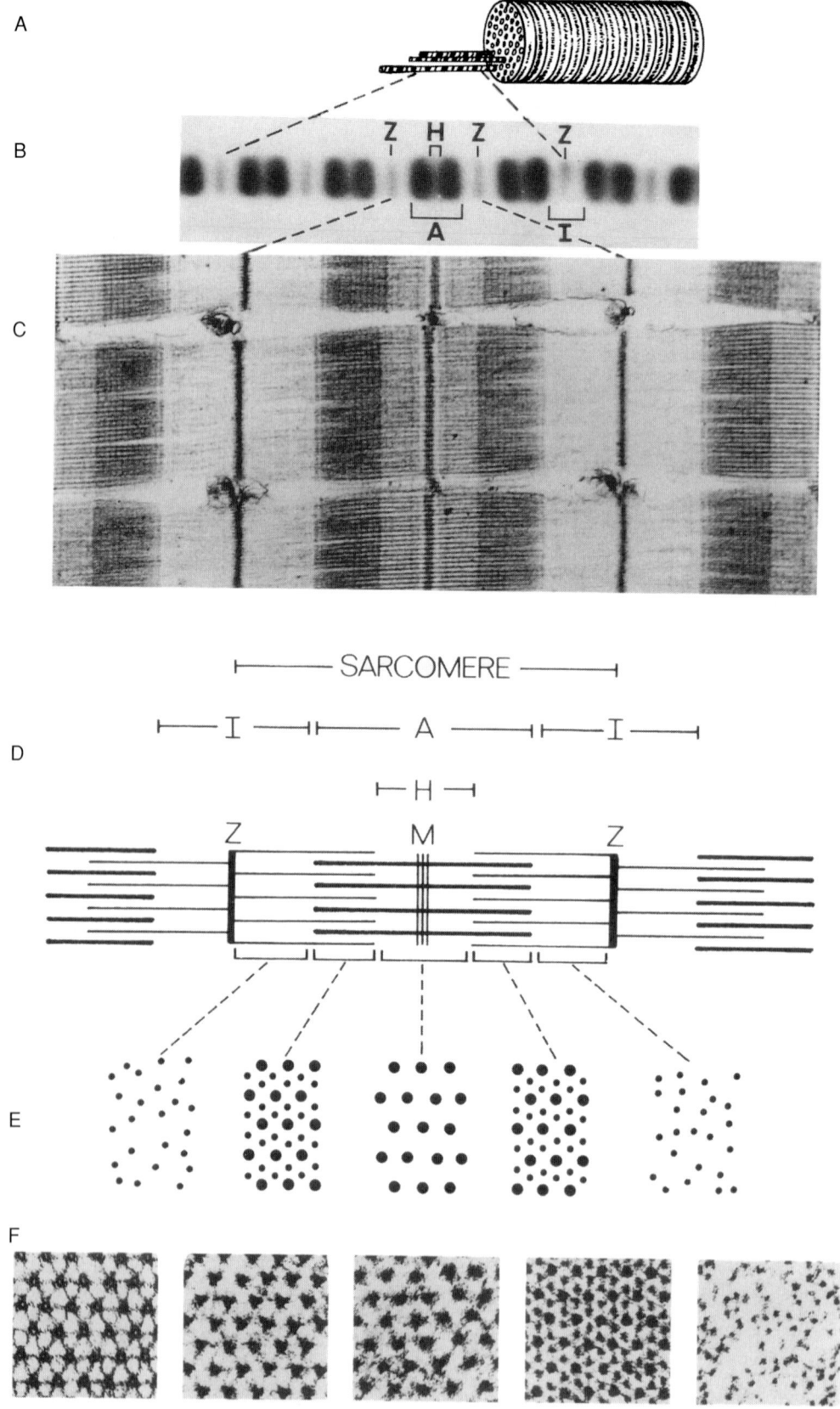

FIGURE 7-1. Origin of the striations in muscle from the arrangement of the myofilaments. *A.* Single muscle fiber with three protruding myofibrils. *B.* Phase-contrast light micrograph of myofibril showing transverse striations. (×5400.) *C.* Electron micrograph of three longitudinally sectioned myofibrils. Transverse stripes in A band are due to myosin-binding proteins and in the I band to troponin. (×23,000.) *(Courtesy of H. E. Huxley.)* *D.* Interpretation of *(B)* and *(C)* in terms of thick (myosin-containing) and thin (actin-containing) filaments arranged in register. *E.* Cross-sectional appearance of sarcomere at different axial levels. *F.* Electron micrographs of transverse sections at different points along the sarcomere. From left to right: the M line, the bare zone, the H zone, the zone of thick and thin filament overlap, the I band. (×120,000.) *(Courtesy of F. A. Pepe.)*

allel to the fiber axis. The fibrils are themselves striated and furthermore are in register, thus producing the striated appearance of the fiber as a whole (Fig. 7-1).

The striation pattern of the myofibril repeats with a periodicity of about 2 to 3 μm. The repeating unit, known as a *sarcomere*, is the fundamental contractile unit of striated muscle. Knowledge of its structure is critical to understanding the molecular mechanism of muscular contraction. The sarcomere is bordered at each end by a dark, narrow (~0.1 μm) line known as the *Z line* (Fig. 7-1B to D). Each Z line bisects a lighter ~1-μm-long *I band* (approximately *isotropic* in polarized light), which is shared between adjacent sarcomeres. At the center of the sarcomere is a dark, 1.6-μm-long *A band* (anisotropic in polarized light), bisected by a less dense *H zone*. In the middle of the H zone is a still lighter region, the *pseudo-H zone* (Fig. 7-1C). Within the pseudo-H zone is a narrow band of higher density (which may show three or more fine stripes) called the *M line* (Fig. 7-1C and D).

This pattern of bands is simply explained in terms of a precisely ordered arrangement of contractile filaments within the myofibril (Fig. 7-1), first clearly observed in ultrathin sections of muscle viewed in the electron microscope[1,2] (Figs. 7-1 and 7-2). The A band contains an array of *thick* (15 nm in diameter) myofilaments, 1.6 μm long, in longitudinal register and running parallel to the fibril axis. Each half I band contains an array of *thin* (~10 nm in diameter) filaments, ~1 μm long, also in longitudinal register. Thin filaments run from their attachment sites at the Z line through the I band and into the A band, where they overlap partially with the thick filaments. The H zone is less dense than the rest of the A band owing to the absence of overlapping thin filaments.

In cross section, the filaments are arranged in a double hexagonal array within the A band[1] (Fig. 7-2), as was first suggested by x-ray diffraction studies of muscle.[3] Only thick filaments are present in the H zone, while in the overlap zone thin filaments are equidistant from the three nearest thick filaments (Figs. 7-1E and F and 7-2). In the I band only thin filaments are present, in a less ordered arrangement than in the A band. The thin filaments are held together lat-

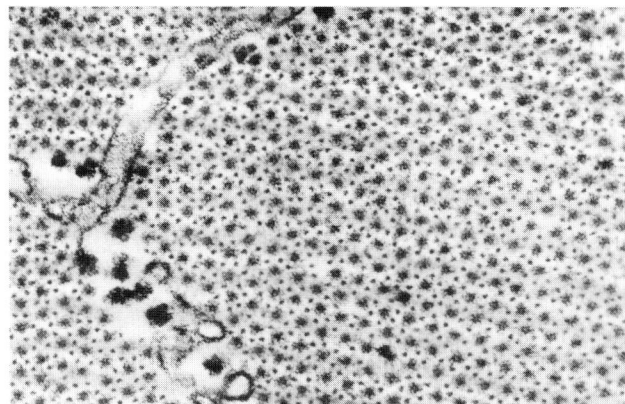

FIGURE 7-2. Electron micrograph of parts of three myofibrils of vertebrate striated muscle seen in transverse section in the overlap zone, illustrating the hexagonal arrangement of thick and thin filaments. (×130,000.) *(Courtesy of H. E. Huxley.)*

erally in a square arrangement by the Z line, while the thick filaments are interconnected by the M line.

Molecular Composition and Function of the Sarcomere

The sarcomere is a complex structure containing, in vertebrate muscle, at least 28 different proteins (Fig. 7-3; Table 7-1). The thick and thin myofilaments are both polymers of noncovalently associated protein molecules. Extraction of myosin and actin results in disappearance of the thick and thin filaments, respectively.[4] Actin and myosin together account for more than 70 percent of myofibrillar protein (actin, 20 percent; myosin, 54 percent[5,6]). The two proteins are responsible for the transduction of chemical energy into mechanical work when a muscle contracts. The actin-myosin complex was early shown to hydrolyze ATP, thus linking these two proteins with the energy source for contraction.[7] It

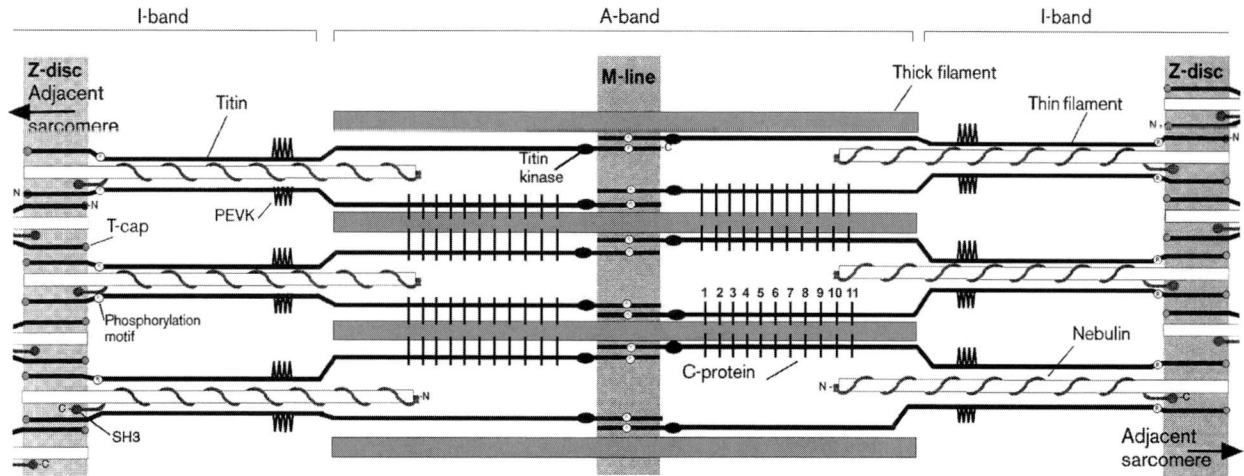

FIGURE 7-3. Schematic diagram of sarcomere summarizing organization and locations of major sarcomeric components. *(From Gregorio CC,* Granzier H, Sorimachi H, et al: Muscle assembly: A titanic achievement? Curr Opin Cell Biol 11:18, 1999. With permission from Elsevier Science.)

Table 7-1. PROPERTIES, LOCATION, AND FUNCTIONS OF THE MAJOR SARCOMERIC PROTEINS OF VERTEBRATE STRIATED MUSCLE[a]

PROTEIN	MW/SUBUNITS/ STRUCTURE/ ALIAS	LOCATION	MAJOR FUNCTIONS AND INTERACTIONS	DISEASE
Actin	42 kDa, globular monomer	Thin filament (~360 molecules), helical polymer	Filament formation, myosin ATPase activation, filament sliding. Binds myosin, tropomyosin, troponin, nebulin, α-actinin.	FHC, NM
α-actinin	190 kDa (homodimer 2 × 95 kDa); CH, spectrin-like, EF hand domains	Z filaments (?) linking actin and titin filaments	Integrates Z line. Binds actin, titin, CapZ, myopalladin, myozenin, myotilin, ZASP/Cypher, synemin.	
CapZ (β-actinin)	68 kDa, heterodimer (36- and 32-kDa subunits), 1 per filament	Caps barbed end of thin filament, in Z line	Length stabilization. Binds actin, α-actinin.	
Desmin/ vimentin	~55 kDa, α-helical core, nonhelical ends	Surrounds and runs between Z lines	Sarcomere strengthening and connection with each other and cell membrane.	Desmin myopathy
FATZ (calsarcin 2, myozenin)	32 kDa	Z line	Binds α-actinin, γ-filamin, telethonin.	
γ filamin	CH domain, Ig repeats	Z line	Binds myozenin, myotilin	
MM creatine kinase	86 kDa, dimer (2 × 43 kDa)	Line M4 and M4' of M line	Buffers [ATP], bridges thick filaments.	
M protein	165 kDa, Ig and Fn domains	Line M1 of M line	Bridges thick filaments. Binds myosin.	
Myomesin	185 kDa, Ig and Fn domains	M line	Binds myosin and titin (forming M-filaments?).	
Myopalladin	145 kDa	Z line	Anchors nebulin in Z line? Binds α-actinin, nebulin, and CARP.	
Myopodin	80–95 kDa	Z line	Bundles actin filaments. May signal between Z line and nucleus.	
Myosin	~520 kDa, hexamer, 2 heavy chains (223 kDa), 4 light chains (~20 kDa)	Thick filament (~300 molecules), helical polymer	Filament formation, ATPase, filament sliding, modulation of contraction. Binds actin, titin, MyBPs, M protein, myomesin.	FHC
MyBP-C (-X) and MyBP-H	140 kDa (C, X), 86 kDa (H) Modular (Ig and Fn domains)	Stripes 3–11 (C, X), 3 (H), 43 nm apart in each half of A band	Myofibrillogenesis, filament stabilization, modulation of contraction. Binds myosin, titin.	FHC
Myotilin	57 kDa	Z line	Binds α-actinin, γ-filamin.	MD
Nebulin (nebulette)	800 kDa (nebulette 109 kDa), single chain. Modular (35–amino acid actin-binding modules)	Extends from Z line (C terminus) to filament tip (N terminus)	Thin-filament length determination and stabilization. Binds actin, tropomyosin, tropomodulin, myopalladin.	NM
Nestin	220–240 kDa, IF protein	Z-line periphery, with desmin	Similar to synemin but mainly in developing muscle.	
Paranemin	180 kDa, IF protein	Z-line periphery, with desmin	Similar to synemin.	
Plectin	High molecular weight, α-helical coiled coil	IFAP, at and between Z lines	Connects Z-line IFs to actin filaments, cell membrane, and organelles. Binds actin, IFs.	MD
Skelemin	~200 kDa, modular structure, splice variant of myomesin	Periphery of M line	Connects myofibrils at M line. Binds myosin, IFs (?), and integrins.	

Table 7-1 (Continued). PROPERTIES, LOCATION, AND FUNCTIONS OF THE MAJOR SARCOMERIC PROTEINS OF VERTEBRATE STRIATED MUSCLE[a]

PROTEIN	MW/SUBUNITS/ STRUCTURE/ ALIAS	LOCATION	MAJOR FUNCTIONS AND INTERACTIONS	DISEASE
Synemin	230 kDa	Z-line periphery; co-polymer with desmin	Links between Z lines and to cell membrane. Binds α-actinin, vinculin.	
Syncoilin	64 kDa, IF protein	Z line and sarcolemma	Links IFs to sarcolemma via dystrophin complex?	
Telethonin (T-cap)	19 kDa	Z line, at N terminus of titin	Binds titin, myozenin, cell membrane K channel.	MD
Titin (connectin)	~3 MDa (single polypeptide). Modular (Ig and Fn domains, PEVK segment)	Extends from Z line (N terminus) to M line (C terminus)	Developmental sarcomeric template, muscle elasticity. Binds myosin, MyBP-C, α-actinin, myomesin, telethonin.	FHC
Tropomodulin (Tmod)	40 kDa, monomer, 1 or 2 per filament	Caps pointed end of thin filament	Thin-filament length stabilization. Binds actin, nebulin, tropomyosin.	
Tropomyosin	65 kDa, coiled-coil dimer of 2 α helices (32 kDa each)	Thin filament, ~50 molecules, 38-nm repeat	Filament stabilization and regulation. Binds actin, troponin, nebulin, tropomodulin.	FHC, NM
Troponin	80 kDa, complex of TnC (18 kDa), TnI (20–24 kDa), TnT (31–36 kDa)	Thin filament, one per tropomyosin, 38-nm repeat	Regulation of contraction. Binds actin, tropomyosin.	FHC
ZASP/Cypher	~32 kDa, PDZ-motif protein	Z line	Binds α actinin.	Myopathy

KEY: CH, calponin homology; MD, muscular dystrophy; NM, nemaline myopathy; FHC, familial hypertrophic cardiomyopathy.
[a] This table lists only the major and/or best-characterized proteins of the vertebrate sarcomere. For details on amorphin, Znin, and Z protein and for references from which the table data were obtained, see text.

was also found that synthetic threads of actomyosin contracted on addition of ATP,[8] thus linking chemical energy with mechanical work.

In addition to myosin, the thick filaments of vertebrate striated muscle contain significant quantities of nonmyosin proteins. These include myosin-binding proteins C, H, and X, which are present in the middle third of each half of the thick filaments, and myomesin, M protein, and creatine kinase, present in the M line. These proteins play primarily a structural role. The thick filaments are also associated along their length with the giant protein titin, which extends beyond the thick filaments and through the I band as far as the Z line. Titin is an elastic protein that appears to function to keep the A band centered and to ensure that equal forces are developed in the two halves of the A band. It also appears to function in development as a molecular template that defines the precise length and organization of the myosin filament. The thin filaments also contain components in addition to actin. The most important are troponin and tropomyosin, which form a complex involved in the regulation of contraction (see Chap. 13) in response to Ca^{2+}. The thin filaments contain, in addition, a second giant myofibrillar protein, nebulin,[9,10] which, like titin, appears to play a role in length determination. α-Actinin, together with at least 10 other proteins, constitutes the Z line, which functions to hold the thin filaments in a regular lateral array and to connect sarcomeres into the linear array of the myofibril. Intermediate filaments and associated proteins attach to the sarcomere at the M and Z lines, forming transverse links between adjacent myofibrils and maintaining them in register with each other across the fiber.

CONTRACTION OF MUSCLE: SLIDING FILAMENTS

It was long thought that actomyosin formed a single set of continuous filaments in each sarcomere and that contraction resulted from the large-scale shortening of the filaments brought about by some sort of internal folding.[11,12] The description of muscle structure given in the preceding pages (resulting from experiments in the early 1950s) suggested a quite different picture. X-ray diffraction patterns of muscle showed that the filaments were in fact present in a *double* hexagonal array,[3] and electron microscopy (EM) revealed that there were indeed two sets of filaments[1] (the actin and myosin filaments), overlapping but not continuous with each other[2] (Fig. 7-4). These results provided the basis for a radical revision of the contractile mechanism. H. E. Huxley and J. Hanson[13] and A. F. Huxley and R. Niedergerke[14] independently suggested that contraction was a result of the sliding of filaments past each other, producing greater overlap of the filaments without a change in their lengths (Fig. 7-5). This *sliding-filament* model was based on light microscopic observations that the A band remained constant in length during contraction, whereas the I band and H zone shortened. Subsequent EM observations, where the filaments were directly resolved, gave strong support to this model.[15] X-ray diffraction studies of living contracting muscle revealed essentially no change in the longitudinal spacings of actin and myosin molecules within the filaments when a muscle shortens,[16–18] thus supporting the view that the filaments remain constant in length when muscle contracts. The sliding-filament model is generally accepted as the mechanism by which muscles contract.

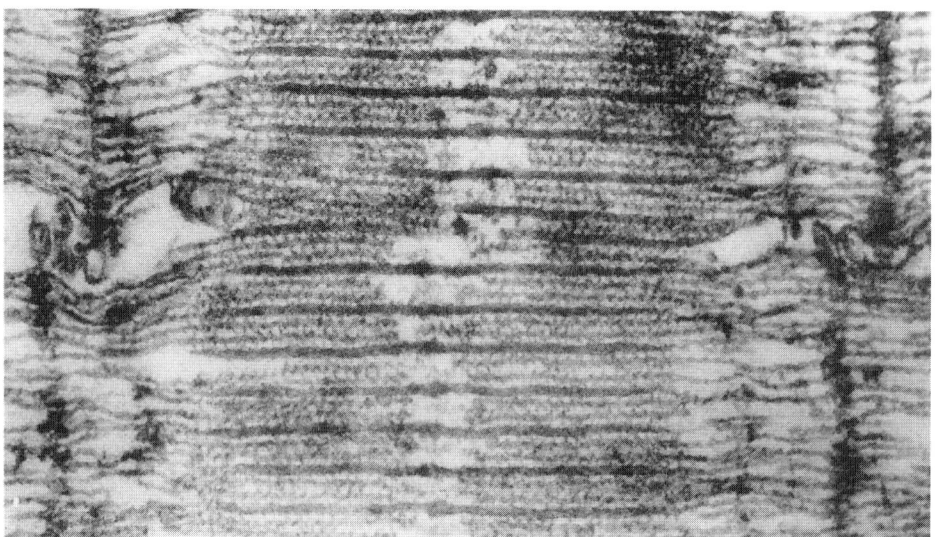

FIGURE 7-4. Electron micrograph of thin longitudinal section of rabbit psoas muscle revealing cross-bridges between thick and thin filaments in the A band. The appearance of two thin filaments between each pair of thick filaments is caused by the plane of section. (×100,000.) *(From Huxley HE: The double array of filaments in cross-striated muscle. J Biophys Biochem Cytol 3:631, 1957. By copyright permission of The Rockefeller University Press.)*

The Cross-Bridge Cycle

In his classic EM study of muscle, H. E. Huxley[2] observed that the thick filaments bore projections (cross-bridges) on their surfaces that formed links with the thin filaments in the region of filament overlap (Fig. 7-4; Color Plate 3e), and suggested that these cross-bridges could provide the mechanical link between thick and thin filaments necessary for sliding. Thus the sliding force could be generated by a change in conformation of the bridges while attached to actin. As the length of the cross-bridge was much less than the distance over which sliding could occur, it was suggested that cross-bridges might act cyclically: attaching to actin, changing conformation (and thus pulling on actin), detaching, then attaching again further along the filament and repeating the cycle.[12,19,20] In this way large-scale movement of filaments would occur by the addition of multiple small-scale cross-bridge movements, which would act to "row" the filaments past each other. This model of the cross-bridge cycle forms the focus of current biochemical, structural, and physiologic studies of the molecular mechanism of muscle contraction (see Chap. 9).

The Thick Filament

The thick filaments of vertebrate skeletal muscle are bipolar, spindle-shaped structures, 1.6 μm in length and ~15 nm in diameter.[21] They have a rough appearance along most of their length due to the presence of projections (the cross-bridges) except for a centrally located "bare zone," which is free of projections (Figs. 7-1C, 7-4, and 7-6). In the intact sarcomere, the bare zones are aligned owing to registration of the filaments, giving rise to a less dense region at the center of the A band in longitudinal section, referred to earlier as the pseudo-H zone.

In cross section, the thick filaments have different appearances, depending on the axial point at which they are sectioned (Fig. 7-1F). In the cross-bridge region, the filaments are roughly circular or polygonal in profile, and the projections appear as an ill-defined halo of lower density surrounding the dense, central backbone. In the bare zone, projections are absent and the backbone is triangular in shape. The backbone is also triangular near the filament tips. Cross sections of the M line show a circular filament backbone with dense bridges (consisting of nonmyosin proteins) radiating from each filament and connecting it to its six neighbors.

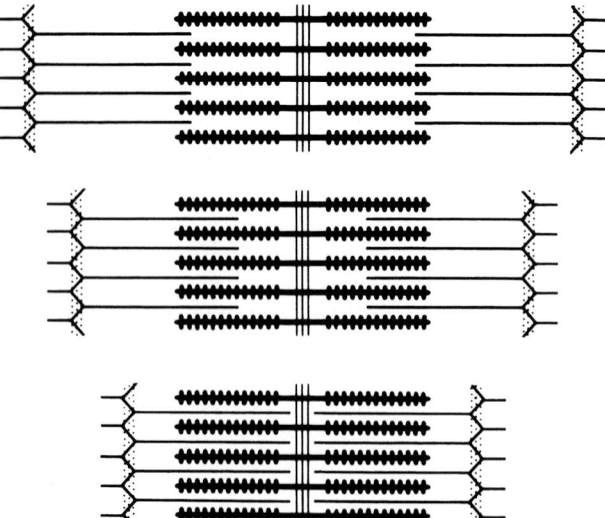

Figure 7-5. The sliding-filament model of muscle contraction. From top to bottom, the transition from the stretched to the contracted state. *(From Offer G: The molecular basis of muscular contraction, in Bull AT, Lagnado JR, Thomas JD, Tipton KF (eds): Companion to Biochemistry: Selected Topics for Further Study. London: Longman, 1974. By copyright permission of Longman Group Ltd.)*

POLYMERIZATION OF MYOSIN TO FORM FILAMENTS

The thick filament is a polymer containing about 300 molecules of the protein myosin II[21–23] together with nonmyosin

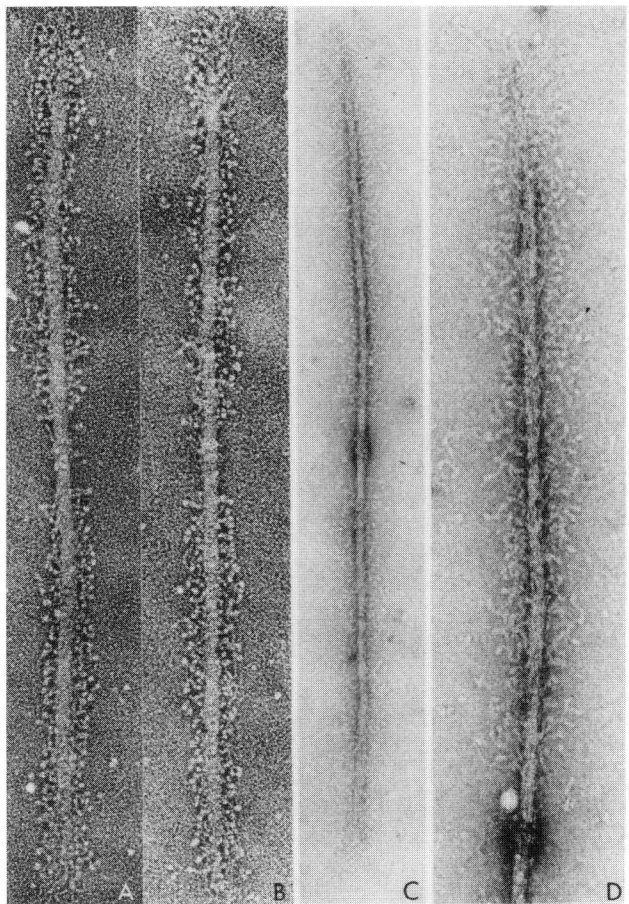

FIGURE 7-6. Native thick filaments from vertebrate skeletal muscle showing projections (cross-bridges) except in the central bare zone (at bottom in enlargement in D). A and B. Rotary shadowed with platinum. *(From Trinick J, Elliott A: Electron microscope studies of thick filaments from vertebrate skeletal muscle. J Mol Biol 131:133, 1979. With permission from Elsevier Science. C and D. Negatively stained with uranyl acetate. (Courtesy of J Trinick, P Knight.) (A, B, and C, ×70,000. D, ×130,000.)*

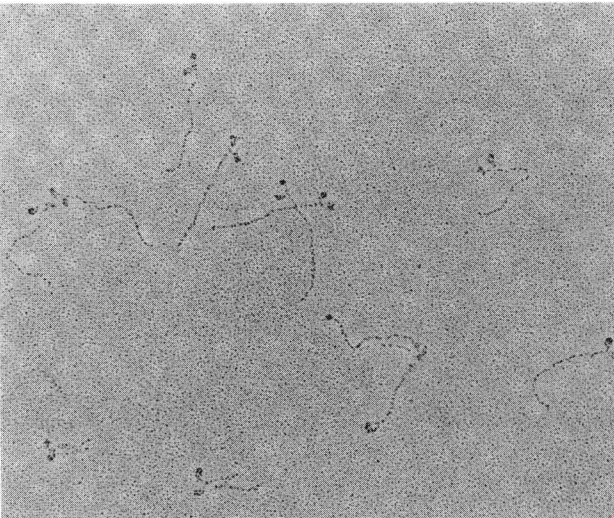

FIGURE 7-7. Electron micrograph of rotary shadowed myosin II molecules. (×100,000.) *(From Flicker PF, Wallimann T, Vibert P, et al: Electron microscopy of scallop myosin: Location of regulatory light chains. J Mol Biol 169:723, 1983. With permission from Elsevier Science.)*

spond to the cross-bridges seen to link thick and thin filaments in sections of muscle (Fig. 7-4) and to the projections seen on the surface of the backbone, giving it its rough appearance (Fig. 7-6).[21,26] The projections on the thick filament are often referred to as cross-bridges whether or not they actually link thick and thin filaments together.

STRUCTURE OF THE MYOSIN MOLECULE

The myosin molecule[23] (Chap. 8) is a hexamer consisting of two identical heavy chains (molecular mass 223 kDa[27]) and two pairs of light chains (molecular mass 15 to 22 kDa,

proteins. When thick filaments are treated with high-ionic-strength solution (e.g., 0.6 M KCl), they dissolve. The myosin molecules in solution consist of two globular "heads" attached by flexible hinges to an elongated and flexible "tail" (Fig. 7-7).[21,22,24]

When the ionic strength of a myosin solution is lowered to the physiologic range (0.15 M), the molecules spontaneously reassemble into filaments that resemble, in all but length, the native structure[21] (Fig. 7-8). The filaments, both short and long, have a central bare zone (0.15 to 0.2 μm long) and are rough along the rest of their length. This structure is readily accounted for by a simple model[21] (Fig. 7-9). The elongated myosin molecules initially associate in a tail-to-tail, antiparallel array (the "tail-only" region accounting for the bare zone), and the filaments elongate by staggered, head-to-tail, parallel addition of molecules at each end, possibly in the form of parallel dimers with a stagger of 43 nm between molecules.[25] The myosin tails form the backbone of the filament (biochemical studies show that the main part of the tail is insoluble at physiologic ionic strength), while the soluble globular regions (the heads) lie at the surface. The heads corre-

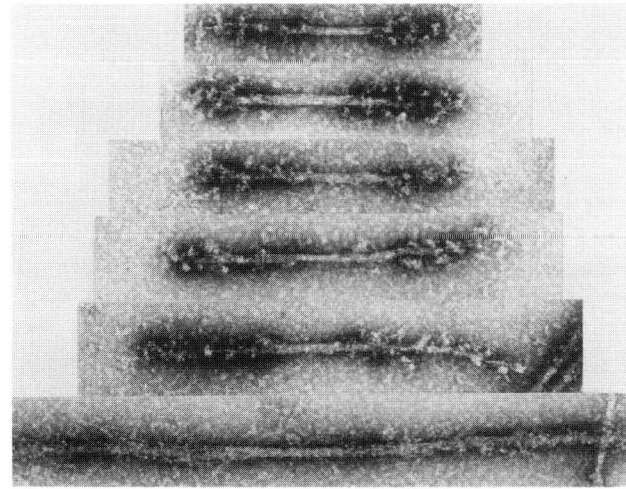

FIGURE 7-8. Electron micrographs of negatively stained synthetic myosin filaments at different stages of growth. (×65,000.) *(From Huxley HE: Electron microscope studies on the structure of natural and synthetic protein filaments from striated muscle. J Mol Biol 7:281, 1963. With permission from Elsevier Science.)*

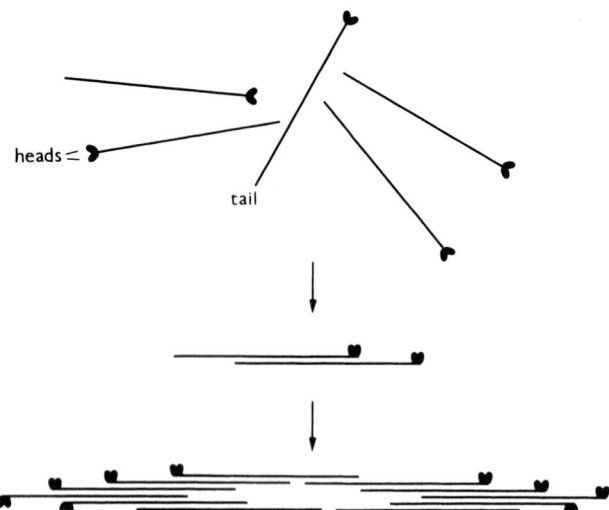

FIGURE 7-9. Model of the assembly of myosin molecules to form thick filaments. *(From Offer G: The molecular basis of muscular contraction, in Bull AT, Lagnado JR, Thomas JD, Tipton KF (eds): Companion to Biochemistry: Selected Topics for Further Study. London: Longman, 1974. By copyright permission of Longman Group Ltd.)*

depending on the source).[23,28] The heavy chains are α-helical for their C-terminal halves apart from the last ~20 residues at the C terminus;[29,30] they twist around each other, forming a stable, double-α-helical coiled-coil tail 155 nm long (Fig. 7-10).[22,24] In its N-terminal half, each heavy chain folds to form one globular, pear-shaped head about 19 nm long and 5 nm wide at its widest.[31] The light chains are of two chemically distinct classes, one of each class being associated with each head.

Myosin is both an enzyme (it hydrolyzes ATP) and a structural protein. Its unusual structure reflects the physical separation of its structural (the myosin tail) and enzymatic (the head) domains. Our understanding of the properties of these domains has been aided by studying fragments of the molecule produced by controlled enzymatic digestion. Digestion may occur near the middle of the tail (Fig. 7-10), producing light meromyosin (LMM), which is almost fully α-helical, and heavy meromyosin (HMM), which consists of the two heads attached to a shorter section of tail. LMM is insoluble at physiologic ionic strength and self-associates to form ordered aggregates.[22] HMM is soluble and has the ability both to hydrolyze ATP and to bind to actin. Myosin can alternatively be digested at the head-tail junction to produce myosin rod (the isolated myosin tail) and two subfragment 1 (S1) molecules (isolated myosin heads) (Fig. 7-10). S1 is soluble and has actin-binding and ATPase activity, while the rod is insoluble at physiologic ionic strength and associates to form paracrystals. Myosin rod can be further digested to form LMM and subfragment 2 (S2) of heavy meromyosin. S2 is more soluble than LMM, indicating a weaker tendency to self-associate.

The energy-transducing (ATPase) activity of myosin thus lies in the two heads. This activity is greatly boosted by interaction of the heads with actin. In contracting muscle, this interaction is coupled to a change in shape of the myosin head, which provides the driving force for filament sliding (see Chaps. 8 and 9). The filament-forming properties of myosin lie in the tail, especially LMM, which self-associates to form the filament backbone. The interactions involved generate a regular helical distribution of myosin heads at the filament surface (see below). S2 associates only weakly with itself or with LMM, allowing the myosin heads considerable flexibility in their interactions with actin.

Structure of the Myosin Head

Each myosin head (S1) has a molecular mass of 130 kDa.[32] S1 has been crystallized and its structure solved by x-ray crystallography[31,33] (see Color Plate 1c and d and Chap. 8). Its heavy chain comprises three domains, which have been detected proteolytically.[34] The three domains are arranged with the largest (50 kDa) segment at the N-terminal end. This is adjacent to the centrally located 25-kDa domain, with the 20-

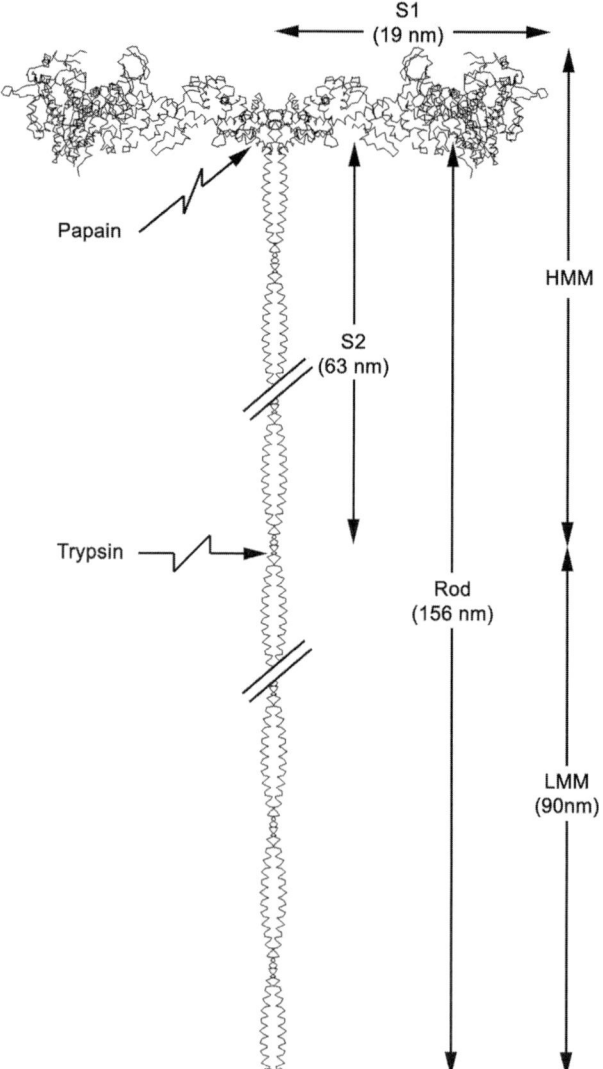

FIGURE 7-10. Diagram of the myosin molecule illustrating the α-helical coiled-coil tail, the folding of each heavy chain to form a globular head, and the principal sites of enzymatic attack by trypsin and papain to form myosin fragments. *(Adapted from Offer G, Knight P: The structure of the head-tail junction of the myosin molecule. J Mol Biol 256:407, 1996. With permission from Elsevier Science.)*

kDa (C-terminal) domain running as an α helix along the narrow neck region of the head, where it associates with the two light chains, to the junction with the tail.[31-33] The 75-kDa (50 + 25 kDa) part of the head is known as the *motor domain*, while the rest of the head, containing the two light chains and the 20-kDa heavy-chain domain, forms the *regulatory domain*, also known as the *lever arm* because of its lever-like function during contraction.[31-33] The ATPase site is 5 nm from the tip of the head and 4 nm away from and opposite to the actin-binding interface of S1.[31,33]

MOLECULAR ARRANGEMENT OF MYOSIN HEADS

Although electron micrographs of isolated thick filaments generally show a disordered array of myosin heads (Fig. 7-6), this is largely an artifact of the preparative method. X-ray diffraction patterns of resting, intact vertebrate muscle reveal that despite a degree of static or dynamic disorder,[36,37] perhaps related to the flexible attachment of the heads, the head origins are organized on a regular, 3D, approximately helical array[16] (Fig. 7-11; Color Plate 2d and e). This is confirmed by EM observations of filaments prepared gently to preserve the helical array (Fig. 7-12).[38-41] In all vertebrate striated muscles, the axial distance between adjacent levels of myosin heads is 14.3 nm and the repeat distance of the helix is three times this (43 nm).[16,42,43] These two characteristic parameters of the head arrangement are identical to periodicities observed in synthetic aggregates of myosin, rod, LMM, and S2, showing that the organization of myosin tails in the backbone dictates that of the heads on the surface.

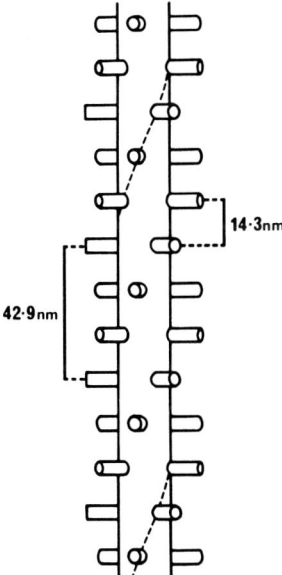

FIGURE 7-11. Schematic diagram of the arrangement of "crossbridges" in the three-stranded vertebrate thick filament. The peg-shaped bridges are purely schematic and should be interpreted to represent a pair of myosin heads, but not their detailed shape or disposition. *(From Offer G: The molecular basis of muscular contraction, in Bull AT, Lagnado JR, Thomas JD, Tipton KF (eds): Companion to Biochemistry: Selected Topics for Further Study. London: Longman, 1974. By copyright permission of Longman Group Ltd.)*

The helical arrangement of myosin heads is multistranded; that is, there are a number (N) of coaxial helices. Computer analysis of electron micrographs of well-ordered, negatively stained filaments shows that N (also referred to as the rotational symmetry) is three in vertebrates (Fig. 7-12D and E), and shadowing shows that the helices are right-handed (Fig. 7-12B and C).[44] The organization of the two heads within a molecule is uncertain. They may be splayed apart axially,[45,46] possibly interacting with heads of axially adjacent molecules in the same long-pitch helix (cf. Fig. 7-12F and G), or they may be parallel to each other (Color Plate 3d).[47,48] The helix appears to be slightly perturbed axially, radially, and azimuthally.[45]

Insights into the general principles of thick-filament structure have come from the study not only of vertebrate but also of invertebrate muscle. The thick filaments of invertebrates share a number of features in common with vertebrate thick filaments.[49] In all cases the myosin heads are spaced axially 14.3 or 14.5 nm apart and are arranged forming right-handed helices.[38,44,50,51] The heads are generally located close to the backbone surface, twisted around the filament, and usually axially splayed,[38,46,52,53] so that adjacent heads may interact with each other.[54] However, in contrast to vertebrate muscle, N varies from four to seven in different invertebrates[51] (Fig. 7-13), and the helical repeat ranges from 38.5 to 48.7 nm.[38,51,55-57] Despite these variations in structure, the local packing of molecules is thought to be very similar, with changes of bond angles and molecular twists being very small from one filament type to another.[56-59] Thus similar myosin-myosin interactions appear to underlie the diverse filament structures found throughout the animal kingdom.

The molecular organization of myosin heads on the thick filament has been studied in greatest detail in invertebrate muscle.[54,60,61] Fitting the atomic structure of S1[31] to the 3D structure of myosin filaments of tarantula muscle determined by EM[38] suggests that the two heads of a myosin molecule run along the helical ridges antiparallel to each other, such that oppositely oriented heads from axially adjacent molecules in a helix interact through contact of the motor domain of a head pointing toward the bare zone with the light-chain domain of the neighboring head pointing toward the Z line (Fig. 7-12G and Color Plate 1c and d).[54,60] This interaction may be important in stabilizing the helical organization present in muscles whose activity is regulated or modulated via their myosin molecules (see below)[60] but may be absent from vertebrate muscle, which is not myosin-regulated.[48]

Change in Organization of Myosin Heads on Activation

The ordered, helical arrangement of myosin heads described above requires the presence of ATP and absence of Ca^{2+} and is thus characteristic of the relaxed state. X-ray evidence indicates that hydrolyzed ATP (ADP.Pi) in the myosin nucleotide site favors helical order in the thick filaments of skeletal muscle.[62] When ATP is depleted (the rigor state), the heads not interacting with actin become disordered and project away from the filament backbone.[63-65] Similar disordering occurs when regulated invertebrate myosin filaments are activated, either by binding of Ca^{2+} to their heads[64] or by phosphory-

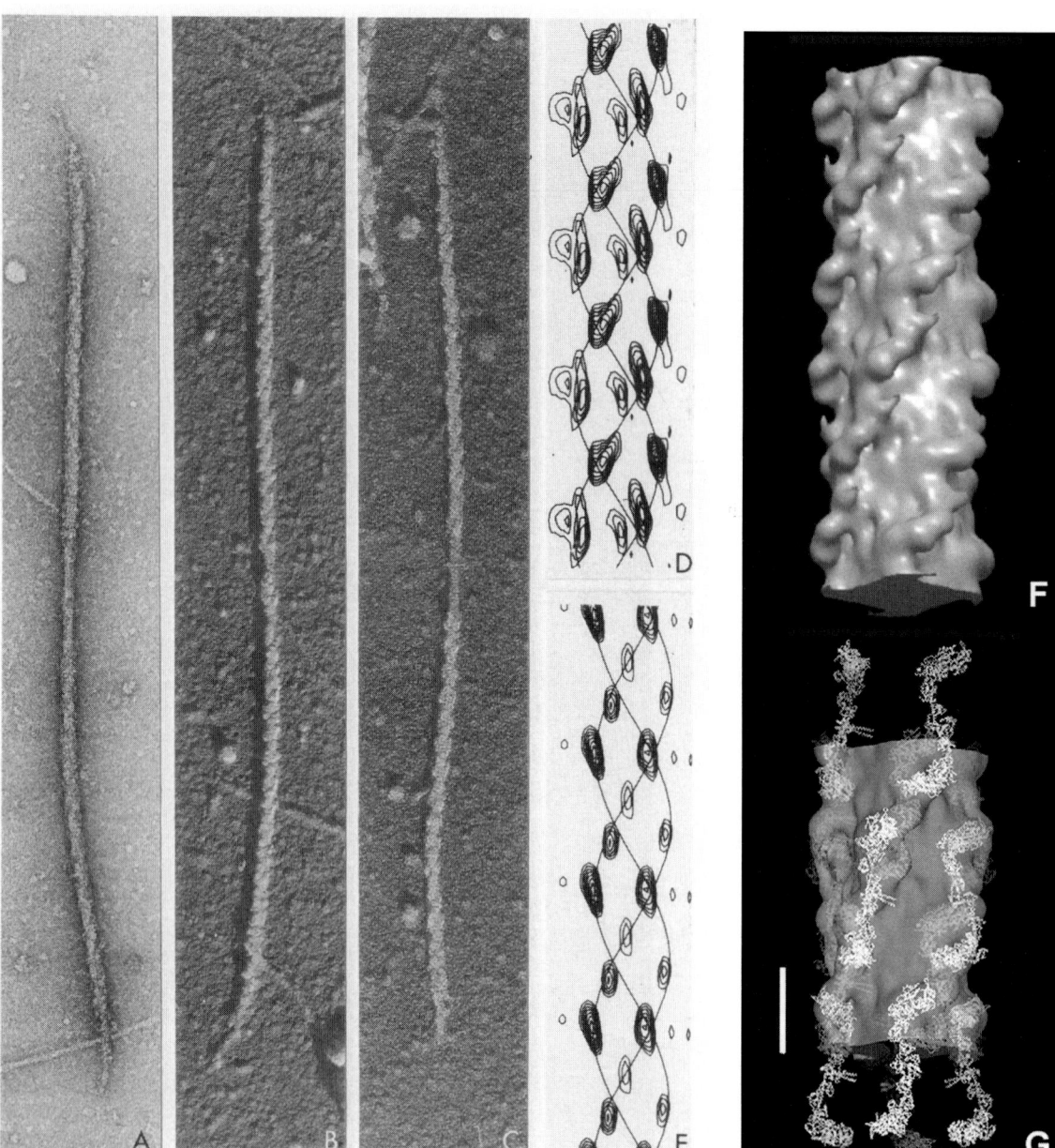

FIGURE 7-12. Electron micrographs, filtered images, and 3D reconstructions of striated muscle thick filaments. *A* to *C.* Vertebrate (frog) filaments: *A.* Negatively stained with uranyl acetate. *B* and *C.* Unidirectionally shadowed with platinum/carbon. The helical appearance is well seen by sighting along the filaments; the right-handed sense is especially clear in *B.* (*A* to *C* courtesy of R. Kensler.) *D* and *E.* Computer filtered images of negatively stained filaments similar to that in *A*, showing myosin cross-bridges every 14.3 nm along three helical strands. *A*, *B*, and *C.* (×92,000.) (*From Kensler RW, Stewart M: Frog skeletal muscle thick filaments are three stranded. J Cell Biol 96:1797, 1983. By copyright permission of The Rockefeller University Press.*) *F.* 3D reconstruction of tarantula myosin filaments showing four helices of myosin heads. (*From Padrón R, Alamo LA, Guerrero JR, et al: Three-dimensional reconstruction of thick filaments from rapidly frozen, freeze-substituted tarantula muscle. J Struct Biol 115:250, 1995. With permission from Elsevier Science.*) *G.* Fitting of atomic model of myosin head[31] to reconstruction shown in F revealing axial splaying of heads.[38] (*From Offer G, Knight PJ, Burgess SA, et al: A new model for the surface arrangement of myosin molecules in tarantula thick filaments. J Mol Biol 298:239, 2000. With permission.*) (A clearer rendition of *G* is seen in Color Plate 3d.) (Bar = 14.5 nm.)

lation of their regulatory light chains.[66] In the case of vertebrate[67] and some invertebrate striated muscles,[68] light-chain phosphorylation does not regulate but does appear to modulate interaction with actin—for example, by potentiating force at submaximal Ca^{2+} levels[67]—and phosphorylation is accompanied by a similar disordering of the myosin helices. X-ray diffraction indicates that the phosphorylation-induced loss of helical ordering is accompanied by a mass movement of the myosin heads of about 6 nm away from the backbone surface.[69] Activated or potentiated heads thus appear to be more loosely associated with the myosin backbone, which may facilitate their interaction with actin during contraction.

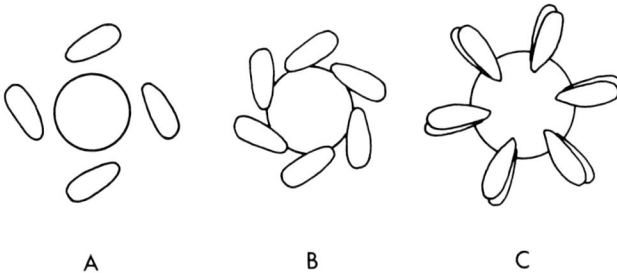

FIGURE 7-13. Cross-sectional views illustrating the diversity of cross-bridge location and configuration in invertebrate myosin filaments (deduced from x-ray diffraction). *A.* Horseshoe crab *(Limulus);* B. lobster *(Homarus);* C. scallop *(Placopecten).* (From Wray JS, Vibert PJ, Cohen C: Diversity of cross-bridge configurations in invertebrate muscles. Nature 257:561, 1975. By copyright permission of Nature Publishing Group.)

STRUCTURE OF THE THICK-FILAMENT BACKBONE

The backbone of the myosin filament consists mainly of staggered, closely packed myosin tails running approximately parallel to the filament axis, as suggested by EM of thick filaments (Fig. 7-6D)[38,70] and by x-ray diffraction of muscle.[59,71] The insolubility of LMM under physiologic conditions indicates that it constitutes the central, most tightly bound portion of the myosin molecule, while the more soluble S2 runs along the surface of the filament, where it is bound less strongly. The detailed packing of the myosin tails within the backbone, however, has been difficult to elucidate because of the extreme length (155 nm), narrow diameter (2 nm), and tight packing of the tails.

Insights into the organization and interactions of myosin tails within the backbone have come from EM and sequence analysis. Synthetic assemblies of myosin and its fragments show that all parts of the myosin molecule affect the structure of the thick filament.[22,25] LMM can adopt many modes of assembly, such as paracrystalline arrays and sheets, generally exhibiting the 43- and 14.3-nm periodicities of the native filament. Myosin rod is less polymorphic, forming sheets or filaments generally with a 14.3-nm repeat. Thus the presence of S2 restricts the interactions of LMM to a narrower range. S2 itself is soluble under physiologic conditions but forms aggregates with a 14.3-nm periodicity at its isoelectric point, suggesting that it interacts only weakly with the thick-filament backbone. Whole myosin molecules form filaments rather than sheets or paracrystals, implying that the heads limit the lateral extent of aggregation.

Sequence analysis of the myosin tail reveals several striking features.[72] The α-helical probability profile is high almost everywhere. The sequence shows a marked seven-residue hydrophobic repeat (Fig. 7-14A to C), consistent with Crick's "knobs-into-holes" model for the stable packing of two helices in a coiled coil [the hydrophobic residues stabilize the structure by interacting with each other in the core of the coiled coil (Fig. 7-14A), while the hydrophilic residues lie at the surface].[73] There is also a larger repeating structural unit with a length of 28 residues, in which a region of peak positive charge is separated from one of peak negative charge by 14 residues (one half zone) (Fig. 7-14B and C). Calculations show that there should be strong charge attractions between tails when they are staggered by an odd multiple of 14 residues and that the attractions should be especially strong when the staggers are 98 or 294 residues, corresponding to displacements of 14.6 and 43.7 nm between adjacent tails. The charge distribution on the myosin tail can thus approximately account for the two fundamental periodicities seen in myosin

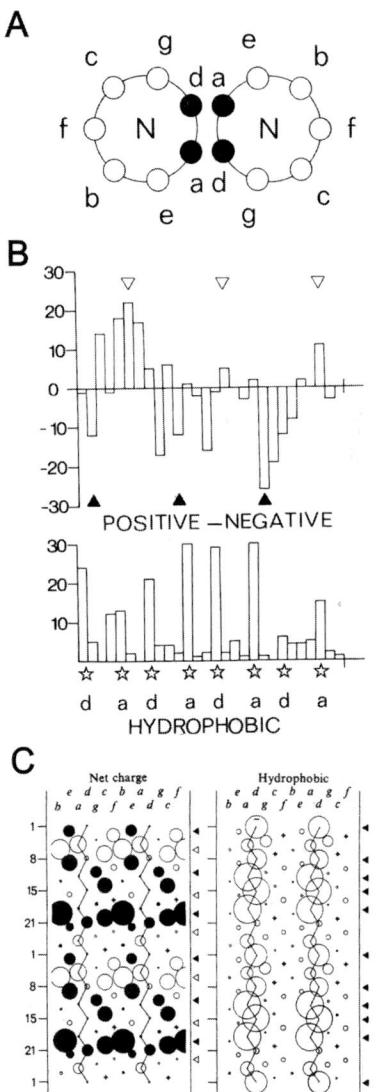

FIGURE 7-14. Periodic distribution of amino acids in the myosin tail. *A.* View down the axis of the two chains in a coiled-coil α helix showing amino acids in one repeat (seven residues) of each chain. Amino acids at *a* and *d* interact along the line of contact, and electrostatic interactions between *e* and *g* stabilize the interaction. *B.* Histograms of amino acid distributions (top, net charge; bottom, hydrophobic residues) in the 28-residue repeats in the myosin tail. *C.* Charge distribution and hydrophobic residues for the averaged 28-residue repeats projected onto a cylinder and unrolled so that each section of sequence appears twice side by side, first on one helix and then on the other. Inner positions *a, d* (see A) are connected by a zig-zag line. Circles (white: positive, black: negative) have radii proportional to the numbers in B. Triangles mark bands of charge. Hydrophobic residues are plotted similarly, with triangles marking major sites. (From McLachlan AD, Karn J: Periodic charge distributions in the myosin rod amino acid sequence match cross-bridge spacings in muscle. Nature 299:226, 1982. With permission from Nature Publishing Group.)

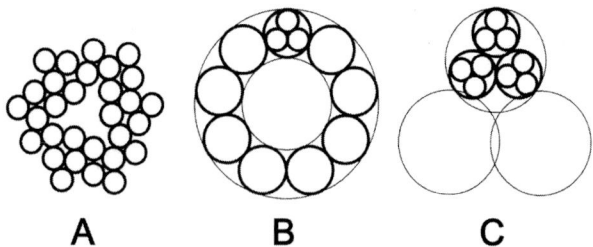

FIGURE 7-15. Hypothetical models for the packing of myosin tails in the vertebrate thick-filament backbone. A. Curved molecular crystalline model, with close-packed myosin tails. B. Simple subfilament model, consisting of nine straight subfilaments, each about 4 nm in diameter and containing three supercoiling tails. C. Myosin tails packed into subfilaments, each containing three molecules, with these subfilaments themselves forming larger subfilaments. This model would be consistent with the fraying shown in Fig. 7-17. (From Chew MW, Squire JM: Packing of α-helical coiled-coil myosin rods in vertebrate muscle thick filaments. J Struct Biol 115:233,1995. With permission from Elsevier Science.)

filaments. This finding suggests that the bonds stabilizing the thick filament are largely electrostatic, as is also implied by the solubility of myosin in high salt solution. The preceding modeling was simplified by averaging the charges around the helix circumference. A more realistic understanding is now possible by 3D modeling of the amino acid side chains.[74]

Experiments on the assembly properties of mutant LMMs suggest that the molecular mechanism of the polymerization of myosin tails to form the backbone is more complex than simple charge complementation, which, instead of being the major driving force in polymerization, may serve to prevent unfavorable interaction geometries by influencing the detailed axial stagger of the interacting molecules.[75,76] C-terminal residues of the myosin tail are nonhelical and mobile and appear to have a major effect on the assembly of myosin tails into the filament backbone,[29,30] possibly functioning as a cement filling the empty spaces remaining after the tail aggregation.[29] A specific sequence near the C terminus of the coiled-coil region of the myosin heavy chain is necessary for the formation of ordered paracrystals.[77]

Although in vitro studies of myosin and its fragments and analysis of their sequences provide a general understanding of filament formation, the mechanism of assembly in vivo remains unknown. Filaments resembling the native structure can be formed synthetically from intact myosin,[21] but their lengths are variable compared with the constant 1.6-μm length observed in vertebrate muscle. Several factors could be important in filament structure and assembly, including the presence of a protein template (titin), the presence of myosin-binding protein C (MyBP-C) or other myosin-binding proteins, and—in invertebrates—a variety of other proteins implicated in thick-filament structure or assembly.[78–81] The list of thick-filament components is still likely to be incomplete.

Models of Backbone Structure

A number of models have been put forward to account for the main features of the backbone structure of myosin filaments.[56–59,82–84] These models use equivalent or quasi-equivalent interactions between myosin tails that are similar between species, with only slight changes in interaction leading to the diverse structures that are found in the animal kingdom.[56–59,82] One set of models, based on x-ray diffraction studies from vertebrate muscle,[71] is built from single myosin tails organized into a curved molecular crystal (Fig. 7-15A). Another, based on x-ray diffraction[56,82] and EM observations[38,70,87,88] of a 4-nm side spacing of backbone subunits, is built from 4-nm-diameter subfilaments (containing varying numbers of myosin molecules), staggered by 14.5 nm, that associate to form the filament (Figs. 7-15B and 7-16). A third set of models, based on EM studies (Fig. 7-17),[89,90] suggests the presence of three larger (6-nm-diameter) subfilaments, possibly built from the smaller ones (Fig. 7-15C).[58,59,83–86] The evidence between these models is still conflicting, and a molecular model integrating both the backbone substructure and the helices of myosin heads is still lacking.

MYOSIN-BINDING PROTEINS

A set of proteins that bind to myosin at regular intervals along the thick filament is found in all vertebrate striated muscles, both cardiac and skeletal (Figs. 7-1C, 7-3, and 7-18), where they were first noted on the basis of x-ray diffraction and EM.[16,92] These additional proteins (up to 15 percent of the thick-filament mass) are absent from smooth, invertebrate, and nonmuscle cells and can thus be considered as specializations of the highly ordered A bands of vertebrates.[91] Biochemically they were detected as persistent

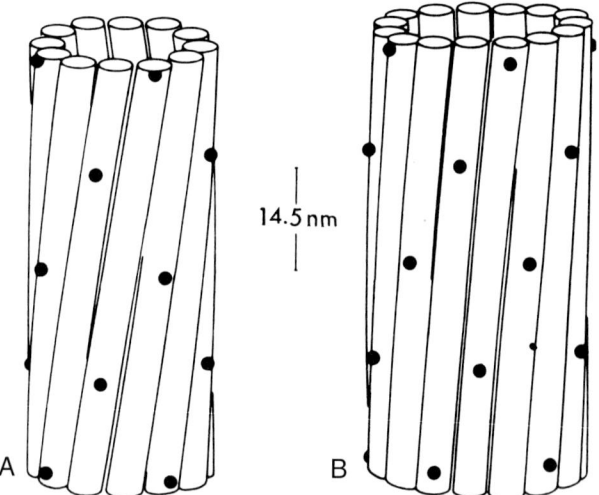

FIGURE 7-16. Models of backbone structure in crustacean thick filaments from fast (A) and slow (B) muscle fibers, based on x-ray diffraction data. The filaments have different diameters, different rotational symmetries (A: N = 4, B: N = 5), and different helical repeats. Nevertheless, the basic structures are very similar: Each consists of 4-nm-diameter subfilaments containing three molecules at any cross-sectional level. The filaments differ in the number (3 N) of subfilaments and slightly in the tilt of the subfilaments, giving rise to the different helical repeats. Black spots represent the positions of cross-bridge origins. (Wray JS: Structure of the backbone in myosin filaments of muscle. Nature 277:37, 1979. By copyright permission of Nature Publishing Group.)

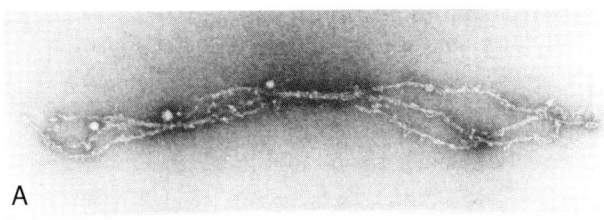

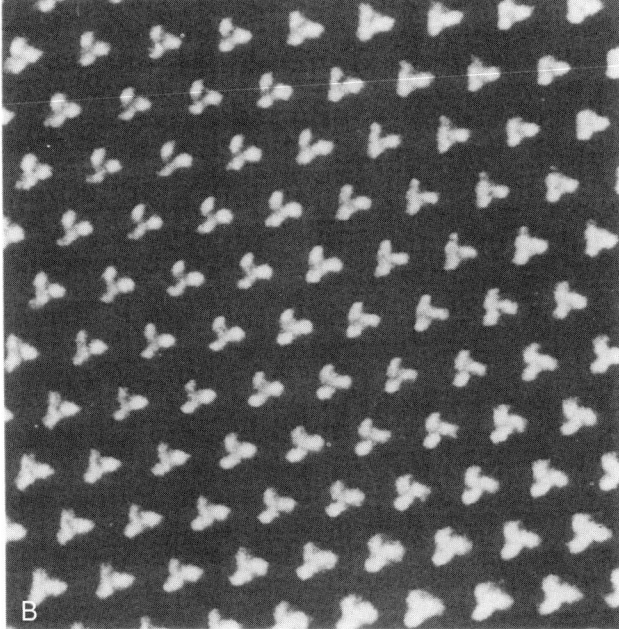

FIGURE 7-17. A. Rat psoas thick filament after treatment with low-ionic-strength buffer, showing fraying of filament into three similar subfilaments in each half. (×50,000.) *(Trinick JA: End filaments. A new structural element of vertebrate skeletal muscle thick filaments. J Mol Biol 151:309, 1981. With permission from Elsevier Science.)* B. Transverse section of fish muscle in the bare zone, showing three subunits in the filament backbone (printed in reverse contrast so that the filaments appear white). (× 220,000.) *(From Luther PK, Munro PMG, Squire JM: Three-dimensional structure of the vertebrate muscle A-band III. M-region structure and myosin filament symmetry. J Mol Biol 151:703; 1981. With permission from Elsevier Science.)*

impurities in myosin preparations, suggesting that they had a high affinity for myosin. The myosin-binding proteins, named alphabetically according to their mobility on SDS polyacrylamide gels,[93] form a closely related family. C protein,[94] or myosin-binding protein C (MyBP-C), is the most abundant and occurs as three distinct isoforms: cardiac, fast (white) skeletal, and slow (red) skeletal (also known as MyBP-X).[91] MyBP-H can be considered a low-molecular-weight isoform of MyBP-C, with which it has sequence homology.

The distribution of MyBP-C, -H, and -X is complex. While only cardiac MyBP-C occurs in cardiac muscle, the distribution of MyBP-C, -X, and -H varies between fiber types and subtypes of skeletal muscle, with one, two, or all three proteins occurring in any one fiber.[91] MyBP-C is found in fast white fibers, often with MyBP-H, but is absent from red fibers. Conversely, slow red muscles have only MyBP-X.[91] At the ultrastructural level, nonmyosin proteins are detected on the thick filament as a series of 11 transverse stripes in the central region of each half of the A band (Figs 7-3 and 7-18), at distances equal to the myosin helical repeat, that is, one stripe for every third level of myosin molecules. The precise positioning of the myosin-binding proteins appears to be dictated by the presence of binding sites on titin at these positions[91] (see "Titin Filaments," below). The distribution of the myosin-binding proteins among these stripes is again complex, varying with fiber type and species. In general, the outer 9 of the 11 stripes (3 to 11) are occupied by a form of MyBP-C or MyBP-H. In rabbit, the simplest pattern occurs in red fibers, which have 9 stripes of MyBP-X.[91] MyBP-C occurs in 8 stripes in fast white fibers, and 7 in fast intermediate fibers. MyBP-H occurs in a single stripe (stripe 3) in fast white and fast intermediate fibers. In all cases the innermost two stripes are apparently occupied by additional myosin-binding proteins that have not yet been identified.

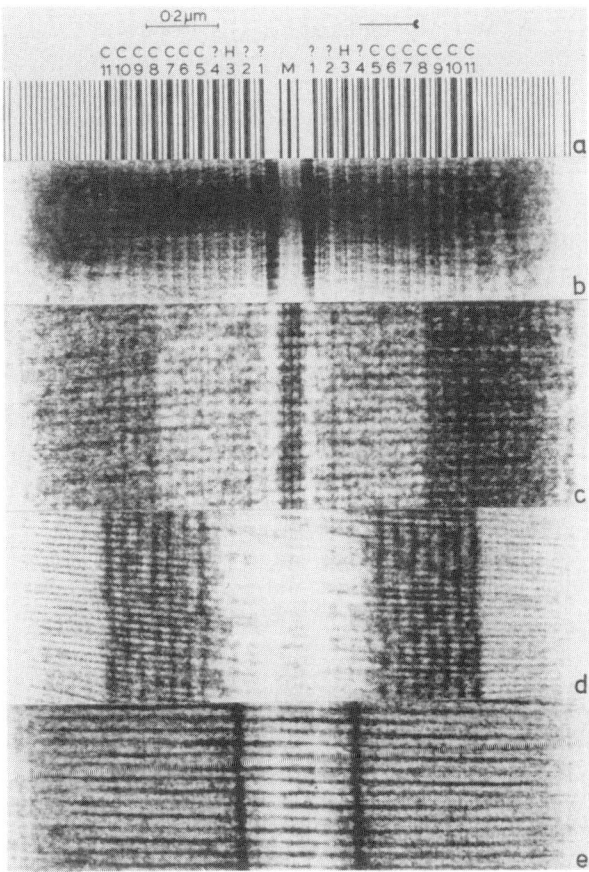

FIGURE 7-18. Nonmyosin components in vertebrate skeletal muscle thick filaments. A. Schematic diagram of 11 stripes of nonmyosin proteins superimposed on array of cross-bridges with 14.3-nm periodicity. B. Negatively stained frog A segment with nonmyosin protein showing as prominent white stripes. C. Positively stained section of frog A band, with nonmyosin proteins showing as narrow dark lines. D. Rabbit muscle with antibodies to C protein labeling stripes 5 to 11. E. Rabbit muscle with antibodies to H-protein labeling stripe 3. All micrographs have the same magnification: The lengths of the A bands appear different because of the variable contrast at the ends. (× 50,000.) *(From Craig R, Megerman J: Electron microscope studies on muscle thick filaments, in Pepe FA, Sanger JW, Nachmias VT (eds): Motility in Cell Function. New York, Academic Press; 1979, p 91.)*

Structure and Interactions with Myosin

MyBP-C and -X are single-chain rod-like molecules with a length of ~40 nm and molecular mass 130 to 150 kDa.[91] The stoichiometry suggests that three molecules of MyBP-C bind to each stripe, one for each of the three coaxial myosin helices. Like several other sarcomeric proteins (titin, myomesin, and M protein), MyBP-C, -X, and -H are made largely from globular immunoglobulin-like (Ig) and fibronectin type III-like (Fn) domains, each containing about 100 amino acids (Fig. 7-19).[91,95] Both types of domain are stable β barrels consisting of 7 antiparallel β sheets. Sequence conservation is limited to the few residues specifying the 3D fold of the barrels, while a higher degree of variability is allowed for the surface residues, thus giving a versatile modular design that can provide distinct ligand-binding properties on the surface.[96] Skeletal MyBP-C and -X (~130 kDa) have 10 such domains, C1 to C10. C1 is flanked amino-terminally by a pro/ala- (PA) rich unique sequence of 50 amino acids, and carboxy-terminally by a 100–amino acid unique sequence called the MyBP-C motif. Cardiac MyBP-C (140 kDa), has an additional Ig domain (C0) preceding the PA sequence.[91] These proteins are well conserved between species and isoforms, conservation being highest at the C terminus. MyBP-H has 4 Ig/Fn domains following a unique N terminus.

The myosin-binding proteins attach to the thick filament via both C- and N-terminal domains (Fig. 7-19). The C terminus binds both to the LMM portion of myosin and to titin, while the N terminus binds to a specific region on myosin S2, close to the myosin head.[97,98] The N terminus of the MyBP-C motif contains three sites, which in the cardiac isoform can be phosphorylated by cAMP-dependent protein kinase,[99] modulating cardiac contractility. Structurally, it has been suggested that MyBP-C may be arranged with its C-terminal end lying along the filament, close to the backbone, while its N terminus runs transversely, accounting for the stripes. In this orientation it could form a collar around the thick filament, holding the heads of every third level of cross-bridges back against the filament backbone,[91,97] or it could project out as flexible arms, possibly, under some conditions, interacting with the neighboring actin filaments.[71]

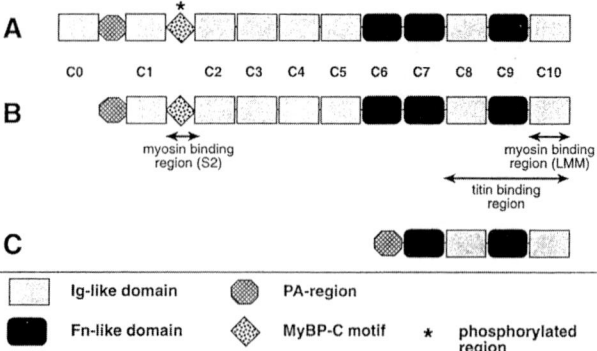

FIGURE 7-19. Domain organization in C-protein isoforms and in the closely related H protein. *A.* Cardiac C protein, *B.* skeletal C protein, *C.* H protein. (From Bennett PM, Fürst DO, Gautel M: The C-protein (myosin binding protein C) family: Regulators of contraction and sarcomere formation? *Rev Physiol Biochem Pharmacol* 138:203, 1999. With permission from Springer-Verlag.)

The confinement of MyBP-C to the middle third of each half of the A band is related to changes in the packing of the underlying myosin tails and the positions of superrepeats in the sequence of titin as one moves from the bare zone to the filament tip[91] (see "Titin Filaments," below). In the first 0.15 μm of myosin heads (no MyBP-C, but ultrastructurally appearing to contain other myosin-binding proteins on stripes 1 and 2), changes in packing occur during the transition from antiparallel to parallel myosin-tail interactions (Fig. 7-9); in the MyBP-C region, where only parallel interactions occur, the myosin packing is approximately constant, producing seven similar MyBP-C binding sites; toward the ends of the filament (no MyBP-C), the packing must again change as the number of molecules in cross section declines toward the tip.[100] The presence of MyBP-C every 43 nm, and not every 14.3 nm in the region of "constant" packing, means that the myosin molecules are not equivalent to each other but are in three different environments, depending on their proximity to a MyBP-C molecule and their binding to a specific part of the underlying titin superrepeat.

Function

The myosin-binding proteins appear to play at least three crucial roles in muscle. MyBP-C is essential to filament formation in myofibrillogenesis; its very precise organization on the thick filament suggests a structural role; and it modulates contractility of cardiac muscle.

MyBP-C is expressed at the earliest times of development, at the same time as titin and myosin. Deletion mutants show that the C-terminal four domains of MyBP-C must be expressed for correct incorporation into the thick filament and correct sarcomere assembly to occur.[101] It appears that during development, a cytoskeletal scaffold consisting first of titin, then myomesin, and finally MyBP-C is formed, and only then does myosin become organized into the repeating sarcomere pattern of mature myofibrils.[102] It was early on suggested that the precision of length determination of the thick filaments might be explained by a vernier mechanism involving coassembly of two components (e.g., myosin and MyBP-C) with slightly different periodicities.[16,91] It now appears unlikely that MyBP-C functions in this way—the strong binding of MyBP-C to myosin suggests that they will have the same periodicity. This conclusion is supported by the small axial extent of MyBP-C (possibly ~20 nm[91]), which appears too short to generate its own ~43-nm periodicity independently of myosin, by the apparent identity of the myosin and MyBP-C periodicities,[103] and most compellingly by the fact that titin appears to be a myosin template, obviating the need for an additional length-determining mechanism (see "Titin Filaments," below).

In addition to its role in development, MyBP-C may also serve a structural role, helping to stabilize the organization of myosin molecules by its multiple thick-filament binding sites. If its N-terminal S2-binding region wraps around the filament,[91,94,97,104] for example, it may help to keep the heads close to the backbone at rest. X-ray diffraction suggests that, during activation, MyBP-C becomes disordered, possibly due to movement of the underlying myosin heads.[91]

MyBP-C also appears to play a role in modulating contractility, apparently limiting shortening velocity and restricting the range of movement of some myosin molecules.[105,106] These constraints are apparently exerted through binding of the N-terminal region of MyBP-C to S2.[97–99] Triphosphorylation of this domain in cardiac MyBP-C by cAMP-dependent protein kinase in response to β-adrenergic stimulation abolishes the S2 interaction, freeing the set of myosin heads close to MyBP-C from the steric constraints it imposes, and increasing contractility.[97,99] Skeletal muscle MyBP-C is not a substrate for such phosphorylation, and these S2/MyBP-C interactions are therefore constitutively on.[97]

The critical importance of MyBP-C in muscle function is reflected most dramatically by its involvement in the class of diseases known as familial hypertrophic cardiomyopathy (FHC) (see "Diseases of the Sarcomere," below). At least 29 mutations have been found in MyBP-C, causing more cases of FHC than any other sarcomeric protein apart from the myosin heavy chain.[91] This is easily understood when one considers the crucial roles played by MyBP-C in both myofibril assembly and cardiac contractile function.

The M Line

STRUCTURE

The striking regularity of filaments in the sarcomere is not a result of the self-assembly properties of their constituent proteins alone but involves specific interactions with a cytoskeletal lattice, which holds them in register.[96] In the case of the thick filaments, this lattice is a structure known as the M line, an ~80-nm-wide transverse band at the center of the A band (Fig. 7-1), which contains protein bridges linking each thick filament to its six neighbors (Fig. 7-20). Intermediate filaments also attach at the M line and run transversely, connecting adjacent myofibrils to each other (see "Intermediate Filaments," below). The M line appears in longitudinal sections of muscle as an electron-dense band with additional fine structure consisting of three to five thin, densely stained lines about 20 nm apart (Figs. 7-1C and 7-18). In the terminology developed to describe the M line, the central line is known as M1, the neighboring strong lines 22 nm on either side of M1 are termed M4 and M4' (Fig. 7-21C), and the additional lines seen in some M lines 22 nm further out are the M6 and M6' lines.[107] These lines, and the underlying density, consist of nonmyosin protein. Additional finer stripes that have been attributed to staining of the antiparallel-packed myosin tails are also seen (Fig. 7-18B).[107]

The detailed structure of the M line varies between fiber types.[96,108,109] Fast (type II) fibers show three lines (M1, M4, and M4'), while slow (type I) fibers have four strong lines (M4, M4', M6, and M6', with M1 absent). Intermediate-speed fibers have all five lines. The consistent presence of M4 lines in all muscles suggests that bridges in this position (see below) are important for the integrity of the A band.[110]

In transverse sections, the M line appears as a hexagonal array of bridges joining each thick filament to its six neighbors (Figs. 7-1F and 7-20).[111–114] A set of such bridges probably corresponds to each of the three main transverse lines seen in longitudinal sections (M1, M4, and M4').[114] Some studies

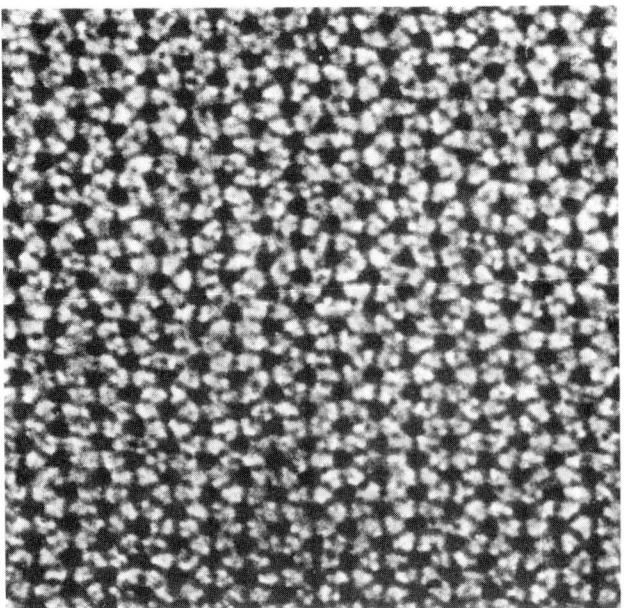

FIGURE 7-20. Transverse section of frog sartorius muscle in the M-line region. (× 125,000.) *(Luther P, Squire J: Three-dimensional structure of the vertebrate muscle M-region. J Mol Biol 125:313, 1978. With permission from Elsevier Science.)*

have suggested the presence of fine "M filaments," 5 nm in diameter, attached to the bridges and running parallel to the thick filaments, these M filaments themselves being attached to each other by finer bridges (Fig. 7-21A,B).[111,112] Another model suggests a structure consisting of a protein collar around the myosin backbone and a network of obliquely oriented struts, which connect at three nodal points between the filaments, giving rise to the three stripes[115] but no M filaments or subsidiary bridges. Some of these differences might arise from the study of different species of muscle.

PROTEIN COMPONENTS AND INTERACTIONS

The M line contains at least three specific M-line proteins—creatine kinase, M protein, and myomesin—in addition to overlapping portions of myosin tails, the C terminus of titin, and skelemin, a peripheral component that may link M lines to intermediate filaments.[96,108]

Creatine kinase[96,116–118] is a dimeric globular protein consisting of two subunits of molecular mass 43 kDa. It buffers cellular ATP and ADP concentrations by catalyzing the reversible exchange of high-energy phosphate bonds between phosphocreatine and ADP, regenerating ATP from ADP produced during contraction.[119] At least five isoforms of creatine kinase exist. MM-CK is a cytosolic form found in several domains of the myofiber where ATP consumption is high. The M line accounts for 5 to 10 percent of the total MM-CK. Antibody labeling suggests that it contributes to the M4 and M4' bridges and thus functions as both a structural protein and an enzyme.

M protein and myomesin are both modular proteins consisting mostly of Fn- and Ig-like domains, as found in MyBP-C and titin (Fig. 7-21F).[96] They have the same core domain

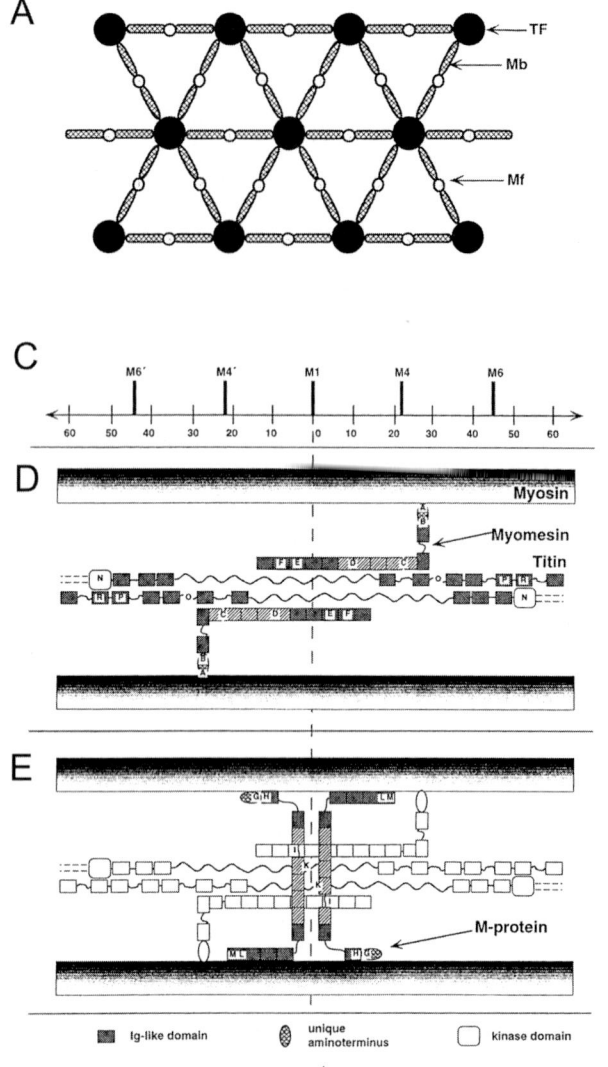
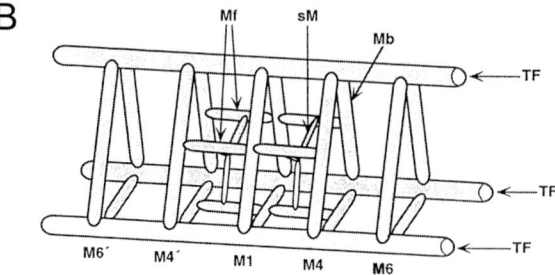
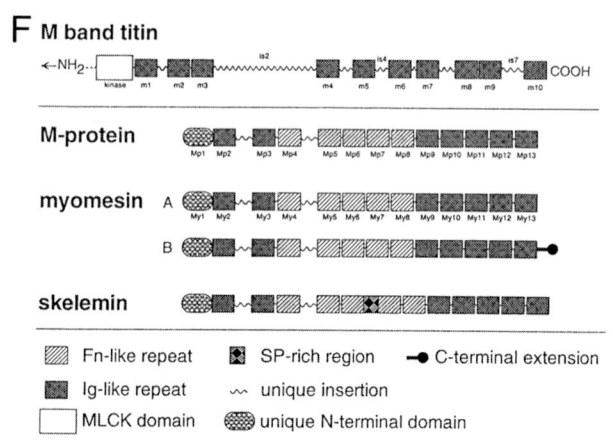

FIGURE 7-21. M-line models. *A.* Transverse view at M4 level, showing thick filaments (TF), M bridges (Mb), and M filaments (Mf). *B.* Suggested 3D model based on electron microscopy; sMs are secondary M bridges. *C.* M-line nomenclature and scale in nanometers. *D* and *E.* Proposed arrangement of titin, myomesin, and M protein based on immuno-electron microscopic observations. *F.* Domain structure of M-line titin, M protein, myomesin, and skelemin. *(From Fürst DO, Obermann WM, van der Ven PF: Structure and assembly of the sarcomeric M band. Rev Physiol Biochem Pharmacol 138:163, 1999. With permission from Springer-Verlag.)*

organization as each other, with >50 percent identical residues, the differences being limited to the C- and N-terminal regions. M protein[120,121] is a flexible ~165-kDa monomer, 36 nm long and 4 nm wide, present only in cardiac and fast skeletal fibers.[122] It interacts with myosin in a phosphorylation-dependent way but not with creatine kinase.[96,123] Antibody labeling suggests that its central region corresponds to the M1 line, with its N- and C-terminal regions organized along neighboring thick filaments (Fig. 7-21E). Thus, in cardiac and fast skeletal muscle (the only muscles having M protein and M1 lines), M protein could provide a link between the thick filaments at M1, in addition to those at M4 and M4', to meet the greater stresses in these muscles.[96] Myomesin[124] is a flexible segmented rod, 50 nm long and 4 nm wide, with a molecular mass of 185 kDa, present in both fast and slow fibers. Its N-terminal region binds to LMM,[125] and its central region interacts with the C-terminal end of titin. The binding of myomesin to titin and myosin suggests that one of its major roles is to link titin molecules to the thick filament.

Skelemin is also built from Fn and Ig domains in an identical order to those in M protein and myomesin. It appears, in fact, to be a splice variant encoded by the same gene as myomesin.[96,126] One unique feature of skelemin is two motifs that have been suggested to be like intermediate filaments, which may specify its incorporation into desmin intermediate filaments encircling the sarcomere at the M line.[127] It is also possible that another unique feature, a serine/proline-rich region, is responsible for the specific targeting of skelemin.[96]

MODEL

The relationship between the proteins and structural components of the M line is not yet known with any certainty.

Based on earlier antibody labeling and protein interaction studies, it was suggested, for example, that the primary bridges at M4 and M4' consisted mainly of creatine kinase[108] or of M protein[109,115] and that myomesin formed a sheath around the thick filaments[109,115] or was the component responsible for the putative M filaments.[109] Recent analysis of protein sequences, the labeling pattern of sequence-specific antibodies, and the binding properties of recombinant fragments suggests the following model (Fig. 7-21B, D, and E).[96] Creatine kinase contributes to the M4 bridges. Titin molecules cross the center of the A band at the M-line/bare zone region, running 60 nm into the neighboring half sarcomere, creating an antiparallel overlap of 120 nm (approximately the length of the bare zone), where they interact with each other. Myomesin molecules from opposite halves of the M line run parallel to the thick filament and titin for most of their length, binding to titin in this region and overlapping with myomesin molecules of opposite polarity from the opposite half sarcomere (Fig. 7-21D). Near its N terminus, myomesin bends perpendicular to the filament axis, extending toward the neighboring thick-filament surface, where it binds to myosin. The complex of myomesin and titin could correspond to the M filaments running parallel to the thick filaments between M4 and M4',[111,112] and the interactions of myomesin with titin and myosin would link the thick filaments to the titin skeleton. The C and N termini of M protein would bind to the surfaces of neighboring myosin filaments, while its central region runs perpendicular to them, forming the M1 bridges and thus an additional, strengthening link between thick filaments in cardiac and fast skeletal fibers, the only places where it is found (Fig. 7-21E).

FUNCTION

The M line plays several roles in the sarcomere. One is to stabilize the transverse and longitudinal order of the thick-filament lattice, which it fulfills by linking neighboring filaments to each other. The high degree of filament order produced in this way (Fig. 7-1C) is important to the rapid and efficient contraction of the sarcomere. Certain vertebrate[128] and many invertebrate muscle fibers have no M line, and filament register is correspondingly less perfect. When a muscle shortens, the interfilament distance increases by as much as 7 nm,[129] suggesting that the M bridges must stretch or change their angle of attachment to the myosin filament.

The presence of creatine kinase suggests that the M line has an enzymatic as well as a structural role, and it has been shown that there is sufficient MM-CK in the M line to supply the immediate needs of the sarcomere in resynthesizing ATP from ADP.[108]

The M line also appears likely to be crucially involved in sarcomere assembly and turnover.[96] Phosphorylation of specific serine residues on myomesin and M protein inhibits their binding to titin and myosin, respectively. It is possible that a single signal-transduction pathway could regulate the interactions of myomesin with titin and of M protein with myosin, facilitating the ordered assembly of the sarcomere in time and space.

Titin Filaments

The presence of a third set of filaments in muscle, in addition to the actin and myosin filaments, was first suggested by the integrity of sarcomeres stretched beyond actin-myosin overlap and of myofibrils from which actin and myosin had been extracted. The subsequent discovery of the giant protein connectin,[9,130,131] now normally referred to as titin, constituting a set of filaments distinct from actin and myosin, provided a molecular explanation of this behavior. Titin plays two crucial roles in muscle: providing a template for the precise organization of myofibrillar proteins during development, and acting as a molecular spring that is responsible for key aspects of the mechanical behavior of muscle. Related molecules have since been found in invertebrate muscles (mini-titins, projectin, kettin, twitchin)[130] and in smooth and nonmuscle cells, where, for example, they may play a role in chromosome mechanics.[132,133]

MOLECULAR STRUCTURE, INTERACTIONS, AND ORGANIZATION

Titin occurs as a single polypeptide chain with a molecular mass of ~3 MDa, containing ~27,000 residues.[134] It is the largest polypeptide known and the third most abundant protein in muscle (~10 percent of myofibrillar mass).[9] The isolated titin molecule is extraordinarily long (~1 μm), thin (4 nm in diameter), and highly flexible. In muscle, single molecules extend the entire length of a half-sarcomere, from Z line to M line (Fig. 7-3). The molecule starts with its N terminus in the Z line (this region of titin was originally thought to be a distinct protein called zeugmatin[135]). Here titin interacts with a 19-kDa protein named telethonin or titin cap (T-cap),[136] a protein that has been implicated in limb-girdle muscular dystrophy type 2G.[137] This is followed by an elastic region 0.7 to 1.5 MDa in mass, depending on isoform, which runs through the I band in parallel with the thin filaments. Finally the C-terminal 2-MDa forms part of the thick filament, where it binds to myosin and to MyBP-C, ending at the M line.[136] At the Z and M lines, titin molecules overlap with those from the neighboring half sarcomere, thus creating a continuous system of filaments throughout the entire myofibril. This, and the binding of numerous myofibrillar proteins to specific titin domains, suggests that titin serves as a molecular blueprint for sarcomere assembly by specifying the precise position of its ligands in each half sarcomere.[9]

Like other myosin-binding proteins, titin has a modular structure, consisting mainly (~90 percent) of Ig- and Fn-like domains, together with a unique domain rich in proline (P), glutamate (E), valine (V), and lysine (K), the so-called PEVK domain (Fig. 7-22).[134,138] Different arrangements of these modules are expressed in different muscle types by differential splicing.[134,139] Fn domains are confined to the A band, where they are arranged with Ig domains in superrepeat patterns.[9,91,140] The I-band region, in contrast, consists of two separate blocks of Ig repeats that are separated by the variable-length PEVK domain.

In the MyBP-C region of the A band, titin has 11 repeats of a pattern of Fn- and Ig-like domains (Ig, 2 Fn, Ig, 3 Fn, Ig, and 3 Fn).[9] With a length of 4 to 4.5 nm per domain, each of the repeats is ~43 nm long. These 11 repeats appear to dictate the positioning of the 11 repeats of myosin-binding proteins (mainly MyBP-C), spaced 43 nm apart along the thick filament (Fig. 7-18). Each repeat contains multiple domains that bind both the myosin tail and MyBP-C. Toward the end of the A band, where the myosin-binding proteins are absent, there are seven repeats consisting of five Fn3 and two Ig domains.

In the I band the tandem Ig domains and PEVK-rich sequences confer extensibility on the titin filament.[134,141] The length of PEVK titin varies by alternative splicing between 163 and 2200 residues and is muscle-specific,[140] giving rise to different mechanical properties in different striated muscle types.[134]

FUNCTION IN MYOFIBRILLOGENESIS

Titin is one of the first myofibrillar proteins to assemble into the nascent myofibril. It is also the only component that extends an entire half sarcomere, interacting with various sarcomeric proteins at specific points along its length, including antiparallel interactions with neighboring titin molecules in the M and Z lines.[142] These facts suggest that titin acts as the key sarcomeric molecular template during development, coordinating the precise assembly of thick and thin filaments from their components and their integration into the sarcomere. This concept is supported by recent antisense and knockout studies in which interference with titin expression results in defective myofibril assembly.[143,144] The highly ordered organization of the sarcomere that appears to be orchestrated by titin is key to the rapid and efficient contraction and relaxation that characterize striated muscle function.

The implication of titin in developmental signal transduction pathways is further evidence of its role in sarcomere assembly. Titin domains within the Z line can be phosphorylated by regulatory kinases, and the M-line region itself contains a serine/threonine kinase domain that can phosphorylate T-cap/telethonin in the Z line. Thus developmental regulatory signals may be relayed between the M and Z ends of titin during myofibril assembly.[9,134,142]

Recently another giant sarcomeric protein resembling titin and involved in sarcomere assembly has been discovered. Obscurin[145] has a molecular mass of 800 kDa and a modular architecture consisting of Ig- and Fn-like domains. A large region resembles the elastic region of titin. Its C terminus contains sequences suggesting a role in signal transduction and also contains domains that interact with the N-terminal Z-line region of titin. The two proteins coassemble during formation of the sarcomere; later, obscurin additionally appears at the M line.

MECHANICAL FUNCTION

The primary function of titin in mature muscle is to act as an elastic element that maintains sarcomere integrity and filament order in the relaxed and active states. Titin elasticity lies specifically in the I-band region and involves two elements in series and with different properties—the Ig and PEVK domains.[146]

Passive tension and slack length of muscle at rest are determined primarily by titin and depend on titin isoform. Fibers with larger titins develop passive tension at longer sarcomere lengths, while smaller isoforms, such as those in cardiac muscle, correlate with higher resting tension.[146] When skeletal muscle is stretched above slack length, it is thought that the Ig region first straightens, with little associated force and without unfolding of the individual Ig modules (Fig. 7-23A). Once taut, further stretch unravels the PEVK domain, requiring substantial force and creating significant levels of passive tension.[146] In highly stretched sarcomeres, unfolding of Ig domains may occur, but this is probably not relevant at physiologic lengths.[141,146] The organization of I-band titin into two domains in series thus contributes to the nonlinear elasticity of striated muscle,

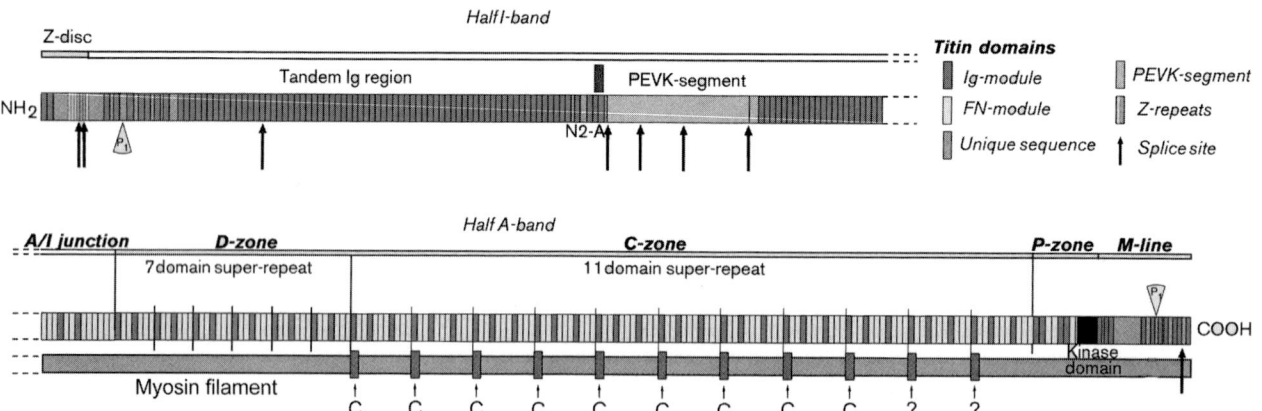

FIGURE 7-22. Modular structure of titin and its relation to (upper): the Z line (Z repeats) and I band (tandem Ig repeats and PEVK segment); and (lower): the myosin filament in the A band (Ig/Fn super-repeats—note positions of nonmyosin proteins on myosin filament) and M line. (Adapted from Gregorio CC, Granzier H, Sorimachi H, et al: Muscle assembly: A titanic achievement? Curr Opin Cell Biol 11:18, 1999. With permission from Elsevier Science.)

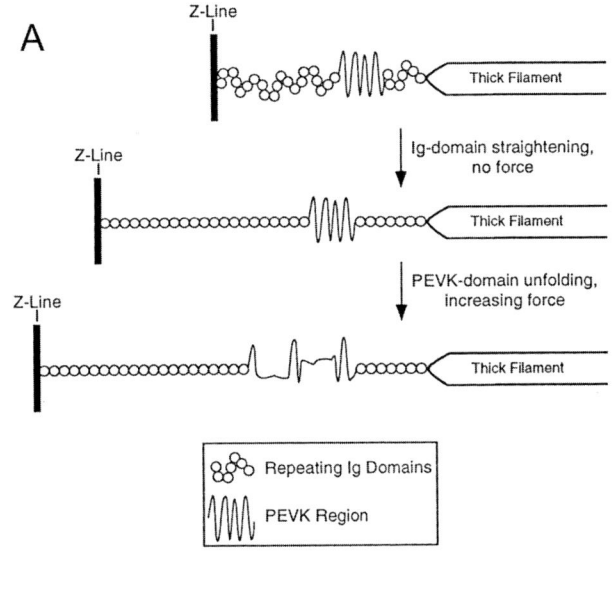

FIGURE 7-23. Models of titin function. A. When a slack sarcomere is stretched, domains containing tandem Ig modules are first straightened, with little increase in tension. Further extension leads to unfolding of the PEVK domain, with exponentially increasing tension. B. Model showing how stretch of titin (stretched spring at right) in unequally contracted sarcomere will tend to recenter thick filaments. (From Horowits R: *The physiological role of titin in striated muscle. Rev Physiol Biochem Pharmacol* 138:57, 1999. With permission from Springer-Verlag.)

allowing limited lengthening with little tension and further extension only with exponentially increasing amounts of tension. The advantage of the former is seen in muscle groups that are stretched when opposing muscles contract: Low resistance allows voluntary movements to occur efficiently. On the other hand, the high levels of passive tension produced at longer lengths help prevent the damage that can occur with excessive stretching.[146]

Titin in cardiac muscle has some unique features.[141,146] It has been suggested that the shorter titin isoform in the heart sets the slack length on the ascending limb of the length/tension curve. This would allow the myocardium to adapt to increased filling with a stronger contraction (Starling's law). The nonlinear elasticity of titin would not impair filling over a limited range but would provide enough diastolic tone to resist overfilling of the heart.[146] An insertion into the I-band region of cardiac titin appears to confer on this isoform an additional spring element.[141] Recruitment of all three elements allows cardiac titin to extend reversibly without unfolding of Ig domains. In addition there is evidence that the insertion also interacts with thin filaments and is necessary for their integrity.[141]

In addition to its influence on the passive mechanical properties of muscle, titin also appears to maintain axial ordering of the filaments in the sarcomere that is critical for the rapid and efficient generation of active tension.[146] In a sarcomere consisting only of two sets of filaments (actin and myosin), no structure would exist to maintain the thick filaments centered in the sarcomere during stretch, as they would not be mechanically linked to the Z line. Titin filaments provide such a centering force, thus maintaining the optimal organization for contraction. Titin may also function to prevent any drop in tension that would occur if thick filaments became uncentered during prolonged contractions (Fig. 7-23B). If the thick filaments overlap more with thin filaments in one half of the sarcomere than in the other during contraction, there will be an instability in force in the two halves due to the unequal number of cross-bridges, and this will be self-propagating as contraction continues. Titin could act to correct this imbalance by exerting greater tension in the longer half sarcomere, where there are fewer cross-bridges. However, during contractions of physiologic duration, only a small movement of the thick filaments from their central position would be expected. Thus the primary ordering function of titin in vivo is to keep the thick filaments centered during passive stretch and to prevent sarcomere asymmetry from accumulating over several contractions by recentering the thick filaments each time a muscle is relaxed.[146]

The Thin Filament

The thin filaments of striated muscle run from the Z line to the edge of the H zone (Fig. 7-1C and D). In vertebrates, they are about 1 μm long and 10 nm in diameter and occupy positions in the filament lattice midway between three thick filaments (Figs. 7-1E and F and 7-2; Color Plate 3e). The major component of the thin filament is actin,[147,148] a key cytoskeletal protein present in virtually all eukaryotic cells. Actin is a globular protein [G actin (G = globular)] with a molecular mass of 42 kDa, which self-associates to form a helical polymer known as F actin (F = filamentous), containing approximately 360 molecules (Fig. 7-24A; Color Plate 1b). Attached at regular intervals to this F-actin backbone are the proteins tropomyosin and troponin[149-151] (Fig. 7-24B and C; Color Plate 3e), which function in the regulation of contraction, and the giant protein nebulin,[9,10,152] which runs the entire length of the filament and is thought to be involved in determining its length. In addition to these bona fide thin-filament proteins, a number of "soluble"' cellular enzymes may also bind to the thin filament.[153]

POLYMERIZATION OF ACTIN TO FORM FILAMENTS

At low ionic strength in vitro, actin[147,148,154] exists in the monomeric G-actin form. G actin is roughly spherical with a diameter of about 5 nm. It is stabilized by the binding of 1 divalent cation and 1 ATP molecule per molecule of actin. When the ionic strength of a G-actin solution is increased to the physiologic range (0.1 M), actin self-associates to form F actin (Figs. 7-24A and 7-25), polymerization being accompanied by hydrolysis of bound ATP to ADP.

The arrangement of monomer subunits in F actin has been determined by x-ray diffraction and EM. The F-actin filament is most simply thought of as two strands of actin subunits twisted around each other to form a double helix (Figs. 7-24A and 7-25).[16,155] The subunits are spaced 5.5 nm apart along each helix, and the two helices are staggered by approximately one-half a repeat (2.7 nm). Each helical strand has 13 to 14 subunits in one turn and crosses over the other every ~37 nm, giving rise to apparent bulges and constrictions in the filament (Fig. 7-24).[16,155,156] Electron micrographs of shadowed filaments show that these "long-pitch" helices are right-handed.[157] The F-actin structure can equally be defined by a left-handed "genetic" helix (a single helix connecting every subunit) with a pitch of 5.9 nm.[155]

F actin is a polar structure, with all the monomers "pointing" in the same direction along the filament axis. Actin polarity is apparent only rarely in electron micrographs of F actin (Fig. 7-25) because of the roughly spherical shape of the actin monomer, but it is readily apparent in the

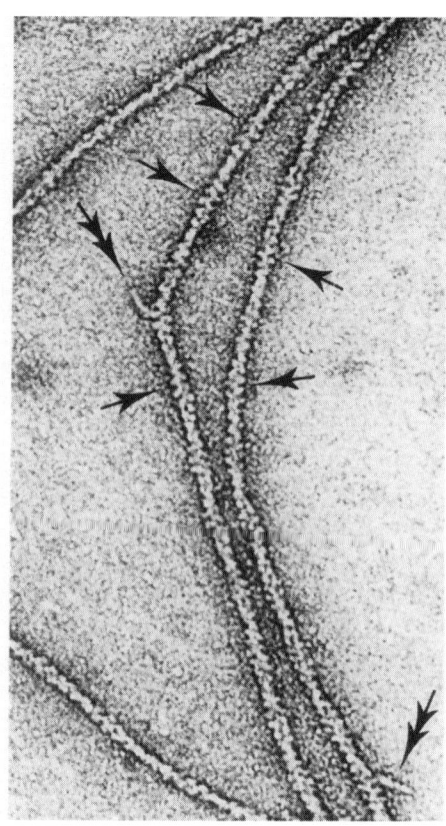

FIGURE 7-25. Negatively stained F-actin filaments. The beaded nature of the filaments, reflecting their assembly from G-actin molecules, is evident. The polarity of the actin subunits is clear in some regions (arrows) and is seen to be opposite to that of attached myosin S1 molecules (double arrows). (× 250,000.) *(From Vibert P, Craig R: Three-dimensional reconstruction of thin filaments decorated with a Ca^{2+}-regulated myosin. J Mol Biol 157:299, 1982. With permission from Elsevier Science.)*

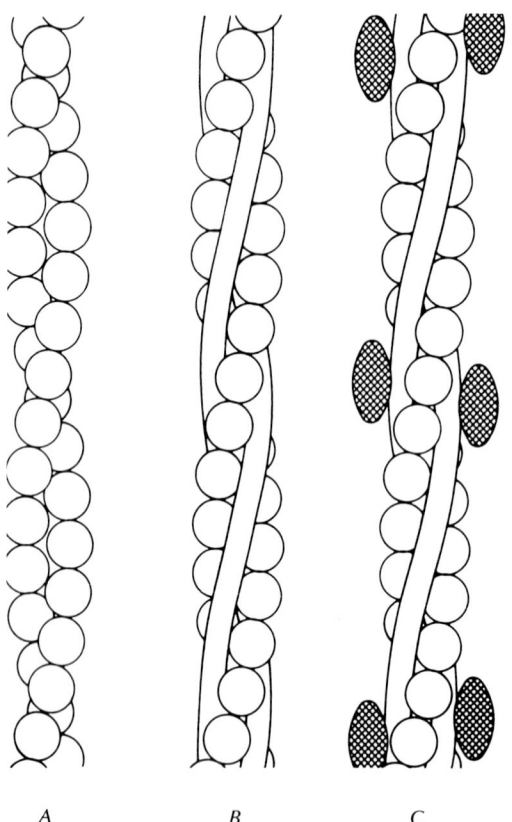

FIGURE 7-24. Schematic diagrams of thin-filament structure. A. F actin (actin subunits are drawn as spheres for simplicity). B. F actin plus tropomyosin. C. F actin–tropomyosin plus troponin. *(From Offer G: The molecular basis of muscular contraction, in Bull AT, Lagnado JR, Thomas JD, Tipton KF (eds): Companion to Biochemistry: Selected Topics for Further Study. London: Longman, 1974. By copyright permission of Longman Group Ltd.)*

atomic resolution model of the filament (Color Plate 1b) and when myosin heads are used to decorate actin filaments, forming a clearly polar, arrowhead structure. The elongated shape of the myosin heads reveals the underlying polarity of the actin molecules to which they are bound (Fig. 7-26).[21,158]

Atomic Structure of G Actin

G actin is a globular protein consisting of a single polypeptide chain containing 375 residues, about one-quarter of which are α-helical, one-quarter β-pleated sheet, and the rest random coil.[83,154] The complete amino acid sequence of actin has been determined, yielding a molecular mass of 41,785 Da. The sequences of diverse actins (e.g., skeletal, cardiac, smooth, and nonmuscle) are strongly conserved but nevertheless functionally unique, the major differences occurring near the N terminus.[159,160] This is probably explained by the fact that actin interacts with numerous other molecules (itself, tropomyosin, troponin, myosin, actin-binding proteins from nonmuscle cells, etc.), necessitating the conservation of many binding sites. Sarcomeric actins form more stable polymers than cytoskeletal actins, in accord with the more permanent structure required in muscle.[160]

Owing to its tendency to polymerize, the first crystal structure of actin was obtained not from pure G actin, but from a 1:1 complex with DNase I, which prevents polymerization.[154,161,162] Using knowledge of the atomic structure of DNase I alone, it was possible to determine the structure of the actin component alone (Fig. 7-27). Later studies produced structures of actin complexed with profilin[163] and segment 1 of gelsolin[164] and most recently of uncomplexed actin.[165] The actin monomer thus revealed has dimensions of approximately $5.5 \times 5.5 \times 3.5$ nm and consists of two major domains of similar size. Each domain can be divided into two subdomains. The smaller domain consists of subdomains 1 and 2, while the larger domain comprises subdomains 3 and 4 (Fig. 7-27; Color Plate 1a). The polypeptide chain follows a very similar course in subdomains 1 and 3, forming a five-stranded β sheet with associated α helices, suggesting that these subdomains may have evolved by gene duplication. Subdomains 2 and 4 may have been inserted subsequently into subdomains 1 and 3, respectively. A molecule of ATP or ADP is located in the cleft between the two domains, with a Ca^{2+} ion (Mg^{2+} in vivo) bound to the β- or β- and γ-phosphate(s). The nucleotide and metal are involved in many interactions with both domains, thus contributing to the stability of the molecule. The chain fold in subdomains 1 and 3 is similar to that in hexokinase and in the N-terminal ATPase fragment of the molecular chaperone, HSC70,[154,161,162] suggesting a common ancestral protein.

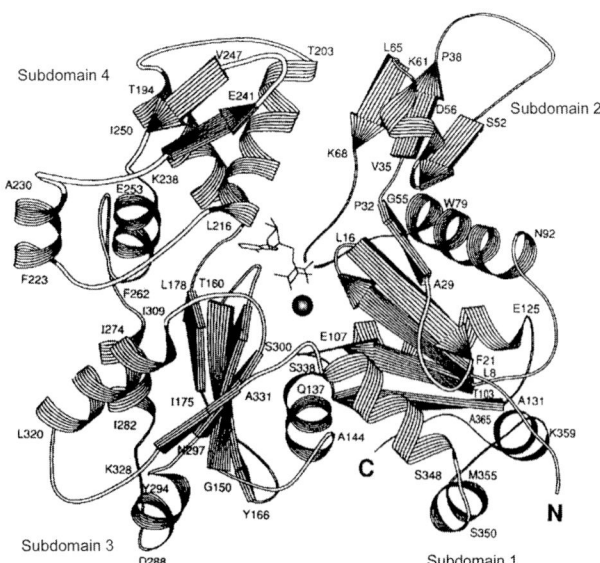

FIGURE 7-27. Schematic representation of the structure of G actin, determined by x-ray crystallography, showing subdomain nomenclature and ATP and Ca^{2+} located in the cleft between the two main domains. *(From Kabsch W, Mannherz HG, Suck D, et al: Atomic structure of the actin:DNase I complex. Nature 347:37, 1990. By copyright permission of Nature Publishing Group.)*

Atomic Model of F Actin

The atomic structure of F actin has not been determined crystallographically because actin filaments do not crystallize. An atomic model of F actin has been deduced, however, by determining the best fit of x-ray diffraction patterns of oriented actin filament gels to patterns computed from models that place the G-actin atomic structure in varying orientations onto the F-actin helix.[162,166–168] The model that best fits the observed diffraction pattern (Fig. 7-28 and Color Plate 1b) has a diameter of ~9.5 nm. The small domain (subdomains 1 and 2) is at high radius and the large domain (subdomains 3 and 4) at a small radius from the filament axis. The large domain is 5.5 nm long and fits naturally along the long-pitch helices. Extensive contacts are made between monomers along these helices, especially between residues in subdomain 3 of one monomer and subdomain 4 of the next. Lesser contacts are also made across the filament axis to molecules in the other long-pitch strand, and it has been proposed that a hydrophobic "plug" stabilizes the filament by extending from subdomains 3 and 4 in one strand into a hydrophobic pocket between two monomers in the opposite strand.[154,166] The shapes of the monomer in the filament and in the actin:DNase I crystal are very similar, although the fit with the gel diffraction data is improved if the domains are allowed to move slightly.[167] Thus G actin undergoes little change in structure when it polymerizes to form F actin except for a small movement of subdomain 2, which may lean over toward subdomain 4, closing the nucleotide pocket between the two main domains. Support for this atomic structure of the filament comes from EM;[169] the model makes an excellent fit with 3D reconstructions computed from negative stain and cryoelectron microscopic micrographs of thin filaments (see Fig. 7-34, below).[170]

The thin filament as pictured above is a rigid structure whose subunits have definite and fixed positions. Several

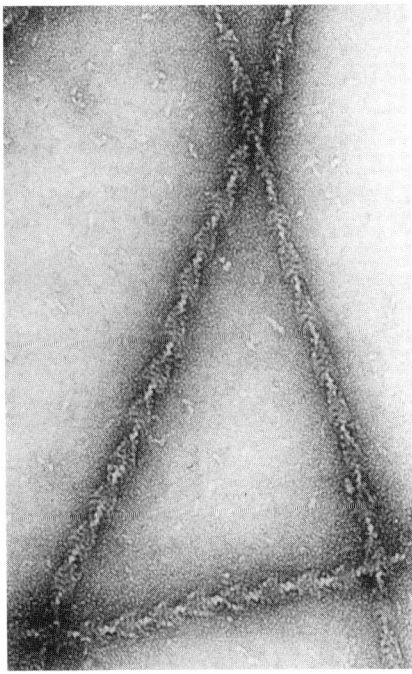

FIGURE 7-26. Electron micrograph of negatively stained actin filaments decorated with myosin S1, forming the arrowhead structure. ($\times 190,000$.)

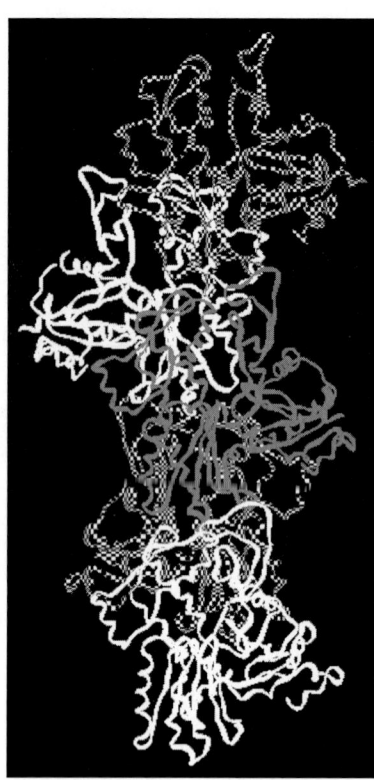

FIGURE 7-28. Atomic model of F actin, showing the C-α positions of five monomers. The end of the filament connecting to the Z line is at the bottom. A clearer representation of this image is shown in Color Plate 1b. (Adapted from image provided courtesy of W. Lehman, based on Holmes KC, Popp D, Gebhard W, Kabsch W: Atomic model of the actin filament. Nature 347:44, 1990. With permission of Nature Publishing Group.)

studies suggest, however, that this is an oversimplification. From its appearance in electron micrographs and from solution studies, it is apparent that F actin is very flexible along its long axis.[171] A different kind of flexibility is evident from the variable distance seen between crossover points of the two actin strands in negatively stained filaments.[156] This kind of variability can be explained if the actin subunits have a constant axial spacing but randomly varying azimuthal separation, deviating by up to ±10 degrees from their helically ideal positions, the disorder being cumulative along the filaments.[172,173] Lateral slipping of the two long-pitch actin strands past each other perpendicular to the filament axis has been suggested as an alternative interpretation of this disorder.[174] Such mobility is also found in actin filaments containing the regulatory proteins troponin and tropomyosin, although it is virtually absent from filaments to which S1 is bound.[173] The variability may be critical to muscle functioning.[173] The helical symmetries of the thick and thin filaments are different, and some flexibility is needed to accommodate the interactions between the two types of filament during force generation. While the S1/S2 and S2/LMM hinges of myosin will play an important part in this, the flexibility of the thin filament may also contribute, and there is indeed evidence for such actin flexibility in intact muscle.[175]

REGULATORY PROTEINS OF THE THIN FILAMENT

Muscle contraction is controlled by the concentration of free Ca^{2+} ions surrounding the myofilaments (see Chaps. 11 to 13). At low levels of Ca^{2+} (10^{-8} M), muscle is relaxed, whereas at high levels (10^{-5} M), it contracts. Control is exercised by regulation of actin-myosin interaction and the concomitant actin-activated ATPase rate of myosin. At low Ca^{2+} levels, myosin interaction with actin is inhibited and the ATPase is low, whereas at high Ca^{2+} levels, myosin interacts with actin and ATPase is high.

In vertebrate striated muscle, contraction is regulated primarily by the thin-filament protein complex of troponin and tropomyosin, which responds to changes in the sarcoplasmic concentration of Ca^{2+} ions released from the SR.[149-151] Tropomyosin is an elongated molecule, associated with seven actin monomers along each long-pitch actin strand (Fig. 7-24B), while troponin is a complex of three subunits that attaches every 38.5 nm along the thin filament to a specific site on each tropomyosin (Fig. 7-24C; Color Plate 3e). The regular spacing of troponin along the thin filament is responsible for periodic cross striations at this interval,[16,155,176] visible especially in the I band in longitudinal sections of muscle (Fig. 7-1C), indicating that in muscle the thin filaments are in longitudinal register. Troponin is the Ca^{2+}-binding component of the complex. In combination with tropomyosin, it regulates contraction by inhibiting actin-myosin interaction at low Ca^{2+} levels, causing relaxation. When Ca^{2+} concentration increases following muscle stimulation, troponin binds Ca^{2+}, releasing the inhibitory effect of troponin-tropomyosin and allowing actin and myosin to interact (with consequent increase in ATPase activity) and contraction to follow.

Tropomyosin, troponin, and the biochemical basis of regulation are discussed in detail in Chap. 13; we focus here on relevant structural features.

Tropomyosin

Tropomyosin[177] is a two-stranded α-helical coiled-coil molecule of molecular mass 65 kDa. Its two chains run parallel to each other with no axial stagger, forming a molecule 41 nm long and 2 nm in diameter. The amino acid sequence of α tropomyosin (284 residues) gives a chain mass of 32,758 Da and conforms to the predictions made by Crick[73] for "knobs-into-holes" packing of α-helical coiled coils, as discussed earlier for the structure of the myosin tail (Fig. 7-14A).

In the thin filament, tropomyosin molecules form two continuous, extended polymers following the two long-pitch helical strands of F-actin subunits, each molecule overlapping with its neighbors at each end by ~2 nm and spanning seven actin monomers, generating a repeat of 38.5 nm (7×5.5 nm) along each actin strand (Fig. 7-24B; Color Plate 3e). EM observation of ordered aggregates of tropomyosin and analysis of the tropomyosin sequence[178,179] reveals a 2.8-nm periodicity arising from a repeating distribution of positively charged, negatively charged, and apolar residues. There are 14 such periods, each about 20 (284/14) residues long and consisting of about 8 residues that are predominantly basic or apolar followed by about 12 residues that are mainly acidic.[178] The 14-fold periodic charge distribution along tropomyosin corresponds to two alternate sets of seven approximately equivalent actin recognition sites, which may be linked to the "off" or "on" states of contraction (see "Changes in Thin-Filament Structure on Activation," below).[178-180] Thus ionic forces producing quasi-equivalent interactions with actin, rather than interactions involving more highly specific sites, play an important role in actin-tropomyosin interaction.[177]

Tropomyosin has been crystallized in a number of forms [181-184] and its structure revealed to 0.7-nm resolution (Fig. 7-29).[184] The molecules appear to overlap head-to-tail with each other by nine residues, forming a region that may be locally modified into an intermeshing globular structure. Throughout the rest of their length, the two α helices of the coiled coil wind around each other continuously, with a coiled-coil pitch that averages 14 nm but varies locally due to local sequence variations.[182,184] Together with the supercoiling of tropomyosin on actin, this leads to seven half turns and seven quasiequivalent actin-binding sites on tropomyosin. The second set of sites mentioned above appears to be much less regular than the first and is not thought to play a major role in the binding of tropomyosin to actin.[182] Observations of tropomyosin crystals and thin filaments suggest that actin plays a part in determining the precise conformation of tropomyosin in muscle (for example, in determining the radius of the supercoil) and that there may be some local unfolding of the α helix in some regions of the molecule. Thus a less regular and less rigid structure than is implied by its α-helical nature may be a more realistic view of tropomyosin in muscle. X-ray crystallography of an 81-residue N-terminal fragment of tropomyosin at atomic resolution adds to this picture.[185] Local clustering of alanine residues is seen to allow slight local staggering of the α helices, leading to specific bends in the molecular axis and providing the flexibility required for the winding of tropomyosin around the thin filament and for changes in its conformation as it moves on actin during regulation.[185,186]

Tropomyosin has several roles in thin-filament function: stabilizing the actin filament, strengthening it and making it less likely to bend or break,[187] and providing a molecular scaffolding for positioning the Ca^{2+}-sensitive troponin molecule on the filament. The troponin-tropomyosin complex regulates actin-myosin interaction, and hence contraction, by moving its position on the F-actin backbone. Because there are only one-seventh as many troponin-tropomyosin complexes as there are actin subunits, the elongated tropomyosin also serves to extend the regulatory influence of the more globular troponin over all seven actin subunits (see "Changes in Thin-Filament Structure on Activation," below).

Troponin

Troponin (~80 kDa) is a complex of three noncovalently linked subunits, TnI, TnT, and TnC, named according to their first identified function. It is an essential component of the Ca^{2+}-regulatory system of vertebrate thin filaments, where it functions, in conjunction with tropomyosin, by allowing or inhibiting actin-myosin interaction.[150,151,188,189] All three components have been sequenced, and their properties and interactions have been widely studied. A detailed discussion appears in Chap. 13. Key features bearing on the structure of the thin filament and on structural changes responsible for regulating contraction are summarized below (see "Changes in Thin-Filament Structure on Activation").

Troponin I. TnI, the inhibitory subunit, is the component that holds troponin together and onto actin by binding to actin, TnC, and TnT, highlighting its central role in muscle regulation.[151,190] The isoforms of vertebrate TnI have molecular masses in the range 20 to 24 kDa and consist of a single polypeptide chain. When bound to F actin, TnI is able to inhibit actin-myosin ATPase in the absence of any of the other subunits. This binding is not responsible for inhibiting actin directly in the native filament, however, because only one TnI is present for seven actins, but it helps to anchor troponin to the thin filament in the absence of Ca^{2+}. TnI's inhibitory function is greatly enhanced if tropomyosin is also present. When Ca^{2+} binds to TnC, the binding of TnI to TnC is strengthened and its binding to actin weakened, support-

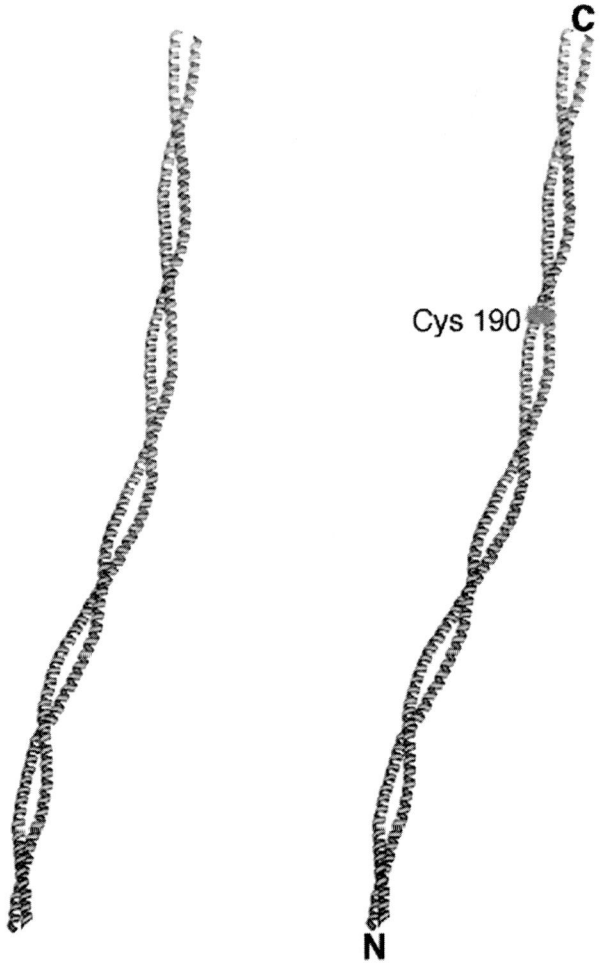

FIGURE 7-29. Stereo view of tropomyosin at 0.7 nm resolution based on x-ray crystallography, showing the two α helices coiling around each other. *(From Whitby FG, Phillips GN Jr: Crystal structure of tropomyosin at 7Å resolution. Proteins 38:49, 2000. Reprinted by permission of Wiley-Liss, Inc., a subsidiary of John Wiley & Sons, Inc.)*

ing the concept that TnI-actin binding acts as a Ca^{2+}-sensitive anchor of Tm-Tn to actin.[151] The crystal structure of TnI has not yet been determined.

Troponin C. TnC is the Ca^{2+}-binding component of troponin.[151] There are a number of isoforms of TnC specific to particular muscle types or stages of development,[191] and these belong to a multigene family of Ca^{2+}-binding proteins.[192] Fast skeletal TnC is a globular protein containing 159 amino acid residues and has a molecular mass of 17,965 Da. TnC can bind to TnI and TnT and possibly also to actin. In the presence of Ca^{2+} ions, TnC removes the inhibition of actin-myosin interaction that TnI imposes on the thin filament—a key feature of muscle regulation. When Ca^{2+} concentration drops again, Ca^{2+} binding by TnC is diminished and the filament reverts to the inhibited state.

All of the proteins of the multigene family to which TnC belongs have at least one EF-hand or helix-loop-helix Ca^{2+}-binding site. Each such site is characterized by a 12-residue Ca^{2+}-binding loop that is interposed between a pair of α helices. Each of the loops is rich in acidic residues that are responsible for the coordination of a single Ca^{2+} ion. Fast skeletal TnC contains four such sites, two high-affinity sites, which are always occupied by Mg^{2+} or Ca^{2+} (Mg^{2+} in the cell), and two low-affinity sites, which bind Ca^{2+} specifically. Binding to the latter regulatory sites occurs only during the increase in cytoplasmic Ca^{2+}, which occurs on muscle activation.

The crystal structure of TnC has been solved to atomic resolution.[151,191,193,194] The molecule is 7.3 nm long and has the shape of a dumbbell, being composed of two globular heads separated by a central α helix (Fig. 7-30; Color Plate 3a). Each of the globular domains contains two of the helix-loop-helix Ca^{2+}-binding sites, the low-affinity sites in the N-terminal domain and the high-affinity sites in the C-terminal domain. Only the high-affinity sites contained Ca^{2+} in the crystal, and there was a significant difference in conformation between the domains occupied and unoccupied by Ca^{2+}. The helices flanking the Ca^{2+}-binding sites lacking Ca^{2+} are nearly parallel to one another (helices A,B and C,D in Fig. 7-30, left), producing a "closed" structure in which the B and C helices are folded down along the central D helix. On Ca^{2+} binding, the helices flanking the Ca^{2+}-binding sites are more perpendicular to one another (helices A,B and C,D in Fig. 7-30, right), and the B and C helices rotate up. This exposes hydrophobic amino acid residues in the central D helix that are thought to interact with TnI, which would enhance TnC-TnI binding. In this model,[151,195] TnI would then bind more weakly to actin (see "Troponin I," above), allowing tropomyosin to move to a new position on actin, resulting in the activated state of the thin filament (see "Changes in Thin-Filament Structure on Activation," below).

Troponin T. TnT is the tropomyosin-binding component of troponin.[151,196] It binds to TnI and TnC of the troponin complex and to tropomyosin and actin of the thin filament, thus functioning as the glue that attaches troponin to the thin filament and makes the filament Ca^{2+}-sensitive. TnT occurs as a wide range of isoforms with molecular mass 31 to 36 kDa. Although TnT has yet to be crystallized, it is known to be an extended molecule with a length of ~18 nm, whose globular C terminus interacts with TnC, TnI, and tropomyosin, while its

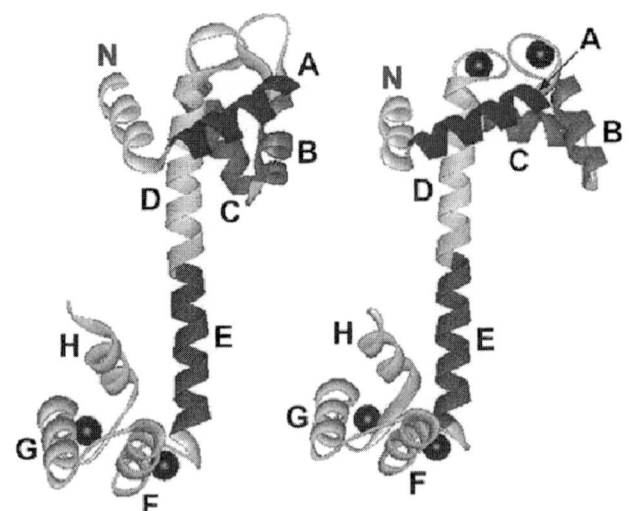

FIGURE 7-30. Ribbon representations of troponin C in low- (left) and high- (right) Ca^{2+} states. Note the two-lobe structure in each case and the upward rotation of helices B and C in high Ca^{2+} compared with low Ca^{2+}, exposing more of helix D. *(From Gordon AM, Homsher E, Regnier M: Regulation of contraction in striated muscle. Physiol Rev 80:853, 2000. With permission.)*

extended N-terminal region lies along, and antiparallel to, the C-terminal half of tropomyosin, including its overlap with the N-terminal region of the neighboring tropomyosin. TnT's ability to bind to tropomyosin is responsible for positioning the troponin complex with its characteristic 38.5-nm periodicity along the thin filament. The large number of TnT isoforms suggests a special significance in contractile regulation and enables the Ca^{2+} response to be fine-tuned.

The troponin complex as a whole is a globular entity with an elongated tail[197] (Fig. 7-31; Color Plate 3e). The entire complex is about 26 nm long and the tail portion 16 nm long and 2 nm wide. Isolated TnT is rod-like, and its dimensions correspond closely to those of the tail portion of the whole troponin complex. The shape and dimensions of TnT indicate that TnI and TnC constitute most of the globular region of troponin. The location of the globular domain of troponin on individual tropomyosin molecules, 10 to 20 nm from one end, is consistent with studies suggesting that the binding region is about one-third of the way along the tropomyosin molecule, in the vicinity of cys 190.[180,198] A plausible picture for the subunits of troponin on tropomyosin has TnC, TnI, and part of TnT binding near cys 190 of tropomyosin while the rest of TnT extends toward the COOH-terminus (Fig. 7-31).

MOLECULAR MODEL OF THE THIN FILAMENT

As we have seen, actin forms the backbone of the thin filament and is arranged in a double helix whose pitch is approximately 37 nm (Figs. 7-24A and 7-28). The detailed organization of troponin and tropomyosin on the actin backbone in native filaments has been elucidated by a combination of x-ray diffraction and EM. The elongated shape of tropomyosin was the first clue that it ran along the two long-pitch actin strands[199] (Fig. 7-24B). This was supported by analysis of

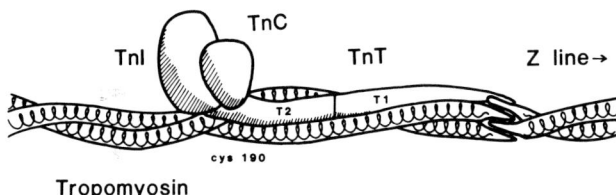

FIGURE 7-31. Diagram of proposed interaction between tropomyosin and troponin deduced from electron microscopy and x-ray diffraction data. T1 and T2 indicate location of two enzymatic fragments of TnT. *(From Flicker PF et al: Troponin and its interactions with tropomyosin. An electron microscope study. J Mol Biol 162:495, 1982. With permission from Elsevier Science.)*

electron micrographs of paracrystals of pure actin compared to those of actin plus tropomyosin and by x-ray diffraction patterns of oriented gels of filaments.[200] With improvements in technique, tropomyosin has more recently been directly observed in electron micrographs of negatively stained thin filaments (Fig. 7-32).[201,202] 3D reconstructions computed from such filaments in the relaxed (low Ca^{2+}) state reveal tropomyosin as a continuous strand of density running along the extreme inner edge of the outer domain of actin, close to its junction with the inner domain (Fig. 7-33).[170,201–203] Computational fitting of the atomic model of F actin (Fig. 7-28) to the reconstruction reveals further detail (Fig. 7-34).[170,202,203] The strands of tropo-myosin are seen to closely approach or contact subdomain 1 of each actin monomer near its junction with subdomain 3. They then bridge over, without touching subdomain 2, to neighboring subdomains 1 and 3 of the next monomer. Crucially, it has been possible to identify several clusters of amino acid residues involved in strong interactions with myosin during the cross-bridge cycle that are covered by the tropomyosin strand (see "Changes in Thin-Filament Structure on Activation," below).

In addition to revealing the position of tropomyosin on actin at near-atomic level, the reconstructions also provide insights into troponin binding and localization, although for technical reasons, this information is less detailed than that on tropomyosin.[204] In the low Ca^{2+} state, troponin is bound to both tropomyosin and actin, apparently acting as a latch that constrains tropomyosin into the myosin-blocking position on actin described above, inhibiting actin-myosin interaction and ATPase activity (in the absence of Ca^{2+} or of troponin, tropomyosin takes up a position on actin that does not interfere with myosin binding).

Changes in Thin-Filament Structure on Activation

The structural mechanism by which the troponin-tropomyosin complex on the thin filament regulates actin-myosin interaction is not yet fully understood. A key model that has guided thinking about this mechanism is the "steric-blocking" model, which proposes that in the relaxed ("off") state, tropomyosin blocks the interaction of actin and myosin by physically cov-

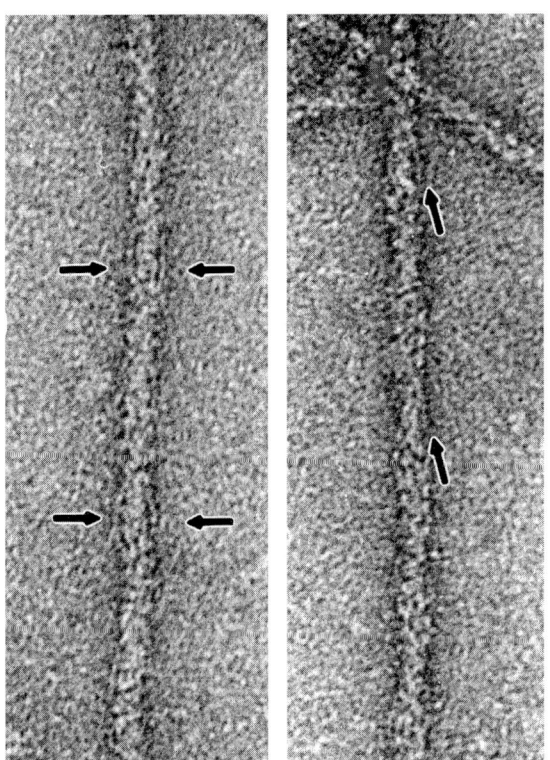

FIGURE 7-32. Electron micrographs of negatively stained thin filaments showing tropomyosin strands (arrows). (× 460,000.) *(From Moody C, Lehman W, Craig R: Caldesmon and the structure of smooth muscle thin filaments: Electron microscopy of isolated thin filaments. J Muscle Res Cell Motil 11:176, 1990. With kind permission of Kluwer Academic Publishers.)*

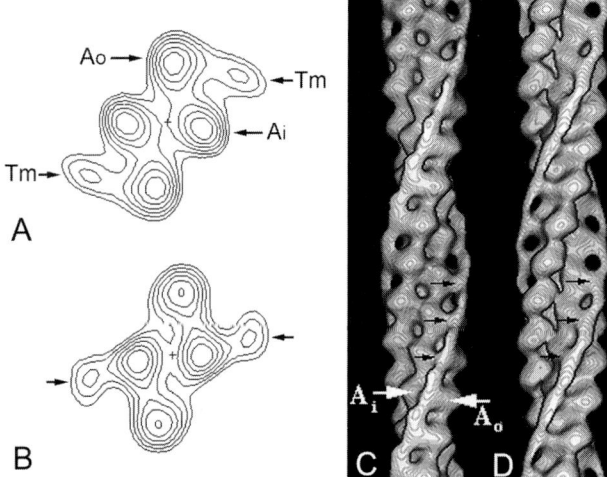

FIGURE 7-33. Three-dimensional reconstructions of thin filaments in high and low Ca^{2+}. A and B are projections down the long-pitch helices of the thin filament, showing actin subunits (Ao, outer domain; Ai, inner domain) in each of the helical strands. In low Ca^{2+} (A), tropomyosin (Tm) attaches to the outer domain, while at high Ca^{2+}, it has moved to the inner domain. C and D are surface views of the same reconstructions, showing tropomyosin as the long strand contacting (black arrows) the outer domain in C (low Ca^{2+}) and the inner domain in D (high Ca^{2+}). *(Adapted from Vibert P, Craig R, Lehman W: Steric model for activation of muscle thin filaments. J Mol Biol 266:8, 1997. With permission from Elsevier Science.)*

ering the myosin-binding site on actin. When muscle is switched "on" (activated), troponin binds Ca^{2+}, leading to a structural change that allows tropomyosin to move to a nonblocking site, thus removing the inhibition.[155] The model was first suggested based on x-ray diffraction observations of relaxed and activated muscle and of thin-filament gels, which showed intensity changes on activation consistent with such a movement.[205–208] Although the model was plausible and appealing, other interpretations remained possible, and it has only been with improvements in EM and image reconstruction methods that evidence directly supporting it has been obtained. As described above, 3D reconstructions of thin filaments[170,201–203] show that tropomyosin in the off state lies over the main myosin-binding site on actin, thereby blocking residues required for myosin interaction. Reconstructions of filaments in the presence of Ca^{2+} reveal that tropomyosin moves azimuthally by approximately 2 nm onto the inner domain of actin (Fig. 7-33),[170,201–203] exposing three of the four clusters of myosin-binding residues on actin that were previously occluded (Fig. 7-34). Strong binding of myosin heads to actin in the absence of ATP causes an additional 1-nm movement of tropomyosin further on to the inner domain, exposing this last cluster as well.[169,170,201–203,209] These observations show directly that the myosin-binding site is indeed physically blocked in the "off" state and exposed in the "on" state, as required by the steric-blocking model, and are consistent with biochemical studies showing that Ca^{2+} alone is insufficient to fully switch on contraction, the binding of myosin heads being required in addition.

A simple structural model emerges from these studies.[170,201–203,210] At low Ca^{2+} levels, tropomyosin physically blocks the strong myosin-binding site on each of the seven actin subunits with which it interacts. Putative nonspecific electrostatic sites of interaction on subdomain-1 are not affected. Thus transient weak interactions of myosin crossbridges with actin that may occur in relaxed muscle would be possible, while transition to a strongly attached, force-producing state would be blocked.[211] At high Ca^{2+}, tropomyosin movement would unblock most of the myosin-binding site, facilitating binding of myosin heads but not fully switching on contraction. Binding of some heads would cause further movement of tropomyosin, fully exposing the myosin-binding site and facilitating the binding of additional heads, cooperatively switching on contraction. This simple model is qualitatively consistent with independently proposed mechanisms involving three regulatory states.[182,212] While the steric model provides a simple structural explanation of regulation, it has been questioned whether the flexibility of tropomyosin is consistent with its moving as a rigid rod over seven actins. It has been suggested that tropomyosin might aid, alternatively, in transmitting changes in actin conformation along the filament (affecting actin's ability to bind myosin), and that tropomyosin movement might be simply an adjustment to this changed conformation, with no role in blocking myosin attachment (see Chap. 13).[177]

The changes in interactions between the troponin subunits, tropomyosin, and actin that lead to this movement of tropomyosin suggest a model in which, in the relaxed state, actin interacts via TnI with the TnC/TnI complex, and TnT anchors the complex to the troponin-binding site on tropomyosin.[151,213] TnI interaction with actin constrains tropomyosin on the outer domain of actin, blocking strong actin-myosin interaction. In the activated state, Ca^{2+} binds to the low-affinity sites on TnC, leading to the "open" TnC structure (see "Troponin C," above). This exposes the central helix in TnC, enhancing binding to TnI, which dissociates from its binding site on actin. This releases the constraint on tropomyosin, allowing it to move to its site on the inner domain of actin, where it no longer blocks myosin binding, thus allowing cross-bridge cycling (Fig. 7-35).[151,204,213] 3D reconstructions revealing troponin[204] support this model.

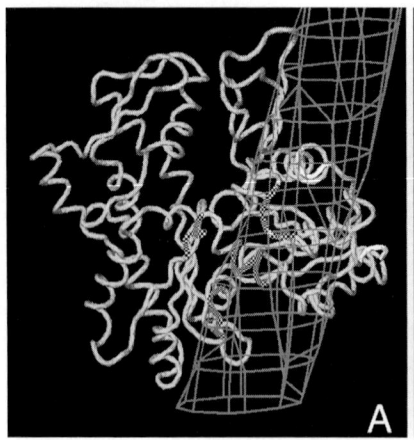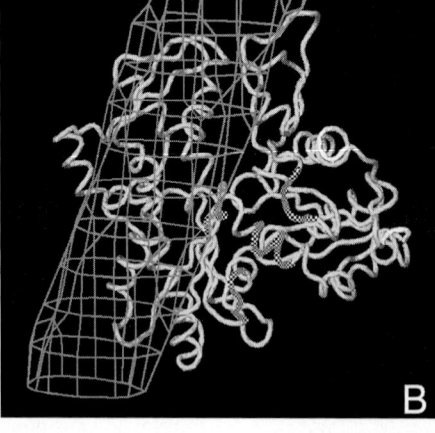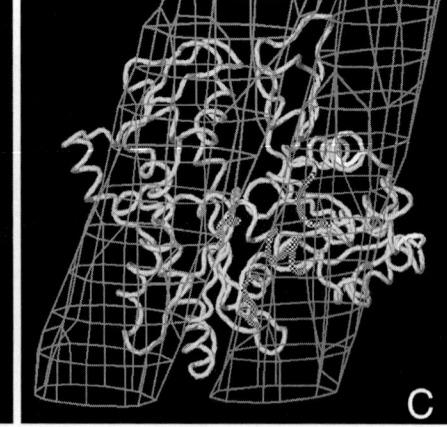

FIGURE 7-34. Location of tropomyosin densities (gray wire cage) on the atomic structure of F actin (white polypeptide chain) based on cryo-EM data. The atomic model of F actin[167] was fitted to the EM reconstruction (similar to Fig. 7-33), and a single actin monomer from the atomic model substituted for actin in the reconstruction; only the tropomyosin density displayed. A. Low-Ca^{2+} tropomyosin lies on the outer domain of actin over clusters of amino acid residues (checkered) involved in myosin binding. B. High-Ca^{2+} tropomyosin has moved to the inner domain, uncovering all but one of the myosin-binding clusters. C. Comparison of the two positions of tropomyosin. (Adapted from Xu C, Craig R, Tobacman L, et al: Tropomyosin positions in regulated thin filaments revealed by cryoelectron microscopy. Biophys J 77:985, 1999. With permission.)

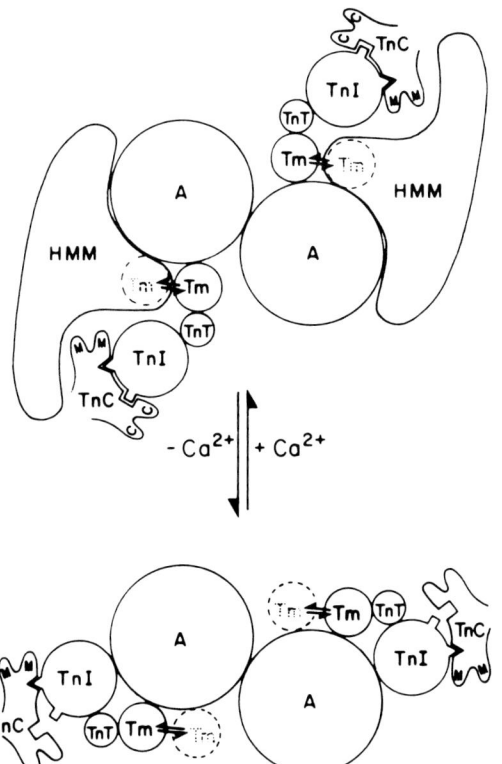

FIGURE 7-35. Schematic diagram of thin filament (cross-sectional view) summarizing biochemical data on interactions that occur between actin, tropomyosin, troponin, and myosin at high and low Ca^{2+}. At low Ca^{2+} (bottom), TnI binds to actin, constraining tropomyosin (Tm) to a position where it sterically blocks actin-myosin (A-HMM) interaction (top). At high Ca^{2+} (top), TnI interacts more strongly with TnC and breaks its contact with actin, allowing tropomyosin to move to its unblocking position and myosin (HMM) to bind. (From Potter JD, Johnson JD: Troponin, in Cheung Y (ed): Calcium and Cell Function. Vol II. New York: Academic Press, 1982; chap 5, p 145. By copyright permission of Academic Press.)

NEBULIN

The thin filaments, like the thick filaments, are also associated with a giant protein that appears to function as a molecular ruler specifying precise filament length.[9,10] Nebulin is an 800-kDa protein specific to skeletal muscle and constituting ~3 percent of myofibrillar mass. Antibody labeling shows that it extends as a single polypeptide along the full length of the thin filament (~0.9 μm), with its C terminal 30 kDa integrated into the Z line and its N terminus at the free end of the thin filaments (Fig. 7-3).[214–218] In cardiac muscle a smaller, closely related protein, nebulette (~109 kDa), sharing extensive structural homology with nebulin's C-terminal region, appears to substitute for nebulin.[219] However, nebulette does not specify cardiac thin-filament length, as it is predicted to extend along only 25 percent of the filament from the Z line.

Like most myofibrillar proteins, nebulin and nebulette have a modular structure (Fig. 7-36A).[218,220] Both are organized into four domains. A short N-terminal domain is followed by a series of 35 amino acid actin-binding repeats, which are linked to a C-terminal Src homology 3 (SH3) domain via a short linker. The C-terminal regions of nebulin and nebulette are identical in domain organization, sharing a family of closely related C-terminal repeats, a serine-rich domain with potential phosphorylation sites, and the SH3 domain.[216] A subgroup of the C-terminal repeats is differentially expressed during development and probably contributes to the anchoring of nebulin in the Z line and to Z-line tissue diversity.[216,218] The SH3 domain is closely related to proteins involved in regulating actin assembly in nonmuscle cells.[218] A third protein, N-RAP,[221] is also related to nebulin and found at the myotendinous junction and intercalated disks. It appears to be part of a complex of proteins that anchors the terminal actin filaments of the myofibril to the cell membrane, functioning in the transmission of force from the myofibrils to the extracellular matrix.

The main part of nebulin (>90 percent) consists almost entirely of multiple copies of the 35-residue motif.[218,220] Sequence analysis suggests that the repeat motifs are likely to be largely α-helical and to interact with both actin and tropomyosin. The central 154 copies are grouped into 22 superrepeats, each containing seven modules. The molecules are apparently oriented along the long-pitch helices of actin, with the 35-residue repeats binding to successive actin subunits and the 7 × 35 residues of one superrepeat spanning the 38.5-nm repeat distance of one regulatory tropomyosin-troponin complex (Fig. 7-36B).

The view that nebulin is a length determinant is suggested by the linear correlation between thin-filament length and the size of nebulin variants generated by alternative splicing in different skeletal muscles.[218,222] Nebulin could regulate length by matching the number of its superrepeats to an equal number of helical repeats of actin.[222] At the free tip of the thin filament, the three N-terminal modules bind to the thin-filament capping protein, tropomodulin (Tmod), suggesting that the two work together to control thin-filament length in skeletal muscle.[217]

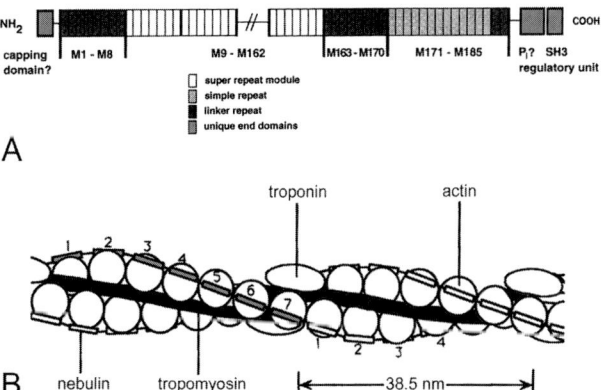

FIGURE 7-36. A. Domain structure of nebulin. (Adapted from Labeit S, Kolmerer B: The complete primary structure of human nebulin and its correlation to muscle structure. J Mol Biol 248:308, 1995. With permission from Elsevier Science.) B. Schematic model of proposed organization of nebulin on thin filament, showing association of one 35–amino acid module with each actin subunit and a superrepeat containing seven modules. (Adapted from Trinick J: Molecular rulers in muscle? Curr Biol 2:75, 1992. With permission from Elsevier Science.)

CAPPING PROTEINS

Actin filaments are major cytoskeletal elements of virtually all eukaryotic cells. Their functioning in intracellular transport and cell motility activities is critically dependent on their ability to polymerize and depolymerize as needed.[223] Polymerization occurs preferentially at the "plus" ("barbed") end of the filament (the end that in striated muscle is at the Z line), and depolymerization occurs more rapidly and polymerization more slowly at the "minus" ("pointed") end (the M-line end) of the filament.[223–225] The dynamic activity of actin filaments in nonmuscle cells is exactly the opposite of the requirements of striated muscle, where rapid and efficient contraction and relaxation depend on a set of relatively permanent, highly organized, linked filaments of defined and constant length. In striated muscle, filament length is stabilized by the binding of "capping" proteins to the filament ends, preventing the addition or removal of actin monomers.[223–225] The Z-line end of the thin filament is capped by the protein CapZ and the M-line end by tropomodulin (Fig. 7-37). Similar proteins perform these functions in nonmuscle cells in situations where more stable filaments are also required (e.g., the erythrocyte membrane skeleton, microvilli of intestinal epithelial cells) or length must temporarily be regulated.[224]

CapZ (β-actinin[226]) is a heterodimeric protein consisting of an α (36-kDa) and a β (32-kDa) subunit. CapZ nucleates actin filament assembly and binds to the barbed end of thin filaments (one copy per filament) with an affinity of ~1 nM, preventing monomer association and disassociation at that end.[224] It has also been shown to interact with α-actinin, providing a mechanism for anchoring CapZ in the Z line in striated muscle.[227] CapZ appears to function early in myofibril assembly, being observed in nascent Z lines before the organization of actin into a striated pattern.[228] It nucleates actin-filament polymerization at the Z line and specifies thin-filament polarity within the sarcomere.[224,228]

Tropomodulin (40 kDa) caps the pointed end of the thin filament, preventing filament growth and maintaining its final length.[224,229] It is present in one to two copies per thin filament.[224] Its high affinity (~1 nM) for the thin-filament tip probably derives from its binding to both actin (through its C-terminal half) and tropomyosin (through its N-terminal half), which it also caps.[224,230] Inhibition of its capping activity in embryonic cardiac myocytes results in dramatic elongation of actin filaments from their free ends and cells that are unable to beat, demonstrating the physiologic importance of capping by tropomodulin.[229] Consistent with its position at the pointed end of the filament, tropomodulin has also been shown to bind to the N terminus of nebulin, located at the filament tip.[217] It has been suggested that these two molecules may act in concert to determine filament length in skeletal muscle. Association of each actin subunit with a nebulin actin-binding module may specify initial thin-filament length. Nebulin's N terminus may then target tropomodulin to the filament tip, where it caps the terminal actin and tropomyosin molecules, thus maintaining this length.[217] Consistent with its involvement in the process of thin-filament assembly, tropomodulin in skeletal muscle myocytes is found in early, nonstriated premyofibrils, suggesting that thin filaments are assembled and capped at both ends first and then integrated into mature myofibrils by rearrangement and alignment.[231] In cardiac muscle, which lacks nebulin, the function of tropomodulin is less clear. It may act primarily to maintain and stabilize the final lengths of the thin filaments after they are assembled and organized into I bands,[230,231] or it may be involved more dynamically in thin-filament formation.[232] Interestingly, it has recently been shown that although thin-filament lengths are stabilized by CapZ and tropomodulin binding, both capping proteins are in fact relatively dynamic, allowing the exchange of actin subunits at both barbed and pointed ends while maintaining stable lengths.[233]

"SOLUBLE" ENZYME BINDING TO THE THIN FILAMENT

In addition to the regular binding of troponin, tropomyosin, nebulin, and capping proteins to the thin filament, there is evi-

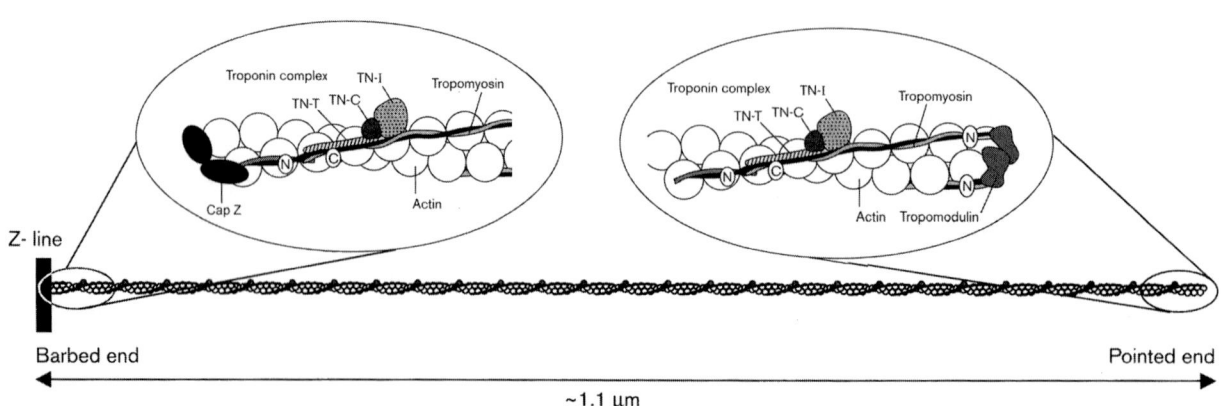

FIGURE 7-37. Schematic representation of the organization of the capping proteins tropomodulin and CapZ on the thin filament. CapZ is shown as a heterodimer with two subunits of similar size. *(Adapted from Fowler VM: Regulation of actin filament length in erythrocytes and striated muscle. Curr Opin Cell Biol 8:86, 1996. With permission from Elsevier Science.)*

dence that several soluble cellular enzymes (mostly glycolytic enzymes) also bind, albeit weakly. Aldolase, glyceraldehyde phosphate dehydrogenase, phosphofructokinase, adenylate kinase, and creatine kinase have all been shown to bind to actin filaments (troponin and tropomyosin may also play a role in this binding) or have been localized in the I bands of striated muscle.[153,234] Some, while not binding directly to the thin filament, may be targeted to the I band by other proteins that do.[235] The binding of glycolytic enzymes to actin filaments in muscle as well as nonmuscle cells may provide a means of modulating cellular metabolism.[236] The binding generally appears to be weak, being reduced or abolished in permeabilized cells,[237] but a significant proportion of these enzymes may be bound in conditions prevailing in the intact cell, while others may not.[238] The amount of binding increases with muscle stimulation.[239]

The Z Line

The striking regularity of the thin filaments in the sarcomere is a result of specific interactions with a cytoskeletal lattice known as the Z line (also called the Z band or Z disk because of its finite thickness). Z lines occur at the ends of the sarcomere, forming the junction between one sarcomere and the next (Fig. 7-1B to D) and the site at which thin-filament polarity reverses.[21] Thin filaments from each half sarcomere are organized at the Z line into a regular tetragonal array that interdigitates with the array from the adjacent half sarcomere and forms links to it. Z lines serve as attachment points and mechanical links not only between thin filaments but also between titin filaments from adjacent sarcomeres, which overlap within the Z line. They thus play a fundamental role in the transmission of force along the myofibril.[240] Z lines are, in addition, attachment sites for inter- mediate filaments that form lateral links with adjacent myofibrils.

STRUCTURE

In longitudinal sections, the Z line appears as either a zigzag pattern or an interdigitation of the thin filaments (Fig. 7-38A). These appearances reflect orthogonal views of the same structure. In transverse section, the Z line has either a square array

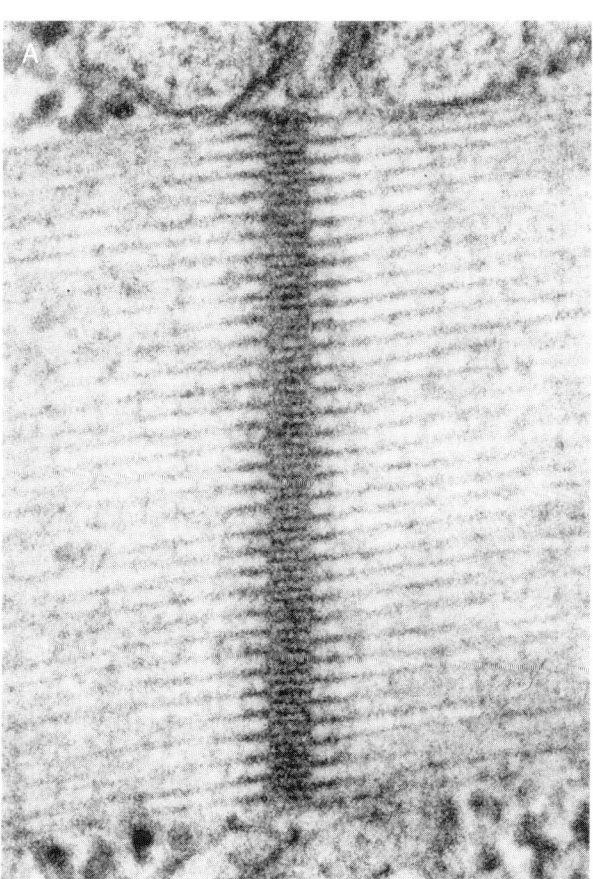
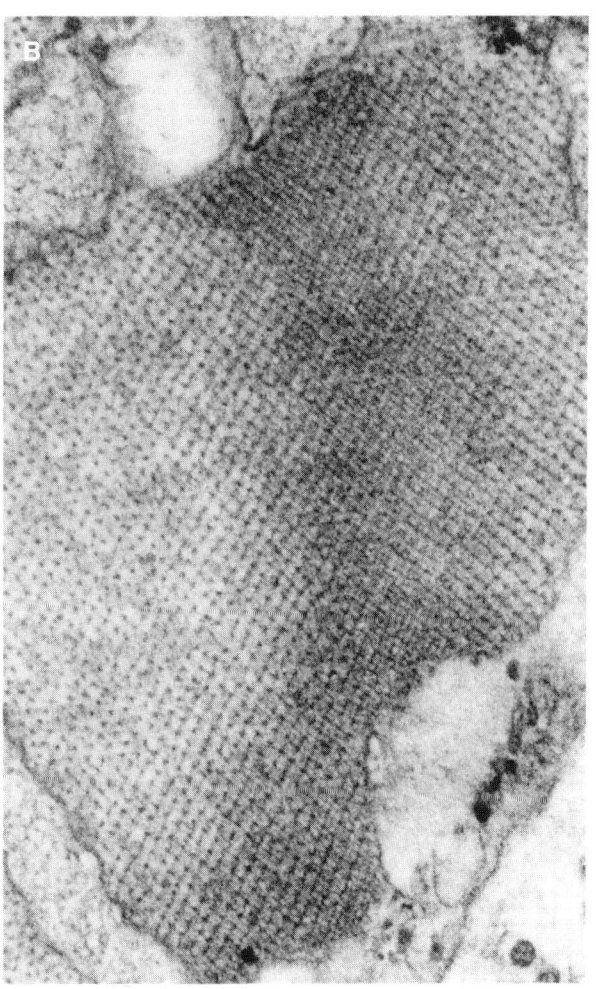

FIGURE 7-38. Z-line structure of frog sartorius muscle observed in electron micrographs of (A) longitudinal section, showing overlapping thin filaments in the Z line extending to either side in the I band, and (B) slightly oblique transverse section, grazing into the I band at left. (A, × 150,000; B, × 90,000.)

or a "basket-weave" appearance, both of which can occur in the same sarcomere[21,241–243] (Fig. 7-38B). The two structures are thought to be closely related[244] and may be related to different physiologic states.[240,245] These appearances show that the thin filaments are not continuous across the Z line but form tetragonal lattices that are offset with respect to each other, such that each thin filament on one side enters the space between four thin filaments from the other. These interpenetrating arrays are connected to each other within the Z line.[241,244,246]

This basic appearance of the Z line varies somewhat from one fiber type and species to another, the differences appearing mainly as variations in Z-line width in longitudinal section (30 to 120 nm).[83,240,244] Fast white muscles have a narrow, "simple" Z line with a single zigzag line connecting the ends of opposing thin filaments, while Z lines in slow muscles are wider, having three or four zigzag lines. The major determinant of Z-line width is the extent of overlap of opposing thin filaments.

COMPOSITION

The Z line contains numerous components, including α-actinin, amorphin, FATZ (myozenin), Znin, Z protein, γ-filamin, ZASP, myotilin, myopodin, and myopalladin in addition to overlapping portions of thin filaments (including actin, CapZ, and nebulin) and of the N terminus of titin filaments, including telethonin [240,247] [it should be noted, however, that the status of some of these proteins as bona fide Z-line components is uncertain (see below)]. In addition, intermediate filaments encircle the periphery of the Z line and link Z lines of adjacent myofibrils together, thus maintaining the striation pattern in register over the whole fiber (see "Intermediate Filaments," below). The properties of some of the main Z-line components are outlined below. Mutations in several of these proteins are associated with a variety of muscular dystrophies and cardiomyopathies, suggesting a central role for the Z line in sarcomere assembly and integrity.[137,248,249]

α-Actinin is the key structural component of the Z line, cross-linking both antiparallel actin filaments and antiparallel titin filaments from abutting half sarcomeres and binding to numerous other Z-line proteins. α-Actinin is an antiparallel homodimer ~35 nm long, with subunit molecular mass of 95 kDa.[240] It is constructed from an N-terminal calponin-homology domain that binds actin, a central rod region composed of repeated spectrin-like triple-helical units, and an EF hand domain. Its dimensions suggest that it might be the bridging protein forming the links (Z filaments) between oppositely polarized thin filaments from neighboring sarcomeres.[246,250] Links between thin filaments of the same polarity are also present and may be due to direct connections between α-actinin molecules along neighboring thin filaments. α-Actinin connects to titin molecules from opposite half-sarcomeres, via two classes of link. Together with its connections to actin, α-actinin thus creates a ternary complex containing titin, actin, α-actinin, and probably several other proteins (see below).[250]

CapZ, the thin-filament barbed end-capping protein, interacts with α-actinin, thus contributing to anchoring the thin filaments in the Z line.[227] It is localized in nascent Z lines during myofibrillogenesis before striations appear and may thus function to organize and stabilize actin filaments during myofibril formation.

Amorphin is an 85-kDa protein thought to be a component of the amorphous Z-line material. It may be the same protein as glycogen phosphorylase,[240] possibly binding to actin as do other enzymes (see "'Soluble' Enzyme Binding to the Thin Filament," above). Znin is an incompletely characterized 300- to 400-kDa protein, possibly a proteolytic fragment of a larger protein, such as titin.[240,247] Z protein is a 55-kDa protein thought to form a tetramer in vivo and localizing to the interior of the Z line.[240]

Myopalladin[251] is a 145-kDa protein that links the C-terminal SH3 domain of nebulin to the EF hand domain of α-actinin, thus anchoring nebulin in the Z line. Myopalladin also binds to the cardiac ankyrin repeat protein (CARP) involved in regulating muscle gene expression. Thus myopalladin may link the regulation of Z-line structure (via α-actinin and nebulin) to that of muscle gene expression (via CARP).[251]

Myopodin[252] is an actin-bundling protein found in the Z line of skeletal and cardiac muscle and also in the cell nucleus. It may play a structural role at the Z line and also participate in signaling between the nucleus and Z line during development and under conditions of cell stress.[252]

Myozenin[253] (also called FATZ or calsarcin-2) is a 32-kDa protein that binds α-actinin, γ-filamin, and telethonin. It may function as an adapter that binds α-actinin or γ-filamin to telethonin or other Z-line proteins, or it may influence the dimerization of these proteins and thus the lateral spacing of thin filaments in the Z line.

Myotilin[254,255] (molecular mass 57 kDa) binds α-actinin and has been implicated in limb-girdle muscular dystrophy type 1A.[249]

Like the other filamin isoforms, γ-filamin has an N-terminal calponin homology domain that binds actin, followed by 24 Ig-like repeats, and a C-terminal domain involved in dimer formation. An insertion in its Ig-like domain 20 interacts directly with myotilin, indirectly anchoring γ-filamin to α-actinin in the Z line.[254]

In addition to the above components, a number of proteins all containing N-terminal PDZ and C-terminal LIM domains have been found associated with the Z line. PDZ motifs are protein-protein interaction domains that often bind to C-terminal peptide sequences, while LIM domains bind to protein kinases. These proteins are thus thought to act as adapter molecules, directing kinases to the cytoskeleton. Their putative role in signaling pathways suggests that they may be involved in muscle development. Several of these proteins (e.g., ZASP[256] and Cypher[248]) bind to α-actinin, localizing these proteins in the Z line, where they play roles in either development or maintenance of Z-line structure.

MODEL

In the most detailed structural study of a Z line carried out so far, using crystallographic averaging techniques, thin filaments from adjacent sarcomeres overlap by ~25 nm, each being linked to its four opposing neighbors by Z filaments thought to contain α-actinin (Fig. 7-39A).[257] These links occur at three points separated by ~15 nm. One pair originates at the center of the Z line and orthogonal pairs emerge 15 nm away in each direction, near the end of each actin filament. This model can account for different width Z lines by simple adjustment of the actin filament overlap and the number of levels of Z links.[244,257] The simplest (narrowest) Z line has minimal actin filament overlap and only two pairs of links originating near the filament ends.[246] Wider Z lines have greater filament overlap, and additional Z-links occur at points spaced half the actin crossover length apart and rotated by 90 degrees.[258] The amount of overlap is set by the requirement that the Z link closest to the M band of one thin filament form a link to the terminus of the opposing thin filament. In addition to these connections between antiparallel filaments, additional links on either side of the center of the Z line may connect thin filaments of the same polarity to each other.[246,257] Tomographic reconstruction of a mammalian Z line also reveals Z filaments that connect interdigitating actin filaments from adjacent sarcomeres via a short additional feature running parallel to the actin filaments.[259] This reconstruction also shows connections between parallel filaments from the same sarcomere in the I band, near to the Z line.

Further insights into Z-line structure come from studies of the sequences, interactions, and antibody labeling patterns of the Z-line components (Fig. 7-39B).[9,136,142,250,260] These studies suggest that titin molecules overlap within the Z line, with their N-terminal 30 kDa located at the edge of the Z line in the adjacent sarcomere, where the first two titin Ig repeats (Z1 and Z2) bind to telethonin (see "Titin Filaments," above). The following 60 kDa of titin span the Z line, overlapping with titin from the adjacent sarcomere. This region of titin contains up to seven copies of a 45-residue "Z repeat," each of which can bind to the carboxy terminus of α-actinin (although this simple one-to-one interaction model has been questioned[261]). Thus α-actinin may function to cross-link not only actin filaments but also antiparallel titin filaments within the Z line. These 45-residue Z repeats are differentially spliced in the central Z-line region of titin. Thus titin molecules may specify Z-line width and internal structure by varying the length of their N-terminal overlap and number of α-actinin binding sites that serve to cross-link titin and thin filaments. Regions of Z-line titin and telethonin are phosphorylated by regulatory kinases, suggesting that the titin N terminus may be involved in controlling fibril assembly. Interestingly, it has also been shown that telethonin binds to a potassium channel likely to be localized in the membrane of the T tubule surrounding the Z line of cardiac myofibrils. It is speculated that this link between myofibril and T tubule may contribute to stretch-dependent regulation of potassium flux in cardiac muscle, providing a "mechanoelectrical feedback" system.[262]

In contrast to actin and titin, which span the Z line, nebulin appears likely to insert only in the periphery, via its C-terminal, SH3-containing domain,[216] which binds to α-actinin via myopalladin.[251] This additional connection to α-actinin further emphasizes the role of α-actinin as the major integrator of Z-line structure, connecting all key components of the Z-line lattice. It is possible that the ending of nebulin at the edge of the Z line determines where tropomyosin binding to actin terminates, and thus where the binding of α-actinin (with which tropomyosin competes) becomes possible. Regulating the amount of titin and actin filament overlap in the Z line and the degree of nebulin insertion is likely to be physiologically important, as the width of the Z line determined in this way (narrow in fast- and wide in slow-twitch fibers) correlates with the mechanical properties of the muscle. In addition to nebulin's links to α actinin, it appears that nebulin modules from the peripheral region of the Z line may also be part of the link to the system of desmin intermediate filaments that encircle Z lines and cross-link adjacent myofibrils. In addition, synemin, a component of these intermediate filaments, also binds directly to α-actinin and to vinculin, a component of the costamere[263] (see "Intermediate Filaments," below). These links could enable the intermediate filaments to directly link all myofibrils to each other and the peripheral layer to the cell membrane,

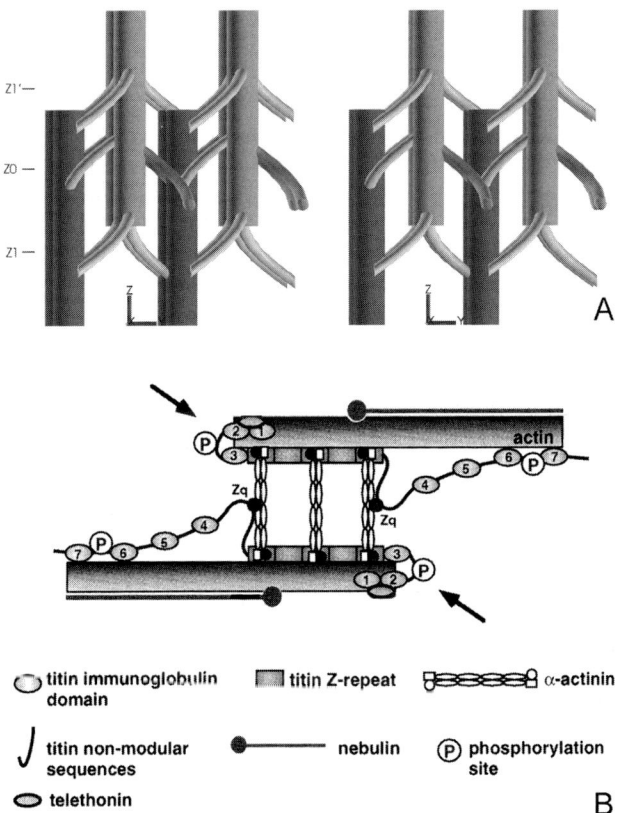

FIGURE 7-39. Models of Z-line structure. A. Stereo view based on 3D reconstruction from tilted sections of intermediate-width Z line of fish muscle. Actin filaments running vertically overlap in the Z line and are connected there by obliquely oriented filaments, probably largely α-actinin. (From Luther PK: Three-dimensional structure of a vertebrate muscle Z-band: Implications for titin and α-actinin binding. J Struct Biol 129:1, 2000. With permission from Elsevier Science.) B. Schematic diagram of suggested actin, α-actinin, titin, nebulin, and telethonin organization, based on sequence and immunoelectron microscopic data. (Modified from Gautel M, Mues A, Young P: Control of sarcomeric assembly: The flow of information on titin. Rev Physiol Biochem Pharmacol 138:97, 1999, to show nebulin molecules extending only part way into the Z line.[216] With permission from Springer-Verlag.)

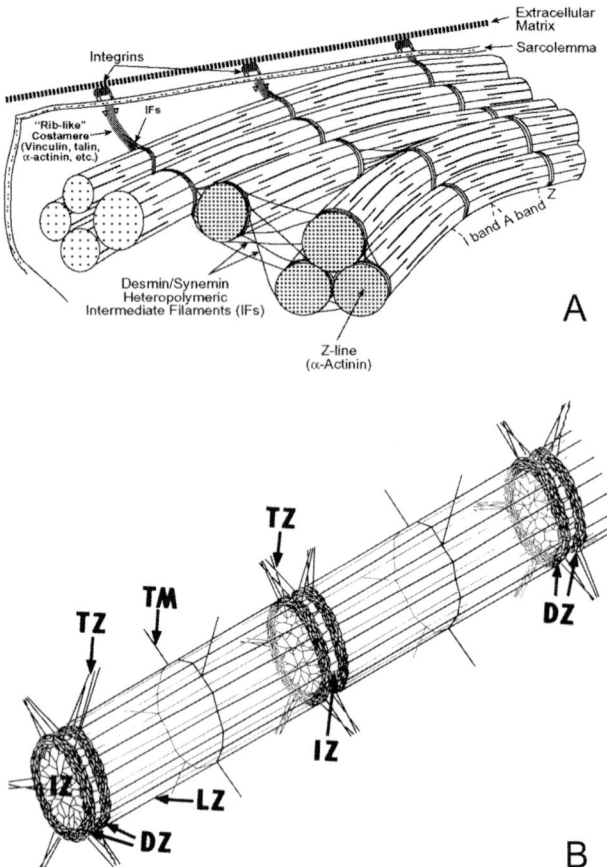

FIGURE 7-40. Schematic diagrams showing intermediate filaments (A) encircling sarcomeres at the Z line and connecting to other sarcomeres and to the cell membrane (*From Bellin RM, Huiatt TW, Critchley DR, et al: Synemin may function to directly link muscle cell intermediate filaments to both myofibrillar Z-lines and costameres. J Biol Chem 276:32330, 2001. With permission.*); (B) encircling and extending from the Z line (TZ) and M line (TM) and extending longitudinally from Z line to Z line (LZ). (*From Wang K, Ramirez-Mitchell R: A network of transverse and longitudinal intermediate filaments is associated with sarcomeres of adult vertebrate skeletal muscle. J Cell Biol 96:562, 1983. By copyright permission of the Rockefeller University Press.*)

thus providing a radial route for transmission of force to the surrounding connective tissue.

Intermediate Filaments

In addition to the cytoskeletal lattices formed by the M and Z lines, which function to organize the thick and thin filaments in three dimensions, a lattice of intermediate filaments 10 nm in diameter attaches to the periphery of the sarcomere, organizing the structure of the muscle cell at the supersarcomeric level (Fig. 7-40). These filaments reinforce and integrate the structure of the cell by forming transverse links between adjacent myofibrils (possibly via attachment to SR or T-tubule membranes), maintaining them in register with each other across the fiber, and by connecting myofibrils to the sarcolemma and the nucleus.[247,264–266]

Intermediate filaments are best detected following extraction of the thick and thin filaments from muscle.[264,265] It is generally agreed that they encircle the myofibril at the Z line,[264] possibly in two closely spaced rings (Fig. 7-40B).[265] A less prominent ring at the M line has also been reported.[265] From the peripheries of these rings emerge transverse filaments connecting myofibrils to each other at neighboring Z and M lines, respectively, and to the sarcolemma at the costamere (Fig. 7-40A).[264] It has also been suggested that 50 to 100 longitudinal filaments span the length of the sarcomere from Z line to Z line (Fig. 7-40B), possibly contributing to transmission of force along the fibril, even through sarcomeres that have been damaged or overstretched.[265] Such myofibrils could therefore still develop force. The identification of the longitudinal and M-line filaments as intermediate filaments has been questioned, however.[264]

The major constituent of the intermediate filaments of mature muscle is desmin, the muscle-specific member of the intermediate-filament family. Vimentin is strongly expressed during development and coexists with desmin in the same filaments, but it disappears in mature muscle. Smaller quantities of the intermediate-filament proteins, synemin, paranemin, and nestin, associate with desmin filaments, while the intermediate-filament-associated protein plectin forms links between intermediate filaments and other cellular structures.[267] All of these proteins colocalize at the Z line and are found in addition at the myotendinous junction and in the postsynaptic area of motor end plates.

Desmin and vimentin (53 to 55 kDa) are typical intermediate-filament proteins. They are characterized by a mostly α-helical central rod domain and have C- and N-terminal nonhelical regions.[267,268] They assemble into nonpolar filaments via their coiled-coil domains, which form the filament core, with their globular regions on the surface. Both proteins are able to form homopolymers, although in vivo they are probably mostly heteropolymeric. Desmin is the first muscle-specific protein to appear during myogenesis, but it does not appear to be essential for muscle development.[266,269] However, postnatally, highly used muscles lacking desmin become susceptible to damage and show severe disruption of structure, consistent with the essential role of intermediate filaments in strengthening cells subject to mechanical stress.[266,269]

Synemin, paranemin, and nestin are additional intermediate-filament proteins that cannot form intermediate filaments on their own but coassemble with desmin or vimentin in muscle cells.[267] Synemin (~230 kDa) occurs at the Z line and contains binding sites for α-actinin and for the costameric protein vinculin.[263] It is thought to anchor intermediate filaments to the Z line by interaction with α-actinin and to costameres at the sarcolemma via interaction with vinculin and/or α-actinin.[263] It may thus play a key role in directly linking all myofibrils of the cell to each other and peripheral myofibrils to the sarcolemma (Fig. 7-40A). Paranemin is a 180-kDa intermediate-filament protein that coassembles with vimentin and desmin in adult and embryonic skeletal and cardiac muscle.[270] Nestin is coexpressed with desmin and vimentin in developing muscle, colocalizing with them at the Z line, but it is postnatally downregulated.[266]

Syncoilin[271] (64 kDa) is an intermediate-filament protein that binds to desmin and to the dystrophin protein complex. It is found at the neuromuscular junction, the sarcolemma, and the Z line. In contrast to most intermediate-filament proteins, syncoilin appears to be highly soluble and not to form filaments. It has therefore been suggested that, rather than associating with desmin to form filaments, it may be involved in organizing the intermediate-filament network and anchoring it to the sarcolemma via the dystrophin protein complex. It may thus play an important role in providing structural support to muscle fibers.

Skelemin[126,127] (~200 kDa) appears to be a splice variant of myomesin (being encoded by the same gene), containing two motifs that have been suggested to be intermediate-filament-like (see "The M Line," above). It appears to be present in the filaments forming rings around the periphery of the M line and also linking the rings in adjacent myofibrils.[127] The myosin-binding ability of skelemin, together with its putative intermediate-filament core-like motifs, could enable it to link myosin filaments at the periphery of the sarcomere to the intermediate-filament cytoskeleton.[127] There is also evidence that skelemin interacts with the cytoplasmic domain of sarcolemmal integrin molecules, thus potentially connecting peripheral myofibrils to the cell membrane at the M line.[272]

Plectin is a member of the plakin family of large (>200-kDa) coiled-coil dimeric linker proteins that function to connect intermediate filaments (via a carboxy-terminal IF binding domain) to other elements of the cytoskeleton (actin filaments and microtubules) and to additional structures such as cell junctions.[273] In muscle, plectin colocalizes with desmin filaments at the Z line and with the links between Z lines.[267,274] Plectin may use its actin-binding capacity to function as a link between the Z line and the encircling intermediate filaments.[266] Plectin is also present in the links between peripheral myofibrils and the sarcolemma[266] and appears additionally to function as a link between myofibrillar desmin filaments and mitochondria, possibly playing a role in mitochondrial positioning and shape.[274] The absence of plectin is associated with muscular dystrophy.[273]

The intermediate filaments and their associated proteins thus play a crucial role in structural integration at the cellular level, strengthening the sarcomere, maintaining myofibrils in register, and transmitting force from the interior of the cell to the extracellular matrix by directly linking all cellular myofibrils to each other and attaching the peripheral layer to the cell membrane.

Diseases of the Sarcomere

Mutations in sarcomeric proteins are the prime cause of a major class of diseases that affect cardiac function. Familial hypertrophic cardiomyopathy (FHC) is an autosomal dominant disease characterized by ventricular hypertrophy, myocyte hypertrophy, and disarray.[275–279] It is the most common cause of sudden cardiac death in the young and a major cause of death in the old. The identification of over 100 mutations in nine sarcomeric proteins in FHC patients implies that FHC is a disease of the sarcomere. The genes encode cardiac thick-, thin-, and titin-filament proteins: the β-myosin heavy chain, α-tropomyosin, troponin T, troponin I, MyBP-C, the myosin regulatory and essential light chains, actin, and titin. Those most commonly implicated are the β-myosin heavy chain, troponin T, and MyBP-C, which together account for two-thirds of all FHC cases. It is speculated that the mutation leads to a poison polypeptide that is incorporated into the sarcomere, leading to altered sarcomere and myocyte structure and exerting a dominant negative effect on sarcomere function. Impaired cardiac function would lead to less efficient pumping by the heart, and it is thought that hypertrophy may result as a compensatory mechanism. The sarcomeric mutations cause a variety of defects, including alterations in myosin ATPase, actin-myosin interaction, cross-bridge kinetics, or Ca^{2+} sensitivity, leading to impaired contraction or relaxation.

As one example we can consider mutations in the cardiac MyBP-C gene, one of the most common causes of FHC.[91] These include point mutations, misspliced or truncated polypeptides, and deletions that disrupt a single domain while leaving the reading frame intact. Some mutants retain thick-filament binding sites at the C terminus (those that bind titin and LMM) and are assembly-competent. Others lack one or more C-terminal domains and do not assemble into the filament. Since cardiac C protein is crucial in myofibril assembly, reduced amounts of functional protein could lead to disturbed myofibril assembly and thus the sarcomere disarray characteristic of FHC. Mutations in the proteins to which MyBP-C binds also lead to FHC. The phosphorylatable N-terminal domain of cardiac MyBP-C binds to a specific region of myosin S2.[98] Mutations in this binding region of S2 are associated with FHC, apparently due to the loss of interaction with MyBP-C. It is suggested that the regulatory function of MyBP-C is mediated by this interaction with S2 and that mutations in S2 may act by altering these interactions.[98]

Other mutations in sarcomeric proteins lead to a variety of other myopathies, including limb-girdle muscular dystrophy type 2G (telethonin),[137] limb-girdle muscular dystrophy type 1A (myotilin),[249] nemaline myopathy (actin, tropomyosin, and nebulin),[280] desmin-related myopathy (desmin),[280] and other myopathies (e.g., plectin[273] and Cypher[248]).

Acknowledgments

This revision was supported by grants AR34711 and HL62468 from the National Institutes of Health (to RC) and from the Howard Hughes Medical Institute and the Venezuelan National Fund for Science, Technology and Innovation (FONACIT) (to RP). We thank Lorenzo Alamo for help with the figures.

List of Abbreviations

ADP	adenosine diphosphate	IFAP	IF-associated protein
AMP	adenosine monophosphate	Ig	immunoglobulin
ATP	adenosine triphosphate	LMM	light meromyosin
ATPase	adenosine triphosphatase	M	mol/L
CARP	cardiac ankyrin repeat protein	MyBP-C (-H, -X)	myosin-binding protein C (H, X)
CK	creatine kinase	Pi	inorganic phosphate
EM	electron microscopy	S1	subfragment 1 (of HMM)
FHC	familial hypertrophic cardiomyopathy	S2	subfragment 2 (of HMM)
Fn	fibronectin	SDS	sodium dodecyl sulfate
HMM	heavy meromyosin	SR	sarcoplasmic reticulum
IF	intermediate filament	TnC (TnI, TnT)	troponin C (I, T)

References

1. Huxley HE: Electron microscope studies of the organization of the filaments in striated muscle. *Biochim Biophys Acta* 12:387, 1953.
2. Huxley HE: The double array of filaments in cross-striated muscle. *J Biophys Biochem Cytol* 3:631, 1957.
3. Huxley HE: X-ray analysis and the problem of muscle. *Proc R Soc Lond [Biol]* 141:59, 1953.
4. Hanson J, Huxley HE: Structural basis of the cross-striations in muscle. *Nature* 172:530, 1953.
5. Huxley HE, Hanson J: Quantitative studies on the structure of cross-striated myofibrils. I. Investigations by interference microscopy. *Biochim Biophys Acta* 23:229, 1957.
6. Hanson J, Huxley HE: Quantitative studies on the structure of cross-striated myofibrils. II. Investigations by biochemical techniques. *Biochim Biophys Acta* 23:250, 1957.
7. Engelhardt WA, Ljubimowa MN: Myosine and adenosinetriphosphatase. *Nature* 144:668, 1939.
8. Szent-Györgyi A: *Chemistry of Muscular Contraction.* New York: Academic Press, 1951.
9. Gregorio CC, Granzier H, Sorimachi H, et al: Muscle assembly: A titanic achievement? *Curr Opin Cell Biol* 11:18, 1999.
10. Horowits R, Luo G, Zhang JQ, et al: Nebulin and nebulin-related proteins in striated muscle. *Adv Biophys* 33:143, 1996.
11. Needham DM: *Machina Carnis.* Cambridge, UK: Cambridge University Press, 1971.
12. Huxley AF: *Reflections on Muscle. The Sherrington Lectures XIV.* Liverpool: Liverpool University Press, 1980.
13. Huxley HE, Hanson J: Changes in the cross-striations of muscle during contraction and stretch and their structural interpretation. *Nature* 173:973, 1954.
14. Huxley AF, Niedergerke R: Structural changes in muscle during contraction. Interference microscopy of living muscle fibres. *Nature* 173:971, 1954.
15. Page SG, Huxley HE: Filament lengths in striated muscle. *J Cell Biol* 19:369, 1963.
16. Huxley HE, Brown W: The low-angle x-ray diagram of vertebrate striated muscle and its behavior during contraction and rigor. *J Mol Biol* 30:383, 1967.
17. Elliott GF, Lowy J, Millman BM: Low angle x-ray diffraction studies of living striated muscle during contraction. *J Mol Biol* 25:31, 1967.
18. Huxley HE, Faruqi AR, Kress M, et al: Time-resolved x-ray diffraction studies of the myosin layer-line reflections during muscle contraction. *J Mol Biol* 158:637, 1982.
19. Huxley AF: Muscle structure and theories of contraction. *Prog Biophys Biophys Chem* 7:255, 1957.
20. Huxley HE: The mechanism of muscular contraction. *Science* 164:1356, 1969.
21. Huxley HE: Electron microscope studies on the structure of natural and synthetic protein filaments from striated muscle. *J Mol Biol* 7:281, 1963.
22. Craig R, Knight P: Myosin molecules, thick filaments and the actin-myosin complex, in Harris R (ed): *Electron Microscopy of Proteins.* Vol 4. London: Academic Press, 1983; p 97.
23. Cooke R: Muscle myosin, skeletal, in Kreis T, Vale R (eds): *Guidebook to the Cytoskeletal and Motor Proteins,* 2d ed. New York: Oxford University Press, 1999; p 421.
24. Lowey S, Slayter HS, Weeds AG, Baker H: Substructure of the myosin molecule. I. Subfragments of myosin by enzymic degradation. *J Mol Biol* 42:1, 1969.
25. Davis JS: Assembly processes in vertebrate skeletal thick filament formation. *Annu Rev Biophys Biophys Chem* 17:217, 1988.
26. Knight P, Trinick J: Structure of the myosin projections on native thick filaments from vertebrate skeletal muscle. *J Mol Biol* 177:461, 1984.
27. Maita T, Yajima E, Nagata S, et al: The primary structure of skeletal muscle myosin heavy chain: IV. Sequence of the rod, and the complete 1,938-residue sequence of the heavy chain. *J Biochem* 110:75, 1991.
28. Warrick HM, Spudich JA: Myosin structure and function in cell motility. *Annu Rev Cell Biol* 3:379, 1987.
29. Kalbitzer HR, Maeda K, Rosch A, et al: C-terminal structure and mobility of rabbit skeletal muscle light meromyosin as studied by one- and two-dimensional ^{1}H NMR spectroscopy and x-ray small-angle scattering. *Biochemistry* 30:8083, 1991.
30. Maeda K, Rosch A, Maeda Y, et al: Rabbit skeletal muscle myosin. Unfolded carboxyl-terminus and its role in molecular assembly. *FEBS Lett* 281:23, 1991.
31. Rayment I, Rypniewski WR, Schmidt-Base K, et al: Three-dimensional structure of myosin subfragment-1: A molecular motor. *Science* 261:50, 1993.
32. Vibert P, Cohen C: Domains, motion and regulation in the myosin head. *J Muscle Res Cell Motil* 9:296, 1988.
33. Dominguez R, Freyzon Y, Trybus KM, et al: Crystal structure of a vertebrate smooth muscle myosin motor domain and its complex with the essential light chain: Visualization of the pre-power stroke state. *Cell* 94:559, 1998.
34. Mornet D, Pantel P, Audemard E, et al: Proteolytic approach to structure and function of actin recognition site in myosin heads. *Biochemistry* 20:2110, 1981.
35. Walker M, Knight P, Trinick J: Negative staining of myosin molecules. *J Mol Biol* 184:535, 1985.
36. Poulsen FR, Lowy J: Small-angle x-ray scattering from myosin heads in relaxed and rigor frog skeletal muscles. *Nature* 303:146, 1983.
37. Wray JS: Structure of relaxed myosin filaments in relation to nucleotide state in vertebrate skeletal muscle. *J Muscle Res Cell Motil* 8:62, 1987.
38. Crowther RA, Padron R, Craig R: Arrangement of the heads of myosin in relaxed thick filaments from tarantula muscle. *J Mol Biol* 184:429, 1985.
39. Stewart M, Kensler RW, Levine RJC: Structure of *Limulus* telson muscle thick filaments. *J Mol Biol* 153:781, 1981.
40. Vibert P, Craig R: Electron microscopy and image analysis of myosin filaments from scallop striated muscle. *J Mol Biol* 165:303, 1983.
41. Morris EP, Squire JM, Fuller GW: Three-dimensional reconstruction of the myosin filaments from *Lethocerus* flight muscle. *J Struct Biol* 107:237, 1991.
42. Matsubara I: Light and x-ray diffraction studies on chick skeletal muscle under controlled physiological conditions. *J Physiol (Lond)* 238:473, 1974.
43. Matsubara I, Millman BM: X-ray diffraction patterns from mammalian heart muscle. *J Mol Biol* 82:527, 1974.
44. Kensler RW, Stewart M: Frog skeletal muscle thick filaments are three-stranded. *J Cell Biol* 96:1797, 1983.
45. Stewart M, Kensler RW: Arrangement of myosin heads in relaxed thick filaments from frog skeletal muscle. *J Mol Biol* 192:831, 1986.
46. Haselgrove JC: A model of myosin crossbridge structure consistent with the low-angle x-ray diffraction pattern of vertebrate muscle. *J Muscle Res Cell Motil* 1:177, 1980.

47. Harford JJ, Squire JM: "Crystalline" myosin cross-bridge array in relaxed bony fish muscle: Low-angle X-ray diffraction from plaice fin muscle and its interpretation. *Biophys J* 50:145, 1986.
48. Eakins F, Al-Khayat H-A, Kensler RW, et al: 3D structure of fish muscle myosin filaments. *J Struct Biol* 137:154, 2002.
49. Squire JM: *Muscle: Design, Diversity, and Disease*. Menlo Park, CA: Benjamin/Cummings, 1986.
50. Kensler RW, Levine RJ: Determination of the handedness of the cross-bridge helix of *Limulus* thick filaments. *J Muscle Res Cell Motil* 3:349, 1982.
51. Wray JS, Vibert PJ, Cohen C: Diversity of cross-bridge configurations in invertebrate muscles. *Nature* 257:561, 1975.
52. Levine RJ, Chantler PD, Kensler RW: Arrangement of myosin heads on *Limulus* thick filaments. *J Cell Biol* 107:1739, 1988.
53. Levine RJ: Evidence for overlapping myosin heads on relaxed thick filaments of fish, frog, and scallop striated muscles. *J Struct Biol* 110:99, 1993.
54. Padrón R, Alamo L, Murgich J, et al: Towards an atomic model of the thick filaments of muscle. *J Mol Biol* 275:35, 1998.
55. Kensler RW, Levine RJC: An electron microscopic and optical diffraction analysis of the structure of *Limulus* telson muscle thick filaments. *J Cell Biol* 92:443, 1982.
56. Wray JS: Structure of the backbone in myosin filaments of muscle. *Nature* 277:37, 1979.
57. Tregear RT, Hoyland J, Sayers AJ: The repeat distance of myosin in the thick filaments of various muscles. *J Mol Biol* 176:417, 1984.
58. Squire JM: General model for the structure of all myosin-containing filaments. *Nature* 233:457, 1971.
59. Squire JM: General model of myosin filament structure. III. Molecular packing arrangements in myosin filaments. *J Mol Biol* 77:291, 1973.
60. Offer G, Knight PJ, Burgess SA, et al: A new model for the surface arrangement of myosin molecules in tarantula thick filaments. *J Mol Biol* 298:239, 2000.
61. Padrón R, Alamo L, Guerrero JR, et al: Three-dimensional reconstruction of thick filaments from rapidly frozen, freeze-substituted tarantula muscle. *J Struct Biol* 115:250, 1995.
62. Xu S, Gu J, Rhodes T, et al: The M.ADP.P(i) state is required for helical order in the thick filaments of skeletal muscle. *Biophys J* 77:2665, 1999.
63. Haselgrove JC: X-ray evidence for conformational changes in the myosin filaments of vertebrate striated muscle. *J Mol Biol* 92:113, 1975.
64. Vibert P, Craig R: Structural changes that occur in scallop myosin filaments upon activation. *J Cell Biol* 101:830, 1985.
65. Padrón R, Craig R: Disorder induced in nonoverlap myosin crossbridges by loss of adenosine triphosphate. *Biophys J* 56:927, 1989.
66. Levine RJ, Chantler PD, Kensler RW: Effects of phosphorylation by myosin light chain kinase on the structure of *Limulus* thick filaments. *J Cell Biol* 113:563, 1991.
67. Levine RJ, Kensler RW, Yang Z, et al: Myosin light chain phosphorylation affects the structure of rabbit skeletal muscle thick filaments. *Biophys J* 71: 898, 1996.
68. Craig R, Padrón R, Kendrick-Jones J: Structural changes accompanying phosphorylation of tarantula muscle myosin filaments. *J Cell Biol* 105:1319, 1987.
69. Padrón R, Panté N, Sosa H, et al: X-ray diffraction study of the structural changes accompanying phosphorylation of tarantula muscle. *J Muscle Res Cell Motil* 12:235, 1991.
70. Levine RJC, Kensler RW, Reedy MC, et al: Structure and paramyosin content of tarantula thick filaments. *J Cell Biol* 97:186, 1983.
71. Chew MW, Squire JM: Packing of α-helical coiled-coil myosin rods in vertebrate muscle thick filaments. *J Struct Biol* 115:233, 1995.
72. McLachlan AD, Karn J: Periodic charge distributions in the myosin rod amino acid sequence match cross-bridge spacings in muscle. *Nature* 299:226, 1982.
73. Crick FHC: The packing of α-helices. Simple coiled-coils. *Acta Cryst* 6:689, 1953.
74. Offer G, Sessions R: Computer modeling of the α-helical coiled coil: Packing of side-chains in the inner core. *J Mol Biol* 249:967, 1995.
75. Atkinson SJ, Stewart M: Molecular interactions in myosin assembly. Role of the 28-residue charge repeat in the rod. *J Mol Biol* 226:7, 1992.
76. Atkinson SJ, Stewart M: Molecular basis of myosin assembly: Coiled-coil interactions and the role of charge periodicities. *J Cell Sci Suppl* 14:7, 1991.
77. Sohn RL, Vikstrom KL, Cohen C, et al: A 29 residue region of the sarcomeric myosin rod is necessary for filament formation. *J Mol Biol* 266:317, 1997.
78. Barral JM, Epstein HF: Protein machines and self assembly in muscle organization. *Bioessays* 21:813, 1999.
79. Ao W, Oilgrim D: *Caenorhabditis elegans* UNC-45 is a component of muscle thick filaments and colocalizes with myosin heavy chain B, but not myosin heavy chain A. *J Cell Biol* 148:375, 2000.
80. Reedy MC, Bullard B, Vigoreaux JO: Flightin is essential for thick filament assembly and sarcomere stability in Drosophila flight muscles. *J Cell Biol* 151:1483, 2000.
81. Standiford DM, Davis MB, Miedema K, et al: Myosin rod protein: A novel thick filament component of Drosophila muscle. *J Mol Biol* 265:40, 1997.
82. Wray JS: Organization of myosin in invertebrate thick filaments, in Twarog BM, Levine RJC, Dewey MM (eds): *Basic Biology of Muscles: A Comparative Approach*. New York: Raven, 1982; p 29.
83. Squire J: *The Structural Basis of Muscular Contraction*. New York: Plenum Press, 1981.
84. Squire J, Cantino M, Chew M, et al: Myosin rod-packing schemes in vertebrate muscle thick filaments. *J Struct Biol* 122:128, 1998.
85. Squire JM: Muscle filament structure and muscle contraction. *Annu Rev Biophys Bioeng* 4:137, 1975.
86. Squire JM: Organization of myosin in the thick filaments of muscle, in Parry DAD, Creamer LK (eds): *Fibrous Proteins. Scientific, Industrial, and Medical Aspects*. Vol 1. London: Academic Press, 1979; p 27.
87. Stewart M, Ashton FT, Lieberson R, et al: The myosin filament. IX. Determination of subfilament positions by computer processing of electron micrographs. *J Mol Biol* 153:381, 1981.
88. O'Brien EJ, Bennett PM, Hanson J: Optical diffraction studies of myofibrillar structure. *Phil Trans R Soc Lond [Biol]* 261:201, 1971.
89. Maw MC, Rowe AJ: Fraying of A-filaments into three subfilaments. *Nature* 286:412, 1980.
90. Trinick JA: End filaments. A new structural element of vertebrate skeletal muscle thick filaments. *J Mol Biol* 151:309, 1981.
91. Bennett PM, Fürst DO, Gautel M: The C-protein (myosin binding protein C) family: Regulators of contraction and sarcomere formation? *Rev Physiol Biochem Pharmacol* 138:203, 1999.
92. Huxley HE: Recent x-ray diffraction and electron microscope studies of striated muscle. *J Gen Physiol* 50(suppl):71, 1967.
93. Starr R, Offer G: Polypeptide chains of intermediate molecular weight in myosin preparations. *FEBS Lett* 15:40, 1971.
94. Offer G, Moos C, Starr R: A new protein of the thick filaments of vertebrate skeletal myofibrils. Extraction, purification and characterization. *J Mol Biol* 74:653, 1973.
95. Kenny PA, Liston EM, Higgins DG: Molecular evolution of immunoglobulin and fibronectin domains in titin and related muscle proteins. *Gene* 232:11, 1999.
96. Fürst DO, Obermann WM, van der Ven PF: Structure and assembly of the sarcomeric M band. *Rev Physiol Biochem Pharmacol* 138:163, 1999.
97. Gruen M, Prinz H, Gautel M: cAPK-phosphorylation controls the interaction of the regulatory domain of cardiac myosin binding protein C with myosin-S2 in an on-off fashion. *FEBS Lett* 453:254, 1999.
98. Gruen M, Gautel M: Mutations in β-myosin S2 that cause familial hypertrophic cardiomyopathy (FHC) abolish the interaction with the regulatory domain of myosin-binding protein-C. *J Mol Biol* 286:933, 1999.
99. Kunst G, Kress KR, Gruen M, et al: Myosin binding protein C, a phosphorylation-dependent force regulator in muscle that controls the attachment of myosin heads by its interaction with myosin S2. *Circ Res* 86:51, 2000.
100. Craig R, Offer G: The location of C-protein in rabbit skeletal muscle. *Proc R Soc Lond [Biol]* 192:451, 1976.
101. Gilbert R, Cohen JA, Pardo S, et al: Identification of the A-band localization domain of myosin binding proteins C and H (MyBP-C, MyBP-H) in skeletal muscle. *J Cell Sci* 112:69, 1999.
102. van der Ven PF, Ehler E, Perriard JC, et al: Thick filament assembly occurs after the formation of a cytoskeletal scaffold. *J Muscle Res Cell Motil* 20:569, 1999.
103. Craig R: Structure of A-segments from frog and rabbit skeletal muscle. *J Mol Biol* 109:69, 1977.
104. Offer G: C-protein and the periodicity in the thick filaments of vertebrate skeletal muscles. *Cold Spring Harbor Symp Quant Biol* 37:87, 1972.
105. Hofmann PA, Hartzell HC, Moss RL: Alterations in Ca^{2+} sensitive tension due to partial extraction of C-protein from rat skinned cardiac myocytes and rabbit skeletal muscle fibers. *J Gen Physiol* 97:1141, 1991.
106. Hofmann PA, Greaser ML, Moss RL: C-protein limits shortening velocity of rabbit skeletal muscle fibres at low levels of Ca^{2+} activation. *J Physiol (Lond)* 439:701, 1991.
107. Sjöström M, Squire JM: Fine structure of the A-band in cryo-sections. The structure of the A-band of human skeletal muscle fibres from ultra-thin cryo-sections negatively stained. *J Mol Biol* 109:49, 1977.
108. Wallimann T, Eppenberger HM: Localization and function of M-line bound creatine kinase. M-band model and creatine phosphate shuttle. *Cell Muscle Motil* 6:239, 1985.
109. Squire JM, Luther PK, Trinick J: Muscle myofibril architecture, in Squire JM, Vibert PJ (eds): *Fibrous Protein Structure*. London: Academic Press, 1987; p 423.
110. Pask HT, Jones KL, Luther PK, et al: M-band structure, M-bridge interactions and contraction speed in vertebrate cardiac muscles. *J Muscle Res Cell Motil* 15:633, 1994.
111. Knappeis GG, Carlsen F: The ultrastructure of the M-line in skeletal muscle. *J Cell Biol* 38:202, 1968.
112. Luther P, Squire J: Three-dimensional structure of the vertebrate muscle M-region. *J Mol Biol* 125:313, 1978.
113. Luther PK, Crowther RA: Three-dimensional reconstruction from tilted sections of fish muscle M-band. *Nature* 307:566, 1984.

114. Crowther RA, Luther PK: Three-dimensional reconstruction from a single oblique section of fish muscle M-band. *Nature* 307:569, 1984.
115. Variano-Marston E, Franzini-Armstrong C, Haselgrove JC: Structure of the M band. *J Electron Microsc Tech* 6:131, 1987.
116. Morimoto K, Harrington WF: Isolation and physical chemical properties of an M-line protein from skeletal muscle. *J Biol Chem* 247:3052, 1972.
117. Turner DC, Wallimann T, Eppenberger HM: A protein that binds specifically to the M-line of skeletal muscle is identified as the muscle form of creatine kinase. *Proc Natl Acad Sci USA* 70:702, 1973.
118. Wallimann T, Turner DC, Eppenberger HM: Localization of creatine kinase isoenzymes in myofibrils. I. Chicken skeletal muscle. *J Cell Biol* 75:297, 1977.
119. Kushmerick MJ: Energy balance in muscle activity: Simulations of ATPase coupled to oxidative phosphorylation and to creatine kinase. *Comp Biochem Physiol B Biochem Mol Biol* 120:109, 1998.
120. Masaki T, Takaiti O: M-protein. *J Biochem (Tokyo)* 75:367, 1974.
121. Trinick J, Lowey S: M-protein from chicken pectoralis muscle: Isolation and characterization. *J Mol Biol* 113:343, 1977.
122. Eppenberger HM, Perriard JC, Rosenberg UB, et al: The Mr 165,000 M-protein myomesin: A specific protein of cross-striated muscle cells. *J Cell Biol* 89:185, 1981.
123. Woodhead JL, Lowey S: An in vitro study of the interactions of skeletal muscle M-protein and creatine kinase with myosin and its subfragments. *J Mol Biol* 168:831, 1983.
124. Grove BK, Kurer V, Lehner C, et al: A new 185,000 dalton skeletal muscle protein detected by antibodies. *J Cell Biol* 98:518, 1984.
125. Obermann WM, Gautel M, Steiner F, et al: The structure of the sarcomeric M band: Localization of defined domains of myomesin, M-protein, and the 250-kD carboxy-terminal region of titin by immunoelectron microscopy. *J Cell Biol* 134:1441, 1996.
126. Steiner F, Weber K, Fürst DO: M band proteins myomesin and skelemin are encoded by the same gene: Analysis of its organization and expression. *Genomics* 56:78, 1999.
127. Price MG, Gomer RH: Skelemin, a cytoskeletal M-disc periphery protein, contains motifs of adhesion/recognition and intermediate filament proteins. *J Biol Chem* 268:21800, 1993.
128. Page SG: A comparison of the fine structures of frog slow and twitch muscle fibres. *J Cell Biol* 26:477, 1965.
129. Elliott GF, Lowy J, Worthington CR: An x-ray and light-diffraction study of the filament lattice of striated muscle in the living state and in rigor. *J Mol Biol* 6:295, 1963.
130. Maruyama K: Comparative aspects of muscle elastic proteins. *Rev Physiol Biochem Pharmacol* 138:1, 1999.
131. Trinick J: Titin as a scaffold and spring. *Curr Biol* 6:258, 1996.
132. Keller TC, Eilertsen K, Higginbotham M, et al: Role of titin in nonmuscle and smooth muscle cells. *Adv Exp Med Biol* 481:265, 2000.
133. Machado C, Andrew DJ: Titin as a chromosomal protein. *Adv Exp Med Biol* 481:221, 2000.
134. Labeit S, Kolmerer B, Linke WA: The giant protein titin. Emerging roles in physiology and pathophysiology. *Circ Res* 80:290, 1997.
135. Turnacioglu KK, Mittal B, Dabiri GA, et al: Zeugmatin is part of the Z-band targeting region of titin. *Cell Struct Funct* 22:73, 1997.
136. Gregorio CC, Trombitas K, Centner T, et al: The NH2 terminus of titin spans the Z-disc: Its interaction with a novel 19-kD ligand (T-cap) is required for sarcomeric integrity. *J Cell Biol* 143:1013, 1998.
137. Moreira ES, Wiltshire TJ, Faulkner G, et al: Limb-girdle muscular dystrophy type 2G is caused by mutations in the gene encoding the sarcomeric protein telethonin. *Nat Genet* 24:163, 2000.
138. Fürst DO, Gautel M: The anatomy of a molecular giant: How the sarcomere cytoskeleton is assembled from immunoglobulin superfamily molecules. *J Mol Cell Cardiol* 27:951, 1995.
139. Freiburg A, Trombitas K, Hell W, et al: Series of exon-skipping events in the elastic spring region of titin as the structural basis for myofibrillar elastic diversity. *Circ Res* 86:1114, 2000.
140. Kolmerer B, Witt CC, Freiburg A, et al: The titin cDNA sequence and partial genomic sequences: Insights into the molecular genetics, cell biology and physiology of the titin filament system. *Rev Physiol Biochem Pharmacol* 138:19, 1999.
141. Linke WA, Rudy DE, Centner T, et al: I-band titin in cardiac muscle is a three-element molecular spring and is critical for maintaining thin filament structure. *J Cell Biol* 146:631, 1999.
142. Gautel M, Mues A, Young P: Control of sarcomeric assembly: The flow of information on titin. *Rev Physiol Biochem Pharmacol* 138:97, 1999.
143. Person V, Kostin S, Suzuki K, et al: Antisense oligonucleotide experiments elucidate the essential role of titin in sarcomerogenesis in adult rat cardiomyocytes in long-term culture. *J Cell Sci* 113:3851, 2000.
144. van der Ven PF, Bartsch JW, Gautel M, et al: A functional knock-out of titin results in defective myofibril assembly. *J Cell Sci* 113:1405, 2000.
145. Young P, Ehler E, Gautel M: Obscurin, a giant sarcomeric Rho guanine nucleotide exchange factor protein involved in sarcomere assembly. *J Cell Biol* 154:123, 2001.
146. Horowits R: The physiological role of titin in striated muscle. *Rev Physiol Biochem Pharmacol* 138:57, 1999.
147. Pollard TD: Actin. *Curr Opin Cell Biol* 2:33, 1990.
148. Sheterline P, Clayton J, Sparrow J: Actin. *Protein Profile* 2:1, 1995.
149. Zot AS, Potter JD: Structural aspects of troponin-tropomyosin regulation of skeletal muscle contraction. *Annu Rev Biophys Biophys Chem* 16:535, 1987.
150. Solaro RJ, Rarick HM: Troponin and tropomyosin. Proteins that switch on and tune in the activity of cardiac myofilaments. *Circ Res* 83:471, 1998.
151. Gordon AM, Homsher E, Regnier M: Regulation and contraction in striated muscle. *Physiol Rev* 80:853, 2000.
152. Wang K, Wright J: Architecture of the sarcomere matrix of skeletal muscle. Immunoelectron microscopic evidence that suggests a set of parallel inextensible nebulin filaments anchored at the Z line. *J Cell Biol* 107:2199, 1988.
153. Clarke FM, Masters CJ: On the association of glycolytic enzymes with structural proteins of skeletal muscle. *Biochim Biophys Acta* 381:37, 1975.
154. Kabsch W, Vandekerckhove J: Structure and function of actin. *Annu Rev Biophys Biomol Struct* 21:49, 1992.
155. O'Brien EJ, Dickens MJ: Actin and thin filaments, in Harris R (ed): *Electron Microscopy of Proteins*. Vol 4. London: Academic Press, 1983; p 1.
156. Hanson J: Axial period of actin filaments. Electron microscope studies. *Nature* 213:353, 1967.
157. Depue RH, Rice RV: F-actin is a right-handed helix. *J Mol Biol* 12:302, 1965.
158. Moore PE, Huxley HE, DeRosier DJ: Three-dimensional reconstruction of F-actin, thin filaments and decorated thin filaments. *J Mol Biol* 50:279, 1970.
159. Herman IM: Actin isoforms. *Curr Opin Cell Biol* 5:48, 1993.
160. Khaitlina SY: Functional specificity of actin isoforms. *Int Rev Cytol* 202:35, 2001.
161. Kabsch W, Mannherz HG, Suck D, et al: Atomic structure of the actin:DNase I complex. *Nature* 347:37, 1990.
162. Holmes KC, Kabsch W: Muscle proteins: Actin. *Curr Opin Struct Biol* 1:270, 1991.
163. Schutt CE, Myslik JC, Rozycki MD, et al: The structure of crystalline profilin-β-actin. *Nature* 365:810, 1993.
164. McLaughlin PJ, Gooch JT, Mannherz H-G, et al: Structure of gelsolin segment 1-actin complex and the mechanism of filament severing. *Nature* 364:685, 1993.
165. Otterbein LR, Graceffa P, Dominguez R: The crystal structure of uncomplexed actin in the ADP state. *Science* 293:708, 2001.
166. Holmes KC, Popp D, Gebhard W, Kabsch W: Atomic model of the actin filament. *Nature* 347:44, 1990.
167. Lorenz M, Popp D, Holmes KC: Refinement of the F-actin model against x-ray fiber diffraction data by the use of a directed mutation algorithm. *J Mol Biol* 234:826, 1993.
168. Tirion MM, ben-Avraham D, Lorenz M, et al: Normal modes as refinement parameters for the F-actin model. *Biophys J* 68:5, 1995.
169. Milligan RA, Whittaker M, Safer D: Molecular structure of F-actin and location of surface binding sites. *Nature* 348:217, 1990.
170. Vibert P, Craig R, Lehman W: Steric model for activation of muscle thin filaments. *J Mol Biol* 266:8, 1997.
171. Oosawa F: The flexibility of F-actin. *Biophys Chem* 11:443, 1980.
172. Egelman EH, Francis N, DeRosier DJ: F-actin is a helix with a random variable twist. *Nature* 298:131, 1982.
173. Stokes DL, DeRosier DJ: The variable twist of actin and its modulation by actin-binding proteins. *J Cell Biol* 104:1005, 1987.
174. Bremer A, Millonig RC, Sutterlin R, et al: The structural basis for the intrinsic disorder of the actin filament: The "lateral slipping" model. *J Cell Biol* 115:689, 1991.
175. Taylor KA, Reedy MC, Cordova L, et al: Three-dimensional reconstruction of rigor insect flight muscle from tilted thin sections. *Nature* 310:285, 1984.
176. Hanson J: Evidence from electron microscope studies on actin paracrystals concerning the origin of the cross-striation in the thin filaments of vertebrate skeletal muscle. *Proc R Soc Lond [Biol]* 183:39, 1973.
177. Perry SV: Vertebrate tropomyosin: Distribution, properties and function. *J Muscle Res Cell Motil* 22:5, 2001.
178. Parry DAD: Analysis of the primary sequence of α-tropomyosin from rabbit skeletal muscle. *J Mol Biol* 98:519, 1975.
179. McLachlan AD, Stewart M: The 14-fold periodicity in α-tropomyosin and the interaction with actin. *J Mol Biol* 103:271, 1976.
180. Hitchcock-DeGregori SE, Varnell TA: Tropomyosin has discrete actin binding sites with sevenfold and fourteenfold periodicities. *J Mol Biol* 214:885, 1990.
181. Phillips GN, Lattman EE, Cummins P, et al: Crystal structure and molecular interactions of tropomyosin. *Nature* 278:413, 1979.
182. Phillips GN, Fillers JP, Cohen C: Tropomyosin crystal structure and muscle regulation. *J Mol Biol* 192:111, 1986.
183. Whitby FG, Kent H, Stewart F, et al: Structure of tropomyosin at 9 Å resolution. *J Mol Biol* 227:441, 1992.
184. Whitby FG, Phillips GN Jr: Crystal structure of tropomyosin at 7 Å resolution. *Proteins* 38:49, 2000.
185. Brown JH, Kim K-H, Jun G, et al: Deciphering the design of the tropomyosin molecule. *Proc Natl Acad Sci USA* 98:8496, 2001.

186. Stewart M: Structural basis for bending tropomyosin around actin in muscle thin filaments. *Proc Natl Acad Sci USA* 98:8165, 2001.
187. Cooper JA: Actin dynamics: Tropomyosin provides stability. *Curr Biol* 12:R523, 2002.
188. Farah CS, Reinach FC: The troponin complex and regulation of muscle contraction. *FASEB J* 9:755, 1995.
189. Gergely J: Molecular switches in troponin, in Sugi H, Pollack G (eds): *Mechanisms of Work Production and Work Absorption in Muscle*. New York: Plenum Press, 1998; p 169.
190. Perry SV: Troponin I: Inhibitor or facilitator. *Mol Cell Biochem* 190:9, 1999.
191. Parmacek MS, Leiden JM: Structure, function, and regulation of troponin C. *Circulation* 84:991, 1991.
192. Kretsinger RH: Structure and evolution of calcium-modulated proteins. *CRC Crit Rev Biochem* 8:119, 1980.
193. Herzberg O, James MNG: Refined crystal structure of troponin C from turkey skeletal muscle at 2.0 Å resolution. *J Mol Biol* 203:761, 1988.
194. Satyshur KA, Rao ST, Pyzalska D, et al: Refined structure of chicken skeletal muscle troponin C in the two-calcium state at 2.0 Å resolution. *J Biol Chem* 263:1628, 1988.
195. Herzberg O, Moult J, James MN: Molecular structure of troponin C and its implications for the Ca^{2+} triggering of muscle contraction. *Methods Enzymol* 139:610, 1987.
196. Perry SV: Troponin T: Genetics, properties and function. *J Muscle Res Cell Motil* 19:575, 1998.
197. Flicker PF, Phillips GN, Cohen C: Troponin and its interactions with tropomyosin. An electron microscope study. *J Mol Biol* 162:495, 1982.
198. Ohtsuki I: Localization of troponin in thin filament and tropomyosin paracrystal. *J Biochem (Tokyo)* 75:753, 1974.
199. Hanson J, Lowy J: The structure of actin filaments and the origin of the axial periodicity in the I-substance of vertebrate striated muscle. *Proc R Soc Lond [Biol]* 160:449, 1964.
200. Hanson J, Lednev V, O'Brien EJ, et al: Structure of the actin containing filaments in vertebrate skeletal muscle. *Cold Spring Harbor Symp Quant Biol* 37:311, 1972.
201. Lehman W, Craig R, Vibert P: Ca^{2+}-induced tropomyosin movement in *Limulus* thin-filaments revealed by three-dimensional reconstruction. *Nature* 368:65, 1994.
202. Lehman W, Vibert P, Uman P, et al: Steric-blocking by tropomyosin visualized in relaxed vertebrate muscle thin filaments. *J Mol Biol* 251:191, 1995.
203. Xu C, Craig R, Tobacman L, et al: Tropomyosin positions in regulated thin filaments revealed by cryoelectron microscopy. *Biophys J* 77:985, 1999.
204. Lehman W, Rosol M, Tobacman LS, et al: Troponin organization on relaxed and activated thin filaments revealed by electron microscopy and three-dimensional reconstruction. *J Mol Biol* 307:739, 2001.
205. Haselgrove JC: X-ray evidence for a conformational change in the actin-containing filaments of vertebrate striated muscle. *Cold Spring Harbor Symp Quant Biol* 37:341, 1972.
206. Huxley HE: Structural changes in the actin- and myosin-containing filaments during contraction. *Cold Spring Harbor Symp Quant Biol* 37:361, 1972.
207. Vibert PJ, Haselgrove JC, Lowy J, et al: Structural changes in actin-containing filaments of muscle. *J Mol Biol* 71:757, 1972.
208. Gillis JM, O'Brien EJ: The effect of calcium ions on the structure of reconstituted muscle thin filaments. *J Mol Biol* 99:445, 1975.
209. Milligan RA, Flicker PF: Structural relationship of actin, myosin, and tropomyosin revealed by cryo-electron microscopy. *J Cell Biol* 105:29, 1987.
210. Craig R, Lehman W: The ultrastructural basis of actin filament regulation, in Thomas DD, dos Remedios CG (eds): *Results and Problems in Cell Differentiation*. Vol 36. *Molecular Interactions of Actin. Actin-Myosin Interaction and Actin-Based Regulation*. Berlin-Heidelberg: Springer-Verlag, p 149, 2002.
211. Chalovich JM: Actin mediated regulation of muscle contraction. *Pharmacol Ther* 55:95, 1992.
212. McKillop DFA, Geeves MA: Regulation of the interaction between actin and myosin subfragment 1: Evidence for three states of the thin filament. *Biophys J* 65:693, 1993.
213. El-Saleh SC, Warber KD, Potter JD: The role of tropomyosin-troponin in the regulation of skeletal muscle contraction. *J Muscle Res Cell Motil* 7:387, 1986.
214. Jin J-P, Wang K: Nebulin as a giant actin-binding template protein in skeletal muscle sarcomere. *FEBS Lett* 281:93, 1991.
215. Wright J, Huang QQ, Wang K: Nebulin is a full-length template of actin filaments in the skeletal muscle sarcomere: An immunoelectron microscopic study of its orientation and span with site-specific monoclonal antibodies. *J Muscle Res Cell Motil* 14:476, 1993.
216. Millevoi S, Trombitas K, Kolmerer B, et al: Characterization of nebulette and nebulin and emerging concepts of their roles for vertebrate Z-discs. *J Mol Biol* 282:111, 1998.
217. McElhinny AS, Kolmerer B, Fowler VM, et al: The N-terminal end of nebulin interacts with tropomodulin at the pointed ends of the thin filaments. *J Biol Chem* 276:583, 2001.
218. Labeit S, Kolmerer B: The complete primary structure of human nebulin and its correlation to muscle structure. *J Mol Biol* 248:308, 1995.
219. Moncman CL, Wang K: Nebulette: A 107 kD nebulin-like protein in cardiac muscle. *Cell Motil Cytoskeleton* 32:205, 1995.
220. Wang K, Knipfer M, Huang QQ, et al: Human skeletal muscle nebulin sequence encodes a blueprint for thin filament architecture. Sequence motifs and affinity profiles of tandem repeats and terminal SH3. *J Biol Chem* 271:4304, 1996.
221. Luo G, Herrera AH, Horowits R: Molecular interactions of N-RAP, a nebulin-related protein of striated muscle myotendon junctions and intercalated disks. *Biochemistry* 38:6135, 1999.
222. Kruger M, Wright J, Wang K: Nebulin as a length regulator of thin filaments of vertebrate skeletal muscles: Correlation of thin filament length, nebulin size, and epitope profile. *J Cell Biol* 115:97, 1991.
223. Cooper JA, Schafer DA: Control of actin assembly and disassembly at filament ends. *Curr Opin Cell Biol* 12:97, 2000.
224. Fowler VM: Regulation of actin filament length in erythrocytes and striated muscle. *Curr Opin Cell Biol* 8:86, 1996.
225. Littlefield R, Fowler VM: Defining actin filament length in striated muscle: Rulers and caps or dynamic stability? *Annu Rev Cell Dev Biol* 14:487, 1998.
226. Maruyama K, Kurokawa H, Oosawa M, et al: β-Actinin is equivalent to Cap Z protein. *J Biol Chem* 265:8712, 1990.
227. Papa I, Astier C, Kwiatek O, et al: α-Actinin-CapZ, an anchoring complex for thin filaments in Z-line. *J Muscle Res Cell Motil* 20:187, 1999.
228. Schafer DA, Hug C, Cooper JA: Inhibition of CapZ during myofibrillogenesis alters assembly of actin filaments. *J Cell Biol* 128:61, 1995.
229. Gregorio CC, Weber A, Bondad M, et al: Requirement of pointed-end capping by tropomodulin to maintain actin filament length in embryonic chick cardiac myocytes. *Nature* 377:83, 1995.
230. Gregorio CC, Fowler VM: Mechanisms of thin filament assembly in embryonic chick cardiac myocytes: Tropomodulin requires tropomyosin for assembly. *J Cell Biol* 129:683, 1995.
231. Almenar-Queralt A, Gregorio CC, Fowler VM: Tropomodulin assembles early in myofibrillogenesis in chick skeletal muscle: Evidence that thin filaments rearrange to form striated myofibrils. *J Cell Sci* 112:1111, 1995.
232. Rudy DE, Yatskievych TA, Antin PB, et al: Assembly of thick, thin, and titin filaments in chick precardiac explants. *Dev Dyn* 221:61, 2001.
233. Littlefield R, Almenar-Queralt A, Fowler VM: Actin dynamics at pointed ends regulates thin filament length in striated muscle. *Nat Cell Biol* 3:544, 2001.
234. Masters C: Interactions between glycolytic enzymes and components of the cytomatrix. *J Cell Biol* 99:222s, 1984.
235. Kraft T, Hornemann T, Stolz M, et al: Coupling of creatine kinase to glycolytic enzymes at the sarcomeric I-band of skeletal muscle: A biochemical study in situ. *J Muscle Res Cell Motil* 21:691, 2000.
236. Pagliaro L, Taylor DL: 2-Deoxyglucose and cytochalasin D modulate aldolase mobility in living 3T3 cells. *J Cell Biol* 118:859, 1992.
237. Wegmann G, Zanolla E, Eppenberger HM, et al: In situ compartmentation of creatine kinase in intact sarcomeric muscle: The acto-myosin overlap zone as a molecular sieve. *J Muscle Res Cell Motil* 13:420, 1992.
238. Brooks SP, Storey KB: Where is the glycolytic complex? A critical evaluation of present data from muscle tissue. *FEBS Lett* 278:135, 1991.
239. Parra J, Pette D: Effects of low-frequency stimulation on soluble and structure-bound activities of hexokinase and phosphofructokinase in rat fast-twitch muscle. *Biochim Biophys Acta* 1251:154, 1995.
240. Vigoreaux JO: The muscle Z band: Lessons in stress management. *J Muscle Res Cell Motil* 15:237, 1994.
241. Knappeis GG, Carlsen F: The ultrastructure of the Z disc in skeletal muscle. *J Cell Biol* 13:323, 1962.
242. Kelly DE: Models of muscle Z-band fine structure based on a looping filament configuration. *J Cell Biol* 34:827, 1967.
243. Franzini-Armstrong C: The structure of a simple Z line. *J Cell Biol* 58:630, 1973.
244. Yamaguchi M, Izumimoto M, Robson RM, et al: Fine structure of wide and narrow vertebrate muscle Z-line. *J Mol Biol* 184:621, 1985.
245. Goldstein MA, Lloyd MH, Schroeter JP, et al: The Z-band lattice in skeletal muscle before, during and after tetanic contraction. *J Muscle Res Cell Motil* 7:527, 1986.
246. Luther PK: Three-dimensional reconstruction of a simple Z-band in fish muscle. *J Cell Biol* 113:1043, 1991.
247. Stromer MH: Immunocytochemistry of the muscle cell cytoskeleton. *Microsc Res Tech* 31:95, 1995.
248. Zhou Q, Chu PH, Huang C, et al: Ablation of Cypher, a PDZ-LIM domain Z-line protein, causes a severe form of congenital myopathy. *J Cell Biol* 155:605, 2001.
249. Hauser MA, Horrigan SK, Salmikangas P, et al: Myotilin is mutated in limb girdle muscular dystrophy 1A. *Hum Mol Genet* 9:2141, 2000.
250. Young P, Ferguson C, Banuelos S, et al: Molecular structure of the sarcomeric Z-disk: Two types of titin interactions lead to an asymmetrical sorting of α-actinin. *EMBO J* 17:1614, 1998.
251. Bang ML, Mudry RE, McElhinny AS, et al: Myopalladin, a novel 145-kilodalton sarcomeric protein with multiple roles in Z-disc and I-band protein assemblies. *J Cell Biol* 153:413, 2001.

252. Weins A, Schwarz K, Faul C, et al: Differentiation- and stress-dependent nuclear cytoplasmic redistribution of myopodin, a novel actin-bundling protein. *J Cell Biol* 155:393, 2001.
253. Takada F, Vander Woude DL, Tong HQ, et al: Myozenin: An α-actinin and γ-filamin-binding protein of skeletal muscle Z lines. *Proc Natl Acad Sci USA* 98:1595, 2001.
254. van der Ven PF, Wiesner S, Salmikangas P, et al: Indications for a novel muscular dystrophy pathway. γ-Filamin, the muscle-specific filamin isoform, interacts with myotilin. *J Cell Biol* 151:235, 2000.
255. Salmikangas P, Mykkanen OM, Gronholm M, et al: Myotilin, a novel sarcomeric protein with two Ig-like domains, is encoded by a candidate gene for limb-girdle muscular dystrophy. *Hum Mol Genet* 8:1329, 1999.
256. Faulkner G, Pallavicini A, Formentin E, et al: ZASP: A new Z-band alternatively spliced PDZ-motif protein. *J Cell Biol* 146:465, 1999.
257. Luther PK: Three-dimensional structure of a vertebrate muscle Z-band: Implications for titin and α-actinin binding. *J Struct Biol* 129:1, 2000.
258. Luther PK, Barry JS, Squire JM: The three-dimensional structure of a vertebrate wide (slow muscle) Z-band: Lessons on Z-band assembly. *J Mol Biol* 315:9, 2002.
259. Schroeter JP, Bretaudiere JP, Sass RL, et al: Three-dimensional structure of the Z band in a normal mammalian skeletal muscle. *J Cell Biol* 133:571, 1996.
260. Gautel M, Goulding D, Bullard B, et al: The central Z-disk region of titin is assembled from a novel repeat in variable copy numbers. *J Cell Sci* 109:2747, 1996.
261. Luther PK, Squire JM: Muscle Z-band ultrastructure: Titin Z-repeats and Z-band periodicities do not match. *J Mol Biol* 319:1157, 2002.
262. Furukawa T, Ono Y, Tsuchiya H, et al: Specific interaction of the potassium channel β-subunit minK with the sarcomeric protein T-cap suggests a T-tubule-myofibril linking system. *J Mol Biol* 313:775, 2001.
263. Bellin RM, Huiatt TW, Critchley DR, et al: Synemin may function to directly link muscle cell intermediate filaments to both myofibrillar Z-lines and costameres. *J Biol Chem* 276:32330, 2001.
264. Stromer MH: Intermediate (10 nm) filaments in muscle, in Goldman RD, Steinert PM (eds): *Cellular and Molecular Biology of Intermediate Filaments.* New York: Plenum Press, 1990; p 19.
265. Wang K, Ramirez-Mitchell R: A network of transverse and longitudinal intermediate filaments is associated with sarcomeres of adult vertebrate skeletal muscle. *J Cell Biol* 96:562, 1983.
265a. Nunzi MG, Franzini-Armstrong C: Trabecular network in adult skeletal muscle. *J Ultrastruct Res* 73:21, 1980.
266. Carlsson L, Thornell LE: Desmin-related myopathies in mice and man. *Acta Physiol Scand* 171:341, 2001.
267. Herrmann H, Aebi U: Intermediate filaments and their associates: Multi-talented structural elements specifying cytoarchitecture and cytodynamics. *Curr Opin Cell Biol* 12:79, 2000.
268. Parry DAD: Structural features of IF proteins, in Kreis T, Vale R (eds): *Guidebook to the Cytoskeletal and Motor Proteins,* 2d ed. New York: Oxford University Press, 1999; p 285.
269. Capetanaki Y, Milner DJ, Weitzer G: Desmin in muscle formation and maintenance: Knockouts and consequences. *Cell Struct Funct* 22:103, 1997.
270. Hemken PM, Bellin RM, Sernett SW, et al: Molecular characteristics of the novel intermediate filament protein paranemin. Sequence reveals EAP-300 and IFAPa-400 are highly homologous to paranemin. *J Biol Chem* 272:32489, 1997.
271. Poon E, Howman EV, Newey SE, et al: Association of syncoilin and desmin: Linking intermediate filament proteins to the dystrophin-associated protein complex. *J Biol Chem* 277:3433, 2002.
272. Reddy KB, Gascard P, Price MG, et al: Identification of an interaction between the M-band protein skelemin and β-integrin subunits. *J Biol Chem* 273:35039, 1998.
273. Fuchs E, Yang Y: Crossroads on cytoskeletal highways. *Cell* 98:547, 1999.
274. Reipert S, Steinbock F, Fischer I, et al: Association of mitochondria with plectin and desmin intermediate filaments in striated muscle. *Exp Cell Res* 252:479, 1999.
275. Marian AJ, Roberts R: The molecular genetic basis for hypertrophic cardiomyopathy. *J Mol Cell Cardiol* 33:655, 2001.
276. Towbin JA: Molecular genetics of hypertrophic cardiomyopathy. *Curr Cardiol Rep* 2:134, 2000.
277. Bonne G, Carrier L, Richard P, et al: Familial hypertrophic cardiomyopathy: From mutations to functional defects. *Circ Res* 83:580, 1998.
278. Watkins H, Seidman JG, Seidman CE: Familial hypertrophic cardiomyopathy: A genetic model of cardiac hypertrophy. *Hum Mol Genet* 4(Spec No):1721, 1995.
279. Townbin JA, Bowles NE: The failing heart. *Nature* 415:227, 2002.
280. Laing NG: Inherited disorders of sarcomeric proteins. *Curr Opin Neurol* 12:513, 1999.

Chapter 8
Mammalian Muscle Myosin

H. LEE SWEENEY
ANNE HOUDUSSE

Structure and Function
   HISTORICAL OVERVIEW
   MYOSIN AND ACTOMYOSIN KINETICS
   DUTY RATIO
   X-RAY STRUCTURE OF THE MYOSIN HEAD
   LEVER-ARM HYPOTHESIS
   CORRELATION BETWEEN STRUCTURAL AND KINETIC STATES
   ACTIN-MYOSIN COMPLEX

Myosin Diversity
   MYOSIN SUPERFAMILY
   MUSCLE MYOSIN HEAVY-CHAIN ISOFORMS
   MYOSIN LIGHT-CHAIN ISOFORMS
   REGULATORY LIGHT-CHAIN PHOSPHORYLATION
   KINETIC DIVERSITY
   HYPERTROPHIC CARDIOMYOPATHY
   IN VITRO EXPRESSION AND ASSAYS OF MYOSIN FUNCTION

Conclusions

The purpose of this chapter is to summarize what is currently known about the structure and function of the molecular motor of muscle, myosin. The last decade has been revolutionary for the myosin field. At the time the previous edition of *Myology* went to press, the first high-resolution structure of myosin had only recently been published, and only two classes of myosin were known to exist. We now have high-resolution structures of the motor domains of several muscle myosins in different structural states, and the structures of several "unconventional" myosins have been solved. Furthermore, the myosin superfamily has grown from two members to nearly twenty. The ability to express and analyze these myosins has developed such that single-molecule mechanical studies are being performed. Our knowledge of the functional diversity of myosin is also growing. There are myosins that can traffic as a single molecule (processive movement) and even myosins that move in the reverse direction. This chapter focuses on the properties of the myosins found in muscle, which are still the best-characterized and understood members of the myosin superfamily.

Structure and Function

HISTORICAL OVERVIEW

Myosin is the force generator of skeletal, cardiac, and smooth muscle. *Myosin* is the name originally used by Kühne[1] in 1859 for his extract from skeletal muscle that contained the contractile material. In 1939, Engelhardt and Lyubimova discovered that myosin had adenosine triphosphatase (ATPase) activity.[2] In 1948, Straub demonstrated that some myosin preparations contained a second protein, which he named *actin*.[3]

The name *myosin* is now applied to a large superfamily of motor proteins. The form isolated from muscle is now referred to as myosin II, or conventional myosin. The nonmuscle form of this same type of myosin is found in nearly all eukaryotic cells. It is the motor that powers cytokinesis, and it plays a role in cellular locomotion and the establishment of cellular polarity during development.[4]

The first insights into its molecular structure came in 1967 with the work of Slayter and Lowey.[5] Based on a combination of hydrodynamics and electron microscopy (EM), it was proposed that the myosin molecule consisted of two globular heads attached to a rod-like tail. This nomenclature is still in use for the myosin molecule. Proteolytic studies[6] provided further details of this structural picture, which is shown in Fig. 8-1. It was later shown that muscle myosin is a hexameric protein consisting of four light chains and two heavy chains[7] (Fig. 8-1). The heavy chains contain the two distinct regions initially described by Slayter and Lowey: the head and the rod. The rod is an α-helical coiled-coil structure approximately 1500 Å long and 20 Å in diameter.[8] Via a flexible linkage,[5,6] the rod connects to the two globular regions, or heads. The rod is necessary for assembly of myosin molecules into filaments. The head is the enzymatic region, containing the site of ATP hydrolysis and actin binding. Biochemical studies[9–11] and the first high-resolution crystal structure[12] identified regions in the myosin heavy-chain head that are involved in nucleotide binding, actin binding, and light-chain binding.

Each of the two heavy chains is approximately 200 kDa.[13] Associated with each of the two heads are two light chains (thus a total of four light chains per myosin molecule). One of the light chains associated with each head is about 18.5 kDa; the other ranges from 16.5 to 24 kDa.[14,15] This light-chain heterogeneity was first demonstrated for vertebrate striated muscle using gel electrophoresis[14] (Fig. 8-2).

The myosin light chains have been referred to by a variety of names over the years. The 18.5-kDa light chain can be dissociated from myosin using DTNB[16] and thus has been called the DTNB light chain. Since it is generally the second largest of the light chains of fast-twitch muscles, it is also known as light chain 2 (LC2). To denote the fact that it is LC2 from fast-twitch muscle, it is referred to as $LC2_f$. This light chain can be phosphorylated[17] and thus has been referred to as the P light chain.[18] In fact, this phosphorylation event forms the on/off switch for smooth and nonmuscle myosin activity; hence it is known as the regulatory light chain.[19] Regulatory light chain (RLC) is the term in current use for this light chain and is used throughout this chapter.

The other class of light chains has been known as the alkali light chains, since treatment of myosin at pH 11 removes them.[20] Using this nomenclature, the two light chains of fast skeletal myosin have been referred to as A1 (21 kDa) and A2 (16.5 kDa).[15] These specific light chains from mammalian fast-twitch muscle have more often been denoted $LC1_f$ and $LC3_f$, respectively (see Fig. 8-2). This class of light chains is most commonly referred to as the *essential light chains*, based

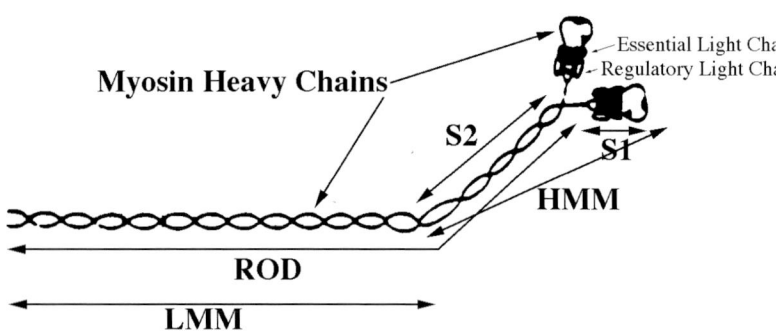

FIGURE 8-1. Representation of the myosin molecule, depicting its subunit structure and the location of the head and rod domains.

on an early observation that they could not be removed without loss of myosin activity.[16] The term *essential light chain* (ELC) is the most general and currently used[21] and is the term used below.

Rotary shadowing, combined with light-chain-specific antibodies, revealed that the regulatory light chain was located at the base of the myosin head, at the junction with the rod[22] (Fig. 8-3). The position of the ELC was less clear, because a number of isoforms have extended N-terminal peptides that interact with actin, including LC1$_f$ of vertebrate skeletal muscle myosin.[23,24]

The myosin molecule is divided into two pieces by limited tryptic or chymotryptic digestion: heavy meromyosin and light meromyosin. The heavy meromyosin (HMM) fragment of MHC (~150 kDa) contains the enzymatically functional head (S1) and N-terminal portion (S2) of the rod (Fig. 8-1). The S1 fragment, or myosin head, can be cleaved from the S2 region by the use of either papain or chymotrypsin.[25] The HMM and S1 proteolytic fragments of all types of muscle myosin have been used extensively for the delineation of actin-myosin kinetics in solution, since they do not aggregate at the low ionic strengths used in such assays.

With further tryptic digestion, the myosin head, or S1 region, can be divided into three subfragments.[26] Moving from the N-terminus, these subfragments are M_r 25,000, 50,000, and 20,000. These tryptic subfragments are created by cleavage of flexible loops that are generally not resolvable in the high-resolution x-ray structures of myosin. The nomenclature derived from myosin proteolysis was adapted by Rayment et al.[12] to describe the subdomains revealed by the high-resolution crystal structure for the skeletal muscle myosin head.

Myosin molecules pack together to form filaments. The C-terminal 300 amino acids of the heavy chains of the molecule are necessary for this filament formation.[27] Higher-order filament assembly is controlled by alternating stretches of positive and negative charges along the rod surface.[28,29] The details of the structure of myosin filaments (known as the thick filaments) are discussed in Chap. 7. The globular myosin heads project from the thick filaments, while the myosin rods form their backbone. Since the myosin head is the site of enzymatic activity and actin binding,[30] the projections arising from the thick filament backbone are sites of these activities. In 1968, Eisenberg and Moos demonstrated that the intrinsic ATPase activity of myosin is enhanced by its interaction with actin.[31]

As presented in Chap. 7, the thick (myosin) and thin (actin) filaments can interdigitate and slide over one another. In 1954, both H. E. Huxley and J. Hanson[32] and A. F. Huxley and R. Niedergerke[33] proposed that active sliding between thick and thin filaments was the mechanism of shortening in mammalian skeletal muscle. Later it became apparent that the projections from the thick filament, often called cross-bridges, interact with actin and split ATP and that the resulting energy is somehow harnessed in the form of mechanical strain, which causes a relative sliding of the thick and thin filaments.

To generate the mechanical strain necessary for filament sliding, H. E. Huxley postulated that the cross-bridge itself might undergo a change in its angle of attachment with actin.[34] Of course, the structural details of how this might occur could not be envisioned. The tilting cross-bridge that was proposed by H. E. Huxley was reborn as a tilting lever arm of myosin[12,35,36] once high-resolution structures of myosin were solved.

MYOSIN AND ACTOMYOSIN KINETICS

Many years of kinetic studies of the actin-myosin interaction have defined an ATP-consuming cycle (Fig. 8-4) that is catalyzed by actin association and contains many more states than have been seen in structural studies.[36,37] The ATPase activity of myosin resides in its conserved motor domain, which interacts with actin, hydrolyzes ATP, and produces the force necessary for movement along actin filaments. During the actomyosin ATPase cycle, weak ($K_d > \mu M$) actin-binding states (ATP and ADP-P$_i$ states) alternate with

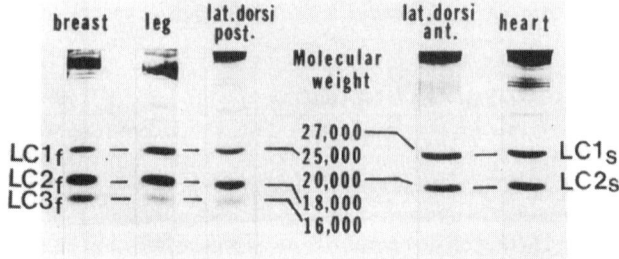

FIGURE 8-2. Light chains from chicken striated muscles. (*From Lowey and Risby.*[14] *Reproduced by permission.*)

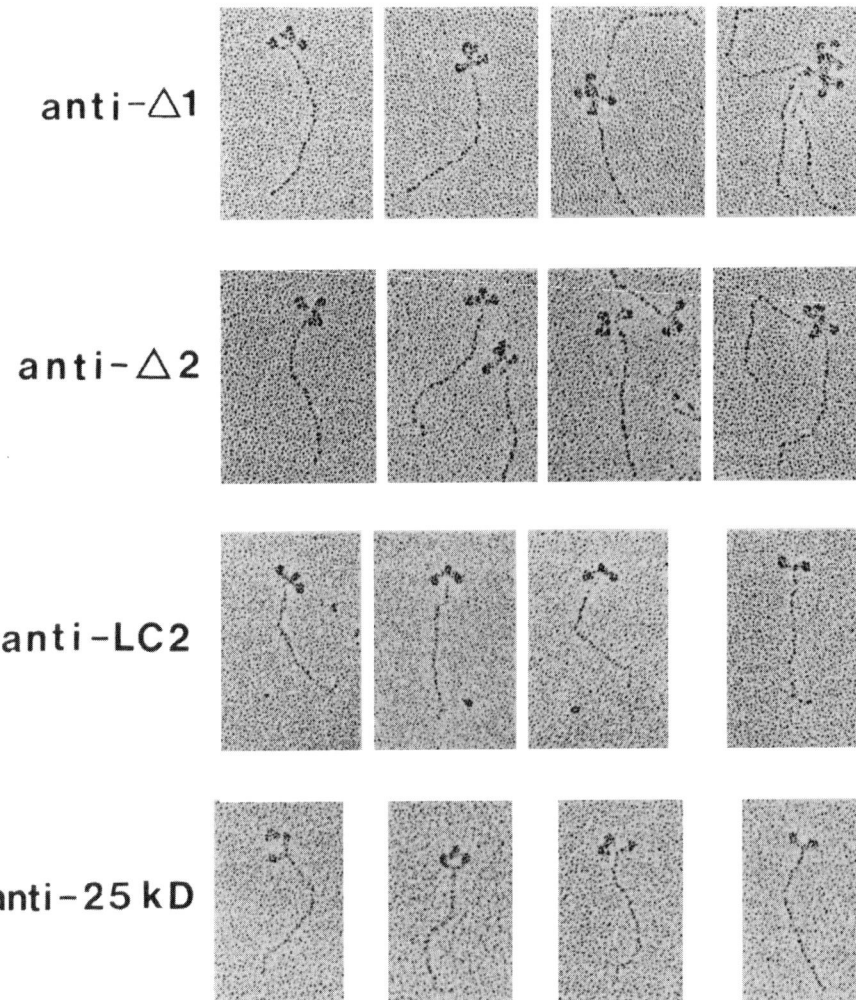

FIGURE 8-3. A composite of fast-twitch skeletal muscle myosin molecules complexed with antibodies specific for either of the two ELCs, LC1$_f$ (anti-Δ1) and LC3$_f$ (anti-Δ2), the RLC (anti-LC2), and the N-terminal 25-kDa peptide of the myosin head (anti–25 kDa). Anti-LC2 is a Fab fragment; two unreacted myosin molecules are shown in the lower right-hand corner for comparison. x150,000. (*Molecules labeled with anti-LC2 anti–25 kDa are reproduced from Winkelmann et al.[22] with permission; the remainder are courtesy of G. S. Waller and D. D. LeBlanc.*)

strong ($K_d \ll \mu M$) actin-binding states (ADP states and nucleotide-free or rigor state).[38] Biochemical, kinetic, and mechanical studies on conventional myosins have established that ATP binding dissociates the actomyosin complex and that ATP hydrolysis is rapid when myosin is not associated with actin. Phosphate release precedes ADP release, and both product release steps are accelerated considerably upon actin binding. Force development occurs when myosin binds strongly to actin and is associated with actin-induced acceleration of phosphate release.

The breakthrough in our understanding of the actin-myosin kinetic cycle came in 1971 with the work of Lymn and Taylor.[38] Their transient kinetic analysis explained the puzzling observation that although myosin could bind tightly to actin only in the absence of ATP, actin greatly accelerated myosin's ATPase activity. Lymn and Taylor demonstrated that although myosin rapidly hydrolyzed ATP in the absence of actin, rapid product release required a transient interaction with actin. Once the P$_i$ and ADP have been released, ATP rapidly rebinds to the actin-bound myosin, causing rapid dissociation. The scheme deduced by Lymn and Taylor[38] is shown below. The authors suggested that this scheme could accommodate the tilting cross-bridge model of force generation if repriming of the myosin occurred upon ATP hydrolysis.

Scheme 1 is as follows:

$$\begin{array}{ccc}
A \cdot M \cdot D \cdot P & \xrightarrow[-D, P]{(4)} & A \cdot M \\
{\scriptstyle (3)} \uparrow {\scriptstyle +A} & & {\scriptstyle +T} \downarrow {\scriptstyle -A} \;(1) \\
M \cdot D \cdot P & \xleftarrow{(2)} & M \cdot T
\end{array}$$

Later work of Eisenberg and collaborators established that myosin could bind either weakly ($K_d > 10^{-6}$ M) or strongly ($K_d < 10^{-5}$ M) to actin, dependent on its nucleotide state.[39] The weak complexes were in rapid equilibrium between bound and dissociated states. This modification of the Lymn and Taylor scheme is depicted below. In this model, force generation occurred during the transition from a weakly bound (A•M•D•P) cross-bridge to a strongly bound (A•M•D) cross-bridge and was associated with the release of inorganic phosphate. Scheme 2 is as follows[39]:

$$\begin{array}{ccccccccc}
M & \rightleftharpoons & M \cdot T & \rightleftharpoons & M \cdot D \cdot P & \rightleftharpoons & M \cdot D & \rightleftharpoons & M \\
\updownarrow & & \updownarrow & & \updownarrow & & \updownarrow & & \updownarrow \\
A \cdot M & \rightleftharpoons & A \cdot M \cdot T & \rightleftharpoons & A \cdot M \cdot D \cdot P & \rightleftharpoons & A \cdot M \cdot D & \rightleftharpoons & A \cdot M
\end{array}$$

$\underbrace{}_{\textit{Weak-binding states}}$ $\underbrace{}_{\textit{Strong-binding states}}$

Further modification of this scheme was proposed by Geeves and collaborators[40] to allow for the formation of a weak actomyosin complex prior to strong binding, regardless of the nucleotide state, as shown in scheme 3, as follows:

$$\begin{array}{ccccccccc}
M & \rightarrow & M \cdot T & \rightarrow & M \cdot D \cdot P & \rightarrow & M \cdot D & \rightarrow & M \quad \textit{Dissociated} \\
\updownarrow & & \updownarrow & & \updownarrow & & \updownarrow & & \updownarrow \\
A \cdot M & \rightarrow & A \cdot M \cdot T & \rightarrow & A \cdot M \cdot D \cdot P & \rightarrow & A \cdot M \cdot D & \rightarrow & A \cdot M \quad \textit{Weak binding (A states)} \\
\updownarrow & & \updownarrow & & \updownarrow & & \updownarrow & & \updownarrow \\
A \cdot M & \rightarrow & A \cdot M \cdot T & \rightarrow & A \cdot M \cdot D \cdot P & \rightarrow & A \cdot M \cdot D & \rightarrow & A \cdot M \quad \textit{Strong binding (R states)}
\end{array}$$

They referred to the weakly bound actin states as "A" states and the strongly bound actin states as "R" states. Later work provided evidence for such transitions,[41] at least in the case of isoforms of myosin II.

Several additional pieces of kinetic evidence require even further modification of this scheme. First, it is clear that hydrolysis requires a structural transition,[42] commonly denoted as from M' to M". (As discussed below, it is now clear that M' is the near-rigor state of myosin, while M" is the transition state.) It is also now clear that phosphate cannot be released from the A•M"•D•P state, so another state must form to allow phosphate release.[37] It is likely but unproven that this state can bind strongly to actin, as indicated in scheme 4. Such a scheme would be consistent with data on single muscle fibers.[43] Following release of phosphate, a strong actin-binding, strong ADP-binding state (A•M•D^S) is formed (but not for fast skeletal myosin II), followed by a strong actin-binding, weak ADP-binding state (A•M•D^W).[44] ADP is released from this state, forming the rigor complex. These modifications are included in scheme 4, below. Note that in this scheme, only the predominant steady-state pathway is shown and not all known possible states. Scheme 4 (the predominant steady-state pathway for the actomyosin ATPase cycle) is as follows:

$$\begin{array}{ccccc}
M' \cdot T & \rightarrow & M'' \cdot T & \rightarrow & M'' \cdot D \cdot P \quad \textit{Dissociated} \\
\updownarrow & & & & \updownarrow \\
A \cdot M' \cdot T & & & & A \cdot M'' \cdot D \cdot P \quad \textit{Weakly bound} \\
\updownarrow & & & & \updownarrow \\
A \cdot M \rightarrow A \cdot M \cdot T & & & & A \cdot M \cdot D \cdot P \rightarrow A \cdot M \cdot D^s \rightarrow A \cdot M \cdot D^W \rightarrow A \cdot M \\
& & & & \textit{Strongly bound}
\end{array}$$

DUTY RATIO

While all forms of myosin have the same kinetic cycle, as pictured in Fig. 8-4, the rates of transition between the states are highly variable. This allows myosin to be "kinetically tuned" for a variety of cellular functions not only by altering the rate at which it proceeds through the ATPase cycle, but also by changing the relative amount of the cycle that myosin spends in the strongly actin-bound (force-generating) states. The ratio of the occupancy of the strong states to the occupancy of the weak + dissociated + strong states is known as the *duty ratio*. Fast skeletal muscle myosin functions in large ensembles within the half sarcomere. Thus, to maximize speed of shortening and power output, this type of myosin has a low duty ratio (i.e., the cross-bridges spend most of the cycle detached or weakly attached). Rapid detachment from the strongly bound states prevents drag on moving cross-bridges. Although more rapid detachment leads to higher shortening velocities, it also causes the isometric

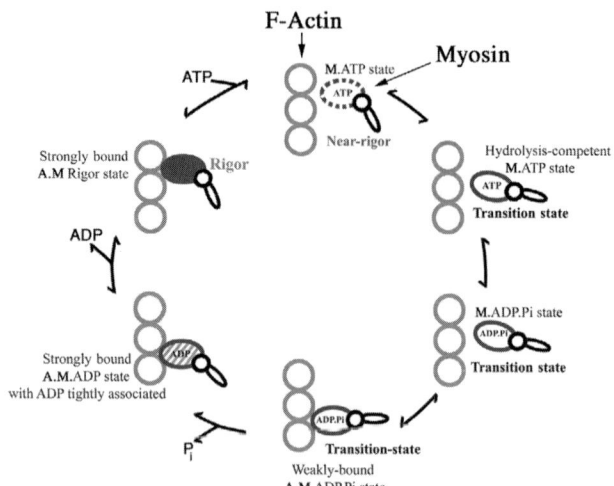

FIGURE 8-4. Simplified version of the actin-myosin ATPase cycle. The individual states shown correspond to states that have been seen in high-resolution structures (x-ray) and/or at lower resolution with cryoelectron microscopy. The high-resolution structures are labeled "Transition state," "Near-rigor" state, and "Rigor," and are discussed in the corresponding text. Force production follows the initial attachment to actin and accompanies phosphate (P_i) release. Repriming of the myosin takes place following ATP-induced detachment of the myosin from actin. A more complete cycle is depicted in scheme 4 (see text).

economy to be low. Thus the myosins of smooth muscle (smooth and nonmuscle) have higher duty ratios and slower speeds of movement than those of skeletal muscle.

The myosins with the highest duty ratios are not those of muscle but those that are capable of moving their cargo as a single molecule.[45] The ability of a single molecule to undergo multiple interactions with actin without releasing from the actin has been termed processivity. The first example of a processive myosin was myosin V.[46] Each head has a duty ratio that approaches unity at high actin concentrations.[45] This ensures that when one head detaches from actin on ATP rebinding, the other head will be in a strong binding state and remain in a strong binding state long enough for the detached head to hydrolyze the ATP and rebind to a more distal actin-binding site. In this manner myosin V can "walk" along an actin filament, as shown further on.

X-RAY STRUCTURE OF THE MYOSIN HEAD

The single biggest advance in the myosin field following the proposal of the sliding-filament theory was the solution of the first high-resolution x-ray structure of myosin in 1992.[12] This structure was of the entire S1 fragment (head) of chicken fast skeletal myosin. While 2½ decades of biochemistry had provided a general picture of what to expect,[47] many of the details were unanticipated. Two key features of the structure generated immediate predictions as to the myosin mechanism. First was the presence of a large cleft (Fig. 8-5) in the middle of the head, which ran from the nucleotide-binding site to the actin interface (identified as

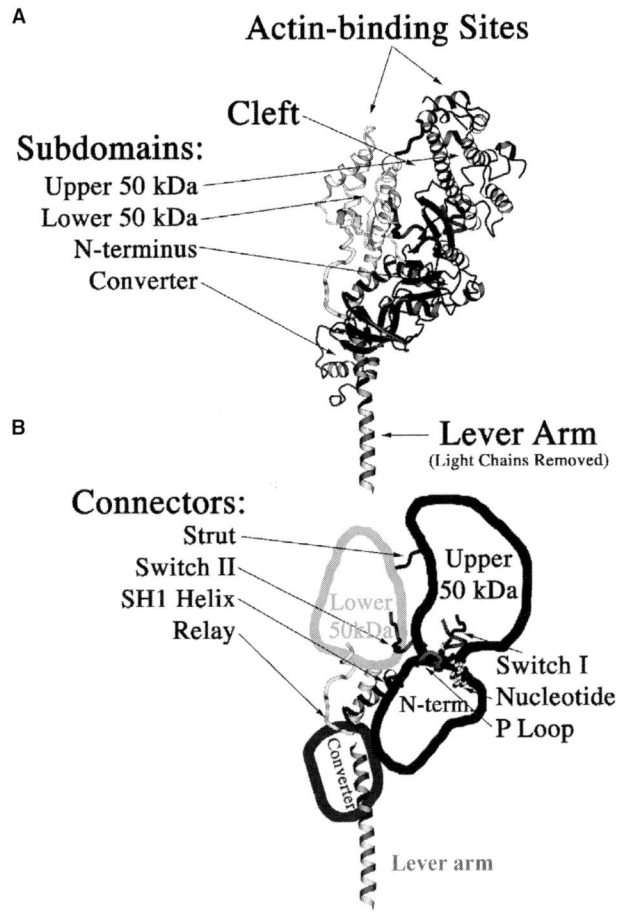

FIGURE 8-5. High-resolution structure of the myosin head. A. A ribbon diagram of the S1 portion of the myosin heavy chain (light chains removed). B. Functional domains and connectors within the myosin head.

such on the basis of earlier cross-linking studies). Rayment et al.[12] suggested that this cleft likely closes when myosin loses its hydrolysis products upon strong binding to actin. Indirect evidence from electron microscopy combined with image reconstruction as well as fluorescent probes located in the cleft supported this prediction.[48,49] A high-resolution structure of a myosin (chicken myosin V) motor without nucleotide for the first time demonstrated that this cleft can indeed close.[50]

The second striking feature and prediction focused on the myosin light chains. The light chains (which are members of the calmodulin superfamily) were bound to the C-terminal portion of the heavy chain, which formed an extended alpha helix. It appeared that the light chains bound to the heavy chain in calmodulin-like conformations and in essence formed a lever arm that could likely amplify small movements within the rest of the head (which Rayment et al.[12] referred to as the *motor domain*). This has come to be known as the lever-arm hypothesis (Fig. 8-6).[35,36] The crystal structures to date support this concept, with the state that hydrolyzes ATP as the beginning of the power stroke and the state that binds ADP or ATP analogues being similar, in lever-arm position, to the final rigor state on actin (see Fig. 8-6 and Color Plate 1).

A recent structure of the unconventional myosin, myosin V, reveals details of the rigor structure of myosin,[50] albeit not bound to actin. It shows major rearrangements of the subdomains and cleft closure in this final rigor state, as compared to the so-called near rigor state, but the lever-arm position does appear to be similar in both instances (see Color Plate 1c and d). This is further supported by energy-transfer measurements[51] that report similar positions of the lever arm in the near-rigor (no actin, but either ADP or no nucleotide) and true actomyosin rigor states. (Thus there is no reversal of the lever-arm swing when ATP binds to myosin attached to actin to induce dissociation.) There is good evidence that myosin II and likely most other members of the myosin superfamily generate movement and force by this mechanism. However, it may not be universal throughout the myosin superfamily, as at least myosin VI appears to use a different mechanism.[52]

Comparison of these structures shows that the myosin motor domain is functionally made up of four major subdomains (Fig. 8-5) linked by four flexible structural connectors (so-called joints) that are highly conserved in sequence[50,53] (see Fig. 8-5B). Thus, as shown in Fig. 8-5, rather than the proteolytic junctions used by Rayment et al.[12] in their original description of subdomains of the motor, the subdomain boundaries have been altered to reflect intersubdomain movements.[50,53] The connectors are found at the periphery of the subdomains and can readily change conformation, in coordination with the movement of the subdomains relative to one another. Among these subdomains, the converter (which leads directly to the lever arm) has by far the greatest potential for movement, since it is connected to the lower 50-kDa and N-terminal subdomains by only two deformable joints (the relay and the SH1 helix, respectively). Rotation of the converter and lever arm can thus amplify relatively small conformational changes of the motor domain. Internal coupled rearrangements of the subdomains allow direct communication between the nucleotide-binding site, the actin-binding interface, and the lever arm. Coupling between the actin- and nucleotide-binding sites is mediated via the large cleft between the upper and lower 50-kDa subdomains that separates the actin-binding site into two distinct subdomains and communicates with the γ-phosphate pocket via a third connector, called Switch II (see Fig. 8-5).

LEVER-ARM HYPOTHESIS

As mentioned above, it had been proposed that force generation by myosin involves a structural change on actin after initially binding and releasing the hydrolysis products. Experimental support for the swinging-lever-arm hypothesis (Fig. 8-6 and Color Plate 1c and d) for myosin force generation comes primarily from two types of studies. First, as discussed below and shown in Fig. 8-7, electron-density maps from cryoelectron microscopy that compare actomyosin either in rigor or with ADP bound to the myosin reveal that, for some myosins, the lever arm moves upon dissociation of ADP.[54,55] Further support comes from in vitro motility and single-molecule mechanical studies showing that the velocity and/or unitary displacement of the myosin are related to lever-arm

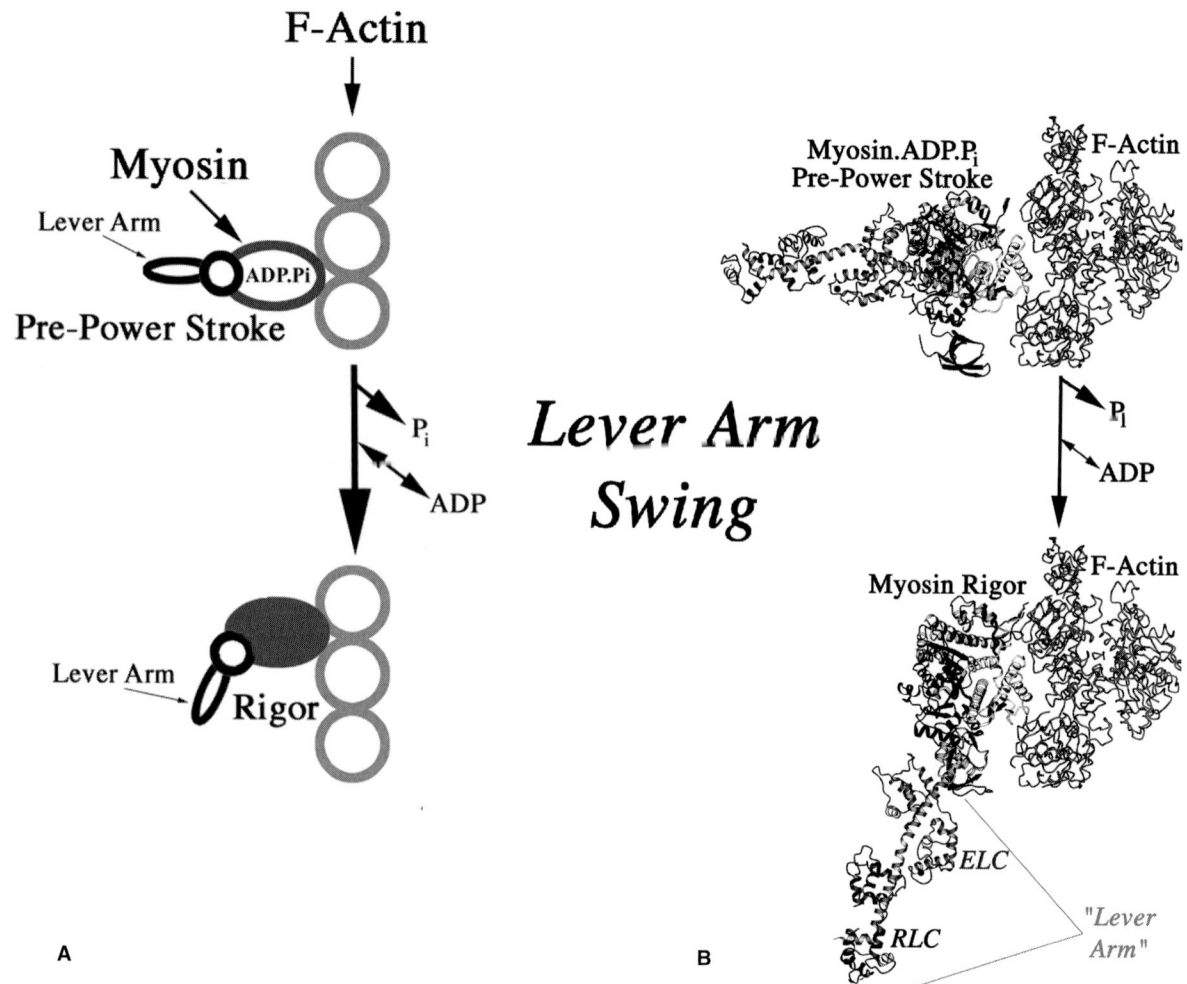

FIGURE 8-6. Structural basis for the myosin lever-arm hypothesis. A. Diagrammatic representation showing that myosin movement occurs due to movement of the light-chain domain (lever arm) when actin catalyzes the release of hydrolysis products from myosin. B. Hypothetical docking of the high-resolution structures of actin and myosin using the myosin pre-power stroke structure from scallop[53] and the rigor structure of chicken myosin V.[50] (See Color Plate 1 for greater detail.)

length.[56–58] While both lines of evidence support a role for swinging of the lever arm in the generation of force and movement, they do not address whether or not force production is directly coupled to lever-arm movement.

Perhaps the earliest evidence for a shape change in the myosin head that can now be interpreted as a lever-arm swing came from EM on insect flight muscle.[59] Two cross-bridge angles were described: 90 degrees (rigor) and 45 degrees (relaxed). More recent work on contracting insect flight muscle—involving rapid activation and freezing, cryo-electron microscopy, and image reconstruction—provided a much better picture of the cross-bridge shapes.[60] These images from intact sarcomere, although subject to interpretation, strongly indicate lever-arm movement.

The displacement of the lever arm deduced by comparing the transition state and near-rigor structures[61,62] formed the initial structural evidence in support of the lever-arm hypothesis.[35,36] However, since neither of those structural states constitutes a force-bearing state when bound to actin (they both have weak affinities for actin), they cannot truly represent extremes of the power stroke. The rigor state of myosin V directly supports the lever-arm hypothesis by revealing that the lever arm's position in a nucleotide-free, strong actin-binding state has indeed moved in the appropriate direction away from the lever-arm position in the transition state[50] (see Color Plate 1).

Correlation between Structural and Kinetic States

High-resolution crystal structures of the myosin head with various nucleotides bound have provided direct visualization of the myosin motor in four distinct conformational states, two of which are shown in Color Plate 1. The first of the structures is known as the *near-rigor structure* and was the state represented in the original chicken myosin II structure of Rayment.[12] This structure has been seen for myosin II with ADP, ATP, and ATP analogues or no nucleotide at the active site.[53,61,63] ATP cannot be hydrolyzed in this state. In the overall actin-myosin ATPase cycle (see Fig. 8-4), it is the state created when ATP binds to myosin and dissociates it from the actin-myosin complex. The second state that was found[53,61,62] is known as the *transition or pre-power stroke state*. This state is formed by structural rearrangements of the near-rigor state and is the state in which ATP is hydrolyzed to form ADP and inorganic phosphate. It is sometimes referred to as the *closed state*, since there is partial cleft closure in this state, as well as trapping of the inorganic phosphate.[35] It is not clear where the third structural state of myosin that was solved fits into the ATPase cycle.[64] It was named the *detached state* and was important in that it made clear the ability of the subdomains of the myosin motor (Fig. 8-5) to move relative to each other. It has been suggested that under negative strain in muscle, formation of this state could lead to rapid detachment from actin.[65] The fourth myosin structural state was found in solving the structure of nucleotide-free myosin V.[50] Based on features of the structure and the kinetic properties of myosin V, it was argued that the motor domain is in a true rigor state. As shown in Color Plate 1, it forms the most extensive interface with actin, closes the cleft, and cannot strongly bind nucleotide. Therefore it is likely that it represents the structural state that all myosins adopt when tightly bound to actin in the absence of nucleotide.

Understanding the chemomechanical coupling in the myosin motor requires assigning structural states to the distinct steps of the actomyosin cycle characterized by kinetic studies. Of the high-resolution myosin structural states described above, all—with the exception of the myosin V rigor state—are states that bind weakly to actin. As already discussed, the transition state likely represents the beginning of the power stroke and the rigor state the end of the power stroke, as shown in Fig. 8-6 and Color Plate 1. In many myosins, a strong actin-binding, strong ADP-binding state precedes the rigor state (Fig. 8-4), which must be followed by a weak ADP-binding state, not shown in Fig. 8-4, that gives rise to rigor upon ADP dissociation.[44] We have little insight into the structural intermediates between the initial weak interaction of the transition state with actin and the release of inorganic phosphate and formation of strong actin binding.

However, there is kinetic evidence for the existence of multiple states.[36] Specifically, there must be formation of an actin.myosin.ADP.P_i state that is distinct from the transition state in order to provide an escape route for the inorganic phosphate. What is yet unclear is the nature of the structural changes that allow strong actin binding that precede the release of phosphate. Studies on muscle fibers suggest that force generation, and thus strong actin binding, occurs prior to phosphate release.[43]

The transition-state structures crystallized when either ATP or ATP analogues are bound to myosin[53,61,62] show that ATP hydrolysis requires interactions between switch II and the γ-phosphate that result in the closure of the γ-phosphate pocket, preventing phosphate release. To avoid steric hindrance, the rigid conformation of switch II in this state must be coupled with precise conformations of both the relay and the SH1 helix that lead to a primed position for the converter and the lever arm, characteristic of the pre-power stroke conformation of the myosin head. Site-directed mutagenesis studies have confirmed that this conformation is essential for ATP hydrolysis and is preceded by a lever-arm movement.[35,66] Hydrolysis of ATP in the myosin motor is thus highly correlated with the priming of the lever arm. Trapping of the phosphate explains the stability of the pre-power stroke conformation until actin binding favors an isomerization that allows phosphate release. This underlies the low intrinsic ATPase activity of myosin in the absence of actin and provides the structural basis for the results of Lymn and Taylor (scheme 1).[38]

The assignment of the "detached" structural state[64] to particular steps of the contractile cycle has been more controversial.[65] The detached state of the myosin head demonstrates that nucleotide binding in the myosin head can favor the unwinding of the SH1 helix and results in very flexible connections between subdomains, providing very loose coupling between the motor domain and the lever arm.[53] This structure thus explains for the first time how two reactive thiols (separated by ~18 Å when the SH1 helix is intact) can be

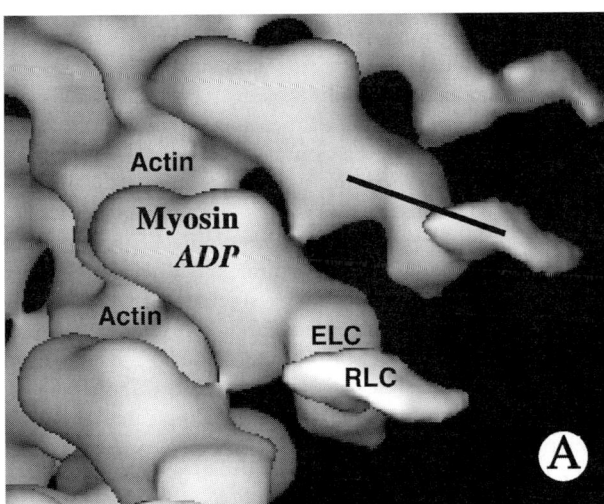 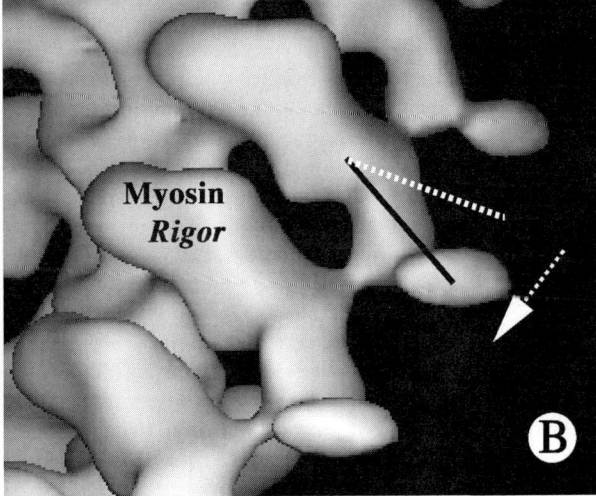

FIGURE 8-7. Cryoelectron microscopy of smooth muscle myosin heads with and without MgADP. *A*. Three-dimensional map of cryoelectron micrograph of recombinant smooth muscle S1 decorating an actin filament in rigor. *B*. Recombinant smooth muscle myosin S1 decorating an actin filament in the presence of MgADP. (*Adapted from Whitaker et al.[54] Reproduced by permission.*)

cross-linked in the presence of nucleotide.[67] Recent kinetic studies show that the cross linking is faster with ATP analogues than with ADP and much slower when no nucleotide is bound in the myosin head.[68] Moreover, strong binding to actin prevents cross linking, whether or not ADP is bound in the myosin head.[69] The internal mobility of the head in the detached state could explain the disorder of SH1 probes observed by fluorescence polarization[70] and EPR studies[71] in skinned fibers following ATP binding. Uncoupling of the converter from the rest of the motor domain leads to multiple orientations of the motor that could favor detachment from actin, prevent any possibility of reverse power stroke, and increase the lifetime of the prehydrolysis state. Delaying reattachment to the actin filament could be particularly important when multiple motors with a low duty ratio need to work efficiently together.

The overall shape of the myosin head strongly bound to actin, as seen in cryoelectron micrographs, has similarities with the crystal structures that define the near-rigor conformation, observed either with ATP analogues bound,[61,63,72] with ADP,[72] or in the absence of nucleotide.[12,72] Similarly, the so-called detached state can be crystallized when either ADP[53] or ATP analogues[64] are bound in the active site. However, since ATP binding and strong binding to actin are mutually exclusive, these studies show that both of these structural states correspond to weak actin-binding states. Kinetic studies also show that binding of either an ADP-containing or nucleotide-free myosin II to F-actin is a two-step process that includes a temperature-dependent conformational change.[73–75] The ADP-containing state that initially interacts with actin binds weakly before undergoing a transition to a strong-binding state. This provides further evidence that none of the high-resolution structures, not even the near rigor state, represent strong actin-binding states. Actin thus must be a major determinant of the myosin conformation in the strong actin-binding states of myosin II.

As already discussed above, myosin V has been crystallized in a "rigor" state in the absence of actin.[50] This was perhaps due to the kinetic tuning that allows myosin V to predominantly occupy strong-binding actin states in the presence of ATP (high duty cycle). In contrast to skeletal myosin II, nucleotide-free myosin V does not undergo any temperature-dependent conformational changes when it binds to actin.[45,50] Based on this and on a number of other important structural changes, the nucleotide-free structure of myosin V likely represents the conformation of the myosin motor domain when it is bound to actin in rigor.

ACTIN-MYOSIN COMPLEX

High-resolution structures of an actin monomer are available,[76,77] as are models for the F-actin filament.[78,79] While there is no high-resolution structure of the actin-myosin complex, there are numerous low-resolution structures of the complex that have been generated from cryoelectron microscopy and image averaging (e.g., Fig. 8-1).[35,44,48,54,55,80,81] What these reveal, as mentioned above, is that the lever arm of myosin II bound to actin in the absence of nucleotide is in a position that is very similar to that in the near-rigor high-resolution structures.[35] However, it is clear that the subdomains of the motor are not in the same position as in the near-rigor structure and that the rigor maps are best fit by a relative movement of the upper and lower 50-kDa subdomains toward each other. This movement is necessary to generate a strong binding interface with actin (see Color Plate 1), as myosin in the near-rigor conformation can bind only weakly to actin (discussed above). Only the myosin V nucleotide-free structure has a closed cleft; thus it fits even the myosin II cryoelectron microscopy maps better than the myosin II near-rigor structures.

A second feature revealed by the EM structures is that for most myosins (Fig. 8-7), there is a state where the lever arm is in an intermediate (between the pre-power stroke and rigor) position and in which the myosin binds strongly to both actin and ADP (Fig. 8-4). In terms of the myosin IIs found in mammalian muscle, this intermediate ADP state exists for the nonmuscle myosin IIs, smooth muscle myosin,[44,54] and the cardiac myosins. Fast skeletal myosin does not populate this state, and the lever-arm position in its rigor state is most similar to the position in the ADP state of smooth muscle myosin II.[82] This intermediate actomyosin ADP state seems to be necessary to allow myosin to bind strongly to both actin and ADP and likely produces a highly strain-dependent ADP release step. For myosins that have weak affinities for ADP when bound to actin (e.g., fast skeletal), this intermediate state either does not exist or is not populated.[44] This is likely an adaptation for speed of shortening, as it creates less strain dependence on the ADP release step, since less movement of the lever arm is required to release ADP.

Myosin Diversity

MYOSIN SUPERFAMILY

The myosin superfamily of motor proteins (Fig. 8-8) is now known to consist of at least 18 distinct classes of related proteins.[83] The cellular function of all of these proteins, and indeed whether or not they all function as motors, has yet to be established. However it is clear that they are involved in many aspects of cellular movement, including cellular locomotion, endocytosis, phagocytosis, and intracellular trafficking.[84,85] A summary of the structural elements of these actin-interacting motors is shown in Fig. 8-9.

Some members of the myosin family of motor proteins can move cargo as single two-headed molecules. The first demonstration of this was with myosin V,[46] which is known to be a vesicle trafficking motor, analogous to kinesin-moving vesicles on a microtubule (Fig. 8-10). The term *processivity* implies that these two-headed motor proteins can move along the actin filament (in the case of myosin V) or along a microtubule (in the case of kinesin) in such a manner that one head is always bound to the filament. If both heads ever dissociated simultaneously, the motor and cargo would diffuse away. While this is optimal for moving a cargo with a small number of motors, it is not the design of a myosin motor optimized for muscle.

Chapter 8. Mammalian Muscle Myosin

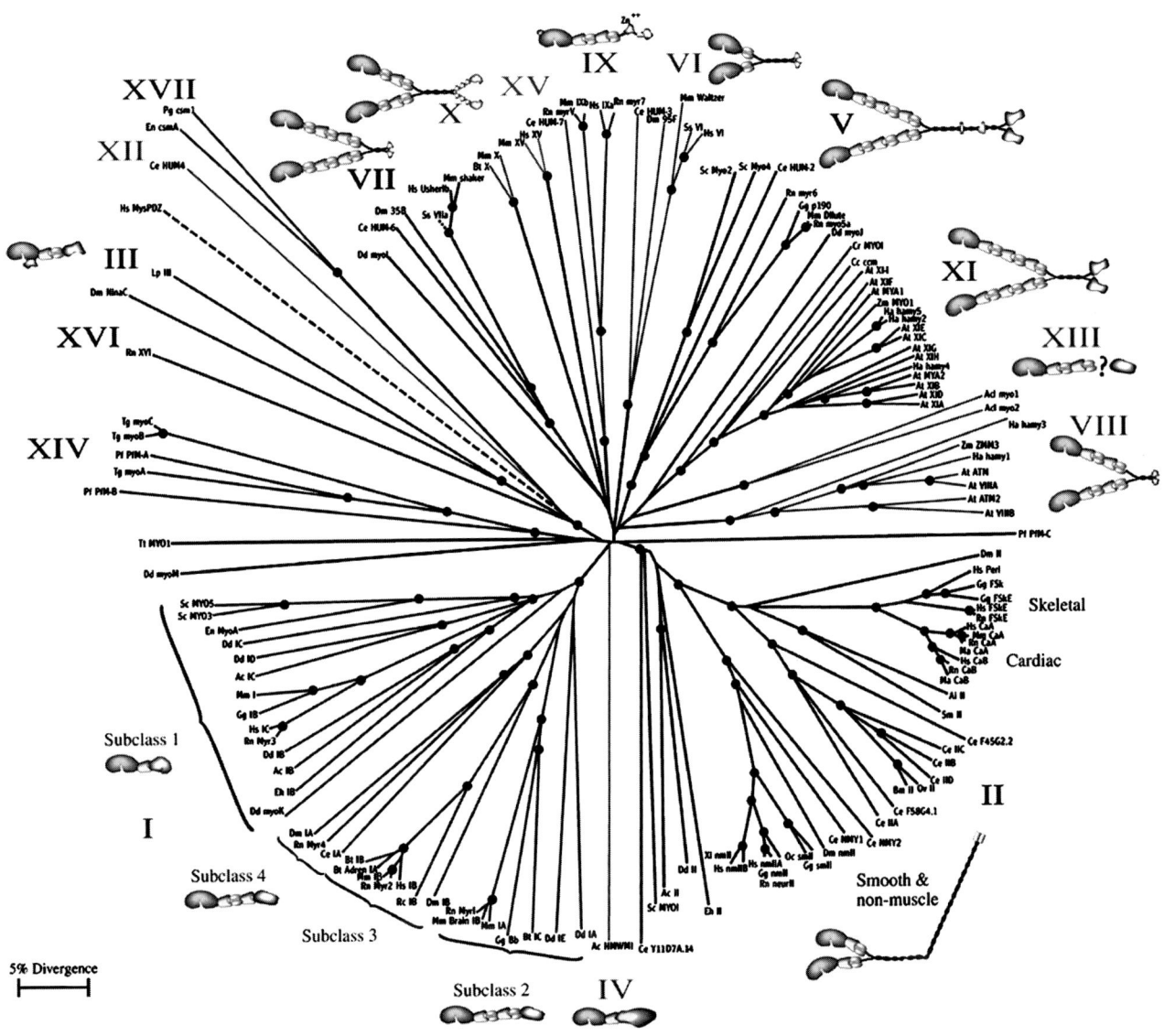

FIGURE 8-8. The myosin superfamily. The evolutionary relationships between the 18 classes of myosin that had been described as of 2002 are shown.

At one time it was thought that all members of the myosin family moved toward the (+) end (barbed end) of an actin filament. In muscle, this means that the myosin heads move toward the Z line. However, one class of myosin, myosin VI, moves in the opposite direction [i.e., toward the (−) end of the actin filament].[88] More recently, there have been conflicting reports as to the directionality of the class IX myosin motors.[89,90]

The most conserved feature within the myosin superfamily is the motor domain itself. The differences that do exist within the motor domains of myosin are primarily restricted to additions/deletions at the N-terminus of the motor and to insertions in loop 2 (the 50/20-kDa loop in myosin II). Myosin VI is a notable exception to this, with two unique insertions within the motor domain. Perhaps the least conserved feature is the C-terminus of the myosin molecule. While all two-headed myosins contain a coiled coil following the light-chain-binding region, the most C-terminal region is different in each class of myosin, likely due to its role in cargo binding. Only the myosin II class appears to have a C-terminal coiled-coil domain that promotes filament formation.

Interestingly, the length of the light-chain/calmodulin-binding region varies within the myosin superfamily and even within the same class of myosin. The range is from one to six binding sites (known as "IQ" motifs).[91] For the unconventional myosins, these sites are mostly occupied by calmodulin, but there are instances of unconventional myosins using the myosin II light chains. For example, each head of chicken myosin V contains two light chains and four calmodulins.[92,93] All myosin II isoforms are thought to use authentic light chains, and all have two IQ motifs (ELC and RLC binding sites).

As discussed earlier in this chapter, the IQ motifs with associated calmodulins/light chains are generally thought to function as a lever arm for the myosin motor. Altering the

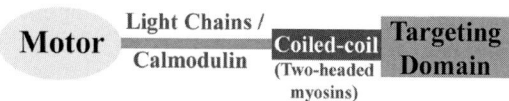

FIGURE 8-9. Structural elements of myosin motors.

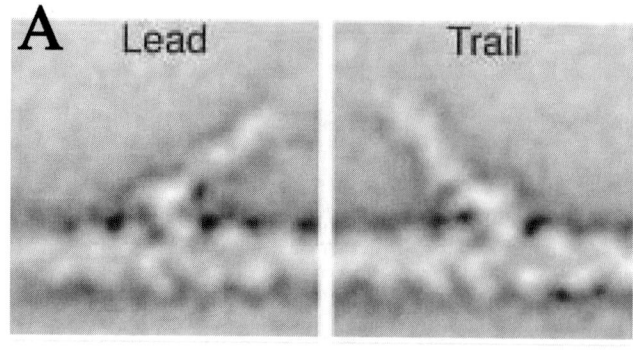

length of the lever arm will change the step size of the myosin movement (see Fig. 8-10) as well as alter the ratio between speed of movement and ATP consumed. However, as pointed out by Howard and Spudich,[94] since the lever arm is likely compliant, lengthening of the lever arm decreases force production.

With the completion of the human genome, it is now clear that there are ~40 different myosin heavy-chain genes in humans, which represent 12 of the myosin classes.[83] A phylogenic tree of the myosin heavy-chain superfamily in humans is shown in Fig. 8-11.

MUSCLE MYOSIN HEAVY-CHAIN ISOFORMS

Mammalian muscle cells express members of four gene families of myosin II heavy chains (fast skeletal, cardiac, smooth, and nonmuscle) and three additional sarcomeric myosin heavy-chain genes (superfast, slow A, and slow B).[95] The fast skeletal locus is composed of six distinct heavy-chain genes. These are embryonic, perinatal (or neonatal), fast type IIa, fast type IIx (or IId), fast type IIb, and extraocular. These myosin heavy-chain forms are expressed only in skeletal muscle. Interestingly, there is no evidence that human muscles ever express the IIb isoform, which is abundant in the muscles of smaller mammals, rodents in particular. [Note that the original use of the type I, IIa, and IIb nomenclature was for histochemical fiber typing by Brooke and Kaiser.[96] It is unfortunate that when three adult fast-twitch myosin heavy chains were found in rodents,[97] it was not known that only two of them were expressed in the corresponding human muscles. Thus the IIb human fibers of Brooke and Kaiser contain the myosin heavy-chain isoform that Schiaffino and colleagues named IIx.] Embryonic and perinatal isoforms are expressed during muscle development and reexpressed in the adult during muscle regeneration.[98] The other heavy chains are expressed in adult muscles, with the order listed above reflecting increasing speed (velocity of shortening and actin-activated ATPase activity) of the myosins that they form. All of the fast skeletal myosin heavy-chain genes are found as part of a multigene locus (on chromosome 17p13 in humans).[98,99] In mammals, there is an additional myosin heavy chain, called *superfast*,[100] that is highly enriched in jaw muscles. This myosin gene is on chromosome 7 in humans.[95] Two additional sarcomeric myosin heavy chains whose distribution of tissue expression and function are unknown have been found on human chromosomes 3 and 20 (slow A and slow B).[95]

The two cardiac heavy-chain genes (α and β) are found in tandem on human chromosome 14q12.[101] These are the only two myosin heavy chains found in cardiac muscle cells, and

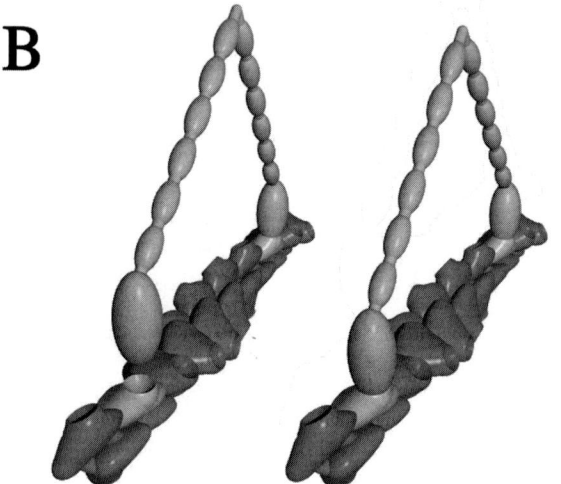

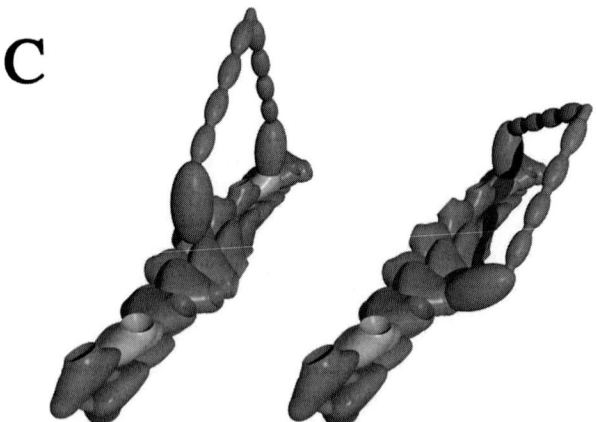

FIGURE 8-10. Myosin V "walks" along actin in 36-nm steps. *A*. Electron microscopy and image enhancement of myosin V directly demonstrates that the two heads (lead and trail) on the same molecule can simultaneously bind to actin sites that are 36 nm apart. Even at low resolution, the lead head appears to be in the transition-state structure, while the trail head is in a state more like near-rigor.[86,87] *B*. Diagrammatic representation of myosin V with its six CaM/light chains taking a 36-nm step on actin. *C*. Diagrammatic representation of a mutant myosin V with only four CaM/light chains per head. This mutant took shorter steps than the wild type (~25 nm), helping to validate the lever-arm hypothesis for myosin movement.[58]

their relative amounts differ with species and developmental stage. In adult humans, the primary isoform is β, whereas in mice it is α. Both heavy chains can be found in skeletal muscles, with β being the myosin heavy chain that is expressed in slow-twitch skeletal muscles. The α expression is much less frequent in skeletal muscle and has been demonstrated only in muscles of the head and neck. In cardiac muscle, coexpression of the two heavy chains leads to three myosin forms—known as V1, V2, and V3—listed in order of decreasing enzymatic activity. VI is an α-α homodimer, V3 is a β-β homodimer, and V2 is a heterodimer between α and β.

Smooth muscles contain multiple splice forms of the smooth muscle myosin heavy chain (human chromosome 16p13)[102] as well as varying amounts of the nonmuscle IIa isoform (human chromosome 22q11.2)[103] (unrelated in any way to fast-twitch IIa other than nomenclature). The nonmuscle IIa isoform is important for sustained tonic contractions, whereas phasic contractions rely on one or more of the smooth muscle heavy-chain isoforms. Vertebrate smooth muscle arose with vertebrate evolution; thus the myosin of smooth muscle is not closely related to the myosins of striated muscles.[83,95] In fact, smooth muscle myosin is closely related to the vertebrate nonmuscle myosin IIs, from which it undoubtedly arose.[83,95] Comparisons of vertebrate smooth muscle isoforms reveal a remarkable level of sequence conservation (>90 percent identity). However, one of the areas of variability is the same as is found in vertebrate sarcomeric myosins, the 25/50-kDa junction (loop 1).[104,105] In fact, different smooth muscle myosin heavy-chain isoforms are created by alternative splicing of exons that code for this region.[106] The other alternatively spliced region in the smooth muscle heavy chain is an alternative insertion at the end of the rod. One possible function of this variability is to alter the type of filament formation.[107,108]

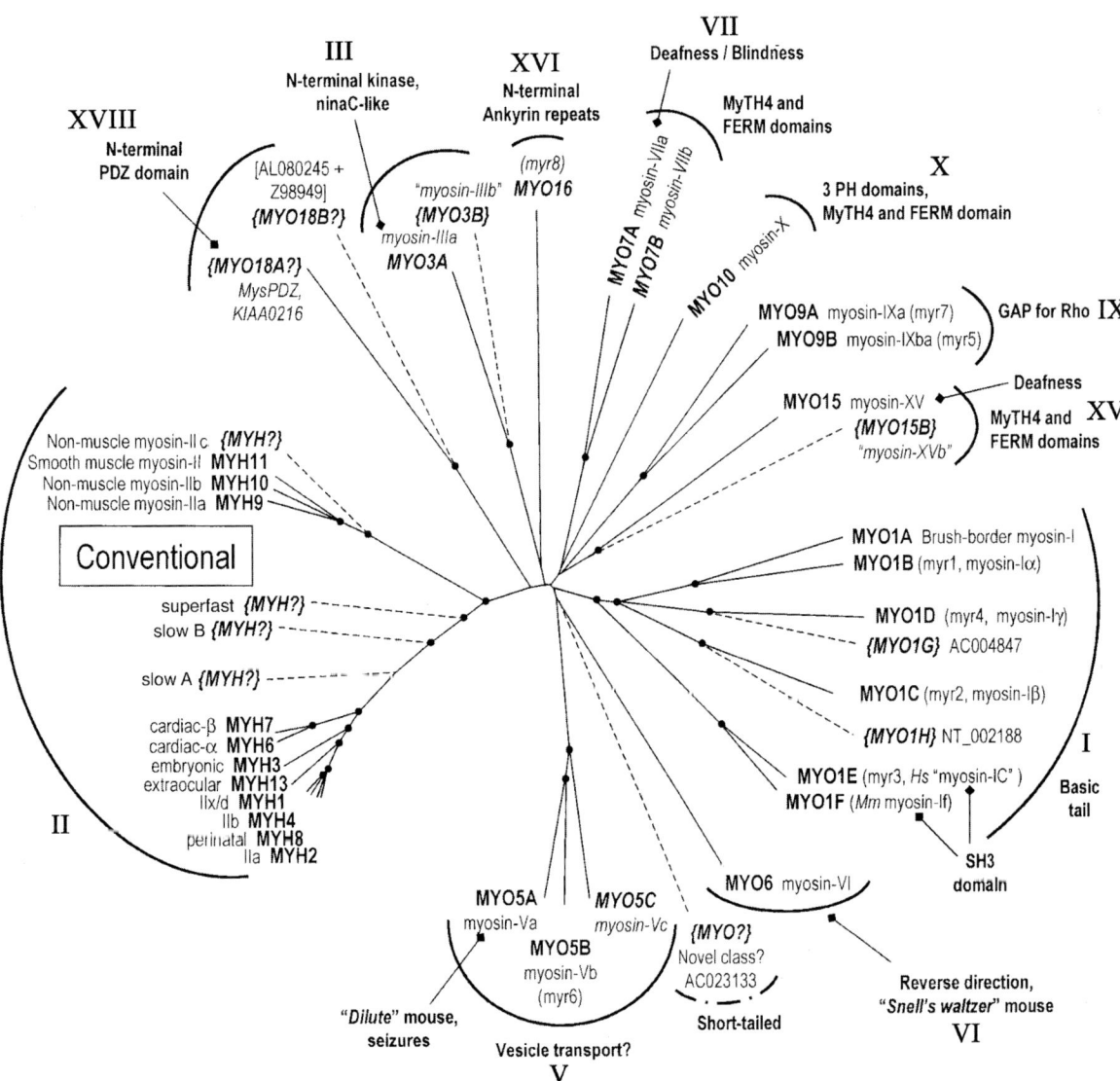

FIGURE 8-11. The human myosin superfamily. (*Adapted from Berget al.*[83] *Reproduced by permission.*)

MYOSIN LIGHT-CHAIN ISOFORMS

Just as there are multiple heavy-chain isoforms expressed in mammalian muscles, there is also a range of myosin light-chain isoforms (Fig. 8-12).[109] There are likely functional differences associated with this light-chain diversity. This can come about in one of two ways. Since the essential light chain (ELC) has direct associations with the converter subdomain, it can potentially affect transitions between structural states. Second, alterations in the interactions of both the ELC and the regulatory light chain (RLC) with the heavy-chain helix can alter the compliance of the lever arm, which will affect all strain-dependent state transitions.[110] Figure 8-12 provides a diagram of the ELC and RLC isoforms found in mammalian muscle.

In comparing the sequences of the essential light-chain isoforms expressed in vertebrate striated muscle versus those of vertebrate smooth/nonmuscle myosins, the striking difference is that all vertebrate striated ELC isoforms (with the exception of LC-3f) have an extended N-terminus,[109] whereas the nonmuscle ELCs (with the exception of LC1-sa, an isoform that is shared between nonmuscle, embryonic smooth, and some slow-twitch skeletal fibers) do not have the N-terminal extension.[109,111] A number of different experimental approaches have led to the conclusion that some part of this N-terminal extension interacts with actin.[112–119] Several lines of evidence[114,115,118] indicate that the interaction is with the C-terminus of actin. One possible consequence of this interaction between the N-terminal domains of all of the striated muscle ELCs except LC3$_f$ and the C-terminus of

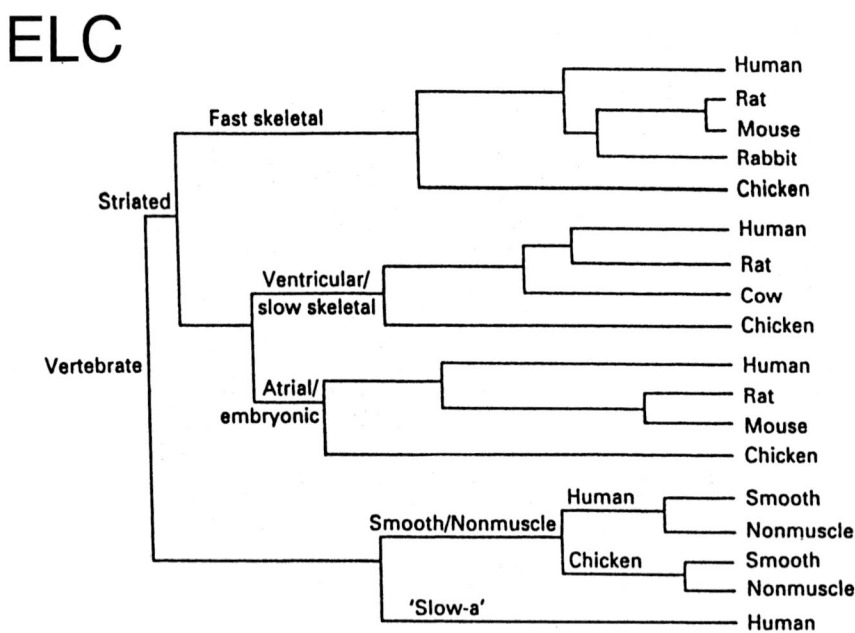

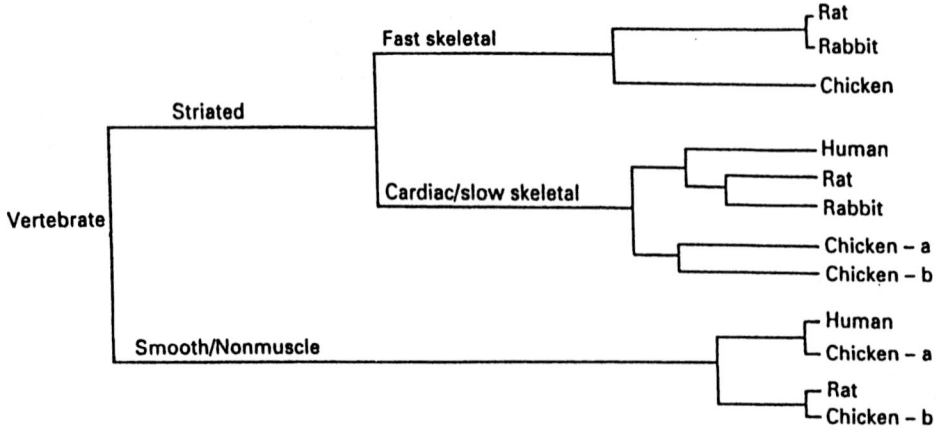

FIGURE 8-12. Evolutionary relationships of the vertebrate myosin light chains. (*Adapted from Collins.*[109] *Reproduced by permission.*)

actin could be to alter the maximal velocity of shortening, as reported by a number of groups.[120–123] Furthermore, other aspects of cross-bridge kinetics (e.g., rate of cross-bridge attachment) could be altered by this tethering.

While a modulatory role for the N-terminal extension of the essential light chain probably exists in muscle contraction, it is interesting to speculate whether or not this role is the only or indeed the primary function of the N-terminal extension. The discovery of an alternative gene product of the striated muscle myosin heavy-chain gene of *Drosophila melanogaster*[124] suggests the possibility of an additional and perhaps more fundamental role for this extended peptide. In addition to multiple myosin heavy-chain isoforms, the *Drosophila* gene encodes a peptide consisting of an N-terminal extension that is highly homologous to that of the ELC, fused to the striated muscle myosin rod (i.e., this N-terminal extension replaces the myosin head). Its purpose may be to provide a tether between thick and thin filaments, as would the N-terminal extension of the ELC in vertebrate striated muscle (and in developing vertebrate smooth muscle). Such a tethering might serve to position thick and thin filaments to facilitate cross-bridge interactions. This may be especially important when the filaments are not in a sarcomeric lattice and may be a possible role for the unusual *Drosophila* gene product in nonmuscle cells. Furthermore, while the purpose of extended light-chain tethering would be to alter cross-bridge kinetics in a mature sarcomere, it could also provide a means of positioning thick and thin filaments during sarcomere assembly. This could be a reason for the lack of $LC3_f$ expression in early muscle development within vertebrates.

REGULATORY LIGHT-CHAIN PHOSPHORYLATION

The cyclic interaction of myosin and actin must be regulated in all muscle and nonmuscle cells that utilize actomyosin-based motility. In all cases, the signal to initiate contraction is an increase in the cytoplasmic calcium concentration. In striated muscle (skeletal and cardiac muscle), regulation is via calcium binding to troponin, the thin filament protein (see Chap. 13).

For nonmuscle and smooth muscle cells, the increase in $[Ca^{2+}]$ leads to activation of myosin II cross-bridges via phosphorylation of one of the myosin light chains.[4,125] The regulatory light chain of nonmuscle and smooth muscle myosin IIs prevents the myosin cross-bridge from binding to actin (hence the term *regulatory*) unless it is phosphorylated at a specific site near its amino-terminus. When intracellular Ca^{2+} concentration rises, Ca^{2+} binds to calmodulin (four ions per molecule), forming a Ca^{2+}-calmodulin complex, which can activate many enzyme systems. One such Ca^{2+}-calmodulin-dependent enzyme system is myosin light-chain kinase (MLCK), which catalyzes the phosphorylation from ATP of a serine residue in the RLC. This phosphorylation negates the inhibitory action of the light chain so that the phosphorylated cross-bridge can repetitively cycle, releasing the hydrolysis products of ATP until the RLC is dephosphorylated by a myosin light-chain phosphatase (MLCP).

While phosphorylation of the RLC is not an on/off switch in striated muscle myosins, it does modulate the actin-myosin activity. The phosphorylation alters the force-calcium relationship (increased calcium sensitivity), increases the rate of force redevelopment, and alters the time course of stretch activation.[126,127] The striated muscles of a number of invertebrates may be dually regulated, requiring both phosphorylation of the myosin light chain and calcium binding to troponin C to be activated.[128]

The RLCs from skeletal muscle and smooth muscle are highly homologous (71 percent similarity and 53 percent identity in sequence). Both RLCs contain a high-affinity divalent cation-binding site near the N-terminus that mutational analysis has demonstrated is necessary for proper binding of the light chain to the myosin II heavy chain.[129] The initiation of smooth muscle contraction must be preceded by serine phosphorylation of the myosin RLC.[125] As mentioned above, although the RLC is also reversibly phosphorylated in vertebrate striated muscle (at a homologous serine), this phosphorylation simply modulates contractile activity.[126] The loss of myosin regulation in striated muscle is due to undetermined alterations in the myosin heavy chain. Additionally, the smooth muscle and skeletal muscle RLCs are not functionally equivalent. The RLC from skeletal muscle myosin (skRLC) is unable to confer regulation to smooth muscle myosin and locks the myosin in the "off" state when substituted for the endogenous smooth muscle RLC (smRLC).[130] Additionally, the smRLC can confer calcium sensitivity to scallop muscle myosin (a Ca^{2+}-regulated myosin), while the skRLC fails to do so.[131] However no RLC can inhibit the activity of vertebrate skeletal muscle myosin.[132]

Phosphorylation of the smooth myosin II RLC promotes unfolding of the myosin (transition from 6S to 10S conformation) as well as turning on the ATPase activity.[133] Mutagenesis studies that have removed and reversed positively charged residues that are immediately N-terminal of the phosphorylatable serine of the smooth muscle myosin II RLC demonstrate that the interactions regulating the folded-to-extended conformational transition in smooth muscle myosin are distinct from those that control ATPase activity.[134–136]

A structure of the dephosphorylated smooth muscle HMM has been obtained by the use of two-dimensional crystals and electron microscopy.[137,138] This structure explains many puzzling observations found in mutagenesis studies that were designed to probe regulation, but it does not make clear the role of the RLC itself. As depicted in Fig. 8-13, the modeled structure shows direct interactions between the two motor domains, which explains why removal of one motor domain from a HMM eliminates most of the regulation.[139] The interaction is between a large component of the actin interface of one motor domain and the converter region of the other. Thus while the actin interface of one head is free to interact with actin, the converter domain of that head is constrained, so that it cannot move out of the ADP.Pi conformation. Thus both heads are trapped in ADP.Pi states, even in the presence of actin. Why phosphorylation of the RLC breaks these head-head interactions is not clear from the structure. One possibility is that flexibility of the light-chain domains is necessary for the head-head interactions to occur. If phosphorylation forms intramolecular interactions within the RLC that alter its interactions with the heavy chain and/or ELC, this could lead to loss of flexibility

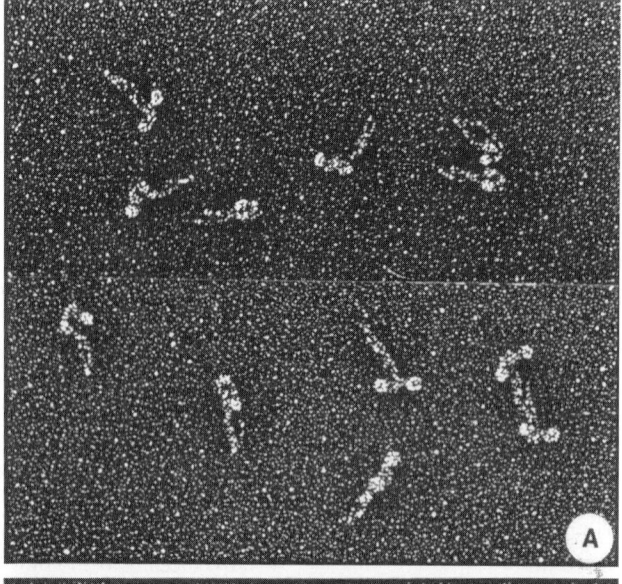

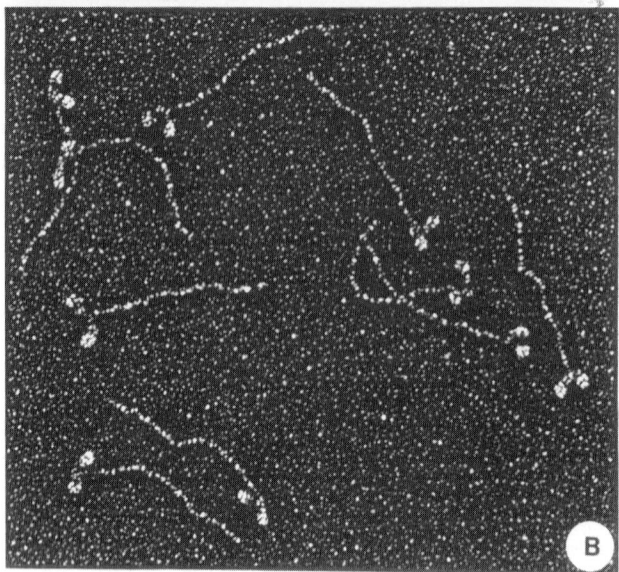

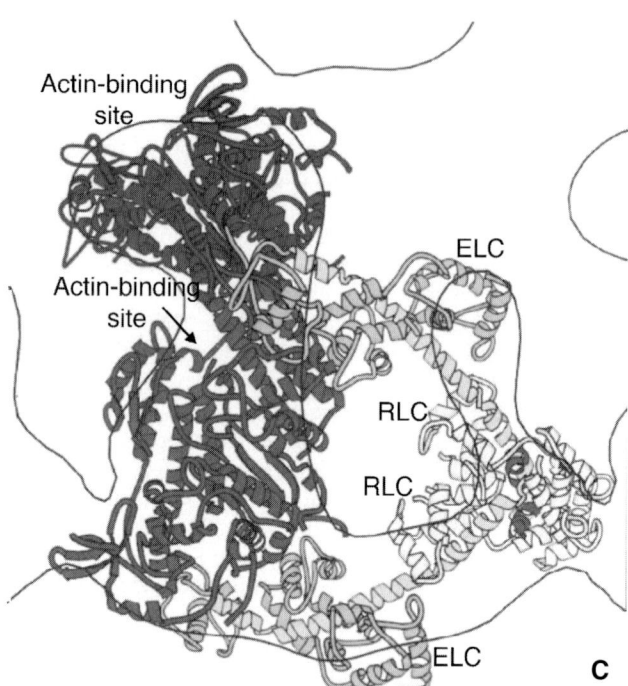

FIGURE 8-13. Structural changes associated with smooth muscle myosin regulation. A. Electron micrographs of rotary-shadowed smooth muscle myosin molecules in the folded ("off" or dephosphorylated) state. B. Rotary-shadowed smooth muscle myosin molecules in the extended ("on" or phosphorylated) state. C. Image reconstruction from electron micrographs of two-dimensional crystals of dephosphorylated smooth muscle myosin. The atomic structure of smooth muscle myosin[62] was made to fit into the electron myographic density. Note the position of the light chains and that the actin interface of one head is opposed against the converter region of the second head, while the actin interface of the second head is unblocked. (A and B courtesy of K. M. Trybus; C adapted from Wendt et al.[138] Reproduced by permission.)

in the light-chain-binding domain (lever arm), breaking the head-head interactions.

Studies of chimeric RLCs composed of the N- or C-terminal half of each skRLC and smRLC indicate that it is the C-terminal half of skRLC that lacks structural elements necessary for phosphorylation-mediated regulation.[130] C-terminal truncation studies on the smooth RLC indicate that this region of the light chain must be present for tight binding[140,141] and normal coupling between ATPase activity and motility[141]; these studies have also shown that it contains a region necessary to confer regulation.[140,141] Mutations in the C-terminal domain are consistent with interactions between the phosphate and C-terminal residues that could provide the type of intramolecular interactions necessary to change the properties of the lever arm, as speculated above.[142]

Another type of myosin II regulation involving the regulatory light chain is found in the myosin II of scallop striated muscle.[143] This regulation involves direct Ca^{2+} binding to the neck region of myosin. The location of the Ca^{2+}-binding site was revealed in the crystal structure of the scallop myosin II neck.[144] Coordination of the Ca^{2+} binding requires contributions from the ELC (primarily), the myosin heavy chain, and the RLC. The RLC contribution involves a glycine residue in the loop between the F and G helices, which is absolutely conserved in regulated myosin RLCs. Removal of this glycine results in loss of regulation, trapping the myosin in the "off" state.[145] This explains earlier results indicating that some conserved elements of the C-terminal region of the RLC were necessary for Ca^{2+} binding.[146] If scallop myosin can form a folded "off" complex similar to the one seen for smooth muscle myosin II, then Ca^{2+} could play the same structural role as phosphorylation of vertebrate smooth/nonmuscle RLCs. The calcium-induced interaction between the ELC and RLC of scallop would reduce the flexibility of the light-chain-binding region, preventing formation of the folded complex.

In the striated muscles of vertebrates, phosphorylation of the myosin II RLC modulates both the rate of force production and the steady-state level at submaximal levels of thin filament activation.[126] This may be explained either by movement of myosin heads away from the thick filament backbone[147] or by a disordering of the heads, which may indicate increased head mobility.[148–150] The mechanism for this effect involves a simple charge alteration via phosphorylation, which is mimicked by altering the fixed charge adjacent to the phosphorylatable serine.[136] This may be analogous to the electrostatic mechanism that accounts for the ability of smRLC phosphorylation to unfold the bent smooth muscle myosin monomer to the extended conformation.

KINETIC DIVERSITY

In moving the skeleton, pumping blood, and controlling movements in the viscera and vasculature, muscle performs mechanical work in animals. Given the large muscle mass of an animal, it is generally considered that the design of muscle must be optimized to perform its function with minimal energy cost and maximal efficiency. In order for this to occur, a number of processes within muscle must be altered in parallel as the functional demand on the muscle is changed. Of central importance is the design of the molecular motor, myosin, which, via its cyclic, ATP-consuming interaction with actin, accounts for most of the energetic cost of muscle contraction.[151]

One might expect that, given the differences in functional demands placed on the three types of mammalian muscle (skeletal, cardiac, and smooth), fundamental differences should exist in the myosin motor isozymes expressed in these tissues if optimization has occurred. Smooth muscle cells must generate forces for prolonged periods of time with little shortening. Thus a myosin capable of generating a high isometric force with low energy cost (high economy) would be optimal. Skeletal muscle is heterogeneous in its myosin isozymes and in the functional demands it faces. Thus the myosin isozymes of skeletal muscle must be based on compromises providing for high economy in muscles that are used in a predominantly isometric pattern and providing high shortening velocities and power outputs with maximal efficiency in muscles that perform shortening work. For cardiac muscle, the demands, and thus the optimal solution, should be similar to those for skeletal muscle in that both economical isometric contractions and efficient but powerful shortening contractions must be generated.

Distinct steps of the cross-bridge cycle seem to be rate-limiting for different contractile parameters of muscle. The dynamic properties of muscle that shape its performance are the rate of force generation, the rate of relaxation, and the velocity at which muscle can shorten. The rate of force generation is limited by the rate of the weak-to-strong transition. The rate of relaxation in most muscles is limited by a combination of the detachment rate of myosin and the rate of removal of calcium from troponin.

The maximum shortening velocity of a muscle is limited by how fast myosin can detach from actin, which, in turn, is limited by the rate of ADP release.[152,153] Numerous studies on isolated skeletal muscle fibers suggest that the composition of fibers in terms of myosin heavy-chain isoforms is the primary determinant of the maximal shortening velocity.[120–122,154,155] However, there is evidence of modulation of velocity by myosin light-chain isoforms[110,120–123] as well as other sarcomeric proteins and structural features.[156,157]

In 1967 Barany observed that, for skeletal muscles taken from a number of different vertebrates and invertebrates, there is a linear relationship between the steady-state actin-myosin ATPase activity in solution and the maximal velocity of shortening of the muscle from which the myosin is extracted.[158] Since these processes are limited by different steps in the cycle, parallel changes in rate constants are occurring, which would tend to keep the rate of steady-state ATPase activity of a muscle proportionate to the maximal shortening velocity, at least for muscles containing the myosin isozymes represented in Barany's study.

The amount of isometric force that a muscle produces will be a function of the percentage of the cross-bridge cycle that myosin spends in the force-producing states (the duty ratio), the unitary force each myosin head produces, and the number of myosin heads acting in parallel. At the level of the individual myosin molecule, it is thought that the unitary force is similar among different muscle myosin isozymes, which leaves only the duty ratio as a variable.[159,160]

While the force per cross-sectional area (and thus the myosin duty ratio) is similar in mammalian skeletal muscle fibers containing a variety of different myosin isozymes (types I, IIa, IIx, and IIb), it is clear that the duty ratio is not an invariant myosin parameter. Evidence that the duty ratios of the muscle myosins are variant is derived from comparisons of the two cardiac myosins and smooth muscle myosin with that of fast skeletal muscle.[159,160] Smooth muscle myosin generates greater force per myosin cross-bridge than does its skeletal muscle counterpart, and it does so by increasing the duty ratio.[159] This likely represents a better compromise for smooth muscle. In the case of rodent cardiac muscle, two predominant myosin isozymes are expressed. The slower of the two (β-cardiac) is common to both slow skeletal and cardiac muscle and produces a force per cross-bridge that is similar to that produced by the fast skeletal isozymes of myosin. The faster of the cardiac isozymes (α-cardiac) produces less force per cross-bridge than other mammalian striated muscle myosins via a shorter duty ratio.[160] Thus the α-cardiac myosin achieves its greater speed at the expense of force.[161] Perhaps the α-cardiac myosin isozyme is a better compromise for the rodent heart when it is working at high heart rates against normal pressures than the β-cardiac form, which is expressed when the heart is working at lower heart rates and against higher pressures.

HYPERTROPHIC CARDIOMYOPATHY

Mutations in cardiac myosin have been shown to cause a disease in humans known as *hypertrophic cardiomyopathy* (HCM). The clinical manifestations of HCM range from asymptomatic disease to severe cardiac failure or sudden cardiac death; they present in the elderly as well as in active, young, otherwise healthy individuals. Sudden death is thought to be due to arrhythmias arising from the ischemia that accompanies the hypertrophy. Genetic analyses have shown that HCM is an autosomal dominant disorder of heart muscle that results from mutations in genes encoding sarcomeric proteins.[162–164] Twelve different disease genes have been identified, ten of which code for sarcomeric proteins: the β-myosin heavy chain,[165] the cardiac myosin essential light chain,[166] the cardiac myosin regulatory light chain,[166] α-tropomyosin,[167] cardiac troponin T,[167] cardiac myosin-binding protein C genes,[168,169] cardiac troponin I,[170] cardiac troponin C,[170a] cardiac actin,[171] and titin.[171a] That mutations in these diverse components of the sarcomere appear to produce a related phenotype suggests that the mutations share functional consequences that lead to a related mode of pathogenesis.

Many different mutations in the β-myosin heavy-chain gene cause HCM. These mutations result in functional alterations in the myosin, the nature of which is still subject to some debate.[172–179] Nevertheless, the consequence of these mutations is likely to be a mistuning of the force-velocity characteristics of the working heart, so that these do not match the rate at which the heart is performing work, thus leading to increased energy demands on the heart. Since HCM can result from a number of distinct myosin mutations, it is likely that the severity of the disease is dependent on the position and nature of the mutation in the molecule.

Mutations in either the ELC or RLC of myosin have been linked to an unusual form of hypertrophic cardiomyopathy that is characterized by hypertrophy of the papillary muscles.[166] The fact that five different mutations, two in the ELC and three in the RLC, all lead to a phenotype that is not seen for any of the other HCM mutations suggests that there is a unique contractile deficit associated with the light-chain muations.[166] Given the function of the papillary muscles, one possibility is that the time course of stretch activation is altered. Strong evidence that these mutations alter stretch activation in the heart and cause disease and that lack of phosphorylation of the RLC can lead to a similar problem is provided in the work of Epstein and colleagues.[180–182]

IN VITRO EXPRESSION AND ASSAYS OF MYOSIN FUNCTION

Prior to the 1980s, all of the biochemistry of muscle myosin II was deduced from soluble proteolytic fragments (S1 and HMM) isolated from muscle, and the mechanical properties of myosin were measured within the sarcomeric context of either intact muscle or single muscle fibers (see Chap. 9). In order to study myosin's mechanical properties outside of the sarcomere, a number of in vitro assays were developed. These technical developments allowed the characterization of the mechanical properties of any myosin, even down to the level of a single molecule. Likewise, the desire to study myosins other than those found in muscle and to introduce specific mutations led to the development of in vitro expression systems for myosin and fragments of myosin.

The first in vitro motility assays used the actin cables from the giant algae *Nitella* as the tracks on which beads coated with myosin could be observed to move.[183] More general assays were developed using synthetic actin filaments, the most important of which is that of Kron and Spudich.[184] In this assay, depicted in Fig. 8-14, myosin is attached to a nitrocellulose-coated glass surface on which fluorescently labeled actin filaments can be induced to move, given ATP and appropriate solution conditions. This assay has allowed the determination of the actin-translocating activity of many types of myosin from a variety of sources.

The first myosin expression system involved expression of whole myosin or fragments of myosin in *Dictyostelium discodium*.[185] While this expression system allowed the characterization of mutations in myosin for the first time, it has been limited to the expression from myosins normally found in *Dictyostelium*. To counter this problem, the baculovirus/SF9 cell-expression system has been used to express myosins of a number of classes from a wide range of eukaryotic sources.[173]

The ability to measure the chemomechanical properties of single myosin molecules is the most recent technical advance to have furthered our understanding of myosin's motor mechanism. Of the assays available, the laser light trap has proven the most useful in the measurement of the unitary displacements and force of single myosin molecules.[186–195] This technique is discussed in greater detail in Chap. 9. The best estimates of the size of the unitary displacement by muscle myosins are on the order of 5 to 10 nm.[186–195] The unitary force estimates are more variable due to compliance in the linkages to the actin and myosin but are on the order of a few piconewtons.

Total internal reflectance microscopy has allowed the visualization of single fluorophores and thus the movement of indi-

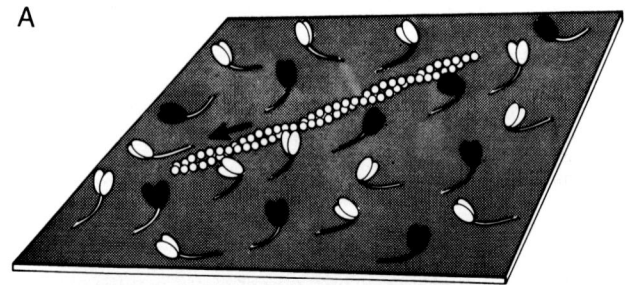

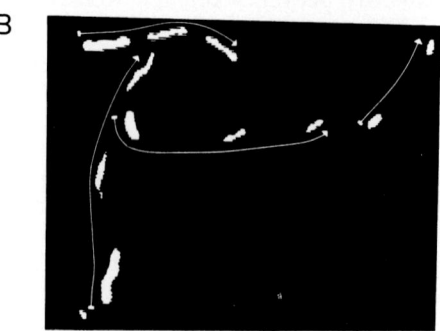

FIGURE 8-14. In vitro motility assay. A. Schematic drawing of myosin-coated surface interacting with an actin filament in the Kron and Spudich[184] assay. B. Myosin or its subfragment is attached to a film of nitrocellulose on a glass cover slip and the movement is observed by video-enhanced fluorescence microscopy. (*Courtesy of D. M. Warshaw.*)

vidual labeled myosin molecules.[196-201] For processive myosins, such as myosins V and VI, this has enabled the visualization of single molecules moving along an actin filament.[202-206] In the future, enzymatic assays coupled to fluorescent substrates/products will allow direct visualization of the chemomechanical coupling of various forms of myosin. Initial attempts of this sort have been published.[196-201]

Conclusions

This chapter does not provide an all-inclusive survey of the myosin literature but instead gives the underpinnings of our current structural and functional understanding of the molecular motor of muscle. Since the last edition of *Myology*, that understanding has advanced tremendously. This is true not only in the detailed structure of the molecule but also in the recognition that muscle myosin is a member of a functionally diverse family of molecular motors. It is now clear that fast skeletal muscle myosin, the molecule on which myosin biochemistry and mechanics were initially based, is highly specialized for the task of speed and power generation within a sarcomeric context. As such, it is merely one end of the myosin spectrum and not the functional prototype for the entire myosin family. Indeed, even within the myosin II class, one finds a tremendous range of functional specialization based on modest structural alterations. The extremes of functional and structural variations as well as cell biological roles across all myosin classes are just beginning to be understood and appreciated.

Acknowledgments

The authors acknowledge grants from the National Institutes of Health and the Muscular Dystrophy Association.

List of Abbreviations

ATP	adenosine triphosphate
ATPase	adenosine triphosphatase
ELC	essential light chain
EM	electron microscopy
HCM	hypertrophic cardiomyopathy
HMM	heavy meromyosin
MLCK	myosin light-chain kinase
MLCP	myosin light-chain phosphatase
RLC	regulatory light chain
skRLC	skeletal muscle myosin regulatory light chain
smRLC	smooth muscle myosin regulatory light chain

References

1. Kühne W: Undtersuchungen über Bewegungen und Veränderungen der contractilen Substanzen. *Arch Anat Physiol Wissensch Med*, p 748, 1859.
2. Engelhardt VA, Lyubimova MN: Myosin and adenosinetriphosphatase. *Nature* 144:668–671, 1939.
3. Straub FB: Actin. *Stud Inst Med Chem Univ Szeged* II:3, 1948.
4. Bresnick AR: Molecular mechanisms of nonmuscle myosin-II regulation. *Curr Opin Cell Biol* 11:26–33, 1999.
5. Slayter HS, Lowey S: Substructure of the myosin molecule as visualized by electron microscopy. *Proc Natl Acad Sci USA* 58:1611, 1967.
6. Lowey S, Slayter HS, Weeds AG, Baker H: Substructure of the myosin molecule: I. Subfragments of myosin by enzymic degradation. *J Mol Biol* 42:1, 1969.
7. Weeds AG, Lowey S: Substructure of the myosin molecule: II. The light chains of myosin. *J Mol Biol* 61:701–725, 1971.
8. Huxley HE: Electron microscope studies on the structure of natural and synthetic protein filaments from striated muscle. *J Mol Biol* 7:281, 1963.
9. Mornet D, Bertrand R, Pantel P, et al: Proteolytic approach to structure and function of actin recognition site in myosin heads. *Biochemistry* 20:2110–2120, 1981.
10. Sutoh K: An actin-binding site on the 20K fragment of myosin subfragment 1. *Biochemistry* 21:4800–4804, 1982.
11. Sutoh K: Mapping of actin-binding sites on the heavy chain of myosin subfragment 1. *Biochemistry* 22:1579–1585, 1983.
12. Rayment I, Rypniewski WR, Schmidt-Bäde K, et al: Three-dimensional structure of myosin subfragment-1: A molecular motor. *Science* 261:50–58, 1993.
13. Bireó NA, Szilágy L, Bálint M: Studies on the helical segment of the myosin molecule. *Cold Spring Harb Symp Quant Biol* 37:55, 1972.
14. Lowey S, Risby D: Light chains from fast and slow muscle myosins. *Nature* 234:81–85, 1971.
15. Frank G, Weeds AG: The amino-acid sequence of the alkali light chains of rabbit skeletal-muscle myosin. *Eur J Biochem* 44:317, 1974.
16. Weeds AG: Light chains of myosin. *Nature* 223:1362, 1969.
17. Perrie WT, Smillie LB, Perry SV: A phosphorylated light chain component of myosin from skeletal muscle. *Biochem J* 135:151, 1973.
18. Morgan M, Perry SV, Ottaway J: Myosin light-chain phosphatase. *Biochem J* 157:687, 1976.
19. Bresnick AR: Molecular mechanisms of nonmuscle myosin-II regulation. *Curr Opin Cell Biol* 11:26–33, 1999.
20. Kominz DR, Carroll WR, Smith EN, Mitchell ER: A subunit of myosin. *Arch Biochem Biophys* 79:191, 1959.
21. Lowey S: The structure of vertebrate muscle myosin, in Engel AG, Franzini-Armstrong C (eds): *Myology*, 2d ed. New York: McGraw-Hill; 1994, pp 485–505.
22. Winkelmann DA, Lowey S, Press JL: Monoclonal antibodies localize changes on myosin heavy chain isozymes during avian myogenesis. *Cell* 34:295–306, 1983.
23. Henry GD, Winstanley MA, Dalgarno DC, et al: Characterization of the actin-binding site on the alkali light chain of myosin. *Biochim Biophys Acta* 830:233–243, 1985.
24. Wade R, Feldman D, Gunning P, Kedes L: Sequence and expression of human myosin alkali light chain isoforms. *Mol Cell Biochem* 87:119–136, 1989.
25. Proteolytic fragments of myosin. *Methods Enzymol* 85, 1982.
26. Mornet D, Bertrand R, Pantel P, et al: Proteolytic approach to structure and function of actin recognition site in myosin heads. *Biochemistry* 20:2110–2120, 1981.
27. Sohn RL, Vikstrom KL, Strauss M, et al: A 29 residue region of the sarcomeric myosin rod is necessary for filament formation. *J Mol Biol* 266:317–330, 1997.
28. McLachlan AD, Karn J: Periodic charge distributions in the myosin rod amino acid sequence match cross-bridge spacings in muscle. *Nature* 299:226–231, 1982.
29. McLachlan AD, Karn J: Periodic features in the amino acid sequence of nematode myosin rod. *J Mol Biol* 164:605–626, 1983.
30. Young M: Studies on the structural basis of the interaction of myosin and actin. *Proc Natl Acad Sci USA* 58:2393, 1967.
31. Eisenberg E, Moos C: The adenosine triphosphatase activity of acto-heavy meromyosin. A kinetic analysis of actin activation. *Biochemistry* 7:1486, 1968.

32. Huxley HE, Hanson J: Changes in the cross-striations of muscle during contraction and stretch and their structural interpretation. *Nature* 173:973, 1954.
33. Huxley AF, Niedergerke R: Structural changes in muscle during contraction. Interference microscopy of living muscle fibres. *Nature* 173:971, 1954.
34. Huxley HE: The mechanism of muscular contraction. *Science* 164:1356–1359, 1969.
35. Rayment I, Holden HM, Whitaker M, et al: Structure of the actin-myosin complex and its implications for muscle contraction. *Science* 261:58–61, 1993.
36. Holmes KC, Geeves MA: Structural mechanism of muscle contraction. *Annu Rev Biochem* 68:687–728, 1999.
37. Houdusse A, Sweeney HL: Myosin motors: Missing structures and hidden springs. *Curr Opin Struct Biol* 11:182–194, 2001.
38. Lymn RW, Taylor EW: Mechanism of adenosine triphosphate hydrolysis by actomyosin. *Biochemistry* 10:4617–4624, 1971.
39. Eisenberg E, Greene LE: The relation of muscle biochemistry to muscle physiology. *Annu Rev Physiol* 42:293–309, 1980.
40. Geeves MA, Goody RS, Gutfreund H: Kinetics of acto-S1 interaction as a guide to a model for the crossbridge cycle. *J Muscle Res Cell Motil* 5:351–361, 1984.
41. Geeves MA, Conibear PB: The role of three-state docking of myosin S1 with actin in force generation. *Biophys J* 68:194S–199S, 1995.
42. Malnasi-Csizmadia A, Pearson DS, Kovacs M, et al: Kinetic resolution of a conformational transition and the ATP hydrolysis step using relaxation methods with a *Dictyostelium* myosin II mutant containing a single tryptophan residue. *Biochemistry* 40:12727–12737, 2001.
43. Dantzig JA, Goldman YE, Millar NC, et al: Reversal of the cross-bridge force-generating transition by photogeneration of phosphate in rabbit psoas muscle fibres. *J Physiol* 451:247–278, 1992.
44. Rosenfeld SS, Xing J, Whithaker M, et al: Kinetic and spectroscopic evidence for three actomyosin:ADP states in smooth muscle. *J Biol Chem* 275:25418–25426, 2000.
45. De La Cruz EM, Wells AL, Rosenfeld SS, et al: The kinetic mechanism of myosin V. *Proc Natl Acad Sci USA* 96:13726–13731, 1999.
46. Mehta AD, Rock RS, Rief M, et al: Myosin V is a processive actin-based motor. *Nature* 400:590–593, 1999.
47. Tokunaga M, Sutoh K, Toyoshima C, Wakabayashi T: Location of the ATPase site of myosin determined by three dimensional electron microscopy. *Nature* 329:635, 1987.
48. Volkman N, Hanein D, Ouyang G, et al: Evidence for cleft closure in actomyosin upon ADP release. *Nat Struct Biol* 7:1147–1155, 2000.
49. Yengo CM, Chrin L, Rovner AS, Berger CL: Intrinsic tryptophan fluorescence identifies specific conformational changes at the actomyosin interface upon actin binding and ADP release. *Biochemistry* 38:14515–14523, 1999.
50. Coureux PD, Wells AL, Menetrey J, et al: A structural state of the myosin V motor without bound nucleotide. *Nature* 425:419–423, 2003.
51. Xiao M, Reifenberger JG, Wells AL, et al: An actin-dependent conformational change in myosin. *Nat Struct Biol* 10:402–408, 2003.
52. Rock RS, Rice SE, Wells AL, et al: Myosin VI is a processive, backwards motor with a large step size. *Proc Natl Acad Sci USA* 98:13655–13659, 2001.
53. Houdusse A, Szent-Györgyi AG, Cohen C: Three conformational states of scallop myosin S1. *Proc Natl Acad Sci USA* 97:11238–11243, 2000.
54. Whitaker M, Wilson-Kubalek EM, Smith JE, et al: A 35-Å movement of smooth muscle myosin on ADP release. *Nature* 378:748–751, 1995.
55. Jontes JD, Wilson-Kubalek EM, Milligan RA: A 32 degree tail swing in brush border myosin I on ADP release. *Nature* 378:751–753, 1995.
56. Uyeda TQ, Abramson PD, Spudich JA: The neck region of the myosin motor domain acts as a lever arm to generate movement. *Proc Natl Acad Sci USA* 93:4459–4464, 1996.
57. Warshaw DM, Guilford WH, Freyzon YM, et al: The light chain binding domain of expressed smooth muscle heavy meromyosin acts as a mechanical lever. *J Biol Chem* 275:37167–37172, 2000.
58. Purcell TJ, Morris C, Spudich JA, Sweeney HL: Role of the lever arm in the processive stepping of myosin V. *Proc Natl Acad Sci USA* 99:14159–14164, 2002.
59. Reedy MK, Holmes KC, Tregear RT: Induced changes in orientation of the cross-bridges of glycerinated insect flight muscle. *Nature* 207:1276–1280, 1965.
60. Taylor KA, Schmitz H, Reedy MC, et al: Tomographic 3D reconstruction of quick-frozen, Ca^{2+}-activated contracting insect flight muscle. *Cell* 99:421–431, 1999.
61. Fisher AJ, Smith CA, Thoden JB, et al: X-ray structures of the myosin motor domain of *Dictyostelium discoideum* complexed with MgADP.BeFx and MgADP.AlF4-. *Biochemistry* 34:8960–8972, 1995.
62. Dominguez R, Freyzon Y, Trybus KM, Cohen C: Crystal structure of a vertebrate smooth muscle myosin motor domain and its complex with the essential light chain: Visualization of the pre-power stroke state. *Cell* 94:559–571, 1998.
63. Bauer CB, Holden HM, Thoden JB, et al: X-ray structures of the apo and MgATP-bound states of *Dictyostelium discoideum* myosin motor domain. *J Biol Chem* 275:38494–38499, 2000.
64. Houdusse A, Kalabokis VN, Himmel D, et al: Atomic structure of scallop myosin subfragment S1 complexed with MgADP: A novel conformation of the myosin head. *Cell* 97:459–470, 1999.
65. Cooke R: Myosin structure: Does the tail wag the dog? *Curr Biol* 9:R773–R775, 1999.
66. Suzuki Y, Yasunaga T, Ohkura R, et al: Swing of the lever arm of a myosin motor at the isomerization and phosphate-release steps. *Nature* 396:380–383, 1998.
67. Wells JA, Yount RG: Reaction of 5,5'-dithiobis(2-nitrobenzoic acid) with myosin subfragment one: Evidence for formation of a single protein disulfide with trapping of metal nucleotide at the active site. *Biochemistry* 19:1711–1717, 1980.
68. Nitao LK, Reisler E: Probing the conformational states of the SH1-SH2 helix in myosin: A cross-linking approach. *Biochemistry* 37:16704–16710, 1998.
69. Nitao LK, Reisler E: Actin and temperature effects on the cross-linking of the SH1-SH2 helix in myosin subfragment 1. *Biophys J* 78:3072–3080, 2000.
70. Berger CL, Craik JS, Trentham DR, et al: Fluorescence polarization from isomers of tetramethylrhodamine at SH-1 in rabbit psoas muscle fibers. *Biophys J* 68:78S–80S, 1995.
71. Thomas DD, Ramachandran S, Roopnarine O, et al: The mechanism of force generation in myosin. A disorder-to-order transition, coupled to internal structural changes. *Biophys J* 68:135S–141S, 1995.
72. Gulick AM, Bauer CB, Thoden JB, Rayment I: X-ray structures of the MgADP, MgATPgammaS, and MgAMPPNP complexes of the *Dictyostelium discoideum* myosin motor domain. *Biochemistry* 36:11619–11628, 1997.
73. Taylor EW: Kinetic studies on the association and dissociation of myosin subfragment-1 and actin. *J Biol Chem* 266:294–302, 1991.
74. Coates JH, Criddle AH, Geeves MA: Pressure-relaxation studies of pyrene-labelled actin and myosin subfragment-1 from rabbit skeletal muscle. *Biochemistry* 232:351–356, 1985.
75. Walker M, Zhang XZ, Jiang W, et al: Observation of transient disorder during myosin subfragment-1 binding to actin by stopped-flow fluorescence and millisecond time resolution electron cryomicroscopy: Evidence that the start of the crossbridge power stroke in muscle has variable geometry. *Proc Natl Acad Sci USA* 96:465–470, 1999.
76. Kabsch W, Mannherz HG, Suck D, et al: Atomic structure of the actin:DNase I complex. *Nature* 347:37–44, 1990.
77. Otterbein LR, Graceffa P, Dominguez R: The crystal structure of uncomplexed actin in the ADP state. *Science* 293:708–711, 2001.
78. Holmes KC, Popp D, Gebhard W, Kabsch W: Atomic model of the actin filament. *Nature* 347:44–49, 1990.
79. Lorenz M, Popp D, Holmes KC: Refinement of the F-actin model against x-ray fiber diffraction data by the use of a directed mutation algorithm. *J Mol Biol* 234:826–836, 1993.
80. Jontes JD, Ostap EM, Pollard TD, Milligan RA: Three-dimensional structure of *Acanthamoeba castellanii* myosin-IB (MIB) determined by cryoelectron microscopy of decorated actin filaments. *J Cell Biol* 141:155–162, 1998.
81. Carragher BO, Cheng N, Wang ZY, et al: Structural invariance of constitutively active and inactive mutants of *Acanthamoeba* myosin IC bound to F-actin in the rigor and ADP-bound states. *Proc Natl Acad Sci USA* 95:15206–15211, 1998.
82. Volkmann N, Ouyang G, Trybus KM, et al: Myosin isoforms show unique conformations in the actin-bound state. *Proc Natl Acad Sci USA* 100:3227–3232, 2003.
83. Berg JS, Powell BC, Cheney RE: A millennial myosin census. *Mol Biol Cell* 12:780–794, 2001.
84. Mermall V, Rost PL, Mooseker MS: Unconventional myosins in cell movement, membrane traffic, and signal transduction. *Science* 279:527–533, 1998.
85. Baker JP, Titus MA: Myosins: Matching functions with motors. *Curr Opin Cell Biol* 10:80–86, 1998.
86. Walker ML, Burgess SA, Sellers JR, et al: Two-headed binding of a processive myosin to F-actin. *Nature* 405:804–807, 2000.
87. Burgess S, Walker M, Wang F, et al: The prepower stroke conformation of myosin V. *J Cell Biol* 159:983–991, 2002.
88. Wells AL, Lin AW, Chen L-Q, et al: Myosin VI is an actin-based motor that moves backwards. *Nature* 401:505–508, 1999.
89. Inoue A, Saito J, Ikebe R, Ikebe M: Myosin IXb is a single-headed minus-end-directed processive motor. *Nat Cell Biol* 4:302–306, 2002.
90. O'Connell CB, Mooseker MS: Native myosin-IXb is a plus-, not a minus-, end-directed motor. *Nat Cell Biol* 5:171–172, 2003.
91. Espreafico EM, Cheney RE, Matteoli M, et al: Primary structure and cellular localization of chicken brain myosin-V (p190), an unconventional myosin with calmodulin light chains. *J Cell Biol* 119:1541–1557, 1992.
92. Espindola FS, Suter DM, Partata LB, et al: The light chain composition of chicken brain myosin-Va: Calmodulin, myosin-II essential light chains, and 8-kDa dynein light chain/PIN. *Cell Motil Cytoskeleton* 47:269–281, 2000.
93. De La Cruz EM, Wells AL, Sweeney HL, Ostap EM: Actin and light chain isoform dependence of myosin V kinetics. *Biochemistry* 39:14196–14202, 2000.
94. Howard J, Spudich JA: Is the lever arm of myosin a molecular elastic element? *Proc Natl Acad Sci USA* 93:4462–4464, 1996.

95. Desjardins PR, Burkman JM, Shrager JB, et al: Evolutionary implications of three novel members of the human sarcomeric myosin heavy chain gene family. *Mol Biol Evol* 19:375–393, 2002.
96. Brooke MH, Kaiser KK: Muscle fiber types: How many and what kind? *Arch Neurol* 23:369, 1970.
97. DiNardi C, Ausoni S, Moretti P, et al: Type 2X myosin heavy chain is coded by a muscle fiber type-specific and developmentally regulated gene. *J Cell Biol* 123:823–835, 1993.
98. Mahdavi V, Strehler EE, Periasamy M, et al: Sarcomeric myosin heavy chain gene family: Organization and pattern of expression, in Emerson FD, Nadal-Ginard B, Siddique MA (eds): *Molecular Biology of Muscle Development*. New York: Liss; 1986, pp 345–361.
99. Weiss A, McDonough D, Wertman B, et al: Organization of human and mouse skeletal myosin heavy chain gene clusters is highly conserved. *Proc Natl Acad Sci USA* 96:2958–2963, 1999.
100. Hoh JF: "Superfast" or masticatory myosin and the evolution of jaw-closing muscles of vertebrates. *J Exp Biol* 205(Pt 15):2203–2210, 2002.
101. Mahdavi V, Chambers AP, Nadal-Ginard B: Cardiac alpha and beta myosin heavy chain genes are organized in tandem. *Proc Natl Acad Sci USA* 81:2626–2630, 1984.
102. Deng Z, Liu P, Marlton P, et al: Smooth muscle myosin heavy chain locus (MYH11) maps to 16p13.13–p13,12 and establishes a new region of conserved synteny between human 16p and mouse 16. *Genomics* 18:156–159, 1993.
103. Saez LJ, Myers JC, Shows TB, Leinwand LA: Human nonmuscle myosin heavy chain mRNA: Generation of diversity through alternative polyadenylation. *Proc Natl Acad Sci USA* 87:1164–1168, 1990.
104. Spudich JA: How molecular motors work. *Nature* 372:515–518, 1994.
105. Sweeney HL, Rosenfeld S, Brown F, et al: Kinetic tuning of myosin via a flexible loop adjacent to the nucleotide binding pocket. *J Biol Chem* 273:6262–6270, 1998.
106. White S, Martin AF, Periasamy M: Identification of a novel smooth muscle myosin heavy chain cDNA: Isoform diversity in the S1 head region. *Am J Physiol* 264:C1252–C1258, 1993.
107. Ikebe M, Komatsu S, Woodhead JL, et al: The tip of the coiled-coil rod determines the filament formation of smooth muscle and nonmuscle myosins. *J Biol Chem* 276:30293–30300, 2001.
108. Rovner AS, Fagnant PM, Lowey S, Trybus KM: The carboxyl-terminal isoforms of smooth muscle myosin heavy chain determine thick filament assembly properties. *J Cell Biol* 156:113–123, 2002.
109. Collins JH: Myosin light chains and troponin C: Structural and evolutionary relationships revealed by amino acid sequence comparisons. *J Muscle Res Cell Motil* 12:3–25, 1991.
110. Lowey S, Waller GS, Trybus KM: Skeletal muscle myosin light chains are essential for physiological speeds of shortening. *Nature* 365:454–456, 1993.
111. Wade R, Feldman D, Gunning P, Kedes L: Sequence and expression of human myosin alkali light chain isoforms. *Mol Cell Biochem* 87:119–136, 1989.
112. Winstanley MA, Trayer IP: Thrombic digestion of myosin alkali light chains. *Biochem Soc Trans* 7:703–704, 1979.
113. Prince HP, Trayer HR, Henry GD, et al: Proton nuclear-magnetic resonance spectroscopy of myosin subfragment 1 isoenzymes. *Eur J Biochem* 121:213–219, 1981.
114. Sutoh K: Identification of myosin-binding sites on the actin sequence. *Biochemistry* 21:3654–3661, 1982.
115. Henry GD, Winstanley MA, Dalgarno DC, et al: Characterization of the actin-binding site on the alkali light chain of myosin. *Biochem Biophys Acta* 830:233–243, 1985.
116. Labbé J-P, Audemard E, Bertrand R, Kassab R: Specific interactions of the alkali light chain 1 in skeletal myosin heads probed by chemical cross-linking. *Biochemistry* 25:8325–8330, 1986.
117. Chaussepied P, Kasprzak AA: Isolation and characterization of the G-actin-myosin head complex *Nature* 342:950–953, 1989.
118. Milligan RA, Whittaker M, Safer D: Molecular structure of F-actin and location of surface binding sites. *Nature* 348:217–221, 1990.
119. L'heureux K, Forne T, Chaussepied P: Interaction and polymerization of the G-actin-myosin head complex: Effect of DNase I. *Biochemistry* 32:10005–10014, 1993.
120. Sweeney HL, Kushmerick MJ, Mabuchi K, et al: Myosin alkali light chain and heavy chain variations correlate with altered shortening velocity of isolated skeletal muscle fibers. *J Biol Chem* 263:9034–9039, 1988.
121. Reiser PJ, Moss RL, Giulian GG, Greaser ML: Shortening velocity in single fibers from adult rabbit soleus muscles is correlated with myosin heavy chain composition. *J Biol Chem* 260:9077–9080, 1985.
122. Bottinelli R, Betto R, Schiaffino S, Reggiani C: Maximum shortening velocity and coexistence of myosin heavy chain isoforms in single skinned fast fibres of rat skeletal muscle. *J Muscle Res Cell Motil* 15:413–419, 1994.
123. Sweeney HL: The N-terminus of the essential light chains of striated muscle myosin modulates muscle shortening. *Biophys J* 68:112s–119s, 1995.
124. Standiford DM, Davis MB, Miedema K, et al: Myosin rod protein: A novel thick filament component of *Drosophila* muscle. *J Mol Biol* 265:40–55, 1997.

125. Trybus KM: Regulation of smooth muscle myosin. *Cell Motil Cytoskeleton* 18:81–85, 1991.
126. Sweeney HL, Bowman BF, Stull JT: Myosin light chain phosphorylation in striated muscle. *Am J Physiol* 264 (*Cell Physiol*) 33:C1085–C1095, 1993.
127. Epstein ND: Cell paper on stretch activation
128. Wang F, Martin BM, Sellers JR: Regulation of actomyosin interactions in *Limulus* muscle proteins. *J Biol Chem* 268:3776–3780, 1993.
129. Reinach FC, Nagai K, Kendrick-Jones J: Site directed mutagenesis of the regulatory light-chain Ca^{+2}/Mg^{+2} binding sites and its role in hybrid myosins. *Nature* 322:80–83, 1986.
130. Trybus KM, Chatman TA: Chimeric regulatory light chains as probes of smooth muscle myosin function. *J Biol Chem* 168:4412–4419, 1993.
131. Chantler PD, Szent-Gyorgyi AG: Regulatory light-chains and scallop myosin, full dissociation, reversibility and co-operative effects. *J Mol Biol* 138:473–492, 1980.
132. Rajasekharan KN, Morita J-I, Mayadevi M, et al: Formation and properties of smooth muscle myosin 20 kDa light chain-skeletal muscle myosin hybrids and photocrosslinking from the maleimidylbenzophenone-labeled light chain to the heavy chain. *Arch Biochem Biophys* 288:584–590, 1991.
133. Onishi H, Wakabayashi T: Electron microscopic studies of myosin molecules from chicken gizzard muscle: The formation of the intramolecular loop in the myosin tail. *J Biochem (Tokyo)* 92:871–879, 1982.
134. Ikebe M, Ikebe R, Kamisoyama H, et al: Function of the NH_2-terminal domain of the regulatory light chain on the regulation of smooth muscle myosin. *J Biol Chem* 269:28173–28180, 1994.
135. Kamisoyama H, Araki Y, Ikebe M: Mutagenesis of the phosphorylation site (serine 19) of smooth muscle myosin regulatory light chain and its effects on the properties of myosin. *Biochemistry* 33:840–847, 1994.
136. Sweeney HL, Yang Z, Zhi G, et al: Charge replacement near the phosphorylatable serine of the myosin regulatory light chain mimics aspects of phosphorylation. *Proc Natl Acad Sci USA* 90:1490–1494, 1994.
137. Wendt T, Taylor D, Messier T, et al: Visualization of head-head interactions in the inhibited state of smooth muscle myosin. *J Cell Biol* 147:1385–1390, 1999.
138. Wendt T, Taylor D, Trybus KM, Taylor K: Three-dimensional image reconstruction of dephosphorylated smooth muscle heavy meromyosin reveals asymmetry in the interaction between myosin heads and subfragment 2. *Proc Natl Acad Sci USA* 98:4361–4366, 2001.
139. Sweeney HL, Chen LQ, Trybus KM: Regulation of asymmetric smooth muscle myosin II molecules. *J Biol Chem* 275:41273–41277, 2000.
140. Ikebe M, Reardon S, Mitani Y, et al: Involvement of the C-terminal residues of the 20,000-dalton light chain of myosin on the regulation of smooth muscle actomyosin. *Proc Natl Acad Sci USA* 91:9096–9100, 1994.
141. Trybus KM, Waller GS, Chatman TA: Coupling of ATPase activity and motility in smooth muscle myosin is mediated by the regulatory light chain. *J Cell Biol* 124:963–969, 1994.
142. Yang Z, Sweeney HL: Restoration of phosphorylation-dependent regulation to the skeletal muscle regulatory light chain. *J Biol Chem* 270:24646–24649, 1995.
143. Kendrick-Jones J, Lehman W, Szent-Gyorgyi AG: Regulation in molluscan muscles. *J Mol Biol* 54:313–326, 1970.
144. Xie X, Harrison DH, Schlichting I, et al: *Nature* 368:306–312, 1994.
145. Jansco A, Szent-Gyorgyi AG: Regulation of scallop myosin by the regulatory light chain depends on a single glycine residue. *Proc Natl Acad Sci USA* 91:8762–8766, 1994.
146. Rowe T, Kendrick-Jones J: The C-terminal helix in subdomain 4 of the regulatory light chain is essential for myosin regulation. *EMBO J* 12:4877–4884, 1993.
147. Metzger JM, Greaser ML, Moss RL: Variations in cross-bridge attachment rate and tension with phosphorylation of myosin in mammalian skinned skeletal muscle fibers: Implications for twitch potentiation in intact muscle. *J Gen Physiol* 93:855–883, 1989.
148. Levine RJ, Kensler RW, Yang Z, et al: Myosin light chain phosphorylation affects the structure of rabbit skeletal muscle thick filaments. *Biophys J* 71:898–907, 1996.
149. Yang Z, Stull JT, Levine RJ, Sweeney HL: Changes in interfilament spacing mimic the effects of myosin regulatory light chain phosphorylation in rabbit psoas fibers. *J Struct Biol* 122:139–148, 1998.
150. Levine RJ, Yang Z, Epstein ND: Structural and functional responses of mammalian thick filaments to alterations in myosin regulatory light chains. *J Struct Biol* 122:149–161, 1998.
151. Reggiani C, Bottinelli R, Stienen GJ: Sarcomeric myosin isoforms: Fine tuning of a molecular motor. *News Physiol Sci* 15:26–33, 2000.
152. Siemankowski RF, Wiseman MO, White HD: ADP dissociation from actomyosin subfragment 1 is sufficiently slow to limit the unloaded shortening velocity in vertebrate muscle. *Proc Natl Acad Sci USA* 82:658–662, 1985.
153. Weiss S, Rossi R, Pellegrino MA, et al: Differing ADP release rates from myosin heavy chain isoforms define the shortening velocity of skeletal muscle fibers. *Biol Chem* 276:45902–45908, 2001.
154. Pellegrino MA, Canepari M, Rossi R, et al: Orthologous myosin isoforms and scaling of shortening velocity with body size in mouse, rat, rabbit and human muscles. *J Physiol* 546:677–689, 2003.

155. Larsson L, Li X, Frontera WR: Effects of aging on shortening velocity and myosin isoform composition in single human skeletal muscle cells. *Am J Physiol* 272:C638–C649, 1997.
156. Moss RL, Diffee GM, Greaser ML: Contractile properties of skeletal muscle fibers in relation to myofibrillar protein isoforms. *Rev Physiol Biochem Pharmacol* 126:1–63, 1995.
157. Bottinelli R: Functional heterogeneity of mammalian single muscle fibres: Do myosin isoforms tell the whole story? *Pflugers Arch* 443:6–17, 2001.
158. Barany M: ATPase activity of myosin correlated with speed of muscle shortening. *J Gen Physiol* 50(suppl):197–218, 1967.
159. Guilford WH, Dupuis DE, Kennedy G, et al: Smooth muscle and skeletal muscle myosins produce similar unitary forces and displacements in the laser trap. *Biophys J* 72:1006–1021, 1997.
160. Palmiter KA, Tyska MJ, Dupuis DE, et al: Kinetic differences at the single molecule level account for the functional diversity of rabbit cardiac myosin isoforms. *J Physiol* 519(Pt 3):669–678, 1999.
161. VanBuren P, Harris DE, Alpert NR, Warshaw DM: Cardiac V1 and V3 myosins differ in their hydrolytic and mechanical activities in vitro. *Circ Res* 77:439–444, 1995.
162. Watkins H, Seidman JG, Seidman CE: Familial hypertrophic cardiomyopathy: A genetic model of cardiac hypertrophy. *Hum Mol Genet* 4:1721–1727, 1995.
163. Bonne G, Carrier L, Richard P, et al: Familial hypertrophic cardiomyopathy: From mutations to functional defects. *Circ Res* 83:580–593, 1998.
164. Arad M, Seidman JG, Seidman CE: Phenotypic diversity in hypertrophic cardiomyopathy. *Hum Mol Genet* 11:2499–2506, 2002.
165. Geisterfer-Lowrance AA, Kass S, Tanigawa G, et al: A molecular basis for familial hypertrophic cardiomyopathy: A beta cardiac myosin heavy chain gene missense mutation. *Cell* 62:999–1006, 1990.
166. Poetter K, Jiang H, Hassanzadeh S, et al: Mutations in either the essential or regulatory light chains of myosin are associated with a rare myopathy in human heart and skeletal muscle. *Nat Genet* 13:63–69, 1996.
167. Thierfelder L, Watkins H, MacRae C, et al: Alpha-tropomyosin and cardiac troponin T mutations cause familial hypertrophic cardiomyopathy: A disease of the sarcomere. *Cell* 77:701–712, 1994.
168. Watkins H, Conner D, Thierfelder L, et al: Mutations in the cardiac myosin binding protein-C gene on chromosome 11 cause familial hypertrophic cardiomyopathy. *Nat Genet* 11:434–437, 1995.
169. Bonne G, Carrier L, Bercovici J, et al: Cardiac myosin binding protein-C gene splice acceptor site mutation is associated with familial hypertrophic cardiomyopathy. *Nat Genet* 11:438–440, 1995.
170. Kimura A, Harada H, Park JE, et al: Mutations in the cardiac troponin I gene associated with hypertrophic cardiomyopathy. *Nat Genet* 16:379–382, 1997.
170a. Hoffman B, Schmidt-Traub H, Perrot A, et al: First mutation in cardiac troponin C, L29Q, in a patient with hypertrophic cardiomyopathy. *Hum Mutat* 17:524, 2001.
171. Olson TM, Doan TP, Kishimoto NY, et al: Inherited and de novo mutations in the cardiac actin gene cause hypertrophic cardiomyopathy. *J Mol Cell Cardiol* 32:1687–1694, 2000.
171a. Satoh M, Takahashi M, Sakamoto T, et al: Structural analysis of the titin gene in hypertrophic cardiomyopathy: Identification of a novel disease gene. *Biochem Biophys Res Commun* 262:411–417, 1999.
172. Cuda G, Fananapazir L, Zhu WS, et al: Skeletal muscle expression and abnormal function of beta-myosin in hypertrophic cardiomyopathy. *J Clin Invest* 91:2861–2865, 1993.
173. Sweeney HL, Straceski AJ, Leinwand LA, et al: Heterologous expression of a cardiomyopathic myosin that is defective in its actin interaction. *J Biol Chem* 269:1603–1605, 1994.
174. Lankford EB, Epstein ND, Fananapazir L, Sweeney HL: Abnormal contractile properties of muscle fibers expressing beta-myosin heavy chain gene mutations in patients with hypertrophic cardiomyopathy. *J Clin Invest* 95:1409–1414, 1995.
175. Cuda G, Fananapazir L, Epstein ND, Sellers JR: The *in vitro* motility activity of beta-cardiac myosin depends on the nature of the beta-myosin heavy chain gene mutation in hypertrophic cardiomyopathy. *J Muscle Res Cell Motil* 18:275–283, 1997.
176. Blanchard E, Seidman C, Seidman JG, et al: Altered crossbridge kinetics in the alphaMHC403/+ mouse model of familial hypertrophic cardiomyopathy. *Circ Res* 84:475–483, 1999.
177. Tyska MJ, Hayes E, Giewat M, et al: Single-molecule mechanics of R403Q cardiac myosin isolated from the mouse model of familial hypertrophic cardiomyopathy. *Circ Res* 86:737–744, 2000.
178. Palmiter KA, Tyska MJ, Haeberle JR, et al: R403Q and L908V mutant beta-cardiac myosin from patients with familial hypertrophic cardio0 myopathy exhibit enhanced mechanical performance at the single molecule level. *J Muscle Res Cell Motil* 21:609–620, 2000.
179. Lowey S: Functional consequences of mutations in the myosin heavy chain at sites implicated in familial hypertrophic cardiomyopathy. *Trends Cardiovasc Med* 12:348–354, 2002.
180. Vemuri R, Lankford EB, Poetter K, et al: The stretch-activation response may be critical to the proper functioning of the mammalian heart. *Proc Natl Acad Sci USA* 96:1048–1053, 1999.
181. Davis JS, Hassanzadeh S, Winitsky S, et al: The overall pattern of cardiac contraction depends on a spatial gradient of myosin regulatory light chain phosphorylation. *Cell* 107:631–641, 2001.
182. Epstein ND, Davis JS: Sensing stretch is fundamental. *Cell* 112:147–150, 2003.
183. Spudich JA, Kron SJ, Sheetz MP: Movement of myosin-coated beads on oriented filaments reconstituted from purified actin. *Nature* 315:584–586, 1985.
184. Kron SJ, Spudich JA: Fluorescent actin filaments move on myosin fixed to a glass surface. *Proc Natl Acad Sci USA* 83:6272–6276, 1986.
185. Manstein DJ, Ruppel KM, Spudich JA: Expression and characterization of a functional myosin head fragment in *Dictyostelium discoideum*. *Science* 246:656–658, 1989.
186. Finer JT, Simmons RM, Spudich JA: Single myosin molecule mechanics: Piconewton forces and nanometre steps. *Nature* 368:113–119, 1994.
187. Veigel C, Bartoo ML, White DC, et al: The stiffness of rabbit skeletal actomyosin cross-bridges determined with an optical tweezers transducer. *Biophys J* 75:1424–1438, 1998.
188. Tanaka H, Ishijima A, Honda M, et al: Orientation dependence of displacements by a single one-headed myosin relative to the actin filament. *Biophys J* 75:1886–1894, 1998.
189. Ishijima A, Kojima H, Funatsu T, et al: Simultaneous observation of individual ATPase and mechanical events by a single myosin molecule during interaction with actin. *Cell* 92(2):161–171, 1998.
190. Kitamura K, Tokunaga M, Iwane AH, Yanagida T: A single myosin head moves along an actin filament with regular steps of 5.3 nanometres. *Nature* 397:129–134, 1999.
191. Veigel C, Coluccio LM, Jontes JD, et al: The motor protein myosin-I produces its working stroke in two steps. *Nature* 398:530–533, 1999.
192. Tyska MJ, Dupuis DE, Guilford WH, et al: Two heads of myosin are better than one for generating force and motion. *Proc Natl Acad Sci USA* 96:4402–4407, 1999.
193. Warshaw DM, Guilford WH, Freyzon Y, et al: The light chain binding domain of expressed smooth muscle heavy meromyosin acts as a mechanical lever. *J Biol Chem* 275:37167–37172, 2000.
194. Tyska MJ, Warshaw DM: The myosin power stroke. *Cell Motil Cytoskeleton* 51:1–15, 2002.
195. Ruegg C, Veigel C, Molloy JE, et al: Molecular motors: Force and movement generated by single myosin II molecules. *News Physiol Sci* 17:213–218, 2002.
196. Funatsu T, Harada Y, Tokunaga M, et al: Imaging of single fluorescent molecules and individual ATP turnovers by single myosin molecules in aqueous solution. *Nature* 374:555–559, 1995.
197. Iwane AH, Funatsu T, Harada Y, et al: Single molecular assay of individual ATP turnover by a myosin-GFP fusion protein expressed in vitro. *FEBS Lett* 407:235–238, 1997.
198. Ishijima A, Kojima H, Funatsu T, et al: Simultaneous observation of individual ATPase and mechanical events by a single myosin molecule during interaction with actin. *Cell* 92:161–171, 1998.
199. Conibear PB, Kuhlman PA, Bagshaw CR: Measurement of ATPase activities of myosin at the level of tracks and single molecules. *Adv Exp Med Biol* 453:15–26, 1998.
200. Bagshaw CR, Conibear PB: Single molecule enzyme kinetics: Application to myosin ATPases. *Biochem Soc Trans* 27:33–37, 1999.
201. Ishii Y, Kitamura K, Tanaka H, Yanagida T: Molecular motors and single-molecule enzymology. *Methods Enzymol* 361:228–245, 2003.
202. Sakamoto T, Amitani I, Yokota E, Ando T: Direct observation of processive movement by individual myosin V molecules. *Biochem Biophys Res Commun* 272:586–590, 2000.
203. Rock RS, Rice SE, Wells AL, et al: Myosin VI is a processive motor with a large step size. *Proc Natl Acad Sci USA* 98:13655–13659, 2001.
204. Nishikawa S, Homma K, Komori Y, et al: Class VI myosin moves processively along actin filaments backward with large steps. *Biochem Biophys Res Commun* 290:311–317, 2002.
205. Forkey JN, Quinlan ME, Shaw MA, et al: Three-dimensional structural dynamics of myosin V by single-molecule fluorescence polarization. *Nature* 422:399–404, 2003.
206. Yildi A, Forkey JN, McKinney SA, et al: Myosin V walks hand-over-hand: Single flourophore imaging with 1.5-nm localization. *Science* 300:2061–2065, 2003.

Chapter 9
Molecular Physiology of the Cross-Bridge Cycle

YALE E. GOLDMAN
EARL HOMSHER

Structure
Working Hypothesis
Muscle Fiber Mechanics
   ISOMETRIC CONTRACTIONS
   LENGTH-TENSION CURVES
   ENERGETICS OF ISOMETRIC CONTRACTIONS
   CONTRACTIONS WITH SHORTENING
   ENERGETICS OF WORKING CONTRACTIONS
   ECCENTRIC CONTRACTIONS
   STIFFNESS
   MECHANICAL TRANSIENTS
   CAGED MOLECULES
Mechanics in Vitro
Summary

The functional outputs of muscles are mechanical force, shortening, and, in some cases, support of other structures. When muscles contract, metabolic energy stored in their cells as adenosine triphosphate (ATP)* is converted into mechanical work. The purpose of this chapter is to explain the mechanism of this energy transduction. A working hypothesis has been developed that is consistent with most of the structural, mechanical, and biochemical evidence accumulated during the past half-century of intensive investigation. We briefly describe the structure of the contractile apparatus, present the widely accepted view of the contraction mechanism, and review the main points of experimental evidence. Nevertheless, points of controversy still exist. Techniques for the detailed investigation of muscle contraction are a prerequisite to understanding the experimental results and are applicable to other examples of cell motility and protein energy transducers. Many of the techniques are also applicable to examining muscle pathology and biopsy material.

Structure

The organelle responsible for contraction, the *myofibril*, and the ultrastructural organization of its contractile protein filaments are described in Chap. 7. By way of review, the myofibril is composed primarily of four contractile proteins: myosin, actin, tropomyosin, and troponin. Muscle myosin is a large molecule (molecular weight 480 kDa) composed of two 220-kDa heavy chains and four ~20-kDa myosin light chains (Fig. 9-1A, Color Plate 1c and d). Each heavy chain has a long (~156-nm) α-helical coiled-coil tail region (S2 and LMM in Fig. 9-1A) and a 16-nm globular head region termed *subfragment 1* (S1, Fig. 9-1B), which constitutes the cross-bridge. A flexible hinge at the head-tail junction allows the S1 to adopt a wide range of angles relative to the tail. About 60 nm along the helical region from the S1 is a second hinge (Fig. 9-1A). Myosin exists in its monomeric form at elevated ionic strengths (500 mM); but at physiologic ionic strengths (~200 mM) the tail regions of approximately 300 myosin molecules polymerize to form the backbone of each 1.6-μm-long thick filament (Fig. 7-6). The S1 cross-bridges (Fig. 9-1B) protruding from the backbone of the filament contain a motor domain (MD) having the adenosine triphosphatase (ATPase) and actin-binding sites that convert chemical energy into mechanical work. S1 also includes the regulatory light chain (RLC) (Fig. 9-1B) and the essential light chain (ELC), which, together with an underlying helix of the heavy chain, constitute the *light-chain domain* (LCD) (Fig 9-1B). Three myosin molecules (six S1 heads) are spaced every 14.3 nm along the filament axis. An antiparallel arrangement of the myosin tails at the center of the thick filaments makes them bipolar (the tails point oppositely on each side) and produces a central area (about 0.15 μm long) termed the *bare* or *pseudo-H zone*, which does not contain S1 heads. Thick filaments are located in the center of the sarcomere in the optically anisotropic A band (Figs. 7-1, 7-3, and 7-4). C-protein is located at discrete intervals along the thick filament in each half of the A band, fulfilling structural and modulatory roles.[1]

Thin filaments (Fig. 9-1C) are helical polymers of actin that extend 1.1 μm from each side of the Z line occupying the optically isotropic I band (Fig. 9-2; see also Chap. 7) and extend into and interdigitate with the thick filaments of the A band. Monomers of actin are 45-kDa globular proteins, leading to the term *G-actin*. When the actin is polymerized, it is called *F (filamentous)-actin*; it is a double-stranded helix 8 nm in diameter. The pitch of the helix is 74 nm, so in longitudinal images the two strands cross over each other every 36 to 40 nm (Fig. 9-1C, Color Plate 1a and b, Chap. 7). In the thin filament, the monomers can also be considered to be wound in a tighter coil, termed the *genetic helix*, with left-handed 5.9-nm and right-handed 5.1-nm pitches. The overall spacing of monomers along the filament axis is 2.7 nm, and each thin filament projecting from the Z line contains approximately 360 monomers. Actin filaments are polarized with slower- and faster-polymerizing ends, termed the *pointed* and *barbed ends*, respectively. The regulatory proteins, troponin (Tn) and tropomyosin (Tm), provide Ca^{2+}-mediated control of contraction and are located on the thin filaments (Fig. 9-1C). Regulation of contraction is discussed in Chap. 13. The barbed ends of the actin filaments insert into the Z line, and the pointed ends are located away from the Z lines. Thus both the thick and thin filaments are structurally polarized. Cross sections of the myofibril in the region of overlap between the thick and thin filaments show that the thin filaments interdigitate with the thick filaments to form a double hexagonal array (see Figs. 7-1 and 7-2). Each thick filament is surrounded by six thin filaments, and each thin filament is surrounded by three thick filaments.

---

*A list of abbreviations used in this chapter is given at the end of the chapter.

Working Hypothesis

The current explanation of energy transduction by actomyosin comprises a hierarchy of theories with increasing detail and diminishing molecular scale. The main hypotheses are as follows: (1) the *sliding filament theory*,[2,3] (2) *cyclic actomyosin interaction*,[4,5] (3) *tilting* of the myosin heads,[6,7] and (4) the *lever-arm hypothesis*.[8,9] When a muscle shortens, the two filaments do not change length appreciably; instead, they *slide* relative to each other. Sliding motions generated within each of the two overlap zones of the sarcomere and in all of the sarcomeres spaced sequentially along a myofibril sum to produce macroscopic shortening of the whole muscle. Thus, the problem of understanding generation of force and shortening of a muscle is reduced to the molecular interactions between the two filaments. Myosin and actin are thought to undergo a cyclic association and dissociation that leads to production of force but still allows sliding to occur. This *cross-bridge cycle* is a sequence of enzymatic reaction steps that are coupled to the binding and splitting of ATP and release of the hydrolysis products, orthophosphate (P_i) and adenosine diphosphate (ADP). A structural change within the myosin head while it is attached to actin is thought to be the direct cause of the filament's sliding, pulling actin toward the center of the sarcomere (Fig. 9-2). During this motion, the whole myosin head probably does not rotate, but the LCD serves as a *lever arm* that rotates to exert the relative pull between the two filaments while the MD stays rigidly attached to actin.

Using the available data, a plausible hypothesis can be proposed for the relationship between the elementary steps in the actomyosin ATPase, the mechanical events, and the structural changes in the proteins leading to force generation and filament sliding.[10,11] In relaxed muscle, most of the myosin S1 heads have ATP or ADP and P_i bound at the active site (Fig. 9-3, states 1 and 2) and wobble freely about the hinge at the head-rod junction. They are prevented from binding strongly to actin by troponin and tropomyosin in the thin filaments. When the muscle is activated, this inhibition is relieved and the myosin-ADP-P_i complex (M•ADP•P_i) attaches to actin. The initial attachment is a *low-affinity*, readily reversible actomyosin-ADP-P_i complex (AM•ADP•P_i, state 3), often designated as a *weakly bound*[12] state. The initial actomyosin complex allows considerable mobility of the head and does not produce a sliding force. An *isomerization* of AM•ADP•P_i (no change of ligands) produces a *strongly bound* actomyosin complex (state 4), which reduces rotational mobility of the MD and probably applies force to the thick filament in the direction of the Z line (downward in Fig. 9-3). P_i then quickly dissociates, forming a force-generating AM•ADP[13] (state 5). A fulcrum (probably near residue Cys^{707} in the MD, Fig. 9-1) translates the stress at the base of the LC domain (lever arm) into a torque, which tends to rotate the neck toward the Z line (downward in Fig. 9-2), transmitting force to the tail of myosin and the filament's backbone.

Whether the LCD moves under the applied stress depends on the mechanical compliance in the head and the mechanical load. If the load is high, the stress is maintained in state 5. If the load can be moved, the filaments slide and the LCD

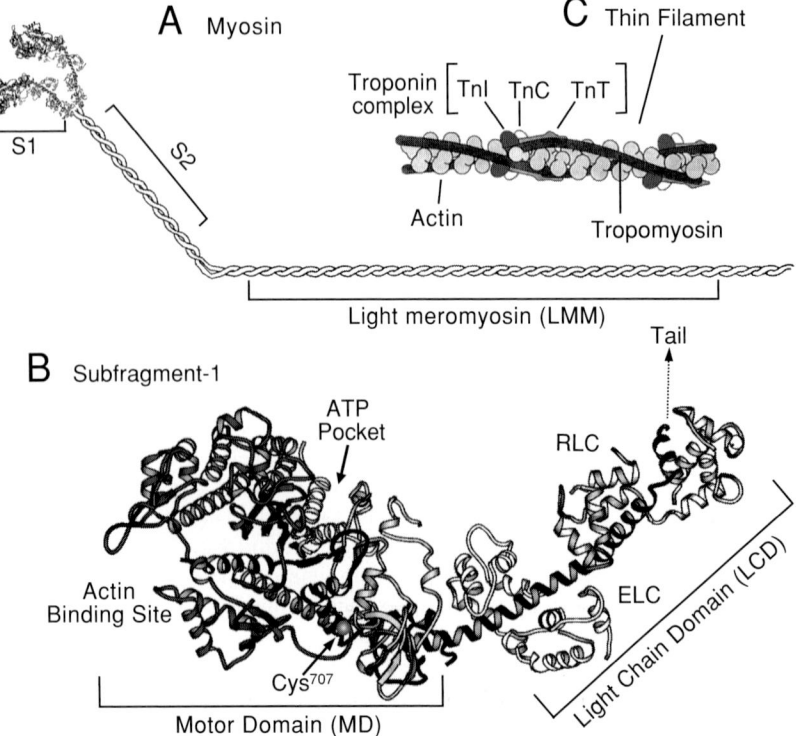

FIGURE 9-1. Structures of the contractile proteins. *A.* Myosin. The two subfragment 1 (S1) heads contain the ATP- and actin-binding sites. The tail is composed of the subfragment 2 (S2) and light mero-myosin (LMM). Heavy meromyosin (HMM) is another fragment containing two S1 heads and S2. *B.* Structure of chicken skeletal myosin S1 in the absence of ATP. The motor domain (MD) of the myosin head contains N-terminal 25-kDa, 50-kDa, and C-terminal 20-kDa peptides ending in an 11-nm α helix (right-hand side). This helix binds the essential light chain (ELC) and regulatory light chain (RLC) making up the light-chain domain (LCD). The C-terminus of S1 is the head-rod junction, which connects through S2 to the thick filament. *C.* Thin filament. Actin monomers polymerize into a double-stranded filament backbone. The regulatory proteins, troponin (Tn) and tropomyosin (Tm), follow the long pitch of this helix. Troponin is composed of three subunits: TnI, TnC, and TnT.

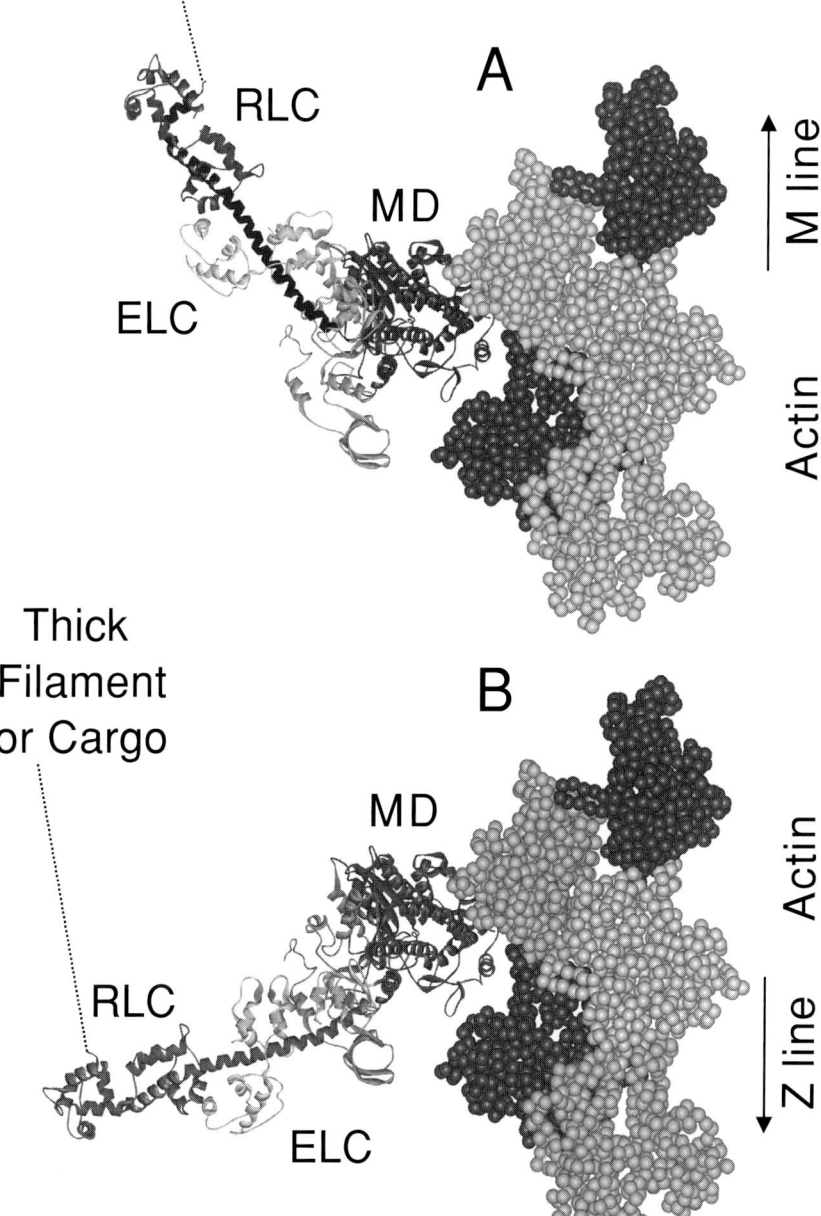

FIGURE 9-2. Actomyosin complex in the putative pre–power stroke (A) and post–power stroke (B) conformations. The coordinates are from (A) Irving et al.[88] and (B) Rayment et al.[8] The motor domain was docked onto actin in the position of chicken skeletal muscle actomyosin in both panels. In A, the heavy-chain residues following Cys[707] and the two light chains were rotated upward by 70 degrees to approximate the conformation of smooth muscle motor domain and ELC in the presence of ADP and VO_4.[17] The region colored tan in Color Plate 1, termed the *converter domain*, is the region of the motor domain that drives the rotation of the LCD and moves with it.

rotates downward (states 5 to 6). ADP dissociates slowly from state 5 but more rapidly from state 6, thus achieving control of the overall ATPase cycle by the load and rate of sliding.[14,15] Filament sliding is followed by ADP release, producing a nucleotide-free state 7 and then rapid ATP binding-induced detachment (7→1). Hydrolysis of ATP to tightly bound ADP and P_i and reversal to reform ATP result in a mixture of M•ATP (state 1) and M•ADP•P_i (state 2) in the detached cross-bridges. Repeated cross-bridge cycles trans-locate myosin and the thick filament toward the Z line, fueled by net hydrolysis of ATP to ADP and P_i.

The crucial structural change that directly causes the force generation and filament sliding is a conformational change in the myosin head from a bent configuration (e.g., states 2 and 3) to a more extended shape[16,17] (state 6, Fig. 9-3). The LCD is thought to function as a lever arm that magnifies the subnanometer structural changes of highly conserved "switch" regions at the active site into several nanometers of motion at the head-rod junction. In this hypothesis, while the MD is bound stereospecifically and rigidly to actin, the lever arm rotates downward to produce force and sliding. The swing is depicted in Fig. 9-3 as a straightening of the angle between two helices (the switch II helix, within the MD, and the long heavy-chain helix within the LCD) around a pivot (⊗) near Cys[707] (see also Color Plate 1c and d). In the diagram, the actual rotation accompanies sliding (5 → 6), as if the myosin rod (S2) linking the head to the backbone of the thick filament were very stiff. However, if the rod is less stiff,

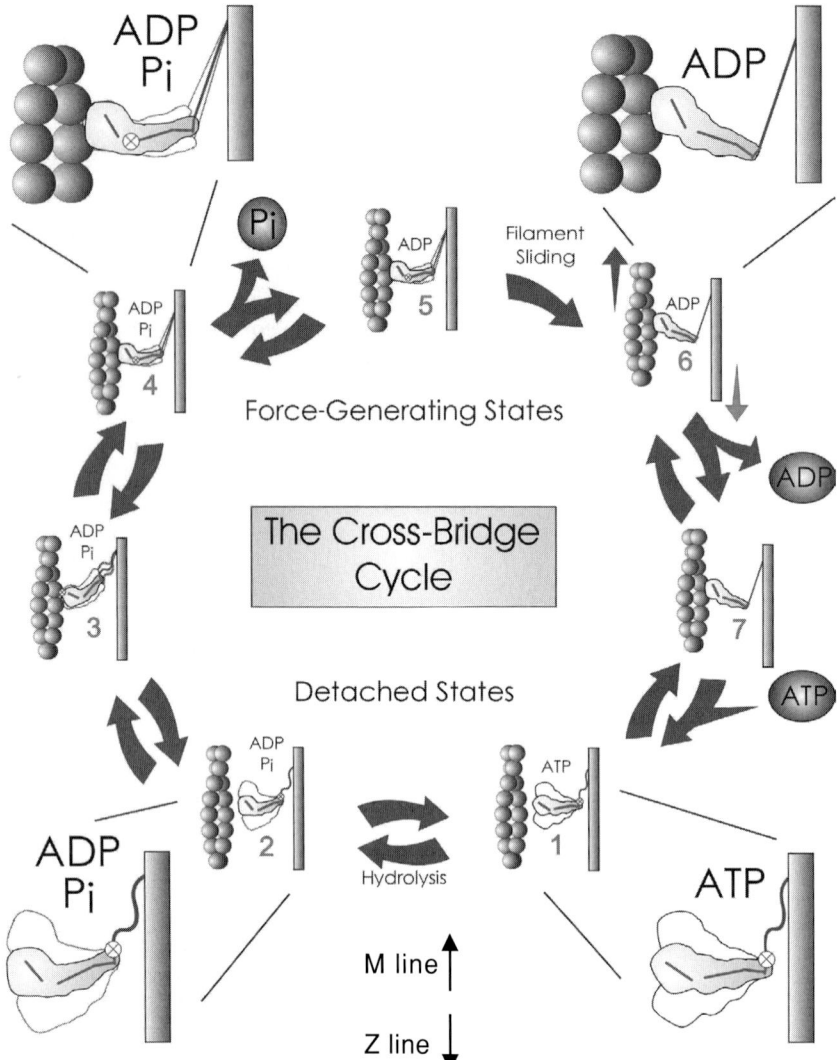

FIGURE 9-3. A hypothesis for actomyosin energy transduction. Shaded balls are actin monomers arranged into filaments, barbed end downward. The myosin head, rod, and thick-filament backbone are shown to the right of actin in each panel. Dashed outlines indicate mobility. Axes of two heavy-chain helices within the S1 are indicated by dark bars, the switch II helix in the motor domain (MD), and the long light-chain domain (LCD) helix. The relative orientations of the two helices change when the head is cocked into the pre–power stroke state (1→2) and during the swing in the power stroke (5→6). Hinges where flexibility enables motion at the head-rod junction (states 1 and 2), between myosin and actin (state 3), and within the head (states 4 and 5) are indicated by ⊗. The larger-scale drawings in the four corners are expanded views of states 1, 2, 4, and 6. Note that the shape of the head and the angle between the helix axes marking the MD and the LCD differ in states 2 and 4 (pre–working stroke) and in states 1 and 6 (post–wozYE: Wag the tail: Structural dynamics of actomyosin. Cell 93:1, 1998. With permission.)

the rotation might be as early as steps 3→4 or 4→5. The term *power stroke* is often applied to the structural change in myosin that produces force, but it should be reserved for transfer of work when the filaments actually slide, not simply to designate generation of force in a muscle held at fixed length. Reversal of the structural change in the head, which primes it for the next cycle, either accompanies ATP hydrolysis, as indicated by the change in angle between the two helices at step 1→2 in Fig. 9-3, or else is an isomerization of M•ATP just before hydrolysis.[18,19]

The hypothesis that the LCD serves as a lever does not rule out a contribution to force generation or filament sliding directly from the weak-to-strong transition (3→4). This step is readily reversible, but it is biased forward by the immediate release of P_i.[13,20] Then the energy liberated in forming the actomyosin bond could make a contribution to the work output, a type of *thermal ratchet* mechanism. Evidence favoring this idea comes from electron micrographic reconstructions of ultrarapidly frozen muscles that have shown the MD to rotate in the correct direction (downward in Fig. 9-3) at the beginning of the working stroke,[21] and from x-ray diffraction[22] and electron spin resonance spectroscopy,[23] which have associated a disorder-to-order transition of the MD with force generation. Whether these motions actually participate in the power stroke or are merely prerequisites for the crucial lever motion is controversial.

The mechanism of energy transduction illustrated in Fig. 9-3 derives support from the structure of the myofibril described above and in Chap. 7, the biochemistry of actomyosin described in Chap. 8, and mechanical and physiological experiments described below. However, some of the steps and motions in this working hypothesis are conjectural or have not been conclusively demonstrated. Combinations of mechanical, biochemical, and structural data in experimental preparations actively transducing energy are required to test the ideas and to interrelate the processes. Most of the remainder of this chapter surveys the physiological and mechanical experimental evidence leading to the ideas in Fig. 9-3.

Muscle Fiber Mechanics

ISOMETRIC CONTRACTIONS

Single living muscle fibers can be immersed in oxygenated physiological solution and mounted between mechanical sensors. One tendon is attached to a motor to control its length while the other tendon is attached to a transducer that measures force, P. An electrical stimulator is used to activate the muscle and a microelectrode records the fiber's membrane potential. When the muscle length is near its rest length, about 2.0 μm (L_0), the resting force (also termed *resting tension*) is small. The result of administering a single stimulus is shown in Fig. 9-4.[24] The electrical activity of skeletal muscle membrane is similar to that of a nerve in that the action potential depolarization is a result of a sudden increase in *sodium current*, while repolarization is caused by sodium channel inactivation and a delayed increase in *potassium current*. Cl⁻ ions, driven into the cell by the membrane depolarization, also contribute to repolarization (see Chap. 10). Initially the membrane potential repolarizes to a value more positive than the resting potential and, over the time course of 5 to 30 ms, approaches the prestimulus resting potential. The resting skeletal muscle membrane is most permeable to chloride ions; Cl⁻ conductance (g_{Cl}) is about twice potassium conductance, while sodium conductance is small (about 0.01 g_{Cl}).[25] Resting potentials are typically −75 to −90 mV.[26] After the stimulus, there is a 5- to 18-ms time interval (the *latent period*) between the beginning of the action potential and the beginning of force development. The signaling events occurring during the latent period are called *excitation-contraction coupling* (E-C coupling; see Chap. 12).

The mechanical response to a single action potential is called a *twitch*; when the muscle is not allowed to shorten, it is called an *isometric twitch* (Fig. 9-4). The duration of this response is dependent on a number of variables, including temperature, animal species, type of muscle, and previous activity (see Chap. 5 for details). For mammalian muscle at 37°C, the twitch lasts 50 to 300 ms and is dependent on the type of muscle involved. The "fast-twitch" muscle fibers (type II) contract and relax in about 50 ms, shorten at a fast rate, and are glycolytic (i.e., they can produce ATP mainly by the conversion of glucose to lactate); while the "slow-twitch" muscle fibers (type I) contract and relax in 200 to 500 ms, shorten at a rate 30 percent of that of type II fibers, and rely on oxidative phosphorylation for production of ATP. The different fiber types express different proteins involved in contraction (myosin, actin, troponin, and tropomyosin) and in E-C coupling.

As temperature is reduced, both the twitch amplitude and duration increase. Figure 9-4 shows that the action potential duration is <5 percent of that of the isometric twitch. Consequently, the refractory period for stimulating another action potential is a small fraction of the twitch duration, and the muscle can be stimulated a number of times during the twitch. When the muscle is stimulated more than once in close succession, the twitches *fuse*, and the amount of force produced increases. The isometric force responses to successive stimuli administered to a slow mammalian muscle (type I) motor unit at successively faster intervals are shown in Fig. 9-5, B to D, respectively.[27] Repetitive stimulation at increasing rates leads to an oscillatory state called an *unfused tetanus* (Fig. 9-5B and C). Repetitive stimulation of mammalian muscles (at 40 to 200 Hz at 35°C) produces a smoothly rising *fused tetanus* (solid lines in Fig. 9-5D). In fast (type II) skeletal muscle, the stimulus frequency required to produce a fused tetanus is greater than that needed for type I fibers. This is a consequence of the higher rate of cross-bridge cycling and calcium pumping by the sarcoplasmic reticulum in fast fibers. When the stimulation ends, the muscle quickly relaxes. In Fig. 9-5, the twitch tension is roughly 25 percent of the tetanic tension, P_0. In mammalian muscles, the twitch tension is often only 10 to 20 percent of P_0. Thus, the frequency of stimulation and the number of motor units firing modulate the force exerted by the muscle.

The amount of force exerted in a single isometric tetanus is remarkable. Amphibian and mammalian skeletal muscles produce a maximal isometric force of ~300 kN of isometric force per square meter of muscle cross-sectional area[28] (3 × 10^{-7} N/μm² or 45 lb/in.²). The maximal force produced by a muscle contraction is proportional to the muscle's cross-sectional area. To estimate the force produced by an individual myosin molecule, consider that there are ~500 thick filaments within each square micrometer of skeletal muscle cross-sectional area and 300 myosin S1 heads per thick filament within each overlap zone.[29] Thus the force exerted per S1 is 2 pN if all the cross-bridges are attached during a tetanus. If only 25 percent are attached at a particular instant, then the force per attached S1 head is 8 pN.

LENGTH-TENSION CURVES

A resting skeletal muscle at a sarcomere length of 2.0 μm exerts relatively little force. Stretching a resting muscle increases the force it exerts, even though the fiber is not stimulated. The dotted and dashed lines in Fig. 9-6 show the *passive forces* exerted by amphibian and mammalian muscle fibers, respectively, as a function of the sarcomere length.[30] This *passive force* is produced by the distention of elastic connective tissue surrounding the muscle fibers and a sarcomeric

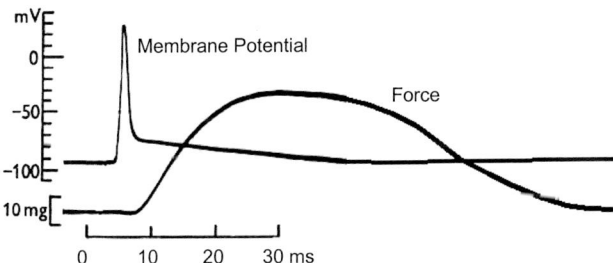

FIGURE 9-4. The recording of the membrane potential and isometric twitch in response to an electrical stimulation of a single frog muscle fiber at 20°C. Note that the action potential precedes the mechanical response with a 3- to 4-ms latent period and that the contractile response of the muscle cell is much longer than the refractory period (5 to 10 ms) of the electrical response. (*Based on data in Hodgkin AL, Horowicz P: The differential action of hypertonic solutions on the twitch and action potential of a muscle fibre. J Physiol 136:17P, 1957. With permission.*)

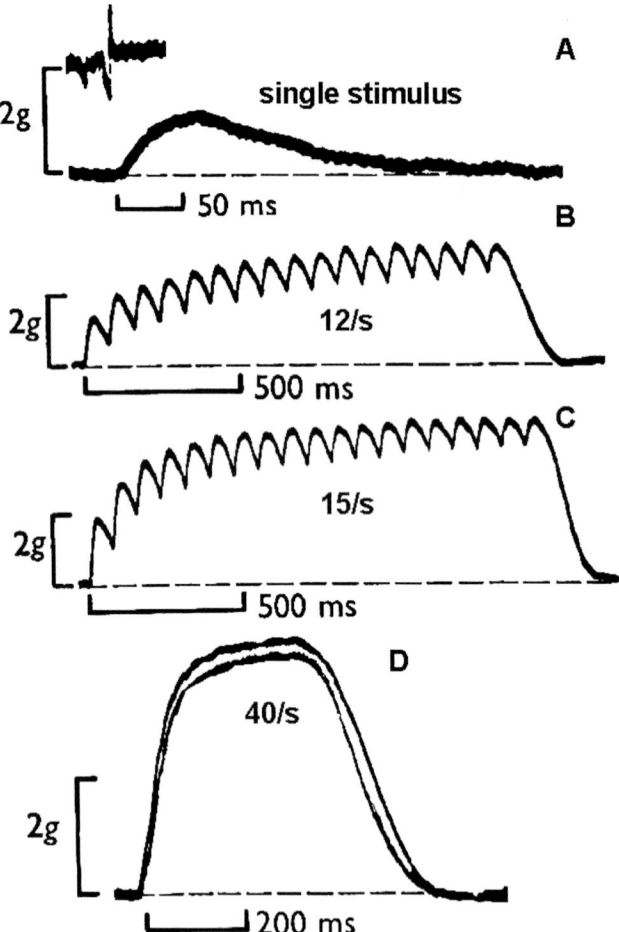

FIGURE 9-5. The mechanical response to single and multiple stimulations of a slow (type I) motor unit of a cat gastrocnemius muscle. The muscle temperature is at 36 to 38°C. Recording A shows an isometric twitch and, above it, the extracellularly recorded compound action potential in response to a single motor neuron action potential. Records B, C, and D show the mechanical responses to motor nerve stimulation at 12, 15, and 40/s. In D, the motor unit was tetanically stimulated for 320 ms; two mechanical records are shown. The larger of the two is the first tetanus and the smaller is that obtained from the 60th tetanus in a series in which the muscle was tetanized every 2 s. The minimal decline in isometric force illustrates the fatigue resistance of this type of muscle. (From Burke RE, Levine DN, Tsairis P, Zajac FE III: *Physiological types and histochemical profiles in motor units of the cat gastrocnemius.* J Physiol 234:723, 1973. With permission.)

protein that anchors adjacent Z lines to the thick filaments. This protein, called *titin* because of its huge size (~3 MDa), acts to position the thick filaments in the center of each sarcomere[31] (see Chap. 7). If a stretched muscle is released, the sarcomeres passively return to the resting length, $L_0 = $ ~2.2 to 2.5 μm. To shorten the fiber further, it must be stimulated. A single stimulus causes an untethered fiber to shorten to about 1.7 to 1.8 μm, and then it stays at this length. Several stimuli given in rapid succession can shorten a muscle fiber to ~1.4 μm. When the stimuli stop, the sarcomere length returns passively toward 1.8 μm. This behavior implies the existence of a "restoring force" that limits shortening of the resting muscle to sarcomere lengths above 1.7 μm. This force may derive from compression of the thick filaments against the Z line during the shortening and/or from either the cytoskeleton or the extracellular matrix.

Contractions in which the muscle length is held rigidly between two fixed supports and thus not allowed to shorten are termed *isometric*. How does active production of isometric force vary with initial muscle length? To examine this length-tension relationship, the resting muscle length is set to 0.6 to 1.7 times L_0. The muscle is then tetanized, and the maximum force is measured during the tetanus at each length. Reliable results are achieved only when sarcomere inhomogeneities are taken into account. The results of this type of experiment on an amphibian muscle fiber are shown in Fig. 9-6 by the solid line.[32] The amount of *active force* produced above the passive force strongly depends on the initial length of the muscle. Maximal *active force* (P_0) is generated at a sarcomere length of ~2.0 to 2.2 μm and declines when the length is set to values either above or below this range. Active force declines to near zero at about 1.3 and 3.6 μm. Skeletal muscles normally work near the peak of the length-tension curve, in the range of ~0.8 to 1.2 L_0 (1.6 to 2.6 μm).

The behavior of the muscle at sarcomere lengths greater than 2.0 μm, termed the *descending limb* of the length-tension curve, is explained by the sliding filament model.[28,32] The important elements in this explanation are that the lengths of the thick and thin filaments do not change at sarcomere lengths >2.0 μm, that the active force exerted during a contraction is proportional to the number of cross-bridges attached to the thin filaments, and that each cross-bridge exerts a unit of force that is largely independent of sarcomere length and is directed to toward the center of the thick filament. At sarcomere lengths >3.6 μm, the thick and thin filaments do not overlap, so it is impossible for cross-bridges to attach to the thin filament and active force is zero. As the sarcomere length is reduced to <3.6 μm, the overlap of the thick and thin filaments increases, and with it the number of cross-bridges able to attach to the thin filaments. Since the cross-bridges are uniformly distributed along the thick filament, isometric force rises in direct proportion to the overlap between the thick and thin filaments, as seen in Fig. 9-6. At 2.2 μm, the overlap between the cross-bridge-bearing regions of the thick filaments and thin filaments is complete, so that force will be maximal. In the length range from 2.2 to 2.0 μm, no additional cross-bridges can form, as the tips of the thin filaments extend into the center of the sarcomere at the "bare zone" of the thick filaments, so the active isometric force over this interval is constant. Maximal overlap in mammalian muscle cells extends to slightly longer lengths (2.4 μm per sarcomere) than in amphibian muscle because mammalian thin filaments are each 1.1 μm long, compared to 1.0 μm in amphibians. The thick filament in all vertebrate striated muscle is 1.65 to 1.7 μm long, and the bare zone is 0.2 μm long.

The mechanism for the force decline at short sarcomere lengths, the *ascending limb* of the length-tension curve, is not quantitatively understood. As sarcomere length decreases below 2.0 μm, the thin filaments from opposite half-sarcomeres begin to collide with one another, perhaps causing a repulsive force. As the sarcomere length is decreased further, the lateral distance between the thick and thin filaments increases (because the muscle fiber volume is constant[33]), perhaps affecting the number of cross-bridges attaching to the thin filament. As the sarcomere length is reduced below

1.8 μm, thin filaments from one side of the sarcomere may disrupt the cross-bridges formed with the thin filaments from the other side of the sarcomere, reducing the number of cross-bridges productively attached to the thin filament. Finally, if the sarcomere length is reduced to 1.65 μm or lower, the Z lines are compressed against the ends of the thick filaments, producing a strong repulsive force. Activation of the muscle is also impaired at very short lengths. Thus active force declines rapidly as sarcomere length decreases below 1.7 μm.

ENERGETICS OF ISOMETRIC CONTRACTIONS

During a contraction, reactions associated with the ionic movements accompanying membrane excitation, calcium release and sequestration, cross-bridge cycling, and phosphorylation of contractile proteins consume energy.[34] Hydrolysis of ATP is the energy source for all of these processes. In isometric contractions, cross-bridge cycling uses 60 to 70 percent of the ATP hydrolysis, intracellular calcium movements 20 to 30 percent, and the remaining processes 5 to 10 percent. It is generally assumed that one ATP is hydrolyzed per cross-bridge power stroke (as in Fig. 9-3; but see Ref. 35).

Energy production during contraction was first characterized by measuring the heat + work (enthalpy) by active amphibian skeletal muscles.[36] The enthalpy produced during the contraction itself (the initial heat) is temporally separate from that produced by the resynthesis of high-energy phosphates, ATP, and creatine phosphate (recovery heat) in amphibian muscle and in slower mammalian muscles. However, in highly oxidative mammalian muscles (e.g., type I skeletal muscle and cardiac muscle), the initial hydrolysis and resynthesis processes are not temporally separated and the resynthesis of high-energy phosphates begins during contraction.[37] The nonspecific nature of enthalpy measurements makes their interpretation difficult. Modern approaches to the study of muscle energetics involve direct measurements of the changes in high-energy phosphates accompanying contraction.[29] Chemical assays on extracts from rapidly frozen muscles, magnetic resonance spectroscopy of intact whole muscle cells, and estimates of ATP resynthesis by oxygen consumption and fluorescence techniques have been used. ATP hydrolysis by contracting permeabilized muscle fibers has been measured chemically after activation by photolysis of caged ATP, with linked-enzyme techniques, and using phosphate- or ADP-binding proteins that report the time course of product release from the myosin heads.[38–40] The amount and time course of energy liberation determined from these different approaches in skeletal muscles have yielded results similar to measurements of the enthalpy production and of high-energy phosphate splitting.

The energy produced during a maintained isometric tetanus, h(t), called the *maintenance heat*, is a function of the duration of tetanic stimulation (t) and is described by the following empirical equation[41]:

$$h(t) = h_a(1 - e^{-\alpha t}) + h_b \bullet t$$

An initial component, the *labile maintenance heat* (LMH), $h_{a'}$ is produced at an exponentially decreasing rate during the first 2 to 5 s of the tetanus. A second term, the *stable maintenance heat* (SMH), h_b, is produced continuously throughout the tetanus. Reactions associated with the release and sequestration of calcium during activation probably produce the LMH and about 30 percent of the SMH.[42] ATP hydrolysis by cycling cross-bridges accounts for the remaining 70 percent.[29] Frog skeletal muscles contracting isometrically at 0°C or mammalian type II skeletal muscles contracting at 10 to 15°C hydrolyze about 1 to 2 ATP molecules per cross-bridge head per second.

The sarcomere length of the muscle, the ambient temperature, and the fiber type all markedly alter the rate of ATP

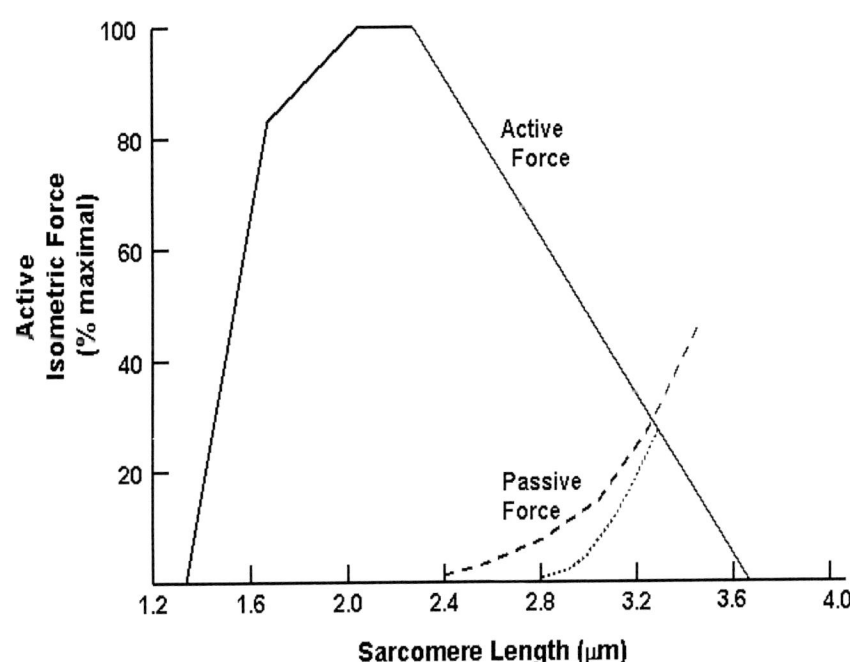

FIGURE 9-6. The length-tension curve from an intact frog single muscle fiber. The solid line plots the isometric active tetanic tension recorded at various sarcomere lengths at 4°C and corrected for sarcomere inhomogeneities.[32] The dotted line is resting or passive tension exerted by the muscle at different sarcomere lengths.[46] The dashed line is resting tension of skinned rabbit psoas muscle fibers.[30]

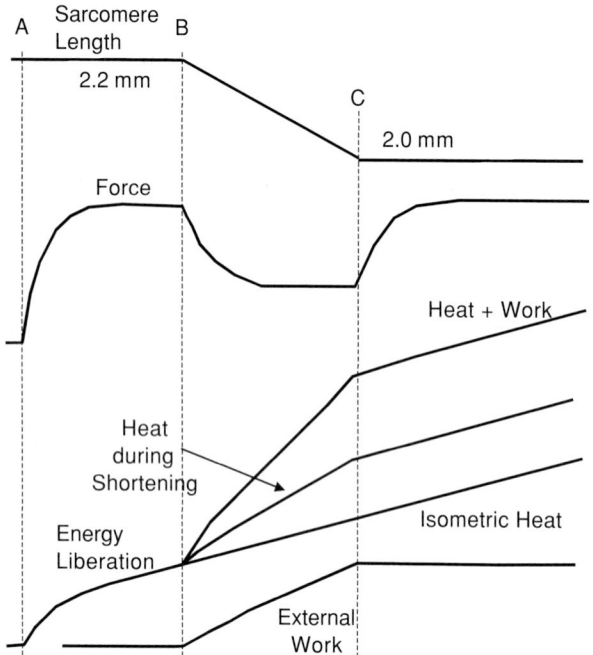

FIGURE 9-7. Sarcomere length, force, energy liberation, and external work done during an isometric tetanus (from time A to B) and during shortening (interval B to C) at a constant velocity less than V_0. Force redevelops to the isometric value after the cessation of shortening. The time from A to C is about 1 s. The energy liberation is given as shortening heat plus external work produced during shortening. The heat + work is directly proportional to the amount of high-energy phosphates utilized by the contracting muscle. (*Based on data from Aubert X: Le couplage energetique de la contraction musculaire. Brussels: Arscia; 1956; and Hill AV: The heat of shortening and the dynamic constants of muscle. Proc R Soc Lon [Biol] 126:136, 1938. With permission.*)

hydrolysis.[29] Increasing the muscle length above optimal reduces the SMH in direct proportion to the decline in filament overlap, whereas there is only a small reduction in the LMH. Reducing the sarcomere length to less than optimal decreases both labile and stable maintenance heat, suggesting an inhibition in muscle activation at shorter sarcomere lengths. Comparisons of muscles containing different fiber types show that the more rapidly contracting muscles have elevated rates of isometric energy consumption.[43] The SMH increases three- to fivefold when temperature is raised by 10°C, whereas the isometric force increases by only ~30 percent in the same temperature range. Warming an amphibian skeletal muscle from 0 to 20°C will increase the rate of ATP hydrolysis by its myosin heads from 1 to 2 s^{-1} to 9 to 50 s^{-1}. The ATP hydrolysis in permeabilized mammalian muscle fibers at 10°C is 2 s^{-1} per S1 head and exhibits a similar dependence on filament overlap and temperature as the isometric heat.[29]

CONTRACTIONS WITH SHORTENING

If a muscle is fully activated, isometrically contracting at fixed length near optimal filament overlap, it produces maximal force P_0. If the load is suddenly reduced to less than P_0, the muscle shortens and reaches a fixed shortening velocity within 5 to 50 ms.[44] This type of contraction is termed an *isotonic contraction*. When the load, P, against which the muscle shortens (termed the *afterload*) is reduced, muscle shortens more rapidly. Conversely, if the isometrically contracting muscle is allowed to shorten at a constant velocity, the force exerted by the muscle falls to a constant value that is inversely dependent on the velocity (see Fig. 9-7: sarcomere length and force recordings). The relationship between force and steady shortening velocity in an activated muscle is hyperbolic and is given by Hill's classic equation,[45] as follows:

$$(P + a)V = b(P_0 - P) \tag{9-1}$$

where P_0 is the isometric force, and a and b are constants in units of force and velocity (muscle lengths per second), respectively (Fig. 9-8). Typical values for a and b in fast amphibian and mammalian type II fiber (at 0 and 15°C, respectively) are 0.25 P_0 and 0.3 to 0.70 L_0/s, respectively.[29] The muscle fiber length, L_0, is usually reported at optimal thick and thin filament overlap (2.2 to 2.5 µm). The shortening occurs by the relative sliding of the thick and thin filaments at the same velocity in all the sarcomeres in the muscle. The total shortening of a myofibril is the sum of the amount of shortening of each overlap zone in series along the myofibril, so the total velocity of muscle shortening is the filament sliding velocity multiplied by the number of overlap zones in series (twice the number of sarcomeres). The speed at which individual thin filaments slide past the thick filaments is given by dividing the sarcomere shortening speed by 2 and the result expressed as µm/(half-sarcomere•s), µm/(hs•s). Velocity of shortening, measured in absolute units (e.g., m/s) from end to end, is increased if the muscle is longer, all other parameters (afterload, contractile protein isoforms, etc.) being the same. The velocity measured in units relative to the muscle length (L_0/s) does not depend on the number of sarcomeres in series.

When the force against which a muscle shortens is zero (unloaded), the velocity is maximal. For frog muscle at 0 to 2°C and mammalian type II fibers at 10°C, the *unloaded short-*

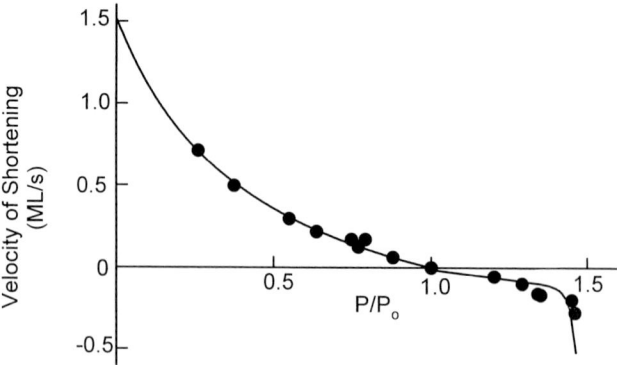

FIGURE 9-8. The force-velocity curve from frog sartorius muscles at 0°C. The maximal isometric force in this case was 190 kN/m^2 and the maximal unloaded shortening velocity was 1.52 muscle lengths per second. The data (shown in filled circles) are the steady-state force during each given velocity of shortening or lengthening of the muscle. (*Data from Aubert X: Le couplage energetique de la contraction musculaire. Brussels: Arscia; 1956. With permission.*)

ening velocity, V_0, is 1.3 to 2.7 L_0/s. The maximal velocity is designated V_0 here instead of V_{max} to avoid confusion with enzymatic rates. Originally, V_0 was estimated by fitting afterload and shortening velocity data to Eq. (9-1).[45] Later Edman[46] introduced a simple method, the *slack test*, to estimate V_0. A quick length change is imposed on the muscle fiber, large enough so that the fiber becomes slack and force is zero. The time required for the muscle to take up this slack while shortening freely gives V_0. Maximum shortening velocities measured using the two test methods are similar.

The force-velocity curve can be understood in molecular terms (Fig. 9-3) as follows: In isometric contractions, cross-bridges attach and exert a constant force during states 4, 5, and 6 (Fig. 9-3). The force is supported by stress in the myosin head and in the S2 rod that links the head to the thick-filament backbone (Figs. 9-1 to 9-3). Force drops to zero when the cross-bridge detaches in steps 7→1. In an isometric contraction, the rate of ADP release is rate-limiting for the cross-bridge ATPase cycle. In mammalian type II fibers at 10°C or amphibian fibers at 0°C, the ADP release rate is 1 to 2 s^{-1}. During shortening, the stress on the cross-bridge is reduced as the filaments slide past each other. Thus, the average force exerted by the attached cross-bridges decreases, relative to the isometric force, when the muscle is shortening. The reduction in stress on the cross-bridge also increases the rate at which ADP release occurs (steps 6→7), thereby accelerating cross-bridge detachment (steps 7→1). This leads to a decrease in the number of cross-bridges attached and contributes to the reduced force exerted during shortening. The accelerated ADP release also increases the rate of the ATP hydrolysis above the isometric rate. The consequent increase of energy liberation with shortening is termed the *Fenn effect* and is an important feature in optimizing the efficiency of contraction[29,47] (see "Energetics of Working Contractions," below).

As the filaments slide, and each attached cross-bridge head moves along with the thin filament (in the downward direction in Fig. 9-3), the stress declines to zero at ~10 nm of displacement. This 10-nm distance of filament sliding generated by an individual cross-bridge is termed the cross-bridge *throw*. At a maximal sliding velocity (V_0) of 5 $\mu m/s$, the filaments slide 10 nm in 2 ms. If the cross-bridge remains attached longer than this time, the stress will become negative, e.g., directed against shortening. This puts a load on the other cross-bridges trying to propel the thin filament and slows shortening. The rate of ADP release from the cross-bridge, the binding of ATP, and detachment from the thin filament (steps 6→7→1 in Fig. 9-3) thus can impose a limit on the shortening velocity.

It is instructive to consider the sarcomere length dependence of shortening velocity. Unlike the isometric force, V_0 does *not* change within the range of sarcomere lengths from 1.7 to 3.1 μm, so that the unloaded shortening velocity is *independent of thick- and thin-filament* overlap.[32,46] Over these sarcomere lengths, the overlap between the thick and thin filaments ranges from 100 to 40 percent. At sarcomere lengths <1.7 μm, V_0 decreases markedly. This occurs presumably because of a resistive force generated as the Z band compresses the thick filaments and as cytoskeletal elements are stretched consequent to the increase in muscle diameter. Thus the unloaded shortening velocity in a maximally activated muscle fiber is independent of the number of cross-bridges pulling on the thin filament. These observations imply that there is no appreciable force retarding shortening other than the cross-bridges themselves. The kinetics of force generation and detachment and the effect of negatively stressed cross-bridges that remain attached farther than their 10-nm throw determine V_0. An analogy to a tug-of-war game applies closely to this result. The number of participants on each side of the center determines the force. But if one team releases the rope completely, the maximum velocity of translation (after the initial, possibly dramatic transient) will be independent of the number of players moving the rope on the opposite side. Thus constant V_0, independent of overlap, provided further support for the hypothesis that the cross-bridges operate as independent force generators.

Shortening velocities of different types of muscle fibers vary over a very wide range. Fibers can be classified according to their size, twitch duration, speed of contraction, balance between aerobic and glycolytic metabolism, and resistance to fatigue. In addition, isoenzymes of the signaling, regulatory, and contractile proteins and the surface area of the sarcoplasmic reticulum membranes are key features that distinguish functional properties of fiber types (see Chaps. 4 and 5). A striking example of this diversity is given by three skeletal muscle fiber types in the toadfish: red and white swimming muscles and superfast muscles of the sound-generating swimbladder, one of the fastest known muscles in vertebrates. Shortening velocities vary 5-fold and twitch durations vary 50-fold among these fish muscle fiber types due to specialized isoforms of myosin, troponin, and sarcoplasmic reticulum Ca-ATPase. The cross-bridge detachment rate in swimbladder is 40-fold faster than in the red muscle, allowing faster relaxation after a twitch and faster filament sliding during shortening contractions but leading to very low force production.[48,49] These specialized features of cross-bridge kinetics are necessary for adaptation to the functional roles of each muscle, and they represent trade-offs in the design of the contractile apparatus.

ENERGETICS OF WORKING CONTRACTIONS

In muscles contracting isometrically or shortening at V_0 (where force = 0), no work is transferred to the external environment. However, at forces between zero and P_0, the muscle does work on the load as it moves. The work done by the muscle is the product of the force exerted and distance shortened. The rate of work production (power output) is the product of the force (P) and the shortening velocity (V) and, by rearrangement of the force-velocity relationship, is given by the following:

$$P \bullet V = P\,b\,(P_0 - P)/(P + a)$$

This relationship is plotted versus V/V_0 in Fig. 9-9. When a muscle shortens, it transfers energy into its load. Hill[50] and others[39,51] have shown that during shortening, the rate of heat production and ATP hydrolysis also increase above the isometric rate. The traces in Fig. 9-7 labeled "Energy Liberation" show the heat produced by a tetanized muscle in the isometric condition [Eq. (9-1), isometric] and when it is allowed to shorten actively at a constant velocity (interval B to C). During shortening, the rate of heat production increases above the isometric rate, producing an excess over the isometric amount called the *shortening heat*. The excess heat is proportional to the distance shortened, to the load, and to the amount of filament overlap.[29] The extra heat persists after the redevelopment of maximal isometric force (Fig. 9-7), so it reflects an increase in ATP hydrolysis during shortening. The total energy produced by the muscle is given by the sum of the isometric heat, the shortening heat, and the work done by the muscle (Fig. 9-7, heat + work). The shortening heat produced in mammalian skeletal muscle is comparable to that in the more fully studied amphibian muscle.[52]

The increased rate of energy liberation during shortening is known as the Fenn effect.[47] Fenn found that when a muscle performed external work in a twitch, the total amount of energy liberated by the muscle increased by the amount of work. This was an extremely important experimental observation, because it implies that the energy liberated in a contraction is controlled by the load. Muscle is not a simple elastic element, like a spring, that stores a fixed amount of energy. Instead, the elementary biochemical rates that govern the ATPase activity and the energetic cost of contraction are regulated to optimize the energy expenditure.

The quantitative relationships for isometric heat, shortening heat, and work shown in Figs. 9-7 and 9-8 imply that, during an isometric contraction, cross-bridges cycle slowly (1 to 2 s^{-1}); during shortening, they cycle more rapidly.[39,51] Thus the kinetics of one or more of the attached cross-bridge transitions must depend on the cross-bridge stress. At high stress, this transition is slow; during shortening, it accelerates. Current evidence indicates that during isometric contraction, all of the steps in the reaction mechanism in Fig. 9-3 except ADP release from state 5 are 8 to 20 times faster than the steady-state turnover of the cross-bridges.[53] Consequently, the rate-limiting step in the cycle is probably an isomerization of state 5 after P_i release, or the release of ADP ($6 \rightarrow 7$).[54] During shortening, this rate-limiting step must accelerate to produce the four- to eightfold increase in energy liberation. The rate of cross-bridge attachment probably also increases at moderate shortening velocities, because appropriately oriented attachment sites on actin are presented to the myosin heads at a higher rate than in an isometric contraction.[5] However, the increased detachment rate due to faster ADP release predominates because the number of cross-bridges attached during contractions is decreased when the muscle is shortening.[55]

ECCENTRIC CONTRACTIONS

A common type of physiological contraction is the forcible lengthening of a muscle while it is activated. This situation (called an *eccentric contraction*) occurs in the quadriceps femoris when a person is walking down stairs and in the biceps brachii when he or she lowers a weight slowly after an arm curl. The rate of lengthening is a negative shortening velocity (Fig. 9-8). During eccentric contractions, the external environment does work on the attached cross-bridges and the force exerted by the muscle is increased above the isometric value (Fig. 9-8 at $V < 0$ and Fig. 9-9).[56] This behavior occurs because the strongly attached cross-bridges are stretched as the sarcomere length increases (storing the energy from the environment). As the negative shortening velocity increases, the force exerted by the muscle increases rapidly up to 1.5 to 2.0 P_0. At higher elongating forces, the velocity of lengthening increases markedly as cross-bridges are forcibly detached from the thin filaments (Fig. 9-8, extreme right).

The energetic consequences of steady stretching of an activated muscle are shown at the left of Fig. 9-9. As the force exerted by the muscle increases at negative shortening velocities, the work done on the muscle increases and the rate of energy liberation decreases markedly. However, in this case the device used to stretch the muscle is doing work on the muscle, and this negative work is converted into heat. Measurements of utilization of high-energy phosphates (ATP and creatine phosphate) during forced lengthening indicate that the rate of ATP hydrolysis is markedly reduced and, under some circumstances, can approach zero.[56,57] The eccentrically contracting muscle still consumes energy, but at a much reduced rate compared to isometric. Intense eccentric exercise in untrained muscles leads to histologic changes, inflammation, and delayed-onset muscle soreness. Training with similar eccentric exercises but not with isometric aerobic training reduces this effect.[58]

The suppression of the ATPase rate during eccentric contractions may be explained as follows: The cross-bridge cycle is probably forced to proceed partially backward (counterclockwise in Fig. 9-3). If a cross-bridge has yet not released P_i, it may detach to form M•ADP•P_i (state 2). Such a cross-bridge could, in principle, attach and detach several times without releasing ADP and P_i. For cross-bridges that have released P_i (state 5), detachment creates a M•ADP state (not shown in Fig. 9-3) from which ADP detaches quite slowly. Such a M•ADP myosin head could in principle reattach to the thin filament, helping to resist the lengthening and absorb the external work.

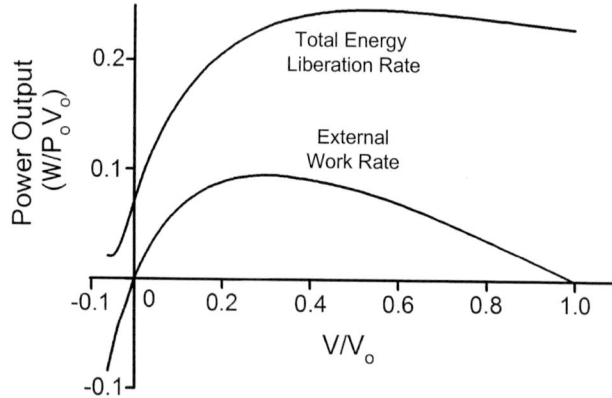

FIGURE 9-9. The rate of total energy liberation and power output as a function of the relative shortening velocity (V/V_0) during shortening or forced lengthening. The plots are based on measurements from frog skeletal muscles contracting at 0 to 4°C. The isometric heat production rate is taken as 0.065 P_0V_0. The rate of heat production during shortening, above the isometric value, is given as $(0.18 P_0 + 0.16 P)\cdot V$ (where P and V are the force and velocity during shortening). The rate of work output is given as $P\cdot V$. During forced lengthening, velocity is negative and no shortening heat is produced. Data from Refs. 51, 56, and 57.

STIFFNESS

When a sudden change in length is applied to an active muscle or muscle fiber, the force changes along with the length change and then recovers toward the value present before the perturbation (Fig. 9-10). The isometric tension is termed T_0 and the tension level immediately after the length step is applied is termed T_1. The ratio of the immediate change in force (T_1 to T_0) to the amount of the length change (ΔL), termed *stiffness*, quantifies the amount of force required to change the length a small known proportion of the overall length (either by stretching or compressing it). The stiffness of a type of material is given quantitatively by its *modulus of elasticity*, also termed *Young's modulus* (E), the ratio of stress (σ, force per unit area, e.g., N/m^2) to strain (ε, change in length per unit length, i.e., dimensionless), σ/ε, e.g., N/m^2. For instance, steel ($E = 200 \times 10^9 \, N/m^2$) is more difficult to stretch by 5 percent than rubber ($E = 20 \times 10^6 \, N/m^2$). The term *elasticity* indicates that the material returns to its original shape after a small stretch or compression. When mechanical elements are arranged parallel to each other, such as strands in a rope, the stiffness of the composite structure is the sum of the stiffnesses of the individual elements.

The reciprocal of stiffness (e.g., $1/E$) is the *compliance*. This concept is useful because when mechanical elements are attached in series, like the links in a chain, the total compliance of the structure is the sum of the elemental compliances. The sarcomeres in a myofibril are arranged in series, so their compliances ($1/E$ for each sarcomere) add. The compliance of a whole myofibril is the sum of the sarcomere compliances in it. The myofibrils in a muscle are parallel to each other, so the stiffness of a whole muscle is the sum of the stiffness of its myofibrils. The cross-bridges within an overlap zone of an individual sarcomere are mechanically parallel to each other, so their force and stiffness add together rather than their compliance. However, compliance of the filament backbones is in series with the cross-bridges (Fig. 7-1).

Relaxed muscle fibers have very low stiffness[59]: $E = 0.2 \times 10^6 \, N/m^2$, because the filaments slide relative to one another very easily at low force.[7] When a muscle dies, on the other hand, it becomes very difficult to stretch because all of the myosin heads attach to actin in the absence of ATP and thus cross-link the two sets of filaments (state 7 of Fig. 9-3 and Chap. 8). This state of a muscle is termed *rigor*. A muscle fiber in rigor is surprisingly stiff: $E = \sim 65 \times 10^6 \, N/m^2$, one-third that of steel.

In an actively contracting muscle fiber, a plot of T_1 (the extreme tension deflection after a length step) versus the magnitude of the length change is termed the T_1 *force-extension curve*. The T_1 curve is nearly linear, indicating that the stiffness of the cross-bridges is a constant, independent of force. The number of myosin heads attached to actin during contraction is intermediate between that in relaxation and in rigor. Each attached cross-bridge adds more stiffness to the muscle fiber (e.g., they are mechanically in parallel), so the stiffness has been used to estimate the proportion of myosin heads attached to actin. If the filament backbones and the mechanical connections to the muscle fiber were much stiffer than the cross-bridges themselves, then the stiffness would be directly proportional to the number of attached cross-bridges. Extensibility of the filament backbones and mechanical connections are termed *series compliance*. The effect of the external connections in stiffness measurements can be effectively removed by detecting the length change (strain) within the muscle itself. However, the compliance of the filament backbones (especially the thin filaments) accounts for approximately half of the total sarcomere compliance, so stiffness measurements need to be corrected for filament compliance. During tetanic contraction of individual intact muscle fibers from the frog, the stiffness is $40 \times 10^6 \, N/m^2$, approximately two-thirds of the value in rigor.[60] After correction for the filament compliance, these values indicate that ~40 percent of the myosin heads are attached during contraction compared to the number in rigor. There is evidence that only half of the rigor cross-bridges contribute stiffness,[61–63] possibly because the extensible part of the cross-bridge is contained in subfragment 2. Thus, the number of cross-bridges attached during a contraction may be only 20 percent of the total,[64,65] and only one of the two heads of each myosin is attached at any instant.[21]

The stiffness of an actively shortening muscle fiber is less than that during an isometric contraction. At V_0, the stiffness is about one-fifth of the isometric value, indicating considerably fewer cross-bridges attached.[55] This result indicates that the detachment rate of cross-bridges is accelerated by filament shortening, as discussed above under "Contractions with Shortening."

MECHANICAL TRANSIENTS

After a quick length change is applied to an active muscle fiber and the force reaches its extreme value, T_1, the force recovers toward the isometric tension value with a complex time course.[66] Tension recovers partly within 2 to 5 ms to a value termed T_2 (Fig. 9-10); it then delays or reverses for 10 to 20 ms and finally recovers to the prestep value over the next 100 to 200 ms. The kinetics of this tension recovery provide remarkably detailed information about the mechanism of contraction and have helped to solidify the power stroke and tilting models of the cross-bridge cycle.[28,67] Study of the kinetics of recovery and readjustment of a dynamic system after a sudden change in its physical or chemical condition is generally referred to as *perturbation analysis*. Sudden changes of mechanical stress and strain imposed on the cross-bridges perturb the steady state. The kinetics of recovery toward the original tension reveal the rates and strain dependence of the force-generating steps of the cross-bridge cycle.

During the quick recovery of force after a small (0.2 to 1 percent) length release, the cross-bridges are partly synchronized while developing force. The stiffness, measured by test length changes imposed various times after the first step, remains constant during the quick force recovery. This behavior indicates that the cross-bridges maintain their attachment to actin while force increases. A tilting motion, such as the downward swing of the LCD shown in Fig. 9-3 (states 5→6), can explain the increased force generation of a cross-bridge while it is attached to an actin. Huxley and Simmons[67] showed that detailed nonlinear behavior of the T_1 to T_2 recovery can be explained by such a structural change after a cross-bridge attaches. A length release corresponding to 4 nm of filament sliding results in T_1 force near zero,[68] indicating that the average strain in the force-bearing cross-bridges is less than 4 nm. At 12-nm release, little force is redeveloped at T_2 either,[68] providing a mechanical indication that the throw of the attached cross-bridge is 12 nm or less, consistent with tilting of the LCD, a 10-nm lever through 60 to 70 degrees (Fig. 9-2).

In fact, several techniques show that the light-chain region of the myosin head does tilt during imposed length changes and during the quick recovery. The mechanical transients must be combined with structural studies to investigate the motions of the myosin head during force generation. Two such structural studies are illustrated in Fig. 9-10. The low-angle scattering of x-rays by a muscle fiber detects periodic structures such as the actin monomers constituting the thin filaments and the cross-bridges. The x-ray reflection on the muscle fiber axis (the meridian) and spaced at 14.3 nm from the center of the pattern is termed M3 because it is the third order of the cross-bridge pitch, 43 nm (Fig. 7-11). The intensity of this reflection [I (M3)] decreases during the recovery of tension from T_1 to T_2 after a quick length release (Fig. 9-10A), indicating a change in the shape of the myosin heads that spreads their electron density along the direction of the filament axes.[69] This change in mass distribution is consistent with tilting motion of the LCD during force generation.

Fluorescent probes have been attached to the regulatory light chain in muscle fibers and their orientation measured using polarized optical detectors. This technique is particularly sensitive to rotational motions. The polarization signal shown during a mechanical transient in Fig. 9-10B, termed $Q_\perp$, deflects during the imposed length change, and it deflects further during the tension recovery. This experiment shows that some of the mechanical compliance in the cross-bridge is located within the S1 head, leading to rotation of the regulatory light chain. The quick tension recovery is also accompanied by tilting of the regulatory light chain. Thus the LCD contributes to both force generation and filament sliding. However, the idea that rotation of the MD provides an additional component (e.g., states 3 → 4 in Fig. 9-3) has not been ruled out[21,22,23,70] (see "Working Hypothesis," above).

CAGED MOLECULES

The relationship between the biochemistry and mechanics of the contractile apparatus has been illuminated by another type of perturbation study: laser photolysis of "caged molecules." These compounds are precursors of substrate or signaling molecules that are relatively inert, but can be cleaved under intense UV irradiation to release the active compound. For instance, caged ATP has a bulky chemical moiety, an orthonitrobenzyl group, bound to the γ-phosphate atom that makes it poorly recognized by myosin. Thus caged ATP can be diffused into a muscle fiber whose membrane has been permeabilized. In the absence of ATP, the muscle fiber stays in rigor. An intense pulse of laser light near 350 nm cleaves the orthonitrobenzyl group, releasing ATP and suddenly initiating cross-bridge cycling.

In Fig. 9-11, the time course of force is shown after release of ATP from caged ATP by a pulse of laser light (ΔATP). Force declines due to prompt cross-bridge detachment (Fig. 9-3, steps 7→1). In the presence of Ca^{2+}, force then rises due to cross-bridge reattachment and the power stroke. The muscle fiber is either held isometric (i) or stretched (s) by 0.3 percent shortly before the ATP is released to determine the strain dependence of these reactions. The amplitude of the transients initiated by laser photorelease of ATP is altered by the prestretch, but the kinetics is very similar in the isometric and stretched recordings. This result indicates that the ATP-induced detachment (7→1) is not markedly strain-dependent. Stiffness also declines promptly on release of ATP (not shown) and remains at a value between the relaxed and rigor levels because a proportion (e.g., 25 percent) of the cross-bridges are attached during the contraction.

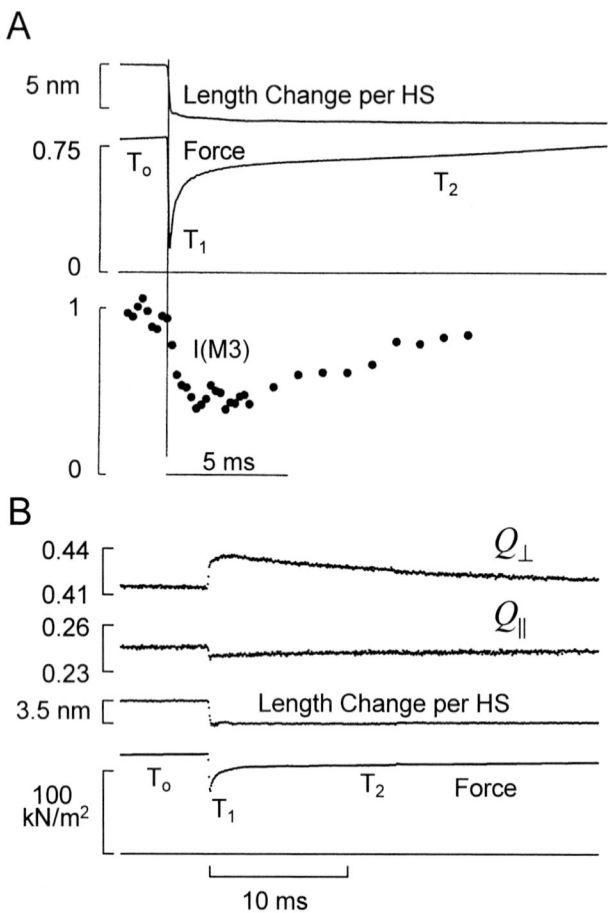

FIGURE 9-10. Mechanical transients recorded in conjunction with structural signals. A. X-ray diffraction experiment on a single intact frog semitendinosus muscle fiber. The muscle is tetanically stimulated at 4°C and a quick 5-nm release per half sarcomere length is applied. Force decreases synchronously with the length change from the isometric value (T_0) to a peak deflection (T_1) and then recovers within a few milliseconds to a quasisteady value (T_2). $T_0 - T_1$ is proportional to stiffness. The intensity of the third-order meridional diffraction peak (M3) indexing on the thick-filament periodicity decreases during the $T_1 \to T_2$ recovery. B. Fluorescence polarization experiment on a glycerol-extracted psoas fiber from rabbit muscle. The regulatory light chain (RLC) was labeled with 6-iodoacetamidotetramethyl rhodamine at Cys^{108}. Signal deflections indicate rotational motions. The probe and RLC rotate during the $T_0 \to T_1$ transition, indicating rotational flexibility within the S1 head, and also during $T_1 \to T_2$, signaling lever-arm tilting during force generation.

Chapter 9. Molecular Physiology of the Cross-Bridge Cycle

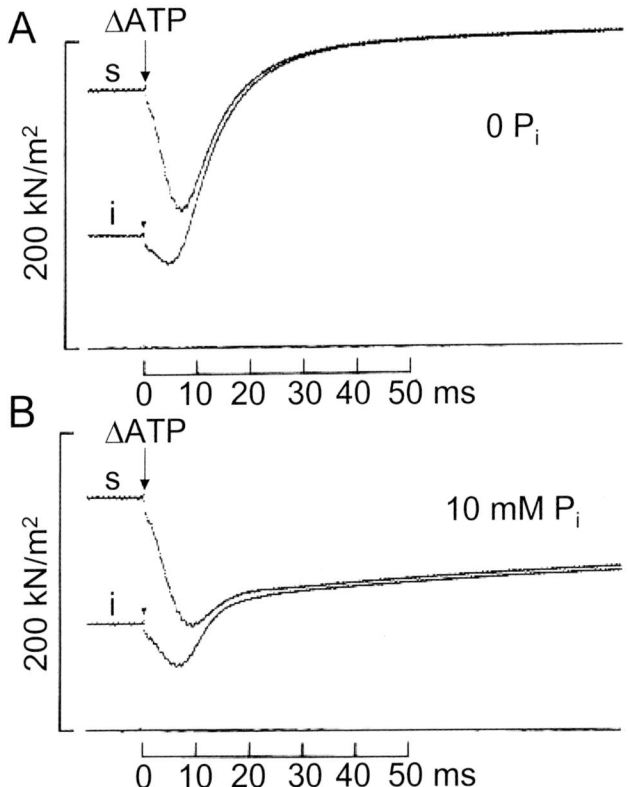

FIGURE 9-11. Tension transients recorded during activation of a glycerol-extracted psoas fiber from rabbit muscle by release of ATP by laser photolysis of caged ATP in the absence and presence of 10-mM P_i. Approximately 800 μM ATP was released from caged ATP at the arrows by single 50-ns, 347-nm laser pulses. Free Ca^{2+} concentration (100 μM) was saturating for activation of the thin-filament regulatory system. For traces labeled i, the muscle fiber was held at a fixed length; for those marked s, the fiber was stretched by 0.5 percent 1 s before the laser pulse. (Data from Goldman YE: Kinetics of the actomyosin ATPase in muscle fibers. Annu Rev Physiol 49:637, 1987.[89] With permission.)

initiated by length steps and chemical steps. These powerful methods provide extensive support for the mechanism of the contractile cycle shown in Fig. 9-3.

Mechanics in Vitro

Individual actin filaments can be visualized by sensitive fluorescence microscopy if they are labeled with an appropriate fluorophore. Often a fluorescent derivative of phalloidin, the mushroom toxin, is used for this purpose because it also stabilizes the filamentous actin and prevents depolymerization. When fluorescent actin is introduced with ATP onto a microscope slide coated with myosin, the actin filaments are seen to glide along their axes at speeds similar to those of active filament sliding in a muscle.[78,79] This recapitulation of movement and force generation from purified protein components in microscopic assays has rapidly advanced the study of the contractile mechanism. Subfragment 1 is the minimum portion of myosin that will propel actin in vitro, proving that the myosin head is the active motor unit. The sliding speeds of thin filaments in this assay are dependent on the [ATP], [ADP], ionic strength, and temperature much as V_0 is in the permeabilized muscle fibers and as predicted by the mechanism of Fig. 9-3. Sliding velocity also varies with myosin-head density, the presence of regulatory proteins on actin, and Ca^{2+} concentration.

An actin filament can be brought within interaction distance of a single myosin molecule by manipulating it in an optical microscope. The technique is termed the *infrared optical trap* or *laser tweezers*. An infrared laser beam is brought to a narrow focus by a high-aperture microscope objective. The high gradient of electromagnetic field near this beam waist draws small particles toward its center. The force is generated by the transfer of momentum between the particle and the photons of the laser beam when they are scattered or refracted. Small (0.5- to 2-μm) refractile beads made of polymer or silica can thus be "trapped" and manipulated by this optical beam. The laser tweezers functions as an energy well holding the bead near the focus (the lowest free energy). If the bead is displaced from this position in any direction, a restoring force acting on the bead increases. A typical measure of the optical trap stiffness is 0.02 pN/nm displacement. This value can be increased markedly (to >7 pN/nm) by increasing the intensity of the laser beam and by using feedback on the position of the optical trap to reduce movement of the bead.[80,81]

A common geometry for measuring the force or displacement due to single actomyosin interactions is shown in Fig. 9-12. The myosin is coated sparsely on "pedestal beads" to raise them above the surface of the microscope slide. Actin is suspended between two smaller beads held in a pair of optical traps. When the myosin binds to the actin and produces its mechanical output, the force generated (in piconewtons) or the deflection of the beads (in nanometers) can be measured (Fig. 9-13). Measurement of the displacement of the bead at low trap stiffness (to estimate the throw of the cross-bridge) yields unitary displacements between 5 and 10 nm per interaction.[80,82,83] This value is close to that expected from crystal

Inclusion of inorganic P_i in the medium bathing the fiber alters the kinetics in this type of experiment (Fig. 9-11B). This effect of P_i is caused by binding of P_i to AM•ADP (state 5), which reverses the force-generating transition coupled to release of P_i from AM•ADP•P_i (step 4 → 5). The steady-state force is also decreased by P_i due to reaction flux (step 5 → 4). These experiments have provided strong evidence that force generation is coupled to release of P_i from AM•ADP•P_i.[71,72] The decline in force due to reversal of P_i release helps to explain rapid fatigue in skeletal muscle (Chap. 5) and decreased cardiac output in myocardial ischemia.[73] Many other caged compounds are available for kinetic studies, such as caged P_i, Ca^{2+}, ATPγS, phenylephrine, etc.[74] Release of substrates or signaling molecules by laser photolysis has also been combined with structural techniques, such as fluorescence polarization[65] and x-ray diffraction,[75] to link alterations of the myosin-head conformation to the enzymatic steps of the ATPase cycle.

Several other types of reaction perturbation have been used to investigate the kinetics and pathway of the cross-bridge cycle. Jumps in temperature[22,76] and pressure[77] alter the steady state and induce mechanical transients analogous to those

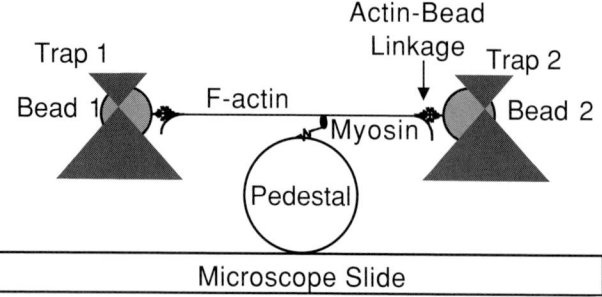

FIGURE 9-12. Three-bead assay for measurement of displacement and force of single actomyosin interactions.

structures of myosin in the presumed pre- and poststroke positions (Fig. 9-2), from the studies of transient kinetics in muscle fibers described above,[66,68] and from changes in sliding velocity and step size in vitro when the length of the neck linker region is altered.[84,85]

The unitary force exerted by the cross-bridge on the thin filament in the optical trap varies between 0.8 and 3.5 pN among different studies.[80,82,86] These values are underestimates of the maximum force generated by an individual cross-bridge due to series mechanical compliance where the beads are attached to the actin. When myosin produces a sliding force, this compliance allows the actin to move several nanometers and the stress and strain of the attached cross-bridge decrease, as in a shortening muscle fiber. Recently, the compliance of the system has been reduced, using a feedback mechanism, to approach the isometric condition more closely.[87] Much larger forces, ranging from 6 to 18 pN, have been measured in this system. It is likely that unitary cross-bridge force in an isometric contraction is on the order of about 8 pN, a value compatible with the force produced by intact muscle fibers if 25 percent of the cross-bridges are attached at any particular instant during a contraction (see "Isometric Contractions," above).

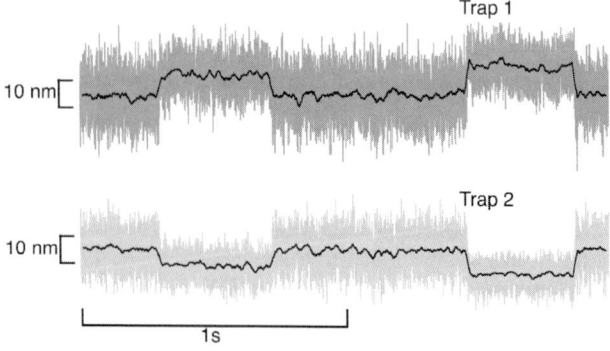

FIGURE 9-13. Individual actomyosin interactions in vitro using an optical trap three-bead assay with position feedback. (*Data from Drs. Y. Takagi and H. Shuman. With permission.*)

With a linear force-extension curve (see "Stiffness," above), the amount of energy that can be transferred from a compliant element to the external environment is $\frac{1}{2}Pd$, where P is the maximal force and d is the maximal extension. If the unitary cross-bridge force is 8 pN and the cross-bridge throw is 10 nm, then the maximal work obtained from a single cross-bridge would be 4×10^{-20} J per ATP hydrolyzed, or 50 percent of the free energy available from ATP hydrolysis under physiologic conditions.[29] This value matches well with the maximum efficiency (work output/energy liberated by ATP splitting = ~50 percent) of muscular contraction. Thus the force of a muscle fiber is explained by adding up the individual forces of its individual myosin heads.

Summary

Physiological and biophysical studies of muscle contraction identify very detailed aspects of the relationship between the mechanics, structural biology, and enzymology of the contractile proteins. Elementary steps of the actomyosin ATPase cycle are correlated well with a mechanical cycle of attachment, force generation, and detachment of myosin heads and actin. Once the myosin head is strongly bound to actin, tilting of the LCD serves as a lever to apply the sliding force. Mechanical experiments on single molecules provide data for the force, translocation distance, sliding velocity, and energy transduction that can be scaled up to explain most aspects of whole-muscle physiology. Thus a fairly complete and integrated picture of the mechanism of contraction from the molecular to the macroscopic level of integration emerges from these studies. As mentioned, many aspects of this mechanism are not certain. Among these points are the number of cross-bridges attached during contraction, the unitary force and throw, whether rotation of the MD contributes to force or sliding, the detailed structural changes at the nucleotide-binding site that cause the lever arm to swing, how actin triggers this motion, and how ATP weakens actomyosin affinity. Further studies on muscle fibers or on single isolated actomyosin complexes that combine mechanical and structural signals will be required to resolve these issues.

Acknowledgments

This work was supported by NIH grants AR26846 and HL15835 to YEG and AR30988 to EH. The optical trap data (Fig. 9-13) were kindly supplied by Dr. Yasuharu Takagi and Dr. Henry Shuman. Ms. Kimberly Vanzi helped with preparation of the manuscript.

List of Abbreviations

ADP	adenosine diphosphate	MD	motor domain
ATP	adenosine triphosphate	P_i	orthophosphate
ATPase	adenosine triphosphatase	RLC	regulatory light chain
E-C	excitation-contraction	SMH	stable maintenance heat
ELC	essential light chain	Tm	tropomyosin
HMM	heavy meromyosin	Tn	troponin
LCD	light-chain domain	TnC	C subunit of Tn
LMH	labile maintenance heat	TnI	I subunit of Tn
LMM	light meromyosin	TnT	T subunit of Tn
M•ADP•P_i	muscle•ADP•P_i complex		

References

1. Bennett PM, Fürst DO, Gautel M: The C-protein (myosin binding protein C) family: Regulators of contraction and sarcomere formation? *Rev Physiol Biochem Pharm* 138:203, 1999.
2. Huxley AF, Niedergerke R: Structural changes in muscle during contraction. *Nature* 173:971, 1954.
3. Huxley HE, Hanson J: Changes in the cross-striations of muscle during contraction and stretch and their structural interpretation. *Nature* 173:973, 1954.
4. Hanson J, Huxley HE: The structural basis of contraction in striated muscle. *Symp Soc Exp Biol* 9:228, 1955.
5. Huxley AF: Muscle structure and theories of contraction. *Prog Biophys Biophys Chem* 7:255, 1957.
6. Huxley HE: The mechanism of muscular contraction: Recent structural studies suggest a revealing model for cross-bridge action at variable filament spacing. *Science* 164:1356, 1969.
7. Huxley AF: Review lecture: Muscular contraction. *J Physiol* 243:1, 1974.
8. Rayment I, Holden HM, Whittaker M, et al: Structure of the actin-myosin complex and its implications for muscle contraction. *Science* 261:58, 1993.
9. Cooke R: Actomyosin interaction in striated muscle. *Physiol Rev* 77:671, 1997.
10. Goldman YE: Wag the tail: Structural dynamics of actomyosin. *Cell* 93:1, 1998.
11. Geeves MA, Holmes KC: Structural mechanism of muscle contraction. *Annu Rev Biochem* 68:687, 1999.
12. Brenner B: Mechanical and structural approaches to correlation of cross-bridge action in muscle with actomyosin ATPase in solution. *Annu Rev Physiol* 49:655, 1987.
13. Dantzig JA, Goldman YE, Millar NC, et al: Reversal of the cross-bridge force-generating transition by photogeneration of phosphate in rabbit psoas muscle fibres. *J Physiol* 451:247, 1992.
14. Dantzig JA, Hibberd MG, Trentham DR, Goldman YE: Cross-bridge kinetics in the presence of MgADP investigated by photolysis of caged ATP in rabbit psoas muscle fibres. *J Physiol* 432:639, 1991.
15. Cremo CR, Geeves MA: Interaction of actin and ADP with the head domain of smooth muscle myosin: Implications for strain-dependent ADP release in smooth muscle. *Biochemistry* 37:1969, 1998.
16. Smith CA, Rayment I: X-ray structure of the magnesium(II)•ADP•vanadate complex of the *Dictyostelium discoideum* myosin motor domain to 1.9 Å resolution. *Biochemistry* 35:5404, 1996.
17. Dominguez R, Freyzon Y, Trybus KM, Cohen C: Crystal structure of a vertebrate smooth muscle myosin motor domain and its complex with the essential light chain: Visualization of the pre-power stroke state. *Cell* 94:559, 1998.
18. Suzuki Y, Yasunaga T, Ohkura R, et al: Swing of the lever arm of a myosin motor at the isomerization and phosphate-release steps. *Nature* 396:380, 1998.
19. Shih WM, Gryczynski Z, Lakowicz JR, Spudich JA: A FRET-based sensor reveals large ATP hydrolysis-induced conformational changes and three distinct states of the molecular motor myosin. *Cell* 102:683, 2000.
20. Webb MR, Hibberd MG, Goldman YE, Trentham DR: Oxygen exchange between P_i in the medium and water during ATP hydrolysis mediated by skinned fibers from rabbit skeletal muscle. Evidence for P_i binding to a force-generating state. *J Biol Chem* 261:15557, 1986.
21. Taylor KA, Schmitz H, Reedy MC, et al: Tomographic 3D reconstruction of quick-frozen, Ca^{2+}-activated contracting insect flight muscle. *Cell* 99:421, 1999.
22. Tsaturyan AK, Bershitsky SY, Burns R, Ferenczi MA: Structural changes in the actin-myosin cross-bridges associated with force generation induced by temperature jump in permeabilized frog muscle fibers. *Biophys J* 77:354, 1999.
23. Ostap EM, Barnett VA, Thomas DD: Resolution of three structural states of spin-labeled myosin in contracting muscle. *Biophys J* 69:177, 1995.
24. Hodgkin AL, Horowicz P: The differential action of hypertonic solutions on the twitch and action potential of a muscle fibre. *J Physiol* 136:17P, 1957.
25. Dulhunty AF: The dependence of membrane potential on extracellular chloride concentration in mammalian skeletal muscle fibres. *J Physiol* 276:67, 1978.
26. Hironaka T, Morimoto S: The resting membrane potential of frog sartorius muscle. *J Physiol* 297:1, 1979.
27. Burke RE, Levine DN, Tsairis P, Zajac FE III: Physiological types and histochemical profiles in motor units of the cat gastrocnemius. *J Physiol* 234:723, 1973.
28. Huxley AF: *Reflections on Muscle*. Princeton, NJ: Princeton University Press; 1980.
29. Woledge RC, Curtin NA, Homsher E: *Energetic Aspects of Muscle Contraction*. London: Academic Press; 1985.
30. Granzier HL, Wang K: Passive tension and stiffness of vertebrate skeletal and insect flight muscles: The contribution of weak cross-bridges and elastic filaments. *Biophys J* 65:2141, 1993.
31. Labeit S, Kolmerer B, Linke WA: The giant protein titin: Emerging roles in physiology and pathophysiology. *Circ Res* 80:290, 1997.
32. Gordon AM, Huxley AF, Julian FJ: The variation in isometric tension with sarcomere length in vertebrate muscle fibres. *J Physiol* 184:170, 1966.
33. April EW: The myofilament lattice: Studies on isolated fibers IV. Lattice equilibria in striated muscle. *J Mechanochem Cell Motil* 3:111, 1975.
34. Homsher E: Muscle enthalpy production and its relationship to actomyosin ATPase. *Annu Rev Physiol* 49:673, 1987.
35. Ishii Y, Ishijima A, Yanagida T: Single molecule nanomanipulation of biomolecules. *Trends Biotechnol* 19:211, 2001.
36. Hill AV: *Trials and Trails in Physiology*. Baltimore: Williams & Wilkins; 1965.
37. Kushmerick MJ: Energetics of muscle contraction, in Peachey LD (ed): *Handbook of Physiology: Skeletal Muscle*. Bethesda, MD: American Physiological Society; 1983, p 189.
38. Ferenczi MA, Homsher E, Trentham DR: The kinetics of magnesium adenosine triphosphate cleavage in skinned muscle fibres of the rabbit. *J Physiol* 352:575, 1984.
39. Sun Y-B, Hilber K, Irving M: Effect of active shortening on the rate of ATP utilisation by rabbit psoas muscle fibres. *J Physiol* 531:781, 2001.
40. He Z-H, Bottinelli R, Pellegrino MA, et al: ATP consumption and efficiency of human single muscle fibers with different myosin isoform composition. *Biophys J* 79:945, 2000.
41. Aubert X: *Le couplage energetique de la contraction musculaire*. Brussels: Arscia; 1956.
42. Homsher E, Mommaerts WFHM, Ricchiuti NV, Wallner A: Activation heat, activation metabolism and tension-related heat in frog semitendinosus muscles. *J Physiol* 220:601, 1972.
43. Bottinelli R, Reggiani C: Human skeletal muscle fibres: Molecular and functional diversity. *Prog Biophys Mol Biol* 73:195, 2000.
44. Podolsky RJ, Nolan AC: Muscle contraction transients, cross-bridge kinetics, and the Fenn effect. *Cold Spring Harbor Symp Quant Biol* 37:661, 1972.
45. Hill AV: The heat of shortening and the dynamic constants of muscle. *Proc R Soc Lon [Biol]* 126:136, 1938.
46. Edman KAP: The velocity of unloaded shortening and its relation to sarcomere length and isometric force in vertebrate muscle fibres. *J Physiol* 291:143, 1979.

47. Fenn WO: A quantitative comparison between the energy liberated and the work performed by the isolated sartorius muscle of the frog. *J Physiol* 58:175, 1923.
48. Rome LC, Syme DA, Hollingworth S, et al: The whistle and the rattle: The design of sound producing muscles. *Proc Natl Acad Sci USA* 93:8095, 1996.
49. Rome LC, Cook C, Syme DA, et al: Trading force for speed: Why superfast crossbridge kinetics leads to superlow forces. *Proc Natl Acad Sci USA* 96:5826, 1999.
50. Hill AV: The effect of load on the heat of shortening of muscle. *Proc R Soc Lon [Biol]* 159:297, 1964.
51. Kushmerick MJ, Davies RE: The chemical energetics of muscle contraction: II. The chemistry, efficiency and power of maximally working sartorius muscles. *Proc R Soc Lon [Biol]* 174:315, 1969.
52. Holroyd SM, Gibbs CL, Luff AR: Shortening heat in slow- and fast-twitch muscles of the rat. *Am J Physiol* 270:C293, 1996.
53. Ma Y-Z, Taylor EW: Kinetic mechanism of myofibril ATPase. *Biophys J* 66:1542, 1994.
54. Sleep JA, Hutton RL: Exchange between inorganic phosphate and adenosine 5'-triphosphate in the medium by actomyosin subfragment 1. *Biochemistry* 19:1276, 1980.
55. Ford LE, Huxley AF, Simmons RM: Tension transients during steady shortening of frog muscle fibres. *J Physiol* 361:131, 1985.
56. Hill AV, Howarth JV: The reversal of chemical reactions in contracting muscle during an applied stretch. *Proc R Soc Lon [Biol]* 151:169, 1959.
57. Curtin NA, Davies RE: Very high tension with very little ATP breakdown by active skeletal muscle. *J Mechanochem Cell Motil* 3:147, 1975.
58. Patel TJ, Cuizon D, Mathieu-Costello O, et al: Increased oxidative capacity does not protect skeletal muscle fibers from eccentric contraction-induced injury. *Am J Physiol* 274:R1300, 1998.
59. Hill DK: Tension due to interaction between the sliding filaments in resting striated muscle. The effect of stimulation. *J Physiol* 199:637, 1968.
60. Linari M, Dobbie I, Reconditi M, et al: The stiffness of skeletal muscle in isometric contraction and rigor: The fraction of myosin heads bound to actin. *Biophys J* 74:2459, 1998.
61. Pate E, Cooke R: Energetics of the actomyosin bond in the filament array of muscle fibers. *Biophys J* 53:561, 1988.
62. Fajer PG, Fajer EA, Brunsvold NJ, Thomas DD: Effects of AMPPNP on the orientation and rotational dynamics of spin-labeled muscle cross-bridges. *Biophys J* 53:513, 1988.
63. Hopkins SC, Sabido-David C, van der Heide UA, et al: Orientation changes of the myosin light chain domain during filament sliding in active and rigor muscle. *J Mol Biol* 318:1275, 2002.
64. Cooke R, Crowder MS, Thomas DD: Orientation of spin labels attached to cross-bridges in contracting muscle fibres. *Nature* 300:776, 1982.
65. Hopkins SC, Sabido-David C, Corrie JET, et al: Fluorescence polarization transients from rhodamine isomers on the myosin regulatory light chain in skeletal muscle fibers. *Biophys J* 74:3093, 1998.
66. Ford LE, Huxley AF, Simmons RM: Tension responses to sudden length change in stimulated frog muscle fibres near slack length. *J Physiol* 269:441, 1977.
67. Huxley AF, Simmons RM: Proposed mechanism of force generation in striated muscle. *Nature* 233:533, 1971.
68. Piazzesi G, Linari M, Reconditi M, et al: Cross-bridge detachment and attachment following a step stretch imposed on active single frog muscle fibres. *J Physiol* 498:3, 1997.
69. Irving M, Lombardi V, Piazzesi G, Ferenczi MA: Myosin head movements are synchronous with the elementary force-generating process in muscle. *Nature* 357:156, 1992.
70. Brenner B: Rapid dissociation and reassociation of actomyosin cross-bridges during force generation: A newly observed facet of cross-bridge action in muscle. *Proc Natl Acad Sci USA* 88:10490, 1991.
71. Hibberd MG, Dantzig JA, Trentham DR, Goldman YE: Phosphate release and force generation in skeletal muscle fibers. *Science* 228:1317, 1985.
72. Cooke R, Pate E: The effects of ADP and phosphate on the contraction of muscle fibers. *Biophys J* 48:789, 1985.
73. Kentish JC: The effects of inorganic phosphate and creatine phosphate on force production in skinned muscles from rat ventricle. *J Physiol* 370:585, 1986.
74. Dantzig JA, Higuchi H, Goldman YE: Studies of molecular motors using caged compounds. *Methods Enzymol* 291:307, 1998.
75. Tsaturyan AK, Bershitsky SY, Burns R, et al: Structural responses to the photolytic release of ATP in frog muscle fibres, observed by time-resolved x-ray diffraction. *J Physiol* 520:681, 1999.
76. Goldman YE, McCray JA, Ranatunga KW: Transient tension changes initiated by laser temperature jumps in rabbit psoas muscle fibres. *J Physiol* 392:71, 1987.
77. Vawda F, Geeves MA, Ranatunga KW: Force generation upon hydrostatic pressure release in tetanized intact frog muscle fibres. *J Muscle Res Cell Motil* 20:477, 1999.
78. Kron SJ, Spudich JA: Fluorescent actin filaments move on myosin fixed to a glass surface. *Proc Natl Acad Sci USA* 83:6272, 1986.
79. Harada Y, Noguchi A, Kishino A, Yanagida T: Sliding movement of single actin filaments on one-headed myosin filaments. *Nature* 326:805, 1987.
80. Finer JT, Simmons RM, Spudich JA: Single myosin molecule mechanics: Piconewton forces and nanometre steps. *Nature* 368:113, 1994.
81. Wang MD, Yin H, Landick R, et al: Stretching DNA with optical tweezers. *Biophys J* 72:1335, 1997.
82. Guilford WH, Dupuis DE, Kennedy G, et al: Smooth muscle and skeletal muscle myosins produce similar unitary forces and displacements in the laser trap. *Biophys J* 72:1006, 1997.
83. Kitamura K, Tokunaga M, Iwane AH, Yanagida T: A single myosin head moves along an actin filament with regular steps of 5.3 nanometres. *Nature* 397:129, 1999.
84. Uyeda TQP, Abramson DP, Spudich JA: The neck region of the myosin motor domain acts as a lever arm to generate movement. *Proc Natl Acad Sci USA* 93:4459, 1996.
85. Warshaw DM, Guilford WH, Freyzon Y, et al: The light chain binding domain of expressed smooth muscle heavy meromyosin acts as a mechanical lever. *J Biol Chem* 275:37167, 2000.
86. Ishijima A, Kojima H, Higuchi H, et al: Multiple- and single-molecule analysis of the actomyosin motor by nanometer-piconewton manipulation with a microneedle: Unitary steps and forces. *Biophys J* 70:383, 1996.
87. Takagi Y, Homsher EE, Goldman YE, Shuman H: Probing the transduction mechanism of rabbit skeletal myosin II under isometric condition using an optical trap. *Biophys J* 82:373a, 2002.
88. Irving M, Piazzesi G, Lucii L, et al: Conformation of the myosin motor during force generation in skeletal muscle. *Nat Struct Biol* 7:482, 2000.
89. Goldman YE: Kinetics of the actomyosin ATPase in muscle fibers. *Annu Rev Physiol* 49:637, 1987.

SECTION 3

The Control of Muscle Fiber Activity

Chapter 10
Ion Channels and Electrical Properties of Skeletal Muscle

KARIN JURKAT-ROTT
FRANK LEHMANN-HORN

The Resting Potential and the Passive Electrical
  Properties of the Membrane
  VOLTAGE-INSENSITIVE CATION CHANNELS SETTING
    THE RESTING POTENTIAL
  VOLTAGE-GATED POTASSIUM CHANNELS MAINTAINING
    THE RESTING POTENTIAL
  CHLORIDE CHANNELS DO NOT CONTRIBUTE TO THE RESTING
    MEMBRANE POTENTIAL
  ACTIVE ION TRANSPORT THROUGH THE SODIUM-POTASSIUM
    PUMP
  THE SODIUM-CALCIUM EXCHANGERS, NCX
  THE CATION-CHLORIDE COTRANSPORTERS
  BISTABILITY OF THE RESTING MEMBRANE POTENTIAL
  PASSIVE ELECTRICAL PROPERTIES OF THE MEMBRANE

The Action Potential—The Regenerative 1-0 Bit
  of Signal Transduction
  CHARACTERISTICS OF THE SKELETAL MUSCLE ACTION POTENTIAL
  CURRENTS CONDUCTED DURING THE ACTION POTENTIAL
  VOLTAGE-GATED ION CHANNELS ESSENTIAL FOR THE
    ACTION POTENTIAL
  THE SPREAD OF ELECTRICAL ACTIVITY

Appendix: The Patch-Clamp Technique
  WHOLE-CELL RECORDING
  SINGLE-CHANNEL RECORDING
  TRANSIENT EXPRESSION SYSTEMS, AS IN OOCYTES
  STABLE EXPRESSION SYSTEMS
  MEASUREMENTS ON NATIVE MUSCLE FIBERS
  POTENTIAL FUTURE TECHNOLOGIES

From the point of view of motor activity, the primary task performed by the electrically excitable membranes of a skeletal muscle fiber is the activation of the contractile machinery in response to signals received from the motor nerve. Motor neuron activity is transferred to the myofibers via the neuromuscular junctions, where action potentials that propagate along the fiber membranes are generated. From there, excitation spreads along the transverse tubular system (TTS) into the depth of the fibers, thereby achieving uniform distribution of activation. This is a prerequisite for synchronization of contraction, which is initiated by intracellular calcium release brought about by direct interaction of channel proteins of TTS and sarcoplasmic reticulum (SR).

This chapter describes electrical properties of the muscle fiber membrane and the molecular basis for maintenance of the resting potential and the generation of the action potential. Common bases for these properties are ion channel proteins and transporters that are equipped with a membrane-spanning ion-conducting pathway and channel gates and are situated in the surface and inner membranes of the muscle fibers. They activate (i.e., open) in response to ligands, transmitters, or voltage changes and inactivate (i.e., close) by a usually intrinsic inactivation process. Voltage-gated channels contain additional voltage-sensing transmembrane segments and are essential for the generation and modification of the action potentials. In contrast, ligand-gated ion channels are essential for setting myoplasmic calcium concentration and establishing signal transduction pathways. Even though the human genome has been sequenced, it is presently not completely clear which genes are expressed in skeletal muscle and how these are tissue-specifically spliced. Therefore the contents of this chapter should be considered only as current general opinion. It may still take several years before more precise knowledge on the exact interplay between these proteins and other regulatory or signaling pathways is available.

The Resting Potential and the Passive Electrical Properties of the Membrane

The normal resting potential serves to keep the ion channels in an activatable state for generating the action potential. In a first approximation, it is determined by the transmembrane potassium and sodium ion gradients and by the membrane conductance, G_m, for these two ions. Numerically, the resting potential can be estimated from the reversal potentials for potassium and sodium—that is, from the potentials of equilibrium at which the net current of these specific ions through the membrane is zero. The reversal potentials can be calculated from the ion gradient across the membrane for each ion.

For potassium, the ion gradient for skeletal muscle fibers is large: The extracellular resting concentration K_o is 3.5 to 5.0 mM and the intracellular concentration K_i is 135 mM.

A list of abbreviations used in this chapter is given at the end of the chapter.

According to the Nernst equation, the reversal potential E_K is then

$$E_K = RT/Fz \ln([K]_o/[K]_i) \quad (10\text{-}1)$$

E_K can be easily calculated as –97 mV for the concentrations given above, a temperature of 37°C, and z = +1, the valence of charge for potassium ions. In excised human intercostal muscle fibers, the resting membrane potential is only –84 mV in both fast and slow fibers.[1] The discrepancy between the two values is based on the conductance of the resting membrane for sodium ions, which is quite small. Using the extra- and intracellular sodium concentrations of 145 and 12 mM, respectively, the reversal potential for sodium E_{Na} can be calculated to be +62 mV. As at the resting potential, the net current must be zero; also, the size of the potassium efflux must be equivalent to the sodium influx. Looking at the difference between membrane potential and reversal potential, the so-called driving force, the potassium ions have a driving force of only $|-97 - (-84)| = 13$ mV, while the sodium ions have a driving force of $|+62 - (-84)| = 146$ mV. Consequently, the conductance ratio of potassium to sodium can be calculated: 146/13 = 11, suggesting that the potassium conductance is 11 times as high as the sodium conductance, making up ~92 percent of the total membrane conductance at rest.

Therefore a reasonable prediction of the resting membrane potential E_m is possible just by solving the equation $I_K = I_{Na}$ with I = U/R and taking into account that the conductance g is the reciprocal of the resistance, g = 1/R: $E_m = (E_{Na} g_{Na} + E_K g_K)/(g_{Na} - g_K)$. The more common form of this equation was developed by Goldman:

$$E_m = RT/F \ln[([K]_o + \alpha[Na]_o)/([K]_i + \alpha[Na]_i)] \quad (10\text{-}2)$$

with $\alpha = P_{Na}/P_K$ being the ratio of the permeabilities P, which are proportional to the conductances and represent the ion flux depending on membrane potential and concentration gradient. The permeability for sodium ions is conferred by voltage-gated sodium channels that randomly open and by nonselective cation channels. The potassium channels with high permeabilities at the resting potential are discussed in the following section.

VOLTAGE-INSENSITIVE CATION CHANNELS SETTING THE RESTING POTENTIAL

The structure of voltage-insensitive channels is generally highly heterogeneous, but those structures contributing to the resting potential of striated muscle are of a limited variety. The pore-forming α subunits basically follow one of two highly conserved structural patterns (Fig. 10-1): A channel domain is formed by two transmembrane segments (2T) connected by an extracellular loop, which dips into the membrane and contains parts of the ion selectivity filter of the single channel pore (1P); or a channel domain is formed by six transmembrane segments (6T) with the loop connecting segments five and six forming parts of the single pore (1P). A functional channel consists of four channel domains, because of their similarity also called repeats I to IV. In the majority of channels, the C- and N-terminals of the α subunits are both situated intracellularly but may contain additional helical segments conveying ligand-binding properties, trafficking signals, or regulatory elements. A functional ion-conducting pore requires coassembly of four α-subunit pore loops. Additional accessory subunits called β, γ, and δ may be required for channels to function properly. These subunits modify expression, trafficking, or gating of the cation channel complex. They do not share a common structure, some having one to several transmembrane segments and others being entirely intra- or extracellular.

Some voltage-insensitive cation channels are selective for specific ions, such as potassium; others conduct more than one monovalent cation, such as potassium *and* sodium; and other cation channels are even less selective. The voltage-gated and voltage-insensitive potassium-selective channels constitute the most diverse class of ion channels with respect to activation, kinetic properties, regulation, pharmacology, and structure so far defined. They not only contribute to the resting membrane potential of cells but also play a role in volume regulation and signal transduction.

Inwardly Rectifying Potassium Channels of the $K_{ir}2.x$ Family Open at Negative Potentials

Much of the membrane conductance responsible for the resting potential of skeletal muscle fibers and other cells is due to the 2T/1P inwardly rectifying potassium channel IRK or K_{ir}, consisting of four α subunits forming a tetramer. Its pore architecture has recently been demonstrated by crystallization of the corresponding *Streptomyces lividans* channel.[2,3] $K_{ir}2.x$ channels conduct inward currents at potentials more negative than the potassium reversal potential, but they do not conduct outward currents at less negative potentials. The conductance of single channels ranges from 23 to 30 pS in symmetrical potassium solutions. Rectification in $K_{ir}2.x$ channels is caused by the binding of intracellular cations, mostly magnesium ions and the ubiquitously cytoplasmic polyamines, to their inner pore. The strong voltage dependence of channel block is associated with transport of potassium ions, which displace blocking polyamines. Therefore, at a given concentration of intracellular potassium, rectification is related to the difference between the membrane potential and the potassium equilibrium potential rather than to the membrane potential itself.[4] The strength of rectification is determined by specific amino acid residues in M2 near the cytoplasmic side of the cell, whereby a negatively charged aspartate confers strong rectification and a neutral asparagine confers weak rectification.[5] Although the N-terminal does not carry an inactivation particle, fast inactivation is conferred by spermine.

The inward-going rectifiers are encoded by the more than 15 genes of the *KCNJ* family. Several potassium channels are expressed in the sarcolemmal and T-tubular membrane of skeletal muscle (see Table 10-1). The major skeletal muscle inward-going rectifier, $K_{ir}2.1$, has a highly conserved TIGYG motif in the pore region, and the absence of the peculiar lysine residue in the N-terminal explains its pH insensitivity. The channel block by Mg^{2+}, spermine, spermidine, and putrescine may be linked to amino acid D172. The RRESEI motif situated in the C-terminal is a candidate for the observed modulation by phosphatases.[6]

In addition to its well-understood role in controlling electrogenesis, $K_{ir}2.1$ is a K^+ sensor. A small increase in extracellular K^+, such as that resulting from the activation of

Chapter 10. Ion Channels and Electrical Properties of Skeletal Muscle

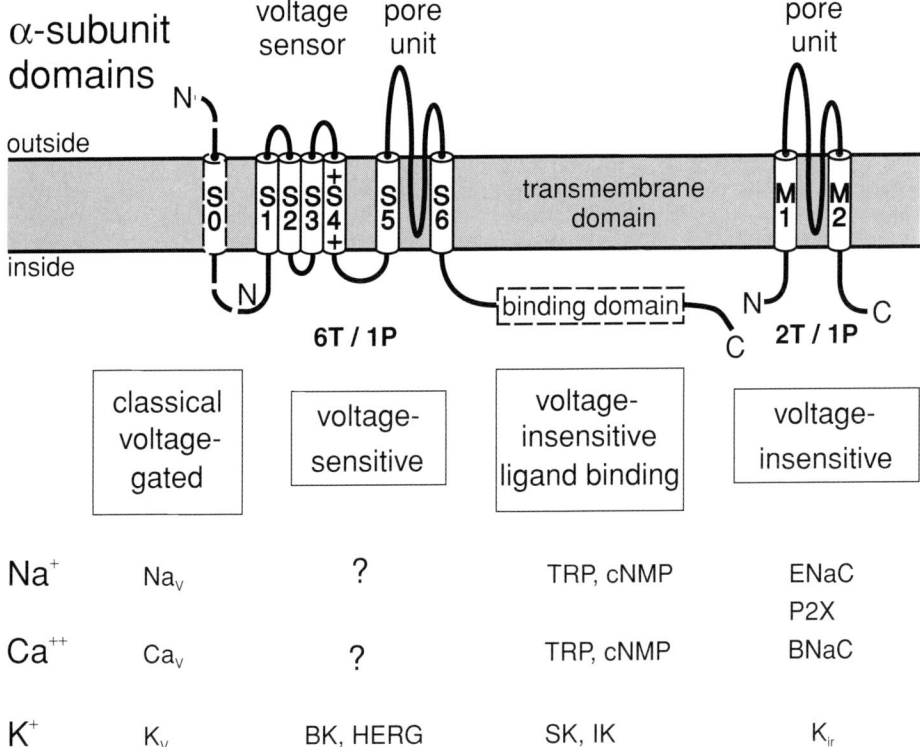

FIGURE 10-1. Diversity of domains forming cation channel α subunits. The simplest domain, typically used for inward-going rectifier potassium channel α subunits, is a pore unit (2T/1P) that consists of two transmembrane segments, M1 and M2; an extracellular loop dipping into the membrane and lining the pore; and intracellular N- and C-terminals. The transmembrane segments are thought to be α helices. All voltage-gated α subunit domains are 6T/1P domains, since they contain a four-transmembrane segment unit, S1 to S4, acting as voltage sensor and the two transmembrane pore units. S4 is the particular voltage-sensing segment that contains positive charges at each third amino acid residue. Ligand-gated cation channel α subunit domains usually possess a C-terminal binding site in addition to the 6T/1P domain. Although some ligand-gated channels—e.g., the calcium-activated SK potassium channel—contain a positively charged S4 segment, they are not voltage-sensitive at all, perhaps due to uncoupling of the sensor and activation gate. BK potassium channels possess an additional S0 segment. Not expressed in skeletal muscle but completing the classification of the α subunit domains are HERG, a potassium channel encoded by the human ether-a-go-go–related gene, which is similar to the *Drosophila* ether-a-go-go gene (eag); IK, a potassium channel with intermediate conductance; cNMP, sodium or calcium channels activated by cyclonucleotide monophosphates such as cGMP; and voltage-insensitive NaC sodium channels of epithelial cells (ENaC) and in free nerve terminals of the brain (BNaC). BNaC was later identified to conduct calcium. Not shown is another group of α subunit domains, 4T/2P, which contain four transmembrane segments and two pore units but do not occur in skeletal muscle.

calcium-activated potassium channels (see below), shifts the reversal potential for K+ toward a more positive value and thereby increases the conductance of $K_{ir}2.1$. This enhanced conductance is sufficient to overcome the depolarizing action of the nonselective cation conductance and shift the membrane potential toward more negative potentials.

Missense mutations cause Andersen syndrome, an autosomal dominant disease characterized by the clinical triad of dyskalemic periodic paralysis, ventricular ectopy, and potential dysmorphic features (see Chap. 46). Apparently the mutant channels are less functional and the remaining genetically normal channels are not able to set the resting membrane potential to the usual value. The less negative resting potential seems to enable the generation of action potentials under normal conditions; however, an additional reduction of the resting value under altered conditions may cause muscle fiber inexcitability.

Inwardly Rectifying Potassium Channels of the $K_{ir}6.x$ Family (K_{ATP}) Open at Energy Depletion

Two skeletal muscle inward-going rectifiers are activated by depletion of intracellular ATP: $K_{ir}6.1$ (or KATP1) and $K_{ir}6.2$ (or KATP2). $K_{ir}6.1$ is ubiquitous, whereas $K_{ir}6.2$ is relatively specific for pancreatic islet cells, brain, and skeletal muscle. The density of these channels in muscle is about as high as that of the voltage-gated potassium channels. Both channels interact in the skeletal muscle with the sulfhydrylurea receptor SUR2B, forming heterooctameric K_{ATP} channel complexes with a $(SUR2B-K_{ir}6.x)_4$ stoichiometry and a tetrameric pore of 76 pS in the fully open state.[7,8] K_{ATP} complexes modulate insulin secretion and are activated by MgADP, cromakalim, pinacidil, and diazoxide, and inhibited by ATP and by sulfonylureas—for example, the antidiabetic drug glibenclamide.[9]

Table 10-1. ION CHANNEL GENES EXPRESSED IN PLASMALEMMA, T TUBULES, AND SARCOPLASMIC RETICULUM OF SKELETAL MUSCLE[a]

Gene	Gene Locus	Channel Protein	Channel Properties	Significance for Muscle Function	Disease
			Voltage-Gated Potassium Channels		
KCNA1	12p13	α subunit Kv1.1	Fast activation, slow inactivation	Maybe modifies resting potential	(Episodic ataxia 1 with myokymia)
KCNA1B	3q26.1	β subunit Kvβ1.1	Acts as fast inactivation ball	Unknown if expressed	
KCNA4	11p14	α subunit Kv1.4	Fast activation, fast inactivation	Maybe modifies action potential	
KCNA7	19q13.3	α subunit Kv1.7	Fast activation, slow inactivation	Maybe modifies resting potential	
KCNA10	1p13-22	α subunit Kv1.8	Fast activation, slow inactivation		
KCNB1	20q13.2	α subunit Kv2.1	Fast activation, slow inactivation		
KCNC1	11p15.1	α subunit Kv3.1	Fast activation, no inactivation	Probably low, since activated at 0 mV	Force reduced in knockout mice
KCNC4	1p21	α subunit Kv3.4	Fast activation, fast inactivation	Maybe modifies action potential	
KCNF1	2p25	β subunit Kv5.1	Modifies Kv2.1	See Kv2.1	
KCNG1	20q13	β subunit Kv6.1			
KCNQ4	1p34	α subunit Kv7.4	Slow activation, slow inactivation	Reduce subthreshold excitability	
KCNQ5	6q14	α subunit Kv7.5	Slow activation, slow inactivation		
			Voltage-Insensitive Potassium Channels		
KCNJ1	11q24	α subunit Kir1.1 (ROMK1)	Inward-going rectifier, activated by ATP	Probably low	(Antenatal Bartter or hyperprostaglandin E syndrome, see also NKCC)
KCNJ2	17q23	α subunit Kir2.1 (IRK1)	Inward-going rectifier	Essential for membrane potential	Andersen syndrome
KCNJ8	12p11.23	α subunit Kir6.1 (K_{ATP1})	Open at ATP depletion	Perhaps maintaining resting potential at subsarcolemmal energy depletion	
KCNJ11	11p15.1	α subunit Kir6.2 (K_{ATP2})	Open at ATP depletion		(Hyperinsulinemic hypoglycemia in infants)
ABCC9	12p12.1	β subunit SUR2 of K_{ATP}	Binds ADP, ATP, and drugs	Interacts with Kir6.1 and Kir6.2	
			Calcium-Activated Potassium Channels		
KCNMA1	10q22-23	α subunit KCa1.1 of maxiK (or BK or SLO)	Voltage-sensitive	Maybe terminating bursts of action potentials, open at high intracellular calcium concentration, i.e., during contraction	Force reduced in −/− mice, abnormally broad action potentials and possible muscle weakness in Drosophila mutants
KCNN2	5q22	α subunit KCa2.2 (SK2)	Insensitive to voltage		
KCNN3	1q21	α subunit KCa2.3 (SK3)	Insensitive to voltage		Upregulated in denervated and myotonic dystrophy fibers
			Nonselective Cation Channels		
P2RX5	17p13	P2X5	Conducts calcium	Differentiation of satellite cells	
TRPV6	7q33-34	TRPV6, CaT1, ECaC2	Calcium inward-going rectifier	Refilling emptied calcium stores (ER)	
TRPM4	19q13	TRPM4	Selective to monovalent cations	Calcium-activated depolarization	
TRPM7	15q21	TRPM7	Outward-going rectifier	Protein kinase with unknown substrates	

Table 10-1 (Continued). ION CHANNEL GENES EXPRESSED IN PLASMALEMMA, T TUBULES, AND SARCOPLASMIC RETICULUM OF SKELETAL MUSCLE[a]

Gene	Gene Locus	Channel Protein	Channel Properties	Significance for Muscle Function	Disease
Voltage-Gated Sodium Channels					
SCN4A	17q23-25	α subunit $Na_v1.4$ M1, SKm1	Major sodium channel of adult muscle, TTX[b]-sensitive	Essential for action potential generation in plasmalemma and T-tubular membrane	Hyperkalemic periodic paralysis, paramyotonia congenita, potassium-aggravated myotonia, hypokalemic periodic paralysis type 2
SCN1B	19q13	β subunit Na_vbeta1	Increases current, accelerates fast inactivation	Potential influence on action potential	(Generalized epilepsy with febrile seizures plus type 1 [GEFS+1])
SCN5A	3p21	α subunit $Na_v1.5$ SKm2	Predominant in fetal muscle, TTX-insensitive	Excitability of fetal muscle	(Long-QT syndrome 3)
SCN6A= SCN7A	2q21-23	α subunit $Na_v1.6$	Probably in denervated muscle, TTX-insensitive	Excitability of denervated muscle	
Voltage-Gated Calcium Channels					
CACNA1H	16p13	$Ca_v3.2$, T-type α1H subunit	Rapid activation and inactivation, small conductance	Transient expression during fetal development	
CACNA1S	1q31-32	$Ca_v1.1$, L-type, DHP receptor, α1S subunit	Major calcium channel of adult muscle	Essential for ECC[c]	Hypokalemic periodic paralysis type 1, malignant hyperthermia 5, dysgenic mice
CACNA2D1	7q21-22	α2/δ subunit	Increases current	Unknown	
CACNB1	17q21-22	β1 subunit	Increases current	Essential for ECC	−/− mice lethal
CACNB3	12q13	β3 subunit			
CACNG1	17q24	γ subunit 1	Increases inactivation	Probably low (−/− mice normal)	
Ligand-Gated Calcium Channels					
RYR1	19q13.1	Ryanodine receptor 1	Calcium release under voltage control	Essential for ECC	Malignant hyperthermia 1, central core disease, −/− mice lethal
RYR3	15q14-15	Ryanodine receptor 3	Calcium-induced calcium release	Probably low (−/− mice normal)	
Voltage-Gated Chloride Channels					
CLCN1	7q32-qter	ClC1, highly muscle-specific	Outward rectifier, deactivating at hyperpolarization	Stabilizes membrane potential due to high conductance	Myotonia congenita Thomsen and Becker
CLCN2	3q27-28	ClC2	Slowly activating inward rectifier	Ubiquitous, reduces fiber swelling	(Idiopathic generalized epilepsy)
CLCN4	Xp22.3	ClC4	Outward rectifier, low pH_o inhibits	Subcellular localization unknown	
CLCN6	1p36	ClC6	Outward rectifier, cAMP-sensitive	Ubiquitous, ER related, role unknown	

[a] Diseases other than those affecting the skeletal muscle are given in brackets.
[b] Tetrodotoxin.
[c] Excitation-contraction coupling.

Under physiologic conditions, that is, with an intracellular ATP concentration in the millimolar range, the channels have a very low open probability. Therefore the functional role of these channels in skeletal muscle is not clear. It appears that during metabolic exhaustion, a subsarcolemmal ATP depletion can occur and open the K_{ATP} channels. Such openings could account for the increased membrane potassium conductance that has been observed.[10] Like a short circuit, the low membrane resistance would reduce membrane excitability, thereby forcing the muscle fibers to rest.[11] The membrane hypo- or inexcitability reduces the energy consumption of the muscle fibers and prevents cell death. Since $K_{ir}6.2$ mutations cause hyperinsulinemic hypoglycemia in infancy and no known muscle malfunction, the malfunction of mutant channels may be compensated by $K_{ir}6.1$.

Drugs that activate K_{ATP} channels, such as cromakalim or pinacidil, hyperpolarize the membrane and reduce its resistance in normal, not energy-depleted muscle fibers.[12] Muscle fibers that are largely depolarized and therefore inexcitable, such as fibers from patients with dyskalemic periodic paralysis, can be easily repolarized by these K_{ATP} channel activators. If the resulting increase in membrane conductance does not exceed a certain value, the fibers can become excitable and contract.[13]

Another inwardly rectifying potassium channel with the same 2T/1P α-subunit structure is activated by intracellular ATP: Kir1.1 (or ROMK1 for renal outermedullary potassium channel), which is present in many tissues, including skeletal muscle.[14] Loss-of-function mutations lead to the antenatal Bartter syndrome, or isolated kidney malfunction characterized by severe renal salt and fluid wasting.[15] Since muscle signs, if any, are secondary to the resulting hypokalemia, ROMK1 is probably insufficiently expressed in the skeletal muscle or of minor importance for it.

Calcium-Activated Potassium Channels Open at High Intracellular [Ca^{2+}]

Calcium-activated potassium channels are activated by high intracellular calcium as a result of cell activity—for example, by calcium influx through voltage-gated calcium channels or by calcium released from intracellular stores. It has been suggested that the binding of Ca^{2+} activates the channel by attenuating the inhibitory activity of the C-terminal.[16]

$K_{Ca}1.1$ is present in adult skeletal muscle and known as the large conductance (>150 pS with symmetrical high potassium concentrations) calcium-activated channel or B_K (B for big), maxi K, or SLO channel. In contrast to all other K_{Ca} channels, $K_{Ca}1.1$ possesses an additional transmembrane segment, called S0, resulting in an extracellular N-terminus. Therefore it is a 7T/1P channel. In contrast to the other K_{Ca} channels, it shows voltage dependence in addition to the calcium sensitivity[17] (Fig. 10-2). A β subunit, Kvβ hslo-β, interacts with $K_{Ca}1.1$ and markedly increases its sensitivity to intracellular calcium.[18] As the β subunit is not present in skeletal muscle, $K_{Ca}1.1$ requires a large depolarization and a high intracellular calcium concentration for channel activation, or conditions that might occur during a burst of action potentials. The hyperpolarizing effect of activation of these channels may terminate the burst and thus reduce development of muscle strength. Functional data on mammalian muscle are missing, but *Drosophila* mutants show abnormally broad action potentials and possible muscle weakness.[19,20]

$K_{Ca}2.1$, $K_{Ca}2.2$, and $K_{Ca}2.3$ are calcium-sensitive potassium channels with small potassium conductance (SK1-3; approximately 10 pS at symmetrical potassium concentrations). They possess a typical 6T/1P α-subunit structure with positive residues in S4 at almost every third amino acid, but do not show voltage-dependent gating. The various SK types are resistant to tetraethylammonium chloride; however, they differ in their affinity to gallamine, d-tubocurarine, scyllatoxin, and the bee venom apamin. $K_{Ca}2.2$ and $K_{Ca}2.3$

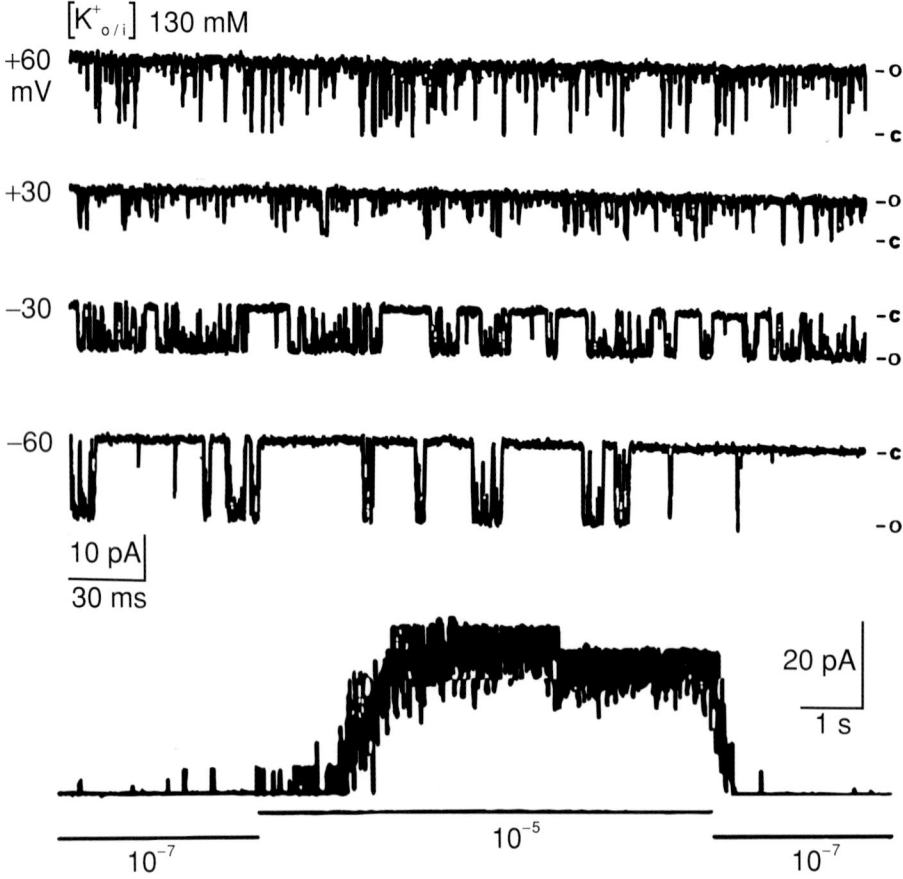

FIGURE 10-2. Single-channel recordings on membrane blebs of human skeletal muscle fibers performed in the bleb-attached mode. The upper four traces show openings and closures of single large-conductance potassium channels for various membrane potentials at symmetrical potassium solution of 130 mM. The channels are predominantly in the closed state (c) at negative potentials and open (o) at positive values, demonstrating their voltage dependence. The single-channel conductance is about 230 pS in the voltage range shown. Note the occurrence of subconductance states. The lower trace reveals the dependence of the channel-open probability on the intracellular [Ca^{2+}]: pCa varied from 7 to 5 and back to 7, justifying the term *calcium-activated potassium currents*. The inside-out patch contained seven channels. Clamp potential zero, physiologic [K$^+$]. (Modified from Lerche et al.[17] Reproduced by permission.)

are present in mature skeletal muscle, the latter at a low level, which is markedly increased in denervated and myotonic dystrophy muscle[21] and involved in the generation of the myotonia that can be blocked by apamin.[22]

Ionotropic P2X Receptors

Many types of excitatory or nonexcitatory cells contain these receptors, particularly peripheral and central neurons and smooth muscle, in cells of immune and hematopoetic origin. P2X receptor subunits are activated by ATP or other nucleotides released into the extracellular milieu. The channels are nonselective for cations, i.e., permeable to Ca^{2+}. Prolonged exposure of slowly inactivating isoforms to ligands leads to dilation of the pore, making it permeable to larger molecules. The receptor channels bear a common topology and are of 2T/1P structure with intracellular N- and C-terminals. The two transmembrane domains are connected by a large extracellular loop that contains 10 conserved cysteines. Like other ion channels, the functional channel is formed by homo- or heterooligomeric assembly of several subunits. The stoichiometry of the assembly is unknown. At least one member of the P2X receptor family, P2X5, is present on satellite cells and is a regulator of skeletal muscle differentiation.[23]

Transient Receptor Potential Channels

The transient receptor potential (TRP) channels have the classic 6TM/1P subunit structure. Neither voltage dependence nor another activation mechanism is a unifying feature. The TRPV (vanilloid receptors) subfamily includes ion channels that are involved in neuronal pain and the sensing of light and heat, osmolarity, and other stimuli. The TRPM (melastatin receptors) subfamily has potential roles in Ca^{2+}-dependent signaling, control of cell-cycle progression, division, or migration, and thermosensation. Several TRP channel proteins are known to form heteromultimers, and their electrophysiologic properties depend on the subunit composition. The multipotent phosphatidylinositol pathway is involved in most TRP regulation, but the details of this regulation are just beginning to be elucidated.

At least the following three TRP channels are expressed in skeletal muscle: TRPV6, TRPM4, and TRPM7. TRPV6 is calcium-selective, is activated by low levels of intracellular free calcium, and is inactivated by higher levels. Unlike many other TRP channels, TRPV6 displays a steeply inward rectifying current-voltage relation, passing most of its current at hyperpolarized potentials. As it is located mainly in the SR, it may coregulate calcium content of the stores. In contrast, TRPM4 is calcium-activated and selective to monovalent cations.[24] Thus, upon opening, these channels depolarize cells from their resting membrane potentials to around 0 mV, thereby raising intracellular sodium and decreasing potassium. TRPM7 is ubiquitously expressed and, uniquely among ion channels, it functions also as a protein kinase, but besides TRPM7 itself, its substrates are unknown. It exhibits a steeply outward rectifying conductance and is inhibited by intracellular magnesium at concentrations above 1 mM. Also, it allows several divalent trace metal cations such as Zn^{2+} to permeate it, which could be of significance for skeletal muscle function.[25]

VOLTAGE-GATED POTASSIUM CHANNELS MAINTAINING THE RESTING POTENTIAL

Some voltage-gated potassium channels operate in the subthreshold range of an action potential and are thought to maintain the resting potential and to modulate electrical excitability. These are mainly the fast and slowly inactivating Kv channels (for an overview of the classification and the characteristics of voltage-gated potassium channels, see the relevant section and Table 10-1).

CHLORIDE CHANNELS DO NOT CONTRIBUTE TO THE RESTING MEMBRANE POTENTIAL

In addition to potassium and sodium ions, chloride ions can also principally contribute to the resting membrane potential. The extended Goldman equation includes the chloride system, but this part of the equation can be neglected for skeletal muscle because the chloride gradient results from simple *passive* distribution in response to the resting membrane potential. This results from the very high chloride conductance, making up ~80 percent of the total membrane conductance at rest. Therefore the chloride reversal potential is equal to the resting potential, and the simplification made in Eq. (10-2) is permissible. Even though chloride ions do not set the resting membrane potential of muscle fibers, their membrane conductance reduces fast potential deviations and thus stabilizes the resting value (see also "ClC1, the major chloride channel of skeletal muscle").

ACTIVE ION TRANSPORT THROUGH THE SODIUM-POTASSIUM PUMP

The Pump Mechanism and Its Effect on Ion Gradients

The sodium-potassium pump, also called the sodium-potassium ATPase or simply the sodium pump, is a membrane-bound protein that requires sodium for phosphorylation and potassium for dephosphorylation. By using the energy from the hydrolysis of one molecule of adenosine triphosphate (ATP), the sodium pump extrudes three sodium ions in exchange for the uptake of two potassium ions. The mechanism of pumping is called "ping-pong" because the transport of sodium and potassium is accomplished by independent half-reactions that occur sequentially (Fig. 10-3). Under physiologic conditions, the pump produces a positive (outward) current that proportionally increases with membrane depolarization until it becomes saturated at a membrane potential of about zero. On the other hand, hyperpolarizations of over −160 mV will reverse the chemical reaction; that is, the pump works as an ATP-synthetase, permitting sodium entry and K^+ extrusion (for review, see Carlsen and Villarin[26]).

The Pump's Electrical Contribution to the Resting Potential

The assymetrical flow of charges effected by the sodium pump contributes directly to the resting membrane potential. We can calculate the amplitude of this contribution by first

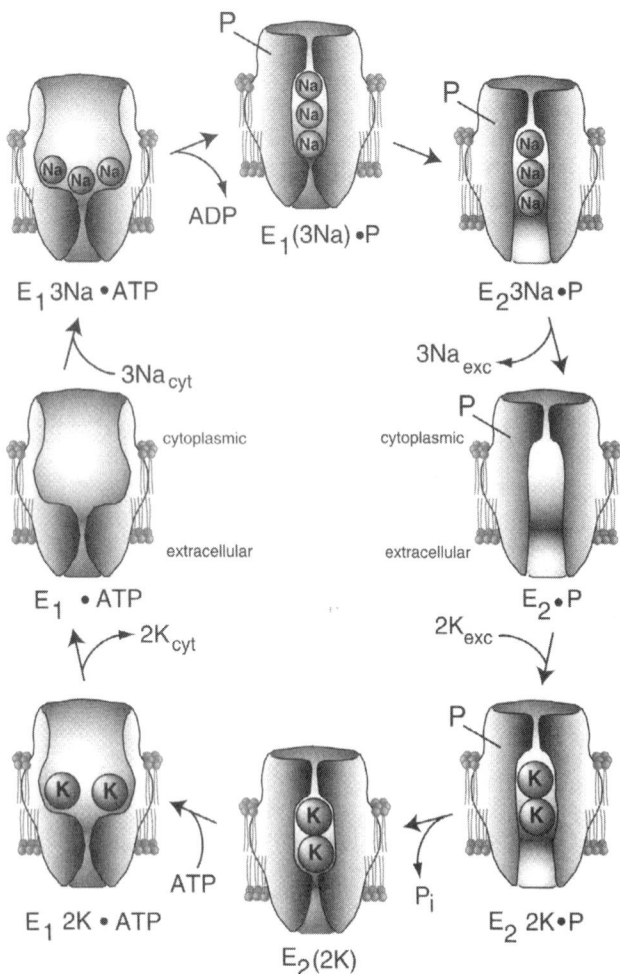

FIGURE 10-3. Ping-pong scheme for pumping cycle of the sodium-potassium pump. Cycle begins at top left, with the enzyme in the form $E_1 3Na \cdot ATP$. (Note that in this rendering the extracellular side is below each enzyme molecule and the cytoplasmic side above.) After a series of reactions, as described in the text, the enzyme is in the form $E_1 \cdot ATP$ (*middle, left*). Three sodium ions from inside the cell enter the pump, and the cycle begins again. (*Adapted from Läuger.[27] Reproduced by permission.*)

assuming that the muscle fiber is at steady state, and we ignore chloride by supposing that it is passively distributed. Since the resting sodium and potassium currents must be compensated by the active pump currents for the two ions, the resting membrane potential is given not by the Goldman equation, but rather by

$$V_m = RT/F \ln[(r [K^+]_e + \alpha [Na^+]_e)/(r [K^+]_i + \alpha [Na^+]_i)] \quad (10\text{-}3)$$

with the permeability ratio $\alpha = P_{Na}/P_K$ and electrogenicity rate $r = 1.5$ (transport ratio of three sodium to two potassium ions). Under physiologic conditions ($\alpha = 0.01$, 37°C), the resting membrane potential is about 3 mV more negative due to pump activity than it would be without. Under pathologic conditions—for example, an increased sodium permeability with α approaching 1—the pump contributes up to 11 mV to the membrane potential. In the T-tubular system of skeletal muscle, the pump activity may reduce the potassium con-

centration to such an extent that the potassium permeability is reduced, α increased, and thus the pump contribution high.[28] This hyperpolarizing effect is abolished as soon as T-tubular potassium is depleted to such an extent that it cannot be bound by the pump, which then becomes unable to cycle.

The ATPase Subunits

The Na^+,K^+-ATPase is an oligomer composed of two major polypeptides, the α and the β subunits (for review, see Blanco and Mercer[29]). The former, a protein containing 10 transmembrane segments, is responsible for the catalytic and transport properties of the enzyme and contains binding sites for cations, ATP, and the inhibitor ouabain (Fig. 10-4). The β subunit, a small polypeptide that crosses the membrane once, is essential for the normal activity of the enzyme and conveys the sodium affinity to the enzyme. In addition, in vertebrate cells, the β subunit may act as a chaperone, stabilizing the correct folding of the α-polypeptide to facilitate its delivery to the plasma membrane. A third protein, a γ subunit possessing a single membrane domain, seems to modify the voltage dependence of potassium activation; it is the substrate for kinases and is tissue-specifically spliced.[30]

Of the many isoforms, $\alpha 1$ in association with the $\beta 1$ subunit is found in nearly every tissue, including skeletal muscle. The $\alpha 2/\beta 2$ complex predominates in skeletal muscle.[31,32] A subunit specifically expressed in skeletal muscle and at a much lower level in heart is $\beta 4$.[33] It exhibits a cellular location and its significance has not yet been clarified.

Patients with McArdle disease exhibit lower levels of 3H-ouabain-binding sites than do control subjects and therefore higher peak increases in plasma potassium in response to exercise.[34] It is not specified whether the decreased exercise capacity is related to a reduction of $\alpha 1$ or $\alpha 2$ subunits. A completely different disease, familial hemiplegic migraine type 2, is caused by loss-of-function mutations in the $\alpha 2$ subunit.[35]

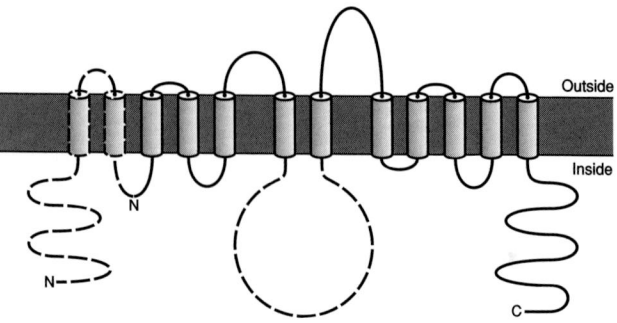

FIGURE 10-4. Scheme of the membrane topology of the α subunits of ion transporters. The protein contains 10 or 12 transmembrane segments, which form α helices. The sodium pump α subunits contain 10 segments; their long intracellular loop possesses the catalytic and transport units of the enzyme and the binding sites for the cations, ATP, and the inhibitor ouabain. The cation-chloride cotransporters NKCC and KCC contain 12 transmembrane segments. They are driven by the sodium gradient established by the sodium pump. They need neither a catalytic unit nor ATP binding sites, and the intracellular loop connecting segments 6 and 7 is short.

Table 10-2. ION TRANSPORTER GENES EXPRESSED IN THE PLASMALEMMAL OR T-TUBULAR MEMBRANE OF SKELETAL MUSCLE[a]

Gene	Gene Locus	Transporter Protein	Transporter Properties	Significance for Muscle Function	Disease
		ATPases			
ATP1A1	1p13	Na$^+$/K$^+$ pump α1 subunit	Transport and catalytic units, bind cations, ATP, and ouabain	Ubiquitous	Ouabain binding sites reduced in McArdle's disease, not specified if α1 or α2
ATP1A2	1q21-23	Na$^+$/K$^+$ pump α2 subunit		Predominates in brain and skeletal muscle	(Loss-of-function mutations cause familial hemiplegic migraine type 2)
ATP1B1	1q22-25	Na$^+$/K$^+$ pump β1 subunit	Na$^+$ affinity, chaperone	Ubiquitous	
ATP1B2	17p13	Na$^+$/K$^+$ pump β2 subunit		Predominates in skeletal muscle	
ATP1B4	Xq24	X/K$^+$ pump β4 subunit		Muscle-specific, unknown function	
FXYD1	19q13	PLM, phospholemman precursor, reacts to insulin, adrenalin	Induces chloride current at hyperpolarization	Predominates in muscle and heart, contraction	
FXYD2	11q23	ATP1G1, Na$^+$/K$^+$ pump γ1 subunit	Involved in ouabain binding	Highly expressed in kidney, muscle	(Renal hypomagnesemia type 2)
		Anion-Anion Exchanger			
SLC4A2	7q35-36	Cl$^-$/HCO$_3^-$ exchange	Electroneutral	Wide distribution	
SLC4A3, int CGG repeat	2q36	Cl$^-$/HCO$_3^-$ exchange	Electroneutral	Cardiac and brain splice variants	
		Cation-Anion Exchanger			
SLC4A4, SLC4A5	4q21	Na$^+$/HCO$_3^-$ exchange, NBC1, NBC2	Electroneutral cotransport	Expression level highest in kidney	(Proximal, renal tubular acidosis)
		Cation-Cation Exchanger			
SLC8A1	2p23-22	NCX1, Na$^+$/Ca^{++} exchange	Extrudes calcium from myoplasm	In oxidative fibers	
SLC8A3	14q24.1	NCX3, Na$^+$/Ca^{++} exchange	Extrudes calcium from myoplasm	In fast glycolytic (type 2B) fibers	
SLC9A6	Xq26.3	NHE6, Na$^+$/H$^+$ exchange, in Northern highest in muscle, brain	Electroneutral transport	Acid-activated sodium uptake into mitochondria	
SLC12A1	15q15-21	NKCC2, Na$^+$/K$^+$/2Cl$^-$ cotransport	Electroneutral		(Antenatal Bartter or hyperprostaglandin E syndrome, see also Kir1.1)
SLC12A2	5q23.3	NKCC1, Na$^+$/K$^+$/2Cl$^-$ cotransport	Electroneutral		
SLC12A4	16q22	KCC1, K$^+$/Cl$^-$ cotransport	Electroneutral	Cell volume regulation	
SLC12A5	20q13.12	KCC2, "neuronal" K$^+$/Cl$^-$ cotransport	Active under isotonic conditions	High expression in muscle, lung	(Renal tubular acidosis)
SLC12A7	5p15.33	KCC4, electroneutral K$^+$/Cl$^-$ cotransport	Active under hypotonic conditions	Highly expressed in muscle	
SLC24A1	15	NCKX1, Na$^+$/K$^+$/Ca^{++} exchange	4Na$^+$ against 1K$^+$ and 1Ca^{++}, dependent on Na$^+$ and K$^+$		
SLC24A3	20	NCKX3, Na$^+$/K$^+$/Ca^{++} exchange			
CA3	8q13-22	Carboanhydrase type 3	H$^+$ transfer		

[a]Diseases other than those affecting the skeletal muscle are given in parentheses.

Acute and Long-Term Regulation of the Sodium Pump

As extracellular potassium is required for pump cycling, tubular potassium depletion blocks the sodium pump, whereas intracellular sodium ions activate it. Exercise translocates preexisting α2/β1 from intracellular stores to the plasma membrane in skeletal muscle within 20 s.[31] This results in the recruitment of additional functional sodium pumps to the cell surface and increased Na^+,K^+-ATPase activity, an effect with a half-life of approximately 20 min.[36] Hormones can elicit their action by directly affecting the pump rate and the number of pump sites and also by modulating the expression of a particular isoform.[37] For example, insulin leads to the same rapid translocation as described for exercise. Long-term alteration of thyroid hormone levels change the amount of α2 mRNA and protein, with a free T4 index giving the highest positive correlation. Hypothyroidism decreases and hyperthyroidism increases 3H-ouabain-binding sites,[38] and these changes may account for the variations in digitalis sensitivity associated with thyroid disorders. Long-term administration of glucocorticoids increases the amount of α2 and β1 mRNA and protein. Chronic hypokalemia, such as that due to potassium-wasting diuretics administered to human individuals, reduces the number of 3H-ouabain-binding sites,[39] probably by α2 and β1 downregulation. In rat muscle, potassium deprivation over 10 days reduces α2 and β2 proteins, particularly in glycolytic fibers.[40]

THE SODIUM-CALCIUM EXCHANGERS, NCX

NCX1 is the primary cardiac mechanism by which calcium is extruded from the cell into the T-tubular system during relaxation. The exchange of 3 Na^+ for 1 Ca^{2+} is powered by the sodium pump. Sodium/calcium exchangers are regulated by extracellular sodium and intracellular calcium concentrations; depending on these, the direction of exchange is reversible (extracellular Ca^{2+} exchanging for intracellular Na^+). NCX proteins consist of 12 membrane-spanning segments, but disulfide bond analysis and cysteine mutagenesis coupled with accessibility studies indicate that nine transmembrane segments are α helices, while the other structures are α repeat regions forming nonhelical reentrant loops.[41] In that model, the pore through which the cations pass is lined by S2, S3, S7, and S8.

NCX1 and NCX3 expression is developmentally regulated as studied in rat muscle.[42] NCX1 peaks shortly after birth, while NCX3 is expressed at low quantities at birth but then increases rapidly during the first weeks of life. NCX2 is abundantly expressed in skeletal muscle.[43] The existence of multiple exchanger isoforms may participate in regulation of calcium homeostasis.

THE CATION-CHLORIDE COTRANSPORTERS

Cation-chloride cotransporters are putative homodimers,[44] each monomer consisting of 10 to 12 transmembrane segments (Fig. 10-4). They mediate the translocation of ions (H^+, Ca^{2+}, Cl^-, and others), and the majority is driven by the sodium gradient established by the sodium pump. Transmembrane domains T3 to T12 are homologous to the large amino acid permease domain. Amino- and carboxyl-terminal domains are located intracellularly, are subject to phosphorylation by protein kinases, and are involved in the regulation of cotransport activity. T2 may possess several splice variants and contributes to ion affinity.[45]

The Sodium-Potassium-Chloride Cotransporter

$Na^+/K^+/2Cl^-$ cotransporters mediate the electroneutral transport of 1 Na^+, 1 K^+, and 2 Cl^- ions across the membrane. There are two closely related genes encoding these cotransporters: NKCC1, often referred to as the secretory $Na^+/K^+/2Cl^-$ cotransporter because of its expression in many secretory epithelia, and NKCC2, the absorptive $Na^+/K^+/2Cl^-$ cotransporter, because of the apical cotransport in the renal thick ascending limb. Both have a 12-transmembrane-segment structure. NKCC1 makes a major contribution to the volume-regulatory potassium uptake induced by hyperosmolarity. It reacts upon changes of intracellular chloride[46] and hypertonicity.[47] NKCC2 loss-of-function mutations cause the antenatal Bartter syndrome, also called hyperprostaglandin E syndrome, which can also result from loss-of-function mutations in Kir1.1. Although the expression rate in skeletal muscle is low, NKCCs are supposed to modulate the bistability of the resting membrane potential of skeletal muscle (see "Bistability of the Resting Membrane Potential," below).

The Potassium-Chloride Cotransporters

KCC1 and KCC3 are expressed in skeletal muscle.[48,49] The relatively wide expression pattern in brain, heart, and the urogenital and digestive tracts indicates a housekeeping role, probably in cell volume regulation. These transporters consist of 12 membrane-spanning segments, a large extracellular loop with potential N-glycosylation sites, and cytoplasmic N- and C-terminal regions with phosphorylation sites. Dephosphorylation activates KCC1 cotransporters, while phosphorylation inactivates them under isotonic conditions (for review, see Delpire and Mount[50]). KCC3 is activated by cell swelling.[51] The chloride gradient is important for the activity.[52] The KCC3 knockout mouse shows abnormal gait already within the first days after birth.[50] These mice present with muscle weakness and only partially myelinated peripheral nerves, comparable to a sensorimotor neuropathy.

BISTABILITY OF THE RESTING MEMBRANE POTENTIAL

The nonlinear properties of the inwardly rectifying potassium channel, $K_{ir}2.1$, can lead to an unstable membrane potential. In particular, a reduction of the extracellular potassium concentration from normal to subnormal values results in either hyperpolarization or depolarization of the fiber, as the current-voltage relationship of $K_{ir}2.1$ is extremely flat under this condition. Transitions between two polarization levels can occur.[53] The more negative polarization depends on the reversal potential E_K, which is large at low extracellular potassium; the less negative polarization level follows the potassium conductance, which is small at low extracellular potassium. If depolarized, the membrane will respond to an increase in extracellular potassium with repolarization because of an increase in potassium conductance, although the reversal potential simultaneously shifts toward less negative values.

Hypertonicity is supposed to support membrane depolarization by enhancing chloride import through the $Na^+/K^+/2Cl^-$ cotransporter and to alter the bistable behavior of mammalian muscle fibers.[54] Addition of bumetanide, a potent inhibitor of the $Na^+/K^+/2Cl^-$ and other cotransporters, and of anthracene-9-carboxylic acid, a blocker of chloride channels, favors membrane hyperpolarization, particularly under hypertonic conditions. $BaCl_2$ or temperature reduction from 35 to 27°C induces depolarization of fibers that are originally hyperpolarized.

PASSIVE ELECTRICAL PROPERTIES OF THE MEMBRANE

A single striated muscle fiber may be approximated by a cylindrical cell of very great length. In this case steady current will flow axially through the conductive myoplasm and exit through various conductive pathways of the membrane systems into the extracellular space. The density of the axial myoplasmic current decreases with increasing distance from the source of excitation because the current has progressively more conductive pathways by which to exit the fiber. If the cell membranes were perfect capacitors with no leakage resistance, the axial current density would be constant and independent of distance. Cell membranes are leaky, however, and as one moves away from the current source, the total membrane resistance decreases inversely with distance from the source while the total axial resistance increases in proportion to the distance from the source. At some distance these two resistances are equal. This distance is referred to as the *space constant*, denoted by the Greek letter lambda. For the simple one-dimensional case considered here, the spatial decrement of the axial current declines in proportion to $e^{-x/\lambda}$, where x is the distance from the current source. In human muscle, λ is of the order of 2 to 2.5 mm.[55]

Specific Membrane Conductance and Steady-State Voltage-Current Density Relationship

The steady-state voltage-current density relationship can be determined by use of three microelectrodes or by sucrose or Vaseline gap in standard solution. The slope of this relationship reflects the total membrane conductance at rest, G_m, which is about 170 $\mu S/cm^2$ at 37°C at the resting potential.[1] Measured in chloride-free bathing solution, the membrane conductance is reduced to approximately the membrane potassium conductance at rest, G_K, of about 40 $\mu S/cm^2$ at the resting potential.[1] The difference of the conductances in chloride-containing and chloride-free solutions is identical with the resting chloride conductance, G_{Cl}. It is about 80 percent of the total membrane conductance of skeletal muscle.

Specific Membrane Resistance and Capacitance— Causes of the Signal Loss over Distance

The membrane potential shifts associated with turning on a current source depend on the capacitative properties of the cell membranes, in particular their time constant, τ_m, which is equal to the product $R_m \cdot C_m$, where R_m is the specific membrane resistance (Ω/cm^2) and C_m is the specific membrane capacitance (F/cm^2). The spreading velocity of the gradual progression of the charging process is given by the approximate relation $v = 2\lambda/\tau_m$.[56]

In human intercostal and quadriceps muscle at rest, R_m is 6.900 Ω/cm^2 and C_m is 3.6 $\mu F/cm^2$.[57] With $\lambda \sim 2.5$ mm as stated above, τ_m is about 25 ms and $v \sim 0.2$ mm/ms. Thus, it takes 10 ms for a subthreshold signal to propagate 2 mm. Such a slow propagation velocity can be found only in curarized muscle, where the end plate potential in response to nerve stimulation is reduced below threshold for initiating propagating action potentials. Under these circumstances, the end plate potential spreads only a few millimeters along the fiber and takes from 5 to 15 ms to reach its peak at these distances from an end plate focus.[58] Because such a slow signal spreading velocity is unrealistic, it is clear that another mechanism for transmission must be present; that is, action potentials must be elicitable in the T-tubular system also.

The Action Potential—The Regenerative 1-0 Bit of Signal Transduction

Motor neuron activity is transmitted to skeletal muscle in the neuromuscular junction, thus generating an all-or-nothing signal, the action potential. It propagates along the surface membrane and also into the transverse tubular system—a set of membrane invaginations projecting deep into the cell. Thus an even distribution of the impulse is warranted (see Chaps. 11, 15, and 16). The ionic basis of the propagated action potential in muscle is similar to that in nerve; action potentials in both tissues result from the presence of time- and voltage-dependent membrane conductances to sodium and potassium ions, as first described by Hodgkin and Huxley for the squid giant axon.[59] In the meantime, the "particles" producing these conductances have been identified as integral membrane proteins called sodium channels and potassium channels.

CHARACTERISTICS OF THE SKELETAL MUSCLE ACTION POTENTIAL

The condition for initiating an action potential is that the net membrane current be inward, in the direction that results in further depolarization and further activation of sodium channels. The potential at which this condition is reached is termed the *threshold potential* and is, under normal conditions, always exceeded by the end plate potential. The upstroke of the action potential is mediated by opening of the voltage-gated sodium channels, which passively conduct a fast sodium inward current in a feedforward mechanism along both the electrical and concentration gradients. Due to the resulting high conductance of the membrane for sodium ions, the membrane potential suddenly depolarizes from the resting value of −84 mV to approximately +25 mV. Immediate repolarization of the membrane to the highly negative resting value is made possible by fast inactivation of the sodium channels, resulting in the usual predominance of the membrane conductance for potassium ions, which may be further supported by the opening of additional potassium channels, called delayed potassium rectifier channels. Specifically in skeletal muscle, repolarization is enforced by a high chloride conductance that buffers the resting membrane potential (Fig. 10-5). After an action potential, the membrane is inexcitable for a short period of time, the so-called refractory period, determined by the kinetics of recovery from inactivation.

CURRENTS CONDUCTED DURING THE ACTION POTENTIAL

The quantitative description of the ionic currents underlying the action potential is derived from experiments in which the membrane potential (V) is electronically controlled ("voltage clamp") and the currents elicited by step changes in V are measured. Ionic currents measured under voltage clamp consist of a rapidly rising inward current carried by sodium and a slower outward current carried by potassium. The success of a voltage-clamp analysis of sodium and potassium currents was first demonstrated by Hodgkin and Huxley,[59] who developed mathematical equations that reproduced the main features of the action potential. The Hodgkin-Huxley equations formed the basis for all kinetic analyses in muscle. The basic equations for sodium and potassium currents, I_{Na} and I_K, for the squid axon are as follows:

$$I_{Na} = \underline{G}_{Na}\, m^3 h\, (V - V_{Na}) \qquad (10\text{-}4)$$

$$I_K = \underline{G}_K\, n^4\, (V - V_K) \qquad (10\text{-}5)$$

where $\underline{G}_{Na}$ and $\underline{G}_K$ are maximum conductances for sodium and potassium and n, m, and h are voltage-dependent probability factors that change exponentially in time with a step change in voltage. The values of n and m are larger at depolarized potentials and describe the increases in I_{Na} and I_K caused by depolarization, while h decreases with depolarization and describes the decline in I_{Na}, called inactivation, that follows the initial increase. Hodgkin and Huxley assumed that inactivation was voltage-dependent and independent of the channel activation process. However, later experiments, first using gating-current measurements[60-62] and then confirmed by single-channel measurements,[63] indicated that sodium channels must undergo several transitions before inactivation begins.

Gating currents are generated by the movement of the voltage sensor in response to membrane depolarization. This movement drives the conformational change in the protein that results in channel activation. Early work on gating currents by Armstrong and Bezanilla[61] showed that, during membrane depolarization, the gating charge became immobilized, or stuck, in the open configuration. This charge immobilization had kinetics identical to those of channel inactivation, suggesting a relationship between the two phenomena.

VOLTAGE-GATED ION CHANNELS ESSENTIAL FOR THE ACTION POTENTIAL

Voltage-gated cation channels have at least one open state and two closed states, one from which the channel can directly be activated (i.e., from the resting state) and one from which it cannot (the inactivated state). This implies that there are at least two gates regulating the opening of the pore, an activation and an inactivation gate, both of which are usually mediated by the α subunit (Fig. 10-6). Activation results from depolarization-induced movements of the highly charged and conserved α-helical S4 segments, and other conformational changes of the protein lead to the opening of the ion-conducting pore. The size and shape of the hydrophobic residues between the positive charges are equally important for the ability of S4 to move.[64] As positive charges are shifted from the intracellular to the extracellular space, a so-called gating current can be measured if the much larger current through the ion-conducting pore is blocked.

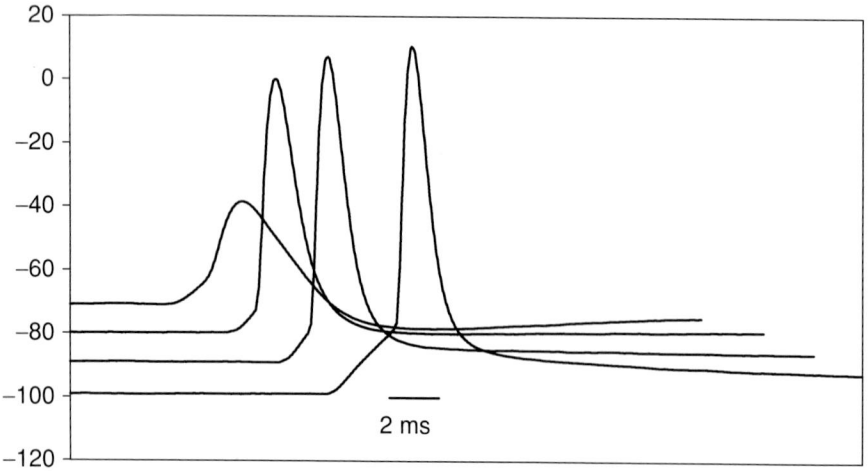

FIGURE 10-5. Action potentials of an excised human skeletal muscle fiber bathed in normal extracellular Bretag's solution containing 3.5 mM potassium. The various potentials from which the action potentials were elicited by a depolarizing step were held by constant current. The zero-current potential was −80 mV. Note that this resting value was reached at the end of the action potential.

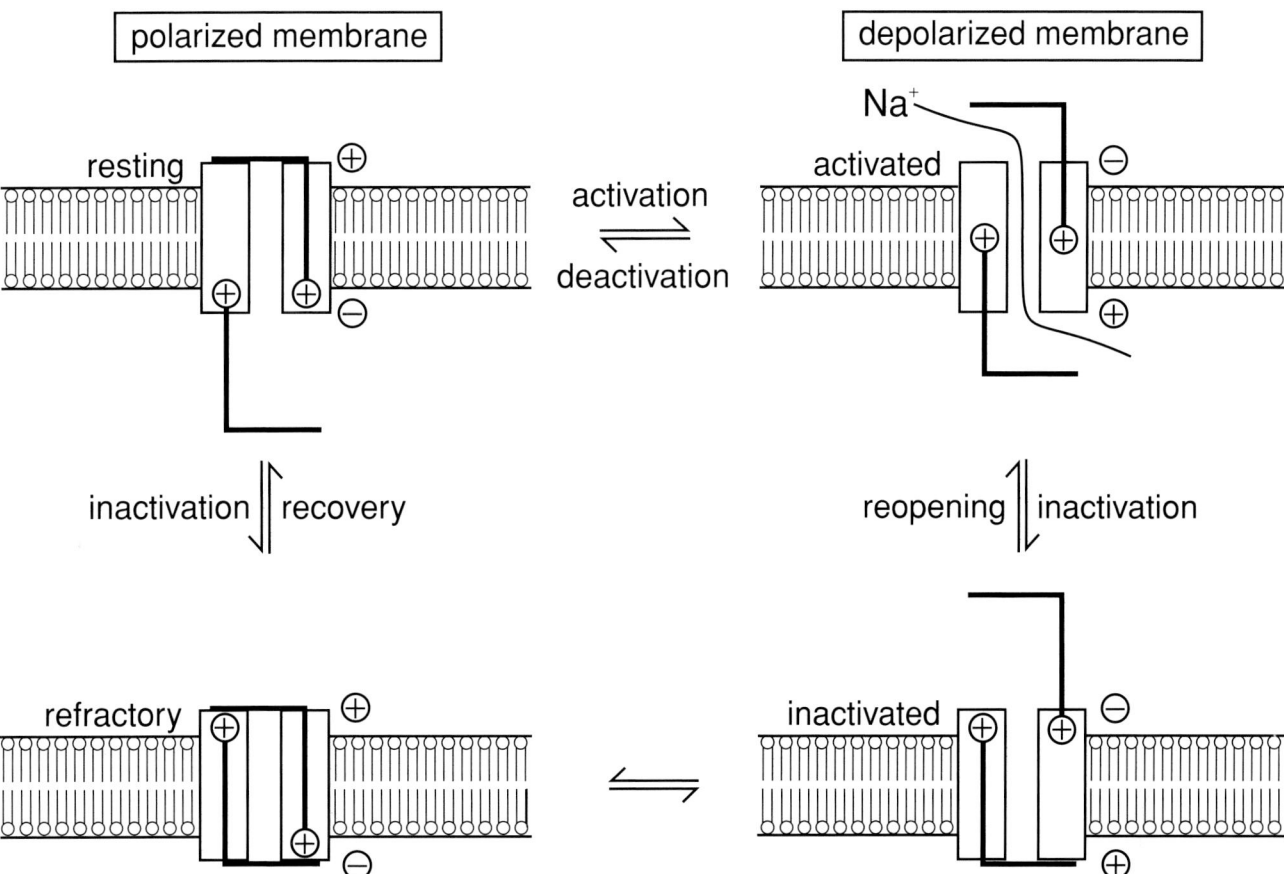

FIGURE 10-6. Scheme of the four potential sodium channel states. The channel opens rapidly upon fast depolarization and then closes to an inactivated (closed) state, from which it reopens very rarely. Repolarization of the membrane leads to recovery from inactivation via a refractory closed state. Activation is again possible from the resting state. There are probably more than one open and at least two inactivated (fast and slow) states (*not shown*). Note that transition from the resting to the inactivated state is also possible without channel opening, particularly during slow depolarization (so-called accommodation).

While activation is a voltage- and time-dependent process, inactivation and the recovery from the inactivated state are dependent on time and voltage. Voltage-gated channels usually display two modes of inactivation, fast and slow. These nonconducting inactivated states are probably mediated by different molecular mechanisms. Fast inactivation describes the rapid and complete decay of currents observed in response to short (millisecond) depolarizations. Slow inactivation occurs when cells are depolarized for seconds or minutes. Recovery from inactivation takes place at membrane repolarization on similar time scales as inactivation itself.

The Voltage-Gated Sodium Channel and Its Regenerative Current

Voltage-gated sodium channels are membrane-spanning proteins responsible for the generation of action potentials in nerve and muscle cells. Membrane depolarization causes a conformational change, called activation, from the resting, closed channel state to the open, ion-conducting state, which is associated with further membrane depolarization (upstroke of the action potential). The channel's intrinsic fast inactivation, which closes the channel within 1 ms, leads to membrane repolarization (downstroke). The precise control of opening and closing of the sodium channel is necessary for the regulation of an action potential and the excitability of nerve and muscle cells.

The sodium channel complex of adult (innervated) skeletal muscle consists of a tissue-specific α subunit, Nav1.4, and a ubiquitously expressed β1 subunit with modifying effects. The α subunit is a tetramic assembly of a series of six transmembrane amphipathic α-helical segments, numbered S1 to S6, connected by both intracellular and extracellular loops, the interlinkers (Fig. 10-7). It contains the ion-conducting pore and determines the main characteristics of the cation channel complex, conveying ion selectivity, voltage sensitivity (S4 segments), pharmacology, and binding characteristics for endogenous and exogenous ligands. Of the 12 genes known to encode four-domain α subunits of voltage-gated sodium channels, *SCN4A* (Table 10-1) is exclusively expressed in the sarcolemmal and the T-tubular membrane. The primary sequence of the channel protein of skeletal muscle is about 200 amino acids shorter than others expressed in brain and heart.

The voltage-sensing part. Of the six transmembrane segments, S1 to S4 are considered to form the voltage-sensing part and S5 and S6 the pore region of the channel.

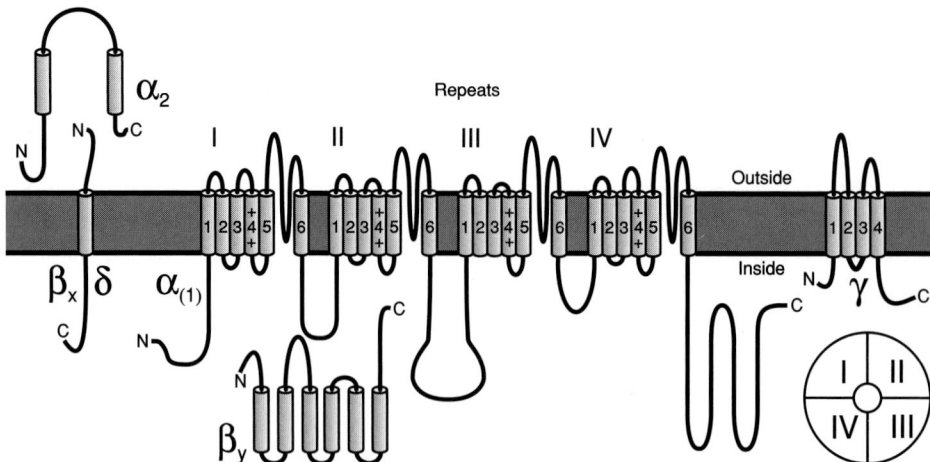

FIGURE 10-7. Scheme of the membrane topology of the voltage-gated cation channels. The $\alpha_{(1)}$ subunit consists of four repeated domains of six transmembrane segments each, including the voltage-sensor unit. When inserted in the membrane, the four domains fold to generate a central pore, as schematically indicated on the right-hand bottom of the figure. The four domains are encoded by a single sodium (or calcium) channel gene, whereas potassium channel genes code for only one domain, so that the channel α subunit is a homotetramer or a heterotetramer if the products of different channel genes assemble. Auxilliary subunits α_2/δ, β_1 to β_n, and γ are optional intracellular, transmembrane, or extracellular proteins. Intracellular β subunits bind to the N- or C-terminal or to an intracellular loop. α_2 is a calcium channel subunit that was misnamed: It was originally thought to possess an ion-conducting pore, as expression in cells devoid of functional calcium channels resulted in an appreciable calcium current. However, this phenomenon can be explained by the drastic increase in expression of endogenous $\alpha_{(1)}$ subunits by coexpression of the α_2/δ subunit.

The S4 segments are characterized by four to eight positively charged residues at every third position (Figs. 10-7 and 10-8). As no other segments carry so many charges, they are the actual sensors of the membrane voltage. Reduction of the steepness of the voltage dependence of activation as a result of replacing the positive charges with neutral or negatively charged residues[65] and microscopic observation of state-dependent localization of residues labeled with fluorescent dyes or antibodies have supported the voltage-sensor hypothesis.[66] Previously the S4 segments were proposed to move in a spiral path ("sliding helix" or "helical screw" model) outward through "canaliculi" of the channel protein, the outer charges becoming exposed on the cell surface while the inner charges become buried in the membrane during activation.[67] Recent evidence suggests a 180-degree rotation of the S4 helices, associated with a slight tilt rather than an outward movement.[68]

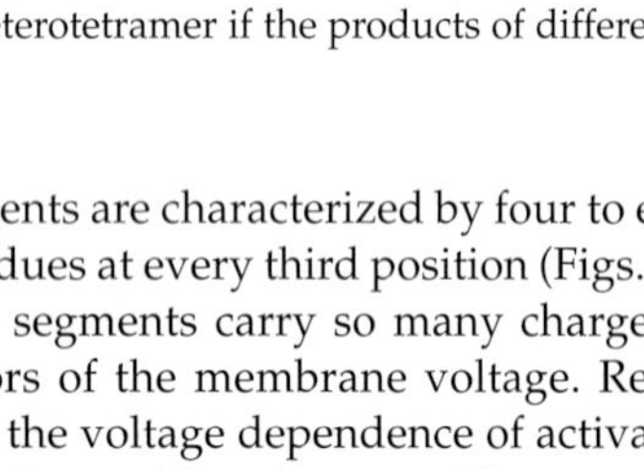

The pore-determining part and the selectivity filter. Segments S5 to S6 surround the ion-conducting pore. Parts of the extracellular S5 to S6 interlinkers dip into the membrane and line the outer vestibule of the pore, thereby forming the selectivity filter. Specific negative charges determine the selectivity for a cation. The permeability of an ion relative to sodium can be measured by substituting for sodium in the external fluid and measuring the change in the reversal potential for current through sodium channels. Measured in this way in skeletal muscle, Li^+ is nearly as permeant as sodium.[71]

Channel activation and deactivation. Membrane depolarization causes sodium channel activation in a positive feedback mechanism along the electrochemical gradient. The channel's intrinsic inactivation occurs within 1 to 2 ms (Fig. 10-9A and B) and leads under unclamped (i.e., natural) conditions to repolarization of the membrane even in the absence of voltage-gated (e.g., delayed) rectifier potassium channels. In the inactivated state, the channel is refractory. The duration of this period of time is regulated by the kinetics of recovery of the channels from inactivation.

Immediate repolarization of the membrane prior to the beginning of inactivation deactivates the channels (i.e., reverse activation). The channel enters the closed state as soon as the fastest S4 segment moves back to its resting position. If not all voltage sensors move back, a variety of closed states can be generated. Slowly inactivating potassium channels will undergo the process of deactivation during the repolarizing phase of the action potential because they are not inactivated at that time. In contrast, voltage-gated sodium channels are usually not deactivated, since they inactivate so rapidly (Fig. 10-9A, C, and E).

FIGURE 10-8. A three-dimensional representation of the voltage-gated sodium channel, based on images published by Sato et al.[69] and adapted from Catterall.[70] The dashed line inserted in the top view of the channel shows the position at which the cross section was taken. The cross section shows the central ion-conducting pore and its intracellular and extracellular connections to the bathing medium (1 to 3 and 2 to 4 via the central pore). Note the canaliculi containing the S4 segments (1 to 3, and 2 to 4, directly), which move and rotate during activation, and their connections to the central pore.

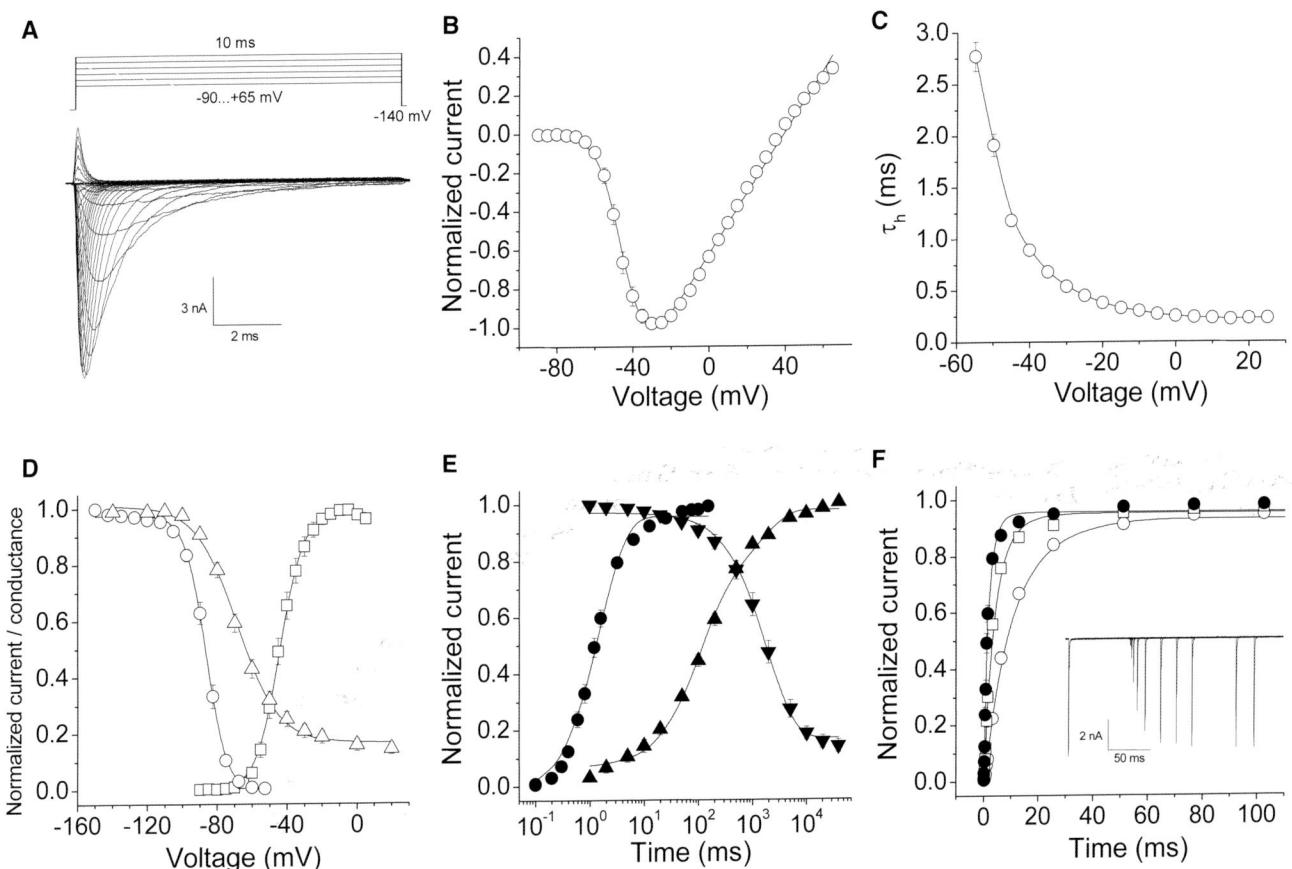

FIGURE 10-9. Whole-cell recordings of sodium currents on HEK cells (transiently or permanently) expressing human Nav1.4 cDNA. A. Sodium currents elicited by a family of depolarizations recorded from tsA201 cells expressing skeletal muscle sodium channel α subunit (bottom) and experimental protocol applied (top). B. Corresponding peak current-voltage relationships. C. Voltage dependence of fast inactivation time constants (τ_h) obtained by a fit of current decay with a monoexponential function. D. Conductance-voltage relationships (open squares); steady-state fast inactivation (open circles) determined from a holding potential of −150 mV using a series of 300-ms prepulses from −150 to −45 mV in 7.5-mV increments prior to the test pulse to −20 mV; cumulative steady-state slow inactivation (open upward-pointing triangles) determined from a holding potential of −140 mV using a series of 30-s prepulses from −140 to +20 mV; channels were let to recover from fast inactivation for 20 ms at −140 mV prior to the test pulse to −20 mV. For all the protocols presented, obtained data were normalized to the maximum and were fit with a Boltzmann function. E. Recovery from fast inactivation (closed circles) determined by a 100-ms depolarization to −20 mV followed by a variable-duration return to the holding potential and a short depolarizing pulse; recovery from slow inactivation (closed upward-pointing triangles) obtained by a 30-s depolarization to −20 mV followed by a variable-duration return to −140 mV and a control depolarizing pulse to record sodium current; entry into slow inactivation (closed downward-pointing triangles) determined by a variable-duration depolarization to −20 mV, followed by a 20-ms step to the holding potential to allow recovery from fast inactivation and a short control pulse to −20 mV. The holding potential was −140 mV for all the protocols. Normalized data were fit with an exponential function. F. Recovery from fast inactivation for holding potentials of −140 mV (closed circles), −120 mV (open squares), and −100 mV (open circles). Inlay demonstrates an example of recovery from fast inactivation at −100 mV. All data are presented as mean ± standard error of the mean. (Modified from Kuzmenkin et al.[91] Reproduced by permission.)

Fast inactivation. The absence of charge movements during inactivation suggested the localization of the inactivation gate to be outside of the membrane. Based on these studies, Armstrong and Bezanilla[61,62] proposed a ball-and-chain model in which the ball, tethered to the cytoplasmic side of the channel by a chain, swings into the inner mouth of the pore, where it binds and blocks the ionic current. Although originally proposed for the sodium channel, this model has quite convincingly been shown for fast-inactivating potassium channels where the pore-blocking ball is part of or attached to the N-terminus (so-called N-type inactivation).[72] For sodium channels, one or more of the cytoplasmic loops that connect the various domains could be involved in fast inactivation. That the loop between domains III and IV is essential was demonstrated by antibodies specifically directed against this region, which slowed fast inactivation.[73] Mutagenesis experiments confirmed the sodium channel III/IV loop as the putative inactivation gate.[74,75] The interaction of the inactivation particle with its receptor is likely to be hydrophobic, and current research focuses on the hydrophobic parts of the putative intracellular orifice of the pore or its surrounding protein parts to be the molecular correlate.[76–78]

Fast inactivation derives most of its voltage dependence from coupling to activation. The conformational changes resulting from depolarization-induced activation increase the rate of inactivation. Although the structural nature of this coupling is unknown, electrophysiologic experiments on naturally occurring mutants revealed that mutations in segment S4 of domain IV selectively affect the voltage dependence of inactivation time constants.[79,80] Because of the resemblance of this III-to-IV loop to the hinged lids of allosteric enzymes controlling substrate access, a slight modification of the ball-and-chain model was proposed. According to this hinged-lid model, the inactivation particle acts as a latch to a catch to be identified, and one of the hinges consists of a pair of glycines situated in the vicinity of the phenylalanine.[74,81] In potassium channels, the S4-to-S5 interlinkers putatively adjacent to the intracellular orifice of the pore may act as the acceptor for the N-type inactivation particle.[82-84] In the sodium channel similar but not identical parts of the supposed S4-to-S5 helices and adjacent amino acids of the transmembrane segments S5 and S6 may form the catch.[76,85,86]

Slow and ultraslow inactivation.
Upon prolonged depolarization, additional inactivation processes also appear, called core-associated or C-type inactivation. This not only is kinetically distinct from fast inactivation (Fig. 10-9E) but also involves different structural elements. Present in almost all voltage-gated cation channels, it is detectable even when fast inactivation has been made impossible (i.e., by removing the inactivation particle).

A slow inactivation process has been described, with time constants for onset and recovery of about 0.5 s.[87] On an even slower time scale, "ultraslow" inactivation, with time constants of a few minutes, has been also described in human muscle fibers.[88] Ultraslow inactivation develops at potentials only slightly less negative than the normal resting potential and therefore is of physiologic significance in muscles that undergo pathologic prolonged depolarization, as in hyper- and hypokalemic periodic paralysis.

Recovery from inactivation.
In principle, transitions from any one state into another are possible, allowing the transition from the resting to the inactivated state at depolarization as well as the same way backward. Forward and backward rate constants for the transitions determine the likelihoods of the various channel states. The likelihood that inactivated voltage-gated sodium channels will directly enter the open state is very low. Instead, the channels are in a refractory state and require repolarization and a certain time for recovery from inactivation until they enter the resting state (Fig. 10-9F).

Steady-state activation and inactivation.
Sodium channel activation is highly dependent on the membrane potential in the way that the steady-state conductance increases steeply with the membrane potential.[59] The relationship between the open probability of the channel, P, and membrane voltage, V_m, can be fit with the Boltzmann equation[89] in order to estimate the number of equivalent gating charges per channel:

$$P = 1/\{1 + \exp[(V_{0.5} - V_m)/k]\} \quad (10\text{-}6)$$

with $V_{0.5}$ being the potential at which half of the channels are activated, and the steepness of the curve being $1/k = -Q/RT$, where Q is the charge transferred and k the slope factor. For the Nav1.4 of macropatches of membrane blebs formed from native normal human muscle, $V_{0.5}$ is -32.0 mV and k is -9.6 mV, equivalent to the movement of 2.7 elementary charges across the membrane.[90]

The steady-state inactivation curve can be fit with the same Boltzmann equation, with the steepness positive. For the Nav1.4 of the same macropatches as above, $V_{0.5}$ and k are -93.7 and 8.4 mV, respectively, equivalent to the movement of 3 e_o across the membrane.[90] Examples for steady-state activation and inactivation curves of human Nav1.4 channels expressed in human embryonic kidney (HEK) cells are shown in Fig. 10-9D.

Single-channel conductance and channel density.
Single-channel recordings have shown that sodium channels possess two conductance levels: zero when the channel is closed and a constant conductance when the channel is open. Following depolarization, there is a brief delay before channels open. After a subsequent short interval, the current jumps back to zero as the channel closes. These intervals are not identical during each depolarization; in fact, the opening and closing of the channel appears to be a random process.[92,93] The channel state has to acquire enough energy to "hop over" an energy barrier to a neighboring position even though the open probability depends on the voltage and is more sensitive to the voltage than an electronic device, such as a transistor. The average behavior of a single channel is remarkably similar in time course to the macroscopic, whole-cell sodium current (compare Figs. 10-9A and 10-10A). It is clear from the single-channel recordings that the open probability for the sodium channel decreases with time during the depolarization.

The conductance of single sodium channels has been determined to be ~3 pS by single-channel recordings.[94] In these measurements, the time to opening after a depolarizing step (first latencies ~0.75 ms) and mean open times (~ 0.4 ms) can also be determined. From these values, rate constants for kinetics of channel state transitions and an alternative method to determine the steady-state activation can be derived. This best demonstrates the potency of the patch-clamp technique to describe the behavior of individual proteins and enables study of the full spectrum of possible channel behavior, ranging from single openings to long-lasting bursts, when a sufficient number of observations are made (Fig. 10-10).

The distribution of sodium channels over the surface of a muscle fiber is not homogeneous, as has been shown by experiments using the "loose patch" voltage-clamp technique.[95] Channel density varies up to threefold over distances of 10 to 30 μm along the fiber surface. Furthermore, the density changes little with time,[96] suggesting that the channels are anchored in the membrane, probably by cytoskeletal structures. There is no indication of a specific location relative either to the sarcomere intervals or to the openings of T tubules, nor is there any information on how closely clustered the channels are.

The β subunits—modulators of expression and channel kinetics.
Quarternary structure and channel function are dependent on additional subunits which may modify voltage sensitivity, kinetics, expression levels, or membrane localization.[97] Of the several genes encoding β subunits,

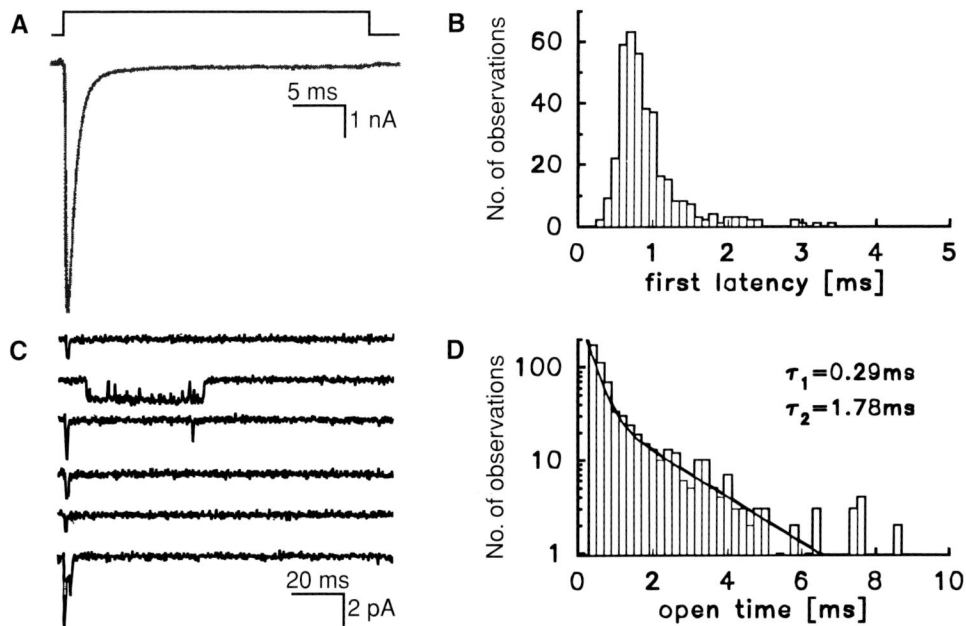

FIGURE 10-10. Whole-cell (A) and single-channel (B, C, D) recordings of sodium currents from normal channels. (A) Representative whole-cell current from transfected HEK 293 cells held at a potential of −85 mV. After a 15-ms prepulse to −120 mV the currents were elicited by an above shown test pulse to −20 mV. (B) Histogram of all first latencies to openings occurring during 500 depolarizations; medians for a larger number of control patches were 0.75 ± 0.07 ms (n = 7). (C) "Single" channel recordings of sodium currents on a membrane patch containing four sodium channels, performed in the bleb-attached mode. Note the burst in the second, and the late reopening in the third trace. (D) Semi-logarithmic histogram of open times of 1000 depolarization steps; the line represents a fit to a second order exponential with time constants indicated. (*Modified after Lerche et al.*[90] *Reproduced by permission.*)

SCN1B and *SCN3B* are expressed in skeletal muscle. They are composed of a transmembrane segment, an extracellular N-terminal, and an intracellular C-terminal and are noncovalently bound to α. In *Xenopus* oocytes, coexpression of *SCN1B* in addition to *SCN4A* increased functional expression and current amplitude, shifted the steady-state activation and inactivation curves toward more negative potentials, and accelerated recovery from inactivation.[98,102] The observation that the sodium channel exhibited a more rapid inactivation when expressed in mammalian cell lines than in *Xenopus* oocytes was originally attributed to the lack of endogenous β-subunit expression in the oocytes. Later, by demonstrating that the rapid kinetics were also found when expressed in cells without endogenous β subunits, post-translational modifications and association of sodium channels with other membrane proteins such as cytoskeletal components have been made responsible for the differences in kinetics.[103–106]

Channel blockers and modifiers. Action potential generation in muscle is prevented when current through sodium channels is blocked by the specific neurotoxins tetrodotoxin (TTX) and saxitoxin (STX). The origin of TTX is liver and ovaries of the puffer fish *Fugu*, whose flesh and testes are an exquisite Japanese dish. Separation of the ovaries from the testes in the hermaphrodite fish is a prerequisite for consumption, a task requiring expertise if the physiologically interested gourmet is to survive. The toxin occludes the external mouth of the pore and is extremely specific, involving very high affinity binding with dissociation constants in the nanomolar range (e.g., 5 nM for TTX and 0.9 nM for STX). In contrast to brain sodium channels, Nav1.4 is also blocked by micro-conotoxins obtained from the piscovorous marine snail *Conus geographus* L.[107] These toxins act at the same site as TTX and STX.[108] Sea anemone toxin (ATX) and α and β scorpion toxins bind to different extracellular parts of the channel and impair fast inactivation or activation.[109]

Local anesthetics such as procaine, lidocaine, and benzocaine block muscle sodium channels.[110] This interesting class of compounds may exhibit "use dependence"—a dependence of the depth of block on the frequency of stimulation. The degree of use dependence varies with the structure (charge and hydrophobicity) of the drug.

As in nerve, increasing external hydrogen ion concentration blocks sodium channels in at least two ways: (1) peak current is reduced and (2) voltage dependence of gating is shifted in the depolarizing direction.[111] As the apparent pKa for this effect is near 5, this block is of little importance in the physiologic pH range but has been useful in formulating hypotheses concerning the nature of the chemical groups glutamates and aspartates, which are important for sodium ion transport.[112]

Of physiologic relevance is the effect of changes in external calcium or magnesium ion concentration. Divalent cations are thought to bind to sites on the membrane surface, and the presence of these positively charged particles provides a surface potential, in addition to the transmembrane potential, on the electric field within the membrane and in particular the field experienced by the voltage-sensitive sodium channels. Changes in divalent ion concentration shift the voltage dependence of the sodium channel activation parameters. This has the effect of changing the threshold potential, so that action potential initiation requires a larger depolarization in a high Ca^{2+} concentration, whereas a smaller depolarization is sufficient in low Ca^{2+}. A twofold change in outside free Ca^{2+} concentration causes a shift in the voltage dependence of the sodium activation parameter of about 7 mV; the shifts stemming from changes in Mg^{2+} concentration are smaller in size.[113]

Voltage-Gated Potassium Channels

Potassium channels constitute the most diverse class of ion channels with respect to activation, kinetic properties, regulation, pharmacology, and structure. Voltage-gated (Kv) potassium channels are activated by membrane depolarization, and, once opened, they conduct potassium ions from inside to outside along the concentration gradient and against the electric field. This outwardly rectifying current leads to repolarization of the surface membrane. Although almost all outward rectifiers (except Kv7.x) exhibit fast activation within a few milliseconds, the historical term *delayed rectifiers* reflects the delay in comparison to the extremely rapid activation of the sodium current. Kv channels inactivate slowly or fast, and the slowly inactivating channels will be deactivated by the membrane repolarization during the second phase of the action potential (i.e., the process of activation will be reversed; fast-inactivating channels may be already inactivated at this time). Besides voltage-gated channels, there is a large spectrum of potassium channels more or less sensitive to membrane potential and activated or blocked by endogenous ligands. Voltage-insensitive potassium channels convey background conductance and therefore determine the resting membrane potential of cells, excitable, such as the skeletal muscle, and nonexcitable. They also play a role in volume regulation and signal transduction.

The Kv channels are the human homologues of Shaker (Kv1.x), Shab (Kv2.x), Shaw (Kv3.x), and Shal (Kv4.x) potassium channel α subunits, first identified in *Drosophila*, and the channel family is still increasing (up to Kv12.x to date). They are found in almost all eukaryotic cells of the animal and plant kingdom and are present not only in nerve or muscle cells, but also in lymphocytes, pancreatic islet cells, and others. In contrast to voltage-gated sodium and calcium channels, a single domain containing six transmembrane segments (6T/1P) (Fig. 10-1) is encoded by a single gene (Kv1.x by *KCNAx*, Kv2.x by *KCNBx*, etc., with $x = 1$ to n), and four gene products form a functional tetrameric α subunit. In nature, some members of the same protein family can assembly to heterotetramers (e.g., Kv1.1 and Kv1.2).

Kv homo- and heterotetramers inactivate at different rates and to a varying extent. The first studied potassium current is the "delayed" outward potassium current, I_K, that shows very slow inactivation.[114] In 1971, Connor and Stevens[115] identified a rapidly inactivating potassium current in the neuronal soma of the *Anisodoris*, I_A, and termed it *A-type potassium current* after the initial letter of the sea snail's name and also in contrast to the typical delayed rectifier current, I_K. Although the historical name A-type current is still in use, it is more and more replaced by the modern term *fast N-type inactivation*, for those Kv channels that contain the intracellular N-term fast-inactivation "ball" and mediate this transient current. Fast N-type inactivation already occurs if one domain of a heterotetrameric channel complex contains the ball and also if just any Kv channel tetramer interacts with a certain intracellular β subunit—for example $Kv\beta_1$—that is capable of fast inactivation.[116]

The typical delayed rectifier potassium currents are conducted by slowly inactivating Kv channels that either do not possess the inactivation ball or are not coexpressed with $Kv\beta_1$. This type of inactivation is called C-type inactivation and is influenced by cations of external and internal solutions that interact with certain amino acids of the ion-conducting pore (foot-in-the-door model of gating[117,118]). The removal of inactivation by a point mutation in the pore leads to the depiction of another term, the P-type (pore type) inactivation.[119]

Fast-inactivating Kv channels. These "A-type" currents with fast "N-type inactivation" operate in the subthreshold range of an action potential and are thought to maintain the resting potential and to modulate electrical excitability. Most of these channels are blocked at low extracellular potassium ion concentration; at 1 to 2 mM there is a ~50 percent reduction in current.[118,120,121] Potassium is bound to a "pocket" at or in the vicinity of the TEA-binding site. The two skeletal muscle channels show the potassium dependency: Kv1.4, which is present in skeletal muscle at only low expression level, shows the highest potassium sensitivity; and Kv3.4, with mRNA levels being five- to sixfold lower in the soleus muscle than in fast muscles.[122] Differential splicing and alternative transcription start sites are utilized to generate a set of Kv3.4 variants in murine skeletal muscle and brain, presumably involved in the regulation of excitability.[123]

Slowly inactivating Kv channels. Slowly inactivating Kv channels support repolarization of the muscle cell membrane during the second phase of an action potential and reduce cell excitability. Until now, only one human disease, episodic ataxia, is known to be caused by mutations in a Kv channel; that is Kv1.1, the Shaker homologue. The channel does not possess an "N-type ball" and therefore slowly inactivates. Kv1.1 is expressed in brain (particularly in the basket cells of the cerebellum), nerve (particularly the motor neuron), cardiac and skeletal muscle, the retina, and the pancreatic islet. The mutations cause episodic ataxia with interictal myokymia (EA-1). The myokymia may be generated by hyperexcitable motor neurons. Although muscle fatigue similar to a myasthenic syndrome was reported for a patient, the significance of Kv1.1 for skeletal muscle function does not seem to be essential. Interestingly, rapid inactivation of Kv1.1 is achieved by the $Kv\beta_1$ subunit,[124] but its expression in skeletal muscle has not been demonstrated so far. Of the Kv1.x family, Kv1.7 and Kv1.8 have been identified in skeletal muscle, but their significance has not been clarified. Of the other Kv families, Kv2.1 and its modifiers Kv5.1 and Kv6.1 as well as Kv3.1 are also present in skeletal muscle. In the Kv3.1 −/− mice, muscle shows slower contraction and relaxation and smaller forces, but these effects are not due to changes in skeletal muscle excitability, but rather dependent on strain.[125] Therefore, the significance of Kv3.1 channels for muscle function remains unclear.

Slowly activating and inactivating Kv channels. In contrast to all other Kv channels, which reach current peaks within 10 to 20 ms following depolarization, only those of the Kv7.x family show slow activation. Of the corresponding *KCNQ* family, a splice variant of the *KCNQ5* mRNA is clearly expressed in skeletal muscle,[126] and likewise *KCNQ4* encoding Kv7.4.[127] Apparently both channel types conduct detectable currents without Kv7.3 channel that forms the "mother" heterotetramers with several other Kv7.x α subunits and is important for trafficking.[128]

The C-terminus of all Kv7.x channels is long compared to other K+ channels and is endowed with distinctive structural domains. Though there is evidence that the C-terminus contains a channel assembly domain and binds calmodulin, its structural and functional significance is not yet known. All Kv7.x channels modify subthreshold membrane excitability. Coexpression of *KCNQ4* and *KCNQ5* with a member of the MiRP (MinK-related protein) protein family forming β subunits has not been reported.

The Voltage-Gated Calcium Channels

Of the many genes (*CACNA-1,S*) encoding α subunits, only one is expressed in the T-tubular membrane of adult skeletal muscle: *CACNA1S* encoding the L-type calcium channel α1 subunit, Cav1.1 (Fig. 10-7). The subclassification α1 was made because a second subunit was originally thought to possess an ion-conducting pore, α2, which later turned out to be a modifying subunit without pore. The term L-type means long-lasting currents according to their inactivation properties, in contrast to the transient (T-type) currents. While L-type (and P-type, *P* for Purkinje cell) channels reveal high thresholds for activation (HVA channels), T-type channels are low-voltage-activated (LVA). All L-type channels, including those in brain and heart and pancreatic islet cells encoded by different genes, are very sensitive to dihydropyridines (DHP, e.g., nifedipine), phenylalkylamines (PAA, e.g., verapamil), and benzothiazepines (BTZ, e.g., diltiazem), which has led to the term *dihydropyridine receptor*, a misnomer, as it suggests ligand activation when in fact the channel is activated by voltage.

The α1 subunit is structurally homologous to the α subunit of sodium channels, being 6T/1P; however, recent biochemical and three-dimensional structural data indicate that functional channels could contain two α1 subunits.[129] As functional studies have not yet been performed, it is not clear whether there are one or two pores in the whole channel complex.

The high selectivity for calcium over sodium is conferred by a group of conserved glutamate residues forming a high-affinity calcium-binding site in the pore exhibiting an apparent dissociation constant of about 700 nM.[130] Nevertheless, the channel conducts a reasonably high sodium current, probably because of the vicinity of a second binding site. When only one of the sites is occupied, which is the case at low concentration, calcium is bound tightly. However, as soon as the probability of double occupancy increases at higher calcium concentration, electrostatic repulsion drastically reduces the time that the ions spend at the site, and calcium flows through the channel along its electrochemical gradient. Therefore, monovalent cations (e.g., sodium) pass the channel in the absence of divalents, micromolar calcium blocks the monovalent current, and millimolar external calcium leads to an almost pure calcium inward current.[131] This binding site is conserved through all α1 subunits of the calcium channel family.

Physiologically, at least two Cav1.1 isoforms are expressed in muscle, the rare 212-kD complete protein and a similar 190-kD truncated form. The 190-kD subunit, comprising 95 percent of total channel population, results by posttranslational proteolysis at amino acid 1690.[132,133] An additional variant has been suggested to exist, at least in postnatal skeletal muscle (see below). As L-type channels can be modulated by cAMP-dependent protein kinase A via certain G_S proteins,[134] further functional alterations have also been demonstrated. The physiologic importance of these alterations is acknowledged for the cardiac channel, but seems questionable for the skeletal muscle.[135] Mutations in Cav1.1 cause hypokalemic periodic paralysis and malignant hyperthermia susceptibility type 5 in humans, and muscular dysgenesis in mice.

So called T-type (transient) LVA calcium channels are encoded by the *CACNA1H* gene. They are expressed in myoblasts just before fusion and mediate an intracellular calcium rise due to a window current at hyperpolarized potentials.[136] They are not found in adult skeletal muscle.

Kinetics and potential dependency of $Ca_v1.1$ channel states. As in voltage-gated sodium channels, depolarization causes $Ca_v1.1$ activation in a positive feedback mechanism along both the concentration gradient and the electric field and increases the open probability until the time-dependent occurrence of channel inactivation during maintained depolarization reduces it, a process that is not intrinsically voltage-dependent. As the time constants for activation are ~60 ms, the currents cannot substantially contribute to the action potential, which lasts only 1 to 2 ms. Additionally, at the peak of the action potential, only a small fraction of the channels can be activated, as indicated by the Boltzman curves for activation and inactivation (Fig. 10-11). It has not been unambiguously clarified whether $Ca_v1.1$ channels conduct calcium during high-frequency discharges of action potentials under physiologic conditions at all or whether the sole function of the channels consists of coupling to the ryanodine receptor to initiate calcium release. The latter function is also voltage-dependent, but the midpoint of half-maximal activation is shifted toward hyperpolarizing potentials by 40 mV compared to the midpoint of current activation (Fig. 10-11). Therefore, Cav1.1 functions as a voltage sensor of excitation-contraction coupling and activator of the ryanodine receptor (RyR1), which releases calcium from the sarcoplasmic reticulum (SR), initiating contraction (see Chap. 12).

Modifying subunits. While voltage-gated sodium and potassium channels consist of α and optional β subunits, only voltage-gated calcium channels consist of additional proteins: α2, β, γ, and δ. The extracellularly located α2 protein is anchored by disulfide bonds to the membrane-spanning α1 subunit,[97,138] and the two proteins are encoded by a single gene. The originally assumed existence of an α2 associated ion-conducting pore can be explained by the drastic increase in expression of endogenous α1 subunits by coexpression of the α2/δ subunit.[139] The α2/δ subunit,

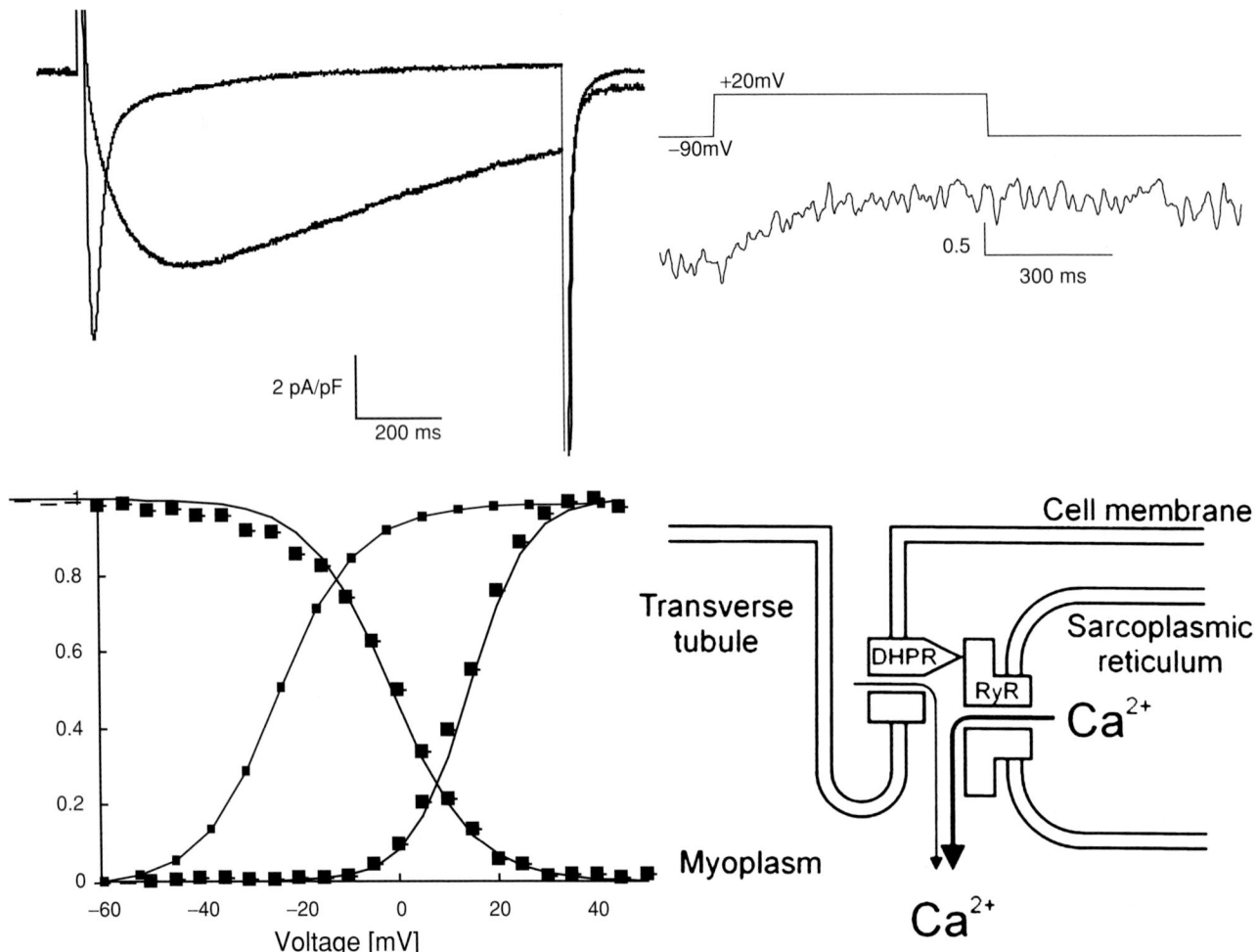

FIGURE 10-11. Whole-cell calcium currents and calcium transient of human myotubes. *Upper left panel*: The myotubes revealed a rapidly activating and inactivating calcium current with a voltage threshold at −20 mV (T-type current) and a slowly activating and inactivating L-type current at +25 mV. *Upper right panel*: Depolarization-induced calcium transient as normalized fluorescent intensity increases elicited from a holding potential of −90 mV. *Lower left panel*: Steady-state activation and inactivation curves of the L-type current (*large squares*) and steady-state activation of calcium transients (*small squares*). Note that the calcium transients occur at much smaller cell depolarizations than the current. *Lower right panel*: The triadic junction between the T-tubular and the sarcoplasmic reticulum. Note the position of the two calcium channels of skeletal muscle—the L-type calcium channel, also called dihydropyridine (DHP) receptor, and the calcium release channel, also called ryanodine receptor—which interact directly during excitation-contraction coupling. (*Modified from Jurkat-Rott et al.[137] Reproduced by permission.*)

which can bind the anticonvulsant drug gabapentin, not only increases α1 expression rates and current density, but also accelerates inactivation kinetics and slightly shifts both steady-state inactivation and activation curves in hyperpolarizing directions.[140]

Coexpression of any of the four β subunits with $α1_A$ markedly increases the number of channel complexes inserted into the membrane and the current amplitude.[141] For $α1_S$, the skeletal muscle variant, β coexpression increased the number of DHP-binding sites and accelerated current activation kinetics, however, without increasing current density.[142,143] Of the four β subunits identified so far, β1 is an intracellular acidic protein and binds to the loop connecting domains I and II of Cav1.1, distinct from the consensus site for the G protein β-γ complex.[144] Besides the intracellular I/II loop, the C-term also seems to act as a binding site for β.[145]

The γ subunits consist of four transmembrane segments, and at least one of them, γ1, is expressed in skeletal muscle. Coexpression of γ1 with the cardiac α1 subunit in amphibian and mammalian cell systems moderately increased calcium current amplitude and inactivation rate. The main effect is a marked shift of the voltage dependence of inactivation in the hyperpolarizing direction.[140,146]

Voltage-Dependent Chloride Channels

Chloride channels are present in the plasma membrane of most cells. They play important roles in cell volume regulation, transepithelial transport, secretion of fluid from secretory glands, and in the stabilization of the resting membrane potential. Of the four superfamilies, the first consists of transmitter-gated chloride channels that are predominantly expressed at inhibitory synapses (i.e., $GABA_A$ and glycine receptor channels mediating chloride influx). The second superfamily consists of the ATP-binding cassette channels, including the cystic fibrosis transmembrane regulator (CFTR). The third is composed of the voltage-gated anion-selective channels (VDAC—e.g., porin type 1 in the plasmalemma and the SR membrane of striated muscle), and the fourth is the large family of voltage-gated chloride channels, present in excitable and epithelial cells. The latter will be elaborated on further, since it contains several members that are expressed in skeletal muscle.

Generally, voltage-dependent chloride channels fulfil a variety of functions depending on their tissue distribution and subcellular localization (for review, see Jentsch et al.[147]). The dimeric channel complex possesses two independent ion-conducting pores, each with a fast opening mechanism of its own, two selectivity filters, and two voltage sensors, and conducts over the whole physiologic voltage range (for review, see Fahlke[148]). Recent cryoelectron microscopy and x-ray studies have elucidated the structure of the channel[149,150] and confirmed the conclusions derived from electrophysiologic results (Fig. 10-12). Of the nine human genes encoding voltage-dependent chloride channels of the *CLCN* family, at least four are expressed in skeletal muscle: the ClC1, specific for skeletal muscle (see below); the ubiquitous ClC2; the acid-activated ClC4; and the intracellular ClC6.

ClC2 is ubiquitously expressed and is the most closely related to ClC1. Both may assemble together as heterodimers, forming voltage- and volume-sensitive channels expressed in skeletal muscle.[151,152] ClC2 channels show a typical chloride over iodide specificity, are blockable by unspecific agents only, and generate an inwardly rectifying current (i.e., there is a chloride extrusion at potentials more negative than the reversal potential). Mutations therein cause idiopathic generalized epilepsy.[153] Knockout mice do not present with muscular symptoms, but rather with retinal degeneration and infertility,[154] so that a loss of function may be compensable by presence of a functional ClC1.

Not much is known on ClC4. It is expressed in skeletal muscle, and one study with the whole-cell patch-clamp technique showed that the channel was activated by external acidic pH. The channel produces a strong outward chloride current with a permeability similar to ClC1. There are consensus sites for phosphorylation by protein kinase A; however, stimulation of PKA had no effect on the currents.[155]

There is evidence that ClC6 is an intracellular chloride channel rather than being located in the plasma membrane. Confocal imaging of transfected cells revealed a similar expression pattern of two splicing variants, ClC6a and ClC6c, to SR Ca^{2+} pump SERCA2b.[156] Therefore these channels do not directly contribute to muscle excitability.

ClC1, the major chloride channel of skeletal muscle.

The encoding gene for this channel, *CLCN1*, is almost exclusively expressed in skeletal muscle.[157] The electrophysiologic identification and characterization of ClC1 at the single-channel level were difficult because its conductance is very low (i.e., near 1 pS, as estimated from noise analysis).[158] The large macroscopic chloride conductance of the skeletal muscle fiber membrane (i.e., 80 percent of the total conductance of the sarcolemma and the T-tubular membrane) must therefore result from an extremely high channel density. The channel is functional without any other subunits and conducts over the whole physiologic voltage range, showing inward rectification in the negative potential range. It is activated upon depolarization, and with hyperpolarizing voltage steps it is deactivated to a nonzero steady-state level (Fig. 10-13). During tetanic muscle excitation the high chloride conductance is thought to be necessary for a fast repolarization of the transverse tubular membrane, which becomes depolarized by potassium accumulation in the tubules. As known from macroscopic experiments,[159,160] the channel can be blocked by external iodide and monocarboxylic aromatic acids. The acid of choice, 9-anthracene carboxylic acid, is effective at low m*M* concentrations.[157,158] Mutations in ClC1 that lower the chloride conductance at the resting poten-

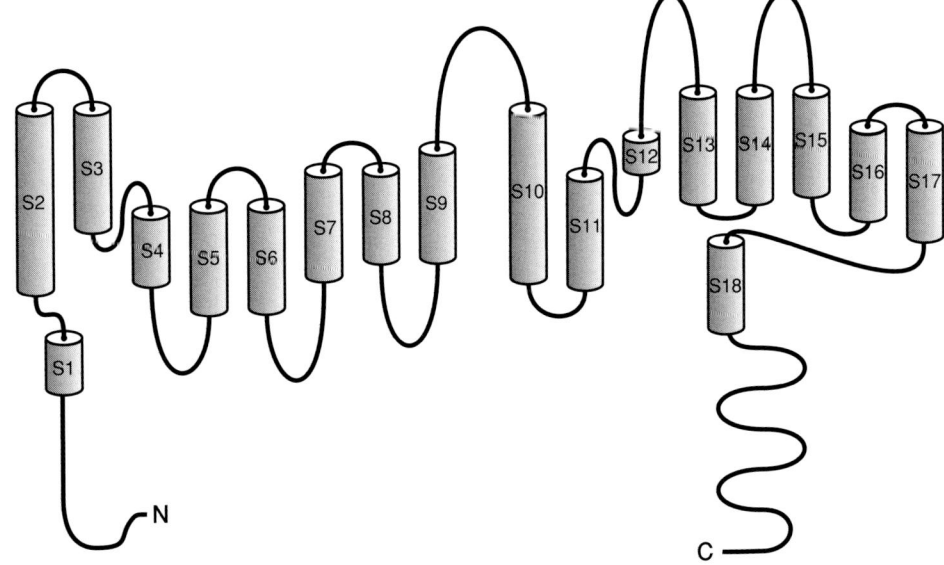

FIGURE 10-12. Membrane topology model of the skeletal muscle chloride channel monomer ClC1, modified from Dutzler et al.[150] The channel complex is a homodimer formed in an antiparallel orientation. ClC1/2 heterodimers are also functional. Each protein contains parts of the two channel pores. The loop connecting segments S7 and S8 is involved in the formation of one pore, and the loop between S13 and S14 and the N-region of S18 form the other pore, supplemented by the corresponding parts of the second protein in an antiparallel formation

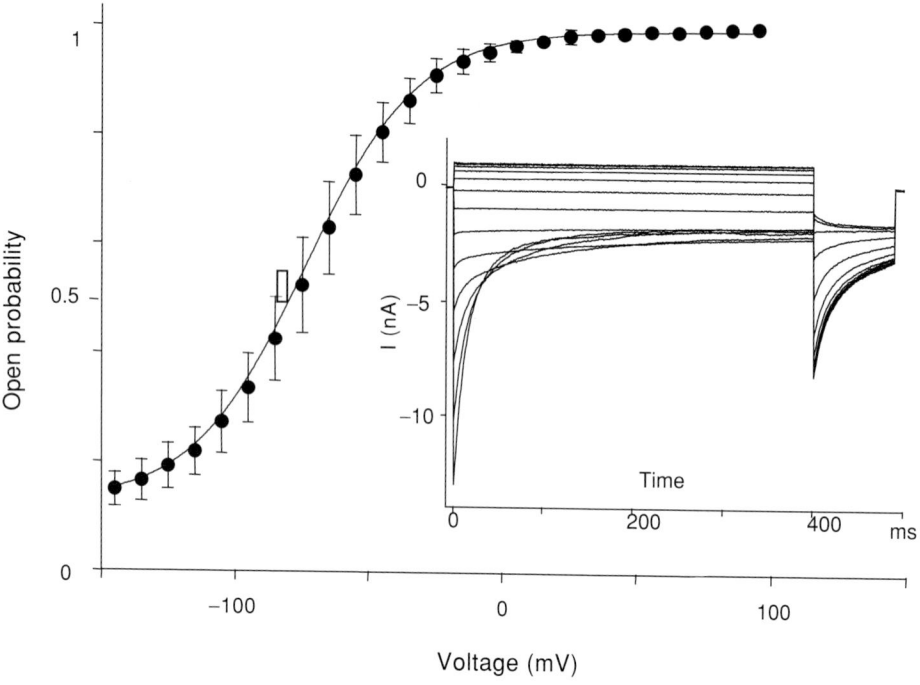

FIGURE 10-13. Behavior of the human ClC-1, the major chloride channel of skeletal muscle, expressed in a mammalian cell line and measured in a symmetrical chloride solution. The channel-open probability depends on the voltage and is high in the physiologic potential range. It is about 40 percent at the resting potential of −80 mV. The inset shows macroscopic currents recorded in the whole-cell mode. They are activated by steps going from a holding potential of 0 mV to potentials over a range of −145 to +95 mV and deactivated after 400 ms by polarization to −105 mV. (*Adapted from Wagner et al.*[161] *Reproduced by permission.*)

tial cause dominant or recessive myotonia congenita[16,158] (see Chap. 4).

THE SPREAD OF ELECTRICAL ACTIVITY

Conduction Velocity

According to mathematical models, the conduction velocity θ of propagated action potentials depends on various fiber parameters: fiber radius a, intracellular resistivity R_i, rate coefficient k for activation of the conductance, excitatory membrane conductance G ~ G_{Na}, and membrane capacitance C_m. The following equation accounts for the delay in the activation process that, in the Hodgkin-Huxley equations, is represented by the third power of m reaction and leads to a realistic approximation of the action potential conduction velocity θ[162]:

$$\theta \propto (a/2R_i)^{1/2} (kG_{Na})^{1/8} C_m^{-5/8} \quad (10\text{-}7)$$

The equation shows that the velocity increases with the square root of the fiber radius a and this is in agreement with the predictions of the wave equation and the cable theory. Children with smaller muscle fiber diameters should exhibit lower action potential conduction velocities than adults for whom values of 3 to 4 m/s have been measured by multichannel recordings using surface electrodes.[163] The equation also shows that only a little increase in speed can be obtained by further increasing the membrane conductance G_{Na}, particularly as a higher sodium channel density also increases the capacitance. The maximum sodium conductance depends on how many channels are available for activation. Therefore not only the channel density but also the resting membrane potential that determines the percentage of channels in the inactivated state is important. The maximum sodium conductance is proportional to a parameter often measured on native muscle fibers, i.e., the maximum rate of rise of an action potential. For human skeletal muscle, maximum rates of about 300 to 400 V/s are reported, as well as peak potentials of +10.5 mV and action potential durations of about 1.3 ms at a membrane potential of −80 mV.[164,165] Under the pathological condition of a transient membrane depolarization of several hours, as in paralytic attacks, or during persistent membrane depolarization, the maximum rate can be reduced to 100 V/s or less, and these slow action potential upstrokes result in a reduced velocity. Indeed, reduced muscle fiber action potential velocities have been reported for patients with hypokalemic periodic paralysis in attack-free intervals and—more pronounced—during paralytic attacks.[166] It is known that the muscular resting membrane potential is slightly reduced between attacks and markedly reduced during attacks.[165,167]

The Role of the T-Tubules

The radial spread of the action potential is mediated by conduction along the TTS. This is made possible by a high density of voltage-gated sodium channels in this structure,[168] producing a regenerative sodium current[169] as theoretical calculations earlier had demanded.[170] Due to the TTS, the action potential of skeletal muscle differs from that of nerve. The most obvious distinction between the nerve and muscle action potentials is the prolonged afterdepolarization of the sarcolemma following a spike. The early part of the afterdepolarization is caused by the spreading of the spike in the depth of the TTS lagging behind the almost synchronized spread of excitation; the late afterdepolarization is caused by an accumulation of potassium ions in the TTS that increases with frequency and duration of repetitive action potentials.[28] The lower sodium channel density in the TTS than in the surface membrane results in a smaller excitatory inward sodium current that could be compensated by the inhibitory outward potassium current. Consequently, the propagation of action potentials in the TTS would be disturbed. To avoid this problem, inwardly rectifying potassium channels that conduct almost no outward current during depolarization are predominantly expressed in the TTS.

Appendix: The Patch-Clamp Technique

Modern research into the properties of ionic channels was initiated by the pioneering work of Hodgkin and Huxley,[59] who utilized the voltage-clamp technique to provide the first detailed description of the ionic basis of the action potential in nerve axons. Their work provided our first look at some of the functional properties of voltage-gated sodium and potassium channels. For the following 50 years, the voltage clamp became the principal tool for the study of channels. Two more recent developments have revolutionized this field. The first of these is the patch-clamp technique, developed by Neher and colleagues,[171] which is a specific application of voltage clamping (Fig. 10-14). The second is the use of molecular cloning techniques to isolate channel genes, thereby determining the primary structure of the channel. By combining the patch clamp with molecular biological techniques, structure-function correlations are rapidly elucidated. A common approach in these studies is the following: Molecular cloning techniques are used to isolate the gene of interest and then either to design or to take advantage of naturally occurring mutations in the primary gene structure that will, it is hoped, produce measurable changes in channel function. Then, a heterologous ("of a different tissue") expression system is used to express the gene product. This expression can be either transient, as in RNA-injected *Xenopus* oocytes,

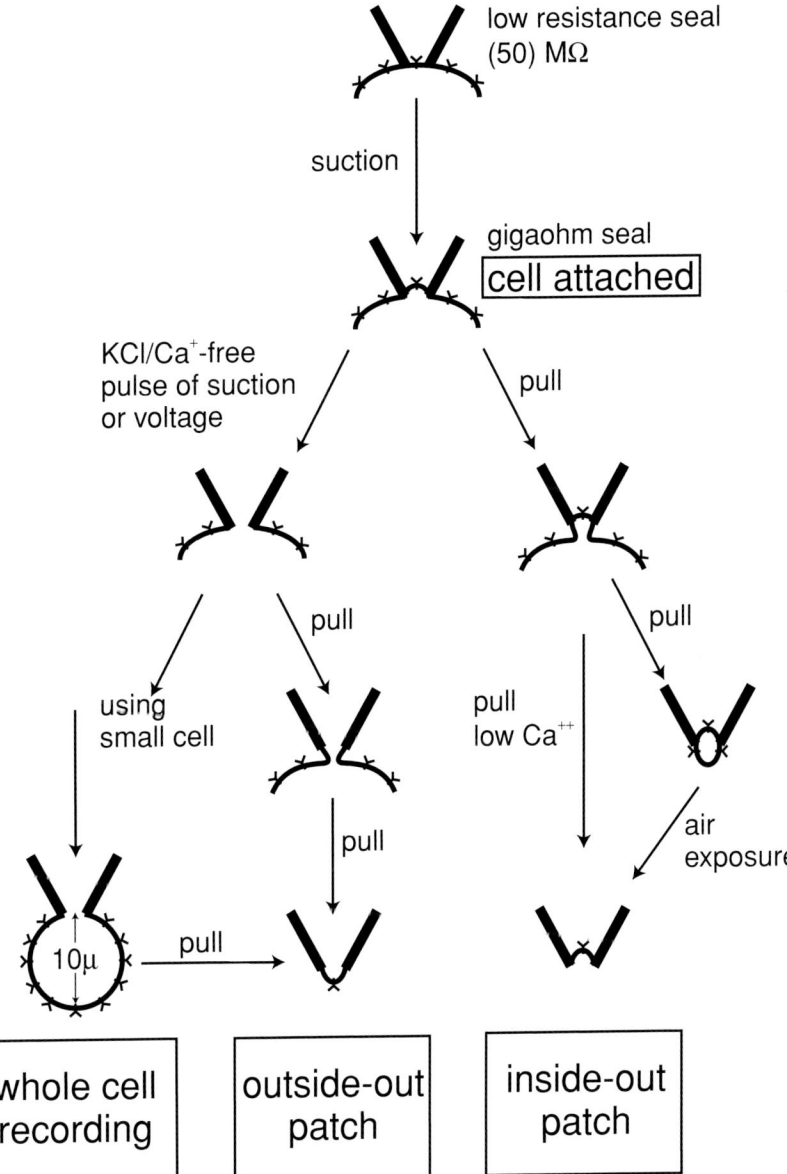

FIGURE 10-14. Schematic representation of the procedures leading to recording configurations. A fine-tipped (about 0.5- to 5-μm in tip diameter) glass patch electrode is used as a current monitor and the voltage in the pipette is held at a desired level. The first step in applying the technique is the formation of a high-resistance seal between the patch electrode and the surface of the cell. Once the seal is established, several recording configurations are available to the investigator, and these fall into two broad categories. On one hand, current flow through the patch of membrane under the electrode tip can be monitored, in which case single-channel currents are usually recorded. Alternatively, for whole-cell recording, the patch of membrane can be disrupted, so that the electrode monitors current flow through the entire cell surface. (Modified from Sakmann and Neher.[172] Reproduced by permission.)

WHOLE-CELL RECORDING

Two methods are available for voltage clamping the entire cell surface and recording macroscopic, or whole-cell, currents: the "classic" whole-cell technique and the nystatin, or perforated-patch, technique.[173–175] To obtain the classic whole-cell recording configuration, a brief suction is applied to the interior of the electrode in order to rupture the patch of membrane under the electrode tip. After this break-in, there will be a low-resistance pathway for current and diffusional flow between the electrode and the cell interior. The cell membrane is voltage-clamped at the pipette potential by virtue of this low-resistance pathway, and the electrode monitors the current flowing across the entire cell surface. The ionic composition of the cytoplasm rapidly equilibrates with the pipette contents, offering a pathway for the control of cellular constituents. For example, to eliminate potassium currents, the pipette can be filled with an isotonic intracellular solution containing Cs salts instead of potassium salts.

Although whole-cell recording can produce highly accurate current recordings, two important limitations are associated with the technique. The first of these is correlated with the resistance in series with the membrane (R_s), which in whole-cell recording is the access resistance between the interior of the pipette and the cytoplasm. The nature of series resistance errors in whole-cell recording has been summarized by Armstrong and Gilly.[176] Briefly, there are three types of errors associated with R_s: (1) The membrane voltage differs from the command voltage by an amount proportional to the magnitude of the current flowing through R_s. (2) The membrane voltage rises exponentially with a time constant approximately equal to R_s times the cell capacitance (C_m). Thus, in the presence of a large R_s, achieving control of the membrane voltage can be a slow process. (3) The recorded current must be filtered, which could severely distort the recorded currents. All of these errors can be minimized by using low-resistance patch electrodes and by using electronic compensating methods.

Another limitation of the whole-cell configuration is that important intracellular regulatory molecules, like cAMP, Ca^{2+}, or guanosine triphosphate (GTP), can diffuse out of the cell through the patch electrode. Thus, the physiologic regulation of these important second messenger substances is disrupted. If one of these second messengers modulates the activity of the channel under study, whole-cell recordings might not reflect the physiologic behavior of the channels. The perforated-patch technique[175] provides a solution to this problem by making it possible to record macroscopic currents with a cell-intact recording configuration. This configuration is obtained by including a pore-forming antibiotic, like nystatin or amphotericin B, in the pipette solution. After a seal is formed on the cell, the antibiotic channels are inserted in the patch of membrane under the electrode tip, thereby providing electrical continuity between the pipette and the cell interior. However, these channels select for monovalent cations and do not allow multivalent ions and other large solute molecules to pass through. Therefore, the intracellular concentration of many second messengers will not be altered during this type of recording. Perforated-patch recordings have been used to record calcium currents without rundown[175,177] and to characterize the response of calcium-dependent potassium and chloride currents to muscarinic receptor activation.[173]

SINGLE-CHANNEL RECORDING

The ability to monitor the activity of a single ionic channel probably represents the most widely used aspect of the patch-clamp technique. After a giga Ω seal between the patch electrode and the cell membrane is formed, the background noise is sufficiently attenuated so that the current flowing through a single ionic channel can be resolved.[171] This configuration of electrode sealed onto the cell has been referred to as a *cell-attached patch recording*. In addition to cell-attached recordings, there are two other configurations that allow single-channel currents to be monitored. If the recording electrode is withdrawn from the cell after a cell-attached patch is formed, the patch of membrane can be excised from the cell with the inside surface of the membrane facing the bath solution; this is called the *inside-out configuration*. An *outside-out* patch can be formed by removing the electrode after entering the whole-cell configuration. One advantage of these cell-free patch recordings is that they provide more accurate control of the membrane potential. In the cell-attached mode, the membrane potential of the patch is equal to the resting potential of the cell minus the pipette potential. Since the resting potential may not be known with certainty or might vary during an experiment, there will be uncertainty in the value of the patch membrane potential. However, in the isolated-patch configurations, the magnitude of the patch potential is equal to the pipette potential and is therefore known with precision. A second advantage is that the experimenter can rapidly exchange the solution on either surface of the patch simply by changing the bath or pipette solution.

TRANSIENT EXPRESSION SYSTEMS, AS IN OOCYTES

Oocytes from *Xenopus laevis* have become a widely used preparation for the expression of cloned ion channel genes. A series of recent papers has reviewed many of the technical aspects of the use of this expression system.[178–183] Isolated *Xenopus* oocytes are capable of translating injected mRNA from a variety of sources and producing biologically active proteins. The mRNA can be extracted from the tissue of interest[181] or it can be synthesized from an isolated clone (cDNA) which codes for the channel protein.[182] The isolated mRNA is pressure-injected into the oocyte through a relatively large-diameter (10-μm) microelectrode. Within a few days, functional channels will be present in the surface membrane of the oocyte and can be studied with various voltage-clamp techniques, including the conventional two-microelectrode voltage clamp and the patch clamp.[183] Several types of ionic channels have now been expressed in oocytes using these techniques (e.g., Noda et al.[184] and Timpe et al.[185]).

STABLE EXPRESSION SYSTEMS

In contrast to transient expression systems like injected *Xenopus* oocytes, stable expression involves the introduction of exogenous DNA into the genome of a cell so that it is transcribed with the cell's DNA and inherited by offspring cells during cell division. One of the obvious advantages of this type of system is that once the cell line is established, studies can be performed on a uniform cell population without reestablishing expression for each experiment (as an example, see a patched HEK cell in Fig. 10-15, right panel). The foreign DNA can be introduced by microinjection, electroporation, viral expression vectors, or transfection using various techniques.[186]

MEASUREMENTS ON NATIVE MUSCLE FIBERS

Because of the gycocalix, no giga Ω seals can be produced on the sarcolemma. However, plasmalemmal blebs can be formed from native fibers by stretching a fiber in the presence of $\geq 10^{-5}$ M [Ca^{2+}] in the bath solution or with enzymatic treatment (Fig. 10-15, left panel). The current through single or few channels situated in the electrically isolated bleb membrane patch can be measured in all modes without fiber contractions.[17,187]

POTENTIAL FUTURE TECHNOLOGIES

Although very powerful, the patch-clamp technique is extremely labor-intensive and thereby limited to 10 to 20 individual cell measurements per day. Therefore, several firms are trying to develop technologies for high-throughput screening. Achieving this goal requires more than just the automation of existing patch-clamp techniques; it requires the development of an entirely new paradigm for making electrophysiological measurements. All developments are based on positioning a cell on a small pore separating two isolated fluid chambers in a manner that requires no manual intervention or micromanipulation. In order to perform whole-cell electrophysiological measurements within this geometry, two criteria must be met. First, a high-resistance seal must form between the cell membrane and peripheral region of the substrate pore. As in the case of patch-clamp electrophysiology, this ensures that the current measured between the two electrodes passes through the cell membrane. Second, for the control of the membrane potential, a low-resistance electrical pathway must form through the cell wall that covers the pore. This latter requirement, in effect, places the associated electrode at the interior of the cell and allows one to clamp the membrane potential over the rest of the cell membrane. Once these criteria have been met, and assuming no manual intervention, it is then possible to conceive of a parallel format in which many wells can be measured simultaneously.

The electrophysiological study of mutant channels expressed in cell systems allows one to characterize the functional alterations and to develop new strategies for the therapy of ion channelopathies, e.g., by testing drugs that are already on the market for other indications, or drugs that could be specifically designed either to block mutant channels that reveal a gain of function, or to activate nonmutant channels that could compensate for channels functionally lost by a mutation.

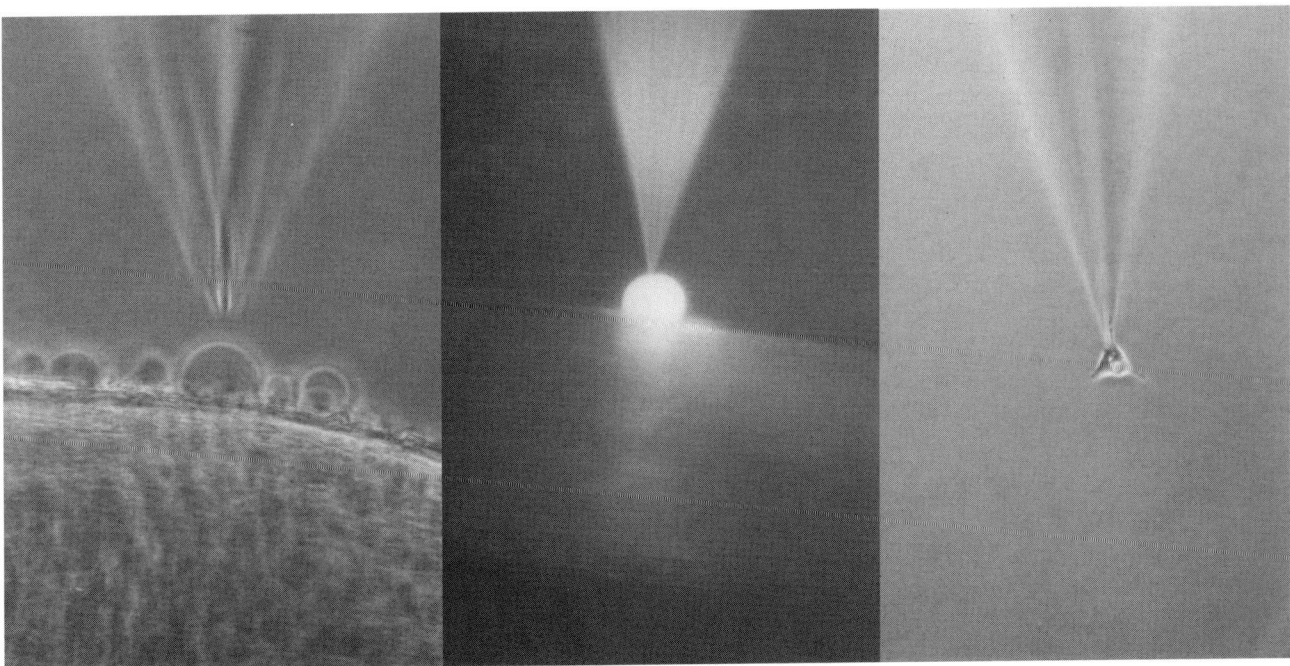

FIGURE 10-15. Measurements on membrane blebs of native human muscle fibers (*left and middle panels*) and measurements on HEK cells (*right panel*). The middle panel shows that lucifer yellow, added to the bathing solution, entered the blebs during their formation and remained within them. The membrane of native HEK and other cultured cells is so clean that giga Ω seals can easily be produced without additional measures. The diameter of a bleb is ~ 2 μm, that of a HEK cell ~ 15 μm.

Additional methods that may help to determine the electrical properties and the structure-function relationships of ion channels are becoming increasingly adapted to study single proteins in their native environment: Total internal reflection fluorescence microscopy (TIRF) makes visualization of fluorescently labeled membrane proteins possible; fluorescent resonance energy transfer (FRET) resolves the relative proximity of molecules beyond the optical limit of a light microscope; and fluorescence recovery after photobleaching (FRAP) determines whether a protein is able to move within a membrane or is tethered to structural components of the cell. In particular, the combination of these techniques with patch clamping will help to explain the mechanisms of channel gating.[188]

Acknowledgments

The chapter is based on the one previously written by Paul Horowicz, Bruce C. Spalding, and Donald R. Matteson. We thank Drs. S. Grissmer, W. Melzer, and R. Rüdel for helpful discussions, U. Richter for drawing the figures, and S. Gabriel for documentary assistance. This work was supported by the German Research Foundation (DFG) (JU470/1) and the network on Excitation-Contraction Coupling and Calcium Signaling in Health and Disease of the IHP Program funded by the European Community.

List of Abbreviations

ATP	adenosine triphosphate	PAA	phenylalkamine
BTZ	benzothiazepine	RyR1	ryanodine receptor
cAMP	cyclic adenosine monophosphate	SR	sarcoplasmic reticulum
CFTR	cystic fibrosis transmembrane regulator	STX	saxitoxin
DHP	dihydropyridine	TRP	transient receptor potential
EA-1	episodic ataxia with interictal myokymia	TTS	transverse tubular system
GTP	guanosine triphosphate	TTX	tetrodotoxin
LVA	low-voltage-activated	VDAC	voltage-gated anion-selective channels

References

1. Lehmann-Horn F, Rüdel R, Ricker K: Membrane defects in paramyotonia congenita (Eulenburg). *Muscle Nerve* 10:633–641, 1987.
2. Armstrong C: The vision of the pore. *Science* 280:56–57, 1998.
3. Doyle DA, Morais-Cabral J, Pfuetzner RA, et al: The structure of the potassium channel: Molecular basis of K+ conduction and selectivity. *Science* 280:69–77, 1998.
4. Guo D, Ramu Y, Klem AM, et al: Mechanism of rectification in inward-rectifier K+ channels. *J Gen Physiol* 121:261–276, 2003.
5. Wei A, Jegla T, Salkoff L: Eight potassium channel families revealed by the *C. elegans* genome project. *Neuropharmacology* 35:805–829, 1996.
6. Kamouchi M, Van den Bremt K, Eggermont J, et al: Modulation of inwardly rectifying potassium channels in cultured bovine pulmonary artery endothelial cells. *J Physiol* 504:545–556, 1997.
7. Ämmälä C, Moorhouse A, Gribble F, et al: Promiscuous coupling between the sulphonylurea receptor and inwardly rectifying potassium channels. *Nature* 379:545–548, 1996.
8. Clement JP IV, Kunjilwar K, Gonzalez G, et al: Association and stoichiometry of K$_{ATP}$ channel subunits. *Neuron* 18:827–838, 1997.
9. Mutations in the gene encoding the inwardly-rectifying renal potassium channel, ROMK, cause the antenatal variant of Bartter syndrome: Evidence for genetic heterogeneity. International Collaborative Study Group for Bartter-like Syndromes. *Hum Mol Genet* 6:17–26, 1997.
10. Davies NW, Standen NB, Stanfield PR: The effect of intracellular pH on ATP-dependent potassium channels of frog skeletal muscle. *J Physiol* 445:549–568, 1992.
11. Spruce AE, Standen NB, Stanfield PR: Studies of the unitary properties of adenosine-5′-triphosphate-regulated potassium channels of frog skeletal muscle. *J Physiol* 382:213–236, 1987.
12. Spuler A, Lehmann-Horn F, Grafe P: Cromakalim (BRL 34915) restores in vitro the membrane potential of depolarized human skeletal muscle fibres. *Naunyn Schmiedebergs Arch Pharmacol* 339:327–331, 1989.
13. Grafe P, Quasthoff S, Strupp M, et al: Enhancement of K+ conductance improves in vitro the contraction force of skeletal muscle in hypokalemic periodic paralysis. *Muscle Nerve* 13:451–457, 1990.
14. Kondo C, Isomoto S, Matsumoto S, et al: Cloning and functional expression of a novel isoform of ROMK inwardly rectifying ATP-dependent K+ channel, ROMK6 (Kir1.1f). *FEBS Lett* 399:122–126, 1996.
15. Jeck N, Derst C, Wischmeyer E, et al: Functional heterogeneity of ROMK mutations linked to hyperprostaglandin E syndrome. *Kidney Int* 59:1803–1811, 2001.
16. Schreiber M, Yuan A, Salkoff L: Transplantable sites confer calcium sensitivity to BK channels. *Nat Neurosci* 2:416–421, 1999.
17. Lerche H, Fahlke C, Iaizzo PA, et al: Characterization of the high-conductance Ca^{2+}-activated K+ channel in adult human skeletal muscle. *Pflügers Arch* 429:738–747, 1995.
18. Tseng-Crank J, Godinot N, Johansen TE, et al: Cloning, expression, and distribution of a Ca^{2+}-activated K+ channel β-subunit from human brain. *Proc Natl Acad Sci USA* 93:9200–9205, 1996.
19. Elkins T, Ganetzky B: The roles of potassium currents in *Drosophila* flight muscles. *J Neurosci* 8:428–434, 1988.
20. Brenner R, Yu JY, Srinivasan K, et al: Complementation of physiological and behavioral defects by a slowpoke Ca^{2+}-activated K+ channel transgene. *J Neurochem* 75:1310–1319, 2000.
21. Renaud JF, Desnuelle C, Schmid-Antomarchi H, et al: Expression of apamin receptor in muscles of patients with myotonic muscular dystrophy. *Nature* 319:678–680, 1986.
22. Behrens MI, Jalil P, Serani A, et al: Possible role of apamin-sensitive K+ channels in myotonic dystrophy. *Muscle Nerve* 17:1264–1270, 1994.
23. Ryten M, Dunn PM, Neary JT, et al: ATP regulates the differentiation of mammalian skeletal muscle by activation of a P2X5 receptor on satellite cells. *J Cell Biol* 158:345–355, 2002.
24. Launay P, Fleig A, Perraud AL, et al: TRPM4 is a Ca^{2+}-activated nonselective cation channel mediating cell membrane depolarization. *Cell* 109:397–407, 2002.
25. Monteilh-Zoller MK, Hermosura MC, Nadler MJ, et al: TRPM7 provides an ion channel mechanism for cellular entry of trace metal ions. *J Gen Physiol* 121:49–60, 2003.
26. Carlsen RC, Villarin JJ: Membrane excitability and calcium homeostasis in exercising skeletal muscle. *Am J Phys Med Rehabil* 81:S28–S39, 2002.
27. Läuger P: Kinetic basis of voltage dependence of the Na,K-pump. *Soc Gen Physiol Ser* 46:303–315, 1991.

28. Almers W: Potassium concentration changes in the transverse tubules of vertebrate skeletal muscle. *Fed Proc* 39:1527–1532, 1980.
29. Blanco G, Mercer RW: Isozymes of the Na-K-ATPase: Heterogeneity in structure, diversity in function. *Am J Physiol* 275:F633–F650, 1998.
30. Crambert G, Fuzesi M, Garty H, et al: Phospholemman (FXYD1) associates with Na,K-ATPase and regulates its transport properties. *Proc Natl Acad Sci USA* 99:11476–11481, 2002.
31. Hundal HS, Marette A, Mitsumoto Y, et al: Insulin induces translocation of the alpha 2 and beta 1 subunits of the Na^+/K^+-ATPase from intracellular compartments to the plasma membrane in mammalian skeletal muscle. *J Biol Chem* 267:5040–5043, 1992.
32. Lavoie L, Levenson R, Martin-Vasallo P, et al: The molar ratios of alpha and beta subunits of the Na^+-K^+-ATPase differ in distinct subcellular membranes from rat skeletal muscle. *Biochemistry* 36:7726–7732, 1997.
33. Pestov NB, Adams G, Shakhparonov MI, et al: Identification of a novel gene of the X,K-ATPase beta-subunit family that is predominantly expressed in skeletal and heart muscles. *FEBS Lett* 456:243–248, 1999.
34. Haller RG, Clausen T, Vissing J: Reduced levels of skeletal muscle Na^+K^+-ATPase in McArdle disease. *Neurology* 50:37–40, 1998.
35. De Fusco M, Marconi R, Silvestri L, et al: Haploinsufficiency of ATP1A2 encoding the Na^+/K^+ pump alpha2 subunit associated with familial hemiplegic migraine type 2. *Nature Genet* 33:192–196, 2003.
36. Juel C, Grunnet L, Holse M, et al: Reversibility of exercise-induced translocation of Na^+-K^+ pump subunits to the plasma membrane in rat skeletal muscle. *Pflügers Arch* 443:212–217, 2001.
37. Ewart HS, Klip A: Hormonal regulation of the Na^+-K^+-ATPase: Mechanisms underlying rapid and sustained changes in pump activity. *Am J Physiol* 269:C295–C311, 1995.
38. Kjeldsen K, Norgaard A, Gotzsche CO, et al: Effect of thyroid function on number of Na-K pumps in human skeletal muscle. *Lancet* 2:8–10, 1984.
39. Dorup I, Skajaa K, Clausen T: A simple and rapid method for the determination of the concentrations of magnesium, sodium, potassium and sodium, potassium pumps in human skeletal muscle. *Clin Sci (Lond)* 74:241–248, 1988.
40. Thompson CB, McDonough AA: Skeletal muscle Na,K-ATPase alpha and beta subunit protein levels respond to hypokalemic challenge with isoform and muscle type specificity. *J Biol Chem* 271:32653–32658, 1996.
41. Nicoll DA, Ottolia M, Philipson KD: Toward a topological model of the NCX1 exchanger. *Ann N Y Acad Sci* 976:11–18, 2002.
42. Fraysse B, Rouaud T, Millour M, et al: Expression of the Na^+/Ca^{2+} exchanger in skeletal muscle. *Am J Physiol Cell Physiol* 280:C146–C154, 2001.
43. Li Z, Matsuoka S, Hryshko LV, et al: Cloning of the NCX2 isoform of the plasma membrane Na^+-Ca^{2+} exchanger. *J Biol Chem* 269:17434–17439, 1994.
44. Moore-Hoon ML, Turner RJ: The structural unit of the secretory Na^+-K^+-$2Cl^-$ cotransporter (NKCC1) is a homodimer. *Biochemistry* 39:3718–3724, 2000.
45. Isenring P, Jacoby SC, Forbush B 3rd: The role of transmembrane domain 2 in cation transport by the Na-K-Cl cotransporter. *Proc Natl Acad Sci USA* 95:7179–7184, 1998.
46. Xu JC, Lytle C, Zhu TT, et al: Molecular cloning and functional expression of the bumetanide-sensitive Na-K-Cl cotransporter. *Proc Natl Acad Sci USA* 91:2201–2205, 1994.
47. Lindinger MI, Hawke TJ, Lipskie SL, et al: K^+ transport and volume regulatory response by NKCC in resting rat hindlimb skeletal muscle. *Cell Physiol Biochem* 12:279–292, 2002.
48. Gillen CM, Brill S, Payne JA, et al: Molecular cloning and functional expression of the K-Cl cotransporter from rabbit, rat, and human. A new member of the cation-chloride cotransporter family. *J Biol Chem* 271:16237–16244, 1996.
49. Pearson MM, Lu J, Mount DB, et al: Localization of the K^+-Cl^- cotransporter, KCC3, in the central and peripheral nervous systems: Expression in the choroid plexus, large neurons and white matter tracts. *Neuroscience* 103:481–491, 2001.
50. Delpire E, Mount DB: Human and murine phenotypes associated with defects in cation-chloride cotransport. *Annu Rev Physiol* 64:803–843, 2002.
51. Mount DB, Gamba G: Renal potassium-chloride cotransporters. *Curr Opin Nephrol Hypertens* 10:685–691, 2001.
52. Lytle C, McManus T: Coordinate modulation of Na-K-2Cl cotransport and K-Cl cotransport by cell volume and chloride. *Am J Physiol Cell Physiol* 283:C1422–C1431, 2002.
53. Nilius B, Droogmans G: Ion channels and their functional role in vascular endothelium. *Physiol Rev* 81:1415–1459, 2001.
54. Geukes Foppen RJ, Van Mil HG, Van Heukelom JS: Effects of chloride transport on bistable behaviour of the membrane potential in mouse skeletal muscle. *J Physiol* 542:181–191, 2002.
55. Kwiecinski H, Lehmann-Horn F, Rüdel R: The resting membrane parameters of human intercostal muscle at low, normal, and high extracellular potassium. *Muscle Nerve* 7:60–65, 1984.
56. Hodgkin AL, Rushton WAH: The electrical constants of a crustacean nerve fibre. *Proc R Soc Lond [Biol]* 133:444, 1946.
57. Lehmann-Horn F, Rüdel R, Dengler R, et al: Membrane defects in paramyotonia congenita with and without myotonia in a warm environment. *Muscle Nerve* 4:396–406, 1981.
58. Fatt P, Katz B: An analysis of the endplate potential recorded with an intra-cellular electrode. *J Physiol* 115:320, 1951.
59. Hodgkin AL, Huxley AF: A quantitative description of membrane current and its application to conduction and excitation in nerve. *J Physiol* 117:500, 1952.
60. Armstrong CM, Bezanilla F: Charge movement associated with the opening and closing of the activation gates of the Na channels. *J Gen Physiol* 63:533–552, 1974.
61. Armstrong CM, Bezanilla F: Inactivation of the sodium channel: II. Gating current experiments. *J Gen Physiol* 70:567–590, 1977.
62. Bezanilla F, Armstrong CM: Inactivation of the sodium channel: I. Sodium current experiments. *J Gen Physiol* 70:549–566, 1977.
63. Aldrich RW, Corey DP, Stevens CF: A reinterpretation of mammalian sodium channel gating based on single channel recording. *Nature* 306:436–441, 1983.
64. Lopez GA, Jan YN, Jan LY: Hydrophobic substitution mutations in the S4 sequence alter voltage-dependent gating in Shaker K^+ channels. *Neuron* 7:327–336, 1991.
65. Stühmer W, Conti F, Suzuki H, et al: Structural parts involved in activation and inactivation of the sodium channel. *Nature* 339:597–603, 1989.
66. Mannuzzu LM, Moronne MM, Isacoff EY: Direct physical measure of conformational rearrangement underlying potassium channel gating. *Science* 271:213–216, 1996.
67. Yang N, George AL Jr, Horn R: Molecular basis of charge movement in voltage-gated sodium channels. *Neuron* 16:113–122, 1996.
68. Cha A, Snyder GE, Selvin PR, et al: Atomic scale movement of the voltage-sensing region in a potassium channel measured via spectroscopy. *Nature* 402:809–813, 1999.
69. Sato C, Ueno Y, Asai K, et al: The voltage-sensitive sodium channel is a bell-shaped molecule with several cavities. *Nature* 409:1047–1051, 2001.
70. Catterall WA: A 3D view of sodium channels. *Nature* 409:988–991, 2001.
71. Campbell DT: Ionic selectivity of the sodium channel of frog skeletal muscle. *J Gen Physiol* 67:295–307, 1976.
72. Hoshi T, Zagotta WN, Aldrich RW: Biophysical and molecular mechanisms of Shaker potassium channel inactivation. *Science* 250:533–538, 1990.
73. Vassilev PM, Scheuer T, Catterall WA: Identification of an intracellular peptide segment involved in sodium channel inactivation. *Science* 241:1658–1661, 1988.
74. West JW, Patton DE, Scheuer T, et al: A cluster of hydrophobic amino acid residues required for fast Na^+-channel inactivation. *Proc Natl Acad Sci USA* 89:10910–10914, 1992.
75. Kellenberger S, Scheuer T, Catterall WA: Movement of the Na^+ channel inactivation gate during inactivation. *J Biol Chem* 271:30971–30979, 1996.
76. Lerche H, Peter W, Fleischhauer R, et al: Role in fast inactivation of the IV/S4–S5 loop of the human muscle Na^+ channel probed by cysteine mutagenesis. *J Physiol* 505:345–352, 1997.
77. McPhee JC, Ragsdale DS, Scheuer T, et al: A critical role for the S4-S5 intracellular loop in domain IV of the sodium channel α-subunit in fast inactivation. *J Biol Chem* 273:1121–1129, 1998.
78. Filatov GN, Nguyen TP, Kraner SD, et al: Inactivation and secondary structure in the D4/S4-5 region of the SkM1 sodium channel. *J Gen Physiol* 111:703–715, 1998.
79. Chahine M, George AL Jr, Zhou M, et al: Sodium channel mutations in paramyotonia congenita uncouple inactivation from activation. *Neuron* 12:281–294, 1994.
80. O'Leary ME, Chen LQ, Kallen RG, et al: A molecular link between activation and inactivation of sodium channels. *J Gen Physiol* 106:641–658, 1995.
81. Patton DE, West JW, Catterall WA, et al: A peptide segment critical for sodium channel inactivation functions as an inactivation gate in a potassium channel. *Neuron* 11:967–974, 1993.
82. Isacoff EY, Jan YN, Jan LY: Putative receptor for the cytoplasmic inactivation gate in the Shaker K^+ channel. *Nature* 353:86–90, 1991.
83. Holmgren M, Jurman ME, Yellen G: N-type inactivation and the S4-S5 region of the Shaker K^+ channel. *J Gen Physiol* 108:195–206, 1996.
84. Shon KJ, Grilley MM, Marsh M, et al: Purification, characterization, synthesis, and cloning of the lockjaw peptide from *Conus purpurascens* venom. *Biochemistry* 34:4913–4918, 1995.
85. McPhee JC, Ragsdale DS, Scheuer T, et al: A critical role for transmembrane segment IVS6 of the sodium channel α subunit in fast inactivation. *J Biol Chem* 270:12025–12034, 1995.
86. Mitrovic N, Lerche H, Heine R, et al: Role in fast inactivation of conserved amino acids in the IV/S4-S5 loop of the human muscle Na^+ channel. *Neurosci Lett* 214:9–12, 1996.
87. Ruff RL: Single-channel basis of slow inactivation of Na^+ channels in rat skeletal muscle. *Am J Physiol* 271:C971–C981, 1996.
88. Todt H, Dudley S-C Jr, Kyle JW, et al: Ultra-slow inactivation in mu1 Na^+ channels is produced by a structural rearrangement of the outer vestibule. *Biophys J* 76:1335–1345, 1999.
89. Almers W: Gating currents and charge movements in excitable membranes. *Rev Physiol Biochem Pharmacol* 82:96–190, 1978.
90. Lerche H, Mitrovic N, Dubowitz V, et al: Paramyotonia congenita: The R1448P Na^+ channel mutation in adult human skeletal muscle. *Ann Neurol* 39:599–608, 1996.

91. Kuzmenkin A, Muncan V, Jurkat-Rott K, et al: Enhanced inactivation and pH sensitivity of Na$^+$ channel mutations causing hypokalaemic periodic paralysis type II. *Brain* 125:835–843, 2002.
92. Colquhoun D, Hawkes AG: Relaxation and fluctuations of membrane currents that flow through drug-operated channels. *Proc R Soc Lond [Biol]* 199:231–262, 1977.
93. Colquhoun D, Hawkes AG: On the stochastic properties of single ion channels. *Proc R Soc Lond [Biol]* 211:205–235, 1981.
94. Franke C, Hatt H: Characteristics of single Na$^+$ channels of adult human skeletal muscle. *Pflügers Arch* 415:399–406, 1990.
95. Chen Q, Kirsch GE, Zhang D, et al: Genetic basis and molecular mechanism for idiopathic ventricular fibrillation. *Nature* 392:293–296, 1998.
96. Angaut-Petit D, McArdle JJ, Mallart A, et al: Electrophysiological and morphological studies of a motor nerve in "motor endplate disease" of the mouse. *Proc R Soc Lond [Biol]* 215:117–125, 1982.
97. Gurnett CA, Campbell KP: Transmembrane auxiliary subunits of voltage-dependent ion channels. *J Biol Chem* 271:27975–27978, 1996.
98. Makita N, Bennett PB Jr, George AL Jr: Voltage-gated Na$^+$ channel β1 subunit mRNA expressed in adult human skeletal muscle, heart, and brain is encoded by a single gene. *J Biol Chem* 269:7571–7578, 1994.
99. Krafte DS, Snutch TP, Leonard JP, et al: Evidence for the involvement of more than one mRNA species in controlling the inactivation process of rat and rabbit brain Na channels expressed in Xenopus oocytes. *J Neurosci* 8:2859–2868, 1988.
100. Krafte DS, Goldin AL, Auld VJ, et al: Inactivation of cloned Na channels expressed in Xenopus oocytes. *J Gen Physiol* 96:689–706, 1990.
101. Isom LL, De Jongh KS, Patton DE, et al: Primary structure and functional expression of the β1 subunit of the rat brain sodium channel. *Science* 256:839–842, 1992.
102. Isom LL, De Jongh KS, Catterall WA: Auxiliary subunits of voltage-gated ion channels. *Neuron* 12:1183–1194, 1994.
103. Isom LL, Scheuer T, Brownstein AB, et al: Functional co-expression of the β1 and type IIA α subunits of sodium channels in a mammalian cell line. *J Biol Chem* 270:3306–3312, 1995.
104. Ji S, Sun W, George AL Jr, et al: Voltage-dependent regulation of modal gating in the rat SkM1 sodium channel expressed in *Xenopus* oocytes. *J Gen Physiol* 104:625–643, 1994.
105. Schreibmayer W, Wallner M, Lotan I: Mechanism of modulation of single sodium channels from skeletal muscle by the β1-subunit from rat brain. *Pflügers Arch* 426:360–362, 1994.
106. Stevens EB, Cox PJ, Shah BS, et al: Tissue distribution and functional expression of the human voltage-gated sodium channel beta3 subunit. *Pflügers Arch* 441:481–488, 2001.
107. Cruz LJ, Gray WR, Olivera BM, et al: Conus geographus toxins that discriminate between neuronal and muscle sodium channels. *J Biol Chem* 260:9280–9288, 1985.
108. Ohizumi Y, Nakamura H, Kobayashi J, et al: Specific inhibition of [3H] saxitoxin binding to skeletal muscle sodium channels by geographutoxin II, a polypeptide channel blocker. *J Biol Chem* 261:6149–6152, 1986.
109. Possani LD, Becerril B, Delepierre M, et al: Scorpion toxins specific for Na$^+$-channels. *Eur J Biochem* 264:287–300, 1999.
110. De Luca A, Proebstle T, Brinkmeier H, et al: The different use dependences of tocainide and benzocaine are correlated with different effects on sodium channel inactivation. *Naunyn Schmiedebergs Arch Pharmacol* 344:596–601, 1991.
111. Hille B: *Ion Channels of Excitable Membranes*. Sunderland, MA: Sinauer; 2001.
112. Khan A, Romantseva L, Lam A, et al: Role of outer ring carboxylates of the rat skeletal muscle sodium channel pore in proton block. *J Physiol* 543:71–84, 2002.
113. Hahin R, Campbell DT: Simple shifts in the voltage dependence of sodium channel gating caused by divalent cations. *J Gen Physiol* 82:785–805, 1983.
114. Nakajima S, Kusano K: Behavior of delayed current under voltage clamp in the supramedullary neurons of puffer. *J Gen Physiol* 49:613–628, 1966.
115. Connor JA, Stevens CF: Voltage clamp studies of a transient outward membrane current in gastropod neural somata. *J Physiol* 213:21–30, 1971.
116. Kukuljan M, Labarca P, Latorre R: Molecular determinants of ion conduction and inactivation in K$^+$ channels. *Am J Physiol* 268:C535–C556, 1995.
117. Grissmer S, Cahalan MD: Divalent ion trapping inside potassium channels of human T lymphocytes. *J Gen Physiol* 93:609–630, 1989.
118. Lopez-Barneo J, Hoshi T, Heinemann SH, et al: Effects of external cations and mutations in the pore region on C-type inactivation of Shaker potassium channels. *Recept Channels* 1:61–71, 1993.
119. De Biasi M, Hartmann HA, Drewe JA, et al: Inactivation determined by a single site in K$^+$ pores. *Pflügers Arch* 422:354–363, 1993.
120. Pardo LA, Heinemann SH, Terlau H, et al: Extracellular K$^+$ specifically modulates a rat brain K$^+$ channel. *Proc Natl Acad Sci USA* 89:2466–2470, 1992.
121. Jäger H, Rauer H, Nguyen AN, et al: Regulation of mammalian Shaker-related K$^+$ channels: Evidence for non-conducting closed and non-conducting inactivated states. *J Physiol* 506:291–301, 1998.
122. Vullhorst D, Klocke R, Bartsch JW, et al: Expression of the potassium channel KV3.4 in mouse skeletal muscle parallels fiber type maturation and depends on excitation pattern. *FEBS Lett* 421:259–262, 1998.
123. Vullhorst D, Jockusch H, Bartsch JW: The genomic basis of K(V)3.4 potassium channel mRNA diversity in mice. *Gene* 264:29–35, 2001.
124. Morales MJ, Castellino RC, Crews AL, et al: A novel beta subunit increases rate of inactivation of specific voltage-gated potassium channel alpha subunits. *J Biol Chem* 270:6272–6277, 1995.
125. Sanchez JA, Ho CS, Vaughan DM, et al: Muscle and motor-skill dysfunction in a K$^+$ channel-deficient mouse are not due to altered muscle excitability or fiber type but depend on the genetic background. *Pflügers Arch* 440:34–41, 2000.
126. Schroeder BC, Hechenberger M, Weinreich F, et al: KCNQ5, a novel potassium channel broadly expressed in brain, mediates M-type currents. *J Biol Chem* 275:24089–24095, 2000.
127. Kubisch C, Schroeder BC, Friedrich T, et al: KCNQ4, a novel potassium channel expressed in sensory outer hair cells, is mutated in dominant deafness. *Cell* 96:437–446, 1999.
128. Cooper EC, Aldape KD, Abosch A, et al: Colocalization and coassembly of two human brain M-type potassium channel subunits that are mutated in epilepsy. *Proc Natl Acad Sci USA* 97:4914–4919, 2000.
129. Wang MC, Velarde G, Ford RC, et al: 3D structure of the skeletal muscle dihydropyridine receptor. *J Mol Biol* 323:85–98, 2002.
130. Yang J, Ellinor PT, Sather WA, et al: Molecular determinants of Ca^{2+} selectivity and ion permeation in L-type Ca^{2+} channels. *Nature* 366:158–161, 1993.
131. Almers W, McCleskey EW, Palade PT: A non-selective cation conductance in frog muscle membrane blocked by micromolar external calcium ions. *J Physiol* 353:565–583, 1984.
132. De Jongh KS, Warner C, Colvin AA, et al: Characterization of the two size forms of the alpha 1 subunit of skeletal muscle L-type calcium channels. *Proc Natl Acad Sci USA* 88:10778–10782, 1991.
133. Beam KG, Adams BA, Niidome T, et al: Function of a truncated dihydropyridine receptor as both voltage sensor and calcium channel. *Nature* 360:169–171, 1992.
134. Yatani A, Wakamori M, Niidome T, et al: Stable expression and coupling of cardiac L-type Ca^{2+} channels with β1-adrenoceptors. *Circ Res* 76:335–342, 1995.
135. Fleig A, Penner R: Silent calcium channels generate excessive tail currents and facilitation of calcium currents in rat skeletal myoballs. *J Physiol* 494:141–153, 1996.
136. Bijlenga P, Liu JH, Espinos E, et al: T-type alpha 1H Ca^{2+} channels are involved in Ca^{2+} signaling during terminal differentiation (fusion) of human myoblasts. *Proc Natl Acad Sci USA* 97:7627–7632, 2000.
137. Jurkat-Rott K, Uetz U, Pika-Hartlaub U, et al: Calcium currents and transients of native and heterologously expressed mutant skeletal muscle DHP receptor α1 subunits (R528H). *FEBS Lett* 423:198–204, 1998.
138. Jay SD, Sharp AH, Kahl SD, et al: Structural characterization of the dihydropyridine-sensitive calcium channel α$_2$-subunit and the associated δ peptides. *J Biol Chem* 266:3287–3293, 1991.
139. Gurnett CA, De Waard M, Campbell KP: Dual function of the voltage-dependent Ca^{2+} channel α2 δ subunit in current stimulation and subunit interaction. *Neuron* 16:431–440, 1996.
140. Singer D, Biel M, Lotan I, et al: The roles of the subunits in the function of the calcium channel. *Science* 253:1553–1557, 1991.
141. Brice NL, Berrow NS, Campbell V, et al: Importance of the different beta subunits in the membrane expression of the alpha1A and alpha2 calcium channel subunits: Studies using a depolarization-sensitive alpha1A antibody. *Eur J Neurosci* 9:749–759, 1997.
142. Lacerda AE, Kim HS, Ruth P, et al: Normalization of current kinetics by interaction between the α$_1$ and β subunits of the skeletal muscle dihydropyridine-sensitive Ca^{2+} channel. *Nature* 352:527–530, 1991.
143. Varadi G, Lory P, Schultz D, et al: Acceleration of activation and inactivation by the β subunit of the skeletal muscle calcium channel. *Nature* 352:159–162, 1991.
144. De Waard M, Liu H, Walker D, et al: Direct binding of G-protein betagamma complex to voltage-dependent calcium channels. *Nature* 385:446–450, 1997.
145. Walker D, Bichet D, Campbell KP, et al: A β4 isoform-specific interaction site in the carboxyl-terminal region of the voltage-dependent Ca^{2+} channel α1A subunit. *J Biol Chem* 273:2361–2367, 1998.
146. Sipos I, Pika-Hartlaub U, Hofmann F, et al: Effects of the dihydropyridine receptor subunits gamma and alpha2delta on the kinetics of heterologously expressed L-type Ca^{2+} channels. *Pflügers Arch* 439:691–699, 2000.
147. Jentsch TJ, Stein V, Weinreich F, et al: Molecular structure and physiological function of chloride channels. *Physiol Rev* 82:503–568, 2002.
148. Fahlke C: Ion permeation and selectivity in ClC-type chloride channels. *Am J Physiol Renal Physiol* 280:F748–F757, 2001.
149. Mindell JA, Maduke M, Miller C, et al: Projection structure of a ClC-type chloride channel at 6.5 A resolution. *Nature* 409:219–223, 2001.
150. Dutzler R, Campbell EB, Cadene M, et al: X-ray structure of a ClC chloride channel at 3.0 A reveals the molecular basis of anion selectivity. *Nature* 415:287–294, 2002.

THE MACROMOLECULAR COMPLEX OF JSR

Limited detergent extraction of jSR extracts the Ca ATPase, but leaves behind a complex set of proteins.[117,118] It is now clear that calsequestrin (CSQ),[118,119] triadin,[44–46,121,122] RyRs,[122,123] and junctin[47] are associated with each other in the jSR (Fig. 11-21A). CSQ is confined to the lumen of the jSR in skeletal and cardiac muscle, despite the continuity of this compartment with the free SR lumen. Yet CSQ is a luminal protein that is easily extracted with EGTA or EDTA under slightly alkaline conditions.[124] Search for a possible targeting signal within the CSQ molecule that may allow it to be retained in the jSR have so far given negative results.[125] Neither phosphorylation sites, nor specific glycosylation, nor the C-terminal region of the molecule are necessary for its location in the jSR.

Deep etching of the jSR reveals elongated links connecting the central loose CSQ network to the SR membrane (Fig. 11-21B).[126] The nature of the CSQ linkage to the jSR membrane has been elucidated through overexpression of junctin and triadin in cardiac muscle. Native jSR cisternae in myocardial cells are flat and the calsequestrin is condensed in periodic densities (Fig. 11-20).[9,10] Overexpression of CSQ results in greatly enlarged SR cisternae with a finely dispersed CSQ content. Although many of the CSQ-containing cisternae are junctional, CSQ is also found in other parts of the SR. Overexpression of junctin and triadin has effects that are similar to each other and opposite to the CSQ effect: The jSR cisternae in this case are narrower than usual and the calsequestrin content is highly aggregated.[127] When overexpressed in combination with calsequestrin, junctin is capable of condensing the calsequestrin in proximity to the membrane, but not elsewhere. Thus triadin and junctin have overlapping roles in clustering and maintaining calsequestrin in the jSR regions.

Based on in vitro interactions and domain analysis, a different role for triadin, as a RyR-DHPR linker, has also been proposed.[44] It is unlikely that a single protein can make a

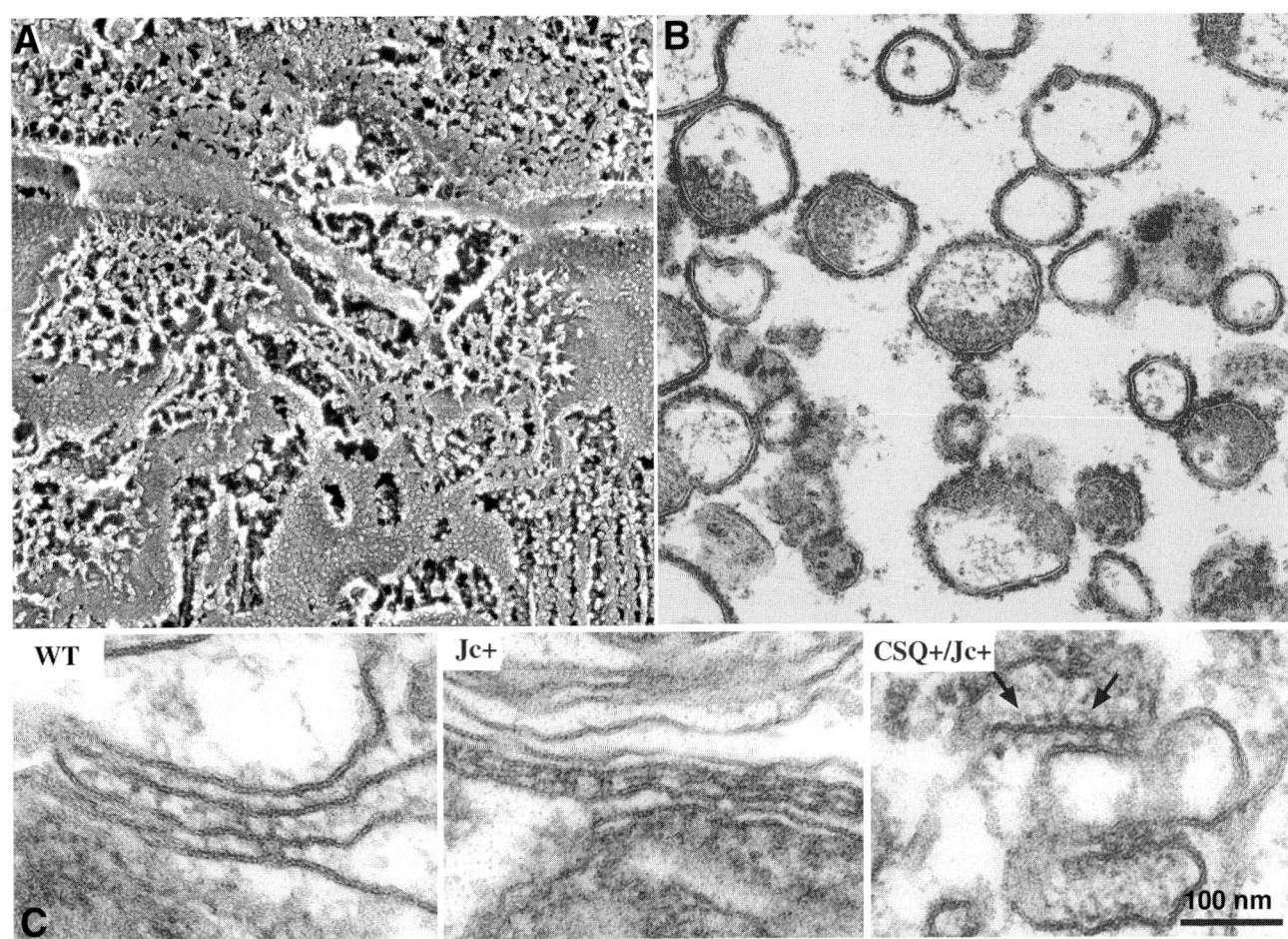

FIGURE 11-21. One of the junctional SR proteins, calsequestrin, is visible within the SR lumen. In deeply etched images of the toadfish swimbladder muscle (A), calsequestrin forms a three-dimensional meshwork. B. In the isolated heavy SR, calsequestrin is clustered in proximity of the feet-bearing SR membrane. The role of junctin in clustering calsequestrin in proximity of the jSR membrane is put in evidence by overexpression of the junctin and calsequestrin in cardiac muscle. A. In a native SR vesicle from the heart of a 1-week-old mouse, calsequestrin is loosely arranged in the SR lumen. B. Overexpression of junctin results in tightening of the calsequestrin disposition. C. Overexpression of calsequestrin and junctin results in widening of the junctional SR cisternae due to a larger amount of calsequestrin, but clustering at the edge of the membrane is still visible. (See Zhang L, Franzini-Armstrong C, Ramesh V, et al: Structural alterations in cardiac calcium release units resulting from overexpression of junctin. J Mol Cell Cardiol 33:233, 2000.)

of the two molecules is essential to the interaction. Interestingly, however, RyR segments that are most effective in allowing channel cross talk are in the same region of the molecule but do not exactly coincide with those that are effective in inducing tetrad formation. The mechanical linkage that allows formation of tetrads and the functional coupling that allows cross talk are thus probably mediated by slightly different but partially overlapping regions of the molecules.[103]

RYR AND DHPR ISOFORMS: FUNCTIONAL ROLE AND LOCATION

Three isoforms of the RyR (RyR1, RyR2, RyR3), with widespread tissue distribution, have been identified in vertebrates and extensively reviewed in the literature.[69,104,105] The α and β isoforms of avian and amphibian muscle are equivalent, although not identical, to RyR1 and RyR3, respectively. The three RyR isoforms have related sequences, which, however, differ largely in two divergent domains (D1 and D2) of the large hydrophilic region forming the foot. The D2 domain is actually missing in RyR3. Skeletal muscle always contains RyR1, but it may also have variable amounts of RyR3, from none to approximately 50 percent of the total. Cardiac muscle has the RyR2 isoform. Invertebrates have a single RyR isoform,[107,108] which probably derives from a common precursor of all three vertebrate forms.[109]

RyR1 is an obligatory component of skeletal muscle because it is the only type that can link to DHPR and sustain skeletal type e-c coupling. Lack of RyR1 results in grave developmental defects, muscle paralysis, and lack of DHPR tetrads. RyR3 does not sustain e-c coupling in the absence of RyR1,[110–112] it does not link to skeletal DHPR,[112] and its absence in mouse has only minor effects on muscle activity.[113]

The position of RyR3 is parajunctional in skeletal muscle: Feet representing this isoform are located at the sides of the junction and thus face toward the myofibrils rather than toward the T tubules (Fig. 11-20B and C). In addition to being parajunctional, RyR3s differ from RyR1s in that they form arrays with different parameters. It is logical to assume that RyR3s are not directly activated by DHPR but are probably regulated by the Ca^{2+} released through the junctional RyR1s.

The single RyR type present in cardiac and invertebrate muscles also has two possible positions relative to the T tubules and to the DHPRs. Some RyRs are located in the jSR membrane facing T tubules, while others either are parajunctional like RyR3, or are present on corbular SR, which may be at a large distance from T tubules and/or surface membrane (Fig. 11-9).

The $\alpha 1$ channel-forming subunit of the DHPR is also muscle-type specific: The $\alpha 1_s$ (also known as $Ca_V 1.1$) is present in skeletal muscle and the $\alpha 1_c$ (also known as $Ca_V 1.2$) in cardiac muscle.[83,84] The two isoforms have different channel kinetic properties and interact differently with RyRs (see Chap. 12).

VARIATIONS IN DHPR/RYR RATIO

The alternate tetrad disposition of skeletal muscle predicts a DHPR/RyR ratio of 2:1 in the junctional membranes of CRUs with maximum possible occupancy of feet by complete tetrads. In avian cardiac muscle, the density of DHPR in the junctional domains of the plasmalemma participating in peripheral couplings also indicates a ratio of DHPR particles to feet of approximately 2:1.[92] Measurements of radiolabeled dihydropyridine and ryanodine binding confirm a 2:1 ratio in rabbit fast-twitch fibers but give lower and variable ratios in other species and muscles.[114–116] The measured DHPR/RyR ratios in a variety of cardiac muscles are also considerably lower than predicted for the avian peripheral couplings. The binding data are not in contradiction with the structural information when one considers the reasons given below.

In skeletal muscle, there are two reasons for observing a DHPR/RyR ratio lower than 2. First, alternate RyR1 are associated with DHPR tetrads, but RyR3 are located in a parajunctional position and do not associate with DHPRs. In muscles with equal amounts of RyR3 and RyR1, the maximum predicted DHPR/RyR ratio is thus 1 rather than 2, and values between 1 and 2 are expected in muscles with various RyR3/RyR2 ratios. A second parameter affecting the DHPR/RyR ratio is the variable occupancy of tetrads by DHPRs. In most cases, tetrad arrays contain "incomplete" tetrads that are located in the appropriate position relative to the feet but miss one or more elements, thus lowering the DHPR/RyR ratio. Given the low affinity between DHPR and RyR, it is expected that in a dynamic view of the junction DHPRs are continuously shifting around from one tetrad to the other.

In cardiac muscle, the overall DHPR/RyR ratio is also affected by two factors. One is the density of DHPRs in the jPl domains, which seems to be much lower in mammalian than in avian myocardium, and the other is the presence of extended (or corbular) jSR, whose feet are not associated with DHPRs. In the fast myocardium of the finch,[10] up to 80 percent of the feet are located in SR cisternae belonging to CRUs that have no DHPR-containing domains (the extended jSR), and other avian muscles have a similar high proportion of extended junctional SR. This effectively lowers the overall DHPR/RyR ratio to very low values even if the ratio at sites of peripheral couplings is close to 2.

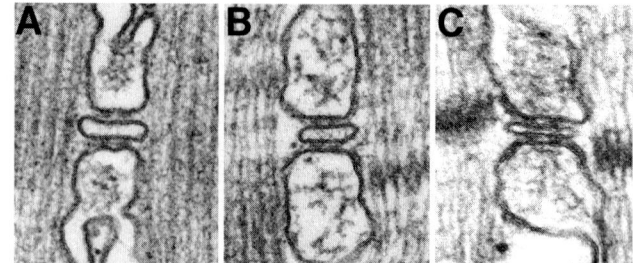

FIGURE 11-20. Thin sections of triads from muscles with different contents of RyR type 3 (or β). The toadfish swimbladder muscle (A) has no RyR3 and presents two rows of junctional feet. The toadfish white tail muscle (B) and the frog leg muscle (C) have a 1:1 ratio of the two types of RyRs. They show two rows of junctional feet and additional rows of parajunctional feet in the adjacent SR membrane. (See Felder E, Franzini-Armstrong C: Type 3 ryanodine receptors of skeletal muscles are segregated in a parajunctional position. Proc Natl Acad Sci USA, 99:1695, 2002.)

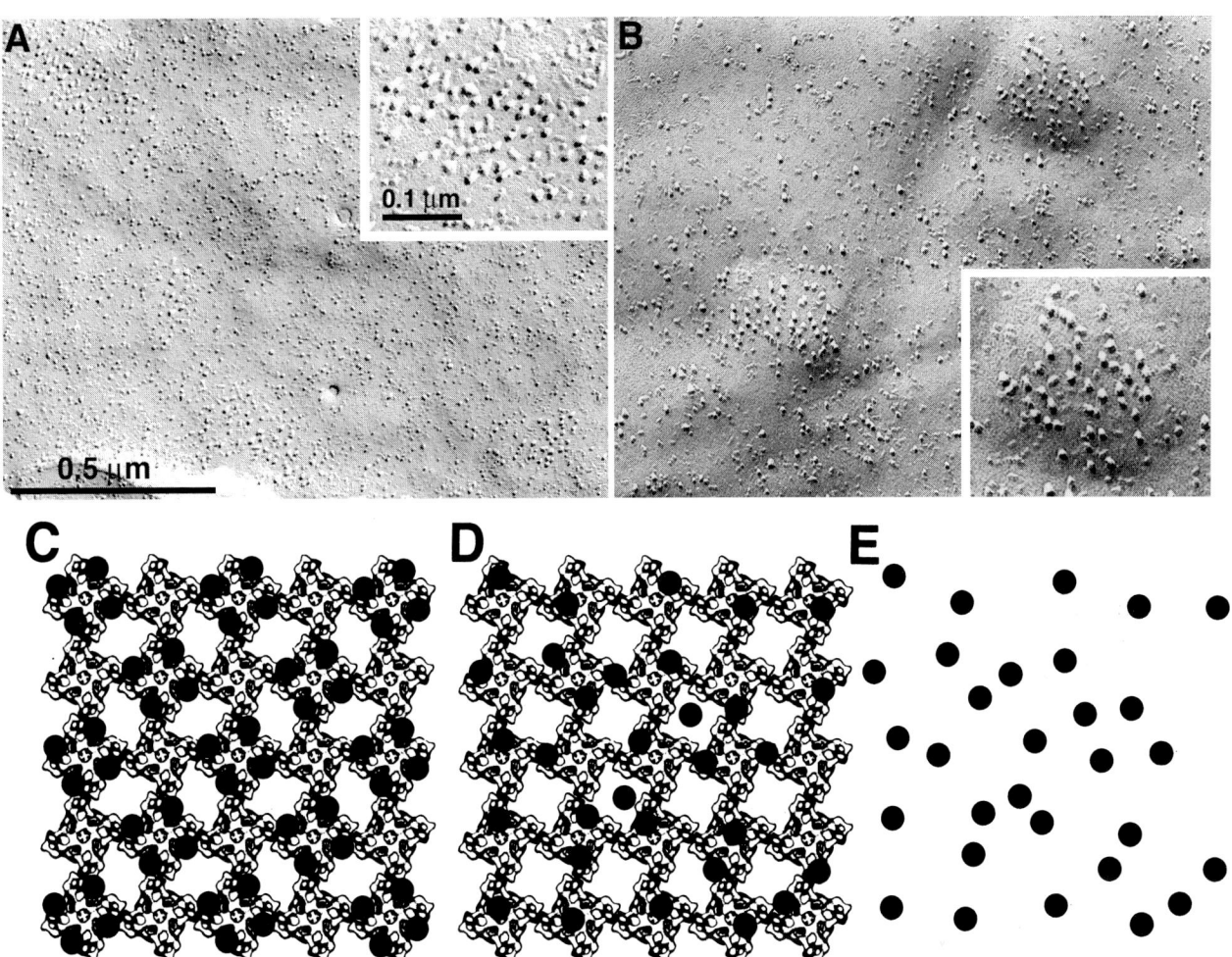

FIGURE 11-19. A and B. DHPRs are clustered at CRUs in vertebrate cardiac (A, from finch ventricle) and invertebrate body (B, from crayfish tail flexor) muscles, but they do not form tetrads. C and D. Models showing RyR-DHPR relationships in skeletal (A), cardiac (B), and dyspedic skeletal (C) muscles. RyRs are represented by four gray balls and each DHPR by one black circle. *(See Protasi F, Franzini-Armstrong C, Allen PD: Role of ryanodine receptors in the assembly of calcium release units in skeletal muscle. J Cell Biol 140:831, 1998.)* *((A) From Protasi F, Sommer JR, and Franzini-Armstrong C, unpublished; (B) from Eastwood AB, Franzini-Armstrong C, Peracchia C: Structure of membranes in crayfish muscle: comparison of phasic and tonic fibers. J Muscle Res Cell Motil 3:273, 1982. With permission.)* *(Parts C–E from Paolini C, Protesi, F, Franzini-Armstrong C, unpublished.)*

this case, proximity of RyR and DHPR is essential, but a close link between the two proteins is not necessary. The basis for the structural and functional dichotomy between skeletal muscle and all others is based on variations in the isoform composition (see below). The RyR-DHPR interaction in skeletal muscle involves bidirectional talk and a direct conformational coupling between the two molecules (see Chap. 12).[96–98] Although numerous examples of channel interactions and their modulations are known, this talk between channels located in two separate membrane systems is novel. Discovery of this molecular interaction in muscle has led to the understanding of other systems in which two sets of membranes exchange information. Most notable is the case of the store-operated channels, in which permeability to calcium of surface membrane channels may be modulated by interaction with RyR.[99] It should be noted that the DHPR-RyR interaction may not be direct but may be mediated by some intermediary protein (see below).

One puzzle remains unexplained: DHPR tetrads are associated with alternate feet, so that every other foot is not connected (Figs. 11-18 and 11-19). The arrangement seems to be common to all vertebrate muscles, and it is also present when tetrads are just beginning to assemble in nascent CRUs.[90] This leaves three possibilities open: Either alternate feet are silent, or they are indirectly activated by Ca^{2+} liberated by the coupled feet,[100,101] or they are activated by a direct interaction with the DHPR coupled feet, as suggested for the cardiac channel.[102,103]

Cardiac-skeletal chimeras for the RyR and DHPR, and peptides derived from them, have been used to define which domains are responsible for cross talk, as described in Chap. 12. From the structural point of view, it is important to note that any combination of RyR and DHPR chimeras that supports DHPR-RyR communication of the skeletal muscle type (i.e., probably direct) also results in the formation of tetrads. This demonstrates that the appropriate relative positioning

units of the feet. The centers of the four tetrad particles are slightly peripheral relative to the centers of the feet subunit and are located approximately above the region of the RyR forming the "clamp," which changes configuration when the channels open.

Identification of the four particles constituting the tetrads with four DHPRs is based on their absence in the dysgenic mouse model, which carries a lethal, null mutation of the skeletal muscle DHPRs. The mutation results in lack of e-c coupling and absence of tetrads, although SR–T tubule junctions with feet and calsequestrin are present. Transfection of cultured dysgenic myotubes with cDNA for skeletal muscle DHPRs restores e-c coupling and tetrads (see Chap. 12).[94] Other data confirming the identification of tetrads as groups of four DHPRs are the location of DHPRs at CRUs in situ,[88–90] and the comparable size of purified DHPRs and of the individual components of j tetrads.[65]

In a skeletal muscle cell line lacking RyRs, DHPRs are associated with sites of peripheral couplings, but are not organized into tetrads (Figs. 11-18C and D). Transfection with cDNA for RyR1 restores DHPR tetrads (Fig. 11-18E and F), confirming that anchorage of DHPRs to the four subunits of RyR is a requisite for tetrad formation.[91] Note that this anchorage is specific to the skeletal DHPR-RyR1 interaction. Other RyR isoforms do not restore DHPR tetrads (see below).

The functional significance of the specific DHPR-RyR link of skeletal muscle that results in the tetrad arrangement of DHPRs is emphasized by a comparison of skeletal on one side with cardiac and invertebrate muscles on the other.

Functionally the two sets of muscles differ in that e-c coupling is independent of Ca^{2+} permeation through the DHPRs in skeletal muscle, while it requires Ca^{2+} currents in cardiac and invertebrate muscles (see Chap. 12). Structurally, the muscles differ because in skeletal muscle the DHPRs are linked to RyRs and thus are arranged into arrays of tetrads (Fig. 11-18),[65,90] while in cardiac and invertebrate muscles tetrads are not present (Fig. 11-19A through D). [92,93] Figure 11-19C through E illustrates the superimposition of DHPR tetrads and RyR subunits that is present in skeletal muscle, the random arrangement of DHPRs superimposed on ordered RyRs in cardiac and invertebrate muscles, and the random arrangement of skeletal DHPRs in the absence of RyR1 in dyspedic muscle.

With the recent publication of the DHPR structure at a fairly high level of resolution,[94a,94b] the relative positioning of DHPRs and RyRs in skeletal muscle is being considered more closely. The model of Fig. 11-19C provides a low-resolution view of the overlapping RyR and DHPR arrays, suggested by a comparison of freeze-fracture, freeze-drying, and thin-sectioning data.

It is thought that skeletal muscle DHPRs act as voltage sensors for the membrane depolarization and that they transmit the effect of depolarization to the RyR via a molecule-to-molecule cross talk, essentially as postulated by Schneider and Chandler.[95] Evidence for this interaction is very strong and is discussed in Chap. 12. In cardiac and invertebrate muscles, on the other hand, it is thought that Ca entering via the DHPR acts as a messenger for the activation of RyR. In

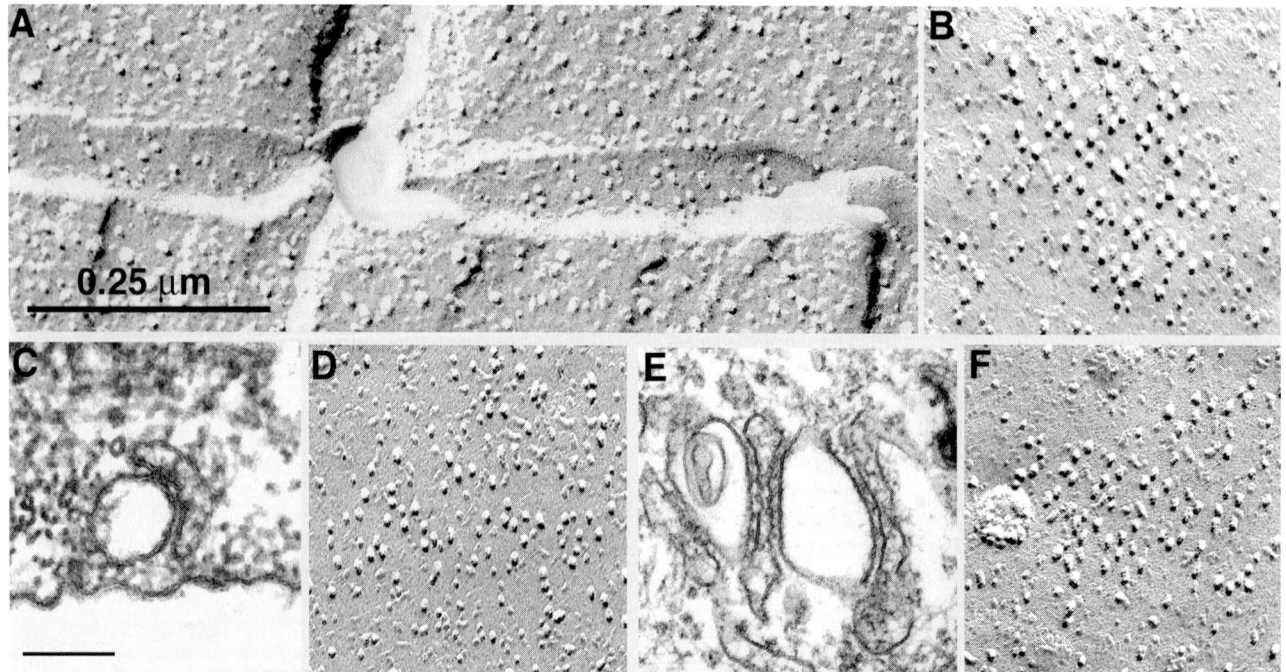

FIGURE 11-18. Freeze-fractures of T tubules (A) and surface membranes (B, D, and F) at sites of CRUs. Tetrads, constituted of four dihydropyridine receptors, occupy the junctional domains of T tubules. (A from fish[65]; B from a mouse skeletal muscle cell line.[90]) Association of DHPRs with RyRs is necessary for the formation of tetrads: In a dyspedic cell resulting from a null mutation for RyR1, feet are absent (C) and DHPRs are clustered at the junctions but do not form tetrads (D). Feet (E) and tetrads (F) are restored by transfection of the dyspedic cells with cDNA for RyR1. (See Protasi F, Franzini-Armstrong C, Allen PD: Role of ryanodine receptors in the assembly of calcium release units in skeletal muscle. J Cell Biol 140:831, 1998.)

porated into a lipid bilayer form Ca^{2+} release channels with a high conductivity[61] and properties similar to the rapid release from heavy SR. A second breakthrough came with the initial isolation of a high-molecular-weight component of the triad[62] and the subsequent purification of a large (30S) macromolecular complex with high affinity for ryanodine from the heavy SR fraction.[63-65] The complex was reconstituted into a Ca^{2+} channel that has the same properties as the in situ Ca^{2+} release channel and whose cytoplasmic domain is identified with the jSR feet. The RyR channel is regulated by Ca^{2+} and a variety of ligands.[66-70]

RyR is a high-molecular-weight (~2.10^6 Da) homotetramer composed of four identical peptides, each with a short hydrophobic domain inserted in the jSR membrane to constitute the channel regions and a large hydrophilic domain in the cytoplasm.[71,72] One foot, with its four subunits, represents the cytoplasmic domain of one RyR (Fig. 11-17A). The intramembrane portion of RyR can be directly visualized within the jSR membrane using the freeze-fracture technique.[65] Three-dimensional reconstructions of the RyR have greatly advanced understanding of this complex molecule and its interactions.[73,74] The cytoplasmic domain of the foot has a complex structure, including four radially arranged low-density regions apparently connecting a central channel with the periphery of the molecule (Fig. 11-17B). The three known types of RyR (see below) differ only slightly in the structure of the cytoplasmic domains.[73-75] Functionally significant domains (e.g., calmodulin and FKBP12-binding regions) have been identified within the tertiary structure, laying the foundation for eventual high-resolution reconstructions (Fig. 11-17B).[75-79] Interestingly, interventions that affect the open state of the channel result in detectable motions of the "clamp" regions of the molecule that are located at the four corners of the foot, far from the intramembrane channel-forming domains (Fig. 11-17C).[80,81] Somewhat similar rearrangement of cytoplasmic domains is induced by calcium regulation in the other ER calcium release channel, the inositol 1,4,5-trisphosphate receptor (IP3R).[82] Thus long-range molecular interactions are probably at the basis of channel regulation, in a manner reminiscent of events in the Ca ATPase (see Chap. 14).

RyRs are responsible for a class of muscle diseases, including malignant hyperthermia, that are characterized by Ca^{2+} leakage from the SR (see Chap. 61).

Structural Relationships between Components of Calcium Release Units

Identification of RyRs with the feet puts the Ca^{2+} release function of the SR in a very convenient location, in proximity to junctional domains of exterior membranes [T tubules (jT) and/or plasmalemma (jPl)] from which the initial signal for e-c coupling is initiated. Transduction of plasmalemma and T-tubule depolarization into a signal for release of Ca^{2+} via the SR RyR is mediated by a second Ca^{2+} channel, the L-type Ca^{2+} channels, or dihydropyridine receptor (DHPR).[83-87] DHPRs are located at high density in jT and jPl domains of both skeletal and cardiac muscles.[88-93]

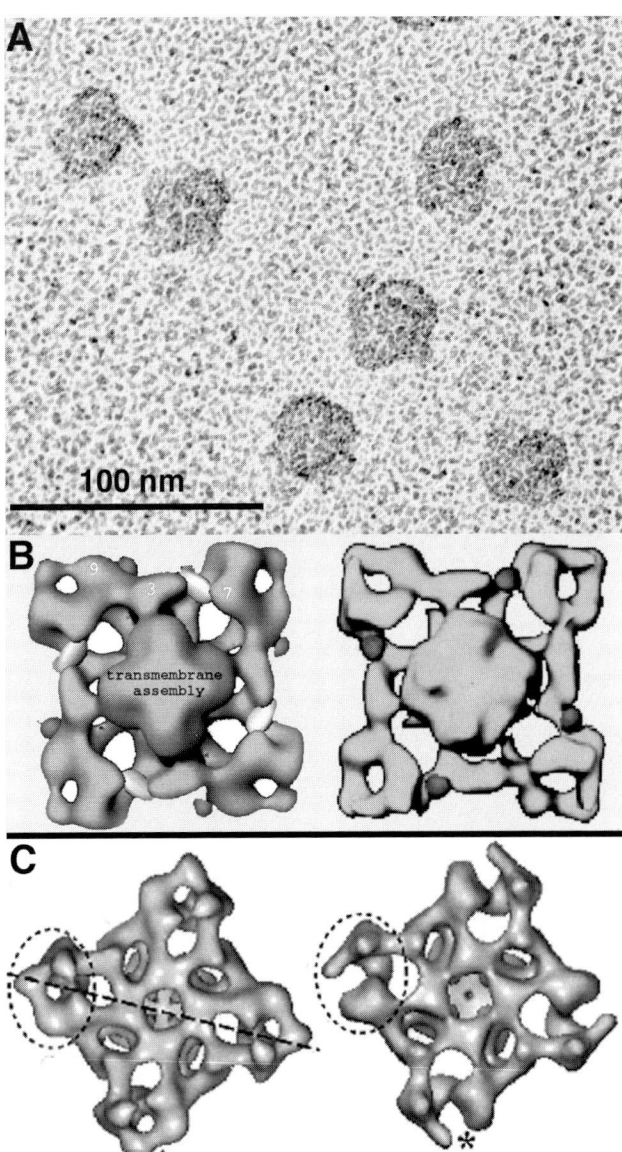

FIGURE 11-17. A. Rotary shadowed images of the purified RyR showing the four large cytoplasmic domains and the raised central transmembrane domain. (See Block BA, Imagawa T, Campbell KP, et al: Structural evidence for direct interaction between the molecular components of the transverse tubules/sarcoplasmic reticulum junction in skeletal muscle. J Cell Biol 107:2587, 1988.) B. Three-dimensional reconstructions of the isolated RyR molecule showing the transmembrane domain and details of the cytoplasmic domains. Sites of interactions with calmodulin and FKBP (white and light-gray spots, respectively, at left) and with imperatoxin (dark-gray spots at right) have been reconstructed.[76,77] C. Reconstructions of the RyR in the open and closed configurations show a large conformational change in the "clamp" domain, which is in the vicinity of the T-tubule membrane.[81]

In freeze-fracture replicas, the jT and jPl membranes are occupied by distinctive tall intramembranous particles, which directly face the jSR membrane covered by feet. Other membrane proteins are mostly excluded from these regions. In skeletal muscle the particles are arranged in groups of four (junctional tetrads) (Fig. 11-18A and B).[65] This positioning is due to a stereospecific interaction with the four sub-

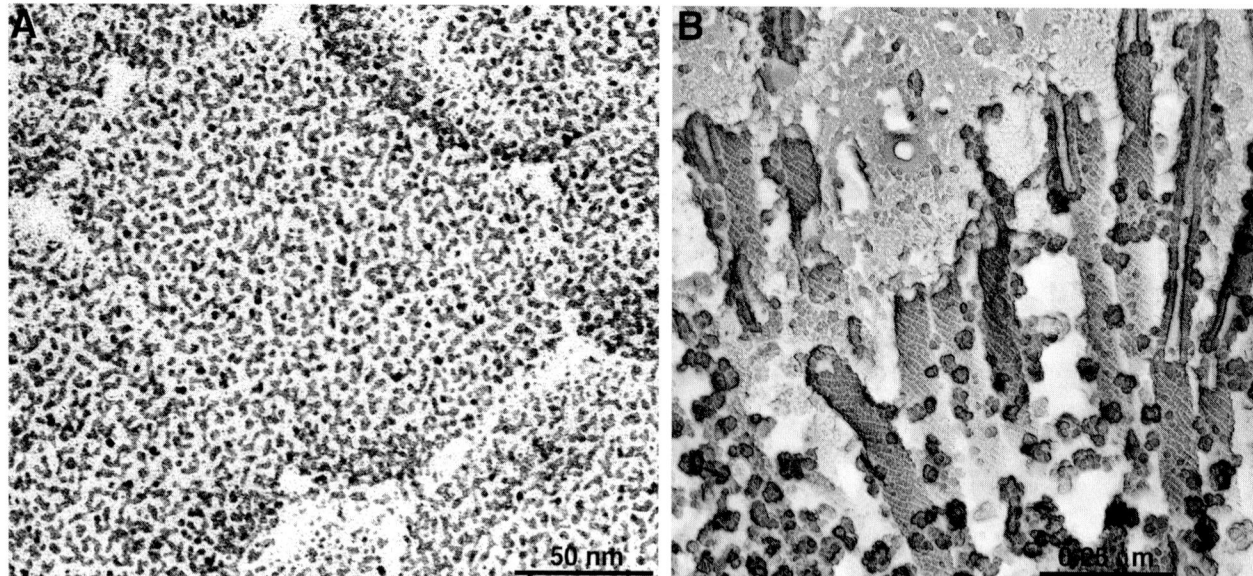

FIGURE 11-15. Surface views of isolated rabbit SR vesicles (A) and in situ SR tubes in a scallop muscle (B). Note different magnification. Each of the small spots in (A) is the cytoplasmic domain of a single Ca^{2+} ATPase molecule. The molecules are disposed without apparent order but may frequently form dimers. In the native SR of scallop muscle (B) the Ca^{2+} ATPase has a semicrystalline arrangement, with rows of ATPase dimers helically arranged around the SR tubes. (See Ferguson DG, Franzini-Armstrong C, Castellani L, et al: Ordered arrays of CaATPase tails on the cytoplasmic surface of isolated sarcoplasmic reticulum. Biophys J 48:597, 1985; Castellani L, Hardwicke P, Franzini-Armstrong C: Effect of Ca^{2+} on the dimeric structure of scallop sarcoplasmic reticulum. J Cell Biol 108:511, 1989.)

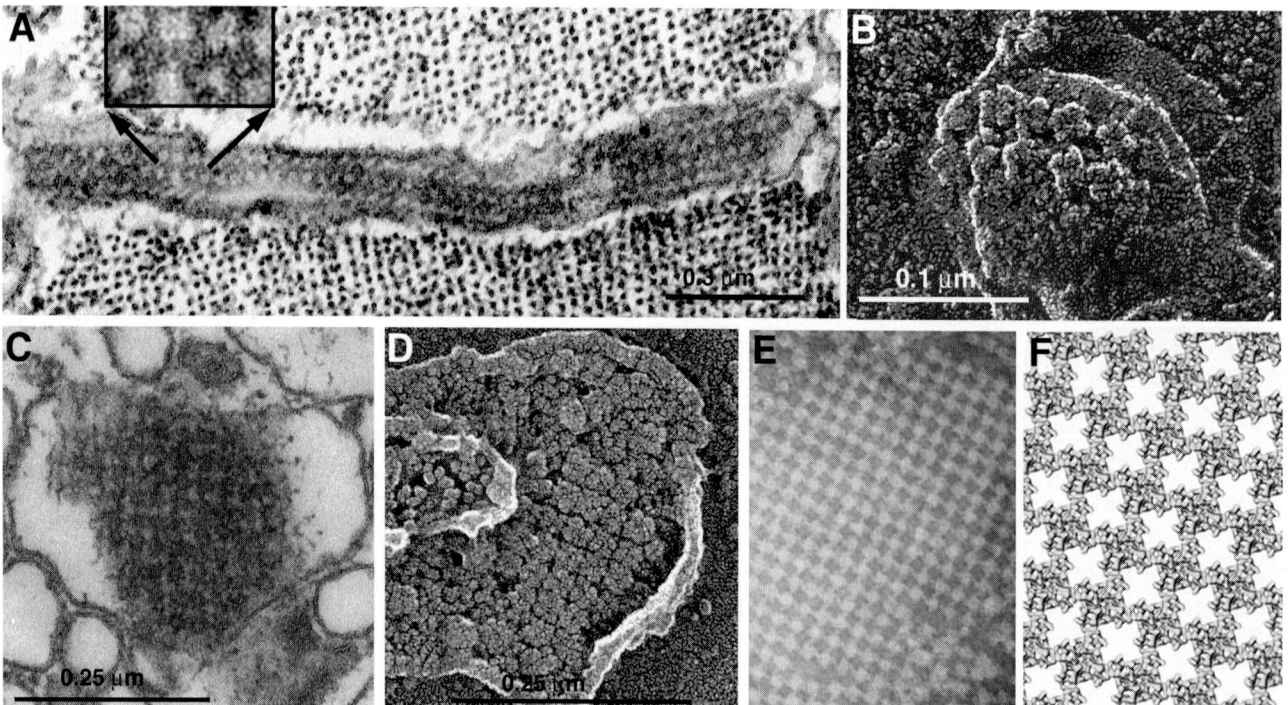

FIGURE 11-16. Dispositions of feet in vivo and in vitro. A and B. In skeletal muscles, feet are disposed in orthogonal arrays in which they abut corner to corner, but with a slight skew. (From Ferguson DG, Schwartz H, and Franzini-Armstrong C: Subunit structure of junctional feet in triads of skeletal muscle. A freeze-drying, rotary-shadowing study. J Cell Biol 99:1735, 1984. With permission.) (Note: the images in B and F are mirror images of the real disposition, which is shown in Fig. 11-19.) C and D. In muscles of arthropods, the arrangement is also tetrameric, but the skew of alternate molecules is slightly different. E. Purified RyRs assemble in vitro into the same orthogonal configuration as in vivo. (From Yin CC, Lai FA: Intrinsic lattice formation by the ryanodine receptor calcium-release channel. Nature New Biol 2:669, 2000. With permission.) F. A model of the disposition of feet constructed with the use of high-resolution images (see Fig. 11-17). (See Protasi F, Takekura H, Wang Y, et al: RYR1 and RYR3 have different roles in the assembly of calcium release units of skeletal muscle. Biophys J 79: 2494–2508, 2000.)

distributed all over the surface of the cell. The proposed identification of square arrays with clusters of aquaporins[50] is confirmed by expression in CHO cells of aquaporin 4, the muscle isoform.[51] The lower protein/lipid ratio of T tubules relative to the plasmalemma is emphasized by the scarcity of intramembrane particles in the nonjunctional (free) T-tubule segments (see Fig. 11-14).

The structure of the junctional domains of plasmalemma and T tubules are described below.

STRUCTURE OF FREE SR

The functional separation of SR into uptake (free SR) and storage-release (jSR) domains has strong structural correlations. The SR ATPase, or Ca^{2+}-pump protein, is distributed evenly over the entire free SR surface but is excluded from the jSR membrane.[52-54] The protein breaks asymmetrically in freeze-fracture replicas, so that particles remain on the cytoplasmic leaflet (Fig. 11-14).[12] This indicates a protein strongly anchored to the cytoplasmic side of the membrane and uniformly oriented in the membrane. Indeed, the protein has large catalytic and phosphorylation domains of the ATPase that protrude into the cytoplasm, forming a large head domain, ten transmembrane helices, and a very minor luminal component (see Chap. 14).

The distribution of ATPase particles in the free SR membrane is uniform; there are no large areas of obviously greater or lesser density. In slower skeletal muscle fibers, in myocardium, and in muscles of invertebrates, however, there may be small bald spots from which the ATPase is excluded. The distribution of particles in the plane of the membrane is extremely irregular although crowded (Fig. 11-15). Comparison of the fractured membrane and the cytoplasmic surface of the SR (Figs. 11-14 and 11-15) shows that each of the intramembrane particles represents a group of two to three ATPases and that the overall density is approximately $30,000/\mu m^2$. Recent studies of vanadate-induced orderly aggregates of Ca^{2+} ATPase (see Chap. 14) and of aggregates in native SR in scallop muscle (Fig. 11-15)[55] indicate that the basic arrangement of the molecules is dimeric, although it is not clear what portion of the protein is dimeric in vivo.

COMPOSITION AND STRUCTURE OF CRUS

The membrane fraction of the muscle homogenate can be separated into four homogeneous subfractions by density gradient centrifugation.[15] The fractions, in order of increasing density, contain T tubules and surface membrane, free SR, jSR, and mitochondria. The jSR fraction, also called heavy SR, derives from the lateral sacs of the triads, and the density of its vesicles is mostly due to the content of calsequestrin, a luminal protein.[15] Calsequestrin has a low affinity, but high capacity for binding Ca^{2+} and is responsible for the high total Ca^{2+} capacity of jSR. A more careful isolation procedure maintains the integrity of triadic junctions.

The membrane limiting jSR vesicles is divided into two domains. One domain comprises the sides of the jSR vesicles that face the myofibrils in situ and is occupied by Ca^{2+} ATPase, being a continuation of the free SR. The second jSR membrane domain contains the feet and faces the T tubules. ATPase does not penetrate into this domain, which instead is occupied by a macromolecular complex, including the feet, involved in communication with the T tubules and in Ca^{2+} movements (Fig. 11-16A to F).

In the heavy SR fraction and in situ, feet protrude from the cytoplasmic surface of the SR (Fig. 11-16B). Each foot is composed of four apparently identical subunits closely associated and surrounding a central depression (tetrafoil). In the native disposition, feet form ordered arrays by interacting approximately corner to corner but with some overlap. The disposition is slightly different in skeletal and invertebrate muscles (compare Figs. 11-16A and B with C and D). In cardiac muscles, feet are part of an ordered array with spacings similar to those in skeletal muscle, but the exact disposition is not known. Feet reconstituted in vitro and in vivo form arrays with parameters identical to those in situ (Fig. 11-16E and F),[56,57] indicating that the arrangement is due to a direct interaction between feet without need for other jSR proteins.

Experiments in the 1980s determined that feet are the cytoplasmic domains of the SR Ca^{2+} release channels, or RyRs. Feet-bearing heavy SR vesicles release Ca^{2+} at rates comparable to those occurring during muscle activation under appropriate conditions, while light SR does not.[58] The rapid leak is activated by Ca^{2+}, is inhibited by magnesium, requires adenine nucleotides for activity, and is initiated by extremely low concentrations of ryanodine, a plant alkaloid for which heavy SR has a high affinity.[59,60] SR vesicles incor-

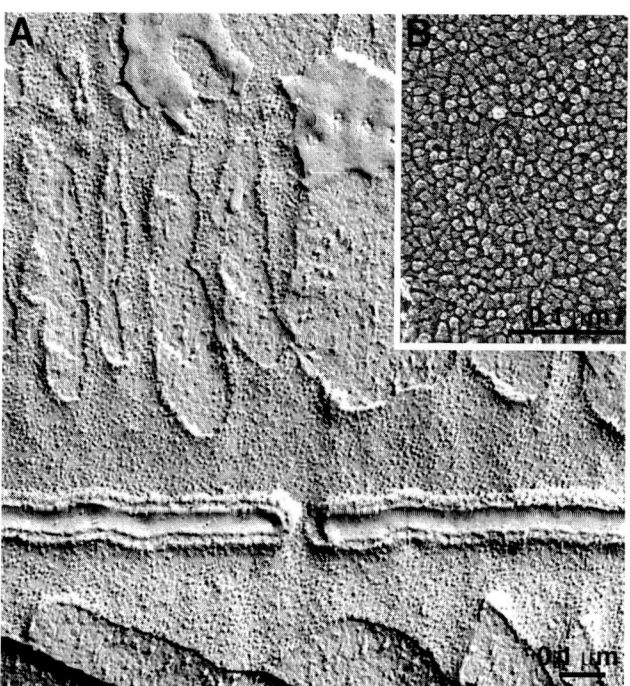

FIGURE 11-14. A. Freeze-fracture showing the even distribution of intramembrane particles representing small clusters of Ca^{2+} ATPase in the free SR membrane. B. Detail in rotary shadow. Each bright spot is constituted of two or three molecules. (See Franzini-Armstrong C, Ferguson DG: Density and disposition of CaATPase in sarcoplasmic reticulum membrane as determined by shadowing techniques. Biophys J 48: 607, 1985.)

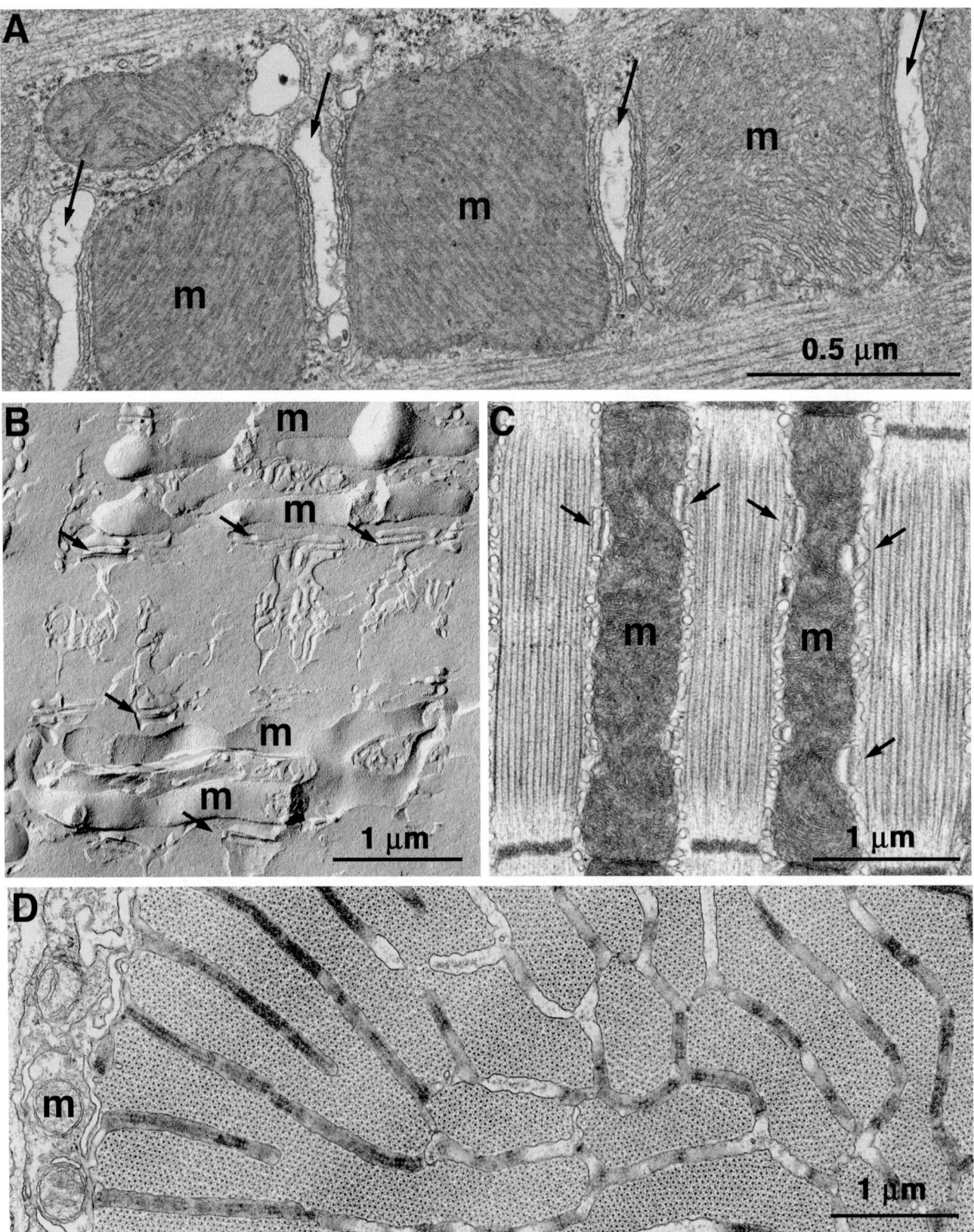

FIGURE 11-13. Mitochondria (m) are often located in close proximity to CRUs (arrows), and as a result they are transiently exposed to high levels of Ca^{2+} during excitation-contraction coupling. A. Cardiac muscle. (From Sharma VK, Ramesh V, Franzini-Armstrong C, Sheu S-S: Transport of Ca from the sarcoplasmic reticulum to mitochondria in rat ventricular myocytes. In "Frontiers of Mitochondrial Research" J Bioenergetics Biomembranes 32:97–104, 2000.) B. Rat "red" muscle fiber in freeze-fracture. C. Dragonfly flight muscle. D. Interestingly, in the very fast acting muscle of the toadfish, mitochondria are segregated at the fiber periphery, at some distance from myofibrils and CRUs.

T tubules have properties and composition similar to those of the surface membrane, but with a different proportion of the corresponding macromolecular structures, such as those associated with pumps and ionic channels and a clearly distinct protein profile (see Chaps. 12 and 19). General roles in ion transport are performed by the free T tubules and probably also by that portion of the membrane in jT tubules which is not directly facing the SR. The SR-associated jT membrane mediates e-c coupling; its content of DHPRs is described below.

Although maintaining a minor complement of generic endoplasmic reticulum (ER) proteins, the two SR domains dedicated to uptake of Ca^{2+} and to its storage and release are mostly composed of the specific proteins dedicated to these specialized tasks. The free SR, with a large surface-to-volume ratio and comprising the large majority of the SR surface area, is dedicated to Ca^{2+} pumping. The free SR membrane is fully occupied by a high density of the Ca^{2+} pump protein or Ca^{2+} ATPase, which is its major component (see Chap. 14). Phospholamban, an intrinsic SR protein, controls the activity of the Ca^{2+} pump in cardiac and slow-twitch skeletal muscle fibers, inhibiting it under basal conditions.[11] The junctional SR, composing CRUs, houses a junctional complex of proteins that include calsequestrin,[15] triadin,[44-46] and junctin[47] in addition to the ryanodine receptor (RyR). A large variety of proteins (calmodulin, FKBP12, Homer) are associated with the RyRs (see Chap. 14).

STRUCTURE OF THE SURFACE MEMBRANE (PLASMALEMMA)

Freeze-fracture replicas reveal intramembrane proteins, and deep-etching unveils the cytoplasmic and/or exterior domains of membrane macromolecules. Alone or in combination, the two techniques are used to define the location and arrangement of membrane components. The exterior membrane of muscle cells is decorated by a large variety of intramembrane particles, representing ionic channels, pumps, receptors, etc.—most of which cannot be given a specific identity because they are randomly disposed. Exceptions are proteins that are identified on the basis of specific location, size, and grouping. The heads of cholinergic receptor molecules are seen as protrusions of the postsynaptic membrane, arranged in orderly parallel rows two abreast at a high concentration.[48] Receptors for excitatory and inhibitory transmitters in arthropod fibers are clearly distinguishable on the basis of their postsynaptic grouping. Gap junctions' connexons are detected as highly ordered arrays of hexagonally arranged proteins, which occupy large membrane patches in differentiating skeletal muscle and in developing and adult cardiac muscle. Aquaporins, the fairly recently identified channels responsible for water permeability, are present in relatively large amounts on the plasmalemma, particularly in fast fibers. They are represented by small tetragonal aggregates of particles, the so-called square arrays,[49] that are

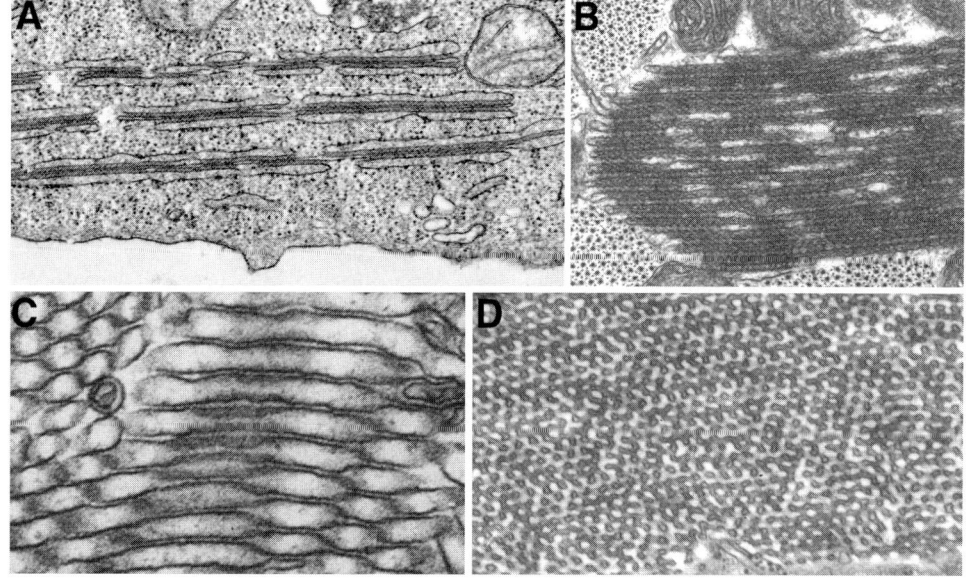

FIGURE 11-12. Unusual dispositions of feet, SR, and T tubules. *A.* Chinese hamster ovary cells expressing ryanodine receptors (RyRs). RyR-decorated ER cisternae face each other. *(See Takekura H, Takeshima H, Nishimura S, et al: Co-expression in CHO cells of two muscle proteins involved in excitation-contraction coupling. J Muscle Res Cell Motil 16:465, 1995.)* *B.* A similar disposition is found in opossum cardiac muscle. *(From Waugh RA, Sommer JR: Lamellar junction and sarcoplasmic reticulum. A specialization of cardiac sarcoplasmic reticulum. J Cell Biol 63:337, 1974. With permission.)* *C.* Tubular aggregates of free SR are induced by either hypoxia or cyanide in rat muscles. *(From Schiaffino S, Severin E, Contini G, et al: Tubular aggregates induced by anoxia in isolated rat skeletal muscle. Lab Invest 37:223, 1977. With permission.)* *D.* T tubules may form extensive "honeycomb" systems in either developing or pathologic muscles. *(From Schotland DL: An electron microscopic investigation of myotonic dystrophy. J Neuropathol Exp Neurol 29:241, 1970. With permission.)*

Diversity of Composition and Molecular Architecture

COMPOSITION OF SURFACE MEMBRANE, FREE T TUBULES, AND FREE SR

Some functions of the membrane system are performed by proteins that are randomly distributed. Some of these distributed functions of the plasmalemma, and the effector molecules involved, include maintenance of constant intracellular ionic composition (sodium, potassium, and Ca^{2+} pumps and exchange mechanisms); water movements (aquaporins); excitability (a variety of voltage-sensitive channels, see Chap. 10); sensitivity to hormones, including importantly insulin (receptors and associated enzymes); and a possible variety of tasks associated with caveolae. In contrast to these, macromolecular assemblies involved in reception of the synaptic signal, cell-to-cell communication via gap junctions (which are present at two stages of muscle differentiation), and e-c coupling are located in specialized membrane domains that are structurally identifiable by electron microscopy. The surface membrane contains clusters of dihydropyridine receptors (DHPRs) involved in excitation-contraction coupling only in the cells that have peripheral couplings (e.g., cardiac muscle, frog tonic fibers, amphioxus and scallop muscles, and skeletal muscle cells at early stages of differentiation).

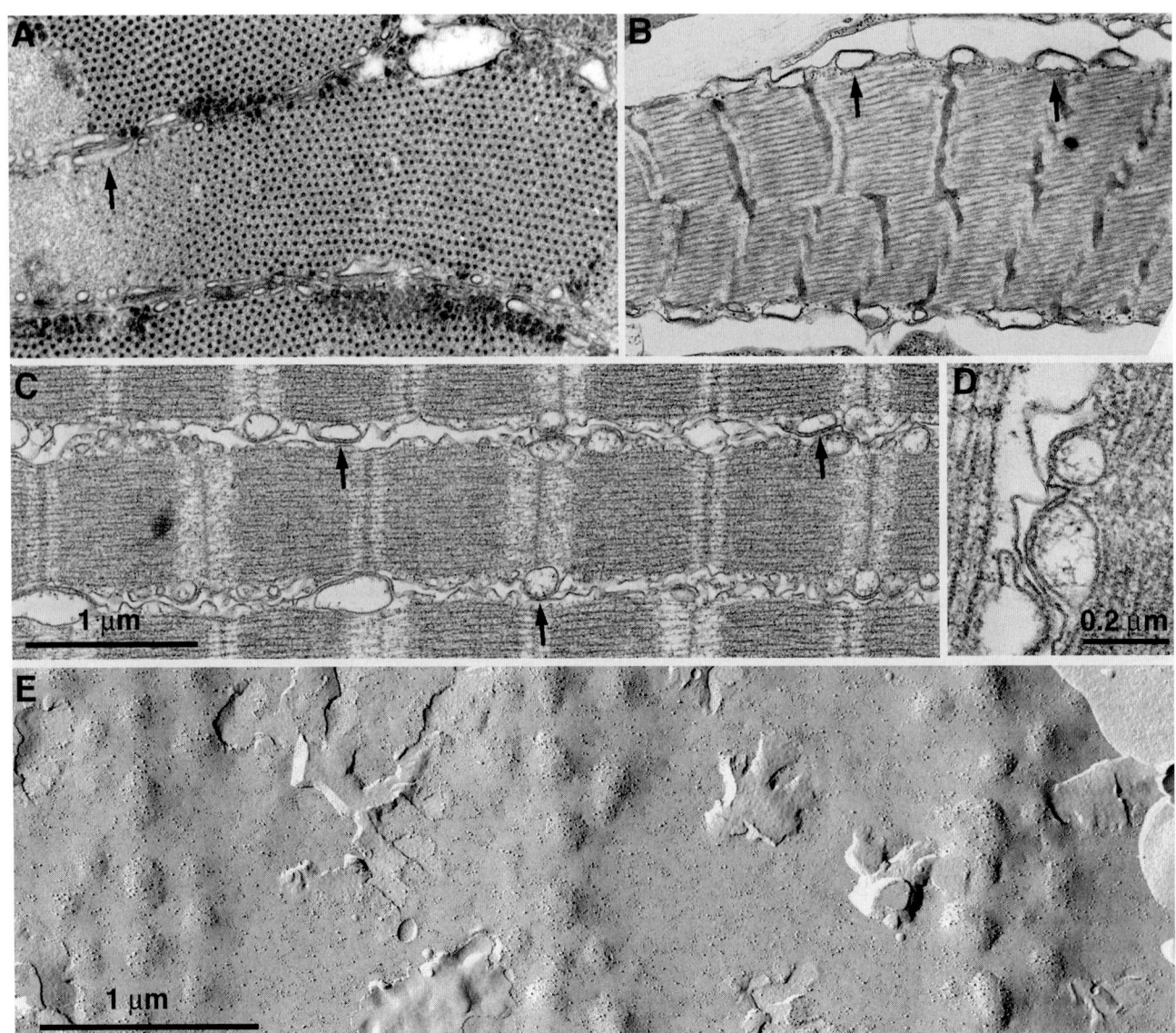

FIGURE 11-11. T tubules are not present in some muscle fibers—e.g., the fast adductor of scallop (A), earthworm body muscle (B), and myotomes of *Amphioxus* (C and D). In all these muscles the diameter of the fiber is small and a single myofibril occupies its center. The SR is present between the myofibrils and the surface membrane and makes junctions, or peripheral couplings, with the latter. Frequent sites of peripheral couplings appear as small dome-shaped patches of membrane located along and on either side of Z lines in a freeze-fracture replica from *Amphioxus* (E). (*See Nunzi MG, Franzini-Armstrong C: The structure of smooth and striated portions of the adductor muscle of the valves in a scallop. J Ultrastruct Res 76:134, 1981.*)

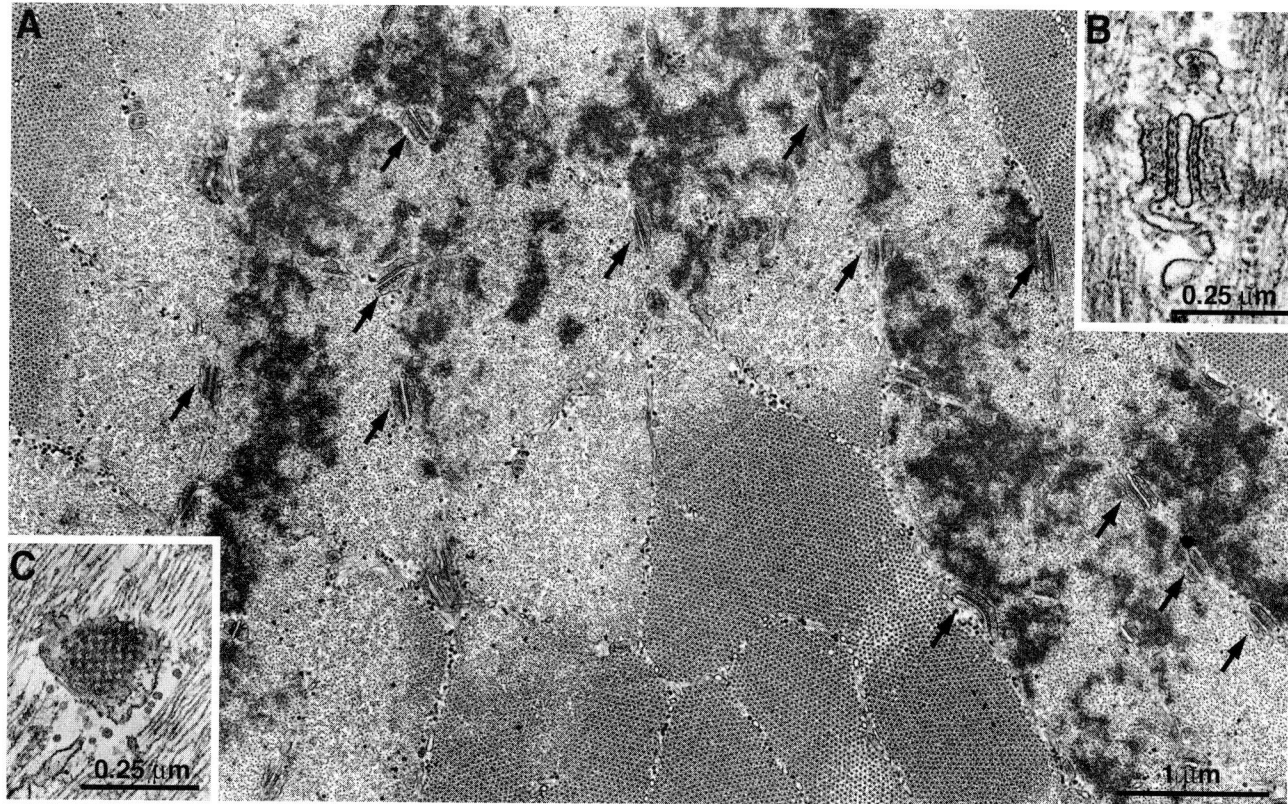

FIGURE 11-10. Cross (A) and longitudinal (B and C) sections of tonic fibers from the frog cruralis muscle. JSR is associated with the T tubules at the level of the Z lines, but the triads are less frequent than in twitch fibers and they have a longitudinal orientation. Orthogonally arranged arrays of feet (B and C) occupy the junctional gap. (Franzini-Armstrong C: Studies of the triad: IV. Structure of the junction in frog slow fibers. J Cell Biol 56:120, 1973.)

pathologic muscles are continuous with large aggregates of membranes derived from an accumulation of caveolae and having a "honeycomb" appearance (Fig. 11-12D, see also Chap. 2).

Another unusual SR disposition is an interesting result of natural adaptation. The extraocular muscles of some fish have been transformed into heat-producing organs.[34] These modified muscle cells are completely filled by tight aggregates of SR sacs interspersed with mitochondria. Heat is produced by futile cycling of Ca^{2+} in the SR, very much as in the case of malignant hyperthermia (see Chap. 61).

THE POSITIONING OF MITOCHONDRIA

Mitochondria take up Ca^{2+} under some conditions.[36] However, the low affinity of these organelles for Ca^{2+} seemed to exclude the possibility of their effectively competing with troponin and other high-affinity Ca^{2+} buffering components of the sarcoplasm. Thus mitochondria were shown to accumulate Ca^{2+} in damaged muscle fibers but not in intact cells.[37] Recently it has become apparent that mitochondria transiently take up Ca^{2+} in a variety of cells under physiologic conditions[38] but that the uptake is strictly dependent on the proximity of the organelles to the source.[39–41]

In muscle cells, the content of mitochondria is related to the metabolic profile and thus indirectly to the pattern of activity (Chap. 5). The positioning of mitochondria in a given muscle cell is highly stereotyped and characteristic for each type of cell in a manner that indicates a possible role in modulating the amplitude of calcium transients. Cardiac muscle, the slow red fibers of leg muscles, and insect flight muscles are noticeable for having a close association of CRUs and mitochondria (Figs. 11-13A to C). The close CRU-mitochondria proximity in cardiac muscle results in Ca^{2+} uptake beat to beat and also following a localized calcium "spark."[42] Mitochondrial calcium uptake has a detectable effect on the rate of relaxation in mitochondria-rich, "red" skeletal muscle.[43] In the fast-acting fibers of the toadfish swimbladder (Fig. 11-13D) on the other hand, mitochondria are strictly segregated in the central core and at the cell periphery, away from myofibrils and CRUs, so that one may predict that little mitochondrial Ca^{2+} uptake is expected in these muscles. This may be appropriate in cells that are required to contract at high frequency for a relatively prolonged period of time.

It should be noted that while mitochondria may take up Ca^{2+} in parallel to the myofibrils and SR during muscle activation, release of Ca^{2+} from them is regulated independently from SR release. Thus mitochondria may influence the time course of contraction and/or relaxation, but do not directly affect e-c coupling events.

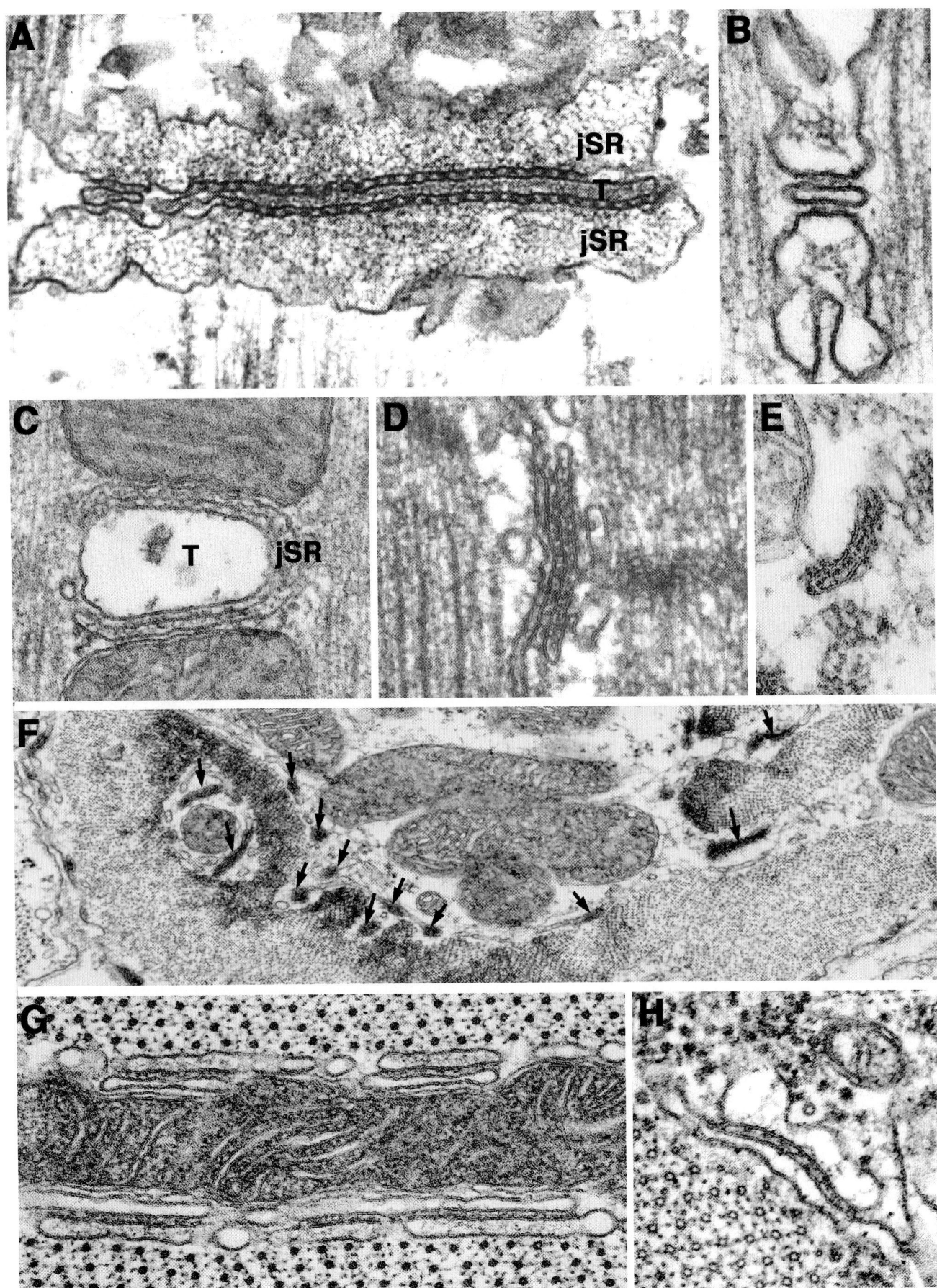

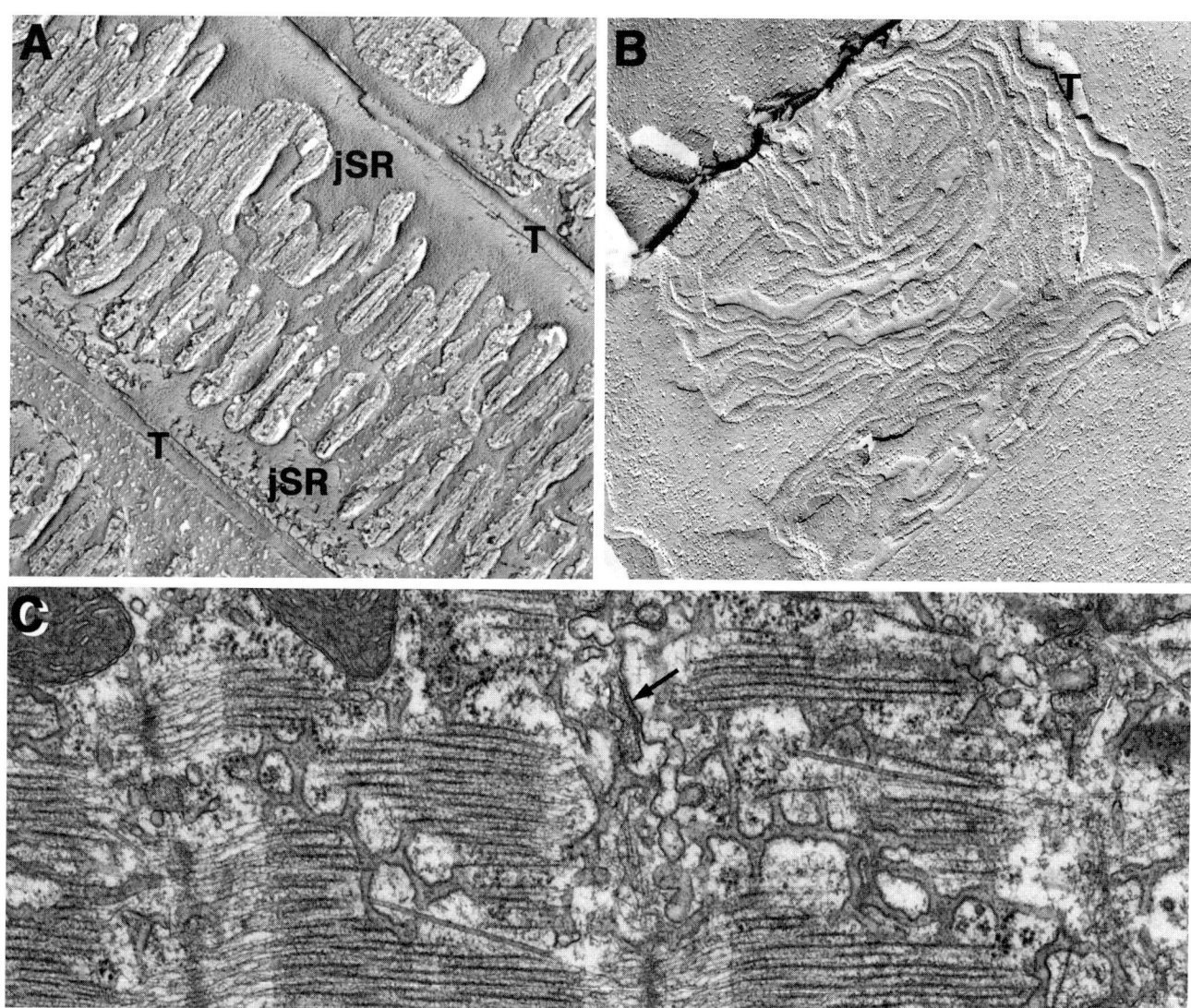

FIGURE 11-8. *A* and *B*. Freeze-fractures from a twitch fiber in a small fish and a tonic fiber in the frog. T tubules (T) separate the SR into segments. The wider jSR cisternae (jSR) are continuous with tubular and fenestrated regions of the SR. *C*. Thin section from cardiac muscle showing the less abundant free SR with wide fenestrations. JSR cisternae (arrow) are smaller than in vertebrate fibers. *See Franzini-Armstrong C: Freeze-fracture of frog slow tonic fibers. Structure of surface and internal membranes. Tissue Cell 16:146, 1984.*

SOME UNUSUAL SR AND T-TUBULE AGGREGATES

Under some pathologic conditions, SR and/or T tubules aggregate into large stacks. Anoxia-induced tubular SR aggregates are shown in Fig. 11-12A. Several layers of flat feet-bearing SR stacks have been observed in opossum cardiac muscle (Fig. 11-12B). A similar configuration is found in nonmuscle cells that have been induced to express the foot protein [or ryanodine receptor (RyR)] and have an excess of feet without the other components of CRUs (Fig. 11-12C). Stacks of CRUs (pentads) are seen in developing and/or denervated muscles. Finally, T tubules in developing and/or

FIGURE 11-9. CRUs are sites of Ca^{2+} release and are composed of jSR cisternae, usually associated with either plasmalemma or T tubules. *A* and *B*. Two views of triads in skeletal muscle, sectioned either parallel (*A*) or perpendicular (*B*) to the T tubule's long axis. Two jSR cisternae face the jT segment. Two rows of feet occupy the narrow junctional gap between the apposed membranes. *C* to *E*. Examples of dyad (jSR and T tubule, *C*), peripheral coupling (jSR and plasmalemma, *D*) and extended junctional SR (EjSR, *E*) from mouse (*C*, *D*) and chicken (*E*) cardiac muscle. All jSR segments contain feet, but the EjSR is not forming a junction. *F*. Arrows point to frequent EjSR segments located at the level of the Z line in chicken cardiac muscle. *G* and *H*. Dyads in arthropod muscle, from dragonfly and Drosophila. (Photo (*H*) Courtesy of E. Polyak.) *(See Franzini-Armstrong C: Studies of the triad: I. Structure of the junction in frog twitch fibers. J Cell Biol 47:488, 1970; Franzini-Armstrong C, Protasi F, Ramesh V: Comparative ultrastructure of calcium release units in skeletal and cardiac muscle. Ann NY Acad Sci 853:20–31, 1998.*

crustacean also have a complex arrangement of surface invaginations comprising several orders of clefts and two classes of tubules: the T and Z tubules (Fig. 11-7B). The T tubules are involved in excitation-contraction coupling; the Z tubules are not,[4] and they differ from the Z tubules in shape and particle content.

T-TUBULE HELICOIDS

High-voltage EM of specifically stained T tubules observed in thick slices of frog skeletal muscle led to the discovery of an unusual disposition of the T network, the T-tubule helicoids.[33] In these, a single T-tubule network provides direct connections between the T systems of adjacent sarcomeres over a short segment of the fiber, much like the exit ramp of a garage. The helicoids are relatively frequent and coincide with vernier arrangements of the cross striation.

FREE SR SHAPES

The free SR is the SR domain responsible for Ca^{2+} uptake; it is not involved in CRUs and is composed of fenestrated, tubular, and junctional regions (Figs. 11-1 and 11-8). The fenestrated regions of the SR are perforated from side to side by fenestrae, or small round openings. Fenestrae have varied sizes and are characteristic for each muscle fiber. The number of openings and extent of fenestrated areas may vary with sarcomere length and fixation. The margins of fenestrated regions of the SR are continuous with tubular regions, where the SR forms individual parallel tubules, usually oriented longitudinally. Fenestrae and the elongated slits between tubules allow direct communication between the fluids bathing myofibrils on the two sides of the SR layers and thus effectively permit diffusion of solutes and relatively rapid equilibration across the fiber. In tonic fibers (Fig. 11-8B) and in cardiac muscle (Fig. 11-8C), the SR is generally more rarefied than in skeletal muscle; this is mostly due to the large size of the fenestrae between the SR elements. In some striated muscles from arthropods, the entire SR is in the form of extended fenestrated sheets (Fig. 11-7D).

The SR forms an extended network, which is continuous across and along the muscle fiber and constitutes a single continuous compartment within each cell. In skeletal muscle, triads interrupt the longitudinal continuity of the SR lumen, so that the SR seems to be divided into separate segments covering all or part of a sarcomere. However, SR bridges bypassing the triads are fairly frequent, thus ensuring longitudinal connections between the segments. The longitudinal continuity of the SR network is most easily seen in cardiac and invertebrate body muscles, where triads and dyads do not delimit sarcomere-related SR segments.

In most cases the SR forms either a single or a double layer between the myofibrils. In muscles with a very rapid cycle of activity, the SR/myofibril ratio is increased by decreasing the myofibril size rather than by adding further layers of SR. However, there are two examples of muscles in which the SR volume is larger than the volume occupied by myofibrils. One is a very fast acting sound-producing muscle of the lobster[34]; the other is a modified extraocular muscle in large fish that acts as a thermogenic organ (see below).[35]

THE SHAPES OF CALCIUM RELEASE UNITS

CRUs take different appearances in various muscles but share common characteristics. The junctional domains of SR (jSR) are associated with feet and are closely apposed through a junctional gap of uniform width, either to junctional domains of plasmalemma (jPl) or to flat segments of T tubules (jT segments) (Fig. 11-9). Triads (Figs. 11-9A and B) have two jSR cisternae; dyads one cisterna (Fig. 11-9C); peripheral couplings are composed of one jSR apposed to the plasmalemma (Fig. 11-9D); and an extended jSR or corbular SR is an SR cisterna with feet but not associated with exterior membranes (Figs. 11-9E and F). The latter type of CRU is present only in cardiac muscle. Peripheral couplings have the same overall structure as triads and dyads and function equally well as Ca^{2+} release units. Corbular SR is present in cells that also have triads/dyads and peripheral couplings. It is thought that in these cells Ca^{2+} release is first initiated in the peripheral couplings and then the effect of the initial Ca^{2+} wave spreads inward, activating the corbular SR.[9,10]

In slow tonic fibers of the frog and in arthropod muscles (Figs. 11-9G and H; Fig. 11-10), the JT segments are in the form of flat round profiles whose surfaces are oriented longitudinally. Thus profiles of T tubules, apposed jSR, and intervening feet are seen to lie parallel to the myofibrils' long axis in longitudinal sections of the muscle fibers and are also visible in cross sections. The jSR sacs are interposed between the jT segments and the myofibrils, forming dyads and triads with the flat SR cisternae.

Some fibers (e.g., frog tonic fibers, ventricular myocardium from several vertebrates, some arthropod fibers) have peripheral couplings between SR and the surface membrane (Fig. 11-9D) in addition to the internal T-SR junctions. Other cells [e.g., atrial myocardium from many vertebrates, muscles from mollusca and worms (Figs. 11-11A and B)] have exclusively peripheral couplings and lack T tubules. An interesting convergence occurs in the myotomes of a chordate, *Amphioxus* sp., or lancelet, and in the fast adductor muscle of the scallop. In the myotomes of these chordates and molluscs, the muscle fibers are essentially the size of a single myofibril, so there is no need for T tubules (Fig. 11-11C). The SR is entirely located between the single myofibril and the plasmalemma, and peripheral couplings, involving junctional domains of SR and surface membrane, are numerous (Fig. 11-11D and E).

◀ FIGURE 11-7 *(continued)* fiber is at 45 degrees. The twin wider bands in (B) are transversely oriented T tubules; the thinner structures are Z tubules, which do not participate in connections with the SR. The T tubules in C have a predominantly longitudinal orientation. D. Electron micrograph of Golgi-stained crab muscle. T tubules are dark gray; the SR is a pale gray. Flat jT cisternae (arrows) are located in correspondence of flat jSR cisternae the same size (double arrow). The free SR is fenestrated. (*See Franzini-Armstrong C, Eastwood AE, Peachey LD: Shape and disposition of clefts, T tubules and sarcoplasmic reticulum in long and short sarcomere fibers. Cell Tissue Res 244:9, 1986.*)

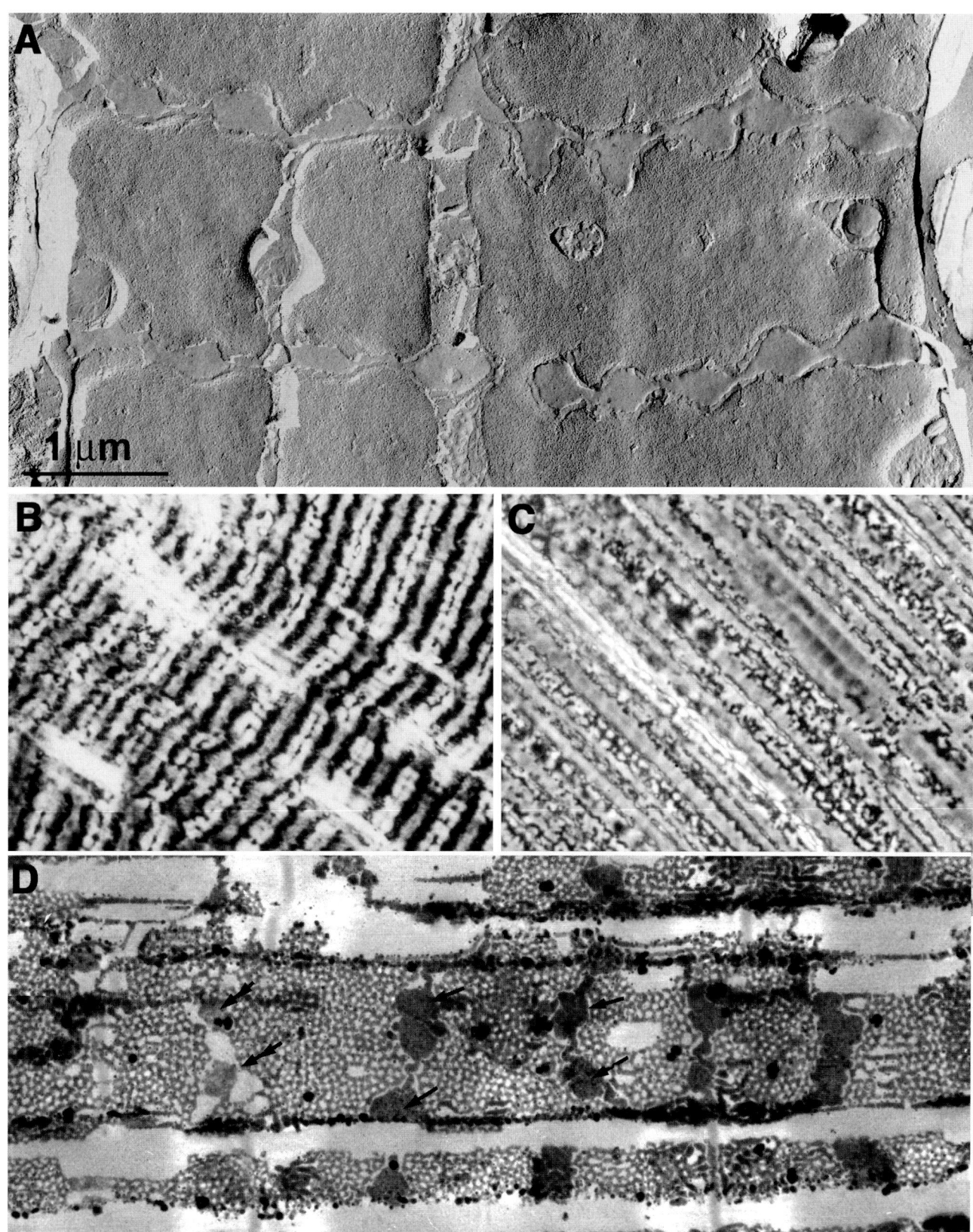

FIGURE 11-7. *A.* Freeze-fracture of a direct flight muscle from the dragonfly. The long axis of the fiber is longitudinal. Two sets of transversely oriented T tubules cross the image from left to right. The T tubules alternate narrow segments (free T) and wide flat cisternae (jT) that face toward the myofibrils. One side of the flat cisternae is associated with a similarly shaped jSR component, forming a dyad. In the background is a mitochondrial membrane. *B* and *C.* Light microscope images of Golgi-infiltrated walking leg muscle from crab (*B*) and tail flexor from crayfish (*C*). The long axis of the

(continued on bottom of next page)

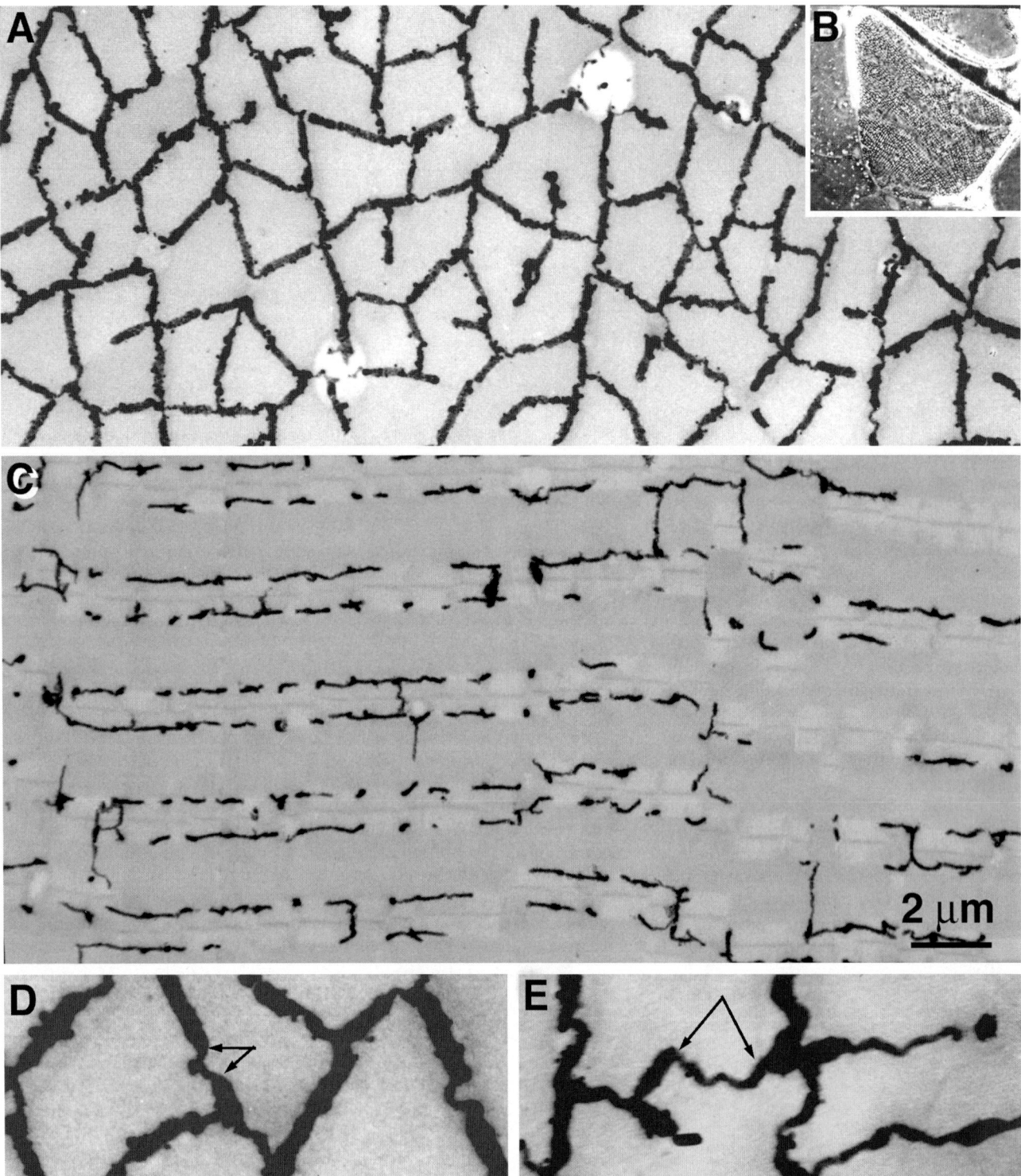

FIGURE 11-6. Golgi stain of skeletal muscles showing dispositions of T tubules. *A* and *B*. Electron micrograph and light microscopic images from cross sections of rat skeletal muscle illustrating the continuity of the transverse T-tubule network. The openings of the network are occupied by myofibrils and lipid droplets (white circular profiles). *C*. Longitudinal section of a muscle from the guinea pig. The transversely oriented T tubules are located at the A-I junctions and run from left to right in the image. Occasional longitudinal extensions connect adjacent levels of T-tubule networks. Longitudinally oriented T tubules are more frequent in differentiating fibers and under pathologic conditions. *D* and *E*. Cross sections of fast-twitch (*D*) and slow-twitch (*E*) muscle fibers from the guinea pig. The T tubules have alternate wider and narrower segments between arrows. The wider segments, or junctional T tubules (jT), are ribbon-like and participate in the formation of triads. JTs constitute a higher proportion of the T network in faster than in slower fibers. (*See Franzini-Armstrong C, Champ C, Ferguson DGJ: Discriminating between fast- and slow-twitch muscle fibres of guinea pig muscle.* Muscle Res Cell Motil *9:403, 1988; Appelt D, Buenviaje B, Champ C, et al: Quantitation of feet content in two types of muscle fibres from hind limbs of the rat.* Tissue Cell *21:783, 1989.)*

regardless of their position relative to the SR. Free and jT segments are of variable length. In general, the faster the fiber, the higher the percentage of T tubules that are junctional (compare Fig. 11-6D and E). Longitudinal extensions of the transverse T networks tend to be totally free.

Arthropod body and flight muscles have a wider range of T-tubule arrangements than skeletal muscle, from strictly transverse networks with few longitudinal connections [in some direct flight muscles (Fig. 11-7A)], to transverse networks with frequent longitudinal connections [some crab muscles (Figs. 11-7B and D)], to a fairly random orientation (some indirect flight muscles), to an almost completely longitudinal arrangement with occasional transverse connections [tail muscle of crayfish (Fig. 11-7C)]. Tonic fibers from

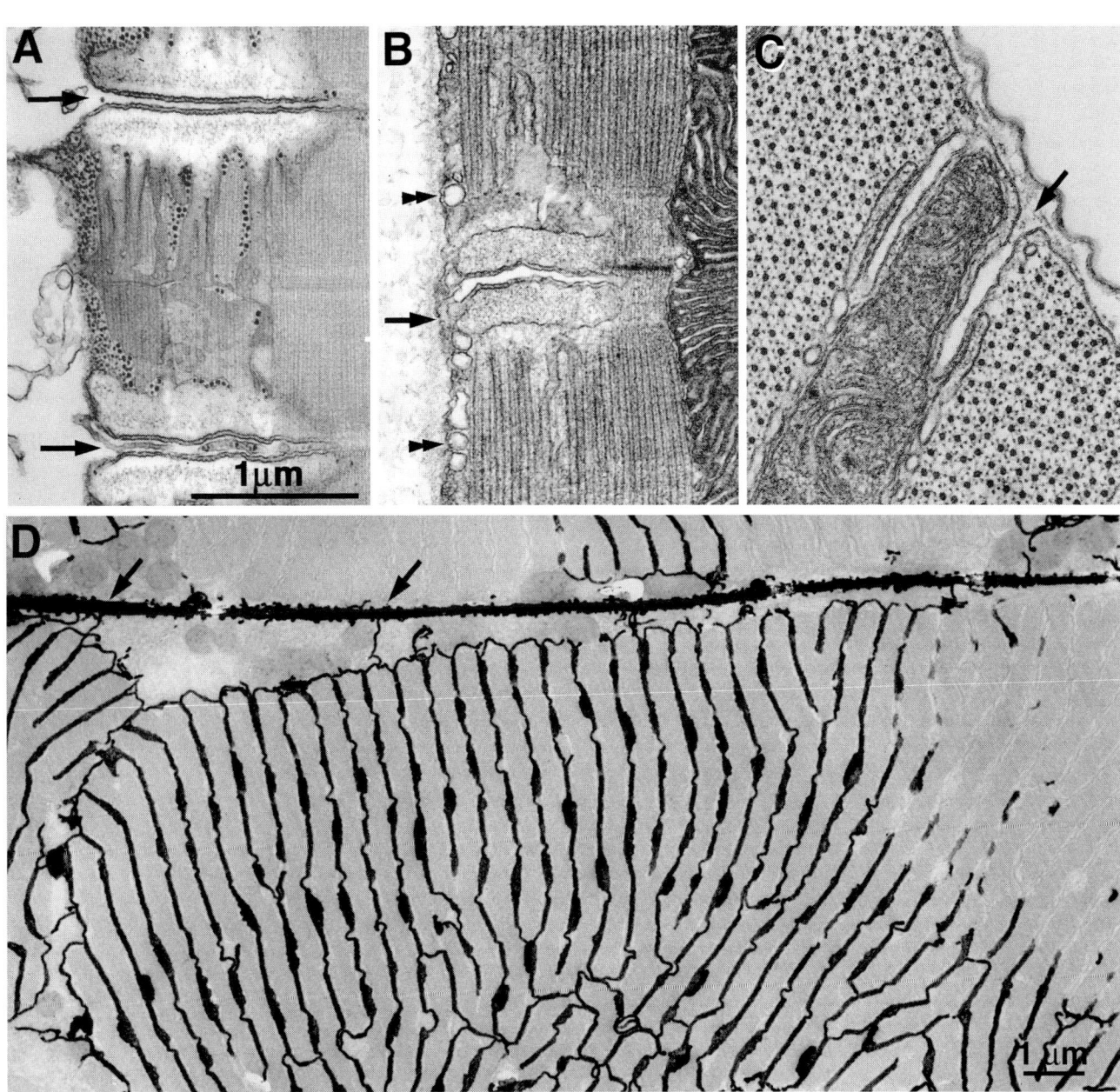

FIGURE 11-5. Direct continuity of T-tubule membrane with the plasmalemma and of the T-tubule lumen with the extracellular spaces (arrows) is illustrated in muscle fibers from a fish (A), a frog (B), and a dragonfly (C). In the frog fiber, the peripheral T-tubule segment is tortuous and the opening is similar to that of a caveolar neck (double arrows). D. The black reaction of Golgi applied to the toadfish swimbladder muscle outlines the T tubules and extracellular spaces with an electron-dense precipitate. The extensive T-tubule network between the thin ribbon-shaped myofibrils is connected to the outside via a circumferential "manifold" and few tortuous tubules (arrows). (See Franzini-Armstrong C, Porter KR: Sarcolemmal invaginations constituting the T-system in fish skeletal muscle. Cell Biol 22:675, 1964; Franzini-Armstrong C: Studies of the triad: I. Structure of the junction in frog twitch fibres. J Cell Biol 47:488-499, 1970; Appelt D, Shen V, Franzini-Armstrong C: Quantitation of Ca ATPase, feet and mitochondria in superfast muscle fibres from the toadfish Opsanus tau. J Muscle Res Cell Motil 12:543, 1991.)

Diversity of Shapes and Dispositions

Shapes and dispositions of SR and T-tubule systems vary little within a single muscle fiber (except for extraocular muscles; see Chap. 6), but they are characteristic for each type of muscle tissue and muscle fiber and are quite different in unrelated species. Varied configurations are assembled using the same basic building blocks, but adapting to fit myofibril parameters and to accommodate for the presence of accessory proteins and the overall functional pattern of the muscle cell. Selective "stains," freeze-fracture, and a combination of light and electron microscopy have been particularly useful in understanding the large-scale structural variations described below.

T-TUBULE OPENINGS

The direct continuity between T tubule and surface membrane is readily seen in insect (Fig. 11-5C)[1] and cardiac muscles and was actually detected in the latter by infiltration with India ink particles as early as the nineteenth century.[4] In most vertebrate muscles, the T tubules open via convoluted tubules and/or caveolae,[27] so the direct connection is rarely seen in thin-section electron microscopy (Fig. 11-5B). This has suggested the possibility of a high access resistance to the T-tubule lumen. Few skeletal muscles have wide direct T-tubule openings (Fig. 11-5C). Golgi stain (Fig. 11-5D),[28] fluorescent probes,[29] and ferritin molecules[30,31] demonstrate continuity between T-tubule and surface membranes and between T-tubule lumen and extracellular fluid in all muscles.

DISPOSITIONS OF THE T-TUBULE NETWORKS

In adult skeletal muscle fibers, the T-tubule networks have an overall transverse orientation; they are continuous across the fiber, completely encircling myofibrils, and are located either at the Z line or at the A-I junction level (Figs. 11-1A and B and Fig. 11-6A and B).[13,17,32] The T-tubule system does not lie in a plane: The tubules meander above and below a mean position (Figs. 11-1A and 11-6C). Deviation from a planar disposition provides extra length for the T tubules, thus allowing expansion of the network when the fibers shorten (and increase in diameter). Indeed, T tubules deviate most from a planar disposition in fibers fixed at long sarcomere lengths. Longitudinally oriented tubules (Fig. 11-6C) extend along the myofibrils and often link adjacent T-tubule networks. Longitudinal extensions are more frequent in cardiac than in skeletal muscle.

JUNCTIONAL AND FREE T TUBULES

T tubules have two shapes that alternate with each other within the transverse network: small tubules with an approximately round cross section and wavy course (free T) and flat tubules [junctional (jT)] that participate in junctions with the jSR (Fig. 11-6D and E). Myocardial T tubules tend to be flat,

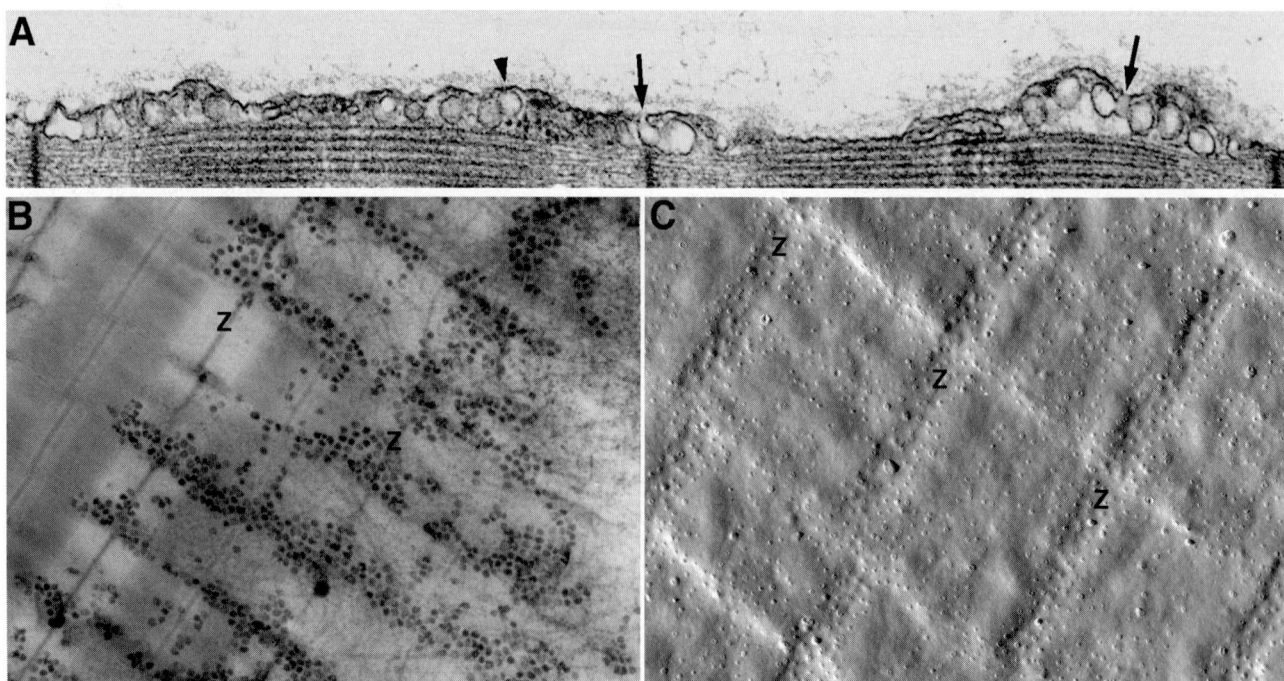

FIGURE 11-4. A. Caveolae (arrowhead) are small, flask-shaped invaginations of the surface membrane. Often two or more caveolae are joined to a common neck opening (arrows). The frequency of caveolae is demonstrated by calcium and lanthanum ions infiltration (B) and by detecting their openings in freeze-fracture replicas (C). Most caveolae are located within broad longitudinal and transverse bands forming a checkerboard pattern. B. High-voltage electron micrograph, courtesy of L. D. Peachey. C. (See Dulhunty AF, Franzini-Armstrong C: The passive electrical properties of frog skeletal muscle fibres at different sarcomere lengths. J Physiol 266:687, 1977.)

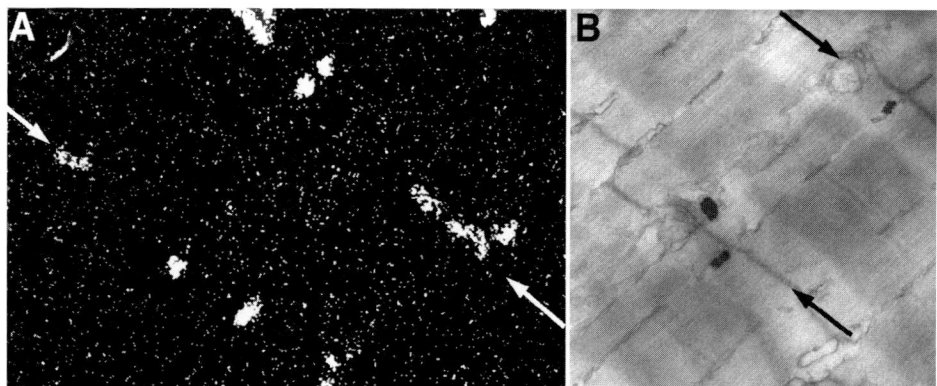

FIGURE 11-2. *A.* The Ca^{2+} content of the SR is revealed by electron microprobe imaging of a cryosection from a rapidly frozen frog fiber. The highest total content of Ca^{2+} is in the lateral sacs of the triad (arrows), where calsequestrin is present. *(From Somlyo AV, Gonzales-Serratos H, Shuman H, et al: Calcium release and ionic changes in the sarcoplasmic reticulum of tetanized muscle: An electron microscope study. J Cell Biol 90:577, 1981. With permission.)* *B.* Accumulation of Ca^{2+} in the SR of a skinned frog muscle fiber in situ is revealed by precipitation with oxalate. *(From Constantin LL, Franzini-Armstrong C, Podolsky RJ: Localization of calcium accumulating structures in striated muscle fibres. Science 147:158, 1965. With permission.)*

T tubules or to the surface membrane. The two facing membranes are separated by a junctional gap of uniform width (approximately 10 nm). The interior of the jSR cisternae is occupied by an electron-dense, periodically condensed content identified as calsequestrin.[15]

In cardiac muscle, SR cisternae analogous to those participating in CRUs but not associated with T tubules are also present in the cells' interior. These cisternae, called corbular SR or extended junctional SR, participate in Ca^{2+} release, presumably by receiving indirect signals from other CRUs.[9,10] Components of the T and SR networks that do not participate in CRUs are called free T and free SR.

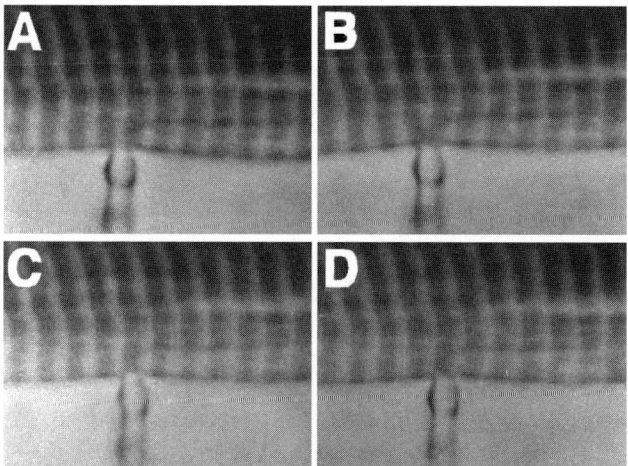

FIGURE 11-3. Local stimulation experiments performed on frog fibers. *A.* A polished pipette is pushed against the surface of a frog fiber, facing the Z line. *B.* A small amount of current is passed, producing a localized depolarization. A localized contraction pulls the two adjacent A bands towards the Z line. This is due to spread of depolarization along the T tubules and release of Ca^{2+} from the adjacent jSR. *C* and *D.* When the pipette is located opposite the A band, contraction cannot be induced. *(From Huxley AF: The Croonian lecture 1967: The activation of striated muscle and its mechanical response. Proc R Soc Lond B 178:1, 1971. With permission.)*

CAVEOLAE

Caveolae are inpocketings of the surface membrane in the form of flask-like vesicles, often clustered around a single narrow neck (Fig. 11-4). Caveolae are fixed elements of the surface membrane; they do not participate in pinocytic activity; and they are quite abundant in some cells (fibroblast, endothelium, most muscle cells). The cytoplasmic surfaces of caveolae are decorated by an array of filaments or strands that form striated coatings identified as caveolin.[21] Cytoplasmic and outer leaflets of the caveolar membrane appear entirely smooth in freeze-fracture. It is not clear whether this is due to lack of large intramembranous protein or to unusual fracturing properties of the selected lipids constituting the caveolar membrane.

In twitch fibers of skeletal muscle, caveolae are preferentially located along circumferential bands: one wider at the level of the I bands, where T-tubule openings are also located, and the other more restricted, opposite the center of the sarcomere. Less prominent longitudinal bands of caveolae mark the interfibrillar spaces (Fig. 11-4). Caveolae increase the surface area of some muscle fibers by 60 to 80 percent. Although this extra membrane would allow stretching of the muscle fibers to about three times rest length without breaking, such stretching never happens in vivo due to constraints imposed by the skeleton. Thus caveolae must have roles other than simply serving as reservoirs of extra membrane (see below and Chap. 19).

The specific shape of caveolae seems to be determined by the interaction of caveolin, an intrinsic protein of the caveolar membrane, with cholesterol and glycosphingolipids, which results in "lipid rafts" with a unique composition and an obligatory small radius of curvature.[22–24] Caveolin 3, the muscle-specific isoform,[25] is associated exclusively with sarcolemmal caveolae in adult muscle. Recruitment of membrane lipids into rafts often initiates signaling events.[26] In this context, caveolae in muscle—and other tissues that are rich in them—may be seen as preformed signaling stations. However, the reason for the abundance of caveolae in muscle remains a mystery.

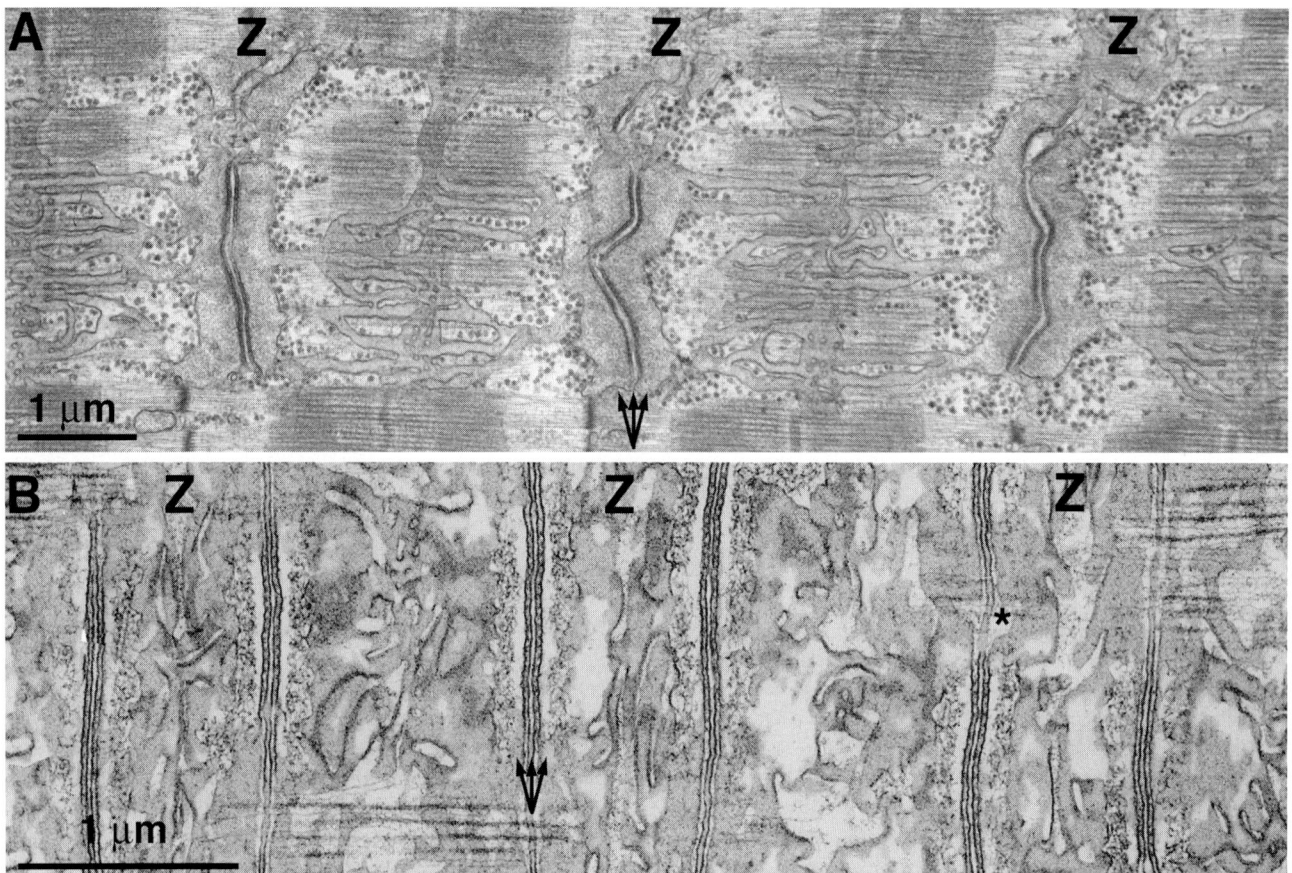

FIGURE 11-1. Longitudinal sections through skeletal muscle fibers of the frog (A) and the toadfish swimbladder (B). The positions of Z lines in the myofibrils are indicated (Z). The sections graze myofibrils and show the layer of sarcoplasmic reticulum surrounding them. Enlarged SR cisternae (junctional, jSR) face two sides of the T tubules, forming a triad (three arrows). Triads are located at the Z lines in the frog and at the A-I junction in the toadfish. *(Photo (A) Courtesy of Dr. E. Castillo de Maruenda.)*

must bring the effect of surface depolarization to the myofibrils within the available time.[4] A second clue came from the passive electrical properties of muscle fibers, indicating either that the surface membrane of a muscle fiber had unexpectedly different properties from that of a nerve fiber or that it was very convoluted. The latter is true; the surface membrane invaginates to form T tubules and caveolae, and the aggregated surface area of these two components fully accounts for the large apparent specific capacitance of a muscle fiber.

"Local stimulation" experiments[4] initiated modern thinking about excitation-contraction (e-c) coupling by showing that depolarization of a small patch of surface membrane leads to local contraction of underlying myofibrils only when depolarization is applied over an area of membrane located at the level of the T-tubule invaginations (Fig. 11-3). In twitch muscle, the contraction initiated by local depolarization of a T-tubule network spreads transversely but not longitudinally with increase in stimulus strength. This could be explained by the spread of the electrical activity along the T-tubule network.

Exposure to and subsequent withdrawal from a low concentration of glycerol induces swelling and vacuolization of T tubules and an interruption of their continuity. The concomitant block of e-c coupling strongly confirms the role of T tubules as important links between surface depolarization and SR Ca^{2+} release.[18]

CA^{2+} RELEASE UNITS

Release of Ca^{2+} from the SR depends upon the transmission of an appropriate signal from the depolarized surface membrane/T tubules to the SR, thus requiring specialized junctions between the two membrane systems. Such junctions are triads, in which a T tubule is sandwiched between two SR cisternae (Fig. 11-1); dyads, in which one SR cisterna forms a junction with the T tubule, and peripheral couplings between the SR and the surface membrane. The three types of junctions have the same structural and molecular components and are collectively called Ca^{2+} release units (CRUs).[1,2,6,9,10,19,20] The SR cisternae that participate in CRUs are called lateral sacs of the triad, terminal cisternae, or junctional SR (jSR). jSR cisternae have a flat surface occupied by small, periodically arranged densities, the feet, and are closely apposed either to corresponding flat surfaces of

Chapter 11

The Membrane Systems of Muscle Cells

CLARA FRANZINI-ARMSTRONG

The Membrane Systems of Muscle Cells—
Definitions and Background
 SARCOPLASMIC RETICULUM AND TRANSVERSE TUBULES
 CA²⁺ RELEASE UNITS
 CAVEOLAE
Diversity of Shapes and Dispositions
 T-TUBULE OPENINGS
 DISPOSITIONS OF THE T-TUBULE NETWORKS
 JUNCTIONAL AND FREE T TUBULES
 T-TUBULE HELICOIDS
 FREE SR SHAPES
 THE SHAPES OF CALCIUM RELEASE UNITS
 SOME UNUSUAL SR AND T-TUBULE AGGREGATES
 THE POSITIONING OF MITOCHONDRIA
Diversity of Composition and Molecular
 Architecture
 COMPOSITION OF SURFACE MEMBRANE, FREE T TUBULES,
   AND FREE SR
 STRUCTURE OF THE SURFACE MEMBRANE (PLASMALEMMA)
 STRUCTURE OF FREE SR
 COMPOSITION AND STRUCTURE OF CRUS
Structural Relationships between Components
 of Calcium Release Units
 RYR AND DHPR ISOFORMS: FUNCTIONAL ROLE AND LOCATION
 VARIATIONS IN DHPR/RYR RATIO
 THE MACROMOLECULAR COMPLEX OF JSR
Morphometry of Muscle Membranes
 and Their Proteins
 MORPHOMETRY OF SR AND T TUBULES
 STRUCTURE-FUNCTION CORRELATIONS

This chapter describes the structure and disposition of the internal membrane systems [sarcoplasmic reticulum (SR)* and mitochondria], of the exterior membranes [surface membrane and its invaginations, caveolae, and transverse (T) tubules], and of the sites of junctions between the SR and exterior membranes [triads, dyads, and peripheral couplings, collectively called Ca²⁺ release units (CRUs)]. SR and exterior membranes are responsible for Ca²⁺ movement and its control in the processes of excitation-contraction coupling (Chap. 12) and relaxation (Chap. 14). The spatial relationship between SR and mitochondria increases the complexity of Ca²⁺ handling. (See Refs. 1 through 12 for general reviews and books covering this subject.)

*A list of abbreviations used in this chapter is given at the end of the chapter.

The Membrane Systems of Muscle Cells—Definitions and Background

SARCOPLASMIC RETICULUM AND TRANSVERSE TUBULES

SR and T tubules are separate but functionally related membrane systems that play distinct roles in the Ca^{2+} movements controlling muscle contraction. T tubules are invaginations of the surface membrane, while the SR is an intracellular membrane system.

The SR was first described as a highly developed form of the smooth endoplasmic reticulum (SER), which is closely wrapped around the myofibril and is differentiated into specialized domains composing groups of three elements, the triads. Triads are located at periodic intervals corresponding to the cross striations of the myofibrils (Fig. 11-1).[13] The special disposition of the SR relative to myofibrils indicates a role in the contractile activity of the muscle fiber. This role, it turns out, is the control of Ca^{2+} movements, and thus of the contraction state, by the active pumping, sequestering, and releasing of Ca^{2+}.[3]

The ATP-dependent Ca^{2+} sequestering activity of the SR and its role in relaxation were initially demonstrated using isolated membrane fractions (see Chap. 14).[14] In skeletal muscle, the SR is an efficient Ca^{2+} sink, so a twitch muscle fiber loses very little Ca^{2+} to the extracellular space even when obliged to contract repeatedly in the absence of extracellular Ca^{2+}. However, under normal in vivo conditions, the SR (at least in frog twitch fibers) is not maximally filled. Thus the Ca^{2+} content of the SR, as seen by deposits of Ca^{2+} oxalate or by electron probe analysis, is less in an intact (Fig. 11-2) than in a damaged or skinned fiber, where the SR has been maximally loaded. The highest total Ca^{2+} content is in the lateral sacs of the triad, where Ca^{2+} is bound to calsequestrin (Fig. 11-2).[15,16] Presumably, however, the free Ca^{2+} concentration is equal throughout the SR. Apart from Ca^{2+}, the lumen of the SR has an ionic composition similar to that of the cytoplasm and different from that of the extracellular space[16] (Fig. 11-2), confirming that it is an intracellular compartment. The amount of Ca^{2+} cycling in and out of the SR during contraction is more than expected from a simple calculation of the requirement to saturate troponin.[16] Internal cycling of Ca^{2+} in vertebrate cardiac and invertebrate muscles is less efficient, and in these muscles a relatively large amount of Ca^{2+} is gained from and subsequently extruded to the extracellular spaces at each cycle of activity.

The T tubules are the central tubular elements of the triads (Fig. 11-1), and they form part of a continuous network that has frequent continuities with the plasmalemma and a transverse orientation in adult skeletal muscles.[17] Initial understanding of the role of T tubules involved interplay of physiologic and morphologic observations. A. V. Hill pointed out that the measurable delay between the surface action potential and the onset of mechanical activity across the whole width of a frog muscle fiber is too short to allow for equilibration by diffusion of an activator substance (say Ca^{2+}) liberated at the fiber periphery by the action potential. The conclusion was that a mechanism faster than diffusion

151. Lorenz C, Pusch M, Jentsch TJ: Heteromultimeric ClC chloride channels with novel properties. *Proc Natl Acad Sci USA* 93:13362–13366, 1996.
152. Weinreich F, Jentsch TJ: Pores formed by single subunits in mixed dimers of different ClC chloride channels. *J Biol Chem* 276:2347–2353, 2001.
153. Haug K, Warnstedt M, Alekov AK, et al: Mutations in CLCN2 encoding a voltage-gated chloride channel are associated with idiopathic generalized epilepsies. *Nature Genet* 33:527–532, 2003.
154. Bosl MR, Stein V, Hübner C, et al: Male germ cells and photoreceptors, both dependent on close cell-cell interactions, degenerate upon ClC-2 Cl⁻ channel disruption. *EMBO J* 20:1289–1299, 2001.
155. Kawasaki M, Fukuma T, Yamauchi K, et al: Identification of an acid-activated Cl⁻ channel from human skeletal muscles. *Am J Physiol* 277: C948–C954, 1999.
156. Buyse G, Trouet D, Voets T, et al: Evidence for the intracellular location of chloride channel (ClC)-type proteins: Co-localization of ClC-6a and ClC-6c with the sarco/endoplasmic-reticulum Ca^{2+} pump SERCA2b. *Biochem J* 330:1015–1021, 1998.
157. Steinmeyer K, Ortland C, Jentsch TJ: Primary structure and functional expression of a developmentally regulated skeletal muscle chloride channel. *Nature* 354:301–304, 1991.
158. Pusch M, Jentsch TJ: Molecular physiology of voltage-gated chloride channels. *Physiol Rev* 74:813–827, 1994.
159. Bryant SH, Morales-Aguilera A: Chloride conductance in normal and myotonic muscle fibres and the action of monocarboxylic aromatic acids. *J Physiol* 219:367–383, 1971.
160. Palade PT, Barchi RL: On the inhibition of muscle membrane chloride conductance by aromatic carboxylic acids. *J Gen Physiol* 69:879–896, 1977.
161. Wagner S, Deymeer F, Kürz LL, et al: The dominant chloride channel mutant G200R causing fluctuating myotonia: Clinical findings, electrophysiology, and channel pathology. *Muscle Nerve* 21:1122–1128, 1998.
162. Hunter PJ, McNaughton PA, Noble D: Analytical models of propagation in excitable cells. *Prog Biophys Mol Biol* 30:99–144, 1975.
163. Huppertz HJ, Disselhorst-Klug C, Silny J, Rau G, Heimann G: Diagnostic yield of noninvasive high spatial resolution electromyography in neuromuscular diseases. *Muscle Nerve* 20:1360–1370, 1997.
164. Lehmann-Horn F, Iaizzo PA: Resealed fiber segments for the study of the pathophysiology of human skeletal muscle. *Muscle Nerve* 13:222–231, 1990.
165. Jurkat-Rott K, Mitrovic N, Hang C, Kuzmenkin A, Iaizzo PA, Herzog J, Lerche H, Nicole S, Vale-Santos JE, Chauveau D, Fontaine B, Lehmann-Horn F: Voltage-sensor sodium channel mutations cause hypokalemic periodic paralysis type 2 by enhanced inactivation and reduced current. *Proc Natl Acad Sci USA* 97:9549–9554, 2000.
166. Links TP, Van der Hoeven JH, Zwarts MJ: Surface EMG and muscle fibre conduction during attacks of hypokalaemic periodic paralysis. *J Neurol Neurosurg Psych* 57:632–634, 1994.
167. Rüdel R, Lehmann-Horn F, Ricker K, Küther G: Hypokalemic periodic paralysis: in vitro investigation of muscle fiber membrane parameters. *Muscle Nerve* 7:110–120, 1984.
168. Jaimovich E, Venosa RA, Shrager P, et al: Density and distribution of tetrodotoxin receptors in normal and detubulated frog sartorius muscle. *J Gen Physiol* 67:399–416, 1976.
169. Adrian RH, Costantin LL, Peachey LD: Radial spread of contraction in frog muscle fibres. *J Physiol* 204:231–257, 1969.
170. Adrian RH, Peachey LD: Reconstruction of the action potential of frog sartorius muscle. *J Physiol* 235:103–131, 1973.
171. Hamill OP, Marty A, Neher E, et al: Improved patch-clamp techniques for high-resolution current recording from cells and cell-free membrane patches. *Pflügers Arch* 391:85–100, 1981.
172. Sakmann B, Neher E: *Single-Channel Recording*. New York: Plenum Press; 1985.
173. Horn R, Marty A: Muscarinic activation of ionic currents measured by a new whole-cell recording method. *J Gen Physiol* 92:145–159, 1988.
174. Rae J, Cooper K, Gates P, et al: Low access resistance perforated patch recordings using amphotericin B. *J Neurosci Methods* 37:15–26, 1991.
175. Horn R, Korn SJ: Prevention of rundown in electrophysiological recording. *Methods Enzymol* 207:149–155, 1992.
176. Armstrong CM, Gilly WF: Access resistance and space clamp problems associated with whole-cell patch clamping. *Methods Enzymol* 207:100–122, 1992.
177. Korn SJ, Horn R: Influence of sodium-calcium exchange on calcium current rundown and the duration of calcium-dependent chloride currents in pituitary cells, studied with whole cell and perforated patch recording. *J Gen Physiol* 94:789–812, 1989.
178. Soreq H, Seidman S: Xenopus oocyte microinjection: From gene to protein. *Methods Enzymol* 207:225–265, 1992.
179. Goldin AL: Maintenance of *Xenopus laevis* and oocyte injection. *Methods Enzymol* 207:266–279, 1992.
180. Goldin AL, Sumikawa K: Preparation of RNA for injection into *Xenopus* oocytes. *Methods Enzymol* 207:279–297, 1992.
181. Snutch TP, Mandel G: Tissue RNA as source of ion channels and receptors. *Methods Enzymol* 207:297–309, 1992.
182. Swanson R, Folander K: In vitro synthesis of RNA for expression of ion channels in *Xenopus* oocytes. *Methods Enzymol* 207:310–319, 1992.
183. Stühmer W: Electrophysiological recording from *Xenopus* oocytes. *Methods Enzymol* 207:319–339, 1992.
184. Noda M, Ikeda T, Suzuki H, et al: Expression of functional sodium channels from cloned cDNA. *Nature* 322:826–828, 1986.
185. Timpe LC, Schwarz TL, Tempel BL, et al: Expression of functional potassium channels from Shaker cDNA in *Xenopus* oocytes. *Nature* 331:143–145, 1988.
186. Claudio T: Stable expression of heterologous multisubunit protein complexes established by calcium phosphate- or lipid-mediated cotransfection. *Methods Enzymol* 207:391–408, 1992.
187. Quasthoff S, Franke C, Hatt H, et al: Two different types of potassium channels in human skeletal muscle activated by potassium channel openers. *Neurosci Lett* 119:191–194, 1990.
188. Lehmann-Horn F, Jurkat-Rott K: Nanotechnology for neuronal ion channels. *J Neurol Neurosurg Psych* 74:1466–1475, 2003

quaternary link involving CSQ, RyR, and DHPR, so only one of the two possibilities is correct.

On the cytoplasmic side of the jSR, feet are associated with and regulated by a variety of cytoplasmic accessory proteins, including Ca^{2+}, calmodulin, PKA, and FKBP12.[68]

Finally, among the recently identified jSR proteins are mitsugumin 29[128,129] and the junctophilin.[130] The important role of junctophilins in the docking event that initiates the formation of CRUs is discussed in Chap. 2. The mitsugumins have been implicated in the control of store-operated calcium channels.[129]

Figure 11-22 illustrates the structural relationship in skeletal muscles between components of SR and T tubules that have to do with the cycling of calcium and that are visible in the electron microscope. The parajunctional RyR3 are not shown.

Morphometry of Muscle Membranes and Their Proteins

Contents of SR and T tubules vary considerably, but not always in concert, between different muscle fibers in a manner that is well related to the fiber properties. Precise knowledge of relative surface areas and volumes of membrane-limited organelles is important in determining structure-function correlations, in understanding fiber types, and in describing pathologic and/or experimentally induced alterations. Local structural variations can be expected and indeed occur frequently along abnormal fibers, particularly with conditions that affect fibers focally. Here much larger samples are required for accurate quantitation, and random samples cannot be considered representative of individual fibers.

MORPHOMETRY OF SR AND T TUBULES

A variety of morphometric/stereological measuring techniques have been used to quantitate muscle membranes, the most successful being computer-aided planimetry and point and intersection counting. With either counting method, the oriented and periodic distributions of organelles are hindrances rather than advantages. The problem has been solved by using judiciously chosen and orientated probes to determine the frequency of profiles and boundary lengths of sectioned organelles.[131] All morphometric approaches may slightly underestimate surface areas and volumes by missing grazing views of organelles.

A major contribution of morphometry has been objective screening for fiber populations (fiber types). Structural parameters relate in a fully logical way to other data from probes used to discriminate between fiber types (i.e., histochemical and immunocytochemical determinations of myosin isoenzymes and physiological measures of contraction speed and fatigability). In general, abundance of SR and T-tubule components is quite closely fitted to the fiber properties. Even within a presumably homogeneous muscle, fibers vary in their content of organelles, forming a continuum, and for an individual organelle, the spectra of variability

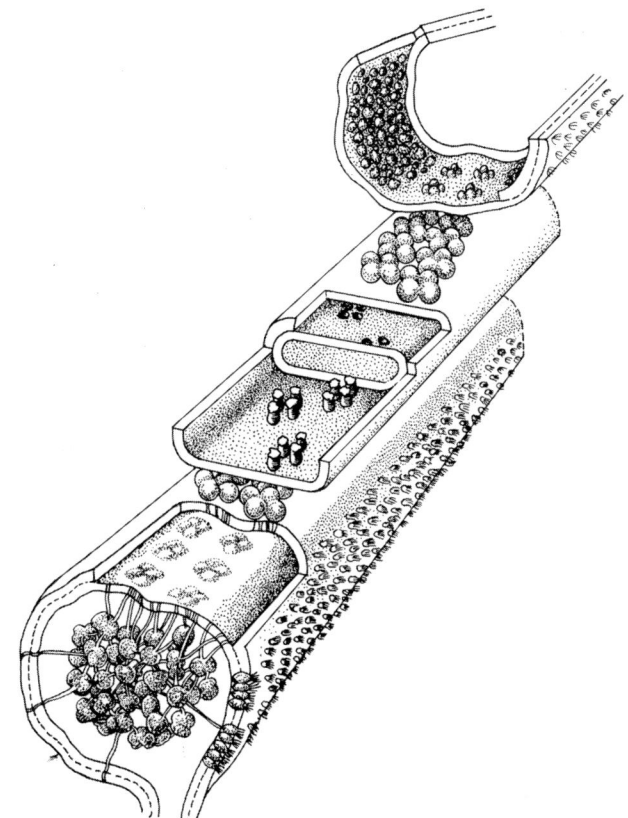

FIGURE 11-22. Schematic drawing of a skeletal muscle triad showing the positioning and relationships of key molecules that can be identified by electron microscopy. The Ca^{2+} ATPase occupies all free SR surfaces. RyRs (feet) and DHPRs organized in tetrads are shown in relationship to each other, with DHPR tetrads associated with alternate RyRs. Calsequestrin in the SR lumen is linked to the SR membrane presumably by triadin/junctin. (See Block B, Leung A, Campbell KP, Franzini-Armstrong C: Structural evidence for direct interaction between the molecular components of the transverse tubules/sarcoplasmic reticulum junction in skeletal muscle. J Cell Biol 107:2587, 1988.)

exhibited by fibers belonging to two groups with different properties (e.g., fast-twitch versus slow-twitch) can overlap. Fiber populations can be discriminated by variant analysis, but assignment of an individual fiber to a population on the basis of its content of one or two organelles has less than a 100 percent chance of being correct. The reason for the above is that a fiber's functional properties are largely determined by its in vivo pattern of activity, which, in turn, is dictated by the firing pattern of its motor neuron (see Chap. 5). The motor neurons innervating muscle fibers of one "type" operate through a hierarchy of firing thresholds, such that motor units recruited at low threshold are active more frequently and for longer periods of time. Firing frequencies of adjacent motor units in the hierarchy vary, resulting in unequal functional properties and structure of fibers in the different motor units along the hierarchy. This is confirmed by the homogeneity of enzymatic content of fibers in the same motor unit, as compared with the variability between fibers of the same general type but from different motor units.[132] Disposition and content of the membrane systems are very sensitive to the innervation and state of activity, and thus they vary in concert with the order of motor unit activation.[133]

STRUCTURE-FUNCTION CORRELATIONS

Interestingly, the contents of various domains of SR and/or T tubules do not vary in precise relationship to each other, and the variations can usually be traced to specific functional requirements. In three different fiber types of guinea pig leg muscles, for example, the overall density of T tubules is approximately the same, but the junctional segments are in considerably higher proportions in fast- than in slow-twitch fibers. As a result, fast fibers have a higher density of junctional feet (RyRs), thus allowing faster Ca^{2+} release in keeping with the faster activation rates, and the content of feet is strictly correlated with the pattern of activity.[134] A second illuminating example is that of superfast muscles used to produce sounds, as in the toadfish swimbladder. In this muscle the junctional regions of T tubules and SR (and thus the density of feet) are only slightly higher than in considerably slower fibers, but the surface area of free SR (and thus the ATPase content of the fibers) is tenfold higher.[135] This can be traced to the requirement for repeated contractions at high frequency, in which reuptake of Ca^{2+} by the SR is the limiting factor even though the muscle may release only limited amounts of Ca^{2+} at each cycle. Finally, a case in the opposite direction is that of the asynchronous flight muscles of some insects, in which the free SR is very scarce while the junctional SR is abundant.[1] These muscles are rapidly activated; thus they need a robust Ca^{2+} release. However, the fibers operate by stretch activation, which does not require synchronous oscillations in cytoplasmic Ca^{2+} content; thus Ca^{2+} uptake does not need to be rapid. Finally, in crayfish, the tail flexor muscles have less free SR than the carpopodite muscles, even though they are faster. Behavioral observations show that the crayfish uses only a few cycles of its rapid tail flip when escaping, presumably because it then has to wait for its relatively scarce SR to accumulate sufficient Ca^{2+} for the following cycles of activity.

List of Abbreviations

CRUs	Ca^{2+} release units	jPl	junctional domains of plasmalemma
CSQ	calsequestrin	jSR	junctional sarcoplasmic reticulum
DHPR	dihydropyridine receptor	jT segments	flat segments of T tubules
e-c	excitation-contraction	RyR	ryanodine receptor
EjSR	extended junctional SR	SER	smooth endoplasmic reticulum
ER	endoplasmic reticulum	SR	sarcoplasmic reticulum
IP3R	inositol 1,4,5-triphosphate receptor	T tubule	transverse tubule

References

1. Smith DS: The organization and function of the sarcoplasmic reticulum and T system of muscle cells. *J Biophys Mol Biol* 16:109, 1966.
2. Page SG: Structure of the sarcoplasmic reticulum in vertebrate muscle. *Br Med Bull* 24:170, 1968.
3. Ebashi S, Endo M: Ca^{2+} and muscle contraction. *Progr Biophys Mol Biol* 18:123, 1968.
4. Huxley AF: The Croonian lecture 1967: The activation of striated muscle and its mechanical response. *Proc R Soc Lond B* 178:1, 1971.
5. Constantin LL: Contractile activation in skeletal muscle. *Prog Biophys Mol Biol* 29:197, 1975.
6. Schneider MF: Membrane charge movement and depolarization contraction coupling. *Annu Rev Physiol* 48:507, 1981.
7. Fleischer S, Inui M: Biochemistry and biophysics of excitation-contraction coupling. *Annu Rev Biophys Chem* 18:333, 1989.
8. Ashley CC, Mulligan IP, Lea TJ: Ca^{2+} and activation mechanisms in skeletal muscle. *Q Rev Biophys* 24:1, 1991.
9. Sommer JR, Johnson EA: Ultrastructure of cardiac muscle, in Burne R (ed): *Handbook of Physiology: The Cardiovascular System*. Vol 1. Baltimore: Williams & Wilkins; 1960, pp 113–186.
10. Sommer JR, Boseen, E. Dalen H: To excite a heart: A bird's view. *Acta Physiol Scand* 142:5, 1991.
11. Johnson RG, Kranias EG (eds): Cardiac sarcoplasmic reticulum function and regulation of contractility. *Ann NY Acad Sci* 853:1–392.
12. Martonosi AN: *The Development of the Sarcoplasmic Reticulum*. Amsterdam: Harwood, 2000; pp 1–618.
13. Porter KR, Palade GF: Studies on the endoplasmic reticulum. III. Its form and distribution in muscle cells. *J Biophys Biochem Cytol* 3:269, 1957.
14. Weber A, Herz R, Reiss I: On the mechanism of the relaxing effect of fragmented sarcoplasmic reticulum. *J Gen Physiol* 46:679, 1963
15. Meissner G: Isolation and characterization of two types of sarcoplasmic reticulum vesicles. *Biochim Biophys Acta* 389:51, 1975.
16. Somlyo AV, Gonzales-Serratos H, Schuman H, et al: Calcium release and ionic changes in the sarcoplasmic reticulum of tetanized muscle: An electron microscope study. *J Cell Biol* 90:577, 1981.
17. Andersson-Cedergren E: Ultrastructure of motor end-plate and sarcoplasmic components of mouse skeletal muscle fiber. *J Ultrastruct Res* (Suppl 11):5, 1959.
18. Krolenko SA, Lucy JA: Reversible vacuolization of T-tubules in skeletal muscle: Mechanisms and implications for cell biology. *Int Rev Cytol* 202:243, 2001.
19. Flucher BE, Franzini-Armstrong C: Formation of junctions involved in excitation-contraction coupling in skeletal and cardiac muscle. *Proc Natl Acad Sci USA* 93:265–278, 1996.
20. Franzini-Armstrong C, Jorgensen AO: Structure and development of e-c coupling units in skeletal muscle. *Annu Rev Physiol* 56:509–534, 1994.
21. Rothberg KG, Heuser JE, Donzell WC, et al: Caveolin, a protein component of caveolae membrane coats. *Cell* 68:673, 1992.
22. Fra AM, Williamson E, Simons K, et al: De novo formation of caveolae in lymphocytes by expression of VIP21-caveolin. *Proc Natl Acad Sci USA* 92:8655, 1995.
23. Fra AM, Masserini M, Polestini P, et al: A photoreactive derivative of ganglioside GM1 specifically cross links VIP21-caveolin on the cell surface. *FEBS Lett* 375:11, 1995.
24. Murata M, Peranen J, Schreiner R, et al: VIP21-caveolin is a cholesterol-binding protein. *Procs Natl Acad Sci USA* 92:10339, 1995.
25. Way M, Parton RG: M-caveolin, a muscle-specific caveolin-related protein. *FEBS Lett* 376:108, 1995.
26. Simons K, Toomre D: Lipid rafts and signal transduction. *Nat Rev Mol Cell Biol* 1:31, 2000.

27. Leeson TS: Sarcolemma, T tubules and subsarcolemmal caveolae: Interrelationship and continuity demonstrated by tannic acid mordating. Can J Zool 56:391, 1978.
28. Veratti E: Investigations on the fine structure of the striated muscle fiber. J Biophys Biochem Cytol 10(4, part 2):3, 1961.
29. Endo M. Entry of fluorescent dyes into the sarcotubular system of the frog muscle. J Physiol 185:224, 1966.
30. Page SG: The organization of the sarcoplasmic reticulum in frog muscle. J Physiol 175:10, 1964.
31. Huxley HE: Evidence for continuity between the central elements of the triad and extracellular space in frog sartorius muscle. Nature 202:1067, 1964.
32. Forbes MS, Sperelakis N: Membrane systems in skeletal muscle of the lizard *Anolis carolinensis*. J Ultrastruct Res 73:245, 1980.
33. Peachey LD, Eisenberg BR: Helicoids in the T system and striations of frog skeletal muscle fibers seen by high voltage electron microscopy. Biophys J 22:145, 1978.
34. Rosenbluth J: Sarcoplasmic reticulum of an unusually fast acting crustacean muscle. J Cell Biol 42:534, 1969.
35. Block BA: Thermogenesis in muscle. Annu Rev Physiol 56:535, 1994.
36. Carafoli E, Gamble RL, Lehninger AL: K$^+$-dependent rebounds and oscillations in respiration-linked movements of Ca^{++} and H$^+$ in rat liver mitochondria. Biochem Biophys Res Commun 21:488, 1965.
37. Somlyo AV, Bond M, Broderick R, Somlyo AP: Calcium and magnesium movements through sarcoplasmic reticulum, endoplasmic reticulum, and mitochondria. Adv Exp Med Biol 232:221, 1988.
38. Rizzuto R, Brini M, Murgia M, et al: Microdomains with high Ca^{2+} close to IP3-sensitive channels that are sensed by neighboring mitochondria. Science 262:744, 1993.
39. Carafoli E, Santella L, Branca D, et al: Generation, control, and processing of cellular calcium signals. Critical Revs Biochem Mol Biol 36:107, 2001.
40. Rizzuto R, Pinton P, Brini M, et al: Mitochondria as biosensors of calcium microdomains. Cell Calcium 26:193, 1999.
41. Pozzan T, Magalhaes P, Rizzuto R: The comeback of mitochondria to calcium signalling. Cell Calcium 28:279, 2000.
42. Pacher P, Thomas AP, Hajnoczky AG: Calcium marks: Miniature calcium signals in single mitochondria driven by ryanodine receptors. Proc Natl Acad Sci USA 99:2380, 2002.
43. Gillis JM. Inhibition of mitochondrial calcium uptake slows down relaxation in mitochondria-rich skeletal muscles. J Muscle Res Cell Motil 18:473, 1997.
44. Caswell AH, Brandt NR, Brunschwig JP, et al: Localization and partial characterization of the oligomeric disulfide-linked molecular weight 95,000 protein (triadin) which binds the ryanodine and dihydropyridine receptors in skeletal muscle triadic vesicles. Biochemistry 30:7507, 1991.
45. Carl SL, Felix K, Caswell AH, et al: Immunolocalization of triadin, DHP receptors, and ryanodine receptors in adult and developing skeletal muscle of rats. Muscle Nerve 18:1232–1243, 1995.
46. Guo W, Jorgensen AO, Campbell KP: Triadin, a linker for calsequestrin and the ryanodine receptor. Soc Gen Physiol Ser 51:19, 1996.
47. Jones LR, Zhang L, Sanborn K, et al: Purification, primary structure and immunological characterization of the 26-K calsequestrin binding protein (junctin) from cardiac sarcoplasmic reticulum. J Biol Chem 270:30787, 1995.
48. Hirokawa N, Heuser JE: Internal and external differentiations of the postsynaptic membrane at the neuromuscular junction. J Neurocytol 11:487, 1982.
49. Ellisman MH, Rash JE, Staehelin LA, et al: Studies of excitable membranes: II. A comparison of specializations at neuromuscular junctions and nonjunctional sarcolemmas of mammalian fast and slow twitch muscle fibers. J Cell Biol 68:752, 1976.
50. Chevalier J, Bourguet J, Hugon JS: Membrane associated particles: Distribution in frog urinary bladder epithelium at rest and after oxytocin treatment. Cell Tissue Res 152:129, 1974.
51. van Hoek AN, Yang B, Kirmiz S, et al: Freeze-fracture analysis of plasma membranes of CHO cells stably expressing aquaporins 1-5. J Membr Biol 165:243, 1998.
52. Jorgensen AO, Kalnins VI, MacLennan DA: Localization of sarcoplasmic reticulum proteins in rat sarcoplasmic reticulum by immunofluorescence. J Cell Biol 80:372, 1979.
53. Franzini-Armstrong C, Ferguson DG: Density and disposition of Ca^{2+} ATPase in SR membrane as determined by shadowing techniques. Biophys J 48:607, 1985.
54. MacLennan D: Molecular tools to elucidate problems in excitation-contraction coupling. Biophys J 58:1355, 1990.
55. Castellani L, Hardwick PMD: Crystalline structure of sarcoplasmic reticulum from scallop. J Cell Biol 97:557, 1983.
56. Yin CC, Lai FA: Intrinsic lattice formation by the ryanodine receptor calcium-release channel. Nature New Biol 2:669, 2000.
57. Takekura H, Takeshima H, Nishimura S, et al: Co-expression in CHO cells of two muscle proteins involved in excitation contraction coupling. J Muscle Res Cell Motil 16:465, 1995.
58. Meissner G, Darling E, Eveleth J: Kinetics of rapid Ca^{2+} release by sarcoplasmic reticulum: Effects of Ca^{2+}, Mg^{2+} and adenine nucleotides. Biochemistry 25:236, 1986.
59. Pessah IN, Waterhouse AL, Casida JE: The calcium-ryanodine receptor complex of skeletal and cardiac muscle. Biochem Biophys Res Commun 128:449, 1985.
60. Fleischer S, Ogunbunmi EM, Dixon MC, et al: Localization of Ca^{2+} release channels with ryanodine in junctional terminal cisternae of sarcoplasmic reticulum of fast skeletal muscle. Proc Natl Acad Sci USA 82:7256, 1985.
61. Smith JS, Coronado R, Meissner G: Single channel measurements of the calcium release channel from skeletal muscle sarcoplasmic reticulum: Activation by Ca^{2+}, ATP and modulation by Mg^{2+}. J Gen Physiol 88:573, 1988.
62. Kawamoto RM, Brunschwig JP, Kun KC, et al: Isolation, characterization and localization of the spanning protein from skeletal muscle. J Cell Biol 103:1405, 1986.
63. Lai TA, Erickson HP, Rousseau E, et al: Purification and reconstitution of the calcium release channel from skeletal muscle. Nature 331:315, 1988.
64. Inui A, Saito A, Fleischer S: Purification of the ryanodine receptor and identity with feet structures of junctional terminal cisternae of SR from fast skeletal muscle. J Biol Chem 262:1740, 1988.
65. Block BA, Imagawa T, Campbell KP, et al: Structural evidence for direct interaction between the molecular components of the transverse tubules/sarcoplasmic reticulum junction in skeletal muscle. J Cell Biol 107:2587, 1988.
66. Fleischer S, Inui M: Biochemistry and biophysics of excitation-contraction coupling. Annu Rev Biophys Biophys Chem 18:333, 1989.
67. Coronado R, Morrissette J, Sukhareva M, et al: Structure and function of ryanodine receptors. Am J Physiol 266:C1485, 1994.
68. Meissner G: Ryanodine receptor/Ca release channels and their regulation by endogenous effectors. Annu Rev Physiol 56:485, 1994.
69. Ogawa Y: Role of ryanodine receptors. Crit Rev Biochem Mol Biol 29:229, 1994.
70. Franzini-Armstrong C, Protasi F: The ryanodine receptor of striated muscles, a complex channel capable of multiple interactions. Physiol Rev 77:699–729, 1997.
71. Takeshima H, Nishimura S, Matsumoto T, et al: Primary structure and expression from complementary DNA of skeletal muscle ryanodine receptor. Nature 339:439, 1989.
72. Zorzato F, Fujii J, Otsu K, et al: Molecular cloning of cDNA encoding human and rabbit forms of the Ca^{2+} release channel (ryanodine receptor) of skeletal muscle sarcoplasmic reticulum. J Biol Chem 265:2244, 1990.
73. Wagenknecht T, Grassucci R, Frank J, et al: Three-dimensional architecture of the calcium channel/foot structure of the sarcoplasmic reticulum. Nature 338:167, 1989.
74. Sharma MR, Penczek P, Grassucci R, et al: Cryo-electron microscopy and image analysis of the cardiac ryanodine receptor. J Biol Chem 273:18429, 1998.
75. Liu Z, Zhang J, Sharma MR, et al: Three-dimensional reconstruction of the recombinant type 3 ryanodine receptor and localization of its amino terminus. Proc Natl Acad Sci USA 98:6104, 2001.
76. Wagenknecht T, Radermacher M, Grassucci R, et al: Locations of calmodulin and FK506-binding protein on the three-dimensional architecture of the skeletal muscle ryanodine receptor. J Biol Chem 272:32463, 1997.
77. Samso M, Trujillo R, Gurrola GB, et al: Three-dimensional location of the imperatoxin A binding site on the ryanodine receptor. J Cell Biol 146:493, 1999.
78. Benacquista BL, Sharma MR, Samso M, et al: Amino acid residues 4425-4621 localized on the three-dimensional structure of the skeletal muscle ryanodine receptor. Biophys J 78:1349, 2000.
79. Stokes DL, Wagenknecht T: Calcium transport across the sarcoplasmic reticulum: Structure and function of Ca2+-ATPase and the ryanodine receptor. Eur J Biochem 267:5274, 2000.
80. Sharma MR, Jeyakumar LH, Fleischer S, et al: Three-dimensional structure of ryanodine receptor isoform three in two conformational states as visualized by cryo-electron microscopy. J Biol Chem 275:9485, 2000.
81. Serysheva II, Schatz M, van Heel M, et al: Structure of the skeletal muscle calcium release channel activated with Ca^{2+} and AMP-PCP. Biophys J 77:1936, 1999.
82. Hamada K, Miyata T, Mayanagi K, et al: Two-state conformational changes in inositol 1, 4, 5-trisphosphate receptor regulated by calcium. J Biol Chem 77:2115, 2002.
83. Campbell KB, Leung AT, Sharp AH: The biochemistry and molecular biology of the dihydropyridine sensitive calcium channel. Trends Neurosci 11:425–430, 1988.
84. Catterall WA: Excitation-contraction coupling in vertebrate skeletal muscle: A tale of two calcium channels. Cell 64:871, 1991.
85. Rios E, Brum G: Involvement of dihydropyridine receptors in excitation-contraction coupling in skeletal muscle. Nature 325:717–720, 1987.
86. Beam KG, Knudson CM, Powell JA: A lethal mutation in mice eliminates the slow calcium current in skeletal muscle cells. Nature 320:168, 1986.
87. Tanabe T, Beam KG, Powell JA, et al: Restoration of excitation-contraction coupling and slow calcium current in dysgenic muscle by dihydropyridine receptor complementary DNA. Nature 336:134, 1988.
88. Jorgensen AO, Shen AC-Y, Arnold W, et al: Subcellular distribution of the 1,4-dihydropyridine receptor in rabbit skeletal muscle in situ: An immunofluorescence and immunogold labeling study. J Cell Biol 109:135, 1989.

89. Carl SL, Felix K, Caswell AH, et al: Immunolocalization of sarcolemmal dihydropyridine receptor and sarcoplasmic reticular triadin and ryanodine receptor in rabbit ventricle and atrium. *J Cell Biol* 129:672–682, 1995.
90. Protasi F, Franzini-Armstrong C, Flucher B: Coordinated incorporation of skeletal muscle dihydropyridine receptors and ryanodine receptors in peripheral couplings of BC3H1 cells. *J Cell Biol* 137:859–870, 1997.
91. Protasi F, Franzini-Armstrong C, Allen PD: Role of ryanodine receptors in the assembly of calcium release units in skeletal muscle. *J Cell Biol* 140:831, 1998.
92. Sun X-H, Protasi F, Takahashi M, et al: Molecular architecture of membranes involved in excitation-contraction coupling of cardiac muscle. *J Cell Biol* 129: 659–673, 1995.
93. Protasi F, Sun X-H, Franzini-Armstrong C: Formation and maturation of calcium release units in developing and adult avian myocardium. *Dev Biol* 173:265–278, 1996.
94. Takekura H, Bennett L, Tanabe T, et al: Restoration of junctional tetrads in dysgenic myotubes by dihydropyridine receptor cDNA. *Biophys J* 67:793, 1994.
94a. Serysheva II, Ludtke SJ, Baker MR, et al: Structure of the voltage-gated L-type Ca^{2+} channel by electron cryomicroscopy. *Proc Natl Acad Sci USA* 99:10370, 2002.
94b. Wolf M, Eberhart A, Glossmann H, et al: Visualization of the domain structure of an L-type Ca^{2+} channel using electron cryo-microscopy. *J Mol Biol* 332:171, 2003.
95. Schneider MF, Chandler WK: Voltage-dependent charge movement in skeletal muscle: A possible step in excitation-contraction coupling. *Nature* 242:244, 1973.
96. Fleig A, Takeshima H, Penner R: Absence of Ca^{2+} current facilitation in skeletal muscle of transgenic mice lacking the type 1 ryanodine receptor. *J Physiol* 496:339, 1996.
97. Nakai J, Dirksen J, Nguyen RT, et al: Enhanced dihydropyridine receptor channel activity in the presence of ryanodine receptor. *Nature* 380:72, 1996.
98. Grabner M, Dirksen RT, Suda N, et al: The II-III loop of the skeletal muscle dihydropyridine receptor is responsible for the bi-directional coupling with the ryanodine receptor. *J Biol Chem* 274:21913, 1999.
99. Kiselyov KI, Shin DM, Wang Y, et al: Gating of store-operated channels by conformational coupling to ryanodine receptors. *Mol Cell* 6:421–431, 2000.
100. Rios E, Pizarro G: Voltage sensor of excitation-contraction coupling in skeletal muscle. *Physiol Rev* 71:849, 1991.
101. Block BA, O'Brien J, Franck J: The role of ryanodine receptor isoforms in the structure and function of vertebrate triads, in Clapham DE, Ehrlich BE (eds): *Organellar Ion Channels and Transporters*. New York: Rockefeller University Press; 1996, p 47.
102. Marx SO, Ondrias K, Marks AR: Coupled gating between individual skeletal muscle calcium release channels (ryanodine receptors). *Science* 281:818, 1998.
103. Marx SO, Gaburjakova J, Gaburjakova M, et al: Coupled gating between cardiac calcium release channels (ryanodine receptors). *Circ Res* 88:1151, 2001.
104. Protasi F, Paolini C, Nakai J, et al: Multiple regions of RYR1 mediate functional and structural interactions with a1s DHPR in skeletal muscle. *Biophys J* 83:3230, 2002.
105. Sorrentino V, Volpe P: Ryanodine receptors: How many, where and why? *Trends Pharmacol Sci* 14:98, 1993.
106. Sutko JL, Airey JA: Ryanodine receptor calcium release channels: Does diversity in form equal diversity in function? *Annu Rev Physiol* 76:1027, 1996.
107. Xu X, Bhat MB, Nishi M, et al: Molecular cloning of cDNA encoding a *Drosophila* ryanodine receptor and functional studies of the carboxyl-terminal calcium release channel. *Biophys J* 78:1270, 2000.
108. Maryon EB, Coronado R, Anderson P: *unc-68* encodes a ryanodine receptor involved in regulating *C. elegans* body-wall muscle contraction. *J Cell Biol* 134:885, 1996.
109. Tunwell REA, Wickenden C, Bertrand BMA, et al: The human cardiac muscle ryanodine receptor-calcium release channel—identification, primary structure and topological analysis. *Biochem J* 318:477, 1996.
110. Airey JA, Baring AMD, Beck CF, et al: Failure to make normal α-ryanodine receptor is an early event associated with the crooked neck dwarf (*cn*) mutation in chicken. *Dev Dyn* 197:169, 1993.
111. Takeshima H, Iino M, Takekura H: Excitation-contraction uncoupling and muscle degeneration in mice lacking functional skeletal muscle ryanodine-receptor gene. *Nature* 369:566, 1994.
112. Protasi F, Takekura H, Wang Y, et al: RYR1 and RYR3 have different roles in the assembly of calcium release units of skeletal muscle. *Biophys J* 79:2494–2508, 2000.
113. Barone V, Bertocchini F, Bottinelli R, et al: Contractile impairment and structural alterations of skeletal muscle from knockout mice lacking type 1 and type 3 ryanodine receptors. *FEBS Lett* 422:160, 1998.
114. Margret A, Damiani E, Tobaldin G: Ratio of dihydropyridine to ryanodine receptors in mammalian and frog twitch muscles in relation to the mechanical hypothesis of excitation-contraction coupling. *Biochem Biophys Res Commun* 197:1303, 1993.
115. Bers DM, Stiffel VM: Ratio of ryanodine and dihydropyridine receptors in cardiac and skeletal muscle, and implications for excitation-contraction coupling. *Am J Physiol* 264:C1587, 1993.
116. Marty L, Robert M, Villaz M, et al: Biochemical evidence for a complex involving dihydropyridine receptor and ryanodine receptor in triad junctions of skeletal muscle. *Proc Natl Acad Sci USA* 91:2270, 1994.
117. Costello B, Chadwick C, Fleischer S: Isolation of the junctional face membrane of sarcoplasmic reticulum. *Methods Enzymol* 157:46, 1988.
118. Motoike HK, Caswell AH, Smilowitz HM: Extraction of junctional complexes from triad junctions of rabbit skeletal muscle. *J Muscle Res Cell Motil* 15:493–504, 1994.
119. MacLennan D, Wong PTS: Isolation of a calcium sequestering protein from the sarcoplasmic reticulum. *Proc Natl Acad Sci USA* 68:1231, 1971.
120. Jorgensen A, Campbell KP: Evidence for the presence of calsequestrin in two structurally different regions of myocardial sarcoplasmic reticulum. *J Cell Biol* 98:1597, 1984.
121. Guo W, Campbell KP: Association of triadin with the ryanodine receptor and calsequestrin in the lumen of the sarcoplasmic reticulum. *J Biol Chem* 270:9027, 1995.
122. Zhang L, Kelley J, Schmeisser YM, et al: Complex formation between junctin, triadin calsequestrin and the ryanodine receptor. Proteins of the cardiac junctional sarcoplasmic reticulum membrane. *J Biol Chem* 272: 23389, 1997.
123. Caswell AH, Motoike HK, Fan H, et al: Location of ryanodine receptor binding site on skeletal muscle triadin. *Biochemistry* 38:90–97, 1999.
124. Duggan PE, Martonosi A: Sarcoplasmic reticulum. IX. The permeability of sarcoplasmic reticulum membranes. *J Gen Physiol* 56:147, 1970.
125. Nori A, Valle G, Massimino ML, et al: Targeting of calsequestrin to the sarcoplasmic reticulum of skeletal muscle upon deletion of its glycosylation site. *Exp Cell Res* 265:104–113, 2001.
126. Franzini-Armstrong C, Kenney L, Varriano-Marston E: The structure of calsequestrin in triads of vertebrate muscle. *J Cell Biol* 105:49–56, 1987.
127. Zhang L, Franzini-Armstrong C, Ramesh V, et al: Structural alterations in cardiac calcium release units resulting from overexpression of junctin. *J Mol Cell Cardiol* 33:233–247, 2000.
128. Kamazaki S, Nishi M, Takeshima H, et al: Abnormal formation of sarcoplasmic reticulum networks and triads during early development of skeletal muscle cells in mitsugumin 29-deficient mice. *Dev Growth Diff* 43:717, 2001.
129. Pen Z, Yang D, Nagari RY, et al: Dysfunction of store-operated calcium channels in muscle cells lacking mitsugumin 29. *Nat Cell Biol* 4:379, 2002.
130. Ito K, Kamazaki S, Sasamoto K, et al: Deficiency of triad junction and contraction in mutant skeletal muscle lacking junctophilin type 1. *J Cell Biol* 154:1059, 2001.
131. Eisenberg BR: Quantitative ultrastructure of mammalian skeletal muscle, in Peachey LD, Adrian RH (eds): *Handbook of Physiology: Skeletal Muscle*. Baltimore: Williams & Wilkins; 1983, pp 73–112.
132. Pette D (ed): *Plasticity of Muscle*. Berlin: de Gruyter; 1980.
133. Eisenberg BR, Salmons S: The reorganization of subcellular structure in muscle undergoing fast-to-slow transformation: A stereological study. *Cell Tissue Res* 220:449, 1981.
134. Franzini-Armstrong C, Ferguson DG, Champ C: Discrimination between fast- and slow-twitch fibres of guinea pig skeletal muscle using the relative surface density of junctional transverse tubules. *J Muscle Res Cell Motil* 9:403, 1988.
135. Appelt D, Shen V, Franzini-Armstrong C: Quantitation of Ca ATPase, feet and mitochondria in superfast muscle fibres from the toadfish, *Opsanus tau*. *J Muscle Res Cell Motil* 12:543, 1991.

Chapter 12
Excitation-Contraction Coupling in Skeletal Muscle

KURT G. BEAM
PAUL HOROWICZ

Contractile Responses to Membrane Depolarization
  ACTIVATION AND INACTIVATION RELATIONS
Voltage-Dependent Charge Movement and SR Calcium Release
  CHARGE MOVEMENT AND DEPOLARIZATION-CONTRACTION COUPLING
  DEPOLARIZATION-INDUCED CALCIUM TRANSIENTS
Molecular Basis of Excitation-Contraction Coupling
  STRUCTURE OF DHPRS AND RYRS
  IDENTIFYING DOMAINS OF DHPRS AND RYRS IMPORTANT FOR EXCITATION-CONTRACTION COUPLING
Summary

This chapter represents an update of the chapter written by the late Paul Horowicz in the second edition of *Myology* (in 1994). The basic physiologic observations that were summarized at that time remain accepted today, and it is instructive to recall that Professor Horowicz began his chapter with a quotation from a much earlier review (1965) by Alexander Sandow[1]:

Excitation-contraction coupling is the function of the muscle fiber in which an electrical depolarization of the plasma membrane initiates a sequence of reactions that causes mechanical activation of the contractile myofibrils lying within the membrane. By far the greatest amount of work on this function has been done on fast skeletal muscle fibers. In this type of muscle, the membrane electrical change is the action potential, and the present evidence indicates that this gives rise to contraction by a sequence of at least two main processes. Firstly, the action potential generates a signal, probably also electrical in nature, which is conducted inwardly by the internal membranous structures of the T system, and which, in effect, rapidly transforms the depolarization at the plasma membrane into an equivalent change in close proximity to the myofibrils. Secondly, this signal causes release from internal stores within the sarcoplasmic reticulum of a chemical agent, very likely the calcium ion, which directly activates contraction in the myofibrils.

By way of explanation, the "fast skeletal muscle fibers" referred to in the quotation above are the same as twitch fibers (both slow-twitch and fast-twitch), which represent the vast majority of vertebrate skeletal muscle. In mammals, slow or tonic fibers are present only as a subset of the extraocular muscle fibers. In modern terms, it is now universally accepted that the initial electrical signal in twitch fibers is sensed by a voltage-gated calcium channel (also known as the dihydropyridine receptor, or DHPR)* and that conformational changes of the DHPR are communicated to the ryanodine receptor (RyR), which functions as a calcium release channel within the sarcoplasmic reticulum. Although we now understand some of the molecular architecture underlying excitation-contraction coupling, the basic description of physiologic function remains unchanged. Therefore the initial part of this chapter contains large segments from the last edition, with short additions that relate the physiologic observations to the molecular architecture. The second part of the chapter discusses the molecular components in greater detail.

Contractile Responses to Membrane Depolarization

ACTIVATION AND INACTIVATION RELATIONS

The adequate stimulus for contraction is depolarization of the transverse (T)-tubule membranes.[2] The tension response of a single muscle fiber is very sensitive to depolarization. Using rapid increases in external potassium ion concentration to simultaneously depolarize the whole fiber, Kuffler[3] clearly showed that a definite threshold depolarization was required before a mechanical response was obtained. If a depolarization above threshold is maintained in twitch fibers, the active tension initially developed soon declines to zero. This behavior is shown in Fig. 12-1A, where a single frog twitch fiber was successively depolarized to varying levels of internal potential by different external potassium concentrations.[4] The characteristic feature of the contractures is an abrupt transition from a plateau, in which the tension fades slowly, to a rapid phase of relaxation. The maximum tension achieved early in the contractures and the slow decline in the plateau in response to the higher K⁺ concentrations were comparable in magnitude to those seen when the fiber was electrically stimulated at rates above the fusion frequency. The fiber gave no response when $[K^+]_o$ was increased to 10 mM, which produced a depolarization below the contraction threshold, and it gave only a small, brief response when $[K^+]_o$ was increased to 20 mM, which depolarized the fiber above the contraction threshold. Another interesting feature about the contractures produced by high external potassium concentrations is that the duration of the plateau and the apparent time constant of the rapid phase of relaxation both shorten progressively as the potassium concentration is increased from 30 to 190 mM. Parenthetically, it should be stated that although the use of elevated $[K^+]_o$ has a long history in the study of excitation-contraction coupling, it remains a valuable tool because it provides the ability to produce spatially uniform changes of membrane potential in intact fibers.

Exposure of a single *Xenopus* tonic slow fiber[5] to elevated $[K^+]_o$ resulted in steady-state, nonzero tensions (Fig. 12-1B) that could be maintained for several minutes unless terminated sooner by removing the potassium. An interesting feature of these contractures is that although the peak tensions

---
*A list of abbreviations used in this chapter is given at the end of the chapter.

are about the same for solutions containing 20, 40, and 80 mM potassium, the final steady tension is lower the higher the external potassium concentration, and partial relaxation from the peak tension occurs when the external potassium is 40 and 80 mM but not when it is 20 mM. The inactivation of excitation-contraction coupling in twitch fibers is reminiscent of the inactivation of ionic current observed for many voltage-gated ion channels. The effects of prolonged depolarization on gating charge movements of the DHPR are discussed under "Complexities of Charge Movement," below. However, the precise molecular correlates within the DHPR that account for the inactivation of excitation-contraction coupling have not yet been identified. The inactivation may represent an important protective mechanism whereby local damage in muscle does not result in prolonged contractures.

The relation between normalized peak tension developed and log $[K^+]_o$ (the activation curve for contraction) for the two types of fibers is given in Fig. 12-2. In the lower part of the curve for both types, tension increases extremely steeply with

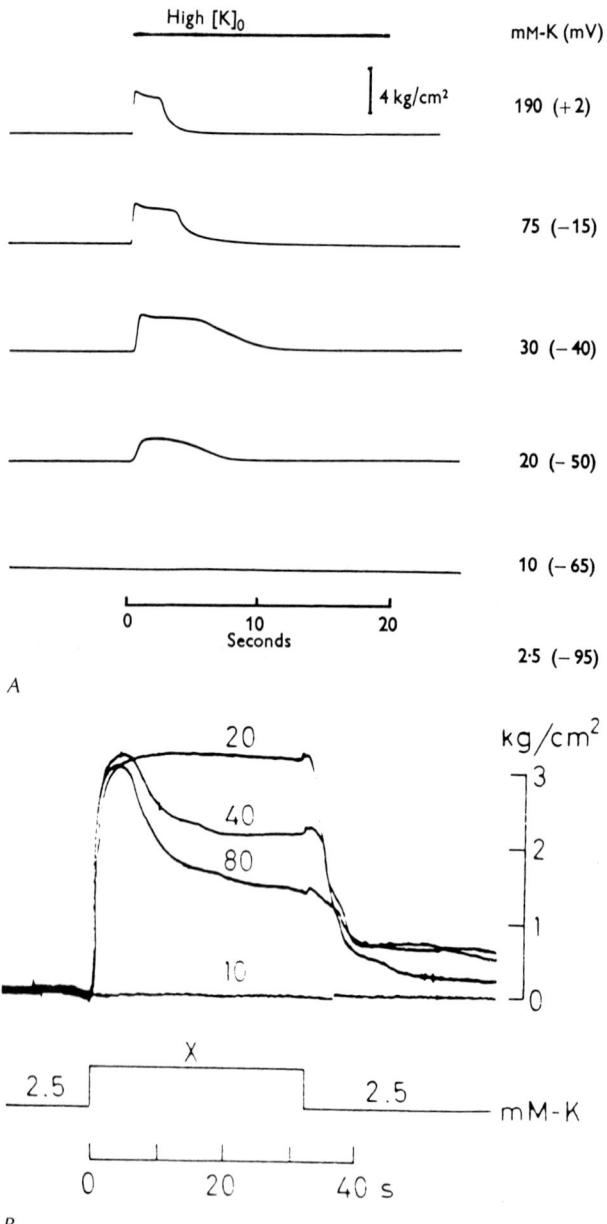

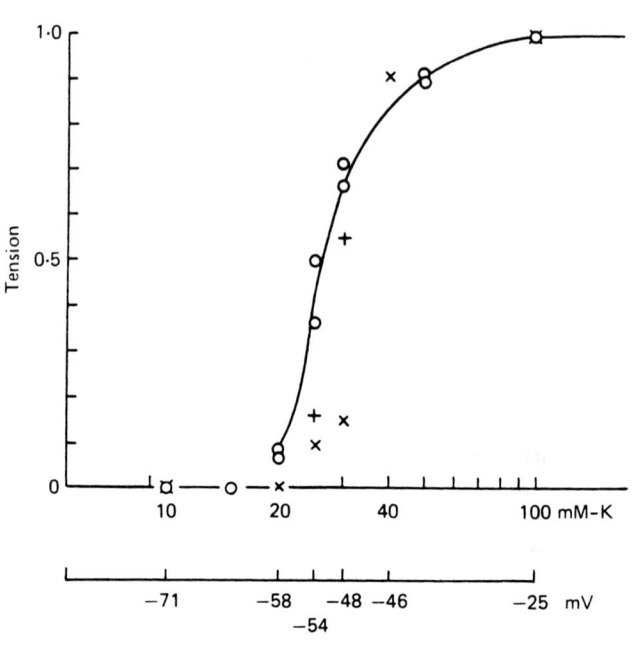

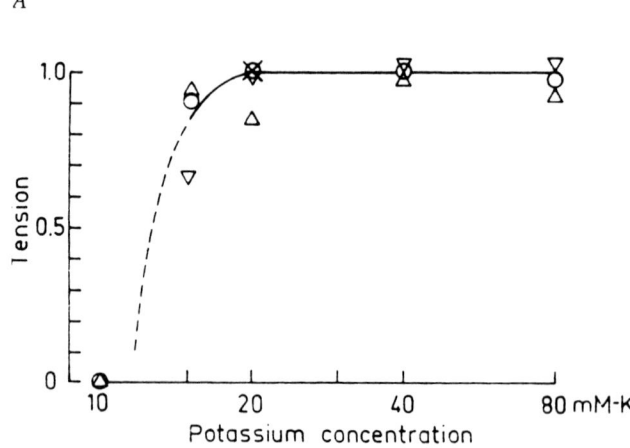

FIGURE 12-1. Tension response to application of high $[K^+]_o$ in twitch and slow amphibian single skeletal muscle fibers. *A.* Single twitch fiber from the semitendinous muscle of *Rana temporaria*. Potassium concentration used and internal potentials are given at right. Temp 21°C. *(From Hodgkin and Horowicz.[4] Reproduced by permission.)* *B.* Single slow fiber from the iliofibularis muscle of *Xenopus laevis*. Potassium concentrations (in mM) are shown above the tension reponses, which are superimposed. Temp. ~22°C. *(From Lännergren.[5] Reproduced by permission.)*

FIGURE 12-2. Relation between normalized peak tension and external potassium concentration or internal potential. *A.* Data from several single twitch fibers isolated from semitendinous muscles of *R. temporaria*. Each symbol represents a different fiber. Maximum tensions between 3.0 and 4.0 kg/cm². Temp 18°C. *(From Hodgkin and Horowicz.[4] Reproduced by permission.)* *B.* Each symbol represents data from a single slow fiber isolated from an iliofibularis muscle of *X. laevis*. Maximum tensions between 3.1 and 5.1 kg/cm2. Temp. ~22°. *(From Lännergren.[5] Reproduced by permission.)*

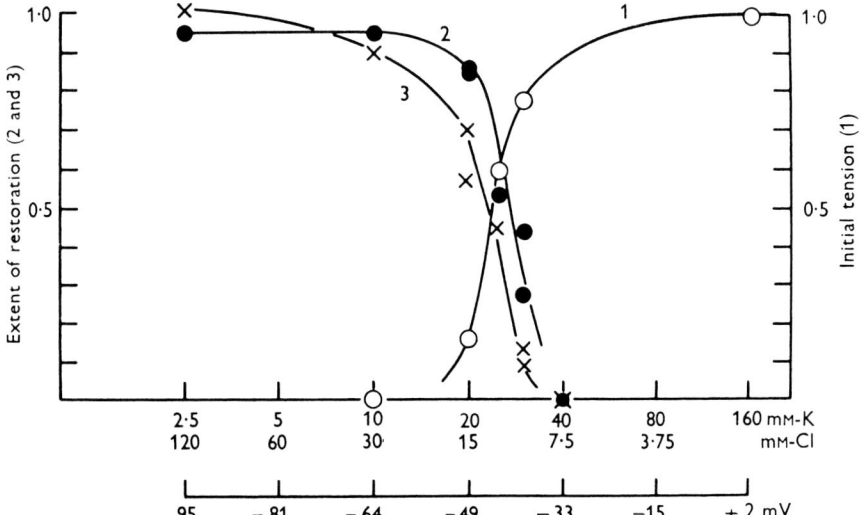

FIGURE 12-3. Relation between external potassium concentration and initial peak tension (curve 1) or degree of restoration (curves 2 and 3). For curve 1, the ordinate is the initial tension on increasing external K+ from 2.5 to x mM, relative to the maximum tension of 4/kg/cm². For curve 2, the ordinate is the tension in 190 mM K+, 2.5 mM Cl⁻ after 1-min recovery in x mM K+, (300/x) mM Cl⁻. For curve 3, the ordinate is the area under the tension-time curve for the same contractures as in curve 2. The ordinates in curves 2 and 3 are given relative to the peak tension or area in the first contraction. The abscissa gives the potassium and chloride concentrations of the test solutions. The lower scale gives the probable values of internal potential. (From Hodgkin and Horowicz.[4] Reproduced by permission.)

potassium concentration. However, for slow fibers, the activation curve is so steep that in one fiber 13.5 mM [K+]$_o$ produced no contraction, whereas 15 mM produced a nearly maximal peak tension. Nevertheless, in neither case is the relation all or none or "nongraded" in nature. The graded tension response as a function of membrane potential is reminiscent of the conductance-versus-potential relationship for voltage-gated ion channels (Chap. 10) and places important constraints on the possible mechanisms of excitation-contraction coupling.

The curve for recovery from inactivation of twitch fibers is compared with the activation curve in Fig. 12-3. To measure recovery from inactivation, the fiber was first immersed in 190 mM K+ to produce a control contracture (followed by relaxation resulting from inactivation). The bath was then changed for 1 min to an intermediate test level of potassium, after which the fiber was reexposed to 190 mM K+ to measure a second contracture as an index of the recovery that had occurred during the prior 1 min. If either the peak tension or the area under the second contracture is plotted as a function of the test K+ concentration, one obtains curves that are very nearly the same, as shown in Fig. 12-3. As an alternative to measuring the recovery from inactivation as just described, one can also measure inactivation[6] by beginning with a fiber in normal physiologic saline and then exposing it to a partially elevated test level of potassium and finally measuring the contracture in response to 190 mM K+. The inactivation curve measured in this way (for example, the filled symbols in Fig. 12-4) is similar to the curve for recovery from inactivation.

Effects of External Ca²⁺ on Activation and Inactivation

Over the years much effort has been devoted to deciphering the role of external Ca²⁺ in excitation-contraction coupling.

One role, conventionally referred to as "the stabilizing action of calcium," can be performed by other divalent cations such as Mg²⁺ and is generally ascribed to adsorption or desorption of the divalent cations to fixed charges on the cell membrane.[7] This phenomenon affects cell membranes generally, with the consequence that removal of all divalents and their unbinding from the fixed charges effectively depolarizes the cell, which in muscle inactivates excitation-contraction coupling.

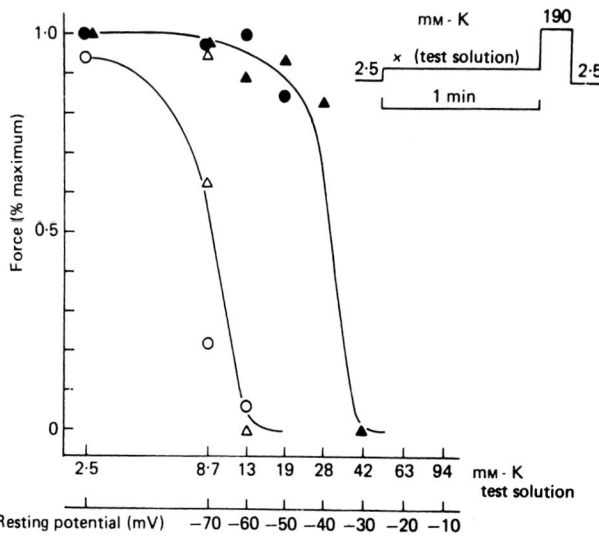

FIGURE 12-4. "Inactivation" curve from two single twitch fibers for two external Ca²⁺ concentrations. The inset shows the experimental procedure. Filled symbols: 3.0 to 3.1 mM Ca²⁺; open symbols: 2.8 to 3.2 mM Mg²⁺, 10⁻⁹ M Ca²⁺. Temp. 20 to 22°C. Fibers isolated from semitendinosus or iliofibularis of *R. temporaria*. (From Lüttgau and Spiecker.[9] Reproduced by permission.)

As long as measures are taken to prevent this membrane destabilization (by elevating Mg^{2+} to compensate for the removal of Ca^{2+}), one can show that external calcium is not required for excitation-contraction coupling in skeletal muscle.[8,9] In the presence of 2.5 to 3.0 mM Mg^{2+}, which stabilizes the membrane potential in low $[Ca^{2+}]_o$, twitch fibers develop maximal tensions even when external Ca^{2+} is reduced to 10^{-9} M in solutions buffered with ethyleneglycol-bis-(2-aminoethylether)-N,N,N',N'-tetraacetic acid (EGTA). More importantly, the activation curve was not measurably affected when external Ca^{2+} was lowered to 10^{-9} M in the presence of Mg^{2+}. In contrast to the activation, the inactivation of excitation-contraction coupling was shifted to more negative internal potentials when external Ca^{2+} was reduced to 10^{-9} M (Fig. 12-4), as also shown by Frankenhaeuser and Lännergren.[6] One consequence of lowering external Ca^{2+} is that the inactivation-versus-potential curve no longer overlaps the activation curve; hence there is a range of external K^+ concentration in which inactivation can occur without prior activation.

The Strength-Duration Relation to Attain Contraction Threshold

Up to this point the mechanical response to a membrane depolarization lasting a few seconds or longer has been considered. However, in order to determine the depolarization required to produce a just detectable mechanical response for pulse durations of less than a few tenths of a second, membrane voltage-clamp techniques have to be employed. The use of these techniques on fibers treated with tetrodotoxin allows the determination of the criteria that an electrical stimulus must satisfy in order to give a contraction in the absence of an action potential as well as examination of the interaction of two brief subthreshold pulses on the excitation process.

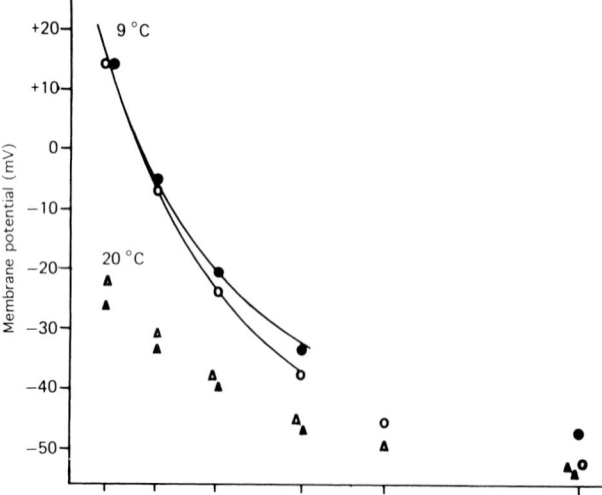

FIGURE 12-5. Comparison of strength-duration durves for twitch and slow muscle fibers. Data points represent means from many single fibers. Slow fibers are represented by open symbols, twitch fibers by filled symbols. Circles are 9°C, triangles are for 20°C. All fibers from warm adapted *R. temporaria*. (From Gilly and Hui.[11] Reproduced by permission.)

The first study of this type was performed by Adrian et al.[10] For pulses shorter than 20 ms, they found that the membrane depolarization required for threshold activation increased as the pulse duration decreased. Figure 12-5 illustrates similar experiments performed by Gilly and Hui[11] for both twitch and slow muscle fibers at two temperatures. At the higher temperature (20°C), there is no significant difference in the strength-duration curve for mechanical activation between the two types of fibers. At the lower temperature (9°C), there is little difference at short pulse durations, but a gradual separation occurs as the pulse durations are lengthened; for a pulse duration of 100 ms, the potential at threshold is about 4 mV more negative in slow than in twitch fibers. The close similarity of the strength-duration curves indicates that the activation processes are basically similar in the two types of fibers. In addition, in the presence of about 11 mM external Mg^{2+}, reducing external Ca^{2+} from 1.8 mM to about 10^{-8} M in EGTA-containing solutions has no effect on the strength-duration curves for either slow or twitch fibers, indicating that, provided sufficient Mg^{2+} is present, extracellular Ca^{2+} plays no measurable specific role in mechanical activation at threshold. The shape of the strength-duration curve reflects the balance between calcium release via RyRs and removal via endogenous calcium buffers and transport into the sarcoplasmic reticulum. Thus, shorter pulses must achieve more depolarized levels in order to activate a sufficient number of RyRs to overcome removal.

Effects of Caffeine

Methylxanthines (typified by caffeine) potentiate tension responses by acting directly on the RyR (see Chap. 14). Caffeine, with a pKa of 0.8, is present almost exclusively as the neutral molecule at physiologic pH, and it readily penetrates the cytoplasm.[12] With frog muscle at room temperatures, caffeine produces potentiation of twitches in the range of concentrations between 0.1 and 2 mM, with no effect on membrane potential and only a 10 percent prolongation of the repolarizing phase of the action potential.[13–15] At higher concentrations (e.g., 3.6 mM), caffeine produces contractures in addition to twitch potentiation. Caffeine does not appear to have any direct effect on the actomyosin system,[16] suggesting that it alters the relation between membrane potential and Ca^{2+} release.[17] In fact, subthreshold concentrations of caffeine potentiate submaximal K^+ contractures—i.e., shifting the relation between $[K^+]_o$ and peak contracture tension.[18] A typical set of results from single fibers illustrating this effect is shown in Fig. 12-6.

An important finding, reported by several investigators, is that caffeine contractures can still occur during exposure to solutions with no added external Ca^{2+} and either with or without added EGTA.[19–21] The main conclusion to be drawn from these results is that the Ca^{2+} source that gives rise to the caffeine-induced contractures is entirely intracellular, and it is generally agreed to be the sarcoplasmic reticulum (SR). In modern terms, caffeine is potentiating the same release pathway (the RyR) that is involved in conventional excitation-contraction coupling, which is independent of external calcium, as described above. Caffeine remains important as a diagnostic tool for identifying RyRs and their physiologic function not only in muscle but also in all other cell types. Of

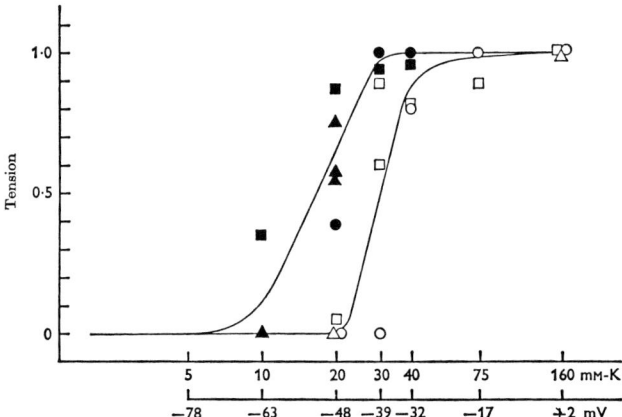

FIGURE 12-6. Normalized peak tension versus external potassium concentration (or internal potential) relation with 1.5 mM caffeine (filled symbols) and with no caffeine (open symbols). Three single twitch fibers from semitendinosus or iliofibularis muscles of *R. temporaria*. Temp. 22 to 23°C. (From Lüttgau and Oetliker.[15] Reproduced by permission.)

special importance is the fact that caffeine is used as an in vitro test for susceptibility to malignant hyperthermia (see Chap. 59).

Voltage-Dependent Charge Movement and SR Calcium Release

Changes in transmembrane potential drive numerous cellular events, such as muscle contraction and increases in sodium and potassium permeability of neuronal membranes (Chap. 10). Some time ago, Hodgkin and Huxley[22] suggested that one possible means for sensing and responding to changes of transmembrane potential could involve specific charged or dipolar molecules within the membrane changing position or orientation when the electric field in the membrane is altered, giving rise to displacement currents in response to changes in transmembrane potential. Because transmembrane potential–dependent physiologic processes are generally sensitive over only a restricted range of internal potentials, one expects to find specific displacement currents in these restricted ranges. Specific charge displacement currents were first demonstrated in muscle by Schneider and Chandler[23] and in nerve by Armstrong and Bezanilla.[24] The major portion of the charge movements in nerve are involved in gating Na⁺ channels,[25] whereas the major portion of the charge movements in muscle, which are much slower than those in nerve, are thought to be a step involved in coupling depolarization to contraction.[23,26,27]

Nonlinear displacement currents (also called charge movement or gating currents) are obtained by reducing the voltage- and time-dependent ionic currents by using poorly permeant ions and specific channel blockers. The linear displacement currents and any remaining small ionic currents are then subtracted from the current transients produced by the voltage pulses. The total charge that moves during the on transient, Q_{on}, evaluated as the time integral of the asymmetry current, is in most instances equal in magnitude but opposite in direction to the total charge that moves during the off transient of the pulse, Q_{off}. The total charge moved Q is related in a sigmoid manner to the membrane potential, which can be approximated by either the sum of two Boltzmann distribution functions or a single such function which, in the present context, can be expressed as $Q = Q_{max}/\{1+ \exp[-(V - V_{1/2})/k]\}$, where Q_{max} is the maximum charge moved at positive internal potentials, $V_{1/2}$ (referred to as mid-potential or transition potential) is the internal potential at which $Q = Q_{max}/2$, and k is a factor that determines the maximum steepness of the function.

CHARGE MOVEMENT AND DEPOLARIZATION-CONTRACTION COUPLING

Evidence was gathered early in support of the notion that muscle membrane charge movement was involved with coupling of depolarization to contraction. For one thing, in fibers held at approximately the normal resting level, there was a general similarity of the voltage dependences of charge movement and activation of contraction. Moreover, it was found that maintained depolarization (which causes the inactivation of contraction) caused the amount of mobile charge to decline, as well as that the reappearance of charge and the ability to contract again have similar time courses under similar conditions.[27–29] A further detailed study of so-called repriming experiments after prolonged depolarization showed that recovery of contraction is affected by potential in the same way as recovery of charge movement.[30] In twitch fibers, the removal of external calcium has similar effects on inactivation of excitation-contraction coupling and on the loss of mobile charge in depolarized fibers.[31,32] In tonic fibers, the mobile charge is much more resistant to immobilization by prolonged depolarization.[33]

Strong support for a link between charge movement and depolarization-contraction coupling was provided by an examination in individual fibers of the amount of charge moved and the threshold for contractile activation, which demonstrated that a relatively fixed amount of charge had to be moved to reach the contractile threshold in response to depolarizations of varying amplitude and duration.[34] A link between muscle charge movement and depolarization-contraction coupling is also supported by observations that similar shifts of the contraction-activation relation (i.e., tension versus V) and the Q-versus-V relation can be produced by altering the ionic composition of the fluids to which muscle fibers are exposed. Increases in pH from 5.5 to 9.0 at constant external Ca^{2+}, elevation of external Ca^{2+} at constant pH, and 8 mM perchlorate shift both curves in the same direction.[35–37] The shifts produced by altering pH and pCa are consistent with surface charge theory.

Studies on mammalian muscle also support the association of muscle charge movements with contractions produced by depolarization. Both contractile activation and charge movement in slow-twitch fibers occur at more negative potentials than they do in fast-twitch fibers,[38,39] and the differences are abolished as the fiber properties change following denervation.[40] Figure 12-7 illustrates membrane currents and intra-

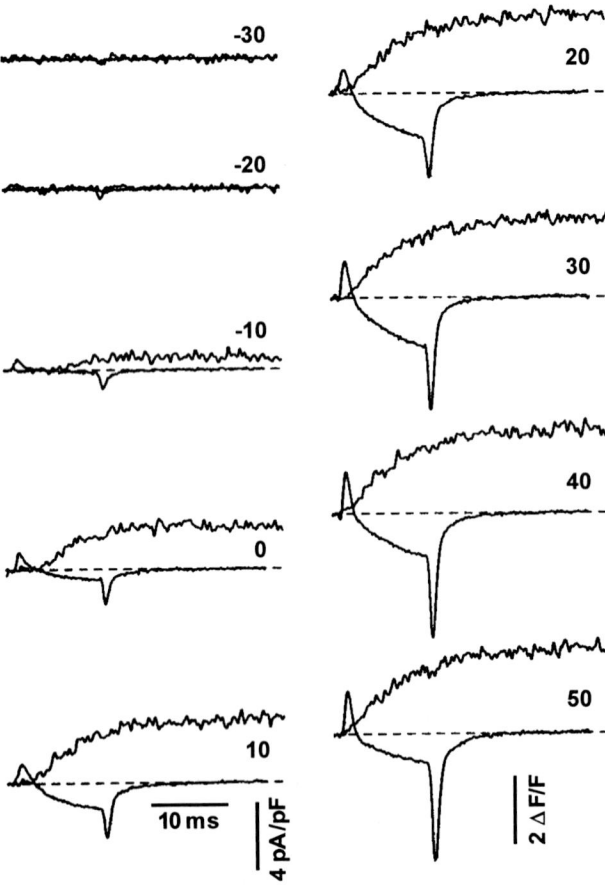

FIGURE 12-7. Membrane currents and intracellular calcium transients measured with the whole-cell technique in a normal mouse myotube. The indicated test pulses followed a −50-mV prepulse to inactivate T-type calcium current (which is expressed in embryonic muscle but not in adult muscle) and to immobilize charge associated with voltage-gated sodium channels. Charge movement (transient upward and downward deflections at the onset and offset of the 15-ms test pulse) was first detected at −20 mV, the intracellular calcium transient (sustained upward deflections) at −10 mV, and inward calcium current at 0 mV. Because the calcium current was not blocked, the OFF charge movement is contaminated by ionic tail current. The patch pipette contained 0.1 mM EGTA and 0.2 mM Fluo-3 as the calcium indicator. (From García et al.[41] Reproduced by permission.)

cellular calcium transients measured simultaneously in a mouse skeletal myotube in primary culture.[41] Charge movements could be detected without blocking the calcium currents, because these currents are slowly activating and quite small (consequently, Q_{on} is fairly well resolved, whereas Q_{off} is contaminated by ionic tail current). The Q_{on} charge movement has the expected properties to be causal for the calcium transient, appearing earlier in both voltage and time, and saturating in amplitude, like the transients, for potentials ≥ 30 mV.

Voltage Sensors in Dihydropyridine Receptor Proteins

Based on molecular analyses, it is now well accepted that the charge movements related to excitation-contraction coupling in skeletal muscle arise from the DHPR. The genesis of this idea was the observation that skeletal muscle contains a large density of high-affinity binding sites for dihydropyridines, which are known to block calcium currents (now termed L-type) in both heart and skeletal muscle. Thus, it was an obvious question of why these sites should exist at such high density, given the strong evidence that external calcium (and thus calcium current) is unnecessary for excitation-contraction coupling in skeletal muscle. An additional conundrum was that micromolar concentrations of dihydropyridines were required to block L-type calcium currents, whereas the binding sites displayed nanomolar affinity. In part, this discrepancy could be accounted for by the fact that the effective concentration for block of cardiac calcium current was found to change from micromolar to nanomolar during prolonged depolarization,[42] the condition expected to apply to homogenized muscle membranes.

This issue was reexamined by Schwartz et al.,[43] who concluded that even in intact frog sartorius muscle, there was an excess number of dihydropyridine-binding sites compared to the number of calcium channels. However, as pointed out by Lamb and Walsh,[44] the number of calcium channels was probably underestimated, owing to an assumption of an unrealistically high probability for calcium channel opening during maximal activation. In a subsequent influential report, Rios and Brum[45] proposed that these high-affinity dihydropyridine receptors in frog skeletal muscle provide the molecular basis for the charge movement that couples depolarization to SR calcium release. This proposal was supported by voltage-clamp studies on cut fibers, which showed that nifedipine, a dihydropyridine, inhibits both the total charge moved and SR calcium release in response to depolarizing pulses and that this inhibition is greater at more depolarized holding potentials.

Arguments remained as to whether there were differences between intact and cut fibers and about whether an identical pool of dihydropyridine receptors functions simultaneously as voltage sensors for both excitation-contraction coupling and L-type Ca^{2+} current. The molecular evidence supporting the idea that dihydropyridine receptors do indeed function simultaneously as voltage sensors for both current and excitation-contraction coupling is presented in the following section.

Complexities of Charge Movement

Fibers maintained at approximately normal resting potentials display charge movements over the range of test potentials associated with activation of contraction. However, charge movements also occur over a much more hyperpolarized range of potentials in persistently depolarized fibers (conditions that would cause inactivation of excitation-contraction coupling).[46–48] The charge movements found in polarized fibers were referred to as charge 1 and those in depolarized fibers as charge 2. In 1987, Brum and Rios[49] reported data from cut fibers supporting the idea that charge 2 manifests mobile charge movement of the voltage sensor between inactivated states, while charge 1 manifests the movement of the voltage sensor between resting and active states when the membrane is polarized and the sensors are primed. However, the interconversion of charge 1 and charge 2 was not observed by all workers,[50,51] perhaps due to differences in experimental conditions.

Experiments on polarized and depolarized fibers demonstrated a link between the effects of Ca^{2+} on charge movements and on the inactivation of contraction. Specifically, in the total absence of calcium and other metal cations (with tetraethylammonium and dimethonium ions being replacements), charge movements of the charge-1 type and calcium release disappeared, with a concomitant increase of charge movements of charge-2 type.[31,32] The potency sequence of the metal cations in restoring charge movements and calcium release is quantitatively similar to the selectivity sequence of the intrapore binding sites of L-type Ca^{2+} channels.

Mutating the pore of the DHPR to cause it to lose its selectivity for calcium has little effect on the voltage dependence of charge movements or calcium release,[52] which suggests that binding within the pore is not involved in the effects of calcium on inactivation of excitation-contraction coupling. Measurements of Q_{off} charge movements with this pore-mutant DHPR (facilitated by the near absence of inward ionic tail current) revealed a component of Q_{off} charge with a dependence on time and voltage suggesting that it represented the return movement of a voltage-sensing structure necessary for channel opening. The magnitude of this additional Q_{off} can be most easily explained under the assumption that all DHPRs undergo the conformational change necessary for channel opening.

An interesting feature of charge movement in normally polarized amphibian muscle is that for depolarizations to levels near the contraction threshold, a "hump" appears on the falling phase of the Q_{on} charge movement, even though Q_{on} decays monotonically for weaker and stronger depolarizations. Based on its kinetics, voltage dependence, and sensitivity to specific pharmacologic manipulations,[53-55] the hump component was categorized as functionally separable and was given the term "Q_γ" (or I_γ) to distinguish it from "Q_β" (or I_β), the major (monotonically decaying) component of Q_{on}. Moreover, it was proposed that the Q_γ component is distinct from the Q_β component and is the necessary and sufficient antecedent for SR Ca^{2+} release. However, other investigators proposed an alternative view in which Q_γ is a consequence rather than an antecedent of SR calcium release and is not a distinct component from Q_β. Those favoring the latter point of view found that interventions that have as their primary action the reduction of SR Ca^{2+} release reduce and alter the I_γ component in a way consistent with its being the consequence rather than the cause of SR release.[56] However, other investigators found that similar interventions did not eliminate the I_γ component.[57] Whatever its precise role in amphibian muscle, Q_γ does not appear to be essential for excitation-coupling because a hump component is not present in charge movement in mammalian skeletal muscle.[58]

DEPOLARIZATION-INDUCED CALCIUM TRANSIENTS

Various methods have been devised to measure the rapid ionized Ca^{2+} transients that follow either action potentials or voltage-clamp pulses. Usually, one or sometimes two Ca^{2+} indicators are introduced into the myoplasm and appropriate optical measurements are made to follow the changes in absorption and/or fluorescence—or in some cases luminescence—that occur when the stimulated, increased myoplasmic Ca^{2+} binds to the indicators. From these optical measurements, estimates can be made of the amplitude and time course of ionized Ca^{2+} response to an imposed stimulus, and from that one can calculate the rate of release from the internal stores. In general, the measurements are influenced by many factors, and the calculations depend to some extent on *in vitro* calibrations, so that, at best, some uncertainties remain. A review of the various procedures used has been published by Baylor and Hollingworth.[59]

By themselves and without further analysis, the measured ionized Ca^{2+} transients have provided important and useful information. However, to analyze more fully how depolarization and the charge movements associated with the voltage sensors in the transverse tubular membranes are linked to the rise of ionized Ca^{2+}, a measure of the rate of Ca^{2+} entry into the myoplasm is required. The ionized Ca^{2+} transients do not directly provide the rate of Ca^{2+} entry, since they represent the integral of the difference between the rate of Ca^{2+} entry and the rate of Ca^{2+} removal from the myoplasmic water.

From consideration of conservation, the rate of Ca^{2+} entry is equal to the rate at which ionized Ca^{2+} is changing plus the rate of Ca^{2+} removal by all sequestering systems present. In general, the rate of Ca^{2+} removal will depend on the measured ionized Ca^{2+} transient in the myoplasm. In various studies, different approaches have been taken to estimate the rate of Ca^{2+} removal. One approach, used by Baylor et al.,[60] has been to calculate the rate of removal based on the *in vitro* measured properties of the known sequestering systems at concentrations assumed to be present in the fiber under investigation. Another approach, originally used by Melzer et al.,[61,62] has been to empirically characterize the rate of Ca^{2+} removal from the decay segments of the ionized Ca^{2+} transient after the calcium entry has been turned off. This was done for a series of voltage-clamp pulses of varying amplitude and duration. This empiric Ca^{2+} removal function was then applied to the entire ionized Ca^{2+} transient to calculate the rate of Ca^{2+} entry during the voltage-clamp pulses on the assumption that the Ca^{2+} removal function was independent of the membrane potential. Klein et al.[63] combined elements of the two approaches in an attempt to obtain a more accurate characterization of the Ca^{2+} removal process.

Some comparative magnitudes can be cited to indicate the critical importance of making such calculations. Baylor and Hollingworth[64] estimated that a single action potential in a mouse fast-twitch fiber produced a peak myoplasmic ionized Ca^{2+} concentration of about $18 \times 10^{-6}\ M$, and that this required a total release of about $3.5 \times 10^{-4}\ M\ Ca^{2+}$, produced by a peak rate of SR Ca^{2+} release of about $200 \times 10^{-6}\ M/ms$. Thus about 95 percent of the estimated quantity of total Ca^{2+} entry is composed of the model-based calculation for calcium removal, indicating the overall magnitudes and strengths of the calcium sequestering systems that have to be accounted for in any quantitative study.

In response to single suprathreshold depolarizing pulses lasting a few hundred milliseconds, the estimated rate of calcium release from the SR in both amphibian[61] and mammalian[65] muscle rapidly reaches a peak value and then declines, with a time constant of a few tens of milliseconds, to a lower nearly steady rate; both the peak and final rates increase as the depolarization is increased (Fig. 12-8). The relatively rapid decline from the peak release to the steady rate has been shown to be due to Ca^{2+}-dependent inactivation of the Ca^{2+} release channels in terminal cisternae.[66,67] In cut fiber preparations, half inactivation of the early peak calcium release component is produced when the myoplasmic ionized calcium concentration is about 3×10^{-7} M.[67] Ca^{2+}-dependent inactivation of Ca^{2+} release confirms the proposal by Baylor et al.[60] to explain the finding that the second action potential in a 100-Hz train produces a much smaller peak rate of calcium release.

For suprathreshold depolarizing pulses, the peak rate of calcium release and the total charge moved increase monotonically with increasing internal potentials up to values of +60 mV, at least in cut fibers, as shown in Fig. 12-9.[68] Nevertheless, it is not clear that transverse tubular charge movement is the only factor determining the peak rate of release through RyRs in the terminal cisternae. Over the years, different diffusible substances have been proposed for involvement in the linkage between depolarization and calcium release. The earliest proposed and the most enduring candidate has been Ca^{2+}. Its role has been studied extensively as

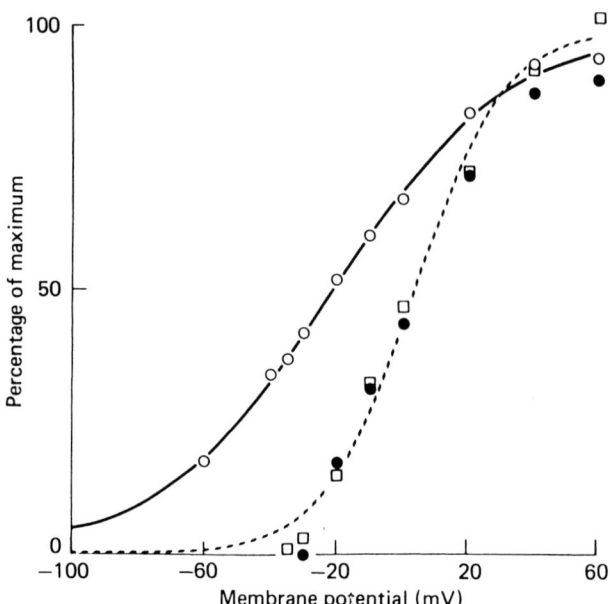

FIGURE 12-9. Comparison of potential dependence of peak rate of calcium release and total intramembranous charge moved. Open circles give Q_{on} versus V plot. Open squares give the peak rate of calcium release versus V plot. Filled circles are $(Q_{on}-Q_{th})/(Q_{max}-Q_{th})$ versus V plot, where Q_{th} is Q_{on} (−35 mV), the amount of charge moved at the threshold potential for calcium release. (*From Schneider and Simon.*[68] *Reproduced by permission.*)

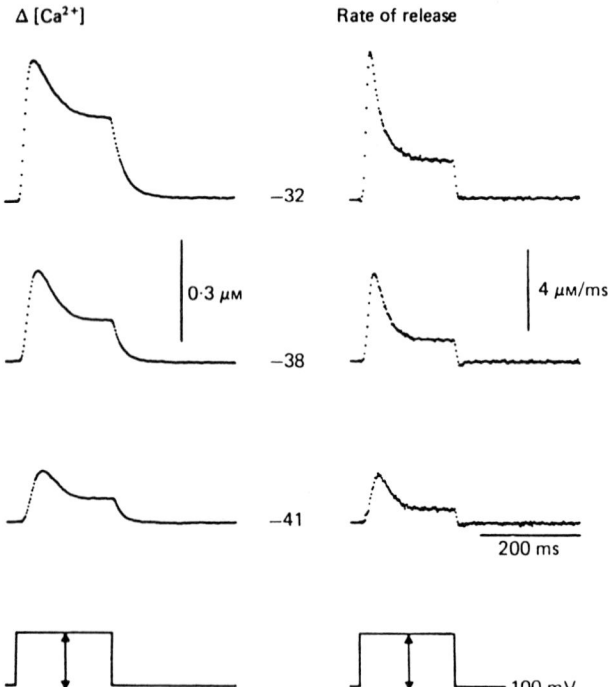

FIGURE 12-8. Time course of the rate of calcium release from SR. Increments in myoplasmic Ca^{2+} concentration in left column and the corresponding calculated rate of calcium release in right column are shown for 200-ms depolarizing steps to indicated potentials (mV) from a holding potential of −100 mV. Rates of release rise to a peak and then decline exponentially to a steady level. Increasing the magnitude of depolarizing pulses increases the magnitude of the rate of calcium release but has little effect on the time course or extent of decline during release. (*From Schneider and Simon.*[66] *Reproduced by permission.*)

Ca^{2+}-induced Ca^{2+} release from the SR in skinned skeletal muscle fibers,[69,70] in vesicles isolated from the SR,[71,72] and with RyRs incorporated into planar lipid bilayers.[73] Nonetheless, the role of Ca^{2+}-induced Ca^{2+} release in normal contractile activation of intact skeletal muscle fibers remains uncertain.

The potential, supplementary contribution of Ca^{2+}-induced Ca^{2+} release to the Ca^{2+} release triggered by depolarization has been debated, on the basis of different experimental findings. In cut fibers, immediately after the injection of millimolar quantities of high-affinity calcium buffers [about 4 mM 1,2-bis[o-aminophenoxy]ethane-N,N,N′,N′-tetraacetic acid (BAPTA) or 2.5 mM fura-2], the usual early peak component of Ca^{2+} release was selectively eliminated.[74] The authors thus concluded that calcium leaving the SR via Ca^{2+}-induced Ca^{2+} release generates the early peak component of the release waveform. By contrast, with intact fibers, when fura-2 is injected to concentrations between 1 and 3 mM, the rate of calcium release from the SR in response to action potentials was increased rather than decreased.[75,76] An increased calcium release in heavily calcium-buffered fibers can be explained by reduction of Ca^{2+}-dependent inactivation of Ca^{2+} release, since the injected Ca^{2+} buffer markedly reduces the myoplasmic ionized calcium concentrations during the stimulated calcium transient.[75] The reasons for these contradictory results are not apparent. Since the rate of calcium release is generally considerably higher for intact fibers compared with cut fibers, one possibility is that local reductions in calcium concentrations by the same concentrations of high-affinity buffers may not be as severe for intact fibers as for cut fibers.

Differences in cytoplasmic factors between the two types of preparation may also be involved.

Localized Calcium Release Events

Over the years, many laboratories have demonstrated that calcium influx from the extracellular space does not contribute directly to the activation of contraction in skeletal muscle.[8,9,77]

Consequently, calcium release from the SR must serve as the source for depolarization-induced myoplasmic calcium transients, and this release must be initiated by events at the terminal cisternae (see Chaps. 11 and 14). The advent of laser confocal microscopy has made it possible to examine the localization and timing of the calcium release process. Of particular importance was the observation in cardiac muscle of localized calcium release events of stereotyped waveform, termed sparks.[78] To measure sparks, the laser beam is scanned repeatedly along a single line or a small area within a muscle cell loaded with a calcium indicator and exposed to conditions (e.g., caffeine, weak depolarization) that cause a small increase in the globally averaged myoplasmic calcium. As the stimulus is made stronger, the rate of occurrence of the sparks increases but the time course of individual sparks is not greatly altered, leading to the idea that summed, quantal release events underlie the global Ca^{2+} transient. Despite this general consensus, there is still no agreement as to how many RyRs contribute to a spark: Owing to large variations in the estimated underlying flux (from about 1.4 up to 30 pA), anywhere from one or two up to as many as sixty RyRs might be involved.[79]

Shortly after being demonstrated in cardiac muscle, similar sparks were observed in response to depolarization of amphibian skeletal muscle.[80,81] Quantal events that are evoked by depolarization and are of sufficient amplitude to be well resolved have not yet been reported for mammalian muscle with an intact surface membrane, although sparks have been described in skinned or permeabilized mammalian fibers.[82,83] Possibly accounting for this difference is that mammalian muscle predominantly expresses only one RyR isoform (RyR1), whereas amphibian muscle expresses approximately equal levels of isoforms homologous to both RyR1 and RyR3.[84]

One important feature of sparks is that they appear to arise nearly exclusively in the vicinity of triads, as is illustrated in Fig. 12-10 for an intact fiber depolarized by a modest ele-

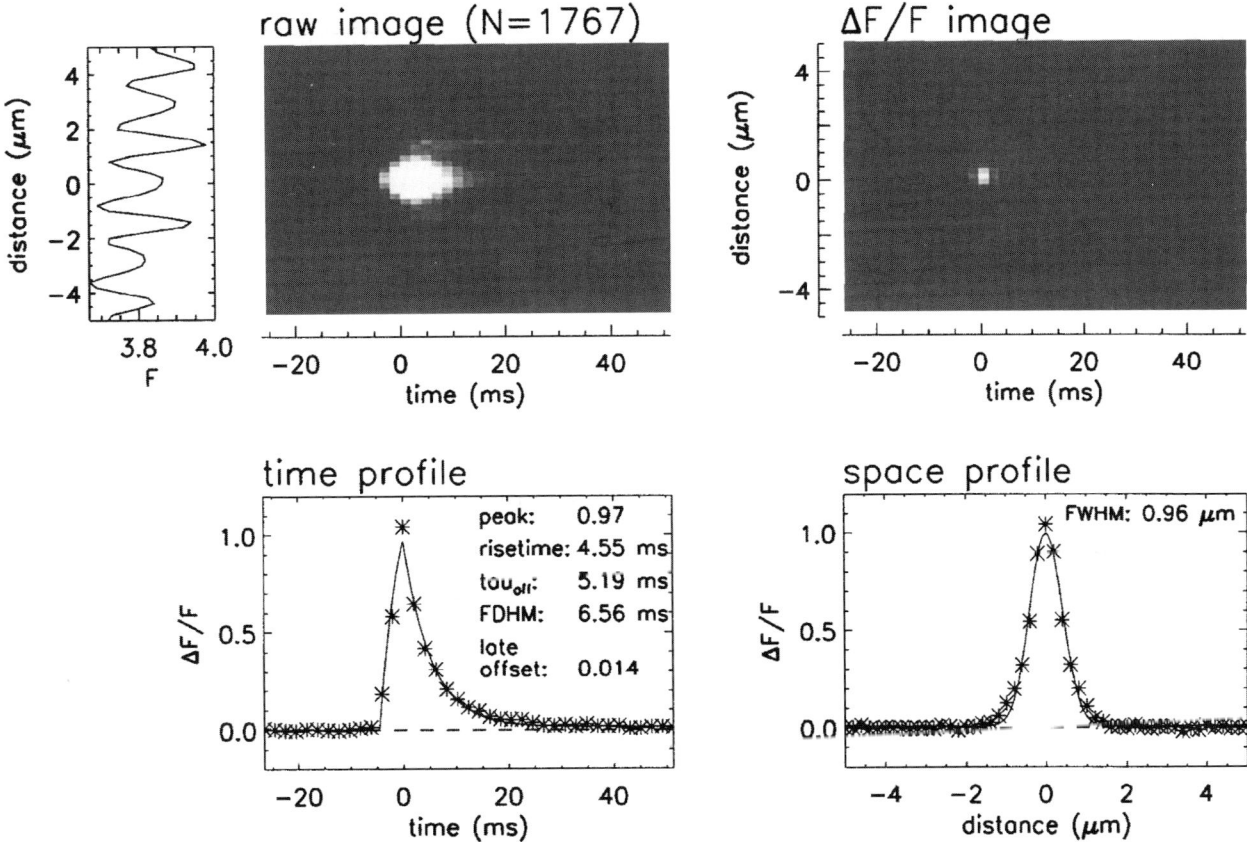

FIGURE 12-10. Averaged image of sparks obtained from a frog intact skeletal muscle fiber depolarized by 13 mM K$^+$. The laser line was repeatedly scanned along a 10.2-μm line parallel to the fiber axis (shown vertically), with successive scans arrayed horizontally. In addition to the averaged spark, the raw image displays alternating thin and thick stripes, with the thick stripes corresponding to Z lines where triads are located in amphibian muscle. The $\Delta F/F$ image emphasizes that the averaged spark in an intact fiber is restricted both spatially and temporally. Based on a model of calcium binding and diffusion, this average spark would result from a current of 2.5 pA flowing for 4.6 ms. (Modified from Hollingworth et al.[85] Reproduced by permission.)

vation of external potassium.[85] This behavior provides confirmation (with much better spatial resolution) of experiments carried out in the late fifties and early sixties on contractile responses to local stimulation.[86] The restricted generation of sparks at triads suggests that the terminal cisternae of the SR are the sole source of calcium release for excitation-contraction coupling, although it has also been argued that an action potential triggers some Ca^{2+} release from a region broader than the T-tubule/SR junction.[87] There is also some uncertainty about the exact shape of sparks in skeletal muscle. In cut fibers, sparks have been described as riding on much longer duration (~100 ms) lower-amplitude events (ridge and ember), which was interpreted to mean that long openings of a few RyRs under the control of voltage (via DHPRs) could lead to the concerted opening of a larger number of RyRs (via Ca^{2+}-induced Ca^{2+} release).[88] However, embers are not evident in intact muscle fibers, where sparks also tend to be much smaller and narrower than in cut or permeabilized fibers.[85]

Measurements of sparks by Klein et al.[89] have provided independent support for the time course of calcium release that had been deduced from globally averaged calcium. Because individual sparks cannot be resolved for other than very weak depolarizations applied from a negative holding potential, the approach taken was to briefly repolarize fibers that were maintained at a depolarized level. This prolonged depolarization caused most of the voltage sensors to enter the inactivated state for excitation-contraction coupling, and the brief repolarization caused a small fraction of these sensors to be reprimed and available to trigger calcium release during a subsequent depolarization to any desired level. Increasing the amplitude of this depolarization caused an increase in the overall spark frequency and a pronounced increase in the clustering of sparks near the onset of the depolarization. Thus, the time course of the probability of spark occurrence agrees well with release waveforms like those illustrated in Fig. 12-8.

Molecular Basis of Excitation-Contraction Coupling

STRUCTURE OF DHPRs AND RyRs

Because excitation-contraction coupling is initiated by an electrical change, the action potential, this process must necessarily involve voltage-sensing structures in the plasma membrane. This idea was first clearly enunciated by Schneider and Chandler,[23] who proposed that the initiation of excitation-contraction coupling involved depolarization-induced conformational changes of these voltage-sensing structures. A priori, voltage-gated ion channels would seem well suited for such a role and, indeed, it is now well accepted that the L-type Ca^{2+} channel, or dihydropyridine receptor, serves this function in skeletal muscle (see Chap. 14). The dihydropyridine receptor is composed of the essential α_{1S} (CaV1.1) subunit and the auxiliary α_2-δ, β, and γ subunits (Fig. 12-11).[90] The gating machinery and ion pore reside within the α_{1S} subunit, which, like other calcium channel α subunits, is a polypeptide having four homologous repeats (I, II, III, and IV) arranged such that the amino and carboxyl terminals as well as the interdomain loops are located in the cytoplasm and such that four repeats are pseudosymmetrically arrayed around a central ion-conducting pore. This subunit is essential for function, since excitation-contraction coupling is absent in mice homozygous for a null mutation of the α_{1S} gene (muscular dysgenesis, mdg).[91] Each of the four repeats of α_{1S} contains six transmembrane α helices (S1 through S6). Conformational changes of the protein (e.g., gating of the ion pore) in response to changes of membrane potential are initiated by the S4 segments, which contain lysine or arginine at every third position. The S5 and S6 segments and their linker of each of the four repeats contribute to the formation of the ion-conducting pore, which can be gated open to allow extracellular Ca^{2+} to enter the myoplasm.

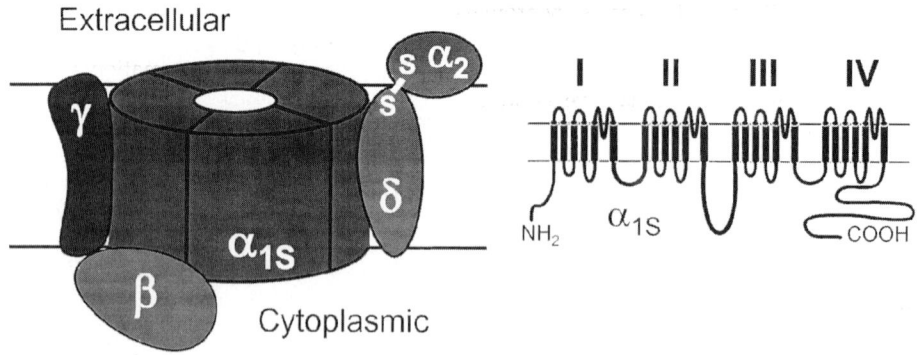

FIGURE 12-11. Subunit composition of the dihydropyridine receptor in skeletal muscle. Except for the general folding topology of the α_{1S} subunit and the fact that the β subunit binds to the I–II cytoplasmic domain of α_{1S}, precise information is lacking about the three-dimensional structure of the protein. Within α_{1S}, the fourth membrane-spanning segment (termed S4) within each of the homology repeats (I through IV) contains positively charged arginine or lysine at every third position. The S4 segments serve as the voltage-sensing structures that initiate conformational changes responsible for excitation-contraction coupling.

The β subunit is entirely cytoplasmic and interacts with the I–II loop of the α_1 subunit. In addition to affecting the gating properties of the assembled channel, the β subunit is essential for effective trafficking of the channel to the plasma membrane. Consequently, excitation-contraction coupling is absent in mice null for the gene encoding the isoform of β (β1) expressed in skeletal muscle.[92] The α_2-δ subunit consists of two disulfide-linked polypeptides, one of which (δ) is thought to span the membrane and the other of which (α_2) is entirely extracellular. The α_2 and δ peptides arise by post-translational cleavage of a single polypeptide. Based on studies of heterologously expressed Ca^{2+} channels, it appears as if the α_2-δ subunit influences the level of expression without much effect on function. The γ subunit, which is predicted to have four membrane-spanning α helices, does not appear to play a major role, since only minor functional alterations occur as a consequence of knocking out the gene encoding the γ subunit in skeletal muscle of mice.[93]

Conformational changes of the DHPR control the intracellular release of Ca^{2+} via RyRs[94] located in the sarcoplasmic reticulum. RyRs are currently known to be encoded by three different genes (RyR1, RyR2, and RyR3)[95–98] and are homotetramers having a mass of $\sim 2 \times 10^6$ D. In addition to RyR1, RyR3 is also present to varying degrees, depending on the muscle in question and the stage of development. However, knockout of RyR1,[99] but not of RyR3,[100] abolishes excitation-contraction coupling, indicating that only RyR1 is essential for this function. In addition, there are no skeletal muscles having only RyR3, whereas there are some having only RyR1.[101] Although the general morphology of the RyRs has been determined from single-particle cryoelectronmicroscopy,[102,103] the folding topology of the monomers is not well known at the current time, except that at the amino terminal, about nine-tenths of each of the four monomers contributes to the "foot" structure visible in thin-section electron micrographs (see Chap. 11) and, at the carboxyl terminal, about one-tenth contributes to the formation of the pore. In mammalian skeletal muscle, RyR1 is the predominantly expressed RyR isoform. Upon purification, it is found to be stoichiometrically associated with the immunophilin-binding protein, FKBP12 (four FKBP12s per RyR).[104] Thus FKBP12 can be considered a subunit, particularly since it stabilizes the full gating transitions. Other accessory proteins of likely importance are calmodulin and homer. Calmodulin has been shown to bind both to RyR1 and to α_{1S} and has been shown to have pronounced functional effects on isolated RyRs; however, its physiologic function *in vivo* remains uncertain.[105,106] Homer, which exists in both short and long forms (the latter of which can dimerize by coiled-coil interactions), has two consensus binding sites (PPXXY) in RyR1 as well as a binding site in the carboxyl terminal of α_{1S} and has pronounced effects on the function of RyR1 reconstituted into planar lipid bilayers.[107] However, the role of homer in vivo remains unknown.

Additional Protein Components of Triad Junctions

In addition to RyR1 and the skeletal DHPR, a number of other proteins have been identified as components of triad junctions (Fig. 12-12). Several of these proteins appear to function together to increase the Ca^{2+} storage capacity within the terminal cisternae adjacent to RyRs. Within the lumen of the SR terminal cisternae, calsequestrin serves as a moderate-affinity (k_D of ~ 1 mM), high-capacity calcium buffer.[108,109] Triadin[110,111] and junctin[112,113] are two integral membrane proteins that are localized to the junctional SR and have been shown to form a complex with calsequestrin and the RyR.[113,114] Based on primary sequence, both triadin[115] and junctin[112] are predicted to have a short amino terminal located in the cytoplasm, a single membrane-spanning segment, and a long, carboxyl-terminal portion located in the lumen of the SR. This carboxyl-terminal domain is much more extensive for triadin (with a mass of 95 kDa for the major isoform) than for junctin (which has a mass of 26 kDa). The topology predicted for triadin on the basis of primary sequence is supported by protease analysis[115] and by peptide-directed antibodies.[116] However, data have also appeared that support an alternative topology in which a substantial portion of the carboxyl-terminal domain is cytoplasmic and interacts with the DHPR.[117] This topology is consistent with the hypothesis that triadin participates in the functional coupling between the DHPR and RyR1.[118] In addition to the 95-kDa isoform of triadin, a 51-kDa isoform has also been identified in skeletal muscle[119] and three other isoforms of triadin have been found in cardiac muscle.[120] All the identified triadin isoforms are conserved in the amino-terminal region but differ in their carboxyl-terminal domains.

Interestingly, junctin arises by alternative splicing of the gene that encodes aspartyl β-hydroxylase, which is also alternatively spliced to produce a third protein, junctate.[121] Junctate (33 kDa) contains the first 78 amino-terminal residues of junctin fused to aspartyl β-hydroxylase. The carboxyl-terminal domain has a high content of acidic residues, is predicted to have a luminal location, and is able to bind ~ 20 Ca^{2+} ions with a k_D of ~ 200 μM. Thus, in addition to calsequestrin, junctate may function as a Ca^{2+} buffer within the lumen of the SR.

It is quite evident that excitation-contraction coupling depends upon the formation of stable junctions between the SR and plasma membrane. Significantly, such junctions are still formed in skeletal muscle cells null for both dihydropyridine receptors and RyRs.[122] Thus, it is necessary to suppose that proteins other than DHPRs and RyRs must be involved in the formation of junctions. Two proteins that might serve this sort of function are mitsugumin29 and junctophilin.[123,124] Both proteins were identified and cloned by producing large numbers of monoclonal antibodies against triad preparations, followed by screening to determine which antibodies interacted with proteins that were both restricted to triads and abundant there. Based on hydropathy, mitsugumin29 (29 kDa, as implied by its name) is predicted to have four membrane-spanning segments with both the amino and carboxyl terminals located in the cytoplasm (i.e., projecting towards the T tubules). Its expression is largely restricted to skeletal muscle and kidney. Mitsugumin29 is related in both primary sequence and general structural features to the synaptophysin family of proteins. Synaptophysin is present in synaptic vesicles and is postulated to be involved in the biogenesis of vesicles

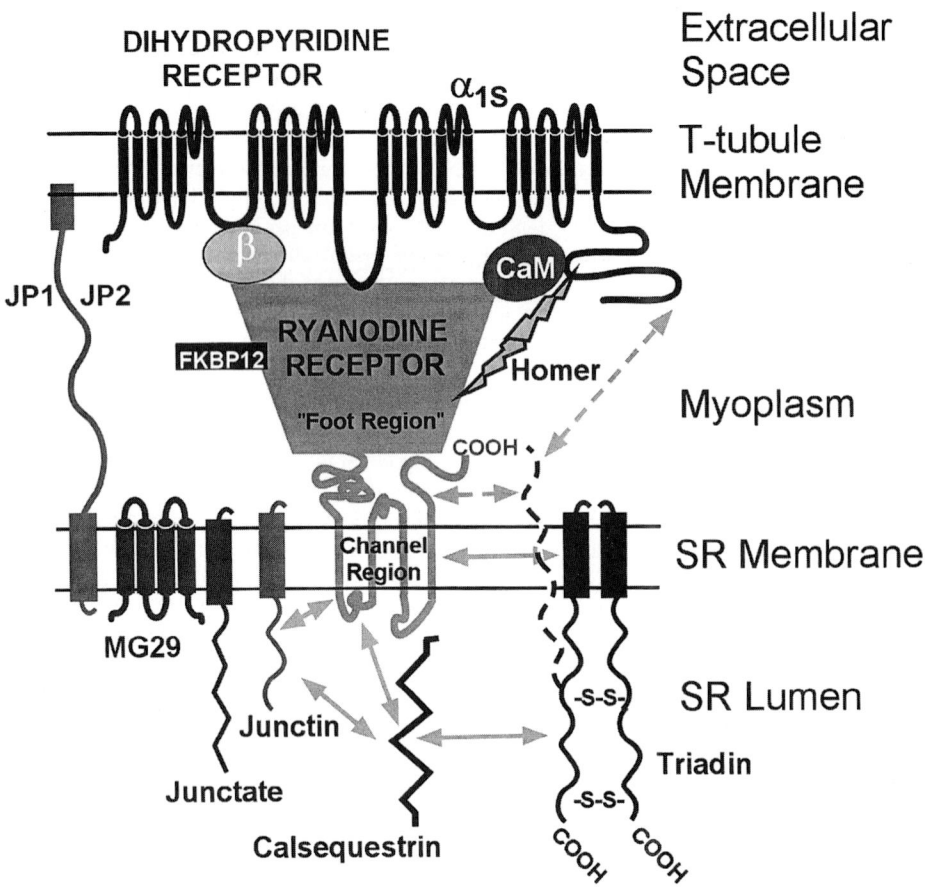

FIGURE 12-12. Schematic diagram of important protein components of the triad junction. Proposed protein-protein interactions are indicated either by direct contact or by double-headed arrows. For simplicity, only the α_{1S} and β subunits are shown for the dihydropyridine receptor. The channel region of the ryanodine receptor is indicated by four transmembrane segments, which is one of the proposed topologies for each monomer of the RyR tetramer. Two of the proposed alternatives have been illustrated for the carboxyl terminal of triadin.

and in their Ca^{2+}-dependent release. Supporting the idea that mitsugumin29 is involved in the formation of junctions, mitsugumin29 knockout mice display ultrastructual alterations of triad junctions and some changes in muscle function.[125] However, the mice are overall quite healthy, indicating that mitsugumin29 is not essential for excitation-contraction coupling.

A more essential role appears to be played by junctophilin, which is currently known to have three isoforms (JP-1, JP-2, and JP-3), all having a mass of ~70 kDa. Junctophilin has a short, hydrophobic carboxyl-terminal domain, which would allow it to be inserted into the ER/SR membrane, and a large cytoplasmic domain containing eight 14-residue "MORN" (membrane occupation and recognition nexus) motifs. Thus, the structure of junctophilin is well suited for the role of providing a physical link between the SR and plasma membrane at triad junctions. Based on mRNA levels, JP-1 and somewhat less JP-2 are expressed in skeletal muscle, whereas cardiac muscle expresses JP-2 at a severalfold higher level than JP-1. JP-3 is mainly found in brain and testis. Knockout of JP-2 resulted in irregular, weak heartbeats and greatly altered morphology of junctional membrane structures in the embryonic heart, with the animals dying by embryonic day 11.5, which is too early to determine whether there are also effects in skeletal muscle.[124] In newborn animals, knockout of JP-1 resulted in a reduced number of triad junctions in all skeletal muscles examined (tongue, jaw, diaphragm, and thigh) as well as a large reduction of dyads in jaw muscles.[126] Moreover, an inability to suckle led to death of these knockout mice shortly after birth, and hindlimb muscles showed altered force generation. These results, together with the observation that JP-1 expression increases postnatally, suggest that JP-1 may be more effective than JP-2 in promoting the formation of triad junctions.

IDENTIFYING DOMAINS OF DHPRs AND RyRs IMPORTANT FOR EXCITATION-CONTRACTION COUPLING

It is almost universally accepted that DHPRs in the T-tubular membrane function as voltage sensors for excitation-contraction coupling, that RyRs in the SR membrane serve as calcium release channels, and that calcium release in response to excitation involves conformational coupling between these two proteins. The idea that DHPRs function as voltage sensors for excitation-contraction coupling was first advanced on the basis of the finding that dihydropyridines could inhibit both voltage-dependent charge movements and depolarization-induced calcium release.[45] Moreover, the arrangement of DHPRs as tetrads in precise register with the four subunits of RyRs (see Chap. 11) provides even more direct evidence of protein-protein links between DHPRs and RyRs. Nonetheless, the identity of these protein-protein links, or even whether they are direct or involve intervening proteins, has not been fully established, despite a large number of studies. These studies have employed various methodologies, each with advantages and limitations, which will be briefly indicated before discussing the results of specific experiments. One approach has been to measure contractions, intracellular Ca^{2+} transients, and membrane currents in cultured myotubes that are derived from wild-type mice or from mice genetically null either for RyR1 (dyspedic mice) or for the α_{1S} (dysgenic mice) or $\beta 1$ ($\beta 1$ knockout) subunits of the DHPR. The expression of cDNAs encoding RyRs or the subunits of the DHPR in these myotubes allows one to analyze the consequences of altering primary amino acid sequence within each of these proteins. A major advantage of this approach is that it provides a physiologically relevant test of the importance of specific regions of primary sequence. A major disadvantage of chimeras is that they do not provide a direct method of distinguishing between several alternatives for why a region might be important for excitation-contraction coupling. For example, the region might be a site of intermolecular contact (e.g., between DHPRs and RyRs) or it might influence the ability of other regions of the protein to participate in intermolecular contacts.

A second approach has been to examine whether the function of purified RyR1 is affected by the application of peptides corresponding to specific regions of α_{1S}. If effects are observed, it implies that the peptides (and perhaps the corresponding regions of α_{1S}) interact with RyR1. However, this approach also has some significant weaknesses, including the absence of clear criteria for whether the state of the isolated RyR1 corresponds to that in vivo, whether the peptides assume conformations similar to those of intact α_{1S}, and whether peptides act at sites of the RyR inaccessible to α_{1S} within intact cells. In addition to the just described functional assays, potential interactions between DHPRs and RyRs have also been assayed by means of biochemical methods. Although these biochemical measurements share some of the weaknesses of the peptide experiments, they have the advantage that they can potentially identify "inert" intermolecular binding sites in addition to those that may be involved in "active" signal transmission between two proteins. Additionally, strong in vitro binding may be less subject to artifacts than effects of peptides on function of isolated RyRs.

As mentioned earlier, excitation-contraction coupling fails in muscle cells genetically null for α_{1S}, β_1, or RyR1. Moreover, voltage-dependent membrane charge movement is greatly reduced and slowly activated L-type Ca^{2+} is absent in dysgenic (null for α_{1S})[91,127] and β_1-null myotubes,[91,92,127] which is not surprising given that both subunits are necessary for surface expression of functional DHPRs. The residual charge movement in dysgenic and β_1-null myotubes appears to reflect the presence of voltage-gated sodium channels and T-type Ca^{2+} channels, since a substantial fraction of this charge is immobilized by pulse protocols that inactivate these channels. By contrast, the bulk of charge movement in normal myotubes is "immobilization-resistant." Expression of cDNA encoding β_{1a} in β_1-null myotubes or α_{1S} in dysgenic myotubes restores skeletal-type excitation-contraction coupling (Ca^{2+}-entry independent), slowly activated L-type Ca^{2+} current, and immobolization-resistant charge movement.[92,127] These results strongly support the hypothesis that the DHPR in skeletal muscle serves as the voltage sensor for excitation-contraction coupling and is responsible for the generation of voltage-dependent charge movement and slow L-type Ca^{2+} current.

Importantly, expression of α_{1C} (the cardiac isoform of the α_1 subunit) in dysgenic myotubes results in the appearance of large (rapidly activated) L-type Ca^{2+} currents and excitation-contraction coupling that is cardiac-type (dependent on Ca^{2+} entry).[128] This result demonstrates that RyR1 can be activated by Ca^{2+} entry under the appropriate conditions, even though this mechanism may not be important in vivo. Additionally, it has provided the basis for a series of experiments utilizing α_{1S}/α_{1C} chimeras in an attempt to identify regions of α_{1S} important for skeletal-type excitation-contraction coupling.

Rather surprisingly, the magnitude of L-type Ca^{2+} currents is greatly reduced in dyspedic myotubes null for RyR1, despite the presence of near normal levels of immobilization-resistant charge movement, an indirect indication (see above) that the surface expression of DHPRs is near normal.[129] Furthermore, expression in dyspedic myotubes of cDNA encoding RyR1 restores both depolarization-induced Ca^{2+} release and the magnitude of Ca^{2+} current. On this basis, it has been postulated that there is bidirectional, functional coupling between DHPRs and RyRs in skeletal muscle: orthograde signaling responsible for excitation-contraction coupling and retrograde signaling responsible for regulating the ability of DHPRs to function as calcium channels (Fig. 12-13). Expression of RyR2 (the cardiac RyR isoform) in dyspedic myotubes fails to restore either excitation-contraction coupling or slowly activating L-type Ca^{2+} current.[130] On this basis, chimeras of RyR1 and RyR2 have been used to identify regions important for bidirectional signaling (see below).

The Alphacentric View of Excitation-Contraction Coupling

The well-defined transmembrane topology of α_1 subunits (Fig. 12-11) greatly facilitated the relatively rational design of α_{1S}/α_{1C} chimeras. In particular, the large cytoplasmic domains (which would be expected to project toward RyRs in the SR) were likely candidates to be important for excitation-contraction coupling. Thus, chimeras were constructed in which the amino-terminal domain, the carboxyl-terminal domain, and the I–II, II–III, and III–IV loops of α_{1C} were replaced singly or in combination by the corresponding region of α_{1S}.[131] These chimeras were expressed in dysgenic myotubes, followed by whole-cell clamping to measure intracellular Ca^{2+} transients in both the presence and absence of extracellular Ca^{2+}. As shown in Fig. 12-14, the replacement of only the II–III loop of α_{1C} by the II–III loop of α_{1S} was sufficient to produce a chimera (CSk3) that supported skeletal-type excitation-contraction coupling. This is evidenced by a large intracellular Ca^{2+} transient in response to depolarization in the absence of extracellular Ca^{2+}, whereas the purely cardiac construct was able to support a Ca^{2+} transient only in the presence of external

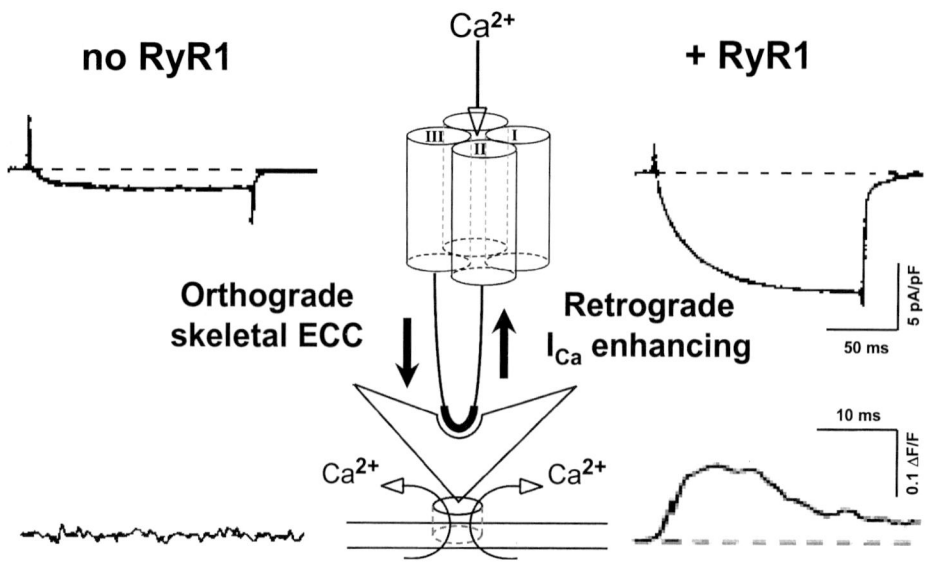

FIGURE 12-13. Calcium currents and calcium transients measured with the whole-cell technique from a dyspedic (no RyR1) myotube and from a dyspedic myotube expressing RyR1 cDNA. Because RyR1 is absent, depolarization does not elicit intracellular calcium release (lower trace) in the dyspedic myotube. Additionally, even though the DHPR (indicated by the four cylinders) is present, depolarization elicits only a small calcium current (upper trace). In the RyR1-expressing myotube, depolarization elicits both calcium release and a large calcium current. On this basis it was proposed that there is both orthograde (excitation-contraction) coupling and retrograde (enhancing DHPR calcium current) coupling between the DHPR and RyR1. Test potential of 30 mV for all traces. (*Modified from Nakai et al.[125] Reproduced by permission.*)

Ca^{2+}. In fact, chimera CSk53, which contained only 46 residues of the α_{1S} II–III loop (the "critical domain"), was able to support robust skeletal-type excitation-contraction coupling, and weak skeletal coupling was supported by chimera CSk58, which contained only 18 skeletal residues (the "minidomain").[132]

The importance of the II–III loop for excitation-contraction coupling, as well as for retrograde signaling, was demonstrated by the chimera SkLC (skeletal-loop-cardiac), which is a kind of inverse of CSk3 in which the II–III loop of α_{1S} has been replaced by that of α_{1C}.[133] In myotubes expressing SkLC, immobilization-resistant charge move-

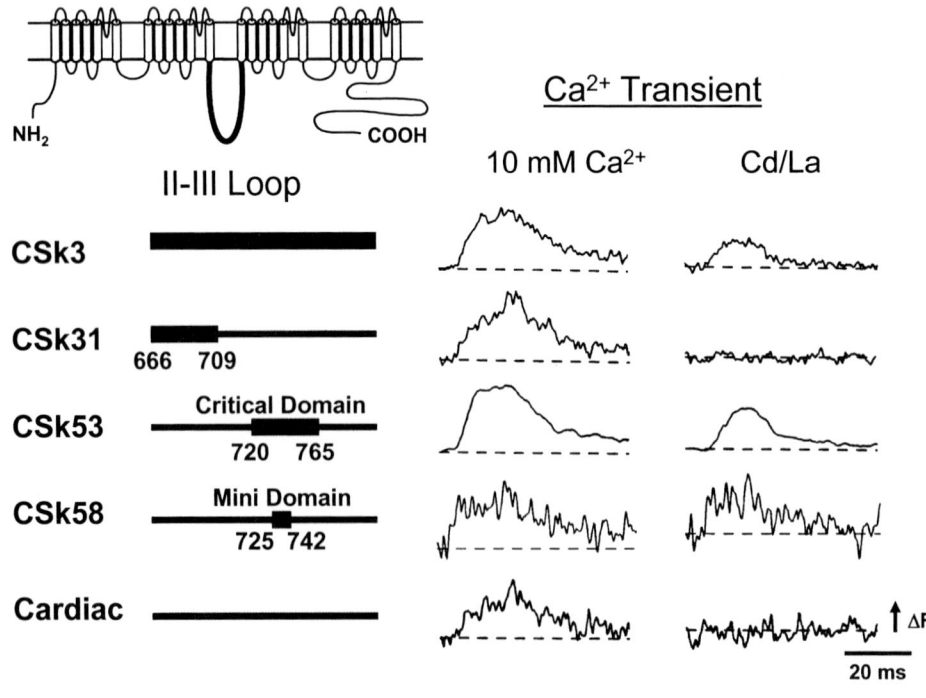

FIGURE 12-14. Identification of a domain within the II–III loop of α_{1S} that is critical for excitation-contraction coupling. cDNAs encoding either the purely cardiac α_1 subunit (α_{1C}) or α_{1C} with all (CSk3) or part of the II–III loop replaced by skeletal (α_{1S}) sequence were expressed in dysgenic myotubes, followed by whole-cell measurements of currents and calcium transients. Thin and thick lines represent cardiac and skeletal sequences, respectively, with the residue numbers indicated for inserted skeletal sequence. Skeletal coupling was strong for CSk3 and CSk53 (all cells gave a measurable transient in Cd/La) and weak for CSk58 (only 25 percent gave a measurable transient in Cd/La). Test potentials were 15 ms to 40 mV (Cardiac, CSk3), 70 mV (CSk53), or 90 mV (CSk58); Cd/La solution contained 2 mM Ca^{2+}, 8 mM Mg^{2+}, 0.5 mM Cd^{2+}, and 0.1 mM La^{3+}. (*Modified from Nakai et al.[132] Reproduced by permission.*)

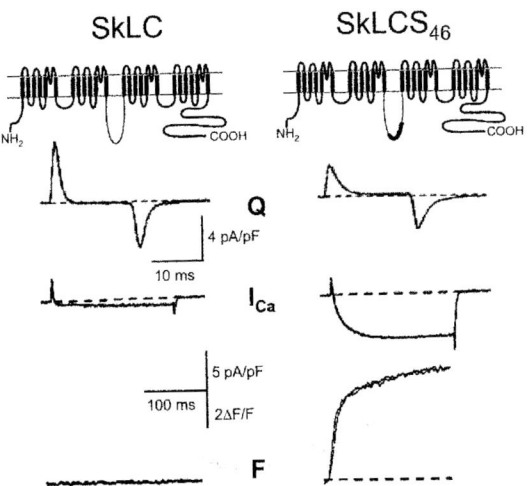

FIGURE 12-15. Charge movements (Q), Ca^{2+} ionic currents (I_{Ca}), and intracellular Ca^{2+} transients (F) in dysgenic myotubes expressing either full-length α_{1S} with the II–III loop replaced by the α_{1C} loop (left: SkLC), or SkLC in which part of the α_{1C} loop was replaced by the critical domain (residues 720–765) of the α_{1S} loop (right: SkLCS46). Test potential was 40 mV (Q), 30 mV (I_{Ca}), or 30 and 80 mV (F, two traces superimposed). Note that the presence of the α_{1C} II–III loop caused SkLC to be uncoupled from RyR1. Thus SkLC behaves in a dysgenic myotube much like α_{1S} in a dyspedic (RyR1-lacking) myotube: Depolarization causes only a small calcium current and fails to elicit calcium release. (Modified from from Grabner et al.[133] Reproduced by permission.)

ment was similar in magnitude to that of the wild-type α_{1S}, whereas L-type Ca^{2+} current was of much reduced amplitude and depolarization-induced Ca^{2+} release was absent (Fig. 12-15). Function like that of wild-type α_{1S} was restored when the 46-residue "critical domain" of the α_{1S} II–III loop was substituted for the corresponding cardiac segment within SkLC (producing the construct labeled "SkLCS46" in Fig. 12-15).

Taken together, the results just described are consistent with the hypothesis that the II–III loop, the critical domain in particular, is a site at which the α_{1S} subunit of the DHPR contacts RyR1 and which serves to control the gating of RyR1 in response to potential across the T-tubular membrane. However, such chimeras would be unable to identify other α_{1S} regions of potential importance if those regions were sufficiently conserved between α_{1S} and α_{1C} to be interchangeable. A specific version of this hypothesis would be to suppose that residues within the critical domain influence the ability of other regions of the DHPR to interact with RyR1. Some support for this idea is provided by results obtained with β-subunit chimeras and α_{1S} constructs bearing deletions of the critical domain; these results are described in the section entitled "The Betacentric View of Excitation-Contraction Coupling."

Application of Peptide Fragments to Isolated RyRs

Based in part on the results obtained in the chimera experiments, a number of laboratories have carried out experiments to determine whether the entire II–III loop or portions thereof activate or inhibit RyR1, as determined by Ca^{2+} fluxes from RyR-containing SR vesicles, by ryanodine binding (as an indirect indication of channel opening), and by single-channel activity after reconstitution in artificial planar lipid bilayers. Figure 12-16 summarizes a number of experiments examining the effects of II–III loop peptides on isolated RyRs. In the earliest work, which examined the effect of the full-length loop produced as a fusion protein, it was found that II–III loops from both α_{1S} and α_{1C} were able to increase ryanodine binding and to activate channels reconstituted into bilayers.[134] Similar activation could also be produced by the amino-terminal half (residues 666–726) of the α_{1S} loop.[135] Although not satisfyingly congruent with the chimera experiments, these results may indicate that in isolation from the rest of the channel, the amino terminal half of both the α_{1C} and α_{1S} II–III loops can assume a structure sufficiently similar to cause activation of RyR1. One group did indeed find activation of RyR1 by peptides corresponding to both the amino-terminal portion of the skeletal II–III loop

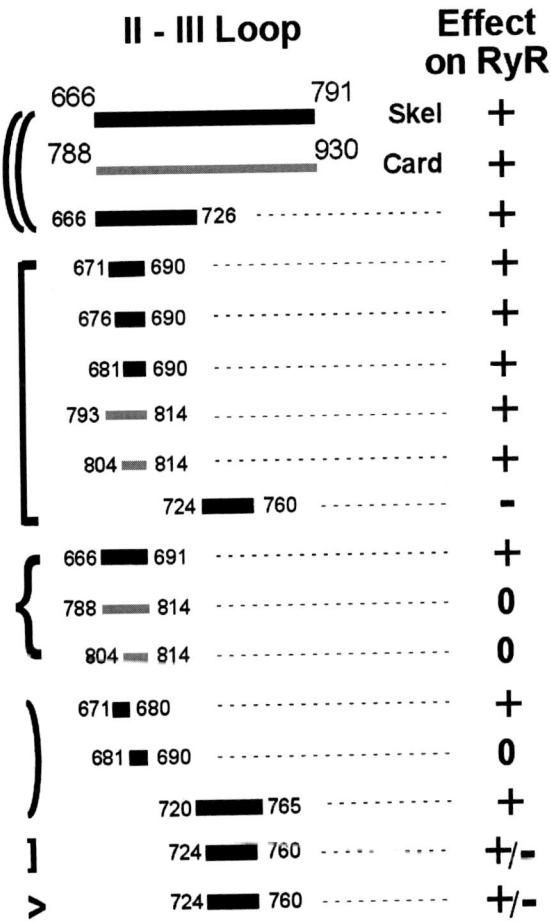

FIGURE 12-16. Effects of II–III loop peptides on ryanodine receptor function, where +, –, and 0 indicate activation, inhibition, or no effect, respectively. The experiments are presented in roughly chronological order: ((Lu et al., 1994, 1995)),[134,135] [El Hayek et al., 1995, 1998; Saiki et al., 1999],[136,137,143] {Gurrola et al., 1999; Zhu et al., 1999},[138,139])Stange et al., 2001(,[144]]Yamamoto et al., 2002[,[145] >Haarman et al., 2003<.[146] The α_{1S} residues 671–690 are frequently referred to as "peptide A" and residues 724–760 as "peptide C."

(e.g., residues 671–690, termed "peptide A") and the amino-terminal portion of the cardiac II–III loop,[136,137] whereas a second group found activation by skeletal but not by cardiac peptides.[138,139] Not only are these results contradictory, but subsequent studies showed that skeletal-type excitation-contraction coupling could be restored in dysgenic myotubes by α_{1S} constructs in which the sequence within the peptide-A region was scrambled, replaced by nonrelated sequence, or deleted entirely.[140–142] Thus, the peptide-A region seems unlikely to play a critical role in excitation-contraction coupling.

In contrast to the activation shown for skeletal peptides corresponding to the amino half of the II–III loop, downstream peptides were found in the earliest studies either to have no effect or to be inhibitory to activation by peptide A.[136,137,143] One of these downstream peptides (residues 724–760, peptide C) corresponds to a portion of the loop contained in the critical domain (residues 720–765), which was found in the chimera experiments (Figs. 12-13 and 12-14) to be important for both excitation-contraction coupling and retrograde signaling. However, subsequent experiments revealed rather different effects of peptides corresponding not only to the peptide-C region but also to the upstream region, which includes peptide A. In particular, these studies revealed that a peptide comprising residues 720–765 caused activation of the skeletal RyR with a cytoplasmic Ca^{2+} concentration of 1 μM,[144] as did a peptide comprising residues 724–760 at a cytoplasmic Ca^{2+} concentration of ≤ 0.03 μM.[145] Haarmann et al.[146] also found activation by the 724–760 peptide. However, a number of discrepancies remain. As one example, the latter group found that the 724–760 peptide was inhibitory for Ca^{2+} of 1 μM, which appears to be at odds with the results of Stange et al.[144] One could imagine that the disparity of results with applied peptides reflects, at least in part, variability in the RyR itself (e.g., phosphorylation state) and variability in the presence of associated proteins. In any event, the peptide experiments have not yet produced a clear picture of the possible function of regions within the II–III loop of α_{1S}.

Domains of RyR1 Important for Excitation-Contraction Coupling

Because expression of RyR1 in dyspedic myotubes (null for endogenous RyR1) restores bidirectional signaling with the DHPR whereas expression of RyR2 does not,[130] chimeras of RyR1 and RyR2 have been used in an attempt to identify regions of RyR1 important for this signaling. An important limitation of this approach is that whereas a relatively well accepted domain structure provides a rational basis for the design of α_1 chimeras, there is no well-defined domain structure for RyRs. About all that can be said is that the pore-forming region of RyRs lies in approximately the carboxyl-most tenth of the protein and that the bulk of the protein forms the cytoplasmically located foot structure visible in thin-section electron microscopy. Additionally, there are regions of high divergence between RyR1 and RyR2, which provide some assistance in the design of chimeras. Despite these limitations, the expression in dyspedic myotubes of cDNAs encoding RyR1/RyR2 chimeras has provided some information about regions of importance for signaling. In the experiment illustrated in Fig. 12-17, calcium currents were measured with the whole-cell technique and excitation-contraction coupling was analyzed by brief (10-ms) current pulses applied to intact myotubes loaded with the calcium indicator Fluo3-AM.[147] Both skeletal-type excitation-contraction coupling (as indicated by a large calcium transient even when the myotube was bathed in a Ca^{2+}-free medium) and retrograde signaling were robust for "R10," which contains RyR1 residues 1635–2636. The chimera "R9," which contains RyR1 residues (2659–3720) adjacent to those of R10, did not support skeletal excitation-contraction coupling

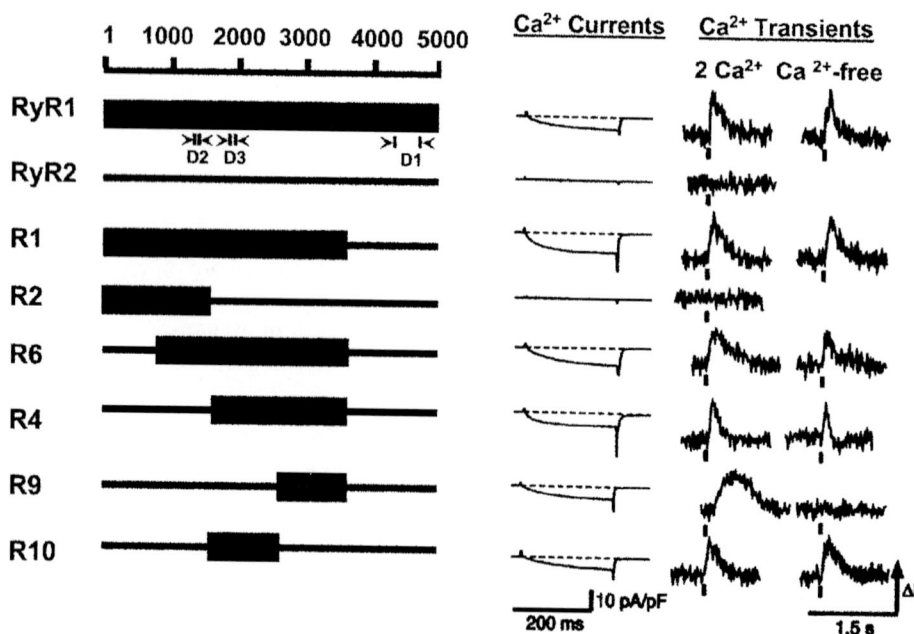

FIGURE 12-17. Expression of chimeric RyRs in dyspedic myotubes. Schematic representation of the RyR chimeras, with regions having skeletal (RyR1) sequence represented by thick lines and regions having cardiac (RyR2) sequence represented by thin lines. RyR1 residues contained in the chimeras were R1: 1–3720; R2: 1–1631; R4: 1635–3720; R6: 812–3720; R9: 2659–3720; R10: 1635–2636. The labels *D1*, *D2*, and *D3* indicate three regions of RyR1 highly divergent from RyR2. Ca^{2+} currents were measured with the whole-cell patch-clamp technique. Ca^{2+} transients were measured in response to 10-ms electrical stimuli applied focally to intact myotubes loaded with Fluo 3-AM. Ca^{2+}-free solution contained Mg^{2+} in equimolar replacement of Ca^{2+}. (Modified from Nakai et al.[147] Reproduced by permission.)

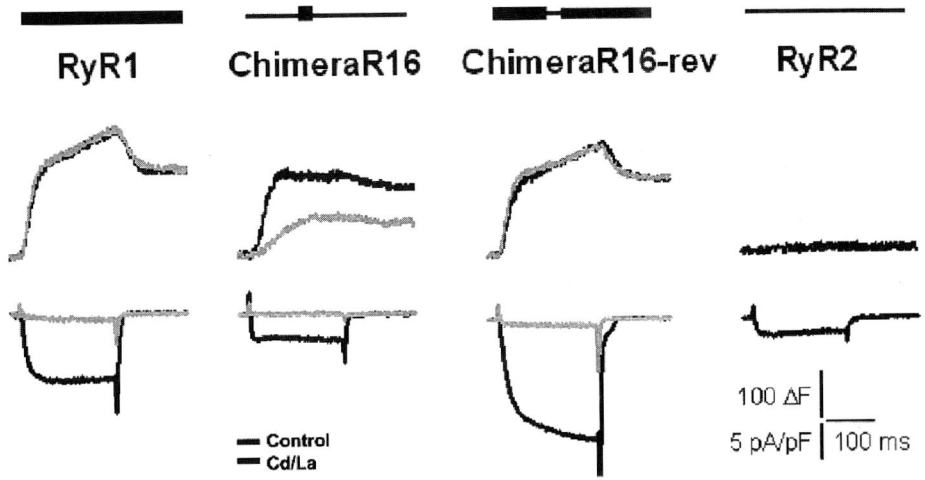

FIGURE 12-18. RyR1 residues 1837–2168 are sufficient for weak skeletal excitation-contraction coupling but are not necessary for strong bidirectional signaling. Thick and thin lines represent RyR1 and RyR2 sequence, respectively. Chimera R16 contained RyR1 residues 1837–2168 substituted into a RyR2 background, whereas Chimera R16-rev had RyR1 residues 1645–2154 replaced by RyR2 sequence. Whole-cell calcium currents (lower row) and transients (middle row) in dyspedic myotubes expressing the indicated constructs are shown for control and after block of Ca^{2+} currents by the addition of 0.5 mM Cd^{2+} and 0.1 mM La^{3+} to the bath. Note that for chimera R16 retrograde coupling was absent and that blocking calcium current partially reduced the transient (weak skeletal excitation-contraction coupling) but not for wild-type RyR1 or chimera R16-rev. Illustrated traces were obtained with 200-ms depolarizations to 40 mV. (*Modified from Proenza et al.*[148] *Reproduced by permission.*)

sufficiently strong to be detected with the protocol used (no transient in the Ca^{2+}-free medium) but was equivalent to R10 with respect to retrograde coupling. Thus, the experiments on RyR1/RyR2 chimeras indicate that two nonoverlapping RyR1 segments can restore substantial function.

The possibility of direct contact between these regions of RyR1 and α_{1S} was tested in yeast two-hybrid experiments (described in the following section), which showed a weak interaction between RyR1 residues 1837–2168 (within the R10 region) and the critical domain of the α_{1S} II–III loop.[148] Moreover, a chimera (R16) containing this region produced weak skeletal-type excitation-contraction coupling, although not retrograde signaling (Fig 12-18). However, this region is clearly not necessary for excitation-contraction coupling, since chimera R16-rev (in which residues 1645–2154 of RyR1 are replaced by RyR2 sequence) was able to mediate strong skeletal excitation-contraction coupling as well as retrograde signaling. Thus, the simplest conclusion from the RyR1/RyR2 chimeras is that multiple regions of RyR1 may be sites of protein-protein interaction necessary for signaling.

The involvement of multiple regions receives additional support from analysis of RyR3-based chimeras, which have two advantages compared to chimeras based on RyR2. The first is that RyR3 chimeras are less apt to display spontaneous, intracellular Ca^{2+} releases than are chimeras based on RyR2 (these spontaneous releases make it difficult to analyze Ca^{2+} release in response to membrane depolarization). Second, RyR3 shows greater divergence from RyR1 than does RyR2, and this allows one to analyze the effects of larger changes in primary sequence. Figure 12-19 illustrates results obtained by expression in dyspedic myotubes of RyR3-based chimeras containing insertions of RyR1 sequence roughly similar to those for the previously discussed RyR2-based chimeras.[149] To assess excitation-contraction coupling, intact myotubes were loaded with the calcium indicator Fluo4-AM and then depolarized by means of 5- to 10-s exposures to elevated external potassium. As a positive control, cells were analyzed only if they produced a Ca^{2+} transient in response to the application of caffeine. Excitation-contraction coupling was then quantified in two ways: as the percentage of caffeine-responsive cells that produced a measurable transient in response to KCl depolarization and as the magnitude of the KCl response in relation to the maximum (caffeine) response: A KCl response with entry of external Ca^{2+} blocked (Cd^{2+} and La^{3+} in the bath) is indicative of skeletal-type excitation-contraction coupling. By both measures, the RyR3-based chimeras give the same general result as the RyR2-based chimeras: Skeletal excitation-contraction coupling is restored by both Ch-9 and Ch-10, which contain nonoverlapping RyR1 sequences (2642–3770 and 1681–2641, respectively). Thus, both the RyR2- and RyR3-based constructs suggest that if there are direct contacts between RyR1 and the DHPR, these may involve multiple regions of RyR1.

One point of apparent discrepancy is that the data in Fig. 12-19 indicate that Ch-9 mediates skeletal excitation-contraction coupling (albeit weak), whereas the data of Fig. 12-18 indicate that R9, the closely related RyR2-based construct, does not. However, it is important to note that the experimental conditions for Fig. 12-19 (5- to 10-s depolarization) differ considerably from those for Fig. 12-18 (10-ms depolarization). Because the change in myoplasmic calcium depends on the integrated rate of release (as well as buffering and uptake), prolonged depolarization would be expected to allow detection of release rates too small to detect during a brief depolarization. Indeed, when assayed under conditions similar to those used for the RyR3-based chimeras, R9 was also found to mediate weak skeletal coupling.[150] Thus, judgments about coupling depend on the sensitivity of

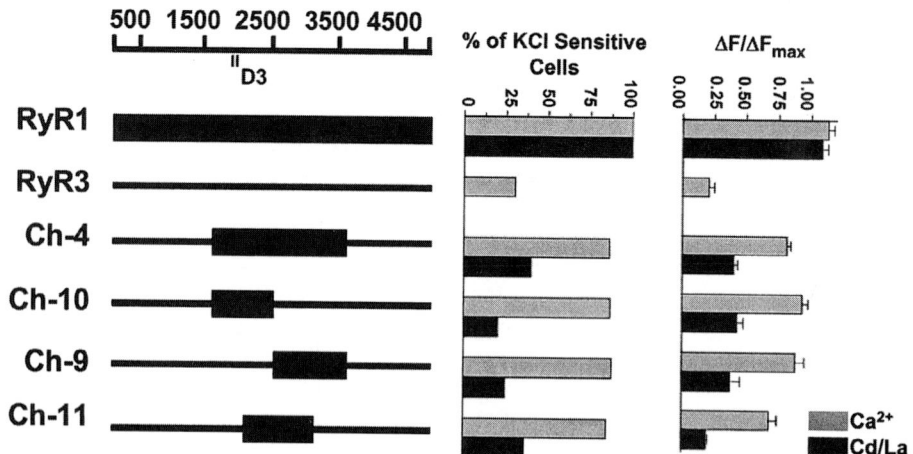

FIGURE 12-19. Comparison of the ability of chimeras composed of RyR1 (thick segments) and RyR3 (thin segments) to restore skeletal excitation-contraction coupling in dyspedic myotubes. Calcium transients were measured in intact myotubes in response to 5- to 10-s exposures to 80 mM K$^+$. The plots give the percentage of caffeine-responsive cells that also gave a measurable response to KCl (center panel) or the magnitude of the KCl response normalized by the magnitude of the caffeine response (right panel). RyR1 residues contained in the chimeras were Ch-4: 1681–3770; Ch-9: 2642–3770; Ch-10:1681–2641; Ch-11: 2218–3223. The Cd/La solution was nominally Ca^{2+}-free and contained 0.5 and 0.1 mM of Cd^{2+} and La^{3+}, respectively. (Modified from Perez et al.[149] Reproduced by permission.)

the assay used. It is also important to note that the various assays applied to myotubes may be useful for rank-ordering constructs but do not provide a linear measure of "coupling efficiency," which might be defined as the average open probability per RyR coupled to a DHPR (or to a DHPR tetrad).

Biochemical Interactions between DHPRs and RyRs

A variety of different techniques have been used to investigate whether specific regions of RyR1 and the DHPR interact with one another in vitro. On the basis of cosedimentation and coimmunoprecipitation, it has been concluded that the DHPR and RyR are present within a molecular complex at triad junctions,[151] although these techniques cannot test whether the two proteins interact directly with one another. Toward this end, a number of studies (Fig. 12-20) have focused on the ability of fragments of the two proteins to interact, motivated in large part by the goal of identifying specific regions whose interaction produces the conformational coupling responsible for bidirectional signaling. In one such study, Lu et al.[135] found that recombinant II–III loop peptide bound to RyR1; of three peptide subfragments (E666–E726, P709–L766, and K733–L791), only E666–E726 was found to measurably displace binding of the full-length loop and to increase ryanodine binding. Additionally, it was found that a recombinant loop bearing the mutation S687A was still able to bind to RyR1 but not to increase ryanodine binding. By way of comparison, expression of full-length α_1 constructs in dysgenic myotubes indicates that the sequence within the region E666–E726 can be significantly altered without eliminating skeletal-type excitation-contraction coupling,[151a] and that a full-length α_{1S} bearing the S687A mutation is able to restore excitation-contraction coupling in dysgenic myotubes.[132,141]

An alternative to examining the interaction of loop peptides with the intact RyR is to determine whether binding occurs between loop peptides and peptide segments of the RyR. With this approach it has been determined that the α_{1S} II–III loop binds to RyR1 residues L922–D1112 but not to the corresponding RyR2 residues.[152] Moreover, the cardiac (α_{1C})

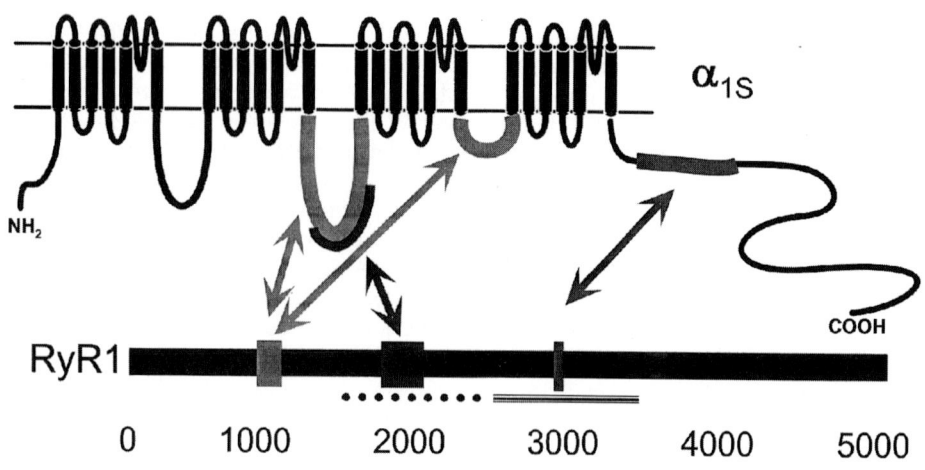

FIGURE 12-20. Biochemical interactions that have been reported to occur between domains of α_{1S} and RyR1. The dotted and striped lines indicate, respectively, the approximate location of RyR1 sequence contained in the chimeras R10 and R9 (see Fig. 12-17).

II–III loop did not bind to RyR1 L922–D1112 and the mutations K677E/K682E within the α_{1S} II–III loop largely eliminated its ability to bind RyR1 L922–D1112. Subsequently, it was found that the α_{1S} III–IV cytoplasmic loop also binds to RyR1 L922–D1112 (but not to the corresponding RyR2 residues at a site that partially overlapped the binding site for the II–III loop).[153] The interaction between the α_{1S} III–IV loop and RyR1 is intriguing, given that a mutation affecting the III–IV loop has been linked to susceptibility for malignant hyperthermia.[154] However, it is worth noting that the ability of the α_{1S} II–III and III–IV loops to bind to RyR1 L922–D1112 and not to the corresponding RyR2 region seems unlikely to account for the inability of RyR2 to restore skeletal-type excitation-contraction coupling in dyspedic myotubes, because such coupling is restored by chimeras containing RyR2 sequence in this region (Fig. 12-17).

An interaction between a segment of the II–III loop and RyR1 has also been suggested on the basis of the yeast two-hybrid technique, which revealed an interaction between the critical domain of α_{1S} (residues 720–765; see Fig. 12-14) and the "R16" region of RyR1 (residues 1837–2168), which lies in the middle of the R10 region that is important for skeletal-type excitation-contraction coupling (see Fig. 12-17).[148] This interaction displayed some of the expected specificity, since the region of α_{1C} corresponding to the α_{1S} critical domain did not interact with the R16 region of RyR1. Moreover, as described above (Fig. 12-18), a chimera composed of the R16 region of RyR1 substituted into RyR2 was able to restore weak skeletal-type excitation-contraction coupling (but not retrograde signaling). However, the ability of chimera R16-rev to mediate strong bidirectional signaling indicates that skeletal sequence in this region of RyR1 is not required for effective signaling.

In addition to the II–III and III–IV loops, it has also been reported that the carboxyl-terminal region of α_{1S} binds to RyR1. The possibility of such an interaction was raised by the demonstration that peptides corresponding to various portions of the α_{1S} carboxyl terminal inhibit ryanodine binding to skeletal and cardiac SR fractions as well as inhibiting the channel activity of RyR1 reconstituted into artificial bilayers.[155] Subsequent experiments with surface plasmon resonance demonstrated that a segment of the carboxyl terminal that is known to be important for the binding of calmodulin to α_{1C} binds to both RyR1 and RyR2.[156] Consistent with the very high conservation between this region of α_{1C} and α_{1S}, a segment of α_{1S} (1393–1527) was found to bind calmodulin and (in the absence of calmodulin) to inhibit ryanodine binding to SR membranes and to bind to a segment of RyR1 (3609–3643).[157] Moreover, RyR1 3609–3643, which is a region important for the binding of calmodulin to the RyR,[105,106] was found to bind to the detergent-solubilized skeletal DHPR. These observations led to the hypothesis that the calmodulin-binding domains of α_{1S} and RyR1 can bind to one another in vivo in a manner that may be modulated by calmodulin. However, if this binding occurs in vivo, it seems unlikely to be a sole determinant for ortho- and retrograde coupling between α_{1S} and RyR1, which appears to depend more directly on other regions of α_{1S} (specifically the II–III loop) and of RyR1 (those more toward the amino terminal than residues 3609–3643). These same regions of α_{1S} and RyR1 also appear to be critical for the formation of DHPR tetrads[150] (Chap. 11). Nonetheless, it remains an important possibility that the regions of α_{1S} and RyR1 identified as interacting biochemically (and summarized in Fig. 12-20) are important for coupling in vivo, but that their interaction depends on the presence of critical sequences elsewhere in both proteins.

The Betacentric View of Excitation-Contraction Coupling

Although the α_{1S} subunit of the DHPR has received much attention in molecular analyses of excitation-contraction coupling, an important role for the β subunit is now also emerging. There are currently four known β-subunit genes, of which only $\beta1$ is highly expressed in skeletal muscle. Knockout of the $\beta1$ gene causes excitation-contraction uncoupling (as in dysgenic muscle), and $\beta1$-null myotubes display a large reduction in calcium current and membrane charge movement (the latter being an indication that trafficking of DHPRs to the plasma membrane is impaired).[92] Specifically, in $\beta1$-null myotubes, depolarization-induced Ca^{2+} transients are absent and only a relatively small amount of charge movement (2.5 nC/μF) is present. This phenotype is an important feature of the $\beta1$-null myotubes because it supports the idea that there is no compensatory upregulation of the other β-subunit genes. Expression in $\beta1$-null myotubes of cDNA encoding $\beta1a$ (the dominant splice variant in skeletal muscle) rescues a near normal phenotype.[158] However, the expression of different β-subunit constructs was found to have decidedly different effects on the DHPR in terms of surface expression (as measured by charge movement), calcium current, and excitation-contraction coupling (as indicated by the magnitude of depolarization-induced calcium transient). Experiments demonstrating these points are illustrated in Fig. 12-21. The expression of $\beta1a$ resulted in appreciable surface expression of DHPRs (maximum charge movment, Q_{max}, of 6.8 nC/μF), large calcium currents (maximum calcium conductance, G_{max}, of 161 pS/pF), and large calcium transients ($\Delta F/F_{max}$ of 3.3). By comparison, expression of $\beta2a$ restored comparable calcium currents (G_{max} of 153 pS/pF) but much smaller calcium transients ($\Delta F/F_{max}$ of 1.1) and little surface expression (Q_{max} of 2.6 nC/μF). Thus, association of α_{1S} with $\beta2a$ appears to produce channels of much higher open probability than association with $\beta1a$.

A number of truncations and chimeras were examined in an attempt to identify structural determinants of these functional differences between $\beta1a$ and $\beta2a$. As one example, truncation of 35 residues from the carboxyl terminal of $\beta1a$ (the construct $\beta1a$-3't) had little effect on surface expression (Q_{max} of 6.4 nC/μF) but greatly reduced both calcium currents (G_{max} of 88 pS/pF) and transients ($\Delta F/F_{max}$ of 0.7), raising the possibility that the carboxyl-terminal region of the $\beta1a$ subunit is involved in signaling between the DHPR and RyR1. Support for this idea is provided by the behavior of a chimera ($\beta2$–$\beta1$) in which the carboxyl-terminal portion of $\beta2a$ was replaced by the corresponding region of $\beta1a$. The $\beta2$–$\beta1$ construct behaved in a manner much like that of wild-type $\beta1a$. Thus, introduction of the $\beta1$ carboxyl terminal into $\beta2a$ appears to introduce a gain of function (excitation-contraction coupling). However, it might also be viewed as a

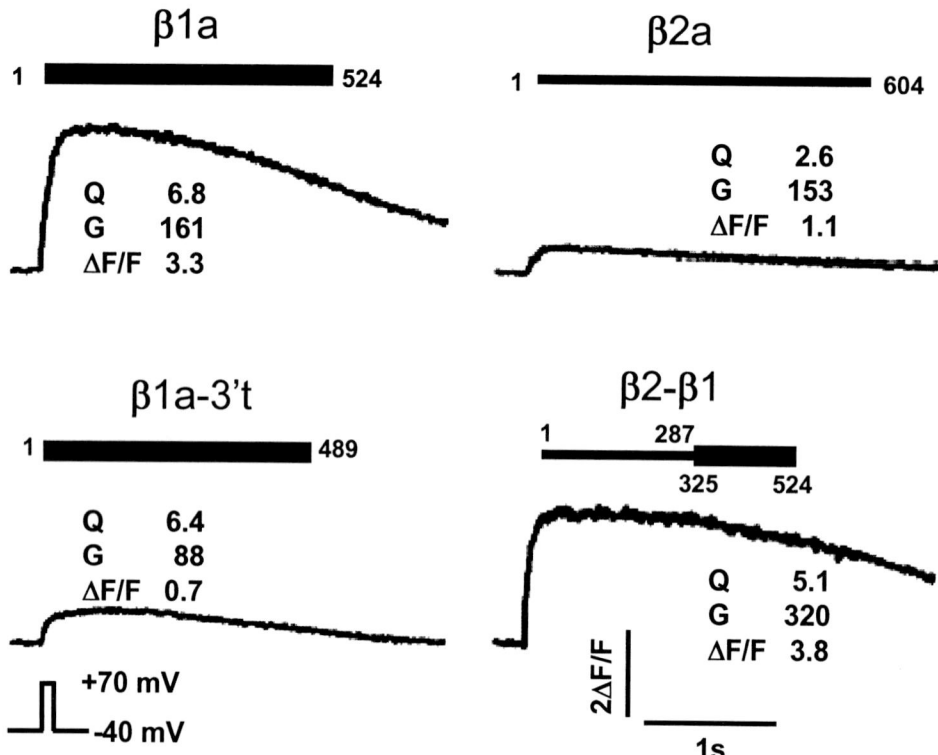

FIGURE 12-21. Representative calcium transients in β1-null myotubes expressing different β-subunit constructs. The composition of the constructs is designated by thick and thin segments for β1a and β2a, respectively, with residue numbers as indicated. Whole-cell clamping was used to measure charge movements, calcium currents, and calcium transients (by laser confocal line scanning). Average values for maximum charge (Q), calcium conductance (G), and calcium transient (ΔF/F) are from Table 1 of Beurg et al. (*Modified from Beurg et al.*[158] *Reproduced by permission.*)

loss of function because the transients produced by wild-type β2a are nearly one-third the size of those for wild-type β1a, which is quite large considering that β2a produces a very low level of DHPR expression in the plasma membrane: Although Q_{max} was 6.8 and 2.6 nC/μF for β1a and β2a, respectively, the value for β2a is only slightly larger than the 2.5 nC/μF found in control β1-null myotubes.

In addition to functioning in excitation-contraction coupling, it has also been suggested that the β subunit may be important for retrograde signaling. Certainly it is clear that β can regulate calcium current independently of RyR1, as is evidenced by the increased calcium current density that result from expressing β2a in myotubes genetically null for both β1 and RyR1.[159] However, such a result does not invalidate the importance of RyR1 in regulating the calcium current via the DHPR, because β1a should have been present in both the absence and presence of RyR1 in experiments like those illustrated in Fig. 12-13. Nonetheless, the effects of β on calcium current in β1- RyR1- double-null myotubes highlights the necessity for caution in ascribing changes in calcium current density to altered "retrograde signaling" as opposed to other sources. Besides playing potential roles in skeletal excitation-contraction coupling and in retrograde signaling, the carboxyl terminal of β1a may also play a role in inhibiting the sensitivity of RyR1 to activation by Ca^{2+} entry.[160]

The potential importance of the β subunit for excitation-contraction coupling has been reinforced by experiments in which $α_{1S}$ constructs bearing deletions in the II–III loop were expressed in dysgenic myotubes. In one approach, two separate cDNAs were expressed, one of which encoded repeats I–II and a proximal portion of the II–III loop and the other of which encoded a distal portion of the loop together with repeats III–IV. Ahern et al.[142] expressed cDNAs encoding $α_{1S}$ residues 1–670 and residues 701–1873; Flucher et al.[161] expressed cDNAs encoding residues 1–670 and residues 691–1873. Despite the fact that the two fragments of $α_{1S}$ examined in both studies were entirely missing the peptide-A region (see Fig. 12-16), they were found able to restore excitation-contraction coupling. Interestingly, the I–II constructs (but not the III–IV constructs) were able to traffic to the plasma membrane and to generate charge movement,[142,161] although not to target to triad junctions.[161] Effects of deletions within the II–III loop have also been examined in single constructs in which the residues just before and just after the deletion were directly linked to one another (Fig. 12-22).[162] As with the double fragment experiments, deletion of residues 671–690 in the single $α_{1S}$ construct did not noticeably alter excitation-contraction coupling. Deletion of residues 720–765 completely abolished coupling, although measurements of charge movements indicated that the protein still trafficked to the membrane. This result is consistent with the importance found for this same region (the "critical domain") in the experiments with $α_{1S}/α_{1C}$ chimeras (see Fig. 12-14).

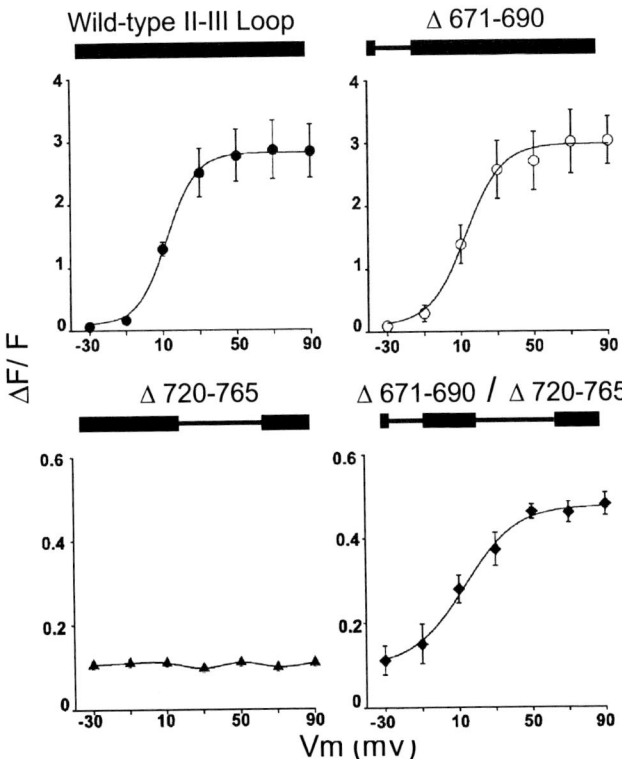

FIGURE 12-22. Voltage dependence of calcium transients in dysgenic myotubes expressing α_{1S} in which the II–III loop either was wild-type or contained deletions. Wild-type sequence is indicated by thick segments and deletions of the indicated residues by thin segments. Outside of the II–III loop, all the constructs had wild-type α_{1S} sequence. The sigmoidal dependence on test potential of the amplitude of the calcium transient is diagnostic of skeletal excitation-contraction coupling. With cardiac coupling, the transients become smaller for very strong depolarizations, which decrease the driving force for calcium entry. Note that the $\Delta F/F$ scales differ in the upper and lower panels. (*Modified from Ahern et al.*[162] *Reproduced by permission.*)

Oddly, when both deletions (671–690, 720–765) were introduced together, a small amount of excitation-contraction coupling was restored ($\Delta F/F_{max}$ about 15 percent of normal). This result implies that some part of the DHPR outside of the critical domain of α_{1S} (β, perhaps) has the potential to engage in the conformational coupling with RyR1 that is necessary for excitation-contraction coupling. However, it is unclear at this point whether the double deletion is revealing an interaction that already exists in native DHPRs (containing wild-type α_{1S}) or if it induces an interaction that does not occur for native DHPRs.

Summary

Many fundamental principles of excitation-contraction coupling in skeletal muscle are known: The process does not require extracellular calcium, it is initiated by charge movements generated within dihydropyridine receptors in the T-tubule membrane, it proceeds via the release of calcium from RyRs in the terminal cisternae of the SR, and it is completed by the interaction of this released calcium with troponin.

Sparks now provide a view of quantal calcium release events occurring at the terminal cisternae, but it is not yet clear whether a few or many RyRs contribute to the production of sparks or why sparks appear to differ greatly between cut and intact amphibian fibers and between amphibian and mammalian fibers. Muscle cells obtained from genetic "knockout" animals have provided new insights into the role of specific proteins in triad junctions, both in the structural formation of the junctions and more functionally in excitation-contraction coupling. Mix-and-match constructions of DHPRs and of RyRs, expressed in appropriate knockout myotubes, have revealed information about regions important for signaling interactions between the two proteins, as have more reductionist approaches involving peptides and biochemical assays.

Within the DHPR, both the II–III loop of α_{1S} and the carboxyl terminal of β1a appear to play important roles in the signaling interactions with RyR1. Neither RyR2 nor RyR3 can functionally substitute for RyR1, but chimeras between RyR1 and either RyR2 or RyR3 give the impression that large regions of RyR1 are important for the signaling interactions with the DHPR. Indeed, it may well be likely that large regions of both RyR1 and the DHPR are involved in the protein-protein interactions underlying signaling and that a search for small regions that are both necessary and sufficient may prove to be fruitless.

It seems likely that continued progress will depend upon a multidisciplinary approach. This avenue can be fruitful not only when the different approaches produce a self-consistent set of results but also when they lead to contradictions. For example, the experiments on peptides prompted experiments in myotubes that ruled out a critical role for the peptide A region of the α_{1S} II–III loop. Obtaining improved resolution of the structure of DHPRs and RyRs will be of critical importance for understanding excitation-contraction coupling. A priori, portions of the RyR1 primary sequence that are present in the region of the foot structure close to T tubules will be candidates for protein-protein interactions with the DHPR.

A decade ago, Professor Horowicz ended this chapter with the statement that "the primary transmission mechanism by which the relevant component of charge movement initiates SR calcium release remains obscure." This statement remains true today. Perhaps the application of diverse techniques to the study of excitation-contraction coupling will allow a more definitive conclusion a decade hence.

Acknowledgments

I thank Clara Franzini-Armstrong, without whose help and patience this chapter would not have been completed.

List of Abbreviations

BAPTA	1,2-bis[o-aminophenoxy] ethane-N,N,N',N'-tetraacetic acid	RyR	ryanodine receptor
DHPR	dihydropyridine receptor	SR	sarcoplasmic reticulum
EGTA	ethyleneglycol-bis-(2-aminoethylether)-N,N,N',N'-tetraacetic acid	T tubule	transverse tubule

References

1. Sandow A: Excitation-contraction coupling in skeletal muscle. *Pharmacol Rev* 17:265, 1965.
2. Huxley AF, Taylor RE: Local activation of striated muscle fibers. *J Physiol (Lond)* 144:426, 1958.
3. Kuffler SW: The relation of electric potential changes to contracture in skeletal muscle. *J Neurophysiol* 9:367, 1946.
4. Hodgkin AL, Horowicz P: Potassium contractures in single muscle fibres. *J Physiol (Lond)* 153:386, 1960.
5. Lännergren J: Contractures of single slow muscle fibres of *Xenopus laevis* elicited by potassium, acetylcholine or choline. *Acta Physiol Scand* 69:362, 1967.
6. Frankenhauser B, Lännergren J: The effect of calcium on the mechanical response of single twitch muscle fibres of *Xenopus laevis*. *Acta Physiol Scand* 69:242, 1967.
7. Hille B: *Ionic Channels of Excitable Membranes*, 3d ed. Sunderland, MA: Sinauer Associates; 2001.
8. Armstrong CM, Bezanilla FM, Horowicz P: Twitches in the presence of ethylene glycol bis-aminoethyl ether)-N,N'-tetracetic acid. *Biochim Biophys Acta* 267:605, 1972.
9. Lüttgau HC, Spiecker W: The effects of calcium deprivation upon mechanical and electrophysiological parameters in skeletal muscle fibres of the frog. *J Physiol (Lond)* 296:411, 1979.
10. Adrian RH, Chandler WK, Hodgkin AL: The kinetics of mechanical activation in frog muscle. *J Physiol (Lond)* 204:207, 1969.
11. Gilly WF, Hui CS: Mechanical activation in slow and twitch skeletal muscle fibres of the frog. *J Physiol (Lond)* 301:137, 1980.
12. Bianchi CP: Kinetics of radiocaffeine uptake and release in frog sartorius. *J Pharmacol Exp Ther* 138:41, 1962.
13. Sandow A, Taylor SR, Preiser H: Role of the action potential in excitation-contraction coupling. *Fed Proc* 24:1116, 1965.
14. Sandow A, Brust M: Caffeine potentiation of twitch tension in frog sartorius muscle. *Biochem Z* 345:232, 1966.
15. Lüttgau HC, Oetliker H: The action of caffeine on the activation of the contractile mechanism in striated mucle fibres. *J Physiol (Lond)* 194:51, 1968.
16. Korey S: Some factors influencing the contractility of a non-conducting fiber preparation. *Biochim Biophys Acta* 4:58, 1950.
17. Kovács L, Szücs G: Effect of caffeine on intramembrane charge movement and calcium transients in cut skeletal muscle fibres of the frog. *J Physiol (Lond)* 341:559, 1983.
18. Foulks JG, Perry FA: Some effects of drugs and ions upon activation and relaxation in striated muscle, in Paul WM, Daniel EE, Kay CM, Monckton G (eds): *Muscle*. New York: Pergamon Press; 1965, pp 185–198.
19. Frank GB: Effects of changes in extracellular calcium concentration on the potassium-induced contracture of frogs skeletal muscle. *J Physiol (Lond)* 151:518, 1960.
20. Fujino M, Fujino S: Die Beziehung zwischen Caffein-Kontraktur und Calcium am Froschskeletmuskel. *Pflugers Arch* 278:478, 1964.
21. Miyamoto Y: Effects of changes in extracellular calcium concentration on the electrical and mechanical responses of an isolated single muscle fibre. *J Fac Sci Hokkaido Univ Ser VI Zool* 51:235, 1963.
22. Hodgkin AL, Huxley AF: A quantitative description of membrane current and its application to conduction and excitation in nerve. *J Physiol (Lond)* 117:500, 1952.
23. Schneider MF, Chandler WK: Voltage dependent charge movement in skeletal muscle: A possible step in excitation-contraction coupling. *Nature* 242:244, 1973.
24. Armstrong CM, Bezanilla FM: Currents related to the movement of the gating particles of the sodium channels. *Nature* 242:459, 1973.
25. Armstrong CM, Bezanilla F: Charge movement associated with the opening and closing of the activation gates of the Na channels. *J Gen Physiol* 63:533, 1974.
26. Chandler WK, Rakowski RF, Schneider MF: A non-linear voltage dependent charge movement in frog skeletal muscle. *J Physiol (Lond)* 254:245, 1976.
27. Chandler WK, Rakowski RF, Schneider MF: Effects of glycerol treatment and maintained depolarization on charge movement in skeletal muscle. *J Physiol (Lond)* 254:285, 1976.
28. Caputo C: The effect of low temperature on the excitation-contraction coupling phenomena of frog single muscle fibres. *J Physiol (Lond)* 223:461, 1972.
29. Caputo C: The time course of potassium contractures of single muscle fibres. *J Physiol (Lond)* 223:483, 1972.
30. Adrian RH, Chandler WK, Rakowski RF: Charge movement and mechanical repriming in skeletal muscle fibres. *J Physiol (Lond)* 254:361, 1976.
31. Brum G, Fitts R, Pizarro G, et al: Voltage sensors of the frog skeletal muscle membrane require calcium to function in excitation-contraction coupling. *J Physiol (Lond)* 398:475, 1988.
32. Pizarro G, Fitts R, Uribe I, Rios E: The voltage sensor of excitation-contraction coupling in skeletal muscle. *J Gen Physiol* 94:405, 1989.
33. Gilly WF, Hui CS: Voltage-dependent charge movement in frog slow muscle fibres. *J Physiol (Lond)* 301:175, 1980.
34. Horowicz P, Schneider MF: Membrane charge moved at contraction thresholds in skeletal muscle fibres. *J Physiol (Lond)* 314:595, 1981.
35. Dörrscheidt-Käfer M: The action of Ca2i, Mg2+, and H+ on the contraction threshold of frog skeletal muscle. *Pflugers Arch* 362:33, 1976.
36. Shlevin HH: Effects of external calcium concentration and pH on charge movement in frog skeletal muscle. *J Physiol (Lond)* 288:129, 1979.
37. Lüttgau HC, Gottschalk G, Kovács L, et al: How perchlorate improves excitation-contraction coupling in skeletal muscle fibers. *Biophys J* 43:247, 1983.
38. Dulhunty AF: Potassium contractures and mechanical activation in mammalian skeletal muscles. *J Membr Biol* 57:223, 1980.
39. Hollingsworth S, Marshall MW: A comparative study of charge movement in rat and frog skeletal muscle fibres. *J Physiol (Lond)* 321:583, 1981.
40. Dulhunty AF, Gage PW: Asymmetrical charge movement in slow- and fast-twitch mammalian muscle fibres in normal and paraplegic rats. *J Physiol (Lond)* 341:213, 1983.
41. García J, Tanabe T, Beam KG: Relationship of calcium transients to calcium currents and charge movements in myotubes expressing skeletal and cardiac DHP receptors. *J Gen Physiol* 103:125, 1994.
42. Bean BP: Nitrendipine block of cardiac calcium channels: High-affinity binding to the inactivated state. *Proc Natl Acad Sci USA* 81:6388, 1984.
43. Schwartz LM, McCleskey EW, Almers W: Dihydropyridine receptors in muscle are voltage-dependent but most are not functional calcium channels. *Nature* 314:747, 1985.
44. Lamb GD, Walsh T: Calcium currents, charge movements and dihydropyridine binding in fast- and slow-twitch muscles of rat and rabbit. *J Physiol (Lond)* 393:595, 1987.
45. Rios E, Brum G: Involvement of dihydropyridine receptors in excitation-contraction coupling in skeletal muscle. *Nature* 325:717, 1987.
46. Adrian RH, Almers W: The voltage dependence of membrane of capacity. *J Physiol (Lond)* 254:317, 1976.
47. Adrian RH, Almers W: Charge movement in the membrane of striated muscle. *J Physiol (Lond)* 254:339, 1976.
48. Schneider MF, Chandler WK: Effects of membrane potential on the capacitance of skeletal muscle fibers. *J Gen Physiol* 67:125, 1976.
49. Brum G, Rios E: Intramembrane charge movement in frog skeletal muscle fibers: Properties of charge 2. *J Physiol (Lond)* 387:489, 1987.
50. Feldmeyer D, Melzer W, Pohl B: Effects of gallopamil on calcium release and intramembrane charge movements in frog skeletal muscle fibers. *J Physiol (Lond)* 421:343, 1990.
51. Lamb GD: Asymmetric charge movement in polarized and depolarized fibres of the rabbit. *J Physiol (Lond)* 383:349, 1987.
52. Dirksen RT, Beam KG: Role of calcium permeation in dihydropyridine receptor function: Insights into channel gating and excitation-contraction coupling. *J Gen Physiol* 114:393, 1999.
53. Adrian RH, Peres A: Charge movement and membrane capacity in frog muscle. *J Physiol (Lond)* 289:83, 1979.
54. Huang, CL-H: Pharmacological separation of charge movement components in frog skeletal muscle. *J Physiol (Lond)* 324:275, 1982.
55. Hui CS, Chandler WK: Intramembranous charge movement in frog cut twitch fibers mounted in a double Vaseline-gap chamber. *J Gen Physiol* 96:257, 1990.

56. Csernoch L, Pizarro G, Uribe I, et al: Interfering with calcium release suppresses I gamma, the "hump" component of intramembranous charge movement in skeletal muscle. *J Gen Physiol* 97:845, 1991.
57. Jong DS, Pape PC, Chandler WK: Effects of sarcoplasmic reticulum (SR) calcium depletion on intramembranous charge movement in frog cut muscle fibers. *J Gen Physiol* 106:659, 1995.
58. Hollingworth S, Marshall MW: A comparative study of charge movement in rat and frog skeletal muscle fibres. *J Physiol (Lond)* 321:583, 1981.
59. Baylor SM, Hollingworth S: Measurement and interpretation of cytoplasmic [Ca^{2+}] signals from calcium-indicator dyes. *News Physiol Sci* 15:19, 2000.
60. Baylor SM, Chandler WK, Marshall MW: Sarcoplasmic reticulum calcium release in frog skeletal muscle fibres estimated from arsenazo III calcium transients. *J Physiol (Lond)* 344:625, 1983.
61. Melzer W, Rios E, Schneider MF: Time course of calcium release and removal in skeletal muscle fibers. *Biophys J* 45:637, 1984.
62. Melzer W, Rios E, Schneider MF: A general procedure for determining the rate of calcium release from the sarcoplasmic reticulum in skeletal muscle fibers. *Biophys J* 51:849, 1987.
63. Klein MG, Simon BJ, Schneider MF: Effects of caffeine on calcium release from the sarcoplasmic reticulum in skeletal muscle fibres. *J Physiol (Lond)* 425:599, 1990.
64. Baylor SM, Hollingworth S: Sarcoplasmic reticulum calcium release compared in slow-twitch and fast-twitch fibres of mouse muscle. *J Physiol (Lond)* 551:125, 2003.
65. Shirokova N, Garcia J, Pizarro G, Rios E: Ca^{2+} release from the sarcoplasmic reticulum compared in amphibian and mammalian skeletal muscle. *J Gen Physiol* 107:1, 1996.
66. Schneider MF, Simon BJ: Inactivation of calcium release from the sarcoplasmic reticulum in frog skeletal muscle. *J Physiol (Lond)* 405:727, 1988.
67. Simon BJ, Klein MG, Schneider MF: Calcium dependence of inactivation of calcium release from the sarcoplasmic reticulum in skeletal muscle fibers. *J Gen Physiol* 97:437, 1991.
68. Melzer W, Schneider MF, Simon BJ, et al: Intramembrane charge movement and calcium release in frog skeletal muscle. *J Physiol (Lond)* 373:481, 1986.
69. Endo M, Tanaka M, Ogawa Y: Calcium induced release of calcium from the sarcoplasmic reticulum of skinned skeletal muscle fibers. *Nature* 228:34, 1970.
70. Ford LE, Podolsky RJ: Regenerative calcium release within muscle cells. *Science* 167:58, 1970.
71. Miyamoto H, Racker E: Mechanism of calcium release from skeletal sarcoplasmic reticulum. *J Membr Biol* 66:193, 1982.
72. Meissner G, Darling E, Eveleth J: Kinetics of rapid Ca^{2+} release by sarcoplasmic reticulum: Effects of Ca^{2+}, Mg^{2+}, and adenine nucleotides. *Biochemistry* 25:236, 1986.
73. Smith JS, Coronado R, Meissner G: Single channel measurements of the calcium release channel from skeletal muscle sarcoplasmic reticulum. *J Gen Physiol* 88:573, 1986.
74. Jacquemond V, Csernoch L, Klein MG, et al: Voltage-gated and calcium-gated calcium release during depolarization of skeletal muscle fibers. *Biophys J* 60:867, 1991.
75. Baylor SM, Hollingworth S: Fura-2 Ca^{2+} transients in frog skeletal muscle fibres. *J Physiol (Lond)* 403:151, 1988.
76. Hollingworth S, Harkins AB, Kurebayashi N, et al: Excitation-contraction coupling in intact frog skeletal muscle fibers injected with mmolar concentrations of fura-2. *Biophys J* 63:224, 1992.
77. Gonzalez-Serratos H, Valle-Aguilera R, Lathrop DA, et al: Slow inward calcium currents have no obvious role in muscle excitation-contraction coupling. *Nature* 298:292, 1982.
78. Cheng H, Lederer WJ, Cannell MB: Calcium sparks: Elementary events underlying excitation-contraction coupling in heart muscle. *Science* 262:740, 1993.
79. Rios E, Brum G: Ca^{2+} release flux underlying Ca^{2+} transients and Ca^{2+} sparks in skeletal muscle. *Front Biosci* 7:d1195, 2002.
80. Tsugorka A, Rios E, Blatter LA: Imaging elementary events of calcium release in skeletal muscle cells. *Science* 269:1723, 1995.
81. Klein MG, Cheng H, Santana LF, et al: Two mechanisms of quantized calcium release in skeletal muscle. *Nature* 379:455, 1996.
82. Kirsch WG, Uttenweiler D, Fink RHA: Spark- and ember-like elementary Ca^{2+} release events in skinned fibres of adult mammalian skeletal muscle. *J Physiol* 537:379, 2001.
83. Zhou J, Brum G, Gonzalez A, et al. Ca^{2+} sparks and embers of mammalian muscle. Properties of the sources. *J Gen Physiol* 122:95, 2003.
84. Schneider MF, Ward CW: Initiation and termination of calcium sparks in skeletal muscle. *Front Biosci* 7:d1212, 2002.
85. Hollingworth S, Peet J, Chandler WK, Baylor SM: Calcium sparks in intact skeletal muscle fibers of the frog. *J Gen Physiol* 118:653, 2001.
86. Huxley AF, Taylor RE: Local activation of striated muscles from the frog and the crab. *J Physiol (Lond)* 135:17P, 1956.
87. DiFranco M, Novo D, Vergara JL: Characterization of the calcium release domains during excitation-contraction coupling in skeletal muscle fibres. *Pflugers Arch* 443:508, 2002.
88. González A, Kirsch WG, Shirokova N, et al: The spark and its ember: Separately gated local components of Ca^{2+} release in skeletal muscle. *J Gen Physiol* 115:139, 2000.
89. Klein MG, Lacampagne A, Schneider MF: Voltage dependence of the pattern and frequency of discrete Ca^{2+} release events after brief repriming in frog skeletal muscle. *Proc Natl Acad Sci USA* 94:11061, 1997.
90. Catterall WA: Structure and regulation of voltage-gated Ca2+ channels. *Annu Rev Cell Dev Biol* 16:521, 2000.
91. Tanabe T, Beam KG, Powell JA, Numa S: Restoration of excitation-contraction coupling and slow calcium current in dysgenic muscle by dihydropyridine receptor complementary DNA. *Nature* 336:134, 1988.
92. Strube C, Beurg M, Powers PA, et al: Reduced Ca^{2+} current, charge movement and absence of Ca^{2+} transients in skeletal muscle deficient in dihydropyridine receptor $\beta 1$ subunit. *Biophys J* 71:2531, 1996.
93. Freise D, Held B, Wissenbach U, et al: Absence of the gamma subunit of the skeletal muscle dihydropyridine receptor increases L-type Ca^{2+} currents and alters channel inactivation properties. *J Biol Chem* 275:14476, 2000.
94. Meissner G: Regulation of mammalian ryanodine receptors. *Front Biosci* 7:d2072, 2002.
95. Takeshima H, Nishimura N, Matsumoto T, et al: Primary structure and expression from complementary DNA of skeletal muscle ryanodine receptor. *Nature* 339:439, 1989.
96. Zorzato F, Fujii J, Otsu K, et al: Molecular cloning of cDNA encoding human and rabbit forms of the Ca^{2+} release channel (ryanodine receptor) of skeletal muscle sarcoplasmic reticulum. *J Biol Chem* 265:2244, 1990.
97. Otsu K, Willard HF, Khanna VK, et al: Molecular cloning of cDNA encoding the Ca^{2+} release channel (ryanodine receptor) of rabbit cardiac muscle sarcoplasmic reticulum. *J Biol Chem* 265:13472, 1990.
98. Giannini G, Clementi E, Ceci R, et al: Expression of a novel ryanodine receptor/Ca^{2+} channel that is regulated by TGFβ. *Science* 257:91, 1992.
99. Takeshima H, Iino M, Takekura H, et al: Excitation-contraction uncoupling and muscular degeneration in mice lacking functional skeletal muscle ryanodine-receptor gene. *Nature* 369:556, 1994.
100. Bertocchini F, Ovitt CE, Conti A, et al: Requirement for the ryanodine receptor type 3 for efficient contraction in neonatal skeletal muscles. *EMBO J* 16:6956, 1997.
101. Sutko JL, Airey JA: Ryanodine receptor Ca2+ release channels: Does diversity in form equal diversity in function? *Physiol Rev* 76:1027, 1996.
102. Wagenknecht T, Radermacher M: Ryanodine receptors: Structure and macromolecular interactions. *Curr Opin Struct Biol* 7:258, 1997.
103. Serysheva II, Schatz M, van Heel M, et al: Structure of the skeletal muscle calcium release channel activated with Ca^{2+} and AMP-PCP. *Biophys J* 77:1936, 1999.
104. Brillantes AB, Ondrias K, Scott A, et al: Stabilization of calcium release channel (ryanodine receptor) function by FK506-binding protein. *Cell* 77:513, 1994.
105. Hamilton SL, Serysheva I, Strasburg GM: Calmodulin and excitation-contraction coupling. *News Physiol Sci* 15:281, 2000.
106. Balshaw DM, Yamaguchi N, Meissner G: Modulation of intracellular calcium-release channels by calmodulin. *J Membr Biol* 185:1, 2002.
107. Feng W, Tu JC, Yang TZ, et al: Homer regulates gain of ryanodine receptor type 1 channel complex. *J Biol Chem* 277:44722, 2002.
108. MacLennan DH, Wong PT: Isolation of a calcium-sequestering protein from sarcoplasmic reticulum. *Proc Natl Acad Sci USA* 68:1231, 1971.
109. MacLennan DH, Campbell KP, Reithmeyer RAF: Calsequestrin. *Calcium Cell Funct* 4:151, 1983.
110. Kim KC, Caswell AH, Talvenheimo JA, Brandt NR: Isolation of a terminal cisterna protein which may link the dihydropyridine receptor to the junctional foot protein in skeletal muscle. *Biochemistry* 29:9281, 1990.
111. Caswell AH, Brandt NR, Brunschwig JP, Purkerson S: Localization and partial characterization of the oligomeric disulfide-linked molecular weight 95,000 protein (triadin) which binds the ryanodine and dihydropyridine receptors in skeletal muscle triadic vesicles. *Biochemistry* 30:7507, 1991.
112. Jones LR, Zhang L, Sanborn K, et al: Purification, primary structure, and immunological characterization of the 26-kDa calsequestrin binding protein (junctin) from cardiac junctional sarcoplasmic reticulum. *J Biol Chem* 270:30787, 1995.
113. Zhang L, Kelley J, Schmeisser G, et al: Complex formation between junctin, triadin, calsequestrin, and the ryanodine receptor. Proteins of the cardiac junctional sarcoplasmic reticulum membrane. *J Biol Chem* 272:23389, 1997.
114. Guo W, Campbell KP: Association of triadin with the ryanodine receptor and calsequestrin in the lumen of the sarcoplasmic reticulum. *J Biol Chem* 270:9027, 1995.
115. Knudson CM, Stang KK, Moomaw CR, et al: Primary structure and topological analysis of a skeletal muscle-specific junctional sarcoplasmic reticulum glycoprotein (triadin). *J Biol Chem* 268:12646, 1993.
116. Marty I, Robert M, Ronjat M, et al: Localization of the N-terminal and C-terminal ends of triadin with respect to the sarcoplasmic reticulum membrane of rabbit skeletal muscle. *Biochem J* 307:769, 1995.
117. Fan H, Brandt NR, Peng M, et al: Binding sites of monoclonal antibodies and dihydropyridine receptor alpha 1 subunit cytoplasmic II-III loop on skeletal muscle triadin fusion peptides. *Biochemistry* 34:14893, 1995.

118. Brandt NR, Caswell AH, Brunschwig J-P, et al: Effects of anti-triadin antibody on Ca^{2+} release from sarcoplasmic reticulum. *FEBS Lett* 299:57, 1992.
119. Marty I, Thevenon D, Scotto C, et al: Cloning and characterization of a new isoform of skeletal muscle triadin. *J Biol Chem* 275:8206, 2000.
120. Guo W, Jorgensen AO, Jones LR, Campbell KP: Biochemical characterization and molecular cloning of cardiac triadin. *J Biol Chem* 271:458, 1996.
121. Treves S, Feriotto G, Moccagatta L, et al: Molecular cloning, expression, functional characterization, chromosomal localization, and gene structure of junctate, a novel integral calcium binding protein of sarco(endo)plasmic reticulum membrane. *J Biol Chem* 275:39555, 2000.
122. Felder E, Protasi F, Hirsch R, et al: Morphology and molecular composition of sarcoplasmic reticulum surface junctions in the absence of DHPR and RyR in mouse skeletal muscle. *Biophys J* 82:3144, 2002.
123. Takeshima H, Shimuta M, Komazaki S, et al: Mitsugumin29, a novel synaptophysin family member from the triad junction in skeletal muscle. *Biochem J* 331:317, 1998.
124. Takeshima H, Komazaki S, Nishi M, et al: Junctophilins: A novel family of junctional membrane complex proteins. *Mol Cell* 6:11, 2000.
125. Nishi M, Komazaki S, Kurebayashi N, et al: Abnormal features in skeletal muscle from mice lacking mitsugumin29. *J Cell Biol* 147:1473, 1999.
126. Ito K, Komazaki S, Sasamoto K, et al: Deficiency of triad junction and contraction in mutant skeletal muscle lacking junctophilin type 1. *J Cell Biol* 154:1059, 2001.
127. Adams BA, Tanabe T, Mikami A, et al: Intramembrane charge movement restored in dysgenic skeletal muscle by injection of dihydropyridine receptor cDNAs. *Nature* 346:569, 1990.
128. Tanabe T, Mikami A, Numa S, Beam KG: Cardiac-type excitation-contraction coupling in dysgenic muscle injected with cardiac dihydropyridine receptor cDNA. *Nature* 344:451, 1990.
129. Nakai J, Dirksen RT, Nguyen HT, et al: Enhanced dihydropyridine receptor channel activity in the presence of ryanodine receptor. *Nature* 380:72–75, 1996.
130. Nakai J, Ogura T, Protasi F, et al: Functional nonequality of the cardiac and skeletal ryanodine receptors. *Proc Natl Acad Sci USA* 94:1019, 1997.
131. Tanabe T, Beam KG, Adams BA, et al: Regions of the skeletal muscle dihydropyridine receptor critical for excitation-contraction coupling. *Nature* 346:567, 1990.
132. Nakai J, Tanabe T, Konno T, et al: Localization in the II-III loop of the dihydropyridine receptor of a sequence critical for excitation-contraction coupling. *J Biol Chem* 273:24983, 1998.
133. Grabner M, Dirksen RT, Suda N, Beam KG: The II-III loop of the skeletal muscle dihydropyridine receptor is responsible for the bi-directional coupling with the ryanodine receptor. *J Biol Chem* 274:21913, 1999.
134. Lu X, Xu L, Meissner G: Activation of the skeletal muscle calcium release channel by a cytoplasmic loop of the dihydropyridine receptor. *J Biol Chem* 269:6511, 1994.
135. Lu X, Xu L, Meissner G: Phosphorylation of dihydropyridine receptor II-III loop peptide regulates skeletal muscle calcium release channel function. Evidence for an essential role of the β-OH group of Ser687. *J Biol Chem* 270:18459, 1995.
136. El-Hayek R, Antoniu B, Wang J, et al: Identification of calcium release-triggering and blocking regions of the II-III loop of the skeletal muscle dihydropyridine receptor. *J Biol Chem* 270:22116, 1995.
137. El-Hayek R, Ikemoto N: Identification of the minimum essential region in the II-III loop of the dihydropyridine receptor α1 subunit required for activation of skeletal muscle-type excitation-contraction coupling. *Biochemistry* 37:7015, 1998.
138. Gurrola GB, Arévalo C, Sreekumar R, et al: Activation of ryanodine receptors by imperatoxin A and a peptide segment of the II-III loop, the dihydropyridine receptor. *J Biol Chem* 274:7879, 1999.
139. Zhu X, Gurrola G, Jiang MT, et al: Conversion of an inactive cardiac dihydropyridine receptor II-III loop segment into forms that activate skeletal ryanodine receptors. *FEBS Lett* 450:221, 1999.
140. Proenza C, Wilkens CM, Beam KG: Excitation-contraction coupling is not affected by scrambled sequence in residues 681-690 of the dihydropyridine receptor II-III loop. *J Biol Chem* 275:29935, 2000.
141. Wilkens CM, Kasielke N, Flucher BE, et al: Excitation-contraction coupling is unaffected by drastic alteration of the sequence surrounding residues L720-L764 of the α_{1S} II-III loop. *Proc Natl Acad Sci USA* 98:5892, 2001.
142. Ahern CA, Arikkath J, Vallejo P, et al: Intramembrane charge movements and excitation–contraction coupling expressed by two-domain fragments of the Ca^{2+} channel. *Proc Natl Acad Sci USA* 98:6935, 2001.
143. Saiki Y, El-Hayek R, Ikemoto N: Involvement of the Glu724-Pro760 region of the dihydropyridine receptor II-III loop in skeletal muscle-type excitation-contraction coupling. *J Biol Chem* 274:7825, 1999.
144. Stange M, Tripathy A, Meissner G: Two domains in dihydropyridine receptor activate the skeletal muscle Ca^{2+} release channel. *Biophys J* 81:1419, 2001.
145. Yamamoto T, Rodriguez J, Ikemoto N: Ca^{2+}-dependent dual functions of peptide C. The peptide corresponding to the Glu724-Pro760 region (the so-called determinant of excitation-contraction coupling) of the dihydropyridine receptor alpha 1 subunit II-III loop. *J Biol Chem* 277:993, 2002.
146. Haarmann CC, Green D, Casarotto MG, et al: The random-coil 'C' fragment of the dihydropyridine receptor II-III loop can activate or inhibit native skeletal ryanodine receptors. *Biochem J* 372:305, 2003.
147. Nakai J, Sekiguchi N, Rando T, et al: Two regions of the ryanodine receptor involved in coupling with L-type Ca^{2+} channels. *J Biol Chem* 273:13403, 1998.
148. Proenza C, O'Brien JJ, Nakai J, et al: Identification of a region of RyR1 that participates in allosteric coupling with the α_{1s} ($Ca_V1.1$) II-III loop. *J Biol Chem* 277:6530, 2002.
149. Perez CF, Voss AN, Pessah IN, Allen PD: RyR1/RyR3 chimeras reveal that multiple domains of RyR1 are involved in skeletal-type E-C coupling. *Biophys J* 84:2655, 2003.
150. Protasi F, Paolini C, Nakai J, et al: Two separate regions of RyR1 participate in the functional and structural interactions with DHPRs that allow skeletal type e-c coupling. *Biophys J* 83:3230, 2002.
151. Marty I, Robert M, Villaz M, et al: Biochemical evidence for a complex involving dihydropyridine receptor and ryanodine receptor in triad junctions of skeletal muscle. *Proc Natl Acad Sci USA* 91:2270, 1994.
151a. Wilkens CH, Kasielke N, Flucher BE, et al: Excitation-contraction coupling is unaffected by drastic alterations of the sequence surrounding residues L720-L764 of the alpha1's II-III loop. *Proc Natl Acad Sci USA* 98:5892, 2001.
152. Leong P, MacLennan DH: A 37-amino acid sequence in the skeletal muscle ryanodine receptor interacts with the cytoplasmic loop between domains II and III in the skeletal muscle dihydropyridine receptor. *J Biol Chem* 273:7791, 1998.
153. Leong P, MacLennan DH: The cytoplasmic loops between domains II and III and domains III and IV in the skeletal muscle dihydropyridine receptor bind to a contiguous site in the skeletal muscle ryanodine receptor. *J Biol Chem* 273:29958, 1998.
154. Monnier N, Procaccio V, Stieglitz P, Lunardi J: Malignant-hyperthermia susceptibility is associated with a mutation of the alpha1-subunit of the human dihydropyridine-sensitive L-type voltage-dependent calcium-channel receptor in skeletal muscle. *Am J Hum Genet* 60:1316, 1997.
155. Slavik KJ, Wang J-P, Aghdasi B, et al: A carboxyl-terminal peptide of the α_1-subunit of the dihydropyridine receptor inhibits Ca^{2+}-release channels. *Am J Physiol* 272:C1475, 1997.
156. Mouton J, Ronjat M, Jona I, et al: Skeletal and cardiac ryanodine receptors bind to the Ca^{2+}-sensor region of dihydropyridine receptor alpha(1C) subunit. *FEBS Lett* 505:441, 2001.
157. Sencer S, Papineni RV, Halling DB, et al: Coupling of RYR1 and L-type calcium channels via calmodulin binding domains. *J Biol Chem* 276:38237, 2001.
158. Beurg M, Ahern CA, Vallejo P, et al: Involvement of the carboxy-terminus region of the dihydropyridine receptor beta1a subunit in excitation-contraction coupling of skeletal muscle. *Biophys J* 77:2953, 1999.
159. Ahern CA, Sheridan DC, Cheng W, et al: Ca^{2+} current and charge movements in skeletal myotubes promoted by the β-subunit of the dihydropyridine receptor in the absence of ryanodine receptor type 1. *Biophys J* 84:942, 2003.
160. Sheridan DC, Cheng W, Ahern CA, et al: Truncation of the carboxyl terminus of the dihydropyridine receptor β1a subunit promotes Ca^{2+} dependent excitation-contraction coupling in skeletal myotubes. *Biophys J* 84:220, 2003.
161. Flucher BE, Weiss RG, Grabner M: Cooperation of two-domain Ca^{2+} channel fragments in triad targeting and restoration of excitation-contraction coupling in skeletal muscle. *Proc Natl Acad Sci USA* 99:10167, 2002.
162. Ahern CA, Bhattacharya D, Mortenson L, Coronado R: A component of excitation-contraction coupling triggered in the absence of the T671-L690 and L720-Q765 regions of the II-III loop of the dihydropyridine receptor α_{1S} pore subunit. *Biophys J* 81:3294, 2001.

Chapter 13
Activation of the Contractile Mechanism by Calcium

SAMUEL VICTOR PERRY

Development of Ideas on the Role of Calcium in Muscle Contraction
  WHOLE INTACT CELLS
  ISOLATED CONTRACTILE SYSTEMS

Special Features of the Magnesium-Activated Actomyosin–Adenosine Triphosphatase System That Enable Its Regulation

Calcium Transients in Muscle

Calcium-Binding Proteins of Muscle

Thin- (I-) Filament Regulation
  TROPOMYOSIN
  TROPONIN COMPLEX
  TROPONIN C
  TROPONIN I
  TROPONIN T

Phosphorylation of the Regulatory Proteins of the Thin Filament of the Myofibril
  TROPOMYOSIN
  TROPONIN I
  TROPONIN T

Thick- (A-) Filament Regulation
  THE LIGHT CHAINS OF MYOSIN
  PHOSPHORYLATION OF THE REGULATORY LIGHT CHAINS
  STRIATED MUSCLE
  VERTEBRATE SMOOTH MUSCLE
  MOLLUSCAN ADDUCTOR MUSCLE

Myosin-Binding Protein C

Parvalbumins

Chromosome Locations of Genes Expressing Regulatory Proteins of the Thin Filaments
  MUTATIONS OF THE REGULATORY PROTEINS

Overview and Concluding Comments

It is now widely accepted that contraction in muscle is a consequence of the activation of the actomyosin adenosine triphosphatase (ATPase) of the contractile structures. This results in the rapid cross-bridge cycling process responsible for tension development (see Chap. 9). Activation of the actomyosin ATPase occurs in all types of striated or smooth muscles when the sarcoplasmic calcium concentration rises from the resting level of approximately 10^{-7} to 10^{-5} M. The rise in intracellular Ca^{2+} concentration follows from its rapid release from intracellular stores, such as the sarcoplasmic reticulum in striated muscle (see Chaps. 11 and 14), which occurs very soon after a stimulus reaches the cell membrane.

This chapter reviews the current understanding of the role of Ca^{2+} in the activation of the actomyosin Mg ATPase. Actomyosin systems in all types of muscle are remarkably similar, and the differences in muscle properties in part depend on the variety of mechanisms that exist for the initiation and modulation of the contractile process. Emphasis is on skeletal muscle, but some discussion of the mechanisms of regulation in other muscle types is necessary to understand the general principles involved in the regulation of the contractile response.

Development of Ideas on the Role of Calcium in Muscle Contraction

WHOLE INTACT CELLS

The first clear indication that Ca^{2+} had a special significance for contraction in the intact muscle fiber was the observation by Kamada and Kinosita[1] that microinjection of solutions containing Ca^{2+} into single fibers of the bicep muscles of frog was more effective than those containing Mg^{2+} in inducing contraction. Independently, similar observations were reported in a more detailed study by Heilbrun and Wiercinski.[2] Since these early studies, an impressive weight of evidence using a variety of techniques involving the use of calcium-sensitive indicators and photoproteins[3-5] has confirmed that on stimulation, the free Ca^{2+} concentration in the muscle cell rises from a resting level of 10^{-7} to 10^{-5} M at the height of contraction.

ISOLATED CONTRACTILE SYSTEMS

Studies on whole cells, however, do not readily yield details about the molecular mechanisms involved in the regulation of contraction. With the development of model contractile systems—such as actomyosin gels and fibers, myofibrils, glycerated fibers, skinned fibers, and more recently reconstituted filaments in motility assays—it has become possible to study tension development with the actomyosin system in a precisely defined environment.

Using such systems, it was demonstrated that a clear correlation exists between tension development and Mg ATPase activity, and attempts were made with them to simulate a complete contractile cycle, i.e., contraction followed by relaxation. The early work, which is reviewed elsewhere,[6,7] in general indicated that relaxation occurred in the model systems when the rate of ATP hydrolysis fell. In these early studies this occurred as a consequence of substrate inhibition obtained by direct addition of the nucleotide itself or by the action of systems such as myokinase or creatine kinase that regenerated the ATP. Relaxation was also obtained in the presence of enzyme inhibitors such as mersalyl and, significantly, on the addition of metal chelators. Early observations were those of Bozler[8] and Watanabe,[9] who reported that relaxation of glycerated fibers could be obtained under conditions in which they would otherwise contract, by the addition of low concentrations of ethylenediaminetetraacetic acid (EDTA).*

---

*A list of abbreviations used in this chapter is given at the end of the chapter.

The special role of Ca^{2+} in the regulation of the ATPase of actomyosin was indicated by the demonstration by Perry and Grey[10] that the Mg ATPase of myofibrils was dramatically inhibited by EDTA at concentrations less than 10% of that of the Mg^{2+} in the system. This implied that it was the removal of low levels of Ca^{2+} and not Mg^{2+} ions from the system that produced inhibition. The first use of EGTA (originally known as glycol complexon), a chelator with a higher affinity for calcium than magnesium, to produce inhibition of the ATPase of myofibrils and crude preparations of actomyosin confirmed that this indeed was the case.[11] Subsequent careful investigations by Weber[12,13] showed that 10^{-6} to 10^{-5} M Ca^{2+} was required for activation of the Mg ATPase and for superprecipitation of crude actomyosin systems and myofibrils.

In parallel with these studies, other investigators examined the nature of the fraction from muscle that produced relaxation effects in muscle preparations more comparable to the intact fiber. The early observation of Bozler,[14] that long-stored and well-washed glycerated fibers lost the ability to relax while their contractile ability remained unimpaired, suggested the existence of a labile relaxing factor. The first clear indication of the presence of such a factor came from the investigation of Marsh,[15] who demonstrated that a supernatant fraction from rabbit muscle homogenate caused the crude myofibrillar fraction of rabbit muscle to relax in the presence of ATP. If this fraction was removed from a muscle homogenate by centrifugation and washing, the subsequent addition of ATP to the crude myofibrillar residues produced the normal contractile response. These experiments clearly indicated that ATP had a role in both the contractile and the relaxation processes.

The fact that relaxation could be induced by a variety of conditions that reduced the Mg ATPase activity stimulated a large number of differing claims regarding the nature of the factor involved. The first report identifying it with the particulate component of the muscle supernatant was that of Kumagi et al.[16] Subsequently, it was shown that the relaxing activity is associated with the sarcoplasmic reticulum (SR), which contains an active calcium pump that is able to reduce the Ca^{2+} concentrations of the sarcoplasm below that required for activation of the Mg ATPase of myofibrils.[17,18] The early work on the calcium-sequestrating properties of the SR are reviewed in detail elsewhere,[19,20] and the current status is discussed in Chap. 14 of this volume.

By 1960 it was clear that the Mg ATPase of myofibrils and crude preparations of actomyosin required traces of calcium for high activity. Reduction of the Ca^{2+} concentration to <10^{-7} M reduced the ATPase to a low level and induced relaxation. The earlier observations that the Mg ATPase of actomyosin reconstituted from purified actin and myosin was not sensitive to calcium[11] implied that myofibrils and crude actomyosin preparations contained some factor or factors that were necessary to sensitize the actomyosin Mg ATPase to calcium. In 1963, Ebashi[21] reported the isolation of a protein fraction from muscle with just these properties. This fraction was very similar to tropomyosin in chemical and physical properties; he named it "natural" tropomyosin to distinguish it from the preparations of tropomyosin isolated by Bailey,[22] which did not possess the ability to sensitize the actomyosin Mg ATPase to Ca^{2+}. Ebashi and Kodama[23] subsequently showed that the so-called natural tropomyosin consisted of tropomyosin and a new protein, which they named troponin, and that both components were essential for Ca^{2+} regulation of the Mg ATPase of skeletal muscle actomyosin.

Special Features of the Magnesium-Activated Actomyosin–Adenosine Triphosphatase System That Enable Its Regulation

The ability of skeletal muscle to develop a high tension in a matter of milliseconds is a consequence of the activation process producing a several hundredfold increase in the rate of ATP hydrolysis over a very short time interval—a situation that is unique in biology. The enzymic properties of myosin have evolved to accommodate these requirements. In resting or contracting muscle, virtually all the substrate for the ATPase is Mg ATP^{2-}, with the free Mg^{2+} concentration being of the order of 1 to 2 mM. Whereas with most enzymes that act on ATP the magnesium complex is a good substrate, this is not the case with pure myosin in the ionic conditions found in the cell. On the other hand, Ca ATP^{2-} is hydrolyzed rapidly by myosin, but it is not a significant substrate in living muscle, as a negligible proportion of the total intracellular ATP will exist in this form even in stimulated muscle.

The fact that in the purified protein system myosin does not become an effective enzyme for the hydrolysis of Mg ATP^{2-} unless actin is present implies that the interaction with this protein in some way, presumably by inducing a conformational change in myosin, modifies the enzymic properties of the molecule. In the absence of other myofibrillar proteins, the Mg ATPase of striated muscle myosin is fully activated by actin in the absence of calcium. The two proteins are in close proximity in adjacent filaments in resting intact muscle, but because of the presence of the regulatory proteins the interaction causing activation of the enzyme does not take place until the Ca^{2+} concentration rises to 10^{-6}–10^{-5} M. The function of the regulatory systems of muscle is to prevent this interaction at low Ca^{2+} concentrations but to facilitate it when the concentration rises. Thus, in the absence of Ca^{2+}, the regulatory protein system of the thin filament in striated muscle acts as an inhibitor of the actomyosin Mg ATPase.

The protein components of the intracellular regulatory systems of muscle and the effects of calcium on them are, particularly in the case of the striated tissue, quite well defined. Nevertheless, the precise way in which they modulate the actin-myosin interaction in striated muscle is still a matter for discussion, although it is clear that troponin and tropomyosin have important roles in this process. The high-resolution structures for both actin and the head of the myosin molecule, myosin subfragment 1 (S1), are known, but a description at the atomic level of the structure of the actomyosin complex in the absence of the regulatory proteins, when it would exhibit high Mg ATPase activity, is not yet available. As yet it has not been possible to produce crystals of the actomyosin complex to enable the atomic structure of actin-myosin interface to be determined by x-ray crystallography. With some uncertainty regarding the regions on the actin and myosin molecules involved in the interaction, the effects of binding on their conformations, and the current lack of a high-resolution atomic structure of the troponin complex, it is not yet possible to explain in precise molecular terms the mode of action of the complex in modulating the interaction.

Probable regions of interaction between actin and myosin can be deduced from a variety of approaches, in particular modeling studies on the atomic structures of the components, cross-linking studies, use of mutants, nuclear magnetic resonance (NMR) studies, etc. (for review and references, see Milligan[24]). It is clear that the interactions between actin and myosin that lead to activation of the Mg ATPase are extensive and complex. It appears that the myosin head spans the junction between two actin monomers in the long-pitch helix of the actin filament. The binding site seems to be centered on hydrophobic interactions involving helices on the actin and myosin surfaces. Around the presumed main binding site on myosin there are loops, which could provide ionic interactions with residues on the actin monomer surface (see Chaps. 7, 8, and 9).

A further aspect to our understanding of the actin-myosin interaction and its regulation is provided by comparing the regulation of contraction in striated and smooth muscles. The similarity of the amino acid sequences and structures of the actin and myosin isoforms present in the two types of muscle strongly suggests that the nature of their interaction and the mechanism of activation of the Mg ATPase are very similar.

Nevertheless, the regulation of the activation of the Mg ATPase in the two types of muscle is fundamentally different. Striated muscle is regulated mainly through the actin filament, involving the troponin complex, whereas vertebrate smooth muscle, from which troponin is absent, is regulated principally via phosphorylation of the myosin filament.

Calcium Transients in Muscle

One of the distinguishing features of the different muscle types is the speed of their response to stimulation, with the time to maximum tension ranging from a few milliseconds in the fastest skeletal muscle up to seconds in the slowest smooth muscle types. This range of response is reflected in the pattern of the calcium transients observed on stimulation of the different muscle types (Fig. 13-1). In all cases the intracellular calcium concentration, as indicated by the signals from the probes, rises before force develops; nevertheless, force persists, although declining, in all cases even when the intracellular calcium concentration has returned to the resting level.

The form of the calcium transient after stimulation of muscle will depend on the ability of the SR to release calcium into the sarcoplasm and pump it back into the cisternae and the calcium buffering powers of the sarcoplasm and myofibril. The local activation experiments of Huxley and Taylor[28] established that activation of contraction originates at the

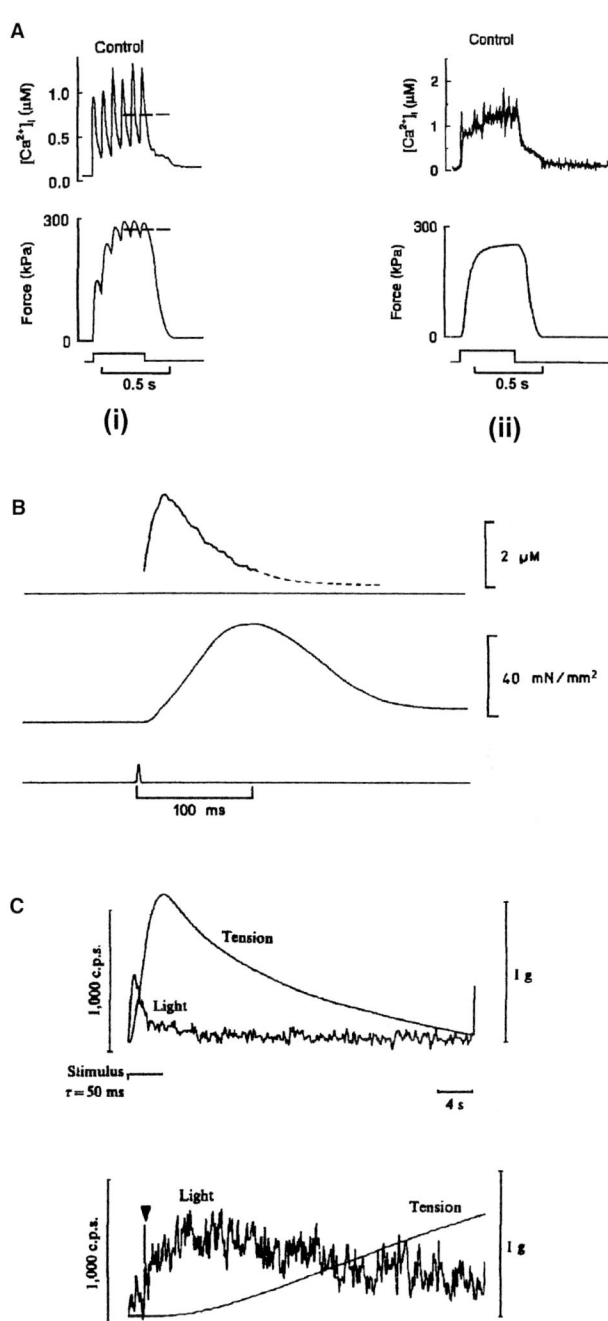

FIGURE 13-1. Calcium transients in different muscle types: A. Skeletal muscle, (i) type I fiber, (ii) type II fiber. Data presented obtained with *Xenopus* muscle at 22°C, although very similar results are obtained with mouse muscle. Ca^{2+} indicator aequorin. *(From Westerblad H, Lannergren J, Allen DG: Slowed relaxation in fatigued skeletal muscle of Xenopus and Mouse. J Gen Physiol 109:385–399, 1997. With permission.)* B. Cardiac muscle. Rat trabeculae at 30°C. Aequorin indicator. Upper curve $[Ca^{2+}]$, lower curve tension. *(From Allen DG, Kurihara S: Calcium transients in mammalian ventricular muscle. Eur Heart J 1(Suppl A):5–15, 1980. With permission.)* C. Smooth muscle. Dog antraval circular smooth muscle at 32 to 35°C. Short-term stimulus (lower figure) compared with long-term stimulus (upper figure). Aequorin indicator. *(From Neering IR, Morgan KG: Use of aequorin to study excitation-contraction coupling in mammalian smooth muscle. Nature 288:285–287, 1980. With permission.)*

level of the Z line in frog skeletal muscle. By introducing into the muscle cell probes such as indo-1, fura-2, Asenazo III, fluoro 3, furaptra, aequorin, etc., which exhibit fluorescence changes on binding to free Ca^{2+}, it is possible to estimate the amount of calcium liberated and demonstrate that in striated muscle Ca^{2+} release from the SR is initiated by depolarization of the t-tubule system (see Ref. 29 for details of earlier literature and the use of computer simulations to estimate the flux of Ca^{2+} between the SR and the myoplasm). Depolarization of the tubular system is sensed by a dihydropyridine receptor, and calcium release takes place through channels in the ryanodine receptor (for reviews, see Refs. 30 and 31). In skeletal muscle, the site of excitation contraction coupling is generally accepted to be at the specialized junctions known as triads between the terminal cisternae of the SR and the t-tubule membrane (for review, see Ref. 32). It was therefore postulated that all the release of Ca^{2+} occurred at the triads close to the Z lines, thus producing a Ca^{2+} gradient along the myofibril to the M-line region. Escobar et al.[33] reported, however, that the initial increase of Ca^{2+} at the M line was not significantly delayed with respect to that at the Z line; they proposed that release of Ca^{2+} occurred along the whole length of the SR. Reexamination of this problem by Hollingworth et al.[34] with frog skeletal muscle fibers imaged with confocal and two-photo microscopy produced no experimental evidence for Ca^{2+} release other than at the Z lines. These authors showed that the peak Ca^{2+} level was within 0.1 μm of the Z line and rose to almost 0.1 mM in 2 ms, whereas the rise in Ca^{2+} concentration at the M line was nearly two orders of magnitude smaller and occurred with a significant delay.

Despite the variation in muscle speed, the systems releasing, pumping, and binding Ca^{2+} in striated muscle regulation are essentially similar in structure. The characteristics of the muscle transients are the consequence of the quantity and quality of the proteins involved in the interaction with calcium, which are unique for each muscle type. Fast-twitch muscle fibers contain more SR containing the "fast" calcium pump SERCA1 and more calcium release units than slow-twitch muscle fibers (see Chaps. 11 and 14). This increases their capacity to release and pump Ca^{2+} from the sarcoplasm. In slow-twitch muscle, the calcium pump is replaced with the less effective isoform SERCA2 and calcium release units are less frequent. Outstanding examples of specialization occur in vertebrate sound-producing muscles such as the swimbladder muscle of the toadfish and the shaker muscles of the rattlesnake,[35] which operate at frequencies much higher than fast locomotory muscles, often exceeding 100 Hz. In the fast synchronous muscle of the toadfish swimbladder, where each release of calcium is followed by contraction and relaxation, the density of the SR is a high fraction (about 0.3) of the fiber volume. The amount of parvalbumin also increases in the sarcoplasm of certain fast skeletal muscles, thereby increasing the Ca^{2+} buffering power of the sarcoplasm and and the speed of relaxation. Differences in the Ca^{2+} response between muscle types are also a consequence of the presence of muscle type–specific isoforms of the protein components of the myofibrillar regulatory system (see later).

Although the form of the calcium transients in different muscle types is fairly well documented, much is still to be learned about the factors that control them. For example, in addition to "global calcium transients" involving thousands of calcium release channels normally involved in activation of contraction, localized release of calcium involving one or a few channels, or "calcium sparks," can also occur. There is evidence that contractile activation in skeletal muscle fibers may involve more than one type of calcium release channel present in the junctional cisternae of the SR, one strictly under the control of membrane potential, the other not. In skeletal muscle, more than one isoform of the ryanodine receptor is present, and structural evidence indicates that not all ryanodine receptors are in close apposition with the dihydropyridine receptors. This suggests that some of the release channels are not under the direct control of the voltage sensors. Calcium itself exhibits feedback properties that presumably are of functional importance. Depending on conditions and muscle type, calcium can have a role in both the inactivation and the induction of calcium release (see Ref. 36 for a review of the factors controlling calcium release).

Calcium-Binding Proteins of Muscle

Any contractile system activated by Ca^{2+} must contain target proteins possessing binding sites that become filled when the Ca^{2+} concentration rises to 10^{-5} M and rapidly lose their calcium when the concentration falls on relaxation. To be effective, such target proteins must bind Ca^{2+} specifically with binding constants in the range of 10^8 to 10^6 M in the presence of Mg^{2+} and K^+ that in muscle cells are at millimolar and decimolar concentrations, respectively.

Three proteins with high affinities for Ca^{2+} that play important roles in the regulation of muscle contraction have so far been identified (Table 13-1). Troponin C (TnC) occurs in striated muscle as the calcium-binding protein component of the troponin complex; the current view is that, at least in vertebrates, it is restricted to striated muscle. On the other hand, calmodulin, an essential component of the myosin light-chain kinase system found in all muscles, is a widely distributed protein involved in a number of other systems in which calcium has a regulatory role. In smooth muscle, where it is of special significance for the regulation of contraction, the amounts of calmodulin are much higher than in skeletal muscle. Parvalbumin is not involved directly in the activation process but may have a modulatory role (see later). Although principally found in muscle cells, parvalbumin also occurs in certain neuronal cells, acting as a slow calcium buffer that may affect the amplitude and time course of intracellular calcium transients after an action potential and hence regulate short-term synaptic plasticity.[37]

The divalent metal-binding properties of vertebrate myosin II are considered to be due to the light chains in the skeletal muscle myosin head. Examination of the amino acid sequences of these light chains indicates that they possess presumptive calcium/magnesium-binding sites. They are, therefore, included in the family of calcium-binding proteins,[38] as they are considered to have evolved from the same primitive gene as the other three proteins listed in Table 13-1. Nevertheless, when separated from myosin, the calcium-

Chapter 13. Activation of the Contractile Mechanism by Calcium

Table 13-1. CALCIUM-BINDING PROTEINS OF SPECIAL SIGNIFICANCE FOR THE REGULATION OF CONTRACTILE ACTIVITY IN MUSCLE

Protein	Molecular Weight	Cell concentration, μM Skeletal	Smooth	No. Sites	Specificity	K_A, M^{-1}	K_{on}, $M^{-1}s^{-1}$	K_{off}, $M^{-1}s^{-1}$
Troponin C[a]								
Skeletal	18000	70	—	2 (I, II)	Ca (specific)	5×10^6	1.15×10^8	23.0
				2 (III, IV)	Ca	5×10^8	3.0×10^8	0.6
					Mg	5×10^4	1×10^{5b}	2.0
Cardiac	18000	70	—	1(II)	Ca (specific)	2×10^6	3.9×10^7	19.6
				2 (III, IV)	Ca	3×10^8	1×10^8	0.3
					Mg	3×10^5	1×10^{5b}	3.3
Calmodulin	16700	3	15–30	4	Ca (specific)	4.2×10^5	1×10^{8b}	238
Parvalbumin	9000–13000	6000	—	2	Ca	2.5×10^8	2.5×10^8	1.0
					Mg	1.1×10^4	6.6×10^4	6.0
Myosin regulatory light chain	18000–20000	400	100–150	1[c]	Ca, Mg	Low		

[a] The affinity of the calcium-specific sites of isolated skeletal and cardiac troponin C is 10 times lower than it is in troponin. Interaction with troponin I increases the affinity of troponin C for Ca^{2+}. (K_A values from Potter et al, 1980[36a], with permission.)
[b] K_{on} was assumed to be 10^8 $M^{-1}s^{-1}$ for Ca^{2+} and 10^5 $M^{-1}s^{-1}$ for Mg^{2+} whenever measurements of K_{off} were not available. In all cases the relation $K_A = K_{on}/K_{off}$ is used to calculate K_{on}. Figures for mammalian muscle (usually rabbit) except for parvalbumin, which is for carp.
[c] The RLCs and ELCs of myosins all fold into dumbell shape with two rudimentary helix-loop-helix structural motifs in each half of the molecule. In all RLCs, site I has retained the ability to bind metal ions. This is most likely to be occupied by Mg^{2+} in vivo (daSilva and Reinach, 1991, Fig. 13-14).

binding constants of the light chains of myosin are quite low compared with those exhibited by the other three proteins listed in Table 13-1.

It is of particular interest that although the essential light chains (ELCs) and regulatory light chains (RLCs) individually have low calcium affinities, the presumptive binding site on the ELC of molluscan adductor myosin becomes a site of high affinity that regulates contraction when stabilized by interactions with residues in the RLC and the heavy chain of intact adductor muscle myosin [see "Thick- (A-) Filament Regulation," below].

There are two main mechanisms for calcium regulation of contraction in muscle: (1) thin or I-filament regulation, which is characteristic of striated muscle and mediated through TnC, and (2) thick- or A-filament regulation, which involves the light chains of myosin and with which calmodulin may or may not, depending on the muscle type, be involved. Calmodulin is essential for activation by calcium of the kinase responsible for the phosphorylation of the myosin RLC, which is particularly important for activation of vertebrate smooth muscle but may also play a modulating role in striated muscle.

Thin- (I-) Filament Regulation

The two myofibrillar components of the major regulatory system in striated muscle, tropomyosin and the troponin complex, are located in the I filament. Figure 13-2 represents a simplified scheme of the structural unit which, assuming the thin filament has a length of 1 μm, occurs as two parallel sequences each of about 26 such units, anchored to the Z membrane of the myofibril. The continuity of the filament is provided by the double helical array of actin monomers stabilized by tropomyosin molecules longitudinally polymerized by head-to-tail interactions and lying in each of the two grooves of the actin filament (Figs. 13-2 and 13-8). The calcium-binding protein of the troponin complex, TnC, is located with the troponin complex along each filament at a periodicity of 38.5 nm, the effective length of the tropo-

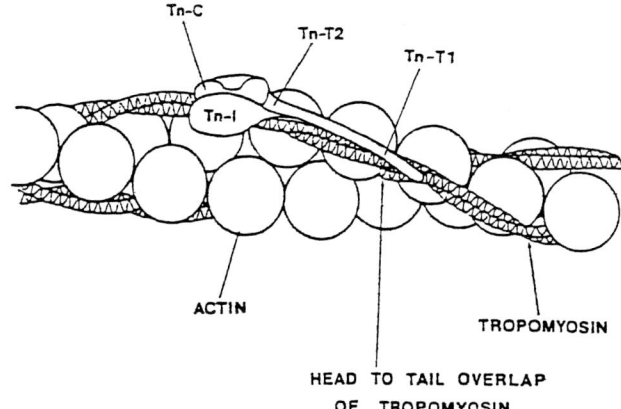

Figure 13-2. Scheme representing the arrangement of the proteins in the thin filament. (See also Color Plate 3e.) TnT extends along about half the length of tropomyosin molecule up to the tropomyosin overlap region, and probably beyond, with the longer cardiac isoform. TnT-T1 and TnT-T2 are the two fragments of TnT (T1 and T2) obtained by chymotryptic digestion of rabbit fast skeletal TnT (see Fig. 13-4). (From Ohtsuki I: Molecular arrangement of troponin T on the thin filament. Biochemistry 86:491, 1979. With permission.) TnC interacts with TnI and both are associated with the C-terminal region of TnT-T2 which is located more centrally along the tropomyosin molecule. (After Heeley DH, Golosinska K, Smillie LB: The effects of troponin T fragments T1 and T2 on the binding of nonpolymerisable tropomyosin to F actin in the presence and absence of troponin I and troponin C. J Biol Chem 262:9971, 1987. With permission.)

myosin molecule. The structural unit therefore consists of one molecule of tropomyosin, M_r 65000; seven actin monomers, each of M_r 42000, and one unit of the troponin complex, M_r about 72000, the precise value varying slightly depending on the isoforms present in different striated muscle fiber types.

X-ray diffraction and EM studies have described in broad molecular terms, but not in atomic detail, how the actomyosin system relates to the other I-filament proteins, tropomyosin, troponin, and nebulin (see Color Plate 3e). The interrelationships of the troponin components are clearly at the heart of this process, but it has not yet been possible to crystallize the complex to obtain this information by x-ray crystallographic methods. The atomic structure of isolated crystallized TnC is available at 2 Å resolution,[39,40] and some progress has been made on the structure of tropomyosin, which has been obtained at a resolution of 7.5 Å.[41] In the case of tropomyosin, the crystals contain too much water to obtain the resolution required to identify individual amino acid residues by x-ray crystallography. Further insight into the structure of the tropomyosin molecule has been obtained from a 2.0-Å resolution study of crystals of an 81-residue N-terminal recombinant fragment.[42] Structural analysis of crystals of intact complexes of the muscle proteins presents further problems for this approach, because the dynamic nature of contractile function will involve conformational changes and movement of the relevant proteins with respect to each other.

TROPOMYOSIN

Tropomyosin is widely distributed in eukaryotes associated with actin filament systems (for review, see Perry[43]). It is most abundant in striated muscle, where it represents about 3 percent of the total protein, for actin filaments are major components of the contractile fibers. The tropomyosin molecule consists of two polypeptide subunits, each containing an identical number of amino acids, which are either identical (homodimer) or nonidentical (heterodimer) in amino acid sequence. In humans and probably vertebrates generally, four genes—TPM1, TPM2, TPM3, and TPM4—are responsible for expressing the subunits of tropomyosin. As a consequence of this multigene pool and the action of alternative promoters and alternative splicing, a large number of tropomyosin isoforms occur. Over 20 isoforms, some of which are tissue-specific, have so far been identified in vertebrates and fall into two main groups. These are the high-molecular-weight group of subunits containing 284 to 281 amino acid residues and the low-molecular-weight group containing 245 to 251 residues. The tropomyosins associated with the contractile structures of striated and smooth muscle fall into the high-molecular-weight group.

The subunit chains are 100 percent α-helical and dimerize as a coiled-coil structure[44] to form the tropomyosin molecule (Fig. 13-3). This structure is stabilized by a strip of nonpolar residues running down the sides of each helical subunit. A slight distortion of the α helices enables them to remain in contact, winding round each other to form the coiled coil, stabilized by the so-called knobs and holes packing arrangement. For this to occur, a nonpolar amino acid must occupy approximately every fourth position in the polypeptide. The sequence of tropomyosin can be considered as a repeat heptapeptide, which largely satisfies these requirements. Important features of the tropomyosin molecule that are fundamental for its function in muscle are its ability to interact with F actin to form a complex and its property of aggregating into long fibrous polymers by head-to-tail interactions. As a consequence of the latter property, tropomyosin molecules form a continuous filament extending along the length of each of the two grooves of the actin filaments (see Chap. 7). In the actin filament, one tropomyosin molecule is associated with seven actin monomers (Fig. 13-2), implying that there are seven sites of interaction distributed along the length of the molecule. Although completely identical repeating regions corresponding to such sites are not present in the polypeptide chain, seven quasiequivalent regions of about 40 amino acids characterized by the distribution of polar and nonpolar amino acids can be identified in the muscle tropomyosins. These are considered to correspond to the actin-binding regions and have been modeled to represent half turns in the coiled coil.[45] According to this model, there would be 3½ turns per molecule of tropomyosin in the structural unit. Recent high-resolution x-ray diffraction studies on tropomyosin crystals, however, indicate that there are three turns per molecule.[41] The significance of this discrepancy is

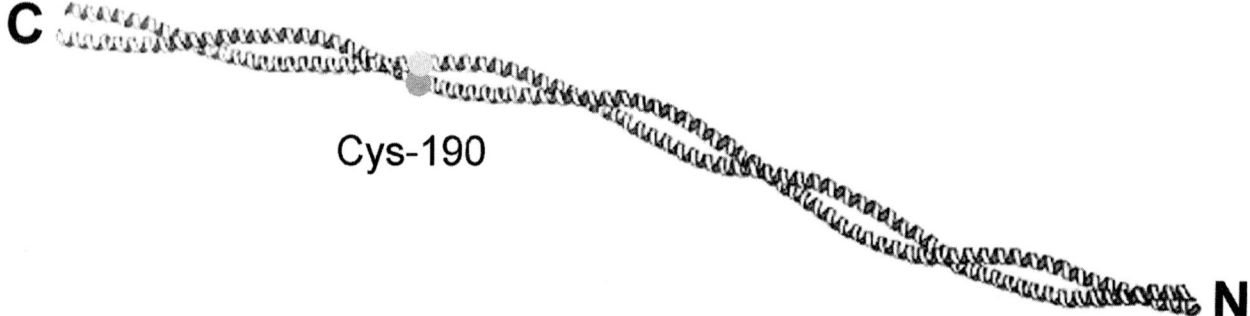

FIGURE 13-3. The α-tropomyosin molecule. Plot at 7 Å resolution of the asymmetrical unit in spermine-induced crystals of α-tropomyosin isolated from porcine ventricles. The gentle bending is similar to that seen in Bailey-type tropomyosin crystals, but the analysis yields local variation in ending angles and radius. Cys 190 is located at similar positions in both subunits as the two polypeptide chains are in register. (From Whitby FG, Phillips GN Jr: Crystal structure of tropomyosin at 7 Å resolution. Proteins 38:49–59, 2000. With permission.)

not clear, but it is possible that the tropomyosin molecule is flexible enough to adapt to the 3½ turns required by the filament model. Although it is usually assumed that α-tropomyosin is a coiled coil structure along the whole of the length of the molecule, recent high resolution studies on peptide fragments have shown that in striated muscle the C-terminal 22 residues do not form a two-stranded coiled coil structure but the helices splay out.[45a] As this conformation is absent from smooth muscle in which troponin is not present, it is suggested that this region is a TnT binding site on tropomyosin.

The major isoforms present in striated muscle are the α- and β-tropomyosin subunits, the products of the TPM1 and TPM2 genes, respectively. The degrees of expression of these genes in a muscle type are affected by a number of factors, such as stage of development, type of innervation, and possibly hormone status,[46] with the result that the relative amounts of α and β subunits vary in the various muscle types. Both subunits, M_r about 33,000, consist of a polypeptide chain of 284 residues but differ in 39 residues. These arise from differences in the regions expressed by exons 2, 6, and 9 (Fig. 13-4) and are mainly conservative, charge differences occurring only at residues 229 and 276.[47,48]

Usually the relative proportions of α tropomyosin are higher in fast skeletal muscle, and skeletal α tropomyosin is the only isoform present in significant amounts in the hearts of small animals. In larger animals β tropomyosin is also found in the heart.[49] When α and β subunits are present in muscle, thermodynamic considerations determine the dimer composition. At physiologic temperatures, the heterodimer, α β, is the preferred form and much of the tropomyosin in striated muscle containing both isoforms is present as the heterodimer. There is some evidence that tropomyosin heterodimers exhibit stronger end-to-end aggregation and bind more strongly to actin.

Although α and β isoforms make up the bulk of tropomyosin in striated muscle, smaller amounts of other isoforms have been reported to be present in some muscles, e.g., the so-called γ and δ tropomyosins, reported particularly in slow-twitch muscles.[50] It is possible that these are products of the TPM3 gene, which is known to be expressed as tropomyosin 3 or slow α tropomyosin, found in adult heart and skeletal muscle of humans. In small animals, such as the rat and rabbit, this isoform is restricted to skeletal muscle, principally to slow-twitch fibers.[51] Tropomyosin from smooth muscles is composed largely of roughly similar amounts of two isoforms known as smooth muscle α and β tropomyosins, as they are also derived from the TPM1 and TPM2 genes, respectively. Although the smooth muscle isoforms are of exactly the same polypeptide chain length, 284 residues, like their skeletal equivalents they are not identical in amino acid sequence as they are produced by a different splicing procedure.

TROPONIN COMPLEX

Unlike tropomyosin, troponin is unique to striated muscle and is the regulatory system that has evolved to control the actomyosin ATPase in that tissue and initiate the cross-bridge cycle to produce an extremely rapid rise in tension. In vertebrate smooth muscle, which has no troponin, the myosin responsible for the mechanochemical process has to be primed by phosphorylation before actin can activate the Mg ATPase. This is a relatively slow process with restricted possibilities for cooperative effects due to the spacing of the

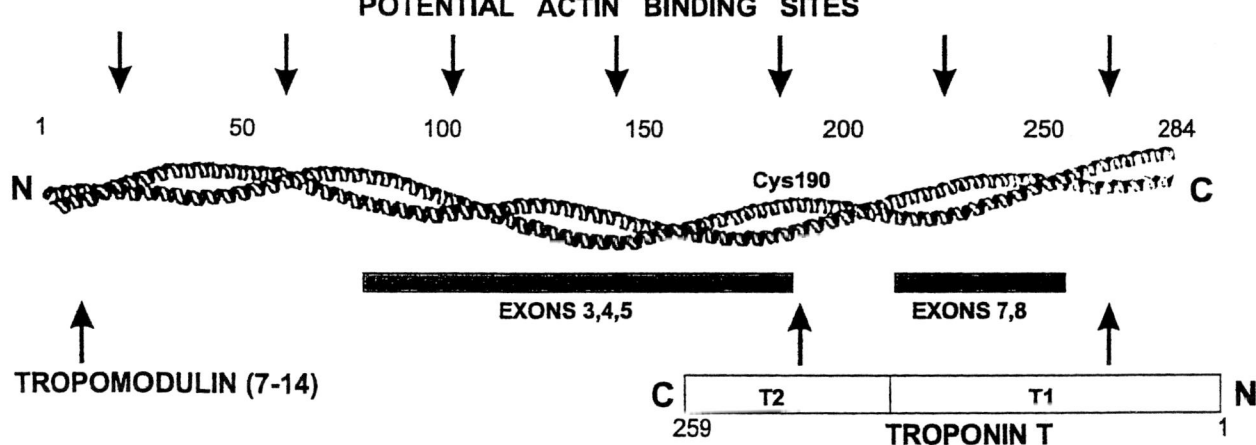

FIGURE 13-4. Scheme illustrating interactions of striated muscle α-tropomyosin with thin-filament proteins. TM molecule as determined by Whitby and Phillips illustrating irregularities in the coiled coil observed in tropomyosin crystals. (From Whitby FG, Phillips GN Jr: Crystal structure of tropomyosin at 7 Å resolution. Proteins 38:49–59, 2000. With permission.) Numbers indicate positions of amino acid residues. N and C are the amino and carboxyl terminals, respectively. Shaded blocks represent regions of exons that are invariant in all tropomyosin isoforms. The binding site illustrated for erythrocyte tropomodulin on human tropomyosin 5 is in a region of strongly conserved tropomyosin isoforms. T1 and T2 represent the chymotryptic fragments of TnT (Otsuki[104]). The binding site for caldesmon is not indicated, as this protein is absent from striated muscle. In smooth muscle a major site has been identified between residues 142 and 227 of tropomyosin with the suggestion of a weaker site at the N-terminus, residues 11 to 127. (Watson et al., J Biol Chem 265:18860, 1990.[46a]) It appears that in striated muscle these regions is at least in part occupied by other proteins. (From Perry SV: Vertebrate tropomyosin: Distribution, properties and function. J Muscle Res Cell Motil 22:5–49, 2001. With permission.)

functional region of the myosin molecule at 14.3 nm along the thick-filament separation. In striated muscle, the myosin is in a form that is instantly activated without covalent modification once it interacts with actin. The troponin in association with tropomyosin in the I filament enables all the actin monomers in the thin filament simultaneously to be rendered able to interact with myosin and activate the Mg ATPase. This occurs when calcium is bound to a molecule of TnC, located every 38.5 nm along the I filament. It is a matter for speculation how the effect of this event is transmitted to actin monomers not in contact with the troponin complex. Each actin monomer has regions of interaction with each of the two adjacent monomers in the single actin filament of which it forms part. It also has points of interaction with two actin monomers in the other filament in the actin double helix.[24] These interactions between actin monomers must play a vital part in facilitating the cooperative response of the whole structural unit of seven actin monomers when calcium binds to a molecule of TnC that is close to one or at most two of the actin subunits.

The troponin complex consists of one molecule each of TnC, troponin I (TnI), and troponin T (TnT)—proteins that are different gene products and that, in isolation, possess markedly different properties that are essential for the function of the complex as a whole in its regulatory capacity. The amino acid sequences of all the troponin components are known, as are their individual properties, and there is some information about their sites of interaction. Nevertheless, in the absence of a high-resolution structure of the complex, the precise manner in which they interact in the presence and absence of calcium is still largely speculative. Whereas the same tropomyosin isoforms are usually expressed in all striated muscles but in varying relative proportions characteristic of the muscle type, this is not the case with troponin. The isoforms of the troponin components expressed in a muscle cell are usually specific for the fiber type and are the products of specific genes. As is the case with tropomyosin, however, the isoform composition of the troponin complex in skeletal muscle depends on a number of factors, such as stage of development, type of innervation, etc. Changes from normal are also seen in dystrophic muscle. The fact that in a mature muscle cell only the isoform of the troponin component characteristic for its type is expressed enables antibodies to be used to identify striated muscle cell types (Fig. 13-5). When muscle is damaged, components of the troponin complex can be detected in serum. The availability of antibodies specific for cardiac TnI and TnT has enabled the development of immunochemical assays on serum to assess myocardial damage, offering advantages over the enzymic assays commonly used.[52]

TROPONIN C

TnC is a protein of about M_r 18000 (Table 13-2) that so far has been isolated only from striated muscles, where it represents about 0.8 percent of the total protein. In a given species it is present in fast and slow skeletal muscles as isoforms that are specific for the muscle fiber type. The slow muscle isoform is identical with the cardiac form and coded by the same gene.[53] Expression of the two forms is controlled by separate single-copy genes, TNNC1 for the slow/cardiac isoform and TNNC2 for the fast skeletal muscle form, which have been cloned and structurally analyzed in the human[54] and other species. It is of interest that small amounts of the slow TnC mRNA have been detected in certain human fibroblasts.[55]

The primary sequence of TnC is characterized by four homologous regions that form the domains responsible for

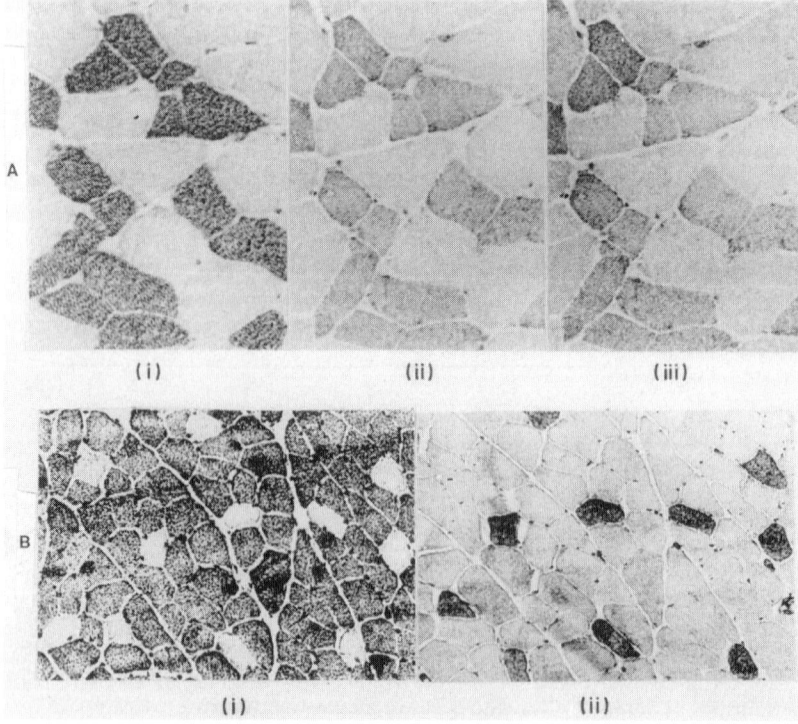

FIGURE 13-5. Localization of the isoforms of the components of the troponin complex in type I and II fibers of mammalian skeletal muscle. Serial sections stained with the antibodies indicated use of the immunoperoxidase sandwich technique. A. Adult human semispinalis capitis muscle; (i) rabbit fast skeletal TnI antibody; (ii) rabbit fast skeletal TnT antibody; (iii) chicken fast skeletal TnC antibody. B. Adult rat gastrocnemius muscle; (i) rabbit fast TnI antibody; (ii) rabbit slow TnI antibody. (From Dhoot GK, Perry SV: Distribution of the polymorphic forms of troponin components and tropomyosin in skeletal muscle. Nature 278:714–718, 1979. With permission.)

Table 13-2. PROPERTIES OF TROPONIN C

1. Present in the troponin complex with equimolar amounts of troponin C and T.
2. Calcium-binding protein of high affinity with Ca^{2+}-specific (regulatory) sites I and II, and Ca^{2+}- and Mg^{2+}-specific (structural) sites III and IV.
3. Present in striated muscle as two isoforms expressed by different genes. The fast skeletal isoform possesses two N-terminal Ca^{2+}-specific sites I and II. In the cardiac isoform only the site corresponding to site II binds Ca^{2+} specifically.
4. Neutralizes inhibition of Mg ATPase of actomyosin produced by troponin I.
5. Forms complex with troponin I that is stable in high urea concentrations and is Ca^{2+}-dependent.
6. Forms complex with troponin T, but the complex is not as stable as that formed with troponin I.
7. Inhibits phosphorylation of skeletal muscle troponin I by phosphorylase kinase and protein kinase A. Does not inhibit phosphorylation of serine 22/23 of cardiac troponin I by protein kinase A.

established that the N-terminal sites I and II are Ca^{2+}-specific, whereas the sites in the C-terminal half of the molecule, sites III and IV, have a higher affinity for Ca^{2+} but also bind Mg^{2+} (Table 13-1) (for review, see Ref. 62).

Although amino acid sequences of the fast and slow cardiac isoforms exhibit considerable homology, they do show one important difference of functional significance. Three aspartic acid residues that are essential for the hexagonal pyramidal coordination cage, at which calcium is bound specifically at site I, are replaced by uncharged amino acids in cardiac TnC.[63] Thus site II is the only specific calcium-binding site on slow/cardiac TnC, but sites III and IV have similar properties to their fast skeletal isoform counterparts.

In resting muscle, sites III and IV will be occupied with magnesium, for the free magnesium ion concentration is probably in the range of 1 to 2 mM. Although the affinity of the C-terminal sites for calcium is greater than that of sites I and II, the latter are considered to be occupied first when muscle is stimulated. This is the consequence of sites III and IV being filled with magnesium in resting muscle and the off rate for magnesium from these sites being too slow to enable them to be replaced with calcium fast enough to account for the contractile response.

Thus the chain of events that leads to muscle contraction is considered to be triggered by the binding of Ca^{2+} at the specific low-affinity sites I and II, which are therefore known as the regulatory sites. Binding is stepwise, with site II occupied first and the affinity of one site being 10 times greater than the other.[64,65] Binding at site II appears to be critical in both isoforms of TnC. Elimination of Ca^{2+} binding at this site in the slow cardiac isoform renders a muscle fiber calcium-insensitive,[66] and replacing site I with site II in this mutant does not restore calcium sensitivity.[67] It has been suggested that site I may modulate the regulatory role of site II in cardiac muscle.

The availability of a high-resolution structure of TnC and the application of multidimensional multinuclear NMR spectroscopy has enabled some progress to be made in describing in atomic terms the early events that lead to the activation of the contractile process (for reviews, see Refs. 68 to 70). The molecule in the crystal and in solution is dumbbell-shaped, with the homologous N- and C-terminal domains arranged at the ends of a central 45-Å helix of amino acid residues (Fig. 13-6 and Color Plate 3a). The extended central helical region linking the two parts of the molecule[39,40] must permit considerable relative movement between them. This would explain the fact that although the x-ray diffraction analysis indicates an extended structure in the crystal, the evidence from fluorescent energy transfer, x-ray diffraction, and cross-linking studies suggests that the molecule is more compact when complexed with TnI. Both C- and N-terminal calcium-binding sites are important for regulatory functions, for fragments containing the regulatory sites will not activate the actomyosin ATPase unless they also contain parts of the high-affinity C-terminal domain. Clearly there are functional interrelationships between these two halves of the molecule.

In the original crystallographic studies of fast skeletal muscle, TnC calcium was absent from sites I and II, whereas sites III and IV in the C-terminal domain were in the Ca_2 form. Despite the homology of sequence the conformations

its Ca^{2+}-binding properties. These domains, which are present in all calcium-binding proteins (Fig. 13-6), were first identified in carp parvalbumin by Kretsinger and Nockolds.[56] They were shown to be present in TnC by Collins et al[57] from sequence homologies with the Ca^{2+}-binding regions of carp parvalbumin. Each domain contains about 30 amino acid residues and consists of a basic structural unit: α helix–calcium-binding loop–α helix; the whole structure is stabilized by interaction between specific hydrophobic side chains in the helices.[58] The calcium-binding sites have been designated I to IV in order along the sequence from the N terminus (Fig. 13-6 and Color Plate 3a–b). Binding studies on TnC from rabbit fast skeletal muscle[59,60] and peptide fragments obtained from it by controlled cleavage[61] have

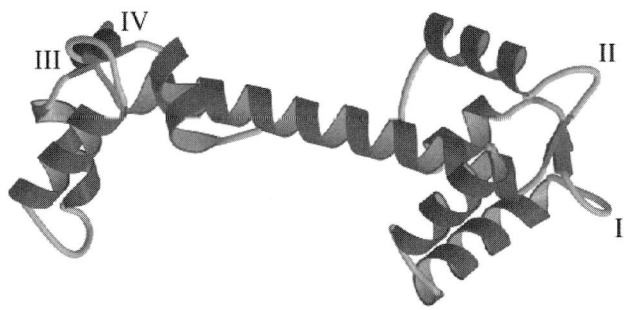

FIGURE 13-6. Crystal structure of troponin C. Ribbon diagram of turkey TnI at 2.0 Å resolution. The N-terminal domain contains the calcium-specific binding sites, I and II, known as the regulatory sites, which fill with calcium to initiate contraction. The C-terminal domain, sometimes referred to as the structural domain, contains sites III and IV, which have an even higher affinity for calcium but will also bind Mg^{2+}. In this crystal, known as the Ca^{2+} form of TnC, sites III and IV are filled with Ca^{2+} (see red spheres in Color Plate 3a). These sites are probably filled with Mg^{2+} in resting muscle. (Coordinates from Herzberg and James.[39] Plotted by Jonathan Parrish. With permission.)

of the N- and C-domains are markedly different in the Ca_2 form of TnC. The N-terminal regulatory sites without bound calcium have fewer exposed hydrophobic residues than C-terminal Ca_2 domain, which contains sites III and IV, is relatively unstructured, and is considered to play a structural role. The binding of Ca_2 to the N-terminal sites results in globular domain with an exposed hydrophobic pocket.[69] The N-terminal domain of fast skeletal TnC consists of five α-helical regions connected by linker peptides. Peptide N is N-terminal, and AB and CD form parts of sites I and II, respectively (Fig. 13-7 and Color Plate 3b). When calcium is bound first in site II and then in site I, helices N, A, and D remain relatively fixed.[68,70] The opening of the structure results from reorientation of helices B and C from almost antiparallel to a perpendicular arrangement which involves motion of up to 15 Å in the case of some residues. A similar arrangement exists in the Ca_2 form of the C-terminal domain. Thus on binding calcium to saturate the regulatory sites, the N-terminal domain takes on a more open structure with exposure of a large hydrophobic surface, similar to the conformation of the C-terminal domain when loaded with divalent cation. It is considered that this hydrophobic surface facilitates interaction with TnI.

Evidence that conformational change involving the relative movement between sites I and II is of importance in calcium regulation has been obtained by site-directed mutagenesis of the fast skeletal muscle TnC gene.[71] A mutant form in which Gln 48 and Gln 82 were replaced with cysteine residues—together with other minor alterations that alone did not affect the properties of TnC—was prepared. In the oxidized form of this mutant, a disulfide bond locks the two N-terminal calcium-binding sites in one position. Significantly, although this mutant can bind calcium, affinity for sites I and II is decreased, but little changed for sites III and IV. Calcium sensitivity of TnC-deficient myofibrils was not restored by the oxidized mutant but was by the wild-type TnC or by the reduced mutant. (For a review of references summarizing the effects of mutations on the physiologic properties of TnC, see Ref. 72).

In the case of cardiac TnC, a consequence of the fact that there is no calcium bound at site I is that the N-terminal domain does not open up when calcium is bound at site II, as is the case with the fast skeletal isoform.[73,74] Thus the conformational change when calcium is bound is much less and there is a substantially reduced exposure of hydrophobic residues. This implies that the nature of the interaction between TnC and TnI may be different in the cardiac and skeletal isoforms and that the difference is of functional significance.

In addition to binding Ca^{2+} with high affinity, another important property of TnC (Table 13-2) is its ability to form a complex with TnI. At low ionic strength, the complex is formed in the absence of Ca^{2+}, but it is strengthened at least 1000-fold by the presence of this cation, with the result that it is not dissociated in 8 M urea.[75] Removal of the Ca^{2+} causes reversible dissociation of the complex in high urea concentrations. This property is the basis of an effective affinity chromatographic method for the isolation of TnI in one step from whole-muscle homogenates.[76] Interaction of TnC with fast skeletal muscle TnI results in inhibition of phosphorylation of the latter protein by phosphorylase kinase and cAMP-dependent protein kinase (see discussion of phosphorylation, below).

TROPONIN I

TnI has so far been identified unambiguously only in striated muscle, from which it can be isolated as a protein that is rather insoluble at pH 7.0 and with an isoelectric point in the region of pH 8 (for review, see Ref. 77). Three isoforms, slow skeletal, fast skeletal, and cardiac, each the product of a separate gene, TNNI1, TNNI2, and TNNI3, respectively, are expressed in mammalian vertebrate muscle. The amino acid sequences of the three isoforms possess considerable homology, exhibiting about 60 percent identity in the rabbit. The skeletal muscle isoforms have ~21000 Mr, with the cardiac isoforms slightly higher at about 24000 Mr due to an additional N-terminal amino acid sequence of ~30 residues. An important phosphorylation site that enables the response to the calcium transients in the heart to be modulated is located in this region (see discussion of phosphorylation, below). In the mature muscle cell, usually only the isoform characteristic of the fiber type is present and its detection by a specific antibody enables the cell to be typed.[78] It is of interest that in developing fetal skeletal and cardiac muscles the slow skeletal isoform is expressed and is replaced in fast skeletal and cardiac muscles by the appropriate isoform when development is complete.[79-81] Both fast and slow isoforms of TnI can be expressed in fibers that normally express only one isoform as a result of cross-innervation, hormonal effects, and pathologic conditions.

The most striking property of TnI (Table 13-3) is its inhibitory action on the Mg ATPase of actomyosin. This effect is

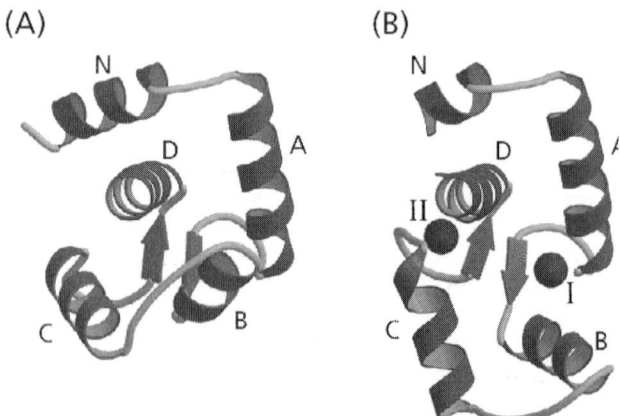

FIGURE 13-7. The calcium-induced change in the N-terminal domain of troponin C. Ribbon diagram of the N-terminal domain of turkey TnC. A. The apo form (A) and the calcium saturated form (B) with Ca^{2+} ions (spheres, see also Color Plate 3b) bound at sites I and II. The helices N, A, and D remain relatively fixed during the calcium-induced transition. The two helices B and C move up to 15 Å and expose a large central core of hydrophobic residues, a proposed TnI binding site. *(From Strynadka NCJ, Cherney M, Sielecki AR, et al: Structural details of a calcium induced molecular switch: X-ray crystallographic analysis of the calcium-saturated N-terminal domain of troponin C at 1.75 Å resolution. J Mol Biol 273:238–258, 1997. With permission. Picture kindly supplied by Jonathan Parrish.)*

Table 13-3. PROPERTIES OF TROPONIN I

1. Expressed in striated muscle by independent genes as three isoforms which are specific for fast skeletal, slow skeletal, and cardiac muscles. Molecular ratios of skeletal muscle isoforms about 21000; cardiac isoforms about 24000.
2. Specific inhibitor of the Mg ATPase of actomyosin. Inhibition much increased by tropomyosin. Both these properties retained by peptides derived from the region represented by residues 96 to 116 in the rapid fast muscle isoform of rabbit TnI.
3. Forms complex with troponin C and calmodulin that is calcium-dependent. Complex with troponin C is stable in high urea concentrations.
4. Interacts with actin.
5. Skeletal isoforms possess sites whose phosphorylation is catalyzed by phosphorylase kinase and protein A kinase. Cardiac troponin possesses a unique phosphorylation site (serines 23 and 24 in human cardiac troponin I), the phosphorylation of which by protein kinase A changes the calcium-binding characteristics of the troponin complex.

---

specific for the Mg ATPase; therefore presumably TnI in some way affects the interaction of actin with myosin that stimulates the Mg ATPase. TnI has inhibitory activity alone, but its effectiveness is much increased by tropomyosin. In vitro with tropomyosin present, maximum inhibition of the actomyosin Mg ATPase can be obtained with molar ratios of actin monomer to TnI, which approaches that of these two proteins in the structural unit of the myofibril, 7:1,[82,83] The fact that under appropriate ionic conditions, and particularly in the presence of Ca^{2+}, TnC neutralizes this inhibition implies that the interaction of TnC and TnI is fundamental to the regulatory process. The nature of the interaction between these proteins has been extensively investigated using a variety of techniques (for review, see Ref. 77), from which it is concluded that TnI is present in the complex in an extended conformation and winds round the dumbbell structure of the TnC with the polypeptide chains of the two proteins running in an antiparallel direction. Nevertheless, due to the unavailability of crystals of TnI or the TnI/C complex, this interaction cannot yet be described in precise atomic terms. (See Ref. 84 for a model of the binary complex.) It has been known for some time from affinity chromatographic studies that the N-terminus, residues 1 to 47, and a more central region known as the inhibitory peptide, residues 96 to 116 of rabbit fast skeletal TnI, are significant sites for the interaction with TnC.[85] From the homology that exists between the amino acid sequences of the cardiac and skeletal isoforms of TnI, it would be expected that the sites of interaction with TnC are similar in all isoforms of TnI. In addition to these well-defined sites, the interactions in the TnI/C complex appear to be extensive. Using a library of 20 residue peptides covering in an overlapping manner the entire sequence of hcTnI, some six sites of interaction have been identified, two of which correspond to those identified by affinity chromatography.[86]

The N-terminal domain of skeletal TnI encompassed by residues 1 to 47 is bound to the C-terminal structural domain of TnC both in the activated and in the inhibited state of the muscle.[87] The marked conformational changes involving the regulatory N-terminal–specific calcium-binding domain of TnC, which results in activation of the Mg ATPase when the calcium concentration rises, must lead to changes in the nature of the interaction with the inhibitory peptide region and possibly other regions of the TnI molecule. The result is that the inhibitory activity of TnI is lost and the actomyosin ATPase activated. Due to the inability to crystallize TnI or the TnI/C complex, the atomic description of the interaction, which is at the heart of the regulatory process, is not yet available. Low resolution studies indicate that the TnI is wrapped around the TnC in a coiled manner (see Ref. 87a for review). By co-crystallizing TnC with peptide fragments of TnI, residues 1–47 and 34–210, the regions where these peptides of TnI interact with cardiac TnC have been established.[87b, 87c] When calcium is bound to the regulatory site of skeletal troponin C, it changes from a "closed" to an "open" confirmation exposing a hydrophobic surface that acts as a binding site for TnI. In the case of the binding of calcium to cardiac TnC the hydrophobic exposure is less. Nevertheless the cardiac TnI binds with the result that the regulatory domains of cardiac and skeletal TnC adopt similar open conformations when bound to cardiac and skeletal TnI, respectively.[87d, 87e]

The inhibitory peptide, and the shorter synthetic duodecapeptide representing residues 104 to 115[88] inhibit the Mg ATPase of actomyosin, a property that is much accentuated by tropomyosin in a similar manner to TnI but about 50 percent as effective as an inhibitor compared to the intact molecule. These facts imply that the interaction of quite a small region of TnI with actin is adequate to prevent activation of the Mg ATPase and thus maintain the state that is characteristic of resting muscle. The general pattern that is emerging from a number of investigations is that the N terminus of TnI, residues 1–40, remains bound to the C domain of TnC in the presence of high and low calcium concentrations. At low calcium concentration, the regulatory site of TnC closes and the inhibitory region of TnI becomes detached and is free to interact with actin resulting in inhibition of the actomyosin MgATPase[88a]

The mechanism described above explains how a single molecule of TnI could control the interaction of an actin monomer (or possibly two adjacent monomers) with myosin. In the myofibril, however, there is only one TnI molecule for every seven actin monomers, all of which must change from the nonactivating to the activating state when muscle is stimulated. In relaxed muscle in the presence of ropomyosin, the inhibitory action of one molecule of TnI is extended to the seven actins of which the structural unit is composed. Despite the evidence for the highly specific inhibitory activity of TnI, current dogma postulates that it is tropomyosin extending alongside the seven actin monomers of the structural unit of the myofibril that regulates the interaction of actin with myosin responsible for the activation of the Mg ATPase. This is the steric hypothesis. In its original form it was postulated[89–91] that in resting muscle tropomyosin blocks the site on myosin with which actin must interact for activation of the Mg ATPase. On stimulation, the tropomyosin is considered to move azimuthally around the actin filament to expose the interaction site with consequent activation of the Mg ATPase. (For references, see Ref. 43.) In recent years, from the analysis of the kinetics of the activation in filament systems and image reconstruction data using wild-type and mutant forms of tropomyosin, a three-state model has been proposed.[92,93] It is proposed that the tropomyosin moves from the blocked B position in resting muscle first to the calcium-induced C, or closed, position, which is then converted to the M, or open, state by myosin binding when the system is fully activated (Fig. 13-8).

Strong evidence that tropomyosin is in some way involved in the activation process is provided by x-ray diffraction studies on whole muscle, which indicate that movement of the tropomyosin polymers in the groove of the actin filament occurs 12 to 17 ms before the mechanical response.[94] Furthermore, this movement when visualized by image reconstruction studies with striated muscle[95] suggests that tropomyosin moves from a position in which it partially blocks the presumptive binding site on actin for myosin to one in which it does not when the system is activated (Fig. 13-9). The fact that under certain ionic conditions in the absence of the troponin complex tropomyosin alone is able to inhibit the Mg ATPase of actomyosin also gives support to a steric blocking role for tropomyosin. Despite this supporting evidence, there are a number of difficulties with the steric hypothesis even in its modified form. It does not offer any satisfactory explanation for the mechanism that results in the movement of the flexible tropomyosin molecule along the whole of its length along the actin filament when TnC binds calcium. Nor does it explain the role of TnI, a protein that has uniquely evolved in striated muscle for the regulation of the activation by actin of the Mg ATPase. In an attempt to explain the role of TnI, it has been suggested it increases the affinity of tropomyosin for actin and thus increases the inhibitory activity of tropomyosin.[96] Another possible explanation for its movement associated with contraction is that tropomyosin does not have a specific blocking role but moves as a consequence of conformational changes that occur in the actin monomers with which it is associated in the thin filament. Cooperative action between the actin monomers is a prerequisite for this explanation. In resting muscle, TnI binding to actin at regular intervals along the thin filament induces conformational changes in the other actins in the structural unit, with the result that they are no longer able to activate the Mg ATPase. On the binding of calcium, TnC displaces TnI from actin, which reverts to the form that can activate the Mg ATPase. According to this explanation the conformational changes in the actin monomer originally bound to the TnI are transmit-

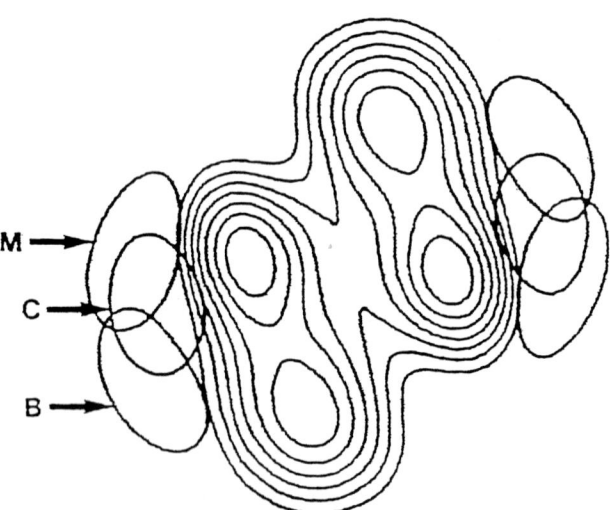

FIGURE 13-8. Relative positions of tropomyosin on the actin filament in the M, B, and C states. F-actin and B- and C-state tropomyosin densities have been merged and plotted as helical projections for comparison with myosin S1 decorated thin filaments. Tropomyosin densities labeled B, C, and M, respectively. Note the three distinct tropomyosin positions and apparent binding contact points on the surface of actin; only the outermost contours of tropomyosin densities are displayed to help demarcate their boundaries. (From Lehman W, Hatch V, Korman V, et al: Tropomyosin and actin isoforms modulate the localisation of tropomyosin strands on actin filaments. J Mol Biol 302:593–606, 2000. With permission.)

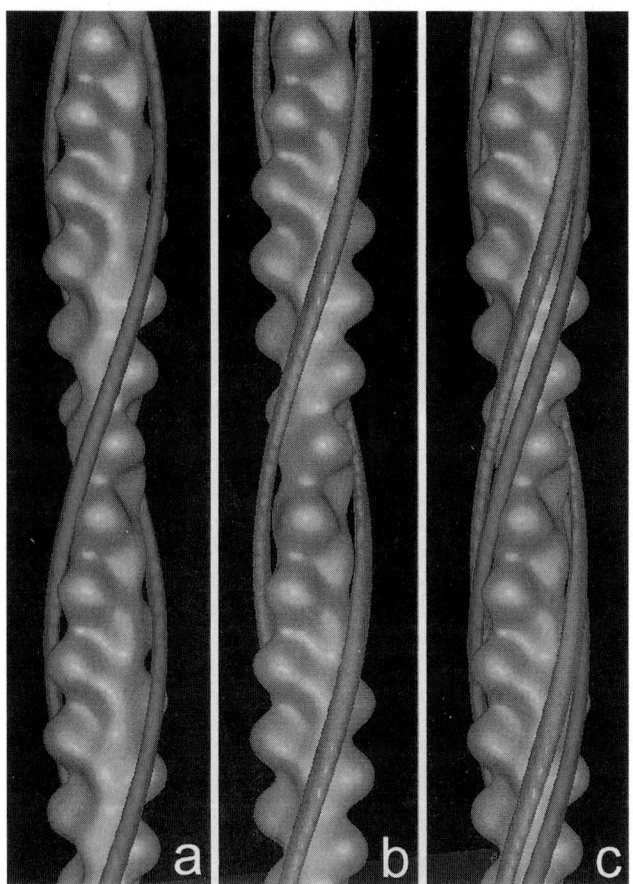

FIGURE 13-9. Position of the tropomyosin molecule on the actin filament in the presence and absence of calcium. (See Color Plate 3e.) Surface views of reconstructions showing tropomyosin superimposed on actin in (A) EGTA, (B) Ca^{2+}. In (C), tropomyosin strands associated with both EGTA and Ca^{2+} are superimposed on actin for comparison. Reconstructions show characteristic bilobed actin. In EGTA the tropomyosin occupies a position on the inner edge of the outer domain of actin, whereas in Ca^{2+} the tropomyosin lies along the outer edge of the inner domain. Surface rendering was carried out by superimposing tropomyosin strand densities obtained by difference analysis on the maps of pure F-actin. (From Xu C, Craig R, Tobacman L, Horowitz R, Lehman W: Tropomyosin positions in regulated thin filaments revealed by cryoelectronmicroscopy. Biophys J 77:985–992, 1999. With permission.)

ted by cooperative effects to the other actin monomers in the structural subunit. The slight changes in position of the amino acid residues at the tropomyosin interaction sites—which occur as a result of conformational changes when actin binds ligands such as TnI and myosin—will require the tropomyosin to adjust its position as a consequence of binding energy considerations. In this hypothesis the role of tropomyosin is to stabilize the actin filament and facilitate cooperativity and hence enable conformation changes to be transmitted between monomers in the filament. These cooperative effects are now well established and can be demonstrated on the binding of TnI, myosin, and caldesmon, ligands that all have the capacity to induce conformational changes in actin (for review, see Ref. 43). Clearly there is uncertainty about the role of tropomyosin in the regulation of the contractile response in striated muscle, which will not be finally resolved until the structures of all the proteins of the thin filament can be described in atomic detail. If the role of tropomyosin is to block the actin-myosin interaction as demanded by the steric hypothesis, this would be unique to striated muscle, for it does not appear to have this role in smooth muscle (see later).

TROPONIN T

Under in vitro conditions, TnC can be shown to neutralize the inhibitory activity of TnI on the actomyosin Mg ATPase in a manner that is calcium-insensitive. Addition of TnT restores calcium sensitivity to the system. Thus all three protein components must be present for troponin to function as a calcium-sensitive regulatory system. TnT is the largest of the troponin components and, like TnI, occurs in three main forms in striated muscle, each the product of separate genes: TNNT1, mainly expressed in slow-twitch skeletal muscle; TNNT2, in cardiac muscle; and TNNT3, in fast-twitch skeletal muscle (Table 13-4) (for review, see Ref. 97).

TnT differs from the two other components of the troponin complex in that, by alternative RNA splicing mechanisms, each gene can give rise to a number of isoforms. These isoforms, which vary in number between species and muscle types, can be distinguished by high-resolution two-dimensional electrophoresis and staining with specific monoclonal antibodies. The TNNT3 gene is particularly susceptible to differential splicing in a region near the N-terminus. Usually four or five isoforms of TnT are identified in vertebrate skeletal and cardiac muscles, although many more in small amounts, have been reported in chicken leg and wing muscles. Four isoforms of fast TnT are detected in human biceps, triceps, pectoralis major, gastrocnemius, and external and internal oblique muscles.[98] Whereas the three higher-molecular-weight forms—HF1, HF2, and HF3—were present in approximately similar amounts, there is significantly less of the lowest-molecular-weight form, HF4, in all these muscles. None of these isoforms could be detected in the human diaphragm, which, like the external and internal oblique muscles, contained three isoforms of slow TnT, HS1, HS2, and HS3. Only the first two of these slow isoforms were present in human biceps, triceps, gastrocnemius, and pectoralis major muscles.

The fact that both fast and slow isoforms of TnT were present in most of the human muscles examined in these studies probably reflects their mixed fiber composition. Although in mature, fully differentiated skeletal fiber types the isoforms present are usually expressed by the gene appropriate for the fiber type, both fast and slow forms may occur in the same skeletal muscle cell. This occurs particularly when the tissue is undergoing transformation, as, for example, during development, after denervation or cross-innervation, and in some dystrophies. A fetal form of fast skeletal TnT is produced by splicing in a mutually exclusive manner two C-terminal exons to produce the α (adult) and β (fetal) forms. There is evidence for an additional fetal form of fast skeletal TnT resulting from the insertion of an eight–amino acid sequence, exon f (Fig. 13-10). A fetal form of the cardiac TnT is produced by a splicing procedure that eliminates a highly acidic 10–amino acid sequence, exon 5, in the N-terminal region. In adult human cardiac muscle, four isoforms have been reported, which are present in different amounts in normal and failing hearts. It is of interest that small amounts of the cardiac isoform are present in some normal human skeletal muscles (for references on TnT gene expression, see Ref. 97). The observation that adult forms of cardiac TnT are restricted to the heart has stimulated interest in using immunologic detection of this protein in serum as an index of myocardial damage.[52]

Most of the structural information available about TnT has been obtained with the fast isoform of rabbit skeletal muscle.[99] It consists of a single polypeptide chain of 259 residues (M_r = 30500) and probably exists as an open asymmetrical molecule. Unlike TnC, which is an acidic protein, TnT resembles TnI in possessing a high isoelectric point, in the region of pH 8.0. At pH 7.0, about 50 percent of the residues are charged and there are no significant stretches of nonpolar amino acids in the sequence. Circular dichroism measurements indicate that there is relatively little ordered structure, although the region represented by residues 71 to 151 is about 80 percent α-helical. So far it has not been possible to crystallize TnT to enable its high-resolution structure to be determined, but from cocrystals with tropomyosin, it has been concluded that the skeletal isoform exists in the myofibril as an extended molecule about 180 Å long and 20 Å wide. The

Table 13-4. PROPERTIES OF TROPONIN T

1. Occurs as a number of isoforms that are usually muscle type specific in mature fibers. Expressed by three genes; slow twitch, *TNNT1*; cardiac, *TNNT2*; and fast twitch, *TNNT3*, which are located on different chromosomes. Exons in the N- and C-terminal regions represent variant regions where differential splicing leads to a number of isoforms including a fetal form, particularly in the fast-twitch muscle.
2. Forms viscous complex with tropomyosin.
3. Forms complex with TnC that is calcium dependent but not stable to high-urea concentration (cf. TnI/TnC complex).
4. Essential component for the inhibitory activity of the troponin complex to be calcium sensitive.
5. Evidence that isoforms may have role in determining calcium sensitivity of muscle fibers.
6. N-terminal serine usually phosphorylated when TnT is isolated.

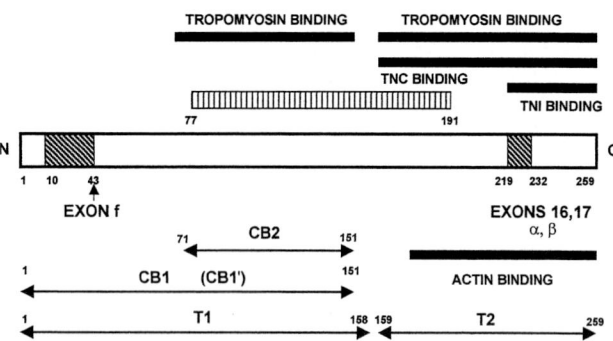

FIGURE 13-10. Interactions of troponin TNT3. Schematic representation of the adult fast skeletal troponin-T molecule based on the polypeptide sequence of the rabbit fast skeletal muscle isoform TnT2f (TNT3 gene). Cross-hatched areas represent variable regions in which alternative mRNA splicing occurs. In the N-terminal variable regions, exons 4, 6, 7, and f may or may not be present in the various fast-TnT isoforms (see Fig. 13-2), whereas exons 16 and 17 are the alternates in the C-terminal variable region. Thick lines represent regions of the TnT polypeptide chain considered to be implicated in interactions with the myofibrillar proteins indicated. Numbers indicate amino acid residue positions based on the sequence of Pearlstone JR, Johstone P, Carpenter MR, et al. The primary structure of rabbit skeletal muscle troponin T. Sequence determination HH2 terminal fragment CB3 and the complete sequence of troponin T. *J Biol Chem* 252:983–989, 1977.[98a] CB1, CB1', and CB2, peptides obtained by cyanogen bromide cleavage. T1 and T2, chymotryptic fragments of rabbit TnT2f. Region of chicken fast-twitch TnT which activates Mg ATPase of actomyosin in the presence of tropomyosin, indicated by IIIIIIIIIII (Oliviera et al[110]). Remarkably, this effect is not obtained with intact TnT. The evidence for actin binding is perhaps not quite so well defined as it is for other proteins that bind to TnT. *(After Perry SV: Vertebrate tropomyosin: Distribution, properties and function. J Muscle Res Cell Motil 22:5–49, 2001. With permission.)*

cardiac isoform is significantly longer, due principally to additional amino acids in the N-terminal region.

Interaction of Troponin T with Tropomyosin

TnT possesses a number of properties (Table 13-4), of which its ability to interact with tropomyosin is of particular interest in view of the postulated role of the latter protein in the regulation of contraction. This property is responsible for the marked increase in viscosity that occurs when troponin and tropomyosin are mixed, for TnT is the only component of the troponin complex for which clear evidence of interaction with tropomyosin exists. Evidence from a variety of investigations indicates that TnT lies in extended conformation alongside the C-terminal half of the tropomyosin molecule, continuing over the interlap region. Two binding regions have been postulated with the TnT and the tropomyosin amino acid chains arranged in an antiparallel manner (Fig. 13-10). Site 1 on rabbit fast skeletal TnT is located in the region represented by residues 71 to 151 and site 2 in that represented by residues 159 to 259. As TnC and TnI both bind in the C-terminal region of TnT, the bulk of the troponin complex is bound in the C-terminal half of the tropomyosin molecule at a regular periodicity of 38.5 Å. Thus TnT acts as a kind of "functional glue" in the regulatory system of striated muscle. It fixes the position of the troponin complex on the actin filament and its probable role is to make the interaction between TnC and TnI, and in consequence the Mg ATPase of the actomyosin system, sensitive to the changes in calcium concentration that occur when striated muscle is stimulated. The fact that in the presence of calcium it binds to TnC probably reflects an aspect of this role, as indeed does the evidence that in some muscle cells—for example, the fast fibers of rabbit—the proportions of the fast TnT isoforms vary, as do the isoforms of tropomyosin present, suggesting expression of the appropriate genes is linked. The tension response to Ca^{2+} concentration in these muscles appears to depend on the isoforms of these two proteins that are present. Fibers expressing primarily the 2f isoform of TnT and α tropomyosin possess a steeper Ca^{2+}/tension curve and are more sensitive to calcium concentration than those in which the TnT1f and TnT3f isoforms and β tropomyosin predominate.[100] The pattern of expression of the isoforms of both proteins alters in the expected way when muscle speed is changed by cross-innervation or direct stimulation. This implies that the isoforms of both proteins play a role in modulating the response of the tissue to calcium liberation on stimulation.

A relationship between TnT and calcium sensitivity also occurs in cardiac muscle for differences in calcium sensitivity and inhibition of force development have been observed with four isoforms of TnT expressed by gene TNNT2 in skinned fiber preparations and with reconstituted actomyosin assays.[100a]

Specific sites for interaction with TnT on the tropomyosin molecule have been identified, and this interaction fixes the position of the troponin complex on the I filament. One region is close to cysteine 190 in α tropomyosin of rabbit skeletal muscle.[101] The peptide obtained on digestion of TnT with cyanogen bromide, consisting of residues 71 to 160, is the only one in the digest that produces a viscosity increase with tropomyosin.[102] It has been suggested that interaction is facilitated by the region of residues 90 to 150 of TnT forming a continuous triple α-helical structure, with the coiled-coil structure of tropomyosin represented by residues 155 to 220.[103] If TnT is subjected to controlled digestion by chymotrypsin,[104] cleavage occurs at tyrosine 158, to give an N-terminal fragment, peptide T1, of M_r = 22000, and a C-terminal fragment, peptide T2, of M_r = 11000.[104–107] As would be expected from the studies on the cyanogen bromide digests, peptide T1 interacts with tropomyosin, but contrary to the findings with the latter digest, so does the smaller C-terminal fragment T2 (Fig. 13-10). This is explained by the fact that on further fragmentation to the peptides obtained on digestion by chymotrypsin or by cyanogen bromide, the T2 fragment loses its property of interaction with tropomyosin. The evidence[108–110] indicates that the highly asymmetrical TnT molecule extends along one-half to one-third of the carboxyl end of tropomyosin and is probably stabilized by coiled-coil interactions at approximately the middle of and at the C-terminal end of the TnT sequence.

A clear role for TnT in the function of the troponin complex has yet to emerge. Recent evidence suggests that at least part of the molecule can modulate the actin-myosin interaction. The Mg ATPase of actomyosin in the presence of tropomyosin, but in the absence of calcium, is activated by up to 30 to 40 percent in the presence of fragment of TnT, corresponding to residues 77 to 191.[110] As this effect is not observed with the whole TnT molecule, it is difficult to relate it to the events that take place in the intact troponin complex. This finding is also difficult to reconcile with reports that the N-terminal region of TnT represented by residues 1–153 or 1–158 inhibits the actomyosin ATPase[110a,110b,113] and implies that much has still to be learned about the role of TnT in the regulatory process.

Interaction of Troponin T with Troponin C

Under ionic conditions comparable to those occurring in the cell, TnT can form a complex with TnC that is Ca^{2+}-sensitive. The Ca^{2+} dependency is not as pronounced as is the case with the TnC/TnI interaction, particularly with cardiac TnT, for example. Electrophoretic studies suggest complex formation with cyanogen bromide peptides derived from the regions consisting of residues 71 to 160 and residues 161 to 185 with TnC.[102] Inhibition of phosphorylation at site 2 (serine 149 or 150) and site 3 (serine 156 or 157) by TnC (see below) supports the view that one point at which TnC interacts is the region of TnT represented approximately by residues 150 to 170.[111] These findings have been extended by interaction studies with the fragment from the C-terminal region, peptide T2.[104,112] Interaction with this region of the molecule of TnT is responsible for conferring Ca^{2+} sensitivity on the Mg ATPase of actomyosin in reconstituted systems[113] and indicates that a major binding site for TnC is located in the C-terminal fragment. Affinity chromatography, sedimentation, and electrophoretic studies indicate that there are two sites of TnC interaction on TnT—namely, at the N- and C-terminal regions of peptide T2 (Fig. 13-10). Blumenschein et al.[114] have confirmed from NMR studies that TnC binding occurs at the N and C terminals of the T2 fragment of TnT. Nevertheless the interaction appears to extend over much of this region, for none of the smaller fragments, such as those obtained by cyanogen bromide digestion of T2, interact with TnC. The interaction of TnC with peptide T2 is Ca^{2+}-sensitive.[107] The observation that when this reaction occurs tropomyosin binding to T2 is disrupted[115] suggests a functional significance for the interactions in this region of the TnT molecule.

Interaction of Troponin T with Troponin I

By the application of affinity chromatographic techniques, it has been shown that T2 but not T1 interacts with TnI.[115,116] On the basis of the binding of a range of partial chymotryptic digestion products of peptide T2, it has been concluded that the TnI interaction site includes residues 223 to 227,[107] although this region is not identical with that proposed by the Smillie group.[115] The inconsistency of these findings may arise from the strongly basic nature of TnI and its ability to complex nonspecifically with acidic peptides.

Phosphorylation of the Regulatory Proteins of the Thin Filament of the Myofibril

On isolation from fresh muscle tropomyosin, TnT and TnI but not TnC contain small amounts of covalently bound phosphate, usually 1 to 2 moles per mole or less. With the exception of cardiac TnI, rapid turnover of this phosphate is not seen during periods of contractile activity, suggesting that the effect of thin-filament phosphorylation is, with the exception of the cardiac isoform, of structural or long-term modulatory significance in striated muscle.

TROPOMYOSIN

The α and β tropomyosin of skeletal and cardiac muscle possess a single site, serine 283, that is phosphorylated by an enzyme considered to be specific, designated tropomyosin kinase. When isolated from adult muscle the α tropomyosin is partially phosphorylated, with higher levels in fetal, skeletal, and cardiac muscles. There is some evidence that phosphorylation enhances polymerization by stabilizing head-to-tail interaction as a result of the formation of salt linkages between phosphate groups and lysine residues on neighboring chains. There is no evidence that tropomyosin phosphorylation modulates calcium sensitivity.

TROPONIN I

When isolated from fresh rabbit skeletal muscle, TnI contains about 0.5 mole phosphate per mole. This is principally located at threonine 11 and serine 116, the sites of phosphorylation by phosphorylase and protein kinase A, respectively, when isolated TnI is incubated with the enzymes. The significance of phosphorylation of these sites is not clear, but the sites are close to regions of high homology in all three isoforms of TnI and are considered to be involved in interaction with TnC (Fig. 13-11). The presence of charged residues of phosphate would be expected to modulate the interaction with TnC and affect binding constants. In the presence of TnC, phosphorylation of fast skeletal TnI is inhibited, implying that in the complex the potential phosphorylation sites are not readily available to enzymes.

Cardiac TnI is much more rapidly phosphorylated by protein kinase A than the skeletal isoform, for in addition to hydroxy amino acids in homologous positions to those in the other isoforms, it possesses two phosphorylation sites (serine 22, 23 in the rabbit and serine 23, 24 in the human) unique to this isoform. These are located on an additional N-terminal peptide extension of about 30 residues present in the vertebrate cardiac TnI isoform. In the normal beating heart, this site is partially phosphorylated; but on adrenaline intervention, both sites become phosphorylated. With protein kinase A in vitro, ordered phosphorylation of the site occurs. The C-terminal of the two serines, residue 24 in the case of the human, is phosphorylated before significant phosphorylation of the adjacent serine occurs. When both sites are phosphorylated, the calcium concentration at which 50 percent activation of the Mg ATPase occurs rises.[117] Thus, by reducing the sensitivity of the cardiac myofibrillar ATPase, phosphorylation of TnI acts as a negative feedback mechanism in response to the rising calcium transients induced by the intervention with adrenaline. It has been suggested that phosphorylation of cardiac TnI also speeds up relaxation, but direct determination on skinned guinea pig trabeculae

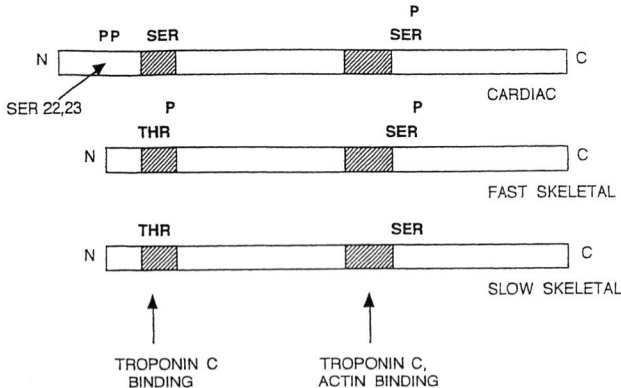

FIGURE 13-11. Phosphorylation sites on the isoforms of troponin I of the rabbit. Schematic representation of the isoforms of TnI present in skeletal and cardiac muscles. Sites in the isoform that have been shown to be phosphorylated when the isoform is isolated from live muscle are indicated by P. The amino acid residues in the shaded areas are very similar in all isoforms. Regions of the isoforms shown to interact with TnC and actin are indicated by brackets. In human cardiac TnI, the N-terminal phosphorylatable sites are Ser23 and Ser24.

suggests that this is not the case.[118] In addition to the sites indicated in Fig. 13-11, cardiac TnI contains a number of other hydroxyamino amino acid residues (rabbit cardiac TnI has 21 in total), some of which may be potential phosphorylation sites in vivo. Phosphorylation of mouse residues ser 43/ser 45 by protein kinase C does not alter calcium sensitivity but decreases the calcium-activated Mg ATPase of actomyosin. There is evidence that these sites are phosphorylated in cardiac myocytes (for references and fuller discussion of TnI phosphorylation, see Ref. 77).

TROPONIN T

The bulk of the covalent phosphate present in troponin preparations is associated with TnT. The major site of the covalent phosphate of the skeletal and cardiac isoforms is Ser1, which is phosphorylated by a specific enzyme, TnT kinase. The function of phosphorylation at this site is unknown, for it does not affect the actomyosin ATPase or its sensitivity to calcium, and the phosphate does not exchange rapidly with the intracellular pool. TnT is an effective substrate for protein kinase C, which acts on a number of sites, particularly in the C-terminal region of the molecule. This results in decreased activity but no change in calcium sensitivity of the actomyosin Mg ATPase. It has been suggest that in vivo phosphorylation of TnT is responsible for the negative inotropic effect on the heart observed with phorbol esters, which activate protein kinases.

Thick- (A-) Filament Regulation

On general grounds it would appear simpler and more effective to control contraction by direct action of Ca^{2+} on the myosin motor. This is the case in more primitive contractile systems containing the unconventional myosins found in nonmuscle cells[119] and that present in the adductor muscle of molluscs. In striated muscle of vertebrates, however, the direct control of the enzyme by calcium binding to the I-filament system is the major mechanism. Presumably control via the thin filament has advantages for a rapidly responding muscle because the cooperative properties of the actin monomers enable an extremely rapid transition between the myosin noninteracting and the myosin interacting states to occur along the whole length of the filament. A feature of the striated muscle systems is that in the absence of the tropomyosin-troponin the myosin and actin readily interact and the complex possesses high Mg ATPase activity. The role of calcium is to regulate this interaction by direct effects on the regulatory protein system present in the thin-filament system as described above. Stimulation of striated muscle is in effect release of the inhibition of the Mg ATPase that exists in relaxed muscle. This is in contrast to the activation that occurs on stimulation in nonstriated muscle systems. When the latter systems are relaxed, the myosin is in a state that will not interact with actin to produce a complex with high Mg ATPase activity. The function of calcium in these muscles is either to have a direct effect by binding to the light chains of myosin or to activate the kinase that phosphorylates the RLC. Both effects results in activation of myosin to form an actomyosin complex of high Mg ATPase activity.

THE LIGHT CHAINS OF MYOSIN

The myosin responsible for muscle contraction, designated myosin II to distinguish it from the unconventional myosins, always has two classes of light chains associated with it. The nomenclature associated with these light chains is somewhat confusing, and a variety of properties such as electrophoretic mobility, function, and solubility properties have been used to distinguish them (see Chaps. 7 and 8 and Ref. 120). In this section, the following terminology—essential light chain, ELC (also referred to in the literature as the alkali light chain, light chain 1, LC1) and regulatory light chain, RLC (also referred to as the DTNB light chain, light chain 2, LC2, phosphorylatable or P light chain)—is used. In striated muscle, the RLC has a molecular weight of about 18000, but in vertebrate smooth muscle it is approximately 20000. Whereas a single isoform of the regulatory light chain is present in rabbit skeletal muscle, two isoforms, P1 and P2, both of which can be phosphorylated, are found in the slow skeletal and cardiac muscles.[121] There is no evidence that each of the two isoforms of the P light chain are present in different cell types.

One of each class of these light chains (Fig. 13-12), both of which exist in a number of isoforms specific for the muscle type and ranging in apparent molecular ratios from 16000 to 27000, are associated with each myosin head. Neither light chain is essential for the ATPase activity of striated muscle myosin, but some loss in activity occurs on removal of the essential light chain, particularly in the case of adductor myosin, hence its name. As they belong to the superfamily of calcium-binding proteins with EF domains that has evolved from the same primitive gene, both light chains preserve the dumbbell-like shape characteristic of TnC—i.e., with two helix-loop-helix structural motifs in each half of the molecule. Although rudimentary calcium-binding domains can be identified in the sequences,[122] the binding properties of the isolated light chains from vertebrate myosin are not adequate for a regulatory role in contraction. Spectroscopic studies have indicated that Ca^{2+}-binding sites on striated muscle myosin, which presumably include those resulting from the light chains, are nonspecific and not competent to play a direct role in regulation (for a review, see Ref. 123). Further, there have been no reports of minor A-filament proteins such as C, H, X, or F proteins possessing Ca^{2+}-binding properties.

The two light chains bind in tandem to the α helix in the neck region of the myosin head to two similar sequences of the so-called IQ motif present in all myosins. The core consensus sequence is IQXXXRGXXXR.[119,124] The C-terminus of the ELC binds to the myosin neck close to the point at which the α helix emerges from the motor domain at a region that shows more variation from the consensus sequence than does the region at which the RLC binds. The latter binds to the myosin α helix below the essential light chain, with contact between the two light chains limited to regions near the calcium-binding loop of the ELC and the linker between domains III and IV of the regulatory light chain. The polarity of both light chains is opposite to that of the myosin heavy chain. In all myosins, the A helix-loop-B helix, which represents domain 1, has retained the ability to bind a metal ion and in vivo is most likely occupied by a Mg ion[125]. It is remarkable that although the structure in the region of the association of the light chains with the myosin neck is very similar in rabbit fast skeletal[126] and molluscan adductor myosin,[124] the regulatory roles of the light chains in myosin activation are not identical in different muscle types. This presumably arises as a consequence of the slightly different amino acid sequences of the light chains in various muscle types. Two different mechanisms of myosin activation by calcium involving the light chains can be distinguished—namely, phosphorylation and direct Ca^{2+} binding.

and catalyzes the phosphorylation of the RLC (Fig. 13-12). Although present in the highest concentrations in muscle, the enzyme is widely distributed and is probably present in all vertebrate cells that contain myosin (for reviews, see Refs. 127 and 128). A notable exception is the adductor muscle of certain molluscs in which the enzyme is not present at a significant level. In all the regulatory light chains from vertebrate muscle so far sequenced there are two adjacent serines at the phosphorylation site, serines 14 and 15 in rabbit fast muscle myosin (Fig. 13-13).

Myosin light chain kinase is most abundant in fast skeletal and smooth muscles, in which tissues the activity per unit wet weight is similar. In the rabbit, slow skeletal muscle kinase activity is about half that in the fast muscle but much higher than in cardiac muscle. Striated muscle also contains a myosin light chain phosphatase, which is responsible for dephosphorylation of myosin after contractile activity. The regulation of smooth muscle phosphorylation is complex and not completely understood. A number of phosphatases that can dephosphorylate myosin are present in smooth muscle,[129] and there is evidence that their regulation is involved in the contractile response of smooth muscle to calcium.

The catalytic unit of myosin light-chain kinase appears to fall into two types, namely that present in skeletal[130] and cardiac muscle[131] with molecular weights in the range 75000–95000 depending on the species and the isoform present. Vertebrate smooth muscle kinase exists in two isoforms, the so-called short kinase with a molecular mass of 150000 and the long myosin light chain kinase mass 210000 (for review, see Ref. 131a). The smooth muscle enzyme is particularly susceptible to proteolysis by endogenous enzymes, which presumably accounts for the range of molecular weights that were earlier reported in the literature. There has been no confirmation of a report that the skeletal enzyme also exists in a high-molecular-weight form. In addition to the catalytic unit, myosin light-chain kinase requires the calcium-binding protein calmodulin for activity. All muscles

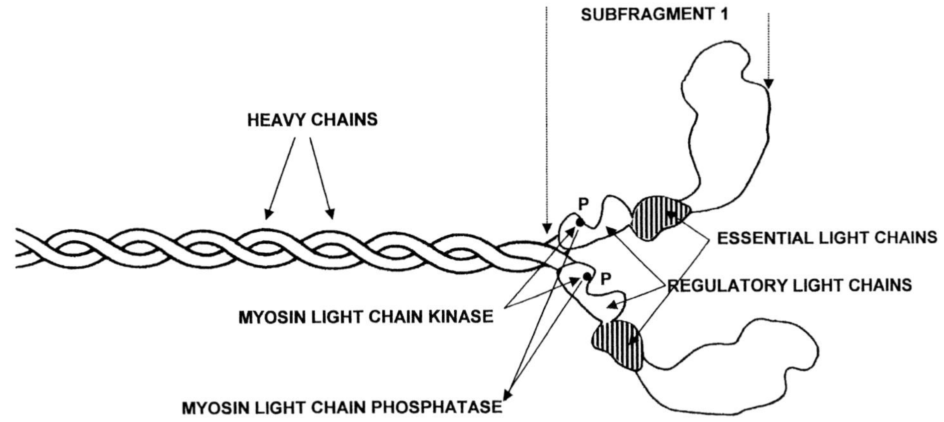

PHOSPHORYLATION OF THE REGULATORY LIGHT CHAINS

All vertebrate muscles contain a specific enzyme, myosin light chain kinase, that is present mainly in the sarcoplasm

FIGURE 13-12. Location of the light chains on the myosin molecule. Schematic representation of the head region of the myosin molecule. The two heavy chains that run the length of the molecule are largely α-helical and exist for much of the tail region as a coiled coil. Each heavy chain, organized in a much less ordered manner, forms one of the two globular heads of the molecule, subfragment 1. The light chains are arranged around the α-helical region of the heavy chain, which forms the neck of subfragment 1 approximately in the manner indicated. See Ref. 126 and Fig. 13-14. P represents the serine residue that is phosphorylated by myosin light-chain kinase.

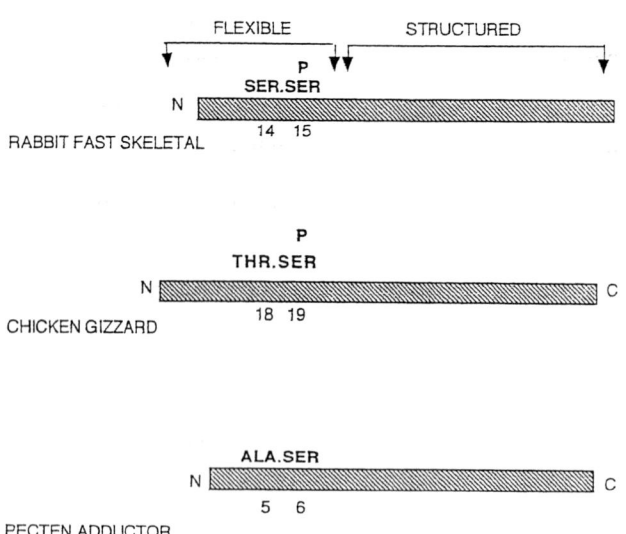

FIGURE 13-13. Schematic representation of the regulatory light chains of myosin. The potential phosphorylation sites are indicated and those most readily phosphorylated marked with P. Amino acid residue positions indicated by numbers.

contain calmodulin, ranging from about 40 to 50 mg/kg fresh weight in a fast muscle such as rabbit longissimus dorsi to 300 to 400 mg/kg fresh weight in vertebrate smooth muscle. There is no evidence that calmodulin is preferentially bound to the myofibril, and much of it is removed from skeletal muscle by low-ionic-strength extracts. Part of the protein is bound to calmodulin-binding proteins such as caldesmon and to various enzyme complexes such as phosphorylase kinase and myosin light-chain kinase. In its presence, when the free Ca^{2+} concentration rises to 10^{-5} M, the kinase catalyzes the phosphorylation of the site on the P light chain.

Both striated and smooth muscle kinases are inactive in the absence of calmodulin and Ca^{2+}. In fast skeletal muscle, the capacity to phosphorylate the RLC is only about 1 to 2 percent of the maximum rate of hydrolysis of ATP by the myofibril. The enzyme shows high specificity for the RLC in the isolated form or in the intact myosin molecule. Immunochemical evidence suggests that the kinases exist as isoforms specific for the striated muscle type.

STRIATED MUSCLE

Actomyosin from striated muscle that is not phosphorylated has high Mg ATPase activity and the effects of phosphorylation obtained in vitro are somewhat variable and sensitive to aging. It does not affect the maximal activation of the ATPase (V_{max}) but does affect the ability of actin to submaximally activate the enzyme, for the K_m for actin is decreased by a factor of about 2.[132] With regulated actomyosin about a twofold increase in Mg ATPase activity can be obtained under conditions of submaximal activation by actin, and the ability to enhance the Mg ATPase was most apparent at low calcium concentrations—i.e., the calcium sensitivity is increased under these conditions. The effects are reversed by treatment with the specific myosin light-chain phosphatase present in muscle. As judged by the effects of controlled proteolysis on skeletal myosin, phosphorylation induces conformational changes in the regulatory and heavy chains. X-ray diffraction studies suggest that in the nonphosphorylated state the myosin heads are held on the filament surface, probably by intermolecular interactions between the myosin molecules. Phosphorylation causes a loss of the helical order and projection of the myosin heads, possibly facilitating movement of the heads to the actin filaments.[132] In skinned skeletal and cardiac muscle fibers, phosphorylation has no effect on maximal calcium activation; but at levels of calcium that produced partial activation, phosphorylation increased isometric force (for references, see Ref. 133). Thus although phosphorylation of the regulatory light chain is not essential for contraction in striated muscle, it increases the sensitivity to calcium at suboptimal calcium concentrations. In this way phosphorylation amplifies the effectiveness of Ca^{2+} release.

It has been suggested[134] that the regulatory light chain phosphorylation has a role in the potentiation of isometric twitch tension observed after a tetanus in fast-twitch muscle (posttetanic potentiation). The precise relationship remains uncertain, for the correlation between RLC phosphorylation and posttetanic potentiation is by no means complete.[135,136]

VERTEBRATE SMOOTH MUSCLE

In striated muscle, actin alone can maximally activate the myosin Mg ATPase, and phosphorylation, which is not essential for contraction, can under certain conditions increase the enzymic activity by a factor of only about 2. In contrast, in vertebrate smooth muscle actin will not activate the myosin Mg ATPase until the RLC (sometimes referred to as the LC 20 in smooth muscle) is phosphorylated. Thus in relaxed smooth muscle the myosin is dephosphorylated, and the phosphorylation by the kinase that is activated by the rise in calcium increases the actin activated Mg ATPase by 50 to 100 times. Chicken gizzard RLC is usually phosphorylated at Ser19, a site that is homologous with Ser15, the residue phosphorylated in the RLC of rabbit fast muscle skeletal myosin. Phosphorylation of the adjacent Thr18 (Fig. 13-13), which can be obtained in vitro with excess kinase, also produces activation. The mechanism for converting vertebrate smooth myosin from a form of the Mg ATPase which cannot be activated by actin to one that can is not understood. The ELC is not essential for this process, which is specific for the smooth myosin RLC and cannot be replaced with fast skeletal myosin RLC. Studies with mutants indicate that substitution of negative charges at the phosphorylation sites only partially mimics the effects of phosphorylation. The C-terminal half of the smooth muscle RLC is particularly important for the activation effect, which must involve interaction with the heavy chain. Thus it appears that the regulatory process in smooth muscle involves changes in the interactions between the RLC and the myosin heavy chain. In some way not understood, the effect of phosphorylation on the conformation of the RLC is conveyed to the motor domain of the myosin head.[124] It has been speculated that phosphorylation induces a change in the gradual bend in the α helix between the two light chains. It would be expected

Chapter 13. Activation of the Contractile Mechanism by Calcium

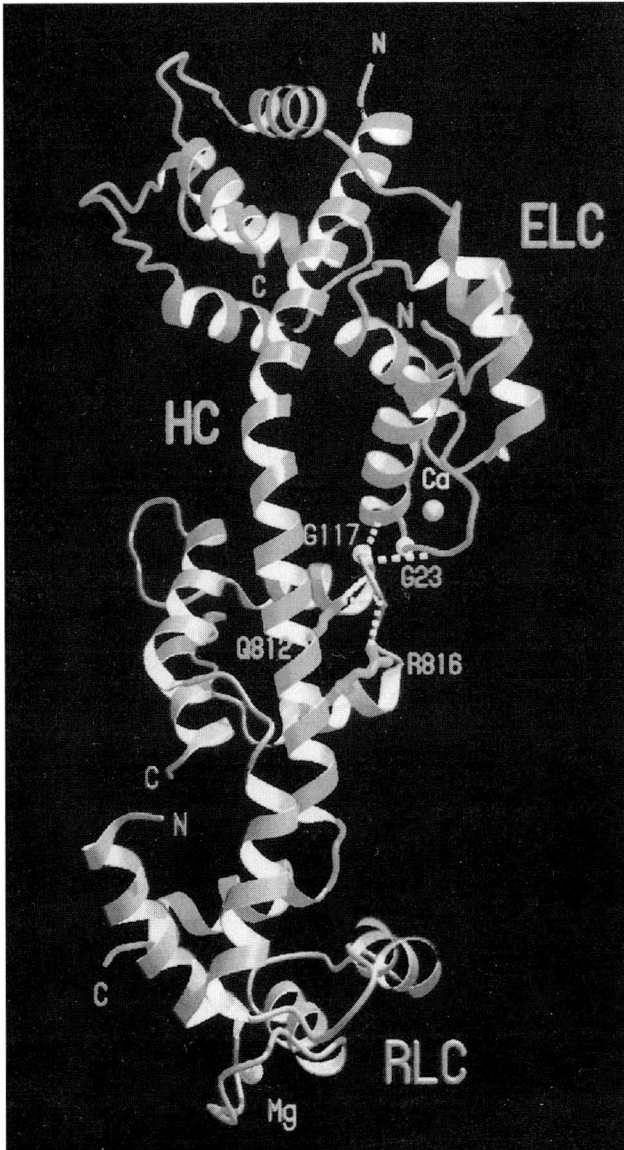

FIGURE 13-14. Ribbon diagram of the overall fold of the light-chain binding region from scallop myosin, the regulatory domain. (See Color Plate 2.) The α-helical heavy chain (Met 773–Ala 840) has one gradual ~40 degree bend in the region between the two light chains and one sharp turn at the C-terminus, involving the residues Trp-Gln-Trp (824–826). The conserved invariant proline is residue 835 of the scallop sequence. The essential light chain (ELC residues Ser1 Pro 154) winds around the N terminal half of this heavy chain, and the regulatory light chain (RLC residues Leu12–Glu 153) interacts with the C-terminal portion. Note that the electron density for Ser 6 of the scallop RLC, which is homologous to phosphorylatable Ser 19 of vertebrate smooth myosin RLC (see Fig. 13-13), is six residues before the first amino acid shown here. A Mg^{2+} ion is shown bound to the divalent cation-binding site in domain 1 of the RLC. The specific calcium-binding site that regulates the activity of scallop myosin is formed by a loop of nine residues of the ELC (bound Ca^{2+}) and stabilized by a number of key linkages involving both heavy-chain and RLC residues (hydrogen bonds). This figure shows that Gly 117, in the linker between domains III and IV of the RLC, forms hydrogen bonds with Phe 20 and Arg 24 of the ELC. These bonds allow very close contact between Gly 117 of the RLC and Gly 23 of the ELC (α-carbons). Gln 812 of the heavy chain forms hydrogen bonds with two residues adjacent to Gly 117 (Met 116

that, as has been reported for phosphorylation of fast striated muscle RLC, phosphorylation increases flexibility at the head-and-neck junction of the myosin molecule, thus permitting the head to project out more from the thick filament and facilitating interaction with actin.

It is generally accepted that phosphorylation of the RLC, which is a consequence of activation of the myosin light-chain kinase by Ca^{2+}, is the primary mechanism for initiating smooth muscle contraction The regulation of contraction, however, in vertebrate smooth muscle is complex, and the understanding is complicated by its ability to exist in the "latch state," in which high force is exerted associated with a slow cross-bridge cycling rate. Other proteins such as caldesmon and calponin are also considered to have a role in the regulation of vertebrate smooth muscle contraction. (For detailed discussion of the relation of phosphorylation to contraction in smooth muscle, see Refs. 137 and 138.)

MOLLUSCAN ADDUCTOR MUSCLE

The myosin present in molluscan adductor smooth muscle is structurally very similar to the myosins of vertebrate striated and smooth muscle containing two light chains corresponding to the ELC and RLC of the vertebrate myosins. The activation of intact scallop myosin Mg ATPase by actin requires the presence of calcium, which binds directly to the head of the myosin molecule and does not involve phosphorylation of the RLC chain, as is the case with vertebrate smooth myosin. Adductor muscle lacks myosin light-chain kinase and the RLC, which has only one serine residue at a site homologous to the phosphorylation sites of the vertebrate myosins (Fig. 13-13), is a poor substrate for the kinase. Removal of the RLC destroys the calcium sensitivity of the Mg ATPase, but some activity is preserved, which is lost when the ELC is subsequently removed. For activation of the scallop actomyosin Mg ATPase by calcium, an unusual calcium-binding site is formed by interactions between both light chains and the heavy chain.[124] The C-terminal half of the ELC binds to the 8.5-nm α helix of the myosin heavy chain close to the point where it emerges from the motor domain. The RLC binds to the C-terminal portion of the α-helical region of the myosin heavy chain just below the ELC. The calcium-binding site is formed by a loop of nine residues in domain 1 of the ELC and stabilized by a number of critical linkages involving both heavy-chain and RLC residues (Fig. 13-14).[120] Gly 117 of the RLC is particularly important in this respect, for vertebrate smooth muscle RLC, in which it is present, can replace scallop RLC in the activation of molluscan Mg ATPase. Fast skeletal RLC, in which this residue is absent, cannot.

It would appear that the more primitive the myosin contractile system, the more dependent its regulation on the action of calcium directly on the motor domain. Uncon-

FIGURE 13-14 *(continued)*
and Asp 118) Arg 816 of the heavy chain also forms a hydrogen bond with Asp 118. *(Data from Xie et al.[124] and presented by Trybus.[120] Figure kindly provided by C. Cohen and M. Silver, Brandeis University.)*

ventional myosins widely involved in intracellular movement bind the calcium-binding protein calmodulin in the region of the consensus sequence IQXXXRQXXXR, located in the neck of the molecule. The consensus sequence is preserved in the myosin II family, but the calmodulin is replaced by the light-chain proteins of similar evolutionary origin but with only rudimentary calcium-binding sites. Although these light chains in solution do not bind calcium to any significant extent, a high-affinity site is produced when they are bound to the myosin heavy chain in adductor myosin. The conformational change that results from binding calcium is in some way conveyed to the myosin motor domain (or to the actin), so that the inhibitory effect is lost. In vertebrate smooth muscle, although its RLC is sufficiently homologous to replace the scallop RLC, actin activation is switched on by the conformational changes produced by phosphorylation at a site close to its N-terminal and near the C-terminal of the heavy-chain α-helix and not by calcium binding. The role of the RLC in the regulation of the actin activation of the Mg ATPase is one of the more striking differences between the various muscle types (Table 13-5). In both vertebrate and molluscan smooth muscles in the resting state, the RLC acts as an inhibitor of the actin activation of the myosin Mg ATPase. This inhibitory property is destroyed when the calcium concentration rises, resulting in either calcium binding or the phosphorylation of the RLC, depending on the smooth muscle type. The RLC chain in striated muscle has lost the inhibitory property but does preserve some modulatory effect on calcium activation; however, the inhibition of the actomyosin interaction is now taken over by the tropomyosin troponin system of the thin filament. Thus the role of calcium in both smooth and striated muscle is to override the inhibitory systems of the thick and thin filaments, respectively, that are active in the resting state. This takes place by mechanisms that are specific for each of the muscle types—namely striated, vertebrate smooth, and invertebrate smooth.

Myosin-Binding Protein C

Myosin-binding protein C (MBPC), previously called the C protein, is located in 7 to 9 of the transverse stripes present in the region of the A band, the C zone, where the myosin cross bridges are found. Associated with MBPC are smaller amounts of related proteins, myosin-binding proteins H and X. There are three isoforms of MBPC, each associated with fast skeletal, slow skeletal, and cardiac muscles and under individual genetic control, which suggests slight differences in function in the different muscle types. The cardiac form is of special interest, as it possesses an additional N-terminal region and three sites phosphorylated by protein kinase A. The role of MBPC is far from clear, but there is evidence that it has a structural role in the formation of thick filaments and myofibrils. The presence of three sites in the cardiac isoform phosphorylated by protein kinase A implies that it may also have a modulatory role. MBPC increases the ATPase of cardiac actomyosin, an effect that requires the presence of the RLC, and which suggests it may have a role in the crossbridge cycle. There is no evidence of calcium binding by the MBPC and its direct involvement in the activation process, but extraction of a major portion of the protein from both skeletal and cardiac skinned fibers increases the calcium sensitivity of contraction. This implies that the MBPC may in some way interact with the regulatory proteins of the I filament system as well as with myosin (for references, see Refs. 139 and 140).

Parvalbumins

Parvalbumins is the name given by Pechere[141] to a homologous group of proteins originally characterized from fish

Table 13-5. RELATIONSHIPS BETWEEN THE PHOSPHORYLATION OF THE REGULATORY LIGHT CHAIN OF MYOSIN AND THE CALCIUM REGULATION OF THE Mg ATPase OF ACTOMYOSIN FROM DIFFERENT MUSCLES

Muscle	Phosphorylation	Calcium Regulation	Regulatory Light-Chain Inhibitory Activity
Molluscan adductor	No	Yes	Yes (calcium relieves)
Vertebrate smooth	Yes (high)	Yes	Yes (phos. relieves)
Vertebrate skeletal	Yes (high)	Yes	No
Vertebrate cardiac	Yes (low)	?	No

Note: Myosins above the dotted line are mainly thick-filament regulated; those below the line are thin-filament regulated.

and amphibian skeletal muscle. They exist in several types, up to six of which have been identified in fish on the basis of their electrophoretic mobilities, and their molecular weights range from 9000 to 13000. Parvalbumin 3 from carp was the first to be described and crystallized,[142] and in any one species of fish several of the components are usually present. The parvalbumins are responsible for the slowly sedimenting fraction in low ionic strength extracts of muscle observed first by Deuticke[143] and later studied intensively by Hamoir and his colleagues.[144] Although the amounts present in fish red muscle are barely significant, it is one of the most abundant proteins in the white muscle, representing 0.7 percent of the wet weight in the carp.

The mammalian genome encodes two isoforms, α and β parvalbumin, which possess 49 percent sequence identity.[145] Significant amounts of α parvalbumin have been found in the muscles of mammals, particularly those of small animals such as the rat, mouse, guinea pig, and chicken, although less than is present in fish muscle. Parvalbumin is also present in GABAergic neurons present in different parts of the brain.[37,146] The organ of Corti is apparently the only site of expression of β parvalbumin in adult animals. The amounts of parvalbumin are much greater in fast-twitch muscles, with the levels highest in type IIB and type IID/2X fibers. Much less parvalbumin is present in type IIA and slow-twitch (type 1) fibers.[147] Levels are very low in larger mammals such as humans and the horse, even in muscles that contain a substantial proportion of type II fibers. For example, mouse gastrocnemius muscle, with its very fast contraction and relaxation times, contains 4.9 g/kg, whereas the much slower deep gluteal muscle of the horse and the vastus and triceps muscles of humans contain less than 1 mg/kg. Cardiac and smooth muscle cells do not stain with parvalbumin antibodies.

The role of the parvalbumins was obscure until it was reported[148] that large amounts of calcium representing about 2 mole per mole were present in the ash obtained from these proteins after incineration. In view of the general similarity of certain properties of the parvalbumins to those of TnC, e.g., UV spectra and amino acid composition, it was suggested that they might be structurally related and had possibly evolved from a common precursor.[148] Direct measurement of binding constants indicated that the parvalbumins bound two molecules of Ca^{2+} with affinities similar to those of the Ca-Mg sites of TnC (sites III and IV). Kretsinger and Nockolds[56] determined the three-dimensional structure of carp parvalbumin 3 and identified the two Ca^{2+} binding domains, the CD and EF regions. Similar domains in a number of proteins that bind calcium with high affinity have now been identified by their characteristic amino acid sequence.

The presence of parvalbumin in the soluble sarcoplasm of fast muscles of fish and amphibia, often at concentrations that are an order of magnitude greater than that of the TnC in the myofibril, raises the question of its role in the excitation process. At the concentration of the free Mg^{2+} ion in resting muscle, the Ca^{2+} binding sites of parvalbumin and the Ca-Mg sites on TnC will be saturated with Mg^{2+}. From computer simulation of the situation, it has been concluded that immediately after a pulse of Ca^{2+} corresponding to that occurring on stimulation of muscle, the regulatory sites I and II of TnC, which are Ca^{2+}-specific, will be 97 percent saturated, but very little Ca^{2+} would be bound to the parvalbumin.[149] After 200 ms, which is comparable to the duration of a twitch in frog sartorius muscle, the Mg^{2+} on the parvalbumin is replaced by Ca^{2+}. This would suggest, at least in muscles with parvalbumin concentrations five times greater than that of the TnC, that parvalbumin acts as a soluble relaxing factor.[149–151] Binding of Ca^{2+} will occur toward the end of the contraction-relaxation cycle, when the Ca^{2+} concentration in the sarcoplasm starts to fall and hence lead to a speeding up of relaxation. There is a good correlation between relaxation speed and the parvalbumin content in mammalian skeletal muscles; despite the relatively lower amounts it has been suggested that parvalbumin plays a similar role in these tissues.[147,152] Evidence for such a role has been obtained by the demonstration that increasing the parvalbumin content of rat soleus[153] and of rat heart[154] by direct gene transfer into the muscle increased relaxation times. The activity pattern of the muscle is an important factor determining the expression of the parvalbumin gene. The fall in levels of parvalbumin in the extensor digitorum longus of the rat that occurs on aging can be reversed by high-intensity exercise,[155] whereas low-frequency stimulation suppresses parvalbumin gene expression.[156]

Chromosome Locations of Genes Expressing Regulatory Proteins of the Thin Filaments

The genes responsible for expressing the muscle regulatory proteins are widely distributed, as they are located on 11 different chromosomes in the human genome (Table 13-6). It is of interest that in no case are the genes expressing the different isoforms of a given protein located on the same chromosome. In certain situations, as during development and cross-innervation, the expression of the fast isoform is stimulated and that of the slow isoform repressed (and vice versa), e.g., with TnI, TnT, α and β tropomyosin. This suggests a reciprocal coupling of gene expression between the isoforms on different chromosomes by a mechanism yet to be determined. Chromosomes 1, 11, and 19 appear to be particularly important for the location of regulatory protein genes. In contrast, only one gene for a regulatory protein is located on each of the remaining 8 chromosomes involved. Where more than than one regulatory protein gene is present on a chromosome, they are usually located close to each other (Table 13-7).

MUTATIONS OF THE REGULATORY PROTEINS

In recent years there has been a steady increase in the number of mutant forms of proteins of the contractile and regulatory systems of muscle that have been shown to be associated with muscular dystrophies. Many of the mutations, which usually involve single amino acid residue replacements, give rise to a common phenotype, familial hypertrophic cardiomyopathy (FHC). This condition is characterized by increased myocardial mass and myocyte and

Table 13-6. CHROMOSOME LOCATIONS OF GENES EXPRESSING THE REGULATORY PROTEINS OF MUSCLE

Tropomyosin	
TPM 1 (α)	15q22.1
TPM2 (β)	9p13.2-p13.1
TPM 3	1q22-23
TPM 4	19p13.1
Troponin C	
TNNC1 (slow twitch /cardiac)	3p21.3-14.3
TNNC2 (fast twitch)	20q12-13.11
Troponin I	
Slow twitch (TNNI1)	1q31.3
Fast twitch (TNNI2)	11p15.5
Cardiac (TNNI3)	19q13.4
Troponin T	
Slow twitch (TNN1)	19q13.4
Cardiac (TNNT2)	1q32
Fast twitch (TNNT3)	11p15.5
Parvalbumin	
PVALB	22q12-13.1
Caldesmon	
CALD1	7q33
Calmodulin	
CALM1	14q24-q31
CALM2	2p21
CALM3	19q13.2-q133

SOURCE: Online Mendelian Inheritance in Man. National Center for Biotechnology Information. USA.

myofibrillar disarray, although the mutations responsible occur in tropomyosin, TnI, TnT, β-cardiac myosin heavy chain, ELC, RLC, myosin-binding protein C, and α-actin. This has led to the suggestion that the mutations of the myofibrillar proteins give rise to a "sarcomeric" disease.[157] It is postulated that mutation of any of these proteins can lead to a change in gene expression, which results in changes in the stoichiometry of expression of the proteins involved in the formation of the sarcomere. Thus mutation in almost any protein component of the sarcomere can produce a common phenotype. In some cases, however, the myopathy takes on a different form—e.g., nemaline myopathy, which is characterized by an accumulation of nemaline bodies, stacked Z lines.

Nemaline myopathy is associated with the Met 9Arg mutation of the TPM3 gene expressed in skeletal muscle[158] nebulin,[159] actin ACTA1,[160] and slow skeletal TnT gene TNNT1.[161] Mutations at different regions of the gene, the human actin gene (ACTA1) for example, can give rise to a range of phenotypes ranging from severe nemaline myopathy to conditions characterized by excess thin filaments outside the sarcomere (for review of the relation between the genotype and phenotype in familial muscle disease, see Ref. 162).

The regulatory proteins involved in calcium regulation, tropomyosin, TnT, and TnI, occur in a number of mutant forms and are usually associated with FHC. (For details of mutations, see reviews in Refs. 43, 97, and 163–165.) In the case of the Asp175Asn mutation of α tropomyosin, increased calcium sensitivity can be demonstrated with skinned fibers from biopsy samples of human vastis lateralis muscle.[166] It is of interest that although FHC is usually associated with mutations of α tropomyosin, no clinical evidence of the disease has been reported in skeletal muscle, where α tropomyosin is often the dominant isoform present.[157] This may imply that the mutation is less easily tolerated by the continuous activity pattern of the heart, or it may be due to the fact that because of the presence of substantial amounts of β tropomyosin in skeletal muscle, the mutant form will be present as a heterodimer with the wild-type β tropomyosin, in which the effects of the mutation are masked.

Overview and Concluding Comments

Although the interaction of actin with myosin which results in the activation of the Mg ATPase of the motor system is triggered by calcium in all types of muscle, the precise mechanism of the calcium effect is specific for the muscle type. In all cases the actomyosin interaction is blocked in the resting state of the muscle. This blocking action is carried out by the troponin-tropomyosin system in striated muscle and by the inhibitory action of the RLC of myosin in smooth muscle. Activation in striated muscle results from the binding of calcium to TnC, which displaces TnI from the inhibitory mode on actin. In smooth muscle, calcium acts directly on the myosin motor, inducing conformational changes in the RLC chain, which eliminates its inhibitory activity. This follows

Table 13-7. LOCATION OF GENES ON CHROMOSOMES THAT CONTAIN GENES FOR MORE THAN ONE MUSCLE REGULATORY PROTEIN

Chromosome 1		Chromosome 11		Chromosome 19	
TMN3	1q22-23	TNNI2 (fast)	11p15.5	TMN4	19p13.1
TNNI1 (slow)	1q31.3	TNNT3 (fast)	11p15.5	TNNI3 (cardiac)	19q13.4
TNNT2 (cardiac)	1q32			TNNT1 (slow)	19q13.4
				CALM 3	19q13.2-13.3

from activation of the light-chain kinase, resulting in phosphorylation of the RLC in vertebrate smooth muscle and by direct binding of calcium to a site involving the myosin heavy chain, the ELC, and the RLC in molluscan adductor myosin. The precise atomic description of how calcium activates the actomyosin ATPase in any of these systems has yet to be determined, but the direct action of calcium at the myosin motor level is perhaps easier to understand than the rapid activation characteristic of fast striated muscle. This takes place via the thin filament, in which the calcium-binding protein TnC is located with a periodicity of 385 Å along the thin filament, one molecule of TnC for every seven actin monomers in the thin filament.

Two major problems exist in our understanding of the regulation of contraction in muscle: (1) the changes that occur at the actin myosin interface that result in Mg ATP becoming an effective substrate and thus initiating the contractile cycle and (2) the mechanism that enables the effect of calcium binding by TnC to be transmitted in striated muscle to the seven actins in the structural unit of the thin filament. The former is still a matter for speculation, whereas it is widely held that the steric hypothesis explains the latter. For full acceptance of the steric hypothesis, there are many questions still to be answered, which require definition at the atomic level of the actin-myosin interaction sites and the relation of the TnI, TnT, and TnC to them. Although the evidence is strong, particularly in striated muscle, that the tropomyosin molecule moves on contraction, the driving force for this movement and how it is transmitted along the molecule from the region on TnC that binds calcium is a matter for discussion.[166a] The evidence of flexibility in the tropomyosin molecule[42,167] suggests that its position on the actin molecule would be determined by local interactions rather than effects transmitted along the tropomyosin molecule. It should be borne in mind that tropomyosin is a widely distributed protein, an invariant component of stable actin filament systems in all vertebrate cell types. The high concentrations in muscle merely reflect the abundance of actin filaments in contractile tissue. One may ask if tropomyosin possesses special properties unique to the actin filaments of striated muscle systems. In this respect, its ability to induce cooperative properties in the actin monomers of the F-actin filament is surely of special significance for muscle function[168] (for review, see Ref. 43).

The regulation of contractile activity in striated muscle involves the interaction of at least six proteins: myosin, actin, tropomyosin, TnI, TnT, and TnC (possibly also nebulin and myosin-binding protein C). This is a very complex system, and its understanding in atomic terms requires a precise description of the regions of the proteins involved in these interactions. But so far, these interaction sites have been identified with certainty in only a few instances. Progress in this field, however, should be rapid with advanced structural studies of the proteins involved and investigation of the effects of mutations, both naturally occurring and induced, on the function of the regulatory system.

Acknowledgments

I am particularly grateful to Valerie Patchell for her skilled assistance in producing this chapter. I would also like to thank Chris Ashley of the Physiological Laboratory, Oxford University, for providing me with records from the literature of calcium transients in different muscle types, and the colleagues who have allowed me to reproduce figures from their work.

List of Abbreviations

ATPase	adenosinetriphosphatase		MBPC	myosin-binding protein C
Mg ATPase	magnesium-activated adenosine triphosphatase		NMR	nuclear magnetic resonance
EDTA	ethylenediaminetetraacetic acid		SR	sarcoplasmic reticulum
EGTA	ethylene glycol-*bis* (*b*-aminoethylether) N, N'-tetraacetic acid		TnC	troponin C
			TnI	troponin I
ELC	essential light chain		TnT	troponin T
RLC	regulatory light chain			

References

1. Kamada T, Kinosita H: Disturbances initiated from naked surface of muscle protoplasm. *Jpn J Zool* 10:469, 1943.
2. Heilbrun LV, Wiercinski FJ: The action of various cations on muscle protoplasm. *J Cell Comp Physiol* 29:15, 1947.
3. Ashley CC, Mulligan IP, Lea TJ: Ca^{2+} and activation mechanisms in skeletal muscle. *Q Rev Biophys* 24:1–73, 1991.
4. Williams AJ, West DJ, Sitsapesan R: Light at the end of the Ca^{2+} release channel tunnel: Structures and mechanisms involved in ion translocation in ryanodine receptor channels. *Q Rev Biophys* 34:61–104, 2001.
5. Caputo C: Calcium release in skeletal muscle: From K^+ contractures to Ca^{2+} sparks. *J Muscle Res Cell Motil* 22:485–504, 2002.
6. Perry SV: Relation between chemical and contractile function and structure in skeletal muscle. *Physiol Rev* 36:1–76, 1956.
7. Needham DM: *Machina Carnis*. London: Cambridge University Press, 1971.
8. Bozler E: Interactions between magnesium, pyrophosphate and the contractile elements. *J Gen Physiol* 38:53, 1954.
9. Watanabe S: Relaxing effects of EDTA on glycerol-treated muscle fibres. *Arch Biochem Biophys* 54:559, 1955.
10. Perry SV, Grey TC: A study of the effects of substrate concentration and certain relaxing factors on the magnesium activated myofibrillar ATPase. *Biochem J* 64:184–192, 1956.
11. Perry SV, Grey TC: Ethylenediaminetetraacetate and the ATPase activity of actomyosin systems. *Biochem J* 64:5, 1956.
12. Weber A: On the role of calcium in the activity of adenosine triphosphate hydrolysis by actomyosin. *J Biol Chem* 234:2764, 1959.

13. Weber A, Winicur S: The role of Ca^{2+} in the superprecipitation of actomyosin. *J Biol Chem* 236:3198, 1961.
14. Bozler E: Mechanism of relaxation in extracted muscle fibres. *Am J Physiol* 167:276, 1951.
15. Marsh BB: The effects of adenosine triphosphate on the fibre volume of a muscle homogenate. *Biochim Biophys Acta* 9:247, 1952.
16. Kumagi H, Ebashi S, Takeda F: Essential relaxing factor in muscle other than myokinase and creatine phosphokinase. *Nature* 176:166, 1955.
17. Ebashi S: Calcium binding activity of vesicular relaxing factor. *J Biochem (Tokyo)* 50:236, 1961.
18. Ebashi S, Lipmann F: ATP-linked concentration of calcium ions in a particulate fraction of rabbit muscle. *J Cell Biol* 14:389, 1962.
19. Hasselbach W: Relaxing factor and the relaxation of muscle. *Prog Biophys* 14:167, 1964.
20. Ebashi S, Endo M: Calcium ion and muscle contraction. *Prog Biophys Mol Biol* 18:123, 1968.
21. Ebashi S: Third component participating in the superprecipitation of natural actomyosin. *Nature* 200:1010, 1963.
22. Bailey K: Tropomyosin: A new asymmetric protein component of the muscle fibril. *Biochem J* 43:271, 1948.
23. Ebashi S, Kodama A: A new protein factor promoting aggregation of tropomyosin. *J Biochem (Tokyo)* 58:107, 1965.
24. Milligan RA: Protein-protein interactions in the rigor actomyosin complex. *Proc Natl Acad Sci USA* 93:21–26, 1996.
25. Westerblad H, Lannergren J, Allen DG: Slowed relaxation in fatigued skeletal muscle of Xenopus and mouse. *J Gen Physiol* 109:385–399, 1997.
26. Allen DG, Kurihara S: Calcium transients in mammalian ventricular muscle. *Eur Heart J* 1(Suppl A):5–15, 1980.
27. Neering IR, Morgan KG: Use of aequorin to study excitation-contraction coupling in mammalian smooth muscle. *Nature* 288:285–287, 1980.
28. Huxley AF, Taylor RE: Local activation of skeletal muscle fibres. *Nature* 144:426–441, 1958.
29. Baylor SM, Chandler WK, Marshall MW: Sarcoplasmic reticulum calcium release in frog skeletal muscle fibres estimated from arsenazo III calcium transients. *J Physiol* 344:625–666, 1983.
30. Rios E, Stern MD: Calcium in close quarters: Microdomain feedback in excitation-contraction coupling and other cell biological phenomena. *Annu Rev Biophys Biomolec Struct* 26:47–82, 1997.
31. Franzini-Armstrong C, Jorgensen AO: Structure and development of E-C coupling units in skeletal muscle. *Annu Rev Physiol* 56:509–534, 1994.
32. Escobar AL, Monck JR, Fernandez JM, et al: Localisation of the site of Ca^{2+} release at the level of a single sarcomere in skeletal muscle fibres. *Nature* 367:739–741, 1994.
33. Leong P, MacLennan DH: Complex interactions between skeletal muscle ryanodine receptor and dihydropyridine receptor proteins. *Biochem Cell Biol* 76:681–694, 1998.
34. Hollingworth S, Soeller C, Baylor SM, et al: Sarcomeric Ca^{2+} gradients during activation of frog skeletal muscle fibres imaged with confocal and two photomicroscopy. *J Physiol* 526:551–560, 2000.
35. Rome LC, Syme DA, Hollingworth S, et al: The whistle and the rattle: The design of sound producing muscles. *Proc Natl Acad Sci USA* 93:8095–8100, 1996.
36. Caputo C: Calcium release in skeletal muscle: From K^+ contractures to Ca^{2+} sparks. *J Muscle Res Cell Motil* 22:485–504; 2001.
36a. Potter TD, Robinson SP, Collins JH et al. The role of Ca^{2+}- and Mg^{2+}-binding sites on troponin and other contractile proteins, in Siegel FL, Carafoli E, Kretsinger RH, et al (eds): *Calcium Binding Proteins: Structure and Function*. Amsterdam, Elsevier/North Holland, 1980; pp 279–280.
37. Caillard O, Moreno H, Schwaller B, et al: Role of the calcium-binding protein parvalbuminin short-term synaptic plasticity. *Proc Natl Acad Sci USA* 97:13372–13377, 2000.
38. Barker HC, Ketcham LK, Dayhoff MO: Evolutionary relationship among calcium binding proteins, in Wasserman RUG, Cordon RA, Carafoli E, et al (eds): *Calcium-Binding Proteins and Calcium Function*. Amsterdam: North-Holland, 1977; pp 73–75.
39. Herzberg O, James MN: Refined crystal structure of troponin C from turkey skeletal muscle at 2 Å resolution. *J Mol Biol* 203:761–779, 1988.
40. Satyshur KA, Rao ST, Pyzalska D, et al: Refined structure of chicken skeletal troponin C in the two calcium state at 2 Å resolution. *J Biol Chem* 263:1628–1647, 1988.
41. Whitby FG, Phillips GN Jr: Crystal structure of tropomyosin at 7 Å resolution. *Proteins* 38:49–59, 2000.
42. Brown JH, Kim K-H, Jun G, et al: Deciphering the design of the tropomyosin molecule. *Proc Natl Acad Sci USA* 98:8496–8501, 2001.
43. Perry SV: Vertebrate tropomyosin: Distribution, properties and function. *J Muscle Res Cell Motil* 22:5–49, 2001.
44. Crick FHC: The Fourier transform of a coiled-coil. *Acta Crystallog* 6:15, 1953.
45. Stewart M, McLachlan AD: Fourteen actin-binding sites on tropomyosin. *Nature* 257:331–333, 1975.
45a. Li Y, Mui S, Brown JH, Strand J, et al. The crystal structure of the C-terminal fragment of striated muscle α-tropomyosin reveals a key troponin T recognition site. *Proc Natl Acad Sci USA*, 99:7378–7383, 2002.
46. Heeley DH, Dhoot DK, Perry SV: Factors determining the subunit composition of tropomyosin in mammalian muscle. *Biochem J* 226:461–468, 1985.
46a. Watson MH, Kuhn AE, Novy RE, et al. Caldesmon binding site on tropomyosin. *J Biol Chem* 265:18860–18866, 1990.
47. Stone D, Smillie LB: The amino acid sequence of rabbit skeletal α-tropomyosin. The NH2 terminal half and complete sequence. *J Biol Chem* 253:1137, 1978.
48. Mak AS, Smillie LB, Stewart GR: A comparison of the amino acid sequences of rabbit skeletal muscle α and β-tropomyosins. *J Biol Chem* 255:3647, 1980.
49. Leger J, Bouveret P, Schwartz K, et al: A comparative study of skeletal and cardiac tropomyosins. *Pflugers Arch* 362:271–277, 1976.
50. Heeley DH, Dhoot DK, Frearson N, et al: The effect of cross innervation on the tropomyosin composition of rabbit skeletal muscle. *FEBS Lett* 152:282–286, 1983.
51. Pieples K, Wieczorek DF: Tropomyosin 3 increases striated muscle diversity. *Biochemistry* 39:8291–8297, 2000.
52. Mair J: Cardiac troponin I and troponin T: Are enzymes still relevant as markers? *Clin Chem Acta* 257:99–115, 1997.
53. Hastings KEM, Emerson CP: cDNA clone analysis of six coregulated mRNAs encoding skeletal muscle contractile proteins. *Proc Natl Acad Sci USA* 79:1553–1557, 1982.
54. Schreier T, Kedes L, Gahlmann R: Cloning, structural analysis and expression of human slow twitch skeletal muscle/cardiac troponin C gene. *J Biol Chem* 265:21247–21253, 1991.
55. Gahlmann R, Kedes L: Cloning structural analysis and expression of the human fast twitch skeletal muscle troponin C. *J Biol Chem* 265:12520–12528, 1990.
56. Kretsinger RH, Nockolds CE: Carp muscle calcium-binding protein: Structure determination and general description. *J Biol Chem* 248:3313, 1973.
57. Collins JH, Potter JD, Horn MJ, et al: The amino acid sequence of rabbit skeletal muscle troponin C: Gene replication and homology with calcium-binding proteins from carp and hake muscle. *FEBS Lett* 36:268, 1973.
58. Kretsinger RH, Barry CD: The predicted structure of the calcium-binding component of troponin. *Biochim Biophys Acta* 405:40, 1975.
59. Potter JD, Gergely J: The calcium and magnesium binding sites on troponin and their role in regulation of myofibrillar ATPase. *J Biol Chem* 250:4268, 1975.
60. Potter TD, Robertson SP, Collins JH, Johnson JS: The role of Ca^{2+} and Mg^{2+} binding sites on troponin and other contractions, in Siegel FL, Carafoli E, Kretsinger RH, et al (eds): *Calcium Binding Proteins: Structure and Function*. Amsterdam: Elsevier/North-Holland, 1980; pp 279–280.
61. Leavis PC, Rosenfeld SS, Gergely J, et al: Proteolytic fragments of troponin C. *J Biol Chem* 253:5452, 1978.
62. Grabarek Z, Tao T, Gergely J: Molecular mechanism of troponin C function. *J Muscle Res Cell Motil* 13:383, 1992.
63. Van Eerd J-P, Takahashi K: Determination of the complete amino acid sequence of bovine troponin C. *Biochemistry* 15:1171, 1976.
64. Li MX, Gagne SM, Tsuda S, et al: Calcium binding to the regulatory domain of skeletal muscle troponin C occurs in a stepwise manner. *Biochemistry* 34:8330–8340, 1995.
65. Li MX, Gagne SM, Spyracopoulos L, et al: NMR studies of Ca^{2+} binding to the regulatory domains of cardiac and E41A skeletal troponin C reveal the importance of site 1 to the energetics of the induced structural changes. *Biochemistry* 36:12519–12525, 1997.
66. Putkey JA, Sweeney HL, Campbell ST: Site directed mutation of the trigger calcium-binding sites in cardiac troponin C. *J Biol Chem* 264:12370–12378, 1989.
67. Sweeney HL, Brito RM, Putkey JA: The low-affinity Ca^{2+} binding site in cardiac/slow muscle troponin C perform distinct functions: Site 1 alone cannot trigger contraction. *Proc Natl Acad Sci USA* 87:9538–9552, 1990.
68. Strynadka NCJ, Cherney M, Sielecki AR, et al: Structural details of a calcium induced molecular switch: X-ray crystallographic analysis of the calcium-saturated N-terminal domain of troponin C at 1.75 Å resolution. *J Mol Biol* 273:238–258, 1997.
69. Gagne SM, Li MX, Mckay RT, et al: The NMR angle on troponin C. *Biochem Cell Biol* 76:302–312, 1998.
70. Strynadka NC, James MNG: Crystal structures of the helix-loop-helix calcium binding proteins. *Ann Rev Biochem* 58:951, 1989.
71. Grabarek Z, Tan R-Y, Wang J, et al: Inhibition of mutant troponin C activity by an intradomain disulphide bond. *Nature (London)* 345:132, 1990.
72. Allhouse LD, Miller T, Li Q, et al: Investigation of a genetically engineered mutant of barnacle troponin C containing a central helix deletion. *Eur J Physiol* 439:67–75, 1999.
73. Sia SK, Li MX, Spyracopoulos L, et al: Structure of cardiac muscle troponin C unexpectedly reveals a closed regulatory domain. *J Biol Chem* 272:18216–18221, 1997.
74. Spyracopoulos L, Li MX, Sia SK, et al: Calcium-induced structural transition in the regulatory domain of human cardiac troponin C. *Biochemistry* 36:12138–12146, 1997.
75. Head JF, Perry SV: The interaction of the calcium binding protein troponin C with bivalent cations and the inhibitory protein, troponin I. *Biochem J* 37:145, 1974.

76. Syska H, Perry SV, Trayer IP: A new method of preparation of troponin I (inhibitory protein) using affinity chromatography. Evidence for three different forms of troponin I in striated muscle. *FEBS Lett* 40:253–257, 1974.
77. Perry SV: Troponin I: Inhibitor or facilitator. *Mol Cell Biochem* 190:9–32, 1999.
78. Dhoot GK, Perry SV: Distribution of the polymorphic forms of troponin components and tropomyosin in skeletal muscle. *Nature* 278:714–718, 1979.
79. Dhoot GK, Perry SV: The components of the troponin complex and development in skeletal muscle. *Exp Cell Res* 127:75–87, 1980.
80. Sabry MA, Dhoot GK: Identification and pattern of expression of a developmental isoforms of troponin I in chicken and rat cardiac muscle. *J Muscle Res Cell Motil* 10:85–91, 1989.
81. Saggin L, Gorza L, Ausoni S, Schiaffino S: Troponin I switching in developing heart. *J Biol Chem* 264:16299–16302, 1989.
82. Perry SV, Cole HA, Head, JF et al: Localisation and mode of action of the inhibitory component of the troponin complex. *Cold Spring Harbor Symp Quant Biol* 37:251–262, 1972.
83. Geeves MA, Chai M, Lehrer SS: Inhibition of actin-myosin subfragment 1 ATPase activity by troponin I and IC: Relationship to thin filament states of muscle. *Biochemistry* 39:9345–9350, 2000.
84. Tung C-S, Wall ME, Gallagher SC, et al: A model of troponin I in complex with troponin C using hybrid experimental data: The inhibitory region is a beta hairpin. *Protein Sci* 9:1312–1326, 2000.
85. Syska HA, Wilkinson JM, Grand RJA, et al: The relationship between biological activity and primary structure of troponin I from white skeletal muscle of the rabbit. *Biochem J* 153:375–387, 1976.
86. Ferrieres G, Pugniere M, Mani JC, et al: Systematic mapping of regions of cardiac troponin I involved in binding to troponin C: N- and C-terminal low affinity contributing regions. *FEBS Lett* 479:99–105, 2000.
87. Luo Y, Lezyk J, Li B, et al: Proximity relationships between residue 6 of troponin I and residues on troponin C. Further evidence for the extended conformation of troponin C in the troponin complex. *Biochemistry* 39:15306–15315, 2000.
87a. Abbott MB, Gaponenko V, Abusamhadneh E, et al: Regulatory domain conformational exchange and linker region flexibility in cardiac troponin C bound to troponin I., *J Biol Chem* 275:20610–20617, 2000.
87b. Vassylyev DG, Takeda S, Wakatsuki S, et al: Crystal structure of troponin C in complex with troponin I fragment at 2.3 Å resolution. *Proc Natl Acad Sci USA* 95:4847–4852, 1998.
87c. Takeda S, Yamashita A, Maeda K, et al: Structure of the core domain of human cardiac troponin in the Ca^{2+}-saturated form. *Nature* 421:35–41, 2003.
87d. Dvoretsky A, Abusamhadneh E, Howarth JW, et al: Solution structure of calcium saturated cardiac troponin C bound to cardiac troponin I. *J Biol Chem* 277:38565–38570, 2002.
87e. Wang X, Li MX and Sykes BD: The structure of the regulatory domain of human cardiac troponin C in complex with human cardiac troponin I 147–163 and bepridil. *J Biol Chem* 277:31124–31133, 2002.
88. Talbot JA, Hodges RS: Synthetic studies on the inhibitory region of rabbit skeletal troponin I. *J Biol Chem* 256:2798–2802, 1981.
88a. Tripet B, De Crescenzo G, Grothe S, et al: Kinetic analysis of the interactions between troponin C (TnC) and troponin I (TnI) binding peptides: evidence for separate binding sites for the "structural" N-terminus and the "regulatory" C-terminus of TnI on TnC. *J Molec. Recognition* 16:37–53, 2003.
89. Haselgrove JC: X-ray evidence for a conformational change in the actin containing filaments of vertebrate striated muscle. *Cold Spring Harbor Symp Quant Biol* 37:341–352, 1972.
90. Huxley HE: Structural changes in the actin- and myosin-containing filaments during contraction. *Cold Spring Harbor Symp Quant Biol* 37:361–378, 1972.
91. Parry DAD, Squire JM: Structural role of tropomyosin in muscle regulation: Analysis of the x-ray diffraction patterns from relaxed and contracting muscles. *J Mol Biol* 75:35–55, 1972.
92. McKillop DFA, Geeves MA: Regulation of the interaction between actin and myosin subfragment 1: Evidence of three states of the thin filament *Biophys J* 65:693–701, 1993.
93. Lehman W, Hatch V, Korman V, et al: Tropomyosin and actin isoforms modulate the localisation of tropomyosin strands on actin filaments. *J Mol Biol* 302:593–606, 2000.
94. Kress, M, Huxley HE, Faruqi AR, Hendrix J: Structural changes during activation of frog muscle studied by time resolved x-ray diffraction. *J Mol Biol* 188:325–342, 1986.
95. Xu C, Craig R, Tobacman L, Horowitz R, Lehman W: Tropomyosin positions in regulated thin filaments revealed by cryoelectronmicroscopy. *Biophys J* 77:985–992, 1999.
96. Eaton BL, Kominz DR, Eisenberg E: Correlation between the inhibition of the acto-heavy meromyosin ATPase and the binding of tropomyosin to F-actin: Effects of Mg^{2+}, KCl, troponin I and troponin C. *Biochemistry* 14:2718–2725, 1975.
97. Perry SV: Troponin T: Genetics, properties and function. *J Muscle Res Cell Motil* 19:575–560, 1998.
98. Sabry MA, Dhoot GK: Identification and patterns of cardiac adult slow and slow skeletal muscle-like embryonic forms of troponin T in developing rat and human skeletal muscles. *J Muscle Res Cell Motil* 12:262, 1991.
98a. Pearlstone JR, Johstone P, Carpenter MR et al. The primary structure of rabbit skeletal muscle troponin T. Sequence determination HH2 terminal fragment CB3 and the complete sequence of troponin T. *J Biol Chem* 252:983–989, 1977.
99. Pearlstone JR, Johnson P, Carpenter MR, et al: Primary structure of rabbit skeletal troponin T. *J Biol Chem* 242:983, 1977.
100. Schachat FH, Diamond MS, Brandt PW: Effect of different troponin T-tropomyosin combinations on thin filament activation *J Mol Biol* 198:551–554, 1987.
100a. Gomes AV, Guzman G, Zhao J, et al: Cardiac troponin I isoforms affect the Ca^{2+}-sensitivity and inhibition of force development. *J Biol Chem* 277:35341–35349, 2002.
101. Phillips GN, Lattma EE, Cummins P, et al: Crystal structure and molecular interactions of tropomyosin. *Nature* 278:413, 1979.
102. Jackson P, Amphlett GW, Perry SV: The interaction with tropomyosin and the primary structure of troponin T. *J Biochem* 1151:85, 1975.
103. Nagano K, Mikamoto K, Matsumura M, Ohtsuki I: Possible formation of a triple-stranded coiled-coil region in tropomyosin–troponin T binding complex. *J Mol Biol* 141:217, 1980.
104. Ohtsuki I: Molecular arrangement of troponin T on the thin filament. *Biochemistry* 86:491, 1979.
105. Tanokura M, Tawada Y, Onoyama Y, et al: Primary structure of chymotryptic subfragments from rabbit skeletal troponin T. *J Biochem (Tokyo)* 90:263, 1981.
106. Pearlstone JR, Smillie LB: Identification of a second binding region on rabbit skeletal troponin T for α-tropomyosin. *FEBS Lett* 128:119, 1981.
107. Tanokura M, Tawada Y, Ono A, Ohtsuki I: Chymotryptic subfragments of troponin T from rabbit skeletal muscle: Interaction with tropomyosin, troponin I and troponin C. *J Biochem (Tokyo)* 93:331, 1983.
108. Mak AS, Smillie LB: Structural interpretation of the two-site binding of troponin on the muscle thin filament. *J Mol Biol* 149:541, 1981.
109. Cabral-Lilly D, Tobacman LS, Mehegan JP, et al: Molecular polarity in tropomyosin-troponin T co-crystals. *Biophys J* 73: 1763, 1997.
110. Oliveira DM, Nakaie CR, Sousa AD, et al: Mapping the domain of troponin T responsible for the activation of actomyosin ATPase activity. *J Biol Chem* 275:27513–27519, 2000.
110a. Tobacman LS, Nihli M, Butters C, et al: The troponin tail domain promotes a conformational state of the thin filament that suppresses myosin activity. *J Biol Chem* 277:27636–27642, 2002.
110b. Maytum R, Geeves MA and Lehrer SS: Modulatory role for the troponin T tail domain in thin filament regulation. *J Biol Chem* 277:29774–29780, 2002.
111. Moir AJG, Cole HA, Perry SV: The phosphorylation sites of troponin T from white skeletal muscle and the effects of interaction with troponin C on their phosphorylation by phosphorylase kinase. *Biochem J* 161:371, 1977.
112. Pearlstone JC, Smillie LB: Troponin T fragments: Physical properties and binding to troponin C. *Can J Biochem* 56:521, 1978.
113. Nakamura S, Yamamoto K, Hashimoto K, Ohtsuki I: Effect of chymotryptic troponin T subfragments on the Ca^{2+} sensitivity of superprecipitation. *J Biochem (Tokyo)* 89:1639, 1981.
114. Blumenschein TMA, Tripet BP, Hodges RS, et al: Mapping of the interacting regions of troponins T and C. *J Biol Chem* 276:36606–36612, 2001.
115. Pearlstone JC, Smillie LB: The binding sites of rabbit troponin I on troponin T. *Can J Biochem* 58:649, 1980.
116. Heeley DH, Golosinska K, Smillie LB: The effects of troponin T fragments T1 and T2 on the binding of nonpolymerisable tropomyosin to F actin in the presence and absence of troponin I and troponin C. *J Biol Chem* 262:9971, 1987.
117. Ray KP, England PJ: Phosphorylation of the inhibitory subunit of troponin and its effect on the calcium dependence of cardiac myofibril adenosine triphosphatase. *FEBS Lett* 70:11, 1976.
118. Johns EC, Simnett SJ, Mulligan IP, et al: Troponin phosphorylation does not increase the rate of relaxation following laser flash photolysis of diazo-2 in guinea pig skinned trabeculae. *Eur J Physiol* 433:842–844, 1997.
119. Cheney RE, Mooseker MS. Unconventional myosins. *Curr Opin Cell Biol* 4:27–35, 1992.
120. Trybus KM: Role of myosin light chains. *J Muscle Res Cell Motil* 15: 587–594, 1994.
121. Westwood SAW, Perry SV: Two forms of the P-light chain of myosin in rabbit and bovine hearts. *FEBS Lett* 142:31, 1982.
122. Collins JH: Homology of myosin DTNB light chains with alkali light chains, troponin C and parvalbumin. *Nature* 259:699, 1976.
123. Kendrick-Jones J, Scholey JM: Myosin linked regulatory systems. *J Muscle Res Cell Motil* 2:347, 1981.
124. Xie X, Harrison DH, Schlichting I, et al: Structure of the regulatory domain of scallop myosin at 2.8 Å resolution. *Nature* 368:306–312, 1994.
125. daSilva ACR, Reinach FC: Calcium binding introduces conformational changes in muscle regulatory proteins. *Trends Biochem Sci* 16:53–57, 1991.

126. Rayment I, Rypniewski WR, Schmidt-Base K, et al: Three dimensional structure of myosin subfragment-1: A molecular motor. *Science* 261:50, 1993.
127. Perry SV, Cole HA, Hudlicka O, et al: The role of myosin light chain kinase in muscle contraction. *Fed Proc* 43:3015, 1984.
128. Stull JT, Nunnally MH, Moore RL, Blumenthal DK: Myosin light chain kinases and myosin phosphorylation in skeletal muscle. *Adv Enzyme Regul* 23:123, 1985.
129. Erdodi F, Ito M, Hartshorne DJ: Myosin light chain phosphatases, in Barany M (ed): *Biochemistry of Smooth Muscle Contraction.* San Diego, CA: Academic Press, 1996; p131.
130. Pires EMV, Perry SV: Purification and properties of myosin light chain kinase from fast skeletal muscle. *Biochem J* 167:1137, 1977.
131. Walsh MP, Vallet B, Autric F, Demaille JG: Purification and characterisation of bovine cardiac calmodulin-dependent myosin light chain kinase. *J Biol Chem* 254:12136, 1979.
131a. Smith L, Parizi-Robinson M, Zhut M-S et al: Properties of long myosin light chain kinase binding to actin in vitro and in vivo. *J Biol Chem* 277:35597–35604, 2002.
132. Pembrick SM: The phosphorylated L2 light chain of skeletal myosin is a modifier of the actomyosin ATPase. *J Biol Chem* 255:8836–8841, 1980.
133. Sweeney HL, Bowman BF, Stull JT: Myosin light chain phosphorylation in vertebrate striated muscle: Regulation and function. *Am J Physiol* 264(Cell Physiol 33):C1085–C1095, 1993.
134. Manning DR, Stull JT: Myosin light chain phosphorylation and phosphorylase A activity in rat extensor digitorum longus muscle. *Biochem Biophys Res Commun* 90:164–170, 1979.
135. Westwood SAW, Hudlicka O, Perry SV: The effect of contractile activity on the phosphorylation of the P light chain of myosin of rabbit skeletal muscle. *Biochem J* 218:841, 1984.
136. Decostre V, Gillis JM, Gailly P: Effect of adrenaline on the post tetanic potentiation in mouse skeletal muscle. *J Muscle Res Cell Motil* 21:247–254, 2000.
137. Barany M. (ed): *Biochemistry of Smooth Muscle Contraction.* New York: Academic Press, 1996; chaps 25–27.
138. Butler TM, Seigman MJ: Control of cross bridge cycling by myosin light chain phosphorylation in mammalian smooth muscle. *Acta Physiol Scand* 164:389–400, 1998.
139. Winegrad S: Cardiac myosin binding protein C. *Circ Res* 84:1117–1126, 1999.
140. Winegrad S: Myosin binding protein C, a potential regulator of cardiac contractility. *Circ Res* 86:6–7, 2000.
141. Pechere JF: Muscular parvalbumins as homologous proteins. *Comp Biochem Physiol* 24:289, 1968.
142. Henrotte JG: A crystalline component of carp myogen precipitating at high ionic strength. *Nature* 176:1221, 1955.
143. Deuticke HJ: Uber die Sedimentations Konstante von Muskelproteinen. *Hoppe-Selyers Z Physiol Chem* 224:216, 1934.
144. Konosu S, Hamoir G, Pechere JF: Carp myogens of white and red muscles. *Biochem J* 96:98, 1965.
145. Henzl MT, Larson JD, Agah S: Influence of monovalent cations on rat α- and β-parvalbumin stabilities. *Biochemistry* 39:5859–5867, 2000.
146. Hermann CW: Parvalbumin, an intracellular calcium-binding protein: Distribution, properties and possible roles in mammalian cells. *Experimentia* 40:910, 1984.
147. Heizman CW, Berchtold MW, Rowlerson AM: Correlation of parvalbumin concentration with relaxation speed. *Proc Natl Acad Sci USA* 79:7243, 1982.
148. Pechere JF, Capony JP, Lars R: The primary structure of the major parvalbumin from hake muscle. *Eur J Biochem* 23:421, 1971.
149. Haiech J, Derencourt J, Pechere JF, et al: Magnesium and calcium binding to parvalbumins: Evidence for differences between parvalbumins and an explanation of their relaxing function. *Biochemistry* 18:2752, 1979.
150. Gillis JM, Thomason D, Lefevre J, et al: Parvalbumins and muscle: A computor simulation study. *J Muscle Res Cell Motil* 3:377–398, 1982.
151. Rall RJ: Role of parvalbumin in skeletal muscle relaxation. *News Physiol Sci* 11:249–255, 1996.
152. Celio MR, Heizmann CW: Calcium binding protein parvalbumin is associated with fast contracting fibres. *Nature* 297:504,1982.
153. Muntener M, Kaser I, Weber J, et al: Increase of skeletal muscle relaxation speed by direct injection of parvalbumin DNA. *Proc Natl Acad Sci USA* 92:6504–6508, 1995.
154. Szatkowski ML, Westfall MV, Gomez CA, et al: In vivo acceleration of heart relaxation performance by parvalbumin gene delivery. *J Clin Invest* 107:191–197, 2001.
155. Cai DQ, Li M, Lee KKH, et al: Parvalbumin expression is down-regulated in rat fast-twitch skeletal muscles during aging. *Arch Biochem Biophys* 387:202–208, 2001.
156. Huber B, Pette D: Dynamics of parvalbumin expression in low-frequency-stimulated fast-twitch muscle. *Eur J Biochem* 236:814–819, 1996.
157. Thierfelder L, Watkins H, MacRae C, et al: α-Tropomyosin and cardiac troponin T mutations cause familial hypertrophic cardiomyopathy: A disease of the sarcomere. *Cell* 77:701–712, 1994.
158. Laing NG, Wilton SD, Akkari PA, et al: A mutation in the α-tropomyosin gene TPM 3 associated with an autosomal dominant nemaline myopathy. *Nat Genet* 9:75–79, 1995.
159. Pelin K, Hilpela P, Donner K, et al: Mutations in the nebulin gene associated with an autosomal recessive nemaline myopathy. *Proc Natl Acad Sci USA* 96:2305–2310, 1999.
160. Nowak KJ, Wattanasirichaigoon D, Goebel HH: Mutations in the skeletal muscle alpha-actin gene in patients with actin myopathy and nemaline myopathy. *Nat Genet* 23:208–212, 1999.
161. Johnston JJ, Kelley RI, Crawford TO, et al: A novel nemaline myopathy in the Amish caused by a mutation in troponin T1. *Am J Hum Genet* 67:814–821, 2000.
162. Marston SB, Hodgkinson JL: Cardiac and skeletal myopathies: Can genotype explain phenotype? *J Muscle Res Cell Motil* 22:1–4, 2001.
163. Elliot K, Watkins H, Redwood CS: Altered regulatory properties of human cardiac troponin I mutants that cause hypertrophic cardiomyopathy. *J Biol Chem* 275:23069–23074, 2000.
164. Bonne G, Carrier L, Richarde P, et al: Familial hypertrophic cardiomyopathy. From mutations to functional effects. *Circ Res* 83:580–593, 1998.
165. Redwood CS, Moolman-Smook JC, Watkins H: Properties of mutant conractile proteins that cause hypertrophic cardiomyopathy. *Cardiovasc Res* 44:20–36, 1999.
166. Bottellini R, Coviello DA, Redwood CS, et al: A mutant tropomyosin that causes hypertrophic myopathy is expressed in vivo and associated with an increased calcium sensitivity. *Circ Res* 82:106–115, 1998.
166a. Perry SV: What is the role of tropomyosin in the regulation of contraction in striated muscle? *J Muscle Res Cell Motil* 24, 2003. In press.
167. Phillips GN Jr, Fillers JP, Cohen C: Tropomyosin crystal structure and muscle regulation. *J Mol Biol* 192:111–131, 1986.
168. Bremel RD, Murray JM, Weber A: Manifestations of cooperative behaviour in the regulated actin filament during actin activated ATP hydrolysis in the presence of calcium. *Cold Spring Harbor Symp Quant Biol* 37:267–275, 1972.

Chapter 14
The Proteins of the Sarcotubular System

KIMBY N. BARTON
DAVID H. MACLENNAN

Introduction
Removal of Ca^{2+} from the Cytosol
  Ca^{2+} PUMPS
Proteins Modulating Ca^{2+} Pumps
  PHOSPHOLAMBAN
  SARCOLIPIN
Release of Ca^{2+} into the Cytosol
  Ca^{2+} RELEASE CHANNELS (RYANODINE RECEPTORS)
Proteins Modulating Ca^{2+} Release Channels
  DIHYDROPYRIDINE RECEPTORS
  DISEASES RESULTING FROM MUTATIONS IN Ca^{2+} RELEASE CHANNELS
  FK-506 BINDING PROTEIN (FKBP12)
  CALMODULIN
Other Integral Membrane Proteins
  TRIADIN
  JUNCTIN
  MITSUGUMIN
  JUNCTOPHILIN
  CALMODULIN-DEPENDENT PROTEIN KINASE
Luminal Proteins
  CALSEQUESTRIN
  CALRETICULIN
  SARCALUMENIN
  HISTIDINE-RICH Ca^{2+}-BINDING PROTEIN
Conclusions

Introduction

Muscle contraction and relaxation are regulated by the concentration of free Ca^{2+} in the sarcoplasm. Ca^{2+} concentrations, in turn, are regulated by the interplay between proteins in two elaborate membranous structures: the sarcoplasmic reticulum (SR)* and transverse (T) tubules[1]; see Chaps. 11 and 12. In this chapter, we describe the functional roles of a variety of proteins in the sarcotubular system that are involved in excitation-contraction (EC) coupling and relaxation. For many of these proteins, primary sequence, molecular genetics, high-resolution crystal structures, and interactions with other proteins involved in Ca^{2+} regulation are well defined. These studies of individual proteins provide molecular insights into the workings of this complex membrane regulatory system.

*A list of abbreviations used in this chapter is given at the end of the chapter.

Removal of Ca^{2+} from the Cytosol

Ca^{2+} PUMPS

The major protein in the longitudinal SR and the nonjunctional face of the terminal cisternae is an ATP-dependent Ca^{2+} ATPase.[2] The function of this protein is to return Ca^{2+} released from the terminal cisternae during EC coupling to the lumen of the SR. In contrast to the passive entry of Ca^{2+} down its electrochemical gradient, removal of Ca^{2+} from the cytoplasm requires the expenditure of chemical energy and has a fixed stoichiometry of two Ca^{2+} ions transported per ATP hydrolyzed. Since contraction/relaxation cycles can occur in less than 100 ms in some muscles, the density of Ca^{2+} pumps must be very high throughout most regions of the SR membrane to account for such rapid relaxation rates.

While high ATPase activity was associated with a "granular" fraction of muscle in 1948[3] and "relaxing factor" activity was found in insoluble muscle fractions in 1951,[2] it was not until the early 1960s that ATP-dependent Ca^{2+} transport activity was described in SR preparations[3,4] and its significance clearly explained.[5,6] The Ca^{2+} ATPase of fast-twitch skeletal muscle SR (SERCA1) was isolated in functional form in 1970 and shown to be a 110-kDa membrane-bound protein.[7] In the 1980s, three homologous *ATP2A* genes were identified and shown to encode three SERCA isoforms and their splice variants.[8-10] SERCA1a is highly expressed in adult fast-twitch skeletal muscle, while SERCA1b is an alternatively spliced variant expressed in fetal and neonatal muscle; SERCA2a is highly expressed in cardiac and slow-twitch muscles, and its splice variant, SERCA2b, is expressed as the "housekeeping" Ca^{2+} pump in smooth muscle and nonmuscle tissues; SERCA3 and its splice variants have a lower Ca^{2+} affinity and might subserve a specialized function in endothelial and epithelial cells.[11,12]

SERCA enzymes are typical of the class of P-type ATPases, which form a phosphoprotein intermediate and undergo conformational changes during the course of ATP hydrolysis (Fig.14-1).[13] Some of the conformational states can be stabilized, either by adjustment of reaction conditions or through mutagenesis, and characterized as intermediates in the overall reaction cycle. The phosphorylated intermediate, E_1PCa_2, can phosphorylate ADP, while E_2P can react only with water. The formation of E_1P requires that both high-affinity Ca^{2+} binding sites be occupied. The enzyme is then phosphorylated by ATP and, concomitantly, the two Ca^{2+} ions are occluded and can no longer exchange with unlabeled Ca^{2+}. The rate-limiting transition to E_2P is accompanied by loss of Ca^{2+} into the lumen, the affinity having fallen by three orders of magnitude. Hydrolysis of E_2P and regeneration of the high-affinity Ca^{2+} binding sites, allowing formation of E_1Ca_2, complete the cycle.

All of the steps in the reaction cycle are reversible.[14] The energy for ATP synthesis does not come from a Ca^{2+} gradient; indeed, solubilized Ca^{2+} ATPase can synthesize ATP if it is first phosphorylated by inorganic phosphate (Pi), followed by the addition of ATP and Ca^{2+}.[15] Reverse phosphorylation of the enzyme by Pi is Mg^{2+}-dependent and occurs only in the absence of Ca^{2+}.[16,17]

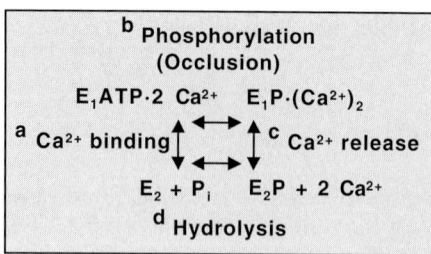

FIGURE 14-1. Conformational states of the Ca^{2+}-ATPase. During the cycle of ATP-dependent Ca^{2+} transport, at least four interconvertible phosphorylated and unphosphorylated conformations have been defined. First, a rise in Ca^{2+} on the cytoplasmic side of the membrane saturates the two high-affinity sites to form $E_1ATP\cdot 2Ca^{2+}$. Second, this activates formation of a phosphoenzyme with ATP, trapping Ca^{2+} within the protein to form the high-energy intermediate $E_1P(Ca^{2+})_2$. Third, in a rate-limiting step to E_2P, the phosphoenzyme loses both its ability to rephosphorylate ADP and its high affinity for Ca^{2+}, and opens its gate to luminal spaces. Fourth, water enters the catalytic site and hydrolyzes the aspartyl phosphate to give the low-energy intermediate $E_2 + P_i$.

Ligand binding studies[18] and kinetic analysis, combined with stoichiometric measurements,[19] have demonstrated that each SERCA1a molecule contains two Ca^{2+}-binding sites. A model of two-step, cooperative binding of Ca^{2+} to the enzyme was proposed, in which binding of the first ion induced a conformational change that would form the second high-affinity site. Kinetic analysis provided evidence for sequential binding of the two Ca^{2+} ions, with the first ion binding more quickly than the second[20] and only one of the two ions exchanging freely with external Ca^{2+}.[21] The order of the binding is believed to be preserved upon translocation,[21] although this conclusion is controversial.[22] H^+ ions are countertransported during the pumping cycle, but the high permeability of the SR membrane to monovalent ions makes it difficult to analyze this process.[23]

Freeze-fracture studies of isolated, longitudinal SR vesicles showed a high density of uniform intramembrane particles.[24] Negative staining of the surface of these vesicles[25] also showed the presence of "headpieces." Both of these features could be associated with the Ca^{2+} pump.[26] The analysis of structure-function relationships of the Ca^{2+} ATPase began in earnest with the cloning of SERCA2a in 1985,[8] since knowledge of the primary sequence permitted prediction of the topology of the enzyme. The cytoplasmic region was predicted to consist of three domains, referred to as the nucleotide-binding, phosphorylation, and transduction domains. Earlier studies of the functional consequences of amino acid derivatization and identification of the aspartyl phosphate and the sequence surrounding it provided support for such predictions. Hydropathy analysis permitted the prediction of ten transmembrane helices, M1 to M10. Amphipathic, negatively charged cytosolic extensions of helices M1 to M5 were proposed to make up a stalk region connecting the cytosolic domains to the transmembrane domain. The transduction domain, located between helices M2 and M3, were predicted to contain seven β-strands, folded into an antiparallel β-sandwich. The nucleotide-binding and phosphorylation domains, located between helices M4 and M5, were predicted to be formed from alternating α-helices and β-sheets. More precise modeling of these domains became possible when haloacid dehalogenase, an enzyme with known crystal structure, was found to have sequence homology with the nucleotide-binding and phosphorylation domains of SERCA1a.[27] Modeling, in which the nucleotide-binding domain splits the phosphorylation domain by erupting from it as a well-defined subdomain, required a revision of the original model.[28]

Two- and three-dimensional crystals of SERCA1a were obtained in the 1980s. Two-dimensional crystals could be formed within the membrane by treatment of rabbit SR vesicles with sodium orthovanadate.[29] Tubular crystallization, combined with frozen-hydrated electron microscopy and helical image reconstruction, allowed the analysis of the structure of SERCA1a at 8 Å by 1998.[30] The headpiece, in which domain densities could be described, was attached to a stalk sector, which, in turn, was associated with a transmembrane domain in which 10 transmembrane helices could be resolved but not clearly assigned.

The potential for expression of mutant forms of SERCA1a or SERCA2a in heterologous cell culture and their functional analysis[31] made it possible to examine the contribution to function of any individual amino acid. The primary screen was, first, measurement of the Ca^{2+} dependence of Ca^{2+} transport in microsomal fractions containing elevated levels of the mutant enzyme to determine whether activity survived and, if activity were present, whether Ca^{2+} affinity or maximal velocity (V_{max}) were affected. If activity were lost, then it was possible to analyze partial reactions. As an example,[32] mutation of a group of hydrophilic and charged amino acids in predicted transmembrane sequences disrupted Ca^{2+} transport. No phosphorylation could be observed from ATP in the presence of Ca^{2+}, but phosphorylation of mutant enzymes from Pi in the absence of Ca^{2+} was normal. In contrast to wild-type, the addition of Ca^{2+} did not prevent phosphorylation from Pi, indicating that these residues, residing in transmembrane helices M4, M5, M6, and M8, contributed to the formation of the Ca^{2+}-binding site. Further analysis of the properties of these mutants permitted assignment of each of the residues to either Ca^{2+}-binding site 1 or site 2[33–36] and indicated that these sites would lie side by side.[13] Alanine scanning mutagenesis of each residue in M4, M5, M6, and M8 expanded the number of amino acids that might be involved in the Ca^{2+}-binding site.[37] In a study of the structure of isolated M6 using nuclear magnetic resonance (NMR) spectroscopy,[38] it became evident that the transmembrane helix was disrupted at the level of the key Ca^{2+}-binding residues. Thus a very clear picture emerged of the Ca^{2+}-binding and translocation domains of SERCA1a.

The various mutants were divided into several classes: V_{max} mutants; Ca^{2+}-binding mutants, apparent Ca^{2+}-affinity mutants (possibly reflecting a shift in E_1-to-E_2 equilibrium); phosphorylation mutants; ATP-binding mutants; conformational change mutants blocked between E_1P and E_2P; conformational change mutants blocked in E_2P dephosphorylation; and uncoupled mutants.[34,39] On the basis of the results of mutagenesis, it was possible to describe the mechanism of Ca^{2+} transport by taking into account the characteristics of the transport process and the structure of the pump.[39] The Ca^{2+}-binding and translocation sites lie in a cavity between M4, M5, M6, and M8, where they are formed by the precise juxtaposition of Ca^{2+}-binding residues located in these four helices. Access to the cavity is controlled by the structure of transmembrane and stalk helices at the cytosolic boundary of the transmembrane domain. It is of particular interest that a cluster of acidic residues lies in this boundary region at the cytosolic ends of M1, M2, and M3.[40] Phosphorylation-induced domain movements will close off cytoplasmic access to the cavity and initiate occlusion. Further long-range, phosphorylation-induced domain movements involving M4, M5, M6, and M8 disrupt the precise placement of the ligands required to form the high-affinity Ca^{2+}-binding sites and open the exit gate, permitting release of weakly bound Ca^{2+} to the lumen. Later conformational changes result in dephosphorylation of E_2P, reopening of the Ca^{2+} entry gate, and reformation of E_1Ca_2, completing the Ca^{2+} transport cycle.

Crystal Structure of SERCA1a

In 2000, the crystal structure of the Ca^{2+} ATPase of SERCA1a, in its Ca^{2+}-bound state, was solved at 2.6 Å resolution, elevating our understanding of the structure and function of a Ca^{2+} pump to a new height,[41] see Color Plate 4a. As predicted, two Ca^{2+} ions, 5.7 Å apart, are bound in the transmembrane domain, which comprises 10 transmembrane helices. The ligands identified in helices M4, M5, M6, and M8 by site-directed mutagenesis are confirmed and new ligands, particularly mutation-sensitive backbone carbonyl groups on helix M4, and a single water molecule, are identified in the Ca^{2+}-binding site. A disruption of the helix in both M4 and M6 forms a Ca^{2+}-binding cavity, as anticipated from an earlier NMR structure of helix M6.[38] Helix M5, located in the center of the molecule, extends as a central mast from the lumen to the cytosolic domain, and M2 also forms an extended helix. A 22-residue conserved loop, joining M6 to M7 (L67), coils among the helices and draws them together with H-bonds. Mutation of residues in this loop reduces Ca^{2+} affinity and V_{max}, reinforcing the strong influence of the L67 sequence on the correct positioning of helix M6.[42] The distance between Asp^{351} in the catalytic center and the bound Ca^{2+} ions is approximately 35 Å.

In the Ca^{2+}-bound E_1Ca_2 conformation, there is no vestibule leading from the cytoplasmic surface to the binding sites within the TM domain, suggesting that the entry pathway is already closed. Hydrophilic residues are located in the upper part of the cavity, and rows of exposed oxygen atoms are formed by the unwinding of helix M4 (Glu-Gly-Leu-Pro^{312}). Closely apposed to M4 is the high concentration of negatively charged residues at the cytosolic surfaces of M1 and M3.[40] A Ca^{2+} ion, entering the channel, may pass through a cavity lined with a high concentration of negative charges to reach sites I and II, and then exit through an area surrounded by M3 and M5, where a ring of oxygen atoms with bound water is formed. Neither pathway is obvious in this conformation, suggesting significant changes in helix packing with a change in conformation.

The cytoplasmic headpiece consists of three well-separated domains: the phosphorylation (P) domain; the nucleotide-binding (N) domain, and the actuator (A) domain, formerly referred to as the transduction domain. The P domain is central and is composed of two noncontiguous sequences that adopt a typical Rossman fold, with the phosphorylation site at Asp^{351} situated in the C-terminal end of the β-strand. Domain N, the largest of the cytoplasmic domains, harbors the ATP-binding site. It comprises a seven-stranded, antiparallel β-sheet sandwiched between two helix bundles. Domain A comprises approximately 110 residues between helices M2 and M3, which form a distorted jellyroll structure, and two short helices formed from the 40 residues of the N terminus that runs into M1. The interaction of the A domain with the helices making up M1, M2, and M3 ensures that conformational changes in the A domain will be transmitted directly to those transmembrane helices.

The N domain, inserted directly after the first strand of the P domain, forms an open cap over the catalytic site in the P domain. In the Ca^{2+}-bound conformation, the apparent ATP binding site is more than 25 Å from Asp^{351}, indicating that Ca^{2+} binding alone is insufficient to produce a phosphorylatable conformation. Domain N must move close to domain P in the phosphorylatable state, possibly to exclude water and stabilize the phosphoenzyme as it is formed.[43]

A crystal structure of SERCA1a in the E_2 conformation, stabilized by thapsigargin, has also been reported.[44] In the kinetic steps between E_2 and E_1Ca_2 the pump binds one Ca^{2+}, undergoes a conformational change, and then binds a second Ca^{2+} cooperatively. In comparison with the E_1Ca_2 conformation, complex changes are observed in the membranous Ca^{2+}-binding site and stalk connections. These are amplified even further by movement of the cytoplasmic domains. The structural correlates of this transition are illustrated in Fig. 14-2. Large-scale movements of the N, P, and A domains occur with little internal change. They are coupled to changes in tilt and position of M1 to M6, but M7 to M10 are almost unmoved. The bottom section of M5, below Glu^{771}, remains fixed, packing against M7, but the middle section, with its cytoplasmic extension bonded to the L67 loop, tilts back, straightening the helix and carrying the top section, an integral part of the P domain, through a 30-degree rotation. The largest movements of Ca^{2+} ligands are in M6, which becomes more helical on binding Ca^{2+}, several ligands rotating through 90 degrees. The M4 helix also tightens, but mainly it moves down by 5 Å, carried by the tilting of M5. The net result is that the dispersed Ca^{2+} ligands come together to form the compact sites seen in E_1Ca_2.

These changes stabilize a new configuration of the surrounding helices, and the effects are transmitted to the P domain, M1, M2, and M3, and to the A domain. Parts of the structure are likely to be thermally labile, the molecule being stabilized in the Ca^{2+} free, E_2 form by interdomain H-bonds and nonpolar interactions and, in the crystal, by thapsigargin. The E_1Ca_2 form is stabilized by multiple ligands to Ca^{2+}. This leads to an open structure which can rearrange further following phosphorylation. The central role of the P domain is clear from its many interactions with N, A, and the membrane and stalk domains, which serve to coordinate the global changes.

The E_2 structure indicates access routes for Ca^{2+}. In this conformation, closure of two lumenal loops, L34 and L78, blocks access from the lumenal side in E_2, but polar and negatively charged amino acids in the cytosolic extensions of M1, M2, and M3 now form into a negatively charged aqueous pocket which extends into the membrane region from the cytosolic side. Glu^{309} lies at the bottom of this charged pocket, blocking access to the main Ca^{2+}-binding sites. A small movement of Glu^{309} might open this entrance and

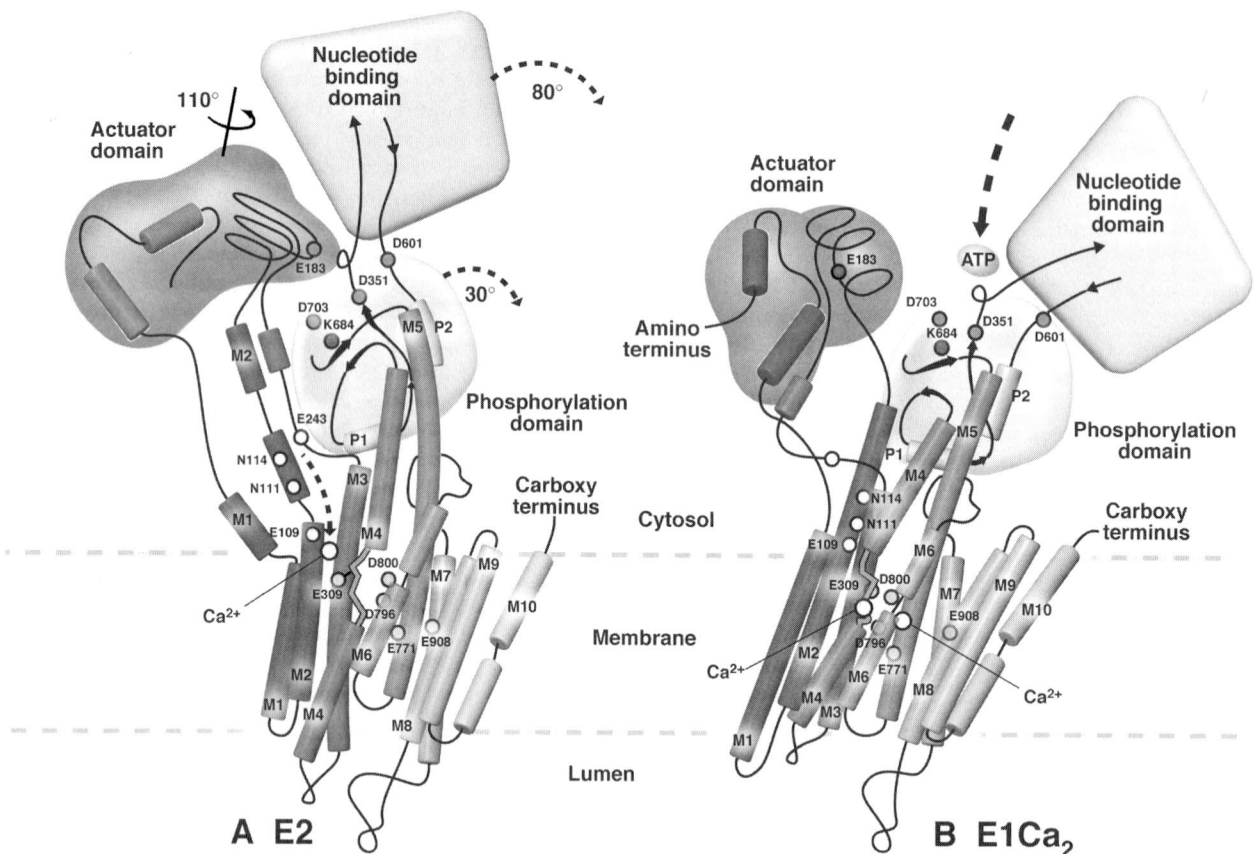

FIGURE 14-2. Structure of the Ca^{2+} pump in the Ca^{2+}-free and Ca^{2+}-bound (E$_1$Ca$_2$) states. Three domains, phosphorylation, nucleotide binding, and actuator, lie in the cytosol. The phosphorylation domain, with the nucleotide-binding domain inserted, connects the tops of transmembrane helices M4 and M5. Additional anchors include two β-strands that continue from these helices and form part of the central β-sheet. This domain includes a cluster of critical catalytic residues: the phosphorylation sites D (aspartic acid) 351, D703, and D601 and K (lysine) 684. Some of the Ca^{2+} ligands on transmembrane helices M4, M5, M6, and M8 and some of the polar or negatively charged residues that line a possible Ca^{2+} entry pathway involving M1, M2, and M3 are shown in relation to bound or unbound Ca^{2+}. A. In the E$_2$ state,[44] entrance to the Ca^{2+} sites is blocked by E (glutamic acid) 309 in M4. The three cytosolic domains form a compact cluster. The actual domain is rotated to meet the phosphorylation domain and carries E183 into the catalytic site, where it may be involved in hydrolysis of E$_2$P. B. In the E$_1$Ca$_2$ state,[41] the cytoplasmic domains have moved apart. ATP can bind in the cleft between N and A, but, because it induces a new conformation, its location is only partly defined. The figure provides only an approximation of the three-dimensional relations. (A) is based on the figures in Ref. 44 with guidance from the model for E$_2$P[41] (1FQU in the protein data bank). (B) is based on Ref. 41 (1EUL). (See Color Plate 4.)

allow Ca^{2+} to enter the binding sites. This would be consistent with a gating role for Glu^{309}.[45] All of these movements illustrate the dynamic interrelationships among key residues and interlinked domains that occur during Ca^{2+} transport.

Proteins Modulating Ca^{2+} Pumps

PHOSPHOLAMBAN

Phospholamban (PLN), a pentameric protein made up of 6-kDa subunits, is highly expressed in the SR of cardiac, smooth, and slow-twitch skeletal muscle. It interacts with—and, at low Ca^{2+} concentrations, reversibly inhibits—the activity of the SERCA2a pump (Fig. 14-3).[46,47] In this role, it is a major regulator of the kinetics of cardiac contractility.[48,49] PLN consists of 52 amino acids organized into three domains. Domain Ia, amino acids 1 to 20, contains sites of regulatory phosphorylation by protein kinase A on Ser[16] and Ca^{2+}-CaM kinase on Thr[17]; domain Ib, amino acids 21 to 30, contains a high proportion of amidated residues; and domain II, amino acids 31 to 52, forms a transmembrane domain. NMR spectroscopy has revealed that PLN is composed of two helices separated by a β-turn involving (Thr)-Ile-Glu-Met-Pro[21].[50–52]

Dephosphorylated PLN inhibits Ca^{2+} transport by interacting directly with SERCA molecules and lowering their apparent affinity for Ca^{2+}. Phosphorylation of PLN is associated with dissociation of the inhibited PLN/SERCA complex and an increase in the apparent affinity of the Ca^{2+} pump for Ca^{2+}, thereby stimulating the rate of Ca^{2+} uptake at low Ca^{2+} concentration. The major effects of phosphorylation of PLN

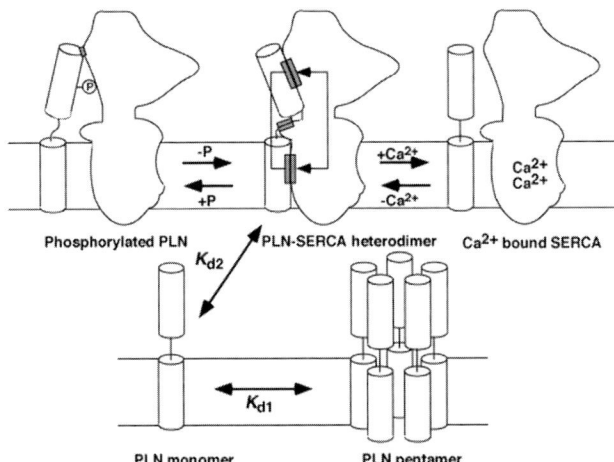

FIGURE 14-3. A model for the reversible inhibition of SERCA2a activity by PLN. Reversible inhibition is proposed to involve dissociation of the PLN pentamer, formation of the inhibited PLN-SERCA2a heterodimer, and dissociation of the heterodimer. Interactions involving the transmembrane domain of PLN inhibit SERCA2a activity and are disrupted by the binding of Ca^{2+} to the transmembrane sequences of SERCA2a. Cytoplasmic interactions involving PLN domain Ia are not considered to be inhibitory. Phosphorylation of the cystolic domain of PLN, however, disrupt the intramembrane inhibitory interactions through long-range interactions within both PLN and SERCA2a. These internal regulatory interactions are represented by arrows connecting at least six sites of inhibitory interaction (shaded).

are an increase in the rate of cardiac relaxation (lusitropic effect) and an increase in cardiac contractility (inotropic effect). Increased contractility is an outcome of increased Ca^{2+} uptake and storage during the relaxation phase, setting the stage for enhanced Ca^{2+} release in the contractile phase.[49,53] Models of the mechanism by which PLN reversibly inhibits SERCA suggest that a reversible physical interaction occurs between the two proteins.

A physical association between the cytosolic domains of PLN and SERCA2a was deduced from the covalent cross-linking of reconstituted purified PLN to SERCA2a, which could be demonstrated only in low Ca^{2+} concentrations, when PLN was dephosphorylated.[54] Further evidence for physical interaction between the two proteins is provided by studies showing that the phosphorylation of PLN results in a nearly twofold decrease in rotational mobility of SERCA2a.[55] Attenuated total-reflection Fourier transform infrared spectroscopy (FTIR) and circular dichroism studies of the Ca^{2+} pump, coreconstituted with PLN, show changes in spectra indicative of an increase in the α-helical stability of the pump. This suggests that the inhibitory regulation of the ATPase by PLN may involve stabilization of helices within the protein.[56]

Physical and functional interactions between PLN and SERCA are mutation-sensitive. The extensive use of site-directed mutagenesis has demonstrated that cytoplasmic interaction sites are formed by charged and hydrophobic amino acids in PLN domain I and by amino acids Lys-Asp-Asp-Lys-Val-Pro^{402} in SERCA2a.[57,58] Transmembrane interactions occur between amino acids on one face of the transmembrane helix of PLN[59] and transmembrane helix 6 of SERCA2a.[60] Structural modeling of the PLN-SERCA1a interaction[61] shows that PLN binds to aa in TM helices M2, M4, and M6 in the E_2 conformation, inhibiting helical rearrangements and the binding of Ca^{2+}. In addition, the cytosolic domain of PLN binds to the N-domain in SERCA1a (Fig. 14.3), presumably blocking its ability to participate in the clustering and dispersion of the cytosolic domains in SERCA1a, which powers conformational changes in the TM domain. To break up this inhibited complex, movement must occur in either SERCA1a or PLN. The binding of Ca^{2+} to SERCA1a triggers, among others, movement of M2 into the PLN binding groove, forcing PLN out of this site. The effect of phosphorylation on PLN structure is not known, but phosphorylation must induce conformational changes in PLN that force it out of its inhibitory site in the inhibited complex.

The physiologic role of PLN has been studied extensively.[46,47,49] Recent studies have focused on animal models. Ablation of the PLN gene in mice has a pronounced inotropic response that cannot be enhanced by isoproterenol.[48] This is manifest by increases in contractility, measured as enhancement of the maximal rates of left ventricular pressure development ($+P/dt$) and decline ($-dP/dt$) and a decrease in the time to half relaxation ($RT_{1/2}$). These manifestations are in line with the view that increased contractility is an outcome of increased Ca^{2+} uptake and storage during the relaxation phase, setting the stage for enhanced Ca^{2+} release in the contractile phase.

The discovery of PLN mutants that are superinhibitory has permitted further evaluation of the physiologic role of such mutants. Mouse lines have been developed that express a variety of superinhibitory PLN point mutations.[62–64] In each of these lines, the maximal rates of left ventricular pressure development and decline were depressed and the time to peak pressure (TPP) and half relaxation was prolonged, suggesting that the hearts from these transgenic animals exhibited depressed systolic and diastolic function. One superinhibitory mutation, V49G, led not only to altered contractility but also to dilated cardiomyopathy and to gender-specific heart failure: Males died within 6 months, while females survived for 18-months. Mutations in PLN that either cause the protein to be degraded (the equivalent of a PLN-null mutation),[64a] or result in chronic inhibition of the Ca^{2+} pump by prevention of phosphorylation of PLN by protein kinase A,[64b] can cause dilated cardiomyopathy in humans. Thus, unlike mice, humans require PLN.

The evidence that PLN can alter SERCA2a function so effectively in a physiologic setting, with dramatic effects on cardiac function and cardiomyopathy, has led to the view that intervention at PLN/SERCA2a interaction sites may be a promising therapeutic approach for heart failure.[65]

SARCOLIPIN

Sarcolipin (SLN) is a low-molecular-weight homologue of PLN that is highly expressed in the same fast-twitch skeletal muscle fibers in rabbits and humans that express SERCA1a (Fig. 14-4).[66–68] In rats, however, there is high expression of SLN in heart and the concentration can be regulated by hormones.[69] Like PLN, SLN is an inhibitor of both SERCA1a

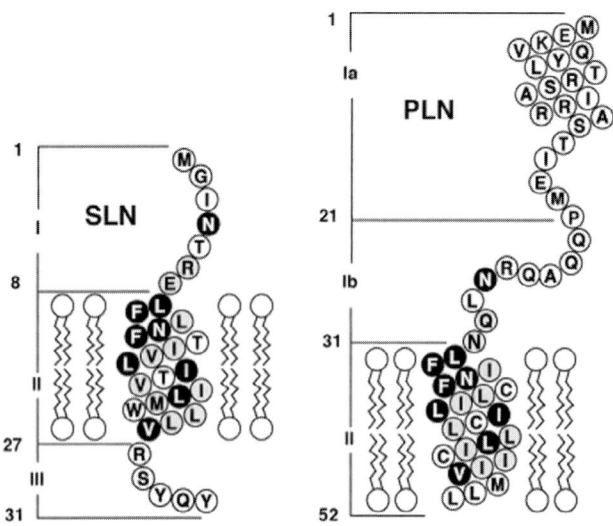

FIGURE 14-4. Similarities between SLN and PLN. Black circles represent identical amino acids and shaded circles represent amino acids conserved between SLN and PLN. Amino acids are indicated in a single-letter code. Domains of SLN and PLN are designated on the left and numbers indicate their positions in the sequence.

and SERCA2a activity at low Ca^{2+} concentrations by reducing the apparent affinity of SERCA molecules for Ca^{2+}.[68,70]

In heterologus cell culture, SLN co-expressed with PLN becomes superinhibitory to SERCA activity.[70] SLN has a higher affinity for PLN than PLN itself, so that, at equal concentrations and at equilibrium, the predominant species in a SLN/PLN mixture is a PLN-SLN heterodimer. SLN can depolymerize PLN pentamers to form SLN-PLN dimers. A ternary PLN-SLN-SERCA complex can be immuno-precipitated by antibodies against either PLN or SLN, indicating that the ternary complex is the most stable complex when all three proteins are expressed together. Biochemistry suggests that SLN can fit into the PLN-binding groove in the E_2 conformation of SERCA1a: modeling of the ternary complex predicts that the PLN-SLN heterodimer can also fit into this groove.[71] The tighter fit creates a higher affinity and the unique C-terminal sequence of SLN adds to the stability by binding to aromatic residues in the luminal loop connecting M1 and M2 helices of SERCA1a. Although a PLN-SLN complex fits snugly into this site, a PLN-PLN complex could not. These studies hint at another level of regulation of SERCA2a by a PLN-SLN complex.

Circular dichroism and solution and solid-state NMR studies of SLN have demonstrated that SLN, like PLN, is predominantly α-helical in structure.[72] Unlike PLN, SLN has only a weak if any propensity to form oligomers.[73]

Release of Ca^{2+} into the Cytosol

Ca^{2+} RELEASE CHANNELS (RYANODINE RECEPTORS)

Early studies showed that Ca^{2+} could induce Ca^{2+} release from preparations that included the terminal cisternae and that Ca^{2+} release could be stimulated by nucleotides and caffeine and inhibited by procain, ruthenium red, and physiologic concentrations of Mg^{2+}.[74–77] The fact that ryanodine alters the properties of the Ca^{2+} release channel at micromolar concentrations[78] led to the use of [^{3}H]-ryanodine for the isolation of the ryanodine receptor (RYR) from homogenates of skeletal muscle.[79–81] The morphologic characteristics of the 2,260 kDa RyR tetramer, made up from 565,000 Da subunits (Fig. 14-5), permitted the identification of the purified protein with the "feet" structures seen at the junction of the terminal cisternae and the transverse tubular membranes, as described in Chap. 11. It is this huge tetrameric SR protein that fills the 15-nm gap between the junctional terminal cisternae of the SR and the T tubule.

The Ca^{2+} release channel is highly cation selective, with an unusually large conductance for monovalent and divalent cations.[82] Unit conductances of 27 and 22 pS for choline and Tris suggest the presence of a large ion-conducting pore.[83] In

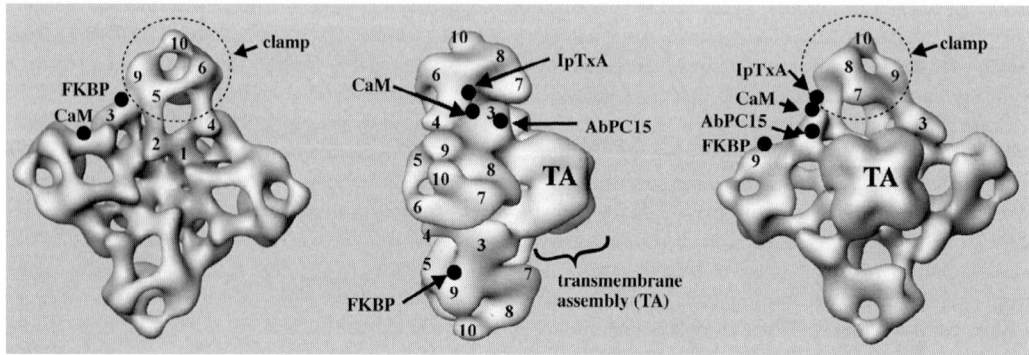

FIGURE 14-5. Solid-body representation of a three-dimensional reconstruction of RyR1. The numbers indicate distinct globular structures that correspond to structural domains, all of which are located in cytoplasmic regions of the protein. The filled circles indicate the locations of ligands as determined by reconstruction of RyR-ligand complexes. CaM, calmodulin; FKBP, FK506-binding protein; IpTxA, imperatoxin A; AbPC15, monoclonal antibody against RyR residues 4425 to 4621; TA, transmembrane assembly. (*From Stokes DL, Wagenknecht T: Calcium transport across the sarcoplasmic reticulum: Structure and function of Ca^{2+}-ATPase and the ryanodine receptor. Eur J Biochem 267:5274–5279, 2000. With permission.*)

the absence of regulatory ligands such as Mg^{2+} and ATP, a bell-shaped curve for Ca^{2+} activation of Ca^{2+} efflux is observed, with Ca^{2+} efflux accelerating as cytosolic Ca^{2+} is raised from 1 to 10 μM and decelerating as it is raised from 10 to 100 μM.[84] These results are consistent with both high-affinity activating and low-affinity inhibitory Ca^{2+}-binding sites. Ca^{2+}-induced Ca^{2+} release is greatly potentiated by mM ATP. In the presence of μM Ca^{2+} and mM ATP, maximal release rates have a first-order rate constant of 20 to 100 s^{-1}. Since a variety of adenine nucleotides also potentiate Ca^{2+} release, activation must occur through binding to an effector site rather than through phosphorylation. Free Mg^{2+} is an inhibitor in the millimolar range, possibly because of competition for the Ca^{2+} site.[85]

Caffeine, ryanodine, and dantrolene are pharmacologic agents with high specificity for RyR channels. Caffeine activates the channel at millimolar concentrations and is widely used in functional studies. Dantrolene closes the channel and is the specific antidote for the excess Ca^{2+} release that initiates episodes of malignant hyperthermia.[86] Ryanodine binds to the open channel with high affinity and converts the channel to an open subconductance state at 1 to 10 μM, but it blocks channel opening in the 100-μM range.[84]

Ca^{2+} release channel genes have been cloned from skeletal (*RYR1*), cardiac (*RYR2*), and nonmuscle sources (*RYR3*), the proteins encoded by these genes containing from 4872 to 5037 amino acids.[87] Transmembrane sequences are found near the C-terminal of each molecule, the number predicted being between 4[88] and 12.[89] Topological analysis suggests that the number of transmembrane helices is 6, but a region of membrane association accurs after amino acid 4300. Therefore, the cytoplasmic component, bridging the gap between T-tubular and SR membranes lies between residues 1 and about 4300.

Proteins Modulating Ca^{2+} Release Channels

DIHYDROPYRIDINE RECEPTORS

Excitation-contraction (EC) coupling in skeletal and cardiac muscle involves a functional interaction between ryanodine receptors, located in the junctional terminal cisternae of the SR, and the α_1 subunit of the voltage-sensitive, dihydropyridine-modulated, slow or L-type Ca^{2+} channels (the dihydropyridine receptor, or DHPR), located in T tubules (Fig. 14-6) (also see Chaps. 11 and 12). A cluster of four DHPR molecules in the transverse tubule of skeletal muscle directly apposes every other ryanodine receptor molecule, with an individual DHPR molecule overlying an individual RyR1 subunit.[90,91] Thus the relative locations of RyR1 and DHPR would permit direct physical interactions between their cytoplasmic domains. Biochemical, physiological and molecular genetic studies show that physical interactions do indeed occur between skeletal muscle RyR1 and DHPR isoforms, leading to both activation of the Ca^{2+} release channel (orthograde interaction) and modulation of the slow Ca^{2+} channel (retrograde interaction).[92] By contrast, there is no indication that direct physical interactions between cardiac RyR2 and DHPR α_1 subunits lead to opening of the cardiac Ca^{2+} release channel.[93] Regulation of Ca^{2+} release is gated by calcium current, not gating charge, in cardiac myocytes.[93] In this case, entry of extracellular Ca^{2+} through the DHPR α_1 subunit induces activation of RyR2 by Ca^{2+}-induced Ca^{2+} release.

The net positive charge on the voltage sensing transmembrane sequence S4 in each of the four repeats of the DHPR α_1 subunit allows it to respond to voltage changes through changes in its conformation.[94] The structural basis for the

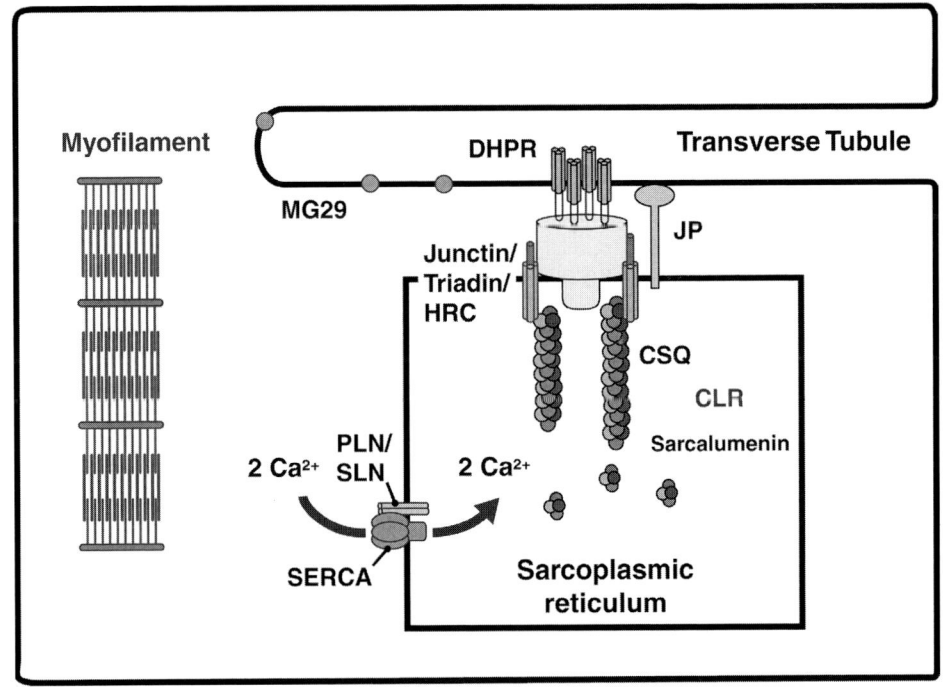

FIGURE 14-6. Schematic representation of a muscle cell, demonstrating the location and topology of some of the proteins responsible for Ca^{2+} cycling and storage.

voltage sensor of a K+ channel has been elucidated (see Color Plate 5).[94a,94b] The mechanism is likely to be the same for the DHPR Ca^{2+} channel. Conformational changes due to voltage-sensing are presumed to be transmitted to RyR1, causing channel opening. The charge movement in the DHPR, which is the probable response to voltage change, precedes Ca^{2+} release, and its block by dihydropyridines also blocks Ca^{2+} release.[95] Presumably, those Ca^{2+} release channels not opened by direct physical interaction are opened by Ca^{2+}-induced Ca^{2+} release. By contrast, there is no indication that direct physical interactions between cardiac RyR2 and DHPR α_1 subunits lead to opening of the cardiac Ca^{2+} release channel.[93] In this case, entry of extracellular Ca^{2+} through the DHPR α_1 subunit induces activation of RyR2 by Ca^{2+}-induced Ca^{2+} release.

The exact site of RyR/DHPR interaction is not clear and the interaction between the two proteins has been the subject of a great deal of research[96] (also see Chap. 12). Expression of $\alpha_{1S}\alpha_{1C}$ chimeras in dysgenic myotubes (which lack endogenous α_1 subunits) has established that skeletal-type EC coupling depends upon the amino acid sequence in the cytoplasmic region between repeats II and III of the skeletal isoform (the II-to-III loop contains amino acids 666 to 791).[97,98] Subsequent studies identified residues 720 to 765 within the II-to-III loop as critical for activation of skeletal-type EC coupling and for retrograde signaling, whereby RyR1 enhances the current density of α_1S.[92,99,100] In vitro observations have indicated that a different region of the II-to-III loop, residues 671 to 690, is important for activation of RyR1, as indicated by ryanodine binding, single-channel activity, and calcium release.[101–103] However, studies of chimeric DHPR with scrambled or deleted sequences of residues 681 to 690 have demonstrated that neither the specific sequence nor the integrity of a cluster of positive charges is essential for EC coupling.[104,105] Surface plasmon resonance studies have provided evidence of a direct interaction between RyR1 and DHPR residues 671 to 690 that was not modulated by Ca^{2+} or Mg^{2+} but was strongly potentiated by FKBP12 and inhibited by rapamycin and FK506.[106] In contrast, this study found no evidence of binding to RyR1 of a peptide sequence from residues 724 to 760. Another study found that a peptide formed from residues 671 to 680 enhanced the submaximal Ca^{2+} activation of Ca^{2+} release channels in experiments using both mono- and divalent ions as current carriers. A peptide formed from residues 671 to 690 showed a bimodal activation/inactivation behavior, indicating a high-affinity activating and low-affinity inactivating binding site.[107]

There is also conflicting evidence with regard to the role of residues 720 to 765. Inclusion of rabbit residues 720 to 764 in an otherwise highly divergent DHPR from the house fly, *Musca domestica*, restored orthograde and retrograde signaling, suggesting that residues 720 to 764 are sufficient to restore bidirectional coupling.[105] These observations are supported by data demonstrating that a peptide formed from residues 720 to 765 specifically activates the Ca^{2+} release channel.[107] Two other studies, however, have suggested that these residues contribute to but are not essential for EC coupling in skeletal muscle,[96,108] and another has suggested that there is no direct physical or functional interaction between these residues and RyR.[106]

DISEASES RESULTING FROM MUTATIONS IN Ca^{2+} RELEASE CHANNELS

Skeletal Muscle

Mutations in *RYR1* have been linked to malignant hyperthermia and central core disease[109] and to central core disease (CCD) with nemaline rod myopathy (Fig. 14-7).[110] *Malignant hyperthermia* (MH) and CCD mutations are clustered in *RYR1* exons 2 to 17 (region 1), 34 to 46 (region 2), and 91 to 102 (region 3).[109,110] The ratio of MH to CCD mutations in region 1 is 5 to 1, in region 2, 8 to 1, and in region 3, 1 to 8. MH mutations are more sensitive to caffeine and halothane activation than wild-type and are more "leaky"; CCD mutant proteins are even more leaky than MH mutations.[111–113] CCD mutations may cause a more severe imbalance in Ca^{2+} regulation than those causing MH. Elevation of resting Ca^{2+} by a very leaky CCD mutant channel may trigger the series of degenerative and compensatory events that lead to core formation in the center of the fiber without affecting the periphery of the muscle cell, where Ca^{2+} homeostasis can be achieved through the intervention of plasma membrane Ca^{2+} pumps and exchangers. However, at least one CCD mutation is not leaky, but rather uncouples EC coupling by disrupting orthograde signaling between the DHPR and RyR1 proteins, without disrupting retrograde signaling between these two proteins.[114]

A functional knockout of the gene encoding the skeletal muscle DHPR (*CACNA1S*) is the basis for muscular dysgenesis in the mouse.[94] This animal model, bearing a specific mutation in an EC coupling component, has played a key role in unraveling the functions of DHPR and RyR proteins and the interactions between them.[115] The homozygous mutation results in the loss of the α_1 subunit of the DHPR, leading to loss of charge movement, Ca^{2+} currents, and EC coupling. Function is restored by transfection of cultured dysgenic mouse myoblasts with cDNA encoding the α_1 subunit of the DHPR.

Mutations in the DHPR have also been linked to MH.[116] In this case, the mutation occurs in the DHPR III to IV loop, which may form a site of physical interaction between the skeletal muscle DHPR and RyR proteins.[117] These observations highlight the fact that proteins in the two membrane systems, the SR and the T tubule, interact closely to regulate Ca^{2+} concentrations in skeletal muscle.

Cardiac Muscle

Mutations in *RYR2* have been linked to arrhythmia and sudden death in humans.[118,119] Catecholaminergic polymorphic ventricular tachycardia (CPVT) occurs in response to stress and in the absence of either structural heart disease or a prolonged QT interval. Juvenile sudden death or stress-induced syncope is present in one-third of cases. Arrhythmogenic right ventricular cardiomyopathy type 2 (ARVD2) is characterized by partial degeneration of the myocardium of the right ventricle, electrical instability, and sudden death. The mutations are located in two regions of the gene that correspond to two cytosolic regulatory regions in *RYR1* that cause MH. Since *RYR2* is not expressed in skeletal muscle, neither MH nor CCD manifests in these diseases. It is probable that

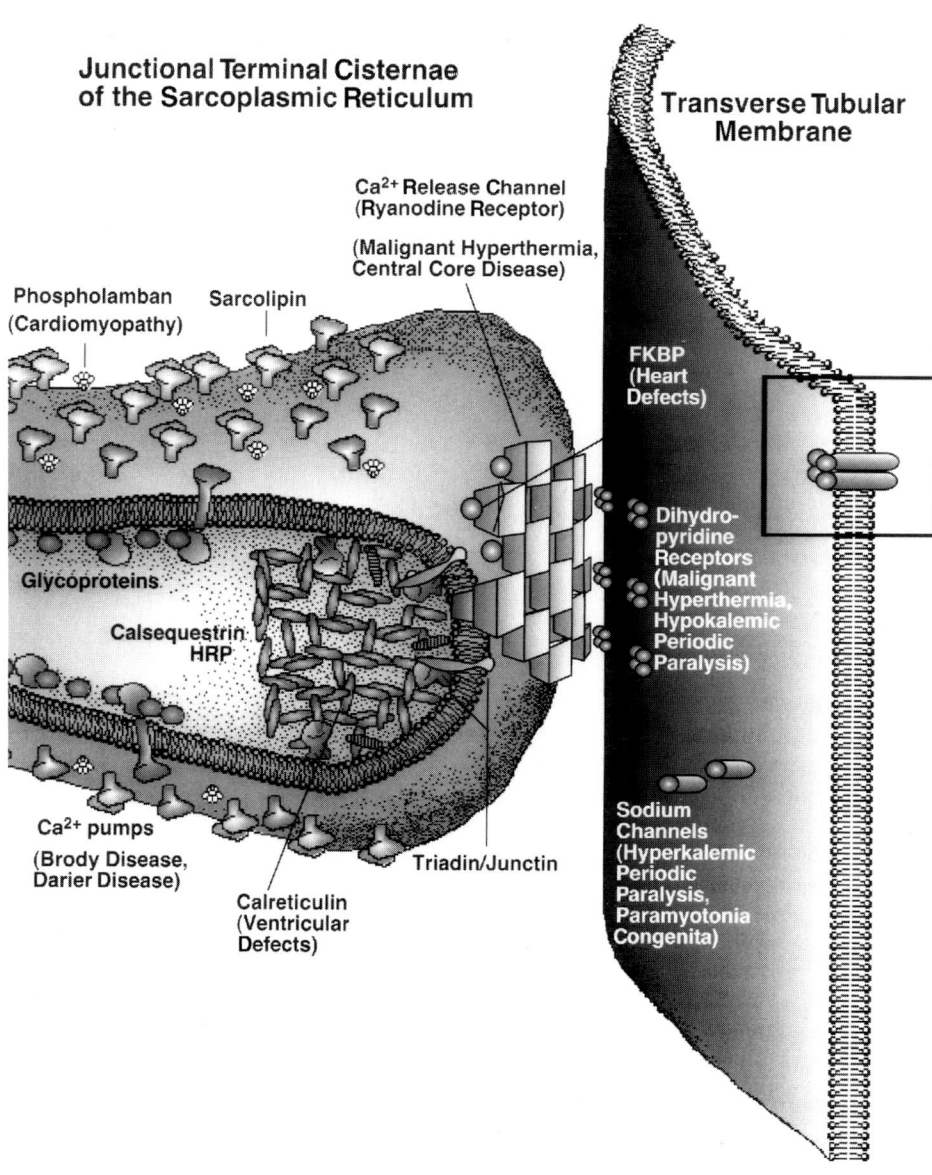

FIGURE 14-7. Muscle diseases associated with proteins in the triad region of the sarcotubular system. Mutations in the skeletal muscle Ca^{2+} release channel (*RYR1*) have been associated with malignant hyperthermia, central core disease, and nemaline rod myopathy; mutations in the cardiac Ca^{2+} release channel (*RYR2*) have been associated with cardiac arrhythmias; mutations in the α_1-subunit of the dihydropyridine receptor (*CACNA1S*) have been associated with malignant hyperthermia and hypokalemic periodic paralysis; mutations in the α-subunit of the sodium channel (*SCN4A*) have been associated with hyperkalemic periodic paralysis, myotonia, and malignant hyperthermia. Mutations in SERCA1 (*ATP2A1*) have been associated with Brody myopathy; mutations in SERCA2 (*ATP2A2*) have been associated with skin defects in Darier disease; mutations in PLN (*PLN*) can induce cardiomyopathy in animal models, as can mutations in FKBP (*FKBP12*) and calsequestrin (*CASQ2*).

CPVT and ARVD2, like MH and CCD, are differentiated phenotypically on the basis of the severity of the alteration in RyR2 channel function.

FK-506 BINDING PROTEIN (FKBP12)

FK506-binding protein (FKBP) is a *cis-trans* peptidyl-prolyl isomerase that binds the immunosuppressant drugs FK506 and rapamycin.[120] FKPB12 is tightly associated with the skeletal muscle RyR1 isoform, and its analogue FKBP12.6 is associated with the cardiac muscle RyR2 isoform. FKBP12 is a 12,000-Da protein that copurifies with RyR in a stoichiometric ratio of four FKBP12 to one RyR tetramer.[121] The interaction between FKBP and RyR1 is essential for the stabilization, activation, and proper functioning of the channel and for coordinated gating of neighboring channels.[122] FKBP, directly visualized by cryoelectron microscopy, is located along the edge of the square-shaped cytoplasmic domain of RyR, at a distance of ~12 nm from the channel-forming domain (Fig. 14-5).[123] An FKBP12-binding domain was mapped to the central regulatory domain of RyR1, between amino acids 2401 and 2480, and the dipeptide Val-Pro^{2462} was shown to be critical for high-affinity interaction.[122] Mutations in this region led to increased gating frequency, suggesting that FKBP12 stabilizes the channel in both the open and closed states.

The physiological roles for FKBP12 and FKBP12.6 have been investigated *in vivo*. Treatment of skinned muscle fibers with FK506, which dissociates FKPB12 from RyR, disrupts EC coupling.[124] Mice in which the gene encoding FKPB12 was disrupted were found to have normal skeletal muscle but to develop dilated cardiomyopathy and ventricular defects, demonstrating a phenotype for FKPB12 deficiency.[125] Cardiac defects have been reported in FKBP12-deficient mice, but the role of FKBP12.6 in cardiac EC coupling remains unclear. The disruption of the FKBP12.6 gene in mice results in cardiac hypertrophy in male mice but not in females.

However, female FKBP12.6-null mice treated with tamoxifen, an estrogen receptor antagonist, develop cardiac hypertrophy similar to that of male mice.[126]

Defective regulation of RyR2 in failing hearts is associated with PKA hyperphosphorylation of the channel, resulting in dissociation of FKBP12.6 and increased sensitivity to Ca^{2+}-dependent activation.[127] This defective regulation results in increased cardiac contractility due to increased EC coupling gain. In failing hearts, this pathway becomes overstimulated, and pathologic consequences may involve depletion of SR Ca^{2+} stores, required for EC coupling, as well as aberrant release of SR Ca^{2+} during diastole, which may serve as a trigger for fatal cardiac arrythmias.

CALMODULIN

Calmodulin (CaM) is a soluble Ca^{2+}-binding protein of 18 kDa that binds to RyR molecules and acts as a Ca^{2+} concentration–dependent modulatory ligand for function of the Ca^{2+} release channel. In vitro studies have shown that CaM binds to RyR with nanomolar affinity and modulates its Ca^{2+}-channel activity by direct protein-protein interactions without involvement of Ca^{2+}-dependent kinases.[82] At resting Ca^{2+} concentrations near 100 nM, CaM binds to RyR1 and acts as a partial agonist. At elevated Ca^{2+} concentrations, such as those measured during a Ca^{2+} transient, CaM inhibits RyR1. RyR1 and RyR3 are activated by Ca^{2+}-free CaM (apoCaM)[128–131] and are inhibited by Ca^{2+}-bound CaM (CaCaM), whereas RyR2 is not activated by apoCaM but is inhibited by CaCaM.[132–134]

Studies using [^{35}S]-labeled CaM show that the tetrameric RyR1 complex binds four CaM molecules in the absence and in the presence of Ca^{2+}, indicating a stoichiometry of one CaM per RyR subunit.[132,134–138] Both apoCaM and CaCaM protect sites after amino acids 3630 and 3637 on RyR1 from trypsin cleavage, but only apoCaM protects sites after amino acids 1982 and 1999 from trypsin.[138a,138b] Both apoCaM and CaCaM bind to two different synthetic peptides representing amino acids 1975–1999 and 3614–3643 of RyR1, but CaCaM has a higher affinity than apoCaM for both peptides. Since disulfide cross-linking shows close proximity between the two CaM-binding sites, CaM appears to bind at a site of intersubunit contact, perhaps with one lobe bound between amino acids 3614 and 3643 on one subunit and the second lobe between amino acids 1975 and 1999 on an adjacent subunit.

Spatial localization of the two forms of CaM, based on cryoelectron microscopy and three-dimensional reconstruction[123], support these results. The target surface for both forms of CaM is situated about 10 nm away from the Ca^{2+}-conducting pore, suggesting that long-range interactions occur between the domain to which CaM is bound and the transmembrane domain of RyR1 which forms the channel pore (Fig. 14-5). This CaM does not dissociate from RyR in response to the oscillating Ca^{2+} concentrations that are responsible for the cycles of contraction-relaxation in skeletal muscle. The location of apoCaM and CaCaM at a critical region for RyR1-DHPR receptor interactions suggests a direct role for CaM in the mechanism of EC coupling.

Other Integral Membrane Proteins

TRIADIN

Triadin was first identified and purified from rabbit skeletal muscle SR as a 95-kDa integral membrane protein localized to skeletal muscle triads (Fig. 14-6).[139] Several triadin isoforms have been identified in skeletal and cardiac muscle, all of which appear to arise from alternative splicing of the same triadin gene.[140–142] The single transmembrane domain of skeletal muscle triadin divides the protein into a short N-terminal cytoplasmic domain and a highly charged C-terminal region, which is located in the lumen of the SR and accounts for the bulk of the molecule. All triadin isoforms in a given species have virtually identical amino acid sequences over their first 250 to 260 residues, which encompass a short N-terminal cytoplasmic region, a membrane-spanning segment, and a highly charged luminal domain.[140,143] The charged luminal domains are basic and are responsible for binding to calsequestrin and RyR.[141–143] Some have suggested that a region of the cytoplasmic domain may also interact with RyR, depending on the Ca^{2+} concentration.[144]

The luminal domain consists of several clusters of amino acids, referred to as KEKE motifs, which have been proposed to facilitate protein-protein interactions by acting as "polar zippers." A specific site of interaction with calsequestrin has been localized to a single KEKE motif of the luminal domain of triadin, from residues 210 to 224.[145] The residues are predicted to form a β-strand, which may tether calsequestrin to the junctional face of the membrane, allowing calsequestrin to sequester Ca^{2+} in the vicinity of the ryanodine receptor during Ca^{2+} uptake and release. Coimmunoprecipitation experiments and fusion-protein binding assays have also demonstrated binding of histidine-rich Ca^{2+}-binding protein to this same KEKE motif.[146]

Transgenic mice with a targeted overexpression of mouse triadin 1 to mouse atrium and ventricle exhibited a benign cardiac hypertrophy and characteristics suggestive of an important role for triadin 1 in the regulation of contractile properties of the heart during EC coupling.[147]

JUNCTIN

Junctin was first identified as a 26-kDa calsequestrin- (CSQ)-binding protein in cardiac and skeletal muscle, and is the major CSQ-binding protein in cardiac SR vesicles (Fig. 14-6).[141] Although junctin and triadin are the products of different genes, the two molecules exhibit structural and functional homology. The 210–amino acid sequence is predicted to form a short N-terminal domain, a transmembrane sequence, and a highly charged luminal domain. Sequence analysis demonstrates significant amino acid sequence homology (greater than 97 percent) in the transmembrane domain and contiguous 61 amino acids of the luminal domain but only 72 to 75 percent homology in the C-terminal region.[148] Junctin appears to bind directly to CSQ, triadin, and RyR. The binding interaction is localized to the luminal domain of junctin that is highly enriched in charged amino acids organized into

KEKE motifs. Junctin and triadin may interact directly in the junctional SR membrane and stabilize a complex that anchors CSQ to RyR. These results suggest that junctin, triadin, CSQ, and RyR form a quaternary complex that may be required for normal regulation of Ca^{2+} release. Indeed, overexpression of junctin in transgenic mice leads to structural alteration in the architecture of the junctional SR, suggesting that junctin alters the packing of CSQ.[149]

MITSUGUMIN

Mitsugumin 29 (MG29) is a 29-kDa protein located specifically in the triad junction of skeletal muscle (Fig. 14-6).[150] The 264 amino acids are predicted to form four transmembrane segments, with cytoplasmic N and C termini. Sequence alignment has revealed that MG29 exhibits a high degree of homology to the synaptophysin family of proteins, a group of membrane proteins presumed to have a role in neurotransmitter release.[151] It has been implicated in the formation of the T-tubule network and in T-tubule–SR (triad) junction formation.[152,153] Mitsugumin 29 isolated from T tubules of mature rabbit skeletal muscle self-associates to form a higher-order hexamer, but it does not appear to associate with other proteins.[154]

MG29 knockout in mice leads to lower twitch forces and morphologic abnormalities of membranes around the triad junction in extensor digitorum longus (EDL) muscle, indicating that MG29 is essential for both refinement of membrane structures and effective EC coupling in the skeletal muscle triad junction.[153] *In vitro* studies in these mice indicate that both EDL and soleus muscles fatigue more easily when compared to controls, probably due to an alteration in calcium homeostasis.[155]

JUNCTOPHILIN

Junctophilin (JP), initially referred to as mitsugumin 72 (MG72), is a 72-kDa protein found in the junctional terminal cisternae (Fig. 14-6).[156] The 661 amino acids comprise a large cytoplasmic region that shows specific affinity for the plasma membrane and a COOH-terminal, membrane-spanning sequence located in the ER/SR membrane.[154] The cytoplasmic region bears homology with proteins that associate with cell-surface membranes and exhibit selective affinity for phospholipids. A 14–amino acid motif, the "MORN" motif (membrane occupation and recognition nexus), is repeated eight times in the NH_2-terminal region.

In mice, at least three JP subtypes are derived from different genes: JP-1 is found predominantly in skeletal muscle; JP-2 is expressed throughout skeletal, cardiac, and smooth muscle cells; and JP-3 is expressed specifically in the brain.[157]

Junctophilin is a strong candidate for the "docking" protein that allows the SR to attach to either surface membranes or T tubules at the beginning of the formation of triads, dyads, and peripheral couplings. Expression of junctophilin in RyR1- and RyR3-deficient myoblasts results in the formation of the triad junction by generating a junctional complex with the cell surface membranes. JP-2 is abundantly expressed in the heart, and mutant mice lacking JP-2 exhibit embryonic lethality. Cardiac myocytes from the mutant mice show deficiency of the junctional membrane complexes and abnormal Ca^{2+} transients.[157]

A JP-1 knockout mouse model showed no milk suckling and mice died shortly after birth.[158] Ultrastructural analysis demonstrated that triad junctions were reduced in number, and that the SR was often structurally abnormal in the skeletal muscle of the mutant mice. Mutant muscle had less contractile force and showed abnormal sensitivity to extracellular Ca^{2+}.

CALMODULIN-DEPENDENT PROTEIN KINASE

A 60-kDa Ca^{2+}-calmodulin-dependent protein kinase (CaMK) has been associated with the terminal cisternae of the SR.[90–92] CaMK is a multifunctional protein kinase shown to phosphorylate a series of proteins in the SR and to regulate their function. Endogenous CaMK phosphorylation of cycling proteins is depressed in heart failure due to myocardial infarction, perhaps leading to abnormalities in SR function and subsequent attenuated cardiac performance.[159]

Luminal Proteins

CALSEQUESTRIN

Calsequestrin (CSQ) is a high-capacity Ca^{2+}-binding protein located in the lumen of the junctional SR in cardiac and skeletal muscle.[160] CSQ sequesters large amounts of Ca^{2+} in the vicinity of the RyR, where it acts as a storage depot for the Ca^{2+} released during muscle contraction, and serves to lower the free Ca^{2+} concentration, reducing the gradient against which the ATPase must pump Ca^{2+}. Two *CASQ* genes encode a fast-twitch skeletal muscle isoform and a cardiac/slow-twitch muscle isoform.[161,162] The mature rabbit skeletal muscle isoform has a mass of 42,435 Da. It binds 40 to 50 moles of Ca^{2+} per mole of protein with a high capacity and a moderate affinity ($Kd \simeq 400\,\mu M$).

CSQ is found in dense, highly concentrated filamentous matrices segregated within the terminal cisternae of the SR, where it appears to be attached to the inner surface of the transmembrane domain of RyR by anchoring proteins, possibly junctin and triadin (see Chap. 11). The formation of the CSQ matrix is likely to result from back-to-back and front-to-front oligomerization of adjacent CSQ molecules (Fig. 14-8 and Color Plate 4c).[163] The site of interaction between triadin and CSQ has been localized to a single KEKE motif comprising 25 amino acids.[145] Overexpression of junctin leads to structural alterations in cardiac Ca^{2+} release units, suggesting that an increase in the expression of junctin can affect the packing of CSQ.[149]

CSQ undergoes Ca^{2+}-induced changes in conformation.[164–167] Transient increases in free luminal Ca^{2+} concentration were observed when Ca^{2+} release was triggered by caffeine in isolated SR vesicles containing CSQ, but not in those from which CSQ was extracted. A loss in responsiveness to Ca^{2+} of heavy SR vesicles that have been deprived of CSQ by treatment with EDTA has been interpreted as evidence of CSQ interaction with RyR. CSQ potentiated

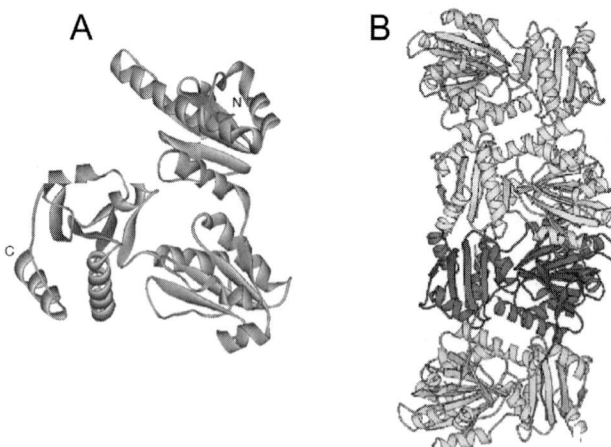

FIGURE 14-8. *A.* A ribbon diagram of CSQ demonstrating the spatial organization of the three thioredoxin-fold domains determined from the crystal structure at 2.6 Å resolution. *B.* Calsequestrin monomers can associate in "front to front" and "back to back" chains, creating additional Ca^{2+}-binding sites in clefts between the individual molecules.[170,171] The highly charged C terminus is disordered in this structure. See Color Plate 4.

[^{3}H]ryanodine binding to solubilized, heavy SR vesicles.[168] Ca^{2+} dependence of [^{3}H]ryanodine binding to solubilized heavy SR was enhanced by CSQ. CSQ dissociation from the junctional face membrane caused a tenfold increase in the duration of ryanodine receptor opening in lipid bilayers, which was reversed when CSQ was added back.[169] In contrast to native receptors, purified channels, depleted of triadin and CSQ, were not inhibited by CSQ, suggesting that CSQ normally reduces RyR activity by binding to triadin or an alternate intermediate protein.

The crystal structure of CSQ (Fig. 14-8 and Color Plate 4b) suggests a mechanism by which CSQ may obtain high-capacity Ca^{2+} binding.[170,171] Three negative thioredoxin-like domains surround a hydrophilic center. At low cation concentration the three domains are stable, probably because of electrostatic repulsion between acidic amino acids on the surface of the individual domains. Trace amounts of cations are able to promote the collapse of the three domains into a compact structure by lowering electrostatic repulsion and by forming intermolecular bridges between the acidic, carboxyl tails. Polymer formation is furthered by an increase in Ca^{2+} concentration. The NH_2-terminal segment of one monomer crosses the dimer interface and wraps itself around the other monomer, leading to a "domain swapping" or "arm exchange" configuration. In between the two dimer interfaces are dense populations of acidic residues, forming electronegative pockets. Calcium coordinates the acidic residues, filling the cavities inside the dimers. The loose association of Ca^{2+} with the surface of the CSQ crystal creates conditions for rapid release of Ca^{2+} from the Ca^{2+}-CSQ complex.

Transgenic mice overexpressing both canine (10-fold overexpression) and murine (20-fold overexpression) cardiac CSQ develop a serious cardiomyopathy. Results suggest that CSQ overexpression is associated with increases in SR Ca^{2+} capacity, but decreases in Ca^{2+}-induced Ca^{2+} release lead to depressed contractility.[172,173]

Nonsense mutations in the cardiac calsequestrin gene, CASQ2, were found in three catecholaminergic polymorphic ventricular tachycardia (CPVT) families.[173a] Two homozygous patients with a complete absence of calsequestrin 2 experienced syncopes before the age of 7. One heterozygous patient experienced syncopes from the age of 11 and another had ventricular arrhythmias at ECG on exercise tests. These observations suggest that CASQ2 mutations produce a severe form of CPVT.

CALRETICULIN

Calreticulin (CLR), a Ca^{2+}-binding protein, was first identified in SR membranes (Fig. 14-6).[66] Since then, it has been isolated from a great variety of cells and is proposed to function as both a molecular chaperone[174] and a buffer to reduce capacitative Ca^{2+} entry into the lumen of the ER.[175] CLR is a minor component of skeletal and cardiac muscle SR membranes. Like CSQ, CLR binds 25 moles of Ca^{2+} per mole of protein, with low affinity, but unlike CSQ it also has a single, high-affinity Ca^{2+}-binding site.[176,177] Ca^{2+}-binding sites are not evident in the primary sequence and may form conformationally. Predictions based on the amino acid sequence indicate that the protein can be divided into three domains.[178] The third, or C domain, containing 37 amino acids, is the most likely to bind Ca^{2+} with high capacity and low affinity. The protein also contains an ER retention signal sequence, KDEL.[161]

The NMR structure of the middle or P domain of CLR has been solved.[179] The P domain is believed to be involved in substrate binding, as part of its chaperone function,[180] and also contains a high-affinity Ca^{2+}-binding site.[181] The amino acid sequence of this domain is highly conserved and is composed in its entire length of multiple copies of short, proline-rich repeat sequences, with the type 1 repeats comprising 17 residues and the type 2 repeats, 14 residues. The NMR structure is consistent with the P domain forming a protrusion from the core of CLR. The best-defined part of this structure is a finger-like loop, the tip of which is proposed to form a protein ligand-binding site, which may bind a cochaperone.[179]

CLR is only a minor component in the adult heart but is highly expressed in cardiovascular tissue during early embryogenesis. It is essential for cardiac development, since disruption of the gene in homozygous mice results in embryonic lethality.[182] The major features of the disruption are failure of absorption of the umbilical hernia, marked decrease in ventricular wall thickness, and deep intratrabecular recesses in the ventricular walls. Impairment of $InsP_3$-dependent Ca^{2+} release and of nuclear import of the NF-AT3 transcription factor, critical for cardiac development, has been demonstrated in cells isolated from the knockout mice. In transgenic mice that overexpress CLR in the heart, postnatally elevated expression of CLR leads to severe cardiac pathology.[183] These data confirm that CLR plays a key role in Ca^{2+} regulatory systems.

SARCALUMENIN

Sarcalumenin exists as two alternatively spliced products of the same gene: an acidic 160-kDa glycoprotein and a 53-kDa glycoprotein, which occur in a ratio of about 1 to 10.[184,185] These proteins are located in the lumen of the longitudinal reticulum and may be associated with the luminal surface of the membrane.[186] The mature 53-kDa glycoprotein is made up of 453 amino acids and 2 moles of [(GlcNAc)2(Man)9]. The cDNA encoding the 160-kDa glycoprotein is identical to that encoding the 53-kDa glycoprotein except that it contains an in-frame insertion of 1308 nucleotides near the 5' end. Thus the two glycoproteins have the same 19–amino acid signal sequence, but a highly acidic amino acid sequence of 436 amino acids is inserted after the signal sequence in the 160-kDa form.

The function of the two glycoproteins is not clear. The 160-kDa form of sarcalumenin has low-affinity, high-capacity Ca^{2+}-binding properties similar to those of CSQ and CLR. This may be a generalized and essential property of all proteins that reside in the lumen of sarco(endo)plasmic reticulum, where the free Ca^{2+} concentration is higher than that of the cytoplasm but lower than that of the extracellular space.[171] Like CSQ, the expression of these glycoproteins is restricted to striated muscle. Their location in the longitudinal reticulum suggests that their function may be to reduce the free Ca^{2+} concentration at the site of Ca^{2+} ejection into the SR lumen, thereby assisting in the overall process of Ca^{2+} pumping.

HISTIDINE-RICH Ca^2-BINDING PROTEIN

In a search for low-density lipoprotein (LDL) receptors, a SR protein was found, unexpectedly, to bind LDL.[187,188] Subsequent staining with $^{45}Ca^{2+}$ and Stains-All revealed that this protein with an apparent mass of 165 kDa is a luminal, acidic Ca^{2+}-binding protein. It is now believed that LDL binding is not a biologically relevant property of this molecule, as there is no access to plasma lipoprotein in the SR. Purification and cloning of the protein revealed several unique features: (1) an N-terminal signal sequence; (2) a middle segment composed of nine tandem repeats of a histidine-rich sequence, HRHRGH, and a stretch of 10 to 11 acidic amino acids; (3) a 13-residue stretch of polyglutamic acid near the C terminus; and (4) a cluster of 14 closely spaced cysteine residues in the C terminus. The acidic repeats are believed to form all or part of the Ca^{2+}-binding domain.

HRC colocalizes with RyR1 on the junctional face of the terminal cisternae and is a substrate for the 60-kDa CaM-dependent protein kinase, located in the same region.[189] Ca^{2+}-sensitive binding of HRC to triadin has been demonstrated.[146] The acidic repeats of HRC are responsible for binding triadin, which occurs in the luminal region of triadin containing the KEKE motif.

Conclusions

In this chapter, we have outlined the ways in which a number of integral and peripheral membrane proteins interact physically and functionally to create a membrane system responsible for Ca^{2+} regulation in muscle cells. Our knowledge concerning each of these proteins is far from complete, and it is certain that a number of additional proteins will be found to contribute to Ca^{2+} regulation and EC coupling as proteomic approaches are used in their identification. We anticipate that many exciting new findings in this field will be described in future editions of this text.

List of Abbreviations

ARVD2	arrhythmogenic right ventricular cardiomyopathy type 2
CaM	calmodulin
CaMK	calmodulin-dependent protein kinase
CCD	central core disease
CLR	calreticulin
CPVT	catecholaminergic polymorphic ventricular tachycardia
CSQ	calsequestrin
DHPR	dihydropyridine receptor
EC	excitation-contraction
EDL	extensor digitorum longus
ER	endoplasmic reticulum
FKBP	FK506-binding protein
FTIR	Fourier transform infrared spectroscopy
$InsP_3$	inositol triphosphate
JP	junctophilin
MH	malignant hyperthermia
NMR	nuclear magnetic resonance
PLN	phospholamban
$RT_{1/2}$	time to half relaxation
RyR	ryanodine receptor
SLN	Sarcolipin
SERCA	Sarco(Endo)plasmic reticulum Ca^{2+} ATPase
SR	sarcoplasmic reticulum
TPP	Time to peak pressure
T tubule	transverse tubule
V_{max}	maximal velocity

References

1. Franzini-Armstrong C, Protasi F: Ryanodine receptors of striated muscles: A complex channel capable of multiple interactions. *Physiol Rev* 77:699–729, 1997.
2. Marsh BB: A factor modifying muscle fibre synaeresis. *Nature* 167:1065–1068, 1951.
3. Hasselbach W, Makinose M: Die Calciumpumpe der Erschlaffungsgrane des Muskels und ihre Abhangigkeit von der ATP. *Biochem Zeitschr* 333:518–528, 1961.
4. Ebashi S, Lipmann F: Adenosinetriphosphate-linked concentration of calcium ions in a particulate fraction of rabbit muscle. *J Cell Biol* 14:389–400, 1962.
5. Ebashi S, Endo M, Otsuki I: Control of muscle contraction. *Q Rev Biophys* 2:351–284, 1969.
6. Hasselbach W: Relaxing factor and the relaxation of muscle. *Prog Biophys* 14:167–222, 1964.
7. MacLennan DH: Purification and properties of an adenosine triphosphatase from sarcoplasmic reticulum. *J Biol Chem* 245:4508–4518, 1970.
8. MacLennan DH, Brandl CJ, Korczak B, Green NM: Amino-acid sequence of a $Ca^{2+} + Mg^{2+}$–dependent ATPase from rabbit muscle sarcoplasmic reticulum deduced from its complementary DNA sequence. *Nature* 316:696–700, 1985.
9. Brandl CJ, Green NM, Korczak B, MacLennan DH: Two Ca^{2+} ATPase genes: Homologies and mechanistic implications of deduced amino acid sequences. *Cell* 44:597–607, 1986.
10. Burk SE, Lytton J, MacLennan DH, Shull GE: cDNA cloning functional expression and mRNA tissue distribution of a third organellar Ca^{2+} pump. *J Biol Chem* 264:18561–18568, 1989.
11. Lytton J, Westlin M, Burk SE, et al: Functional comparisons between isoforms of the sarcoplasmic or endoplasmic reticulum family of calcium pumps. *J Biol Chem* 267:14483–14489, 1992.
12. Wu KD, Lytton J: Molecular cloning and quantification of sarcoplasmic reticulum Ca^{2+}-ATPase isoforms in rat muscles. *Am J Physiol* 264:C333–C341, 1993.
13. MacLennan DH, Rice WJ, Green NM: The mechanism of Ca^{2+} transport by sarco(endo)plasmic reticulum Ca^{2+}-ATPases. *J Biol Chem* 272:28815–28818, 1997.
14. Makinose M, Hasselbach W: ATP synthesis by the reverse of the sarcoplasmic calcium pump. *FEBS Lett* 12:271–272, 1971.
15. Knowles AF, Racker E: Formation of adenosine triphosphate from Pi and adenosine diphosphate by purified Ca^{2+}-adenosine triphosphatase *J Biol Chem* 250:1949–1951, 1975.
16. Kanazawa T, Boyer PD: Occurrence and characteristics of a rapid exchange of phosphate oxygens catalyzed by sarcoplasmic reticulum vesicles. *J Biol Chem* 248:3163–3172, 1973.
17. Masuda H, de Meis L: Phosphorylation of the sarcoplasmic reticulum membrane by orthophosphate: Inhibition by calcium ions. *Biochemistry* 12:4581–4585, 1974.
18. Meissner G: ATP and Ca^{2+} binding by the Ca^{2+} pump protein of sarcoplasmic reticulum. *Biochim Biophys Acta* 298:906–926, 1973.
19. Inesi G, Kurzmack M, Coan C, Lewis DE: Cooperative calcium binding and ATPase activation in sarcoplasmic reticulum vesicles. *J Biol Chem* 255:3025–3031, 1980.
20. Dupont Y: Low-temperature studies of the sarcoplasmic reticulum calcium pump: Mechanisms of calcium binding. *Biochim Biophys Acta* 688:75–87, 1982.
21. Inesi G: Sequential mechanism of calcium binding and translocation in sarcoplasmic reticulum adenosine triphosphatase. *J Biol Chem* 262:16338–16342, 1987.
22. Canet D, Forge V, Guillain F, Mintz E: Ca^{2+} translocation across sarcoplasmic reticulum ATPase randomizes the two transported ions. *J Biol Chem* 271:20566–20572, 1996.
23. Levy D, Seigneuret M, Bluzat A, Rigaud JL: Evidence for proton countertransport by the sarcoplasmic reticulum Ca^{2+}-ATPase during calcium transport in reconstituted proteoliposomes with low ionic permeability. *J Biol Chem* 265:19524–19534, 1990.
24. Deamer DW, Baskin RJ: Ultrastructure of sarcoplasmic reticulum preparations. *J Cell Biol* 42:296–307, 1969.
25. Inesi G, Asai H: Trypsin digestion of fragmented sarcoplasmic reticulum. *Arch Biochem Biophys* 126:469–477, 1968.
26. Stewart PS, MacLennan DH: Surface particles of sarcoplasmic reticulum membranes: Structural features of the adenosine triphosphatase. *J Biol Chem* 249:985–993, 1974.
27. Aravind L, Tatusov RL, Wolf YI, et al: Evidence for massive gene exchange between archaeal and bacterial hyperthermophiles. *Trends Genet* 14:442–444, 1998.
28. Stokes DL, Green NM: Modeling a dehalogenase fold into the 8 Å density map for Ca^{2+}-ATPase defines a new domain structure. *Biophys J* 78:1765–1776, 2000.
29. Dux L, Martonosi A: Two-dimensional arrays of proteins in sarcoplasmic reticulum and purified Ca^{2+}-ATPase vesicles treated with vanadate. *J Biol Chem* 258: 2599–2603, 1983.
30. Zhang P, Toyoshima C, Yonekura K, et al: Structure of the calcium pump from sarcoplasmic reticulum at 8 Å resolution. *Nature* 392:835–839, 1998.
31. Maruyama K, MacLennan DH: Mutation of aspartic acid-351 lysine-352 and lysine-515 alters the Ca^{2+} transport activity of the Ca^{2+}-ATPase expressed in COS-1 cells. *Proc Natl Acad Sci USA* 85:3314–3318, 1988.
32. Clarke DM, Loo TW, Inesi G, MacLennan DH: Location of high affinity Ca^{2+}-binding sites within the predicted transmembrane domain of the sarcoplasmic reticulum Ca^{2+}-ATPase. *Nature* 339:476–478, 1989.
33. Andersen JP, Vilsen B: Functional consequences of alterations to Glu309 Glu771 and Asp800 in the Ca^{2+}-ATPase of sarcoplasmic reticulum. *J Biol Chem* 267:19383–19387, 1992.
34. Andersen JP: Dissection of the functional domains of the sarcoplasmic reticulum Ca^{2+}-ATPase by site-directed mutagenesis. *Biosci Rep* 15:243–261, 1995.
35. Vilsen B, Andersen JP: CrATP-induced Ca^{2+} occlusion in mutants of the Ca^{2+}-ATPase of sarcoplasmic reticulum. *J Biol Chem* 267:25739–25743, 1992.
36. Skerjanc IS, Toyofuku T, Richardson C, MacLennan DH: Mutation of glutamate 309 to glutamine alters one Ca^{2+}-binding site in the Ca^{2+}-ATPase of sarcoplasmic reticulum expressed in Sf9 cells. *J Biol Chem* 268:15944–15950, 1993.
37. Rice WJ, MacLennan DH: Scanning mutagenesis reveals a similar pattern of mutation sensitivity in transmembrane sequences M4 M5 and M6 but not in M8 of the Ca^{2+}-ATPase of sarcoplasmic reticulum (SERCA1a). *J Biol Chem* 271: 31412–31419, 1996.
38. Soulie S, Neumann JM, Berthomieu C, et al: NMR conformational study of the sixth transmembrane segment of sarcoplasmic reticulum Ca^{2+}-ATPase. *Biochemistry* 38:5813–5821, 1999.
39. MacLennan DH, Clarke DM, Loo TW, Skerjanc IS: Site-directed mutagenesis of the Ca^{2+} ATPase of sarcoplasmic reticulum. *Acta Physiol Scand Suppl* 607:141–150, 1992.
40. Clarke DM, Maruyama K, Loo TW, et al: Functional consequences of glutamate aspartate glutamine and asparagine mutations in the stalk sector of the Ca^{2+}-ATPase of sarcoplasmic reticulum. *J Biol Chem* 264:11246–11251, 1989.
41. Toyoshima C, Nakasako M, Nomura H, Ogawa H: Crystal structure of the calcium pump of sarcoplasmic reticulum at 26 Å resolution. *Nature* 405:647–655, 2000.
42. Zhang Z, Lewis D, Sumbilla C, et al: The role of the M6–M7 loop (L67) in stabilization of the phosphorylation and Ca^{2+} binding domains of the sarcoplasmic reticulum Ca^{2+}-ATPase (SERCA). *J Biol Chem* 276:15232–15239, 2001.
43. Hua S, Ma H, Lewis D, et al: Functional role of "N" (nucleotide) and "P" (phosphorylation) domain interactions in the sarcoplasmic reticulum (SERCA) ATPase. *Biochemistry* 41:2264–2272, 2002.
44. Toyoshima C, Nomura H: Structural changes in the calcium pump accompanying the dissociation of calcium. *Nature* 418:605–611, 2002.
45. Vilsen B, Andersen JP: Mutation to the glutamate in the fourth membrane segment of Na+K+-ATPase and Ca^{2+}-ATPase affects cation binding from both sides of the membrane and destabilizes the occluded enzyme forms. *Biochemistry* 37:10961–10971, 1998.
46. Tada M, Kadoma M: Regulation of the Ca^{2+} pump ATPase by cAMP-dependent phosphorylation of phospholamban. *Bioessays* 10:157–163, 1989.
47. Simmerman HK, Jones LR: Phospholamban: Protein structure mechanism of action and role in cardiac function. *Physiol Rev* 78:921–947, 1998.
48. Luo W, Grupp IL, Harrer J, et al: Targeted ablation of the phospholamban gene is associated with markedly enhanced myocardial contractility and loss of beta-agonist stimulation. *Circ Res* 75:401–409, 1994.
49. MacLennan, DH, Kranias EG: Phospholamban—a crucial regulator of cardiac contractility. *Nature Rev Mol Cell Biol* 4:566–577, 2003.
50. Mortishire-Smith RJ, Pitzenberger SM, Burke CJ, et al: Solution structure of the cytoplasmic domain of phospholamban: Phosphorylation leads to a local perturbation in secondary structure. *Biochemistry* 34:7603–7613, 1995.
51. Pollesello P, Annila A, Ovaska M: Structure of the 1–36 amino-terminal fragment of human phospholamban by nuclear magnetic resonance and modeling of the phospholamban pentamer. *Biophys J* 76:1784–1795, 1999.
52. Lamberth S, Schmid H, Muenchbach M, et al: NMR solution structure of phospholamban. *Helv Chim Acta* 83:2141–2152, 2000.
53. Bers DM: *Excitation–Contraction Coupling and Cardiac Contractile Force*. Amsterdam: Kluwer, 2001.
54. James P, Inui M, Tada M, et al: Nature and site of phospholamban regulation of the Ca^{2+} pump of sarcoplasmic reticulum. *Nature* 342: 90–92, 1989.
55. Negash S, Chen LT, Bigelow DJ, Squier TC: Phosphorylation of phospholamban by cAMP-dependent protein kinase enhances interactions between Ca-ATPase polypeptide chains in cardiac sarcoplasmic reticulum membranes. *Biochemistry* 35:11247–11259, 1996.
56. Tatulian SA, Chen B, Li J, et al: The inhibitory action of phospholamban involves stabilization of α-helices within the Ca-ATPase. *Biochemistry* 41:741–751, 2002.
57. Toyofuku T, Kurzydlowski K, Tada M, MacLennan DH: Amino acids Glu2 to Ile18 in the cytoplasmic domain of phospholamban are essential for functional association with the Ca^{2+}-ATPase of sarcoplasmic reticulum. *J Biol Chem* 269:3088–3094, 1994.

58. Toyofuku T, Kurzydlowski K, Tada M, MacLennan DH: Amino acids Lys–Asp–Asp–Lys–Pro–Val402 in the Ca^{2+}-ATPase of cardiac sarcoplasmic reticulum are critical for functional association with phospholamban. *J Biol Chem* 269:22929–22932, 1994.
59. Kimura Y, Kurzydlowski K, Tada M, MacLennan DH: Phospholamban inhibitory function is activated by depolymerization. *J Biol Chem* 272:15061–15064, 1997.
60. Asahi M, Kimura Y, Kurzydlowski K, et al: Transmembrane helix M6 in sarco(endo)plasmic reticulum Ca^{2+}-ATPase forms a functional interaction site with phospholamban: Evidence for physical interactions at other sites. *J Biol Chem* 274:32855–32862, 1999.
61. Toyoshima C, Asahi M, Sugita Y, et al: Modeling of the inhibitory interaction of phospholamban with the Ca^{2+} ATPase. *Proc Natl Acad Sci USA* 100:467–472, 2003.
62. Zhai J, Schmidt AG, Hoit BD, et al: Cardiac-specific overexpression of a superinhibitory pentameric phospholamban mutant enhances inhibition of cardiac function in vivo. *J Biol Chem* 275:10538–10544, 2000.
63. Zvaritch E, Backx PH, Jirik F, et al: The transgenic expression of highly inhibitory monomeric forms of phospholamban in mouse heart impairs cardiac contractility. *J Biol Chem* 275:14985–14991, 2000.
64. Haghighi K, Schmidt AG, Hoit BD, et al: Superinhibition of sarcoplasmic reticulum function by phospholamban induces cardiac contractile failure. *J Biol Chem* 276:24145–24152, 2001.
64a. Schmitt JP, Kamisago M, Asahi M, et al: Dilated cardiomyopathy and heart failure caused by a mutation in phospholamban. *Science* 299: 1410–1413, 2003.
64b. Haghighi K, Kolokathis F, Pater L, et al: Human phospholamban null results in lethal dilated cardiomyopathy revealing a critical difference between mouse and human. *J Clin Invest* 111:869–876, 2003.
65. Minamisawa S, Hoshijima M, Chu G, et al: Chronic phospholamban-sarcoplasmic reticulum calcium ATPase interaction is the critical calcium cycling defect in dilated cardiomyopathy. *Cell* 99:313–322, 1999.
66. MacLennan DH, Yip CC, Iles GH, Seeman P: Isolation of sarcoplasmic rectaculum proteins in *The Mechanism of Muscle Contraction*. Vol 37. Cold Spring Harbor, NY: Cold Spring Harbor Laboratory Press, 1972; pp 469–478.
67. Odermatt A, Taschner PE, Scherer SW, et al: Characterization of the gene encoding human sarcolipin (SLN), a proteolipid associated with SERCA1: Absence of structural mutations in five patients with Brody disease. *Genomics* 45:541–553, 1997.
68. Odermatt A, Becker S, Khanna VK, et al: Sarcolipin regulates the activity of SERCA1, the fast-twitch skeletal muscle sarcoplasmic reticulum Ca^{2+}-ATPase. *J Biol Chem* 273:12360–12369, 1998.
69. Gayan-Ramirez G, Vanzeir L, Wuytack F, Decramer M: Corticosteroids decrease mRNA levels of SERCA pumps whereas they increase sarcolipin mRNA in the rat diaphragm. *J Physiol* 524(Pt 2):387–397, 2000.
70. Asahi M, Kurzydlowski K, Tada M, MacLennan DH: Sarcolipin inhibits polymerization of phospholamban to induce superinhibition of sarco(endo)plasmic reticulum Ca^{2+}-ATPases (SERCAs). *J Biol Chem* 24:24, 2002.
71. Asahi M, Sugita Y, Kurzydlowski K, et al: Sarcolipin regulates sarco(endo)plasmic reticulum Ca^{2+}-ATPase (SERCA1a) by binding to transmembrane helices directly or through phospholamban. *Proc Natl Acad Sci USA* 100:5040–5045, 2003.
72. Mascioni A, Karim C, Barany G, et al: Structure and orientation of sarcolipin in lipid environments. *Biochemistry* 41:475–482, 2002.
73. Hellstern S, Pegoraro S, Karim CB, et al: Sarcolipin the shorter homologue of phospholamban forms oligomeric structures in detergent micelles and in liposomes. *J Biol Chem* 276:30845–30852, 2001.
74. Ogawa Y, Ebashi S: Ca-releasing action of beta gamma-methylene adenosine triphosphate on fragmented sarcoplasmic reticulum. *J Biochem (Tokyo)* 80:1149–1157, 1976.
75. Morii H, Tonomura Y: The gating behavior of a channel for Ca^{2+}-induced Ca^{2+} release in fragmented sarcoplasmic reticulum. *J Biochem (Tokyo)* 93: 1271–1285, 1983.
76. Meissner G: Adenine nucleotide stimulation of Ca^{2+}-induced Ca^{2+} release in sarcoplasmic reticulum. *J Biol Chem* 259:2365–2374, 1984.
77. Ikemoto N, Ronjat M, Meszaros LG: Kinetic analysis of excitation-contraction coupling. *J Bioenerg Biomembr* 21:247–266, 1989.
78. Fleischer S, Ogunbunmi EM, Dixon MC, Fleer EA: Localization of Ca^{2+} release channels with ryanodine in junctional terminal cisternae of sarcoplasmic reticulum of fast skeletal muscle. *Proc Natl Acad Sci USA* 82:7256–7259, 1985.
79. Inui M, Saito A, Fleischer S: Purification of the ryanodine receptor and identity with feet structures of junctional terminal cisternae of sarcoplasmic reticulum from fast skeletal muscle. *J Biol Chem* 262:1740–1747, 1987.
80. Imagawa T, Smith JS, Coronado R, Campbell KP: Purified ryanodine receptor from skeletal muscle sarcoplasmic reticulum is the Ca^{2+}-permeable pore of the calcium release channel. *J Biol Chem* 262:16636–16643, 1987.
81. Lai FA, Erickson H, Block BA, Meissner G: Evidence for a junctional feet-ryanodine receptor complex from sarcoplasmic reticulum. *Biochem Biophys Res Commun* 143:704–709, 1987.

82. Meissner G: Ryanodine receptor/Ca^{2+} release channels and their regulation by endogenous effectors. *Annu Rev Physiol* 56:485–508, 1994.
83. Smith JS, Coronado R, Meissner G: Sarcoplasmic reticulum contains adenine nucleotide–activated calcium channels. *Nature* 316:446–449, 1985.
84. Coronado R, Morrissette J, Sukhareva M, Vaughan DM: Structure and function of ryanodine receptors. *Am J Physiol* 266:C1485–C1504, 1994.
85. Lamb GD, Stephenson DG: Effects of intracellular pH and [Mg^{2+}] on excitation-contraction coupling in skeletal muscle fibres of the rat. *J Physiol* 478:331–339, 1994.
86. Harrison GG: Malignant hyperthermia: Dantrolene—dynamics and kinetics. *Br J Anaesth* 60:279–286, 1998.
87. Sorrentino V, Volpe P: Ryanodine receptors: How many, where, and why? *Trends Pharmacol Sci* 14:98–103, 1993.
88. Takeshima H, Nishimura S, Matsumoto T, et al: Primary structure and expression from complementary DNA of skeletal muscle ryanodine receptor. *Nature* 339:439–445, 1989.
89. Zorzato F, Fujii J, Otsu K, et al: Molecular cloning of cDNA encoding human and rabbit forms of the Ca^{2+} release channel (ryanodine receptor) of skeletal muscle sarcoplasmic reticulum. *J Biol Chem* 265:2244–2256, 1990.
89a. Du GG, Sandhu B, Khanna VK, et al: Topology of the Ca^{2+} release channel of skeletal muscle sarcoplasmic reticulum (RyR1). *Proc Natl Acad Sci USA* 99:16725–16730, 2002.
90. Block BA, Imagawa T, Campbell KP, Franzini-Armstrong C: Structural evidence for direct interaction between the molecular components of the transverse tubule/sarcoplasmic reticulum junction in skeletal muscle. *J Cell Biol* 107:2587–2600, 1988.
91. Block BA, O'Brien J, Meissner G: Characterization of the sarcoplasmic reticulum proteins in the thermogenic muscles of fish. *J Cell Biol* 127: 1275–1287, 1994.
92. Nakai J, Dirksen RT, Nguyen HT, et al: Enhanced dihydropyridine receptor channel activity in the presence of ryanodine receptor. *Nature* 380: 72–75, 1996.
93. Nabauer M, Callewaert G, Cleemann L, Morad M: Regulation of calcium release is gated by calcium current not gating charge in cardiac myocytes. *Science* 244:800–803, 1989.
94. Tanabe T, Beam KG, Powell JA, Numa S: Restoration of excitation-contraction coupling and slow calcium current in dysgenic muscle by dihydropyridine receptor complementary DNA. *Nature* 336:134–139, 1988.
94a. Jiang Y, Lee A, Chen J, et al: X-ray structure of a voltage-dependent K$^+$ channel. *Nature* 423:33–41, 2003.
94b. Jiang Y, Ruta V, Chen J, et al: The principle of gating charge movement in a voltage-dependent K$^+$ channel. *Nature* 423:42–8, 2003.
95. Rios E, Pizarro G, Stefani E: Charge movement and the nature of signal transduction in skeletal muscle excitation-contraction coupling. *Annu Rev Physiol* 54:109–133, 1992.
96. Proenza C, O'Brien J, Nakai J, et al: Identification of a region of RyR1 that participates in allosteric coupling with the alpha(1S) (Ca(V)11) II–III loop. *J Biol Chem* 277:6530–6535, 2002.
97. Tanabe T, Mikami A, Numa S, Beam KG: Cardiac-type excitation-contraction coupling in dysgenic skeletal muscle injected with cardiac dihydropyridine receptor cDNA. *Nature* 344:451–453, 1990.
98. Tanabe T, Beam KG, Adams BA, et al: Regions of the skeletal muscle dihydropyridine receptor critical for excitation-contraction coupling. *Nature* 346:567–569, 1990.
99. Nakai J, Tanabe T, Konno T, et al: Localization in the II–III loop of the dihydropyridine receptor of a sequence critical for excitation-contraction coupling. *J Biol Chem* 273:24983–24986, 1998.
100. Grabner M, Dirksen RT, Suda N, Beam KG: The II–III loop of the skeletal muscle dihydropyridine receptor is responsible for the bi-directional coupling with the ryanodine receptor. *J Biol Chem* 274:21913–21919, 1999.
101. el-Hayek R, Antoniu B, Wang J, et al: Identification of calcium release-triggering and blocking regions of the II–III loop of the skeletal muscle dihydropyridine receptor. *J Biol Chem* 270:22116–22118, 1995.
102. Dulhunty AF, Laver DR, Gallant EM, et al: Activation and inhibition of skeletal RyR channels by a part of the skeletal DHPR II–III loop: Effects of DHPR Ser687 and FKBP12. *Biophys J* 77:189–203, 1999.
103. Casarotto MG, Gibson F, Pace SM, et al: A structural requirement for activation of skeletal ryanodine receptors by peptides of the dihydropyridine receptor II–III loop. *J Biol Chem* 275:11631–11637, 2000.
104. Proenza C, Wilkens CM, Beam KG: Excitation-contraction coupling is not affected by scrambled sequence in residues 681–690 of the dihydropyridine receptor II–III loop. *J Biol Chem* 275:29935–29937, 2000.
105. Wilkens CM, Kasielke N, Flucher BE, et al: Excitation-contraction coupling is unaffected by drastic alteration of the sequence surrounding residues L720–L764 of the α 1S II–III loop. *Proc Natl Acad Sci USA* 98:5892–5897, 2001.
106. O'Reilly FM, Robert M, Jona I, et al: FKBP12 modulation of the binding of the skeletal ryanodine receptor onto the II–III loop of the dihydropyridine receptor. *Biophys J* 82:145–155, 2002.
107. Stange M, Tripathy A, Meissner G: Two domains in dihydropyridine receptor activate the skeletal muscle Ca^{2+} release channel. *Biophys J* 81: 1419–1429, 2001.

108. Ahern CA, Bhattacharya D, Mortenson L, Coronado R: A component of excitation-contraction coupling triggered in the absence of the T671–L690 and L720–Q765 regions of the II–III loop of the dihydropyridine receptor α (1s) pore subunit. *Biophys J* 81:3294–3307, 2001.
109. Loke J, MacLennan DH: Malignant hyperthermia and central core disease: Disorders of Ca^{2+} release channels. *Am J Med* 104:470–486, 1998.
110. Monnier N, Romero NB, Lerale J, et al: Familial and sporadic forms of central core disease are associated with mutations in the C-terminal domain of the skeletal muscle ryanodine receptor. *Hum Mol Genet* 10:2581–2592, 2001.
111. Tong J, McCarthy TV, MacLennan DH: Measurement of resting cytosolic Ca^{2+} concentrations and Ca^{2+} store size in HEK-293 cells transfected with malignant hyperthermia or central core disease mutant Ca^{2+} release channels. *J Biol Chem* 274:693–702, 1999.
112. Lynch PJ, Tong J, Lehane M, et al: A mutation in the transmembrane/luminal domain of the ryanodine receptor is associated with abnormal Ca^{2+} release channel function and severe central core disease. *Proc Natl Acad Sci USA* 96:4164–4169, 1999.
113. Avila G, Dirksen RT: Functional effects of central core disease mutations in the cytoplasmic region of the skeletal muscle ryanodine receptor. *J Gen Physiol* 118:277–290, 2001.
114. Avila G, O'Brien JJ, Dirksen RT: Excitation-contraction uncoupling by a human central core disease mutation in the ryanodine receptor. *Proc Natl Acad Sci USA* 98:4215–4220, 2001.
115. Protasi F, Franzini-Armstrong C, Allen PD: Role of ryanodine receptors in the assembly of calcium release units in skeletal muscle. *J Cell Biol* 140:831–842, 1998.
116. Monnier N, Procaccio V, Stieglitz P, Lunardi J: Malignant-hyperthermia susceptibility is associated with a mutation of the α 1-subunit of the human dihydropyridine-sensitive L-type voltage-dependent calcium-channel receptor in skeletal muscle. *Am J Hum Genet* 60:1316–1325, 1997.
117. Leong P, MacLennan DH: The cytoplasmic loops between domains II and III and domains III and IV in the skeletal muscle dihydropyridine receptor bind to a contiguous site in the skeletal muscle ryanodine receptor. *J Biol Chem* 273:29958–29964, 1998.
118. Tiso N, Stephan DA, Nava A, et al: Identification of mutations in the cardiac ryanodine receptor gene in families affected with arrhythmogenic right ventricular cardiomyopathy type 2 (ARVD2). *Hum Mol Genet* 10:189–194, 2001.
119. Priori SG, Napolitano C, Tiso N, et al: Mutations in the cardiac ryanodine receptor gene (hRyR2) underlie catecholaminergic polymorphic ventricular tachycardia. *Circulation* 103:196–200, 2001.
120. Jayaraman T, Brillantes AM, Timerman AP, et al: FK506 binding protein associated with the calcium release channel (ryanodine receptor). *J Biol Chem* 267:9474–9477, 1992.
121. Qi Y, Ogunbunmi EM, Freund EA, et al: FK-binding protein is associated with the ryanodine receptor of skeletal muscle in vertebrate animals. *J Biol Chem* 273:34813–34819, 1998.
122. Gaburjakova M, Gaburjakova J, Reiken S, et al: FKBP12 binding modulates ryanodine receptor channel gating. *J Biol Chem* 276:16931–16935, 2001.
123. Wagenknecht T, Radermacher M, Grassucci R, et al: Locations of calmodulin and FK506-binding protein on the three-dimensional architecture of the skeletal muscle ryanodine receptor. *J Biol Chem* 272:32463–32471, 1997.
124. Lamb GD, Stephenson DG: Effects of FK506 and rapamycin on excitation-contraction coupling in skeletal muscle fibres of the rat. *J Physiol (Lond)* 494:569–576, 1996.
125. Shou W, Aghdasi B, Armstrong DL, et al: Cardiac defects and altered ryanodine receptor function in mice lacking FKBP12. *Nature* 391:489–492, 1998.
126. Xin HB, Senbonmatsu T, Cheng DS, et al: Oestrogen protects FKBP126 null mice from cardiac hypertrophy. *Nature* 416:334–338, 2002.
127. Marx SO, Reiken S, Hisamatsu Y, et al: PKA phosphorylation dissociates FKBP126 from the calcium release channel (ryanodine receptor): Defective regulation in failing hearts. *Cell* 101:365–376, 2002.
128. Meissner G: Evidence of a role for calmodulin in the regulation of calcium release from skeletal muscle sarcoplasmic reticulum. *Biochemistry* 25:244–251, 1986.
129. Tripathy A, Xu L, Mann G, Meissner G: Calmodulin activation and inhibition of skeletal muscle Ca^{2+} release channel (ryanodine receptor). *Biophys J* 69:106–119, 1995.
130. Chen SR, Li X, Ebisawa K, Zhang L: Functional characterization of the recombinant type 3 Ca^{2+} release channel (ryanodine receptor) expressed in HEK293 cells. *J Biol Chem* 272:24234–24246, 1997.
131. Fruen BR, Mickelson JR, Louis CF: Dantrolene inhibition of sarcoplasmic reticulum Ca^{2+} release by direct and specific action at skeletal muscle ryanodine receptors. *J Biol Chem* 272:26965–26971, 1997.
132. Fruen BR, Bardy JM, Byrem TM, et al: Differential Ca^{2+} sensitivity of skeletal and cardiac muscle ryanodine receptors in the presence of calmodulin. *Am J Physiol Cell Physiol* 279:C724–C733, 2000.
133. Meissner G, Henderson JS: Rapid calcium release from cardiac sarcoplasmic reticulum vesicles is dependent on Ca^{2+} and is modulated by Mg^{2+} adenine nucleotide and calmodulin. *J Biol Chem* 262:3065–3073, 1987.
134. Balshaw DM, Xu L, Yamaguchi N, et al: Calmodulin binding and inhibition of cardiac muscle calcium release channel (ryanodine receptor). *J Biol Chem* 276:20144–20153, 2001.
135. Moore CP, Rodney G, Zhang JZ, et al: Apocalmodulin and Ca^{2+} calmodulin bind to the same region on the skeletal muscle Ca^{2+} release channel. *Biochemistry* 38:8532–8537, 1999.
136. Rodney GG, Krol J, Williams B, et al: The carboxy-terminal calcium binding sites of calmodulin control calmodulin's switch from an activator to an inhibitor of RYR1. *Biochemistry* 40:12430–12435, 2001.
137. Rodney GG, Moore CP, Williams BY, et al: Calcium binding to calmodulin leads to an N-terminal shift in its binding site on the ryanodine receptor. *J Biol Chem* 276:2069–2074, 2001.
138. Yamaguchi N, Xin C, Meissner G: Identification of apocalmodulin and Ca^{2+}-calmodulin regulatory domain in skeletal muscle Ca^{2+} release channel ryanodine receptor. *J Biol Chem* 276:22579–22585, 2001.
138a. Rodney GG, Williams BY, Strasburg GM, et al: Regulation of RYR1 activity by Ca^{2+} and calmodulin. *Biochemistry* 39:7807–7812, 2000.
138b. Zhang H, Zhang JZ, Danila CI, Hamilton SL: A noncontiguous, intersubunit binding site for calmodulin on the skeletal muscle Ca^{2+} release channel. *J Biol Chem* 278:8348–8355, 2003.
139. Kim KC, Caswell AH, Talvenheimo JA, Brandt NR: Isolation of a terminal cisterna protein which may link the dihydropyridine receptor to the junctional foot protein in junctional skeletal muscle. *Biochemistry* 29:9281–9289, 1990.
140. Guo W, Campbell KP: Association of triadin with the ryanodine receptor and calsequestrin in the lumen of the sarcoplasmic reticulum. *J Biol Chem* 270:9027–9030, 1995.
141. Zhang L, Kelley J, Schmeisser G, et al: Complex formation between junctin triadin calsequestrin and the ryanodine receptor proteins of the cardiac junctional sarcoplasmic reticulum membrane. *J Biol Chem* 272:23389–23397, 1997.
142. Kobayashi YM, Jones LR: Identification of triadin 1 as the predominant triadin isoform expressed in mammalian myocardium. *J Biol Chem* 274:28660–28668, 1999.
143. Knudson CM, Stang KK, Moomaw CR, et al: Primary structure and topological analysis of a skeletal muscle-specific junctional sarcoplasmic reticulum glycoprotein (triadin). *J Biol Chem* 268:12646–12654, 1993.
144. Groh S, Marty I, Ottolia M, et al: Functional interaction of the cytoplasmic domain of triadin with the skeletal ryanodine receptor. *J Biol Chem* 274:12278–12283, 1999.
145. Kobayashi YM, Alseikhan BA, Jones LR: Localization and characterization of the calsequestrin-binding domain of triadin 1: Evidence for a charged beta-strand in mediating the protein-protein interaction. *J Biol Chem* 275:17639–17646, 2000.
146. Lee HG, Kang H, Kim DH, Park WJ: Interaction of HRC (histidine-rich Ca^{2+}-binding protein) and triadin in the lumen of sarcoplasmic reticulum. *J Biol Chem* 276:39533–39538, 2001.
147. Kirchhefer U, Neumann J, Baba HA, et al: Cardiac hypertrophy and impaired relaxation in transgenic mice overexpressing triadin 1. *J Biol Chem* 276:4142–4149, 2001.
148. Wetzel GT, Ding S, Chen F: Molecular cloning of junctin from human and developing rabbit heart. *Mol Genet Metab* 69:252–258, 2000.
149. Zhang L, Franzini-Armstrong C, Ramesh V, Jones LR: Structural alterations in cardiac calcium release units resulting from overexpression of junctin. *J Mol Cell Cardiol* 33:233–247, 2001.
150. Takeshima H, Shimuta M, Komazaki S, et al: Mitsugumin29 a novel synaptophysin family member from the triad junction in skeletal muscle. *Biochem J* 331:317–322, 1998.
151. O'Connor V, Duggan M, Siebert A, et al: Molecular approaches to neurotransmitter release. *Ann NY Acad Sci* 733:290–297, 1994.
152. Yuan SH, Arnold W, Jorgensen AO: Biogenesis of transverse tubules and triads: Immunolocalization of the 14-dihydropyridine receptor TS28 and the ryanodine receptor in rabbit skeletal muscle developing in situ. *J Cell Biol* 112:289–301, 1991.
153. Nishi M, Komazaki S, Kurebayashi N, et al: Abnormal features in skeletal muscle from mice lacking mitsugumin29. *J Cell Biol* 147:1473–1480, 1999.
154. Brandt NR, Franklin G, Brunschwig JP, Caswell AH: The role of mitsugumin 29 in transverse tubules of rabbit skeletal muscle. *Arch Biochem Biophys* 385:406–409, 2001.
155. Nagaraj RY, Nosek CM, Brotto MA, et al: Increased susceptibility to fatigue of slow- and fast-twitch muscles from mice lacking the MG29 gene. *Physiol Genom* 4:43–49, 2000.
156. Nagaraj RY, Bhat MB, Nishi M, et al: Co-expression of ryanodine receptor and MG29 (a novel triad junction protein) in CHO cells. *Biophys J* 76:A470, 1999.
157. Takeshima H, Komazaki S, Nishi M, et al: Junctophilins: A novel family of junctional membrane complex proteins. *Mol Cell* 6:11–22, 2000.
158. Ito K, Komazaki S, Sasamoto K, et al: Deficiency of triad junction and contraction in mutant skeletal muscle lacking junctophilin type 1. *J Cell Biol* 154:1059–1067, 2001.
159. Netticadan T, Temsah RM, Kawabata K, Dhalla NS: Sarcoplasmic reticulum Ca^{2+}/calmodulin-dependent protein kinase is altered in heart failure. *Circ Res* 86:596–605, 2000.

160. MacLennan DH, Wong PT: Isolation of a calcium-sequestering protein from sarcoplasmic reticulum. *Proc Natl Acad Sci USA* 68:1231–1235, 1971.
161. Fliegel L, Ohnishi M, Carpenter MR, et al: Amino acid sequence of rabbit fast-twitch skeletal muscle calsequestrin deduced from cDNA and peptide sequencing. *Proc Natl Acad Sci USA* 84:1167–1171, 1987.
162. Scott BT, Simmerman HK, Collins JH, et al: Complete amino acid sequence of canine cardiac calsequestrin deduced by cDNA cloning. *J Biol Chem* 263:8958–8964, 1988.
163. Gatti G, Trifari S, Mesaeli N, et al: Head-to-tail oligomerization of calsequestrin: A novel mechanism for heterogeneous distribution of endoplasmic reticulum luminal proteins. *J Cell Biol* 154:525–534, 2001.
164. Cozens B, Reithmeier RA: Size and shape of rabbit skeletal muscle calsequestrin. *J Biol Chem* 259:6248–6252, 1984.
165. Aaron BM, Oikawa K, Reithmeier RA, Sykes BD: Characterization of skeletal muscle calsequestrin by 1H NMR spectroscopy. *J Biol Chem* 259:11876–11881, 1984.
166. Slupsky JR, Ohnishi M, Carpenter MR, Reithmeier RA: Characterization of cardiac calsequestrin. *Biochemistry* 26:6539–6544, 1987.
167. Ohnishi M, Reithmeier RA: Terbium-binding properties of calsequestrin from skeletal muscle sarcoplasmic reticulum. *Biochim Biophys Acta* 915:180–187, 1987.
168. Ohkura M, Furukawa K, Fujimori H, et al: Dual regulation of the skeletal muscle ryanodine receptor by triadin and calsequestrin. *Biochemistry* 37:12987–12993, 1998.
169. Beard NA, Sakowska MM, Dulhunty AF, Laver DR: Calsequestrin is an inhibitor of skeletal muscle ryanodine receptor calcium release channels. *Biophys J* 82:310–320, 2002.
170. Wang S, Trumble WR, Liao H, et al: Crystal structure of calsequestrin from rabbit skeletal muscle sarcoplasmic reticulum [see comments]. *Nat Struct Biol* 5:476–483, 1998.
171. MacLennan DH, Reithmeier RA: Ion tamers. *Nat Struct Biol* 5:409–411, 1998.
172. Jones LR, Suzuki YJ, Wang W, et al: Regulation of Ca^{2+} signaling in transgenic mouse cardiac myocytes overexpressing calsequestrin. *J Clin Invest* 101:1385–1393, 1998.
173. Sato Y, Ferguson DG, Sako H, et al: Cardiac-specific overexpression of mouse cardiac calsequestrin is associated with depressed cardiovascular function and hypertrophy in transgenic mice. *J Biol Chem* 273:28470–28477, 1998.
173a. Postma AV, Denjoy I, Hoorntje TM, et al: Absence of calsequestrin 2 causes severe forms of catecholaminergic polymorphic ventricular tachycardia. *Circ Res* 91:21–26, 2002.
174. Michalak M, Corbett EF, Mesaeli N, et al: Calreticulin: One protein one gene many functions. *Biochem J* 344(Pt 2):281–292, 1999.
175. Xu W, Longo FJ, Wintermantel MR, et al: Calreticulin modulates capacitative Ca^{2+} influx by controlling the extent of inositol 145-trisphosphate-induced Ca^{2+} store depletion. *J Biol Chem* 275:36676–36682, 2000.
176. Ostwald TJ, MacLennan DH, Dorrington KJ: Effects of cation binding on the conformation of calsequestrin and the high affinity calcium-binding protein of sarcoplasmic reticulum. *J Biol Chem* 249:5867–5871, 1974.
177. Ostwald TJ, MacLennan DH: Isolation of a high affinity calcium-binding protein from sarcoplasmic reticulum. *J Biol Chem* 249:974–979, 1974.
178. Nash PD, Opas M, Michalak M: Calreticulin: Not just another calcium-binding protein. *Mol Cell Biochem* 135:71–78, 1994.
179. Ellgaard L, Riek R, Herrmann T, et al: NMR structure of the calreticulin P-domain. *Proc Natl Acad Sci USA* 98:3133–3138, 2001.
180. Vassilakos A, Michalak M, Lehrman MA, Williams DB: Oligosaccharide binding characteristics of the molecular chaperones calnexin and calreticulin. *Biochemistry* 37:3480–3490, 1998.
181. Baksh S, Michalak M: Expression of calreticulin in *Escherichia coli* and identification of its Ca^{2+} binding domains. *J Biol Chem* 266:21458–21465, 1991.
182. Mesaeli N, Nakamura K, Zvaritch E, et al: Calreticulin is essential for cardiac development. *J Cell Biol* 144:857–868, 1999.
183. Nakamura K, Robertson M, Liu G, et al: Complete heart block and sudden death in mice overexpressing calreticulin. *J Clin Invest* 107:1245–1253, 2001.
184. Leberer E, Charuk JH, Clarke DM, et al: Molecular cloning and expression of cDNA encoding the 53000-dalton glycoprotein of rabbit skeletal muscle sarcoplasmic reticulum. *J Biol Chem* 264:3484–3493, 1989.
185. Leberer E, Charuk JH, Green NM, MacLennan DH: Molecular cloning and expression of cDNA encoding a lumenal calcium binding glycoprotein from sarcoplasmic reticulum. *Proc Natl Acad Sci USA* 86:6047–6051, 1989.
186. Leberer E, Timms BG, Campbell KP, MacLennan DH: Purification calcium binding properties and ultrastructural localization of the 53000- and 160000 (sarcalumenin)-dalton glycoproteins of the sarcoplasmic reticulum. *J Biol Chem* 265:10118–10124, 1990.
187. Hofmann SL, Goldstein JL, Orth K, et al: Molecular cloning of a histidine-rich Ca^{2+}-binding protein of sarcoplasmic reticulum that contains highly conserved repeated elements. *J Biol Chem* 264:18083–18090, 1989.
188. Hofmann SL, Brown MS, Lee E, et al: Purification of a sarcoplasmic reticulum protein that binds Ca^{2+} and plasma lipoproteins. *J Biol Chem* 264:8260–8270, 1989.
189. Damiani E, Picello E, Saggin L, Margreth A: Identification of triadin and of histidine-rich Ca^{2+}-binding protein as substrates of 60 kDa calmodulin-dependent protein kinase in junctional terminal cisternae of sarcoplasmic reticulum of rabbit fast muscle. *Biochem Biophys Res Commun* 209:457–465, 1995.
190. Stokes DL, Wagenknecht T: Calcium transport across the sarcoplasmic reticulum: Structure and function of Ca^{2+}-ATPase and the ryanodine receptor. *Eur J Biochem* 267:5274–5279, 2000.

SECTION 4

Neuromuscular Transmission

Chapter 15
The Neuromuscular Junction
ANDREW G. ENGEL

Definition and History
Patterns of Motor Innervation
The Presynaptic Region
 THE NERVE TERMINAL
 THE EXOCYTOTIC MACHINERY
 THE SNARE COMPLEX, SYNAPTOTAGMIN, AND OTHER PROTEINS
  IMPLICATED IN EXOCYTOSIS
 CYTOSKELETAL COMPONENTS OF THE NERVE TERMINAL ABOVE
  THE ACTIVE ZONES
 THE ACTIVE ZONE
 THE VOLTAGE-GATED CA^{2+} CHANNELS
 MORPHOLOGIC CORRELATES OF QUANTAL TRANSMITTER RELEASE
 ENDOCYTOTIC EVENTS AND THE FORMATION OF NEW SYNAPTIC
  VESICLES
The Synaptic Space
The Synaptic Basal Lamina
The Postsynaptic Region
 THE JUNCTIONAL FOLDS
 THE ACETYLCHOLINE RECEPTOR
 CYTOSKELETAL COMPONENTS
 THE JUNCTIONAL SARCOPLASM
Synaptogenesis
 TROPHIC INTERACTIONS
Synaptic Plasticity

Definition and History

Definition

The neuromuscular junction (NMJ)* is a chemical synapse that is anatomically and functionally differentiated for the transmission of a signal from the motor nerve terminal to a circumscribed postsynaptic region on the muscle fiber. The number and position of NMJs on the muscle fiber, the configuration of the nerve terminals within the NMJ, and the complexity of the postsynaptic region in a junction can vary according to phylum and species, between different muscles

*A list of abbreviations used in this chapter is given at the end of the chapter.

in a given species, and between different fibers in a given muscle. Despite these differences, all NMJs have five principal components: (1) a Schwann cell process forming a cap above that portion of the nerve terminal that does not face the postsynaptic region; (2) a nerve terminal containing the neurotransmitter; (3) a synaptic space lined with basement membrane; (4) a postsynaptic membrane containing the receptor for the neurotransmitter; and (5) junctional sarcoplasm, which provides structural and metabolic support for the postsynaptic region (Fig. 15-1). In vertebrate voluntary muscle the neurotransmitter is acetylcholine (ACh), the receptor is the nicotinic ACh receptor (AChR), and the synaptic space contains ACh esterase (AChE).

Early Light Microscopic Studies

Kühne,[1,2] Hinsey,[3] Couteaux,[4–6] and Anderson-Cedergren[7] have reviewed early anatomic studies of the NMJ. Most of these were based on visualization of the intramuscular nerves and nerve terminals. The gold impregnation method devised by Conheim in 1867, the methylene blue stain employed by Ehrlich in 1885, and the silver impregnation procedure introduced by Bielschowsky in 1904 were used for this purpose. The earliest study of the NMJ, however, was in 1840, when Doyère noted that, in a minute slow-moving arthropod (*Milnesium tardigradum*), the intramuscular nerve fibers ended on conical protuberances on the muscle fibers. In 1847 Wagner noted that intramuscular nerve fibers arose from larger branches and lost their myelin sheath before contacting the muscle fiber. Rouget, in 1862, described plate-like (*en plaque*) nerve terminals composed of round and oval loops in reptiles, birds, and mammals.

In 1870 Kühne[1] observed that at the frog NMJ the myelinated nerve fiber divided into short first-order branches forming a terminal brush, or *Endbüschel*. The branches lost their myelin sheath and then extended in a direction parallel to the muscle fiber, dividing and giving off branches that again coursed in a nearly parallel direction (Fig. 15-2A). Kühne's gold impregnation techniques gave amazingly clear images of the NMJ. However, he noted that, in studies of the NMJ, "the greatest possible delicacy in manipulation is required for the subject is one of the most difficult in whole range of microscopic art, and is one also on which histologists are not, as yet, by any means unanimous." Controversies at that time pertained to the source and position of the junctional nuclei, whether the nerve terminal penetrated the sarcolemma, and the "*Borstensaum*," or bristles, at the fringe of the junction. Kühne incorrectly assumed that the nerve fiber penetrated the sarcolemma after it lost its myelin sheath. The *Borstensaum*, demonstrated by Kühne with silver and combined silver-gold impregnation procedures, consisted of rod-like or palisading structures at the outer margin of the

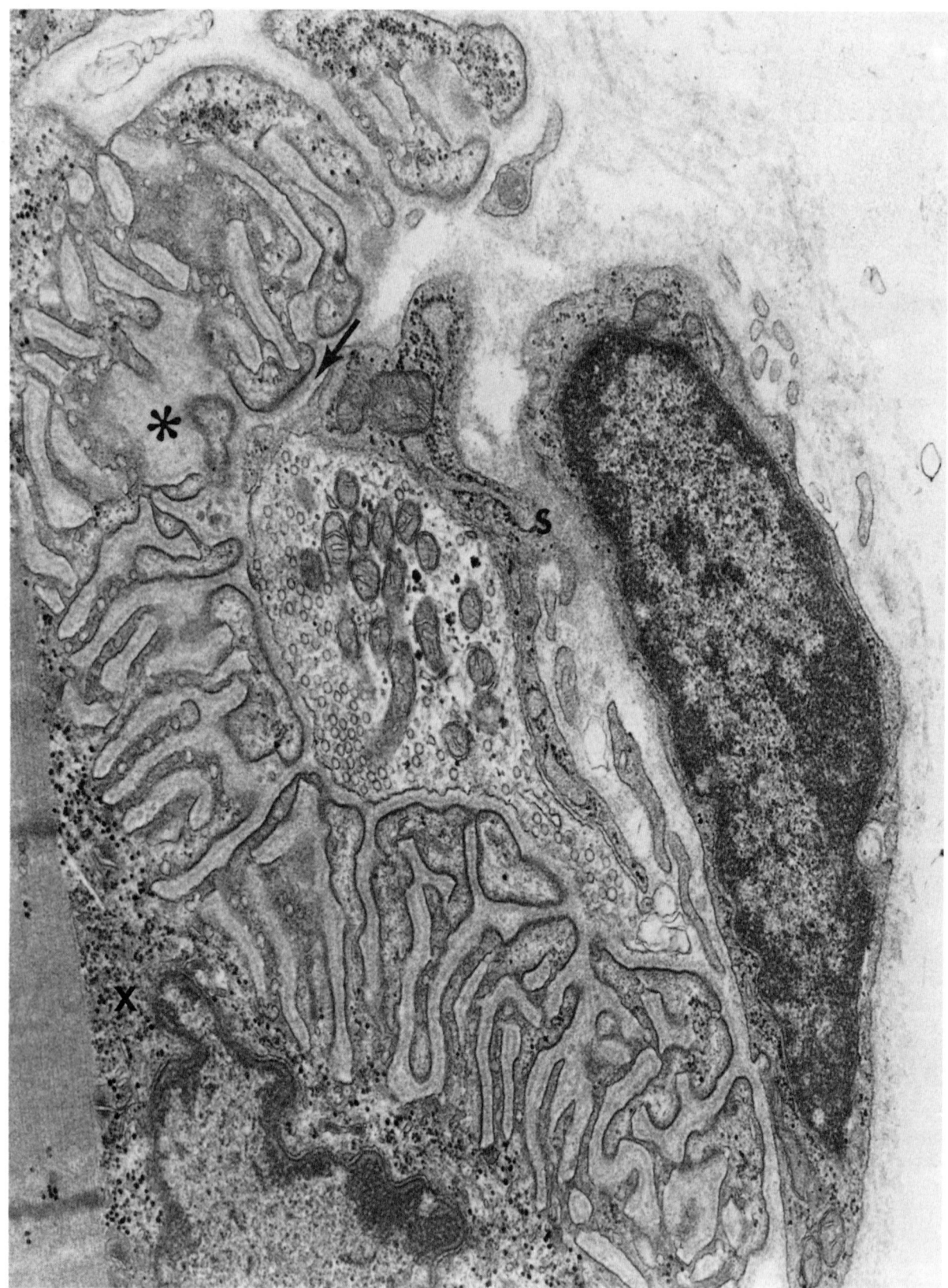

FIGURE 15-1. Electron micrograph of normal human NMJ. The right side of the nerve terminal is covered by a Schwann cell (S); the left side of the terminal faces the postsynaptic region of clefts and folds. Junctional sarcoplasm (X) contains glycogen granules, ribosomes, small tubular profiles, and nucleus. The arrow and asterisk mark primary and secondary synaptic clefts, respectively. (×30,600.) *(Engel AG, Handbook of Clinical Neurology, vol 41, part II. New York: North-Holland; 1979, pp 95–145. With permission.)*

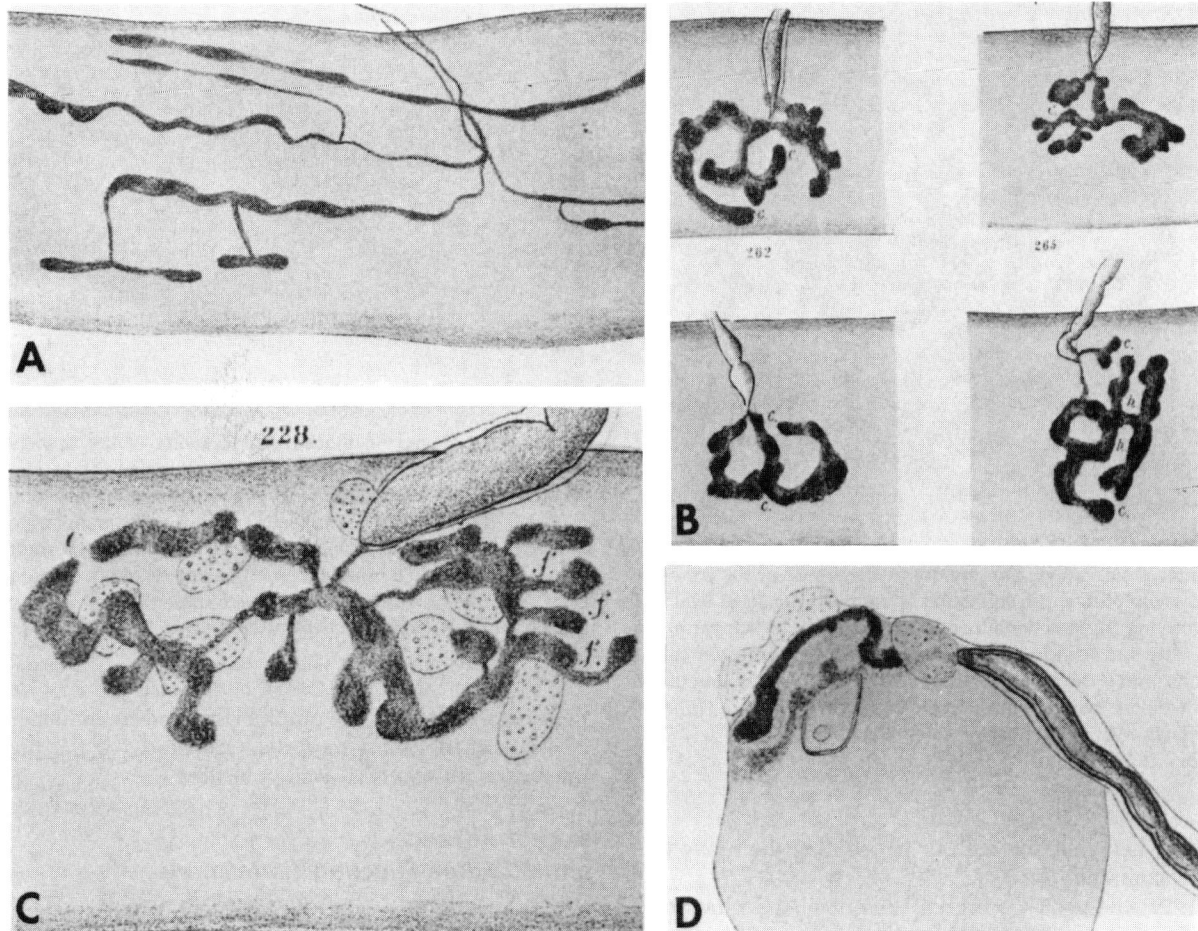

FIGURE 15-2. Kühne's drawings of NMJs. The illustrations show linear (*Endbüschel*) nerve endings on frog (*A*) and plate-like (*en plaque*) nerve endings on guinea pig (*B, D*) and rabbit (*C*) muscle fibers. The termination of the myelin sheath near the junction is clearly seen in *B, C,* and *D*. The stippled nuclear profiles in *C* and *D* are probably associated with Schwann cells. Kühne's drawings were not accompanied by scale bars. The reader may estimate the magnification by assuming that the muscle fiber diameters range from 50 to 100 μm, that the longest junction depicted in *A* extends for several hundred microns, and that the long diameters of the junctions in *B, C,* and *D* range from 30 to 60 μm. (Kühne W, *Z Biol* 23:1, 1887.[2])

junction that persisted even after a long period of denervation[8] (Fig. 15-3). Thus, Kühne's *Borstensaum* probably represents the subneural apparatus. Finally, in 1887, in an article accompanied by 324 colored illustrations, Kühne described the comparative anatomy of motor nerve endings in many vertebrate species[2] (Fig. 15-2). This work showed not only plate-like and end-brush terminals but also grape-like terminals, although Kühne regarded the latter as atypical or immature endings. Two years later, however, Tschiriew described the grape-like terminals (*terminaisons en grappe*) in different vertebrate species[9] (Fig. 15-4).

Applying the recently described methylene blue staining technique, Dogiel in 1890 accurately depicted the branching of intramuscular nerves (Fig. 15-5) and the different types of NMJs in amphibians (Fig. 15-6A) and reptiles (Fig. 15-6B).[10] The macroscopic branching of nerves in human muscles was first described by Frohse in 1898.[11] Frohse's illustrations clearly show that in some muscles (e.g., biceps and lateral rectus) most intramuscular nerve fibers end near the center of the muscle, that in some muscles nerves terminate at different levels (e.g., sartorius), and that some intramuscular nerves reach the tendons (Fig. 15-7). During the first half of the twentieth century the finer branching patterns of nerves and the disposition of nerve terminals in muscle were further investigated in amphibians,[12,13] reptiles,[14,15] and mammals,[16] but these studies yielded no additional insights into the structure of the NMJ. In 1947, however, Couteaux obtained an excellent light microscopic view of the subneural apparatus in different species with the Janus B green stain.[4] Four years later Couteaux and Taxi localized AChE by enzyme cytochemistry at the NMJ. The reaction product delineated the synaptic space, and AChE reactivity persisted after denervation.[5,17] Couteaux concluded that AChE is "chiefly located at the lamellae of the subneural apparatus, situated at the frontier of axoplasm and sarcoplasm." In 1955, however, Couteaux still thought that the Schwann cell covered the entire nerve terminal separating axoplasm from sarcoplasm.[5]

Early Ultrastructural Studies

In 1954 Palade[18] and Robertson[19] published abstracts on the fine structure of the NMJ. Palade established that the nerve

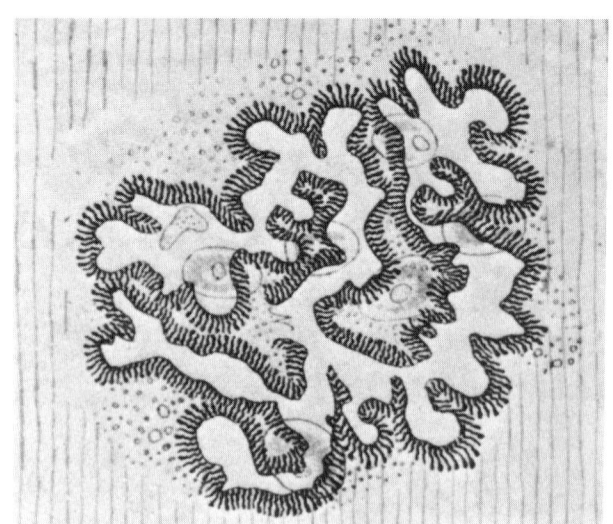

FIGURE 15-3. Kühne's drawings of a lizard hindlimb end plate 22 days after denervation. The bristles at the fringe of the junction (*Borstensaum*) outline the subneural apparatus. The large oval nuclei overlying the junctional region are probably of Schwann cell origin. The fine vertical lines on the muscle fiber represent cross-striations; if the striations were spaced at 2 μm, the junctional region would extend over a distance of 50 μm. Compare Kühne's *Borstensaum* with the pattern of junctional folds in Fig. 15-8. (*Kühne W, Z Biol 19:501, 1883.*[8])

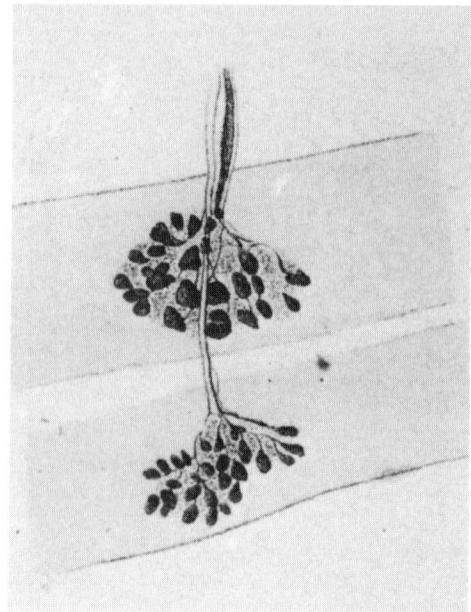

FIGURE 15-4. Tschiriew's drawing of grapelike *(en grappe)* nerve endings on salamander muscle fibers. (*Tschiriew MS, Arch Physiol Norm Pathol, 2nd series, 6:89, 1879.*[9])

terminal contained numerous synaptic vesicles, that the Schwann cell capped but did not surround the nerve terminal, and that Couteaux's subneural apparatus consisted of junctional folds. Robertson also described the junctional folds but thought that the axoplasmic processes extended inside a very thin sarcolemma. In 1955 De Robertis and Bennett recognized synaptic vesicles in frog sympathetic ganglia and in the earthworm nerve cord.[20] In addition, they drew attention to a "submicroscopic filamentary component" in the presynaptic region where the vesicles were found. These findings were particularly relevant to the physiologic studies of Fatt and Katz[21] in 1952 and del Castillo and Katz[22] in 1954, which established that either the spontaneous[21] or nerve impulse–induced[22] release of ACh from the nerve terminal occurs in discrete packets, or quanta. On the basis of the electron microscopic findings, del Castillo and Katz could now postulate that the quantum resides in the synaptic vesicle and that the vesicle loses its content in an all-or-none manner when colliding with or penetrating the nerve terminal membrane.[23]

In 1959 Anderson-Cedergren described the ultrastructure of the mouse NMJ and provided a three-dimensional reconstruction of the junction from serial sections.[7] During the next decade, other electron microscopic studies detailed the fine structure of the amphibian[24] and mammalian[25–27] NMJs, and in 1971 a morphometric study of the human intercostal muscle NMJ was published.[28]

Further Advances and Structure-Function Correlations

Between 1971 and 1979, combined physiologic, conventional electron microscopic, and freeze-fracture electron microscopic studies provided overwhelming evidence that quantal release is associated with synaptic vesicle exocytosis and that the exocytotic event is topographically related to a specialized active zone of the presynaptic membrane. By now the critical role of calcium for the exocytotic release of neurotransmitters had been generally accepted,[29–31] and it was further inferred that the intramembrane particles associated with the active zone may represent the voltage-sensitive calcium channel of the presynaptic membrane (for reviews, see Refs. 29 and 32 to 34). Despite these studies, alternatives to the vesicular hypothesis, postulating that quantal release occurs through "vesigates"[32] or "synaptopores,"[33] were still promulgated but were not generally accepted.[34]

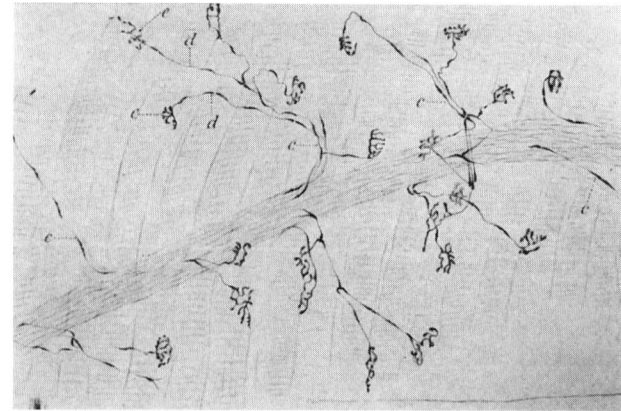

FIGURE 15-5. Dogiel's camera lucida drawing of the branches of intramuscular nerves in salamander muscle visualized by supravistal staining with methylene blue. An intramuscular nerve bundle traverses the field from lower left to upper right, giving off small branches (c) that divide into single nerve fibers (d), which form terminals (e) on individual muscle fibers. The muscle fibers course vertically. The fine horizontal lines on the muscle fibers suggest cross-striations. (*Dogiel AS, Arch Mikrosk Anat 35:305, 1890.*[10])

Chapter 15. The Neuromuscular Junction

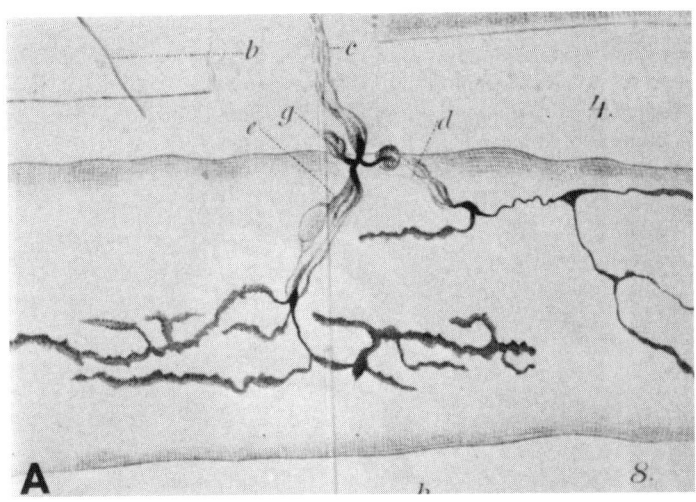
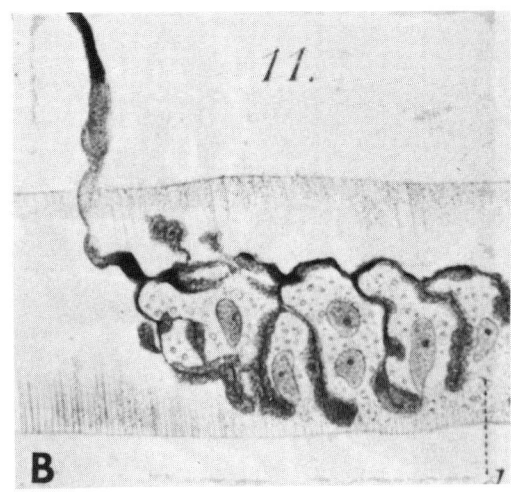

FIGURE 15-6. Dogiel's camera lucida drawings of a supravitally stained *Endbüschel* nerve terminal on a frog muscle fiber (A) and of an *en plaque* nerve terminal on a lizard muscle fiber (B) (Dogiel AS, Arch Mikrosk Anat 35:305, 1890.[10])

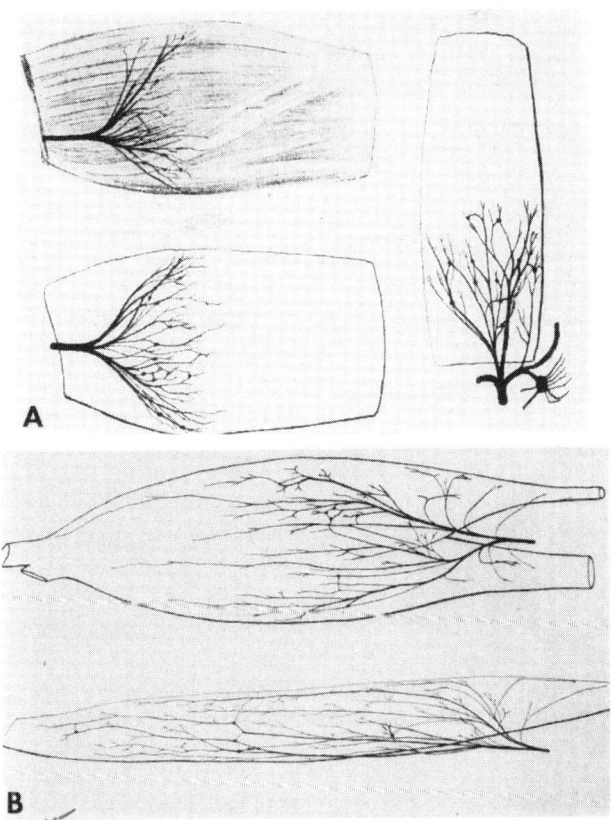

FIGURE 15-7. Frohse's illustrations of the macroscopic branching of intramuscular nerves. A. Clockwise from upper left shows nerves in medial, inferior, and lateral rectus muscles. The intramuscular nerves end in the equatorial region of the extraocular muscles. Many nerves end near the center of the biceps muscle. The branch of the oculomotor nerve to the ciliary ganglion is also shown. Frohse's drawings do not demonstrate those nerve fibers that provide a distributed innervation to some of the extraocular muscle fibers. B. Biceps (top) and sartorius (bottom) muscles. (Frohse F, Anat Anz 14:321, 1898.[11])

Between 1967 and 1979, AChR was localized on the postsynaptic membrane with fluorescent,[35,36] radioactive,[37–39] and peroxidase-labeled[40] α-bungarotoxin (BGT). The topographic distribution of BGT-binding sites on the junctional folds corresponded to that of large intramembrane particles revealed by freeze-fracture.[41–43] Electrophysiologic estimates and autoradiographic studies with iodine 125 (^{125}I)–labeled BGT[39] of the AChR packing density on the junctional folds were in agreement with results obtained in ultrarapidly frozen, deep-etched, and rotary-shadowed preparations of the NMJ.[44,45]

The association of AChE with the synaptic basal lamina was established by several measures (for review, see Chap. 18). Since 1976, increasing attention has been directed to the critical role of the synaptic basal lamina in NMJ development and regeneration[46] and its ability to specify the molecular architecture of the pre- and postsynaptic membrane (for review, see Chap. 20).

Since 1976, the components of the NMJ and of other synapses have been investigated by conventional[47,48] and high-voltage[49,50] transmission electron microscopy; by the quick-freeze, deep-etch, and rotary-shadow techniques[44,51–55]; and by immunocytochemisty[54,56–59]; and remarkable views of the NMJ have been obtained by scanning electron microscopy[60–63] (Fig. 15-8). Finally, with the advent of confocal microscopy, the disposition of the active zones at the frog NMJ has been imaged with fluorescent ω-conotoxin,[64,65] and recycling of the synaptic vesicles has been visualized with fluorescent dyes.[66] Serial observation of the same NMJ labeled with fluorescent dyes in living animals by means of reflected light confocal microscopy has provided a novel approach to follow synaptic maturation and maintenance[67,68] and receptor dynamics.[69] Recent studies of synaptic vesicle–associated proteins have yielded insights into the molecular events associated with synaptic vesicle exocytosis and endocytosis.[70,71] Remarkable electron microscope tomography studies of the active zone demonstrated an exquisitely precise spatial relationship and structural linkage between

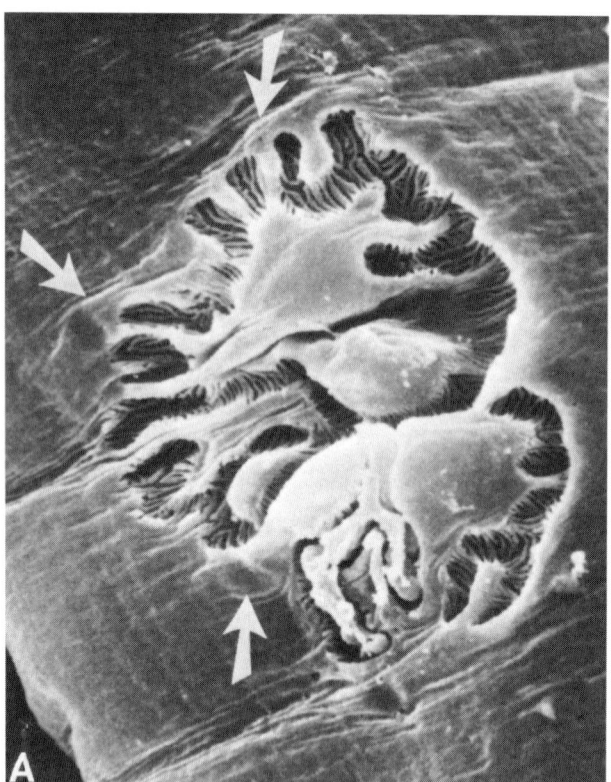 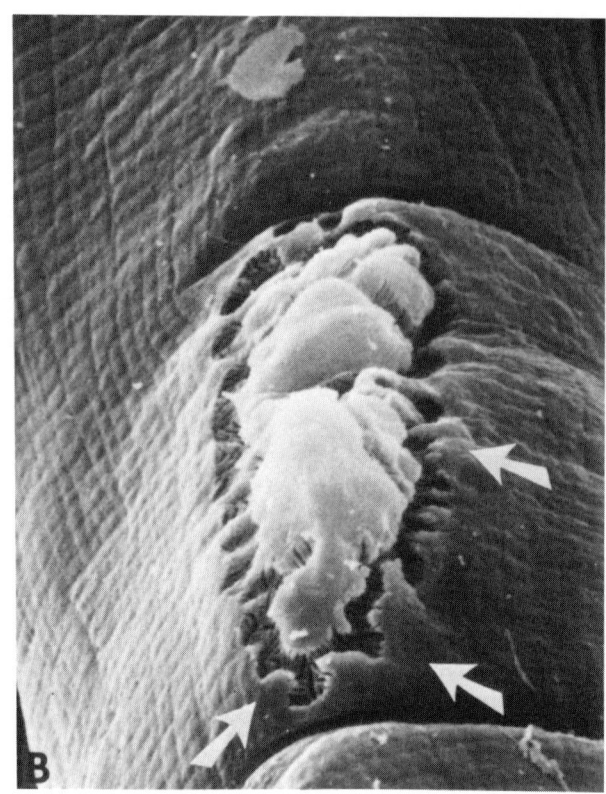

FIGURE 15-8. Scanning electron micrographs of NMJs on mouse extensor digitorum longus muscle. The elliptically shaped NMJ is surrounded by a raised area, marked with arrows. This corresponds to the junctional sarcoplasm. The junctional folds are nicely shown in the synaptic gutter (compare with Fig. 15-3). These micrographs were prepared by Dr. M. A. Fahim. (*Fahim MA et al, Neuroscience* 13:227, 1984. With permission.)

the synaptic vesicles and calcium channels. (See section below "The Active Zone.") Finally, combined biophysical, crystallographic, molecular genetic, and patch-clamp studies of AChR are revealing with increasing precision how AChR subserves signal transduction at the NMJ.[72–74]

Patterns of Motor Innervation

Mature muscle receives a topographic projection of nerve fibers from its motor neuron pool.[75] The rostrocaudal axis of the motor pool is systematically mapped onto the rostrocaudal axis of the muscle. This is associated with segmental ordering of axons in the nerve and may be aided by axonal guidance at branch points in the nerve and by positional labels within the muscle.[76]

The nerve trunks that enter muscle carry both motor and sensory fibers. The motor nerve fibers terminate on extrafusal muscle fibers; β motor nerve fibers terminate on both extra- and intrafusal muscle fibers; and γ motor nerve fibers terminate on intrafusal muscle fibers. The sensory nerves are destined to reach intrafusal and Golgi tendon end organs. In normal mature muscle, a single extrafusal muscle fiber receives its innervation from a single motor neuron, but each motor neuron supplies more than one muscle fiber. The motor neuron and the muscle fibers innervated by it constitute the motor unit. A nerve fiber from a given motor neuron divides into its terminal branches close to the muscle fibers it inner-

vates, but not all fibers in a motor unit are immediately adjacent to each other. In focally innervated muscles, preterminal axons tend to course perpendicularly to the long axis of the muscle fibers[77]; in muscles with distributed innervation, preterminal axons tend to run parallel to the direction of the muscle fibers.[78]

Focal, Distributed, and Myoseptal Innervation

Focally innervated muscle fibers have single NMJs near their center. This, however, does not imply that all NMJs in a focally innervated muscle are in the central, or equatorial, region of the muscle (Fig. 15-7). There are two reasons for this: (1) Not all muscle fibers in a given muscle extend through the entire length of the muscle and (2) muscle fibers may run parallel (e.g., biceps) or obliquely (e.g., rectus femoris) to the long axis of the muscle. Focally innervated muscle fibers are fast phasic fibers: The end plate potential triggers an all-or-none muscle fiber action potential.

A muscle fiber that receives a distributed innervation has multiple NMJs positioned on its surface at regular intervals. The number of junctions per fiber may be as small as two to five, as in the slow fibers of the frog cruralis muscle,[79] or considerably higher, as in the avian anterior latissimus dorsi muscle.

Muscle fibers receiving distributed innervation are either slow tonic fibers whose end plate potential propagates electrotonically without triggering an all-or-none action potential (e.g., avian anterior latissimus dorsi fibers); or fast phasic fibers (e.g., frog sartorius fibers[80]). Cross-reinnervation studies during development indicate that the pattern of synaptic sites on muscle fibers is determined by the nerve fibers.[75,81]

In most mammalian muscles all extrafusal fibers are focally innervated. Distributed innervation in mammalian muscles occurs in (1) intrafusal fibers (see Ref. 78 and Chap. 21) and (2) a relatively small proportion of extrafusal fibers in extraocular,[16,82–87] facial, laryngeal, and lingual[14,82] muscles.

Myoseptal innervation, most frequently observed in myotomes of the lowest vertebrates (e.g., *Cyclotomes*), consists of basket-like nerve endings applied close to the origin and insertion of muscle fibers. This innervation becomes less important in higher vertebrates but still persists in some of the myotomal tail muscles of tadpoles and reptiles. Myoseptal innervation was first illustrated by Retzius in 1892[88] but was thought to be associated with stretch receptors[15,83] until Mackay[89] and Cöers[82] demonstrated its motor character. This type of innervation has not been thoroughly investigated in recent years.

Types of Nerve Endings

Plate-like (en plaque) nerve endings form round or elliptical loops on the muscle fiber surface (Figs. 15-2B to D, 15-6B, and 15-8). On mature muscle fibers the diameter of the innervated zone ranges from 10 to 80 μm with an average of 33 μm, and is proportionate to the muscle fiber diameter.[82] Plate-like endings occur with focal or distributed innervation and generate a propagated action potential. Plate-like terminals are the most common moiety in mammals and reptiles, but also occur in birds and lower vertebrates.[2]

Grape-like (en grappe) nerve endings consist of a spray of fine varicose filaments that end in minute expansions[9,90] (Fig. 15-4). They are typically found in birds and reptiles on "slow tonic fibers" with distributed innervation that cannot propagate an action potential, but they may also occur on focally innervated fibers, and not all muscle fibers with distributed innervation have grape-like terminals.[75,83,90,91] Cöers emphasizes that the distinction between grape- and plate-like terminals was originally based on gold or silver impregnation methods and that the configuration of the nerve endings cannot be used to identify mammalian muscle fibers that cannot propagate an action potential.[82] This argument is supported by a recent methylene blue study of rat diaphragm end plates: White (type 2B) fibers had grape-like terminals, red (type 1) fibers had plate-like terminals, and intermediate (type 2A) fibers had intermediate-type terminals.[92] Thus, grape-like endings were found on those mammalian fibers with the shortest contraction times, and all fibers in the rat diaphragm propagate an action potential.

End-brush (Endbüschel) nerve endings consist of long, slender branches, most of which course parallel to the long axis of the muscle fiber for several hundred microns (Figs. 15-2A and 15-6A). They are commonly observed in frogs and turtles and generate propagated muscle fiber action potentials. At these junctions the active zones and junctional folds course perpendicularly to the long axis of the nerve terminals. This highly oriented arrangement is particularly favorable for anatomic and physiologic studies.

Basket nerve endings are associated with myoseptal innervation, as described above. The comparative anatomy of the myoseptal nerve endings in different species has not been adequately investigated to date.

Trail nerve endings are found on multiply innervated bag$_2$- and chain-type intrafusal muscle fibers supplied by motor nerve fibers. The terminal axons consist of fine branches bearing varicose dilations. The trail endings are concentrated in the juxtaequatorial region of the spindle (see Chap. 21).

The Presynaptic Region

The preterminal myelinated nerve fiber is surrounded by a sheath of perineural epithelial cells (Henle's sheath), which is partially surrounded by fibroblasts and other connective tissue elements (Fig. 15-9A and B). The myelinated nerve fibers and Henle's sheath are covered by basement membrane, but the fibroblasts are not. Sparse collagen fibrils traverse the spaces between the myelinated nerve fiber and Henle's sheath and between Henle's sheath and the fibroblasts. Within a few microns of the NMJ the myelin sheath ends abruptly at the last node of Ranvier (Fig. 15-9A and B). Between the last node of Ranvier and the NMJ, the terminal axon is enveloped by the Schwann cell, which is surrounded by Henle's sheath (Fig. 15-9A to E). A 10- to 30-nm gap intervenes between the axolemma and the Schwann cell plasma membrane, and a distance of 0.1 to about 1.0 μm separates the outer Schwann cell surface from Henle's sheath. Henle's sheath ends abruptly a short distance above the NMJ[26] (Fig. 15-9A to C), but the Schwann cell extends to cover that aspect of the nerve terminal that does not face the postsynaptic region (Fig. 15-9B and C). At some nerve terminals the Schwann cell also sends finger-like extensions into the synaptic space. These extensions recur at regular intervals at frog[24,93] but not mammalian NMJs. The basement membrane overlying the Schwann cell laterally becomes continuous with the nonsynaptic basement membrane of the muscle fiber; medially it merges with the synaptic basement membrane (Figs. 15-1 and 15-9C). Therefore only basement membrane separates the synaptic from the extracellular space.

The Schwann cell process over lying the terminal axon and nerve terminal contains numerous microfilaments, smooth and rough endoplasmic reticulum, mitochondria, and, depending on the plane of the section, the cell's nucleus (Figs. 15-1 and 15-9A).

The terminal axon contains neurofilaments, microtubules, smooth endoplasmic reticulum, a variable number of mitochondria, and a few synaptic vesicles (Fig. 15-9).

THE NERVE TERMINAL

The nerve terminal contains abundant small synaptic vesicles with clear contents, fewer giant synaptic vesicles with clear contents, coated vesicles, dense-core vesicles, mitochondria, and a varying complement of neurofilaments, microtubules, smooth endoplasmic reticulum, glycogen granules, lysosomal structures, and larger canaliculi and cisternae (Figs. 15-1 and 15-10 through 15-12). The relative abundance of the subcellular components in nerve terminals can vary within a given NMJ and from junction to junction; it may also vary with stage of development, aging, and neural activity.

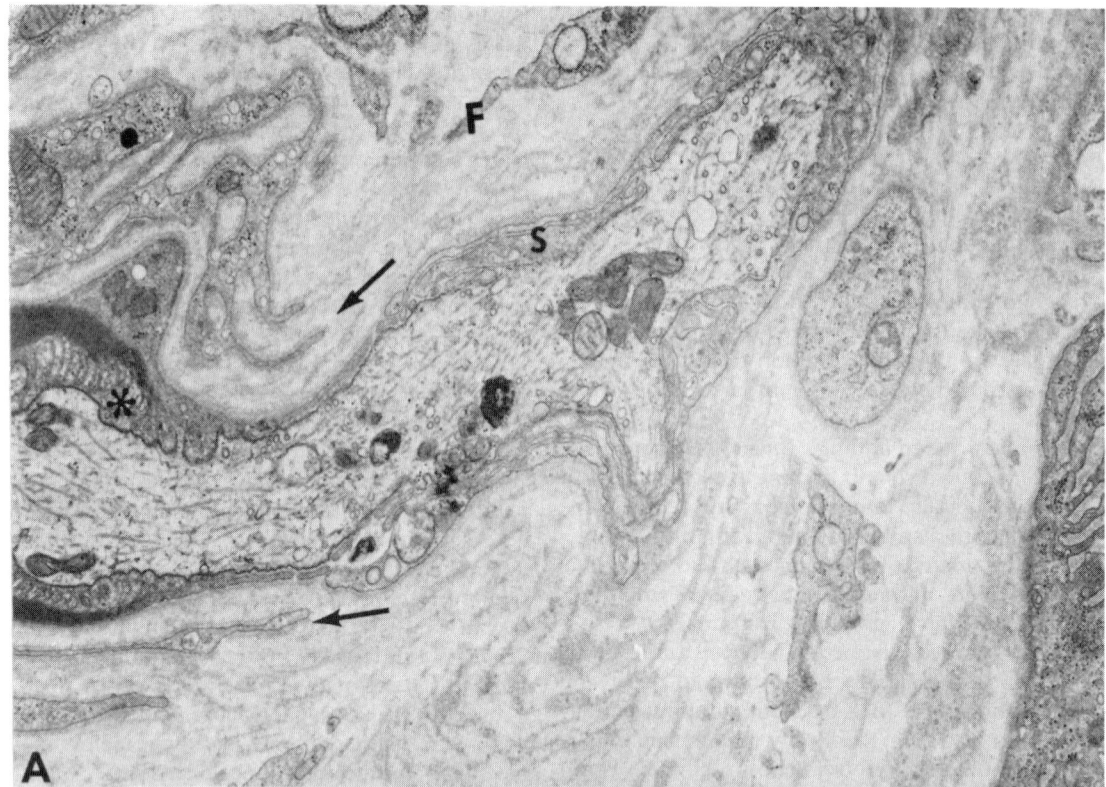
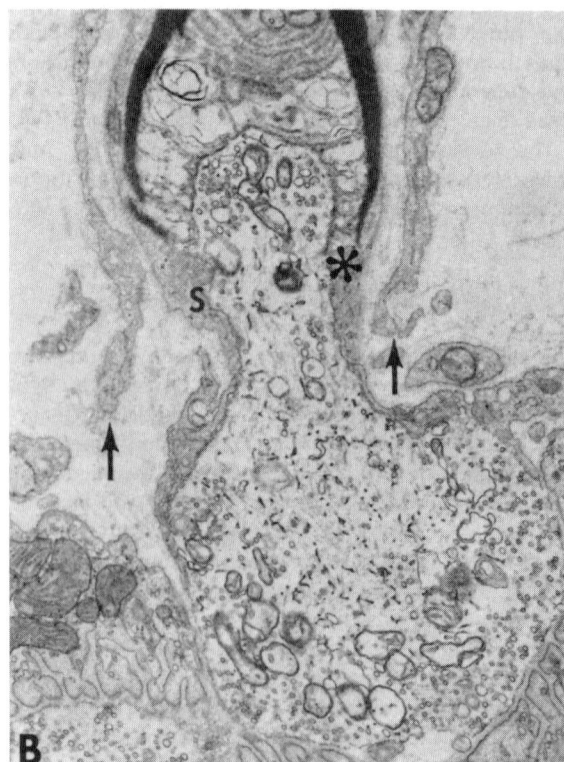
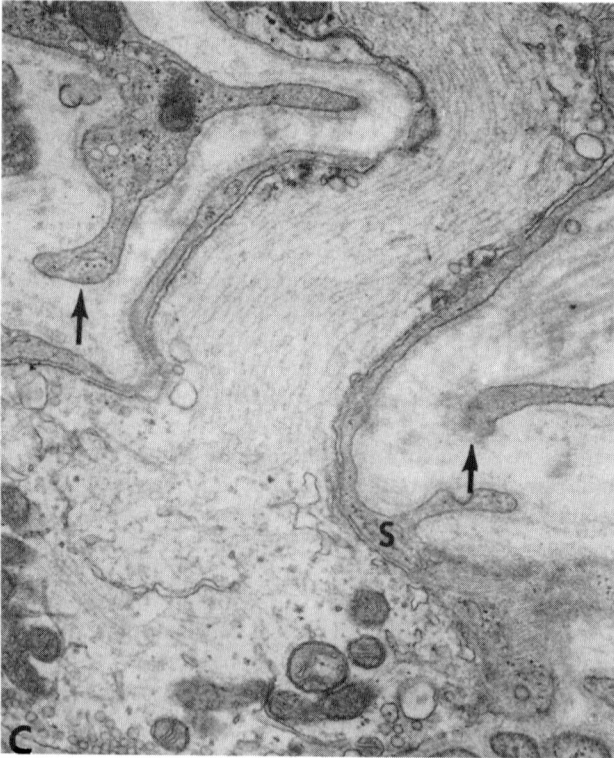

FIGURE 15-9. Approach of the preterminal nerve fiber to the NMJ. A. The myelin sheath ends abruptly at the last node of Ranvier (asterisk). The rest of the preterminal nerve fiber is surrounded by Schwann cell processes (S). Henle's sheath terminates shortly beyond the last node of Ranvier (arrows). The preterminal axon contains mitochondria, neurofilaments, and sparse synaptic vesicles. It approaches but does not reach the junctional region at the right of the field. Layers of basal lamina cover the Schwann cells, surround Henle's sheath, and form multiple layers in the space surrounding the preterminal nerve. The fibroblast process (F) is not surrounded by basement membrane. B. The NMJ appears almost immediately after the last node of Ranvier (asterisk). Henle's sheath (arrows) terminates between the last node of Ranvier and the NMJ. C. The unmyelinated preterminal axon courses for a few micrometers before it reaches the NMJ. Henle's sheath ends abruptly just above the NMJ (arrows). In B and C, the Schwann cell process (S) extends to cover that aspect of the nerve terminal not facing the postsynaptic region. (A, ×13,600; B, ×11,900; C, ×23,300.)

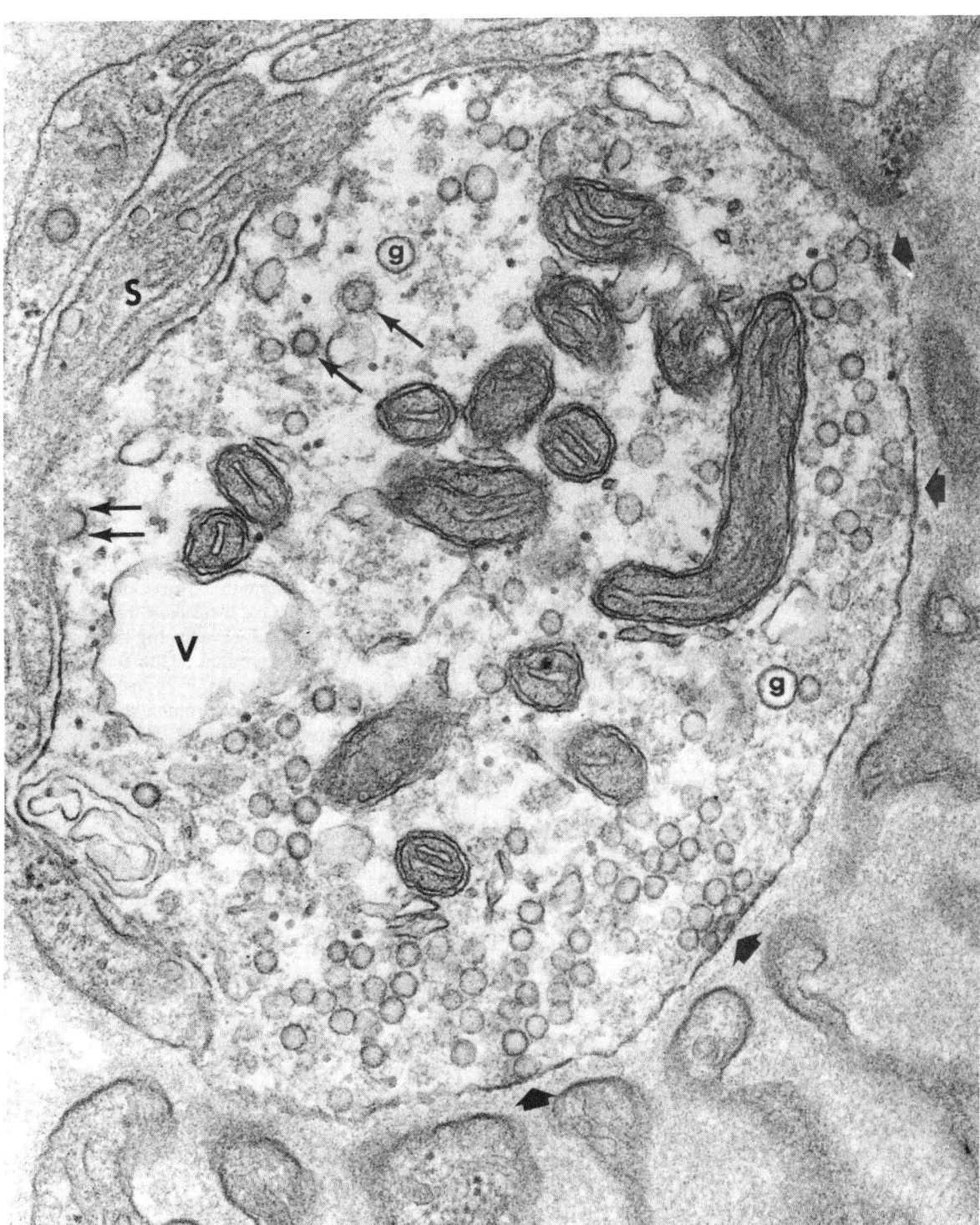

FIGURE 15-10. Nerve terminal in rat gastrocnemius NMJ. The synaptic vesicles are concentrated near the presynaptic membrane; the mitochondria cluster near the center of the nerve terminal. A few giant synaptic vesicles (g) and coated vesicles (arrows) are present. A coated pit (double arrows) is budding from axolemma covered by Schwann cell (S). The nerve terminal also contains glycogen granules, canaliculi, a small vacuole (V), and an amorphous or finely granular matrix. Solid arrows indicate four active zones that consist of dense spots on the inner surface of the presynaptic membrane and associated synaptic vesicles. The active zones are in register with the secondary synaptic clefts. Also note dense membrane specializations on the terminal expansions of the junctional folds. (×63,000.)

vesicles have been replaced by cisternae.[95] Similar vesicles also appear in frog nerve terminals treated with vinblastine.[96] The giant vesicles could arise from coalescence of smaller vesicles,[96] or they may represent intermediates of membrane recycling.[94] The appearance of giant vesicles after prolonged transmitter release has been correlated with that of giant miniature end plate potentials (MEPPs).[94] This suggests that each giant vesicle contains multiple ACh quanta, and that either the giant vesicle or its parent structure can concentrate ACh from the cytosol.

Coated Vesicles

Few vesicles in the rested nerve terminal are coated by fuzzy material[25,97,98] (Figs. 15-10 through 15-12). In quick-freeze, deep-etch, rotary-shadow preparations, the coat consists of a polyhedral surface lattice.[99] The coated vesicles arise from endocytotic pits in the axolemma (Figs. 15-10 and 15-11) and pinch off from even those regions of the axolemma covered by Schwann cell processes[100] (Fig. 15-10). The coated vesicles are also the first ones to pinch off from the axolemma and take up an extracellular marker when the nerve is tetanically stimulated in tracer-containing media,[100,101] and they proliferate in the terminal when ACh secretion is accelerated.[95,100] Under these conditions they merge with or bud from cisternae and canaliculi within the nerve terminal[101] (Fig. 15-13).

The polygonal network of the coated vesicles is made up of clathrin heavy and light chains.[102] These chains are present in the three-legged building blocks (triskelions) of the polygons. Within the network the centers and legs of triskelions become the corners and edges of the polygons, respectively.[103] Disassembly of the triskelions and denuding of the vesicles is induced by a cytosolic uncoating enzyme. This enzyme is an ATPase that interacts with clathrin light chains.[103] Immunocytochemical[104] and biochemical[105] studies localize clathrin in the nerve terminal in the lattice of the coated vesicles and in a "soluble" form in the axoplasmic matrix.

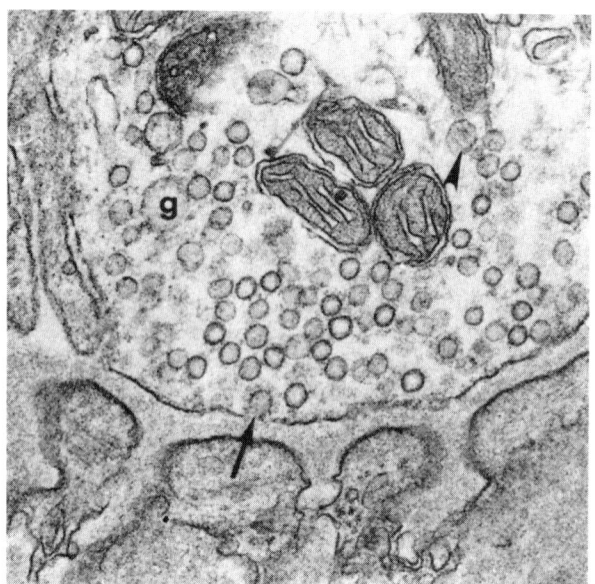

FIGURE 15-11. A portion of a nerve terminal and underlying postsynaptic region in rat forelimb muscle. Note coated vesicle budding from the presynaptic membrane (arrow), giant synaptic vesicle (g), and dense-core vesicle (arrowhead). (×51,800.)

Morphometric studies of human and rat NMJs in the resting state indicate that mitochondria account for approximately 15 percent of the nerve terminal volume, and there are 50 to 70 synaptic vesicles per square micron of the nerve terminal area.

Giant Synaptic Vesicles

In the rested nerve terminal a small proportion of the synaptic vesicles are two to three times larger than the average synaptic vesicle (Figs. 15-10 through 15-12). These giant vesicles increase in number during recovery from tetanic stimulation[94] or after exposure to lanthanum, when most synaptic

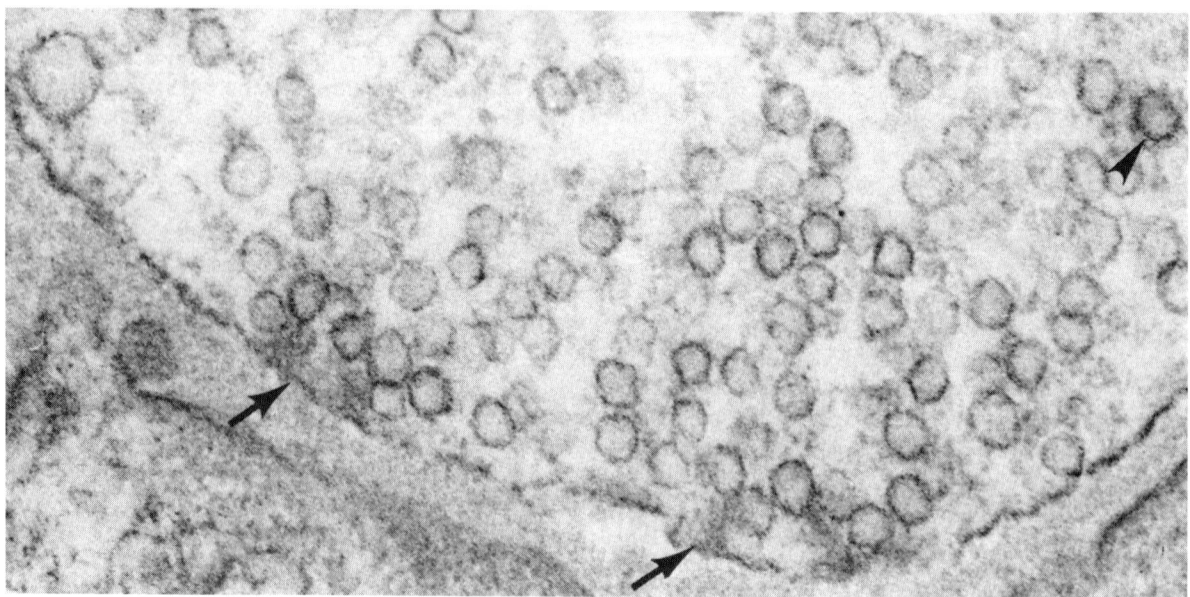

FIGURE 15-12. Nerve terminal in human external intercostal muscle. Arrows indicate two active zones. The dense material on the cytoplasmic surface of the active zones surrounds the associated synaptic vesicles. Arrowhead points to coated vesicle. (×101,000.)

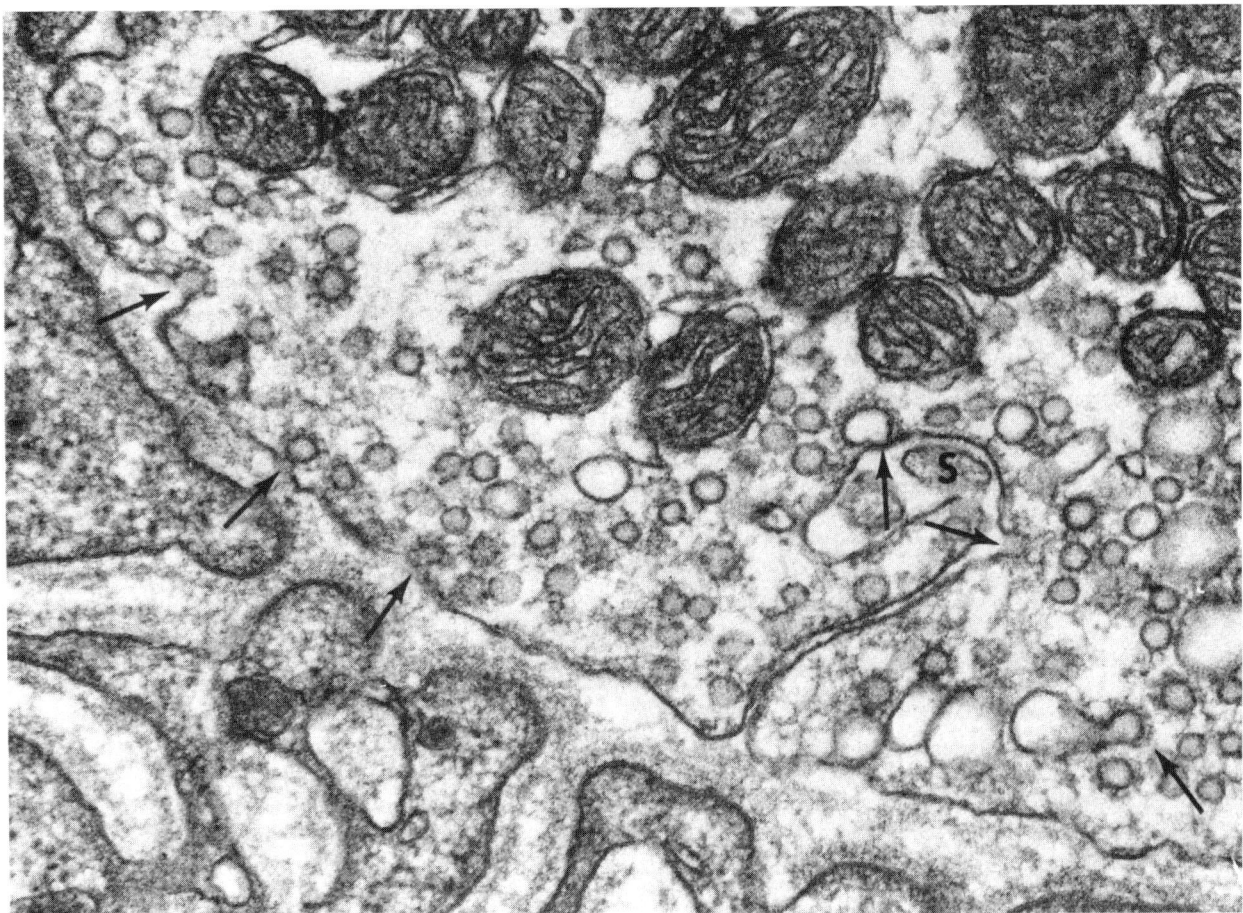

FIGURE 15-13. Rat diaphragm NMJ immersed in a dilute aldehyde fixative during electrical stimulation. Coated vesicles are forming at several regions of the presynaptic membrane (arrows), including the invaginated region that surrounds a Schwann cell process (S). Other coated vesicles are free in the axoplasm or coalesce with larger vacuoles or cisternae. (×100,000.) This micrograph was prepared by Dr. John Heuser. (Heuser JE, Reese TS, in Handbook of Physiology—The Nervous System, vol 1. Bethesda, MD: American Physiological Society; 1977, pp 261–294. With permission.[107])

Dense-Core Vesicles

Normal nerve terminals contain sparse, randomly distributed vesicles with dense cores in their confines whose diameters are 1.5- to 2-fold larger than the diameters of the small clear synaptic vesicles (Fig. 15-11). These vesicles are morphologically and biochemically related to the secretory granules of endocrine cells. Dense-core vesicles are relatively abundant in nerve growth cones and sprouts and in regenerating nerve terminals.[106] In different parts of the nervous system the dense-core vesicles contain neuropeptides, condensed proteins, and small nonprotein molecules. The presence of dense-core vesicles in adrenergic nerve terminals has been correlated with catecholamine-associated fluorescence.[106,107] At the NMJ, the dense-core vesicles may contain agrin, calcitonin gene–related peptide (CGRP),[108,109] and probably other neuroactive substances that can modify synaptic structure and function. Dense-core vesicles possess a vacuolar proton pump but lack synaptotagmin, synaptobrevin, and synapsin. Their release from the nerve terminal is regulated by calcium and Munc18-1[110] and modulated by synaptotagmin[111] and, in *Drosophila*, by a calcium-activated protein for secretion (CAPS).[112] The release mechanism differs from that for the small synaptic vesicles in several respects: The release is not preferentially at the active zones,[113] the rate of release is not enhanced by α-latrotoxin,[109,114] and the release mechanism is relatively slow, occurring after about 50 ms of high-frequency stimulation that results in a gradual increase of calcium concentration in the depth of the nerve terminal.[114,115] Following exocytosis, the dense-core vesicles are recycled, but their refilling requires a passage through the Golgi system.[116]

Small Clear Synaptic Vesicles

The smooth-surfaced clear synaptic vesicles with a mean diameter of 50 to 60 nm represent the predominant vesicle species in the nerve terminal[28,117]; from here onward they are referred to simply as *synaptic vesicles*. The lumens of the synaptic vesicles contain ACh, adenosine triphosphate (ATP), guanosine trihosphate (GTP), a relatively high concentration of calcium and magnesium ions, and a vesicle-specific proteoglycan.[118–121] The vesicles are more abundant near the presynaptic membrane than elsewhere in the terminal, whereas mitochondria and other organelles are concentrated in the center and upper parts of the terminal[7,24,25] (Figs. 15-1 and 15-10). The synaptic vesicles tend to be focused over dense spots on the presynaptic membrane (Figs. 15-10 and 15-12) that are part of the active zones, where synaptic vesicles exocytose their contents into the synaptic space.[20,24,43,122,123]

Synaptic vesicle precursors, associated with different sets of synaptic vesicle proteins, are produced in the body of the anterior horn cell and then are carried to nerve terminals by kinesin-like motors via fast axonal transport[124–127] by means of tubulovesicular organelles.[128] Further maturation of the vesicle precursors and their packaging with ACh occurs within the nerve terminal. A reduced number of synaptic vesicles, associated with a decrease in the number of readily releasable quanta, occurs in a congenital myasthenic syndrome. The putative cause of the syndrome is impaired axonal transport of synaptic vesicle components to the nerve terminal (see Chap. 66).

The functions and activities of the synaptic vesicles include (1) the concentrative uptake and storage of ACh, (2) movement to and docking at the active zones, (3) fusion with the presynaptic membrane to release ACh by exocytosis, and (4) recycling.[70,71,116,129] During recycling, the vesicles are retrieved from the presynaptic membrane and then recharged with ACh. Performance of these tasks requires the interaction of highly specialized vesicular, cytosolic, and target membrane proteins.

ACh uptake. The synthesis of ACh from choline and acetate takes place in the cytoplasm of the nerve terminal in a reaction catalyzed by choline acetyltransferase (ChAT). Uptake of the newly formed ACh into the synaptic vesicles is mediated by a vacuolar proton-pump ATPase that lowers the intravesicular pH and drives ACh uptake through the vesicular ACh transporter (VAChT).[130–132] The same VAChT transiently exports ACh from the nerve terminal when, due to exocytosis, the inner surface of the vesicular membrane is exposed to the synaptic space.

The entire coding region of the *VACHT* gene is contained in the first intron of the *CHAT* gene, and the two genes share common regulatory elements for transcription.[133] The structural information that specifically targets VAChT to the synaptic vesicles resides within the cytoplasmic C-terminal domain of VAChT. An isoform of VAChT, VMAT2, is targeted to the large, dense-core synaptic vesicles, where it subserves the concentrative uptake of neuroactive substances other than ACh.[134] Mutations in *CHAT* cause a highly disabling congenital myasthenic syndrome associated with abrupt episodes of apnea[135] (see Chap. 66).

Synaptic vesicles move from a reserve pool to dock at the active zones. Synapsin I, a vesicle-specific phosphoprotein, links synaptic vesicles to the cytoskeleton in the reserve pool of vesicles above the active zones. Synapsins II and III subserve similar roles in different sets of neurons.[55,59,70,136–138] Although partly homologous, the three synapsins are encoded by three distinct genes and a and b isoforms of each synapsin arise from differential splicing of their primary transcripts. Vesicle-binding proteins for synapsin include Ca^{2+}-calmodulin-dependent protein kinase II (CaM kinase II), c-src, and possibly other proteins. Synapsin I also binds to cytoskeletal actin, spectrin, and tubulin and thus anchors the vesicles to the cytoskeleton. In addition, synapsin I promotes the polymerization of actin monomers into actin filaments and the formation of thick bundles of actin filaments.

Four sites on synapsin I are substrates for phosphorylation by different protein kinases. Phosphorylation by a cAMP-dependent protein kinase A of a conserved serine in the N-terminal domain of all synapsins promotes neurite growth in the developing nervous system.[139]

Phosphorylation of synapsin I by synaptic vesicle–associated CaM kinase II has at least three effects[140]: (1) It reduces the affinity of synapsin I for CaM kinase II and causes synapsin to dissociate from the vesicles,[58] (2) it inhibits the effect of synapsin I on the polymerization of monomeric actin, and (3) it abrogates the ability of synapsin I to bundle actin filaments. Once freed from cytoskeletal constraints, the synaptic vesicles are transported from the deeper regions of the nerve terminal to the proximity of the active zones by kinesin motors on microtubule tracks. From here, myosin motors on actin tracks move them to the active zones.[141] Staurosporine, an inhibitor of a wide spectrum of protein kinases, impairs movement of the synaptic vesicles from the reserve pool to the active zones.[142]

The synaptic vesicles must be docked as well as primed for release at the active zones for efficient exocytotic release by Ca^{2+}. It was previously thought that docking was due to the formation of a complex between synaptobrevin on the synaptic vesicles and syntaxin and SNAP-25 on the presynaptic membrane. However, cleavage of these three proteins by clostridial neurotoxins or deletion of syntaxin in *Drosophila* does not prevent vesicle docking.[143] More recent studies indicate that the interaction of vesicular synaptotagmin with neurexin and the voltage-gated Ca^{2+} channel on the presynaptic membrane play a role in vesicle docking (see "The Voltage-Gated Ca^{2+} Channels," below).

THE EXOCYTOTIC MACHINERY

Ca^{2+}-regulated exocytosis of the synaptic vesicles involves the coordinated interaction of highly conserved proteins located on the synaptic vesicle, in the cytosol, and on the presynaptic membrane. The key proteins involved include (1) synaptobrevin and synaptotagmin, associated with the synaptic vesicles; (2) NSF (N-ethylmaleimide-sensitive ATPase) and α-SNAP (soluble NSF attachment protein) in the cytosol; and (3) syntaxin, SNAP-25 (synaptic vesicle associated protein of 25 kDa), and voltage-gated Ca^{2+} channels associated with the presynaptic membrane (Fig. 15-14). Because isoforms of several of these and of other exocytosis-related proteins play a universal role in vesicle–target membrane fusion in eukaryotic cells, the specificity of the docking and fusion process at the different vesicle–target membrane sites in eukaryotic cells must depend on the specificity of receptors on the vesicular and target membranes and presence of other accessory molecules.[144]

THE SNARE COMPLEX, SYNAPTOTAGMIN, AND OTHER PROTEINS IMPLICATED IN EXOCYTOSIS

The SNARE complex. Vesicular synaptobrevin, together with presynaptic membrane syntaxin and SNAP-25, serves as a receptor for α-SNAP. Therefore, synaptobrevin is referred to as a v-SNARE (vesicular SNAP receptor), and syntaxin and SNAP-25 are called t-SNAREs (target-membrane SNAP receptors).[143] The requirement of t- and v-SNAREs for exocytosis is revealed by effects of clostridial neurotoxins,

Botulinum toxins B, D, F, and G and tetanus toxin cleave synaptobrevin; botulinum toxins A and E cleave SNAP-25; and botulinum toxin C cleaves syntaxin.[145,146] In each case, the result is an arrest of exocytosis.

Biophysical,[147–150] quick-freeze/deep-etch electron microscopy,[151] and crystallographic[152] studies have elucidated the structure and function of the SNARE complexes.[153–155] The cytoplasmic portion of each SNARE protein contains repeats of seven amino acids that can assume an α-helical conformation. Monomeric SNAREs are largely unstructured; after combining with each other, they become highly α-helical, assume a coiled-coil configuration, and acquire enhanced thermodynamic stability.

Assembly of the t- and v-SNAREs occurs in three steps. First, monomeric SNAP-25, anchored to the presynaptic membrane by palmitoyl side chains, binds two molecules of syntaxin and the complex assumes a coiled-coil configuration. Second, the v-SNARE synaptobrevin binds to the preassembled t-SNAREs by displacing one of the two syntaxin molecules bound to SNAP-25. The entire complex is now a coiled coil in which α helices are strongly held together by hydrophobic interactions. The complex has been imaged as a 12- to 14-nm-long and ~2-nm-wide cylindrical bundle, with the N-termini of each component at one end and the C-termini at the other end. Third, the complex is stabilized by complexin, a small soluble neuronal protein that binds to the complex in an antiparallel α-helical conformation to seal the groove between synaptobrevin and syntaxin[156] (see Fig. 15-14). Because the v-SNAREs and t-SNAREs are anchored in two different membranes facing each other, the formation of SNARE complexes, or "SNARE pins," brings vesicle and target membranes into very close proximity. This, together with a strong basic charge at the C-terminal end of the SNARE pins, may provide the driving force behind membrane fusion.[152] Multiple SNARE pins are probably needed to trigger fusion of a single synaptic vesicle, and the pins likely are arranged in a ring-like structure at the contact point.[157] Indeed, when v- and t-SNAREs are reconstituted into separate liposomal vesicles, they assemble to form SNARE pins that link adjacent vesicles; but the fusion process is inefficient, indicating that one or more additional factors participate in exocytosis in vivo after the SNARE pins are assembled.[157]

Synaptotagmin I. Synaptotagmin I, a 65-kDa molecule, belongs to a large family of membrane proteins involved in membrane fusion in brain and other organs.[158] Synaptotagmin I has a short, glycosylated intravesicular N-terminal domain, a transmembrane domain, and a cytoplasmic domain that harbors two Ca^{2+} regulatory C2 domains (C2A and C2B) connected by a short linker and separated from the transmembrane domain by a highly charged sequence.

The C2A domain binds phospholipids and two Ca^{2+} ions held in position by five negatively charged aspartate residues on two peptide loops.[159] The Ca^{2+} concentration for half-maximal binding (EC50) is 200 μM, a concentration attained only in close proximity to the active zones. When the C2A domain binds Ca^{2+}, it acquires a large positive electrostatic potential and then binds syntaxin.[160] Two synaptotagmin molecules, binding 4 Ca^{2+}, are required to initiate vesicle fusion.[160a] Both syntaxin and synaptotagmin are highly associated with the presynaptic voltage-gated Ca^{2+} channels.[161]

The C2B domain of synaptotagmin binds AP2 (see "Endocytotic Events and the Formation of New Synaptic Vesicles," below), β-SNAP (which, like α-SNAP, binds to NSF), polyinositol phosphates, and the vesicular protein SV2A.[158,162] Ca^{2+} inhibits the interaction between SV2A and synaptotagmin, with an EC50 of 10 μM. The C-terminus of synaptotagmin binds neurexin, the presynaptic membrane receptor for α-

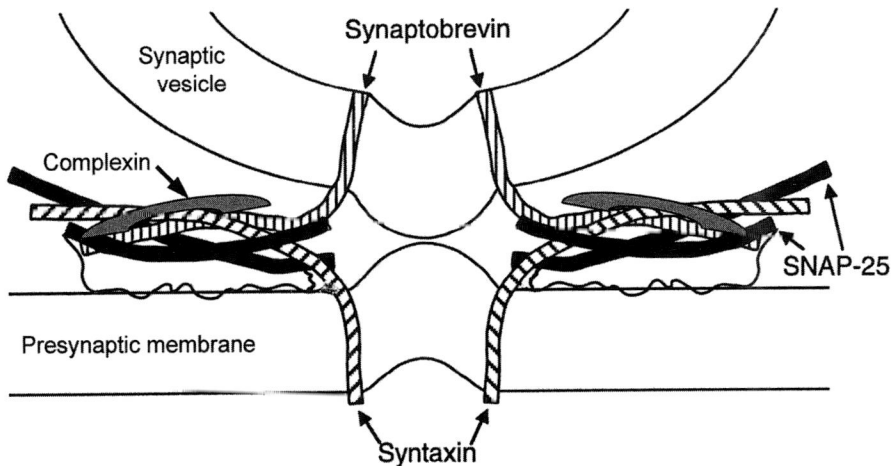

FIGURE 15-14. A possible model of the SNARE complex formed between the v-SNARE synaptobrevin and the t-SNAREs syntaxin and SNAP-25. Two complexes are imaged. Synaptobrevin and syntaxin are anchored by transmembrane regions in the lipid bilayer of the synaptic vesicle (above) and presynaptic membrane (below), respectively. SNAP-25 is linked to the presynaptic membrane by a polypeptide chain (indicated by a thin undulating line). The complex is stabilized by complexin, which binds in an α-helical conformation to seal the groove between synaptobrevin and syntaxin. The cytoplasmic domains of the v- and t-SNAREs form a coiled coil that pulls the synaptic vesicle and the presynaptic membrane into close proximity. Impending fusion is suggested by bulging regions of the vesicular and presynaptic membranes. This diagram is based on models proposed in Refs. 152, 156, and 157.

latrotoxin (the active component of black widow spider venom that causes massive exocytosis). Finally, an unknown region of synaptotagmin binds Munc13.[158] In mutant mice deficient in synaptotagmin, the Ca^{2+}-dependent evoked synaptic response is severely depressed. Consequently, the animals die shortly after birth.[163]

Synaptotagmin binds to the voltage-gated Ca^{2+} channel, as well as to syntaxin and neurexin, which in turn are attached to the presynaptic Ca^{2+} channel.[161,164] Hence, synaptotagmin could also participate in docking. Activation of synaptotagmin by Ca^{2+} likely triggers exocytosis.[158,165]

Steps in exocytosis. On the basis of recent studies, vesicle exocytosis can be postulated to involve the following steps:

1. Partial and reversible assembly of the SNARE complex primes docked synaptic vesicles for exocytosis prior to arrival of the Ca^{2+} trigger.[166]
2. Following Ca^{2+} ingress into the nerve terminal, Ca^{2+} binds to the C2A and C2B domains of synaptotagmin, enabling it to oligomerize and to bind to phospholipids, syntaxin, and SNAP-25.[167–169]
3. Vesicular and target membranes are brought into close proximity by Ca^{2+}-activated synaptotagmin.
4. Syntaxin and SNAP-25 now firmly engage synaptobrevin to complete formation of the SNARE complex.
5. The completed SNARE complex brings the opposing vesicular and presynaptic membranes into contact, which initiates membrane fusion in a probabilistic manner.[170]

Following exocytosis, the SNARE pins remain attached to the cytoplasmic surface of the presynaptic membrane. NSF and α-SNAP cause disassembly of the SNARE pins, and the energy required to separate the pins comes from the hydrolysis of ATP by NSF. According to this scheme, the main function of NSF/SNAP is to make the SNARE components available for another round of exocytosis.[157]

Other Proteins Implicated in Modulating Exocytosis

Munc18, tomosyn, and amysin. Munc18 (also known as n-sec1) competitively inhibits the assembly of t-SNAREs by binding to syntaxin with high affinity.[171] Another protein, tomosyn, displaces Munc18 from syntaxin and, in turn, can be displaced by synaptobrevin.[172,173] This suggests that Munc18 inhibits SNARE assembly in the resting state and that removal of this inhibition by tomosyn permits initial assembly of the SNARE complex. Amysin, a recently recognized soluble protein, may play a role similar to that of Munc-18 by forming complexes with syntaxin and SNAP-25 to inhibit SNARE formation.[174]

Munc13, RIM, CAST, and bassoon. All four proteins are present in the active zone matrix. Munc13 contains C1 and C2 domains and exists in different isoforms. It is required for Ca^{2+}-dependent vesicle fusion[175]; this effect may be owing to its acting as a priming factor that opens syntaxin.[176] RIM (Rab interacting molecule) has zinc-finger and C2 domains and interacts with Munc13 through one of its zinc-finger domains. *RIM*-null animals show a severe defect in spontaneous or evoked vesicle release but can dock vesicles at the active zone. This suggests that RIM is also important for priming the docked vesicles.[175] CAST binds directly to RIM and indirectly to Munc13, forming a ternary complex. Bassoon, another protein present in the active zone matrix, also associates with this complex. Thus, a network of protein-protein interactions exists in the active zone matrix.[177]

Rab3a, Rabphilin-3A, and RIM. Rab3A, a small GTP-binding protein, is also implicated in synaptic vesicle docking and fusion.[178] The Rab proteins belong to the p21ras superfamily, whose members regulate membrane fusion-fission events by cycling between membrane-bound and membrane-free states. When attached to a synaptic vesicle, rab3a binds GTP. Rab3a-GTP binds rabphilin-3A, a cytosolic protein with zinc-finger and C2 domains, and RIM.[179] Both rabphilin3a and RIM bind to rab3a through sequences contained in their zinc-finger domains.

At the time of exocytosis, activation of a GTPase converts rab3A-GTP to rab3A-GDP, whereupon both rab3a-GDP and rabphilin-3a dissociate from the synaptic vesicle.[179–181] Subsequently, rab3a-GDP becomes attached to another synaptic vesicle and recaptures GTP by nucleotide exchange. Evidence to date suggests that rab3a decreases the probability of quantal release,[182] that RIM promotes transmitter release,[179] and that rabphilin-3A plays a regulatory role in both exocytosis and endocytosis.[183]

SV2. SV2 is a protein found in synaptic vesicles and endocrine cells. It is present in two major (SV2A and SV2B) isoforms and one minor isoform (SV2C). As noted above, SV2A interacts with the C2B domain of synaptotagmin in the absence of Ca^{2+}. The major phosphorylation site of SV2 is at its cytoplasmic amino terminus, and phosphorylation increases its affinity for synaptotagmin.[184] Neurons lacking both SV2 isoforms show increased Ca^{2+}-dependent transmitter release.[185] A recent study suggests that SV2 modulates the formation of protein complexes required for fusion and therefore the progression of vesicles to a fusion-competent state.[186]

Synaptophysin. Synaptophysin, a 38-kDa glycoprotein, is the most abundant integral membrane protein of the synaptic vesicles.[187] It has properties of a cation-selective channel, with higher selectivity for K^+ than other cations, but is impermeable to Ca^{2+}.[188] It is phosphorylated by a tyrosine kinase,[189] interacts with a subunit of the vacuolar proton pump,[190] and may interact with synaptobrevin during exocytosis.[191] When overexpressed at the *Xenopus* NMJ, synaptophysin increases the frequency of spontaneous quantal release and augments the number of quanta released by nerve impulse.[192] In the yeast two-hybrid system, synaptophysin interacts with the AP1-adaptor protein γ adaptin and may thus play a role in endocytosis. However, synaptophysin-null mice show no functional or morphologic abnormality.[193]

Cysteine string protein (CSP), heat-shock protein 70 (Hsc70), and SGT chaperone complex. These three proteins interact with each other to form a stable trimeric complex located on the surface of the synaptic vesicles. The complex functions as an ATP-dependent chaperone reactivating denatured substrates.[194]

CSP itself is a 34-kDa protein anchored via palmitoyl groups to the synaptic vesicle so that its C- and N-termini are cytoplasmic.[195,196] CSP harbors an N-terminal J domain, characteristic of heat-shock proteins, and a central multiply palmitoylated string of cysteine residues. By increasing the ATPase activity of Hsc70, CSP cochaperones with Hsc70 to promote the formation or dissociation of protein complexes and to regulate conformational changes in proteins.[197,198] CSP also binds to the P/Q type Ca^{2+} channel with high affinity[199] and interacts with synaptotagmin.[200] In *Drosophila* mutants lacking CSP, the exocytotic machinery is preserved but calcium entry into the nerve terminal, calcium activation of exocytosis, or both are impaired.[201] Injection of CSP into the chick ciliary neuron increases the Ca^{2+} current owing to recruitment of dormant Ca^{2+} channels.[202]

CYTOSKELETAL COMPONENTS OF THE NERVE TERMINAL ABOVE THE ACTIVE ZONES

Quick-freeze, deep-etch electron microscopy shows that the main cytoskeletal elements in the nerve terminal consist of actin filaments and microtubules.[51,52,55,203] The actin filaments honeycomb the nerve terminal. They are most closely packed adjacent to the synaptic membrane, and become more sparse with distance from the membrane. Those filaments terminating against the active zone tend to be perpendicularly oriented to the presynaptic membrane. The filaments are straight, often intersect, and extend from vesicle to vesicle and from vesicle to presynaptic membrane. The actin filaments are linked by approximately 30-nm-long filaments to the synaptic vesicles, the linking filaments representing single synapsin I molecules. Synapsin I molecules also link microtubules to the synaptic vesicles and cross-link the microtubules.[55] A similar cytoskeletal network exists in Purkinje cell dendrites[203] (Fig. 15-15).

THE ACTIVE ZONE

The active zone is an anatomically differentiated region of the presynaptic membrane that is topographically related to the exocytosis of synaptic vesicles. The position of the active zone in the nerve terminal is marked by a dense spot that contains particles interconnected by fibrils in a matrix above which synaptic vesicles tend to cluster (Figs. 15-10 through 15-12). The matrix material, which is soluble above pH 8, contains proteins involved in exocytosis of synaptic vesicles and membrane retrieval.[204] That transmitter release occurs near active zones has been proposed by early studies of both central[205] and neuromuscular[20,24] synapses.

At the NMJ of fast-twitch frog muscle fibers, the active zones recur at regular intervals, so that in longitudinal sections each zone is positioned above a secondary synaptic cleft that is flanked by two junctional folds. The long axis of each active zone is perpendicular to the long axis of the nerve terminal.[24,41,100,107,122,123] These features are clearly shown by freeze-fracture studies (Fig. 15-16). The precise alignment of the active zones of the nerve terminal with the crests of the junctional folds is also shown by dual immunofluorescence localization of the active zones with ω-conotoxin and of AChR with α-bungarotoxin.[64,65] Treatment with proteolytic enzymes results in displacement and disorganization of the active zones and clustering of the active zone particles.[206] This implies that the precise alignment of the active zones on the presynaptic membrane depends, at least in part, on the basal lamina.

Freeze-fracture studies of the presynaptic membrane show additional features in the active zone. These are best observed on the protoplasmic (P) face of the fractured membrane. In the fast-twitch frog muscle fiber the presynaptic membrane P face displays a ribbon-like convexity corresponding to the

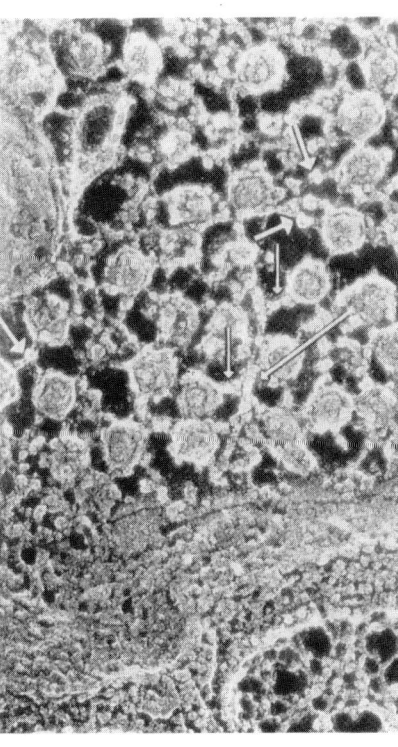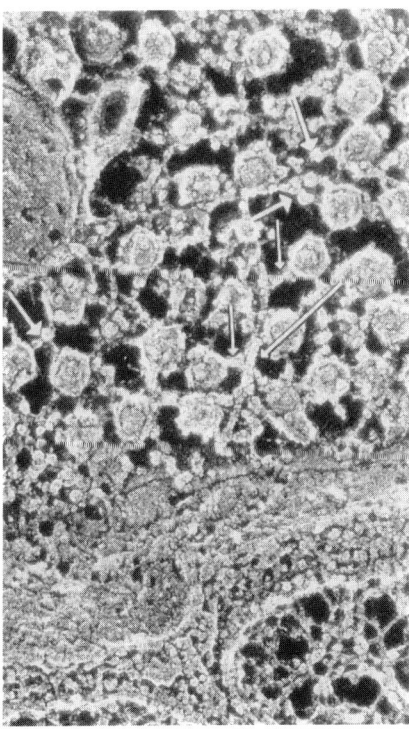

FIGURE 15-15. Stereo-pair electron micrographs of quick-frozen, deep-etched, rotary-shadowed frog NMJ. The cytoskeletal network inside the nerve terminal reveals short strands (20 to 30 nm) (short arrows) between actin filaments (long arrows). There are also short linking strands (30 to 60 nm) between the synaptic vesicles (thick arrows). Frequently globular structures are observed in the middle of linking strands between synaptic vesicles (thick arrows). (×135,000.) These micrographs were prepared by Dr. Nobutaka Hirokawa. (Hirokawa et al, *J Cell Biol*, 108:111, 1989. With permission.)

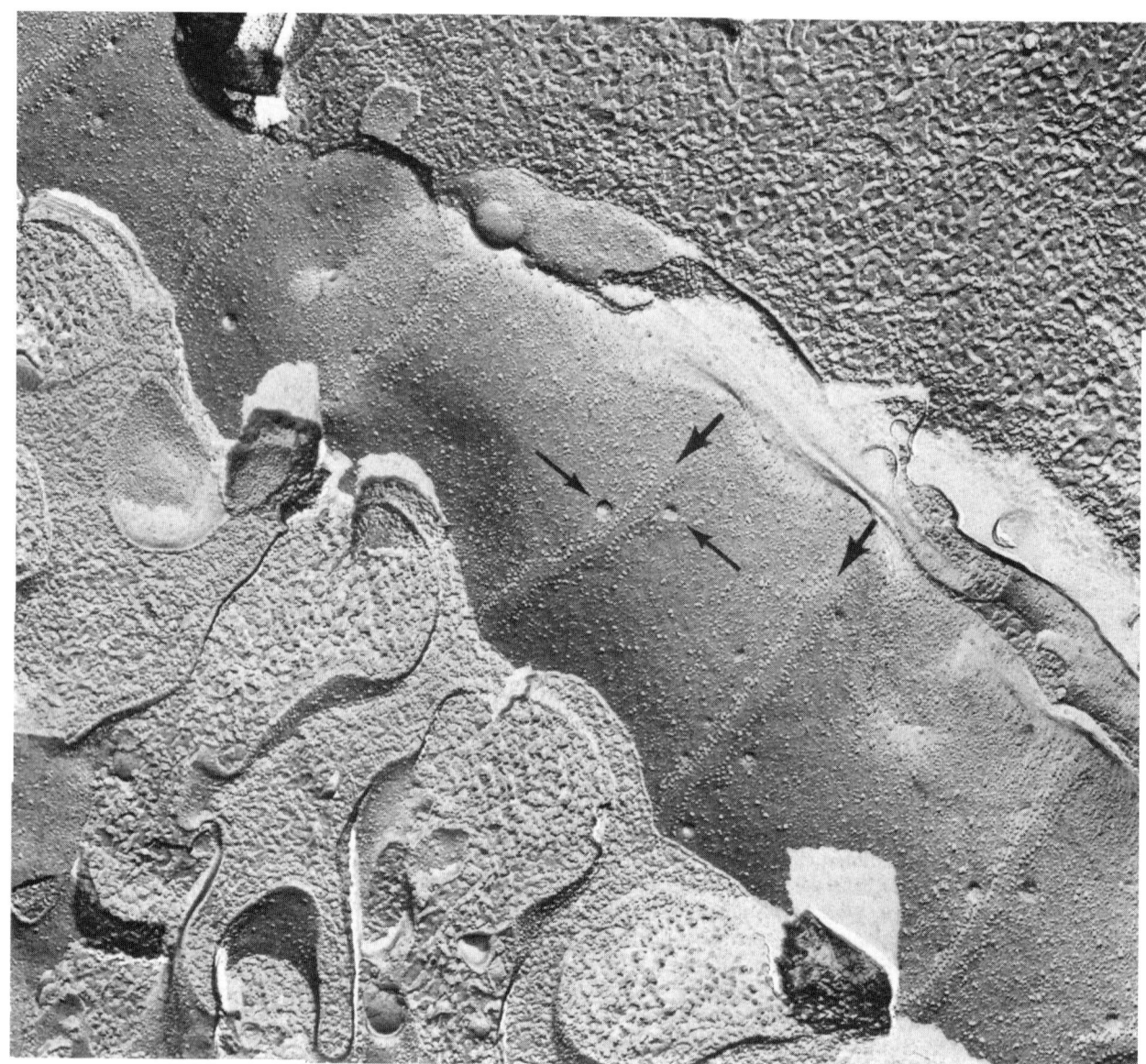

FIGURE 15-16. Freeze-fractured frog NMJ stimulated during fixation in dilute aldehyde fixative. The fracture exposes a large expanse of the presynaptic membrane P face. The active zones consist of a convex ridge flanked on each side by a double parallel row of large intramembrane particles (heavy arrows). The active zones are perpendicularly oriented to the long axis of the nerve terminal and are in register with the secondary synaptic clefts. Dimples adjacent to the active zones (light arrows) indicate exocytotic events that had occurred in the course of stimulation. Only occasional dimples can be observed near the active zones in the resting frog nerve terminal. (×55,000.) This micrograph was prepared by Dr. John Heuser. (Heuser JE et al, J Neurocytol 3:109, 1974. With permission.[41])

dense bar seen within the terminal by conventional transmission electron microscopy. The convexity is flanked on each side by a double parallel row of large (10 to 12 nm) intramembrane particles that represent voltage-gated Ca^{2+} channels[41,43,207] (Fig. 15-16).

A recent and remarkable electron microscopic tomography new P study by McMahan and coworkers of the active zone of the frog cutaneous pectoris muscle revealed with great clarity both a particular relationship and a structural linkage between the docked synaptic vesicles and the presynaptic Ca^{2+} channels and related macromolecules[208] (Fig. 15-17). According to this study, individual active zones are flanked on each side by a row of docked vesicles that flank the Ca^{2+} channels, which flank the ribbon-like convexity of the presynaptic membrane. Running in the center of the convexity are a series of ~75-nm-long "beams" whose orthogonal lateral extensions, or "ribs," associate with docked vesicles, about three ribs reaching each vesicle. The individual ribs are separated from the presynaptic membrane by a ≤7-nm gap that is bridged at intervals by "pegs," with one or two pegs connecting each rib to regions of the membrane containing macromolecules that include the Ca^{2+} channel. While the molecular identity of the components of the active zone scaffold are not yet known, the Ca^{2+} channels could be components of the pegs, and the ribs may contain proteins, such as syntaxin and synaptotagmin, that mediate the effects of Ca^{2+} on vesicle fusion.

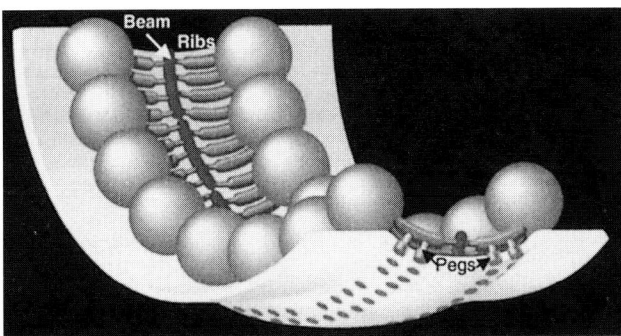

FIGURE 15-17. Arrangement of structures at the active zone based on electron microscopic tomography studies by McMahan and coworkers. (*Nature 409:479–484, 2001. Reproduced by permission.*[208])

The mammalian NMJ is less elongated and more convoluted than the linear NMJ on the fast-twitch frog muscle fiber. At the mammalian NMJ, the active zones retain the relationship to the underlying junctional folds but are shorter and less regularly disposed, and the convexity between the double parallel rows of particles is usually absent[42,209,210] (Figs. 15-18 and 15-19). The presynaptic membrane curves more steeply and irregularly at the mammalian than at the frog NMJ. However, the area of the mammalian membrane can still be determined by stereometric analysis.[211] Using this approach, Fukunaga and coworkers[210] found that in human external intercostal muscle presynaptic membranes, the average density of active zones was $2.6/\mu m^2$, the density of active zone particles was $51/\mu m^2$, the average active zone had 5 particles per row, and, on the average, there were 19 particles per active zone. The same investigators obtained essentially identical values in freeze-fractured presynaptic membranes of the mouse diaphragm.[212] Freeze-fracture studies of physiologically characterized frog NMJs reveal a positive correlation between estimated total active zone length and total number of active zone particles per junction with quantal release from the same junctions.[213]

THE VOLTAGE-GATED CA^{2+} CHANNELS

The voltage-gated Ca^{2+} channels open when the presynaptic membrane is depolarized by the nerve action potential. The resultant Ca^{2+} entry peaks within 200 μs and lasts ~800 μs.[214] During this time, the docked vesicles are engulfed in microdomains in which the Ca^{2+} concentration reaches ~200 to 300 μM.[161] A synaptic vesicle within 20 nm from a Ca^{2+} channel can exocytose with high probability within a few hundred microseconds if the local Ca^{2+} concentration rises above 100 μM. It is estimated that exocytosis of a single vesicle requires the opening of >60 calcium channels and the entry of ~13,000 Ca^{2+} ions into the nerve terminal.[215]

The voltage-gated Ca^{2+} channels at mammalian NMJs are predominantly of the P/Q type; a lesser number of L-type channels has been detected at the mouse NMJ,[216] and N-type Ca^{2+} channels are transiently expressed at the neonatal rat NMJ.[217] The P/Q channels consist of a pore-forming α_{1A} subunit, a partly extracellular $\alpha_2\delta$ subunit, a transmembrane γ subunit, and an intracellular β subunit. P/Q channels differ from N-type channels, which contain an α_{1B} subunit, and from L-type channels, which contain α_{1C} or α_{1D} subunits. Unlike the N- and L-type channels, the P/Q channels are selectively sensitive to ω-agatoxin IVA (<10 nM for the P-

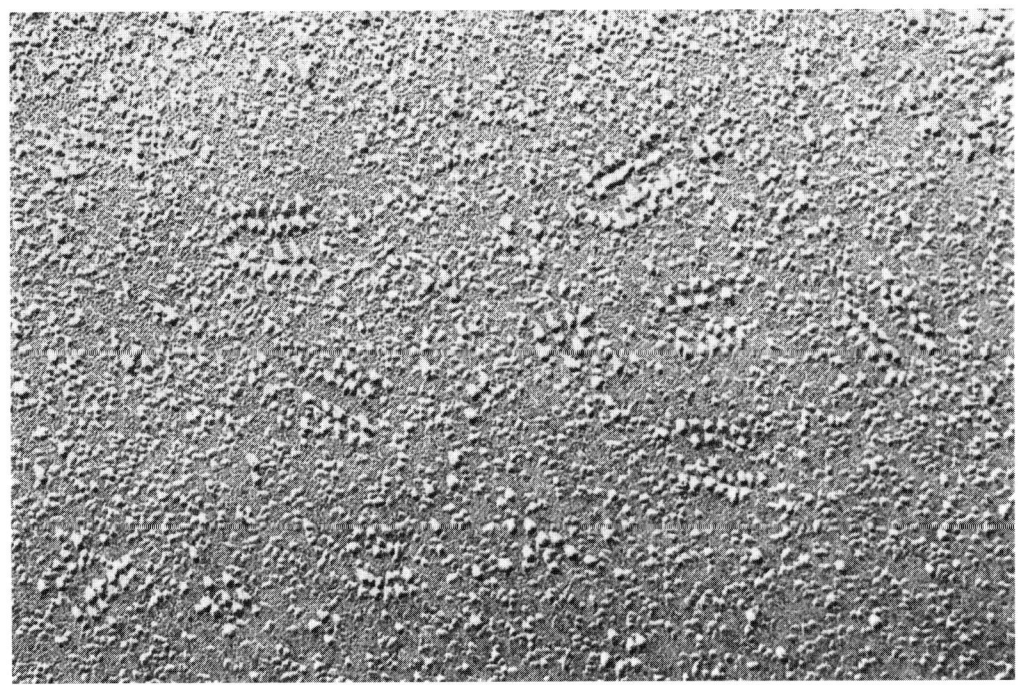

FIGURE 15-18. Freeze-fractured presynaptic membrane P face from mouse diaphragm muscle viewed from the direction of the underlying muscle fiber. The active zones are represented by double parallel rows of large (10 to 12 nm) intramembrane particles. The rows are short and irregularly oriented and are not adjacent to a central ridge (compare with active zones at the frog fast-twitch NMJ in Fig 15-16). (×105,000.)

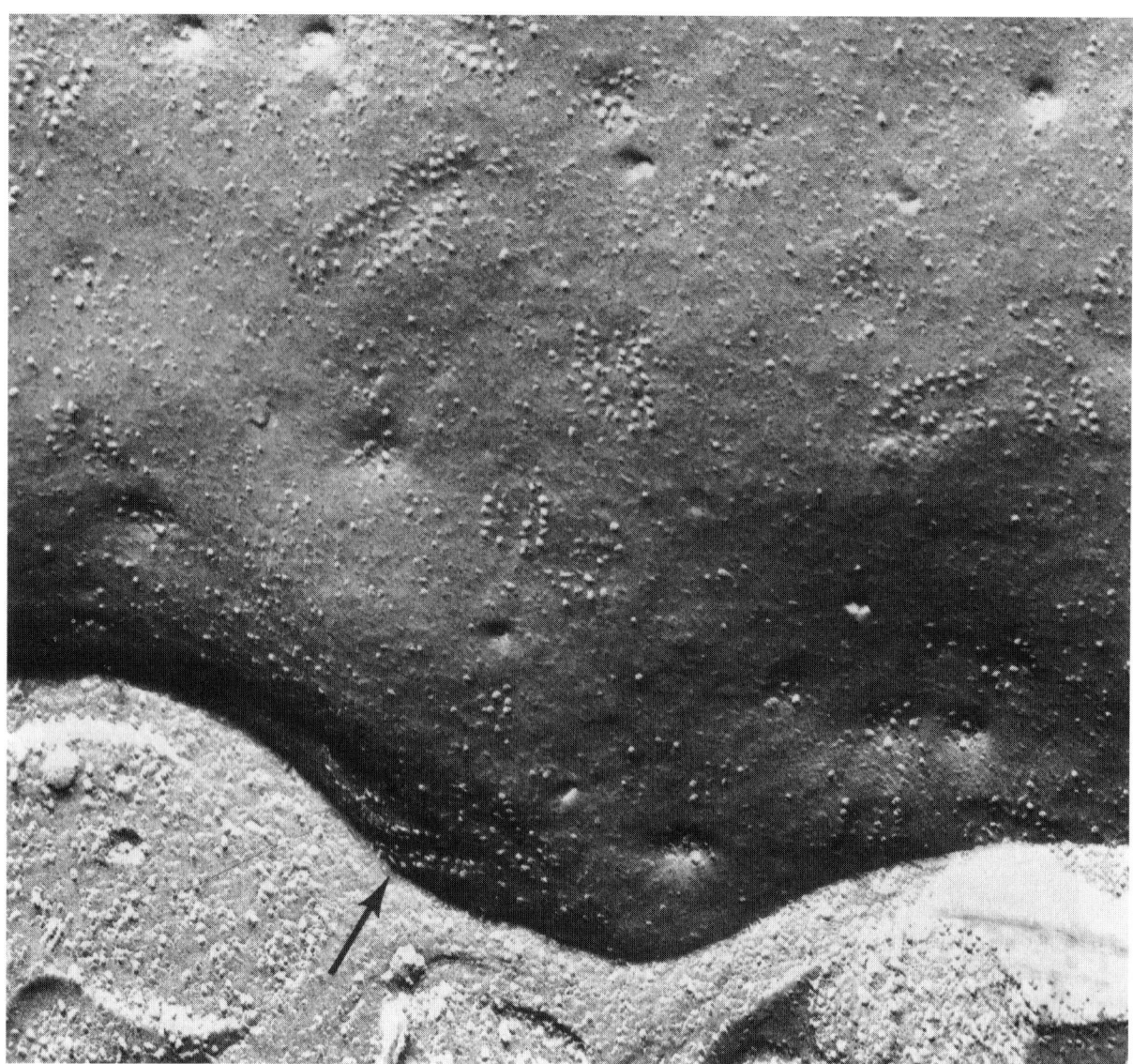

FIGURE 15-19. Freeze-fractured NMJ from human external intercostal muscle. The fracture displays a large expanse of the presynaptic membrane, traverses the synaptic space, and cross-fractures three junctional folds. Numerous active zones are present on the presynaptic membrane. Dimples on the membrane may represent exocytotic or endocytotic events occurring during fixation. One active zone at the lower border of the presynaptic membrane is in register with the underlying secondary synaptic cleft. (×121,000.)

type channel and >10 nM for the Q-type channel) but are insensitive to dihydropyridines.[218] All types of α_1 subunits are composed of four conserved and homologous transmembrane domains (I to IV) linked by nonconserved intracellular hydrophilic loops. The cytoplasmic loop (L_{II-III}) between homologous domains II and III of the α_{1A} subunit of the P/Q channel interacts in a Ca^{2+}-dependent manner with t-SNAREs syntaxin and SNAP-25,[219] vesicular synaptotagmin,[220] and CSP.[199] Each molecule binds to a specific "synprint" (an acronym for synaptic protein interaction) sequence on the L_{II-III} loop. The sequential and Ca^{2+}-dependent interactions of the t-SNAREs and synaptotagmin with Ca^{2+} synprints may play a role in the cascade of reactions leading to vesicle docking and fusion.[161]

An immune-mediated downregulation of the number of presynaptic voltage-gated Ca^{2+} channels results in the Lambert-Eaton myasthenic syndrome (see Chap. 65). An electrophysiologically similar syndrome also occurs in a congenital setting. Here the defect could reside in the presynaptic voltage-gated Ca^{2+} channels, in any of the SNARE components, or in other molecules that regulate exocytosis (see Chap. 66).

Voltage-gated K$^+$ channels of the presynaptic membrane. At mammalian motor nerve endings, the voltage-gated Na$^+$ channels disappear between the last node of Ranvier and the point where the terminal axon becomes associated with the NMJ (see Fig. 15-9). Therefore the presynaptic membrane harbors K$^+$ and Ca^{2+} channels, but not Na$^+$ channels,[221,222] and the depolarizing current that reaches the presynaptic membrane originates from a preterminal nerve branch. The voltage-gated K$^+$ channels of the presynaptic membrane are rapidly acting delayed rectifiers that close the voltage-gated Ca^{2+} channels by restoring the resting membrane potential. Consequently, a deficiency of the presynaptic K+ channels, as in patients with neuromyotonia (see Chap. 47), or their blockage by 3,4-diaminopyridine, prolong Ca^{2+} influx into the depolarized nerve terminal and enhance quantal release (see Chaps. 65 and 66).

MORPHOLOGIC CORRELATES OF QUANTAL TRANSMITTER RELEASE

Quantal ACh Release Is Associated with Synaptic Vesicle Exocytosis

Depolarization of the nerve terminal by lanthanum[95] or facilitation of quantal release by black widow spider venom[223] markedly accelerates quantal ACh release, as shown by a marked increase of the MEPP frequency. After a prolonged period of increased quantal release, the nerve terminal increases in size, while the MEPPs become less frequent and then disappear. These events can be correlated with a decrease and disappearance of synaptic vesicles from the nerve terminal. After a long period of exposure to lanthanum, many cisternae and small vacuoles and numerous coated vesicles appear in the nerve terminal.[95]

Electric stimulation of the frog nerve terminal at 10 Hz for 1 min causes a 30 percent decrease in synaptic vesicle density, which is balanced by a corresponding increase in presynaptic membrane length. If stimulation is continued for 15 min, synaptic vesicle density decreases by 60 percent and numerous membrane-bound cisternae appear within the nerve terminal.[100] After a 15-min rest, the synaptic vesicles reappear and the cisternae become less numerous. If stimulation occurs in the presence of peroxidase, the marker appears in coated vesicles, larger cisternae, and synaptic vesicles in this sequence.[100] Finally, evidence for synaptic vesicle exocytosis and endocytosis has been obtained by the stimulation of nerve terminals containing synaptic vesicles labeled with a fluorescent, lipid-soluble dye.[66,224,225] These experiments are consistent with the notion that ACh quanta reside in synaptic vesicles, that quantal release is by vesicle exocytosis, that membrane added to the axolemma during exocytosis is retrieved by endocytosis (Fig. 15-13), and that cisternae and vacuoles in the nerve terminal represent transient membrane storage sites (Fig. 15-13).

In another study, stimulation of the frog nerve terminal for 3 to 4.5 h at 2 Hz significantly decreased the MEPP amplitude and quantal release without depleting the synaptic vesicles. Stimulation for 20 min at 10 Hz not only reduced the MEPP amplitude but also depleted the synaptic vesicles.[226] These findings are still consistent with the vesicle hypothesis but indicate that during prolonged low-frequency stimulation the resynthesis or packaging of ACh diminishes before the formation of new synaptic vesicles is affected. This can also be inferred from the lack of synaptic vesicle depletion when vesicular ACh stores are reduced by stimulation in the presence of hemicholinium-3.[227]

Further evidence that synaptic vesicle exocytosis accompanies quantal release has come from capturing synaptic vesicle openings during stimulated transmitter release by (1) immersion of the NMJ in a dilute aldehyde fixative during electrical stimulation[41] (Fig. 15-16); (2) immersion of the NMJ in cool, dilute fixative containing sucrose or 20 mM KCl[228]; and (3) pretreatment of the NMJ with 4-aminopyridine (an agent that augments quantal release by nerve impulse), followed by a single electric shock, followed by ultra-rapid freezing of the NMJ within a few ms, followed either by freeze-fracture (Fig. 15-20) or by freeze-substitution fixation and thin sectioning[101,229–231] (Fig. 15-21). Under these conditions, exocytotic figures appear immediately adjacent to the active zones. These images are omega-shaped in thin sections (Fig. 15-21) and appear as dimples in the freeze-fractured presynaptic membrane P-face (Figs. 15-16 and 15-20).

In the presence of 4-aminopyridine, a single electric shock discharges 3000 to 6000 synaptic vesicles from each nerve terminal. Exocytosis begins as soon as 2.5 ms after the stimulus, the vesicles fuse with the axolemma at the same time as the quanta are released, and the number of exocytotic figures corresponds to the estimated number of quanta released.[230,232] Membrane sites where exocytosis had occurred are marked by clusters of two to four large intramembrane particles that derive from the concave cytoplasmic fracture face of the original synaptic vesicle[230,231] (Fig. 15-20). This is excellent evidence that the synaptic vesicles collapse into the presynaptic membrane rather than open and close at the same site.[230] The same conclusion can be reached from the fact that stimulation of sympathetic ganglia during fixation results in a selective depletion of those vesicles aligned at the active zones, for if the vesicles reformed at the same site where they opened, their number should increase rather than decrease near the active zones.[233] Finally, there is convincing immunocytochemical evidence that synaptic vesicle membrane-specific antigens become incorporated into the presynaptic membrane when vesicle exocytosis is stimulated.[59,234,235]

ENDOCYTOTIC EVENTS AND THE FORMATION OF NEW SYNAPTIC VESICLES

Following exocytosis of ACh, the membrane of the synaptic vesicle is retrieved from the presynaptic membrane. Paradoxically, the rate of endocytosis is reduced by the increased cytosolic Ca^{2+} concentration that occurs immediately after prolonged or repetitive stimulation.[236] Two major mechanisms of vesicle retrieval have been proposed. The classic model postulates clathrin-mediated endocytotic uptake of the vesicular membrane either directly from the presynaptic membrane or from endosomal intermediates and away from the sites into which the vesicles collapsed during exocytosis.[99,100] Consistent with this is the increase in coated vesicles in the nerve terminal after increased transmitter release (Fig. 15-13). The clathrin-independent, or "kiss-and-run," model instead postulates rapid closure of a transient exocytotic fusion pore. This model allows the vesicle to retain its identity and remain in the pool of vesicles near the active zone.[234,235] According to proponents of the kiss-and-run hypothesis, clathrin-dependent endocytosis occurs only after severe and exhaustive stimulation, whereas rapid, direct retrieval of the vesicles predominates under most physiologic conditions. More recent evidence suggests that both endocytotic mechanisms might operate simultaneously, with vesicles retrieved by a clathrin-dependent

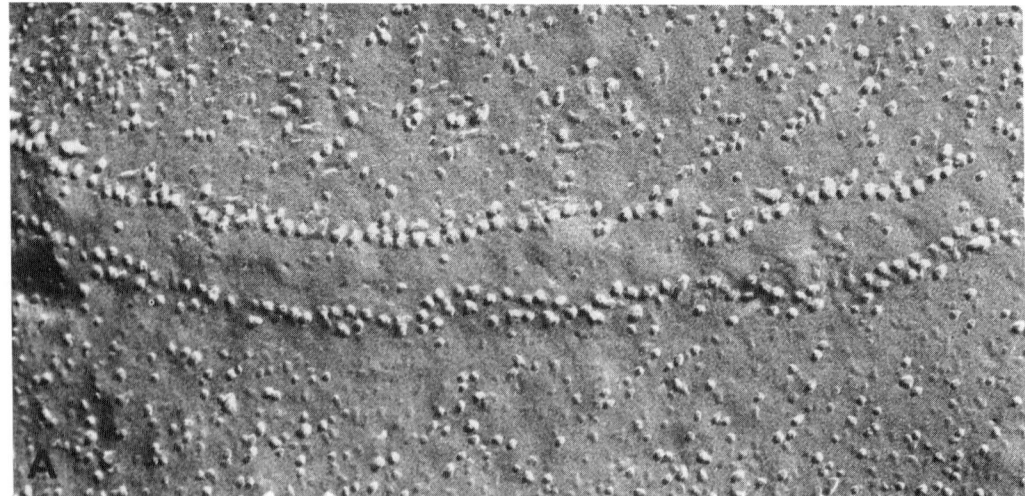
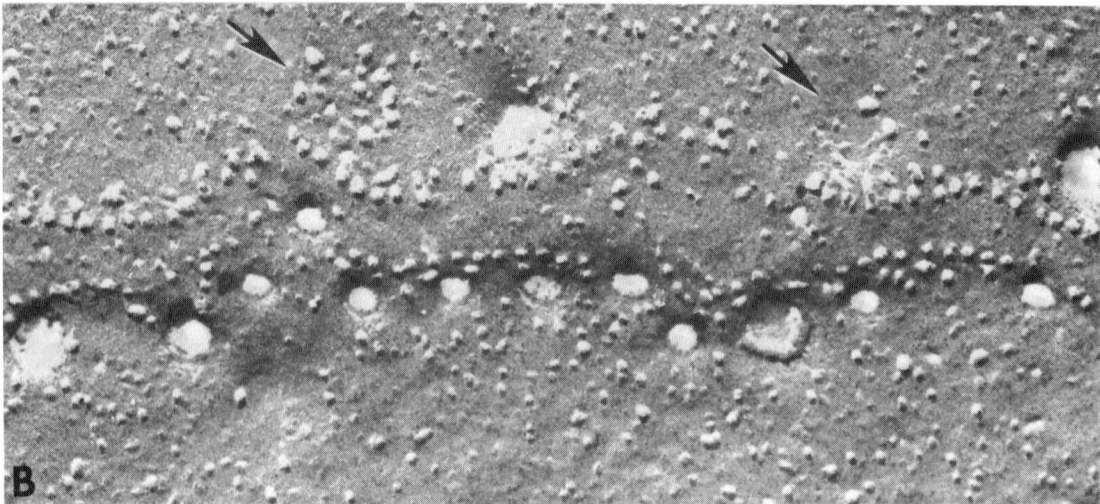

FIGURE 15-20. *A.* Presynaptic membrane P face of frog NMJ exposed to 1 mM 4-aminopyridine and 10 mM Ca^{2+} for 30 min and then given a single stimulus 3 ms before ultrarapid freezing. No exocytotic dimples can be observed adjacent to the active zones at this time. *B.* The presynaptic membrane P face of an active zone from a nerve terminal treated like that in *A*, but given one nerve stimulus 5 ms before freezing. Many exocytotic dimples now appear along the edges of the active zone. The two areas marked by arrows indicate vesicles that have collapsed flat after opening; these display a cluster of two or more large intramembrane particles like those found on the concave cytoplasmic fracture face of intact synaptic vesicles. (*A*, ×143,000; *B*, ×164,000.) These micrographs were prepared by Dr. John Heuser. (Heuser JE et al, *J Cell Biol* 81:275, 1979. With permission.[230])

endocytosis joining the reserve pool, and vesicles retrieved at their release sites accruing to the readily releasable pool of vesicles at the active zone.[237]

The major steps in the clathrin-mediated endocytotic pathway are now well understood.[238,239] First, the adaptor protein AP2 is recruited to the synaptic vesicle–derived patch of the presynaptic membrane; this results from the binding of AP2 to the C2b domain of vesicular synaptotagmin. Next, AP2 molecules form a lattice over the patch and recruit three-legged clathrin building blocks (triskelions).[102,103] Another adaptor protein, AP180, also promotes clathrin cage formation and, in addition, regulates the size of the synaptic vesicle and quanta by defining the amount of presynaptic membrane retrieved into clathrin cages during endocytosis.[240] In a process that requires ATP hydrolysis and GTP, the triskelions assemble into a polygonal network that invaginates the membrane patch so that it becomes a coated pit.[238,239] Complete separation of the coated pit from the presynaptic membrane begins with the amphiphysin-assisted assembly of dynamin molecules at the neck of the coated pit.[241,242] The dynamin molecules first form a choke ring, and then effect fission of the coated pit in a GTP-dependent way. In the last step, an uncoating ATPase denudes the internalized vesicle by dismantling its clathrin coat.[103]

The Synaptic Space

The synaptic space is situated between the presynaptic and postsynaptic membranes. The space is somewhat arbitrarily divided into a primary and a number of secondary clefts. The primary cleft is limited by the presynaptic membrane on

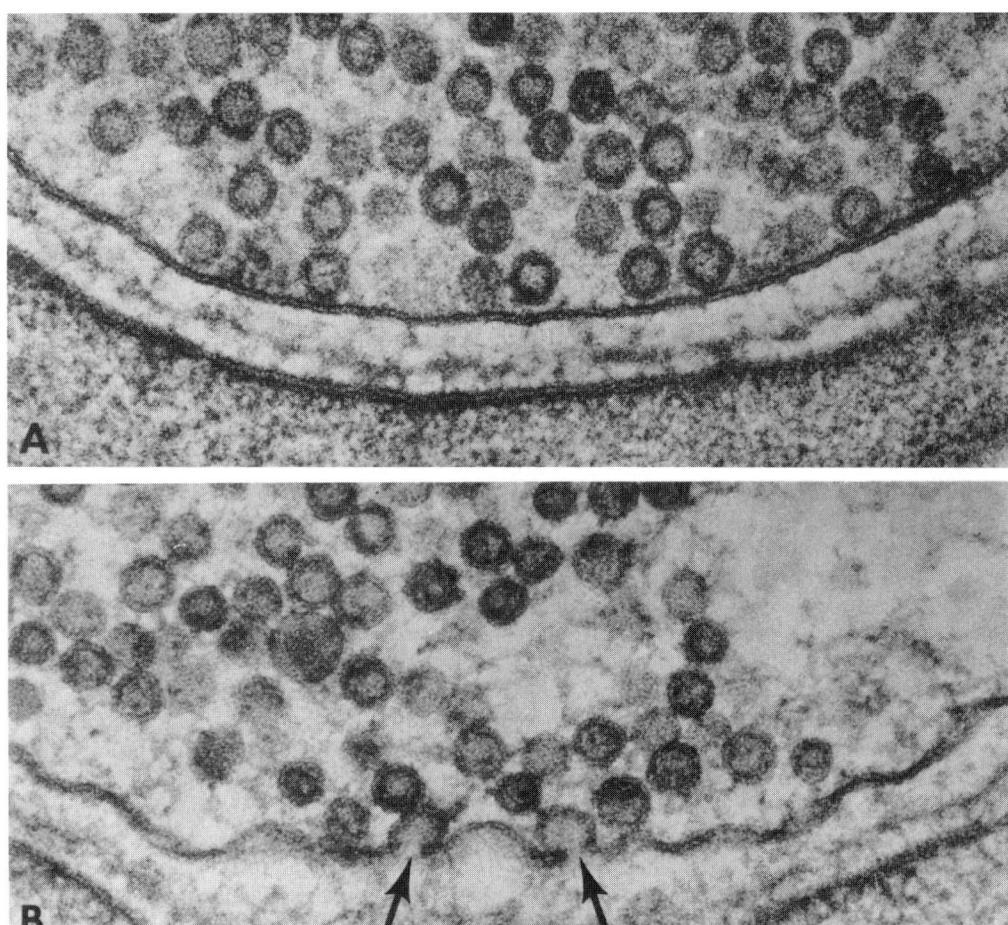

FIGURE 15-21. Frog NMJ *(A)* at rest and *(B)* after stimulation in 4-aminopyridine before ultrarapid freezing followed by freeze substitution fixation. The stimulated nerve terminal is sectioned through the active zone. It displays two omega-shaped exocytotic images (arrows) and many pockets. The smaller of these pockets have the same diameter and curvature as synaptic vesicles. The larger, shallower pockets look like collapsing vesicles. In both *A* and *B* the synaptic space shows a central, feathery layer of basal lamina connected by lateral extensions to the pre- and postsynaptic membranes. (×153,000.) These micrographs were prepared by Dr. John Heuser. *(Heuser JE, Reese TS, J Cell Biol 88:564, 1981. With permission.[231])*

one side and, on the opposite side, by an imaginary plane tangential to the terminal expansions of the junctional folds (Figs. 15-1, 15-10, and 15-11). It is approximately 70 nm wide, and its length is coextensive with that of the presynaptic membrane. The primary cleft lacks lateral boundaries except basement membrane and therefore communicates with the extracellular space. The secondary clefts are spaces between the junctional folds, and each secondary cleft communicates with the primary cleft (Figs. 15-1, 15-10, 15-13, 15-16, and 15-19). In the frog NMJ, the openings of the secondary clefts are in register with the overlying presynaptic membrane active zones (Fig. 15-16). A similar arrangement also exists at the mammalian NMJ[210] (Fig. 15-19). Finger-like extensions of Schwann cell cytoplasm cover small segments of the presynaptic membrane, isolating it from the synaptic space. These extensions appear at varying intervals between the active zones and are more frequent and regularly spaced at the frog than at the mammalian NMJ. The transverse tubules of the muscle fiber extend to and open into the secondary synaptic clefts.[243]

The Synaptic Basal Lamina

In conventionally fixed and embedded NMJs, a layer of basement membrane covers both the pre- and postsynaptic membranes (Figs. 15-1 and 15-10). A different image appears with quick freezing followed either by freeze-substitution fixation and thin sectioning (Fig. 15-21) or by freeze-fracture, deep-etching, and rotary shadowing (Fig. 15-22). The center of the synaptic cleft is occupied by a feathery 10- to 15-nm lamina from which wisps of material extend laterally toward both the pre- and postsynaptic membranes. In the primary synaptic cleft, these extensions form bridges between the two opposed membranes[51] (Figs. 15-21 and 15-22).

The synaptic basal lamina plays an important role in NMJ development and regeneration and in specifying the molecular architecture and physiologic properties of the pre- and postsynaptic membranes (see Chap. 20). Thus, the synaptic basal lamina contains factors that guide regenerating nerve terminals to previously denervated NMJs, induce physio-

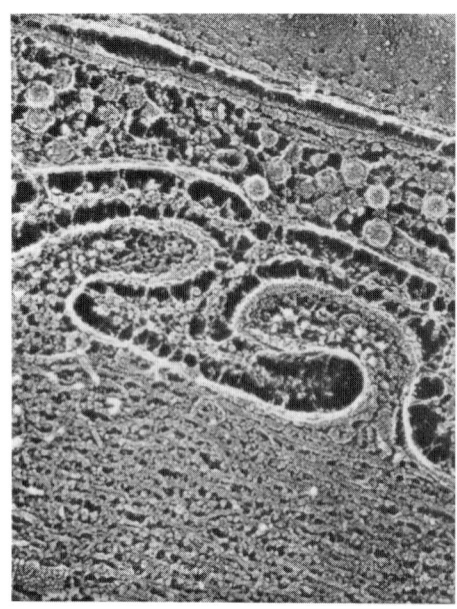 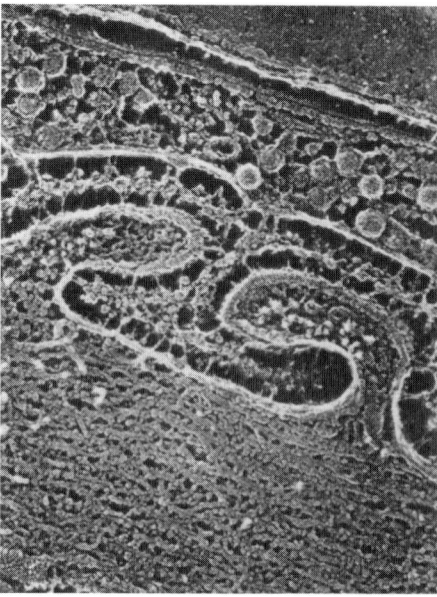

FIGURE 15-22. Stereo-pair electron micrographs of cross-fractured, deep-etched, and rotary-shadowed frog NMJ with vesicle containing nerve above and muscle cytoplasm below the convoluted synaptic space. The center of the synaptic space is occupied by basal lamina with lateral extensions toward both the pre- and postsynaptic membranes. (×80,000.) These micrographs were prepared by Dr. John Heuser. [Heuser JE, in Taxi J (ed): Ontogenesis and Functional Mechanism of Peripheral Synapses. New York: Elsevier/North Holland; 1980, pp 139–155. With permission.[51]]

logic and morphologic maturation of the nerve terminal even in the absence of the muscle fiber, and induce regeneration of the junctional folds and insertion of AChR into the folds even in the absence of the nerve terminal.[108,244–247]

The inductive and regulatory properties of the synaptic basal lamina must depend on its molecular components. The synapse-specific components of the basal lamina include laminins, asymmetrical AChE collagens α3–α5(IV), heparan sulfate proteoglycan, β-N-acetylgalactosamine (βGalNAc)-terminated glycoconjugates, and nerve-derived agrin and neuregulin/ARIA.[248–250] Agrin and neuregulin are discussed further below, under "Trophic Interactions."

Asymmetrical AChE. The synaptic basal lamina harbors the EP-specific asymmetrical species of AChE at a density of ~2000 to 3000/μm[251] (Fig. 15-23). Asymmetrical AChE consists of one, two, or three homotetrameric catalytic subunits (AChE$_T$) attached to a collagenic tail subunit formed by the triple-helical association of three collagen-like strands, ColQ.[252] ColQ has two major functions: (1) to bind tetramers of AChE$_T$ and (2) to attach the enzyme to the synaptic basal lamina. An N-terminal proline-rich attachment domain binds AChE$_T$.[253] Anchorage of the asymmetrical enzyme in the synaptic space is assured by two cationic heparan sulfate proteoglycan–binding domains within the collagen domain[254] as well as by residues in the C-terminal domain.[255,256] The tail subunit is anchored to the synaptic basal lamina by two binding partners: the heparan sulfate proteoglycan perlecan,[257] which, in turn, binds to dystroglycan, and the extracellular domain of the muscle-specific kinase (MuSK).[258] Association with these binding partners predicts close proximity of the extracellular asymmetrical enzyme to the postsynaptic membrane.

Synaptic laminins. Laminins are cruciform, heterotrimeric ~1000-kDa glycoproteins composed of a central α unit and flanking β and γ subunits. The three identified NMJ-specific laminins—laminin-4 (α2β2γ1), laminin-9 (α4β2γ1), and laminin-11 (α5β2γ1)—contain β2 subunits associated with different α and γ subunits. Laminin 9 is restricted to the primary synaptic cleft, whereas laminin 11 lines both the primary and secondary clefts. Laminins play multiple roles in the development and maintenance of the NMJ, as follows:

1. Extrajunctional laminins, and probably tenascin and fibronectin, together with junctional laminin 4, guide growing axons to the NMJ, where junctional laminin 11 stops axon growth.[249]
2. Laminin 11 actively prevents Schwann cells from entering the synaptic cleft.[259]

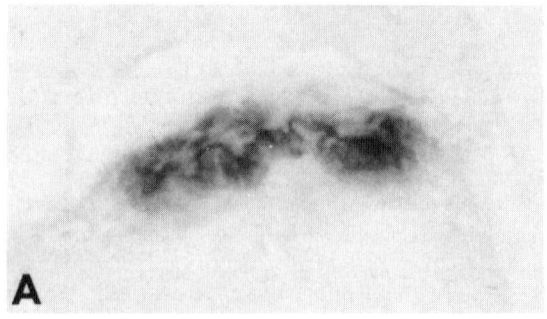
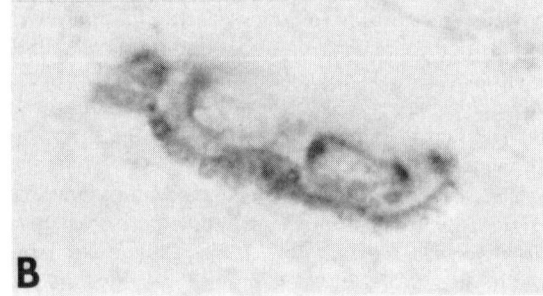

FIGURE 15-23. Immunoperoxidase staining with monoclonal anti-AChE antibodies of (A) human and (B) monkey NMJ. The association of AChE with the basal lamina is well established (see Chap. 20), but cannot be inferred from the light microscopic localization of the enzyme. (×2300.) (Fambrough DM, Engel AG, Rosenberry TL, Proc Natl Acad Sci USA, 79:1078, 1982. With permission.)

3. Both synaptic and extrasynaptic laminins bind to α-dystroglycan (α-DG), the extracellular component of the dystrophin/utrophin-associated transmembrane glycoprotein complex that links the extracellular matrix to the intracellular cytoskeleton. The attachment of synaptic laminins to the postsynaptic cytoskeleton may contribute to the immobilization of AChR at the NMJ.[260]
4. Junctional laminin 4 and extrajunctional laminin 2 (α2β1γ1) bind to the N-terminal domain of agrin and anchor it to the basal lamina.[261]
5. Laminin 1, present in very early muscle development, induces clustering of both α-DG[262] and AChR[263] independently of agrin. This could be a supplemental pathway for AChR clustering during myogenesis, but it does not occur at the mature NMJ.[263]
6. Mice with targeted deletion of the β2-laminin gene fail to express the β2 and α5 subunits of laminin and show simplified terminal branching of presynaptic motor axons, paucity of presynaptic active zones, no clustering of the synaptic vesicles at the active zones, and decreased spontaneous and evoked quantal release.[249,264] Homozygous mutants are weak, suffer from severe proteinuria, and die 15 to 25 days after birth.

The Postsynaptic Region

THE JUNCTIONAL FOLDS

The postsynaptic region consists of junctional folds and junctional sarcoplasm (Figs. 15-1 and 15-24). Junctional folds are found at no other synapse except the NMJ. At synapses that lack junctional folds, the surface areas of the pre- and postsynaptic membranes are essentially identical. The junctional folds produce a severalfold amplification of the postsynaptic surface. For example, morphometric studies of human external intercostal[28] and rat limb muscles[117,265] show that the mean ratio of postsynaptic to presynaptic membrane areas ranges from 8:1 to 10:1 and the mean postsynaptic membrane profile density ranges from 5.8 to 6.4 $\mu m/\mu m^2$. Because the junctional folds are separated by secondary synaptic clefts, they also increase the volume of the synaptic space.

The degree of development, complexity, and dimensions of the junctional folds vary according to species, stage of development, type of innervation, type of nerve ending, and muscle fiber type. For example, junctional folds are absent at newly formed NMJs (Fig. 15-25) and are relatively shallow or absent on multiply innervated muscle fibers (e.g., some extrafusal fibers in extraocular, facial, lingual, and laryngeal muscles and some intrafusal fibers).[75,86] In mammals, fast-twitch (type 2B) muscle fibers have better developed junctional folds than slow-twitch (type 1) muscle fibers, but in humans these differences are difficult to discern.[266]

The three-dimensional disposition of the junctional folds can be determined from serial sections[7] or by scanning electron microscopy.[61–63,267,268] At the linear frog NMJ the folds appear as a series of parallel ridges perpendicular to the long axis of the synaptic gutter. The folds become narrow and shallow at the end of the synaptic gutter and are irregular near the entry of the axon into the synaptic grove.[61] At the mammalian NMJ the junctional folds lack regular orientation with respect to the long axis of the muscle fiber,[7,62] but the crests of the folds still tend to be oriented more or less perpendicularly to the long axis of the irregularly curving synaptic gutter[63,267] (Figs. 15-8A and 15-26).

The junctional folds contain a varying complement of pinocytotic and other vesicles, small tubules and cisternae, microtubules, finer filaments, scattered ribosomes, and infrequent glycogen granules (Figs. 15-1 and 15-24). Some of the tubulovesicular structures in the folds are secondary lysosomes.[269] Coated vesicles appear in the junctional sarcoplasm during synaptogenesis, but are absent from the mature junctional folds.

The sarcolemma lining the terminal expansions of the junctional folds is packed with AChRs ($10,000/\mu m^2$)[39] and also contains rapsyn, integrins, MuSK, ErbB receptors, and N-acetylgalactosaminyl transferase.[270] The troughs of the junctional folds are enriched in neural cell adhesion molecules (NCAM) and in voltage-sensitive Na^+ channels. The Na^+ channels are tethered to the membrane by ankyrin G and β-spectrin,[271,272] and are linked to the cytoskeleton by syntrophins.[273] The cytoskeletal components of the folds include utrophin as well as dystrophin, both linked to isoforms of dystrobrevin and syntrophin, and via β- and α-dystroglycans to the extracellular matrix[108,270,271,274] (Fig. 15-27).

Functional significance of the junctional folds. The junctional folds enhance the safety margin of neuromuscular transmission by three mechanisms: (1) The terminal expansions and upper part of the stalks of the folds are "parking lots" for AChRs, increasing the surface harboring AChR about threefold over that available at synapses without junctional folds.[266] (2) The folds increase the series resistance of the postsynaptic membrane, and thus enhance the depolarization produced by the EPP.[275] (3) A high concentration of AChRs on crests of the folds[39] and on sodium channels in the depth of the folds[271,276] ensures that the depolarizing effect of the EPP is greatest where the sodium channels are concentrated at high density.[275,277] The combined effects of these mechanisms increase the safety factor of neuromuscular transmission at least two- to fourfold.

THE ACETYLCHOLINE RECEPTOR

The postsynaptic membrane on the terminal expansions of the junctional folds is thicker and denser than elsewhere, and its cytoplasmic surface is lined by a 20- to 40-nm layer of fuzzy material (Figs. 15-1 and 15-24). This subsynaptic density corresponds to the location of AChR and its cytoskeletal supporting elements.

AChR localizes with ^{125}I-BGT[278] or peroxidase-labeled BGT[279] on the terminal expansions, where the electron-dense thickened portions of the folds are located. At the mouse NMJ, the maximal concentration of BGT-binding sites is close to $20,000/\mu m^2$, indicating the presence of half as many AChR molecules per unit membrane area.[39] The binding-site density on the junctional folds decreases to 3 percent of the

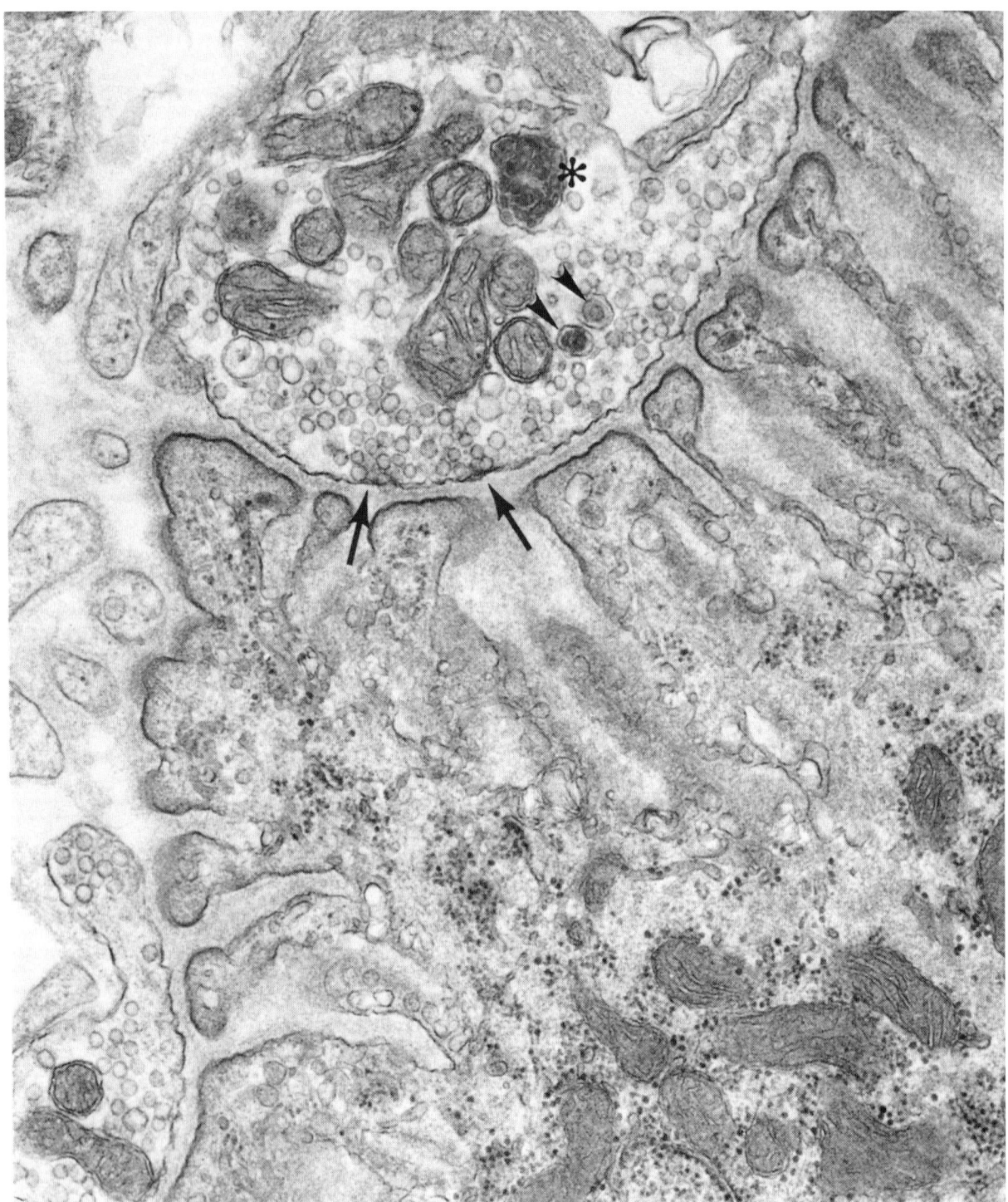

FIGURE 15-24, Normal NMJ in rat gastrocnemius muscle. In the nerve terminal, note dense-core vesicles (arrowheads), agglutinated vesicles surrounded by membrane (asterisk), and active zones in register with secondary synaptic clefts (arrows). The dense postsynaptic specializations are easily recognized on the terminal expansions of the junctional folds. Numerous microtubules, other tubular and vesicular structures, ribosomes, and pinocytotic vesicles can be observed in the junctional folds. The junctional sarcoplasm contains abundant mitochondria, ribosomes, rough- and smooth-surfaced ER, microtubules, and abundant microfilaments. (×40,400.)

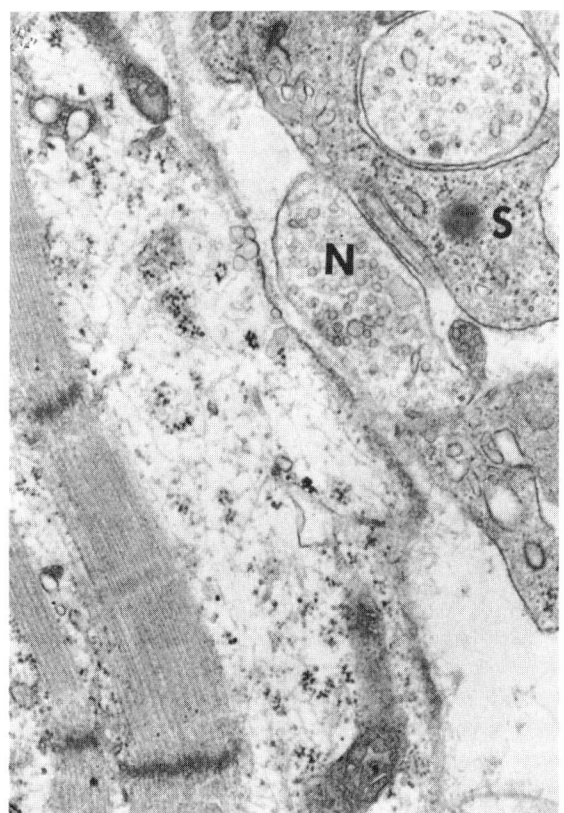

FIGURE 15-25. Developing NMJ in 11-day chick embryo intercostal muscle. The nerve terminal (N) is applied against a simple postsynaptic region. Postsynaptic membrane specialization has already appeared, and traces of basement membrane can be observed on the junctional and extrajunctional surface of the muscle fiber. The junctional cytoplasm contains few ribosomes, mitochondria, and fine filaments. At upper right, Schwann cell (S) surrounds another nerve terminal. (×25,000.) *(Freeman SS, Engel AG, Drachmann DD, Ann NY Acad Sci 274:46, 1976. With permission.)*

At the human external intercostal NMJ, approximately 30 percent of the postsynaptic membrane reacts for AChR.[279] The length of the postsynaptic membrane reacting for AChR normalized by the length of the primary synaptic cleft gives a measure, or index, of the relative abundance of AChR at a NMJ. At the normal human NMJ, the average AChR index is close to 3.[279] This means that the junctional folds increase the ACh-receptive membrane surface for each nerve terminal and each active zone. If the junctional folds are absent, as is the case at some NMJs, the AChR index must be ≤1 and the ACh-receptive surface per nerve terminal, and per active zone, is only one-third or less of that found at NMJs with well-developed junctional folds.

Freeze-fracture studies of the NMJ demonstrate large (10- to 12-nm) intramembrane particles packed in double parallel rows on the P-face of the junctional folds[41–43,50,209] (Figs. 15-30 and 15-31). This arrangement is probably secondary to dimerization of AChRs through their δ subunit.[283] The distribution of the particles is like that of BGT-binding sites, but the maximal particle density is one-half of that expected from ^{125}I-BGT-binding studies. However, the superior quick-freeze, deep-etch, rotary replication method reveals the expected maximal particle concentration of $10,000/\mu m^2$ on

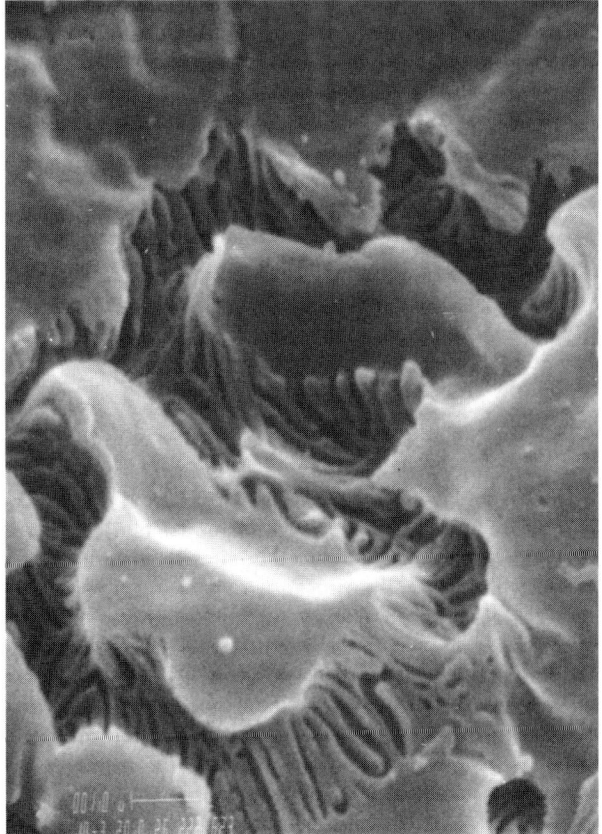

FIGURE 15-26. Scanning electron micrograph of mouse extensor digitorum muscle. The junctional folds tend to run perpendicularly to the long axis of the irregularly curving synaptic gutter. Where the gutter turns sharply or branches, the folds become irregularly oriented. (×10,000.) This micrograph was prepared by Dr. M. A. Fahim. *(Fahim MA et al, J Neurocytol 12:13, 1983. With permission.[63])*

peak value halfway down the folds and is only 4 percent of the peak value on the extrajunctional muscle fiber surface at a distance of 1 μm from the edge of the nerve terminal.[280] Although the autoradiographic method cannot exclude the presence of a small amount of presynaptic AChR, at least 95 percent of NMJ AChR is postsynaptic.[39] Further, no BGT binding is found on the nerve terminal when it is dissociated from the postsynaptic region.[281]

The localization of AChR with peroxidase-labeled BGT gives better light microscopic (Fig. 15-28) and ultrastructural (Fig. 15-29) resolution than autoradiography with ^{125}I-BGT. The peroxidase method reveals AChR on the terminal expansions of the junctional folds and for a variable distance along the stalks of the folds[40] (Fig. 15-29). Fainter reaction product also appears on the presynaptic membrane and Schwann cell processes facing reactive segments of the junctional folds. The staining of Schwann cell processes strongly suggests that any presynaptic localization is a diffusion artifact. That localization of extracellular antigens by the immunoperoxidase procedure is associated with diffusion artifact is now well established.[282]

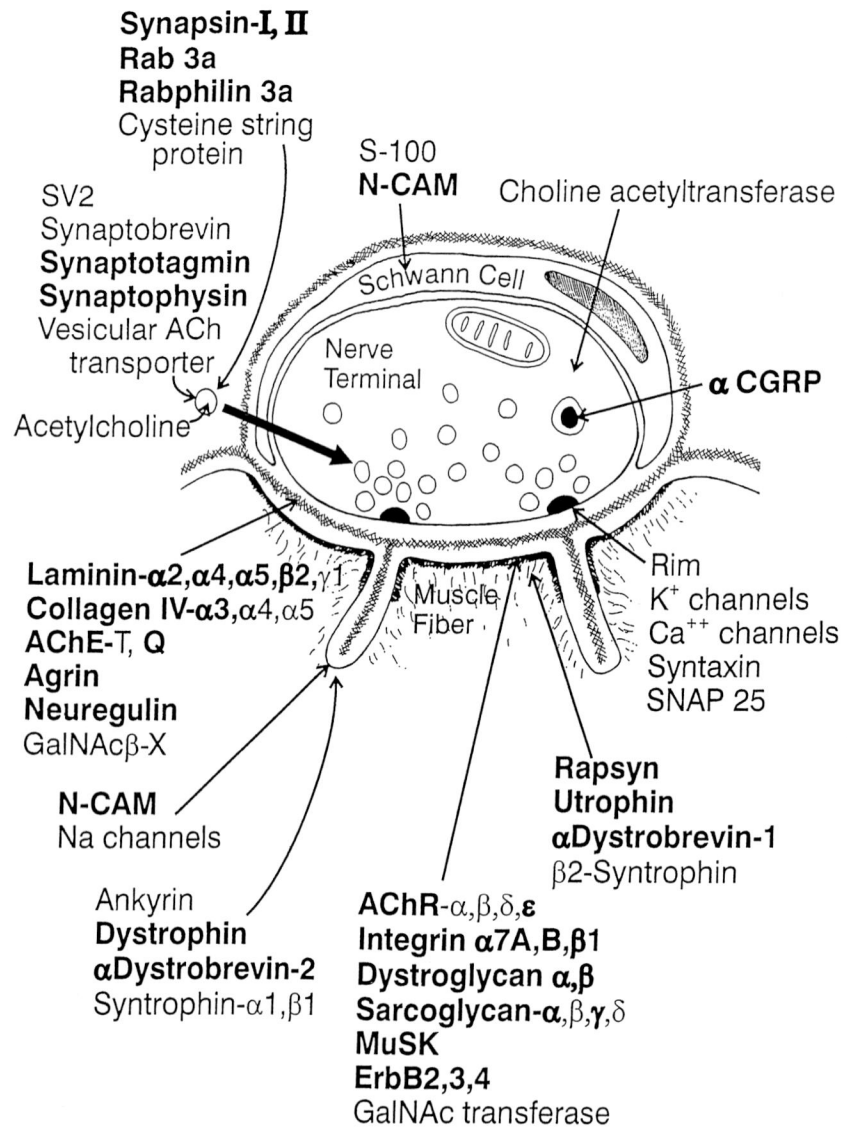

FIGURE 15-27. Key molecular components of the neuromuscular junction. Those components for which knockout mice have been generated are indicated in boldface. Additional components are described in the text. (From Sanes et al: J Physiol (Paris) 92:167–172, 1998. Reproduced by permission.[274])

the outside surface of the postsynaptic membrane at the Torpedo electroplaque synapse[44] (Fig. 15-32) and at the rat,[45,52] snake, and frog[52] NMJ. This value corresponds to the best autoradiographic and electrophysiologic estimates of the peak AChR packing density.[39,44]

At least three other membrane specializations are associated with densely packed AChRs: (1) The overlying basal lamina always contains a heparan sulfate proteoglycan,[284] (2) cholesterol is excluded from membrane domains containing densely packed AChR,[285] and (3) at both the mouse and Torpedo postsynaptic membranes tannic acid–mediated negative staining reveals bar-like projections attached to the cytoplasmic surface of AChR.[286] These projections are alkali-extractable[286,287] and immunostain for rapsyn, which cross-links AChRs[57] (see "Cytoskeletal Components," below). The molecular structure of AChR is considered in Chap. 17.

Structure-Function Correlations

The positioning of the presynaptic active zones in relation to the junctional folds (Figs. 15-16, 15-19, and 15-30), the density (10,000/μm^2) and distribution of AChRs on the terminal expansions of the junctional folds, and the lower density (2000 to 3000/μm^2) but uniform distribution of AChE throughout the synaptic basal lamina provide for effective interaction between the ACh quantum and a disk-like region of the postsynaptic membrane. These features form the basis of the "saturating disk model" of neuromuscular transmission.[39,251] ACh concentration is highest at the exocytotic site and gradually decreases as ACh spreads in the synaptic space. By the time ACh reaches the junctional folds, its average concentration (about 3 mM) is still sufficiently high to swamp AChE and also hinder the action of AChE by substrate inhibition. ACh needs to spread over a distance of only

0.3 μm along the top and the same distance down the side of the folds before it encounters the number of AChRs it can saturate. These factors favor the occurrence of most collisions between ACh and AChR within a few microseconds after quantal release and account for the short rise time of the quantal conductance change. After ACh dissociates from AChR, it diffuses laterally into the primary and radially into the secondary clefts and its concentration decreases. The depths of the secondary clefts, with sparse AChR (Figs. 15-29 through 15-31) and abundant AChE, serve as culs de sac for trapping and hydrolyzing ACh and for trapping choline, so that most of it can be taken up by the nerve terminal. Further, as mentioned above under "Functional Significance of the Junctional Folds," the alternating arrangement of voltage-sensitive sodium channels in the troughs and of AChR on the crests of the junctional folds facilitates the initiation of the action potential.[271]

The small size of the saturating disks of AChR assures that they do not overlap and that only a small proportion of all available disks is saturated with ACh when up to several hundred quanta are released by a nerve impulse. Since the active zone sites that release ACh are discrete and vary from impulse to impulse,[41,107,230,231] different sets of disks become saturated on repetitive stimulation. This prevents desensitization of AChR from continued exposure to ACh.

CYTOSKELETAL COMPONENTS

The junctional folds contain numerous cytoskeletal elements.[108,288] Some of these are topographically related to the AChR macromolecules, whereas others may confer rigidity on the folds. The following cytoskeletal proteins have been immunocytochemically localized to the postsynaptic region: rapsyn[57,289,290] (discussed above); α1-, β1-, and β2-syntrophins[291–293]; α-dystrobrevins-1 and -2[294,295]; tropomyosin 2[296]; actin[56]; talin[297]; vinculin[54,298]; an isoform of β-spectrin[299]; paxilin[300]; filamin[54]; α-actinin[54]; a lamin B–related protein[301]; ankyrin G[271,272]; desmin[302,303]; α-tubulin[304]; dystrophin[305,306]; utrophin[306,307]; and plectin[308] (Fig. 15-27). β-Amyloid precursor protein and amyloid-β protein are also present in the postsynaptic region, but their relation to the cytoskeleton and their functional significance is unclear.[309,310] The precise architectural organization of the cytoskeleton in the junctional folds has not been determined.

Although the above components are concentrated at the NMJ, all except rapsyn and utrophin normally are also present extrajunctionally. Rapsyn, the effector molecule of the agrin signaling pathway (discussed below, under "Agrin and Its Receptors and Effectors"), is present in a 1:1 stoichiometry with AChR. Rapsyn appears early in synaptogenesis, and cross-links AChR at the NMJ.[311] The molecule has distinct domains for membrane targeting, self-association, and AChR clustering.[312] Rapsyn is attached to the sarcolemma as well as to the subsynaptic cytoskeleton by binding to the cytoplasmic tail of β-dystroglycan.[313] The clustering of AChR by rapsyn depends on its coiled-coil domain near the C-terminus of rapsyn.[314] Mutations in rapsyn cause AChR deficiency at the NMJ and result in a congenital myasthenic syndrome[315] (see also Chap. 66). Utrophin, an autosomal dystrophin homologue, is closely associated with AChR on the crests of the junctional folds, while dystrophin and Na+

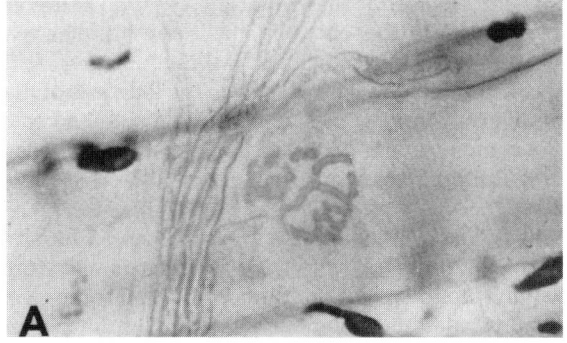
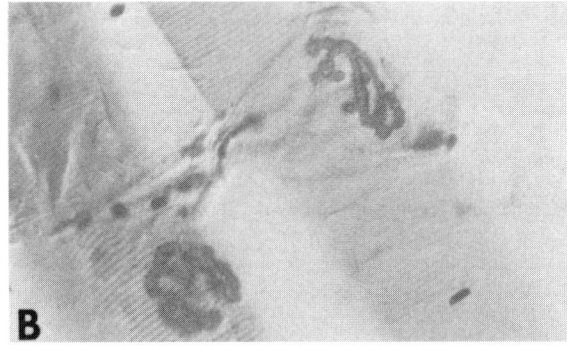
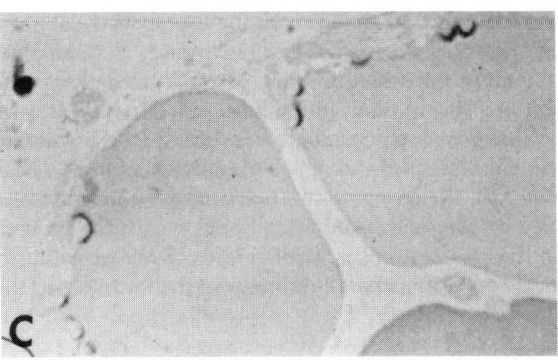
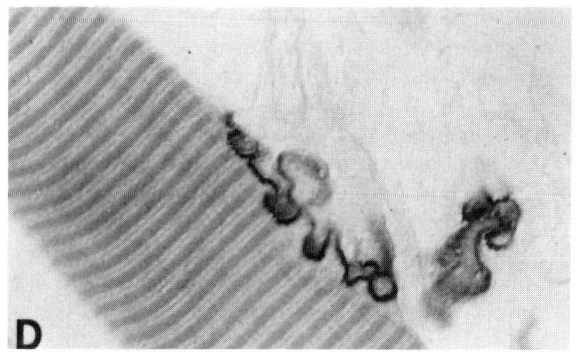

FIGURE 15-28. Light microscopic visualization of NMJ AChR on dissected muscle fibers (A, B) and in transverse (C) and longitudinal (D) sections before (A) and after (B, C, D) osmication. The AChR reactive sites outline the subneural apparatus, but the localization of the reaction product cannot be inferred from light microscopic observations. Nerve fibers near end plates are also observed in A, B, and D. (A, B ×400; C, D ×1000.) (Engel AG et al, Neurology 27:307, 1977. With permission.[279])

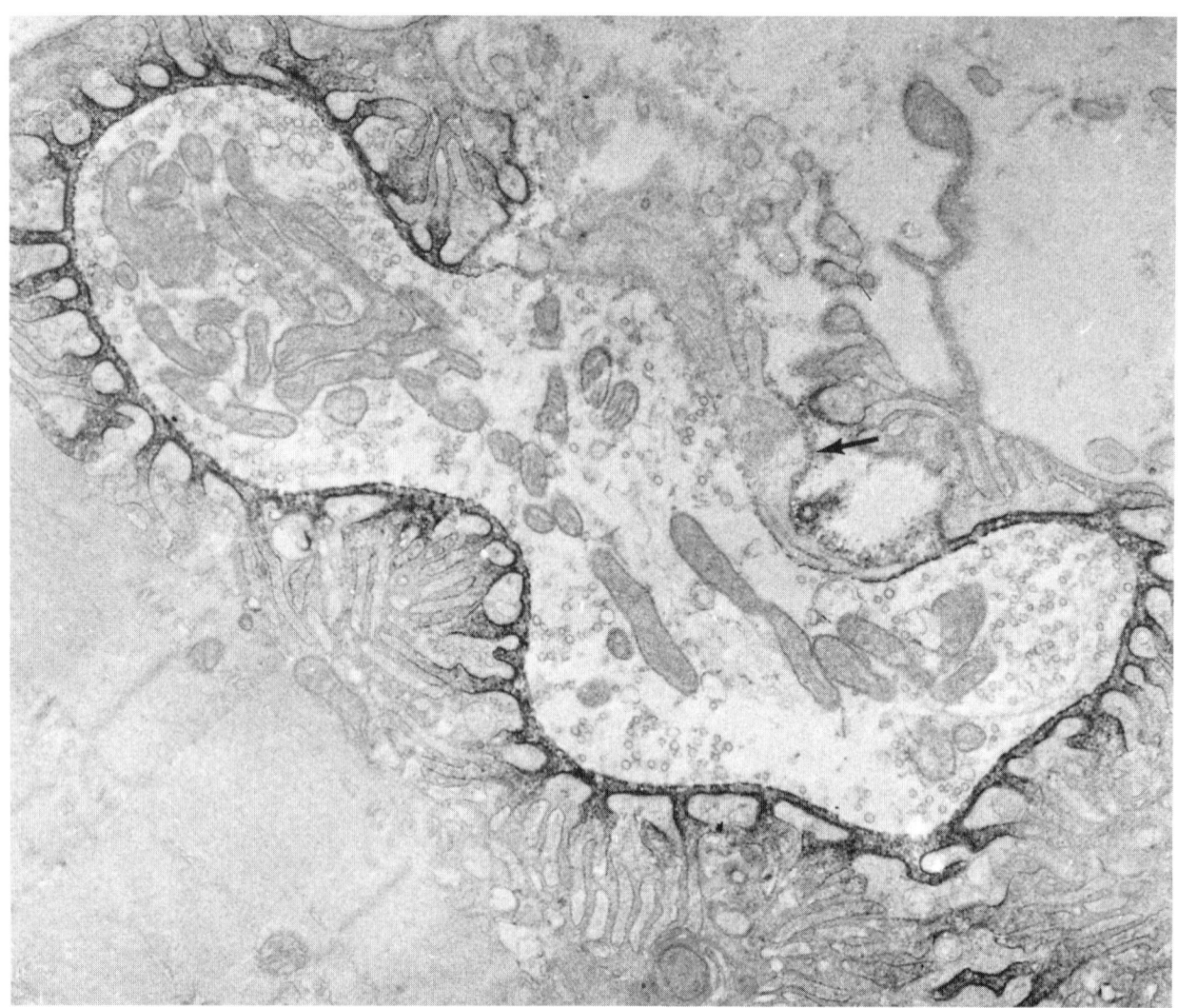

FIGURE 15-29. Ultrastructural localization of AChR with peroxidase-labeled BGT at the rat forelimb digit extensor NMJ. The electron-dense reaction product is localized on the terminal expansion of the junctional folds and extends on the stalks of the folds. Reaction product is also accumulating in the synaptic space and stains the adjacent presynaptic membrane. The presynaptic staining is most intense where this membrane faces the most intensely reacting portions of the junctional folds. Also note faint staining on the surface of a Schwann cell process (arrow). The presynaptic staining represents a diffusion artifact. (×18,400.) (Engel AG et al, Neurology 27:307, 1977. With permission.[279])

channels, together with β-spectrin and G-ankyrin, are concentrated in the depth of the folds.[272,316] Dystrophin is linked to the actin cytoskeleton and also to the extracellular matrix via the cytoplasmic tail of β-dystroglycan; it also associates with α1- and β1-syntrophins and with α-dystrobrevin-2.[293,295] Syntrophins bind the neuronal form of nitric oxide synthase (nNOS) as well as Na^+ channels and therefore act as modular adaptor proteins.[292] Since the density of AChR is not affected in patients with Duchenne dystrophy,[317] dystrophin does not participate in AChR clustering. Dystrophin, however, may regulate turnover of AChR, for in the dystrophin-deficient *mdx* mouse the turnover of AChR is accelerated ($t_{1/2}$ ~3 to 5 days instead of ~10 days).[318] Utrophin, like dystrophin, is linked to the actin cytoskeleton and to the extracellular matrix via β-dystroglycan,[319,320] and it also associates with β1- and β2-syntrophins[291] and α-dystrobrevin-1. The associations of utrophin with cytoskeletal proteins suggest that it plays an important role in the organization of the postsynaptic region and in clustering AChRs on the junctional folds. Utrophin expression at the NMJ is reduced when the density of AChRs at the NMJ is reduced, as in autoimmune myasthenia gravis and in congenital myasthenic syndromes in which AChR expression is reduced.[321] Utrophin-null mice, however, show only mild AChR deficiency and somewhat simplified junctional folds but no decrease in the packing density of AChR.[322,323]

At the mammalian NMJ, high-voltage electron microscopy demonstrates 10-nm filaments that run parallel and at a distance of 50 nm from the AChR-rich portion of the postsynaptic membrane. A network of "connecting" filaments extends from the "parallel" filaments to the dense postsynaptic membrane.[50] The quick-freeze, deep-etch, rotary replication procedure has been applied to the study of the subsynaptic cytoskeleton of the *Torpedo* electroplaque[44] and frog, snake, and rat NMJ.[44,52,298] This approach reveals a submembranous meshwork of short, thin strands that connects with more deeply positioned intermediate filaments coursing parallel to the postsynaptic folds[52,298] (Fig. 15-33). If paclitaxel (Taxol) is also used during the preparatory procedure, microtubules are often observed among the intermediate filaments.[52] The thin strands and intermediate filaments in these preparations correspond to the "connecting" and "parallel" filaments, respectively, observed by high-voltage electron microscopy.

Although the biochemical identity and precise connections of the subsynaptic cytoskeleton are still not fully understood, the following scheme appears probable at the present time:

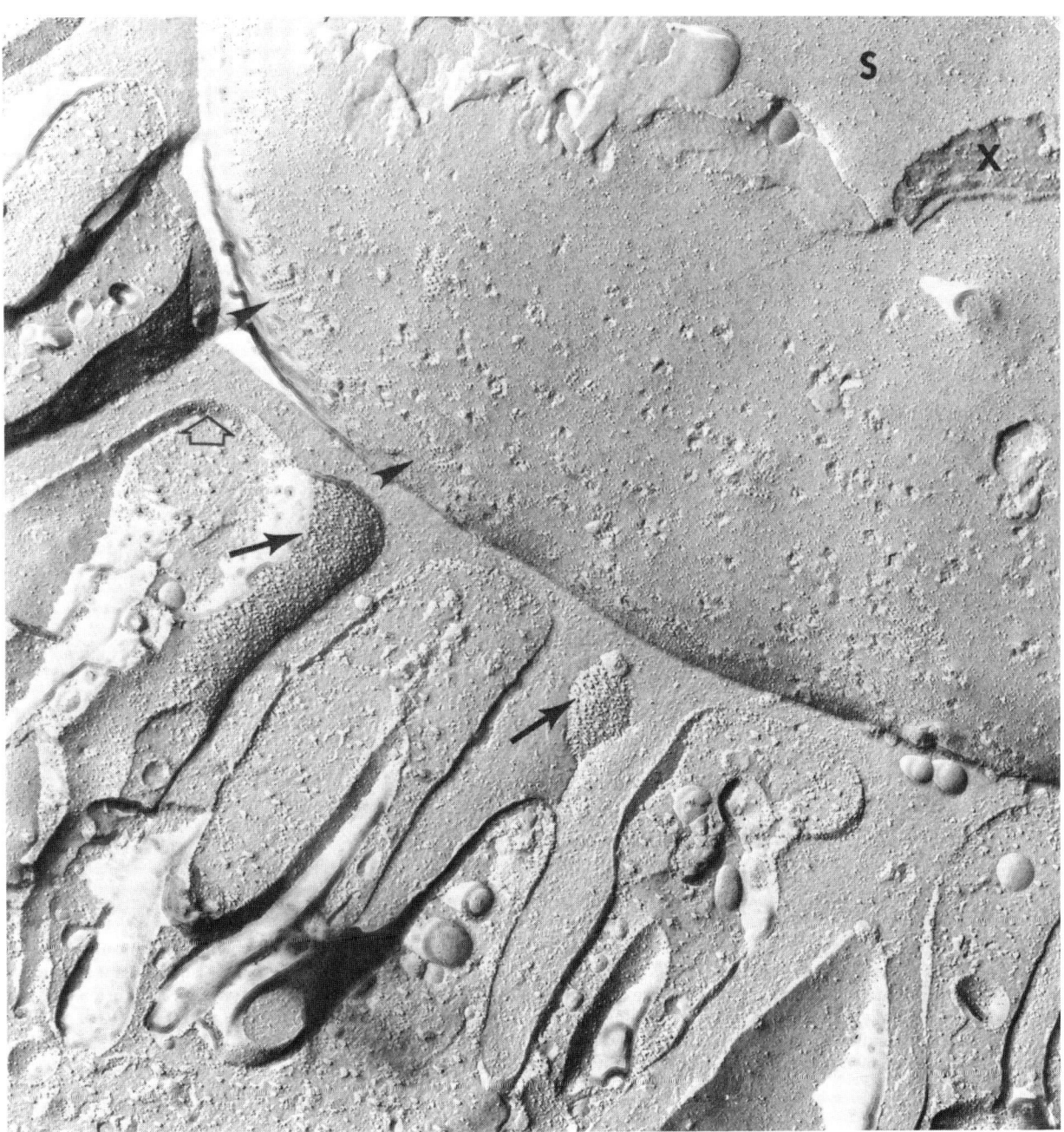

FIGURE 15-30. Freeze-fractured human external intercostal NMJ. The fracture plane traverses Schwann cell P face (S) and interior (X), axon terminal P face, synaptic cleft, and P faces and E faces and interior of junctional folds. The presynaptic membrane P face displays numerous active zones and exocytotic or endocytotic dimples. The upper portion of the exposed presynaptic membrane was covered by Schwann cell before fracture and does not display active zones or dimples. A number of active zones are in register with the secondary clefts (arrowheads). AChRs are represented by densely packed large particles on P faces of junctional folds (arrows) and corresponding pits in the E faces of the folds (open arrow). The AChR particles tend to course in double rows and extend more than halfway down the stalk of a junctional fold. (×50,000.) *(Fukunaga H et al, Muscle Nerve 5:686, 1982. With permission.)*

1. The AChRs are kept in compact arrays by a cross-linking network. This includes rapsyn, which links AChRs via β-dystroglycan to utrophin, which is linked to actin, β2-syntrophin, and dystrobrevin.
2. The cross-linking network is in contact with and is probably stabilized by a network of β-spectrin tetramers, which, in turn, are linked to actin oligomers.[299] These components may be part of the 20- to 40-nm-thick layer of fuzzy material that lines the AChR-rich portions of the postsynaptic membrane in routine preparations.
3. The meshwork of fine filaments is supported by a network of intermediate filaments and microtubules located in the deeper regions of the junctional folds.

THE JUNCTIONAL SARCOPLASM

In a longitudinally oriented fiber and with the NMJ on the upper surface of the fiber, the junctional sarcoplasm is limited inferiorly by the myofibrils (Figs. 15-1 and 15-34D); superiorly it extends to the base of the junctional folds and is continuous with it (Figs. 15-1 and 15-24) and/or is limited by sarcolemma between adjacent junctional regions (Fig. 15-34D). In the scanning electron microscope, the presence of junctional sarcoplasm is indicated by a mound-like elevation beneath and/or around the synaptic gutter[267] (Fig. 15-26). The amount of junctional sarcoplasm differs between different NMJs and even between different regions at a given NMJ.

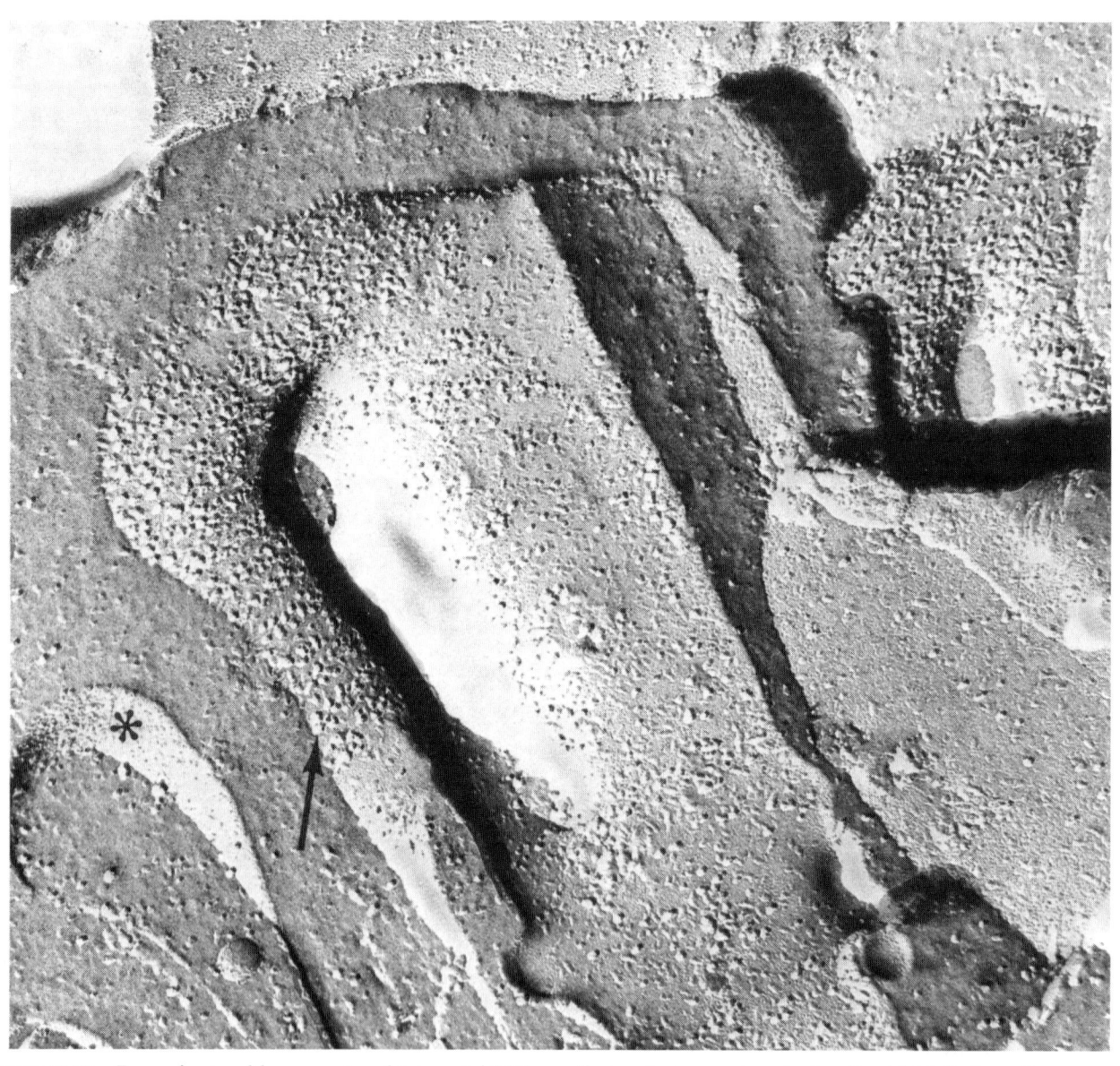

FIGURE 15-31. Freeze-fractured human external intercostal NMJ. Receptor particles exposed on P faces of two junctional folds are packed in double parallel rows. The fold in the center displays particles on its terminal expansion and its stalk (arrow). The E face of the terminal expansion of a junctional fold displays pits corresponding to the AChR particles (asterisk). (×103,000.) *(Engel AG, Fumagalli G: Ciba Foundation Symposium 90:197, 1982. With permission.)*

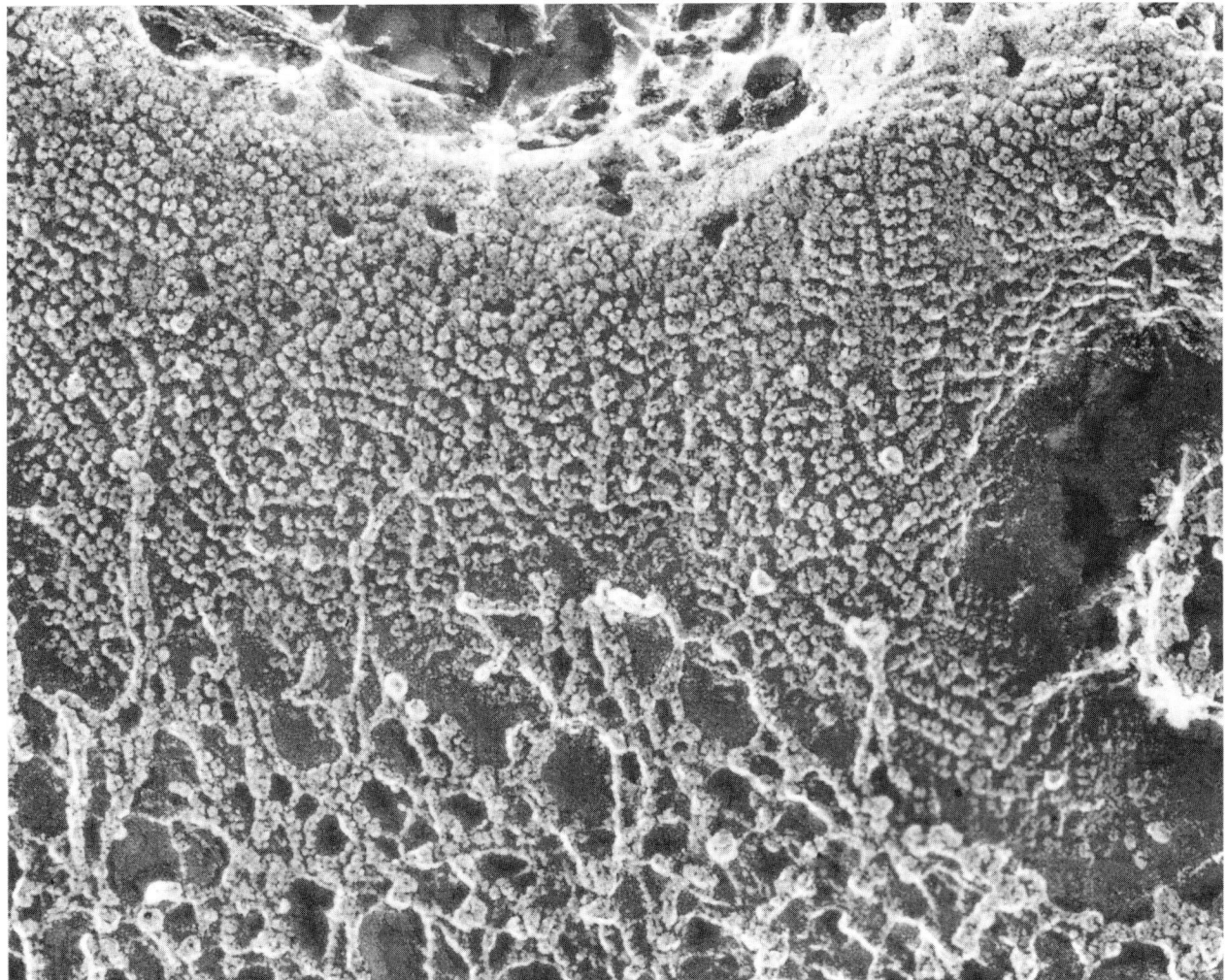

FIGURE 15-32. Organization of AChR in quick-frozen, deep-etched, and rotary-replicated *Torpedo* postsynaptic membrane. The figure provides a panoramic view of the membrane. At the lower portion of the figure, the membrane is obscured by lacelike basal lamina. At the right, this basal lamina forms a ring as it dips down into a dark postsynaptic invagination. The AChRs form linear arrays or occur as dimers and tetramers. (×203,000.) This micrograph was prepared by Dr. John Heuser. *(Heuser JE, Salpeter SR, J Cell Biol 82:150, 1979. With permission.[44])*

The junctional sarcoplasm contains a varying complement of mitochondria, smooth and rough endoplasmic reticulum, Golgi cisternae, lysosomal structures, small clear vesicles, microtubules, intermediate filaments, and scattered glycogen granules (Fig. 15-24). The region is traversed by transverse tubules (T tubules) that open into the secondary synaptic clefts. The known metabolic functions of the junctional sarcoplasm include the synthesis and degradation of AChR, synthesis of the end plate–specific species of AChE, and regulation of the subsynaptic ionic milieu. Multiple nuclei are adjacent to the junctional sarcoplasm at each NMJ or intermingle with it (Fig. 15-1). At the mature NMJ, subsynaptic nuclei are specialized to selectively transcribe mRNA for AChR subunits and for other NMJ-specific proteins.[324–326] In mature muscle fibers, AChR gene expression is spatially restricted to the subsynaptic nuclei.[326] The junctional sarcoplasm is also immunoreactive for cellular prion protein, ApoE, ubiquitin, superoxide dismutase, transforming growth factor β1, and interleukins 1α, 1β, and 6.[310] The biological significance of these proteins at the NMJ is not known.

AChR Synthesis and Degradation

AChR synthesis has not been studied in detail at the mature NMJ; however, it probably resembles that described in model cell systems (see reviews by Green[327] and by Keller and Taylor[328]). AChR subunit messenger RNAs are inserted into endoplasmic reticulum (ER) membrane; the nascent peptides within the ER are cotranslationally glycosylated and undergo initial rapid folding. The nascent peptides are protected against degradation by chaperones, such as calnexin. Next, slower folding reactions and other types of processing, such as disulfide bond formation and proline isomerization, take place to allow oligomerization with other subunits. Amino acids positioned at homologous sites at subunit interfaces direct partnering during assembly of the pentameric receptor.

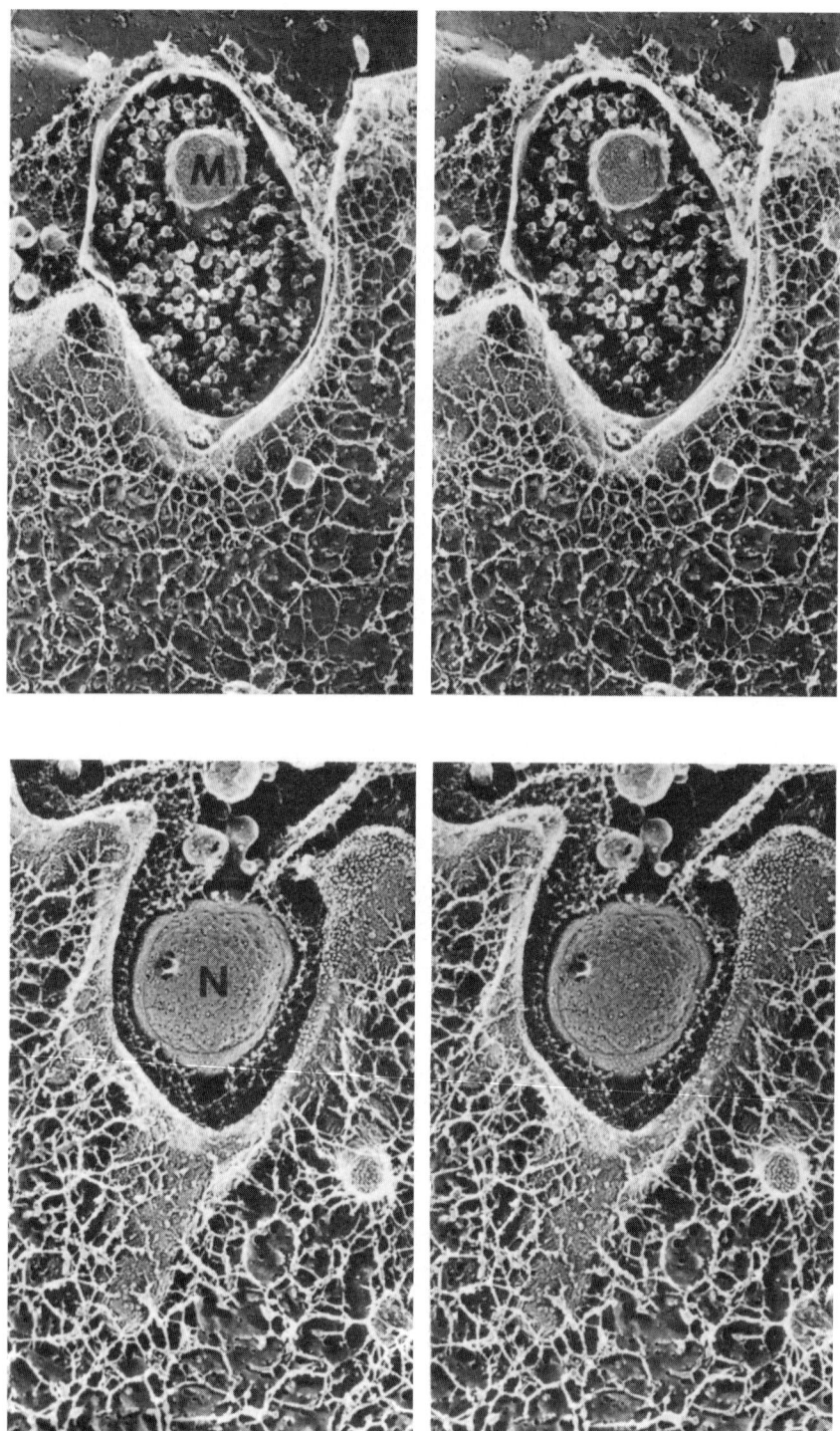

FIGURE 15-33. Stereo-pair electron micrographs of freeze-etched, rotary-replicated *Torpedo* electroplaque synapse. In the upper panel the nerve terminal is cross-fractured and the synaptic space has collapsed. In the lower panel the fracture plane traverses the P face of the nerve terminal and the synaptic space persists. This space contains a layer of basal lamina connected by delicate strands with the pre- and postsynaptic membranes. Both upper and lower panels display the subsynaptic meshwork of fine filaments connected to underlying intermediate filaments. M = mitochodrion, N = nerve terminal. (Upper panel, ×17,000; lower panel, ×23,000.) These micrographs were prepared by Dr. John Heuser. *(Heuser JE, Salpeter SR, J Cell Biol 82:150, 1979. With permission.[44])*

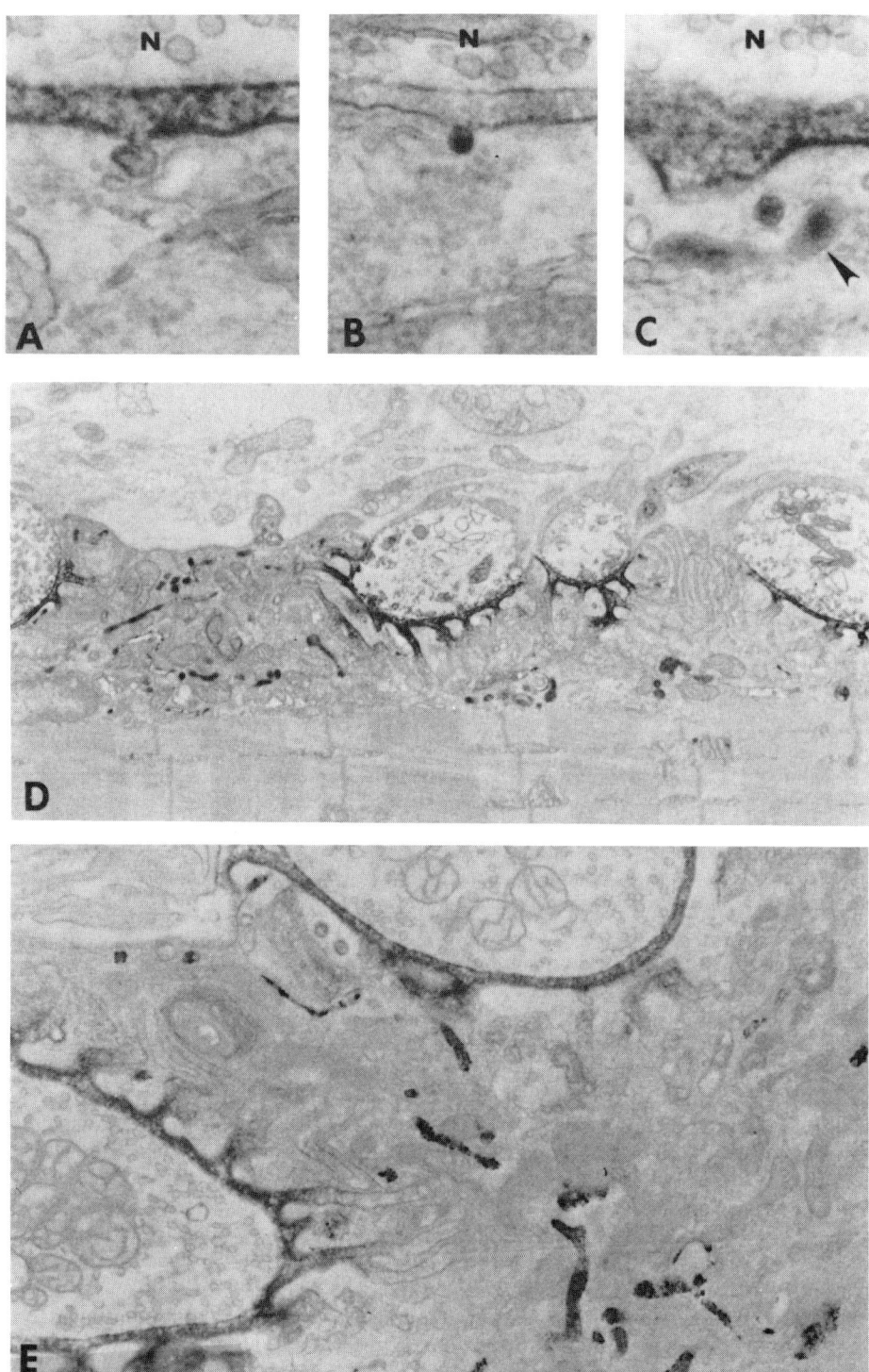

FIGURE 15-34. Ultrastructural study of the internalization of peroxidase-labeled BGT binding to AChR at the rat NMJ. In A, B, and C the nerve terminal (N) is positioned above the synaptic space. Within a few hours after labeling (A, B, C), AChR is noted in endocytotic invaginations of the postsynaptic membrane and in tubulovesicular structures (arrowhead in C). Twenty-four hours after labeling (D), abundant internalized label is present in tubulovesicular structures and larger cisternae in the junctional sarcoplasm. E. Double localization of acid phosphatase and peroxidase 24 h after intramuscular injection of labeled BGT. Punctate and highly electron-dense acid phosphatase reaction product (lead phosphate) is clearly distinguishable from the diffuse and less electron-dense peroxidase reaction product (osmium black). Nearly all tubulovesicular structures and cisternae are doubly stained. There is no acid phosphatase reaction product in the synaptic space. (A, B, C, ×75,000; D, ×11,300; E, ×25,100.) (Fumagalli G et al, J Neuropathol Exp Neurol 41:567, 1982. With permission.[269])

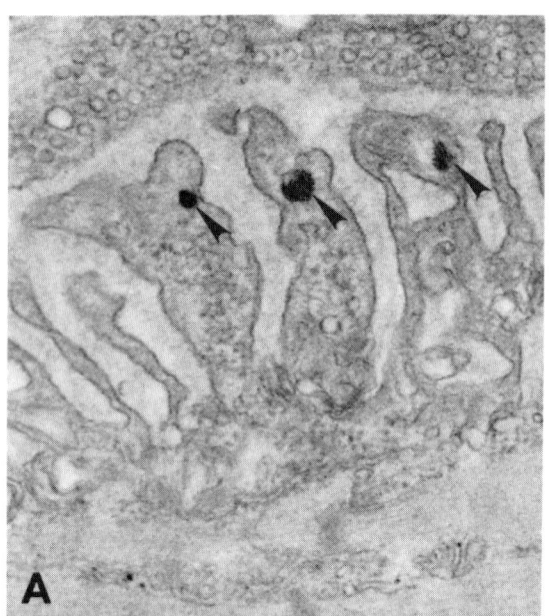
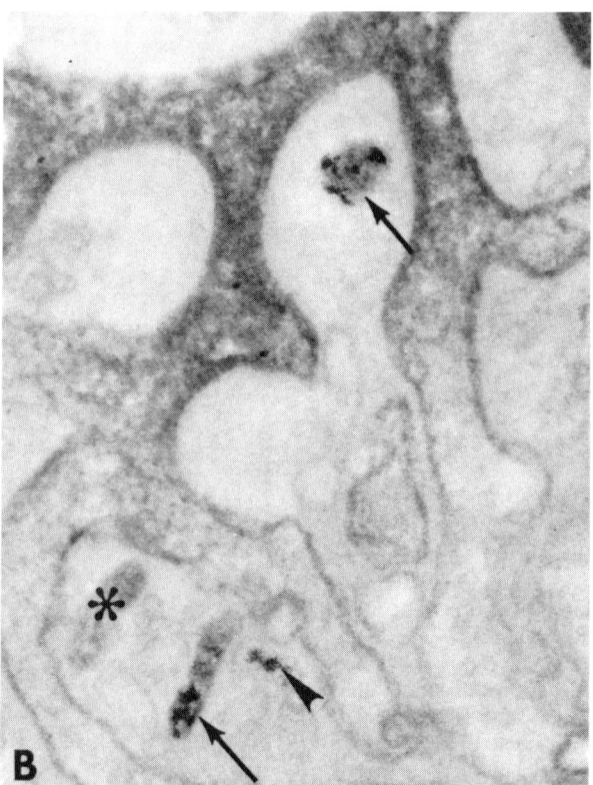

FIGURE 15-35. A. Rat NMJ reacted for acid phosphatase. Punctate and highly electron-dense reaction product is present in lysosomal vesicles in the junctional folds, very close to the postsynaptic membrane (arrowheads). B. Double localization of acid phosphatase and peroxidase 24 h after intramuscular injection of peroxidase-labeled BGT. Note the coexistence of acid phosphatase and peroxidase reaction products in vesicles and tubules in the junctional folds (arrows). One tubule reacts only for peroxidase (asterisk); one vesicle reacts only for acid phosphatase (arrowhead). (A, ×45,800; B, ×101,000.) (Fumagalli G et al, J Neuropathol Exp Neurol 41:567, 1982. With permission.[269])

The assembly process is not very efficient; it extends over 2 to 3 h, and only 20 to 30 percent of the synthesized subunits are assembled. The assembled receptor exits the ER to pass through Golgi cisternae and reaches the surface membrane along the secretory pathway on lipid rafts.[329] Unassembled subunits and intermediates dissociate from calnexin, become polyubiquinated at exposed lysines, enter the cytoplasm, and are degraded in proteasomes.

Recent ingenious studies investigated the manner in which assembled AChRs are inserted and maintained in the postsynaptic membrane: Observation of NMJs of living mice by reflected-light confocal microscopy over several days was combined with periodic laser-flash-induced unbinding of fluorescent BGTs from AChRs.[69] These studies revealed that (1) extrajunctional receptors migrate into the postsynaptic membrane; (2) receptors within the postsynaptic membrane migrate from one spot to another, both directly and by moving in and out of the membrane; and (3) AChRs are maintained for only ~8 h in any one spot. Thus during their 8- to 14-day half-lives at the mature NMJ, AChRs display a remarkable wanderlust. In mice lacking α-dystrobrevin, the rates of AChR turnover and intermingling are increased some four- to fivefold. Thus, α-dystrobrevin emerges as a critical regulator of AChR mobility and turnover.[69]

The macroscopic half-life of AChR at the mature NMJ is approximately 8 to 14 days.[330,331] The loss of labeled AChR is monoexponential, indicating that the probability of degradation is the same for all NMJ AChRs. If any receptors turn over more rapidly than others, then their number must be less than 50 sites per square micron.[330] AChR removal occurs randomly at a given NMJ[332] and on a given junctional fold.[269] AChR degradation after denervation is discussed below, under "Trophic Interactions."

When rat forelimb NMJ AChR is labeled in vivo with peroxidase-labeled BGT, the degradative pathway of AChR can be monitored by electron microscopy.[269] Membrane segments containing AChR are internalized by endocytotic invagination (Fig. 15-34A to C). The labeled vesicles merge with other membrane-bound vesicles, tubules, saccules, or cisternae within the junctional folds, and in the junctional sarcoplasm (Fig. 15-34C and D). Most of the membrane-bound structures containing the internalized label are lysosomes that react for acid phosphatase as well as the internalized AChR (Figs. 15-34E and 15-35), and a lysosomal network composed of tubules and vesicles can be observed throughout the junctional folds (Fig. 15-35A) and junctional sarcoplasm. These morphologic findings indicate that NMJ AChR is internalized by endocytosis and is then rapidly transferred to the lysosomal system, where it can be degraded.[269]

Synaptogenesis

The developing NMJ provides an unusually favorable system for correlating morphologic and physiologic parameters of development, for investigating trophic interactions between nerve and muscle, and for exploring the developmental regulation and the regulatory effects of the basal lamina, AChR, and AChE. Since 1966, the development of chick,[333–335] frog,[77] Xenopus,[336] rat,[335,337–339] mouse,[278] and human[340,341] NMJ has been studied in vivo. NMJ formation has also been investigated in organ cultures of fetal rat intercostal muscle[342] and in cocultures of fetal spinal cord and skeletal muscle obtained from the chick,[343] Xenopus,[344] and mouse.[345] Recent reviews summarize current understanding of the development of NMJ.[68,346]

General Principles

Developing muscles are penetrated by unmyelinated nerve fibers shortly before myoblasts fuse to form myotubes.[337] The earliest nerve-muscle contacts occur soon after the appearance of myotubes. The pre- and postnatal developmental steps are similar in different species, but their onset and the intervals between them vary.[77,336,340,341,347] For example, in human muscles,[341] primitive NMJs appear between the sixth and tenth week; but in mouse[278] and rat[339] muscles, NMJs appear between the 14th and 16th days of embryonic life.

In focally innervated muscles (e.g., the rat diaphragm), the initial synaptic contact occurs at random along the length of the short myotube. As a result of subsequent bidirectional longitudinal growth of the myotube, the initial synaptic site eventually falls close to the center of the mature muscle fiber. As development proceeds, each synapse receives polyaxonal innervation that is lost during the latter part of embryonic life and in the early postnatal period.[78] In muscles that receive a distributed innervation (e.g., the chick anterior latissimus dorsi), a series of synaptic contacts are established along the length of the early myotube, but the distance between individual synaptic contacts is always greater than 170 μm; each junctional site subsequently receives polyaxonal innervation and then loses it, so that eventually all synaptic contacts on the mature muscle fiber are supplied by a single motor neuron. As the fiber becomes elongated, the spacing between the NMJs increases.[335]

The Structural Development of the NMJ

Kelly and Zacks clearly described NMJ formation in rat intercostal muscle from day 16 in utero to day 10 postpartum.[338] On day 16, groups of primitive myotubes are in close apposition to clusters of axons. Early axon-myotube contacts are marked by a shallow depression and a local thickening of the myotube membrane, and traces of basal lamina appear in the rudimentary synaptic space. The axon terminals contain few clear and some dense-core synaptic vesicles.

On day 18 larger myotubes surrounded by and fusing with smaller myotubes and myoblasts are mutually innervated by clusters of axons. The axon terminals contain an increased number of synaptic vesicles. The synaptic gaps are 50 to 90 nm wide and are partially filled with basal lamina. AChE activity becomes detectable at the primitive NMJ.

On day 22, when birth occurs, adjacent small and large muscle fibers are mutually innervated by terminal axon networks covered by Schwann cells. The synaptic vesicles are relatively abundant, but dense-core vesicles are sparse. The primary synaptic clefts are short and the secondary clefts are rudimentary or absent. Incipient junctional sarcoplasm appears beneath or to one side of the postsynaptic membrane.

Ten days postpartum, some NMJs begin to look mature. Axon terminals covered by Schwann cells lie in individual synaptic gutters. The junctional sarcoplasm is more abundant and contains nuclei that are distributed between neighboring synaptic clefts.

With continued maturation, the synaptic site becomes larger, the ramifications of individual nerve terminals increase, the synaptic gutters become deeper, and the junctional folds become more elaborate.[347]

Structure-Function Correlations

The morphologic development of the NMJ has been correlated with changes in the packing density, metabolic stability, and gating properties of AChR, alterations in AChE, differentiation of the basal lamina, and changes in neuromuscular transmission.[46,278,339,342] The description below summarizes the findings at the developing rat and mouse NMJ.

Neuromuscular transmission begins on day 14 or 15 in utero. AChR accumulates at the NMJ 1 or 2 days later, and patches of thickened basal lamina are associated with the accumulating AChR. The initial packing density of AChR is about one-third of that found at the adult NMJ. The AChR turnover rate is as fast as at extrajunctional sites. Synaptic AChE appears 1 or 2 days after AChR begins to accumulate.

Between day 16 in utero and birth, the AChR half-life increases from about 1 day to 8 to 14 days, the half-life found at the mature NMJ. Junctional AChR increases and extrajunctional AChR gradually disappears.[348,349] Basal lamina covers the entire synaptic space; synapse-specific basal lamina antigens appear, and some extrasynaptic basal lamina antigens are cleared from the synaptic space.[46]

Polyaxonal innervation of the junctions peaks about day 17 and then begins to decline.[339] The quantum content (m) of the end plate potential (EPP) and the MEPP frequency are low and remain low until birth. This can be attributed to the relative smallness of the nerve terminal and lack of available quanta for release.[350] The duration of the MEPP and EPP is prolonged because the open time of the AChR ion channel is also prolonged.[351] This is due to the presence of γ-AChR, which has a lower conductance but longer open time than the mature ε-AChR.[352,353] The polyaxonal innervation and prolonged EPP facilitate synaptic transmission and compensate for the low m.[354]

During the first postnatal week, the junctions are still multiply innervated and show relatively little change. The MEPP frequency and m remain low.[278] During the second postnatal week, the postsynaptic surface increases rapidly. Junctional folds develop, and the fraction of the postsynaptic membrane occupied by AChR decreases. Polyaxonal innervation is now rapidly eliminated, so that the number of nerve terminals per

NMJ decreases. The MEPP frequency and m increase, due to an increase in nerve terminal size. The EPP and MEPP duration decrease, due to replacement of a γ-AChR by ε-AChR with a concomitant decrease in the open time and increase in the conductance of the AChR channel.[278,352,353]

Between the second postnatal week and adult life, the nerve terminals enlarge, the postsynaptic membrane surface increases 2-fold, and the AChR-enriched membrane area increases 1.6-fold. The continuing enlargement of the junction is proportional to the increase in muscle fiber diameter and is associated with an increase of m.[278,349] The enlargement of the nerve terminal is proportionate to the enlargement of the synaptic gutter. Repeated visualization of AChR at the same NMJ shows that previously labeled AChR spread apart in the membrane and new AChR are intercalated throughout the enlarging postsynaptic area.[355] Growth of the NMJ is not monotonic, however, for some nerve terminals retract and synaptic branches shorten as net lengthening proceeds.[356]

TROPHIC INTERACTIONS

The sequential changes in the structure, molecular architecture, and function of the developing NMJ imply trophic interactions between the various synaptic elements. Earlier studies of these interactions were based on examination of (1) the electrical activities of muscle cells in culture contacted by nerve growth cones, or patch-clamp recordings from the vicinity of nerve growth cones using excised membrane patches containing AChRs; (2) the effects of neural tissue extracts on cultured muscle cells; (3) the effects of selective ablation of pre- or postsynaptic components on synaptic regeneration; and (4) ectopic synapse formation, which occurs when a muscle containing a preimplanted foreign nerve has its own nerve cut. The initial studies have now been extended by identification of a number of trophic factors and the genes encoding them. A detailed account of the trophic interactions at the NMJ is beyond the scope of this chapter. Trophic interactions at the NMJ are considered further in several recent reviews.[68,346,357–359] Only a brief summary of selected topics is presented here.

Agrin and Its Receptors and Effectors

Agrin, a multidomain proteoglycan, named for its ability to aggregate AChR, is critically important in the organization and maintenance of the synapse.[360] Agrin occurs in different N- and C-terminal isoforms. Long and short N-terminal isoforms (LN and SN agrin) arise from different transcriptional start sites followed by a common sequence (Fig. 15-36). The amino terminus of LN agrin is essential for secretion of agrin into the extracellular matrix of the NMJ. SN agrin is expressed only in the central nervous system, where it is anchored to neuronal membranes through mediation of its unique amino terminus.[361] The secreted C-terminal z+ isoform of LN agrin induces postsynaptic differentiation by effecting accumulation of AChR, neuregulin receptors, rapsyn, and utrophin in the postsynaptic region and of neuregulin and AChE in the synaptic basal lamina.[362–365] Agrin-null mice have severely disorganized NMJs with sparse, scattered AChR clusters, motor nerve branches forming no terminals, and undifferentiated presynaptic regions.[366] Figure 15-36 is a schematic drawing of the agrin molecule, its binding domains, and molecules known to associate with agrin.[68,358,359,361,362,367] Muscle expresses a z-minus isoform of agrin,[368] which is 1000- to 10,000-fold less active than z+ agrin.[369]

NCAM, heparin-binding growth-associated molecule (HP-GAM), βGalNAc, integrins, and laminins all potentiate the agrin-induced aggregation of AChR[363,370–372] but are not the principal agrin receptors. Because agrin binds to α-DG,[373,374] initially α-DG was thought to be the principal agrin receptor. However, some agrin mutants can cluster

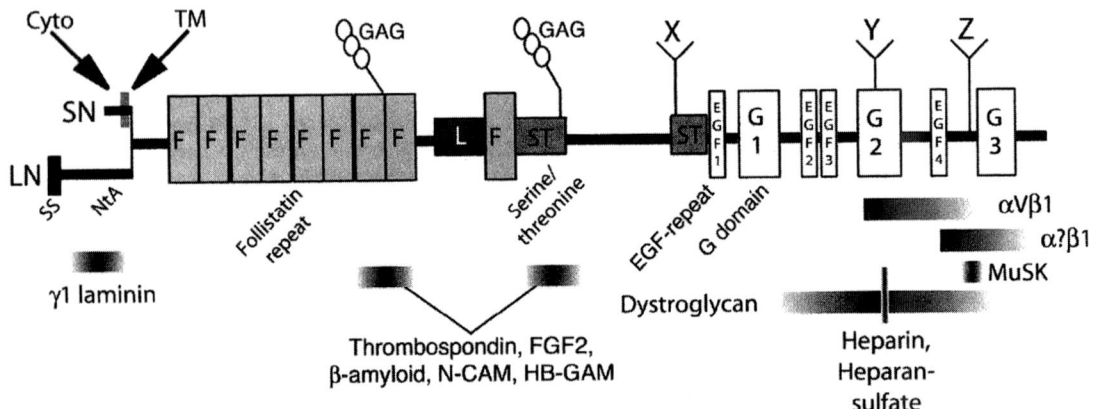

FIGURE 15-36. The agrin protein and its interactions. The domain structure of agrin is shown at the top. SN and LN are distinct N-termini encoded by unique exons and are respectively responsible for insertion into the NMJ basal lamina and for anchoring agrin in neuronal membranes in the brain. LN has a signal peptide and a laminin-binding domain (NtA). F, follistatin repeats; GAG, sites of glycosaminoglycan addition; L, laminin III domain; ST, serine/threonine-rich regions; EGFs, epidermal growth factor–like repeats; G, laminin type G domains; X, Y, and Z are sites of alternative splicing. Shaded boxes indicate their region of interaction with the agrin protein. Growing neurites adhere to G2 via αVβ1 integrin, to EGF4 via a distinct β1 integrin, and to a third N-terminal site.[301] Proteins interacting with agrin are shown at the bottom. FGF, fibroblast growth factor. (From Burgess et al: J Neurochem 83:271–284, 2002. Reproduced by permission.[361])

AChR without binding to α-DG or bind to α-DG but without clustering AChR.[362] Subsequent studies implicated MuSK, a muscle-specific transmembrane protein with intrinsic tyrosine kinase activity, as the main agrin receptor. MuSK is expressed in close association with AChR in developing muscle, and agrin is responsible for its aggregation, phosphorylation, and dimerization at the NMJ.[375] MuSK aggregation, in turn, is accompanied by accumulation of β-2 laminins and of AChE in the synaptic space. MuSK knockout mice closely resemble agrin knockout mice in that they lack differentiated NMJs, but myotubes cultured from the MuSK-deficient mice do not respond to agrin.[376,377] However, agrin does not bind to MuSK directly, but via a receptor complex that includes MuSK and a hypothetical muscle-associated specificity component, MASC.[376,378]

Rapsyn induces clustering of AChR by binding it to a postsynaptic scaffold.[379] Rapsyn knockout mice cluster AChR poorly and fail to accumulate dystroglycan, utrophin, and ErbB receptors at the NMJ. Thus, rapsyn is an effector of agrin-induced clustering. The absence of rapsyn, however, does not abrogate the accumulation of MuSK, β2-laminins, and AChE at the NMJs, nor does it abolish synapse-specific transcription by the junctional nuclei.[363,380,381] This suggests that agrin acts on the MuSK/MASC complex, causing MuSK to cluster postsynaptically, and that a MuSK scaffold, acting together with rapsyn, induces clustering of AChR, ErbB receptors, dystroglycan, and utrophin.[362,363]

The MuSK ectodomain mediates the rapsyn-dependent aggregation of AChR via a still unidentified rapsyn-associated transmembrane linker (RATL), while the MuSK endodomain phosphorylates β and δ subunits of AChR via src-like kinases[377,378,381] in a rapsyn-dependent manner.[382] Phosphorylation of AChR stabilizes and promotes the cytoskeletal linkage of the AChR aggregates.[359] In a hypothetical model, MuSK also uses rapsyn to recruit utrophin, dystroglycan, and ErbB receptors to the synapse. This model assigns both a signaling and a structural role to MuSK in synapse formation.[363]

A recent study proposes that stimulation of MuSK by agrin leads to activation of Cdc-42 and Rac (members of the Rho family of monomeric GTPases), which subsequently activate PAK (a p21 activated kinase). Disheveled (Dvl) then interacts with MuSK and PAK, forming a signaling scaffold required for AChR clustering.[382a]

Other studies have revealed that AChR clusters first appear in central regions of developing noninnervated myotubes in a MuSK- and rapsyn-dependent but agrin-independent manner (prepatterning). After the arrival of the nerve terminal, agrin together with its postsynaptic effectors causes further clustering and stabilization of AChRs in the synaptic region.[383,384] Moreover, AChRs themselves are required for agrin-induced clustering of rapsyn and of some other postsynaptic proteins.[385,386]

Regulation of Synapse-Specific Transcription

Two major candidates for regulation of synapse-specific transcription have emerged. The first, α-calcitonin gene–related peptide (αCGRP), is stored and released from dense-core vesicles of the motor nerve terminal.[109] CGRP increases the synthesis and membrane insertion of AChR in cultured myotubes in a cAMP-dependent manner.[387,388] However, αCGRP-null mice have normal NMJs and show no phenotypic abnormality.[389]

The second candidate to regulate synapse-specific transcription is neuregulin (previously called ARIA, for AChR-inducing activity), an isoform produced by the nr-1 gene. Neuregulin, like agrin, is a motor nerve–derived trophic factor and a member of a family of growth factors that are differentially distributed among functionally distinct classes of neurons.[390,391] Mice homozygous for deletion of neuregulin die before birth; heterozygous animals survive, but with NMJs deficient in AChR and with a reduced safety margin of neuromuscular transmission.[392] The postsynaptic receptor for neuregulin is formed by ErbB2, ErbB3, and ErbB4, members of the 185-kDa epidermal growth factor–related transmembrane receptor tyrosine kinases.[378,393,394] In cultured muscle cells, liganded ErbB receptors activate mitogen-activated protein (MAP) kinases.[395,396] These, in turn, phosphorylate a heterodimeric GA-binding protein (GABPα/β), a member of the Ets-binding family, which serves as a transcription activating factor.[397] Phosphorylated GABPα/β binds to a specific neuregulin response element designated as the Ets-binding site, or N-box, in the promoter regions of genes coding for utrophin and AChE and for the AChR δ and ε and possibly α subunits.[389,397–400] Figure 15-37 shows a proposed scheme of the neuregulin signaling at the NMJ.

A direct or exclusive role of neuregulin in controlling synapse-specific transcription has been questioned for two main reasons: (1) Neuregulin exerts a strong mitogenic effect on Schwann cells, which, in turn, are required for differentiation of the nerve terminal. Thus, the effect on synapse-specific transcription could in part be mediated by factors residing in Schwann cells. (2) Muscle also synthesizes neuregulin that can act downstream of agrin. Consistent with this, agrin in and of itself can augment AChR gene transcription in cultured myotubes via ErbB receptors. Thus, agrin can enhance postsynaptic transcription independent of neuregulin released from the nerve terminal.[346] Whether postsynaptic transcription is stimulated by nerve-released neuregulin, by agrin acting on muscle-derived neuregulin, or both, there is good evidence that the resultant binding of Ets factors GABPα/β to the N-box enhances transcription of selected postsynaptic genes: (1) Missense mutations in the N-box of the AChR ε subunit reduce AChR transcription at the NMJ and result in a congenital myasthenic syndrome[401,402] (see also Chap. 66). (2) Transgenic mice harboring a dominant-negative Ets mutation, which blocks binding of GABPα/β to the N-box, show a ≥50 percent decrease in expression of genes for the AChR ε subunit, AChE, β2-laminin, and utrophin A, and a ~30 percent decrease in expression of the gene for the AChR α subunit; utrophin B, MuSK, and the rapsyn gene expressions are unaffected.[403] Neuregulin also has other inductive functions at the NMJ. One of these is to promote the accumulation of voltage-gated Na$^+$ channels in the depths of synaptic clefts.[270]

Shortly after neuregulin appears at the developing NMJ, fetal AChRs containing the γ subunit (γ-AChRs) are replaced by adult AChRs harboring the ε subunit (ε-AChRs). Continued expression of the ε subunit at the NMJ depends on the presence of neuregulin in the synaptic basal lamina[270,404] or activation of muscle neuregulin by agrin.

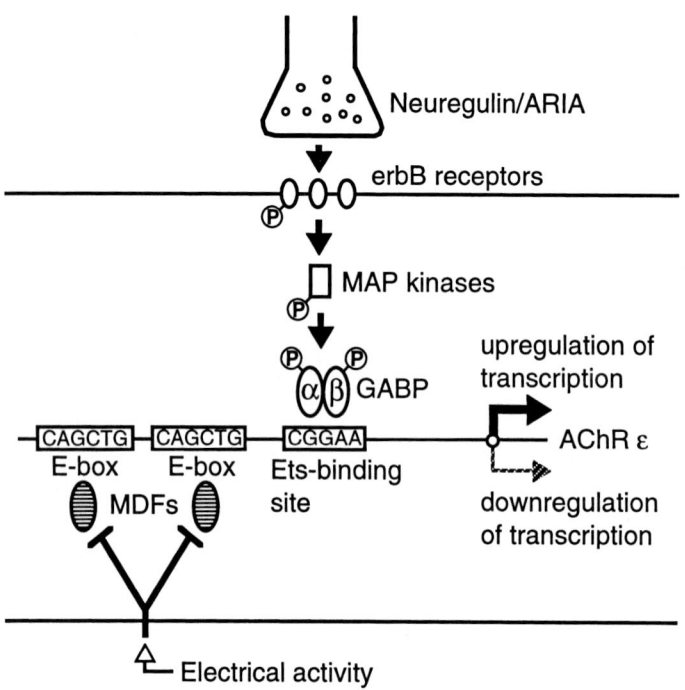

FIGURE 15-37. Scheme showing proposed upregulation of AChR transcription by subsynaptic nuclei by the neuregulin/ARIA signaling pathway and the downregulation of AChR transcription at extrasynaptic nuclei by electrical activity. Neuregulin/ARIA released from the nerve terminal binds to and activates the ErbB family receptor tyrosine kinases on the muscle cell membrane, which then activate a mitogen-activated protein (MAP) kinase signaling cascade. MAP kinases phosphorylate the GABPα/β, which activates transcription of the AChR ε subunit gene by binding to the Ets-binding site in the promoter region of the ε subunit gene. Electrical activity of the innervated muscle causes phosphorylation of the myogenic differentiation factor (MDF) myogenin by protein kinase C. This, in turn, abrogates the ability of myogenin to stimulate the transcription of AChR subunit genes at extrasynaptic nuclei. There is now evidence that the signaling cascade can also be initiated by agrin acting on muscle-derived neuregulin. (*From Ohno et al. Neuromuscul Disord 9:131–135, 1999. Reproduced by permission.*[401])

The Metabolic Stability of NMJ AChR

The metabolic stability of NMJ AChR (i.e., its half-life) depends on innervation. At the mature innervated NMJ, the AChR half-life is about 8 to 14 days, while extrajunctional AChR on myotubes or in denervated muscle is only about 1 day.[331,405] At the denervated NMJ, the degradation of the preexisting AChR accelerates to a half-life of 3 days but returns to normal with reinnervation. Newly synthesized AChRs incorporated into the denervated NMJ have a half-life of about 1 day, and their degradation rate is not slowed down by reinnervation.[331]

The stabilizing effect of innervation on AChR turnover is mediated by activity-dependent calcium influx into the muscle fiber. Stabilization of the turnover of junctional but not of extrajunctional AChR can be induced in the absence of activity if muscles are treated with the calcium ionophore A23187. Conversely, the activity-dependent stabilization of AChR is prevented if the muscle is stimulated in the presence of calcium channel blockers.[406]

Regulation of the Distribution and Kinetic Properties of AChR

Two heterooligomeric forms of muscle AChR exist: an immature extrajunctional form made up of $\alpha_2\beta\delta\gamma$ subunits (γ-AChR) and a mature junctional form consisting of $\alpha_2\beta\delta\varepsilon$ subunits (ε-AChR). γ-AChR has a lower conductance and longer mean open time than AChR. Before innervation, γ-AChR is diffusely distributed over the entire fiber surface; during early synapse formation, γ-AChR is concentrated at the NMJ and disappears from the extrajunctional sites. Subsequently (during the first 14 postnatal days in the rat), γ-AChR is replaced by ε-AChR at the NMJ.[407–409] Experimental studies have defined several regulatory influences underlying the appearance of ε-AChR at the NMJ and the disappearance of γ-AChR from the rest of the muscle fiber.[353] These influences act transiently as neural imprinting signals or continuously as inhibitory signals, and they affect the different AChR subunit genes differently. The following interactions have been identified[353]:

1. Neural agrin causes aggregation of AChR at the NMJ during early synapse formation and maintains this influence after it becomes imprinted on the basal lamina.[410]
2. A neural imprinting influence activates transcription by α, β, δ, and ε subunit genes at NMJ nuclei and also renders these nuclei independent of myogenic control signals. γ-Subunit gene expression at NMJ nuclei remains susceptible to myogenic and neural control signals.

3. Neural inhibiting factor acting on extrajunctional nuclei and electrical activity of the muscle fiber repress extrajunctional α-, β-, γ-, and δ-subunit gene transcription.
4. A neural imprinting signal activates transcription of the ε-subunit gene at NMJ nuclei, and the ε-subunit gene then becomes independent from other control mechanisms.
5. The γ-subunit gene is regulated by a myogenic influence, a neural inhibitory factor, and electrical activity. A neural influence inhibits γ-subunit gene transcription at NMJ nuclei. The neural inhibitory factor requires the presence of the nerve terminal, appears to be released by the clear synaptic vesicles, and could be ACh, ATP, a proteoglycan, or some other factor.

The net result is that the α-, β-, and δ-subunit genes are permanently activated at NMJ nuclei by a neural imprinting influence but remain subject to regulation by electrical activity and a neural inhibitory factor at extrajunctional nuclei.

The differential regulation of AChR subunit genes by a variety of signals is likely to be mediated by transcriptional factors acting on regulatory elements in the AChR subunit genes. MyoD1 sequence motifs—present in α-, δ-, and γ-subunit genes—may serve as cis-acting regulatory elements. Myogenin and MyoD bind directly to α- and γ-subunit enhancers, and the regulatory sequences of both genes contain two MyoD-binding sites.[405,411] Myogenin, MyoD, and Myf-5 transcript levels decrease during innervation, and this precedes decreases in the corresponding AChR mRNAs,[405] while increases in MRF4 transcript levels during development precede the expression of ε mRNA.[412] However, in the rat, the levels of α-, δ-, and γ-subunit transcripts correlate only weakly with changes in the level of myogenin mRNA and do not correlate with levels of MyoD1 mRNA.[353]

AChE Expression at the NMJ

Prior to innervation, the asymmetrical collagen-tailed form of AChE is formed along the entire muscle fiber. Within a few days after innervation there is increased synthesis and accumulation of this AChE at the NMJ and a decreased synthesis of extrajunctional AChE. AChE transcripts diffuse for only a short distance from their nuclei of origin.[405] This suggests preferential transcription of AChE by subsynaptic nuclei and repression of AChE transcription by extrajunctional nuclei. The neural factor that augments AChE synthesis at the synapse is probably agrin,[108] likely acting in combination with neuregulin. If an ectopic synapse is denervated just at it is beginning to form and the muscle is stimulated, AChE still appears at the synaptic site. This indicates transfer of the neural signal to the basal lamina early during synaptogenesis and that muscle activity is also required for the appearance of AChE at the synaptic site.[354]

The above findings imply that activity and neural trophic factors work in concert during different stages of synaptogenesis.[46,413] Activity itself renders the denervated fiber refractory to innervation, but once innervation has taken place, activity is required for the appearance of AChE, metabolic stabilization of AChR, decrease of the AChR ion channel open time, and growth of junctional folds. Neural trophic factors are responsible for the early clustering of AChR at the synaptic site and induce synaptic differentiation of the basal lamina.

These neural factors leave an "imprint" or "imprints" on the basal lamina and possibly the muscle fiber, which allow subsequent activity to exert its effect on AChE, AChR, and synaptic architecture and enable the basal lamina to bind AChE, and to play a key role in synaptic regeneration.[46,108,413]

Synaptic Plasticity

Synaptic plasticity is evidenced by (1) the appearance and disappearance of polyaxonal inputs at the developing NMJ; (2) the sequential changes that occur in the fine structure and molecular architecture of nerve terminal, basal lamina, and postsynaptic region at the developing and regenerating NMJ; (3) the appearance of collateral, ultraterminal, and intraterminal nerve sprouts in response to a variety of stimuli; and (4) remodeling of the NMJ during life and with aging. The sequential changes during synaptogenesis were discussed in the previous section. This section considers some aspects of the removal of polyaxonal innervation, nerve sprouting, and NMJ remodeling.

The Withdrawal of Polyaxonal Innervation

The exact sequence of events associated with the withdrawal of some axon terminals from NMJs that receive multiple axons is still not fully understood. It has been generally accepted that axons from inappropriate segments of the spinal cord are withdrawn, that motor neuron death accompanies withdrawal of incorrect projections from motor neuron pools, and that loss of polyaxonal innervation of synaptic sites accompanies motor neuron death.[75,414,415] However, morphometric study of the mouse spinal cord cannot account for the prenatal loss of polyaxonal innervation by anterior horn cell death.[416] Further, in mammals and birds, postnatal loss of polyaxonal innervation occurs even after correct spatial relationship between motor neuron pools and muscles has been established. At this time there is a decrease in the number of muscle fibers per motor unit but not in the number of motor units per muscle.[417–419] Therefore the late loss of polyaxonal innervation results from the elimination of collateral sprouts rather than motor neuron cell death.[418]

Various structural alterations have been described in axons withdrawing from nerve terminals. Simple retraction of the nerve terminal has been suggested by light microscopic studies,[419–421] but engulfment of the nerve terminal by Schwann cell and changes suggesting axotomy have been observed in an ultrastructural study.[422] Degenerative changes in nerve terminals in multiply innervated soleus NMJs have been reported after indirect electrical stimulation in vitro in the presence of calcium. This effect was prevented by protease inhibitors.[423] Additional ultrastructural studies are required to define the sequence of morphologic events associated with elimination of polyneuronal innervation from the NMJ.

The factors that control withdrawal of the polyneuronal innervation are still not fully understood. Activity or electrical stimulation hastens and inactivity retards the elimination of polyaxonal innervation.[354,420,424] This suggests that inactive muscle releases a trophic "nerve growth factor" that maintains innervation and/or promotes nerve sprouting.[75,354] O'Brien et al. suggest that activity hastens the elimination of multiple innervation through the release of proteolytic enzymes from muscle that attack susceptible nerve terminals.[423] Oppenheim suggests that axonal branches compete for a soluble trophic factor released from muscle.[425] Sequential in vivo observation of BGT-labeled NMJ during the elimination of polyaxonal innervation reveals that AChR depletion of postsynaptic regions precedes the withdrawal of axon terminals from these regions. This might indicate that alterations in the postsynaptic region predetermine synaptic reorganization.[426] Alternatively, a given postsynaptic region fails to support an overlying nerve terminal because more dominant nerve terminals have enticed trophic factors away from that postsynaptic region.[427]

Nerve Sprouting

Excellent morphologic studies of nerve sprouting in denervated muscles were published more than three decades ago.[428–431] Hoffman distinguished between two types of sprouting: (1) ultraterminal, arising from nerve terminals at one NMJ and extending to a nearby denervated NMJ, and (2) collateral, arising from a preterminal nerve fiber at a node of Ranvier and reaching its target through the empty endoneurial sheath of the degenerated axon.[429] Reinnervation begins from ultraterminal branches because collateral sprouts can enter empty endoneurial sheaths only after Wallerian degeneration has taken place. Hoffman noted that growth of a foreign nerve implanted into a muscle was increased by denervating the muscle, and that growth of a foreign nerve into an innervated muscle was enhanced by denervation of a nearby muscle, suggesting a humoral mechanism for nerve growth.[431] Hoffman also found that an ether-soluble factor extracted from myelin stimulated collateral sprouting and postulated that such a factor is released from degenerating nerves.[428]

A third type of sprouting has been referred to as intraterminal sprouting.[432] This is a form of ultraterminal sprouting within the confines of a single NMJ. It may be a feature of local synaptic regeneration with aging, or may occur in pathologic states. The term *intraterminal sprouting* is misleading because an ultraterminal nerve sprout from a NMJ on a given muscle fiber can establish a new synaptic contact on the same muscle fiber, but outside the confines of the original NMJ. This is the case in myasthenia gravis,[28,433,434] some congenital myasthenic syndromes (see Chap. 66), and botulinum intoxication.[435]

Partial denervation of a corresponding contralateral muscle can induce intranodal and preterminal sprouting and increase in end plate size.[436] Ultraterminal sprouting can occur with inactivity without any loss of innervation. It has been observed in hereditary motor end plate disease of the mouse,[437] where the inactivity is attributed to a failure of the nerve action potential to invade the nerve terminal[438]; after local botulinum[435] or tetanus[439] injection into muscle; in human botulism; after prolonged tetrodotoxin blockade of nerve conduction[440] or curarization of AChR[441]; and in inactive winter frogs.[441] Direct electrical stimulation prevents motor nerve sprouting in botulinum poisoned mouse soleus muscle.[442] All these observations support the notion that a humoral factor released by inactive muscle stimulates ultraterminal nerve sprouting.

Candidates for muscle-derived sprouting activity. The local administration of ciliary neurotrophic factor induces intranodal and terminal sprouting; this effect is potentiated by basic fibroblast growth factor, but treatment with the latter alone does not induce sprouting.[443] The subcutaneous injection of minute amounts of insulin-like growth factors induces nerve sprouting in innervated adult muscle. These growth factors are excellent candidates for muscle-derived sprouting activity because their mRNA levels in adult muscle increase severalfold after denervation or paralysis.[444]

Remodeling of the NMJ

Remodeling of the NMJ during life is also a sign of plasticity in the nervous system.[445] A small proportion of the NMJs in normal human muscle have abnormal conformations. These include postsynaptic regions without nerve terminals, nerve terminals engorged by neurofilaments, abnormally small nerve terminals that fail to occupy the entire synaptic gutter, focal degeneration of the junctional folds, and abnormally simple postsynaptic regions that have no or only sparse and shallow synaptic clefts.[446] These alterations probably reflect the wear and tear of NMJ in the normal state.

Conformational changes similar to those noted in normal human muscle and a decrease in synaptic vesicle density have been observed in aging mice.[447] Scanning electron microscopy shows increase in the total length and number of side branches of the synaptic gutter in the old mice.[63] These morphologic changes are associated with a decrease in NMJ AChR in some but not other muscles, with a decrease in the MEPP frequency and an increase in m.[447]

In the rat, the complexity of the NMJ increases with age and is associated with adaptation of terminal axons.[448] In diaphragm NMJs of aged rats, m,[449] ACh released per nerve impulse,[450] NMJ AChR,[451] and the safety margin of neuromuscular transmission all decrease.[450]

Repeated in vivo visualization of NMJs in adult mice reveals that about 15 percent of the NMJ in gastrocnemius and 44 percent of the NMJ in soleus alters its configuration over 3 to 6 months. This suggests that remodeling of the NMJ increases with impulse activity.[452] Similar types of observations on the slow-twitch pectineus muscle of the mouse show that the nerve terminal is the dynamic entity, continually changing shape on a scale of microns, with nerve terminal outgrowths preceding the appearance of new AChR-positive postsynaptic regions. These alterations involve about 1 to 2 percent of the junctional area per month, but with relatively small permanent changes.[453]

Acknowledgments

I thank Drs. John Heuser, M. A. Fahim, Norman Robbins, Nobutaka Hirokawa, Josh Sanes, and Uel J. McMahan for permission to reproduce figures in this chapter. Ms. Cleo Schaefer provided expert assistance in the preparation of the manuscript.

List of Abbreviations

αCGRP	α-calcitonin gene–related peptide	GTP	guanosine triphosphate
ACh	acetylcholine	HB-GAM	heparin-binding growth-associated molecule
AChE	acetylcholinesterase		
AChR	acetylcholine receptor	m	quantum content of EPP
α-DG	α-dystroglycan	MAP	mitogen-activated protein
ApoE	apolipoprotein E	MASC	muscle-associated specificity component
ATP	adenosine triphosphate	MEPP	miniature end plate potential
BGT	α-bungarotoxin	MuSK	muscle-specific kinase
ARIA	acetylcholine receptor–inducing activity	NCAM	neural cell adhesion molecule
cAMP	cyclic adenosine monophosphate	NMJ	neuromuscular junction
CAPS	calcium-activated protein for secretion	nNOS	neuroanal nitric oxide synthase
CGRP	calcitonin gene–related peptide	NSF	N-ethylmaleimide-sensitive ATPase
ChAT	choline acetyltransferase	RATL	rapsyn-associated transmembrane linker
EPP	end plate potential	SNAP	soluble NSF attachment protein
ER	endoplasmic reticulum	T tubule	transverse tubule
GABP	GA-binding protein	VAChT	vesicular ACh transporter

References

1. Kühne W. The mode of termination of nerve fibre in muscle, in Strickler S (ed): *Manual of Human and Comparative Histology*. London: The New Sydenham Society, 1870, pp 202–234.
2. Kühne W: Neue Untersuchungen über die motorische Nervenendigungen. *Z Biol* 23:1–148, 1887.
3. Hinsey JC: The innervation of skeletal muscle. *Physiol Rev* 14:514–585, 1934.
4. Couteaux R: Contribution à l'étude de la synapse myoneurale. *Rev Can Biol* 6:563–711, 1947.
5. Couteaux R: Localization of cholinesterases at neuromuscular junctions. *Int Rev Cytol* 4:335–375, 1955.
6. Couteaux R: Motor end plate structure, in Bourne GH (ed): *The Structure and Function of Muscle*, 2d ed. New York: Academic Press; 1973, pp 483–530.
7. Anderson-Cedergren E: Ultrastructure of the motor end-plate and sarcoplasmic components of mouse skeletal muscle fiber as revealed by three-dimensional reconstructions from serial sections. *J Ultrastruct Res* 1(suppl):1–191, 1959.
8. Kühne W: Der Verbindung der Nervenscheiden mit dem Sarkolemm. *Z Biol* 19:501–534, 1883.
9. Tschiriew MS: Sur les terminaisons nerveuses dans les muscle striés. *Arch Physiol Norm Pathol* 6:89–116, 1879.
10. Dogiel AS: Methylenblautinktion der motorischen Nervenendigungen in den Muskeln der Amphibien und Reptilien. *Arch Mikrosk Anat* 35:305–320, 1890.
11. Frohse F: Ueber die Verzwegung der Nerven zu und in den menschlichen Muskeln. *Anat Anz* 14:321–343, 1898.
12. Kulchitsky N: Nerve endings in the muscles of the frog. *J Anat* 59:1–17, 1924.
13. Mather V, Hines M: Studies in the innervation of skeletal muscle: V. The limb muscles of the newt, *Triturus torosus*. *Am J Anat* 54:177–201, 1934.
14. Hines M: Studies in the innervation of skeletal muscle. IV. Of certain muscles of the boa constrictor. *J Comp Neurol* 56:105–133, 1932.
15. Tiegs OW: A study by degeneration methods of the innervation of muscles of a lizard (*Epernia*). *J Anat* 66:300–322, 1932.
16. Feindel W, Hinshaw JR, Weddell G: The pattern of innervation in mammalian striated muscle. *J Anat* 86:35–48, 1952.
17. Couteaux R, Taxi J: Recherches histochimiques sur la distribution des activities cholinesterasiques au niveau de la synapse myo-neurale. *Arch Anat Microsc Morphol Exp* 41:352–392, 1952.
18. Palade GE, Palay SL: Electron microscope observations of interneuronal and neuromuscular synapses (abstr). *Anat Rec* 118:335–336, 1954.
19. Robertson JA: Electron microscope observation on a reptilian neuromuscular junction (abstr). *Anat Rec* 118:346, 1954.
20. De Robertis EDP, Bennett HS: Some features of the submicroscopic morphology of synapses in frog and earthworm. *J Biophys Biochem Cytol* 1:47–58, 1955.
21. Fatt P, Katz B: Spontaneous subthreshold activity at motor nerve endings. *J Physiol (Lond)* 117:109–128, 1952.
22. del Castillo J, Katz B: Quantal components of the end-plate potential. *J Physiol (Lond)* 124:560–573, 1954.
23. del Castillo J, Katz B: Local activity at a depolarized nerve-muscle junction. *J Physiol (Lond)* 128:396–411, 1955.
24. Birks R, Huxley HE, Katz B: The fine structure of the neuromuscular junction in the frog. *J Physiol (Lond)* 150:134–144, 1960.
25. Düring M: Über die Feinstruktur der motorischen Endplatte von höheren Wirbeltieren. *Z Zellforsch Mikroskop Anat* 81:74–90, 1967.
26. Saito A, Zacks SI: Ultrastructure of Schwann and perineural sheaths at the mouse neuromuscular junction. *Anat Rec* 164:379–390, 1969.
27. Padykula HA, Gauthier GF: The ultrastructure of the neuromuscular junctions of mammalian red, white, and intermediate skeletal fibers. *J Cell Biol* 46:27–41, 1970.
28. Engel AG, Santa T: Histometric analysis of the ultrastructure of the neuromuscular junction in myasthenia gravis and in the myasthenic syndrome. *Ann N Y Acad Sci* 183:46–63, 1971.
29. Llinas RR, Heuser JE: Depolarization-release coupling systems in neurons. *Neurosci Res Program Bull* 15:555–687, 1977.
30. Miledi R, Parker I: Calcium transients recorded with arsenazo III in the presynaptic terminal of the squid giant synapse. *Proc R Soc Lond [Biol]* 212:197–211, 1981.
31. Charlton MP, Smith SJ, Zucker RS: Role of presynaptic calcium ions and channels in synaptic facilitation and depression at the squid giant synapse. *J Physiol (Lond)* 323:173–193, 1982.
32. Tauc L: Nonvesicular release of neurotransmitter. *Physiol Rev* 62:857–893, 1982.
33. Morel N, Manaranche R, Gulik-Krzywicki T, et al: Ultrastructural changes and transmitter release induced by depolarization of cholinergic synaptosomes. A freeze-fracture study of a synaptosomal fraction from *Torpedo* electric organ. *J Ultrastruct Res* 70:347–362, 1980.
34. Reichardt LF, Kelly RB: A molecular description of nerve terminal function. *Annu Rev Biochem* 52:871–926, 1983.
35. Anderson MJ, Cohen MW: Nerve-induced and spontaneous redistribution of acetylcholine receptors on cultured muscle cells. *J Physiol (Lond)* 268:757–773, 1977.
36. Bourgeoise JP, Tsuji S, Bouquet P: Localization of the cholinergic receptor by immunofluorescence in eel electroplax. *FEBS Lett* 16:92–94, 1971.
37. Fertuk HC, Salpeter MM: Localization of acetylcholine receptor by ^{125}I-labelled α-bungarotoxin binding at mouse motor endplates. *Proc Natl Acad Sci USA* 71:1376–1378, 1974.
38. Lee CY, Tseng LF, Chiu TH: Influence of denervation on localization of neurotoxins from elapid venoms in rat diaphragm. *Nature* 215:1177–1178, 1967.
39. Matthews-Bellinger J, Salpeter MM: Distribution of acetylcholine receptors at frog neuromuscular junctions with a discussion of some physiological implications. *J Physiol (Lond)* 279:197–213, 1978.
40. Daniels MP, Vogel Z: Immunoperoxidase staining of α-bungarotoxin binding sites in muscle end-plates shows distribution of acetylcholine receptors. *Nature* 254:339–341, 1975.
41. Heuser JE, Reese TS, Landis DMD: Functional changes in frog neuromuscular junctions studied with freeze-fracture. *J Neurocytol* 3:109–131, 1974.
42. Rash JE, Ellisman MH: Studies of excitable membranes. I. Macromolecular specializations of the neuromuscular junction and the non-junctional sarcolemma. *J Cell Biol* 63:567–586, 1974.
43. Dreyer F, Peper K, Akert K, et al: Ultrastructure of the "active zone" on the frog neuromuscular junction. *Brain Res* 62:373–380, 1973.
44. Heuser JE, Salpeter SR: Organization of acetylcholine receptors in quick-frozen, deep-etched, and rotary-replicated *Torpedo* postsynaptic membrane. *J Cell Biol* 82:150–173, 1979.
45. Grohovaz F, Limbrick AR, Miledi R: Acetylcholine receptors at the rat neuromuscular junction as revealed by deep etching. *Proc R Soc Lond [Biol]* 215:147–154, 1982.
46. Sanes JR, Chiu AY: The basal lamina of the neuromuscular junction. *Cold Spring Harbor Symp Quant Biol* 48:667–678, 1983.

47. Gary EG: Synaptic vesicles and microtubules in frog motor endplates. *Proc R Soc Lond [Biol]* 203:219–227, 1978.
48. Couteaux R: Structure of the subsynaptic sarcoplasm in the interfolds of the frog neuromuscular junction. *J Neurocytol* 10:947–962, 1981.
49. Peng HB: Cytoskeletal organization of the presynaptic nerve terminal and the acetylcholine receptor cluster in cell cultures. *J Cell Biol* 97:489–498, 1983.
50. Ellisman MH, Rash JE, Staehlin LA, et al: Studies of excitable membranes. II. A comparison of specializations at neuromuscular junctions and nonjunctional sarcolemmas of mammalian fast and slow twitch muscle fibers. *J Cell Biol* 68:752–774, 1976.
51. Heuser JE: 3-D visualization of membrane and cytoplasmic specializations at the frog neuromuscular junction, in Taxi J (ed): *Ontogenesis and Functional Mechanisms of Peripheral Synapses*. New York: Elsevier/North Holland; 1980, pp 139–155.
52. Hirokawa N, Heuser JE: Internal and external differentiations of the postsynaptic membrane at the neuromuscular junction. *J Neurocytol* 11:487–510, 1982.
53. Gulley RL, Reese TS: Cytoskeletal organization of the postsynaptic complex. *J Cell Biol* 91:298–302, 1981.
54. Bloch RJ, Hall ZW: Cytoskeletal components of the vertebrate neuromuscular junction: Vinculin, α-actinin, and filamin. *J Cell Biol* 97:217–223, 1983.
55. Hirokawa N, Sobue K, Kanda K, et al: The cytoskeletal architecture of the presynaptic terminal and molecular structure of synapsin. *J Cell Biol* 108:111–126, 1989.
56. Hall ZW, Lubit BW, Schwartz JH: Cytoplasmic actin in postsynaptic structures at the neuromuscular junction. *J Cell Biol* 90:789–792, 1981.
57. Sealock R, Wray BE, Froehner SC: Ultrastructural localization of the M_r 43,000 protein and the acetylcholine receptor at *Torpedo* postsynaptic membranes using monoclonal antibodies. *J Cell Biol* 98:2239–2244, 1984.
58. Tarelli FT, Bossi M, Fesce R, et al: Synapsin I partially dissociates from synaptic vesicles during exocytosis induced by electrical stimulation. *Neuron* 9:1143–1153, 1992.
59. Valtorta F, Villa A, Jahn R, et al: Localization of synapsin I at the frog neuromuscular junction. *Neuroscience* 24:593–603, 1988.
60. Evan AP, Dail WG, Dammrose D, et al: Scanning electron microscopy of cell surfaces following removal of extracellular material. *Anat Rec* 185:433–446, 1976.
61. Shotton DM, Heuser JE, Reese BS, et al: Postsynaptic membrane folds at the frog neuromuscular junction visualized by scanning electron microscopy. *Neuroscience* 4:427–435, 1979.
62. Desaki J, Uehara Y: The overall morphology of neuromuscular junctions as revealed by scanning electron microscopy. *J Neurocytol* 10:101–110, 1981.
63. Fahim MA, Holley JA, Robbins N: Scanning and light microscopic study of age changes at a neuromuscular junction in the mouse. *J Neurocytol* 12:13–25, 1983.
64. Tarelli FT, Passafaro M, Clementi F, et al: Presynaptic localization of omega-conotoxin-sensitive calcium channels at the frog neuromuscular junction. *Brain Res* 547:331–334, 1991.
65. Robitaille R, Adler EM, Charlton MP: Strategic location of calcium channels at transmitter release sites of frog neuromuscular synapses. *Neuron* 5:773–779, 1990.
66. Betz WJ, Bewick GS: Optical analysis of synaptic vesicle recycling at the frog neuromuscular junction. *Science* 255:200–203, 1992.
67. Marques MJ, Conchello JA, Lichtman JW: From plaque to pretzel: Fold formation and acetylcholine receptor loss at the developing neuromuscular junction. *J Neurosci* 20:3663–3675, 2000.
68. Sanes JR, Lichtman JW: Induction, assembly, maturation and maintenance of a postsynaptic apparatus. *Nature Rev Neurosci* 2:791–805, 2001.
69. Akaaboune M, Grady RM, Turney S, et al: Neurotransmitter receptor dynamics studied in vivo by reversible photo-unbinding of fluorescent ligands. *Neuron* 34:865–876, 2002.
70. Südhof TC, Jahn R: Proteins of synaptic vesicles involved in exocytosis and membrane recycling. *Neuron* 6:665–677, 1991.
71. Greengard P, Valtorta F, Czernik AJ, et al: Synaptic vesicle phosphoproteins and regulation of synaptic vesicle function. *Science* 259:780–785, 1993.
72. Miyazawa A, Fujiyoshy Y, Unwin N: Nicotinic acetylcholine receptor at 4.6Å resolution: Transverse tunnels in the channel wall. *J Mol Biol* 288:765–786, 1999.
73. Unwin N, Miyazawa A, Li J, et al: Activation of the nicotinic acetylcholine receptor involves a switch in conformation of the α subunits. *J Mol Biol* 319:1165–1176, 2002.
74. Brejc K, van Dijk WV, Schuurmans M, et al: Crystal structure of ACh-binding protein reveals the ligand-binding domain of nicotinic receptors. *Nature* 411:269–276, 2001.
75. Bennett MR: Development of neuromuscular synapses. *Physiol Rev* 63:915–1048, 1983.
76. Laskowski MB, Sanes JR: Topographic mapping of motor pools onto skeletal muscles. *J Neurosci* 7:252–260, 1987.
77. Letinsky MS, Morrison-Graham K: Structure of developing frog neuromuscular junctions. *J Neurocytol* 9:321–342, 1980.
78. Bennett MR, Pettigrew AG: The formation of synapses in striated muscle during development. *J Physiol (Lond)* 241:515–545, 1974.
79. Verma V, Reese TS: Structure and distribution of neuromuscular junctions on slow muscle fibers in the frog. *Neuroscience* 12:647–662, 1984.
80. Katz B, Kuffler SW: Multiple motor innervation of the frog's sartorius muscle. *J Neurophysiol* 4:209–223, 1941.
81. Bennett MR, Pettigrew AG: The formation of synapses in reinnervated and cross-reinnervated striated muscle during development. *J Physiol (Lond)* 241:547–573, 1974.
82. Cöers C: Structure and organization of the myoneural junction. *Int Rev Cytol* 22:239–267, 1967.
83. Tiegs OW: Innervation of voluntary muscle. *Physiol Rev* 33:90–144, 1953.
84. Namba T, Nakamura T, Grob D: Motor nerve endings in human extraocular muscle. *Neurology* 18:403–407, 1968.
85. Teräväinen H: Electron microscopic and histochemical observations on different types of nerve endings in the extraocular muscles of the rat. *Z Zellforsch Mikroskop Anat* 90:372–388, 1968.
86. Pachter BR: Rat extraocular muscle: I. Three dimensional cytoarchitecture, component fibre populations and innervation. *J Anat* 137:143–159, 1983.
87. Peachey LD, Takeichi M, Nag AC: Muscle fiber types and innervation in adult cat extraocular muscles, in Milhorat AT (ed): *Exploratory Concepts in Muscular Dystrophy: II. Control Mechanisms*. Amsterdam: Excerpta Medica; 1974, pp 246–254.
88. Retzius G: Zur Kenntnis der motorischen Nervenendigungen. *Biol Untersuch (NS)* 3:41–52, 1892.
89. Mackay B, Peters A: Terminal innervation of segmental muscle fibers. *Bibl Anat* 2:182–193, 1961.
90. McMahan UJ, Spitzer JJ, Peper K: Visual identification of nerve terminals in living isolated skeletal muscle. *Proc R Soc Lond [Biol]* 181:421–430, 1972.
91. Hess A: Vertebrate slow muscle fibers. *Physiol Rev* 50:40–62, 1970.
92. Korneliussen H, Waerhaug O: Three morphological types of motor nerve terminals in the rat diaphragm, and their possible innervation of different muscle fiber types. *Z Anat Entwickl Gesch* 140:73–84, 1973.
93. Birks R, Katz B, Miledi R: Physiological and structural changes at the amphibian myoneural junction, in the course of nerve degeneration. *J Physiol (Lond)* 150:145–168, 1960.
94. Heuser JE: A possible origin of the "giant" spontaneous potentials that occur after prolonged transmitter release at frog neuromuscular junctions. *J Physiol (Lond)* 239:106–108, 1974.
95. Heuser JE, Miledi R: Effect of lanthanum ions on function and structure of frog neuromuscular junctions. *Proc R Soc Lond [Biol]* 179:247–260, 1971.
96. Pécot-Dechavassine M, Couteaux R: Modifications structurales des terminaisons motrices des muscles de grenouille soumis à l'action de la vinblastine. *C R Seances Acad Sci [D]* 280:1099–1101, 1975.
97. Nickel E, Vogel A, Waser PG: Coated Vesicles in der Umgebung der neuromuskularen Synapsen. *Z Zellforsch Mikroskop Anat* 78:261–266, 1967.
98. Zacks SI, Saito A: Uptake of exogenous horseradish peroxidase by coated vesicles in mouse neuromuscular junctions. *J Histochem Cytochem* 17:161–170, 1969.
99. Heuser JE: Three-dimensional visualization of coated vesicle formation in fibroblasts. *J Cell Biol* 84:560–583, 1980.
100. Heuser JE, Reese TS: Evidence for recycling of synaptic vesicle membrane during transmitter release at the frog neuromuscular junction. *J Cell Biol* 57:315–344, 1973.
101. Heuser JE: Synaptic vesicle exocytosis and recycling during transmitter discharge from the neuromuscular junction, in Silverstein SC (ed): *Transport of Macromolecules in Cellular Systems*. Berlin: Dahlem Konferenzen; 1978, pp 445–464.
102. Ungewickell E: First clue to biological role of clathrin light chains. *Nature* 311:213, 1984.
103. Schmidt SL, Braell WA, Schlossman DM, et al: A role for clathrin light chains in the recognition of clathrin cages by "uncoating ATPase." *Nature* 311:228–231, 1984.
104. Cheng TPO, Byrd FI, Whitaker JN, et al: Immunocytochemical localization of coated vesicles protein in rodent nervous system. *J Cell Biol* 86:624–633, 1980.
105. Cheng TPO, Wood JG: Compartmentalization of clathrin in synaptic terminals. *Brain Res* 239:210–212, 1982.
106. De Iraldi AP, De Robertis E: The neurotubular system of the axon and the origin of granulated and non-granulated vesicles in regenerating nerves. *Z Zellforsch Mikroskop Anat* 87:330–344, 1968.
107. Heuser JE, Reese TS: Structure of the synapse, in Pappenheimer JR (ed): *Handbook of Physiology—The Nervous System*. Bethesda, MD: American Physiological Society; 1977, pp 261–294.
108. Hall ZW, Sanes JR: Synaptic structure and development: The neuromuscular junction. *Cell* 72(suppl):99–121, 1993.
109. Matteoli M, Haimann C, Torri-Tarrelli F, et al: Differential effect of alpha-latrotoxin on exocytosis of acetylcholine-containing small synaptic vesicles and CGRP-containing large dense-core vesicles at the frog neuromuscular junction. *Proc Natl Acad Sci USA* 85:7366–7370, 1988.
110. Voets T, Toonen RF, Brian EC, et al: Munc18-1 promotes large dense-core vesicle docking. *Neuron* 31:581–591, 2001.
111. Wang C-T, Grishanin R, Earles CA, et al: Synaptotagmin modulation of fusion pore kinetics in regulated exocytosis of dense-core vesicles. *Science* 294:1111–1115, 2001.
112. Renden R, Berwin B, Davis W, et al: *Drosophila* CAPS is an essential gene that regulates dense-core vesicle release and synaptic vesicle fusion. *Neuron* 31:421–437, 2001.

113. Pow DV, Morris XY: Dendrites and hypothalamic magnocellular neurons release neurohypophyseal peptides. *Neuroscience* 32:435–439, 1989.
114. De Camilli P, Jahn R: Pathways to regulated exocytosis of neurons. *Annu Rev Physiol* 52:625–645, 1990.
115. Smith S, Augustine GJ: Calcium ions, active zones and synaptic transmitter release. *Trends Neurosci* 11:458–465, 1988.
116. Jessell TM, Kandel ER: Synaptic transmission: A bidirectional and self-modifiable form of cell-cell communication. *Cell* 72(suppl):1–30, 1993.
117. Engel AG, Tsujihata M, Lindstrom JM, et al: The motor endplate in myasthenia gravis and in experimental autoimmune myasthenia gravis: A quantitative ultrastructural study. *Ann N Y Acad Sci* 274:60–79, 1976.
118. Whittaker VP: The structure and function of cholinergic synaptic vesicles. *Biochem Soc Trans* 12:561–576, 1984.
119. Wagner JA, Carlson SC, Kelly RB: Chemical and physical characterization of cholinergic synaptic vesicles. *Biochemistry* 17:1199–1206, 1978.
120. Stadler H, Kiene ML: Synaptic vesicles in electromotoneurones: II. Heterogeneity of populations is expressed in uptake properties; exocytosis and insertion of a core proteoglycan into the extracellular matrix. *EMBO J* 6:2217–2221, 1987.
121. Volnandt W, Zimmermann H: Acetylcholine, ATP, and proteoglycan are common to synaptic vesicles isolated from the electric organ of eel and electric catfish as well as from rat diaphragm. *J Neurochem* 47:1449–1462, 1986.
122. Couteaux R, Pécot-Dechavassine M: Vésicules synaptiques et poches au niveau des zones actives de la jonction neuromusculaire. *C R Seances Acad Sci [D]* 271:2346–2349, 1970.
123. Couteaux R, Pécot-Dechavassine M: Les zones spécialisées des membranes présynaptiques. *C R Seances Acad Sci [D]* 278:291–293, 1974.
124. Böőj S, Larsson P-A, Dahllöf A-G, et al: Axonal transport of synapsin I and cholinergic synaptic vesicle-like material. Further immunohistochemical evidence for transport of axonal cholinergic transmitter vesicles in motor neurons. *Acta Physiol Scand* 128:155–165, 1986.
125. Kiene L-M, Stadler H: Synaptic vesicles in electromotoneurones. I. Axonal transport, site of transmitter uptake and processing of a core proteoglycan during maturation. *EMBO J* 6:2209–2215, 1987.
126. Llinás R, Sugimori M, Lin J-W, et al: ATP-dependent directional movement of rat synaptic vesicles injected into the presynaptic terminal of squid giant synapse. *Proc Natl Acad Sci USA* 86:5656–5660, 1989.
127. Okada Y, Yamazaki H, Sekine-Aizawa Y, et al: The neuron-specific kinesin superfamily protein KIF1A is a unique monomeric motor for anterograde axonal transport of synaptic vesicle precursors. *Cell* 81:769–780, 1995.
128. Nakata T, Terada S, Hirokawa N: Visualization of the dynamics of synaptic vesicle and plasma membrane proteins in living axons. *J Cell Biol* 140:659–674, 1998.
129. Kelly RB: Storage and release of neurotransmitters. *Cell* 72(suppl):43–53, 1993.
130. McMahon HT, Nicholls DG: The bioenergetics of neurotransmitter release. *Biochim Biophys Acta* 1059:243–264, 1991.
131. Parsons SM, Carter RS, Koenigsberger R, et al: Transport in the cholinergic synaptic vesicle. *Fed Proc* 41:2765–2768, 1982.
132. Anderson DC, King SC, Parsons SM: Proton gradient linkage to active uptake of [^{3}H]acetylcholine by *Torpedo* electric organ synaptic vesicles. *Biochemistry* 21:3037–3043, 1982.
133. Eiden LE: The cholinergic gene locus. *J Neurochem* 70:2227–2240, 1998.
134. Varochi H, Eriksson A: The cytoplasmic tail of the vesicular acetylcholine transporter contains a synaptic vesicle targeting signal. *J Biol Chem* 273:9094–9098, 1998.
135. Ohno K, Tsujino A, Brengman JM, et al: Choline acetyltransferase mutations cause myasthenic syndrome associated with episodic apnea in humans. *Proc Natl Acad Sci USA* 98:2017–2022, 2001.
136. Valtorta F, Benfenati F, Greengard P: Structure and function of the synapsins. *J Biol Chem* 267:7195–7198, 1992.
137. Hosaka M, Südhof TC: Synapsin III, a novel synapsin with an unusual regulation by Ca^{2+}. *J Biol Chem* 273:13371–13374, 1998.
138. Hilfiker S, Pieribone VA, Czernik AJ, et al: Synapsins as regulators of neurotransmitter release. *Philos Trans R Soc Lond [Biol]* 354:269–279, 1999.
139. Kao H-T, Song H-J, Porton B, et al: A protein kinase A-dependent molecular switch in synapsins regulates neurite outgrowth. *Nature Neurosci* 5:431–437, 2002.
140. Benfenati F, Valtorta F, Rubenstein JL, et al: Synaptic vesicle associated Ca^{2+}/calmodulin-dependent kinase II is a binding protein for synapsin I. *Nature* 359:417–420, 1992.
141. Bi G-Q, Morris RL, Liao G, et al: Kinesin- and myosin-driven steps of vesicle recruitment for Ca^{2+}-regulated exocytosis. *J Cell Biol* 138:999–1008, 1997.
142. Becherer U, Guatimosism C, Betz WJ: Effects of staurosporine on exocytosis and endocytosis at frog motor nerve terminals. *J Neurosci* 217:782–787, 2001.
143. Robinson L, Martin TFJ: Docking and fusion in cell biology. *Curr Opin Cell Biol* 10:483–492, 1998.
144. Scales SJ, Chen YA, Yoo BY, et al: Snares contribute to specificity of membrane fusion. *Neuron* 26:457–464, 2000.
145. Jahn R, Hanson PI, Otto H, et al: Botulinum and tetanus neurotoxins: Emerging tools for the study of membrane fusion. *Cold Spring Harb Symp Quant Biol* 40:329–335, 1995.
146. Südhof TC: The synaptic vesicle cycle: A cascade of protein-protein interactions. *Nature* 375:645–653, 1995.
147. Lin RC, Scheller RH: Structural organization of the synaptic exocytosis core complex. *Neuron* 19:1087–1094, 1997.
148. Fasshauer D, Bruns D, Shen B, et al: A structural change occurs upon binding of syntaxin to SNAP-25. *J Biol Chem* 272:4582–4590, 1997.
149. Fasshauer D, Eliason WK, Brunger AT, et al: Identification of the minimal core of the synaptic SNARE complex sufficient for reversible assembly and disassembly. *Biochemistry* 37:10354–10362, 1997.
150. Fasshauer D, Otto H, Eliason WK, et al: Structural changes are associated with soluble N-ethylmaleimide-sensitive fusion protein attachment protein receptor complex formation. *J Biol Chem* 272:28036–28041, 1997.
151. Hanson PI, Roth R, Morisaki H, et al: Structure and conformational changes in NSF and its membrane receptor complexes visualized by quick-freeze/deep-etch electron microscopy. *Cell* 90:523–525, 1997.
152. Sutton RB, Fasshauer D, Jahn R, et al: Crystal structure of a SNARE complex involved in synaptic exocytosis at 2.4 Å resolution. *Nature* 395:347–353, 1998.
153. Götte M, von Mollard FG: A new beat for the SNARE drum. *Trends Cell Biol* 8:215–218, 1998.
154. Jahn R, Hanson PI: SNAREs line up in new environment. *Nature* 393:14–15, 1998.
155. Weis WI, Scheller RH: SNARE the rod, coil the complex. *Nature* 395:328–329, 1998.
156. Chen X, Tomchick DR, Kovrigin E, et al: Three-dimensional structure of the complexin/SNARE complex. *Neuron* 33:397–409, 2002.
157. Weber T, Zemelman BV, McNew JA, et al: SNAREpins: Minimal machinery for membrane fusion. *Cell* 92:759–772, 1998.
158. Südhof TC, Rizo J: Synaptotagmins: C_2-domain proteins that regulate membrane traffic. *Neuron* 17:379–388, 1996.
159. Shao X, Davletov BA, Sutton RB, et al: Bipartite Ca^{2+}-binding motif in C_2 domains of synaptotagmin and protein kinase C. *Science* 273:248–251, 1996.
160. Shao X, Li C, Fernandez I, et al: Synaptotagmin-syntaxin interaction: The C_2 domain as a Ca^{2+} dependent electrostatic switch. *Neuron* 18:133–142, 1997.
160a. Stevens CF, Sullivan JM: The synaptotagmin C2A domain is part of the calcium sensor controlling fast synaptic transmission. *Neuron* 39:299–308, 2003.
161. Sheng Z-H, Westenbroek RE, Catterall WA: Physical link and functional coupling of presynaptic calcium channels and the synaptic docking/fusion machinery. *J Bioenerg Biomembr* 30:335–345, 1998.
162. Schivell AE, Batchelor RH, Bajjalieh SM: Isoform-specific, calcium-regulated interaction of the synaptic vesicle proteins SV2 and synaptotagmin. *J Biol Chem* 271:27770–27775, 1996.
163. Geppert M, Goda Y, Hammer RE, et al: Synaptotagmin I: A major Ca^{2+} sensor for transmitter release at a central synapse. *Cell* 79:717–727, 1994.
164. Rettig J, Heinemann C, Ashery U, et al: Alteration of Ca^{2+} dependence of neurotransmitter release by disruption of Ca^{2+} channel/syntaxin interaction. *J Neurosci* 17:6647–6656, 1997.
165. Söllner T, Whitehart S, Brunner M, et al: SNAP receptors implicated in vesicle targeting and fusion. *Nature* 362:318–324, 1993.
166. Chen YA, Scales SJ, Scheller RH: Sequential SNARE assembly underlies priming and triggering of exocytosis. *Neuron* 30:151–170, 2001.
167. Desai RC, Vyas B, Earles CA, et al: The C2B domain of synaptotagmin is a Ca^{2+}-sensing module essential for exocytosis. *J Cell Biol* 150:1125–1135, 2000.
168. Zhang X, Kim-Miller MJ, Fukuda M, et al: Ca^{2+}-dependent synaptotagmin binding to SNAP-25 is essential for Ca^{2+}-triggered exocytosis. *Neuron* 34:599–611, 2002.
169. Yoshihara M, Littleton JT: Synaptotagmin functions as a calcium sensor to synchronize neurotransmitter release. *Neuron* 36:897–908, 2002.
170. Hu K, Carroll J, Fedorovich S, et al: Vesicular restriction suggests a role for calcium in membrane fusion. *Nature* 415:646–650, 2000.
171. Pevsner J, Hsu SC, Braun JE, et al: Specificity and regulation of a synaptic vesicle docking complex. *Neuron* 13:353–361, 1994.
172. Masuda ES, Huang BCB, Fischer JM, et al: Tomosyn binds t-SNARE proteins via a VAMP-like coiled coil. *Neuron* 21:479–480, 1998.
173. Fujita Y, Shirataki H, Sakisaka T, et al: Tomosyn: A syntaxin-1-binding protein that forms a novel complex in the neurotransmitter release process. *Neuron* 20:905–915, 1998.
174. Scales SJ, Hesser BA, Masuda ES, et al: Amysin, a novel syntaxin-binding protein that may regulate SNARE complex assembly. *J Biol Chem* 277:28271–28279, 2003.
175. Martin TFJ: Prime movers of synaptic vesicle exocytosis. *Neuron* 34:9–12, 2003.
176. Rettig J, Neher E: Emerging roles of presynaptic proteins in Ca^{++}-triggered exocytosis. *Science* 298:781–785, 2002.
177. Ohtsuka T, Akao-Rikitsu E, Inoue K, et al: CAST: A novel protein of the cytomatrix at the active zone of synapses that forms a ternary complex with RIM12 and Munc13-1. *J Cell Biol* 158:577–590, 2002.
178. Monck JR, Fernandez J: The exocytotic fusion pore. *J Cell Biol* 119:1395–1404, 1992.
179. Wang Y, Okamoto M, Schmitz F, et al: RIM is a putative Rab3 effector in regulating synaptic vesicle fusion. *Nature* 388:593–598, 1997.

180. von Mollard FG, Südhof TC, Jahn R: A small GTP-binding protein dissociates from synaptic vesicles during exocytosis. *Nature* 349:79–81, 1991.
181. Bean AJ, Scheller RH: Better late than never: A role for Rabs late in exocytosis. *Neuron* 19:751–754, 1997.
182. Geppert M, Goda Y, Stevens CF, et al: The small GTP-binding protein Rab3A regulates a late step in synaptic vesicle fusion. *Nature* 387:810–814, 1997.
183. Burns ME, Sasaki T, Augustine GJ: Rabphilin-3A: A multifunctional regulator of synaptic vesicle traffic. *J Gen Physiol* 111:243–255, 1998.
184. Pyle R, Schivell AE, Hikada H, et al: Phosphorylation of synaptic vesicle protein 2 modulates binding to synaptotagmin. *J Biol Chem* 275:17195–17200, 2000.
185. Janz R, Goda Y, Geppert M, et al: SV2A and SV2B function as redundant Ca^{2+} regulators in neurotransmitter release. *Neuron* 24:1003–1016, 1999.
186. Xu T, Bajjalieh SM: SV2 modulates the size of the readily releasable pool of secretory vesicles. *Nature Cell Biol* 3:691–698, 2001.
187. Wiedenmann B, Franke WW: Identification and localization of synaptophysin, an integral membrane glycoprotein of M_r 38,000 characteristic of presynaptic vesicles. *Cell* 41:1017–1028, 1985.
188. Ginzel D, Shoshan-Barmatz V: The synaptic vesicle protein synaptophysin: Purification and characterization of its channel activity. *Biophys J* 83:3223–3229, 2002.
189. Jena BP, Webster P, Geibel JP, et al: Localization of SH-PTP1 to synaptic vesicles: A possible role in neurotransmission. *Cell Biol Int Rep* 21:469–475, 1997.
190. Siebert A, Lottspeich F, Nelson N, et al: Purification of the synaptic vesicle binding protein physophilin. Identification as 39-kDa subunit of the vacuolar H(+)-ATPase. *J Biol Chem* 269:28329–28334, 1994.
191. Washbourne P, Schiavo G, Montecucco C: Vesicle-associated membrane protein-2 (synaptobrevin-2) forms a complex with synaptophysin. *Biochem J* 305:721–724, 1995.
192. Alder J, Kanki H, Valtorta F, et al: Overexpression of synaptophysin enhances neurotransmitter release at *Xenopus* neuromuscular junctions. *J Neurosci* 15:511–519, 1995.
193. Eshkind LG, Leube RE: Mice lacking synaptophysin reproduce and form typical synaptic vesicles. *Cell Tissue Res* 282:423–433, 1995.
194. Tobaben S, Thakur P, Fernàdez-Chacón R, et al: A trimeric protein complex functions as a synaptic chaperone machine. *Neuron* 31:987–999, 2001.
195. Calakos N, Scheller RH: Synaptic vesicle biogenesis, docking, and fusion: A molecular description. *Physiol Rev* 76:1–29, 1996.
196. Buchner E, Gundersen CB: The DnaJ-like cysteine ring protein and exocytotic neurotransmitter release. *Trends Neurosci* 20:223–227, 1997.
197. Braun JEA, Wilbanks SM, Scheller RH: The cysteine string secretory vesicle protein activates Hsc70 ATPase. *J Biol Chem* 271:25989–25993, 1996.
198. Chamberlain LH, Burgoyne RD: The molecular chaperone function of cysteine string proteins. *J Biol Chem* 272:31420–31426, 1997.
199. Leveque C, Pupier S, Marqueze B, et al: Interaction of cysteine string proteins with the $\alpha_1 A$ subunit of the P/Q type calcium channel. *Proc Natl Acad Sci USA* 273:13488–13492, 1998.
200. Evans GJ, Morgan A: Phosphorylation-dependent interaction of the synaptic vesicle proteins cysteine string protein and synaptotagmin I. *Biochem J* 364:343–347, 2002.
201. Ranjan R, Bronk P, Zinsmaier KE: Cysteine string protein is required for calcium secretion coupling of evoked neurotransmission in *Drosophila* but not for vesicle recycling. *J Neurosci* 18:956–964, 1998.
202. Chen S, Zheng X, Schulze KL, et al: Enhancement of presynaptic current by cysteine string protein. *J Physiol (Lond)* 538:383–389, 2002.
203. Landis DMD, Reese TS: Cytoplasmic organization in cerebellar dendritic spines. *J Cell Biol* 97:1169–1178, 1983.
204. Phillips GR, Huang JK, Wang Y, et al: The presynaptic particle web: Ultrastructure, composition, dissolution, and reconstitution. *Neuron* 32:63–77, 2001.
205. Palay SL: The morphology of synapses in the central nervous system. *Exp Cell Res* 5(suppl):275–293, 1958.
206. Nystrom RR, Ko C-P: Disruption of active zones in frog neuromuscular junctions following treatment with proteolytic enzymes. *J Neurocytol* 17:63–71, 1988.
207. Ceccarelli B, Hurlbut WP: Vesicle hypothesis of the release of quanta of acetylcholine. *Physiol Rev* 60:396–441, 1980.
208. Harlow ML, Ress D, Stoschek A, et al: The architecture of active zone material at the frog's neuromuscular junction. *Nature* 409:479–484, 2001.
209. Rash JE: Ultrastructure of normal and myasthenic endplates, in Albuquerque EX, Eldefrawi AT (eds): *Myasthenia Gravis*. London: Chapman and Hall; 1983, pp 395–421.
210. Fukunaga H, Engel AG, Osame M, et al: Paucity and disorganization of presynaptic membrane active zones in the Lambert-Eaton myasthenic syndrome. *Muscle Nerve* 5:686–697, 1982.
211. Engel AG, Fukunaga H, Osame M: Stereometric estimation of the area of the freeze-fractured membrane. *Muscle Nerve* 5:682–685, 1982.
212. Fukunaga H, Engel AG, Lang B, et al: Passive transfer of Lambert-Eaton myasthenic syndrome with IgG from man to mouse depletes the presynaptic membrane active zones. *Proc Natl Acad Sci USA* 80:7636–7640, 1983.
213. Propst JW, Ko C-P: Correlation between active zone ultrastructure and synaptic function studied by freeze-fracture of physiologically identified neuromuscular junctions. *J Neurosci* 7:3654–3664, 1987.
214. Llinas RR, Sugimori M, Silver RB: The concept of calcium concentration microdomains in synaptic transmission. *Neuropharmacology* 34:1443–1451, 1995.
215. Borst JGG, Sakmann B: Calcium influx and transmitter release in a fast CNS synapse. *Nature* 383:431–434, 1996.
216. Urbano FJ, Uchitel OD: L-type calcium channels unmasked by cell-permeant Ca^{2+} buffer at mouse motor nerve terminals. *Pflugers Arch* 437:523–528, 1999.
217. Siri MDR, Uchitel OD: Calcium channels coupled to neurotransmitter release at neonatal rat neuromuscular junctions. *J Physiol (Lond)* 514:533–540, 1999.
218. Birnbaumer L, Campbell KP, Catterall WA, et al: The naming of voltage-gated calcium channels. *Neuron* 13:505–506, 1994.
219. Rettig J, Sheng Z-H, Kim DK, et al: Isoform-specific interaction of the α_{1A} subunits of brain Ca^{2+} channels with the presynaptic proteins syntaxin and SNAP-25. *Proc Natl Acad Sci USA* 93:7363–7368, 1996.
220. Charvin N, Leveque C, Walker D, et al: Direct interaction of the calcium sensor protein synaptotagmin I with a cytoplasmic domain of the α_{1A} subunit of the P/Q-type calcium channel. *EMBO J* 16:4591–4596, 1997.
221. Boudier JL, Jover E, Cau P: Autoradiographic localization of voltage-dependent sodium channels on the mouse neuromuscular junction using ^{125}I-α scorpion toxin. I. Preferential labeling of glial cells on the presynaptic side. *J Neurosci* 8:1469–1478, 1988.
222. Brigant JL, Mallart A: Presynaptic currents in mouse motor endings. *J Physiol (Lond)* 333:619–636, 1982.
223. Clark AW, Hurlbut WP, Mauro A: Changes in the fine structure of the neuromuscular junction of the frog caused by black widow spider venom. *J Cell Biol* 52:1–14, 1972.
224. Betz WJ, Bewick GS: Optical monitoring of transmitter release and synaptic vesicle recycling at the frog neuromuscular junction. *J Physiol (Lond)* 460:287–309, 1993.
225. Betz WJ, Mao F, Bewick GS: Activity-dependent fluorescent staining and destaining of living vertebrate motor nerve terminals. *J Neurosci* 12:363–375, 1992.
226. Ceccarelli B, Hurlbut WP, Mauro A: Turnover of transmitter and synaptic vesicles at the frog neuromuscular junction. *J Cell Biol* 57:499–524, 1973.
227. Gorio A, Hurlbut WP, Ceccarelli B: Acetylcholine compartments in mouse diaphragm: A comparison of the effects of black widow spider venom, electrical stimulation, and high concentration of potassium. *J Cell Biol* 78:716–733, 1978.
228. Pecot-Dechavassine M: Synaptic vesicle openings captured by cooling and related to transmitter release at the frog neuromuscular junction. *Biol Cell* 46:43–50, 1982.
229. Heuser JE: Synaptic vesicle exocytosis revealed in quick-frozen frog neuromuscular junctions treated with 4-aminopyridine and given a single electrical shock, in Cowan M, Ferendelli JA (eds): *Neuroscience Symposia*. Bethesda, MD: Society for Neuroscience; 1977, pp 215–239.
230. Heuser JE, Reese TS, Dennis MJ, et al: Synaptic vesicle exocytosis captured by quick freezing and correlated with quantal transmitter release. *J Cell Biol* 81:275–300, 1979.
231. Heuser JE, Reese TS: Structural changes after transmitter release at the frog neuromuscular junction. *J Cell Biol* 88:564–580, 1981.
232. Torri-Tarelli F, Grohovaz F, Fesce R, et al: Temporal coincidence between synaptic vesicle fusion and quantal secretion of acetylcholine. *J Cell Biol* 101:1386–1399, 1985.
233. Dickinson-Nelson A, Reese TS: Structural changes during transmitter release at synapses in the frog sympathetic ganglion. *J Neurosci* 3:42–52, 1983.
234. von Wedel RJ, Carlson SS, Kelly RB: Transfer of synaptic vesicle antigens to the presynaptic plasma membrane during exocytosis. *Proc Natl Acad Sci USA* 78:1014–1018, 1981.
235. Valtorta F, Jahn R, Fesce R, et al: Synaptophysin (p38) at the frog neuromuscular junction: Its incorporation into the axolemma and recycling after intense quantal secretion. *J Cell Biol* 107:2719–2730, 1988.
236. Matthews G: Neurotransmitter release. *Annu Rev Neurosci* 19:219–233, 1996.
237. Wilkinson RS, Cole JC: Resolving the Heuser-Ceccarelli debate. *Trends Neurosci* 24:195–197, 2001.
238. De Camilli P, Takei K: Molecular mechanisms in synaptic vesicle endocytosis and recycling. *Neuron* 16:481–486, 1996.
239. Brodin L, Löw P, Gad H, et al: Sustained neurotransmitter release: New molecular clues. *Eur J Neurosci* 9:2503–2511, 1997.
240. Zhang B, Koh YH, Beckstead RB, et al: Synaptic vesicle size and number are regulated by a clathrin adaptor protein required for endocytosis. *Neuron* 21:1465–1475, 1998.
241. David C, McPherson PS, Mundigl O, et al: A role of amphiphysin in synaptic vesicle endocytosis suggested by its binding to dynamin in nerve terminals. *Proc Natl Acad Sci USA* 93:331–335, 1996.
242. Wigge P, McMahon HT, Vallis Y, et al: Amphiphysin heterodimers: Potential role in clathrin-mediated endocytosis. *Mol Biol Cell* 8:2003–2015, 1997.

243. Zacks SI, Saito A: Direct connections between the T-system and the subneural apparatus in mouse neuromuscular junctions demonstrated by lanthanum. *J Histochem Cytochem* 18:302–304, 1970.
244. Sanes JR, Marshall LM, McMahan UJ: Reinnervation of muscle fiber basal lamina after removal of myofibers. Differentiation of axons at original synaptic sites. *J Cell Biol* 78:176–198, 1978.
245. Glicksman MA, Sanes JR: Differentiation of motor nerve terminals in the absence of muscle fibers. *J Neurocytol* 12:661–671, 1983.
246. Burden SJ, Sargent PB, McMahan UJ: Acetylcholine receptors accumulate at original synaptic sites in the absence of the nerve. *J Cell Biol* 82:412–425, 1979.
247. McMahan UJ, Slater CR: The influence of basal lamina on the accumulation of acetylcholine receptors at synaptic sites in regenerating muscle. *J Cell Biol* 98:1453–1473, 1984.
248. Sanes JR: The synaptic cleft of the neuromuscular junction. *Semin Dev Biol* 6:163–173, 1995.
249. Patton BL, Miner JL, Chiu AY, et al: Distribution and function of laminins in the neuromuscular system of developing, adult, and mutant mice. *J Cell Biol* 139:1507–1521, 1997.
250. Meier T, Masciulli F, Moore C, et al: Agrin can mediate acetylcholine receptor gene expression in muscle by aggregation of muscle-derived neuregulins. *J Cell Biol* 141:715–726, 1998.
251. Salpeter MM: Vertebrate neuromuscular junctions: General morphology, molecular organization, and functional consequences, in Salpeter MM (ed): *The Vertebrate Neuromuscular Junction*. New York: Liss; 1987, pp 1–54.
252. Massoulié J, Pezzementi L, Bon S, et al: Molecular and cellular biology of cholinesterases. *Prog Neurobiol* 41:31–91, 1993.
253. Bon S, Coussen F, Massoulié J: Quaternary associations of acetylcholinesterase: II. The polyproline attachment domain of the collagen tail. *J Biol Chem* 272:3016–3021, 1997.
254. Deprez PN, Inestrosa NC: Two heparin-binding domains are present on the collagenic tail of asymmetric acetylcholinesterase. *J Biol Chem* 270:11043–11046, 1995.
255. Ohno K, Engel AG, Brengman JM, et al: The spectrum of mutations causing endplate acetylcholinesterase deficiency. *Ann Neurol* 47:162–170, 2000.
256. Kimbell LM, Ohno K, Rotundo RL, et al: Transplanting mutant human collagenic tailed acetylcholinesterase onto the frog neuromuscular junction: Evidence for an attachment defect in a congenital myasthenic syndrome (abstr). *Mol Biol Cell* 12(suppl):161a, 2001.
257. Arikawa-Hirasawa E, Rossi SG, Rotundo RL, et al: Absence of acetylcholinesterase at the neuromuscular junction of perlecan-null mice. *Nature Neurosci* 5:119–123, 2002.
258. Legay C, Strochlic L, Lambergeon M, et al: Collagen-tailed forms of acetylcholinesterase are anchored to the basal lamina by a dual mechanism involving perlecan and MuSK (abstr). *Mol Biol Cell* 13:394a–395a, 2002.
259. Patton BL, Chiu AY, Sanes JR: Synaptic laminin prevents glial entry into the synaptic cleft. *Nature* 393:698–701, 1998.
260. Jacobson C, Montanaro F, Lindenbaum MH, et al: α-Dystroglycan functions in acetylcholine receptor aggregation but is not a coreceptor for agrin-Musk signaling. *J Neurosci* 18:6340–6348, 1998.
261. Denzer AJ, Brandenberger R, Gesemann M, et al: Agrin binds to the nerve-muscle basal lamina via laminin. *J Cell Biol* 137:671–683, 1997.
262. Cohen MW, Jacobson C, Yurchenko PD, et al: Laminin-induced clustering of dystroglycan on embryonic muscle cells: Comparison with agrin induced clustering. *J Cell Biol* 136:1047–1058, 1997.
263. Sugiyama JE, Glass DJ, Yancopoulos GD, et al: Laminin-induced acetylcholine receptor clustering: An alternative pathway. *J Cell Biol* 139:181–191, 1997.
264. Noakes PG, Gautam M, Mudd J, et al: Aberrant differentiation of neuromuscular junctions in mice lacking s-laminin β2. *Nature* 374:258–262, 1995.
265. Santa T, Engel AG: Histometric analysis of neuromuscular junction ultrastructure in rat red, white and intermediate muscle fibers, in Desmedt JE (ed): *New Developments in Electromyography and Clinical Neurophysiology*. Basel: Karger; 1973, pp 41–54.
266. Engel AG: Quantitative morphological studies of muscle, in Engel AG, Franzini-Armstrong C (eds): *Myology*, 2nd ed. New York: McGraw-Hill; 1994, pp 1018–1045.
267. Fahim MA, Holley JA, Robbins N: Scanning electron microscopic comparison of neuromuscular junctions of slow and fast twitch mouse muscles. *Neuroscience* 13:227–235, 1984.
268. Ogata T, Yamasaki Y: The three-dimensional structure of motor end-plates in different fiber types of rat intercostal muscle. A scanning electron-microscopic study. *Cell Tissue Res* 241:465–472, 1985.
269. Fumagalli G, Engel AG, Lindstrom J: Ultrastructural aspects of acetylcholine receptor turnover at the normal end-plate and in autoimmune myasthenia gravis. *J Neuropathol Exp Neurol* 41:567–579, 1982.
270. Fischbach GD, Rosen KM: ARIA: A neuromuscular junction neuregulin. *Annu Rev Neurosci* 20:429–458, 1997.
271. Flucher BE, Daniels MP: Distribution of Na$^+$ channels and ankyrin in neuromuscular junctions is complementary to that of acetylcholine receptors and the 43 kD protein. *Neuron* 3:163–175, 1989.
272. Wood SJ, Slater CR: β–Spectrin is colocalized with both voltage-gated sodium channels and ankyrin G at the adult rat neuromuscular junction. *J Cell Biol* 140:675–684, 1998.
273. Gee SH, Madhavan R, Levinson SR, et al: Interaction of muscle and brain sodium channels with multiple members of the syntrophin family of dystrophin-associated proteins. *J Neurosci* 18:128–137, 1998.
274. Sanes JR, Apel ED, Burgess RW, et al: Development of the neuromuscular junction: Genetic analysis in mice. *J Physiol (Paris)* 92:167–172, 1998.
275. Martin AR: Amplification of neuromuscular transmission by postjunctional folds. *Proc R Soc Lond [Biol]* 258:321–326, 1994.
276. Ruff RL: Sodium channel slow inactivation and the distribution of sodium channels on skeletal muscle fibres enable the performance properties of different skeletal muscle fiber types. *Acta Physiol Scand* 156:159–168, 1996.
277. Wood SJ, Slater CP: Safety factor at the neuromuscular junction. *Prog Neurobiol* 64:393–429, 2001.
278. Matthews-Bellinger JA, Salpeter MM: Fine structural distribution of acetylcholine receptors at developing mouse neuromuscular junctions. *J Neurosci* 3:644–657, 1983.
279. Engel AG, Lindstrom JM, Lambert EH, et al: Ultrastructural localization of the acetylcholine receptor in myasthenia gravis and in its experimental autoimmune model. *Neurology* 27:307–315, 1977.
280. Fertuck HC, Salpeter MM: Quantitation of junctional and extrajunctional acetylcholine receptors by electron microscope autoradiography after ^{125}I-α-bungarotoxin binding at mouse neuromuscular junctions. *J Cell Biol* 69:144–158, 1976.
281. Jones SW, Salpeter MM: Absence of [^{125}I]α-bungarotoxin binding to motor nerve terminals of frog, lizard and mouse muscle. *J Neurosci* 3:326–331, 1983.
282. Courtoy PJ, Picton DH, Farquhar MG: Resolution and limitations of the immunoperoxidase procedure in localization of extracellular matrix antigens. *J Histochem Cytochem* 31:945–951, 1983.
283. Brisson A, Unwin PNT: Tubular crystals of acetylcholine receptor. *J Cell Biol* 99:1202–1211, 1984.
284. Anderson MJ, Fambrough DM: Aggregates of acetylcholine receptors are associated with plaques of basal lamina heparan sulfate proteoglycan on the surface of skeletal muscle fibers. *J Cell Biol* 97:1396–1411, 1983.
285. Pumplin DW, Bloch RJ: Lipid domains of acetylcholine receptor clusters detected with saponin and filipin. *J Cell Biol* 97:1043–1054, 1983.
286. Sealock R: Visualization at the mouse neuromuscular junction of a submembrane structure in common with *Torpedo* postsynaptic membranes. *J Neurosci* 2:918–923, 1982.
287. Cartaud J, Sobel A, Rousselet A, et al: Consequences of alkaline treatment for the ultrastructure of the acetylcholine-receptor-rich membranes from *Torpedo marmorata* electric organ. *J Cell Biol* 90:418–426, 1981.
288. Froehner SC: The submembrane machinery for nicotinic acetylcholine receptor clustering. *J Cell Biol* 114:1–7, 1991.
289. LaRochelle WJ, Witzemann V, Fiedler W, et al: Developmental expression of the 43K and 58K postsynaptic membrane proteins and nicotinic acetylcholine receptors in *Torpedo* electrocytes. *J Neurosci* 10:3460–3467, 1990.
290. Krikorian JG, Bloch RJ: Treatments that extract the 43K protein from acetylcholine receptor clusters modify the conformation of cytoplasmic domains of all subunits of the receptor. *J Biol Chem* 267:9118–9128, 1992.
291. Ahn AH, Freener CA, Gussoni E, et al: The three human syntrophin genes are expressed in diverse tissues, have distinct chromosmal localizations, and each bind to dystrophin and its relatives. *J Biol Chem* 271:2724–2730, 1996.
292. Froehner SC, Adams ME, Peters MF, et al: Syntrophins: Modular adapter proteins at the neuromuscular junction and the sarcolemma, in Froehner SC, Bennett V (eds): *Cytoskeletal Regulation and Membrane Function*. New York: Rockefeller University Press; 1997, pp 197–207.
293. Peters MF, Adams ME, Froehner SC: Differential association of syntrophin pairs with the dystrophin complex. *J Cell Biol* 138:81–93, 1997.
294. Newey SA, Gramolini AO, Wu J, et al: A novel mechanism for modulating synaptic gene expression: Differential localization of α-dystrobrevin transcripts in skeletal muscle. *Mol Cell Neurosci* 17:127–140, 2001.
295. Enigk RE, Maimone MM: Cellular and molecular properties of α-dystrobrevin in skeletal muscle. *Front Biosci* 6:d53–d64, 2001.
296. Marazzi G, Bard F, Klymkowsky MW, et al: Microinjection of a monoclonal antibody against a 37-kD protein (tropomyosin 2) prevents the formation of new acetylcholine receptor clusters. *J Cell Biol* 1097:2337–2344, 1989.
297. Sealock R, Paschal B, Beckerle M, et al: Talin is a postsynaptic component of the rat neuromuscular junction. *Exp Cell Res* 163:143–150, 1986.
298. Yorifuji H, Hirokawa N: Cytoskeletal architecture of neuromuscular junction: I. Localization of vinculin. *J Electron Microsc Tech* 12:160–171, 1989.
299. Bloch RJ, Morrow JS: An unusual β-spectrin associated with clustered acetylcholine receptors. *J Cell Biol* 108:481–493, 1989.
300. Turner C, Kramarcy N, Sealock R, et al: Localization of paxilin, a focal adhesion protein, to smooth muscle dense plaques and the myotendinous and neuromuscular junction of skeletal muscle. *Exp Cell Res* 192:651–655, 1991.

301. Cartaud A, Courvalin JC, Ludosky MA, et al: Presence of protein immunologically related to lamin B in the postsynaptic membrane of *Torpedo marmorata* electrocyte. *J Cell Biol* 109:1745–1752, 1989.
302. Sealock R, Murnane AA, Pauline D, et al: Immunochemical identification of desmin in the *Torpedo* postsynaptic membranes and at the rat neuromuscular junction. *Synapse* 3:315–324, 1989.
303. Askanas V, Bornemann A, Engel WK: Immunocytochemical localization of desmin at human neuromuscular junctions. *Neurology* 40:949–953, 1990.
304. Jasmin BJ, Cartaud J: Compartmentalization of cold-stable and acetylated microtubules in the subsynaptic domain of chick skeletal muscle fiber. *Nature* 344:673–675, 1990.
305. Sealock R, Butler MH, Kramarcy NR, et al: Localization of dystrophin relative to acetylcholine receptor domains in electric tissue and adult and cultured skeletal muscle. *J Cell Biol* 113:1133–1144, 1991.
306. Bewick GS, Nicholson LVB, Young C, et al: Different distributions of dystrophin and related proteins at nerve-muscle junctions. *Neuroreport* 3:857–860, 1992.
307. Khurana TS, Hoffman EP, Kunkel LM: Identification of a chromosome 6-encoded dystrophin-related protein. *J Biol Chem* 256:16717–16720, 1990.
308. Banwell BL, Russel J, Fukudome T, et al: Myopathy, myasthenic syndrome, and epidermolysis bullosa simplex due to plectin deficiency. *J Neuropathol Exp Neurol* 58:832–846, 1999.
309. Askanas V, Engel WK, Alvarez RB: Strong immunoreactivity of β-amyloid precursor protein, including the β-amyloid protein sequence, at human neuromuscular junctions. *Neurosci Lett* 143:96–100, 1992.
310. Askanas V, Engel WK, Alvarez RB: Fourteen newly recognized proteins at the human neuromuscular junctions—and their nonjunctional accumulation in inclusion body myositis. *Ann N Y Acad Sci* 841:28–56, 1998.
311. Mitra K, McCarthy MP, Stroud RM: Three-dimensional structure of the nicotinic acetylcholine receptor and location of the major associated 43-kD cytoskeletal protein, determined at 22 Å by low dose electron microscopy and x-ray diffraction to 12.5 Å. *J Cell Biol* 109:755–774, 1989.
312. Ramarao MK, Cohen JB: Mechanism of nicotinic acetylcholine receptor cluster formation by rapsyn. *Proc Natl Acad Sci USA* 95:4007–4012, 1998.
313. Cartaud A, Coutant S, Petrucci TC, et al: Evidence for in situ and in vitro association between β-dystroglycan and the subsynaptic 43K rapsyn protein. Consequence for acetylcholine receptor clustering at the synapse. *J Biol Chem* 273:11321–11326, 1998.
314. Bartoli M, Ramarao MK, Cohen JB: Interactions of the rapsyn RING-H2 domain with dystroglycan. *J Biol Chem* 276:24911–24917, 2001.
315. Ohno K, Engel AG, Shen X-M, et al: Rapsyn mutations in humans cause endplate acetylcholine receptor deficiency and myasthenic syndrome. *Am J Hum Genet* 70:875–885, 2002.
316. Bewick GS, Young C, Slater CR: Spatial relationships of utrophin, dystrophin, β-dystroglycan and β-spectrin to acetylcholine receptor clusters during postnatal maturation of the rat neuromuscular junction. *J Neurocytol* 25:367–379, 1996.
317. Sakakibara H, Engel AG, Lambert EH: Duchenne dystrophy: Ultrastructural localization of the acetylcholine receptor and intracellular microelectrode studies of neuromuscular transmission. *Neurology* 27:741–745, 1977.
318. Xu R, Salpeter MM: Acetylcholine receptor in innervated muscles of dystrophic mdx mice degrade as after denervation. *J Neurosci* 17:8194–8200, 1997.
319. Matsumura K, Ervasti JM, Ohlendieck K, et al: Association of dystrophin-related protein with dystrophin-associated proteins in mdx mouse muscle. *Nature* 360:588–591, 1992.
320. Ervasti JM, Campbell KP: A role for the dystrophin-glycoprotein complex as a transmembrane linker between laminin and actin. *J Cell Biol* 122:809–823, 1993.
321. Slater CR, Young C, Wood SJ, et al: Utrophin abundance is reduced at neuromuscular junctions of patients with both inherited and acquired acetylcholine receptor deficiencies. *Brain* 120:1513–1531, 1997.
322. Deconinck AE, Potter AC, Tinsley JM, et al: Postsynaptic abnormalities at the neuromuscular junction of utrophin-deficient mice. *J Cell Biol* 136:883–894, 1997.
323. Grady RM, Merlie JP, Sanes JR: Subtle neuromuscular defects in utrophin-deficient mice. *J Cell Biol* 136:871–882, 1997.
324. Klarsfeld A, Bessereau J-L, Salmon A-M, et al: An acetylcholine receptor α-subunit promoter conferring preferential synaptic expression in muscle of transgenic mice. *EMBO J* 10:625–632, 1991.
325. Sanes JR, Johnson YR, Kotzbauer PT, et al: Selective expression of an acetylcholine receptor-lacZ transgene in synaptic nuclei of adult muscle fibers. *Development* 113:1181–1191, 1991.
326. Simon AM, Hoppe P, Burden SJ: Spatial restriction of AChR gene expression to subsynaptic nuclei. *Development* 114:545–553, 1992.
327. Green WN: Ion channel assembly: Creating structures that function. *J Gen Physiol* 113:163–169, 1999.
328. Keller SH, Taylor P: Determinants responsible for assembly of the nicotinic acetylcholine receptor. *J Gen Physiol* 113:171–176, 1999.
329. Marchand S, Devillers-Thiéry A, Pons S, et al: Rapsyn escorts the nicotinic acetylcholine receptor along the exocytic pathway via association with lipid rafts. *J Neurosci* 22:8891–8901, 2002.
330. Salpeter MM, Harris R: Distribution and turnover rate of acetylcholine receptors throughout the junction function folds at a vertebrate neuromuscular junction. *J Cell Biol* 96:1781–1785, 1983.
331. Shyng S-L, Salpeter MM: Effect of reinnervation on the degradation rate of junctional acetylcholine receptors synthesized in denervated skeletal muscles. *J Neurosci* 10:3905–3915, 1990.
332. Weinberg CB, Reiness CG, Hall EW: Topographical segregation of old and new acetylcholine receptors at developing ectopic endplates in adult rat muscle. *J Cell Biol* 88:215–218, 1981.
333. Hirano H: Ultrastructural study of the morphogenesis of the neuromuscular junction in the skeletal muscle of the chick. *Z Zellforsch Mikroskop Anat* 79:198–208, 1967.
334. Atsumi S: The histogenesis of motor neurons with special reference to the correlation of their endplate formation. I. The development of endplates in the intercostal muscle in the chick embryo. *Acta Anat* 80:161–182, 1971.
335. Bennett MR, Pettigrew A: The formation of synapses in striated muscle during development. *J Physiol (Lond)* 241:515–545, 1974.
336. Kullberg RW, Lentz TL, Cohen MW: Development of the myotomal neuromuscular junction in *Xenopus laevis*: An electrophysiological and fine-structural study. *Dev Biol* 60:101–129, 1977.
337. Teräväinen H: Development of the myoneural junction in the rat. *Z Zellforsch Mikroskop Anat* 87:249–265, 1968.
338. Kelly AM, Zacks SI: The fine structure of motor end-plate myogenesis. *J Cell Biol* 42:154–169, 1969.
339. Dennis MJ, Ziskind-Conhaim L, Harris AJ: Development of neuromuscular junctions in rat embryos. *Dev Biol* 81:266–279, 1981.
340. Blechschmidt E, Daikoku SH: Die Entstehung der motorischen Innervation in der menschlichen Zungenmuskulatur. Elektronenmikroskopie der embryonalen Endplatte. *Acta Anat* 63:179–198, 1966.
341. Juntunen J, Teräväinen H: Structural development of myoneural junctions in the human embryo. *Histochemie* 32:107–112, 1972.
342. Ziskind-Conhaim L, Dennis MJ: Development of rat neuromuscular junctions in organ culture. *Dev Biol* 85:243–251, 1981.
343. Frank E, Fischbach GD: Early events in neuromuscular junction formation in vitro. *J Cell Biol* 83:143–158, 1979.
344. Anderson MJ, Cohen MW, Zorychta E: Effects of innervation on the distribution of acetylcholine receptors on cultured muscle cells. *J Physiol (Lond)* 268:731–756, 1977.
345. Crain SM, Peterson ER: Development of neural connections in culture. *Ann N Y Acad Sci* 228:6–34, 1974.
346. Sanes JR, Lichtman JW: Development of the vertebrate neuromuscular junction. *Annu Rev Neurosci* 22:389–442, 1999.
347. Juntunen J: Morphogenesis of the cholinergic synapse in striated muscle. *Prog Brain Res* 49:351–358, 1979.
348. Bevan S, Steinbach JH: The distribution of alpha-bungarotoxin binding sites on mammalian skeletal muscle developing "in vivo." *J Physiol (Lond)* 267:195–213, 1977.
349. Steinbach JH: Developmental changes on acetylcholine receptor aggregates in rat skeletal neuromuscular junctions. *Dev Biol* 84:267–276, 1981.
350. Bennett MR, Florin T: A statistical analysis of the release of acetylcholine at newly formed synapses in striated muscle. *J Physiol (Lond)* 238:93–107, 1974.
351. Michler A, Sakmann B: Receptor stability and channel conversion in the subsynaptic membrane of the developing mammalian neuromuscular junction. *Dev Biol* 80:1–17, 1980.
352. Gu Y, Hall ZW: Immunological evidence for a change in subunits of the acetylcholine receptor in developing and denervated rat muscle. *Neuron* 1:117–125, 1988.
353. Sakmann B, Witzemann V, Brenner H: Developmental changes in acetylcholine receptor channel structure and function as a model for synaptic plasticity. *Fidia Foundation Neuroscience Award Lectures* 6:51–103, 1992.
354. Lomo T: What controls the development of neuromuscular junctions. *Trends Neurosci* 3:126–129, 1980.
355. Balice-Gordon RJ, Lichtman JW: In vivo visualization of the growth of pre- and post-synaptic elements of neuromuscular junctions in the mouse. *J Neurosci* 10:894–908, 1990.
356. Hill RR, Robbins N: Mode of enlargement of young mouse neuromuscular junctions observed repeatedly in vivo with visualization of pre- and postsynaptic borders. *J Neurocytol* 20:183–194, 1991.
357. Davis GW, Eaton B, Paradis S: Synapse formation revisited. *Nature Neurosci* 4:558–560, 2001.
358. Burden SJ: Building the vertebrate neuromuscular junction. *J Neurobiol* 53:501–511, 2002.
359. Willman R, Fuhrer C: Neuromuscular synaptogenesis. *Cell Mol Life Sci* 59:1296–1316, 2002.
360. McMahan UJ: The agrin hypothesis. *Cold Spring Harb Symp Quant Biol* 55:407–418, 1990.
361. Burgess RW, Dickman DK, Nunez L, et al: Mapping sites responsible for agrin interactions with neurons. eg. *J Neurochem* 83:271–274, 2002.
362. Glass DJ, Yancopoulos GD: Sequential roles of agrin, Musk and rapsyn during neuromuscular junction formation. *Curr Opin Neurobiol* 7:379–384, 1997.

363. Sanes JR, Apel ED, Gautam M, et al: Agrin receptors at the skeletal neuromuscular junction. *Ann N Y Acad Sci* 841:1–13, 1998.
364. Burden SJ: The formation of neuromuscular synapses. *Genes Dev* 12:133–148, 1998.
365. Meier T, Hauser DM, Chiquet M, et al: Neural agrin induces ectopic postsynaptic specializations in innervated muscle fibers. *J Neurosci* 17:6534–6544, 1997.
366. Gautam M, Noakes PG, Moscoso L, et al: Defective neuromuscular synaptogenesis in agrin-deficient mutant mice. *Cell* 85:525–535, 1996.
367. Reist NE, Magill C, McMahan UJ, et al: Agrin-like molecules at synaptic sites in normal, denervated, and damaged skeletal muscles. *J Cell Biol* 105:2457–2469, 1987.
368. Ferns MJ, Hall ZW: How many agrins does it take to make a synapse? *Cell* 70:1–3, 1992.
369. Gesemann M, Denzer AJ, Ruegg MA: Acetylcholine receptor aggregating activity of agrin isoforms and mapping of the active site. *J Cell Biol* 128:625–636, 1995.
370. Martin PT, Sanes JR: Integrins mediate adhesion to agrin and modulate agrin signaling. *Development* 124:3909–3917, 1997.
371. Burkin DJ, Gu M, Hodges BL, et al: A functional role for specific spliced variants of the α7β1 integrin in acetylcholine receptor clustering. *J Cell Biol* 143:1067–1075, 1998.
372. Ruegg MA, Bixby JL: Agrin orchestrates synaptic differentiation at the vertebrate neuromuscular junction. *Trends Neurosci* 21:22–27, 1998.
373. Sugiyama JE, Bowen DC, Hall ZW: Dystroglycan binds nerve and muscle agrin. *Neuron* 13:103–115, 1994.
374. Campanelli JT, Roberds SL, Campbell KP, et al: A role for dystrophin-associated glycoproteins and utrophin in agrin-induced AChR clustering. *Cell* 77:663–674, 1994.
375. Valenzuela DM, Stitt TN, Distefano PS, et al: Receptor tyrosine kinase specific for the skeletal muscle lineage: Expression in embryonic muscle, at the neuromuscular junction, and after injury. *Neuron* 15:573–584, 1995.
376. Glass DJ, Bowen DC, Stitt TN, et al: Agrin acts via MuSK receptor complex. *Cell* 85:513–523, 1996.
377. Glass DJ, Apel ED, Shah H, et al: Kinase domain of the muscle-specific receptor tyrosine kinase is sufficient for phosphorylation but not clustering of acetylcholine receptors: Required role for the MuSK ectodomain? *Proc Natl Acad Sci USA* 94:8848–8853, 1997.
378. Meier T, Wallace BG: Formation of the neuromuscular junction. *Bioessays* 20:819–829, 1998.
379. Froehner SC, Luetje CW, Scotland PB, et al: The postsynaptic 43K protein clusters muscle nicotinic acetylcholine receptors in *Xenopus* oocytes. *Neuron* 5:403–410, 1990.
380. Gautam M, Noakes PG, Mudd J, et al: Failure of postsynaptic specialization to develop at neuromuscular junctions of rapsyn-deficient mice. *Nature* 377:232–236, 1995.
381. Apel ED, Glass DJ, Moscosco LM, et al: Rapsyn is required for MuSK signaling and recruits synaptic components to a MuSK-containing scaffold. *Neuron* 18:623–625, 1997.
382. Lee YI, Swope SL, Ferns MJ: Rapsyn's C-terminal domain mediates MuSK-induced phosphorylation of the AChR (abstr). *Mol Biol Cell* 13:395a, 2002.
382a. Luo ZG, Wang Q, Zhou JZ, et al: regulation of AChR clustering by disheveled interacting with MuSK and PAKI. *Neuron* 35:489–505, 2002.
383. Yang X, Arber S, William C, et al: Patterning of muscle acetylcholine receptor gene expression in the absence of motor innervation. *Neuron* 30:399–410, 2001.
384. Lin W, Burgess RW, Dominguez B, et al: Distinct roles of nerve and muscle in postsynaptic differentiation of the neuromuscular synapse. *Nature* 410:1057–1064, 2001.
385. Marangi PA, Forsayeth JR, Mittaud P, et al: Acetylcholine receptors are required for agrin-induced clustering of postsynaptic proteins. *EMBO J* 20:7060–7073, 2001.
386. Ono F, Higashijima S, Shcherbatko A, et al: Paralytic zebrafish lacking acetylcholine receptors fail to localize rapsyn clusters to the synapse. *J Neurosci* 21:5439–5448, 2001.
387. New HV, Mudge AW: Calcitonin gene-related peptide regulates muscle acetylcholine receptor synthesis. *Nature* 323:809–811, 1986.
388. Fontaine B, Klarsfeld A, Changeux J-P: Calcitonin-gene related peptide and muscle activity regulate acetylcholine receptor α-subunit mRNA levels by distinct intracellular pathways. *J Cell Biol* 105:1337–1342, 1987.
389. Lu JT, Son Y-J, Lee J, et al: Mice lacking α-calcitonin gene-related peptide exhibit normal cardiovascular regulation and neuromuscular development. *Mol Cell Neurosci* 14:99–120, 1999.
390. Falls DL, Rosen KM, Corfas G, et al: ARIA, a protein that stimulates acetylcholine receptor synthesis, is a member of the Neu ligand family. *Cell* 72:801–815, 1993.
391. Sandrock AW, Goodearl ADJ, Yin Q-W, et al: ARIA is concentrated in nerve terminals at neuromuscular junctions and at other synapses. *J Neurosci* 15:6124–6136, 1995.
392. Sandrock AW, Dryer SE, Rosen KM, et al: Maintenance of acetylcholine receptor number by neuregulins at the neuromuscular junction in vivo. *Science* 276:599–603, 1997.
393. Jo SA, Zhu X, Marchionni MA, et al: Neuregulins are concentrated at nerve-muscle synapses and activate ACh-receptor gene expression. *Nature* 373:158–161, 1995.
394. Lemke G: Neuregulins in development. *Mol Cell Neurosci* 7:247–262, 1996.
395. Si J, Luo Z, Mei L: Induction of acetylcholine receptor gene expression by ARIA requires activation of mitogen-activated protein kinase. *J Biol Chem* 271:19752–19759, 1996.
396. Altiok N, Altiok K, Changeux J-P: Heregulin-stimulated acetylcholine receptor gene expression in muscle—Requirement for MAP kinase and evidence for parallel inhibitory pathway independent electrical activity. *EMBO J* 16:717–725, 1997.
397. Schaffer L, Duckert N, Huchet-Dymanus M, et al: Ets related transcription factor in synaptic expression of the nicotinic acetylcholine receptor. *EMBO J* 17:3078–3090, 1998.
398. Fromm L, Burden SJ: Synapse-specific and neuregulin-induced transcription require an Ets site that binds GABPα/GAPBβ. *Genes Dev* 12:3074–3083, 1998.
399. Koike S, Schaeffer L, Changeux J-P: Identification of a DNA element determining synaptic expression of the mouse acetylcholine receptor delta-subunit gene. *Proc Natl Acad Sci USA* 92:10624–10628, 1995.
400. Duclert A, Savatier N, Schaeffer L, et al: Identification of an element crucial for the sub-synaptic expression of the acetylcholine receptor epsilon-subunit gene. *J Biol Chem* 271:17433–17438, 1996.
401. Ohno K, Anlar B, Engel AG: Congenital myasthenic syndrome caused by a mutation in the Ets-binding site of the promoter region of the acetylcholine receptor ε subunit gene. *Neuromuscul Disord* 9:131–135, 1999.
402. Nichols PR, Croxen R, Vincent A, et al: Mutation of the acetylcholine receptor ε-subunit promoter in congenital myasthenic syndrome. *Ann Neurol* 45:439–443, 1999.
403. de Kerchove d'Exaerde A, Cartaud J, Ravel-Chapuis A, et al: Expression of mutant Ets proteins at the neuromuscular synapse causes alterations in morphology and gene expression. *EMBO Rep* 3:1075–1081, 2002.
404. Sapru MK, Florance SK, Kirk C, et al: Identification of a protein-tyrosine kinase phosphatase response element in the nicotinic acetylcholine receptor ε subunit gene: Regulatory role of an Ets transcription factor. *Proc Natl Acad Sci USA* 95:1289–1294, 1998.
405. Salpeter MM, Buonanno A, Eftimie R, et al: Regulation of molecules at the neuromuscular junction, in Kelly AM, Blau HM (eds): *Neuromuscular Development and Disease*. New York: Raven Press; 1992, pp 251–283.
406. Rotzler S, Schramek H, Brenner HR: Metabolic stabilization of end-plate acetylcholine receptors regulated by Ca^{2+} influx associated with muscle activity. *Nature* 349:337–339, 1991.
407. Sakmann B, Brenner HR: Change in synaptic channel gating during neuromuscular development. *Nature* 276:401–402, 1978.
408. Mishina M, Takai T, Imoto K, et al: Molecular distinction between fetal and adult forms of muscle acetylcholine receptor. *Nature* 321:406–411, 1986.
409. Schuetze SM, Role LW: Developmental regulation of nicotinic acetylcholine receptors. *Annu Rev Neurosci* 10:403–457, 1987.
410. Wallace BG, Nitkin RM, Reist NE, et al: Aggregates of acetylcholinesterase induced by acetylcholine receptor-aggregating factor. *Nature* 315:574–577, 1985.
411. Buonanno A, Lautens L: Regulation of nicotinic acetylcholine receptor gene transcription by myogenin and MyoD. *J Cell Biochem* 15C:22, 1991.
412. Martinou JC, Merlie JP: Nerve-dependent modulation of acetylcholine receptor ε-subunit gene expression. *J Neurosci* 11:1291–1299, 1991.
413. Lomo T: Trophic factors and postsynaptic activity in synapse formation. *Nature* 305:576, 1983.
414. Bennett MR, Raftos J: The formation and regression of synapses during the reinnervation of axolotl striated muscles. *J Physiol (Lond)* 265:261–295, 1977.
415. Miyata Y, Yoshioka K: Selective elimination of motor nerve terminals in the rat soleus muscle during development. *J Physiol (Lond)* 309:631–646, 1980.
416. Banker BQ: Physiologic death of neurons in the developing anterior horn of the mouse, in Rowland LP (ed): *Human Motor Neuron Diseases*. New York: Raven Press; 1982, pp 473–485.
417. Mark RF: Synaptic repression at neuromuscular junctions. *Physiol Rev* 60:355–395, 1980.
418. McGrath PA, Bennett MR: Development of the synaptic connections between different segmental motoneurons and striated muscles in an axolotl limb. *Dev Biol* 69:133–145, 1979.
419. Korneliussen H, Jansen JKS: Morphological aspects of the elimination of polyneuronal innervation of skeletal muscle fibres in new-born rats. *J Neurocytol* 5:591–604, 1976.
420. O'Brien RAD, Östberg JC, Vrbova G: Observations on the elimination of polyneuronal innervation in developing mammalian skeletal muscle. *J Physiol (Lond)* 282:571–582, 1978.
421. Morrison-Graham K: An anatomical and electrophysiological study of synapse elimination at the developing frog neuromuscular junction. *Dev Biol* 99:298–311, 1983.

422. Rosenthal JL, Taraskevich PS: Reduction of multiaxonal innervation at the neuromuscular junction of the rat during development. *J Physiol (Lond)* 270:299–310, 1977.
423. O'Brien RAD, Östberg AJC, Vrbova G: Protease inhibitors reduce the loss of nerve terminals induced by activity and calcium on developing rat soleus muscles in vitro. *Neuroscience* 12:637–646, 1984.
424. O'Brien RAD: A difference in transmitter release between surviving and non-surviving nerve terminals in developing rat skeletal muscles. *J Physiol (Lond)* 371:89P–90P, 1981.
425. Oppenheim RW: Cell death during development of the nervous system. *Annu Rev Neurosci* 14:453–501, 1991.
426. Balice-Gordon RJ, Lichtman JW: In vivo observations of pre- and postsynaptic changes during transition from multiple to single innervation at developing neuromuscular junctions. *J Neurosci* 13:834–855, 1993.
427. Rich MM, Lichtman JW: In vivo visualization of pre- and postsynaptic changes during synapse elimination in reinnervated mouse muscle. *J Neurosci* 9:1781–1805, 1989.
428. Hoffman H: Local re-innervation in partially denervated muscle: A histophysiological study. *Aust J Exp Biol Med Sci* 28:383–397, 1950.
429. Hoffman H: Fate of interrupted nerve-fibers regenerating into partially denervated muscles. *Aust J Exp Biol Med Sci* 29:211–219, 1951.
430. Edds MV: Collateral regeneration of residual motor axons in partially denervated muscles. *J Exp Zool* 113:517–552, 1950.
431. Hoffman H: A study of the factors influencing innervation of muscles by implanted nerves. *Aust J Exp Biol Med Sci* 29:289–308, 1951.
432. Wernig A, Anzil AP, Bieser A: Formation and regression of synaptic contacts in the adult muscle, in Flohr H, Precht W (eds): *Lesion Induced Plasticity in Sensori-motor Systems*. Berlin: Springer-Verlag; 1981, pp 38–50.
433. Engel AG, Santa T: Motor end-plate fine structure. Quantitative analysis in disorders of neuromuscular transmission, in Desmedt JE (ed): *New Developments in Electromyography and Clinical Neurophysiology*. Basel: Karger; 1973, pp 196–228.
434. Bowden REM, Duchen LW: The anatomy and pathology of the neuromuscular junction, in Zaimis E (ed): *Neuromuscular Junction*. New York: Springer-Verlag; 1976, pp 23–29.
435. Duchen LW: An electron microscopic study of the changes induced by botulinum toxin in the motor end-plates of slow and fast skeletal muscle fibres of the mouse. *J Neurol Sci* 14:47–60, 1971.
436. Pachter BR, Eberstein A: Nerve sprouting and endplate growth induced in normal muscle by contralateral partial denervation of rat plantaris. *Brain Res* 560:311–314, 1991.
437. Duchen LW: Hereditary motor end-plate disease in the mouse: Light and electron microscopic studies. *J Neurol Neurosurg Psychiatry* 33:238–250, 1970.
438. Duchen LW, Stefani E: Electrophysiologic studies of neuromuscular transmission in hereditary "motor end-plate" disease in the mouse. *J Physiol (Lond)* 212:535–548, 1971.
439. Duchen LW, Tonge DA: The effects of tetanus toxin on neuromuscular transmission and on the morphology of motor end-plates in slow and fast skeletal muscle of the mouse. *J Physiol (Lond)* 228:157–172, 1973.
440. Brown MC, Ironton R: Motor neuron sprouting induced by prolonged tetrodotoxin block of nerve action potentials. *Nature* 265:459–461, 1977.
441. Wernig A, Pecot-Dechavassine M, Stover H: Sprouting and regression of nerve at the frog neuromuscular junction in normal conditions and after prolonged paralysis with curare. *J Neurocytol* 9:277–303, 1980.
442. Brown MC, Goodwin GM, Ironton R: Prevention of motor nerve sprouting in botulinum toxin poisoned mouse soleus muscles by direct stimulation of the mouse. *J Physiol (Lond)* 267:42P–43P, 1977.
443. Gurney ME, Yamamoto H, Kwon Y: Induction of motor neuron sprouting in vivo by ciliary neurotrophic factor and basic fibroblast growth factor. *J Neurosci* 12:3241–3247, 1992.
444. Caroni P, Grandes P: Nerve sprouting in innervated adult skeletal muscle induced by exposure to elevated levels of insulin-like growth factors. *J Cell Biol* 110:1307–1317, 1990.
445. Young JZ: Growth and plasticity in the nervous system. *Proc R Soc Lond [Biol]* 139:18–37, 1952.
446. Engel AG, Tsujihata M, Jerusalem F: Quantitative assessment of motor end-plate ultrastructure in normal and diseased muscle, in Dyck PJ, Thomas PK, Lambert EH (eds): *Peripheral Neuropathy*. Philadelphia: Saunders; 1975, pp 1404–1415.
447. Banker BQ, Kelly SS, Robbins N: Neuromuscular transmission and correlative morphology in young and old mice. *J Physiol (Lond)* 339:355–375, 1983.
448. Tweedle CD, Stephens KE: Development of complexity in motor nerve endings at the rat neuromuscular junction. *Neuroscience* 6:1657–1662, 1981.
449. Kelly SS: The effect of age on neuromuscular transmission. *J Physiol (Lond)* 274:51–62, 1978.
450. Smith DO: Acetylcholine storage, release and leakage at the neuromuscular junction of mature adults and aged rats. *J Physiol (Lond)* 347:161–176, 1984.
451. Courtney S, Steinbach JH: Age changes in neuromuscular junction morphology and acetylcholine receptor distribution on rat skeletal muscle fibers. *J Physiol (Lond)* 320:435–447, 1981.
452. Wigston DJ: Repeated in vivo visualization of neuromuscular junctions in adult mouse lateral gastrocnemius. *J Neurosci* 10:1753–1761, 1990.
453. Hill RR, Robbins N, Fang ZP: Plasticity of presynaptic and postsynaptic elements of neuromuscular junctions repeatedly observed in living adult mice. *J Neurocytol* 20:165–182, 1991.

Chapter 16
Neuromuscular Transmission

KARL L. MAGLEBY

Introduction
   MECHANISM OF NEUROMUSCULAR TRANSMISSION
   ELECTROPHYSIOLOGIC MEASUREMENTS OF NEUROMUSCULAR TRANSMISSION

Presynaptic Aspects of Neuromuscular Transmission
   BRIEF OVERVIEW OF TRANSMITTER RELEASE
   QUANTAL RELEASE OF TRANSMITTER
   SHORT-TERM SYNAPTIC PLASTICITY
   NONQUANTAL RELEASE OF TRANSMITTER
   RELEASE PROTEINS AND FEEDBACK SYSTEMS

Postsynaptic Aspects of Neuromuscular Transmission
   OVERVIEW
   ACETYLCHOLINE RECEPTOR
   GENERATION OF END PLATE CURRENTS
   DESENSITIZATION

Safety Factor in Neuromuscular Transmission
Conclusion

Introduction

The purpose of this chapter is to summarize current knowledge about the mechanism of skeletal neuromuscular transmission. A general overview is presented first, then a brief discussion of methods used to measure neuromuscular transmission, followed by more detailed discussions of pre- and postsynaptic mechanisms and safety factor. Emphasis is on the general process of neuromuscular transmission rather than on the fine details of the various steps. The interested reader may wish to consult some of the excellent reviews of neuromuscular transmission for a more in-depth overview.[1-12]

MECHANISM OF NEUROMUSCULAR TRANSMISSION

The general mechanism of neuromuscular transmission is clearly established and well supported by experimental evidence.[11,13] It may be summarized as follows:

1. An action potential propagating down the motor axon invades and depolarizes the presynaptic nerve terminal.
2. Voltage-dependent calcium channels in the presynaptic nerve terminal open in response to the depolarization.
3. Ca^{2+} moves down its electrochemical gradient through the calcium channels into the nerve terminal from the extracellular solution.
4. The influx of Ca^{2+} leads to a transient increase in transmitter release by increasing the probability that the synaptic vesicles in the nerve terminal will fuse with the presynaptic membrane.
5. Approximately 50 synaptic vesicles in humans and 200 in frogs fuse with the presynaptic membrane, releasing their quantal packets of acetylcholine (ACh)* into the synaptic cleft. Each quantal packet consists of about 6000 to 10,000 molecules of ACh.
6. The released ACh diffuses toward the postsynaptic (muscle) membrane and the edges of the synaptic cleft. In the process it is bound by ACh receptors (AChR) on the muscle membrane and is also hydrolyzed by acetylcholinesterase (AChE).
7. About 50,000 AChRs with bound ACh in humans and 250,000 in frogs undergo a conformational change and open their channels.
8. The AChR channels, which have an effective open time of 1 to 2 ms, are permeable to Na^+, K^+, and, to a lesser extent, Ca^{2+}. More Na^+ moves through the open channels into the muscle fiber than K^+ moves out, which leads to a net influx of positive charge that depolarizes the fiber, producing the end plate potential (EPP). The net current that flows through the open AChR channels is called the end plate current.
9. When the EPP depolarizes the membrane of the muscle fiber to threshold, an action potential is generated in the muscle membrane that propagates in both directions in the muscle fiber away from the end plate, leading to contraction. In rat skeletal muscle, the resting membrane potential is about −75 mV and the threshold about −63 mV.[6]
10. The Ca^{2+} that enters the nerve terminal is sequestered and eventually extruded; choline from the hydrolyzed ACh is taken up by the nerve terminal for resynthesis into ACh; filled synaptic vesicles containing ACh are positioned at the release sites; and the synaptic vesicles and/or membrane of the empty synaptic vesicles is recycled.

ELECTROPHYSIOLOGIC MEASUREMENTS OF NEUROMUSCULAR TRANSMISSION

Steps 1 to 5 and 10 above constitute the presynaptic aspects of neuromuscular transmission, which are mainly concerned with the mechanism of transmitter release. Steps 6 to 9 constitute the postsynaptic aspects, which are mainly concerned with the process by which released ACh leads to depolarization of the muscle membrane. Electrophysiologic studies of both pre- and postsynaptic mechanisms typically use the flow of current through the AChR channels (end plate current) or the EPP it generates to measure the process under study. For presynaptic studies, the end plate current or EPP is used as an assay of the amount of transmitter released.[14,15] For postsynaptic studies, the end plate current is used to

---

*A list of abbreviations used in this chapter is given at the end of the chapter.

measure the time course of conductance change at the end plate.[16,17] In addition, the patch-clamp technique[18,19] is used to study the properties of the individual ion channels involved in both the presynaptic and postsynaptic aspects of neuromuscular transmission. This section briefly describes how EPPs and end plate currents are measured. The patch-clamp technique is described in a later section, where the properties of the AChR are considered.

The Neuromuscular Preparation and Intracellular Recording

A schematic diagram of the classic neuromuscular preparation[20] is presented in Fig. 16-1A. In this experiment, muscle twitch was prevented by increasing $[Mg^{2+}]_o$ to 15 mM to decrease transmitter release to reduce EPP amplitude far below threshold. The nerve was stimulated with a short (0.1-ms) pulse, and the resulting EPP was recorded with a microelectrode inserted into the muscle fiber in the region of the end plate. The EPP, which was about 3 mV in amplitude, is shown in the oscilloscope tracing in Fig. 16-1B. Also present are three smaller miniature end plate potentials (MEPP) with amplitudes of about 0.3 mV. The EPP and MEPPs shown in Fig. 16-1B represent changes in voltage across the muscle membrane in the region of the end plate.

Measuring Changes in Transmitter Release with EPP Amplitude

Under conditions where postsynaptic sensitivity remains constant and EPP amplitudes do not exceed about 10 mV, changes in EPP amplitude give a good measure of changes in the number of quantal packets of transmitter released.[14,15,21] If the EPP amplitude exceeds about 10 mV, changes in transmitter release are underestimated as a result of the nonlinear summation of unit potentials unless corrections are applied.[22]

Measuring End Plate Current with Voltage Clamp

The magnitude and time course of the EPP is a function of both the magnitude and time course of the ACh-induced current through receptor channels at the end plate and the resistance and capacitance of the muscle cell membrane.[20] Simply stated, the rising phase of the EPP mainly represents the charging up of the muscle fiber membrane within a few millimeters of the end plate by the end plate current (positive ions are added to the inside of the muscle), and the falling phase represents the decay of the positive charge through the muscle membrane and down the muscle fiber away from the end plate region. As the EPP only indirectly reflects the underlying AChR channel activity because of the resistance and capacitance of the muscle fiber, study of postsynaptic mechanism is best done with end plate currents and single-channel currents, both of which give a direct measure of current through the receptor channels.

End plate currents are measured by inserting a current-injecting microelectrode into the muscle fiber near the end plate region in addition to the voltage-measuring microelectrode. Amplifiers are arranged so that, for every net positive (or negative) charge that enters the muscle fiber through the end plate channels, the current electrode removes a positive (or negative) change from the muscle fiber. The removed charge is a direct measure of the current through the end plate, and the membrane potential of the fiber remains constant (clamped) because there is no net change in charge inside the muscle fiber.[23] No current flows through the membrane capacitance because there is no change in voltage.

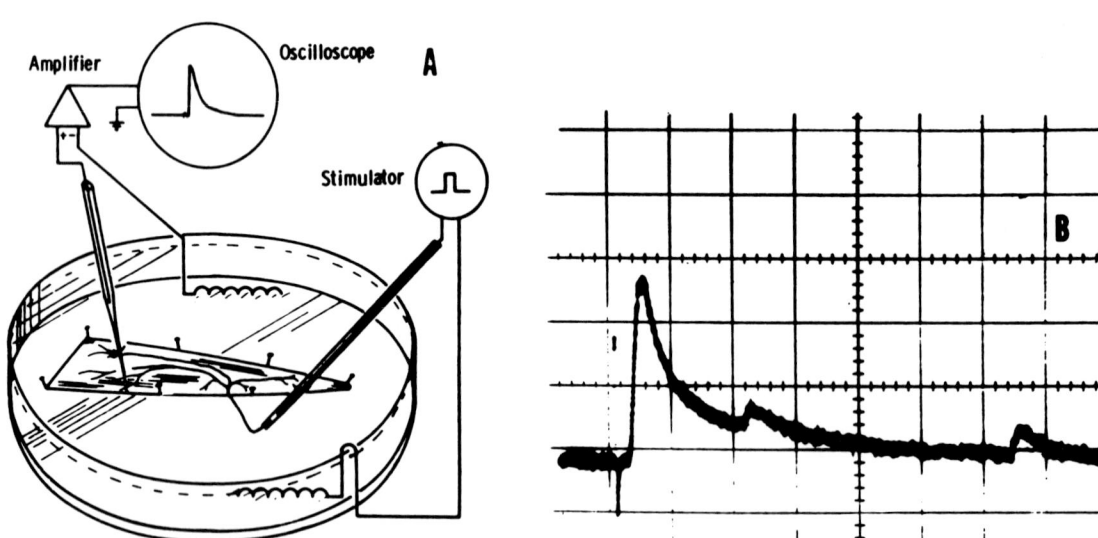

FIGURE 16-1. Intracellular recordings of an EPP from a frog sartorius muscle. A. A microelectrode is inserted into a muscle fiber at the region of the end plate. The potential difference between the tip of the microelectrode in the muscle cell and a reference wire in the bathing solution is amplified and displayed on an oscilloscope. The nerve is stimulated with 0.1-ms current pulses through a suction electrode. B. Oscilloscope tracing of an EPP. Muscle twitch was prevented by decreasing transmitter release by raising $[Mg^{2+}]_o$ to 15 mM. Stimulation of the nerve at the time indicated by the downward-going shock artifact released about nine quantal packets of transmitter, which generated an EPP about 3 mV in amplitude. The smaller potentials on the tail of the EPP are MEPPs that result from the release of single quantal packets of transmitter. Horizontal divisions: 5 ms; vertical divisions: 1 mV. (From Barrett EF, Magleby KL, in Goldberg AM, Hanin I (eds): Biology of Cholinergic Function. New York: Raven Press, 1976, pp 29–100. With permission.)

Chapter 16. Neuromuscular Transmission

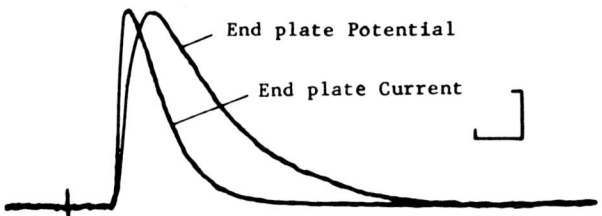

FIGURE 16-2. Superposition of an EPP and an end plate current. The end plate current gives a direct measure of the current that flows through the ACh-activated receptor channels. The EPP reflects the change in membrane potential within a few millimeters of the end plate that results from the end plate current when the cell is not voltage-clamped. The EPP has slower rise and decay times because of the time required to charge and discharge the muscle membrane. See Takeuchi and Takeuchi[23] for earlier experiments of this type. Horizontal bar: 2 ms; vertical bar: 40 nA (end plate current), 1 mV (EPP). End plate current and EPP from separate experiments with different levels of transmitter release. The end plate current is inverted from the normal convention of plotting inward currents downward. (From Barrett EF, Magleby KL, in Goldberg AM, Hanin I (eds): Biology of Cholinergic Function. New York: Raven Press, 1976, pp 29–100. With permission.)

Figure 16-2 shows a comparison of the time course of an EPP and the end plate current. The EPP rises and decays more slowly because of the resistance and capacitance of the muscle membrane.

Presynaptic Aspects of Neuromuscular Transmission

BRIEF OVERVIEW OF TRANSMITTER RELEASE

The nerve terminal, which forms the presynaptic part of the neuromuscular junction, is composed of 500 to 1000 repeating synaptic units in the frog. Each has an active zone (dense band) with about 20 synaptic vesicles along each side. The synaptic vesicles contain ACh.[24] There are also large membrane particles associated with the active zone. These particles likely represent voltage-gated calcium channels (see Refs. 25 to 28 and Chap. 15, on the structure of the neuromuscular junction). Upon depolarization of the nerve, Ca^{2+} enters the nerve terminal through the calcium channels at the region of the active zone[27] and promotes fusion of about 50 synaptic vesicles in humans[29] and 200 in frogs with the presynaptic membrane. The contents of the synaptic vesicles are then released by exocytosis.[30–33] Most of the release is over within a millisecond, as the calcium channels close shortly after the nerve action potential,[34] and the Ca^{2+} that entered rapidly diffuses away from the release sites and is sequestered.[35–37]

QUANTAL RELEASE OF TRANSMITTER

It is well established that transmitter release evoked by action potentials in the nerve terminal occurs in integral multiples of quantal packets of about 6000 to 10,000 ACh molecules each.[15,38–40] Each packet is released from a highly localized region of the nerve terminal, mainly, but not entirely, independent of other packets,[5] in a very brief (less than 0.2 ms) period of time.[41] Under normal physiologic conditions, about 20 to 200 such packets, depending on the species and junction, are released with each nerve impulse, giving rise to an EPP that typically exceeds threshold for generation of an action potential in the muscle fiber.[6] Occasionally, a quantal packet of transmitter is released at random, giving rise to a miniature end plate potential (MEPP). Each quantal packet of transmitter represents the contents of one synaptic vesicle released into the synaptic cleft.[12,25,42–45]

The quantal nature of transmitter release becomes readily apparent when transmitter release is reduced by increasing the $[Mg^{2+}]_o$ and/or reducing the $[Ca^{2+}]_o$. This is shown in Fig. 16-3, which presents seven superimposed oscilloscope tracings. The downward inflection at the start of each trace is a shock artifact indicating when the nerve was stimulated. Notice that the EPP amplitude fluctuates in quantal steps of about 0.3 mV and that the number of quanta released by each impulse varies from impulse to impulse. One of the seven trials was a failure in which no quanta were released. One quantum was released in each of two trials, two quanta were released in each of three trials, and three quanta were released in one trial. In addition, during one trial a spontaneous MEPP occurred with amplitude similar to the quantal steps in the EPP amplitudes. Notice also that there is a variation in the latency of release from trial to trial.

The quantal fluctuation in EPP amplitude and the fluctuation in the latency of release from trial to trial is consistent with a statistical model for quantal transmitter release first proposed by Del Castillo and Katz[15] and extensively developed by Barrett and Stevens.[39,46] The nerve terminal is

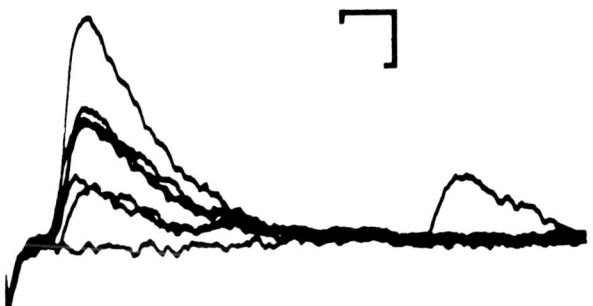

FIGURE 16-3. Quantal fluctuations in transmitter release. Intracellular recording from frog sartorius muscle under conditions of greatly reduced transmitter release obtained by raising $[Mg^{2+}]_o$ to 5 mM and reducing $[Ca^{2+}]_o$ to 0.5 mM. The responses obtained by stimulating the nerve seven consecutive times are superimposed. The EPP amplitude fluctuated from trial to trial in quantal steps of similar amplitude to the spontaneously occurring MEPP at the right of the figure. Three quanta were released in one trial, two quanta were released in three trials, one quantum was released in two trials, and one trial was a failure in which no quanta were released. The average quantal content of these seven trials was 1.57. Horizontal bar: 2.5 ms. Vertical bar: 0.3 mV. See Del Castillo and Katz[15] for first experiments of this type. (From Barrett EF, Magleby KL, in Goldberg AM, Hanin I (eds): Biology of Cholinergic Function. New York: Raven Press, 1976, pp 29–100. With permission.)

assumed to contain a number of quanta, n, available for release, with a probability p of release. The number of quanta released by a nerve impulse, m or quantal content, is then given by $m = np$. Under resting conditions, p is very small, so only an occasional quantum is released, giving rise to a MEPP. Following an action potential in the nerve terminal, the probability of release is greatly increased for about 1 ms because of the entry of Ca^{2+}, evoking the release of many quanta during this brief period, giving rise to an EPP. Quanta are released independently in this hypothesis, and the number available for release, n (see below), can be depleted but is replenished given sufficient time between nerve impulses.

This model predicts that the variation in the number of quanta released by each impulse from trial to trial should be described by the binomial distribution or approximately by the Poisson distribution if the number released is small compared to n. It also predicts that the latency to release of the first quantum following an action potential should vary randomly. In general, the experimental data meet these predictions, although close examination reveals some discrepancies, such as interactions between the release of quanta.[5,47,48]

Physiologic Correlates of the Statistical Parameters n and p

Assuming that the quantal response results from the contents of a synaptic vesicle dumped into the synaptic cleft, then it might be thought that the statistical parameter n in the quantal hypothesis could be related to synaptic vesicles and the parameter p to the probability that the vesicles are released. However, the basis of n and p is more complex. Nerve terminals contain far more vesicles (200,000 to 400,000) than estimates of n (100 to 2000), and the numbers of active zones (4000 to 30,000) may not directly indicate n.[47,49–51] As discussed further on, vesicles must first be docked and then primed at the active zones before their contents can be released.[7,52,53] It may be speculated that n, the release sites, may be a subset of the number of active zones (the number of functional active zones),[54–56] and that this number may change with the experimental conditions. The statistical parameter p has values of 0.1 to near 1 in the presence of Ca^{2+} for mammalian terminals and 0.1 to 0.5 for frog[49] and may be a function of the average number of docked vesicles at each active zone and the probability that an action potential releases the docked vesicles.[45,55] Estimates of p and the readily releasable pool of synaptic vesicles (see below) for human end plate are 0.15 and 326, respectively.[29]

Estimating Quantal Size

In terms of the quantal hypothesis, a MEPP represents the response to the release of a single quantal packet of transmitter and thus serves as a convenient measure of quantal size. The distribution of quantal size, as determined from the distribution of MEPP amplitudes at a single motor end plate, typically has a major component that is well described by a gaussian distribution.[57] In addition, there are often occasional "giant" MEPPs with amplitudes several times the mean amplitude, and in some preparations there is a class of small MEPPs that gives rise to an additional distribution of MEPP amplitudes.[58] Although mean MEPP amplitude generally gives a good measure of quantal size, MEPP amplitude and quantal size are not necessarily the same at regenerating neuromuscular junctions.[58]

It has been suggested that the class of small MEPPs represents subunits of quanta such that the classic MEPPs (the ones described by the gaussian distribution) are composed of integral numbers of subunits.[58] Such a hypothesis seems unlikely, since comparisons between numbers of synaptic vesicles and quanta released suggest one synaptic vesicle per quantum[5,9,50,59,60] rather than the 7 to 15 required if the physical basis for the subunit were a synaptic vesicle. MEPPs also appear uniquantal at central synapses.[61]

Synaptic Delay

The period of time between the arrival of an action potential in the presynaptic nerve terminal and the start of the postsynaptic response in the muscle cell is the synaptic delay.[13] At 20°C the minimal synaptic delay is about 0.5 ms, the average delay is about 1 ms, and some delays extend to several milliseconds.[62] Synaptic delay has both pre- and postsynaptic components: the time required for the nerve terminal to release quantal packets into the synaptic cleft after depolarization by the presynaptic action potential and the time required for the ACh to diffuse to the postsynaptic side, to bind to receptors, and for the receptors to open their channels. Diffusion across the cleft and reaction time for binding and opening of the receptor channels is less than about 0.15 ms.[62] Thus, synaptic delay is mainly of presynaptic origin. Part of the presynaptic component of synaptic delay represents the time required for calcium channels to open after an action potential.[34] The variation in synaptic delay from trial to trial could arise from expected random variation in the kinetics of opening of calcium channels and fluctuations in the time required for the calcium-activated transmitter-releasing machinery to release quanta of transmitter.

Calcium Evokes Transmitter Release

Ca^{2+} acts inside the terminal Katz and Miledi[13] presented a systematic series of experiments that suggested the entry of Ca^{2+} into the nerve terminal at the time of the nerve impulse is what leads to evoked quantal transmitter release. Ca^{2+} is required in the extracellular solution for evoked transmitter release and is sufficient for release in the absence of other cations. Action potentials propagate into the nerve terminals in the absence of extracellular Ca^{2+} but fail to evoke EPPs, and Ca^{2+} must enter the nerve terminal for release to occur. Increasing intracellular Ca^{2+} in the nerve terminal by photolysis of caged Ca^{2+} compounds elicits transmitter release.[63] Release thus requires an elevation in intracellular Ca^{2+}.

Fourth-power relationship. Dodge and Rahamimoff[64] quantified the relationship between $[Ca^{2+}]_o$ and evoked transmitter release at the frog neuromuscular junction. Results are shown in Fig. 16-4A and B. For low $[Ca^{2+}]_o$ there is a fourth-power relationship between $[Ca^{2+}]_o$ and the number of quanta of transmitter released by each nerve impulse, and this fourth-power relationship holds to the very lowest Ca^{2+} concentrations.[65] Similar experiments give a power of about 2.6 in rat,[66] up to 4 in squid,[67] 3 to 5 in crayfish,[68] and

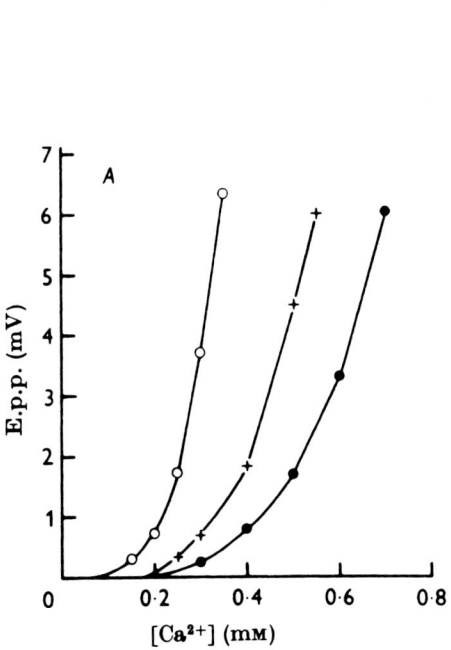
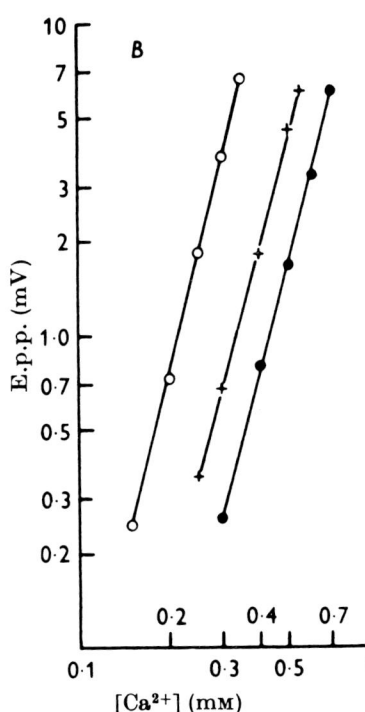

FIGURE 16-4. Effect of $[Ca^{2+}]_o$ on EPP amplitude. Data at three different $[Mg^{2+}]_o$: open circles, 0.5 mM; plus symbols, 2 mM; filled circles, 4 mM. A. Linear plot. B. Double-logarithmic plot. Under the conditions of the experiments the mean number of quanta of transmitter released by each nerve impulse would be proportional to EPP amplitude. There is an approximate fourth-power relationship between $[Ca^{2+}]_o$ and transmittter release. (From Dodge FA, Rahamimoff R: Co-operative action a calcium ions in transmitter release at the neuromuscular junction. J Physiol (Lond) 193:419, 1967. With permission.)

3.5 at a calyx synapse.[54] While the power relationship between MEPP frequency and intracellular Ca^{2+} is 3 to 4 in crayfish, it is closer to being linear in frog.[69]

Dodge and Rahamimoff interpreted their results to suggest that four Ca^{2+} must bind at some site for the release of a quantum of transmitter. At higher $[Ca^{2+}]$, the proposed release sites start to become saturated, so that the relationship between $[Ca^{2+}]_o$ and the number of quanta of transmitter released is closer to linear and eventually saturates. This is expected on the basis of the fourth-power hypothesis, so the observation of a linear relationship between $[Ca^{2+}]_o$ and release does not exclude their model unless it can be shown that the $[Ca^{2+}]$ at the sites of action was sufficiently low that saturation was not occurring. The problem of determining the number of Ca^{2+} ions required to act cooperatively at the site of action is further complicated by the fact that the concentration of Ca^{2+} will be high close to open calcium channels and will fall off rapidly with distance.[35,70,71]

Properties of calcium channels. The Ca^{2+} that activates release enters the nerve terminal through specific voltage-dependent calcium channels that can be different in different types of nerve cells and in different animals.[70,72,73] Calcium channels in presynaptic nerve terminals of mammalian neuromuscular junctions involved in evoked transmitter release are mainly of the P/Q type,[74-76] those in lizard of the N type,[77] those in a calyx synapse of the P type,[78] and those in amphibians of mainly the N type,[79] with a small contribution of L type.[80] At the mammalian neuromuscular junction, channels of the L and N types can contribute to spontaneous but not evoked release.[76]

The presynaptic calcium channels open with a delay following depolarization and do not inactivate in squid[34] but can inactivate at a calyx synapse.[81] The calcium channels start to open at the peak of the action potential and reach their maximum conductance at about the time that the fast falling phase of the action potential has reached the resting membrane potential.[34] The slow kinetics of the calcium channels together with the fact that the greatest electrical driving force on Ca^{2+} to enter the nerve terminal occurs after the AP returns to the resting potential (tail current) would also contribute to the synaptic delay because of the late entry of Ca^{2+}.

Ca^{2+} domains and the removal of Ca^{2+} from the release sites. The short millisecond duration of the Ca^{2+} current into the nerve terminal following an action potential[34] and the resulting short duration of transmitter release[62] suggest that the effective lifetime of the free Ca^{2+} at the release sites is less than a few milliseconds. The Ca^{2+} that enters forms microdomains of elevated Ca^{2+} in the nerve terminal just above the open Ca^{2+} channels, with concentrations of Ca^{2+} reaching 100 μM or more.[71] This microdomain would then initially disperse into the nerve terminal by diffusion,[9,35,70,82,83] but the extent and effectiveness of diffusion would depend on any possible compartmentalization in the nerve terminal in the immediate area. Estimates of intracellular Ca^{2+} required to obtain the evoked release rates observed experimentally are 2 to 5 μM in chromaffin cells,[84] < 10 μM at the calyx of Held,[85] and > 100 μM in bipolar cells in goldfish retina[86] and in amphibian nerve-muscle cultures.[87]

After the initial diffusion away from the release sites, secondary uptake or removal of Ca^{2+} would be by binding to mobile and fixed Ca^{2+} buffers, uptake by smooth endoplasmic reticulum and mitochondria, and direct extrusion from the nerve terminal.[82,88-93] Due to the rapid buffering, less than 0.1 to 2 percent of the Ca^{2+} entering the cell will remain free.[35] Mitochondria are further from the release sites, have a lower affinity than the nonmitochondrial ATP-dependent component, and have a very high capacity, equivalent to a total cytosolic Ca^{2+} load of ~ 1 mM.[88] Mitochondria can serve as a backup Ca^{2+} sequestering system when the Ca^{2+} load becomes elevated, as can occur with repetitive stimulation.[93–95]

The Ca^{2+} that enters the terminal, even though buffered and sequestered in the endoplasmic reticulum and mitochondria, eventually has to be extruded back across the nerve terminal membrane to the extracellular space. The plasmalemmal Ca^{2+} pump, which is activated by increased intracellular Ca^{2+}, moves Ca^{2+} out of the cell using the hydrolysis of ATP as an energy source. In addition to the Ca^{2+} pump, Na^+/Ca^{2+} exchangers couple the influx of 3 Na^+ with the efflux of 1 Ca^{2+}. These two active processes function to restore the free intracellular Ca^{2+} to about 0.1 μM.[96]

Ca^{2+} substitutes and antagonists. Ca^{2+}, Sr^{2+}, and Ba^{2+} readily enter the nerve terminal through the voltage-sensitive calcium channels.[97] Sr^{2+} will substitute for Ca^{2+} in evoked transmitter release but is much less potent. For example, for the same molar concentrations, the release in Sr^{2+} is only about 1 to 6 percent[98] the expected release in Ca^{2+}. Ba^{2+} is even less effective than Sr^{2+} in maintaining evoked transmitter release,[99,100] and Ba^{2+} can antagonize the entry of Ca^{2+} into the nerve terminal.[101] Mg^{2+}, Mn^{2+}, Co^{2+}, and La^{3+} act as calcium antagonists, most likely by inhibiting the entry of Ca^{2+}.[49,97,102] Thus, the Mg-induced parallel shift in the curves relating Ca^{2+} to EPP amplitude shown in Fig. 16-4 probably results from Mg^{2+} blocking Ca^{2+} entry.

Mechanism of Transmitter Release

Fusion pore and exocytosis proteins. Action potentials in the nerve terminal evoke transmitter release through the opening of Ca^{2+} channels and not from direct effects on the release mechanism.[103] Evoked transmitter release is related to the third to fourth power of $[Ca^{2+}]_o$ (Fig. 16-4) and Ca^{2+} entry into the nerve terminal,[54,104] suggesting that evoked release is related to the fourth power of $[Ca^{2+}]$ at the release sites. The Ca^{2+}-dependent steps in the release process leading to the exocytosis of a synaptic vesicle at neuroendocrine cells can be modeled by a sequence of 2 to 4 Ca^{2+}-binding steps followed by a rate-limiting exocytosis step.[105] The mechanics of the exocytotic fusion step involved in fusion of the large secretory granules (vesicles) with the surface membrane in mast cells have been defined through simultaneous measurements of membrane capacitance together with vesicle diameter or conductance.[31,106,107] These measurements have shown that the first step in exocytosis in mast cells is the formation of an aqueous fusion pore[107] with an initial pore conductance of about 230 pS.

The fusion pore would form at the area of contact of the secretory vesicle with the surface membrane, passing through both membranes to connect the interior of the secretory vesicle to the exterior of the cell. After forming, the fusion pore can flicker closed and open a number of times or expand to allow exocytosis of the secretory vesicle contents. Swelling of the secretory vesicle occurs after the formation of the fusion pore, but is not required to expand the fusion pore for exocytosis.[108]

At least nine families of synaptic vesicle proteins, many of which are expressed in multiple isoforms, are associated with synaptic vesicles and the release process.[72,109,110] The Ca^{2+}-dependent process leading to the fusion pore and exocytosis most likely involves SNARE proteins (Vamp/synaptobrevin, syntaxin, and SNAP-25), the syntaxin-binding protein munc18a, rab3 and rab3 effector proteins, and the Ca^{2+}-binding protein synaptotagmin.[3,83,109–111] In one highly simplified version of exocytosis, the synaptic vesicle first *docks* at the release site in the active zone using rab and rab effector proteins. Displacement of munc18a then allows the synaptobrevin and synaptotagmin on the synaptic vesicle membrane to associate with syntaxin 1 and SNAP-25 on the plasma membrane, forcing the membranes together and forming a *primed* complex. The binding of Ca^{2+} to synaptotagmin then triggers membrane fusion, leading to the fusion pore and exocytosis. In model systems, the voltage-dependent Ca^{2+} channels that provide the influx of Ca^{2+} to trigger the release process are associated with and appear to be directly modulated by the syntaxin/synaptotagmin complex.[72] It may be that Ca^{2+} channels are inhibited if they are not associated with docked vesicles.[72]

The synaptic vesicle cycle. Synaptic vesicles that release their contents by exocytosis are replenished by an elaborate process of synaptic vesicle trafficking.[2,3,53,60,111–113] The vesicular membrane can be retrieved by endocytosis, which involves total fusion with the plasma membrane, followed by clathrin coating, budding, retrieval, and then uncoating. Synaptic vesicles may also fuse temporarily long enough to release their contents and then detach relatively intact (kiss-and-run mechanism). The large numbers of synaptic vesicles not directly located at the active zone represent the reserve pool of vesicles. Vesicles from the reserve pool can be mobilized toward the active zones for docking and priming. Mobilization from the reserve pool to the readily releasable pool is facilitated by stimulation and starts after about 10 s. The docked and primed vesicles represent the readily releasable pool of vesicles[60]—those that can be released in a few seconds by very high frequency stimulation. At the neuromuscular junction, the readily releasable pool represents only ~2 percent of the total vesicles in the nerve terminal. Two endocytotic recycling routes are available. Incorporation of dyes into the synaptic vesicles indicates that some vesicles recycle directly into the readily releasable pool in < 1 min, while others are internalized and recycle into the reserve pool in 5 to 10 min.[112]

SHORT-TERM SYNAPTIC PLASTICITY

Facilitation, Augmentation, Potentiation, and Depression

EPP amplitude following each nerve impulse is not constant but varies as a function of the frequency and duration of stimulation.[114] These changes in EPP amplitude generally result from changes in the number of quanta of transmitter released from the nerve terminal,[5,14,21,115] although quantal size (MEPP amplitude) can change during prolonged stimulation[116] and also in the presence of esterase inhibitors.[117] Stimulation-induced changes in transmitter release are typically studied by conditioning the nerve terminal with trains of impulses and then applying testing impulses to follow the resulting changes in transmitter release. Studies of this type suggest that the changes in release can be divided into a number of components or processes. Increases in transmitter release include augmentation, potentiation (tetanic and posttetanic potentiation, or PTP), and first and second components of facilitation. Some marked differences in the kinetic properties and ionic specificities of these four components suggest that they are separable and can act somewhat independently of one another.[99,118] For example, a small amount of Ba^{2+} in the bathing solution increases the magnitude of augmentation while having little effect on potentiation, whereas Sr^{2+} increases the magnitude and time constant of decay of the second component of facilitation while having little effect on augmentation or potentiation.[99] Decreases in transmitter release with repetitive stimulation are generally referred to as depression, which can be divided into fast (5 to 7 s) and slow (tens of seconds to minutes) components, based on the time course of recovery.[118,119]

Table 16-1 summarizes the properties of the processes that underlie stimulation-induced changes in transmitter release. The magnitudes of the processes after one impulse and approximate time courses are indicated.

Experimental Demonstration of Facilitation, Augmentation, Potentiation, and Depression

Low quantal content. The processes that act to increase transmitter release are most easily observed when transmitter release is greatly reduced by decreasing $[Ca^{2+}]_o$ and/or increasing $[Mg^{2+}]_o$, so that depression is not obviously present.[118] Figure 16-5A plots stimulation-induced changes in transmitter release under such conditions of low quantal content. In this experiment the nerve was first stimulated once every 5 s to establish a control response. At this slow stimulation rate, the amount of transmitter released by each nerve impulse (measured as changes in EPP amplitude) remained relatively constant. The nerve was then stimulated at a rate of 20 impulses per second for 15 s. EPP amplitudes increased progressively during the train to about 14 times the control level. The increase is the result of facilitation, augmentation, and potentiation.[99,120] Testing impulses applied after the train in a series of trials (so that only a few testing impulses were applied in any trial immediately after the train) indicate a return of EPP amplitude to the control level. This decay can be described by four exponentially decaying components: a first component of facilitation that decays with a time constant of 50 ms, a second component of facilitation that decays with a time constant of about 500 ms, augmentation that decays with a time constant of about 7 s, and potentiation that decays with a time constant of about 50 s (details in Zengel and Magleby[120]). The approximate periods over which facilitation, augmentation, and potentiation decay as well as the relative contributions to the decay are indicated.

Normal quantal content. Depression is most easily observed under physiologic conditions in which the level of transmitter release is not reduced.[118] Figure 16-5B plots stimulation-induced changes in transmitter release under conditions of normal quantal content. The nerve was first stimulated once every 10 s to establish a control response. The nerve was then stimulated at 100 impulses per second for 9 s. Transmitter release first increased and then decreased. The increase in this type of experiment is classically called facilitation but is most likely the result of the combined actions of facilitation, augmentation, and potentiation. The decrease below the control level is classically called depression but most likely represents depression superimposed on at least some of the processes that act to increase transmitter release.[45,121] Testing impulses applied once every 10 s after the train indicated a slow recovery and then an increase in EPP amplitude to about two times the control level, followed by a slow return to the baseline level. This increased release after the train has classically been called posttetanic potentiation. Because there is no reason to think that it is any different from a potentiation that builds up during the train, it is called potentiation here.[118,122] The apparent delayed onset of potentiation in experiments of this type most likely reflects the recovery from depression and not the properties of potentiation.[118]

Table 16-1. PROCESSES UNDERLYING STIMULATION-INDUCED CHANGES IN TRANSMITTER RELEASE

Process	Magnitude for One Impulse[a]	Time Constant of Decay
Components of increased release		
Facilitation		
First component	0.8	50 ms
Second component	0.12	300 ms
Augmentation	0.01[b]	7 s
Potentiation	0.01	20 s to minutes
Components of decreased release		
Depression		
Fast component	0.15	5 s
Slow component	0.001	minutes[b]

[a]For components of increased release, magnitude is the fractional increase in release over control; a magnitude of 0.8 increases release 80 percent. Time constant is the time to decay to 37 percent of the initial magnitude of increased release. For components of decreased release, magnitude is the fractional decrease in release below the control; a magnitude of 0.1 decreases release 10 percent. Time constant is the time to recover to 37 percent of the initial magnitude of decreased release.
[b]Increases with repetitive stimulation.

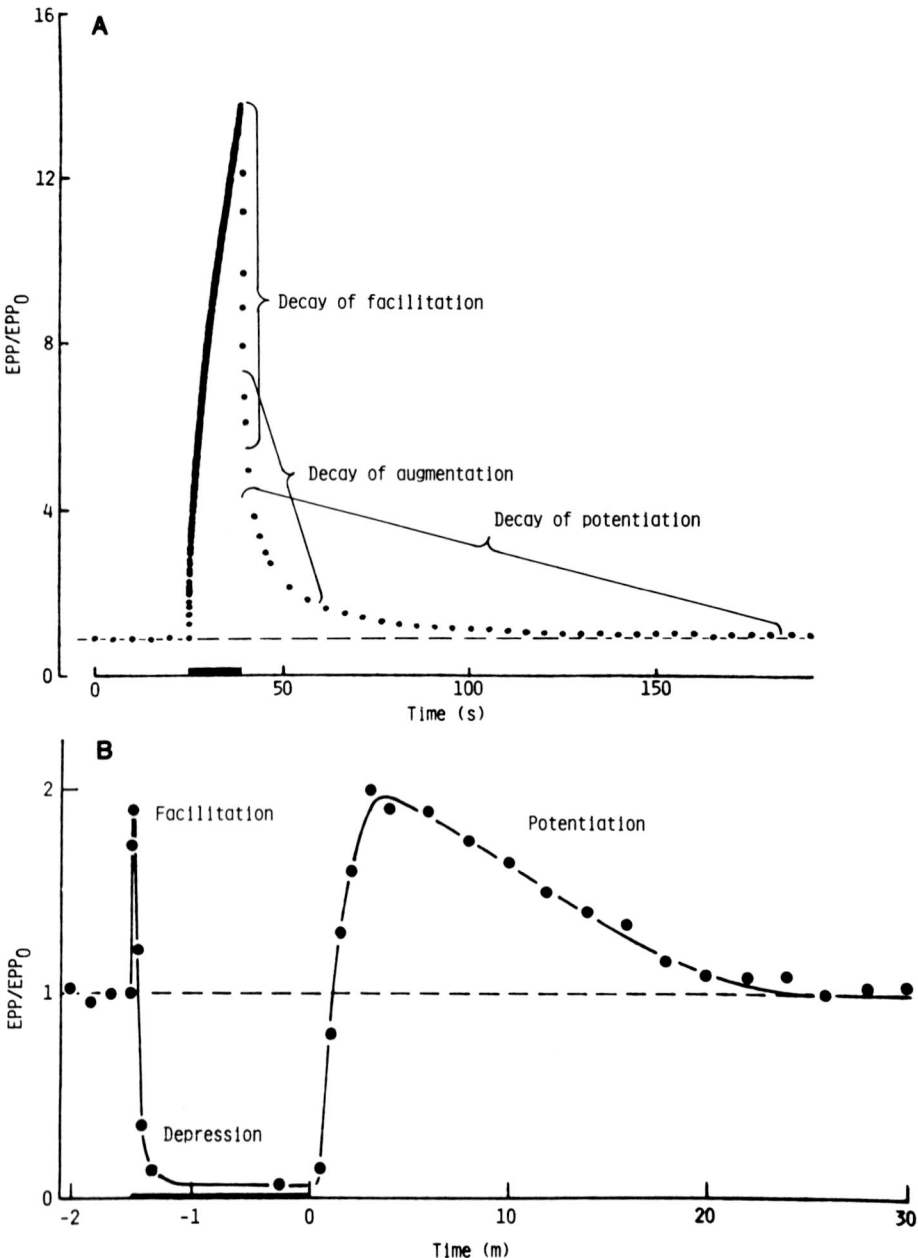

FIGURE 16-5. Changes in EPP amplitude with repetitive stimulation. A. Conditions of reduced quantal content (5 mM Mg^{2+}, 0.5 mM Ca^{2+}). Each point plots average EPP amplitude divided by control EPP amplitude. The nerve was first stimulated once every 5 s to establish the control response. The nerve was then stimulated at 20 impulses per second for 300 impulses during the time indicated by the horizontal bar. EPP amplitudes increased over 14-fold during the train. Test EPP amplitudes then decayed after the train. Only a few test impulses were given in any single trial. The increase in EPP amplitudes during the train is the result of the buildup of facilitation, augmentation, and potentiation. The approximate decay of these components after the train is indicated. *(From Zengel JE, Magleby KL: Augmentation and facilitation of transmitter release. A quantitative description at the frog neuromuscular junction. J Gen Physiol 80: 583, 1982. With permission from The Rockefeller University Press.)* B. Conditions of normal levels of transmitter release. The nerve was stimulated once every 10 s to establish a control response. The nerve was then stimulated at 100 impulses per second for 90 s. Test impulses were then applied at a slow rate after the tetanus. Facilitation (which also includes some augmentation and potentiation), depression, and potentiation (posttetanic potentiation) are observed under these conditions. Curare 3 µM was present. *(From Barrett EF, Magleby KL, in Goldberg AM, Hanin I (eds): Biology of Cholinergic Function. New York: Raven Press, 1976, pp 29–100. With permission.)*

Accounting for Short-Term Synaptic Plasticity under Conditions of Low Quantal Content

Magleby and Zengel[122] have shown that the kinetic properties of potentiation, augmentation, and the two components of facilitation are sufficient to account for stimulation-induced changes in transmitter release under conditions of low quantal content when depression is not obvious. Results are shown in Fig. 16-6. The large dots in Fig. 16-6A (which overlap and form thick lines) plot EPP amplitudes during conditioning trains of 10 and 20 impulses per second. The continuous lines, which superimpose the 10-impulses-per-second data and give a reasonable description of the 20-impulses-per-second data, are the calculated increases in transmitter release from the combined effects of potentiation, augmentation, and the two components of facilitation. Figure 16-6B, C, and D plots the calculated changes in facilitation (the first and second components are combined for ease of presentation), augmentation, and potentiation for each stimulation rate. Facilitation increases rapidly during the first second of the train and then remains constant, while augmentation and potentiation increase throughout the train. The effect of doubling the stimulation rate on the components can be seen.

The large dots in Fig. 16-6E (which overlap and form a thick line during the train) plot the increase in EPP amplitudes during and after the 10-impulses-per-second stimulation on a slower time base. The smaller plotted dots, which superimpose the experimental data and are not readily visible, are the calculated increase and decrease in EPP ampli-

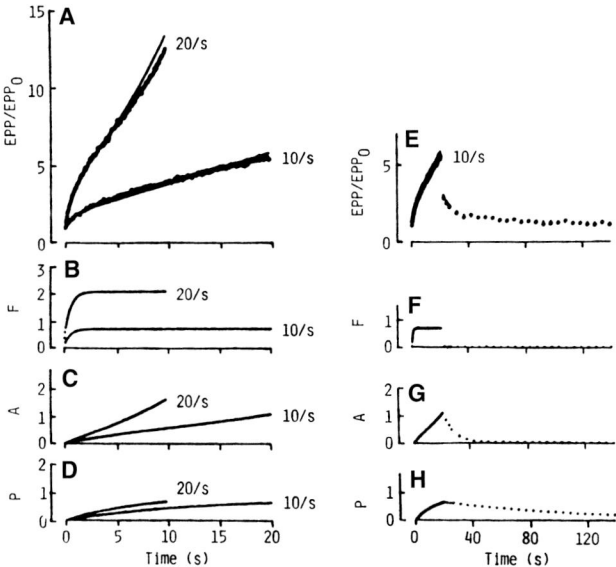

FIGURE 16-6. Accounting for stimulation-induced changes in transmitter release under conditions of low quantal content (5 mM Mg^{2+}, 0.5 mM Ca^{2+}). *A.* Change in EPP amplitudes during repetitive stimulation at 10 and 20 impulses per second. EPP amplitudes are plotted as large filled circles that overlap to form a thick line. The thin lines plot predicted EPP amplitudes during the trains, assuming that potentiation, augmentation, and the first and second components of facilitation are responsible for stimulation-induced changes in transmitter release. For most of the duration of the trains, the predicted response overlaps the observed and is not visible. *B, C, D.* The calculated changes in facilitation (F), augmentation (A), and potentiation (P) during the trains at the two frequencies. *E.* Change in EPP amplitudes during and after the 10/s train. Observed EPP amplitudes are plotted as large filled circles that overlap during the train, forming a thick line, and appear as separated dots for the test EPP amplitudes after the train. Predicted EPP amplitudes during and after the train are superimposed on the data and are not visible because of the excellent agreement. *F, G, H.* The calculated rise during and decay after the 10/s train for facilitation, augmentation, and potentiation. (From Magleby KL, Zengel JE: *A quantitative description of stimulation-induced changes in transmitter release at the frog neuromuscular junction.* J Gen Physiol 80:613, 1982. With permission from The Rockefeller University Press.)

tudes during and after the train. Figure 16-6F, G, and H presents the calculated increase and decrease in facilitation, augmentation, and potentiation during and after the train. Facilitation decays to insignificant levels within about a second after the train, augmentation decays in about 20 s, and potentiation decays over many tens of seconds. Details of the specific models used to describe the data may be found in Magleby and Zengel.[122] The main conclusion to be drawn from the experiments shown in Fig. 16-6 is that the kinetic properties of potentiation, augmentation, and the two components of facilitation are sufficient to account for stimulation-induced changes in transmitter release under conditions of low quantal contents. The kinetic properties of the components are the same during and after the train. Notice especially that all components contribute to the increased transmitter release during the train and for varying periods after the train.

Lambert-Eaton (Myasthenic) Syndrome

A characteristic feature of Lambert-Eaton syndrome (an autoimmune disorder) is that there is a delayed onset and progressive development of strength during a maximal voluntary contraction. This effect is associated with decreased EPP amplitudes in the resting state and a progressive increase in EPP amplitude and surface recorded muscle action potentials during repetitive stimulation.[123] Lambert-Eaton syndrome results from a reduced number of the Ca^{2+} channels at the active zones.[26,124–127] The reduction in Ca^{2+} channels results because the patients develop an antibody that downregulates the P/Q-type Ca^{2+} channels.[128–130] Less Ca^{2+} channels would lead to less Ca^{2+} entry. It might be suggested, then, that the progressive increase in transmitter release in Lambert-Eaton syndrome results from an increase in the facilitation, augmentation, and potentiation that occurs at low levels of Ca^{2+} entry and transmitter release, as shown in Fig. 16-6.

Facilitation, Augmentation, and Potentiation of MEPP Frequency

In addition to increasing EPP amplitude, repetitive stimulation of the nerve also leads to an increase in MEPP frequency (residual or asynchronous release).[5,49,131] MEPP frequency is typically about 0.1 to 1 per second in the resting state in vitro and increases to about 10 per second during 10 s of stimulation at 20 impulses per second under conditions of low quantal content. Facilitation, augmentation, and potentiation of MEPP frequency have been demonstrated and have kinetic properties and ionic specificities similar to stimulation-induced changes in EPP amplitude.[132] These similarities suggest that similar mechanisms underlie stimulation-induced increases in these two types of quantal transmitter release. Spontaneous increases of MEPP frequency are not typically present in the resting state in vivo,[133] perhaps because the nerve terminals are healthier and the resting level of Ca^{2+} in the terminals is lower.

Mechanisms of Short-Term Synaptic Plasticity

The observation that the components of stimulation-induced increases in transmitter release retain and express their properties in the intervals between nerve impulses during repetitive stimulation and in the absence of nerve impulses after a conditioning train, as indicated by studies on MEPP frequency,[131,132] suggests that potentiation, augmentation, and the two components of facilitation arise from residual changes in some factor or factors in the nerve terminal that affect transmitter release. One such factor may be Ca^{2+}, as it does accumulate and then decay in nerve terminals during and following repetitive stimulation.[55,134–137] Katz and Miledi[138] found that facilitation of transmitter release to a second nerve impulse required that Ca^{2+} be present during the first impulse. They suggested that residual calcium remaining in the nerve terminal from the first impulse combined with the Ca^{2+} that entered with the second impulse and facilitated transmitter release. This "residual-calcium hypothesis" has served as a working hypothesis for stimulation-induced increases in transmitter release, because facilitation, augmentation, and potentiation all appear to require and/or be related to the accumulation and decay of Ca^{2+} in the nerve terminal.[37,63,90,134,139–145]

Residual-calcium hypothesis. The residual-calcium hypothesis states that stimulation-induced increases in transmitter release (facilitation, augmentation, and potentiation) result from the buildup and decay of residual Ca^{2+} at the release sites during and following repetitive stimulation. This residual Ca^{2+} then combines with the Ca^{2+} that enters through the voltage-dependent Ca^{2+} channels to facilitate release. Although attractive, the residual-Ca^{2+} hypothesis is too simple to account for all the observed experimental observations.[45,55,132,144] Assuming that quantal transmitter release is proportional to the fourth power of Ca^{2+} at the release sites,[54,64–68] the predicted MEPP frequency at the end of a train is easily calculated from the observed increase in EPP amplitudes. When this is done, the predicted MEPP frequency of 150 per second after 100 conditioning impulses is 15 times greater than the experimentally observed MEPP frequency of 10 per second.[132] If a linear relationship between [Ca]$_i$ and transmitter release is assumed, the predicted MEPP frequency of 6000 per second is 600 times the observed MEPP frequency. Thus neither a fourth power residual-Ca^{2+} model nor a linear residual-Ca^{2+} model can account for all forms of transmitter release. This conclusion is consistent with the experimental observations of a fourth power relationship between Ca^{2+} and EPP amplitude[64] and a linear relationship between Ca^{2+} and MEEP frequency.[69]

Residual-factor hypothesis. An alternative possibility for stimulation-induced increases in transmitter release is that repetitive stimulation (most likely acting through Ca^{2+} or other ions) triggers changes in different factors in the nerve terminal that affect release, such that the different components of transmitter release reflect the time courses of changes in these factors in addition to the time course of removal of Ca^{2+} from the release sites. It follows from this hypothesis that Ca^{2+} would be acting on sites in addition to the sites involved in the rapid evoked release of transmitter immediately after an action potential. If the different factors act jointly to increase transmitter release, such as, for example, through changes in the size of the readily releasable pool of vesicles and through changes in the probability that the vesicles will be released, then some of the components of transmitter release might be expected to have a multiplicative relationship, as has been observed.[118,122,146]

Support for such a "residual-factor or multiple-site hypothesis" comes from the observations that evoked release tends to be fourth power with Ca^{2+} (see above), while facilitation, augmentation, and potentiation tend to be linear with Ca^{2+} in some cases and for some models, suggesting different sites and/or mechanisms for evoked and enhanced release.[55] There may be at least three sites involved: a low-affinity site for evoked release, an intermediate-affinity site for the F1 and F2 components of facilitation, and a higher-affinity site for augmentation and potentiation. In support of multiple sites, computational studies show that facilitation can be modeled with a secondary site.[147] The different time courses of facilitation, augmentation, and potentiation are likely to reflect, at least in part, the time course of removal of Ca^{2+} from the nerve terminal, as the decay of Ca^{2+} roughly approximates the decays of these processes.[55,134–137]

The decay of potentiation may reflect the slow efflux of tetanically accumulated mitochondrial Ca^{2+}.[143] The decay of augmentation may reflect the removal of Ca^{2+} from the nerve terminal by extrusion by a Ca^{2+} pump and Na/Ca^{2+} exchanger.[55] Augmentation is not an inverse of depression resulting from a depletion of vesicles, as augmentation can increase at the same time that depression is increasing.[121] Consistent with this observation, augmentation is a potentiation of the exocytotic process, not an increase in the pool size.[148] The decay of the two components of facilitation may reflect the unbinding of Ca^{2+} from one or more secondary sites and/or the diffusion of Ca^{2+} away from the active zones by both free diffusion and mobile buffers.[55]

Properties of Depression

Some of the properties of depression of transmitter release were presented in Table 16-1 and Fig. 16-5B. The time course of recovery from depression can occur with two quite different time courses, depending on the experimental conditions. If the conditioning stimulation consists of one or a few impulses under conditions of normal or increased quantal contents, recovery from depression is approximately exponential, with a time constant of about 5 s.[119] This is the case whether depression represents a 15 percent reduction in transmitter release after a single conditioning impulse or a 50 percent reduction after five conditioning impulses. Following conditioning trains of several hundred impulses, depression recovers with a time course of tens of seconds to minutes,[118,149,150] as shown in Fig. 16-5B.

Mechanism of Depression

Depression may result from a depletion of the immediately available store of transmitter[119]: Depression is associated with high levels of transmitter release (Fig. 16-5); it increases with the amount of transmitter release,[119] and synaptic vesicles are depleted during repetitive stimulation.[25,111] Although depression is associated with a decrease in the statistical parameter n of the quantal hypothesis,[151] there also appears to be a decrease in p.[152] Depression is observed when the Ca^{2+} current that enters with each impulse remains constant, suggesting that depression is not due to decreased calcium entry.[153] The Ca^{2+} that enters may facilitate the mobilization of synaptic vesicles to replace those that have been released.[154,155] The increased Ca^{2+} may also enhance the release of recently replaced vesicles.[156] Depression is not a decrease in facilitation[157] or augmentation[121] below control levels.

NONQUANTAL RELEASE OF TRANSMITTER

In addition to the quantal release of transmitter, there is nonquantal release that originates either from the nerve terminal or from structures closely associated with the end plate region.[158] The nonquantal release, about 10^6 molecules of ACh per second per end plate, is several hundred times greater in the resting state than the release associated with the spontaneous release of quanta at a rate of about 1 per second. However, as the nonquantal release occurs at a steady rate in a diffuse manner over the end plate region, it has little if any depolarizing effect on the membrane potential unless the esterases are blocked. The nonquantal release is inhibited by glutamate and ATP.[159,160] It has been suggested that nonquantal release may arise, at least in part, from the transient incorporation of the vesicular acetylcholine transport system into the nerve terminal membrane during the exocytotic release of quantal acetylcholine,[161] but measurements of ACh from the active zones suggest this may not be the source for the release.[162] Nonquantal release may regulate factors through a calcium-dependent mechanism that maintains the resting membrane potential of muscle fibers.[163]

RELEASE PROTEINS AND FEEDBACK SYSTEMS

The last decade has resulted in tremendous progress towards identifying a large number of proteins involved in vesicle recycling[3,163] and transmitter release.[109] The process is rendered more difficult than might be expected because of the numerous isoforms and possible overlapping functions, but a systematic attack will eventually strip the nerve terminal of its secrets. Central to understanding the mechanism of release will be to further characterize the feedback systems involved.[164] Increasing evidence suggests that muscarinic receptors on the nerve terminal have two opposing actions, to both facilitate and inhibit release, perhaps terminating the release process itself.[165–169] Transmitter release is also modulated by purinergic systems (inhibition at low concentrations)[170] and high concentrations of adrenergic agents (enhanced release and also block of AChR channels).[171,172]

Postsynaptic Aspects of Neuromuscular Transmission

OVERVIEW

Following stimulation of the nerve, about 50 quantal packets of ACh in humans and 200 in frogs, each containing 6000 to 10,000 molecules of ACh, are released into the synaptic cleft. The released ACh binds to AChRs on the postsynaptic membrane, is hydrolyzed by AChE, and perhaps some molecules escape from the cleft by diffusion. In the process, about 50,000 AChRs (humans) and 250,000 AChRs (frogs) with two bound molecules of ACh open their channels for an average effective duration of about 1 ms. Na^+, K^+, and to a lesser extent Ca^{2+} pass through each open channel. There is a net influx of positive charge into the muscle cell, thus depolarizing it. If the muscle cell is depolarized sufficiently to generate an action potential, which is generally the case, the muscle fiber contracts. The activated AChRs close their channels and lose their bound ACh. Depending on the experimental conditions, the released ACh may bind to and open additional channels before it is lost from the synaptic cleft through hydrolysis and diffusion.

Because most of the activated AChRs have closed their channels by the time the action potential in the muscle cell is completed, any current through the few remaining open ACh-activated channels is not sufficient to generate a second action potential. Thus, each nerve-evoked end plate current generates a single action potential in the muscle cell. In the following sections the properties of AChRs are first examined and then the specific events that occur during the generation of end plate currents are considered.

ACETYLCHOLINE RECEPTOR

The AChR in the skeletal muscle membrane is a large glycoprotein (molecular weight of about 290,000 kDa) that is formed of five homologous subunits that form a central pore (channel) through which ions can flow.[173,174] In adult innervated muscle about 95 to 98 percent of the AChRs have the adult subunit composition of α, α, β, δ, and ε, and 2 to 5 percent have the embryonic composition with a γ subunit replacing the ε subunit. The predominance of the two types of AChRs is reversed in both embryonic and denervated adult muscle, with about 80 to 85 percent of the AChRs having the embryonic composition and about 15 to 20 percent having the adult composition.[175–180] Recordings from the AChR channels and antibody binding suggest that the two types of channels are not segregated on the basis of whether they are located in the junctional or extrajunctional regions.[175]

The study of the properties of AChRs is often divided into two aspects. The first is the permeability of the receptor channel to various ions (selectivity). The second is the kinetics of opening and closing (gating).

Permeability of the AChR Channel

Under physiologic conditions, the major ions[181] that would pass through the AChR channel are Na^+ and K^+ and to a lesser extent Ca^{2+} and Mg^{2+}; the channel appears impermeable to Cl^-. The magnitude and direction of the current through the end plate depends on the membrane potential. At −90 mV, the current is inward mainly because of the net influx of Na^+ and to a lesser extent Ca^{2+}. At about −4 mV (the reversal potential), there is no net current; the charge carried by the net influx of Na^+ and Ca^{2+} would equal the charge carried by the net efflux of K^+. At potentials more positive than the reversal potential the end plate current is outward.[16]

The AChR channel appears to be a water-filled pore, with the smallest cross sections of the open channel not less than about 0.65 × 0.65 nm. Many small organic cations can pass through the channel. Some, such as ammonium, are more permeable than Na^+. Cs^+, Rb^+, K^+, and Li^+ pass through the channel with permeability ratios that do not differ from Na^+ by more than 30 percent. Mg^{2+}, Ca^{2+}, Sr^{2+}, Ba^{2+}, Mn^{2+}, Co^{2+}, Ni^{2+}, Zn^{2+}, and Cd^{2+}, although permeable, are only about 13 to 26 percent as permeable as Na^+.[182,183]

Studies using site-directed mutagenesis to change the charge of negatively charged and glutamine residues neighboring the second transmembrane segment (M2) of the ACh receptor subunits have indicated that the conductance and selectivity are controlled, at least in part, by three rings of negative charge located at the extracellular, intermediate, and cytoplasmic areas of the channel.[179] The conductance of the channel (which gives a measure of the ease with which ions flow through the channel) decreased as the net numbers of negative charges decreased, and the effect was greatest when the charge was changed in the intermediate ring.[179] The observation that single mutations in the intermediate ring could have relatively large effects on the selectivity of the channel towards various cations led Konno et al.[176] to suggest that the selectivity filter of the AChR channels is made up, at least in part, by the side chains of the amino acids forming the intermediate ring. The rings of negative charge provide an explanation for the observation that anions do not pass through the channel. In summary, the AChR channel is a water-filled pore with three rings of negative charge. The pore is permeable to most small cations and impermeable to Cl^-.

Activation of AChRs

The binding of ACh to the ACh receptor initiates a conformational change that opens the channel.[17,184–186] The kinetic gating mechanism that describes the conformational changes can be summarized by the expansion of a model initially proposed by Del Costillo and Katz,[184] shown in scheme 1 below:

$$R \underset{k_{-1}}{\overset{[ACh]k_{+1}}{\rightleftarrows}} AChR \underset{k_{-2}}{\overset{[ACh]k_{+2}}{\rightleftarrows}} ACh_2R$$

$$\alpha'' \updownarrow \beta'' \qquad \alpha' \updownarrow \beta' \qquad \alpha \updownarrow \beta \qquad (1)$$

$$R^* \underset{k'_{-1}}{\overset{[ACh]k'_{+1}}{\rightleftarrows}} AChR^* \underset{k'_{-2}}{\overset{[ACh]k'_{+2}}{\rightleftarrows}} ACh_2R^*$$

where R is the receptor with closed channel and no bound ACh; AChR and ACh_2R are receptors with one and two ACh molecules bound, respectively; $AChR^*$ and $ACh2R^*$ indicate that the receptor has opened its channel; k_{+1}, k_{+2}, k'_{+1}, and k'_{+2} are the forward binding rate constants for ACh; k_{-1}, k_{-2}, k'_{-1}, and k'_{-2} are the unbinding rate constants; and α and β, α' and β', and α'' and β'' are the rate constants for the paired closing and opening conformational changes associated with the indicated closings and openings of the channel.[17,187–189]

In terms of scheme I, the AChR can open its channel with zero,[190] one, or two molecules of ACh. However, openings with zero or one bound ACh are infrequent, so that the conformational change associated with the opening of the channel is typically associated with the binding of two ACh molecules at the external interfaces of the α/δ and the α/ε (or α/γ) subunits. The binding of (typically) two ACh molecules to initiate opening would be consistent with the observations of Hill slopes typically approaching two for activation of AChRs.

Once open to the doubly liganded state, the channel typically closes and reopens two to three times, causing a burst of activity[187,191] before the bound ACh dissociates. The duration of this burst of activity (burst duration) is also referred to as *effective* channel open time (see following sections), and determines the time course of the exponential decay of the end plate currents. The mean burst duration is about 0.5 ms for a membrane potential of +50 mV and about 1.8 ms at −150 mV.[17] Magleby and Stevens[17] could account for the voltage sensitivity of the decay of the end plate current by assuming that the action of ACh in the synaptic cleft is brief and that the gating part of the receptor that undergoes or triggers the conformational changes associated with channel opening and closing has a dipole moment. Consequently, the ease with which the channel opens and closes (given by the rate constants β and α) would depend on the membrane potential and the associated electric field through the membrane. Currents through single AChRs (see below) verify the expected increases in mean channel open time and burst duration with hyperpolarization, due to a slowing of channel closing rate α.[18,192,193] The same data show that the opening rate β is relatively voltage independent.

In summary, the AChR channel opens with a conformational change after typically binding two molecules of ACh. Mean burst duration (effective open time) increases as the membrane potential is made more negative, because the conformational change associated with channel closing becomes slower.

Recording from Single AChR Channels

In 1976 Neher and Sakmann published recordings of currents flowing through single AChR channels.[18] (This study and additional work gained them the Nobel prize in Physiology and Medicine in 1991.) A micropipette with a tip of a few microns was pushed against the surface of a muscle fiber. The micropipette contained bathing solution and agonist. A low-noise current amplifier connected to the pipette measured the current that flowed through the channels in the membrane patch under the pipette. Results obtained for three different agonists (suberyldicholine, ACh, and carbachol) are shown in Fig. 16-7. The steps in downward-going currents of about 3 to 5 pA (10^{-12} A) shown in each record are currents through individual channels. Notice that observed channel open time (the duration of the downward-going steps) depends on the agonist used. Channels typically stayed open longer in suberyldicholine than in carbachol; ACh gave intermediate open times. Two channels were often open simultaneously in suberyldicholine, as indicated by two steps of unit height.

The channels opened by ACh in these records have effective open times considerably longer than the 1 ms typically stated for the following reasons. The data were collected at a decreased temperature (8°C), which increases open-channel lifetimes[17,192]; the membrane was hyperpolarized to −120 mV, which also increases open-channel lifetimes[194]; and the recordings were made from AChRs in denervated skeletal muscle, which have open-channel lifetimes about three to five times longer than AChRs in innervated skeletal muscle.[175] These effects are multiplicative and account for the mean channel open lifetime of about 26 ms for ACh.

By applying suction to the patch pipette, it is possible to seal the membrane to the pipette under appropriate conditions and greatly improve the signal-to-noise ratio.[195] Seals of several gigaohms (giga-seal technique) can be obtained, allowing the current-measuring amplifier connected to the pipette to also clamp the membrane voltage of the patch to a specified level. The patch of membrane sealed to the pipette can be excised from the cell simply by withdrawing the pipette. With this patch-clamp technique, it is possible to

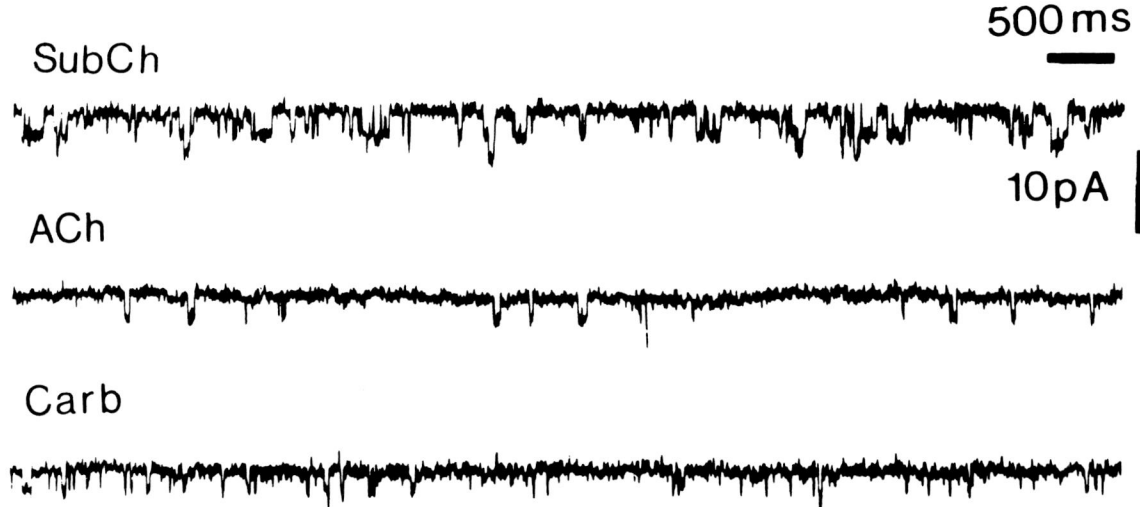

FIGURE 16-7. Currents through single extrajunctional AChR channels in frog muscle at 8°C. Downward-going current steps represent a channel opening and upward-going steps back to the control level represent channel closing. Two channels are occasionally open at once, as indicated by a second step downward after a first step. Channels typically stay open longer in suberyldicholine (SubCh) than in ACh. In contrast, channel open times are briefer in carbachol (Carb) than in ACh. The channels were activated with 2×10^{-7} M SubCh, 2×10^{-6} M ACh, 6×10^{-5} M Carb. *(From Neher E, Sakmann B: Single-channel currents recorded from membrane of denervated frog muscle fibres. Nature (Lond) 260:799, 1976. With permission from Macmillan Journals Limited.)*

record from single channels in excised patches of membranes for hours while controlling the composition of the solution at the normal intracellular side of the membrane. Records from AChR channels in the perisynaptic membrane of the frog cutaneous pectoris muscle using this giga-seal technique are shown in Fig. 16-8A. Notice that the amplitudes of the single-channel currents increase with membrane hyperpolarization. (Downward currents indicate channel opening.) A plot of amplitude versus voltage in Fig. 16-8B gives a single-channel conductance of 32 pS. An apparent increase in channel open time with hyperpolarization is also apparent in Fig. 16-8A. Four AChR channels were active in the membrane patch for the record in Fig. 16-8C, recorded from cultured rat muscle cells. Notice that the current steps from the different channels are of similar amplitude. The actual time required for the transition between the open and shut states for the AChR channel is too fast to measure, but is less than 10 μs. For the record in Figs. 16-7 and 16-8 the AChRs were continuously exposed to the agonist in the recording pipette. Consequently, the channels opened and closed repeatedly.

In agreement with scheme 1, the distribution of shut intervals recorded from single ACh receptor channels is mainly described by the sum of three exponentials, suggesting at least three closed-channel states, and the distribution of open intervals is mainly described by two exponential components suggesting two open states.[187,191,196] Kinetic analysis indicates that most openings are to the double liganded state, which has a lifetime of about 1 ms. Infrequent openings to the singly liganded state had a lifetime of about 0.1 ms. The binding of ACh is within the range of being diffusion limited (~1×10^8 M^{-1} s^{-1}). The binding rates for ACh show little voltage dependence, indicating that they are outside of the electric field of the membrane, consistent with structural studies which place the binding site well above the membrane in the extracellular domain.[197,198] Scheme 1 has served both as a useful working hypothesis for the gating of AChR as well as a starting point to show that the gating can be more complex.[188,193,199–205]

Bursting Kinetics of ACh Receptors

A consistent feature of high-resolution current records from single AChRs is that openings of AChR channels typically occur in bursts of several openings,[187,189,191,206–209] and this is still the case when the concentration of ACh is low. Figure 16-9 shows a burst of three openings. For continuous agonist application, the bursts of activity are grouped into clusters.[210] Bursts occur when the channel typically opens and closes several times between ACh_2R and ACh_2R^* in scheme 1 without losing its bound ACh.[207] Bursting suggests that ß, the rate constant for channel opening, is larger than the rate of loss of ACh.[211] Estimates for the opening rate constant ß range from about 5000 to 60,000/s.[187,188,192] With diffusion-limited binding of ACh and about 1 mM ACh in the synaptic cleft immediately following quantal release, the forward rates for k_{+1} and k_{+2} would fall in the range of 100,000/s, assuming binding in the range 10^8 $M^{-1}s^{-1}$. Thus, the time required for the conformational change can be a limiting factor in the activation of the receptor, as suggested by Magleby and Stevens.[17]

Studies on AChRs carried out before about 1981 did not detect the brief closings during the bursts of activity, like the burst shown in Fig. 16-9, because of the limited frequency response of both the single-channel recordings[18] and noise analysis.[194] The brief closings were also not detected in the decay of end plate currents, because the end plate current reflects the activity of many channels, which would average out the brief closings. In these earlier studies (and in present

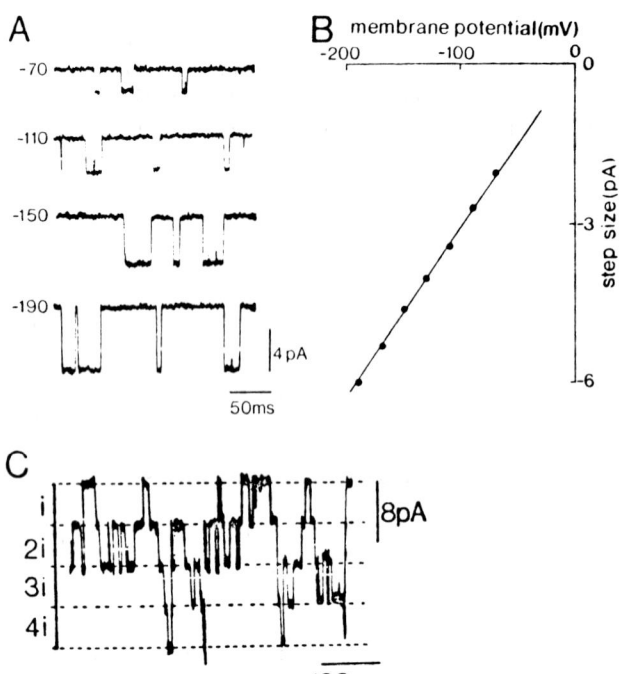

FIGURE 16-8. Properties of single AChR channels. A. Increase in single-channel current amplitudes and apparent open times with increasing hyperpolarization for ACh channels in the perisynaptic membrane of cutaneous pectoris muscle of frog. 50 nM SubCh. Downward-going currents represent channel opening. B. Plot of single-channel current amplitude against membrane potential. The straight line represents a single-channel conductance of 32 pS. C. Currents recorded from AChR channels in myotubes: 1 μM ACh, −140 mV membrane potential. The stepwise fluctuation in current results from zero to four channels being open at different times. (From Hamill OP, Marty A, Neher E, et al.: Improved patch-clamp techniques for high-resolution current recording from cells and cell-free membrane patches. Pflugers Arch 391:85–100, 1981. With permission.)

measured under voltage clamp. The variation in the current, which reflects random variations in the number of channels open at any time, can be analyzed in terms of assumed molecular mechanisms to obtain estimates of single-channel conductance and mean channel open time.[194,212] Because of limited frequency response, it should be assumed that burst duration (rather than mean channel open time) is the parameter being measured with noise analysis unless there is evidence to exclude this assumption. If bursts consist of more than one opening, the noise spectrum will have two components (if the frequency response of the recording system is adequate), reflecting burst duration and mean channel open time.

Channel Blockers

Once the AChR channel is open, a variety of agents appear to enter and block the channel. Local anesthetics, decamethonium, d-tubocurarine, ACh, amphetamine, ephedrine, quinidine, and fluoxetine all appear capable of doing so in addition to their other well-known effects.[172,192,213–217,217a,217b] Single-channel recordings in the presence of high concentrations of channel-blocking drugs that can rapidly enter and exit the channel often show rapid transitions between the blocked and open states, reflecting the blocking and unblocking of the channel by the blocking agent; the channel cannot close and release its agonist when it is blocked but must become unblocked first; although the duration of individual channel openings is shortened, the effective channel open time is essentially unaltered.[213] By contrast, channel blockers that are slow to exit from the channel, such as quinidine or fluoxetine, shorten both individual channel openings and the effective channel open time.[217a,217b] The latter agents, also known as long-lived open-channel blockers, are useful in the treatment of the slow-channel congenital myasthenic syndromes (also see Chap. 66).

studies with limited frequency response), each burst of openings would be detected as a single opening. Thus, what was reported as open-channel lifetime in the earlier studies represents burst duration. While the distinction between burst duration and actual channel open time is important in understanding receptor kinetics, the functionally important parameter is burst duration, as this determines the effective duration that the channel is open for a double occupancy of the receptor by ACh. When filtering is heavy so as to obscure the brief closings (flickers), as in the earlier papers, it should be kept in mind that the measured "open-channel lifetime" typically refers to burst duration, and consequently will be referred to as effective mean channel open time in this chapter.

Estimating Mean Channel Open Time, Burst Duration, and Single-Channel Conductance from Fluctuation Analysis

Estimates of single-channel properties can also be made in a more indirect manner called noise, or fluctuation, analysis. In experiments of this type, ACh is applied to the end plate region and the resulting current through the end plate is

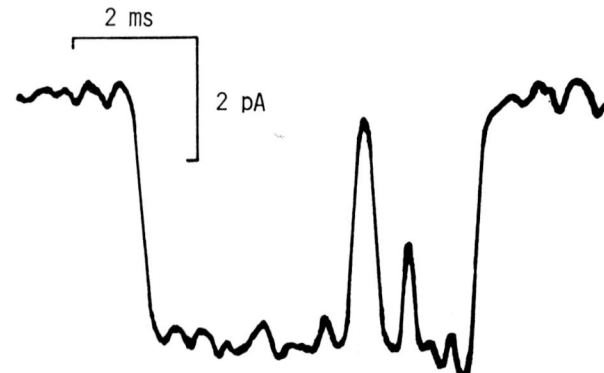

FIGURE 16-9. Single-channel current from and AChR channels in the perisynaptic region of frog cutaneous pectoris muscle. 20 nM SubCh, −128 mV membrane potential. Downward current represents channel opening. The record consists of a burst of channel activity consisting of three brief openings. The second closing during the burst does not appear to be complete because of the limited frequency response of the recording system. (From Colquhoun D, Sakmann B: Fluctuations in the microsecond time range of the current through single acetylcholine receptor ion channels. Nature 294:464–466, 1981. With permission from Macmillan Journals Limited.)

Receptor Properties at Human End Plate

Noise analysis for human intercostal muscle end plates clamped to −80 mV near room temperature[29,218,219] gives an effective mean channel open lifetime (burst duration) of 2.3 ms and a single-channel conductance of 32 pS. Miniature end plate current amplitude is 3.8 nA, and the time constant of decay of miniature end plate currents is 3.3 ms.[29] A quantal packet of transmitter, which gives rise to a miniature end plate current, would open about 1400 channels. These values are similar to the values typically found at rat and frog neuromuscular junctions.

Measurements of single-channel properties from human cultured myotubes using the patch-clamp technique with low time resolution recording gave an effective mean channel open time (burst duration) of about 8.2 ms.[219] This can be compared to the effective mean open times (burst duration) of 2.3 to 3.3 ms determined from innervated adult human muscle from noise analysis and the decay of end plate currents (see above). Thus, as in other vertebrates, AChRs in noninnervated human muscle close their channels about three to four times slower than AChR channels in innervated adult human skeletal muscle.

Direct measurement of single-channel properties of ACh receptors at end plates of isolated human intercostal muscle indicates a conductance of ~60 pS, a mean single-channel open time of ~1 ms, and a mean burst duration of ~2.6 ms.[209] Thus, the channel typically opens two to three times for each burst of activity, mainly by transitions between ACh_2R and ACh_2R^* in scheme 1. A number of naturally occurring myasthenic syndromes alter the kinetic properties of AChRs. In slow-channel syndromes, prolonged and/or repeated openings lead to greatly prolonged burst duration, while in fast-channel syndromes, the numbers of openings per burst are decreased, leading to decreased burst durations.[220–222] Since the decay of end plate currents mainly reflects the termination of the bursts of channel activity (see below), slow-channel syndromes give rise to prolonged end plate currents and fast-channel syndromes give rise to shortened end plate currents.[222]

GENERATION OF END PLATE CURRENTS

The mechanism of generation and decay of end plate currents is well understood.[6,16,17] ACh released from the presynaptic nerve terminal diffuses to the AChRs on the postsynaptic membrane. ACh binds to the receptors, which open their channels over a period of time of 200 to 300 μs. Unbound ACh is rapidly hydrolyzed and some is lost by diffusion, so that there is little free ACh in the synaptic cleft at the peak of the end plate current. The opened channels typically close and reopen several times, creating a burst of activity with a mean duration of 2 to 3 ms, before closing and losing their bound ACh. Closing with loss of ACh occurs in a random manner, leading to an exponential decay in the number of open channels. Because the ACh-induced current through the end plate is proportional to the number of open channels, the end plate current also decays exponentially.

When the acetylcholine esterase is inhibited[220] or missing, as in a myasthenic syndrome,[221,223] some of the ACh that is released from the receptors after they close their channels rebinds to the same or different AChRs, thus initiating additional bursts of openings and prolonging the duration of the end plate currents and potentials.[220,222] The following sections examine the various steps involved in the generation of end plate currents.

Saturating Disk Model for Receptor Activation

AChRs are packed at a density of about 6000 to 10,000 receptors per μm^2 on the tops of the junctional folds of the muscle membrane across from the release sites on the presynaptic nerve terminal.[224–227] Because of the narrow synaptic cleft, the high density of AChRs, and the high affinity of AChRs for ACh, the saturating disk model for receptor activation proposes that the released molecules of ACh bind to the first available free receptors as they diffuse in the synaptic cleft away from the release site. On this basis, it has been calculated that the receptors directly across from the quantal release sites would become saturated to a radius of about 0.3 μM with two bound ACh molecules each, within about 40 μs after the release of the 10,000 molecules of ACh from the quantal packet of transmitter. Beyond this radius there would be few receptors with bound ACh.[224–227] The efficiency of capture of released ACh is so high that about 75 percent of each quantal packet of ACh released from the nerve is captured by receptors.[228]

The synaptic folds beneath the nerve terminal, which decrease the efficiency of the capture of ACh,[229] serve a threefold purpose[230–234]: (1) to provide low-resistance conductance pathways to supply current (Na^+) to the AChR channels to generate the EPP; (2) to provide low-resistance conductance pathways to supply current (Na^+) to the voltage-dependent Na^+ channels involved in the generation of the action potential, and (3) to provide additional membrane surface to increase the effective density of Na^+ channels at the end plate. The voltage-dependent Na^+ channels involved in generation of the action potential are concentrated about 25-fold at the end plate and about fivefold within 100 μm of the end plate, when compared to areas away from the end plate.[232]

Factors Determining the Rising Phase of End Plate Currents

The rising phase of end plate currents (about 100 μs at 25°C in the frog sartorius muscle) (Fig. 16-2) reflects conduction time for the action potential along the nerve terminal and the time dispersion of quantal transmitter release as well as receptor activation time. Miniature end plate currents, which result from the release of single quanta of transmitter, rise in 100 to 200 μs.[234,235] The rising phase is probably not determined by diffusion alone but also reflects the time required for ACh binding and the conformational change associated with channel opening.[224,227,229,236] The contribution of diffusion to the rising phase would be more significant at lower receptor density where the diffusion distances are greater,[227] and also at higher temperatures where the binding and conformational changes becomes progressively faster when compared to diffusion.[192]

Factors Determining the Decaying Phase of End Plate Currents

Active esterase. Magleby and Stevens[16,17] proposed that the exponential decay of end plate currents reflects the closing of the channels opened by the brief pulse of ACh from the nerve. If this is the case, the time constant of decay of the miniature end plate currents and end plate currents should be the same as the measured effective mean channel open times (burst durations). The time constant of decay of miniature end plate currents and end plate currents has been found to be similar[194] to or somewhat longer[29,218] than the measured channel open lifetimes determined from noise analysis or burst durations determined from single channels. End plate currents that decay more slowly than predicted from measured channel open times could result if some of the ACh released when the receptors close their channels rebinds to the same or different receptors, thus leading to additional bursts of channel opening.[220]

The above results suggest, then, that the decay of the end plate currents when the esterase is active is determined mainly by the termination of bursts of activity, but that some repeated binding and bursting may occur. Thus, the time constant of decay of end plate currents is equal to or somewhat longer than effective mean channel open time (mean burst duration).

Inhibited esterase. When the AChE is inhibited, the time course of decay of end plate currents is markedly prolonged, as shown in Fig. 16-10. Diffusion rather than hydrolysis now becomes the major means of clearing the synaptic cleft of ACh. As the ACh diffuses from the synaptic cleft, it repeatedly binds to and activates receptors, greatly prolonging the time course of the end plate current.[220,226] The time course of decay of end plate currents now reflects both receptor kinetics and the delayed diffusion of ACh from the cleft.

Excess Receptors

A nerve-evoked end plate current activates only about 10 percent of the receptors at the end plate. Pennefather and Quastel[228] found, as might be expected for a large excess of receptors, that blocking 50 percent of the receptors when the AChE was active reduced miniature end plate current amplitude by only about 20 percent. When the esterase was inhibited, blocking 50 percent of the receptors had even less of an

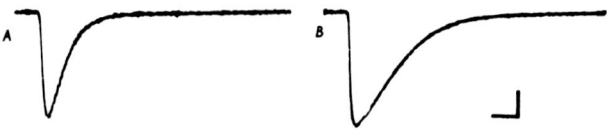

FIGURE 16-10. Effect of blocking AChE with prostigmine on the time course of end plate currents recorded under voltage clamp from the frog sartorius nerve-muscle preparation. *A.* Without prostigmine. *B.* With 3-μM prostigmine. The time constant of decay of the endplate currents increased from 1.4 to 3.1 ms after exposure to prostigmine. Horizontal bar: 2 ms. Vertical bar: 200 nA. (*From Magleby KL, Terrar D: Factors affecting the time course of decay of endplate currents: A possible cooperative action of acetylcholine on receptors at the frog neuromuscular junction. J Physiol (Lond) 244:467–495, 1975. With permission.*)

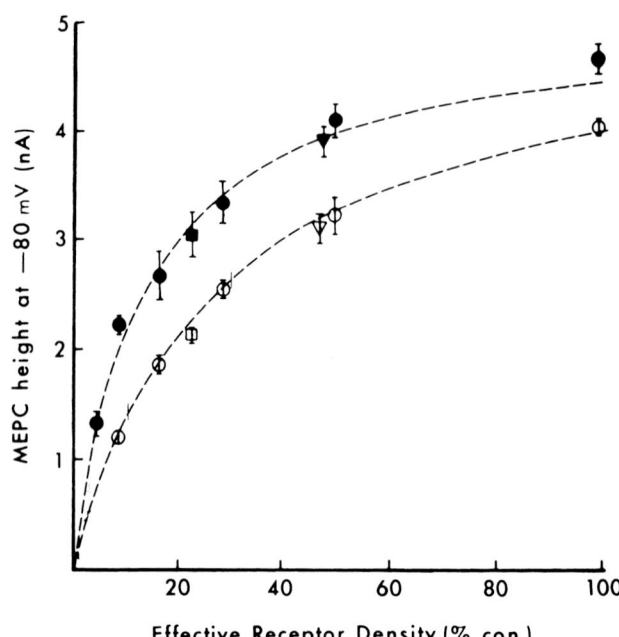

FIGURE 16-11. Relationship between the functional receptor density and the amplitude of miniature end plate currents (MEPC height) in mouse diaphragm. Open symbols: active AChE. Closed symbols: inhibited AChE with paraoxon. Notice that a large percentage of the receptors have to be blocked before there is an appreciable decrease in MEPC amplitude. This suggests that there is normally a large excess of receptors at the end plate. (*From Pennefather P, Quastel DMJ: Relation between subsynaptic receptor blockade and response to quantal transmitter at the mouse neuromuscular junction. J Gen Physiol 78:313, 1981. With permission from the Rockefeller University Press.*)

effect, reducing miniature end plate current amplitudes by only about 12 percent. This relationship between receptor blockade and reduction in response is shown in Fig. 16-11. These results suggest that if some of the receptors are blocked, free ACh has a high probability of diffusing to the next available receptor before it is hydrolyzed. Blocking the esterase increases this probability even further.

DESENSITIZATION

General Properties

When AChRs are exposed to ACh or other agonists for extended periods of time, the receptors become inactive or desensitized and no longer open their channels in the presence of agonist.[193,206,237–239] The desensitized state is a nonconducting state with a high affinity for agonist. Desensitization is not due to block of the channel by ACh.[239] Desensitization probably consists of a number of processes with time course ranging from milliseconds to many seconds. Our concern here is with those processes of desensitization that may be relevant to neuromuscular transmission.

Desensitization of AChRs

Using single-channel recording to study desensitization, Auerbach and Akk[239] found that a single channel desensi-

$$\begin{array}{ccccc}
& [ACh]\ 2.2\times 10^8 M^{-1}s^{-1} & & [ACh]\ 1.1\times 10^8 M^{-1}s^{-1} & \\
R & \underset{\leftarrow}{\to} & AChR & \underset{\leftarrow}{\to} & ACh_2R \\
& 18{,}000\ s^{-1} & & 36{,}000\ s^{-1} & \\
& & & 1200\ s^{-1}\ \updownarrow\ 50{,}000\ s^{-1} & \\
4s^{-1}\ \updownarrow\ {\sim}0.005\ s^{-1} & & & ACh_2R^* & \quad(2)\\
& & & 0.01\ s^{-1}\ \updownarrow\ 4\ s^{-1} & \\
& [ACh]\ 2.9\times 10^9 M^{-1}s^{-1} & & [ACh]\ 5.7\times 10^8 M^{-1}s^{-1} & \\
R^{**} & \underset{\leftarrow}{\to} & AChR^{**} & \underset{\leftarrow}{\to} & ACh_2R^{**} \\
& 23\ s^{-1} & & 46\ s^{-1} &
\end{array}$$

tizes after about 10 s of activity when exposed to 1 μM ACh and after about 300 ms of activity when exposed to 100 μM ACh. They found that the product of the duration of channel activity before desensitization with the open probability of the channel remained a constant at ~285 ms, consistent with the idea that the channels desensitize at a slow rate of 3.5/s from the open state. If the mean open time is ~1 ms, then a channel would open and close about 285 times before desensitization. Recovery from desensitization occurred at a rate of ~4/s in the absence of ACh. Thus, in the absence of ACh, any desensitized receptors fully recover in ~12 s.

Auerbach and Akk[239] could account for their data with a simple cyclic model of desensitization[237] in which open channels can desensitize, and once desensitized, can lose their bound ACh and then recover to the normal unliganded state, as shown in Scheme 2 below, where R, R*, and R** are the closed, open, and desensitized forms of the receptor, respectively. In terms of scheme 2, the recovery from desensitization would be slowed or prevented in the presence of ACh, because ACh would rebind to the desensitized states, as shown in the diagram.

Does Desensitization Occur in Vivo?

To investigate whether desensitization might occur during normal neuromuscular transmission, Magleby and Pallotta[117] used nerve-released transmitter to study desensitization at the neuromuscular junction. They found that even with 400 million channel openings elicited by 1000 impulses of stimulation delivered at 33 Hz (for a total of 30 s of stimulation) there was no detectable desensitization. With 2 to 10 million AChRs per end plate, each channel on average would have opened 40 to 200 times. These observations of no desensitization are consistent with the observations of Auerbach and Akk,[239] because there would be time during the 30-s train for recovery from desensitization, if it occurred.

The observations of Magleby and Pallotta[117] suggest that under physiological conditions and stimulation rates when the esterase is active, desensitization is not a significant factor acting to reduce EPP amplitudes. Because sustained stimulation rates in humans during voluntary contractions are usually less than 20 to 30 s,[240] the same conclusion may apply to humans. For artificial high-frequency stimulation, however, desensitization may occur when the esterase is active.[117]

When the esterase is inhibited, desensitization readily develops during conditioning trains at the frog neuromuscular junction, and this is still the case for only partial inhibition of the esterase and stimulation rates as low as 5 per second.[117] Desensitization is not the result of an increased number of channel openings when the esterase is inhibited, as desensitization is observed with inhibited esterase after as few as 30 million channel openings (compared with lack of desensitization with 400 million openings when the esterase is active).

The more rapid desensitization to nerve-released transmitter in the presence of esterase inhibitors is inconsistent with simple cyclic models for desensitization of the type shown in scheme 2. Magleby and Pallotta[117] used pairs of impulses for nerve-released transmitter to explore the inconsistency. It was found that desensitization occurred if receptors were exposed to ACh a second time within 5 to 25 ms after being exposed a first time. Even very brief pulses of ACh were sufficient to induce desensitization during this critical period. Based on these results, Magleby and Pallotta[117] suggested that desensitization (to nerve-released transmitter) involves a two-step process, with both steps requiring ACh. In the first step, ACh converts some receptors to a desensitizable state with a lifetime of less than about 30 ms; in the second step, ACh desensitizes the desensitizable state. In support of the two-step model for desensitization, Sakmann and coworkers,[210] in a study of the kinetics of open and shut intervals of the ACh channel, found evidence of two closed-channel states related to desensitization with lifetimes of about 180 ms and 33 s at 12°C. If correction is made for the lower temperature of their experiment, the lifetimes of their two desensitized states would be consistent with the desensitizable and desensitized states in the two-step scheme for desensitization. Additional states would be needed in scheme 2 to account for the two-step observations of Magleby and Pallotta.[117]

Safety Factor in Neuromuscular Transmission

As initiation of muscle contraction in each individual fiber is all or none, EPPs that give subthreshold depolarizations are of little use. In order for a muscle fiber to contract, the EPP must exceed threshold for generation of an action potential. If the EPP amplitude is much larger than is necessary to generate an action potential, then the safety factor[6] is large. Paton and Waud[241] have studied the safety factor in neuromuscular transmission in limb muscles of cat and dog by examining what percentage of receptors had to be blocked for neuromuscular transmission to fail (measured as a change in twitch height to motor nerve stimulation with single impulses). They found that about 75 percent of the receptors had to be blocked before there was any decrease in twitch height and that 92 percent of the receptors had to be blocked to decrease twitch tension to insignificant levels (Fig. 16-12). Their observations suggest that the end plates have 4 to 12 times more receptors than needed for successful neuromuscular transmission, that is, for the EPP to exceed threshold.

Diaphragm muscle is even more resistant to receptor block.[242] From Fig. 16-11 it can be seen that blocking 75 percent of the receptors might be expected to reduce EPP amplitude to about 63 percent of their amplitude and that blocking 92 percent of the receptors might be expected to reduce EPP amplitudes to about 30 percent of their amplitude if nonlinear summation of unit potentials is ignored.[22] Defining safety factor as (the number of receptor channels opened at an end plate following nerve stimulation) divided by (the number that have to be opened to depolarize the muscle fiber to threshold) gives a typical safety factor for neuromuscular transmission in fibers in mammalian limb muscles[6] of from 1.7 to 5.0.

Although such a safety factor seems more than adequate for a single nerve stimulus, muscle contraction is generally produced by trains of impulses, and EPP amplitudes typically decrease (fade or run down) during repetitive stimulation under physiologic conditions. For example, for the rat diaphragm in vitro, the safety factor is about 3 for steady-state stimulation at 10 per second, compared with about 7 for single impulses.[243] Nevertheless, it appears that the safety factor is sufficient, even during maximal sustained voluntary contractions, to prevent failure of neuromuscular transmission.[244] Endurance exercise training in rats can increase quantal content 30 percent and decrease the rate of rundown.[245]

In summary, skeletal neuromuscular junctions have excess receptors, and the nerve also releases more quantal packets of ACh than are necessary to depolarize the muscle fiber to threshold. The excess receptors and excess ACh give rise to a safety factor; that is, the number of activated AChRs can be greatly reduced to 8 to 25 percent of their normal number *or* the number of quantal packets of transmitter release can be reduced several times without reducing the EPP amplitudes below threshold for generation of an action potential in the muscle cell. During trains of impulses the amount of transmitter released by each nerve impulse is decreased and the safety factor is reduced, but neuromuscular transmission does not usually fail.

Why Neuromuscular Transmission at End Plates with Reduced Numbers of Receptors Is Especially Sensitive to d-Tubocurarine and Can Be Helped with AChE Inhibitors

End plates in patients with myasthenia gravis have about 10 to 30 percent of the normal number of AChRs,[246,247] and consequently do not have the large excess of receptors found at normal end plates. Although the morphology of the end plate region in patients with myasthenia gravis is often changed[246] so that direct comparisons should perhaps not be made to normal end plates, the data in Fig. 16-12 suggest that with this reduced number of receptors the EPP amplitudes at many end plates would be below threshold and that there would be little safety factor at the functional end plates. The decrease in transmitter release that occurs during sustained efforts (depression) would then lead to failure of neuromuscular transmission at many additional end plates.

Patients with myasthenia gravis would be expected to be especially sensitive to paralysis from receptor blockers such as d-tubocurarine because their end plates have few if any excess receptors. If receptors have the same properties as myasthenic and normal end plates, as appears to be the case,[248] a given concentration of curare would block the same percentage of receptors at both normal and myasthenic end plates. Blocking 75 percent of the receptors at normal end plates would reduce end plate currents only to about 60 percent of their normal amplitude (Fig. 16-11) and have little or no effect on neuromuscular transmission (Fig. 16-12). In contrast, blocking 75 percent of the receptors at end plates that had only 10 to 30 percent of the normal number of receptors would reduce available receptors to about 2.5 to 7.5 percent of the normal level and reduce end plate currents to about 10 to 30 percent of their amplitudes in the normal state (Fig. 16-11). This would lead to a failure of neuromuscular transmission in most fibers, as most EPP amplitudes would now be below threshold. Thus, a dose of curare that would have little effect in normal patients could lead to almost complete paralysis in patients with reduced numbers of receptors at their end plates.

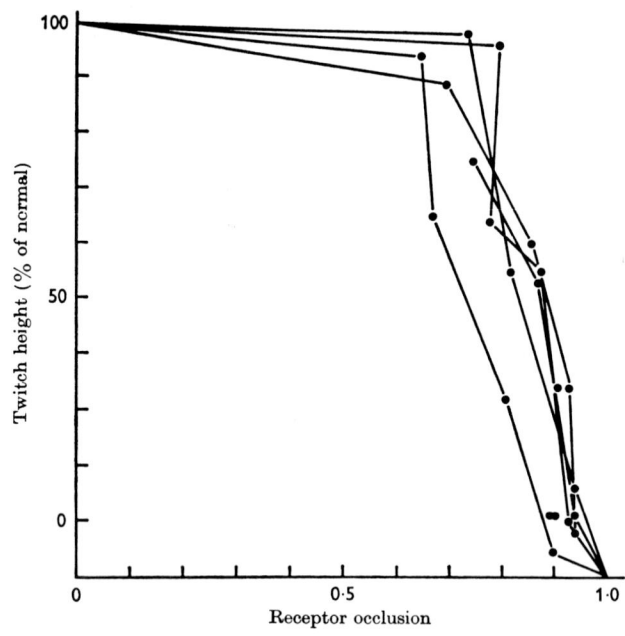

FIGURE 16-12. Relationship between degree of AChR occlusion by a competitive receptor blocking agent, and twitch height in mammalian skeletal muscle. Twitch height is a measure of muscle contraction resulting from stimulation of the motor nerve to the muscle. Note that over 60 percent of the receptors have to be blocked before there is a decrease in twitch height, indicating the onset of failure of neuromuscular transmission in some fibers. (From Paton WDM, Waud DR: The margin of safety of neuromuscular transmission. *J Physiol (Lond)* 191:59, 1967. With permission.)

Inhibition of the acetylcholine esterase often restores neuromuscular transmission at end plates with reduced numbers of receptors resulting from myasthenia gravis or curare blockade. When the esterase is inhibited, ACh is no longer rapidly hydrolyzed but is lost from the synaptic cleft by diffusion. Consequently, the released ACh binds and opens channels repeatedly as it diffuses from the synaptic cleft. The released ACh can then diffuse to functional receptors farther away from the release sites than would be possible if the esterase were active. Both these factors would increase the effective number of receptors, the number of channel openings, and the size of the EPP.

In addition to its main action of competitive block of ACh-binding sites on the receptor and some direct blocking of end plate channels,[215] both of which lead to a reduction of end plate currents, curare also leads to a greater rundown of end plate currents and EPP amplitudes during trains of impulses.[249] For example, at rat diaphragm, EPP amplitudes are reduced to about 60 percent of their amplitude to single stimuli after 20 impulses at 150 Hz. In the presence of 1.1×10^{-6} g/mL curare, the rundown is greater and EPP amplitudes are reduced to about 20 percent of their amplitudes for the same stimulation.[249] The greater rundown is not caused by voltage-dependent channel blockade by curare,[249] but is likely to be a prejunctional effect of curare on receptors that decrease the rate of transmitter mobilization.[250,251] This greater rundown would act to further decrease the safety factor in the presence of d-tubocurarine.

Conclusion

Because of the rapid progress toward understanding the molecular basis of neuromuscular transmission, it seems likely that most of the various proteins involved in the process will be characterized over the next decade. Characterizing the function of these proteins will lead to more detailed questions being asked and further understanding of the mechanism of neuromuscular transmission.

Acknowledgments

Supported in part by grants from the National Institute of Health and the Muscular Dystrophy Association.

List of Abbreviations

ACh	acetylcholine
AChE	acetylcholinesterase
AChR	acetylcholine receptor
EDL	extensor digitorum longus
EPP	end plate potential
MEPP	miniature end plate potential
PTP	posttetanic potentiation

References

1. Atwood HL, Karunanithi S. Diversification of synaptic strength: Presynaptic elements. *Nat Rev Neurosci* 3:497–516, 2002.
2. Schneider SW. Kiss and run mechanism in exocytosis. *J Membr Biol* 181:67–76, 2001.
3. Augustine GJ, Burns ME, DeBello WM, et al: Proteins involved in synaptic vesicle trafficking. *J Physiol (Lond)* 520:33–41, 1999.
4. Hilfiker S, Pieribone VA, Czernik AJ, et al: Synapsins as regulators of neurotransmitter release. *Philos Trans R Soc Lond B Biol Sci* 354:269–279, 1999.
5. Van der Kloot W, Molgo J: Quantal acetylcholine release at the vertebrate neuromuscular junction. *Physiol Rev* 74:899–991, 1994.
6. Wood SJ, Slater CR: Safety factor at the neuromuscular junction. *Prog Neurobiol* 64:393–429, 2001.
7. Augustine GJ, Burns ME, DeBello WM, et al: Exocytosis: Proteins and perturbations. *Annu Rev Pharmacol Toxicol* 36:659–701, 1996.
8. Ruff RL: Electrophysiology of postsynaptic activation. *Ann N Y Acad Sci* 841:57–70, 1998.
9. Zucker RS, Kullmann DM, Bennett M: Release of neurotransmitters, in Zigmond MJ, Bloom FE, Landis SC, et al (eds): *Fundamental Neuroscience*. New York: Academic Press, 1999; pp 155–192.
10. Boonyapisit K, Kaminski HJ, Ruff RL: Disorders of neuromuscular junction ion channels. *Am J Med* 106:97–113, 1999.
11. Martin AR: Principles of neuromuscular transmission. *Hosp Pract* 27:147–158, 1992.
12. Ceccarelli B, Hurlbut WP: Vesicle hypothesis of the release quanta of acetylcholine. *Physiol Rev* 60:396–441, 1980.
13. Katz B: *The Release of Neural Transmitter Substances*. Liverpool: England University Press, 1969.
14. Del Castillo J, Katz B: Statistical factors involved in neuromuscular facilitation and depression. *J Physiol (Lond)* 124:574–585, 1954.
15. Del Castillo J, Katz B: Quantal components of endplate potentials. *J Physiol (Lond)* 257:560, 1954.
16. Magleby KL, Stevens CF: The effect of voltage on the time course of end-plate currents. *J Physiol (Lond)* 223:151–171, 1972.
17. Magleby KL, Stevens CF: A quantitative description of end-plate currents. *J Physiol (Lond)* 223:173–197, 1972.
18. Neher E, Sakmann B: Single-channel currents recorded from membrane of denervated frog muscle fibres. *Nature* 260:799–802, 1976.
19. Sakmann B, Neher E: *Single-Channel Recording*. New York: Plenum Press, 1995.
20. Fatt P, Katz B: An analysis of the end-plate potential recorded with an intra-cellular electrode. *J Physiol (Lond)* 115:320–370, 1951.
21. Magleby KL, Zengel JE: Augmentation. A process that acts to increase transmitter release at the frog neuromuscular junction. *J Physiol (Lond)* 257:449–470, 1976.
22. McLachlan EM, Martin AR: Non-linear summation of end-plate potentials in the frog and mouse. *J Physiol (Lond)* 311:307–324, 1981.
23. Takeuchi A, Takeuchi N: Active phase of frog's endplate potential. *J Neurophysiol* 22:395, 1959.
24. Whittaker VP: The cell and molecular biology of the cholinergic synapse: Twenty years of progress, in Aquilonius SM, Gillberg PG (eds): *Progress in Brain Research* 84. New York: Elsevier, 1990; pp 419–436.
25. Heuser JE, Reese TS: Evidence for recycling of synaptic vesicle membrane during transmitter release at the frog neuromuscular junction. *J Cell Biol* 57:315–344, 1973.

26. Pumplin DW, Reese TS, Llinas R: Are the presynaptic membrane particles the calcium channels? *Proc Natl Acad Sci USA* 78:7210–7213, 1981.
27. Robitaille R, Adler EM, Charlton MP: Strategic location of calcium channels at transmitter release sites of frog neuromuscular synapses. *Neuron* 5:773–779, 1990.
28. Harlow ML, Ress D, Stoschek A, et al: The architecture of active zone material at the frog's neuromuscular junction. *Nature* 409:479–484, 2001.
29. Engel AG, Walls TJ, Nagel A, Uchitel O: Newly recognized congenital myasthenic syndromes: I. Congenital paucity of synaptic vesicles and reduced quantal release. II. High-conductance fast-channel syndrome. III. Abnormal acetylcholine receptor (AChR) interaction with acetylcholine. IV. AChR deficiency and short channel-open time. *Prog Brain Res* 84:125–137, 1990.
30. Heuser JE, Reese TS: Evidence for recycling of synaptic vesicle membrane during transmitter release at the frog neuromuscular junction. *J Cell Biol* 57:315–344, 1973.
31. Breckenridge LJ, Almers W: Final steps in exocytosis observed in a cell with giant secretory granules. *Proc Natl Acad Sci USA* 84:1945–1949, 1987.
32. Betz WJ, Mao F, Bewick GS: Activity-dependent fluorescent staining and destaining of living vertebrate motor nerve terminals. *J Neurosci* 12:363–375, 1992.
33. Zenisek D, Steyer JA, Almers W: Transport, capture and exocytosis of single synaptic vesicles at active zones. *Nature* 406:849–854, 2000.
34. Llinas R, Steinberg IZ, Walton K: Presynaptic calcium currents in squid giant synapse. *Biophys J* 33:289–321, 1981.
35. Neher E: Vesicle pools and Ca^{2+} microdomains: New tools for understanding their roles in neurotransmitter release. *Neuron* 20:389–399, 1998.
36. Helmchen F, Borst JG, Sakmann B: Calcium dynamics associated with a single action potential in a CNS presynaptic terminal. *Biophys J* 72:1458–1471, 1997.
37. Feller MB, Delaney KR, Tank DW: Presynaptic calcium dynamics at the frog retinotectal synapse. *J Neurophysiol* 76:381–400, 1996.
38. Katz B, Miledi R: Spontaneous and evoked activity of motor nerve endings in calcium Ringer. *J Physiol* 203:689–706, 1969.
39. Barrett EF, Stevens CF: Quantal independence and uniformity of presynaptic release kinetics at the frog neuromuscular junction. *J Physiol (Lond)* 227:665–689, 1972.
40. Kuffler SW, Yoshikami D: The number of transmitter molecules in a quantum: An estimate from iontophoretic application of acetylcholine at the neuromuscular synapse. *J Physiol (Lond)* 251:465–482, 1975.
41. Del Castillo J, Katz B: Localization of active spots within the neuromuscular junction of the frog. *J Physiol (Lond)* 132:630, 1956.
42. Rash JE, Walrond JP, Morita M: Structural and functional correlates of synaptic transmission in the vertebrate neuromuscular junction. *J Electron Microsc Technol* 10:153–185, 1988.
43. Südhof TC, Petrenko AG, Whittaker VP, Jahn R: Molecular approaches to synaptic vesicle exocytosis. *Progr Brain Res* 98:235–240, 1993.
44. Whittaker VP, Luqmani YA: False transmitters in the cholinergic system: implications for the vesicle theory of transmitter storage and release. *Gen Pharmacol* 11:7–14, 1980.
45. Regehr WG, Stevens CF: Physiology of synaptic transmission and short-term plasticity, in Cowan WM, Südhof TC, Stevens CF (eds): *Synapses*. Baltimore: Johns Hopkins University Press, 2001; pp 135–175.
46. Barrett EF, Stevens CF: The kinetics of transmitter release at the frog neuromuscular junction. *J Physiol (Lond)* 227:691–708, 1972.
47. Steinbach JH, Stevens CF: Neuromuscular transmission in frog neurobiology, in Llinas R, Precht W (eds): *Frog Neurobiology*. Berlin: Springer-Verlag, 1976; pp 33–92.
48. Day NC, Wood SJ, Ince PG, et al: Differential localization of voltage-dependent calcium channel α_1 subunits at the human and rat neuromuscular junction. *J Neurosci* 17:6226–6235, 1997.
49. Barrett EF, Magleby KL: Physiology of cholinergic transmission, in Goldberg AM, Hanin I (eds): *Biology of Cholinergic Function*. New York: Raven Press; 1976, pp 29–100.
50. Heuser JE, Reese TS, Dennis MJ, et al: Synaptic vesicle exocytosis captured by quick freezing and correlated with quantal transmitter release. *J Cell Biol* 81:275–300, 1979.
51. Katz B, Miledi R: Estimates of quantal content during "chemical potentiation" of transmitter release. *Proc R Soc Lond B Biol Sci* 205:369–378, 1979.
52. Schweizer FE, Betz H, Augustine GJ: From vesicle docking to endocytosis: Intermediate reactions of exocytosis. *Neuron* 14:689–696, 1995.
53. Südhof TC, Scheller RH: Mechanisms and regulation of neurotransmitter release, in Cowan WM, Stevens CF (eds): *Synapses*. Baltimore: Johns Hopkins University Press, 2000; pp 177–215.
54. Schneggenburger R, Meyer AC, Neher E: Released fraction and total size of a pool of immediately available transmitter quanta at a calyx synapse. *Neuron* 23:399–409, 1999.
55. Zucker RS, Regehr WG: Short-term synaptic plasticity. *Annu Rev Physiol* 64:355–405, 2002.
56. Meyer AC, Neher E, Schneggenburger R: Estimation of quantal size and number of functional active zones at the calyx of held synapse by nonstationary EPSC variance analysis. *J Neurosci* 21:7889–7900, 2001.

57. Magleby KL, Miller DC: Is the quantum of transmitter release composed of subunits? A critical analysis in the mouse and frog. *J Physiol (Lond)* 311:267–287, 1981.
58. Erxleben C, Kriebel ME: Subunit composition of the spontaneous miniature end-plate currents at the mouse neuromuscular junction. *J Physiol* 400:659–676, 1988.
59. Hurlbut WP, Iezzi N, Fesce R, Ceccarelli B: Correlation between quantal secretion and vesicle loss at the frog neuromuscular junction. *J Physiol* 425:501–526, 1990.
60. Schikorski T, Stevens CF: Morphological correlates of functionally defined synaptic vesicle populations. *Nat Neurosci* 4:391–395, 2001.
61. Frerking M, Borges S, Wilson M: Are some minis multiquantal? *J Neurophysiol* 78:1293–1304, 1997.
62. Katz B, Miledi R: The measurements of synaptic delay, and the time course of acetylcholine release at the neuromuscular junction. *Proc R Soc Lond (Biol) Sci* 161:483, 1965.
63. Mulkey RM, Zucker RS: Calcium released by photolysis of DM-nitrophen triggers transmitter release at the crayfish neuromuscular junction. *J Physiol (Lond)* 462:243–260, 1993.
64. Dodge FAJ, Rahamimoff R: Co-operative action of calcium ions in transmitter release at the neuromuscular junction. *J Physiol (Lond)* 193:419–432, 1967.
65. Andreu R, Barrett EF: Calcium dependence of evoked transmitter release at very low quantal contents at the frog neuromuscular junction. *J Physiol (Lond)* 308:79–97, 1980.
66. Hubbard JI, Jones SF, Landau EM: On the mechanism by which calcium and magnesium affect the release of transmitter by nerve impulses. *J Physiol* 196:75–86, 1968.
67. Augustine GJ, Charlton MP: Calcium dependence of presynaptic calcium current and post-synaptic response at the squid giant synapse. *J Physiol (Lond)* 381:619–640, 1986.
68. Lando L, Zucker RS: Ca^{2+} cooperativity in neurosecretion measured using photolabile Ca^{2+} chelators. *J Neurophysiol* 72:825–830, 1994.
69. Angleson JK, Betz WJ: Intraterminal Ca^{2+} and spontaneous transmitter release at the frog neuromuscular junction. *J Neurophysiol* 85:287–294, 2001.
70. Smith SJ, Augustine GJ: Calcium ions, active zones and synaptic transmitter release. *Trends Neurosci* 11:458–464, 1988.
71. Llinas R, Sugimori M, Silver RB: Microdomains of high calcium concentration in a presynaptic terminal. *Science* 256:677–679, 1992.
72. Atlas D: Functional and physical coupling of voltage-sensitive calcium channels with exocytotic proteins: Ramifications for the secretion mechanism. *J Neurochemistry*, 77:972–985, 2001.
73. Sher E, Biancardi E, Passafaro M, Clementi F: Physiopathology of neuronal voltage-operated calcium channels. *FASEB J* 5:2677–2683, 1991.
74. Protti DA, Reisin R, Mackinley TA, Uchitel OD: Calcium channel blockers and transmitter release at the normal human neuromuscular junction. *Neurology* 46:1391–1396, 1996.
75. Katz E, Protti DA, Ferro PA, et al: Effects of Ca^{2+} channel blocker neurotoxins on transmitter release and presynaptic currents at the mouse neuromuscular junction. *Br J Pharmacol* 121:1531–1540, 1997.
76. Losavio A, Muchnik S: Spontaneous acetylcholine release in mammalian neuromuscular junctions. *Am J Physiol* 273:C1835–C1841, 1997.
77. David G, Barrett JN, Barrett EF: Stimulation-induced changes in $[Ca^{2+}]$ in lizard motor nerve terminals. *J Physiol (Lond)* 504:83–96, 1997.
78. Forsythe ID, Tsujimoto T, Barnes-Davies M, et al: Inactivation of presynaptic calcium current contributes to synaptic depression at a fast central synapse. *Neuron* 20:797–807, 1998.
79. Thaler C, Li W, Brehm P: Calcium channel isoforms underlying synaptic transmission at embryonic *Xenopus* neuromuscular junctions. *J Neurosci* 21:412–422, 2001.
80. Sand O, Chen BM, Grinnell AD: Contribution of L-type Ca^{2+} channels to evoked transmitter release in cultured *Xenopus* nerve-muscle synapses. *J Physiol* 536:21–33, 2001.
81. Cuttle MF, Rusznak Z, Wong AY, et al: Modulation of a presynaptic hyperpolarization-activated cationic current (I(h)) at an excitatory synaptic terminal in the rat auditory brainstem. *J Physiol (Lond)* 534:733–744, 2001.
82. Klingauf J, Neher E: Modeling buffered Ca^{2+} diffusion near the membrane: Implications for secretion in neuroendocrine cells. *Biophys J* 72:674–690, 1997.
83. Augustine GJ: How does calcium trigger neurotransmitter release? *Curr Opin Neurobiol* 11:320–326, 2001.
84. Chow RH, Klingauf J, Neher E: Time course of Ca^{2+} concentration triggering exocytosis in neuroendocrine cells. *Proc Natl Acad Sci USA* 91:12765–12769, 1994.
85. Schneggenburger R, Neher E: Intracellular calcium dependence of transmitter release rates at a fast central synapse. *Nature* 406:889–893, 2000.
86. Mennerick S, Matthews G: Ultrafast exocytosis elicited by calcium current in synaptic terminals of retinal bipolar neurons. *Neuron* 17:1241–1249, 1996.
87. Yazejian B, Sun XP, Grinnell AD: Tracking presynaptic Ca^{2+} dynamics during neurotransmitter release with Ca^{2+}-activated K^+ channels. *Nat Neurosci* 3:566–571, 2000.

88. Xu T, Naraghi M, Kang H, Neher E: Kinetic studies of Ca^{2+} binding and Ca^{2+} clearance in the cytosol of adrenal chromaffin cells. *Biophys J* 73:532–545, 1997.
89. Rozov A, Burnashev N, Sakmann B, Neher E: Transmitter release modulation by intracellular Ca^{2+} buffers in facilitating and depressing nerve terminals of pyramidal cells in layer 2/3 of the rat neocortex indicates a target cell-specific difference in presynaptic calcium dynamics. *J Physiol (Lond)* 531:807–826, 2001.
90. Tang Y, Schlumpberger T, Kim T, et al: Effects of mobile buffers on facilitation: Experimental and computational studies. *Biophys J* 78:2735–2751, 2000.
91. Augustine GJ, Charlton MP, Smith SJ: Calcium action in synaptic transmitter release. *Annu Rev Neurosci* 10:633–693, 1987.
92. Albrecht MA, Colegrove SL, Friel DD: Differential regulation of endoplasmic reticulum Ca^{2+} uptake and release rates accounts for multiple modes of Ca^{2+}-induced Ca^{2+} release. *J Gen Physiol* 119:211–233, 2002.
93. Friel DD: Mitochondria as regulators of stimulus-evoked calcium signals in neurons. *Cell Calcium* 28:307–316, 2000.
94. David G, Barrett JN, Barrett EF: Evidence that mitochondria buffer physiological Ca^{2+} loads in lizard motor nerve terminals. *J Physiol (Lond)* 509:59–65, 1998.
95. Zenisek D, Matthews G: The role of mitochondria in presynaptic calcium handling at a ribbon synapse. *Neuron* 25:229–237, 2000.
96. Kostyuk P, Verkhratsky A: Calcium stores in neurons and glia. *Neuroscience* 63:381–404, 1994.
97. Katz B, Miledi R: Tetrodotoxin-resistant electric activity in presynaptic terminals. *J Physiol (Lond)* 203:459–487, 1969.
98. Meiri U, Rahamimoff R: Activation of transmitter release by strontium and calcium ions at the neuromuscular junction. *J Physiol (Lond)* 215:709–726, 1971.
99. Zengel JE, Magleby KL: Differential effects of Ba^{2+}, Sr^{2+}, and Ca^{2+} on stimulation-induced changes in transmitter release at the frog neuromuscular junction. *J Gen Physiol* 76:175–211, 1980.
100. Quastel DM, Saint DA: Transmitter release at mouse motor nerve terminals mediated by temporary accumulation of intracellular barium. *J Physiol (Lond)* 406:55–73, 1988.
101. Silinsky EM: Antagonism of calcium currents and neurotransmitter release by barium ions at frog motor nerve endings. *Br J Pharmacol* 129:360–366, 2000.
102. Nachshen DA, Blaustein MP: Some properties of potassium-stimulated calcium influx in presynaptic nerve endings. *J Gen Physiol* 76:709–728, 1980.
103. Mulkey RM, Zucker RS: Action potentials must admit calcium to evoke transmitter release. *Nature* 350:153–155, 1991.
104. Sakaba T, Neher E: Quantitative relationship between transmitter release and calcium current at the calyx of held synapse. *J Neurosci* 21:462–476, 2001.
105. Heinemann C, Chow RH, Neher E, Zucker RS: Kinetics of the secretory response in bovine chromaffin cells following flash photolysis of caged Ca^{2+}. *Biophys J* 67:2546–2557, 1994.
106. Zimmerberg J, Curran M, Cohen FS, Brodwick M: Simultaneous electrical and optical measurements show that membrane fusion precedes secretory granule swelling during exocytosis of beige mouse mast cells. *Proc Natl Acad Sci USA* 84:1585–1589, 1987.
107. Breckenridge LJ, Almers W: Currents through the fusion pore that forms during exocytosis of a secretory vesicle. *Nature* 328:814–817, 1987.
108. Monk J, Oberhauser A, deToledo G, Fernandez JM: Is swelling of the secretory granule matrix the force that dilates the exocytotic fusion pore? *Biophys J* 59:39, 1991.
109. Südhof TC, Scheller RH: Mechanism and regulation of neurotransmitter release, in Cowan WM, Stevens CF (eds): *Synapses*. Baltimore: Johns Hopkins University Press; 2001, pp 177–215.
110. Scales SJ, Finley MFA, Scheller RH: Fusion without SNAREs? *Science* 294:1015–1016, 2001.
111. Betz WJ, Angleson JK: The synaptic vesicle cycle. *Annu Rev Physiol* 60:347–363, 1998.
112. Richards DA, Guatimosim C, Betz WJ: Two endocytic recycling routes selectively fill two vesicle pools in frog motor nerve terminals. *Neuron* 27:551–559, 2000.
113. Rosenmund C, Sigler A, Augustin A, et al: Differential control of vesicle priming and short-term plasticity by Munc13 isoforms. *Neuron* 33:411–424, 2002.
114. Magleby KL: Short-term changes in synaptic efficacy, in Edelman GM, Gall WE, Cowan WM (eds): *Synaptic Function*. New York: Wiley; 1987, pp 21–56.
115. Magleby KL, Zengel JE: Stimulation-induced factors which affect augmentation and potentiation of trasnmitter release at the neuromuscular junction. *J Physiol (Lond)* 260:687–717, 1976.
116. Doherty P, Hawgood BJ, Smith IC: Changes in miniature end-plate potentials due to moderate hypertonicity at the frog neuromuscular junction. *J Physiol (Lond)* 376:1–11, 1986.
117. Magleby KL, Pallotta BS: A study of desensitization of acetylcholine receptors using nerve-released transmitter in the frog. *J Physiol (Lond)* 316:225–250, 1981.
118. Magleby KL: The effect of tetanic and post-tetanic potentiation on facilitation of transmitter release at the frog neuromuscular junction. *J Physiol (Lond)* 234:353–371, 1973.
119. Takeuchi A: The long-lasting depression in neuromuscular transmission of frog. *J Physiol (Tokyo)* 8:102–113, 1958.
120. Zengel JE, Magleby KL: Augmentation and facilitation of transmitter release. A quantitative description at the frog neuromuscular junction. *J Gen Physiol* 80:583–611, 1982.
121. Magleby KL, Zengel JE: Long term changes in augmentation, potentiation, and depression of transmitter release as a function of repeated synaptic activity at the frog neuromuscular junction. *J Physiol (Lond)* 257:471–494, 1976.
122. Magleby KL, Zengel JE: A quantitative description of stimulation-induced changes in transmitter release at the frog neuromuscular junction. *J Gen Physiol* 80:613–638, 1982.
123. Elmqvist D, Lambert EH: Detailed analysis of neuromuscular transmission in a patient with the myasthenic syndrome sometimes associated with bronchogenic carcinoma. *Mayo Clin Proc* 43:689–713, 1968.
124. Adler EM, Augustine GJ, Duffy SN, Charlton MP: Alien intracellular calcium chelators attenuate neurotransmitter release at the squid giant synapse. *J Neurosci* 11:1496–1507, 1991.
125. Engel AG: Review of evidence for loss of motor nerve terminal calcium channels in Lambert-Eaton myasthenic syndrome. *Ann N Y Acad Sci* 635:246–258, 1991.
126. Engel AG, Nagel A, Fukuoka T, et al: Motor nerve terminal calcium channels in Lambert-Eaton myasthenic syndrome. Morphologic evidence for depletion and that the depletion is mediated by autoantibodies. *Ann N Y Acad Sci* 560:278–290, 1989.
127. Fukunaga H, Engel AG, Osame M, Lambert EH: Paucity and disorganization of presynaptic membrane active zone in the Lambert-Eaton myasthenic syndrome. *Muscle Nerve* 5:686, 1982.
128. Satoh Y, Hirashima N, Tokumaru H, et al: Lambert-Eaton syndrome antibodies inhibit acetylcholine release and P/Q-type Ca^{2+} channels in electric ray nerve endings. *J Physiol (Lond)* 508:427–438, 1998.
129. Kim YI, Neher E: IgG from patients with Lambert-Eaton syndrome blocks voltage-dependent calcium channels. *Science* 239:405–408, 1988.
130. Kim YI, Nam TS, Kim SH, et al: Specificity of the Lambert-Eaton syndrome antibodies. Downregulation of P/Q-type calcium channels in bovine adrenal chromaffin cells. *Ann N Y Acad Sci* 841:677–683, 1998.
131. Erulkar SD, Rahamimoff R: The role of calcium ions in tetanic and post-tetanic increase of miniature end-plate potential frequency. *J Physiol (Lond)* 278:501–511, 1978.
132. Zengel JE, Magleby KL: Changes in miniature endplate potential frequency during repetitive nerve stimulation in the presence of Ca^{2+}, Ba^{2+}, and Sr^{2+} at the frog neuromuscular junction. *J Gen Physiol* 77:503–529, 1981.
133. Blight AR, Precht W: Miniature endplate potentials related to neuronal injury. *Brain Res* 238:233–238, 1982.
134. Delaney KR, Zucker RS, Tank DW: Calcium in motor nerve terminals associated with posttetanic potentiation. *J Neurosci* 9:3558–3567, 1989.
135. Zucker RS: Short-term synaptic plasticity. *Annu Rev Neurosci* 12:13–31, 1989.
136. Mulkey RM, Zucker RS: Posttetanic potentiation at the crayfish neuromuscular junction is dependent on both intracellular calcium and sodium ion accumulation. *J Neurosci* 12:4327–4336, 1992.
137. Zucker RS: Calcium- and activity-dependent synaptic plasticity. *Curr Opin Neurobiol* 9:305–313, 1999.
138. Katz B, Miledi R: The role of calcium in neuromuscular facilitation. *J Physiol (Lond)* 195:481–492, 1968.
139. Dudel J: Inhibition of Ca^{2+} inflow at nerve terminals of frog muscle blocks facilitation while phasic transmitter release is still considerable. *Pflugers Arch* 415:566–574, 1990.
140. Nussinovitch I, Rahamimoff R: Ionic basis of tetanic and post-tetanic potentiation at a mammalian neuromuscular junction. *J Physiol (Lond)* 396:435–455, 1988.
141. Tank DW, Regehr WG, Delaney KR: A quantitative analysis of presynaptic calcium dynamics that contribute to short-term enhancement. *J Neurosci* 15:7940–7952, 1995.
142. Kamiya H, Zucker RS: Residual Ca^{2+} and short-term synaptic plasticity. *Nature* 371:603–606, 1994.
143. Tang Y, Zucker RS: Mitochondrial involvement in post-tetanic potentiation of synaptic transmission. *Neuron* 18:483–491, 1997.
144. Delaney KR, Tank DW: A quantitative measurement of the dependence of short-term synaptic enhancement on presynaptic residual calcium. *J Neurosci* 14:5885–5902, 1994.
145. Dittman JS, Kreitzer AC, Regehr WG: Interplay between facilitation, depression, and residual calcium at three presynaptic terminals. *J Neurosci* 20:1374–1385, 2000.
146. Bain AI, Quastel DM: Multiplicative and additive Ca^{2+}-dependent components of facilitation at mouse endplates. *J Physiol (Lond)* 455:383–405, 1992.
147. Tang Y, Schlumpberger T, Kim T, et al: Effects of mobile buffers on facilitation: Experimental and computational studies. *Biophys J* 78:2735–2751, 2000.
148. Stevens CF, Wesseling JF: Augmentation is a potentiation of the exocytotic process. *Neuron* 22:139–146, 1999.

149. Lass Y, Halevi Y, Landau EM, Gitter S: A new model for transmitter mobilization in the frog neuromuscular junction. *Pflugers Arch* 343:157–163, 1973.
150. Rosenthal J: Post-tetanic potentiation at the neuromuscular junction of the frog. *J Physiol (Lond)* 203:121–133, 1969.
151. Glavinovic MI: Change of statistical parameters of transmitter release during various kinetic tests in unparalysed voltage-clamped rat diaphragm. *J Physiol (Lond)* 290:481–497, 1979.
152. Christensen BN, Martin AR: Estimates of probability of transmitter release at the mammalian neuromuscular junction. *J Physiol (Lond)* 210:933–945, 1970.
153. Charlton MP, Smith SJ, Zucker RS: Role of presynaptic calcium ions and channels in synaptic facilitation and depression at the squid giant synapse. *J Physiol (Lond)* 323:173–193, 1982.
154. Stevens CF, Wesseling JF: Activity-dependent modulation of the rate at which synaptic vesicles become available to undergo exocytosis. *Neuron* 21:415–424, 1998.
155. Wang LY, Kaczmarek LK: High-frequency firing helps replenish the readily releasable pool of synaptic vesicles. *Nature* 394:384–388, 1998.
156. Wu LG, Borst JG, Sakmann B: R-type Ca^{2+} currents evoke transmitter release at a rat central synapse. *Proc Natl Acad Sci USA* 95:4720–4725, 1998.
157. Mallart A, Martin AR: The relation between quantum content and facilitation at the neuromuscular junction of the frog. *J Physiol (Lond)* 196:593–604, 1968.
158. Katz B, Miledi R: Transmitter leakage from motor nerve endings. *Proc R Soc Lond B Biol Sci* 196:59–72, 1977.
159. Malomuzh AI, Mukhtarov MR, Urazaev AK, et al: Effect of glutamate on spontaneous secretion of acetylcholine in the nerve-muscle synapse in rats. *Ross Fiziol Zh Im I M Sechenova* 87:492–498, 2001.
160. Galkin AV, Giniatullin RA, Mukhtarov MR, et al: ATP but not adenosine inhibits nonquantal acetylcholine release at the mouse neuromuscular junction. *Eur J Neurosci* 13:2047–2053, 2001.
161. Zemkova H, Vyskocil F, Edwards C: The effects of nerve terminal activity on non-quantal release of acetylcholine at the mouse neuromuscular junction. *J Physiol* 423:631–640, 1990.
162. Meriney SD, Young SH, Grinnell AD: Constraints on the interpretation of nonquantal acetylcholine release from frog neuromuscular junctions. *Proc Natl Acad Sci USA* 86:2098–2102, 1989.
163. Bray JJ, Forrest JW, Hubbard JI: Evidence for the role of non-quantal acetylcholine in the maintenance of the membrane potential of rat skeletal muscle. *J Physiol* 326:285–296, 1982.
164. MacDermott AB, Role LW, Siegelbaum SA: Presynaptic ionotropic receptors and the control of transmitter release. *Annu Rev Neurosci* 22:443–485, 1999.
165. Slutsky I, Silman I, Parnas I, Parnas H: Presynaptic M(2) muscarinic receptors are involved in controlling the kinetics of ACh release at the frog neuromuscular junction. *J Physiol (Lond)* 536:717–725, 2001.
166. Parnas H, Segel L, Dudel J, Parnas I: Autoreceptors, membrane potential and the regulation of transmitter release. *Trends Neurosci* 23:60–68, 2000.
167. Yusim K, Parnas H, Segel LA: Theory for the feedback inhibition of fast release of neurotransmitter. *Bull Math Biol* 62:717–757, 2000.
168. Ilouz N, Branski L, Parnis J, et al: Depolarization affects the binding properties of muscarinic acetylcholine receptors and their interaction with proteins of the exocytic apparatus. *J Biol Chem* 274:29519–29528, 1999.
169. Ravin R, Parnas H, Spira ME, Parnas I: Partial uncoupling of neurotransmitter release from $[Ca^{2+}]_i$ by membrane hyperpolarization. *J Neurophysiol* 81:3044–3053, 1999.
170. Henning RH: Purinoceptors in neuromuscular transmission. *Pharmacol Ther* 74:115–128, 1997.
171. Sieb JP, Engel AG: Ephedrine: Effects on neuromuscular transmission. *Brain Res* 623:167–171, 1993.
172. Bouzat C: Ephedrine blocks wild-type and long-lived mutant acetylcholine receptor channels. *Neuroreport* 8:317–321, 1996.
173. Stroud RM, McCarthy MP, Shuster M: Nicotinic acetylcholine receptor superfamily of ligand-gated ion channels. *Biochemistry* 29:11009–11023, 1990.
174. Galzi JL, Ravah F, Bessis A: Functional architecture of the nicotinic acetylcholine receptor: From electric organ to brain. *Annu Rev Pharmacol* 31:37, 1991.
175. Brehm P, Henderson L: Regulation of acetylcholine receptor channel function during development of skeletal muscle. *Dev Biol* 129:1–11, 1988.
176. Konno T, Busch C, Von Kitzing E, et al: Rings of anionic amino acids as structural determinants of ion selectivity in the acetylcholine receptor channel. *Proc R Soc Lond B Biol Sci* 244:69–79, 1991.
177. Jackson MB, Imoto K, Mishina M, et al: Spontaneous and agonist-induced openings of an acetylcholine receptor channel composed of bovine muscle α-, β- and δ-subunits. *Pflugers Arch* 417:129–135, 1990.
178. Fukuda K, Kubo T, Maeda A, et al: Selective effector coupling of muscarinic acetylcholine receptor subtypes. *Trends Pharmacol Sci Suppl* 4–10, 1989.
179. Imoto K, Busch C, Sakmann B, et al: Rings of negatively charged amino acids determine the acetylcholine receptor channel conductance. *Nature* 335:645–648, 1988.
180. Mishina M, Takai T, Imoto K, et al: Molecular distinction between fetal and adult forms of muscle acetylcholine receptor. *Nature* 321:406–411, 1986.
181. Takeuchi N: Some properties of conductance changes at the end-plate membrane during the action of acetylcholine. *J Physiol (Lond)* 167:128, 1963.
182. Dwyer TM, Adams DJ, Hille B: The permeability of the endplate channel to organic cations in frog muscle. *J Gen Physiol* 75:469–492, 1980.
183. Adams DJ, Dwyer TM, Hille B: The permeability of endplate channels to monovalent and divalent metal cations. *J Gen Physiol* 75:493–510, 1980.
184. Del Castillo J, Katz B: Interaction at endplate receptors between different choline derivatives. *Proc R Soc Lond (Biol)* 146:369, 1957.
185. Cymes GD, Grosman C, Auerbach A: Structure of the transition state of gating in the acetylcholine receptor channel pore: A phi-value analysis. *Biochemistry* 41:5548–5555, 2002.
186. Grosman C, Zhou M, Auerbach A: Mapping the conformational wave of acetylcholine receptor channel gating. *Nature* 403:773–776, 2000.
187. Colquhoun D, Sakmann B: Fast events in single-channel currents activated by acetylcholine and its analogues at the frog muscle end-plate. *J Physiol* 369:501–557, 1985.
188. Salamone FN, Zhou M, Auerbach A: A re-examination of adult mouse nicotinic acetylcholine receptor channel activation kinetics. *J Physiol (Lond)* 516:315–330, 1999.
189. Bouzat C, Gumilar F, del Carmen EM, Sine SM: Subunit-selective contribution to channel gating of the M4 domain of the nicotinic receptor. *Biophys J* 82:1920–1929, 2002.
190. Jackson MB: Kinetics of unliganded acetylcholine receptor channel gating. *Biophys J* 49:663–672, 1986.
191. Colquhoun D, Sakmann B: Fluctuations in the microsecond time range of the current through single acetylcholine receptor ion channels. *Nature* 294:464–466, 1981.
192. Sine SM, Claudio T, Sigworth FJ: Activation of *Torpedo* acetylcholine receptors expressed in mouse fibroblasts. Single channel current kinetics reveal distinct agonist binding affinities. *J Gen Physiol* 96:395–437, 1990.
193. Auerbach A, Sigurdson W, Chen J, Akk G: Voltage dependence of mouse acetylcholine receptor gating: Different charge movements in di-, mono- and unliganded receptors. *J Physiol (Lond)* 494:155–170, 1996.
194. Anderson CR, Stevens CF: Voltage clamp analysis of acetylcholine produced end-plate current fluctuations at frog neuromuscular junction. *J Physiol (Lond)* 235:655–691, 1973.
195. Hamill OP, Marty A, Neher E, et al: Improved patch-clamp techniques for high-resolution current recording from cells and cell-free membrane patches. *Pflugers Arch* 391:85–100, 1981.
196. Ohno K, Wang HL, Milone M, et al: Congenital myasthenic syndrome caused by decreased agonist binding affinity due to a mutation in the acetylcholine receptor ε subunit. *Neuron* 17:157–170, 1996.
197. Harel M, Kasher R, Nicolas A, et al: The binding site of acetylcholine receptor as visualized in the x-ray structure of a complex between α-bungarotoxin and a mimotope peptide. *Neuron* 32:265–275, 2001.
198. Brejc K, van Dijk WJ, Klaassen RV, et al: Crystal structure of an ACh-binding protein reveals the ligand-binding domain of nicotinic receptors. *Nature* 411:269–276, 2001.
199. Grosman C, Auerbach A: The dissociation of acetylcholine from open nicotinic receptor channels. *Proc Natl Acad Sci USA* 98:14102–14107, 2001.
200. Grosman C, Auerbach A: Asymmetric and independent contribution of the second transmembrane segment 12' residues to diliganded gating of acetylcholine receptor channels: A single-channel study with choline as the agonist. *J Gen Physiol* 115:637–651, 2000.
201. Akk G, Auerbach A: Activation of muscle nicotinic acetylcholine receptor channels by nicotinic and muscarinic agonists. *Br J Pharmacol* 128:1467–1476, 1999.
202. Wang HL, Ohno K, Milone M, et al: Fundamental gating mechanism of nicotinic receptor channel revealed by mutation causing a congenital myasthenic syndrome. *J Gen Physiol* 116:449–462, 2000.
203. Kreienkamp HJ, Maeda RK, Sine SM, Taylor P: Intersubunit contacts governing assembly of the mammalian nicotinic acetylcholine receptor. *Neuron* 14:635–644, 1995.
204. Bouzat C, Barrantes F, Sine S: Nicotinic receptor fourth transmembrane domain: Hydrogen bonding by conserved threonine contributes to channel gating kinetics. *J Gen Physiol* 115:663–672, 2000.
205. Colquhoun D: Binding, gating, affinity and efficacy: The interpretation of structure-activity relationships for agonists and of the effects of mutating receptors. *Br J Pharmacol* 125:924–947, 1998.
206. Cachelin AB, Colquhoun D: Desensitization of the acetylcholine receptor of frog end-plates measured in a Vaseline-gap voltage clamp. *J Physiol (Lond)* 415:159–188, 1989.
207. Colquhoun D, Hawkes AG: On the stochastic properties of single ion channels. *Proc R Soc Lond B Biol Sci* 211:205–235, 1981.
208. Grosman C, Salamone FN, Sine SM, Auerbach A: The extracellular linker of muscle acetylcholine receptor channels is a gating control element. *J Gen Physiol* 116:327–340, 2000.
209. Milone M, Wang H-L, Ohno K, et al: Mode switching kinetics produced by a naturally occurring mutation in the cytoplasmic loop of the human acetylcholine receptor ε subunit. *Neuron* 20:575–588, 1998.

210. Sakmann B, Patlak J, Neher E: Single acetylcholine-activated channels show burst-kinetics in presence of desensitizing concentrations of agonist. *Nature* 286:71–73, 1980.
211. Ogden DC, Colquhoun D: The efficacy of agonists at the frog neuromuscular junction studied with single channel recording. *Pflugers Arch* 399:246–248, 1983.
212. Silberberg SD, Magleby KL: Preventing errors when estimating single channel properties from the analysis of current fluctuations. *Biophys J* 65:1570–1584, 1993.
213. Neher E, Steinbach JH: Local anaesthetics transiently block currents through single acetylcholine-receptor channels. *J Physiol (Lond)* 277:153–176, 1978.
214. Adams PR, Sakmann B: Decamethonium both opens and blocks endplate channels. *Proc Natl Acad Sci USA* 75:2994–2998, 1978.
215. Colquhoun D, Dreyer F, Sheridan RE: The actions of tubocurarine at the frog neuromuscular junction. *J Physiol (Lond)* 293:247–284, 1979.
216. Spitzmaul GF, Esandi MC, Bouzat C: Amphetamine acts as a channel blocker of the acetylcholine receptor. *Neuroreport* 10:2175–2181, 1999.
217. Milone M, Engel, AG: Block of the endplate acetylcholine receptor channel by the sympathomimetic agents ephedrine, pseudoephedrine, and albuterol. *Brain Res* 740:346–352, 1996.
217a. Fukudome T, Ohno K, Brengman JM, Engel AG: Quinidine normalizes the open-duration of slow-channel mutants of the acetylcholine receptor. *Neuroreport* 9:1907–1911, 1998.
217b. Harper CM, Engel AG, Fukudome T, et al: Treatment of slow-channel myasthenic syndrome with fluoxetine (abstr). *Neurology* 58 (Suppl 3): A329, 2002.
218. Cull-Candy SG, Miledi R, Trautmann A: End-plate currents and acetylcholine noise at normal and myasthenic human end-plates. *J Physiol (Lond)* 287:247–265, 1979.
219. Adams DJ, Bevan S: Some properties of acetylcholine receptors in human cultured myotubes. *Proc R Soc Lond B Biol Sci* 224:183–196, 1985.
220. Magleby KL, Terrar DA: Factors affecting the time course of decay of end-plate currents: A possible cooperative action of acetylcholine on receptors at the frog neuromuscular junction. *J Physiol (Lond)* 244:467–495, 1975.
221. Engel AG, Lambert EH, Mulder DM, et al: Recently recognized congenital myasthenic syndromes: (a) End-plate acetylcholine (ACh) esterase deficiency (b) putative abnormality of the ACh induced ion channel (c) putative defect of ACh resynthesis or mobilization-clinical features, ultrastructure and cytochemistry. *Ann N Y Acad Sci* 377:614–639, 1981.
222. Engel AG, Ohno K, Sine SM: Congenital myasthenic syndromes: Progress over the past decade. *Muscle Nerve* 27:4–25, 2003.
223. Engel AG, Lambert EH, Gomez MR: A new myasthenic syndrome with end-plate acetylcholinesterase deficiency, small nerve terminals, and reduced acetylcholine release. *Ann Neurol* 1:315–330, 1977.
224. Stiles JR, Bartol TM, Salpeter MM, et al: Synaptic variability: New insights from reconstructions and Monte Carlo simulations with MCell in synapses, in Cowan WM, Sudhof TC, Stevens CF (eds): *Synapses*. Baltimore: Johns Hopkins University Press; 2001, pp 681–731.
225. Salpeter MM: Vertebrate neuromuscular junctions: General morphology, molecular organization, and functional consequences, in *The Vertebrate Neuromuscular Junction*. New York: Liss, 1987.
226. Land BR, Harris WV, Salpeter EE, Salpeter MM: Diffusion and binding constants for acetylcholine derived from the falling phase of miniature endplate currents. *Proc Natl Acad Sci USA* 81:1594–1598, 1984.
227. Land BR, Salpeter EE, Salpeter MM: Acetylcholine receptor site density affects the rising phase of miniature endplate currents. *Proc Natl Acad Sci USA* 77:3736–3740, 1980.
228. Pennefather P, Quastel DM: Relation between subsynaptic receptor blockade and response to quantal transmitter at the mouse neuromuscular junction. *J Gen Physiol* 78:313–344, 1981.
229. Bartol TM Jr, Land BR, Salpeter EE, Salpeter MM: Monte Carlo simulation of miniature endplate current generation in the vertebrate neuromuscular junction. *Biophys J* 59:1290–1307, 1991.
230. Martin AR: Amplification of neuromuscular transmission by postjunctional folds. *Proc R Soc Lond B Biol Sci* 258:321–326, 1994.
231. Wood SJ, Slater CR: The contribution of postsynaptic folds to the safety factor for neuromuscular transmission in rat fast- and slow-twitch muscles. *J Physiol (Lond)* 500:165–176, 1997.
232. Caldwell JH, Campbell DT, Beam KG: Na channel distribution in vertebrate skeletal muscle. *J Gen Physiol* 87:907–932, 1986.
233. Wood SJ, Slater CR: Beta-spectrin is colocalized with both voltage-gated sodium channels and ankyrin G at the adult rat neuromuscular junction. *J Cell Biol* 140:675–684, 1998.
234. Stiles JR, Van Helden D, Bartol TM Jr, et al: Miniature endplate current rise times less than 100 microseconds from improved dual recordings can be modeled with passive acetylcholine diffusion from a synaptic vesicle. *Proc Natl Acad Sci USA* 93:5747–5752, 1996.
235. Dwyer TM: The rising phase of the miniature endplate current at the frog neuromuscular junction. *Biochim Biophys Acta* 646:51–60, 1981.
236. Land BR, Salpeter EE, Salpeter MM: Kinetic parameters for acetylcholine interaction in intact neuromuscular junction. *Proc Natl Acad Sci USA* 78:7200–7204, 1981.
237. Katz B, Thesleff S: A study of "desensitization" produced by acetylcholine at the motor endplate. *J Physiol (Lond)* 138:63–80, 1957.
238. Jahn K, Mohammadi B, Krampfl K, et al: Deactivation and desensitization of mouse embryonic- and adult-type nicotinic receptor channel currents. *Neurosci Lett* 307:89–92, 2001.
239. Auerbach A, Akk G: Desensitization of mouse nicotinic acetylcholine receptor channels. A two-gate mechanism. *J Gen Physiol* 112:181–197, 1998.
240. Grimby L, Hannerz J: Firing rate and recruitment order of toe extensor motor units in different modes of voluntary contraction. *J Physiol (Lond)* 264:865–879, 1977.
241. Paton WD, Waud DR: The margin of safety of neuromuscular transmission. *J Physiol (Lond)* 191:59–90, 1967.
242. Waud BE, Waud DR: The margin of safety of neuromuscular transmission in the muscle of the diaphragm. *Anesthesiology* 37:417–422, 1972.
243. Kelly RB, Deutsch JW, Carlson SS, Wagner JA: Biochemistry of neurotransmitter release. *Annu Rev Neurosci* 2:399–446, 1979.
244. Bigland-Ritchie B, Kukulka CG, et al: The absence of neuromuscular transmission failure in sustained maximal voluntary contractions. *J Physiol (Lond)* 330:265–278, 1982.
245. Desaulniers P, Lavoie PA, Gardiner PF: Habitual exercise enhances neuromuscular transmission efficacy of rat soleus muscle in situ. *J Appl Physiol* 90:1041–1048, 2001.
246. Engel A: Myasthenia gravis, in Vinken PJ, Bruyn GW, Ringel SP (eds): *Handbook Clinical Neurology*, Amsterdam: North-Holland; 1980, pp 94–145.
247. Fambrough DM, Drachman DB, Satyamurti S: Neuromuscular junction in myasthenia gravis: Decreased acetylcholine receptors. *Science* 182:293–295, 1973.
248. Cull-Candy SG, Miledi R, Trautmann A: End-plate currents and acetylcholine noise at normal and myasthenic human end-plates. *J Physiol (Lond)* 287:247–265, 1979.
249. Magleby KL, Pallotta BS, Terrar DA: The effect of (+)-tubocurarine on neuromuscular transmission during repetitive stimulation in the rat, mouse, and frog. *J Physiol (Lond)* 312:97–113, 1981.
250. Harborne AJ, Bowman WC, Marshall IG: Effects of tubocurarine on endplate current rundown and quantal content during rapid nerve stimulation in the snake. *Clin Exp Pharmacol Physiol* 15:479–490, 1988.
251. Wilson HI, Nicholson GM: Presynaptic snake β-neurotoxins produce tetanic fade and endplate potential run-down during neuromuscular blockade in mouse diaphragm. *Naunyn Schmiedebergs Arch Pharmacol* 356:626–634, 1997.

Chapter 17
Nicotinic Acetylcholine Receptors: Structure, Function, and Antigenicity

JON M. LINDSTROM

Scope
Historical Perspective
AChRs: Members of a Gene Superfamily
Subtypes of AChRs
Evolution of AChRs
Structures of AChR Proteins
  SEQUENCES OF AChR SUBUNITS
  SIZE AND SHAPE OF AChRs
  THE ACh-BINDING SITE
  THE CATION CHANNEL AND ITS GATE
Muscle AChR Function
Neuronal AChR Function
  AChR KNOCKOUT AND KNOCK-IN MICE
  NEURONAL AChRs IN NONNEURONAL TISSUES
  DISEASES ASSOCIATED WITH NEURONAL AChRs
  NICOTINE AND TOBACCO USE
AChR Synthesis
AChR Destruction
Regulation of AChR Expression
Myasthenia Gravis (MG) Results from an Antibody-Mediated Autoimmune Response to Muscle AChRs
Antigenic Structure of Muscle AChRs
  ANTIBODY EPITOPES
  T-CELL EPITOPES
Specific Immunosuppressive Therapies for EAMG

Scope

The primary function of nicotinic acetylcholine receptors (AChRs*) in skeletal muscles is to open a cation channel through the postsynaptic membrane in response to binding acetylcholine (ACh) released from the nerve ending. This process amplifies the small current required for conduction along the small myelinated motor neuron axon sufficiently to trigger an action potential in the large multinucleate muscle fiber. This chapter describes what is known about the structure and function of AChRs, their synthesis and destruction in normal muscle, their antigenic structure, the autoimmune response to muscle AChRs that causes myasthenia gravis (MG), and its animal model, experimental autoimmune myasthenia gravis (EAMG). The chapter also outlines specific immunosuppressive therapies dependent on various aspects of the antigenic structure being tested on EAMG. Neuronal AChRs are also briefly discussed.

Especially relevant chapters in this volume include Chap. 19, on the subcortical cytoskeleton and the plasma membrane, which discusses the anchoring of AChRs in the postsynaptic membrane to the cytoskeleton; Chap. 20, on the extracellular matrix, which discusses how AChRs are localized at the neuromuscular junction during development; Chap. 15, which describes the complex architecture of the neuromuscular junction, allowing for efficient transmission; Chap. 16, which explains the electrophysiologic aspects of neuromuscular transmission; Chap. 66, which describes MG in detail; and Chap. 68, which describes congenital myasthenic syndromes, many of which result from mutations in AChRs.

For more details, the reader may wish to consult several recent books and journals reviewing AChR structure and function,[1-4] MG, and EAMG.[5-8]

Historical Perspective

Electrophysiologic studies initially identified AChRs as ACh-gated cation channels at neuromuscular junctions (see Chap. 16 on neuromuscular transmission). Electrophysiologic studies now routinely resolve AChR function to the gating of single AChR molecule channels.

The initial barriers to structural studies of AChRs were the low amount of AChR (2×10^7 AChRs per end plate[9]—which is huge as synapses go, but there is only one synapse per muscle fiber) and the low affinity and specificity of small-molecule antagonists such as curare for binding to muscle AChRs. These barriers were overcome by the discovery that the electric organs of electric eels and rays provided abundant sources of highly enriched AChRs and that peptide venom toxins from cobras and kraits bound nearly irreversibly to these AChRs. *Torpedo californica* electric organ evolved from muscle through the loss of contractile proteins and the gain of 10^5 synapses per multinucleate electrocyte, resulting in more than 100 mg of AChR per kilogram of organ.[10] α Bungarotoxin (αBgt) labeled with ^{125}I provided a means for quantifying AChRs.[10] The use of αBgt bearing fluorescent or peroxidase labels provided a means for localizing AChRs by light or electron microscopy (Chap. 15). Cobra toxin was useful for affinity purifying these AChRs.[10,11]

Discovery that MG was caused by an antibody-mediated autoimmune response to muscle AChRs followed immediately after the initial purification of AChRs in 1973, when animals immunized with AChR were found to develop EAMG.[11] This provided an animal model for studying pathologic mechanisms and specific therapies for MG, and it led to both an immunodiagnostic assay for MG and an emphasis on immunosuppressive therapies.[7]

Monoclonal antibodies (mAbs) to muscle AChRs were initially developed as model autoantibodies.[12] These led to the

---
*A list of abbreviations used in this chapter is given at the end of the chapter.

discovery of the pathologically important main immunogenic region (MIR). The mAbs also provided tools for localizing AChRs and studying their structures.[13]

Studies of muscle AChRs led to studies of neuronal AChRs.[14] At about the same time, low-stringency hybridization with muscle AChR α subunit cDNAs identified cDNAs for neuronal AChR subunits, and immunoaffinity chromatography with mAbs to the MIR on muscle α subunits purified neuronal AChRs. Now 17 AChR subunits have been identified that can assemble to form many AChR subtypes.[1–3] Neuronal AChRs[1] have gained most attention because they mediate addiction to tobacco through the agonist effects of nicotine,[15] resulting in a huge impact on public health (250 million premature deaths by the year 2000[16]). AChRs are the predominant excitatory neurotransmitter receptors in the periphery but a distant second to glutamate in the central nervous system. However, interesting physiologic roles are being discovered for neuronal AChRs, and they are being investigated as drug targets.[17] Neuronal AChRs are also being discovered in nonneuronal tissues,[18] including muscle.[19]

Despite the large amounts of AChR that can be purified from fish electric organs, no one has succeeded in making three-dimensional crystals suitable for structural determination. Electron crystallographic analysis of two-dimensional crystals has led to low-resolution (4.6-Å) images[20] of electric organ AChRs as well as images of AChRs with mAbs bound to their MIRs.[21] Recently (2001), atomic resolution (2.7-Å) images of the extracellular domain of a protein closely related to a neuronal AChR became available[22] when it was discovered that a mollusc glial cell secretes this water-soluble ACh-binding protein to modulate cholinergic transmission between neurons.[23] These images account very well for the overall shape of the extracellular domain and the orientation of the MIR determined by electron crystallography[20,21] and for structure of the ACh-binding site inferred from affinity labeling studies and studies of site-specific mutagenesis.[2] Substituted cysteine accessibility method studies[3] and other mutagenesis and affinity labeling studies[2] provide evidence for the amino acids that form the cation channel lining and gate, but the electron crystallographic studies of electric organ AChRs are not yet sufficiently refined to accurately image these structures. Structural knowledge about muscle AChRs is sufficiently refined to permit interpretation of the functional effects of many of the amazingly large numbers of mutations in muscle AChR subunits (greater than 60) that have been discovered to account for many congenital myasthenic syndromes (Chap. 68).

AChRs: Members of a Gene Superfamily

AChRs are cation-selective (i.e., excitatory) neurotransmitter receptors formed from five homologous subunits organized around a central cation channel.

Sequence homologies reveal that other families of neurotransmitter receptor subunits evolved from the same common ancestor as did AChRs.[3,24] The primordial receptor was presumably a homopentamer, which, through repeated gene duplications and mutations, gave rise to the complex families of receptors recognized today. These include AChRs (with 17 known types of subunits), another excitatory receptor, the $5HT_3$ serotonin receptor (with two known types of subunits),[25] as well as two types of inhibitory receptors (with anion-selective channels). $GABA_A$ receptors (with 17 known types of subunits)[26] and glycine receptors (with 5 known types of subunits)[27] both form chloride-selective channels. All of these receptors can form many potential subtypes, defined by the combination of five subunits in each. Among all of these receptors, a relatively small number of subtypes predominate.[28,29] Some subtypes predominate in particular regions. Some subtypes change during development. And sometimes, single neurons express several different subtypes.

Despite all of this variety, there is a common basic structure and, perhaps resembling the evolution of these receptor families, remarkably few amino acid changes are required to change some fundamental properties. For example, changing only three amino acids in the channel lining regions of each subunit of a homomeric α7 AChR to amino acids conserved in $GABA_A$ and glycine receptors changed its channel selectivity from cations to anions, and reciprocal changes have also been reported in $5\text{-}HT_{3A}$ and glycine receptors.[25,30] As examples, the N-terminal extracellular domains of α4, α7, α8, or β2 AChR subunits can be expressed in chimeras with the remaining C-terminal part of a $5HT_3$ subunit and used to express various chimeric AChRs with ACh-binding sites gating the opening of $5HT_3$ channels.[31–33]

Subtypes of AChRs

Some of the major AChR subtypes are depicted in Fig. 17-1. All of these subtypes are formed from combinations of homologous subunits whose structures are depicted in Fig. 17-2. The symmetrical distribution of five homologous subunits around a central cation channel represented in Fig. 17-1 indicates that all of the subunits contribute to the lining of the channel (and therefore contribute to its ion selectivity) and that all participate in and influence the subtle general conformation changes associated with activation and desensitization.

There are only two subtypes of muscle AChRs. One is a fetal subtype that is diffusely expressed all over the myotube surface before innervation and after denervation. It is characterized by a channel open time of about 10 ms and a turnover time of 10 to 20 h.[35] It has the subunit arrangement around the channel α1, γ, α1, δ, β1.[3] The adult form of muscle AChR differs by substitution of the γ subunit with an ε subunit. The adult subtype is expressed in dense arrays at the tips of folds in the mature postsynaptic membrane (Chap. 15). The channel of an activated adult muscle AChR flickers open for only about a millisecond, and the protein turns over with a half-time of many days.[35,36] ACh-binding sites are depicted at the interface between the "plus" side of α1 subunits and the "minus" side of γ, δ, or ε subunits. Because both of the adjacent subunits contribute to the site, the two ACh binding sites in a muscle AChR differ in their affinities for ACh and other ligands.[37] Figure 17-1 also

Chapter 17. Nicotinic Acetylcholine Receptors: Structure, Function, and Antigenicity

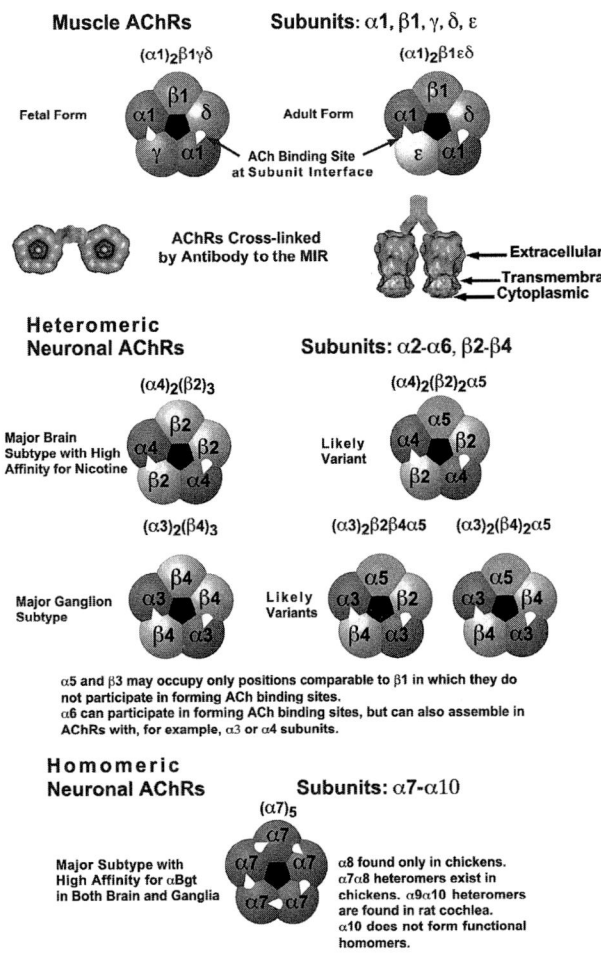

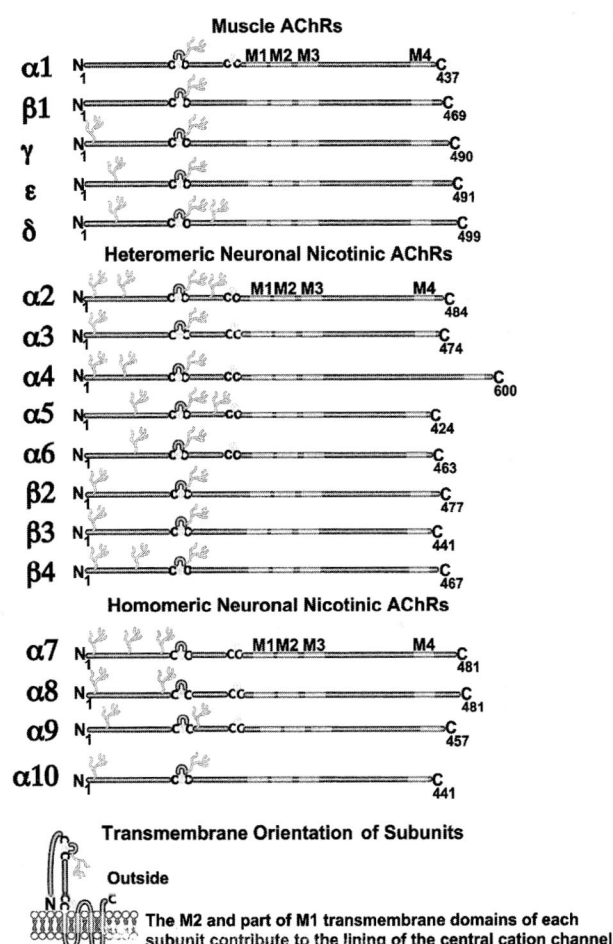

between $\alpha 2$, $\alpha 3$, or $\alpha 4$ subunits and $\beta 2$ or $\beta 4$ subunits, and both subunits contribute to the site.[28] Thus, an $(\alpha 4)_2(\beta 2)_3$ AChR has two identical ACh-binding sites. The subunit position comparable to that of $\beta 1$ of muscle AChRs, a subunit position that is not involved in forming an ACh-binding site, can be occupied (in various subtypes, it is thought) by $\beta 2$, $\beta 4$, $\beta 3$, or $\alpha 5$ subunits. Apparently, $\beta 1$, $\beta 3$, and $\alpha 5$ can occupy this position only. Subunits in this position can influence agonist potency, efficacy, and channel selectivity.[40,41] Although $\beta 2$ and $\beta 4$ subunits can substitute for $\beta 1$ in expressed cloned muscle AChRs, this is thought not to occur in vivo.[42,43] Chicken $\beta 2$ subunits can even function efficiently

FIGURE 17-1. AChR subtypes. AChR subtypes are defined by their subunit compositions. The arrangement of subunits around the central cation channel is known for muscle-type AChRs[3] and inferred by neuronal AChRs based largely on principles established with muscle type AChRs.[7] ACh binding sites are depicted at the interface between the "+" side of α subunits and the "-" side of α, δ, ε, $\beta 2$, or $\beta 4$ subunits. Subunits $\beta 1$, $\beta 3$, and $\alpha 5$ are depicted as occupying positions that do not participate in forming ACh-binding sites. All subunits are expected to contribute to the structure of the channel and to participate in and influence the concerted conformation changes involved in activation and desensitization. The top and side views of two muscle AChRs cross-linked by an antibody to the MIR are shown. This uses a cartoon representation of the mAb and the 9.5 Å resolution image of electric organ AChR determined by electron crystallography.[34] (Modified from Lindstrom J: Acetylcholine receptors and myasthenia. Muscle Nerve 23:453–477, 2000. With permission.)

depicts the top and side views of two muscle AChRs cross-linked by an antibody to the MIR, which links the extracellular tips of adjacent $\alpha 1$ subunits.[21]

Heteromeric neuronal AChRs are formed from subunits $\alpha 2$ to $\alpha 6$ in combination with subunits $\beta 2$ to $\beta 4$.[2,28] Unlike muscle AChRs, this group of AChRs does not bind αBgt. There are many potential subtypes, but a few predominate. In brain, AChRs with high affinity for nicotine are composed of $\alpha 4$ and $\beta 2$ subunits.[38,39] Ten to twenty percent of these also have $\alpha 5$ subunits.[40] The ACh-binding sites form at interfaces

FIGURE 17-2. Homologous sequences of AChR subunits. Prominent features shared by AChR subunits are indicated. These include some features shared by all receptors in the superfamily: A signal sequence at the N-terminal end is cleaved during translation, leaving the mature sequence shown, a disulfide linked loop in the N-terminal large extracellular domain between cysteines homologous to 128 and 142 of $\alpha 1$ subunits, glycosylation sites in the large extracellular domain, and four transmembrane domains numbered M1 to M4. AChR α subunits contain a disulfide bond between adjacent cysteines corresponding to 192 and 193 of the $\alpha 1$ sequence. This is part of the ACh-binding site region. (Modified from Lindstrom J: Acetylcholine receptors and myasthenia. Muscl Nerve 23:453–477, 2000. With permission.) The actual aligned sequences of all rat AChR subunits except $\alpha 10$ are shown in Ref. 28.

in combination with insect α subunits.[44] The major postsynaptic AChR subtype of autonomic ganglia is thought to consist of α3 and β4 subunits, but such neurons also express β2 and α5 subunits and a mixture of heteromeric α3 AChR subtypes, as well as homomeric α7 AChRs.[28,45] The α2 AChRs are minor subtypes in rodent brains, but this may not be true in primates.[46] α6 AChRs are expressed in only limited regions (e.g., substantia nigra, ventral tegmental area, and locus ceruleus) but may play significant roles in Parkinson disease and addiction to nicotine.[47–50] Although α6 can form AChRs in combination with β4 subunits, the addition of β3 as well results in more efficient expression.[51] Some expression of α6 in AChRs with α3 or α4 subunits seems likely. In the locus ceruleus, for example, adjacent neurons can express different complex mixtures of AChR subunits.[52] Some subtypes are probably intended for postsynaptic roles at dendrites, while others may be intended for presynaptic roles in facilitating transmitter release or extrasynaptic roles, perhaps of a trophic nature. The many physiologic roles of neuronal AChRs are still being determined. There are clearly many more subtypes and physiologic roles than in the case of muscle AChRs. A single AChR subtype (α7) has been found in presynaptic, postsynaptic, and extrasynaptic roles, so there is no simple correlation between neuronal AChR subtype and functional role.[28]

Homomeric AChRs can be formed from α7, α8, and α9 subunits.[2,28] Like muscle AChRs, these bind αBgt, but with much lower affinity. Although α7 is sometimes found in heteromeric AChRs with α8 subunits, α8 subunits have been found only in chickens. While α7 is found alone in some central and peripheral neurons (as well as in some nonneuronal tissues), and also often in neurons that express heteromeric AChRs, α9 functions much more effectively in combination with α10.[52,53] Both α9 and α10 are found in cochlear inner hair cells but also in both B and T lymphocytes and other nonneuronal tissues.[54,55]

The variety of properties of AChR subtypes allows them to undertake many functional roles. Muscle AChRs are nonselective cation channels with ohmic conductance properties (Chap. 16). By contrast, all neuronal AChRs exhibit inward rectification (i.e., the channel does not conduct at depolarizing membrane potentials[28,56]). All neuronal AChRs tend to be more Ca^{2+}-permeable than are muscle AChRs, and some neuronal AChRs, such as α7 AChRs, are nearly as Ca^{2+}-permeable as are NMDA forms of ionotropic glutamate receptor.[57] The inward rectification and calcium permeability may both result from glutamate residues in the channel, which bind intracellular polyamines when a positive current flows from inside to out, thereby causing rectification.[56] The high calcium permeability of neuronal AChRs allows them to use Ca^{2+} as a second messenger. For example, Ca^{2+} influx through the postsynaptic α9α10 AChRs of cochlear hair cells triggers Ca^{2+}-sensitive K^+ channels to produce a net inhibitory effect.[58] Neuronal AChRs have been found in postsynaptic roles (where they mediate synaptic transmission),[59] presynaptic roles (where they modulate transmission by facilitating transmitter release),[60,61] and extrasynaptic locations (where they may have a trophic role).[56] Agonist effects of choline on α7 AChRs, unlike other subtypes, may permit it to function in some unique trophic roles.[60,62] Brain α4β2 AChRs have much higher affinity for ACh than other subtypes, and they have often been implicated to have presynaptic roles.[63] The high affinity may be important if, as suspected, volume transmission[64] occurs in the brain (i.e., ACh acts as a paracrine factor on many synapses to facilitate transmission). By contrast, at neuromuscular junctions, the ACh is released directly on AChRs in millimolar concentrations, and the net process is intended to turn high current flow on and off quickly to ensure rapid repeated neuromuscular transmission (Chap. 16).

The evolutionary significance of the many AChR subtypes (and the similar variety of many other receptors) may reflect the occasional usefulness of various AChR properties for particular functional roles, but this is not always obvious. In the case of muscle AChRs, for example, the fetal subtype's long channel open time, diffuse localization, and rapid turnover seem appropriate to its role in responding to the initial stimulation from the growth cones of incoming motor nerve axons.[65] However, the fact is that another neurotransmitter-gated cation channel could fulfill the need for rapid signaling between nerves and muscles, and in insects, glutamate receptors are used for neuromuscular transmission.[66] There can be more subtle interspecies differences. For example, in humans with congenital myasthenic syndromes, mutations in the ε subunits of adult AChRs are more frequent than in other subunits, apparently because expression of the fetal subtype with γ subunits is induced and partially compensates for loss of adult AChRs (Chap. 68). However, in mice, knockout mutations that eliminate the function of ε subunits are perinatally lethal.[65]

Evolution of AChRs

AChRs and other receptors in its superfamily are thought to have evolved from a primordial homomeric receptor.[24]

In the nematode worm *Caenorhabditis elegans*, there is an α7-like AChR.[67] Remarkably, there are 42 AChR subunit–like genes in this genome.[68] This should allow for the expression of an altogether luxuriant supply of AChR subtypes, especially since there are fewer than 300 neurons in the *C. elegans* nervous system.

In insects, AChRs are the predominant excitatory receptor in the central nervous system, and ionotropic glutamate receptors (from a different gene superfamily) are the neurotransmitter receptors at neuromuscular junctions; whereas in mammals, the situation is reversed.[66] Thus, what is important for neuromuscular transmission and certain other functions is the rapid signaling possible with a transmitter-gated ion channel. The type of that receptor is an accidental evolutionary choice in early multicellular organisms.

The structure of muscle-type AChRs had evolved to a fairly perfected state well over 400 million years ago, when we last shared a common ancestor with marine elasmobranchs. The amino acid sequences of α1 subunits of AChRs from the electric organ of *Torpedo californica* and human muscle are 80 percent identical.[69] The other muscle AChR subunits are less well conserved. In all AChR subunits, the signature disulfide-linked loop and the M2 transmembrane domain lining domain are the most highly conserved, while the M1 and M3 transmembrane domains are nearly as well conserved, and the large cytoplasmic domain is by far the least conserved.[28] It has been argued that the structure of the muscle AChR is nearly ideal for its functional role.[70] Studies of congenital myopathies due to single amino acid changes here and there throughout the sequences of muscle AChR subunits (Chap. 68) have confirmed that mutations that either decrease or increase the affinity for ACh or increase or decrease the channel-opening time are detrimental, often resulting in large pleotropic changes in the number of AChRs and the morphology of the neuromuscular junction as well as impairing neuromuscular transmission and thereby causing weakness and excessive fatigability.

Structures of AChR Proteins

SEQUENCES OF AChR SUBUNITS

Figure 17-3 illustrates the highly conserved sequences of α1 subunits from six different species. Figure 17-4 illustrates the substantial but lower conservation among δ subunit sequences from the same six species.

All AChR subunits share several features of their sequences, as depicted diagrammatically for all AChR subunits in Fig. 17-2 and by amino acid sequences for α1 and δ subunits in Figs. 17-3 and 17-4.[2,3,28] An N-terminal signal sequence is removed during translation. A large N-terminal extracellular domain of about 220 amino acids contains a disulfide-linked loop that is characteristic of the subunits of all receptors in this superfamily. In α1 subunits, it extends from cysteine 128 to 142. This sequence is among the most conserved of all AChR subunit sequences. In all but α7-10 there is an N-glycosylation site at 141. All AChRs are glycosylated in their extracellular domains, and many are glycosylated more than once. Three closely spaced, highly conserved, largely α-helical transmembrane sequences (M1 to M3) extend between the large extracellular domain and the large cytoplasmic domain. The N-terminal third of M1 and one side of M2 form each subunit's contribution to the lining of the cation channel.[3,72] The large cytoplasmic domain of 110 to 270 amino acids is the most variable in sequence between subunits and between species. This region in muscle AChRs is involved in interacting with a 43,000 Da extrinsic membrane protein termed rapsyn.[73] Similar proteins linking other AChR subtypes to the cytoskeleton and participating in their transportation and localization are being identified.[74] The large cytoplasmic domain also contains phosphorylation sites and perhaps other sequences thought to be involved in regulating the rate of desensitization[75-77] and probably other properties, such as localization and turnover, as well as intracellular transport.[78] A fourth transmembrane domain (M4) of about 20 amino acids extends from the large cytoplasmic domain to the extracellular surface, leading to a 10- to 20-amino acid extracellular sequence. In the case of human α4 subunits, the C-terminal end of the α4 sequence has been found to form a site through which binding of estrogen enhances AChR function by three- to sevenfold, while it inhibits the responses of α3β2 AChRs.[79,80] No functional role for the C-terminal sequence is known in other subunits.

α Subunits are defined by the presence of a disulfide-linked adjacent cysteine pair homologous to α192,193 of α1 subunits. In all α subunits except α5, this is thought to contribute to the AChR-binding site. These cysteines (when the disulfide bond between them is reduced) were the targets of the first affinity labels developed for AChRs.[3] Three loops of amino acids in α1 subunits have been found to contribute to the ACh-binding site by affinity labeling and mutagenesis studies.[2,3] These define the "plus" interface of α subunits and are thought to form the ACh-binding sites in combination with another three loops of amino acids in the "minus" interface of γ, δ, ε, β2, β4, or α7 to 9 subunits.[81]

The MIR is recognized by rat mAbs to muscle and electric organ AChR, which compete for binding to human muscle AChRs with more than half of the autoantibodies from MG patients.[82,83] It is located at the extracellular tips of α1 subunits and angled away from the central axis of the AChR, so that a single antibody cannot cross-link the two α1 subunits in an AChR molecule but can efficiently link adjacent AChRs.[21] These mAbs also cross-react with human α3 and α5 subunits.[84] Sequences suggest that they should also cross-react with β3 subunits, but this has not been tested. The antigenicity of the MIR depends on its native conformation. α1 Amino acids 66 to 76 contribute to the binding of mAbs to the MIR, and 68 and 71 are especially important to binding of mAbs.[85]

SIZE AND SHAPE OF AChRs

Electron crystallography of two-dimensional helical crystalline arrays of AChRs in fragments of *Torpedo* electric organ membranes have revealed the structure of this AChR and the rapsyn bound beneath it to a resolution of 4.6 Å, as shown in Fig. 17-5.[4,86] This is sufficient resolution to recognize the basic size and shape common to all AChRs and to begin to identify secondary structures like α helices, but it is insufficient for atomic-resolution identification of individual amino acids, ACh-binding-site components, channel linings, or gates. It is sufficient to identify overall conformation changes in the angles between the barrel stave–like subunits arranged around the central channel as the channel changes conformation from resting to activated to desensitized conformations during incubation with agonists.

The *Torpedo* AChR is about 80 Å in diameter and 120 Å long, with 65 Å extending on the extracellular surface, 40 Å crossing the lipid bilayer, and 15 Å extending beneath the bilayer into the cytoplasm.[4,86] The large cytoplasmic domain contacts the rapsyn molecule beneath it through a lattice of finger-like projections that provide a lateral, possibly selective pathway for ion access to flow through the central cation channel. This vaguely resembles the lateral access between the T1-S1 linker and the T1 domain above β subunits of potassium channels for cation flow through the central channel.[87] The extracellular vestibule of the AChR channel is about 25 Å thick (see the 9.5-Å resolution top and side views[34] in the top part of Fig. 17-1). The actual lumen of the channel is quite narrow, sufficient only for rapid flow of hydrated cations (perhaps 7 Å square). The gate of the channel is depicted by Unwin[4,34,86] as

(1)	HUMAN
(2)	MOUSE
(3)	CALF
(4)	CHICKEN
(5)	XENOPUS
(6)	TORPEDO

```
         MEPWPLLLLFSLCSAGLVLG
         MELSTVLLLLGLSSAGLVLG
         MEPRPLLLLGLCSAGLVLG
         MELCRVLLLIFSAAGPALC
         MDYTASCLIFLFIAAGTVFG
         MILCSYWHVGLVLLLFSCCGLVLG
```

N terminus

```
    SEHETRLVAKLFKDYSSVVRPVEDHRQVVEVTVGLQLIQLINVDEVNQIVTTNVRLKQGDVYNLKWNPDDYGGVKKIHIPSEKIWRPDLVLYNNADGDFAIVKFTKVLLQYTGHITWTPPAIFKSYCEIIV
(1) SEHETRLVAKLFEDYSSVVRPVEDHREIQVTVGLQLIQLINVDEVNQIVTTNVRLKQQWVDYNLKWNPDDYGGVKKIHIPSEKIWRPDVVLYNNADGDFAIVKFTKVLLDYTGHITWTPPAIFKSYCEIIV
(2) SEHETRLVAKLFEDYSSVVRPVEDHRQAVEVTVGLQLIQLINVDEVNQIVTTNVRLKQQWVDYNLKWNPDDYGGVKKIHIPSEKIWRPDVVLYNNADGDFAIVKFTKVLLDYTGHITWTPPAIFKSYCEIIV
(3) YEHETRLVDDLFREYSKVVRPVENHRDAVVNVGLQLIQLINVDEVNQIVTTNVRLKQGDVINLKWNPDDYGGIKKIRIPSDDIWRPDLVLYNNADGDFAIVKYTKVLLEHTGHITWTPPAIFKSYCEIIV
(4) TDHETRLIGDLFANYNKVVRPVETYKDQVVVTVGLQLIQLINVDEVNQIVSTNIREKQGVWRDVNLKWDPAKYGGVKKIRIPSSDVWRPDLVLYNNADGDFAIVKFTKKVLLEYTGKITWTPPAIFKSYCEIIV
(5) SEHETRLVAKLENYNKVIRPVEHHTHFVDITVGLQLIQLISVDEVNQIVTTNVRLKQQWVDYRLRWNPADYGGIKKIRLPSDDVWLPDLVLYNNADGDFAIVHMIKLLLDYTGKLMWTPPAIFKSYCEIIV
```

```
                                                              ACh                                                     M1                            M2
    THFPFDEQNCSMKLGTWTYDGSVVAINPESDQPDLSNFMESGEWVIKESRGWKHSVTYSCCPDTPYLDITYHFVMQRLPLYFIVNVIIPCLLFSFLTGLVFYLPTDSGEKMTLSISVLLSLTVFLLVIVELI
(1) THFPFDEQNCSMKLGIWTYDGSVVAINPESDDPDLSNFMESGEWVIKESRGWKHWVYYACCPDTPYLDITYHFIMQRLPLYFIVNVIIPCLLFSFLTGLVFYLPTDSGEKMTLSISVLLSLTVFLLLISKIV
(2) THFPFDEQNCSMKLGIWTYDGSVVAINPESDQPDLSNFMESGEWVIKEARGWKHWVFYSCCPDTPYLDITYHFVMQRLPLYFIVNVIIPCLLFSFLTGLVFYLPTDSGEKMTLSISVLLSLTVFLLLISKIV
(3) TYFPFDQQNCSMKLGTWTYDGTMVVVINPESDRPDLSNFMESGEWVMKYTRGWKHWVYYTCCPDTPYLDITYHFLMQRLPLYFIVNVIIPCLLFSFLTGLVFYLPTDSGEKMTLSISVLLSLTVFLLLISKIV
(4) TYFPFDVQNCMKFGTWTYDGSLLVLNIPERDRPDLSNFMASGEWVMKFTRGWKHWIYYNCCDKPYPDITYHFILMSGKLPYEIVNIIPCLLFSFLTGLVFYLPTDSGEKMTLSISVLLSLTVFLLLISKIV
(5) THFPFDQQNCTMKFNIWTYDGTKVSLHSESDRPDLSTEMESGEWVIMQYVWRKIFDTRGWKHWWFYYTCCDPTPYLDITYHFIMQRIPLYFIVNVIPCLFSFLTGLVFYLPTDSGEKMTLSISVLLSLTVFLLVIVELI
```

M3

```
    PSTSSAVPLTIGKYMLFTMVIAISIIIVIVVINTHHRSPSTHVMPNWVRKVFIDTIPNIMFFSTMKRPSREKQDKKIFTEDIDISGKPGPPPMGFHSPLIKHPEVKSAIEGIKYIAETMKSDQESNNA
(1) PSTSSAVPLTIGKYMLFTMVFVIFSTIIIVVEVFLAVFAGRLIELNQQG.
(2) PSTSSAVPLTIGKYMLFTMVFVIFSTIIVVEVFLAVFAGRLIELHQQG.
(3) PSTSSAVPLTIGKYMLFTMVFVIASIIIVVNALAVFAGRLIELNQQG.
(4) PSTSSAVPLIGKFVAMNKFGIWTLAVFCIVGLIVFAGRLIELNQQG.
(5) PSTSSAVPLIGKQPQKTFAEEMDISHISGKLGPAAVTYQSPALKNPDVKSAIEGIKYIAETMKSDQESNKAS
(6) PSTSSAVPLIGKQPQKTFADDIDLSGKQVTGEVIFQTPLIKNPDVKSAIEGIKYIAIEHIKSDEESSNNA
```

```
    AEWKYVAMVDHILLGVFMLVCIIGTLAVFAGRLIELNQQG.
(1) EEWKYVAMVIDHILLGVFMLVCLIGTLAVFAGRLIELHQQG.
(2) EEWKYVAMVIDHILAVFFMVCLIGTLAVFAGRLIELNQQG.
(3) DEWKFVAMVIDHILLAVFMTVCVIGTLAVFAGRLIELNQQG.
(4) EEWKYVAAMVIDHLLCVFMLICIIGTLAVFAGRIIEMMQE.
(5) EEWKYVAMVIDHLLCVFMLICIIGTLVSVFAGRLIELSQEG.
```

human	Schoepfer et al., 1988	FEBS Letters 226:235
mouse	Boulter et al., 1987	PNAS 84:7763
calf	Noda et al., 1983	Nature 305:818
chicken	Nef et al., 1988	EMBO J 7:595
Xenopus	Baldwin et al., 1988	J Cell Bio 460:469
Torpedo	Noda et al., 1982	Nature 299:793

FIGURE 17-3. Homologies among muscle AChR α1 subunits. (From Luther MA, Schoepfer R, Whiting P, et al: A muscle acetylcholine receptor is expressed in the human cerebellar medulloblastoma cell line TE671. J Neurosci 9:1082–1096, 1989. With permission.)

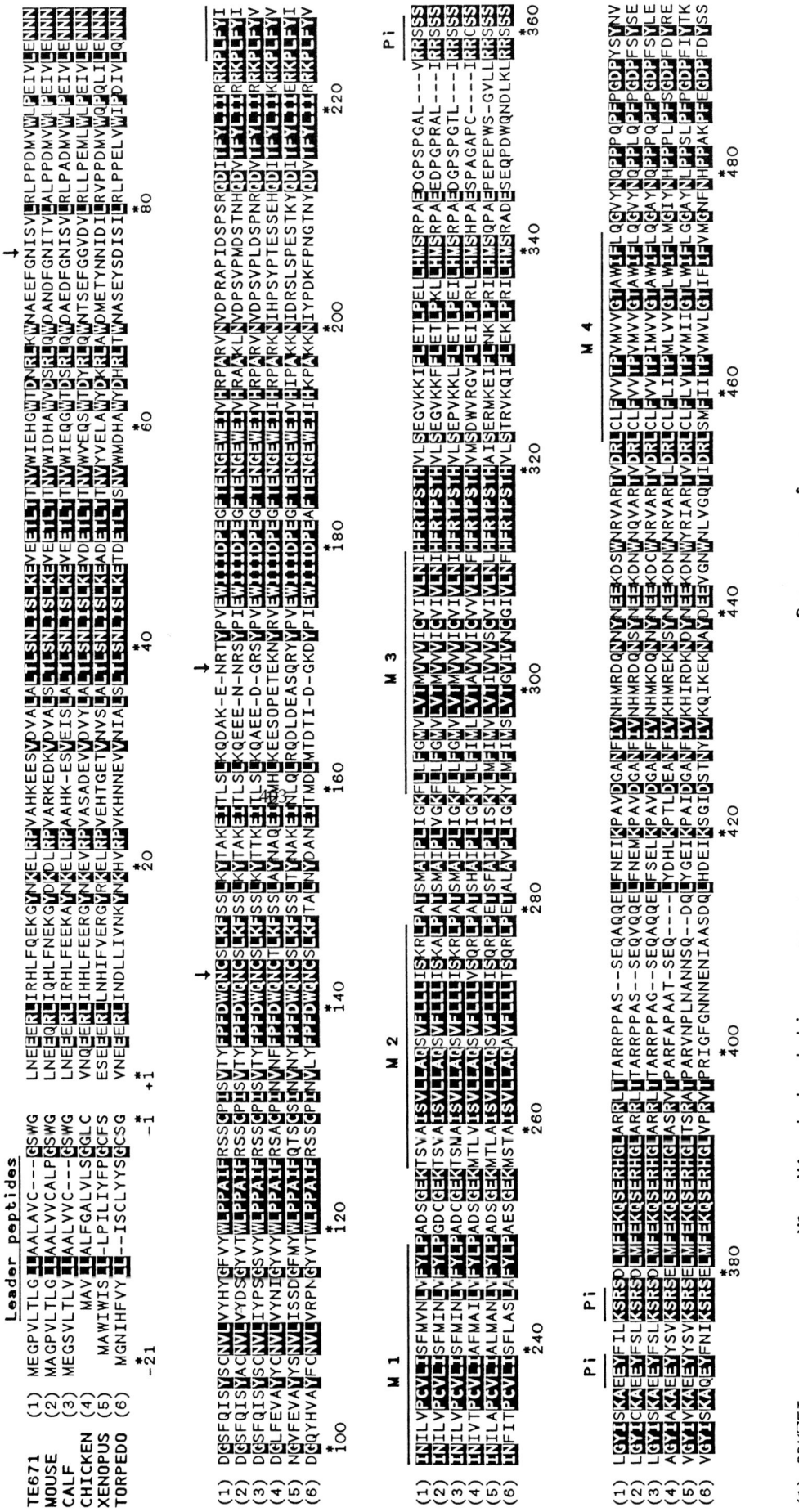

FIGURE 17-4. Homologies among muscle AChR δ subunits. (From Luther MA, Schoepfer R, Whiting P, et al: A muscle acetylcholine receptor is expressed in the human cerebellar medulloblastoma cell line TE671. J Neurosci 9:1082–1096, 1989. With permission.) TE671 is the name of a human rhabdomyosarcoma cell line from which this δ subunit cDNA and the human α1 cDNA in the previous figure were cloned.

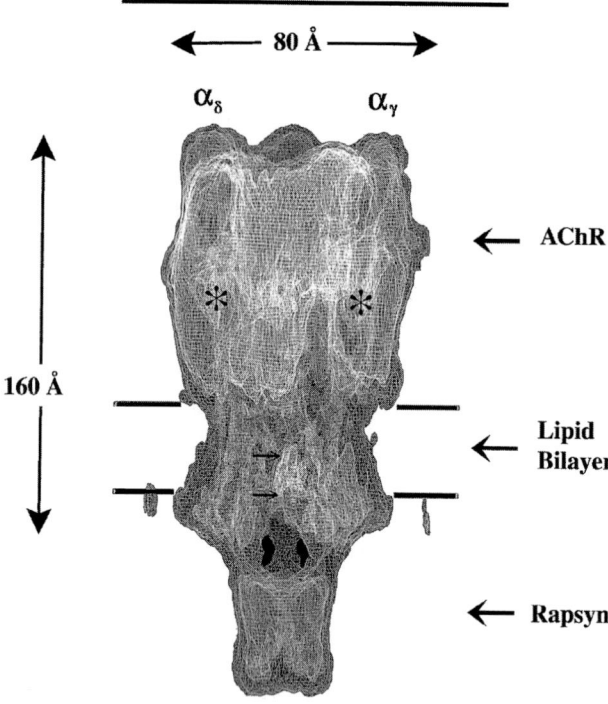

FIGURE 17-5. *Torpedo* electric organ muscle type AChR at 4.6 Å resolution. (*Modified from Unwin N: Nicotinic acetylcholine receptor and the structural basis of fast synaptic transmission. Phil Trans R Soc Lond B 1404:1813–1829, 2000. With permission.*) Asterisks indicate putative ACh-binding sites.

in the center of the transmembrane domain region, but Karlin and coworkers have provided compelling data using the substituted cysteine accessibility method, arguing that the channel is at the cytoplasmic end of the channel, adjacent to or including the highly conserved part of the sequence between M1 and M2.[72]

An atomic-resolution image of the extracellular domain of AChRs, and thus, basically, all the members of their superfamily, has recently been provided by the discovery of a remarkable gift of nature.[22,23] It was found that snail glia modulated transmission at cholinergic synapses by secreting a water-soluble ACh-binding protein.[23] This seems an odd way to modulate transmission, since the ability of ACh esterase to rapidly hydrolyze ACh would seem to make this approach superfluous. However, this evolutionary quirk provides a water-soluble assembled extracellular domain comparable to that of α7 AChRs. Efficiently expressing assembled water-soluble forms of the extracellular domains of α7 had thus far eluded investigators trying to work back by design from cloned α7 AChR.[88] The ACh binding protein from snails was readily expressed in large amounts in yeast, and its crystal structure was determined by x-ray crystallography.[22] A similar quirk of nature in which bacteria were found to express a protein equivalent to the central pore region of K^+ channels led to the easy high-level expression

and crystal structure determination of this protein.[89] Sufficient amounts (hundreds of milligrams) of *Torpedo* electric organ AChRs have long been available, but the mixture of hydrophilic large extracellular domains and hydrophobic transmembrane domains embedded in large detergent micelles prevented formation of three-dimensional crystals suitable for x-ray diffraction crystallography.

Figure 17-6 shows the top and side views of an assembled pentamer of the glial ACh-binding protein (with a positively charged buffer component in the ACh-binding site) as well as a side view of a single monomer on which the MIR, α-subunit ACh-binding site double cysteine, and the signature cysteine loop are labeled.[22] The sequence that would correspond to the MIR on α1 subunits is near the N terminus, angled away from the central axis (as expected), and consists of a tight loop that could account for the conformation dependence of antibody binding to this region. However, there is very little homology in sequence between the ACh-binding protein sequence and the MIR sequence of α1, so the conformation of the actual MIR on α1 is probably significantly different from this part of the ACh-binding protein. The ACh-binding site double cysteine projects from the "plus" side of the subunit to participate in forming an ACh-binding site at the subunit interface about halfway up the extracellular domain. The site includes elements of three loops on the positive interface and another three on the negative interface, which had been identified by affinity labeling and mutagenesis studies. Snake venom toxins like αBgt (8000 to 9000 Da) are large, flat molecules that might occlude 800 to 1200 Å^2 of surface contact area, corresponding to about a 30 × 30-Å square centered on the binding site.[90] Although this might cover about a third of the gross area in the side view projection and an antibody bound to the MIR might occlude at least as large an area,[91] the relative positions and orientations of the MIR and ACh-binding site as well as models of αBgt binding to the ACh-binding protein[92] reveal why both αBgt and antibodies to the MIR can bind simultaneously to muscle AChRs.[82,83] Presumably only the tip of one of the three fingers of αBgt interacts directly with the ACh site.[92] As in the binding sites between a Fab fragment of an antibody and a protein, where one or a few amino acids can play a dominant role in binding despite a large contact area,[91] a few amino acids of αBgt and a few of the AChR are known to predominate in binding,[92] and binding of a small cholinergic ligand, like ACh, can compete with αBgt for binding. The large size of αBgt accounts for its slow rate of binding and its high affinity. The cysteine loop on the ACh binding protein[22] was found to be located near what would be the surface of the lipid bilayer or the surface of the transmembrane region of an AChR protein. The loop sequence in the ACh-binding protein is not well conserved. It is more hydrophilic than in AChRs. This may be part of the secret of the water-solubility of this protein, but it could also indicate that the conformation of the loop in the binding protein does not reflect that in AChRs. For example, a proline in the loop, which is conserved in all AChR subunits, is missing in the ACh-binding protein. Mutating this proline to glycine disrupted assembly of all muscle AChR subunits by affecting the "minus" face and, in the case of β and α subunits, also prevented transport to the surface of assembled AChRs.[81]

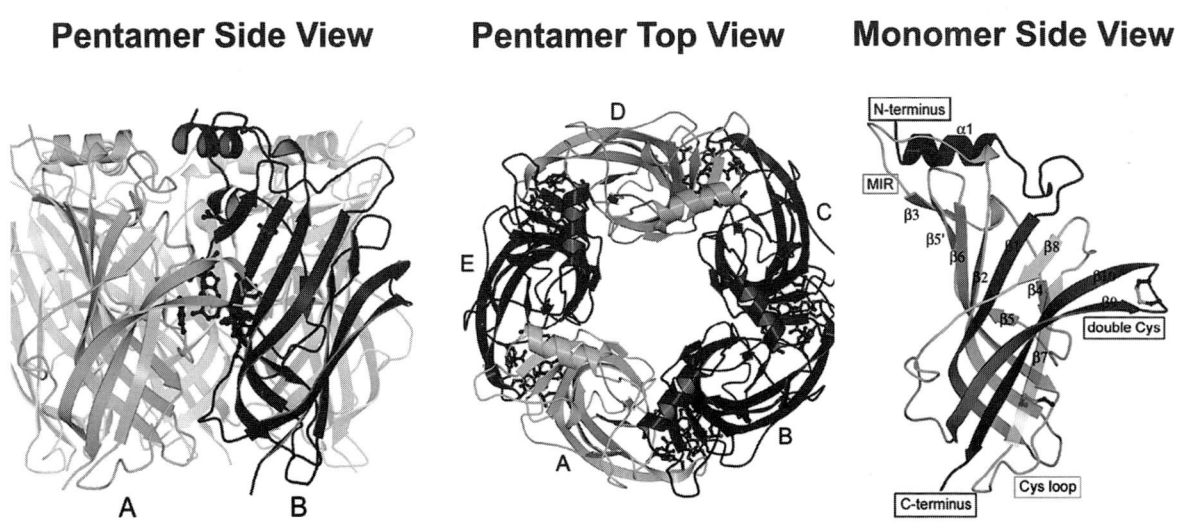

FIGURE 17-6. Crystal structure of 2.7 Å resolution of a snail glial ACh-binding protein reveals the structure of AChR extracellular domains. (*Modified from Brejc K, van Dijk WJ, Klassen R, et al: Crystal structure of an ACh-binding protein reveals the ligand-binding domain of nicotinic receptors. Nature 411: 269–276, 2001. With permission.*)

The crystal structure of the ACh-binding protein provides tremendous revelations about the basic structures of AChRs and related receptors; however, there are limitations. The structure of the signature loop or other areas might be modified to facilitate assembly in the absence of connection to the membrane and/or to form a water-soluble protein. Even if cocrystals with cholinergic ligands were prepared, it is not clear whether this protein would exhibit conformation changes associated with activation and desensitization that would be characteristic of AChRs. The precise structures of ACh-binding sites, characteristic of various AChR subtypes required to design ideal subtype-specific drugs, await structure determinations of these subtypes. The structure of the sequence corresponding to the MIR on the ACh-binding protein would not bind mAbs to the MIR. And, of course, the ACh-binding protein lacks the ion channel, gate, and the highly varied large cytoplasmic domain structures of real AChRs.

THE ACh-BINDING SITE

In heteromeric AChRs, such as muscle AChRs, there are two ACh-binding sites,[2,3] while in homomeric AChRs, such as α7 AChRs, there are five.[93] The small amount of energy to be had from binding ($K_D \geq \mu M$) a small (146-Da) molecule like ACh likely requires the presence of a second site to derive sufficient energy to alter the conformational equilibrium in a large AChR protein (~3×10^5 Da).[70] Even then, the AChR must be relatively a cocked pistol, readily tripped into small conformation changes.

Changes of amino acids in or near the ACh-binding site can alter binding affinity.[2] Such a mutation is responsible for a congenital myasthenic syndrome. Increased ACh affinity results in excessive AChR activation and impairs neuromuscular transmission.[94] Mutations that reduce affinity impair transmission by insufficient activation.[95]

Mutations far from the ACh-binding site (typically in the middle of the M2 channel lining sequence) also increase agonist potency and can so destabilize the conformation changes between the resting and open states that these can be triggered by binding of ligands with very little affinity (such as choline)[96] or ligands with higher affinity but little or no efficacy that might otherwise be antagonists.[97] In these mutants the channel can spontaneously open and remain open for prolonged periods. Such mutations cause various congenital myasthenic syndromes involving excitotoxic damage to muscle due to excess Ca^{2+} influx (Chap. 68).[98] This disrupts postsynaptic morphology and reduces the number of AChRs. Fetal exposure to nicotine is thought to be lethal to developing hippocampal neurons due to excitotoxicity. In this case excessive activation of α7 AChRs is thought to lead to excess Ca^{2+} influx at a developmental stage when hippocampal neurons produce insufficient calbindin to buffer the influx.[99]

It has been argued that the two ACh-binding sites in a muscle AChR should differ in affinity, one having much lower affinity than the other ($K_D = mM$ versus μM), in order to ensure rapid onset and termination of channel opening.[70] During an end plate potential, ACh is present in the synaptic cleft at concentrations up to the millimolar range for less than a millisecond.[100]

Exposure to agonists for long periods results in desensitization. Desensitization is a change in both the conformation of the extracellular domain[101] and the channel,[72] which results in higher agonist binding affinity but a closed channel. In normal neuromuscular transmission, desensitization is not an issue. However, ACh esterase inhibitors given to treat MG (by increasing the concentration and duration of ACh to compensate for the loss of functional AChRs) can, at excessive doses, further impair transmission by causing accumulation of desensitized AChRs (Chap. 66). Nerve gas agents and insecticides that act by inhibiting ACh esterase can have similar effects.[102] The agonist surgical muscle relaxant succinylcholine has a similar component to its action. Nicotine in tobacco users can be present in the serum for many hours ($t_{1/2}$ for clearance is around 2 h) at an average concentration around 0.2 μM and rise to near μM concentrations briefly after inhalation of tobacco smoke.[103] The low affinity of muscle AChRs for nicotine prevents much effect on neuromuscular transmission, but the many effects of nicotine on behavior (addiction, tolerance, anxiolysis, cognitive enhancement) result from a complex mixture of activation, desensitization, and upregulation effects on a wide range of neuronal AChR subtypes.[15,28] The five ACh-binding sites of a homomeric AChR, combined with the occurrence of desensitization—which if it occurs in any one of the sites probably blocks conductance—probably accounts for the rapid and very potent desensitization characteristic of these AChRs.[104]

Both affinity labeling studies of AChRs[2,3] and the structure of the ACh-binding protein[22] reveal that the ACh-binding site does not contain negatively charged amino acids to bind positively charged ligands like ACh. The active site of ACh esterase is similar in this respect.[105,106] These ACh-binding sites are rich in aromatic amino acids, and it is thought that interaction between π electrons on these ring structures and the positively charged amines accounts for binding for this part of the ligands.

Tetramethylammonium is a weak AChR agonist, so binding of a quaternary amine is of itself sufficient to activate AChRs. The composition of the ACh site by amino acids in three loops from each of the subunits at their interface may be critical to initiating movement along the subunit interface. Bivalent ligands, such as decamethonium, probably do not link the two ACh sites, but (as revealed by crystal structure studies with ACh esterase)[107] do link the ACh site and a peripheral anionic site nearby. Antagonists are often multivalent quaternary amines, and hydrophobic components can contribute to their binding affinity. Many antagonists may be very low efficacy agonists, which, on binding, might cause little or inappropriate movement within or around the binding site.

The ACh-binding sites (half way up the extracellular domain)[22] are far removed from the channel gate they regulate.[72] Cryoelectronmicroscopic studies suggest that slight shifts in the angles of rod-like subunits around the channel produce an iris-like regulation of the channel opening.[4] The transition from the resting to the activated state is associated with subtle rotations in all five subunits which alter the shape of the channel. Resolution of such structural studies is not yet sufficient to determine the conformation changes initiated at the ACh-binding site by agonists, how these differ from those initiated by partial agonists, or how antagonists interact at multiple sites to stabilize the resting state. Nor is resolution sufficient to understand how these conformation changes are propagated from the site to the channel gate. The structure of the closed gate is different in the resting and desensitized states.[72] There may well be several different desensitized states.[107] There also appear to be several different open channel states, which differ in conductance and duration.

THE CATION CHANNEL AND ITS GATE

The substituted cysteine accessibility method has provided valuable information about the amino acids that line the AChR cation channel and form its gate and how these change between resting, open, and desensitized states.[3,72] In this method, successive amino acids along a transmembrane domain such as M1 or M2 are individually replaced by cysteine. This introduces a small free thiol group, usually without disrupting the function of the AChR. Then a sulfhydryl reagent which contains a positively charged amino group [e.g., 2-aminoethyl methanethiosulfonate (MTSEA)] is used, which can rapidly covalently react with ionized thiolates in aqueous environments. If MTSEA has access to the substituted cysteine in the channel lining when the reagent is added outside or inside the cell, with or without agonist, then covalently attached MTSEA blocks the channel. The substituted cysteine accessibility method revealed that the AChR cation channel is lined by M2 and the N-terminal third of M1, and that much of these domains appear to be amphipathic α helices (because about every fourth amino acid was accessible to MTSEA). In the resting state, MTSEA applied from outside the cell could react with cysteines substituted to nearly the cytoplasmic surface at a gate located between G240 and T244. In the desensitized state, nearly half of the channel is occluded in a region extending from G240 to L251.

Other mutagenesis and labeling studies have also helped define the structure of the channel.[2] These studies suggest that the upper α-helical part of the channel acts as a water pore, whereas the lower component may not be α-helical. Polar or charged rings of amino acids around the lining of the channel formed by homologous amino acids from each subunit form the selectivity filter.

Most congenital myasthenic syndrome mutations, which are characterized by long channel openings, are found in hydrophobic amino acids of the M2 region (Chap. 65). These mutations (e.g., αV249F, βV266M, εL269F, and εT264P) destabilize the resting channel and stabilize the open channel as well as altering agonist potency and enhancing desensitization. In addition, distant mutations near the end of the large cytoplasmic domain also cause myasthenic syndromes with altered channel-opening properties.[110] The observation that mutations in several subunits for the ACh-binding site stabilize the open state reflects the global conformation changes involved in AChR activation and desensitization.

Muscle AChR Function

AChRs at neuromuscular junctions are specialized for rapid signaling (Fig. 17-7). The architecture of the neuromuscular junction is specialized to ensure reliable signaling through great amplification of the current involved in the motor nerve action potential to ensure efficient triggering of an action potential in the large muscle fiber. The architecture ensures that an excess of ACh is released at high concentration from active zones adjacent to an excess of AChRs concentrated at the tips of synaptic folds and then rapidly removed. Depolarization of the nerve ending releases enough quanta of

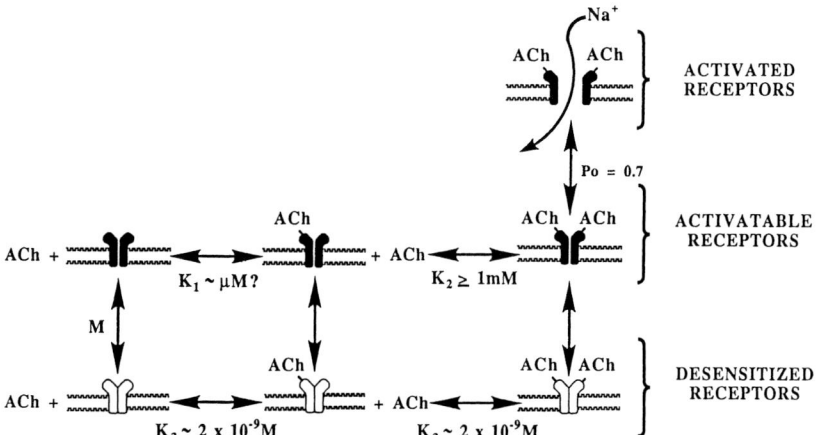

FIGURE 17-7. Allosteric model of AChR activation and desensitization. The parameters shown were determined for the human extrajunctional AChRs of the TE671 cell line.[112] The doubly liganded activatable AChR has a high probability of being open (Po = 0.7). One of the sites of the resting form has moderate affinity for ACh ($K_1 = \mu M$), but the other site has quite low affinity ($K_2 \geq 1$ mM), and it is the rapid binding and unbinding at this site that most critically regulates triggering of the AChR after it has been cocked by higher-affinity binding at the other site. The desensitized state of the AChR has much higher affinity ($K_3 = 3 \times 10^{-9}$ M), so that at equilibrium in the presence of moderate concentrations of ACh, all AChRs would be desensitized. The allosteric constant ($M = 4 \times 10^{-5}$) is such that at rest in the absence of ACh virtually none of the AChR is desensitized. Human extrajunctional AChRs in TE671 cells differ from the junctional AChRs in *Torpedo* in having longer closed times, slower onset and offset of desensitization, equal antagonist affinity for both sites (the two sites from *Torpedo* differ 100-fold in affinity for curare), and much lower affinity for αBgt (the time constant for dissociation is 6 versus 60 h). The single channel conductance for AChRs in TE671 cells is 45 pS.[71] A majority of channel openings are brief (65 percent have a time constant of 0.82 ms) and a minority are longer (35 percent have a time constant of 3.3 ms).

ACh (e.g., ~60, each containing ~10^4 ACh molecules) to produce a peak concentration in the synaptic cleft of ~0.5 mM.[100] Some ACh is hydrolyzed by esterase in the synaptic cleft before it reaches the AChR. Binding of ACh to the AChR is very fast, limited only by the rate of diffusion. Both ACh-binding sites must be bound to provide sufficient energy to efficiently drive the conformational change associated with channel opening. Improbable opening with a single or no ACh-binding site liganded also ensures against potentially excitotoxic cation leakage. The activation conformation change occurs quickly (within 50 μs). The two ACh sites differ in affinity.[70,113] The relatively high affinity site ($K_D \sim 5$ mM) may serve like cocking a pistol to prime the AChR for rapid binding or unbinding at the lower-affinity site ($K_D \sim 3$ mM). After ACh dissociates from AChRs at neuromuscular junctions, it is rapidly destroyed by ACh esterase concentrated in the folds of the synaptic membrane. Thus, most AChRs in an area of postsynaptic membrane exposed to ACh open only once or twice for a period of 1 to 2 ms. Extrajunctional muscle AChRs open for longer durations (~10 ms) and have a higher probability of prolonged bursts of activity. This permits more net current flow per AChR at the low AChR densities of AChRs in muscle fibers before innervation or after denervation. When the channel is open, current flows passively at 50,000 ions per millisecond. This large current flow reflects the basic functional role of AChRs in neuromuscular transmission: to amplify the motor nerve action potential to ensure transmission. The channel is not very selective among small cations, and will allow the slower passage of cations the size of ACh. The passage of cations toward an equilibrium potential of about 0 mV causes depolarization of the postsynaptic membrane (from its resting potential ~ −70 mV) which spreads electrotonically along the postsynaptic membrane to areas in the folds of the membrane where voltage-sensitive sodium channels are concentrated. If sufficient AChRs are activated, an action potential is triggered and neuromuscular transmission is complete.

AChRs exposed to agonists for seconds or longer exhibit desensitization. After opening and closing repeatedly in a burst of activity, an AChR will assume a desensitized conformation characterized by a closed channel more occluded than in the resting state,[72] by higher affinity for agonists reflecting conformation changes in the extracellular domain,[111] and by global conformation changes reflected by a slight (<10-degree) tilt of the δ and α subunits.[114] This is not an issue in normal neuromuscular transmission. In the absence of agonists, AChRs recover from desensitization in seconds or minutes. More prolonged exposure to higher concentrations of agonists may produce more profound and less reversible desensitized states. Passive uptake and rerelease by cells of a tertiary amine like nicotine (which can cross membrane when in an unprotonated form and accumulate in acidic compartments) can also result in sustained reversible desensitization. Protracted desensitization may be very important for some affects of nicotine on neuronal AChRs but does not seem to affect muscle AChRs at the concentrations of nicotine caused by tobacco use.

Neuronal AChR Function

By contrast with the involvement of AChRs in neuromuscular transmission, most neuronal AChRs do not seem to be involved in such a simple postsynaptic role in transmission.[115–118] The α3 AChRs have a rather straightforward postsynaptic role in autonomic ganglionic transmission.[117] However, even there, matters are complex and not well understood. These neurons typically express α3, α5, α7, β2, and β4 subunits. These are assembled into α7 homomers and a variety of α3 subtypes, among which (α3)$_2$(β4)$_3$ AChRs may predominate but (α3)$_2$(β4)α5, (α3)$_2$(β2)$_3$, (α3)$_2$β2β4α5, and other subtypes may be present.[49] The α3 AChRs usually mediate synaptic transmission, but, at certain developmental stages in the chick ciliary ganglion, transmission can occur through either α3 AChRs or α7 AChRs.[53] In these neurons α7 AChRs are present in large amounts perisynaptically in an unusual calyx synapse. In this case, the physiologic role of α7 AChR may be to detect the average rate of transmission for trophic regulatory purposes.[62] High-frequency transmission could lead to the buildup of choline (from ACh hydrolysis), which selectively activates α7 AChRs, allowing Ca^{2+} entry and second-messenger pathway activation. The precise localization and physiologic role of α7 AChRs in the general case of mammalian autonomic ganglia is not known. Cardiac ganglia and superior cervical ganglia may contain previously unknown α7-containing AChRs.[119] In the central nervous system, the physiologic role of many AChRs is to facilitate release of a wide variety of neurotransmitters.[116] It is unclear to what extent these presynaptic AChRs are activated by ACh released directly on the presynaptic AChRs or by volume transmission.[64] Brain synapses in general correspond in size to a tiny fraction of a neuromuscular junction, and the normal probability of transmission is closer to 0.1 than 1.0.

AChR KNOCKOUT AND KNOCK-IN MICE

A good way to get a general overview of the physiologic roles of neuronal AChRs is to study mice in which a particular AChR subunit has been eliminated by genetically "knocking it out" or replaced by a hyperfunctional mutant form that has been genetically "knocked in." Thus far, little has been published on conditional knockout AChR mice in which AChRs in only certain regions are eliminated or where expression is eliminated in response to a drug treatment after normal development.

Mice lacking the α3 subunit lack autonomic ganglionic transmission.[120] They die shortly after birth. Prominent features are megacystis (inflamed urinary bladder) and mydriasis (widely dilated ocular pupils).

Mice lacking the α4 subunit lose most high-affinity nicotine binding throughout their brains, lose nicotine-induced antinociception, and exhibit increased anxiety.[121,122] A potential problem with any knockout mouse is that, during development, adaptive changes may be made to the loss of a subunit, which could cause underestimation of its normal physiologic role. Native α4 was replaced with a mutant α4 in which a conserved leucine in the middle of M2 was replaced with a serine.[123] Like α7 L247T mutants, this α4 mutation was excessively active and highly excitotoxic. The EC$_{50}$ for ACh and nicotine was shifted 30-fold (from 1.2 to 0.04 μM for ACh), and 10 μM choline (a concentration found in cerebrospinal fluid) caused 20 percent maximum activation. Both mutant homozygous and heterozygous mice died, but a heterozygote with some of the neo cassette involved in making the mutant survived because this reduced expression of the mutant AChR. These mice lost dopaminergic neurons in the substantia nigra and exhibited altered motor behavior and motor learning. They also exhibited increased anxiety. A problem with knock-in of excitotoxic mutations is that it exaggerates the physiologic role of an AChR subunit, so that, for example, in a dopaminergic neuron that expresses several AChR subtypes including both α4 and α6, the presence of a toxic α4 kills the neuron. In other neurons, mutant α4 continues to function, but at an exaggerated level that can also alter development.

Knockout of α6 has been reported,[48] but behavioral studies have not been reported yet. These may prove interesting both in the case of addiction to nicotine and in Parkinson disease, because α6 AChRs probably play important roles in modulating the release of dopamine.

Knockout of α7 produced little evident behavioral phenotype despite the widespread expression of α7 in both the central and peripheral nervous systems.[124] These animals did exhibit altered cardiac baroreflexes,[125] and their breeding is impaired. However, knock-in of an excitotoxic hyperactive α7 L250T mutant had a pronounced phenotype characterized in homozygotes by increased neural apoptosis and death within a day of birth.[126] Overall, the α7 knock-in was less severe than the α4 knock-in. The α7 knock-in heterozygotes were phenotypically normal.

Knockout of α9 prevented cochlear efferent stimulation, as expected from its postsynaptic role there.[127]

Knockout of β2 altered some learning behaviors, caused increased neuronal cell death with age, prevented nicotine-induced antinociception, and prevented nicotine reinforcement (addiction).[128]

Knockout of β4 produced viable mice, suggesting that β2 must have replaced β4 in α3 autonomic neurons. However, when both β2 and β4 were knocked out, the effects resembled those of the α3 knockout and were even more severe.[129]

Knockout of β3 altered motor activity and decreased anxiety.[130] The β3 and α6 are rare AChR subunits, often being found together in dopaminergic neurons involved in motor control and Parkinson disease (e.g., substantia nigra) and in nicotine reinforcement and addiction (e.g., ventral tegmental area and locus ceruleus).[28] Much more is likely to be learned about the physiologic roles of α3, α6, and other AChR subunits from further studies of knockout mice.

NEURONAL AChRs IN NONNEURONAL TISSUES

Neuronal AChR subunits including α7 have been found to be expressed in fetal and denervated muscle.[18] Their physiologic role there is unclear. It is not critical, since neuromuscular transmission appears to develop normally in α7 knockout mice.[124] The increased Ca^{2+} permeability of α7 may be useful in some initial trophic interactions during the formation of neuromuscular junctions. Alternatively, there may be some cross talk in the gene regulation of AChR subunit expression, and the expression of neuronal AChRs may be inconsequential.

Human keratinocytes have been found to express a variety of neuronal AChRs (especially α3 AChRs) and to synthesize and release ACh.[131,132] ACh inhibits keratinocyte mobility in cell cultures, and it is thought that cytokine effects of ACh may have some role in wound healing. Thus far, these effects have not been investigated in knockout mice. An autoimmune response to α9 AChRs has been found in pemphigus.[55]

Neuronal AChRs (especially α3 AChRs) have been detected at low concentrations in endothelial cells of blood vessels[133] and in bronchial epithelial cells,[134] where they appear to regulate cell shape and motility. Nicotine has been reported to stimulate angiogenesis and promote tumor growth and atherosclerosis at concentrations that are pathophysiologically relevant.[135] The α7 AChRs have also been detected in several other fetal primate lung cells, and these were upregulated by prenatal nicotine exposure.[136] This also altered lung development, resulting in hypoplasia, reduced alveolar surface complexity, and increased collagen.

Some AChR expression has been found in the immune system. Thymus cells have been found to express α3 AChRs.[137] Both α9 and α10 have been found in both B and T lymphocytes.[54]

DISEASES ASSOCIATED WITH NEURONAL AChRs

Autoimmune responses have recently been discovered to both α3[138] and α9 AChRs.[55] These have not been studied in the detail with which the autoimmune response to α1 AChRs in myasthenia gravis (MG) has been studied.[7] Autoantibodies to α3 AChRs have been implicated in causing autoimmune autonomic neuropathies by impairing transmission through autonomic ganglia. Autoantibodies have been detected in these patients, which bind to α3 AChRs but not to α1 AChRs.[138] Autoantibodies to α9 AChRs have been detected in pemphigus patients, along with autoantibodies to desmoglien.[55] Pemphigus is a disease of skin adhesion, and several neuronal AChR subtypes have been found in keratinocytes, where they modulate motility and adhesion. It would not be surprising if in the future autoantibodies to α7 AChRs were found to be associated with autonomic, reproductive, or other diseases. Nor would it be surprising to discover that autoantibodies to α3 AChRs had effects on vascular[133] or bronchial[134] endothelia, where small amounts of these AChRs have also been detected.

A priori, one might not expect antibody-mediated autoimmune responses to be important in central neuronal diseases because one might expect that the blood-brain barrier would prevent access of serum antibodies to brain AChRs. However, antibody-mediated autoimmune responses to several glutamate receptor subtypes have been found to be associated with both Rasmussen encephalitis and forms of cerebellar degeneration.[139–142] Rabbits immunized with bacterially expressed glutamate receptor proteins developed a fatal Rasmussen-like epilepsy,[139] much as rabbits immunized with the first electric organ AChRs purified developed EAMG.[11] These autoantibodies (unlike those in MG, but like those in Graves disease) can act as agonists and are excitotoxic.[140–142] This appears to be because antibodies bound away from the glutamate-binding site cross-link the two extracellular domains of the receptor, presumably causing a conformation change similar to that caused by glutamate binding at the interface between these lobes. These precedents suggest that it is not impossible that autoantibodies to brain AChRs might be able to produce central pathologic effects.

Autosomal dominant nocturnal frontal lobe epilepsy (ADNFLE) has been found in association with mutations in both α4[143] and β2[144,145] AChR subunits; however, thus far, nothing like the large numbers of mutations in muscle AChR subunits in congenital myasthenic syndromes (CMS) (Chap. 65)[98] have been found, nor has the ADNFLE pathology been so elegantly characterized as has that of CMS patients.[98] Two mutations (S248F and 776 ins 3) have been found in the M2 channel lining domain of α4 subunits.[142] These result in net reduced α4β2 AChR function.[146–148] They are also associated with a use-dependent potentiation of AChR function from an initial very low level to a somewhat higher level characterized by faster desensitization, slower recovery from desensitization, less inward rectification, no Ca^{2+} permeability, and altered single-channel conductance.[148,149] It is known that one physiologic role of α4β2 AChR is to facilitate release of the inhibitory transmitter GABA,[60] and it is thought that reduced activity of α4β2 AChRs might cause the neuronal hyperactivity of epilepsy by reducing GABA release.[148] Curiously, two different mutations associated with ADNFLE have been found at the same position in the β2 subunit M2 region (V287M and V287L), both of which increase α4β2A ChR function.[144,145] These mutations increase ACh sensitivity tenfold, reduce desensitization, and prolong channel opening, much as occurs in slow-channel CMS patients.[98] A direct excitotoxic effect of the β2 mutations might be expected to account for epilepsy in this case. It has been suggested that all α4- and β2-subunit ADNFLE mutations might share a common effect on the regulation of α4β2 AchR function by Ca^{2+}.[149] The large number of mutations found in muscle AChRs,[98] ACh esterase,[150] choline acetyltransferase,[151] and no doubt other proteins to account for many different congenital myasthenic syndromes suggests that there may be an equally large array of mutations associated with neuronal AChRs and neuronal cholinergic transmission. The large variety of AChR subtypes and functional roles further suggests that these mutations may be associated with a wide array of phenotypes.

There are a number of other diseases known in which changes in AChRs occur and in which AChRs may provide a drug target. However, at this time no other diseases have been reported in which AChRs are the primary cause of the disease. Of course, if addiction to tobacco counts as a disease, then this depends directly on AChRs, and its prevalence and mortality dwarfs all other neurologic diseases.[15,16] That is discussed further on.

Parkinson disease is associated with a loss of AChRs in the substantia nigra. Death of cells in this region is thought to account for the movement difficulties characteristic of this disease. The α6 AChRs are particularly prominent in these dopaminergic neurons. AChRs can facilitate dopamine release.[152–154] Treatment of this region with antisense mRNA to α6 produced movement defects.[155] Tobacco use (and by implication nicotine) is known to be protective against the occurrence of Parkinson disease.[156] In tissue culture, several neuroprotective effects of nicotine have been discovered: These involve various AChR subtypes in protection against glutamate excitotoxicity,[157] loss of neurotrophic factors,[158] and Aβ amyloid neurotoxicity.[157]

Alzheimer disease is associated with loss of AChRs, especially of α4 more than α3 or α7.[159,160] The neuronal loss associated with this dementing disease is accompanied by formation of plaques of the Aβ fragment of the amyloid precursor protein and with neurofibrillary tangles. Through an allosteric site, Aβ has been found to very potently inhibit α7 AChR function.[161] It was less potent as an inhibitor of α4β2. It is controversial whether Aβ inhibits binding of αBgt to α7.[161,163] It may be that this depends on the size of the Aβ aggregates used. Monomeric Aβ clearly does not bind to the ACh-binding site, but sufficiently large aggregates bound to an allosteric site might overlap the large surface area occluded by bound αBgt. It might be that polymeric aggregates of Aβ would very efficiently cross-link α7 AChRs on the cell surface, since each AChR would have five binding sites and tens or hundreds of Aβ1-42 peptides in an aggregate would provide very avid binding. Then, just as in MG, where autoantibodies to muscle AChRs cross-link muscle AChRs and thereby facilitate their internalization and lysosomal destruction,[7] Aβ cross-linked α7 AChRs might internalize, leading to accumulation of Aβ in lysosomal compartments. It has been hypothesized that, rather than aggregating extracellularly, Aβ may accumulate within neurons, leaving plaques when the neurons die and disintegrate.[165] In mice engineered to overexpress Aβ1-42 as a model of Alzheimer disease, there is an increase in the amount of α7.[166] It has been reported that treating such mice with nicotine causes an 80 percent reduction in Aβ plaques.[164] β-Amyloid activates a mitogen-activated protein kinase cascade through α7 AChRs.[166] Nicotine acting through α7 AChRs protects against Aβ amyloid toxicity through a signaling cascade that involves phosphatidylinositol 3 kinase.[157] All of these α7 effects are new, and some are controversial. All show AChRs acting in more complex ways than normally expected from the physiologic roles of α1 AChRs. It remains to be seen whether AChRs play a passive role in Alzheimer disease, with their loss simply subsequent to the loss of neurons, or whether AChRs play a more central role in the pathology. Loss of α4β2 AChRs accounts for the loss of high-affinity nicotine-binding sites seen in Alzheimer disease,[159,160,167] and aged mice lacking α4β2 AChRs subsequent to knockout of β2 subunits show excessive neuronal loss.[168] Both the neuroprotective effects and cognitive enhancing effects of nicotine have spurred some interest in developing specific AChR agonists for therapy of Alzheimer disease.[169] If the allosteric effects of Aβ1-42 on AChRs were to prove a significant component of the pathology in this disease, the allosteric site might be a useful drug target. Galantamine is a newly approved drug for therapy of Alzheimer disease. Like the other approved drugs, it is an inhibitor of ACh esterase, but it is also active at an allosteric site on AChRs to promote function.[170]

Tourette syndrome in children is associated with tics and compulsive behavior. Both nicotine (an agonist)[171] and mecamylamine (a channel-blocking antagonist)[172] have proven beneficial in reducing the incidence and severity of these tics. Since both chronic application of nicotine in a patch and an AChR antagonist have the same effect, it seems likely that inhibiting the tics depends on either accumulating desensitized AChRs or directly blocking AChRs.

There may be some association between AChRs and schizophrenia.[173] About 90 percent of schizophrenics are heavy smokers, as if they were trying to self-medicate. Yet the number of their α4 AChRs is not as increased as would be expected from their tobacco use. A dinucleotide polymorphism near the α7 gene was reported to be associated with schizophrenics and their close relatives, who also exhibit a decrease in the normal inhibition of the response evoked to the second of paired auditory stimuli. However, this is controversial.

AChRs have been suggested as drug targets in several other cases, including attention deficit disorder, chronic pain, anxiety, cognitive enhancement, and some inflammatory bowel disorders (e.g., smoking is protective against ulcerative colitis and nicotine shows some therapeutic benefit, whereas smoking exacerbates Crohn disease).[169]

NICOTINE AND TOBACCO USE

By far the biggest medical problem involving AChRs is addiction to tobacco, for which nicotine effects on AChRs are directly responsible.[15] AChRs containing β2 subunits appear especially important for the development of addiction.[128] Nicotine has many effects on behavior, heart rate, blood pressure, weight,[103] and, in certain circumstances, angiogenesis, atherosclerosis, and tumor growth.[134,175] However, the direct effects of nicotine are probably not responsible for most of the 400,000 premature deaths per year in the United States resulting from tobacco use.[15,16]

Nicotine and other addictive drugs are thought to share a common pathway, mediated by dopamine release in the striatum, which pathologically modifies reward-based learning behavior to produce addiction.[176] Addiction to tobacco involves complex behavioral components in addition to nicotine and is not easily treated by nicotine replacement alone. The behavioral effects of nicotine are complex, both because of the many AChR subtypes and varied neural systems with which they are associated and because of the complex pattern in which tobacco users administer nicotine.

Nicotine rapidly crosses cell membranes because it is a tertiary amine. Its half-time for clearance from serum is about 2 h.[103] A tobacco user can transiently make his or her brain nearly micromolar in nicotine within a few seconds of inhaling. Gradually, serum nicotine concentration builds up to a level of about 0.2 μM for many hours. The nicotine concentrations required to half maximally activate many AChR subtypes are in the micromolar range.[28] However, lower sustained activation might facilitate transmitter release presynaptically, enhance responses to endogenous ACh, or alter AChR-mediated trophic effects. Much lower sustained concentrations of nicotine or other cholinergic agonists are required to desensitize AChRs than are required to efficiently acutely activate them.

Prolonged exposure to 0.2 μM nicotine is very effective at desensitizing α4β2, α4α6β2, and α7 AChRs, whereas α3β2 and α3α6β2 AChRs are relatively resistant to desensitization (at least in part reflecting their lower affinity for nicotine).[51,177,178] Accumulation of nicotine in some cells (such as *Xenopus* oocytes) followed by slow release can give the appearance of permanent inactivation, whereas in other cell types or in the case of quaternary amino agonists that cannot passively accumulate within cells, only reversible desensitization is seen.[179]

Prolonged exposure to nicotine also causes an increase in the amount of AChRs. Nicotine at 0.2 μM can upregulate the amount of some neuronal AChRs, but at least a 1000-fold higher concentration is required for much effect on human muscle AChRs.[71] The α4 AChRs are more easily and extensively upregulated than are the α3 or α7 AChRs,[180,181] and α3β2 AChRs are much more sensitive to upregulation than are α3β4 AChRs.[182] The mechanisms of upregulation are being actively investigated. They include increased assembly of AChRs and decreased internalization and degradation. Which mechanisms are involved, to what extent, and whether the upregulated AChRs are sustained in the surface membrane differ according to AChR subtype, species, and the type of cell in which they are being expressed. Some upregulation can be detected with some antagonists,[182] perhaps reflecting their very limited partial agonist activity.

It may be that some of the pleasurable addictive effects of nicotine are mediated by the transient high-dose boluses of nicotine associated with puffing on cigarettes, activating lower-affinity α3 and α6 AChRs, and are not easily replaced by the slow, sustained release of low levels of nicotineby patches. Sustained low concentrations of nicotine that desensitize α4 or α7 AChRs may produce other nicotine effects, including the development of tolerance to some of nicotine's unpleasant effects in nonsmokers (such as nausea).

AChR Synthesis

The most detailed initial studies of AChR synthesis were initially conducted in the mouse myoblast-like cells line BC3H1 and primarily concerned α1 subunits because mAbs and αBgt provided good probes for this subunit.[183] The ability to transfect nonmuscle cell lines with combinations of AChR subunits, fragments of subunits, mutated subunits, and rapsyn permitted further characterization of the processes of subunit synthesis, conformational maturation, and assembly.[184–186] These processes and transport of assembled AChRs to their proper location in the surface membrane and stabilization there require association with many proteins that are still being defined.[187–188] There is general agreement about many aspects of these processes, but others remain controversial.[189] Studies of synthesis of muscle AChRs are far advanced compared to those of neuronal AChRs, but many aspects are likely to be common to all AChRs. Some features of muscle AChR synthesis are depicted in Fig. 17-8 and are described below.

All AChR subunits have an N-terminal signal sequence that binds to a signal recognition protein in the endoplasmic reticulum, targeting the N-terminal part of the mature AChR subunit sequence across the endoplasmic reticulum membrane to form the large extracellular domain.[192] The signal sequence is cleaved as translation proceeds. Glycosylation at specific asparagines occurs as translation proceeds.[193] Signals intrinsic to the sequence cause the formation of additional transmembrane domains as synthesis proceeds. During this stage subunits are associated with chaperone proteins like calnexin which assist in their maturation, prevent assembly with immature subunits, and stabilize them against degradation.[187,194] Unassembled subunits, are rapidly degraded.[193] After synthesis and before assembly with other subunits, conformational maturation occurs. In α1 subunits, this is marked by the acquisition of a near native conformation of the MIR (which permits conformation-dependent mAbs to bind) and by acquisition of a near native conformation of the ACh-binding region (which permits αBgt to bind, although small cholinergic ligands do not bind with high affinity until ACh-binding sites form at subunit interfaces after assembly of appropriate subunit dimers).[190,195,196] Part of this conformational maturation is formation of the disulfide bond forming the signature loop.[193] Sequences in the extracellular domain have been identified that are important in forming the initial specific interactions in assembling AChR subunits.[184] Since all of the subunits have basically homologous structures and some, like β2, can assemble properly in several positions (e.g., both at the positive α4 interface to form an ACh-binding site and at the negative side of α4 in the case of the β2 subunit of α4β2 AChRs, which occupies a position equivalent to β1), assembly is a long and difficult process requiring 1 to 3 h compared to the 15 to 30 min required for conformational maturation or the 1 to 2 min required for synthesis. Because the order of subunits around the cation channel is $\alpha 1 \gamma \alpha 1 \delta \beta 1$,[3] γ or ε subunits must be able to associate both with the "plus" side of α1 subunits to form ACh-binding sites and with the "minus" side. If cells are transfected only with α1 and γ, both α1γ dimers, α1γα1 trimers, and α1γα1γ tetramers form, but the tetramer is an artifact resulting from the absence of δ and β1.[197] Only α1δ dimers form when these two subunits are coexpressed. In the presence of all of the muscle AChR subunits, it is thought that formation of α1γ dimers and α1δ dimers followed by assembly with β1 leads to α1γα1δβ1 pentamers.[187]

Assembled AChRs, like other membrane and secreted proteins,[198] are transported to the Golgi apparatus, where their sugar groups are modified prior to export to the surface membrane. Proper N-glycosylation promotes conformational maturation and is required for surface membrane expression.[199,200] The signature disulfide-linked loop structure is also involved in surface expression, since mutation of cysteines 128 or 142 permits subunit assembly, but the assembled AChRs are retained within the cell.[201] An endoplasmic reticulum retention signal has been mapped on the α1 subunit.[187] It is obscured in the channel vestibule as the AChR is assembled. A retention signal was mapped to R313K314 in the large cytoplasmic domain of α1 where γ COP binds to retain the subunit in the endoplasmic reticulum.[188] Attachment of ubiquitin would normally target an unassembled subunit for destruction in the proteosome, but if the ER retention signal is mutated and the mutant α1 is expressed in a cell line defective in ubiquitination, then unassembled α1 is expressed on the cell surface.

Posttranslational modifications in AChR subunits other than glycosylation are also important. Phosphorylation at some serines and tyrosines in the large cytoplasmic domain[202] and covalent attachment of lipid[203] are known to occur. Phosphorylation plays roles in subunit assembly, AChR aggregation, regulation of desensitization, and perhaps other effects.

In muscle before innervation or after denervation, AChR synthesis proceeds at a high rate and more than half of the

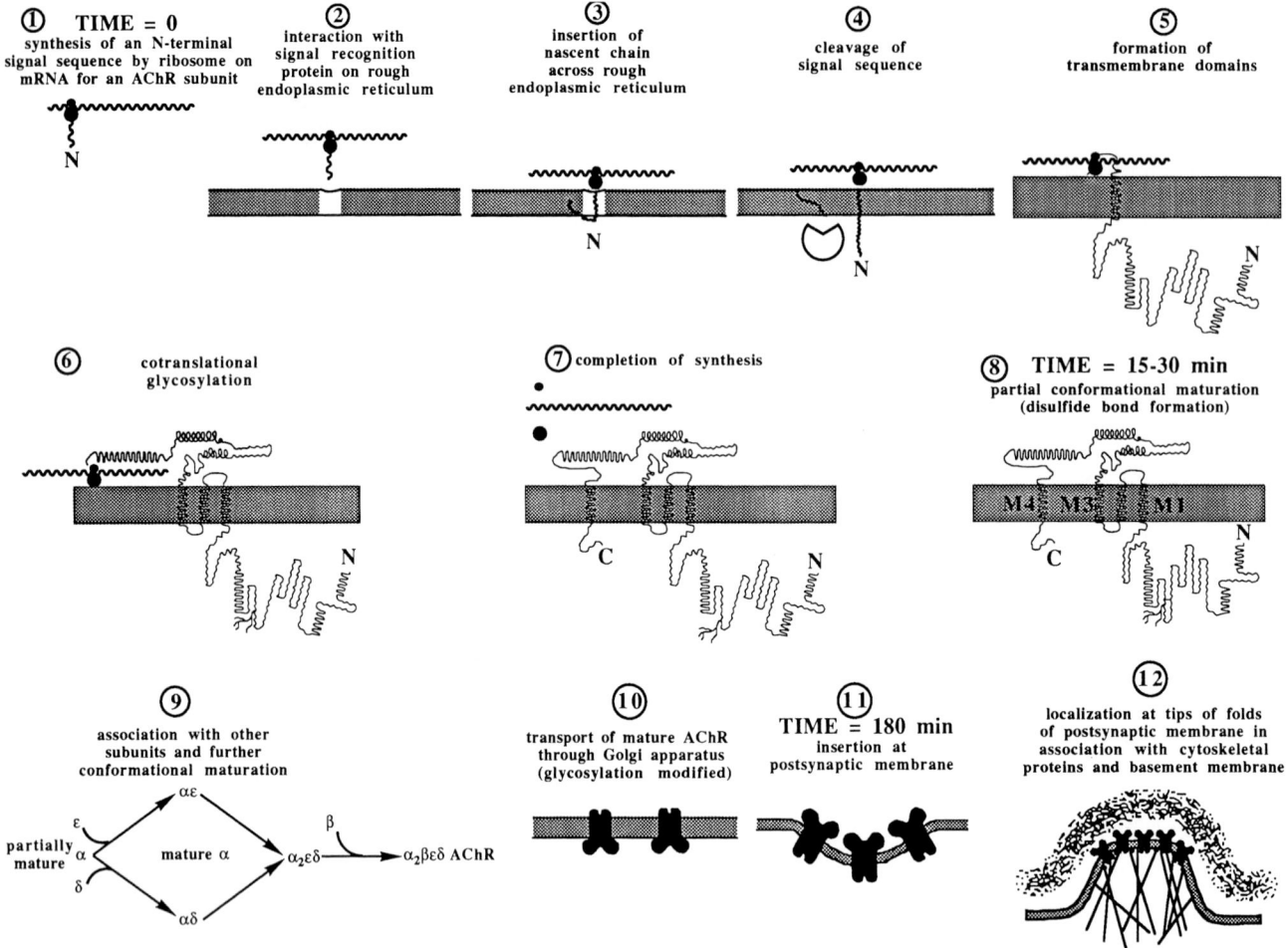

FIGURE 17-8. Model for some aspects of AChR synthesis. The overall time course is modeled from Ref. 183. The pathways of subunit assembly are adapted from Refs. 190 and 191.

AChR is intracellular on the way to or from the surface membrane. At mature neuromuscular junctions, the rate of turnover is much lower and synthesis is confined to the endoplasmic reticulum near nuclei adjacent to the synapse.[65] Once in the surface membrane at a mature junction, muscle AChRs associate on their cytoplasmic surface with rapsyn and are anchored through it to the cytoskeleton. Neuronal AChRs face more complex trafficking problems, sometimes involving transport to distant locations in synaptic endings. Rapsyn is not involved, but the proteins involved are beginning to be identified.[74]

AChR Destruction

AChRs are thought to be destroyed by a process of endocytosis and lysosomal proteolysis, as depicted in Fig. 17-9.[204] AChRs at mature neuromuscular junctions turn over much more slowly ($t_{1/2}$ = 5 to 7 days) than do extrajunctional AChRs in fetal or denervated muscle ($t_{1/2}$ = 20 h).[205] Cross-linking of AChRs by antibodies enhances the rate of destruction two- to threefold, contributing to the loss of AChRs in MG, where this process is termed antigenic modulation.[206–210] Endocytosis involves cytoskeletal elements, requires energy, and is not closely linked to the proteolytic process, so that internalization continues even if lysosomal proteolysis is inhibited.[211] Amino acids resulting from AChR degradation are excreted from the cells, starting about 90 min after internalization is initiated.[204]

Regulation of AChR Expression

Regulation of specific AChR subtype expression, the rate of expression, and the localization of expression is controlled by many factors during the development of the neuromuscular junction. These have been worked out in significant detail.[65] This provides a model for developmental studies of neuronal AChRs and other neurotransmitter receptors. Neuronal AChR subtypes are just being defined and localized.[28] Promotor analysis of neuronal AChR subunits is under way.[212]

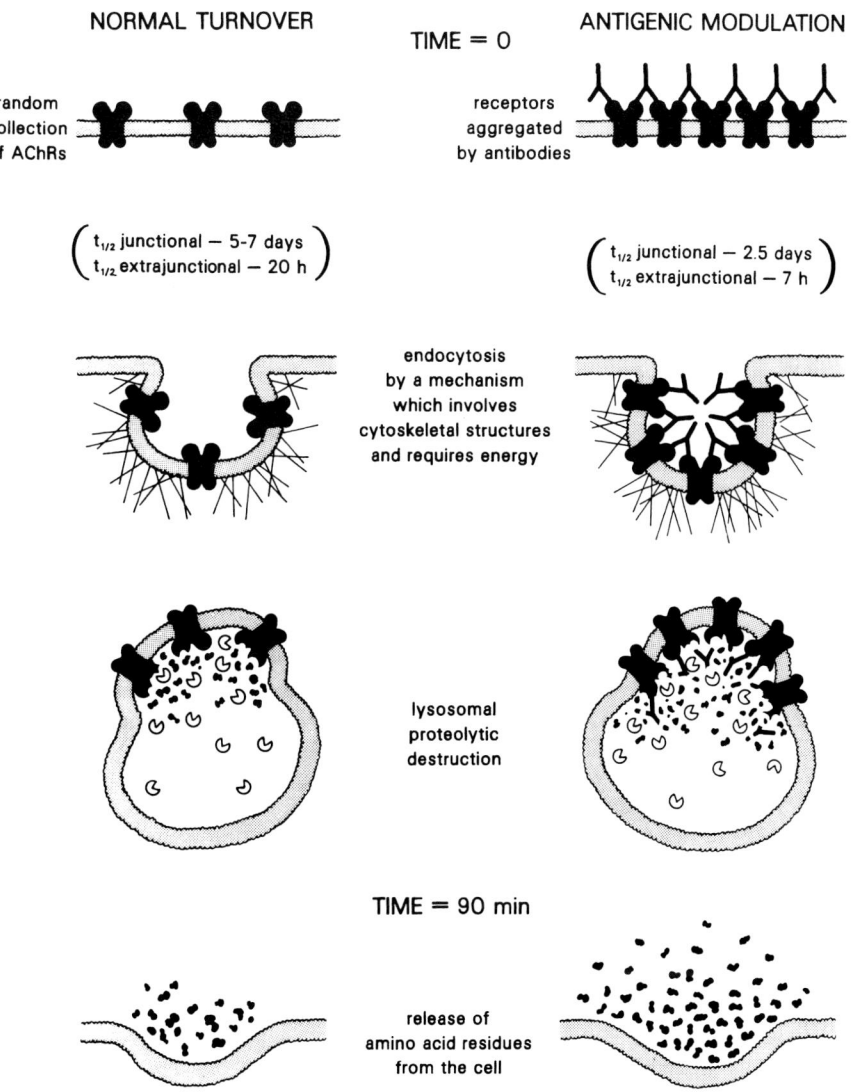

FIGURE 17-9. Model for the mechanism of destruction of AChRs in the normal case and in MG where antigenic modulation is initiated by cross-linking of AChRs with antibodies.

Myasthenia Gravis (MG) Results from an Antibody-Mediated Autoimmune Response to Muscle AChRs

Chapter 64 describes MG in detail. The points to be made in this and the following sections are that the characteristic muscular weakness and fatigability of MG results from an antibody-mediated autoimmune response to $\alpha 1$ AChRs, that the antigenic structure is known in some detail (although some important questions remain), that the antigenic structure explains some important pathologic activities of autoantibodies to AChRs, and that aspects of the antigenic structure of AChRs may be exploited to develop specific immunosuppressive therapies.

The autoimmune response to $\alpha 1$ AChRs in MG impairs neuromuscular transmission by reducing the number of functional AChRs and disrupting the organization of the postsynaptic membrane.[7] Experimental autoimmune MG (EAMG) is induced by immunizing animals with purified AChR. EAMG provides an accurate model for the mechanisms impairing transmission in MG. The specificities of the autoantibodies produced in MG and EAMG are similar, suggesting that in MG the endogenous immunogen that initiates and sustains the autoimmune response is AChR rather than a cross-reacting antigen with limited similarity. MG can be induced in some rheumatoid arthritis patients by treatment with penicillamine, but this form of MG remits after cessation of penicillamine treatment (which may act by chemically modifying the AChR to make it more immunogenic).[213] This observation and the observation that rats not initially killed by EAMG will slowly recover unless repeatedly immunized show that it is not easy to ignite a self-sustaining autoimmune response to AChR. EAMG (and MG) can be passively transferred by antibodies. Even though this massive immune assault consumes enough AChRs from neuromuscular junctions to induce EAMG if given in adjuvant, rats that survive acute passive EAMG recover completely.[214,215] In order to maintain an autoimmune response to AChRs for years in a human MG patient, it seems likely that there must be a continuing source of modified or aberrantly expressed AChRs, perhaps resulting from some sort of infection. In dogs with MG, remission occurs after an average of 6.4 months and MG continues for prolonged periods only in dogs with neoplasia.[216] Thus, the source of immunogen for MG in canines (infection?) is usually resolved much more rapidly than in humans.

One important mechanism by which autoantibodies cause AChR loss in MG and EAMG is complement-mediated focal lysis of the postsynaptic membrane at the end plate due to antibodies bound to the extracellular surface of AChRs.[217] Phagocyte-mediated destruction that depends on bound antibodies is an important mechanism in passive EAMG, but is transient due to regulation of the release of chemotactic fragments of complement and is not a significant component of the pathology in MG.[218] Focal lysis may contribute substantially to the morphologic disruption of the postsynaptic membrane. It may also be a necessary prerequisite before antigenic modulation can contribute substantially to AChR loss, since if complement activity is inhibited, most of the AChRs in rat muscle can be labeled by passive transfer of antibodies without impairing transmission. This observation further illustrates that the small fraction of autoantibodies that bind to or near the ACh-binding site or otherwise directly impair AChR function do not contribute much to impairment of transmission in most patients.

Another important mechanism by which autoantibodies cause AChR loss in MG and EAMG is antigenic modulation.[206-208] This depends on antibodies that can cross-link adjacent AChRs and thereby facilitate endocytosis. Antibodies that do not cross-link AChRs and monovalent Fab fragments do not cause antigenic modulation.

In MG and EAMG, many of the remaining AChRs have antibodies bound.[214] In response to loss of 50 to 75 percent of total AChRs, transcription of AChR subunits increases,[219] and in response to focal destruction of the postsynaptic regions, the end plates may remodel.[218]

Antigenic Structure of Muscle AChRs

The autoimmune response to AChRs depends both on B lymphocytes that give rise to antibody-producing cells and on T-helper lymphocytes that activate the differentiation and proliferation of B cells through release of lymphokines.[220] B- and T-cell epitopes are different. The antigen receptors through which B cells are activated are surface IgM molecules with the same variable regions as the IgG antibodies secreted by plasma cells derived from these B cells. The epitopes recognized by the antibodies may include amino acids from distant parts of the AChR sequence that are juxtaposed only in the native conformation of the AChR and epitopes formed by contiguous amino acid sequences that are not so dependent on the native conformation. The only pathologically significant B-cell epitopes are those on the extracellular surface of the AChR. T-helper cell epitopes are peptide fragments less than 20 amino acids long. These come from AChRs digested by antigen-presenting cells (either "professional" antigen-presenting cells such as dendritic cells, "interested amateurs" such as B cells directed at AChRs, or other cell types, possibly including some previously unsuspected source of immunogen in MG). T-cell epitopes are exhibited on the surface of antigen-presenting cells bound to the surface of class II MHC antigen-presenting proteins. These peptides do not reflect the native conformation of the AChR, and pathologically significant fragments could be derived from any part of the AChR molecule. There is no specific relationship between the T cells and the B cells they help[221] except in the case where the B cells themselves present the antigen. Normally, only the proximity to the antigen at the same time brings these cell types within the range of the lymphokines by which they communicate while their antigen receptors are activated.

ANTIBODY EPITOPES

Immunization with native $\alpha 1$ AChRs provokes antibodies directed primarily at the extracellular surface, whereas immunization with denatured subunits provokes antibodies directed primarily at the cytoplasmic surface.[222,223] This is because there is a highly immunogenic epitope that depends on the native conformation of the extracellular surface (the MIR), and when this is denatured, the only epitopes remaining that can also be recognized in the native AChR are on the cytoplasmic surface.[7,83] This suggests that the extracellular domain is normally more conformationally constrained than the cytoplasmic surface (and this may be reflected in the greater sequence variability in the large cytoplasmic domain). Using synthetic peptides as immunogens, it is possible to induce antibodies to many parts of the AChR sequence, but many of these will not bind to the native conformation of the AChR because the sequence is buried or in an unrecognizable conformation.[223]

MAbs from rats and mice immunized with AChRs have provided excellent structural probes and model autoantibodies.[7,83] Their binding sites have been mapped by binding to subunits, subunit fragments, synthetic peptides, mutated AChRs, and by competitive binding with other mAbs. Half or more of the mAbs to native $\alpha 1$ AChRs are directed at the MIR.[83] Such mAbs compete with each other for binding and prevent the binding of more than half of the autoantibodies from MG patients. This shows that the antibodies bind to overlapping regions but not necessarily to identical epitopes. MAbs bind to the extracellular tips of $\alpha 1$ subunits at an angle away from the central axis of the AChR, which prevents them from cross-linking the two $\alpha 1$ subunits in an AChR molecule, but which ideally positions them to cross-link adjacent AChRs and thereby trigger antigenic modulation.[21] Thus, the fundamental pathologic significance of the MIR derives from the basic antigenic structure: (1) It is highly immunogenic (perhaps because it has a novel shape easily accessible on the protein surface and is present in two copies per AChR to provide avid binding and stimulation of B-cell receptors); (2) it is on the extracellular surface so that antibodies can bind to it and fix complement (and since AChRs are packed solidly in a semicrystalline array at the tips of junctional folds, this also promotes focal lysis); and (3) it promotes AChR cross-linking to trigger antigenic modulation. MAbs to the MIR do not directly inhibit AChR function.[224] Some mAbs to the MIR weakly bind peptides with the sequence α66-76.[83] In vitro mutagenesis and binding of mAbs to mutant *Torpedo* AChRs shows that α68 and 71 are critical to the binding of both MIR mAbs that bind synthetic peptides and MIR mAbs that bind only to mature α1.[85] Some mAbs to the MIR on α1 bind very well to human α3 and α5 subunits, which have similar α66-76 sequences, but these mAbs do not recognize denatured α3, even though they do recognize denatured α1.[84] Antisera from MG patients do not bind significantly to human α3 AChRs, and human autoantibodies to α3 do not bind to α1.[138] Thus, the MIR epitopes recognized by rats and humans are not identical, even though they are close enough that antibodies to them compete for binding.

Prominent epitopes on the cytoplasmic surfaces of α1 subunits and other subunits have been determined using antisera and mAbs (e.g., α161-165, α341-347, α359-365, α368-375).[223] These epitopes are pathologically irrelevant because autoantibodies cannot bind to them in vivo.

The spectrum of autoantibodies to AChRs produced by MG patients is dominated by the MIR but includes other parts of the AChR and closely resembles the spectrum seen in animals immunized with AChR or dogs with idiopathic MG.[82,225] The spectrum is stable in a patient over several years. Many MG sera react better with extrajunctional AChRs than with junctional AChRs.[226] This may reflect both the facts that the endogenous immunogen has γ subunits and that these may be more immunogenic because they are not usually expressed in adults. One unusual MG patient serum was found to be specific for γ, bound only to the α1γ ACh-binding site, and thereby inhibited function.[226,227] Rare mothers have been found who make autoantibodies to γ subunits that potently block AChR function.[228] These have no effect on the mother (because her muscle AChRs have ε subunits), but they paralyze or kill fetuses, causing arthrogryposis multiplex congenita.

T-CELL EPITOPES

α1 Subunits also predominate in the T-cell response to AChRs, but epitopes have been found on all subunits.[229,230] Several α1 T-cell epitopes seem to predominate in MG, but various laboratories do not quite agree on which these are (candidates include α1 48-67, 75-90, 101-137, 149-156, 304-322, and 419-437). In Lewis rats, α1 100-116 is a dominant T-cell epitope, but in other rat strains, other α1 epitopes dominate (e.g., α1 172-205 in brown Norway or 52-70 in buffalo rats).[231]

Because, before an AChR epitope can be recognized by the antigen receptor of a T-helper cell, it must first be recognized by an MHC class II antigen-presenting protein,[220] the proteolytic processing mechanisms of the presenting cell and the binding properties of the various MHC class II proteins restrict what can be recognized by T cells.[232] This may be reflected in part by the higher incidence of HLA-A1, B8, and DR3 class II MHC determinants in young-onset Caucasian MG patients.[233,234] Inbred mice become resistant to EAMG after a single amino acid change in the I-A_B protein.[235,236] The human α1 sequence 144-156 is recognized only when it is presented by HLA-DR4 class II protein variants with glycine at position 86 and not by a variant with valine in this position.[233] If humans were as inbred as some mouse strains, and if AChRs had only one or two epitopes, MG would be a much more genetically constrained disease than is actually the case.

Specific Immunosuppressive Therapies for EAMG

Several approaches have been investigated in hopes of taking advantage of the known identity of the antigen and its antigenic structure in order to provide specific immunosuppressive therapy for EAMG and MG. None has yet shown sufficient promise on EAMG to be properly evaluated in a controlled trial on canine or human MG.

Mucosal tolerance induction by means of feeding or nasal spraying with purified electric organ AChR,[237,238] bacterially expressed human AChR denatured subunits,[239,241] or synthetic AChR peptides[242,243] has proven effective at inhibiting the development of EAMG; in some cases, mucosal treatment has been reported to inhibit ongoing EAMG.[238-241] Such approaches have been successful on many model autoimmune diseases but thus far have had very little success in clinical trials.[244] The conventional theory is that antigen applied in these ways inhibit the T-cell response in two ways.[244] At low doses, suppressor T cells are induced that release suppressive lymphokines that inhibit bystander T cells within range of the suppressor cell and the antigen. High doses of antigen are thought to delete reactive lymphocytes. In addition, or alternatively, the immune response may be diverted from making pathologically significant antibodies to the extracellular surface to instead making irrelevant antibodies to AChR cytoplasmic domains.[239] Mechanisms have been studied in detail using purified *Torpedo* electric organ AChR as antigen.[238] The studies that have reported the most enthusiastic results have used just bacterially expressed human α1 subunit extracellular domains.[240,241] Others found it necessary to include both extracellular and cytoplasmic domains of all human muscle AChR subunits.[239] Bacterial expression has thus far been the only practical approach to producing large amounts of human subunits, and it has the advantage that the subunits are denatured, so that it is unlikely that B lymphocytes to the MIR or other extracellular epitopes would be stimulated. It has the disadvantage that contamination with potent bacterial immunogens is difficult to avoid and that denatured subunits may not be processed for antigen presentation, as native subunits might be.[246] Potentially, genetically modified food plants[247] could be used to produce antigen or a gene therapy approach could be used to produce antigen in the patient.[248]

Native extracellular domain fragments of α1 subunits have recently been expressed in yeast.[249,250] These may be useful for specific plasmapheresis and immunodiagnostic assays as well as for structural studies.

Fab fragments of mAbs to the MIR have been expressed in bacteria and investigated for their ability to treat passively transferred EAMG.[251,252] The theory is that the Fab will compete for binding with autoantibodies to the MIR and inhibit both antigenic modulation (because it is monovalent) and complement fixation (because it lacks the Fc region). The theory works in vitro. In vivo, the Fab is rapidly cleared. Even if the clearance rate is reduced by conjugating with ethylene glycol or other tricks, it would seem likely that large amounts of Fab would be required at great expense to get an effect that would not be permanent and could also be limited by an immune response to the Fab. A clever variation on the Fab theme is the demonstration that injection of papain protected against passive transfer of EAMG by a MIR mAb by cleaving the mAb into Fabs in vivo.[253]

A synthetic mimotope of the MIR was selected using a mAb and shown to prevent passively transferred EAMG by competing for the binding of a mAb to the MIR.[254] This would not work in humans if the precise epitope of the mAb used to select the mimotope were not the same as the MIR epitopes recognized by human autoantibodies to the MIR. In any case, mimotopes of much higher affinity will have to be derived. Then they will have to be tested on chronic EAMG. Even if the mimotopes were not rapidly cleared or did not aggregate and actually stimulated the immune response to AChRs, prolonged therapy with such mimotopes might prove very expensive. However, if variations on acute therapies by such mimotopes could produce a lasting inhibition of the B-cell response to the MIR, such therapies might prove very useful.

Blalock and coworkers have presented the theory that a peptide with a sequence corresponding to what would be encoded by a nucleotide complementary to the sequence encoding a native peptide would bind to the native peptide and would provoke the formation of antibodies that act as anti-idiotype antibodies against the native peptide.[255–257] All this sounds quite unlikely, but they have published extensively on it and have some data that appear to be consistent with this theory. They reported that vaccination of rats with a peptide complementary to the *Torpedo* AChR α1 sequence 61 to 67 (which contributes to the MIR) inhibited development of EAMG.[255] This seems incredible, because most mAbs to the MIR have little or no affinity for even the complete denatured sequence of α1[7,83]; therefore, why would a complementary peptide to a denatured peptide produce anti-idiotype antibodies to autoantibodies directed at a conformation-dependent epitope? They also report that a mAb to the complementary peptide prevents EAMG.[256] This is surprising, because MIR mAbs do not have a single idiotype (because a group of adjacent, overlapping epitopes forms the region).[83,258] Further, they report that vaccination of rats with a complementary peptide against a predominant T-cell epitope in Lewis rats (α1 100-116) reduced the severity of EAMG in Lewis rats.[257] Different α1 epitopes predominate in other rat strains[231] and humans,[229,230] so it would not be expected that the same vaccine would work in humans even if the proposed mechanism of action were correct. All of these reports concerned inhibition of induction of EAMG rather than the therapy of ongoing EAMG. Some of the reported effects might conceivably reflect artifacts of preimmunization, reducing the adjuvant effects in subsequent AChR immunizations. In any case, the studies of mucosal immunosuppressive therapies also reveal how much more difficult it is to treat chronic EAMG than to prevent EAMG.[237,239]

In vitro modeling of a specific immunosuppressive therapy has begun, using genetically engineered antigen-presenting cells.[259,260] The plan is to transfect the patients' antigen-presenting cells so that they (1) express both the antigen and a protein to which it is coupled, ensuring efficient processing and presentation; (2) express Fas L, which induces apoptosis of Fas-expressing activated T-cells; and (3) express a truncated form of the Fas-associated death domain to inhibit Fas L from killing the presenting cell. This complex approach works in vitro with either influenza hemagglutinin[259] or the extracellular domain of *Torpedo* AChR α1 subunits as antigen.[260] It remains to be seen if this approach will work in vivo on EAMG or other model autoimmune diseases.

In the future, these or other specific immunosuppressive therapies may progress to the point where they seem very effective at treating ongoing EAMG in rats. Then testing these therapies on idiopathic canine MG[225] may be a logical next step. However, this would require a well-controlled clinical study, since the natural course of canine MG is toward spontaneous remission over 6 months,[216] by contrast with the many-year time course of human MG.[261] In fact, it is a problem that therapies now in frequent use for MG, such as thymectomy, have never been validated by a clinical trial.[262]

A real revolution in our approaches to specific immunosuppressive therapy of MG may await some revolution in our understanding of the pathologic mechanisms involved in initiating and sustaining the autoimmune response to AChR in MG. Then, much as the realization that *Helicobacter pylori* rather than stress really causes ulcers led to antibiotic therapy for this disease,[263] understanding what sustains the autoimmune response in MG might lead to antimicrobial or other radically different specific immunosuppressive therapies.

List of Abbreviations

αBgt	α bungarotoxin
ACh	acetylcholine
AChR	acetylcholine receptor
EAMG	experimental autoimmune MG
GABA	gamma-aminobutyric acid
mAb	monoclonal antibody
MG	myasthenia gravis
MIR	main immunogenic region

References

1. Clementi F, Fornasari D, Gotti C (Eds): *Neuronal Nicotinic Receptors. Handbook of Experimental Pharmacology.* New York: Springer Verlag; 2000.
2. Corringer PJ, Le Novere N, Changeux JP: Nicotinic receptors at the amino acid level. *Ann Rev Pharmacol Toxicol* 40:431–458, 2000.
3. Karlin A: Emerging structure of the nicotinic acetylcholine receptors. *Nat Rev Neurosci* 3:102–114, 2002.
4. Unwin N: Nicotinic acetylcholine receptor and the structural basis of fast synaptic transmission. *Phil Trans R Soc Lond B* 1404:1813–1829, 2000.
5. Conti-Fine B, Protti M, Bellone M, et al: *Myasthenia Gravis: The Immunobiology of an Autoimmune Disease.* Austin, TX: Landes, 1997.
6. Engel A (ed): *Myasthenia Gravis and Myasthenic Disorders.* New York: Oxford University Press, 1999.
7. Lindstrom J: Acetylcholine receptors and myasthenia. *Muscl Nerve* 23:453–477, 2000.
8. Richman D (ed): Myasthenia gravis and related diseases. *Ann NY Acad Sci* 841:1998.
9. Fambrough D, Drachmann D, Satyamurti S: Neuromuscular junction in myasthenia gravis: Decreased acetylcholine receptors. *Science* 182:293–295, 1973.
10. Lindstrom J, Einarson B, Tzartos SJ: Production and assay of antibodies to acetylcholine receptors. *Methods Enzymol* 74:432–460, 1981.
11. Patrick J, Lindstrom J: Autoimmune response to acetylcholine receptor. *Science* 180:871–872, 1973.
12. Tzartos SJ, Lindstrom JM: Monoclonal antibodies used to probe acetylcholine receptor structure: Localization of the main immunogenic region and detection of similarities between subunits. *Proc Natl Acad Sci USA* 77:755–759, 1980.
13. Lindstrom J: Neuronal nicotinic acetylcholine receptors, in Narahashi T (ed): *Ion Channels.* Vol 4. New York: Plenum Press, 1996; pp 377–450.
14. Lindstrom J: Purification and cloning of nicotinic acetylcholine receptors, in Arneric S, Brioni D (eds): *Neuronal Nicotinic Receptors: Pharmacology and Therapeutic Opportunities.* New York: Wiley, 1999.
15. Dani JA, Ji D, Zhou F-M: Synaptic plasticity and nicotine addiction. *Neuron* 31:349–352, 2001.
16. Peto R, Chen Z, Boreham J: Tobacco—the growing epidemic. *Nat Med* 5:15–17, 1999.
17. Lloyd GK, Williams M: Neuronal nicotinic acetylcholine receptors as novel drug targets. *J Pharmacol Exp Ther* 292:461–467, 2000.
18. Grando S, Horton R: The keratinocyte cholinergic system with acetylcholine as an epidermal cytotransmitter. *Curr Opin Dermatol* 4:262–268, 1997.
19. Romano SJ, Pugh PC, McIntosh J, et al: Neuronal-type acetylcholine receptors and regulation of α7 gene expression in vertebrate skeletal muscle. *J Neurobiol* 32:69–80, 1997.
20. Miyazawa A, Fujiyoshi Y, Stowell M, et al: Nicotinic acetylcholine receptor at 4.6 angstrom resolution: Transverse tunnels in the channel wall. *J Mol Biol* 288:765–786, 1999.
21. Beroukhim R, Unwin N: 3-Dimensional location of the main immunogenic region of the acetylcholine-receptor. *Neuron* 15:323–331, 1995.
22. Brejc K, van Dijk WJ, Klassen R., et al: Crystal structure of an ACh-binding protein reveals the ligand-binding domain of nicotinic receptors. *Nature* 411:269–276, 2001.
23. Smit AB, Syed NI, Schaap D, et al: A glia-derived acetylcholine-binding protein that modulates synaptic transmission. *Nature* 411:261–268, 2001.
24. Lenovere N, Changeux JP: Molecular evolution of the nicotinic acetylcholine-receptor—An example of multigene family in excitable cells. *J Mol Evol* 40:155–172, 1995.
25. Gunthorpe MJ, Lummis SCR: Conversion of the ion selectivity of the 5-HT3A receptor from cationic to anionic reveals a conserved feature of the ligand-gated ion channel superfamily. *J Biol Chem* 276:10977–10983, 2001.
26. Hevers W, Luddens H: The diversity of GABA(A) receptors—Pharmacological and electrophysiological properties of GABA(A) channel subtypes. *Mol Neurobiol* 18:35–86, 1998.
27. Betz H, Kuhse J, Schmeedin V, et al: Structure and functions of inhibitory and excitatory glycine receptors. *Ann NY Acad Sci* 868:667–676, 1999.
28. Lindstrom J: The structures of neuronal nicotinic receptors, in Clementi F, Fornasari D, Gotti C (eds): *Handbook of Experimental Pharmacology.* New York: Springer-Verlag; 2000, pp 101–162.
29. McKernan R, Whiting P: Which $GABA_A$-receptor subtypes really occur in the brain? *Trends Neurosci* 19:139–143, 1996.
30. Galzi JL, Devillersthiery A, Hussy N, et al: Mutations in the channel domain of a neuronal nicotinic receptor convert ion selectivity from cationic to anionic. *Nature* 359:500–505, 1992.
31. Eisele JL, Bertrand S, Galzi JL, et al: Chimeric nicotinic serotonergic receptor combines distinct ligand-binding and channel specificities. *Nature* 366:479–483, 1993.
32. Cooper ST, Millar NS: Host cell-specific folding of the neuronal nicotinic receptor α8 subunit. *J Neurochem* 70:2585–2593, 1998.
33. Cooper ST, Harkness P, Baker E, et al: Up-regulation of cell-surface α4β2 neuronal nicotinic receptors by lower temperature and expression of chimeric subunits. *J Biol Chem* 274:27145–27152, 1999.
34. Unwin N: Neurotransmitter action—Opening of ligand-gated ion channels. *Cell* 72:31–41, 1993.
35. Gu Y, Franco A, Gardner P, et al: Properties of embryonic and adult muscle acetylcholine-receptors transiently expressed in cos cells. *Neuron* 5:147–157, 1990.
36. Bougat C, Bren N, Sine SM: Structural basis of the different gating kinetics of fetal and adult acetylcholine receptors. *Neuron* 13:1395–1402, 1994.
37. Prince RJ, Sine SM: Acetylcholine and epibatidine binding to muscle acetylcholine receptors distinguish between concerted and uncoupled models. *J Biol Chem* 274:19623–19629, 1999.
38. Whiting PJ, Lindstrom JM: Characterization of bovine and human neuronal nicotinic acetylcholine-receptors using monoclonal-antibodies. *J Neurosci* 8:3395–3404, 1988.
39. Flores CM, Davila-Garcia MI, Ulrich Y, et al: Differential regulation of neuronal nicotinic receptor binding sites following chronic nicotine administration. *J Neurochem* 69:2216–2219, 1997.
40. Gerzanich V, Wang F, Kurystov A, et al: α5 subunit alters desensitization, pharmacology, Ca^{2+} permeability and Ca^{2+} modulation of human neuronal α3 nicotinic receptors. *J Pharmacol Exp Ther* 286:311–320, 1998.
41. Forsayeth JR, Kobrin E: Formation of oligomers containing the β3 and β4 subunits of the rat nicotinic receptor. *J Neurosci* 17:1531–1538, 1997.
42. Duvoisin R, Deneris E, Patrick J, Heinemann S: The functional diversity of the neuronal nicotinic receptors is increased by a novel subunit: β4. *Neuron* 3:487–496, 1989.
43. Deneris E, Connolly J, Boulter J, et al: Primary structure and expression of α2: A novel subunit of neuronal nicotinic receptors. *Neuron* 1:45–54, 1988.
44. Bertrand D, Ballivet M, Gomez M, et al: Physiological properties of neuronal nicotinic receptors reconstituted from the vertebrate β2 subunit and *Drosophila* α subunits. *Eur J Neurosci* 6:869–875, 1994.
45. Conroy WG, Berg DK: Neurons can maintain multiple classes of nicotinic acetylcholine receptors distinguished by different subunit compositions. *J Biol Chem* 270:4424–4431, 1995.
46. Han ZY, Le Novere N, Zoli M, et al: Localization of nAChR subunit mRNAs in the brain of *Macaca mulatta*. *Eur J Neurosci* 12:3664–3674, 2000.
47. Le Novere N, Zoli M, Lena C, et al: Involvement of α6 nicotinic receptor subunit in nicotine-elicited locomotion, demonstrated by in vivo antisense oligonucleotide infusion. *Neuroreport* 10:2497–2501, 1999.
48. Champtiaux N, Han Z-Y, Bessis A, et al: Distribution and pharmacology of α6-containing nicotinic acetylcholine receptors analyzed with mutant mice. *J Neurosci* 22:1208–1217, 2002.
49. Kulak J, McIntosh J, Quik M: Loss of nicotinic receptors in monkey striatum after 1-methyl-4-phenyl-1,2,3,6-tetrahydropyridine treatment is due to a decline in α-conotoxin MII sites. *Mol Pharmacol* 61:230–238, 2002.
50. Kulak J, Sum J, Musachio J, et al: 5-Iodo-A-85380 binds to α conotoxin MII-sensitive nicotinic receptors (nAChRs) as well as α4β2 subtypes. *J Neurochem* 81:403–406, 2002.
51. Kuryatov A, Olale F, Cooper J, et al: Human α6 AChR subtypes: Subunit composition, assembly, and pharmacological responses. *Neuropharmacology* 39:2570–2590, 2000.
52. Lena C, d'Exaerde AD, Cordero-Erausquin M, et al: Diversity and distribution of nicotinic acetylcholine receptors in the locus ceruleus neurons. *Proc Natl Acad Sci USA* 96:12126–12131, 1999.
53. Elgoyhen AB, Vetter DE, Katz E, et al: Alpha 10: A determinant of nicotinic cholinergic receptor function in mammalian vestibular and cochlear mechanosensory hair cells. *Proc Natl Acad Sci USA* 98:3501–3506, 2001.
54. Lustig LR, Peng H, Hiel H, et al: Molecular cloning and mapping of the human nicotinic acetylcholine receptor α10 (CHRNA10). *Genomics* 73:272–283, 2001.
55. Grando S: Autoimmunity to keratinocyte acetylcholine receptors in pemphigus. *Dermatology* 201:290–295, 2000.
56. Haghighi AP, Cooper E: A molecular link between inward rectification and calcium permeability of neuronal nicotinic acetylcholine α3β4 and α4β2 receptors. *J Neurosci* 20:529–541, 2000.
57. Seguela P, Wadiche J, Dineley-Miller K, et al: Molecular cloning, functional properties, and distribution of rat brain-α7: A nicotinic cation channel highly permeable to calcium. *J Neurosci* 13:596–604, 1993.
58. Fuchs PA: Synaptic transmission at vertebrate hair cells. *Curr Opin Neurobiol* 6:514–519, 1996.
59. Ullian EM, McIntosh JM, Sargent PB: Rapid synaptic transmission in the avian ciliary ganglion is mediated by two distinct classes of nicotinic receptors. *J Neurosci* 17:7210–7219, 1997.
60. Alkondon M, Pereira EFR, Eisenberg HM, et al: Choline and selective antagonists identify two subtypes of nicotinic acetylcholine receptors that modulate GABA release from CA1 interneurons in rat hippocampal slices. *J Neurosci* 19:2693–2705, 1999.
61. Radcliffe KA, Dani JA: Nicotinic stimulation produces multiple forms of increased glutamatergic synaptic transmission. *J Neurosci* 18:7075–7083, 1998.
62. Shoop RD, Chang KT, Ellisman MH, et al: Synaptically driven calcium transients via nicotinic receptors on somatic spines. *J Neurosci* 21:771–781, 2001.

63. Sharples CGV, Kaiser S, Soliakov L, et al: UB-165: A novel nicotinic agonist with subtype selectivity implicates the α4β2 subtype in the modulation of dopamine release from rat striatal synaptosomes. *J Neurosci* 20:2783–2791, 2000.
64. Zoli M, Jansson A, Sykova E, et al: Volume transmission in the CNS and its relevance for neuropsychopharmacology. *Trends Pharmacol Sci* 20:142–150, 1999.
65. Sanes JR, Lichtman JW: Development of the vertebrate neuromuscular junction. *Annu Rev Neurosci* 22:389–442, 1999.
66. Gundlefinger E, Schuk Z: Insect nicotinic acetylcholine receptors: Genes, structure, physiological and pharmacological properties, in Clementi F, Fornasari D, Gotti C (eds): *Neuronal Nicotinic receptors. Handbook of Experimental Pharmacology*, New York: Springer Verlag; 2000, pp 497–516.
67. Treinen M, Chalfie M: A mutated acetylcholine-receptor subunit causes neuronal degeneration in *C. elegans*. *Neuron* 14:871–877, 1995.
68. Bargmann CI: Neurobiology of the *Caenorhabditis elegans* genome. *Science* 282:2028–2033, 1998.
69. Noda M, Furutani Y, Takahashi H, et al: Cloning and sequence-analysis of calf cDNA and human genomic DNA encoding alpha-subunit precursor of muscle acetylcholine-receptor. *Nature* 305:818–823, 1983.
70. Jackson MB: Perfection of a synaptic receptor—Kinetics and energetics of the acetylcholine-receptor. *Proc Natl Acad Sci USA* 86:2199–2203, 1989.
71. Luther MA, Schoepfer R, Whiting P, et al: A muscle acetylcholine receptor is expressed in the human cerebellar medulloblastoma cell line TE671. *J Neurosci* 9:1082–1096, 1989.
72. Wilson GG, Karlin A: Acetylcholine receptor channel structure in the resting, open, and desensitized states probed with the substituted-cysteine-accessibility method. *Proc Natl Acad Sci USA* 98:1241–1248, 2001.
73. Maimone MM, Merlie JP: Interaction of the 43-kDa postsynaptic protein with all subunits of the muscle nicotinic acetylcholine receptor. *Neuron* 11:53–66, 1993.
74. Conroy W, Liu ZL, Nai Q, et al: PDZ-containing proteins provide a functional postsynaptic scaffold for nicotinic receptors in neurons. *Neuron* 38:759–771, 2003.
75. Miles K, Huganir RL: Regulation of nicotinic acetylcholine receptors by protein phosphorylation. *Mol Neurobiol* 2:91–124, 1988.
76. Fenster CP, Beckman ML, Parker JC, et al: Regulation of α4β2 nicotinic receptor desensitization by calcium and protein kinase C. *Mol Pharmacol* 55:432–443, 1999.
77. Mohamed AS, Rivas-Plata KA, Kraas JR, et al: Src-class kinases act within the agrin/MuSK pathway to regulate acetylcholine receptor phosphorylation, cytoskeletal anchoring, and clustering. *J Neurosci* 21:3806–3818, 2001.
78. Williams BM, Temburni MK, Levey MS, et al: The long internal loop of the α3 subunit targets nAChRs to subdomains within individual synapses on neurons in vivo. *Nat Neurosci* 1:557–562, 1998.
79. Paradiso K, Zhang J, Steinbach J: The C terminus of the human nicotinic α4β2 receptor forms a binding site required for potentiation by an estrogenic steroid. *J Neuroscience* 21:6561–6568, 2001.
80. Curtis L, Buisson B, Bertrand S, et al: Potentiation of the human α4β2 neuronal nicotinic acetycholine receptor by estradiol. *Mol Pharmacol* 61:127–135, 2002.
81. Fu DX, Sine SM: Asymmetric contribution of the conserved disulfide loop to subunit oligomerization and assembly of the nicotinic acetylcholine receptor. *J Biol Chem* 271:31479–31484, 1996.
82. Tzartos SJ, Seybold ME, Lindstrom JM: Specificities of antibodies to acetylcholine receptors in sera from myasthenia gravis patients measured by monoclonal antibodies. *Proc Natl Acad Sci USA* 79:188–192, 1982.
83. Tzartos SJ, Barkas T, Cung MT, et al: Anatomy of the antigenic structure of a large membrane autoantigen, the muscle-type nicotinic acetylcholine receptor. *Immunol Rev* 163:89–120, 1998.
84. Wang F, Gerzanich V, Wells GB, et al: Assembly of human neuronal nicotinic receptor α5 subunits with α3, β2, and β4 subunits. *J Biol Chem* 271:17656–17665, 1996.
85. Saedi MS, Anand R, Conroy WG, et al: Determination of amino acids critical to the main immunogenic region of intact acetylcholine receptors by in vitro mutagenesis. *FEBS Lett* 267:55–59, 1990.
86. Miyazawa A, Fujiyoshi Y, Unwin N: Structure and gating mechanism of the acetylcholine receptor pore. *Nature* 424:949–955, 2003.
87. Zhou M, Morais-Cabral JH, Mann S, et al: Potassium channel receptor site for the inactivation gate and quaternary amine inhibitors. *Nature* 411:657–661, 2001.
88. Wells GB, Anand R, Wang F, et al: Water-soluble nicotinic acetylcholine receptor formed by α7 subunit extracellular domains. *J Biol Chem* 273:964–973, 1998.
89. Doyle DA, Cabral JM, Pfuetzner RA, et al: The structure of the potassium channel: Molecular basis of K+ conduction and selectivity. *Science* 280:69–77, 1998.
90. Malany S, Osaka H, Sine SM, et al: Orientation of α-neurotoxin at the subunit interfaces of the nicotinic acetylcholine receptor. *Biochemistry* 39:15388–15398, 2000.
91. Laver WG, Air GM, Webster RG, et al: Epitopes on protein antigens—Misconceptions and realities. *Cell* 61:553–556, 1990.
92. Harel M, Kasher R, Nicholas A, et al: The binding site of acetylcholine receptor as visualized in the x-ray structure of a complex between α bungarotoxin and a mimotope peptide. *Neuron* 32:265–275, 2001.
93. Palma E, Bertrand S, Binzoni T, et al: Neuronal nicotinic α7 receptor expressed in *Xenopus* oocytes presents five putative binding sites for methyllycaconitine. *J Physiol (Lond)* 491:151–161.
94. Sine SM, Ohno K, Bouzat C, et al: Mutation of the acetylcholine receptor α subunit causes a slow-channel myasthenic syndrome by enhancing agonist binding affinity. *Neuron* 15:229–239, 1995.
95. Ohno K, Wang HL, Milone M, et al: Congenital myasthenic syndrome caused by decreased agonist binding affinity due to a mutation in the acetylcholine receptor ε subunit. *Neuron* 17:157–170, 1996.
96. Zhou M, Engel AG, Auerbach A: Serum choline activates mutant acetylcholine receptors that cause slow channel congenital myasthenic syndromes. *Proc Natl Acad Sci USA* 96:10466–10471, 1999.
97. Bertrand D, Devillers-Thiery A, Revah F, et al: Unconventional pharmacology of a neuronal nicotinic receptor mutated in the channel domain. *Proc Natl Acad Sci USA* 89:1261–1265, 1992.
98. Engel AG, Ohno K, Sine SM.: Congenital myasthenic syndromes—Recent advances. *Arch Neurol* 56:163–157, 1999.
99. Berger F, Gage FH, Vijayaraghavan S: Nicotinic receptor-induced apoptotic cell death of hippocampal progenitor cells. *J Neurosci* 18:6871–6881, 1998.
100. Kuffler S, Yoshikami D: The number of transmitter molecules in a quantum. *J Physiol* 251:465–482, 1975.
101. Bohler S, Gay S, Bertrand S, et al: Desensitization of neuronal nicotinic receptors conferred by N-terminal segments of the β2 subunit. *Biochemistry* 40:2066–2074, 2001.
102. Gunderson CH, Lehmann CR, Sidell FR, et al: Nerve agents—A review. *Neurology* 42:946–950, 1992.
103. Benowitz N: Pharmacology of nicotine: Addiction and therapeutics. *Annu Rev Pharmacol Toxicol* 36:597–613, 1996.
104. Papke RL, Meyer E, Nutter T, et al: α7 receptor-selective agonists and modes of α7 receptor activation. *Eur J Pharmacol* 393:179–195, 2000.
105. Sussman JL, Harel M, Frolow F, et al: Atomic structure of acetylcholinesterase from *Torpedo californica*—A prototypic acetylcholine-binding protein. *Science* 253:872–879, 1991.
106. Harel M, Schalk I, Ehretsabatier L, et al: Quaternary ligand-binding to aromatic residues in the active-site gorge of acetylcholinesterase. *Proc Natl Acad Sci USA* 90:9031–9035, 1993.
107. Edelstein SJ, Schaad O, Changeux JP: Single binding versus single channel recordings: A new approach to study ionotropic receptors. *Biochemistry* 36:13755–13760, 1997.
108. Ohno K, Hutchinson DO, Milone M, et al: Congenital myasthenic syndrome caused by prolonged acetylcholine-receptor channel openings due to a mutation in the m2 domain of the ε subunit. *Proc Natl Acad Sci USA* 92:758–762, 1995.
109. Milone M, Wang HL, Ohno K, et al: Slow-channel myasthenic syndrome caused by enhanced activation, desensitization, and agonist binding affinity attributable to mutation in the M2 domain of the acetylcholine receptor α subunit. *J Neurosci* 17:5651–5665, 1997.
110. Milone M, Wang HL, Ohno K, et al: Mode switching kinetics produced by a naturally occurring mutation in the cytoplasmic loop of the human acetylcholine receptor ε subunit. *Neuron* 20:575–588, 1998.
111. Changeux JP: Functional architecture and dynamics of the nicotinic acetylcholine receptor: An allosteric ligand-gated ion channel, in *Fidia Research Foundation: Neuroscience Award Lectures, 1988–1989*. 4:21–168, 1990.
112. Sine SM: Functional properties of human skeletal muscle acetylcholine receptors expressed by the TE671 cell line. *J Biol Chem* 263:18052–18062, 1988.
113. Sine SM, Claudio T, Sigworth F: Activation of *Torpedo* acetylcholine receptors expressed in mouse fibroblasts. *J Gen Physiol* 96:395–437, 1990.
114. Unwin N, Toyoshima C, Kubalek E: Arrangement of the acetylcholine receptor subunits in the resting and desensitized states determined by cryoelectron microscopy of crystallized *Torpedo* postsynaptic membranes. *J Cell Biol* 107:1123–1138, 1988.
115. Sargent P: The distribution of neuronal nicotinic acetylcholine receptors. in Clementi F, Fornasari D, Gotti C (eds): *Neuronal Nicotinic Receptors. Handbook Experimental Pharmacology*, New York: Springer Verlag; 2000, pp 163–192.
116. Kaiser S, Soliokov L, Wonnacott S: Presynaptic neuronal nicotinic receptors: Pharmacology, heterogenity and cellular mechanisms, in Clementi F, Fornasari D, Gotti C (eds): *Neuronal Nicotinic Receptors. Handbook of Experimental Pharmacology*, New York: Springer Verlag; 2000, pp 192–212.
117. Berg D, Shoop R, Chang K, et al: Nicotinic acetylcholine receptors in ganglionic transmission, in Clementi F, Fornasari D, Gotti C (eds): *Neuronal Nicotinic Receptors. Handbook of Experimental Pharmacology*, New York: Springer Verlag; 2000, pp 247–270.
118. Albuquerque E, Periera E, Alkondon M, et al: Neuronal nicotinic receptors and synaptic transmission in the mammalian central nervous system, in Clementi F, Fornasari D, Gotti C (eds): *Neuronal Nicotinic Receptors. Handbook of Experimental Pharmacology*, New York: Springer Verlag; 2000, pp 237–358.

119. Cuevas J, Roth A, Berg D: Two distinct classes of functional α7 containing nicotinic receptor on rat superior cervical ganglion neurons. *J Physiol* 525:735–746, 2000.

120. Xu W, Gelber S, Orr-Urtreger A, et al: Megacystis, mydriasis, and ion channel defect in mice lacking the α3 neuronal nicotinic acetylcholine receptor. *Proc Natl Acad Sci USA* 96:5746–5751, 1999.

121. Marubio LM, Arroyo-Jimenez MD, Cordero-Erausquin M, et al: Reduced antinociception in mice lacking α3 neuronal nicotinic receptor subunits. *Nature* 398:805–810, 1999.

122. Ross SA, Wong JYF, Clifford JJ, et al: Phenotypic characterization of an α4 neuronal nicotinic acetylcholine receptor subunit knock-out mouse. *J Neurosci* 20:6431–6441, 2000.

123. Labarca C, Schwarz J, Deshpande P, et al: Point mutant mice with hypersensitive α4 nicotinic receptors show dopaminergic deficits and increased anxiety. *Proc Natl Acad Sci USA* 98:2786–2791, 2001.

124. Orr-Urtreger A, Goldner FM, Saeki I, et al: Mice deficient in the α7 neuronal nicotinic acetylcholine receptor lack α-bungarotoxin binding sites and hippocampal fast nicotinic currents. *J Neurosci* 17:9165–9171, 1997.

125. Franceschini D, Orr-Urtreger A, Yu W, et al: Altered baroreflex responses in α7 deficient mice. *Behav Brain Res* 113:3–10, 2000.

126. Orr-Urtreger A, Broide RS, Kasten MR, et al: Mice homozygous for the L250T mutation in the α7 nicotinic acetylcholine receptor show increased neuronal apoptosis and die within 1 day of birth. *J Neurochem* 74:2154–2166, 2000.

127. Vetter DE, Liberman MC, Mann J, et al: Role of α9 nicotinic ACh receptor subunits in the development and function of cochlear efferent innervation. *Neuron* 23:93–103, 1999.

128. Picciotto MR, Caldarone BJ, King SL, et al: Nicotinic receptors in the brain: Links between molecular biology and behavior. *Neuropsychopharmacology* 22:451–465, 2000.

129. Xu W, Orr-Urtreger A, Nigro F, et al: Multiorgan autonomic dysfunction in mice lacking the β2 and the β4 subunits of neuronal nicotinic acetylcholine receptors. *J Neurosci* 19:9298–9305, 1999.

130. Allen R, Cui C, Heinemann S: Gene targeted knock out of the β3 neuronal nicotinic acetylcholine receptor subunit. *Soc Neurosci Abstr* 24:1341, 1998.

131. Grando S, Horton R: The keratinocyte cholinergic system with acetylcholine as an epidermal cytotransmitter. *Curr Opin Dermatol* 4:262–268, 1997.

132. Zia SH, Ndoye A, Lee TX, et al: Receptor-mediated inhibition of keratinocyte migration by nicotine involves modulations of calcium influx and intracellular concentration. *J Pharmacol Exp Ther* 293:973–981, 2000.

133. Macklin K, Maus A, Pereira E, et al: Human vascular endothelial cells express functional nicotinic acetylcholine receptors. *J Pharmacol Exp Ther* 287:435–439, 1998.

134. Maus A, Pereira E, Karachunski P, et al: Human and rodent bronchial epithelial cells also express functional nicotinic acetylcholine receptors. *Mol Pharmacol* 54:779–788, 1998.

135. Heeschen C, Jang J, Weis M, et al: Nicotine stimulates angiogenesis and promotes tumor growth and atherosclerosis. *Nat Med* 7:833–839, 2001.

136. Sekhon HS, Jia YB, Raab R, et al: Prenatal nicotine increases pulmonary α7 nicotinic receptor expression and alters fetal lung development in monkeys. *J Clin Invest* 103:637–647, 1999.

137. Mihovilovic M, Denning S, Mai Y, et al: Thymocytes and cultured thymic epithelial cells express transcripts encoding α3, α5 and β4 subunits of neuronal nicotinic acetylcholine receptors: Preferential transcription of the α3 and β4 genes by immature CD4+8 plus thymocytes. *J Neuroimmunol* 79:176–184, 1997.

138. Vernino S, Low PA, Fealey RD, et al: Autoantibodies to ganglionic acetyl choline receptors in autoimmune autonomic neuropathies. *N Engl J Med* 343:847–855, 2000.

139. Rogers SW, Andrews PI, Gahring LC, et al: Autoantibodies to glutamate-receptor Glur3 in Rasmussen's encephalitis. *Science* 265:648–651, 1994.

140. Rogers SW, Twyman RE, Gahring LC: The role of autoimmunity to glutamate receptors in neurological disease. *Mol Med Today* 2:76–81, 1996.

141. Gahring LC, Rogers SW: Autoimmunity to glutamate receptors in Rasmussen's encephalitis. A rare finding or the tip of an iceberg? *Neuroscientist* 4:373–379, 1998.

142. Carlson NG, Gahring LC, Rogers SW: Identification of the amino acids on a neuronal glutamate receptor recognized by an autoantibody from a patient with paraneoplastic syndrome. *J Neurosci Res* 63:480–485, 2001.

143. Steinlein OK: Neuronal nicotinic receptors in human epilepsy. *Eur J Pharmacol* 393:243–247, 2000.

144. De Fusco M, Becchetti A, Patrignani A, et al: The nicotinic receptor β2 subunit is mutant in nocturnal frontal lobe epilepsy. *Nat Genet* 26:275–276, 2000.

145. Phillips HA, Favre I, Kirkpatrick M, et al: CHRNB2 is the second acetylcholine receptor subunit associated with autosomal dominant nocturnal frontal lobe epilepsy. *Am J Hum Gen* 68:225–231, 2001.

146. Steinlein OK, Mulley JC, Propping P, et al: A missense mutation in the neuronal nicotinic acetylcholine-receptor α4 subunit is associated with autosomal-dominant nocturnal frontal-lobe epilepsy. *Nat Genet* 11:201–203, 1995.

147. Steinlein OK, Magnusson A, Stoodt J, et al: An insertion mutation of the CHRNA4 gene in a family with autosomal dominant nocturnal frontal lobe epilepsy. *Hum Mol Gen* 6:943–947, 1997.

148. Kuryatov A, Gerzanich V, Nelson M, et al: Mutation causing autosomal dominant nocturnal frontal lobe epilepsy alters Ca^{2+} permeability, conductance, and gating of human α4β2 nicotinic acetylcholine receptors. *J Neurosci* 17:9035–9047, 1997.

149. Rodrigues-Pinquet N, Jia L, Li M, et al: Five ADNFLE mutations reduce the Ca^{2+} dependence of the mammalian α4β2 acetylcholine response. *J Physiol* 550.1:11–26, 2003.

150. Ohno K, Brengman J, Tsujino A, et al: Human endplate acetylcholinesterase deficiency caused by mutations in the collagen-like tail subunit (ColQ) of the asymmetric enzyme. *Proc Natl Acad Sci USA* 95:9654–9659, 1998.

151. Ohno K, Tsujino A, Brengman JM, et al: Choline acetyltransferase mutations cause myasthenic syndrome associated with episodic apnea in humans. *Proc Natl Acad Sci USA* 98:2017–2022, 2001.

152. Le Novere N, Zoli M, Changeux JP: Neuronal nicotinic receptor α6 subunit mRNA is selectively concentrated in catecholaminergic nuclei of the rat brain. *Eur J Neurosci* 8:2428–2439, 1996.

153. Goldner FM, Dineley KT, Patrick JW: Immunohistochemical localization of the nicotinic acetylcholine receptor subunit α6 to dopaminergic neurons in the substantia nigra and ventral tegmental area. *Neuroreport* 8:2739–2742, 1997.

154. Quik M, Polonskaya Y, Gillespie A, et al: Differential alterations in nicotinic receptor α6 and β3 subunit messenger RNAs in monkey substantia nigra after nigrostriatal degeneration. *Neuroscience* 100:63–72, 2000.

155. Le Novere N, Zoli M, Lena C, et al: Involvement of α6 nicotinic receptor subunit in nicotine-elicited locomotion, demonstrated by in vivo antisense oligonucleotide infusion. *Neuroreport* 10:2497–2501, 1999.

156. Balfour DJK, Fagerstrom KO: Pharmacology of nicotine and its therapeutic use in smoking cessation and neurodegenerative disorders. *Pharmacol Ther* 72:51–81, 1996.

157. Kihara T, Shimohama S, Sawada H, et al: α7 nicotinic receptor transduces signals to phosphatidylinositol 3-kinase to block a β-amyloid-induced neurotoxicity. *J Biol Chem* 276:13541–13546, 2001.

158. Belluardo N, Mudo G, Blum M, et al: Central nicotinic receptors, neurotrophic factors and neuroprotection. *Behav Brain Res* 113:21–34, 2000.

159. Perry E, Martin-Ruiz C, Lee M, et al: Nicotinic receptor subtypes in human brain ageing, Alzheimer and Lewy body diseases. *Eur J Pharmacol* 393:215–222, 2000.

160. Weavers A, Witter B, Moser N, et al: Classical Alzheimer features and cholinergic dysfunction: Towards a unifying hypothesis? *Acta Neurol Scand* 102(Suppl):176, 2000.

161. Liu QS, Kawai H, Berg DK: β-amyloid peptide blocks the response of α7-containing nicotinic receptors on hippocampal neurons. *Proc Natl Acad Sci USA* 98:4734–4739, 2001.

162. Wang HY, Lee DHS, Davis CB, et al: Amyloid peptide Aβ(1-42) binds selectively and with picomolar affinity to α7 nicotinic acetylcholine receptors. *J Neurochem* 75:1155–1161, 2000.

163. Wang HY, Lee DHS, D'Andrea MR, et al: β-amyloid(1-42) binds to α7 nicotinic acetylcholine receptor with high affinity—Implications for Alzheimer's disease pathology. *J Biol Chem* 275:5626–5632, 2000.

164. Nordberg A, Hillstrom-Lindahl E, Lee M, et al: Chronic nicotine treatment reduces β amyloidosis in the brain of a mouse model of Alzheimer's disease. *J Neurochem* 81:655–658, 2002.

165. D'Andrea MR, Nagele RG, Wang HY, et al: Evidence that neurons accumulating amyloid can undergo lysis to form amyloid plaques in Alzheimer's disease. *Histopathology* 38:120–134, 2001.

166. Dineley KT, Westerman M, Bui D, et al: β-amyloid activates the mitogen-activated protein kinase cascade via hippocampal α7 nicotinic acetylcholine receptors; In vitro and in vivo mechanisms related to Alzheimer's disease. *J Neurosci* 21:4125–4133, 2001.

167. Whitehouse P, Martino A, Marcus K, et al: Reductions in acetylcholine and nicotine binding in several degenerative diseases. *Arch Neurol* 45:722–724, 1988.

168. Zoli M, Picciotto MR, Ferrari R, et al: Increased neurodegeneration during aging in mice lacking high-affinity nicotine receptors. *EMBO J* 18:1235–1244, 1999.

169. Lloyd GK, Williams M: Neuronal nicotinic acetylcholine receptors as novel drug targets. *J Pharmacol Exp Ther* 292:461–467, 2000.

170. Santos M, Alkondon M, Pereira E, et al: The nicotinic allosteric potentiating ligand galantamine facilitates synaptic transmission in the mammalian central nervous system. *Mol Pharmacol* 61:1222–1234, 2002.

171. Sanberg PR, Silver AA, Shytle RD, et al: Nicotine for the treatment of Tourette's syndrome. *Pharmacol Ther* 74:21–25, 1997.

172. Silver AA, Shytle RD, Sanberg PR: Mecamylamine in Tourette's syndrome: A two-year retrospective case study. *J Child Adolesc Psychopharmacol* 10:59–68, 2000.

173. Leonard S, Breese C, Adams C, et al: Smoking and schizophrenia: Abnormal nicotinic receptor statement. *Eur J Pharmacol* 393:237–242, 2000.

174. Neves-Pereira M, Bassett AS, Honer WG, et al: No evidence for linkage of the CHRNA7 gene region in Canadian schizophrenia families. *Am J Med Genet* 81:361–363, 1998.

175. Codignola A, Tarroni P, Cattaneo MG, et al: Serotonin release and cell proliferation are under the control of α-bungarotoxin-sensitive nicotinic receptors in small-cell lung-carcinoma cell lines. *FEBS Lett* 342:286–290, 1994.

176. Di Chiara G: Role of dopamine in the behavioural actions of nicotine related to addiction. *Eur J Pharmacol* 393:295–314, 2000.
177. Olale F, Gerzanich V, Kuryatov A, et al: Chronic nicotine exposure differentially affects the function of human α3, α4, and α7 neuronal nicotinic receptor subtypes. *J Pharmacol Exp Ther* 283:675–683, 1997.
178. Kuryatov A, Olale FA, Choi C, et al: Acetylcholine receptor extracellular domain determines sensitivity to nicotine-induced inactivation. *Eur J Pharmacol* 393:11–21, 2000.
179. Jia L, Flotildes K, Li M, et al: Nicotine trapping causes the persistent desensitization of α4β2 nicotinic receptors expressed in oocytes. *J Neurochem* 84:753–766, 2003.
180. Peng X, Gerzanich V, Anand R, et al: Nicotine-induced increase in neuronal nicotinic receptors results from a decrease in the rate of receptor turnover. *Mol Pharmacol* 46:523–530, 1994.
181. Peng X, Gerzanich V, Anand R, et al: Chronic nicotine treatment up-regulates α3 and α7 acetylcholine receptor subtypes expressed by the human neuroblastoma cell line SH-SY5Y. *Mol Pharmacol* 51:776–784, 1997.
182. Wang F, Nelson ME, Kuryatov A, et al: Chronic nicotine treatment up-regulates human α3 β2 but not α3 β4 acetylcholine receptors stably transfected in human embryonic kidney cells. *J Biol Chem* 273:28721–28732, 1998.
183. Merlie J, Sebbane R, Gardner S, et al: The regulation of acetylcholine receptor expression in mammalian muscle. *Cold Spring Harbor Symp Quant Biol* 48:135–146.
184. Wang ZZ, Hardy SF, Hall ZW: Assembly of the nicotinic acetylcholine receptor—The first transmembrane domains of truncated α and δ subunits are required for heterodimer formation in vivo. *J Biol Chem* 271: 27575–27584, 1996.
185. Wang ZZ, Mathias A, Gautam M, et al: Metabolic stabilization of muscle nicotinic acetylcholine receptor by rapsyn. *J Neurosci* 19:1998–2007, 1999.
186. Ramanathan VK, Hall ZW: Altered glycosylation sites of the δ subunit of the acetylcholine receptor (AChR) reduce α δ association and receptor assembly. *J Biol Chem* 274:20513–20520, 1999.
187. Wang J-M, Zhang L, Yao Y, et al: A transmembrane model governs the surface trafficking of nicotinic acetylcholine recptors, *Nat Neurosci* 5: 963–970, 2002.
188. Keller SH, Lindstrom J, Ellisman M, et al: Adjacent basic amino acid residues recognized by the COPI complex and ubiquitination govern endoplasmic reticulum to cell surface trafficking of the nicotinic acetylcholine receptor α subunit. *J Biol Chem* 276:18384–18391, 2001.
189. Green WN: Perspective—Ion channel assembly: Creating structures that function. *J Gen Physiol* 113:163–169, 1999.
190. Saedi MS, Conroy WG, Lindstrom J: Assembly of *Torpedo* acetylcholine receptors in *Xenopus* oocytes. *J Cell Biol* 112:1007–1015, 1991.
191. Claudio T, Paulson HL, Green WN, et al: Fibroblasts transfected with *Torpedo* acetylcholine receptor β subunit, γ subunit, and δ subunit cDNAs express functional receptors when infected with a retroviral α recombinant. *J Cell Biol* 108:2277–2290, 1989.
192. Smith MM, Lindstrom J, Merlie JP: Formation of the α-bungarotoxin binding site and assembly of the nicotinic acetylcholine receptor subunits occur in the endoplasmic reticulum. *J Biol Chem* 262:4367–4376, 1987.
193. Blount P, Merlie JP: Mutational analysis of muscle nicotinic acetylcholine receptor subunit assembly. *J Cell Biol* 111:2613–2622, 1990.
194. Blount P, Merlie JP: Bip associates with newly synthesized subunits of the mouse muscle nicotinic receptor. *J Cell Biol* 113:1125–1132, 1991.
195. Blount P, Merlie JP: Molecular-basis of the two nonequivalent ligand-binding sites of the muscle nicotinic acetylcholine receptor. *Neuron* 3:349–357, 1989.
196. Blount P, Smith MM, Merlie JP: Assembly intermediates of the mouse muscle nicotinic acetylcholine receptor in stably transfected fibroblasts. *J Cell Biol* 111:2601–2611, 1990.
197. Kreienkamp HJ, Maeda RK, Sine SM, et al: Intersubunit contacts governing assembly of the mammalian nicotinic acetylcholine-receptor. *Neuron* 14:635–644, 1995.
198. Helenius A, Aebi M: Intracellular functions of N-linked glycans. *Science* 291:2364–2369, 2001.
199. Sumikawa K, Miledi R: Assembly and n-glycosylation of all ACh receptor subunits are required for their efficient insertion into plasma membranes. *Mol Brain Res* 5:183–192, 1989.
200. Gehle VM, Walcott EC, Nishizaki T, et al: N-glycosylation at the conserved sites ensures the statement of properly folded functional ACh receptors. *Mol Brain Res* 45:219–229, 1997.
201. Sumikawa K, Gehle VM: Assembly of mutant subunits of the nicotinic acetylcholine receptor lacking the conserved disulfide loop structure. *J Biol Chem* 267:6286–6290, 1992.
202. Swope SL, Moss SJ, Raymond LA, et al: Regulation of ligand-gated ion channels by protein phosphorylation. *Adv Second Messenger Phosphoprotein Res* 33:49–78, 1999.
203. Olson EN, Glaser L, Merlie JP: α and β subunits of the nicotinic acetylcholine receptor contain covalently bound lipid. *J Biol Chem* 259:5364–5367, 1984.
204. Pumplin DW, Fambrough DM: Turnover of acetylcholine receptors in skeletal muscle. *Annu Rev Physiol* 44:319–335, 1982.
205. Gu Y, Franco A, Gardner PD, et al: Properties of embryonic and adult muscle acetylcholine-receptors transiently expressed in cos cells. *Neuron* 5:147–157, 1990.
206. Heinemann S, Bevan S, Kullberg R, et al: Modulation of the acetylcholine receptor by anti-receptor antibody. *Proc Natl Acad Sci USA* 74:3090–3094, 1977.
207. Drachman DB, Angus CW, Adams RN, et al: Myasthenic antibodies cross-link acetylcholine receptors to accelerate degradation. *N Engl J Med* 298:1116–1122, 1978.
208. Lindstrom J, Einarson B: Antigenic modulation and receptor loss in experimental auto-immune myasthenia gravis. *Muscle Nerve* 2:173–179, 1979.
209. Merlie JP, Heinemann S, Einarson B, et al: Degradation of acetylcholine receptor in diaphragms of rats with experimental auto-immune myasthenia gravis. *J Biol Chem* 254:6328–6332, 1979.
210. Merlie JP, Heinemann S, Lindstrom JM: Acetylcholine-receptor degradation in adult rat diaphragms in organ culture and the effect of anti-acetylcholine receptor antibodies. *J Biol Chem* 254:6320–6327, 1979.
211. Libby P, Bursztajn S, Goldberg AL: Degradation of the acetylcholine receptor in cultured muscle cells—Selective inhibitors and the fate of undegraded receptors. *Cell* 19:481–491, 1980.
212. Watanabe H, Zoli M, Changeux JP: Promoter analysis of the neuronal nicotinic acetylcholine receptor α4 gene: Methylation and expression of the transgene. *Eur J Neurosci* 10:2244–2253, 1998.
213. Penn AS, Low BW, Jaffe IA, et al: Drug-induced autoimmune myasthenia gravis. *Ann NY Acad Sci* 841:433–449, 1998.
214. Lindstrom J, Einarson B, Lennon V, et al: Pathological mechanisms in EAMG. I: Immunogenicity of syngeneic muscle acetylcholine receptor and quantitative extraction of receptor and antibody-receptor complexes from muscles of rats with experimental autoimmune myasthenia gravis. *J Exp Med* 144:726–738, 1976.
215. Lindstrom J, Engel A, Seybold M, et al: Pathological mechanisms in EAMG. II: Passive transfer of experimental autoimmune myasthenia gravis in rats with anti-acetylcholine receptor antibodies. *J Exp Med* 144:739–753, 1976.
216. Shelton D, Lindstrom J: Spontaneous remission in canine myasthenia gravis: Implications for assessing human MG therapies. *Neurology* 57:2139–2141, 2001.
217. Sahashi K, Engel AG, Lambert EH, et al: Ultrastructural localization of the terminal and lytic 9th complement component (C9) at the motor endplate in myasthenia gravis. *J Neuropathol Exp Neurol* 39:160–172, 1980.
218. Engel AG: Myasthenia gravis and myasthenic syndromes. *Ann Neurol* 16:519–534, 1984.
219. Asher O, Kues WA, Witzemann V, et al: Increased gene-expression of acetylcholine-receptor and myogenic factors in passively transferred experimental autoimmune myasthenia gravis. *J Immunol* 151:6442–6450, 1993.
220. Hohlfeld R, Wekerle H: The immunopathogenesis of myasthenia gravis, in Engel A (ed): *Myasthenia Gravis and Myasthenic Disorders*. Contemporary Neurology Series. New York: Oxford University Press, 1999; 87–110.
221. Yeh TM, Krolick KA: T-cells reactive with a small synthetic peptide of the acetylcholine-receptor can provide help for a clonotypically heterogeneous antibody-response and subsequently impaired muscle function. *J Immunol* 144:1654–1660, 1990.
222. Froehner SC: Identification of exposed and buried determinants of the membrane-bound acetylcholine-receptor from *Torpedo californica*. *Biochemistry* 20:4905–4915, 1981.
223. Das MK, Lindstrom J: Epitope mapping of antibodies to acetylcholine receptor-α subunits using peptides synthesized on polypropylene pegs. *Biochemistry* 30:2470–2477, 1991.
224. Blatt Y, Montal MS, Lindstrom JM, et al: Monoclonal-antibodies specific to the β-subunit and γ-subunit of the *Torpedo* acetylcholine receptor inhibit single-channel activity. *J Neurosci* 6:481–486, 1986.
225. Shelton GD, Cardinet GH, Lindstrom JM: Canine and human myasthenia gravis autoantibodies recognize similar regions on the acetylcholine-receptor. *Neurology* 38:1417–1423, 1988.
226. Weinberg CB, Hall ZW: Antibodies from patients with myasthenia gravis recognize determinants unique to extrajunctional acetylcholine receptors. *Proc Natl Acad Sci USA* 76:504–508, 1979.
227. Burges J, Wray DW, Pizzighella S, et al: A myasthenia gravis plasma immunoglobulin reduces miniature endplate potentials at human endplates in vitro. *Muscle Nerve* 13:407–413, 1990.
228. Jacobson L, Polizzi A, Morriss-Kay G, et al: Plasma from human mothers of fetuses with severe arthrogryposis multiplex congenita causes deformities in mice. *J Clin Invest* 103:1031–1038, 1999.
229. Conti-Fine BM, Navaneetham D, Karachunski PI, et al: T cell recognition of the acetylcholine receptor in myasthenia gravis. *Ann NY Acad Sci* 841:283–308, 1998.
230. Beeson D, Bond AP, Corlett L, et al: Thymus, thymoma, and specific T cells in myasthenia gravis. *Ann Acad Sci* 841:371–387, 1998.
231. Fujii Y, Lindstrom J: Specificity of the t-cell immune-response to acetylcholine-receptor in experimental autoimmune myasthenia gravis—Response to subunits and synthetic peptides. *J Immunol* 140:1830–1837, 1988.

232. Raju R, Spack E, David C: Acetylcholine receptor peptide recognition in HLA DR3-transgenic mice: In vivo responses correlate with MHC-peptide binding. *J Immunol* 167:1118–1124, 2001.
233. Ong B, Willcox N, Wordsworth P, et al: Critical role for the val/gly86 HLA-DR-beta dimorphism in autoantigen presentation to human T cells. *Proc Natl Acad Sci USA* 88:7343–7347, 1991.
234. Yang H, Goluoszko E, David C, et al: Mapping myasthenia gravis-associated T cell epitopes on human acetylcholine receptors in HLA transgenic mice. *J Clin Invest* 109:1111–1120, 2002.
235. Christadoss P, Lindstrom JM, Melvold RW, et al: Mutation at IA beta-chain prevents experimental autoimmune myasthenia gravis. *Immunogenetics* 21:33–38, 1985.
236. Christadoss P, Poussin M, Deng CS: Animal models of myasthenia gravis. *Clin Immunol* 94:75–87, 2000.
237. Drachman DB, Okumura S, Adams RN, et al: Oral tolerance in myasthenia gravis. *Ann Acad Sci* 778:258–272, 1996.
238. Xiao BG, Link H: Mucosal tolerance: A two-edged sword to prevent and treat autoimmune diseases. *Clin Immunol Immunopathol* 85:119–128, 1997.
239. Lindstrom J, Peng X, Kuryatov A, et al: Molecular and antigenic structure of nicotinic acetylcholine receptors. *Ann Acad Sci* 841:71–86, 1998.
240. Im SH, Barchan D, Fuchs S, et al: Mechanism of nasal tolerance induced by a recombinant fragment of acetylcholine receptor for treatment of experimental myasthenia gravis. *J Neuroimmunol* 111:161–168, 2000.
241. Im SH, Barchan D, Souroujon MC, et al: Role of tolerogen conformation in induction of oral tolerance in experimental autoimmune myasthenia gravis. *J Immunol* 165:3599–3605, 2000.
242. Karachunski PI, Ostlie NS, Okita DK, et al: Subcutaneous administration of T-epitope sequences of the acetylcholine receptor prevents experimental myasthenia gravis. *J Neuroimmunol* 93:108–121, 1999.
243. Zhang GX, Shi FD, Zhu J, et al: Synthetic peptides fail to induce nasal tolerance to experimental autoimmune myasthenia gravis. *J Neuroimmunol* 85:96–101, 1998.
244. Krause I, Blank M, Shoenfeld Y: Immunomodulation of experimental autoimmune diseases via oral tolerance. *Crit Rev Immunol* 20:1–16, 2000.
245. Shi FD, Li HL, Wang HB, et al: Mechanisms of nasal tolerance induction in experimental autoimmune myasthenia gravis: Identification of regulatory cells. *J Immunol* 162: 5757–5763, 1999.
246. Diethelm-Okita B, Wells GB, Kuryatov A, et al: Response of CD4(+) T cells from myasthenic patients and healthy subjects of biosynthetic and synthetic sequences of the nicotinic acetylcholine receptor. *J Autoimmun* 11:191–203, 1998.
247. Ma SW, Zhao DL, Yin ZQ, et al: Transgenic plants expressing autoantigens fed to mice to induce oral immune tolerance. *Nat Med* 3:793–796, 1997.
248. Roy K, Mao HQ, Huang SK, et al: Oral gene delivery with chitosan-DNA nanoparticles generates immunologic protection in a murine model of peanut allergy. *Nat Med* 5:387–391, 1999.
249. Yao Y, Wang J, Viroonchatapan N, et al: Yeast expression and NMR analysis of the extracellular domain of muscle nicotinic acetylcholine receptor α subunit. *J Biol Chem* 277:12613–12621, 2002.
250. Psaridi-Linardaki K, Mamalaki A, Remoundos M, et al: The expression of soluble ligand- and antibody-binding extracellular domain of human muscle acetylcholine receptor α subunit in yeast *Pichia pastoris*. Role of glycosylation in α-bungarotoxin binding. *J Biol Chem* 277: 26980–26986, 2002.
251. Tsantili P, Tzartos SJ, Mamalaki A: High affinity single-chain Fv antibody fragments protecting the human nicotinic acetylcholine receptor. *J Neuroimmunol* 94:15–27, 1999.
252. Papanastasiou D, Poulas K, Kokla A, et al: Prevention of passively transferred experimental autoimmune myasthenia gravis by Fab fragments of monoclonal antibodies directed against the main immunogenic region of the acetylcholine receptor. *J Neuroimmunol* 104:124–132, 2000.
253. Poulas K, Tsouloufis T, Tzartos SJ: Treatment of passively transferred experimental autoimmune myasthenia gravis using papain. *Clin Exp Immunol* 120:363–368, 2000.
254. Venkatesh N, Im SH, Balass M, et al: Prevention of passively transferred experimental autoimmune myasthenia gravis by a phage library-derived cyclic peptide. *Proc Natl Acad Sci USA* 97:761–766, 2000.
255. Araga S, Leboeuf RD, Blalock JE: Prevention of experimental autoimmune myasthenia gravis by manipulation of the immune network with a complementary peptide for the acetylcholine receptor. *Proc Natl Acad Sci USA* 90:8747–8751, 1993.
256. Araga S, Galin FS, Kishimoto M, et al: Prevention of experimental autoimmune myasthenia gravis by a monoclonal antibody to a complementary peptide for the main immunogenic region of the acetylcholine receptor. *J Immunol* 157:386–392, 1996.
257. Araga S, Xu LK, Nakashima K, et al: A peptide vaccine that prevents experimental autoimmune myasthenia gravis by specifically blocking T cell help. *FASEB J* 14:185–196, 2000.
258. Killen JA, Hochschwender SM, Lindstrom JM: The main immunogenic region of acetylcholine receptors does not provoke the formation of antibodies of a predominant idiotype. *J Neuroimmunol* 9:229–241, 1985.
259. Wu B, Wu JM, Miagkov A, et al: Specific immunotherapy by genetically engineered APCs: The "guided missile" strategy. *J Immunol* 166: 4773–4779, 2001.
260. Wu JM, Wu B, Miagkov A, et al: Specific immunotherapy of experimental myasthenia gravis in vitro: The "guided missile" strategy. *Cell Immunol* 208:137–147, 2001.
261. Grob D, Brunner NG, Namba T: The natural course of myasthenia gravis and effect of therapeutic measures. *Ann Acad Sci* 377:652–669,1981.
262. Kissel JT, Franklin GM: Treatment of myasthenia gravis—A call to arms. *Neurology* 55:3–4, 2000.
263. Faller G, Steininger H, Kranzlein J, et al: Antigastric autoantibodies in *Helicobacter pylori* infection: Implications of histological and clinical parameters of gastritis. *Gut* 41:619–623, 1997.

Chapter 18

Function and Molecular Structure of Acetylcholinesterase

RICHARD L. ROTUNDO

Structure of Cholinesterases
  THREE-DIMENSIONAL STRUCTURE OF THE CATALYTIC SUBUNIT
  CLASSIFICATION OF ACETYLCHOLINESTERASE FORMS
  PHYSICAL PROPERTIES OF ACETYLCHOLINESTERASE
  STRUCTURE OF THE NONCATALYTIC SUBUNITS ASSOCIATED WITH ACETYLCHOLINESTERASE

Molecular Biology of Cholinesterases
  PRIMARY STRUCTURE OF ACETYLCHOLINESTERASE DEDUCED BY MOLECULAR CLONING
  STRUCTURE OF THE ACETYLCHOLINESTERASE GENE
  EXPRESSION AND LOCALIZATION OF ACETYLCHOLINESTERASE mRNAs
  TRANSCRIPTIONAL CONTROL OF THE ACETYLCHOLINESTERASE GENE

Function of Acetylcholinesterase
  ENZYMATIC MECHANISMS
  MODELING THE ROLE OF ACETYLCHOLINESTERASE AT THE NEUROMUSCULAR JUNCTION
  METHODS FOR DETECTING, LOCALIZING, AND QUANTITATING ACETYLCHOLINESTERASE

Tissue Distribution, Metabolism, and Regulation of Acetylcholinesterase
  CELLULAR DISTRIBUTION OF ACETYLCHOLINESTERASE FORMS
  BIOSYNTHESIS OF ACETYLCHOLINESTERASE
  REGULATION OF ACETYLCHOLINESTERASE SYNTHESIS AND LOCALIZATION
  TURNOVER OF ACETYLCHOLINESTERASE

Acetylcholinesterase (AChE)* is an essential component of the vertebrate neuromuscular junction and other cholinergic synapses in the central and peripheral nervous systems, where it is in part responsible for terminating neurotransmission. Acute inhibition of AChE—by either nerve gases, organophosphate-type pesticides, or certain snake toxins—can rapidly be fatal. Our understanding of the structure, function, and regulation of AChE has grown rapidly during the past decade, owing to advances in the cell and molecular biology of AChE, the cloning and sequencing of its gene and cDNA, and the elucidation of the crystal structure of the protein. Additional studies have elucidated the structure of the noncatalytic subunits associated with several oligomeric forms of the enzyme; more recently, the molecular mechanisms responsible for transporting and localizing the enzyme to the neuromuscular junction have been determined. Together, these studies have given us a very good picture of the functional aspects of AChE at the neuromuscular junction and details of the events leading from its synthesis in the myoplasm immediately beneath the synapse through its assembly and eventual attachment to the synaptic basal lamina interposed between the muscle fiber and the nerve terminal.

All AChE catalytic subunits are glycoproteins containing between 10 and 15 percent of their mass as covalently linked oligosaccharides. Two distinct classes of AChE are present in skeletal muscle:

1. The homomeric or globular forms, consisting of monomers, dimers, or tetramers of catalytic subunits. They exist as soluble, hydrophilic forms or as amphiphilic (hydrophobic) forms that can associate with membranes through their attachment to a noncatalytic transmembrane subunit or the addition of a glycolipid anchor.
2. The heteromeric, asymmetrical, or collagen-tailed forms, consisting of one to three tetramers of catalytic subunits linked by disulfide bonds to a collagen-like tail that attaches the catalytic subunits to the basal lamina.

In the muscles of most mammals, there is a much higher concentration of the collagen-tailed AChE at the motor end plate region, and it is this form of AChE that is active in terminating neuromuscular transmission. In humans as well as most other species examined, collagen-tailed AChE has also been detected at non–end plate regions, but its function at these sites, if any, is not known. The catalytic AChE subunits of all vertebrate species are encoded by a single gene. The structural diversity of the family of AChE forms arises in part via alternative mRNA processing (see next section). However, in higher vertebrates, all of the AChE forms expressed in neuronal cells and muscle arise through post-translational modifications of a common catalytic subunit and association with other noncatalytic subunits.

Although active AChE molecules are found throughout the length of muscle fibers, the highest concentrations are clearly located at sites of nerve-muscle contact. Biochemical analyses at the single-fiber level indicate that noninnervated regions of skeletal muscle fibers have only about 2 to 3 percent of the AChE levels measured in innervated segments. The molecular mechanisms involved in the selective accumulation of AChE on the synaptic basal lamina are just now becoming apparent and clearly involve several different mechanisms, including (1) selective expression of AChE mRNA in innervated regions of skeletal muscle fibers, (2) localized translation of the AChE mRNA, (3) selective transport and localization of the AChE molecules to the overlying extracellular regions of the muscle fiber, and (4) selective retention of the collagen-tailed AChE molecules on the synaptic basal lamina, possibly via covalent interactions with the extracellular matrix.

During the past few years significant progress has been made in understanding the regulation of AChE expression at the molecular level, as well as identifying the additional molecules involved in targeting and retaining AChE at the appropriate sites of function. However, we still need to learn more about how the necessary molecules involved in synaptic transmission are synthesized in the appropriate amounts, targeted to their correct locations, and retained in a functional state until replaced. Ultimately, an understanding of how important components of synapses, such as

*A list of abbreviations used in this chapter is given at the end of the chapter.

AChE, are regulated will lead to a fundamental understanding of how the synapses are formed, maintained, and regulated in all electrically excitable cells.

Structure of Cholinesterases

Although the importance of AChE in neuromuscular transmission was recognized early on, the extraordinary complexity of this enzyme was not appreciated until the 1970s, when several laboratories—including those of Massoulié,[1,2] Rosenberry,[3] Silman,[4] and Taylor[5]—published a series of papers describing its physicochemical nature. Since then, studies from many laboratories on many organisms have shown that the cholinesterases comprise families of structurally related oligomeric forms.[6] Several of these forms also have unique properties related to their particular cellular locations. Amino acid sequences of AChE and butyrylcholinesterase (BuChE) from several species together with an x-ray crystallographic structure of AChE now suggest that the cholinesterases constitute a family of serine hydrolases quite distinct from the serine proteases.[7,8] Elucidation of the structure of additional members of the cholinesterase family has provided many new insights into the intricate functional and evolutionary relationships within this group of proteins.

THREE-DIMENSIONAL STRUCTURE OF THE CATALYTIC SUBUNIT

The determination of the three-dimensional structure of the AChE catalytic subunit by x-ray crystallography[9] confirmed some expectations but also revealed unpredicted features of the enzyme molecule (Fig. 18-1). Early hydrodynamic studies of the enzyme had indicated that the catalytic subunits were globular in shape, and this was confirmed by the structural data indicating that the AChE monomer is an ellipsoidal protein measuring approximately 45 by 60 by 65 Å. However, based upon many kinetic and chemical studies, the active site of the enzyme was believed to consist of an "esteratic site" containing the active-site serine and an "anionic site" to which the choline portion of ACh would bind. By analogy to the serine proteases, both sites would be located in a fold or pocket on the surface of the enzyme molecule. However, the crystal structure now shows the active site to reside at the base of what has now been termed the *active-site gorge*.[9,10] This gorge extends approximately 20 Å into the center of the catalytic subunit and is lined with 14 aromatic amino acids, making this a very hydrophobic tunnel. The tunnel widens at the base and contains the *catalytic triad*, consisting of the active-site serine (Ser_{200}), glutamic acid (E_{327}), and a histidine (H_{440}) residue. The numbering of the residues refers to the position of the amino acids in the *Torpedo* (electric ray) AChE sequence. The peripheral site, previously defined by pharmacologic and chemical studies and thought to be an allosteric site responsible for substrate inhibition as well as a ligand site for certain charged bisquaternary ligands, now appears to consist of a series of negatively charged residues located on the surface of the catalytic subunit near the opening of the active-site gorge. This site is also the binding site for the snake α-neurotoxins known as fasciculins, highly folded proteins of 61 amino acids and containing eight cysteines forming four disulfide bridges.[11] For a more detailed discussion of the structure of the catalytic subunit, the reader is referred to a volume on cholinesterase function.[12]

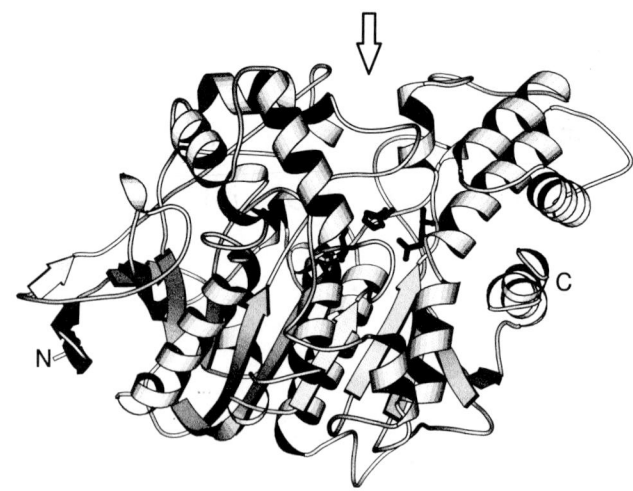

FIGURE 18-1. Structure of the AChE catalytic subunit. This ribbon model of the globular AChE catalytic subunit, derived from x-ray crystallographic data, shows the active-site gorge (arrow) viewed from the side. The polypeptide is ellipsoidal in shape and measures approximately 45 × 60 × 65 Å. The three amino acids that form the catalytic triad, serine 200, glutamic acid 327, and histidine 440, are shown in bold. (Illustration courtesy of Dr. Joel Sussman.) (*From Sussman JL, Harel M, Frolow F, et al: Atomic structure of acetylcholinesterase from Torpedo californica: A prototypic acetylcholine-binding protein. Science 253:872–879, 1991. With permission.*)

CLASSIFICATION OF ACETYLCHOLINESTERASE FORMS

Most of our early knowledge concerning the structure of AChE derives from studies of the enzyme isolated from the electroplax of electric eels and rays.[6,13,14] These electric organs are actually derived during embryonic development by specialization of certain muscle cells.[15] The cells of the electric organ are disk-like in shape and form stacks, much like the plates in a battery. Up to 30 percent of their surface plasma membrane forms the synapses that are homologous to the neuromuscular junctions of higher vertebrates. Most of the findings concerning the molecular forms of AChE in the electroplax are applicable to all other vertebrate species, including humans.

The multiple oligomeric forms of AChE are classified according to their subunit structure (Fig. 18-2). These forms can be separated by gel chromatography or by ultracentrifugation. However, it is also useful to consider them in terms of their physical properties and subcellular location. With regard to structure, the AChEs are classified into globular, or G, forms and asymmetrical, collagen-tailed, or A, forms. The globular forms, G_1, G_2, and G_4, are monomer,

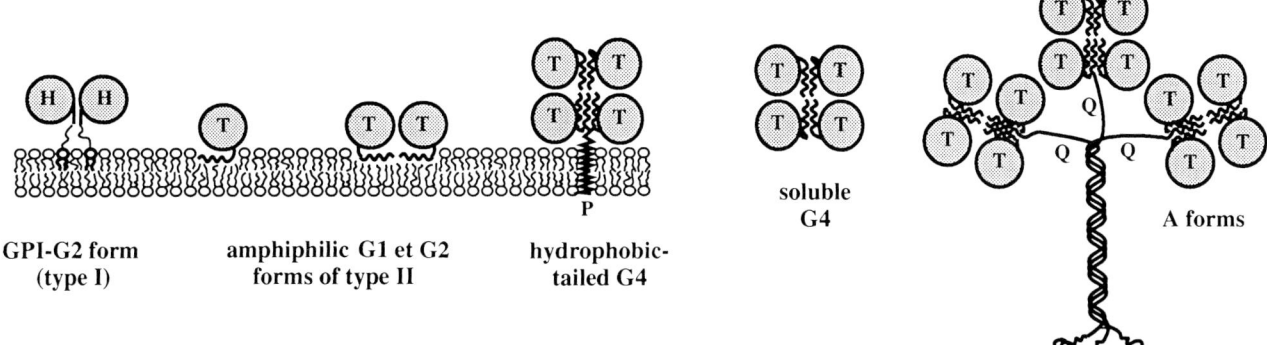

FIGURE 18-2. Classification of the oligomeric forms of acetylcholinesterase. The major forms of AChE found in vertebrates can be classified into globular (G) and collagen-tailed or asymmetrical (A) forms. The nomenclature refers to the type of subunit followed by a number designating the number of catalytic subunits in the oligomer. Only the catalytic subunit possessing the carboxyl terminus encoded by exon 5 (H subunit) can associate with the glycolipid anchor. All the remaining forms consist of varying numbers of catalytic subunits with the carboxy terminus encoded by exon 6 that can associate with other structural subunits such as the collagen-like tail (Q) or a hydrophobic lipid-containing peptide (P), or be secreted unmodified as soluble G4 or G2 forms. There is now some evidence for hydrophobic (amphiphilic) forms of the T subunit; however, the nature of the hydrophobic domain has not yet been elucidated. (*From Massoulié J, Sussman JH, Doctor BP, et al: Recommendations for nomenclature in cholinesterases, in Shafferman A, Velan B (eds): Multidisciplinary Approaches to Cholinesterase Functions. New York: Plenum Press; 1992. With permission.*)

dimer, and tetramer, respectively, of enzymatically active subunits. The subscript accompanying the letter designation refers to the number of catalytic subunits in the oligomer. The molecular weights of the catalytic subunits are around 70 to 76 kDa in most species, except in birds, where the subunits are around 100 to 115 kDa. In humans, the monomer molecular weight is approximately 72,000. Each subunit contains several asparagine-linked oligosaccharides, and each subunit has a single catalytic site.

The globular forms consist of two different classes of catalytic subunits encoded by separate transcripts (see "Structure of the Acetylcholinesterase Gene," below). The amphiphilic (hydrophobic or H form) dimeric AChE form, found in the nervous systems of insects and elasmobranchs and on cells of the erythroid and lymphoid cell lineages in higher vertebrates, contains a glycolipid covalently linked to the cysteinyl residue at the carboxyl terminus. The carboxyl terminus of this polypeptide is encoded by exon 5 in the human gene (Fig. 18-3) and adds 37 amino acids to the polypeptide chain, of which all but two are removed during processing prior to addition of the glycolipid anchor. Only this subset of AChE dimers has so far been found to contain the glycolipid-type posttranslational modification.

All remaining AChE oligomeric forms consist of the catalytic subunit translated from the alternatively spliced mRNA, including exon 6, to give the A-T form of the enzyme, which can encode a carboxyl terminus with a cysteinyl residue capable of either (1) attaching to the assembled collagen-like tail subunits, or (2) attaching to a small 20-kDa hydrophobic peptide with a transmembrane domain that

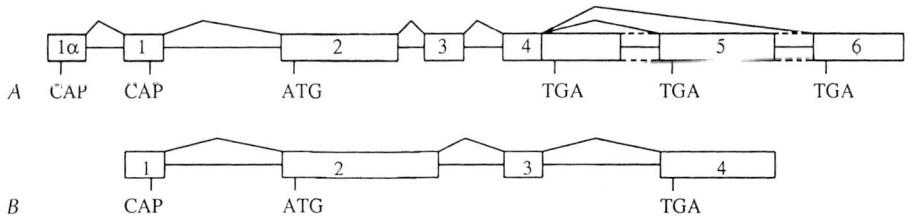

FIGURE 18-3. Structure of the human AChE and BuChE genes. The exonic sequences present in the spliced transcripts are depicted as open boxes in numerical order of their appearance in the genomic sequence. Intron sequences are depicted as single lines. *A.* Human acetylcholinesterase gene. Transcription can be initiated from either of two cap sites designated as exons 1 and 1α, with over 90 percent of the transcripts beginning with exon 1. Three alternatively spliced variants are encoded by this gene, including the read-through 3′ portion encoded in exon 4. The included exons for the alternative transcripts are illustrated connected by angled lines. Alternative exon 5 encodes the carboxyl-terminal amino acids of the hydrophobic or amphiphilic AChE subunit (H subunit), and exon 6 encodes the carboxyl terminus of the catalytic subunit capable of associating with the collagen-like tail and other structural subunits (T subunit). *B.* Human BuChE gene. Only one variant of the BuChE catalytic subunit has been found to date, and it corresponds to the AChE T-subunit form. The sequences encoded by exon 2 in the BuChE gene correspond to the amino acids encoded in exons 2 and 3 of the AChE gene. This "fused" exon is also found in the AChE gene of the electric ray and birds. (*AChE gene structure from Li Y, Camp S, Rachinsky TL, et al: Gene structure of mammalian acetylcholinesterase. J Biol Chem 266:23083–23090, 1991. With permission. BuChE gene structure from Arpagaus M, Kott M, Vatis KP, et al: Structure of the gene for human butyrylcholinesterase. Evidence for single copy. Biochemistry 29:124–131, 1990. With permission.*)

serves to anchor the tetramers to the surface plasma membrane of nerve cells, or (3) perhaps be directly modified with covalently bound phospholipids. Many details of the post-translational modifications of the AChE catalytic subunits still need to be elucidated before our knowledge of their structural diversity will be complete.

The asymmetrical forms of AChE consist of one to three tetramers (G_4 units) covalently linked to a collagen-like "tail." The tail is a partial triple helix involving three polypeptide chains rich in proline and glycine, as is typical of collagen, with an amino terminus that can bind to the catalytic subunits and a carboxyl terminus, predicted to be globular, which contains the localization domain. The collagen-tailed forms are designated A_4, A_8, and A_{12}, depending upon the number of catalytic subunits. Not all collagen-tailed forms are so neatly arranged, though, for in some species subunits other than the catalytic ones may be present. Studies on the collagen-tailed AChE of Torpedo electroplax show that each molecule may contain a noncatalytic 100,000-kDa peptide in addition to the collagen-like tail subunits[16,17]; studies of the avian collagen-tailed AChE have even found covalently attached BuChE.[18] These other subunits could be structural, as suggested by recent studies on the electric ray enzyme, or they may have some as yet unknown function. The collagen-tailed AChE forms are also defined by their sensitivity to collagenase, which removes the tail portion. The collagen-like tail is essential for attaching the cholinesterase molecules to the extracellular matrix (basal lamina), particularly at the neuromuscular junction. In all tissues where collagen-tailed AChE forms are found, the major species is the A_{12} form, with only small amounts of the A_8 and A_4 forms being detected. It is not yet clear whether A_8 and A_4 forms are stable and functionally significant or merely intermediates in the degradation pathway of the A_{12} molecules.

PHYSICAL PROPERTIES OF ACETYLCHOLINESTERASE

As a group, the AChE forms exhibit a variety of physical characteristics related to their oligomeric structure, posttranslational modifications, and subcellular localization. Dimeric and tetrameric forms of AChE are found to some extent in serum of higher vertebrates and can also be extracted from many tissues with aqueous buffers. These are hydrophilic, globular forms referred to as "soluble" or "low salt" extractable AChE. For the most part, however, detergents are needed to solubilize the enzyme molecules from tissue homogenates, indicating that they are either membrane-bound or sequestered within the lumina of intracellular organelles. In general, the detergent-solubilized amphiphilic forms of AChE aggregate upon removal of the detergent as a result of interactions between exposed hydrophobic domains. The best-studied example of this type of AChE is the dimeric form isolated from human erythrocyte membranes.[19,20] The tetrameric AChE isolated from neuronal tissue also belongs to this category; however, it is attached to the membrane via a 20-kDa hydrophobic peptide while the dimeric form from erythrocytes has a glycolipid anchor (see later sections).

Another class of AChE consists of the high-salt extractable forms found almost exclusively in muscle tissue in higher vertebrates. All the collagen-tailed forms fall into this category. Once solubilized, the collagen-tailed AChE forms require high salt concentrations to remain in solution. If the ionic strength is lowered—for example, by dialysis—the collagen-tailed AChE molecules aggregate even in the presence of detergents. When the collagen-like tails are removed by collagenase digestion, the collagen-tailed AChE forms lose their ability to aggregate, indicating that this property is conferred by the tailpiece. Electron microscopy of negatively stained AChE aggregates reveals clusters of molecules attached by their tails. Aggregation of collagen-tailed AChE is promoted by highly charged molecules such as heparan sulfate, chondroitin sulfate, and hyaluronic acid.[21] The ability to bind to proteoglycans, which are normal constituents of basal lamina, may reflect in part the mechanism of attachment of collagen-tailed forms to the cell surface.

Even following extensive extraction of muscle tissue with high-salt and detergent buffers, approximately 10 to 20 percent of the total AChE remains insoluble. Treatment with collagenase, however, can detach this activity from the insoluble extracellular matrix. When preparations of rat or frog muscle are treated with collagenase, all histochemically detectable enzyme activity is lost from the neuromuscular junctions.[22,23] The AChE solubilized only by collagenase digestion appears to be fragments of collagen-tailed AChE molecules that probably were covalently attached to skeletal muscle basal lamina.[24,25] A possible mechanism for this covalent attachment is enzymatically catalyzed cross-linking of amino groups of lysyl residues present both in the tail peptides and in the collagen and other proteins of the extracellular matrix. A second possible mode of attachment could be disulfide bonding of one or more of the 30 cysteinyl residues in the carboxyl terminus of the collagen-like tail with other cysteinyl residues present in the extracellular matrix. These two modes of attachment are not mutually exclusive.

STRUCTURE OF THE NONCATALYTIC SUBUNITS ASSOCIATED WITH ACETYLCHOLINESTERASE

Two noncatalytic subunits have been found covalently attached to the AChE catalytic subunits. The first is the well-described collagenic tail that associates with three tetramers to give rise to the collagen-tailed forms. The primary sequence encoding 455 amino acids has been deduced from the cloned cDNAs in several species, including Torpedo,[26] rat,[27] human,[28] and chicken.[29] Several distinct domains can be discerned, including a very hydrophilic amino-terminus segment that contains the proline-rich attachment domain (PRAD) necessary for covalent attachment of the peptide chain to the catalytic subunits; the triple-helical collagenic domain with cysteines at either end, which can form stabilizing interchain disulfide bonds; and a carboxyl terminus consisting of about 180 amino acids, including a long hydrophilic segment and a distal region containing 10 cysteines that is predicted to form a globular domain. The triple-helical region contains two heparan sulfate–binding sites that may be involved in electrostatic interactions between the collagenic tail and the extracellular matrix,[30] while the carboxyl-terminus globular domain is essential for localizing and attaching the molecule to the synaptic basal lamina.[28,31–33]

The second noncatalytic subunit that can be attached to the $AChE_T$ subunit tetramer is an apparent 20-kDa hydrophobic peptide first described by Inestrosa et al. in 1987[33a] and shown to be expressed predominantly in nervous tissues. Subsequent cloning of the cDNA showed that it encoded a 154–amino acid peptide with a predicted transmembrane domain and a short 31–amino acid cytoplasmic domain.[34] The amino terminus contained a predicted proline-rich domain that was highly homologous to the PRAD found in the collagenic tail sequence. Thus the amino-terminus domain is most likely responsible for covalent attachment to the tetramers, while the transmembrane domain acts as an anchor to retain the enzyme on the plasma membrane. This protein is discussed in more detail in later sections.

Molecular Biology of Cholinesterases

Increasing knowledge of the primary structure of the protein and the molecular basis for the entire family of AChE and BuChE oligomeric forms has gone hand in hand with elucidation of the structures of the AChE and BuChE genes. Nucleotide sequences of AChE genes constitute the database for inferring how these enzymes arose during evolution. Studies on AChE gene promoter regions are revealing how different forms are expressed in different tissues. Analysis of the amino acid sequences of naturally occurring variants of the cholinesterases has shown how these mutants produce their known phenotypes, and analysis of genetically engineered variants has provided insights into the molecular details of catalysis and subunit assembly. We can now expect continued rapid progress toward an understanding of how these genes are regulated and what additional roles these proteins may play in the developing and mature nervous system.

PRIMARY STRUCTURE OF ACETYLCHOLINESTERASE DEDUCED BY MOLECULAR CLONING

The first glimpse of the primary structure of the AChE catalytic subunit came from the deduced amino acid sequence obtained from cDNA clones encoding the enzyme from the electric ray.[35,36] These cDNAs predicted a protein of around 575 amino acids exclusive of the leader peptide, with several potential N-glycosylation sites, in full agreement with the known biochemical information. These initial findings were quickly followed by the isolation and sequencing of cDNA clones encoding the mouse AChE,[37] the human AChE,[38] and the human BuChE.[39] Since then, cholinesterases from numerous species of vertebrates and invertebrates have been cloned and sequenced. All of these cholinesterases share a high level of identity in amino acid sequence, especially in certain regions of the protein that contribute to the active site and domains responsible for attachment to the collagen-like tail. Because these highly conserved regions are the most likely to be involved in catalysis, intra- and interchain disulfide bond formation, subunit assembly, and membrane targeting, the deduced sequences could also predict functions of specific residues in the polypeptide chain. Some of the predictions have been tested and confirmed by site-directed mutagenesis and expression of the mutated proteins in heterologous cell expression systems.

Sequence of the Collagen-like Tail

A subset of AChE catalytic subunits in vertebrates have a noncatalytic collagen-like tail, and it is this collagen-tailed form of the enzyme that is associated with the neuromuscular junction and regulated by nerve-muscle interactions. The primary sequence of the collagen-like tail subunit has been deduced from cloned cDNAs encoding the protein in the electric ray.[40] The cDNA predicts a sequence of 531 amino acids, including the peptide leader sequence, which is cleaved cotranslationally. The polypeptide contains three functional domains: (1) an amino-terminal region that attaches to the catalytic subunits via an interchain disulfide bond; (2) a central collagen-like region rich in glycine, proline, lysine, and arginine; and (3) a carboxyl-terminus region containing 10 cysteine residues, which may be involved in anchoring the protein in the synaptic basal lamina. Coexpression of the cDNA encoding the collagen-tailed subunit in COS cells with cDNA encoding the catalytic subunit of AChE results in assembly of the collagen-tailed form of the enzyme, indicating that coexpression of the two classes of subunits is sufficient to ensure assembly of the collagen-tailed molecules. Details of the interactions between this form of AChE and the synaptic basal lamina are described in later sections.

Sequence of the Prima (P) Subunit

The hydrophobic noncatalytic subunit that anchors the tetrameric AChE form to the plasma membrane of many neurons has recently been cloned and sequenced.[34] The cDNAs from mouse and human are very similar, differing by 14 amino acids. The 154–amino acid peptide encodes a polypeptide predicted to be a type 1 transmembrane glycoprotein with an extracellular domain of about 90 amino acids and a cytoplasmic domain of 31 amino acids, which does not appear to be necessary for either membrane targeting or association with the catalytic subunits. Coexpression of the catalytic subunit together with this peptide results in tetramers being targeted to the cell surface rather than being secreted and thus is necessary for the membrane anchoring of the catalytic subunits. This peptide is most highly expressed in the central nervous system, where the major form of the enzyme is the membrane-associated tetramer.

STRUCTURE OF THE ACETYLCHOLINESTERASE GENE

AChE is encoded by a single gene in all vertebrate species. In humans, the AChE locus is located on chromosome 7p22.[41] The structures of the human AChE[42] and BuChE genes[39] are illustrated diagrammatically in Fig. 18-3. There is considerable similarity among all cholinesterase genes, including those of *Drosophila*, *Torpedo*, chicken, mouse, and human[8,43,44], indicating considerable conservation during evolution. The present discussion will focus on the mammalian gene. One of the most surprising results from recent studies was that deletion of the mouse AChE thus creating a null mutant[45,46] had a relatively mild phenotype, unlike what happens in organisms that have a single cholinesterase gene such as Drosophila and other insects. The explanation most likely is that much of the critical function of AChE in acetylcholine hydrolysis has been taken over by butyrylcholinesterase in the AChE null mouse[47]. This argument is strengthened by the observations that treatment of the AChE null mice with BuChE inhibitors is rapidly lethal, whereas in normal mice they have little or no effect[45].

Most of the coding sequence (535 out of 575 amino acids; 93 percent) of the human AChE catalytic subunit is contained within three exons designated as E2, E3, and E4 (Fig. 18-3). These three coding exons are shared by all oligomeric forms of the enzyme. Variations in the carboxyl terminal amino acids occurs via alternative splicing events which select either of the additional exons 5 or 6, or a read-through sequence in the downstream portion of exon 4. Inclusion of alternative exon 5 adds 30 amino acids at the carboxyl terminus, 28 of which are cleaved during posttranslational processing, to produce a two amino acid extension which can attach to the glycophospholipid anchor, thereby conferring hydrophobicity and the capacity to integrate into lipid bilayers. Alternative exon 6 encodes the 40 amino acid carboxyl terminus capable of associating with either the collagen-like tail or the 20 kDa "P" peptide (Prima), that associates with the plasma membrane through its transmembrane domain. The amino acid sequence encoded by the read-through in exon 4 is predicted to encode a catalytic subunit similar to the form capable of attaching to the collagen-like tail. However, the absence of certain essential cystein residues predicts that this form of the enzyme would be a secreted monomeric species. While the mRNA encoding this putative catalytic subunit has been detected in several tissues examined, including hematopoietic tissues and brain, it is not clear whether it is translated into a functional protein molecule.

The structure of the human BuChE gene is remarkably similar to the AChE gene, to the point of having conserved the same intron-exon boundaries[39] (Fig. 18-3B). However, it also retains some features of the gene found in elasmobranchs, including the single large exon 2 containing most of the coding region. In mammalian AChE, this exon has been interrupted by an intervening sequence to give exons 2 and 3. No hydrophobic variants of the BuChE catalytic subunit have been found, and this observation is supported by the genomic sequence information. In the human BuChE gene exon 4 is homologous to the exon 6 sequence of the AChE gene, which encodes the amino acids required for assembly with the collagen-like tail.

EXPRESSION AND LOCALIZATION OF ACETYLCHOLINESTERASE mRNAs

Regulation of AChE mRNA expression involves both temporal and tissue-specific factors during embryogenesis as well as mechanisms for maintaining appropriate levels of expression in the mature differentiated cells. Although the tissue distribution and cell-type expression of the AChE enzyme has been studied for many years using histochemical and immunocytochemical procedures (see later sections), which clearly requires the expression of AChE mRNA, only recently have the necessary cellular and molecular probes become available for detailed studies on the expression of the AChE transcript.

Higher vertebrates appear to express only the transcripts encoding the catalytic subunit capable of assembling with the collagen-like tail or the 20-kDa peptide in nerves and muscle.[37] In multinucleated skeletal muscle fibers, the mRNAs encoding AChE are translated on the rough endoplasmic reticulum surrounding the nucleus that transcribed them.[48,49] This functional compartmentalization of AChE expression is important because it provides a molecular mechanism for localized control of the AChE gene in mature skeletal muscle fibers. Using a very sensitive polymerase chain reaction (PCR)–based assay to quantitate AChE mRNA levels in segments of single skeletal muscle fibers, Jasmin et al.[50] and Michelle et al.[51] have shown that the AChE mRNA is highly concentrated in the junctional regions of the fibers, whereas the transcripts are rare in the noninnervated regions. This has also been shown by in situ hybridization.[52] These observations suggest that local regulatory factors influenced by the presence of the nerve act to increase expression of this gene either by increasing transcription or stabilizing AChE mRNA in the junctional region.

It is possible that increased local transcription alone is not sufficient to account for the increased expression of AChE mRNA at the neuromuscular junction. Other regulatory events may come into play, including posttranscriptional control of the AChE message.[53] For example, in a muscle cell line, the increases in AChE mRNA after myotube formation can be accounted for by a mechanism increasing the stability of the mRNA. The change in message stability appears to be linked to protein synthesis, because inhibition of protein synthesis by cycloheximide increases AChE mRNA half-life in myoblasts, suggesting rapid turnover of a destabilizing protein. However, to date, these observations have been made only in a muscle cell line and have not yet been observed in mature adult muscle fibers. Thus the relative contributions of each possible level of AChE mRNA regulation to the final amounts found in innervated and noninnervated regions of muscle fibers still remain to be determined.

TRANSCRIPTIONAL CONTROL OF THE ACETYCLCHOLINESTERASE GENE

The promoter regions necessary for regulating expression of the AChE gene have been studied mostly in mouse[54,55] and rat,[56,57] although there is some information on the promoter regions of *Torpedo*,[58] humans,[59,60] and chickens[61] as well. Transcriptional control elements 5-prime of the transcription start site include several E-box elements for muscle-specific factors such as myogenin and MyoD as well as more general *cis*-acting elements such as SP1- and SP2-binding site. Recent studies, however, have pointed to an important role for regulatory elements located within the intron following the first coding region exon, including two N-box elements. These N-box elements are responsive to the Ets family of transcription factors, which are, in turn, activated by neuregulins, neurotrophic factors produced and released by motor neurons as well as many other cell types. The Ets family of transcription factors is essential for differentiation of the neuromuscular junction[62] and for junctional expression of the acetylcholine receptor (AChR) and AChE genes.[63,64] It thus appears that (1) transcriptional elements associated with the myogenic factors are responsible for the initiation of transcription of the AChE gene during muscle differentiation and (2) transcriptional elements associated with the Ets transcription factors maintain the AChE gene active in innervated regions of muscle fibers after muscle activity–coupled events downregulate the enzyme in noninnervated fiber regions.

Function of Acetylcholinesterase

Although the principal known function of AChE is to hydrolyze acetylcholine (ACh) released at cholinergic synapses in the central and peripheral nervous systems, the widespread distribution of the enzyme in noncholinergic cells—such as cells of the erythroid and lymphoid lineages—and at developmental stages when no cholinergic innervation is evident has led to speculations about possible alternative functions. Several studies have suggested the possibility of a peptidase activity associated with AChE, but this was recently shown to be due to contaminating proteases. More interesting is the possibility that AChE may act as a cell surface adhesion or recognition molecule. This unproven speculation is based upon the amino acid sequence similarity between AChE and two *Drosophila* neural cell adhesion molecules, the occurrence of the unique HNK1 epitope (a characteristic of some types of cell surface adhesion molecules) on certain forms of AChE in the central nervous system, and the presence of AChE and BuChE in noncholinergic cells in the developing vertebrate nervous system.[8] There has been some evidence for a cell adhesion role for AChE during neuronal development; evidence for this has always been indirect, and in all cases alternative explanations are possible. Thus the question still remains an open one pending more conclusive data. However, it is clear that deletion of the AChE gene through homologous recombination in mice leads to a fairly mild phenotype of muscle weakness and constant shivering.[45] Had AChE a major role to play in neuronal cell adhesion, one would expect a more severe phenotype. AChE may also have a neuromodulatory role in specific regions of the central nervous system because it is secreted in a stimulus-coupled manner from neurons in the substantia nigra,[65] but the functional significance of AChE, once it is released, is unclear. Our focus here is on the "classic" function of AChE, namely the hydrolysis of the neurotransmitter acetylcholine.

ENZYMATIC MECHANISMS

Until recently, AChE (E.C. 3.1.1.7) was classified in the family of serine esterases, which also includes trypsin, chymotrypsin, plasminogen activator, aromatic amino acid esterase, and many other enzymes. These enzymes are characterized by having serine as part of the catalytic site, the hydroxyl group of serine participating in the formation of the enzyme-substrate complex. However, recent studies on the structure and primary amino acid sequence of the cholinesterases now place them in a separate family that also includes a number of serine hydrolases in organisms as distantly related as slime molds and fungi.[8]

Although ACh is the principal substrate for AChE, the enzyme also hydrolyzes other choline esters, albeit at much reduced rates. Conversely, several other esterases can hydrolyze ACh in addition to their natural substrates, and this reaction, too, occurs at a much slower rate. Thanks to the cloning of AChE and the elucidation of its three-dimensional structure, together with extensive studies using site-directed mutagenesis, the functions of most of the amino acids involved in catalysis are now known. Thus the precise mechanisms of catalysis are now almost completely understood. In brief, it is now thought that ACh initially binds to a charged region, the peripheral anionic site, on the surface of the catalytic subunit near the opening of the active-site gorge and then "glides" down the hydrophobic gorge to reach an expanded pocket at the base containing the catalytic amino acid triad (Ser_{200}, H_{440}, and E_{327}). The oxygen atom on the free hydroxyl group of serine reacts with the α-carbon on the acetate portion of the substrate, forming an acetylated enzyme intermediate and liberating the choline molecule. The acetylated enzyme, in turn, reacts with water to give acetic acid and a regenerated enzyme molecule. The Michaelis constant of the overall reaction is about 60 μM. This reaction is one of the fastest of any known enzyme. The turnover number for AChE has been determined for several different species and ranges from about 1 to 4×10^7 moles of ACh hydrolyzed per mole of enzyme per hour.[66] This translates to about five molecules of ACh hydrolyzed per millisecond per active site.

In the multimeric forms of AChE, each subunit behaves independently. Each subunit has one active site, and there are no allosteric interactions between subunits. The enzyme exhibits substrate inhibition at ACh concentrations above 1 mM. This has been attributed to binding of an ACh molecule to an acylated enzyme intermediate, retarding the liberation of acetate and regeneration of the active enzyme.[67]

The enzymatic mechanisms of BuChE (also referred to as *pseudocholinesterase*) are very similar to those described above except that BuChE does not exhibit substrate inhibition when ACh is used as a substrate. This enzyme preferentially hydrolyzes butyrylcholine and several other choline esters.

Inhibitors of Acetylcholinesterase

Inhibition of AChE at the neuromuscular junction substantially increases the lifetime of ACh in the synaptic cleft. The first effects are an increase in the amplitude and decay time of the synaptic response due to activation of a larger area of the postsynaptic membrane and repeated activations of AChR until ACh leaves the synaptic space by diffusion. This effect is superseded rapidly by desensitization of receptors and consequent blockade of neuromuscular transmission. However, anticholinesterase drugs have proven important in treatment of myasthenia gravis (see Chap. 64). In myasthenia gravis, a shortage of AChRs results in an end plate current insufficient to trigger a much higher action potential, and consequent failure of neuromuscular transmission. Carefully titrated dosages of an anticholinesterase drug can increase the concentration of ACh in the synaptic cleft just enough to potentiate neuromuscular transmission beneficially. Obviously the dosage must be carefully regulated to avoid neuromuscular blockade.

Perhaps the most interesting naturally occurring inhibitors of AChE are the 61–amino acid fasciculin peptides—members of the α-neurotoxin family, which includes α-bungarotoxin, isolated from the venom of the African green mamba snake—called fasciculins because they make the muscle fibers twitch when applied. These peptide neurotoxins contain eight cysteine residues that form four disulfide bonds, making this peptide a very tightly wound molecule.[10] Fasciculin 1 and 2 differ by only one amino acid but differ significantly in their binding affinities for mammalian AChE. The half-life of dissociation of fasciculin 2 (Fas 2) is almost 5 days, making this an extremely useful inhibitor. It has been iodinated and used as a radioactive probe for quantitative electron microscopy autoradiography to visualize and quantitate the distribution of AChE molecules[68] and has been conjugated with fluorophores to produce extremely useful fluorescent probes of AChE.[69,70] A high-resolution image of a mouse neuromuscular junction stained with rhodamine α-bungarotoxin to visualize acetylcholine receptors and Oregon green fasciculin 2 to visualize AChE is shown in Fig. 18-6.

AChE inhibitors are also effective insecticides. Unlike vertebrates, insects use glutamate, and not ACh, as the excitatory transmitter at the neuromuscular junction. However, ACh is a major neurotransmitter in the insect central nervous system, where it is ubiquitous, occurring throughout the cortex and neuropil of the brain and ganglia. Genetic studies with the fruit fly, *Drosophila melanogaster*, indicate that AChE is encoded by a single gene.[71] Mutations in this gene (called *Ace mutations*) can result in the absence of AChE enzyme activity and are lethal. Clever genetic manipulations have been used to generate genetically mosaic flies with some normal tissue mixed with some tissue lacking AChE.[71] In these flies, various neurologic abnormalities have been described, linking AChE function with proper function of various neuronal circuits. Anticholinesterase insecticides presumably mimic the lethal Ace mutations through interference with neuronal functions.

Vertebrates are relatively resistant to many anticholinesterase insecticides for two reasons. First, there is a high concentration of BuChE in blood. Like AChE, this enzyme hydrolyzes ACh efficiently, although it prefers other choline esters, and most of the AChE inhibitors also inhibit BuChE. Thus, BuChE serves as a buffer, interacting with the poison and lowering its effective concentration at the neuromuscular junctions. Second, some of the insecticides do not easily gain access to vertebrate tissue except as a result of accidental ingestion. Cases of anticholinesterase poisoning have occurred with tragic regularity, particularly in underdeveloped countries. A repeated scenario involves undernourished peasants eating seed grain that has been treated with an anticholinesterase such as parathion.

Other anticholinesterase drugs have been developed for use as "nerve gases" for chemical warfare. Such drugs are designed to penetrate the skin and inhibit AChE irreversibly in both peripheral and central nervous systems. Some of these compounds have proven to be valuable tools for exploring the distribution of AChE molecules at neuromuscular junctions and for examining the mechanisms for renewal of synaptic AChE.

Agonist-Induced End Plate Myopathy

Chronic blockade of neuromuscular AChE precipitates a myopathic condition in end plate regions of the affected muscles. This condition was first described by Ariens et al.,[72] who noted that inhibition of junctional AChE led to muscle necrosis that could be prevented by simultaneous blockade of AChRs with curare. This phenomenon has been studied by Engel et al.,[73] Dettbarn and colleagues,[74] and Salpeter and colleagues.[75,76] Salpeter et al. found that diisopropyl fluorophosphate (DFP) blockade of end plate AChE led to very rapid myopathic changes confined to the end plate regions of the affected muscle fibers. Within a few hours, sarcoplasmic reticulum (SR) in the end plate region became dilated and Z disks degenerated. These signs of damage were most severe in the junctional cytoplasm and decreased in severity with increasing distance from the junction (Fig. 18-4).

This led to the hypothesis that the absence of functional AChE results in ACh excess in the synaptic cleft, causing excessive activation of AChRs. The ionic channels opened in response to ACh allow the passage of not only sodium and potassium ions but also calcium ions from the extracellular fluid, where the calcium ion concentration (about 1 mM) is about four orders of magnitude greater than in cytosol of relaxed muscle. The entry of excess calcium, caused by overstimulation of AChRs, triggers the activation of calcium-dependent proteases that attack the Z disks preferentially.[77,78] The excess calcium also overloads the SR, causing swelling. Direct proof of calcium accumulation in the end plate region was obtained recently by Kawabuchi.[79] An end plate myopathy resembling that induced by anticholinesterase also occurs in the slow-channel congenital myasthenic syndrome and in patients with congenital AChE deficiency (see Chap. 66).

This hypothesis explains a variety of observations about the agonist-induced myopathy. The damage resulting from blockade of AChE is not observed if AChRs are not activated during the period of blockade. Thus, denervation or blockade of AChR function by α-bungarotoxin or curare (all conditions eliminating AChR activation) will prevent the damage. Agonist-induced myopathy also occurs in organ culture of skeletal muscle in the presence of carbamylcholine, a nonhydrolyzable cholinergic agonist. This damage mimicked that observed in vivo following DFP inhibition of AChE. In the organ culture situation it was possible to show that extracellular calcium was required for development of the myopathy. Furthermore, leupeptin, an inhibitor of the calcium ion–stimulated protease system, greatly reduced damage to Z disks but did not prevent swelling of the SR. On the other hand, quercetin, an inhibitor of calcium ion transport in the SR, significantly reduced the swelling of the SR without preventing damage to Z disks. Finally, Salpeter and colleagues, citing published observations that dystrophic muscle might be characterized by permanently elevated calcium-dependent proteases, investigated the possibility that dystrophic muscle might be more sensitive to agonist-induced myopathy than normal muscle. Their observations on agonist-induced myopathy at normal versus dystrophic mouse muscles in organ culture were consistent with this idea.

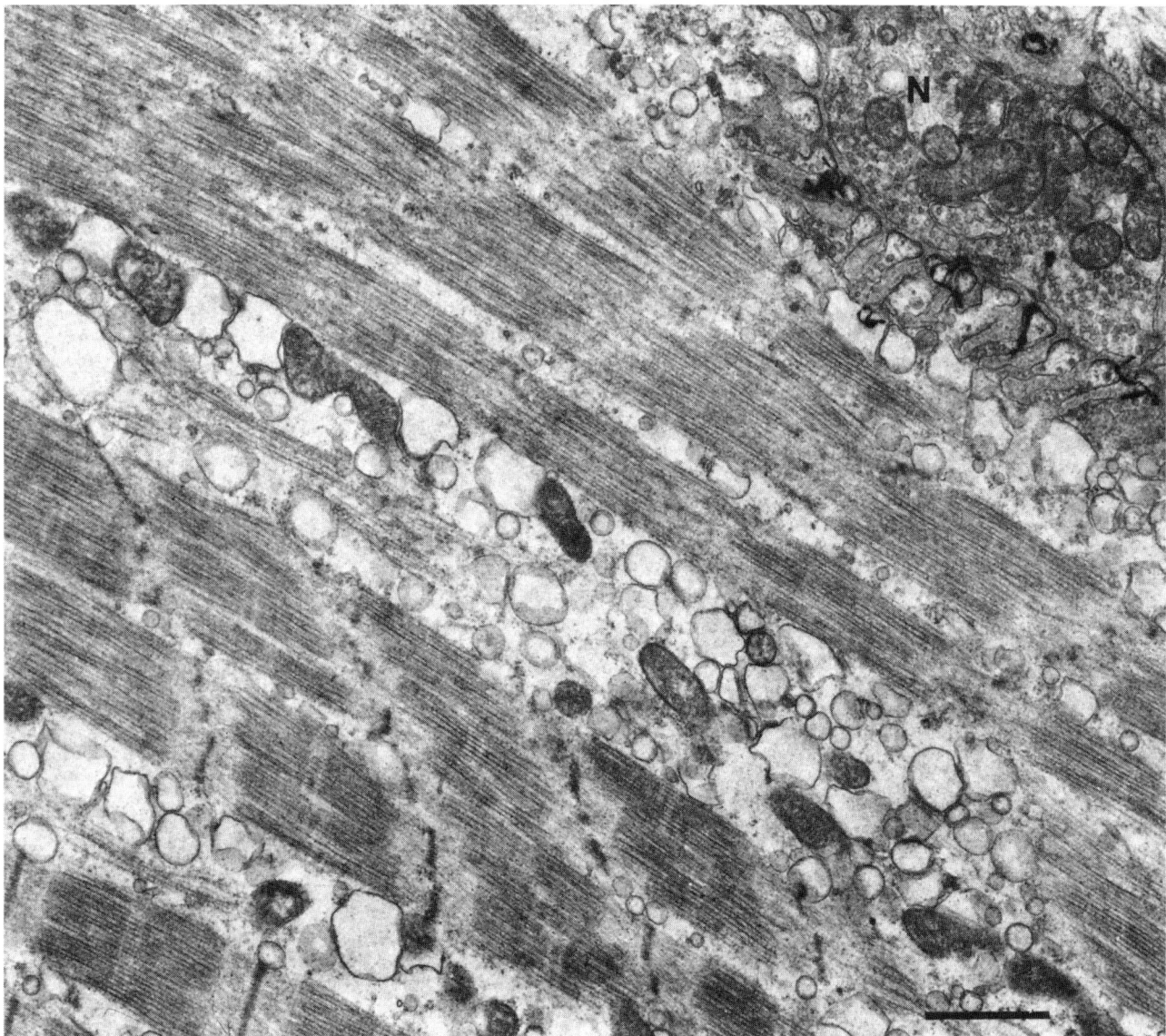

FIGURE 18-4. Autoradiograph of end plate region following inactivation of esterases with [^{3}H] DFP. Note gradation in severity of damage to Z disks from the neuromuscular junction (upper right) into the sarcoplasm. N = nerve terminal. (Magnification bar is 1 μm.)

(From Salpeter MM: Electron microscope radioautography as a quantitative tool in enzyme cytochemistry: I. The distribution of acetylcholinesterase at motor end plates of a vertebrate twitch muscle. J Cell Biol 32:379, 1967. With permission.)

Congenital Myasthenia with End Plate AChE Deficiency

Congenital myasthenia with end plate AChE deficiency was first reported in 1977 by Engel,[80] who was treating a patient who appeared to have almost normal expression of AChE catalytic activity but completely lacked the enzyme at the neuromuscular junction. Detailed biochemical and morphologic studies of the muscle showed that the tissue lacked the collagen-tailed form of AChE. Analysis of the AChE transcripts from several patients showed that the catalytic subunit was normal; thus the problem was not the lack of an appropriate enzyme subunit. Subsequent cloning and sequencing of the ColQ cDNAs clearly showed that the problem was with the noncatalytic subunit.[28,31,32] Mutations varied from premature termination codons resulting in truncations in ColQ near the amino-terminus translation polypeptides that could induce tetramerization of the $AChE_T$ subunits to single amino acid substitutions that in some cases completely prevented binding of the ColQ to the synaptic basal lamina. These studies not only disclosed the molecular basis for this disorder but also provided conclusive evidence that the ColQ portion of the molecule is what confers the ability of AChE to localize to the basal lamina (see also Chap. 66).

MODELING THE ROLE OF ACETYLCHOLINESTERASE AT THE NEUROMUSCULAR JUNCTION

Mathematical models in biology are generated to test whether our concepts and parametric measurements are sufficiently self-consistent and complete to explain our observations. Several such models have been developed to account for events at the neuromuscular junction.[81–84b] These models test the assumption that the time course and magnitude of the end plate current during neuromuscular transmission or of the miniature end plate current caused by the spontaneous release of a single ACh quantum can be modeled accurately. The models incorporate the parameters of chemical reaction of ACh with AChRs and AChE and reasonable values for the number of ACh molecules released per quantum, the spatial density of AChRs and of AChE, the diffusion rate of ACh in the synaptic cleft, and the geometry of the synaptic cleft. Perhaps the most interesting conclusion from the models insofar as AChE is concerned is that they readily explain the paradoxical interposition of AChE in the cleft between the ACh release sites on the nerve terminal and the AChRs on the muscle and the order of magnitude faster rate constant for association of ACh with AChE than with AChR. The models further suggest that substrate inhibition of AChE is not very significant during neuromuscular transmission. Rather, it appears to be simply a biologically insignificant consequence of the molecular mechanism of ACh hydrolysis.

A comforting aspect of the models is that they account for most experimental results. This suggests that our present understanding of the parameters of neuromuscular transmission may be quite adequate. They confirm the effectiveness of AChE in the junction and explain the failure of AChE to prevent access of ACh to the receptor sites. Finally, the models suggest that the details of structure of the synaptic cleft, aside from distance of nerve terminal from postsynaptic membrane, are not important in determining the total duration of the end plate current. On the other hand, the junctional folds are important because they increase the surface into which AChRs can be packed and, by presenting a high-resistance pathway, augment the amplitude of the voltage response to reach the voltage-gated sodium channels concentrated in the troughs of the folds.[84a,84b] Moreover, the folds may salvage products accumulating in the cleft during neuromuscular transmission, i.e., acetate, hydrogen ions, choline, and potassium. When AChE is blocked by inhibitors, the models acquire very much greater sensitivity to exact synaptic morphology. This may be understood by considering that in the absence of AChE, the rate of diffusion of ACh from the synaptic cleft (which, of course, depends upon cleft morphology) becomes a more significant component in terminating the response.

METHODS FOR DETECTING, LOCALIZING, AND QUANTITATING ACETYLCHOLINESTERASE

Many methods for measuring AChE activity have been developed over the years. Most of these are based upon the use of chromogenic substrates or radioactively labeled ACh. The most common colorimetric assay is that of Ellman et al.,[85] which employs acetylthiocholine as a substrate. The hydrolysis of acetylthiocholine yields thiocholine, which, in turn, reacts with the sulfhydryl reagent dithiobisnitrobenzoic acid (DTNB) to form a yellow product. The intensity of the resulting color is proportional to the amount of acetylthiocholine hydrolyzed, and the results are expressed in terms of millimoles substrate hydrolyzed per unit time. The radiometric assays employ either ^{3}H- or ^{14}C-labeled ACh with the label on the acetyl group.[86] Following hydrolysis of ACh, labeled acetate is extracted and counted in a liquid scintillation counter. Alternatively, unreacted ACh can be extracted from the reaction mixture with sodium tetraphenylboron and the remaining labeled acetic acid counted. A third assay method, which is rarely used, involves titrating the acetic acid resulting from the hydrolysis of ACh with a weak or dilute base.

Although all enzymatic assays for AChE employ either ACh or an ACh analogue as substrate, this alone is not sufficient to ensure the specificity of the reaction. As mentioned in earlier sections, several other enzymes are capable of hydrolyzing ACh in addition to their natural substrates. The specificity of the AChE assay is thus contingent on the demonstration that these other enzymes contribute negligibly if at all to the hydrolysis of ACh. This is accomplished through the use of selective inhibitors, often incorporated directly into the reaction mixture. Neostigmine or physostigmine (eserine) is often used to discriminate between cholinesterases and nonspecific esterases capable of hydrolyzing ACh; this drug selectively inhibits all cholinesterases. Fortunately, the presence of interfering nonspecific esterases is rarely a problem. Somewhat more of a problem is the presence of BuChE, which in some tissues can account for more than half of the cholinesterase enzyme activity. In this case tetraisopropylpyrophosphoramide (Iso-OMPA), a specific irreversible inhibitor of BuChE, can be added before assay. The rate of ACh hydrolysis in the presence of this inhibitor can then taken to be the true measure of AChE activity.

Several procedures have been developed for the histochemical localization of AChE and BuChE in tissues at the light and electron microscope levels. The most specific of these procedures, using acetyl- or butyrylthiocholine iodide as the substrate, were developed by Koelle and Friedenwald[87] and Karnovsky and Roots.[88] Readers interested in the specifics of the chemical reactions in these procedures should consult Tsuji.[89] Both these methods take advantage of the fact that thiocholine (a product of enzymatic cleavage of acetylthiocholine) is an SH-radical that can form complexes with certain heavy metals such as copper. In the Koelle method (Fig. 18-5), the thiocholine reacts with copper glycine to form a white precipitate that, upon treatment with ammonium sulfide, yields a black precipitate easily visualized in the light microscope. The reaction of Karnovsky and Roots yields a thiocholine copper ferricyanide complex with a reddish-brown tint. The products of both reactions involve heavy metals, hence are electron-dense and can be seen with an electron microscope. It should be noted that the histochemical procedures for AChE localization are subject to the same limitations of specificity as the enzymatic assays. Thus, appropriate inhibitors of nonspecific esterases or BuChE must be included in the reaction solutions.

Now that AChE has been purified to homogeneity from several different species—including the electric eel,[90–92] ray,[5] chicken,[93] and human[94]—antibodies are now available for immunocytochemical localization of AChE (Fig. 18-5).[94] Immunocytochemical techniques depend on the formation of a precipitate and thus always pose the problem of diffusion of reaction products away from the site of esterase activity. These problems can be circumvented by the use of fluorescent secondary antibodies, or by biotinylating the anti-AChE antibody followed by fluorescent streptavidin. While these

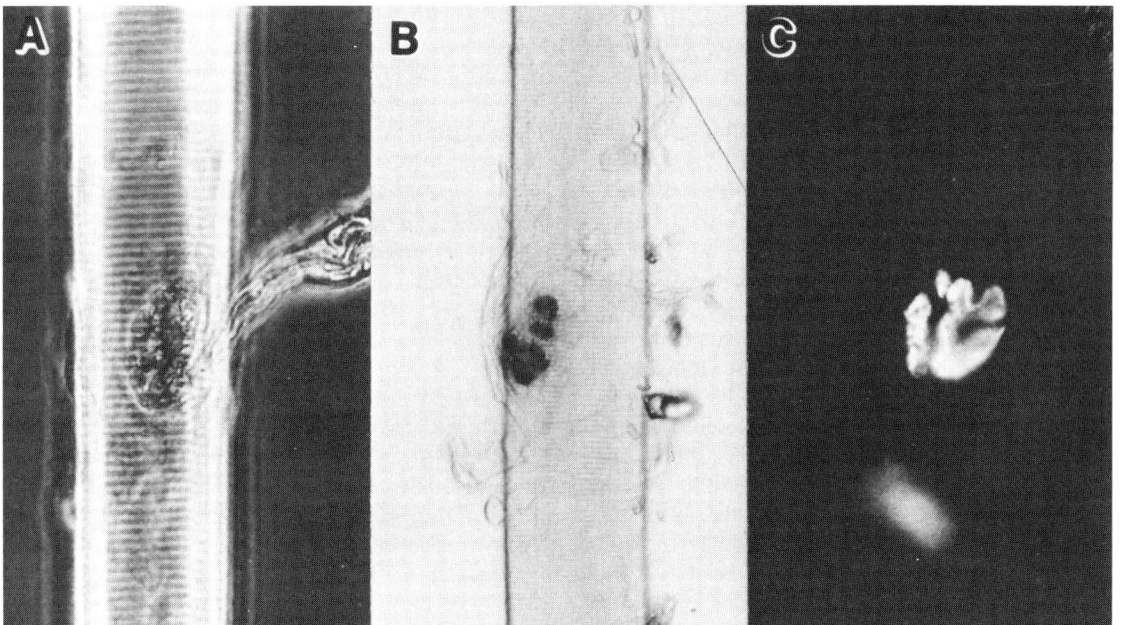

FIGURE 18-5. Single human muscle fiber end plate regions. *A.* Phase micrograph showing attachment of myelinated axon to muscle fiber. *B.* Fiber with neuromuscular junction heavily stained by the Koelle method for AChE. *C.* Immunofluorescence micrograph showing fluorescence resulting from anti-AChE antibody bound to junctional AChE and revealed by a fluorescent-labeled second antibody directed against the first.

immunofluorescence methods require their own specific sets of controls, such as labeling with nonspecific monoclonal antibodies or preimmune serum, they are generally more specific than the cytochemical procedures. Recently, the development of fasciculin 2, a highly specific fluorescent toxin[69] that binds AChE, has almost eliminated the problem of specificity and produced high-resolution localization of the enzyme at cholinergic synapses (Fig. 18-6).

One important and as yet unanswered question regarding the histochemical procedures for locating AChE is to what extent the appearance and persistence of the reaction product depend on its location in or on the cell. Does the reaction product depend on other molecules in its environs for its precipitation? And, hence, does the staining reveal only a particular subset of AChE molecules? These questions can now be answered using combinations of histochemical and immunofluorescence techniques.

Tissue Distribution, Metabolism, and Regulation of Acetylcholinesterase

CELLULAR DISTRIBUTION OF ACETYLCHOLINESTERASE FORMS

Acetylcholinesterase Forms in Muscle

Smooth muscle and cardiac muscle are devoid of the collagen-tailed AChE forms even though the muscle cells are in contact

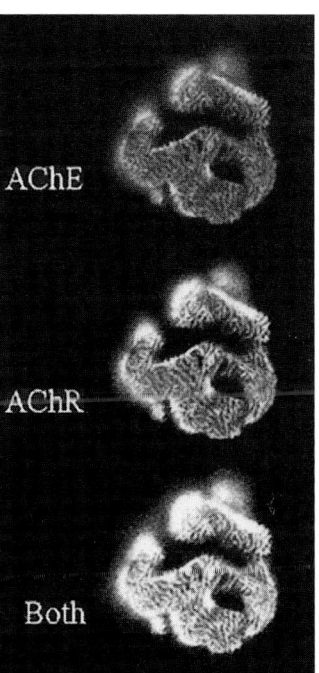

FIGURE 18-6. Mouse neuromuscular junction stained with fluorescent toxins. Single teased mouse gastrocnemius muscle fibers were incubated with rhodamine-conjugated fasciculin 2 to label the AChE (upper panel) and with Oregon Green α-bungarotoxin to label the acetylcholine receptors (middle panel). Superimposition of the two images (lower panel) illustrates the high degree of colocalization at the neuromuscular junction. (*Image by H. Pu and R. Rotundo. With permission.*)

with an extensive extracellular matrix. These muscle types exhibit primarily the dimeric (G_2) and tetrameric (G_4) forms, with smaller amounts of the monomeric form also present. The AChEs in these tissues have not been well characterized; hence, little is known about their subcellular location, solubility characteristics, and relation to nerve terminals.

The oligomeric forms of AChE in skeletal muscles have been more extensively studied, especially in higher vertebrates, with respect to both muscle type and localization.[6,8] Not all muscle types exhibit the same patterns of AChE forms, although in all skeletal muscles both collagen-tailed and globular forms are present to varying degrees. It should be noted, however, that because all studies have been conducted on whole muscles we cannot ascribe a particular pattern of AChE forms to any individual muscle fiber type except in those muscles in mammals and birds that consist predominantly of a single fiber type. As a rule, muscles containing predominantly fast-twitch fibers, such as the posterior latissimus dorsi in the chicken or the gastrocnemius in the rat, contain predominantly the collagen-tailed A_{12} form of AChE and lesser amounts of globular forms. On the other hand, muscles containing predominantly slow fiber types contain a much lower proportion of the collagen-tailed AChE forms. Some muscles, such as the rat diaphragm, have all the oligomeric forms, with collagen-tailed AChE accounting for 25 to 30 percent of the total. In many cases, systematic solubilization procedures have not been performed to distinguish between soluble and membrane-bound globular forms. In most instances these distinctions are not yet clear, because one must also take into consideration the intracellular versus extracellular distribution of these molecules (see below in this section). However the possible molecular basis for these differences in fiber-type expression has recently been elucidated by Krejci and colleagues, who showed that fast muscles express higher levels of ColQ and that this tends to be more highly localized at sites of nerve-muscle contact, whereas slow muscle fibers tend to have lower levels of ColQ, and this is expressed more widely throughout the fiber length.[94a]

Differences in the relative abundance of AChE oligomeric forms may occur along the length of individual muscle fibers. In most higher vertebrates, the collagen-tailed AChE forms appear concentrated at the neuromuscular junction,[95] although they are present in extrajunctional regions as well. The ratio of junctional to extrajunctional collagen-tailed AChE varies widely from one species to another. In human intercostal muscle there may be little if any difference in the relative abundance of these high-molecular-weight forms in innervated and uninnervated regions of muscle.[96] However, the possible contribution of AChE localized at the myotendinous junctions was not taken into consideration in these studies.

Up to this point, we have discussed the many forms of AChE with little specific reference to their subcellular location. Although the most detailed studies on the distribution of AChE localization have been done using cultured muscle cells, a sufficient number of quantitative studies have used whole muscle to permit some generalization. Virtually all studies are in agreement that about one-half or more of the total AChE present in muscle is located intracellularly. These studies employ assays designed to distinguish between intracellular and extracellular enzyme molecules by use of membrane-permeant and membrane-impermeant inhibitors.[97] Localizations of intracellular AChE determined at the electron microscopic level include the rough endoplasmic reticulum (RER), Golgi apparatus, vesicular structures, and occasionally the nuclear membrane.[98,99] The enzyme is also found within the sarcoplasmic reticulum and in the T-tubule system, which is continuous with the external plasma membrane. Within the limits of available techniques, there is little if any cytoplasmic AChE. Based on metabolic studies, the intracellular AChE consists almost entirely of newly synthesized enzyme molecules at various stages of assembly, processing, and transport to the plasma membrane. The predominant intracellular forms of AChE are the globular forms. However, small amounts of the collagen-tailed enzyme molecules are also present. A more detailed account of their interrelationships is presented in the section on biosynthesis, below.

Extracellular AChE can be quantified by treating a portion of muscle with echothiophate iodide, a membrane-impermeant inhibitor, and comparing the pattern of AChE forms with those from untreated muscle. The most detailed study of this type has been done by Younkin et al.,[100] who quantified the intracellular and extracellular AChE forms in innervated and uninnervated regions of the rat diaphragm. All oligomeric forms of AChE—except the monomeric form, which is entirely intracellular—are found in both intracellular and extracellular compartments. Some of the globular forms are associated with the plasma membrane, with their active site oriented toward the cell exterior. All the extracellular collagen-tailed forms are probably associated with the basement membrane that surrounds each muscle fiber. In addition, a certain proportion of the enzyme molecules may be secreted into the body fluids. Many if not most AChE molecules are located outside the neuromuscular junction. Their function, if any, is not known.

Relation of Forms to the Organization of the Neuromuscular Junction

It is apparent from histochemical staining of skeletal muscle that there is a relatively high concentration of AChE at neuromuscular junctions. A far more quantitative determination has been accomplished by Salpeter and colleagues, using autoradiography following labeling of AChE with [^{32}P]DFP.[101,102]

Salpeter et al. and later in collaboration with Anglister have combined this labeling strategy with electron microscopic autoradiography to determine that the AChE activity is distributed throughout the synaptic cleft and secondary folds of the neuromuscular junction. The number of enzymatic sites at the neuromuscular junction varies considerably depending on the species[103,104] and can range from a low of about 600 active sites per square micrometer in the frog to about 2500/μm^2 in the mouse. Yet in all cases there is a surplus of catalytic sites over what is necessary to ensure complete hydrolysis of acetylcholine during neuromuscular transmission. Although many lines of evidence point to the basal lamina as a site of attachment of AChE at the neuromuscular junction, the most graphic demonstration of this was accomplished by McMahan and coworkers,[105] who found that, in the frog cutaneous pectoris muscle, both muscle and nerve terminal could be removed by freezing a portion of the muscle and cutting the nerve, leaving only empty basal lamina sheaths and surrounding extracellular matrix. The basal lamina, which formerly was located at neuromuscular junctions, could still be stained histochemically for AChE. These studies all showed that at least a part of the junctional AChE is incorporated into synaptic basal lamina. It may be that this AChE is relatively stable metabolically and that it would thus account for the fact that former neuromuscular junctions can remain positive in histochemical staining for AChE for many months following denervation of the muscle. More recent immunofluorescence studies using specific antibodies against AChE have shown that most if not all of the AChE at the neuromuscular junction is tightly associated with the synaptic basal lamina and most likely covalently attached.[106,107] Homogenizations using a variety of techniques as well as extraction using high- and low-ionic-strength buffers as well as the chaotropic agents, such as 6 M guanidine HCl or 8 M urea, followed by immunofluorescence localization, all showed that the enzyme remains tightly associated with the basal lamina. Thus it is likely that all of the AChE localized at the sites of nerve-muscle contact is the collagen-tailed form.

There is evidence for other types of cholinesterases at the neuromuscular junction and possibly serine proteases as well, but their function and distributions are poorly understood. Because AChE occurs in pre- and postsynaptic cells, both at the synapse and elsewhere, it is extremely difficult to assign a particular subcellular location to any given form of AChE unequivocally. A major difficulty in quantitatively determining the AChE forms at sites of nerve-muscle contact is our inability to isolate the neuromuscular junctions in pure form. To date, our best estimates of the types and relative abundance of AChE forms at the neuromuscular junction in skeletal muscle derive from studies in chicken, rat, and human, where individual muscles have been dissected into end plate–rich and end plate–free regions. In the rat, the collagen-tailed AChE forms are greatly enriched at the sites of nerve-muscle contact. Rat diaphragm, for example, contains approximately 60 percent of the collagen-tailed AChE concentrated at the neuromuscular junction. If the area of the neuromuscular junction represents 0.1 percent of the total surface area of the muscle fiber, then the junction is increased 1500-fold over the rest of the fiber.

Some biochemical analyses of human and chicken muscles suggest that even the collagen-tailed forms are distributed over the entire muscle surface, although they are present at higher concentrations at the neuromuscular junction. However, in some instances there appears to be little if any increase in the collagen-tailed forms of AChE in regions of nerve-muscle contact. In fact, in the chicken there is no correlation between the amount of synaptic specialization and the occurrence of collagen-tailed AChE. The multiply innervated anterior latissimus dorsi muscles in the chicken have only a few percent of total AChE as the collagen-tailed form, whereas in the singly innervated posterior latissimus dorsi muscles the vast majority of the AChE is the collagen-tailed form.[108,109] In spite of all these observations, it must be emphasized that regardless of the extraction procedures used, most if not all of the junctional AChE remains associated with the synaptic basal lamina. Thus far, the one common denominator that has emerged is the association of the collagen-tailed AChE molecules with the basal lamina and their extraction from tissues with high-ionic-strength buffers. In most cases, all the expressed forms of the enzyme are distributed throughout the length of the muscle fiber even though a high concentration of AChE accumulates at sites of nerve-muscle contact. However, see further discussion below.

Association of the Collagen-Tailed Forms with the Extracellular Matrix

Studies using membrane fractions enriched in synapses isolated from the electric organs of the ray indicated that purified collagen-tailed AChE can attach after the original AChE has been removed by treatment with high-salt buffers. These studies suggested that the electroplax synapses, which are homologous to the neuromuscular junction of higher vertebrates, have associated with them molecules capable of binding collagen-tailed AChE. The tail portion of the collagen-tailed AChE can also bind to certain proteoglycans such as chondroitin sulfate and hyaluronic acid[110] as well as to collagen-binding proteins such as fibronectin.[111] The binding of AChE to certain lipids and glycolipids has also been demonstrated. In some cases, covalent bonds can form between the tail of AChE and extracellular matrix molecules such as fibronectin or possibly even collagen. Thus, several possible mechanisms for the attachment of collagen-tailed AChE to the basal lamina can be demonstrated in vitro.

However, it should be emphasized that all of the above studies employed biochemical approaches to either solubilize AChE or determine binding to extracellular matrix fractions or molecules. In all cases studied, 10 to 25 percent of the enzyme could not be solubilized from skeletal muscle using extraction buffers. As already mentioned, a recent study designed to re-examine the question of AChE attachment to the synaptic basal lamina employed anti-AChE monoclonal antibodies and indirect immunofluorescence to determine the distribution of AChE molecules on the basal lamina following extraction. Several extraction procedures including high-ionic-strength buffers, heparin, or chaotropic agents, such as 8 M urea or 4 M guanidine hydrochloride, failed to remove the AChE associated with the neuromuscular junctions, although most muscle AChE was solubilized.[112] Thus, the junctional forms of AChE are very tightly associated with the extracellular matrix, most likely by covalent attachment.

The strongest evidence for the unique presence of the collagen-tailed AChE form at the neuromuscular junction comes from genetic studies on mice and humans. Recent studies using mice whose *ColQ* gene has been deleted by homologous recombination[113] and human patients with mutations in the *ColQ* gene[28,31,32] have provided convincing evidence that the collagen-tailed form of the enzyme is the predominant if not unique form of AChE at the neuromuscular junction. In all cases, removal of the ColQ subunit leads to a complete absence of AChE at the synapse. Had other forms of AChE been able to localize to the sites of nerve-muscle contact in significant amounts, they would have been detected using the sensitive immunofluorescence methods employed in those studies.

The question now becomes: How does the collagen-tailed AChE form become localized to the neuromuscular junction? While the presence of high levels of AChE mRNA in the subsynaptic cytoplasm, as well as higher levels of the protein, suggests that higher levels of local synthesis are occurring, these observations still do not explain the higher levels of the enzyme associated with the extracellular matrix. Since the collagen-tailed AChE form is a secreted molecule, it must be locally released and then associate with some component of the extracellular matrix. The first evidence that this might be the case was experiments showing that incubation of purified avian collagen-tailed AChE with frozen sections of frog muscle resulted in the attachment of the avian enzyme to the frog neuromuscular junction.[114] These studies provided the first evidence for a specific AChE acceptor site on the synaptic basal lamina. The identity of this site became clear several years later when a series of studies showed that perlecan, a heparan sulfate proteoglycan that colocalizes with AChE, was the most likely acceptor molecule. The collagen-tailed AChE form binds to perlecan both in vitro and on live cells[69] and is capable of being transported to the sites of nerve contact on the surface of a tissue-cultured myotube. Eliminating the expression of either dystroglycan or perlecan in muscle results in the complete elimination of AChE from the synaptic basal lamina, even though an intact ColQ is attached to the catalytic subunits and all other known components of the neuromuscular junction are normally expressed and assembled.[115,116]

Acetylcholinesterase Forms in Neural Tissues

Less information is available concerning the neuronal forms of AChE, largely because of the heterogeneity of the tissues extracted for study. The major AChE forms in neural tissues, such as in brain and sciatic nerve, are dimeric and tetrameric molecules, occasionally with smaller amounts of the monomeric and collagen-tailed forms. The relative abundance of each molecular form depends upon the tissue and the species. In lower vertebrates, collagen-tailed AChE is present in all neural tissues, whereas in higher vertebrates it is frequently absent. In the rat and chicken, it is found in motor nerves but not sensory ones. It is absent from brain in rats but present in small amounts in the optic tectum of the chicken. In all species examined, including humans, the predominant form in brain is the membrane-associated G_4 tetramer. This form is anchored to the plasma membrane via a hydrophobic 154–amino acid glycopeptide,[34] as was described in earlier sections. The molecular forms of AChE in the peripheral nervous system of humans are yet to be described in similar detail, but are most likely very much like the brain tetramer if not identical.

The axoplasmic transport of AChE in peripheral nerves has been studied extensively, although few studies have included examination of the transport of individual molecular forms. It is now clear that the various forms do not travel down the axon at the same rate. The monomeric and dimeric species move with the slow components of transport or not at all, indicating that a large portion is stationary.[117,118] A much larger fraction of the tetrameric AChE and all the collagen-tailed AChE appear to move with the fast components of axoplasmic transport. It should be noted, however, that when the collagen-tailed AChE is found in nerves, it contributes only a very small percentage of the total enzyme present.[117,119]

One important question arises: What if any is the contribution of neuronal AChE to the neuromuscular junction? The detailed electron microscopic autoradiographic studies of Salpeter and colleagues indicate that at least a small portion of the total junctional enzyme is associated with the presynaptic plasma membrane. It has not yet been possible to determine the forms of the enzyme associated with the nerve terminal in species other than the electric ray, where it is possible to purify nerve endings. In this case the only AChE form associated with the nerve terminal is the glycolipid-anchored dimeric form of the enzyme. More important is the possible deposition of collagen-tailed AChE molecules, synthesized by the neurons and transported toward the periphery. That this can indeed occur has recently been shown in the frog. Using a procedure that causes complete degeneration of the muscle while preserving intact the basal lamina and site of nerve-muscle contact, Anglister showed that the nerve can restore the AChE localized on the synaptic basal lamina.[120] However, given the small quantities of collagen-tailed AChE present in nerves compared to muscle, it is unlikely that the neuronal enzyme contributes significantly to AChE at the end plate. Estimates comparing collagen-tailed AChE in muscle and nerve suggest that it would require about 6 months for the sciatic nerve to transport collagen-tailed enzyme molecules equivalent to those found in muscle, a value substantially greater than the known recovery time of AChE at reinnervated neuromuscular junctions.

Acetylcholinesterase Forms in Blood

All vertebrate species examined to date have AChE circulating in the blood, either soluble in the plasma, associated with erythrocytes, or both. Most ACh hydrolyzing activity present in the blood is due to BuChE or nonspecific esterases; hence care must be taken to distinguish between the various molecular species. In humans, the dimeric hydrophobic form of AChE is found in the plasma membrane of erythrocytes[19,29]; in other mammals, both dimeric and tetrameric forms are found.[8] Depending upon the species, varying proportions of all globular AChE forms are found soluble in plasma.

The AChE forms found in blood are likely to derive from several sources. Adrenal chromaffin cells and neurons can release the enzyme into the blood or the cerebral spinal fluid. Muscle cells secrete AChE, at least in tissue culture. Dystrophic chickens have higher levels of plasma AChE than control, as do chickens that have had the pectoral muscles denervated, suggesting that degenerating muscle may contribute as well. The origin of the erythrocyte AChE is unknown. The number of AChE molecules per erythrocyte, estimated at about 200 to 300, is far below what one might expect for a membrane protein. In fact, this number of enzyme molecules could be reasonably explained by a single "leaky" gene transcribing one to several mRNA molecules, each in turn being translated for a couple of hours. An interesting alternative hypothesis has been proposed by Rosenberry,[121] who suggested that the erythrocyte AChE could be picked up from smooth muscle or other cells in the vasculature. This idea receives support from the observation that AChE molecules can spontaneously translocate from erythrocyte membrane to synthetic phospholipid vesicles when these are mixed together in suspension.[122] Regardless of origin, the functional roles of serum and erythrocyte AChE are unknown.

A very small percentage of humans lack BuChE in blood but are not distinguished by any obvious defect. However, when such individuals are given succinylcholine, which is a routine procedure for major surgery, these patients hydrolyze the succinylcholine extremely slowly and generally remain paralyzed and require artificial respiration for hours before they regain neuromuscular transmission.

BIOSYNTHESIS OF ACETYLCHOLINESTERASE

All AChE forms are glycoproteins; hence the events of biosynthesis and intracellular transport resemble those of other plasma membrane and secretory proteins. Detailed studies of the synthesis and metabolism of AChE have been done only with cultured muscle cells. The AChE molecules are synthesized on rough endoplasmic reticulum (ER) and sequestered within its lumen. Glycosylation of AChE most likely occurs cotranslationally, during elongation of polypeptide chains, which explains why partially glycosylated AChE polypeptides are not found in the cells. Assembly of globular AChE forms occurs within minutes after synthesis, yielding catalytically active dimers and tetramers. These are subsequently transported to the Golgi apparatus, where further modification of the asparagine-linked carbohydrate groups occurs. The mature molecules are then transported to the surface of the muscle fiber, where they are either released as secretory molecules or retained on the plasma membrane as cell surface molecules. The transit time of the globular forms from site of synthesis to the cell surface is approximately 2 to 3 h in cultured muscle cells.[97,123,124]

The posttranslational events related to processing of the glycolipid-anchored form of AChE probably occur in the RER within 1 to 3 min following translation of the catalytic subunit. The glycolipid anchor is a complex structure consisting of multiple carbohydrate residues, some with covalently attached lipids, and an ethanolamine moiety that links the complex to the terminal cysteinyl residue of AChE. The structure of the glycolipid anchor associated with human erythrocyte AChE has been determined.[125] This portion of the molecule appears to be synthesized in the rough endoplasmic reticulum as a large precursor. Following translation of the AChE catalytic subunit, the 28 carboxy-terminal residues are cleaved and the glycolipid anchor is transferred intact to the terminal amino acid residue. For reasons that are as yet unknown, only a dimeric form of AChE is associated with the glycolipid anchor. The hydrophobic tetrameric G_4 form found in the nervous systems of higher vertebrates appears to be associated with a 20-kDa lipid-linked polypeptide,[126,127] but this particular posttranslational modification of AChE has not yet been characterized in detail.

The synthesis and assembly of the collagen-tailed AChE forms are somewhat more complex. Unlike the globular forms, the collagen-tailed AChE appears only much later in the biosynthetic pathway, approximately 1.5 to 2 h after the assembly of the dimers and tetramers.[124] The collagen-tailed AChE is most likely assembled in the Golgi apparatus from component parts assembled in the rough ER. Shortly after assembly, the tailed form of AChE is externalized on the muscle fiber surface, where it rapidly becomes attached to the extracellular matrix. Krejci et al.[40] have shown that coexpression of the collagen-like tail subunits with the catalytic subunits in a cell line that does not normally express AChE resulted in assembly of collagen-tailed AChE forms. These studies prove that coexpression of the catalytic and collagen-tailed mRNAs in the same cell is sufficient to ensure proper assembly of the collagen-tailed forms of the enzyme.

As discussed in the earlier section on AChE mRNA localization, the transcripts encoding the catalytic subunit tend to localize and are preferentially around the nucleus of origin.[48,49] The newly synthesized AChE monomers are also assembled and processed in the organelles surrounding the nucleus that encoded the transcript. Recent studies have shown that AChE associated with the extracellular matrix of tissue-cultured myotubes accumulates in clusters, and that those clusters are located directly over the nuclei.[128] Furthermore, experiments using mosaic quail-mouse myotubes and species-specific antibodies to localize the AChE molecules on the cell surface by immunofluorescence indicate that the locally translated and assembled AChE oligomers are preferentially targeted to the regions of the cell surface overlying the nucleus of origin. Together, these studies suggest a plausible mechanism for AChE accumulation at sites of nerve-muscle contact where the availability of AChE mRNA for translation would allow for local synthesis, assembly, and transport of AChE to the cell surface where the enzyme can rapidly attach to the overlying extracellular matrix. Since AChE mRNA is preferentially expressed in the subsynaptic sarcoplasm,[50] this alone could ensure adequate numbers of AChE molecules in the synaptic cleft.

REGULATION OF ACETYLCHOLINESTERASE SYNTHESIS AND LOCALIZATION

The regulation of AChE may occur at multiple levels. One level is transcriptional control, control of how and when the AChE gene becomes transcriptionally active in each tissue and the rate at which the mRNA is transcribed. A second level of regulation involves the many posttranscriptional events leading up to the translation of AChE RNAs, including the alternative splicing that generates alternative catalytic subunits. There is some evidence for translational control steps, but many details still need to be worked out to confirm this as a physiologically significant mechanism. The subsequent posttranslational events, including assembly of the AChE polypeptides and posttranslational modifications, such as glycosylation, glycolipid addition, and activation of the molecules to produce catalytically active enzyme, could all become potential regulatory points under certain circumstances. Finally, a third level of regulation might govern transport to the appropriate subcellular locations and maintenance of the various molecular forms of AChE at their sites of function. We are still just beginning to understand these various steps in expression of AChE, and our understanding of regulatory controls remains fragmentary.

It is clear that AChE is expressed very early during myogenesis. AChE is present in myoblasts and even perhaps presumptive myoblasts. Following fusion of myoblasts to form multinucleated myotubes, there is a large increase in the levels of AChE activity, expressed on a per-nucleus basis. Prior to cell fusion of cultured muscle cells, only the globular forms of AChE are expressed. Following the formation of myotubes and the onset of spontaneous muscle activity, the collagen-tailed form of AChE appears. That muscle activity is a necessary prerequisite for collagen-tailed AChE biosynthesis and/or assembly can be demonstrated by treating the cells with drugs that block either the AChRs or sodium channels.[129–131] Under these conditions, the collagen-tailed forms of AChE disappear, whereas the globular forms are only slightly affected. Innervation is not required for the appearance of any molecular form, because in tissue culture all forms of the enzyme are synthesized and assembled in the absence of nerves. However, innervation can exert a profound influence on the amounts of AChE synthesized, the relative abundance of each molecular form, and their sites of accumulation on the muscle cell surface.

The regulation of AChE synthesis in whole muscle has, for the most part, been studied using denervated or reinnervated in vivo preparations.[6,8] This approach has demonstrated an important role for the nerve in the localization of AChE at the neuromuscular junction. In fact, in the absence of muscle fibers, the motor neurons can deposit AChE on the synaptic basal lamina. However, the denervation approach does not allow for a quantitative assessment of the contributions of nerves and muscle, as both cell types contain substantial amounts of AChE.

Denervation of muscle in almost all species results in the loss of histochemically detectable AChE from the neuromuscular junction (which may take months) and the disappearance of the collagen-tailed forms of the enzyme (which is usually much quicker, of the order of days).[95,132,133] Both reappear upon reinnervation. When the muscle is reinnervated at a site distant from the original neuromuscular junction, a new synapse forms and AChE activity accumulates after about 1 week.[134] Coincident with the appearance of histochemically detectable enzyme is the accumulation of the collagen-tailed forms of AChE.[135] At the same time, collagen-tailed forms of AChE also accumulate at the old neuromuscular junction, which is not innervated, thus showing that the presence of the nerve is not necessary for the accumulation of AChE at the neuromuscular junction once the mature synapse has formed.

These results demonstrate the ability of the muscle to generate at least a large fraction of total end plate AChE and to deposit it in approximately the correct location even in the absence of a nearby nerve terminal. Clearly, some vestige of the former neuromuscular connection is involved in this, and it seems likely that this matter is related to differentiated synaptic basal lamina (see Chap. 20). Further information about the specification of sites for deposition of synaptic AChE has come from the experiments of Lomo and Slater.[136] Using the rat soleus muscle, these investigators have shown that only a transient contact of motor nerve endings and denervated muscle fibers is required for determining the site of AChE deposition. In fact, the contact can be shorter than the time required to establish functional neuromuscular connections (about 2 days). However, the actual deposition of AChE at those contact sites occurs about a week later and only if the muscle fiber is stimulated to contract. The stimulation can come from innervation elsewhere, or from electrical stimulation with implanted electrodes. These experiments suggest an essential role of muscle activity in end plate AChE deposition.

TURNOVER OF ACETYLCHOLINESTERASE

Very little is known about the turnover of cell surface ACh molecules beyond the observation that they are replaced. In cultured muscle cells, the plasma membrane–bound dimers and tetramers are degraded by a process exhibiting first-order decay kinetics and a $t_{1/2}$ of about 50 h. Probably these molecules are internalized and degraded in lysosomes, but the details of the process have not been well documented.[97] Only one study to date has quantitatively determined the half-life of the junctional AChE in vivo. Using mouse sternomastoid muscle, Kasprzak and Salpeter labeled the end plate AChE with [^{3}H]-DFP and determined the loss of AChE by quantitative autoradiography.[137] Their results indicate that the half-life of the junctional AChE is approximately 20 days at the normal innervated end plate, which is approximately twice as long as the half-life of the end plate AChRs.

The globular and collagen-tailed AChE forms are probably degraded by different mechanisms, as the former are predominantly membrane-bound whereas the latter are mostly in the extracellular matrix. In most species, denervation results in the loss of collagen-tailed forms of AChE from muscle.[6,8] The rate of disappearance varies from one species to another. In the rat, complete loss of the enzyme can occur over a period of several days, whereas in some other animals it can persist for at least several months after degeneration of the nerve terminals. Several factors are likely to be involved in the loss of junctional AChE, including local proteolysis and lack of replacement.[138] In some species, however, the collagen-tailed forms will persist for some time and can actually increase, as in the rabbit. Much additional work needs to be done before our understanding is complete.

Acknowledgments

This work was supported by grants from the National Institutes of Health and the Muscular Dystrophy Association to Richard Rotundo. A special acknowledgment goes to Dr. Douglas Fambrough, who contributed to the first edition and revision of this chapter.

List of Abbreviations

ACh	acetylcholine	Fas-2	fasciculin 2
AChE	acetylcholinesterase	Iso-OMPA	tetraisopropylpyrophosphoramide
AChR	acetylcholine receptor	P peptide	transmembrane anchor peptide for AChE
BuChE	butyrylcholinesterase	PCR	polymerase chain reaction
ColQ	collagenic tail subunit of AChE	PRAD	proline-rich attachment domain
DFP	diisopropyl fluorophosphate	RER	rough endoplasmic reticulum
DTNB	dithiobisnitrobenzoic acid	SR	sarcoplasmic reticulum
ER	endoplasmic reticulum		

References

1. Massoulié J, Rieger F: L'acetylcholinesterase des organes electriques de poissons (Torpille et gymnote); Complexes membranaires. *Eur J Biochem* 11:441, 1969.
2. Massoulié J, Rieger F, Bon S: Especes acetylcholinesterasiques globulaires et allongees des organes electriques de poissons. *Eur J Biochem* 21:542, 1971.
3. Rosenberry TL, Richarson JM: Structure of 18S and 14S acetylcholinesterase. Identification of collagen-like subunits that are linked by disulfide bonds to catalytic subunits. *Biochemistry* 16:3550, 1977.
4. Dudai Y, Herberg M, Silman I: Molecular structures of acetylcholinesterase from electric organ tissue of the electric eel. *Proc Natl Acad Sci USA* 70:2473, 1973.
5. Lwebuga-Mukasa JS, Lappi S, Taylor P: Molecular forms of acetylcholinesterase from *Torpedo californica*: Their relationship to synaptic membranes. *Biochemistry* 15:1425, 1976.
6. Massoulié J, Bon S: The molecular forms of cholinesterase and acetylcholinesterase in vertebrates. *Annu Rev Neurosci* 5:57, 1982.
7. Sussman JL, Silman I: Acetylcholinesterase: Structure and use as a model for specific cation-protein interactions. *Curr Opin Struct Biol* 2:721–729, 1992.
8. Massoulié J, Pezzementi L, Bon S, et al: Molecular and cellular biology of cholinesterases. *Prog Neurobiol* 41:31–91, 1993.
9. Sussman JL, Harel M, Frolow F, et al: Atomic structure of acetylcholinesterase from *Torpedo californica*: A prototypic acetylcholine-binding protein. *Science* 253:872–879, 1991.
10. Raves ML, Harel M, Pang Y-P, et al: 3D structure of acetylcholinesterase complexed with the nootropic alkaloid, (-)-huperzine. *Nat Struct Biol* 4:57–63, 1997.
11. le Du MH, Marchot P, Bougis PE, Fontecilla-Camps C: 1.9 Å resolution structure of fasciculin 1, an anti-acetylcholinesterase toxin from green mamba snake venom. *J Biol Chem* 267:22122–22130, 1992.
12. Shafferman A, Velan B (eds): *Multidisciplinary Approaches to Cholinesterase Functions*. New York: Plenum Press; 1992.
13. Massoulié J: The polymorphism of cholinesterase and its physiological significance. *Trends Biochem Sci* 5:160, 1980.
14. Rosenberry TL: Acetylcholinesterase. *Adv Enzymol* 43:103, 1975.
15. Couteaux R: Differentiation of synaptic areas. *Proc R Soc Lond [Biol]* 158:457, 1963.
16. Lee SL, Heinemann S, Taylor P: Structural characterization of the asymetric (17 + 13) S forms of acetylcholinesterase from *Torpedo*. I. Analysis of subunit composition. *J Biol Chem* 257:12283, 1982.
17. Lee S, Taylor P: Structural characterization of the asymmetric (17 + 13) S species of acetylcholinesterase from *Torpedo*. II. Component peptides obtained by selective proteolysis and disulfide bond reduction. *J Biol Chem* 257:12292, 1982.
18. Tsim KWK, Randall WR, Barnard EA: An asymmetric form of muscle acetylcholinesterase contains three subunit types and two enzymic activities in one molecule. *Proc Natl Acad Sci USA* 85:1262–1266, 1988.
19. Ott P, Jenny B, Brodbeck U: Multiple molecular forms of purified human erythrocyte acetylcholinesterase. *Eur J Biochem* 57:469, 1975.
20. Rosenberry TL, Scoggin DM: Structure of the human erythrocyte acetylcholinesterase. Characterization of intersubunit disulfide bonding and detergent interactions. *J Biol Chem* 299:5643, 1984.
21. Bon S, Cartaud J, Massoulié J: The dependence of acetylcholinesterase aggregation at low ionic strength upon a polyanionic component. *Eur J Biochem* 85:1–14, 1978.
22. Hall ZW, Kelly RB: Enzymatic detachment of endplate acetylcholinesterase from muscle. *Nat N Biol* 232:62, 1971.
23. Betz W, Sakmann B: Effects of proteolytic enzymes on function and structure of frog neuromuscular junctions. *J Physiol (London)* 230:673, 1973.
24. Rossi SR, Rotundo RL: Localization of "non-extractable" acetylcholinesterase to the vertebrate neuromuscular junction. *J Biol Chem* 268:19152–19159, 1993.
25. Rossi SR, Rotundo RL: Transient interactions between collagen-tailed acetylcholinesterase and sulfated proteoglycans prior to immobilization on the extracellular matrix. *J Biol Chem* 271:1979–1987, 1996.
26. Krejci E, Coussen F, Duval N, et al: Primary structure of a collagenic tail peptide of *Torpedo* acetylcholinesterase: Co-expression with catalytic subunit induces production of collagen-tailed forms in transfected cells. *EMBO J* 10:1285–1293, 1991.
27. Krejci E, Thomine S, Boschetti N, et al: The mammalian gene of acetylcholinesterase-associated collagen. *J Biol Chem* 272:22840–22847, 1997.
28. Ohno K, Brengman J, Tsujino A, Engel AG: Human endplate acetylcholinesterase deficiency caused by mutations in the collagen-like tail subunit (ColQ) of the asymmetric enzyme. *Proc Natl Acad Sci USA* 95:9654–9659, 1998.
29. W.R. Randall, personal communication.
30. Deprez PN, Inestrosa NC: Two heparin-binding domains are present on the collagenic tail of asymmetric acetylcholinesterase. *J Biol Chem* 270:11043–11046, 1995.
31. Ohno K, Engel AG, Brengman J, et al:. The spectrum of mutations causing end-plate acetylcholinesterase deficiency. *Ann Neurol* 47:162–170, 2000.
32. Donger C, Krejci E, Serradell AP, et al: Mutation in the human acetylcholinesterase-associated collagen gene, COLQ, is responsible for congenital myasthenic syndrome with end-plate acetylcholinesterase deficiency (type Ic). *Am J Hum Genet* 63:967–975, 1998.
33. Kimbell LM, Ohno K, Engel AG, et al: C-terminal and heparin binding domains of ColQ are both essential for anchoring acetylcholinesterase at the synapse. *J Biol Chem* 279:10997–11005, 2004.
33a. Inestrosa NC, Roberts WL, Marshall TL, et al: Acetylcholinesterase from bovine caudate nucleus is attached to membranes by a novel subunit distinct from those of acetylcholinesterase in other tissues. *J Biol Chem* 262:4441–4444, 1987.
34. Perrier AL, Massoulié J, Krejci E: PRiMA: The membrane anchor of acetylcholinesterase in the brain. *Neuron* 33:275–285, 2000.
35. Schumacher M, Camp SJ, Maulet Y, et al: Primary structure of *Torpedo californica* acetylcholinesterase deduced from its cDNA sequence. *Nature* 319:407–409, 1986.
36. Sikorav J-L, Krejci E, Massoulié J: cDNA sequence of *Torpedo marmorata* acetylcholinesterase: Primary structure of the precursor of a catalytic subunit; Existence of multiple 5'-untranslated regions. *EMBO J* 6:1865–1873, 1987.
37. Rachinsky TL, Camp S, Li Y, et al: Molecular cloning of mouse acetylcholinesterase: Tissue distribution of alternatively spliced mRNA species. *Neuron* 5:317–327, 1990.
38. Soreq H, Ben-Aziz R, Prody CA, et al: Molecular cloning and construction of the coding region of human acetylcholinesterase reveals a g+c-rich attenuating structure. *Proc Natl Acad Sci USA* 87:9688–9692, 1990.
39. Arpagaus M, Kott M, Vatis KP, et al: Structure of the gene for human butyrylcholinesterase. Evidence for single copy. *Biochemistry* 29:124–131, 1990.
40. Krejci E, Coussen F, Duval N, et al: Primary structure of a collagenic tail peptide of *Torpedo* acetylcholinesterase: Co-expression with catalytic subunit induces the production of collagen-tailed forms in transfected cells. *EMBO J* 10:1285–1293, 1991.
41. Getman DK, Eubanks JH, Camp S, et al: The human gene encoding acetylcholinesterase is located on the long arm of chromosome 7. *Am J Hum Genet* 51:170–177, 1992.
42. Li Y, Camp S, Rachinsky TL, et al: Gene structure of mammalian acetylcholinesterase. *J Biol Chem* 266:23083–23090, 1991.
43. Taylor P: The cholinesterases. *J Biol Chem* 266:4025–4028, 1991.
44. Taylor P: *Impact of Recombinant DNA Technology and Protein Structure Determination on Past and Future Studies on Acetylcholinesterase*. New York: Plenum Press; 1992.

45. Xie W, Stribley JA, Chatonnet A, et al: Postnatal developmental delay and supersensitivity to organophosphate in gene-targeted mice lacking acetylcholinesterase. *J Pharmacol Exp Ther* 293:896–902, 2000.
46. Li B, Stribley JA, Ticu A, et al: Abundant tissue butyrylcholinesterase and its possible function in the acetylcholinesterase knockout mouse. *J Neurochem* 75:1320–1331, 2000.
47. Mesulam MM, Guillozet A, Shaw P, et al: Acetylcholinesterase knockouts establish central cholinergic pathways and can use butyrylcholinesterase to hydrolyze acetylcholine. *Neuroscience* 110:627–639, 2002.
48. Rotundo RL: Nucleus-specific translation and assembly of acetylcholinesterase in multinucleated muscle cells. *J Cell Biol* 110:715–719, 1990.
49. Tsim KWK, Greenberg I, Rimer M, et al: Transcripts for AChR and AChE show distribution differences in cultured chick muscle cells. *J Cell Biol* 118:1201–1212, 1992.
50. Jasmin BJ, Lee RK, Rotundo RL: Compartmentalization of acetylcholinesterase mRNA and enzyme at the vertebrate neuromuscular junction. *Neuron* 11:467–477, 1993.
51. Michel RN, Vu CQ, Tetzlaff W, Jasmin BJ: Neural regulation of acetylcholinesterase mRNAs at mammalian neuromuscular synapses. *J Cell Biol* 127:1061–1069, 1994.
52. Legay C, Huchet M, Massoulié J, Changeux JP: Developmental regulation of acetylcholinesterase transcripts in the mouse diaphragm: Alternative splicing and focalization. *Eur J Neurosci* 7:1803–1809, 1995.
53. Fuentes ME, Taylor P: Control of acetylcholinesterase gene expression during myogenesis. *Neuron* 10:679–687, 1993.
54. Li Y, Camp S, Rachinsky TL, et al: Promoter elements and transcriptional control of the mouse acetylcholinesterase gene. *J Biol Chem* 268:3563–3572, 1993.
55. Mutero A, Camp S, Taylor P: Promoter elements of the mouse acetylcholinesterase gene. Transcriptional regulation during muscle differentiation. *J Biol Chem* 270:1866–1872, 1995.
56. Boudreau-Lariviere C, Chan RY, Wu J, Jasmin BJ: Molecular mechanisms underlying the activity-linked alterations in acetylcholinesterase mRNAs in developing versus adult rat skeletal muscles. *J Neurochem* 74:2250–2258, 2000.
57. Angus LM, Chan RY, Jasmin BJ: Role of intronic E- and N-box motifs in the transcriptional induction of the acetylcholinesterase gene during myogenic differentiation. *J Biol Chem* 276:17603–17609, 2001.
58. Ekstrom TJ, Klump WM, Getman D, et al: Promoter elements and transcriptional regulation of the acetylcholinesterase gene. *DNA Cell Biol* 12:63–72, 1993.
59. Getman DK, Mutero A, Inoue K, Taylor P: Transcription factor repression and activation of the human acetylcholinesterase gene. *J Biol Chem* 270:23511–23519, 1995.
60. Ben Aziz-Aloya R, Sternfeld M, Soreq H: Promoter elements and alternative splicing in the human ACHE gene. *Prog Brain Res* 98:147–153, 1993.
61. W.R. Randall, personal communication.
62. Briguet A, Ruegg MA: The Ets transcription factor GABP is required for postsynaptic differentiation in vivo. *J Neurosci* 20:5989–5996, 2000.
63. Schaeffer L, Duclert N, Huchet-Dymanus M, Changeux JP: Implication of a multisubunit Ets-related transcription factor in synaptic expression of the nicotinic acetylcholine receptor. *EMBO J* 17:3078–3090, 1998.
64. Angus LM, Chan RY, Jasmin BJ: Role of intronic E- and N-box motifs in the transcriptional induction of the acetylcholinesterase gene during myogenic differentiation. *J Biol Chem* 276:17603–17609, 2001.
65. Greenfield S: Acetylcholinesterase may have novel functions in the brain. *Trends Neurosci* 7:364–368, 1984.
66. Vigny M, Bon S, Massoulié J, Leterrier F: Active-site catalytic efficiency of acetylcholinesterase molecular forms in *Electrophorus*, *Torpedo*, rat, and chicken. *Eur J Biochem* 85:317, 1978.
67. Rosenberry TL, Bernhard SA: Studies of catalysis by acetylcholinesterase. Synergistic effects of inhibitors during the hydrolysis of acetic acid esters. *Biochemistry* 11:4309, 1972.
68. Anglister L, Eichler J, Szabo M, et al: ^{125}I-labeled fasciculin 2: A new tool for quantitation of acetylcholinesterase densities at synaptic site by EM-autoradiography. *J Neurosci Methods* 81:63–71, 1998.
69. Peng HB, Xie H, Rossi SG, Rotundo RL: Acetylcholinesterase clustering at the neuromuscular junction involves perlecan and dystroglycan. *J Cell Biol* 145:911–921, 1999.
70. Arikawa-Hirasawa E, Rossi SG, Rotundo RL, Yamada Y: Absence of acetylcholinesterase at the neuromuscular junctions of perlecan-null mice. *Nat Neurosci* 5:119–123, 2002.
71. Hall AC, Tompkins L, Kyriacou CP, et al: Higher behavior in *Drosophila* analyzed with mutations that disrupt the structure and function of the nervous system, in Siddiqi O (ed): *Development and Neurobiology of Drosophila*. New York: Plenum Press; 1980, pp 425–455.
72. Ariens AT, Meeter E, Wolthius R, Van Benthem RMJ: Reversible necrosis at the end-plate region in striated muscles of the rat poisoned with cholinesterase inhibitors. *Experientia* 25:57, 1969.
73. Engel AG, Lambert EH, Mulder DM, et al: A newly recognized congenital myasthenic syndrome attributed to a prolonged open time of the acetylcholine-induced ion channel. *Ann Neurol* 11:553, 1982.
74. Wecker L, Kiauta T, Dettbarn WD: Relationship between acetylcholinesterase inhibition and the development of a myopathy. *J Pharmacol Exp Ther* 206:97, 1979.
75. Salpeter MM, Kasprzak H, Feng H, Fertuck H: Endplates after esterase inactivation in vivo: Correlation between esterase concentration, functional response and fine structure. *J Neurocytol* 8:95, 1978.
76. Salpeter MM, Leonard JP, Kasprzak H: Agonist-induced postsynaptic myopathy. *Neurosci Comment* 1:73, 1982.
77. Reddy MK, Etlinger JD, Foschman DA, et al: Removal of Z lines and α-actinin from isolated myofibrils by a calcium activated neutral protease. *J Biol Chem* 250:4278, 1975.
78. Sugita H, Ishiura S, Suzuki K, Imahori K: Ca^{++}-activated neutral protease and its inhibitors: In vitro effect on intact myofibrils. *Muscle Nerve* 3:335, 1980.
79. Kawabuchi M: Neostigmine myopathy is a calcium mediated myopathy initially affecting the motor end-plate. *J Neuropathol Exp Neurol* 41:298, 1982.
80. Engel AG, Lambert EH, Gomez MR: A new myasthenic syndrome with end-plate acetylcholinesterase deficiency, small nerve terminals, and reduced acetylcholine release. *Ann Neurol* 1:315–330, 1977.
81. Rosenberry TL: Quantitative simulation of endplate currents at neuromuscular junctions based on the reaction of acetylcholine with acetylcholine receptor and acetylcholinesterase. *Biophys J* 26:263, 1979.
82. Wathey JC, Nass MM, Lester HA: Numerical reconstruction of the quantal event at nicotinic synapses. *Biophys J* 27:145, 1979.
83. Adams PR: Aspects of synaptic potential generation, in Pinsker HM, Willis WD Jr (eds): *Information Processing in the Nervous System*. New York: Raven Press; 1980, pp 109–124.
84. Land BR, Salpeter EE, Salpeter MM: Kinetic parameters for acetylcholine interacting in intact neuromuscular junction. *Proc Natl Acad Sci USA* 78:7200, 1981.
84a. Martin AR: Amplification of neuromuscular transmission by postjunctional folds. *Proc R Soc Lond [Biol]* 258:321–326, 1994.
84b. Wood SJ, Slater CP: Safety factor at the neuromuscular junction. *Prog Neurobiol* 64:393–429, 2001.
85. Ellman GL, Courtney KD, Andres V Jr, Featherstone RM: A new and rapid colorimetric determination of acetylcholinesterase activity. *Biochem Pharmacol* 7:88, 1961.
86. Johnson CD, Russell RL: A rapid, simple radiometric assay for cholinesterase, suitable for multiple determinations. *Anal Biochem* 64:229, 1975.
87. Koelle GB, Friedenwald JS: A histochemical method for localizing cholinesterase activity. *Proc Soc Exp Biol Med* 70:617, 1949.
88. Karnovsky MJ, Roots L: A "direct coloring" thiocholine method for cholinesterase. *Cytochemistry* 12:219, 1964.
89. Tsuji S: On the chemical basis of thiocholine methods for demonstration of acetylcholinesterase activities. *Histochemistry* 42:99, 1974.
90. Dudai Y, Silman I, Shinitzky M, Blumberg S: Purification by affinity chromatography of the molecular forms of acetylcholinesterase present in fresh electric organ tissue of electric eel. *Proc Natl Acad Sci USA* 69:2400, 1972.
91. Rosenberry TL, Chang HW, Chen YT: Purification of acetylcholinesterase by affinity chromatography and determination of active site stoichiometry. *J Biol Chem* 247:1555, 1972.
92. Massoulié J, Bon S: Affinity chromatography of acetylcholinesterase: The importance of hydrophobic interactions. *Eur J Biochem* 68:531, 1976.
93. Rotundo RL: Purification and properties of the membrane bound form of acetylcholinesterase from chicken brain: Evidence for two distinct polypeptide chains. *J Biol Chem* 259:13186, 1984.
94. Fambrough DM, Engel AG, Rosenberry TL: Acetylcholinesterase of human erythrocytes and neuromuscular junctions: Homologies revealed by monoclonal antibodies. *Proc Natl Acad Sci USA* 79:1078, 1982.
94a. Krejci E, Legay C, Thomine S, et al: Differences in expression of acetylcholinesterase and collagen Q control the distribution and oligomerization of the collagen-tailed forms in fast and slow muscles. *J Neurosci* 19:10672–10679, 1999.
95. Hall ZW: Multiple forms of acetylcholinesterase and their distribution in endplate and non-endplate regions of rat diaphragm muscle. *J Neurobiol* 4:343, 1973.
96. Carson S, Bon S, Vigny M, et al: Distribution of acetylcholinesterase molecular forms in neural and non-neural sections of human muscle. *FEBS Lett* 97:348, 1979.
97. Rotundo RL, Fambrough DM: Synthesis, transport, and fate of acetylcholinesterase in cultured chick embryo muscle cultures. *Cell* 22:583, 1980.
98. Tennyson VM, Brzin M, Kremzner LT: Acetylcholinesterase activity in the myotube and muscle satellite cell of the fetal rabbit—An electron microscopic-cytochemical and biochemical study. *J Histochem Cytochem* 21:634, 1973.
99. Sawyer HR, Golder TK, Neiberg PS, Wilson BW: Ultrastructural localization of acetylcholinesterase in cultured cells. I. Embryo muscle. *J Histochem Cytochem* 24:969, 1976.
100. Younkin SG, Rosenstein C, Collins PL, Rosenberry TL: Cellular localization of the molecular forms of acetylcholinesterase in rat diaphragm. *J Biol Chem* 257:13630, 1982.

101. Salpeter MM: Electron microscope radioautography as a quantitative tool in enzyme cytochemistry. I. The distribution of acetylcholinesterase at motor end plates of a vertebrate twitch muscle. *J Cell Biol* 32:379, 1967.
102. Rogers AW, Darzynkiewicz A, Ostrowski K, et al: Quantitative studies on enzymes in structures in striated muscles by labeled inhibitor methods. I. The number of acetylcholinesterase molecules and of other DFP-reactive sites at motor endplates measured by radioautography. *J Cell Biol* 41:655, 1969.
103. Barnard EA, Wieckowski T, Chiu TH: Cholinergic receptor molecules and cholinesterase molecules at mouse skeletal muscle junctions. *Nature* 234:207, 1971.
104. Anglister L, Stiles JR, Salpeter MM: Acetylcholinesterase density and turnover number at frog neuromuscular junctions, with modeling of their role in synaptic function. *Neuron* 12:783–794, 1994.
105. McMahan UJ, Sanes JR, Marshall LM: Cholinesterase is associated with the basal lamina at the neuromuscular junction. *Nature* 271:172, 1978.
106. Rossi SR, Rotundo RL: Localization of "non-extractable" acetylcholinesterase to the vertebrate neuromuscular junction. *J Biol Chem* 268:19152–19159, 1993.
107. Rossi SR, Rotundo RL: Transient interactions between collagen-tailed acetylcholinesterase and sulfated proteoglycans prior to immobilization on the extracellular matrix. *J Biol Chem* 271:1979–1987, 1996.
108. Silman I, Lyles JM, Barnard EA: Intrinsic forms of acetylcholinesterase in skeletal muscle. *FEBS Lett* 94:166, 1978.
109. Lyles JM, Barnard EA: Disappearance of the "end plate" form of acetylcholinesterase for a slow tonic muscle. *FEBS Lett* 109:9, 1980.
110. Bon S, Cartaud J, Massoulié J: The dependence of acetylcholinesterase aggregation at low ionic strength upon a polyanionic component. *Eur J Biochem* 85:1, 1978.
111. Emmerling MR, Johnson CD, Mosher DF, et al: Cross-linking and binding of fibronectin with asymmetric acetylcholinesterase. *Biochemistry* 20:3242, 1981.
112. Rossi SGR, Rotundo RL: Localization of "non-extractable" acetylcholinesterase to the vertebrate neuromuscular junction. *J Biol Chem* 268:19152–19159, 1993.
113. Feng G, Krejci E, Molgo J, et al: Genetic analysis of collagen Q: Roles in acetylcholinesterase and butyrylcholinesterase assembly and in synaptic structure and function. *J Cell Biol* 144:1349–1360, 1999.
114. Rotundo RL, Rossi SG, Anglister L: Transplantation of quail collagen-tailed acetylcholinesterase molecules on to the frog neuromuscular synapse. *J Cell Biol* 136:367–374, 1997.
115. Jacobson C, Côté P, Rossi SG, et al: The dystroglycan complex is necessary for stabilization of acetylcholine receptor clusters at neuromuscular junctions and formation of the synaptic basal lamina. *J Cell Biol* 152:435–450, 2001.
116. Arikawa-Hirasawa E, Rossi SG, Rotundo RL, Yamada Y: Absence of acetylcholinesterase at the neuromuscular junctions of perlecan-null mice. *Nat Neurosci* 5:119–123, 2002.
117. DiGiamberardino L, Couraud JY: Rapid accumulation of high molecular weight acetylcholinesterase in transected sciatic nerve. *Nature* 271:170, 1978.
118. Brimijoin S, Wiermaa MJ: Rapid orthograde and retrograde axonal transport of acetylcholinesterase as characterized by the stop-flow technique. *J Physiol* 285:129, 1978.
119. Fernandez HL, Duell JM, Festoff BW: Cellular distribution of 16S acetylcholinesterase. *J Neurochem* 32:581, 1979.
120. Anglister L: Acetylcholinesterase from the motor nerve terminal accumulates on the basal lamina of the myofiber. *J Cell Biol* 115:755–764, 1991.
121. T. L. Rosenberry, personal communication.
122. Bouma SR, Drislane FW, Huestis WH: Selective extraction of membrane-bound proteins by phospholipid vesicles. *J Biol Chem* 252:6759, 1977.
123. Rotundo RL, Fambrough DM: Secretion of acetylcholinesterase: Relation to acetylcholine receptor metabolism. *Cell* 22:595, 1980.
124. Rotundo RL: Asymmetric acetylcholinesterase is assembled in the Golgi apparatus. *Proc Natl Acad Sci USA* 81:479, 1984.
125. Roberts WL, Santikarn S, Reinhold VN, Rosenberry TL: Structural characterization of the glycoinositide phospholipid membrane anchor of human acetylcholinesterase by fast bombardment mass spectroscopy. *J Biol Chem* 263:18776–18784, 1988.
126. Inestrosa NC, Roberts WL, Marshall TL, Rosenberry TL: Acetylcholinesterase from bovine caudate nucleus is attached to membranes by a novel subunit distinct from those of acetylcholinesterases in other tissues. *J Biol Chem* 262:4441–4444, 1987.
127. Inestrosa NC, Perelman A: Distribution and anchoring of molecular forms of acetylcholinesterase. *Trends Pharmacol Sci* 10:325, 1989.
128. Rossi SG, Rotundo RL: Cell surface acetylcholinesterase molecules on multinucleated myotubes are clustered over the nucleus of origin. *J Cell Biol* 119:1657–1667, 1992.
129. Rieger F, Koenig J, Vigny M: Spontaneous contractile activity and the presence of the 16S form of acetylcholinesterase in rat muscle cells in culture. Reversible suppressive action of tetrodotoxin. *Dev Biol* 76:358, 1980.
130. Rubin LL, Schuetze SM, Weill CL, Fischbach GD: Regulation of acetylcholinesterase appearance at neuro-muscular junctions in vivo. *Nature* 283:264, 1980.
131. Fernandez-Valle C, Rotundo RL: Regulation of acetylcholinesterase synthesis and assembly by muscle activity: Effects of tetrodotoxin. *J Biol Chem* 264:14043–14049, 1989.
132. Vigny M, Koenig J, Rieger F: The motor endplate specific form of acetylcholinesterase: Appearance during embryogenesis and reinnervation of rat muscle. *J Neurochem* 27:1347, 1976.
133. Sketelj J, McNamee MG, Wilson BW: Effect of denervation of the molecular forms of acetylcholinesterase in normal and dystrophic chicken muscles. *Exp Neurol* 60:624, 1978.
134. Guth L, Zalewski AA: Disposition of cholinesterase following implantation of nerve into innervated and denervated muscle. *Exp Neurol* 7:316, 1963.
135. Weinberg CB, Sanes JR, Hall ZW: Formation of neuromuscular junctions in adult rats: Accumulation of acetylcholine receptors, acetylcholinesterase, and components of synaptic basal lamina. *Dev Biol* 84:255, 1981.
136. Lomo T, Slater CR: Control of junctional acetylcholinesterase by neural and muscular influences in the rat. *J Physiol (London)* 303:191, 1980.
137. Kasprzak H, Salpeter MM: Recovery of acetylcholinesterase at intact neuromuscular junctions after in vivo inactivation with diisopropylfluorophosphate. *J Neurosci* 5:951–955, 1985.
138. Fernandez HL, Duell MJ: Protease inhibitors reduce effects of denervation on muscle endplate acetylcholinesterase. *J Neurochem* 35:1166, 1980.
139. Massoulié J, Sussman JL, Doctor BP, et al: Recommendations for nomenclature in cholinesterases, in Shafferman A, Velan B (eds): *Multidisciplinary Approaches to Cholinesterase Functions*. New York: Plenum Press; 1992

SECTION 5

Muscle as a Tissue

Chapter 19a

The Cytoskeleton: Maintenance of Muscle Fiber Integrity

CLARA FRANZINI-ARMSTRONG
ALAN R. HORWITZ

The Muscle Fiber Cytoskeleton
  THE SUBSARCOLEMMAL NETWORK AND THE TRANSVERSE
    CONNECTING SYSTEM
The Complex Structure of Costameres
  THE MYOTENDINOUS AND NEUROMUSCULAR JUNCTIONS
The Integrins
  GENERAL PROPERTIES OF INTEGRINS
  INTEGRINS OF SKELETAL MUSCLE
  FUNCTIONS OF SPECIFIC MEMBERS OF THE $\beta 1$ INTEGRIN FAMILY
Microtubules
Other Structural Connections

In skeletal muscle fibers, the cytoskeleton plays a major structural and supportive mechanical role in the organization of the cross striations in the coordinated transmission of force longitudinally at the fiber ends via the myotendinous junction and in connections between myofibrils and sarcolemma. In this chapter, the term *sarcolemma* is applied to the two stratified structures of the cell surface that consist of the basal lamina and the lipid bilayer and are undercoated by the subsarcolemmal actin network.[1]

Myofibrils assemble in proximity to each other, but independently, during myogenesis (see Chap. 2) and are not well aligned laterally in the early stages. However, in the mature myofiber, the bands of adjacent myofibrils are well aligned in the resting muscle and defects of the cross striation are not frequent. When a fiber is highly stretched, a condition that is not permissible in situ, considerable shearing of the bands occurs, but the myofibrils are still connected and return to their original positions when the fiber is released. It is clear that an organizational system must be responsible for the precise lateral alignment of the myofibrils. Fixation protocols for electron microscopy, other than those routinely used, reveal a filamentous network connecting sarcolemma to peripheral myofibrils and continuing internally into the muscle fiber,[2,3] corresponding to the insoluble Z-disk scaffold that remains after the extraction of most proteins.[4]

Ingenious experiments[3] have shown that skeletal muscle fibers can transmit tension laterally to adjacent fibers in the muscle via the intervening connective tissue. This means that when the fibers contract, they exert a pull not only on the connective tissue of the tendon but also, to a lesser extent, on the connective tissue of the endomysium. In acute muscle injury, tearing occurs not only at the myotendinous junction but also on a transverse plane.[5] A similar lateral transmission of force has also been proposed for cardiac muscle,[6] implying the existence of lateral connections through which the myofibrils can transmit tension sequentially to the sarcolemma and to the extracellular matrix. Indeed, specific sites of transverse tension transmission are identified when fibers are greatly shortened.[7,8] In addition, the subplasmalemmal cytoskeleton provides an overall diffuse protective system that is anchored into the sarcolemma. Failure of this diffuse system and of the lateral connections is probably at the basis of the injury that occurs in some types of muscular dystrophy. The longitudinal transmission of force from the muscle fiber end to the bone via the connective tissue of the tendon also requires a link from the myofibril to the extracellular matrix at the elaborate myotendinous junctions. This chapter covers the structural and molecular organization of the skeletal muscle cytoskeletal network and its connection to the plasmalemma. Chapter 20 defines the extracellular matrix and its connections to the plasmalemma from the extracellular side. An excellent review article covering the relationship between myofibrillar scaffolding and the fiber cytoskeleton has recently been published.[9]

The Muscle Fiber Cytoskeleton

The cytoskeleton of muscle fibers has four components: a subsarcolemmal network that mediates the attachment of several cytoskeletal proteins to the sarcolemma; a transverse connecting system anchored on the subsarcolemmal network and through it to the sarcolemma on one side and to the myofibrils internally; the protein complex that connects the ends of the myofibrils to the sarcolemmal folds at the myotendinous junction; and longitudinally arranged microtubules running parallel to and between the myofibrils.

THE SUBSARCOLEMMAL NETWORK AND THE TRANSVERSE CONNECTING SYSTEM

A fine meshwork of varying density lies immediately below the plasma membrane.[10] It is absent at the sites where caveolae provide internal anchorage and is particularly dense at the myotendinous and neuromuscular junctions (see Chap. 15) as well as at sites connecting the transverse networks to the sarcolemma. The latter sites, called costameres, and their connections to the transverse cytoskeletal network have been most precisely defined.[7,9–11] It is becoming apparent that the Z disks of the myofibrils—with their structural meshwork of α-actinin, their link with the myofibrillar α-actin, and their peripheral association with the cytoplasmic γ-actin (also see Chaps. 7, 31, and 43)[12,13]—are the center of a supramolecular complex that links the myofibrils to the intermediate filament network and to the actin-based cytoskeleton of the muscle cell. This network has a structure-protecting function, so it is also called the *transverse connecting system*. Within the plasmalemma, three different multimolecular complexes coexist: the focal adhesion type, the dystrophin/utrophin–based type, and the spectrin-based membrane skeleton systems.[9,11,14,15] The importance of the network and of the costameres is underlined by the numerous diseases that have become associated with the failure of links in this system (see Chap. 19b).[16]

The Intermediate Filament Network

Intermediate (10 nm in diameter) filaments form a cage around each of the myofibrils, with a prominent transverse cytoskeletal network surrounding the myofibrils at the Z disks and longitudinal connections.[17,18] In adult muscle, the network is composed mainly of desmin, with a molecular mass of 53 kDa,[18,19] which forms a poorly soluble cytoskeleton. In cross sections of muscle fibers at the Z-disk level, desmin filaments form a meshwork around each myofibril and then radiate laterally toward costameres at the edge of the fiber.[3,4,20] Although the major location of desmin is at the level of the Z disk, desmin filaments also extend longitudinally between the myofibrils and toward the plasmalemma, so that the whole network constitutes a complete three-dimensional mesh (Fig. 19a-1) (see also Chap. 2).[17,20] Intermediate filaments are responsible for cell resistance to mechanical stress[21]; thus one may expect that the intermediate filament network is largely responsible for fiber integrity and transmission of lateral force. Interestingly, knocking desmin out by expressing a defective version of the molecule in cultured cells[22] or by an engineered knockout[23] does not alter the myofibril alignment. It is not clear whether cytokeratins, which are also present in parallel to desmin, may not in part substitute for its function.[24] In addition, it is possible that cultured cells do not contract strongly enough to disrupt their structure in the absence of desmin, whereas disruption of the muscular architecture is observed in mice lacking desmin.[25] Indeed, highly used muscles do show disruption of the muscular architecture, as observed in mice lacking desmin.[23,25]

A second component of the transverse network is plectin, an intermediate filament linker.[21] Plectin is a long, slender

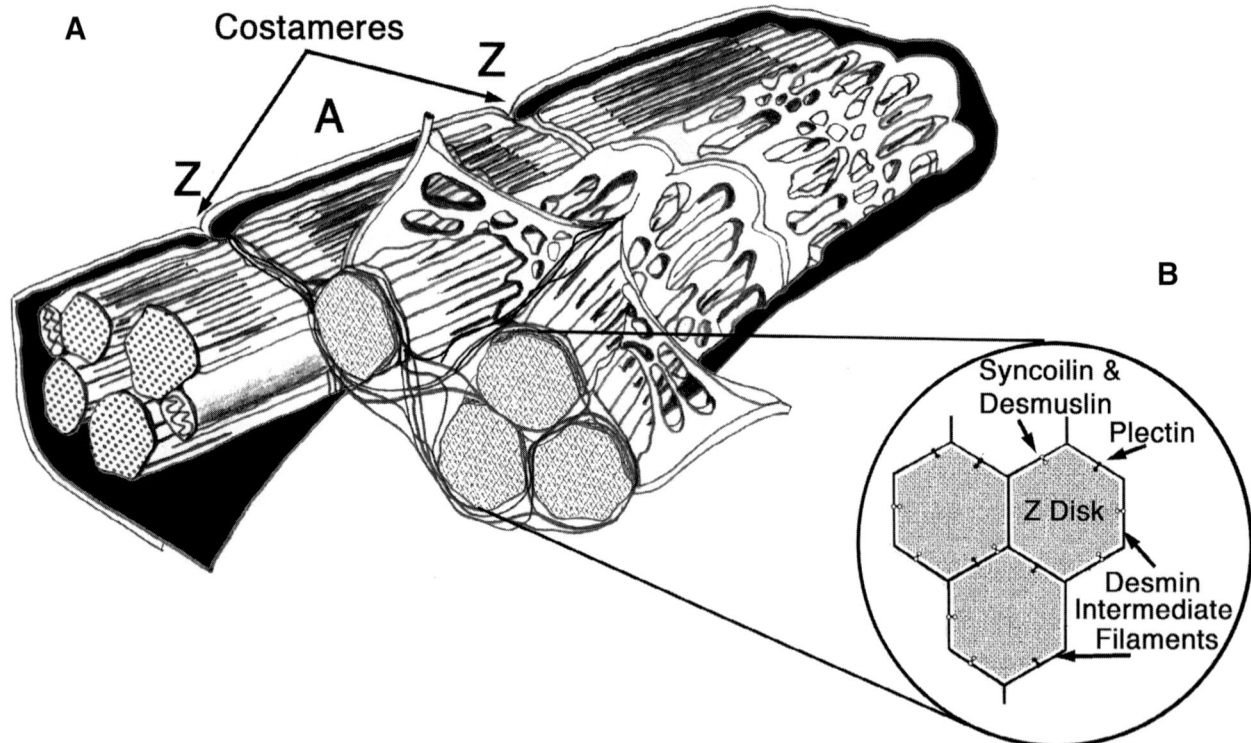

FIGURE 19a-1. The transverse connecting system. *A.* Desmin intermediate filaments (*thin dark lines*) surround the myofibrils at the level of the Z disks and extend to the sarcolemma, where they connect into a protein complex forming the costamere. The intermediate filaments constitute part of the transverse connecting network that keeps the myofibril in alignment during contraction and anchors them to the sarcolemma. *B.* At the level of the Z disks, plectin, syncoilin, and desmuslin connect the intermediate filament networks with the edges of the Z disks. (*The drawing in A is based on Lazarides and Hubbard.[18] With permission.*)

protein with a molecular mass >500 kDa and a spectrin-like actin-binding domain at its N-terminus.[26] It also has a vimentin-binding site at its C-terminus and is known to bind to various intermediate filaments, including desmin[27,28] and microtubules. It immunolocalizes to the Z disks and costameres[26] and is thought to link desmin to the Z disks, perhaps via its γ-actin,[26–29] and to the peripheral cytoskeleton. Association of plectin with Z disks is a prerequisite for the formation of the intermyofibrillar desmin cytoskeleton.[29] Clearly plectin plays a major role in the linking of intermediate filaments and in cytoskeletal dynamics[30]; this is of great importance to maintaining the stability of muscle fiber as well as skin epithelium.[31,32] Interestingly, plectin distribution, unlike that of other Z line-associated proteins (synemin and paranemin), is not affected by the absence of desmin in desmin knockout mice, suggesting the presence of other intermediate filament proteins.[23]

The complexity of the system is greatly increased by the possible link between the desmin network and two actin-based molecular complexes, one being the actin-dystrophin system (see below). Dystrophin (and its analogue utrophin) and dystrophin-associated proteins (DAP)* are defined more fully in Chaps. 19b and 34. They are proteins that connect subcortical actin to a transmembrane glycoprotein complex. The newly discovered proteins syncoilin and desmuslin are putative intermediate filament proteins that interact with desmin and α-dystrobrevin, a member of the dystrophin-associated protein complex.[33,34] Syncoilin is found at the neuromuscular junction, sarcolemma, and Z lines, and, like plectin, it is thought to be important for the integrity of muscle fiber.[14]

Links between the Cytoskeleton and the Extracellular Matrix

Protection of the plasmalemma from mechanical stress. Lipid molecules composing the plasmalemma are associated by hydrophobic bonds to form the cell membrane that serves as a barrier between the intra- and extracellular compartments. The lipid bilayer is mechanically weak and must be protected from destruction during contraction, when the muscle fibers rapidly change shape.[35] Mechanical protection is afforded by the internal actin network and the external basal lamina. The need for prevention of slipping or bulging of these two protective layers is obviated by their strong attachment to each other across the plasmalemma at costameres and light attachment between costameres, either by the complex of dystrophin and sarcoglycans; or by the complex of a related protein, utrophin, and the dystroglycan and sarcoglycan complex; or via members of the integrin family.[9–11] One integrity-maintaining system can in part compensate for a failure in the other.[36,37]

Folding of the sarcolemma. Muscle fibers change their length during contraction, while myofibrils maintain a basically constant volume.[38] The constant volume of the myofibril lattice is also maintained during passive changes in length.[39] This occurs through an increase in cross-sectional area of the whole fiber and of the individual myofibrils, resulting in larger interfilament distances at short sarcomere lengths. Simple geometric considerations indicate that the amount of membrane needed to cover the fiber surface at shorter length is smaller than that at longer lengths. However, the surface area of the sarcolemma does not change as the fiber shortens. Thus, in a fiber below resting length, the sarcolemma is in excess and folds (or "festoons")[3] appear, much as happens when one pulls up one's sleeve (Fig. 19a-2) (see also Chap. 3, Fig. 3-3). At very long sarcomere lengths, which can be obtained experimentally by passively stretching the relaxed muscle, the surface area is larger than at rest length, and the extra plasmalemmal surface is provided by the opening of caveolae.[40] Some muscles do not allow the fibers to be stretched to these long lengths even under experimental conditions because the connective tissue breaks.

Interestingly, the sarcolemmal folds that appear at short sarcomere lengths are specifically constrained at the level of the Z disks and to a lesser extent also at the M lines (Figs. 19a-2 and 19a-3). This indicates that the fiber's cross-sectional area is to some extent constrained from expanding at the level of the Z disks and also, less strongly, at the level of the M lines. The transverse connecting system, constituted of intermediate filaments and connecting proteins, is responsible for this restraint (Figs. 19a-1 and 19a-3). In fibers that have shortened a great deal, either through experimental manipulations or by being exposed to fixatives while unrestrained, the sarcolemma forms a wide festooning, with deep troughs at the Z disks.[2,3]

If the fibers lost water during contraction, the fiber would lose volume and the sarcolemma's folds would be collapsed rather than festooned. However, this does not happen despite the presence of relatively large numbers of aquaporin-4—water-selective membrane channels that are present in fast skeletal muscle fibers but are rare in slow fibers and cardiac cells.[41,42] The "square arrays," first described in freeze-fracture replicas from muscle and glia,[43] have been identified as aquaporin clusters. However, aquaporin-4 expression does not confer enhanced water permeability when the muscle fibers are tested osmotically.[44]

The Complex Structure of Costameres

Costameres (or equivalent structures)[7,9,11] and the transverse network described at the beginning of this chapter are responsible for constraining the sarcolemma at the level of the Z disks. The network and its connection to the surface membrane are the sites of lateral force transmission.[45] At the plasmalemma, these sites were initially recognized to be equivalent (but not identical) in composition and function to the focal adhesion plaques linking stress fibers to extracellular matrix (ECM) in fibroblasts[46] and to be closely related to the myotendinous junctions. Now they are known to be far more complex, and their structure is beginning to be well understood at the molecular level. The lateral adhesions were called *costameres* because of their rib-like appearance over the surface of the muscle fiber when outlined by immunolabeling

---

*A list of abbreviations used in this chapter is given at the end of the chapter.

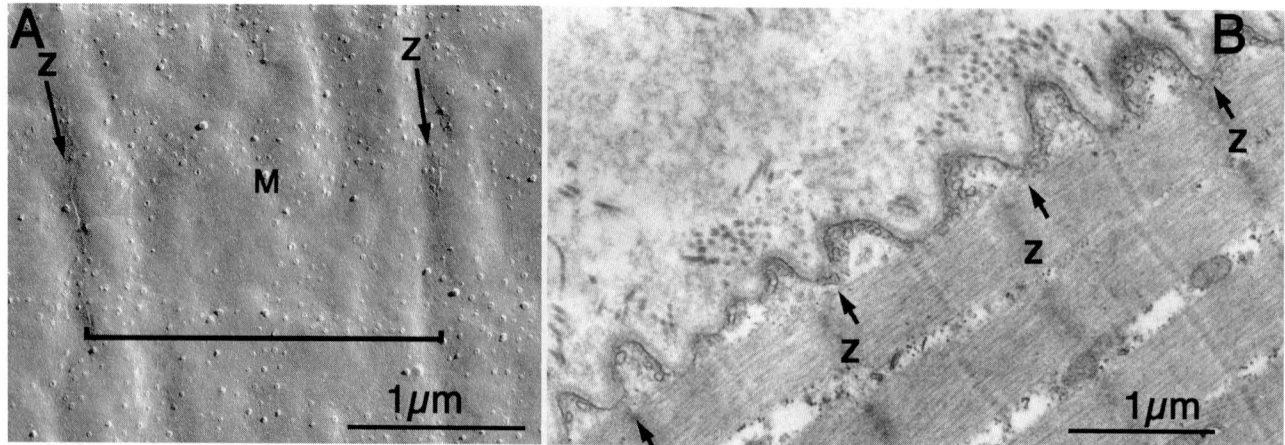

FIGURE 19a-2. Ridges and festoons. When the muscle fiber shortens below a certain length (below the resting length for most muscles), the sarcolemma (plasma membrane and basal lamina) forms folds and ridges. In the freeze-fracture image (A) from the frog, the length of one sarcomere from Z line to Z line is shown. The surface membrane bulges out in ridges that run circumferentially on the fiber surface but are restrained at the Z-disk level, where a groove appears, and also, less prominently, at the M line. The human muscle fiber (B) is fixed at much shorter sarcomeric lengths and its surface bulges out noticeably, forming festoons. As in A, the sarcolemma is restrained at or in proximity to the Z lines (arrows) and the M lines. (Image in B courtesy of A. G. Engel.)

for one of the component proteins (Fig. 19a-4), and the name has been extended to include adhesion sites on the lateral plasmalemma, where clusters of proteins are located regardless of their shape.[45–47]

Three separate sets of proteins were separately found to be located at costameres or equivalent structures. One set comprises ankyrin, vinculin, talin, and vimentin, with integrin as the transmembrane link; a second set includes members of the spectrin family; and the third set involves dystrophin and DAPs.[7,45–58] The last are fully described in Chap. 19b. The costamere contains γ-actin and very small amounts of α- and β-actin; the two sets of costameric proteins are both anchored on actin filaments.[55] Melusin, a novel protein interacting with integrin,[59] as well as syncoilin, desmuslin, dysbindin, and the intermediate filament cross-linker plectin are also present; their possible locations are indicated in Figs. 19a-1 and 19a-5 (see also Chap. 19b).[9,11,34] Note, however, that question marks are still present in this model, indicating incomplete information. Due to their location at the level of the sarcomeric Z disks, costameres have been considered to provide lateral connections between the Z disks of peripheral myofibrils and the extracellular matrix via intramembrane proteins. In some muscle fibers this is probably true, since the Z disks of peripheral myofibrils are directly associated with the plasmalemma by a dense matrix. In other fibers, however, myofibrils are separated from the plasmalemma by relatively large distances (1 μm or more), and the link across that intervening space is visible only indirectly. It is thought that in most muscles the subplasmalemmal complex of the costameres either directly or via its actin component is associated with the transverse intermediate filament network located at the Z lines, thus providing a less direct connection from the myofibril to the plasmalemma (Fig. 19a-5). An equivalent link is present in smooth muscle.[60] The connection might be via plectin for the vinculin-talin proteins and via desmuslin or syncoilin for the dystrophin complex (Fig. 19a-5) (see also Chap. 19b).[7]

The links that associate desmin filaments and the dystrophin system[61–66] with the costameres provide for mechanical continuity between the transverse cytoskeletal network

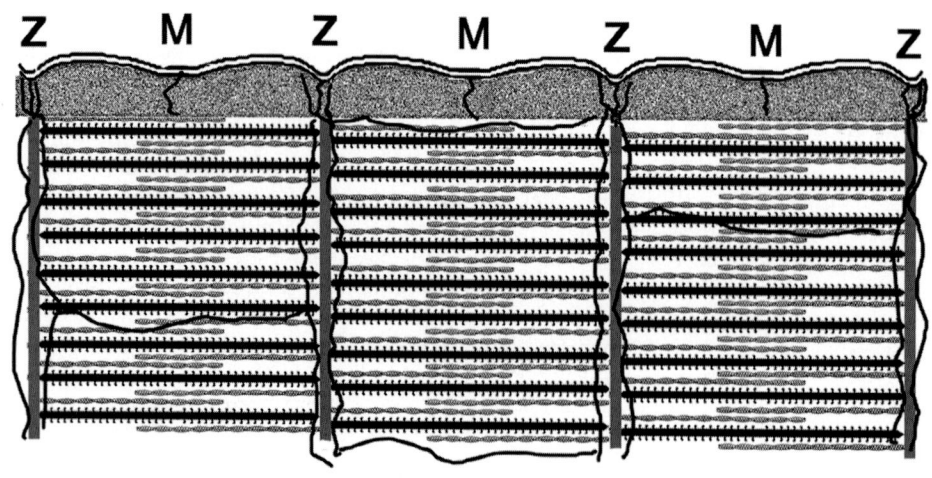

FIGURE 19a-3. The transverse connecting system of intermediate filaments and its connections to the sarcolemma (at costameres) are thought to be responsible for restraining the sarcolemma at the Z and M lines, so that when the fiber shortens to ~1.6-μm sarcomere length (in the drawing), the sarcolemma bulges out.

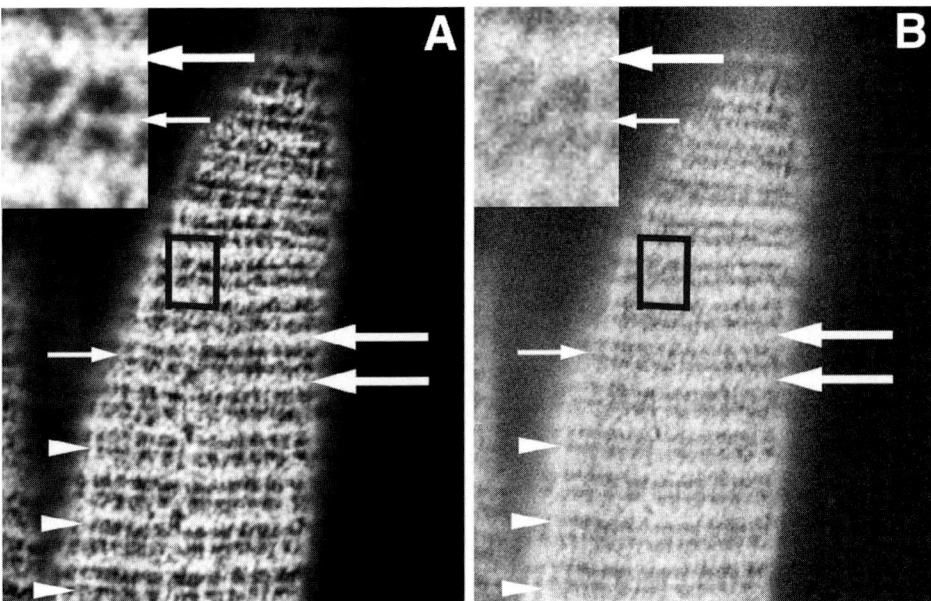

FIGURE 19a-4. Proteins of the adhesion complexes are mostly clustered along transverse subplasmalemmal bands called costameres. A frozen section grazing the surface of a rat EDL muscle fiber was double labeled for β-spectrin (A) and for dystrophin (B). The two proteins colocalize along wide costameres at the Z-line level (*large arrows*) and thinner costameres at the M line (*arrowheads and small arrows*). Both proteins are also present, at lower density, along longitudinally oriented bands, probably marking intermyofibrillar spaces. In this fast-twitch muscle fiber, dystrophin is present at low density between costameres but β-spectrin is not. (From Williams and Bloch.[49] Reproduced by permission.)

and the surface membrane.[62] By fixing laminin in the basal lamina to the subsarcolemmal actin network and then to the transverse network via further transmembrane connections, the whole system is set to prevent mechanical injury of the lipid bilayers during contraction.[16,61] The term *fixation bolt* has been coined to indicate the mechanical properties of the complex composed of either dystrophin or the closely related utrophin and the transmembrane proteins constituting the dystroglycans (see Chap. 19b).[35] The large number of muscle defects associated with failure of this protective system is a clear indication of its importance (see Chap. 19b). Lack of dystrophin in the *mdx* mouse is linked to a specific

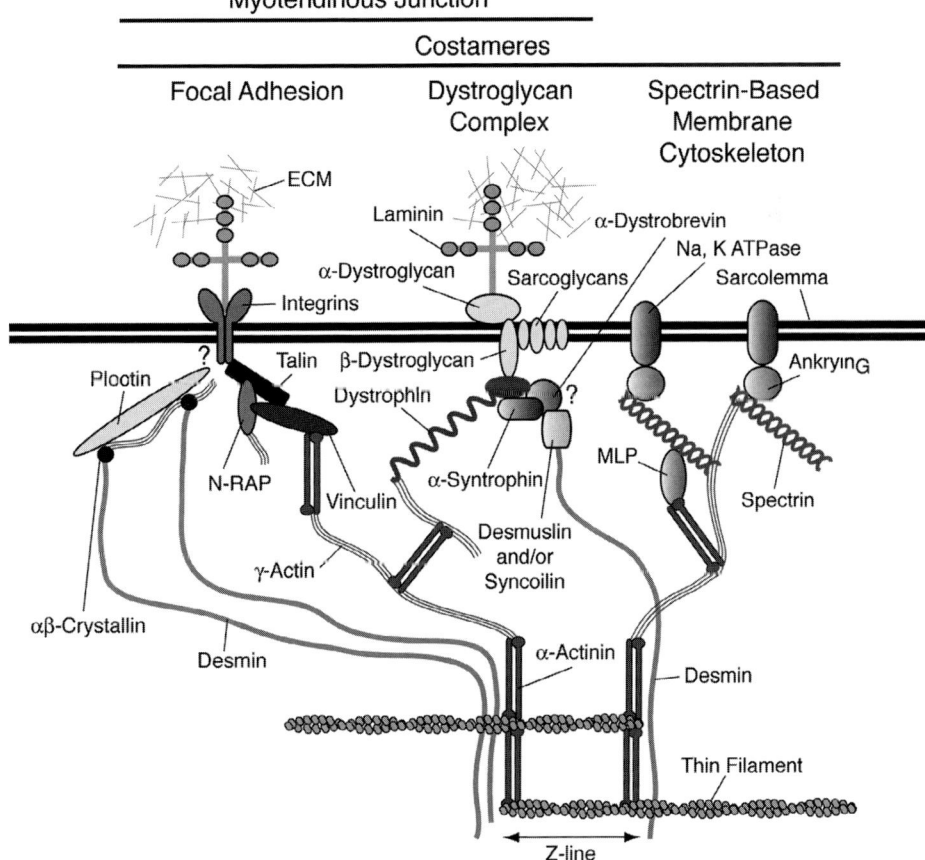

FIGURE 19a-5. Diagram of the macromolecular complexes that stabilize the subplasmalemmal cytoskeleton and connect it to the extracellular matrix on one side (mostly at costameres) and to the transverse network on the other. It has become apparent that the actin filament and the desmin filament systems in the muscle fibers are extensively interconnected. At the edges of the fiber, the connections continue into transmembrane links (via integrins and the dystroglycan-sarcoglycan complex). These connections are essential to the integrity of the muscle fiber. In addition, the spectrin-actin subplasmalemmal cytoskeleton also contributes to the maintenance of the sarcolemma's integrity. The latter is located at costameres in fast-twitch fibers, but it is more diffuse in slow-twitch fibers. Some details of the dystrophin-sarcoglycan complex differ from the model of Fig. 19b-1. MLP, muscle LIM protein; N-RAP, rebulin-related anchoring protein. (From Clark et al.[9] Reproduced by permission.)

rearrangement of subplasmalemmal cytoskeletal components, indicating interactions, perhaps indirectly, between the components of the subplasmalemmal network, particularly at the costameres.[67] However, although modern diagrams indicate the possibility of an interconnection via common interactions with actin and/or desmin filaments (Fig. 19a-5), the precise spatial relationship between the various systems is not established.

Costamere components—integrin and its associated proteins and the dystrophin complex—are not exclusively limited to the level of the Z disk but may extend over part of the adjacent I band and even to the M line; they are located at the neuromuscular junction's T tubules of cardiac muscle[68–71] and are also components of cell adhesion sites in other cells.[60] The disposition is fiber type–specific and affected by innervation. In fast-twitch fibers of the rat, spectrin is located exclusively at the Z lines and dystrophin at the Z lines and elsewhere.[72] In slow-twitch fibers, both molecules are diffused throughout the sarcolemma and costameres are not detected by immunolabeling; the fast fibers lose their sarcomeric organization after denervation.[73] The differences in organization of the sarcolemma may underlie the differential susceptibility of fast and slow myofibers to dystrophinopathies. In addition, adhesion sites are not always in the form of costameres, particularly in developing muscle, where small adhesion sites are uniformly distributed over the fiber surface and there is no visible actin focus under the plasmalemma.[74]

In addition to the integrin- and dystrophin-based systems, the subsarcolemmal cytoskeleton is also anchored to the sarcolemma via spectrin (Figs. 19a-4 and 19a-5), which, in turn, is connected to intramembrane proteins such as the Na,K-ATPase,[7] but not to the extracellular matrix. The spectrin link is present both at costameres and elsewhere. Questions of redundancy and/or functional integration between the various complexes that provide links across the plasmalemma are briefly discussed in a recent review.[75]

THE MYOTENDINOUS AND NEUROMUSCULAR JUNCTIONS

Myotendinous and neuromuscular junctions (MTJs and NMJs) are two functionally distinct compartments of the subsarcolemmal and extracellular matrix domains that contain variants of the sub- and transsarcolemmal components and of the extracellular matrix described above.[76] The NMJ is specialized for maintaining a high local density of the acetylcholine receptors (AChRs) and acetylcholinesterase and to maintain close proximity with motor nerve terminals. Actin filaments may serve to connect small AChR clusters to each other, stabilizing their positions in the postjunctional membrane.[71] Dystrophin, utrophin, and spectrin are highly expressed on the junctional folds and likely help to stabilize them (see also Chaps. 15 and 20).[77–80] Dystrophin is more difficult to remove from the postjunctional cytoskeleton than other proteins, indicating a unique association.[81]

The MTJ is the site of longitudinal force transmission from the ends of the myofibrils to the tendons, and this obviously is a site that requires extreme structural stability. It is a specialized region of the fiber, with deep membrane infoldings that offer interaction over a large surface area (Fig. 19a-6). Vinculin, talin, integrin, fibronectin, and collagen as well as dystrophin are present at the MTJs.[82–89] Dystrophic muscle

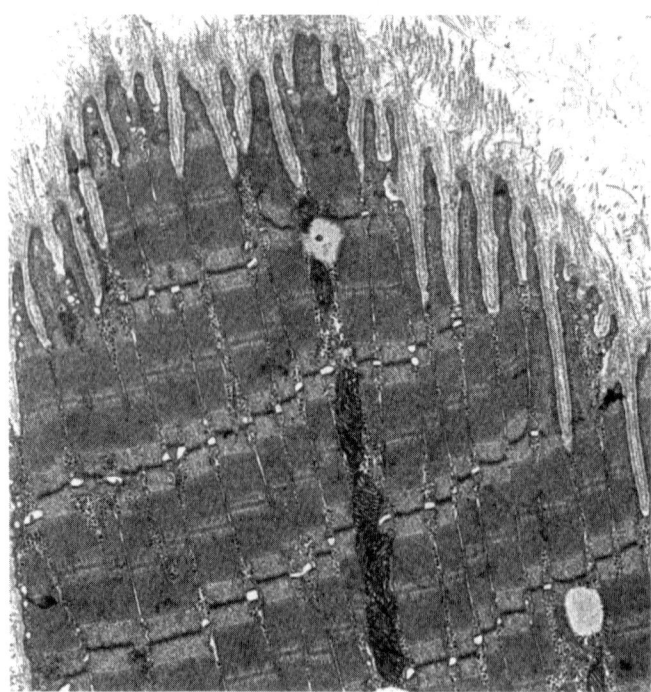
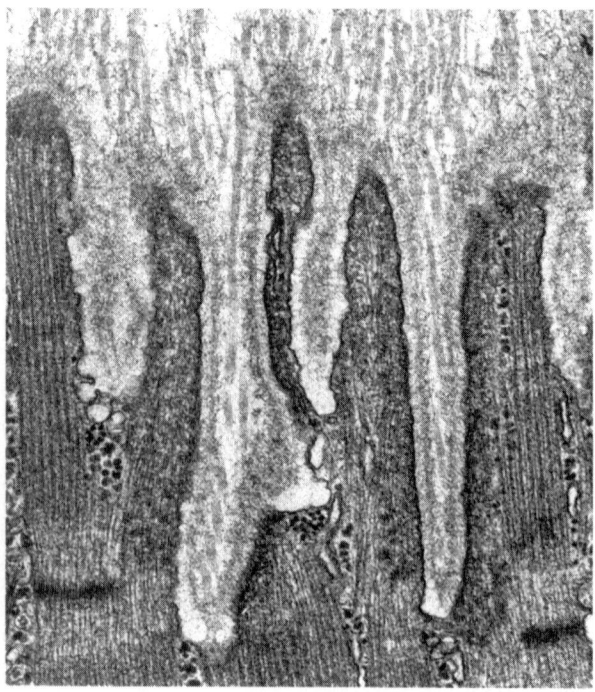

FIGURE 19a-6. The myotendinous junction provides a mechanically strong structural link between the ends of the myofibrils and the connective tissue of the tendon. Deep membrane invaginations enhance the connections. The myotendinous junctions contain the same macromolecular complex as the costameres, but with several isoform variants. This example is from a frog muscle.

sustains injury at the MTJ as well as at the fibers' lateral surfaces.[5,90,90a] However, the differential responses of the lateral surfaces and of the MTJ in muscle fibers lacking dystrophin[5,90,90a] indicate that the transplasmalemmal links provided by the complexes to which these two proteins belong have different roles in different regions of the fiber surface.

During myogenesis, the myofibrils initially do not span the entire myotube length but terminate laterally into the sarcolemma at focal adhesion sites containing vinculin (Fig. 19a-7).[74] As the myofibrils lengthen, their adhesion sites migrate toward the ends of the cells and eventually come together at the MTJ. Deposition of extracellular matrix components precedes that of the subcortical cytoskeleton, so that, in a sense, the extracellular matrix prepares the eventual myotendinous sites for the arrival of the myofibrillar ends.[86] The mechanism for the gradual formation of invaginations at the MTJ has not been identified.[87]

β1-Integrin plays a major role in stabilizing myofibrillogenesis by allowing the adhesion of myofibrillar ends through associating with different α subunits at various stages. The initial isoform is α3; as myofibrils become striated, α3 disappears,[58] to be replaced by α7 at the adult MTJ.[88] Mice with a targeted inactivation of the α7 gene show lack of digit-like extensions into collagen fiber and develop a form of muscular dystrophy that primarily affects the MTJ.[91] This confirms the significance of the link between integrin and laminin.[9,89,92]

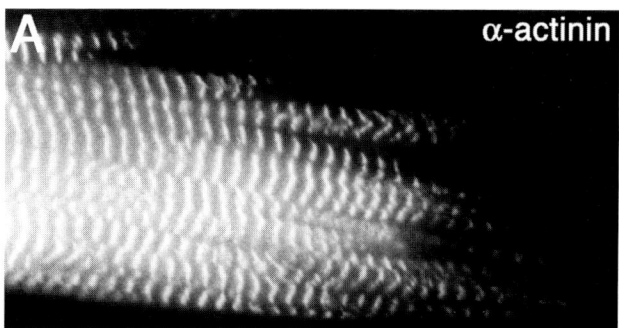

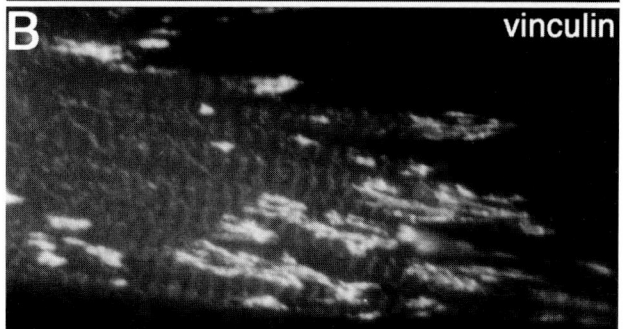

FIGURE 19a-7. Development of the myotendinous junction. Cultured avian muscle, labeled with antibodies against α-actinin (in A, to mark the Z disks) and vinculin (B). The ends of developing myofibrils are individually associated with the sarcolemma along the fiber edges through fixation bolts containing, among others, vinculin and talin (see also Fig. 19a-5). Later the ends of the myofibrils coalesce into the myotendinous junction. (*Courtesy of K. Ojima and H. Holtzer.*)

The Integrins

Most cell surface adhesion molecules can be categorized into several classes based on sequence homology or function. These are the integrin, cadherin, selectin, immunoglobulin (which includes the neural cell adhesion molecule, or NCAM), lectin, and glycosyltransferase families. Of these, integrin only is discussed here, owing to its role in the connection between the subcortical cytoskeleton and the extracellular matrix.

GENERAL PROPERTIES OF INTEGRINS

The integrins are a major superfamily of heterodimeric cell surface receptors for ECM and other cell surface receptors. They also bind to components of the cytoskeleton and thus both act as a transmembrane linkage system that connects cells or the ECM and play a role in transmembrane signaling.[75,93–106] Integrins are heterodimers, each containing a single α and β subunit; the specificity resides largely in the α subunits. Over 20 integrin combinations are currently well established.[100,102] Some integrins bind a single ligand, others bind multiple ligands, and there is redundancy in ligand specificity. It is interesting that the binding specificity of a particular integrin may depend on the cell type expressing it.[102,103] For example, the α2β1 integrin on platelets is specific for collagen, whereas it recognizes both collagen and laminin on other cells.[101] The structure of a prototype integrin has been published, along with potential mechanisms by which it is activated by ligand binding or by cytoplasmic proteins.[103,104]

The arginine-glycine-aspartate (RGD) sequence was first identified in fibronectin[107] as a common motif recognized in many integrin ligands and counterreceptors; however, other sequences are also recognized, and some molecules, like laminin and fibronectin, have multiple binding domains. The integrin specificity among different RGD-containing ligands is due to flanking sequences and the conformation of the RGD sequence in the protein.[108,109]

The associations of integrin with the cytoskeleton have been studied extensively.[110] In vivo and in vitro binding assays demonstrate binding of integrins to a large number of different molecules, including talin and α-actinin,[105,111–113] which reside in adhesion plaques in fibroblasts and costameres in skeletal and cardiac muscle (Fig. 19a-5).[9,11]

In addition to their structural function, integrins also participate in signal transduction and initiate signaling cascades that regulate proliferation, differentiation, migration, and survival.[100,101,105,106] For example, muscle differentiation is modulated by the interactions of antibodies with the integrin β subunit[114] The signaling is mediated by conformational changes that induce phosphorylation of key adapter proteins.[106]

INTEGRINS OF SKELETAL MUSCLE

Muscle has played a special role in integrin research because it was among the first systems in which integrins were discovered and characterized. Integrins play a prominent role in the formation and stabilization of junctional regions of muscle,[115–117] help organize nascent myofibrils,[64] participate in secondary myogenesis,[118,119] serve as a control point for muscle differentiation,[114] and mediate myoblast migration.[120] Initial immunofluorescence studies showed $\beta 1$ integrins to be present at myotendinous and neuromuscular junctions. Correspondingly, $\beta 1$ integrins were seen in adhesion plaque–like structures near the myotube and myoblast tips in cultured muscle and are also prominent at the ends of myotubes and other cell surface sites where myofibrils terminate, as well as on acetylcholine receptor clusters induced by a variety of different agents.[115,121] It is now clear that integrins are present on the lateral surfaces of muscle fibers, mostly at costameres (Fig. 19a-5). However, there are differences between fast- and slow-twitch muscle, the latter having $\beta 1$ integrin along the entire myotube as well as in junctional areas—a difference that arises early in differentiation.[115,122] The $\alpha 7\beta 1$ variant of integrin is the major integrin in adult muscle cells. It is responsible for specific adhesion to laminin,[99,101,123] for the integrity of the NMJs and MTJs, and for the lateral association of muscle fibers across the intervening extracellular matrix in adult muscle.[9,11,91,92,99,100] It is thus not surprising that it has a beneficial effect on the viability of dystrophic muscle and that its absence causes a novel form of dystrophy.[35,91] Posttranslational modifications affect the integrin's adhesion function.[124,125]

FUNCTIONS OF SPECIFIC MEMBERS OF THE $\beta 1$ INTEGRIN FAMILY

Of the integrin α subunits, the $\alpha 7$ integrin (originally called the H36 antigen) is particularly interesting because its expression is restricted to only a few cell types, including skeletal and cardiac muscle, melanoma cell lines, and sensory ganglia.[118,126–128] It functions as a receptor for laminin, and its amino acid sequence has considerable homology to the $\alpha 6$ subunit, another laminin receptor in the $\beta 1$ family.[99,100] Two waves of fusion and terminal differentiation accompany myogenesis (see Chap. 2). The initial event, primary myogenesis, is accompanied by a near synchronous fusion of myoblasts that produces the initial small primary myotubes. Secondary myogenesis is due to proliferation and differentiation of myoblasts derived from a distinct lineage. These secondary myoblasts align along the primary myotubes, where they proliferate and then fuse to form the secondary myotubes (see Chap. 4). The majority of the muscle mass is produced by secondary myogenesis, which proceeds gradually over an extended period. The expression of the $\alpha 7$ subunit is complex and appears to be related to the events of secondary myogenesis.[114,129,130] It is initially seen on primary myoblasts well after terminal differentiation has been initiated. In contrast, both the myoblasts and their precursors that participate in secondary myogenesis express the $\alpha 7$ subunit, with the level increasing following terminal differentiation.[131,132] The appearance of laminin corresponds with the expression of $\alpha 7$ subunit on secondary myoblasts. This correlation, along with the effect of laminin in enhancing myoblast proliferation, suggests that the proliferation of secondary myoblasts may be regulated via interaction of laminin with the $\alpha 7\beta 1$ integrin.[118,133–135] Other functions for the $\alpha 7$ subunit are suggested by a mutant myogenic cell line that expresses low levels of the $\alpha 7$ subunit; these cells neither interact nor fuse.[118] The correlation between early expression of $\alpha 7\beta 1$ integrin in secondary myotubes and its higher expression level in slow fibers (see above) has not been explored.

The $\alpha 4$ subunit and its cell surface counterreceptor VCAM-1 also appear to play a prominent role in secondary myogenesis: The primary myotubes are $\alpha 4$-positive shortly after their formation; in contrast, little $\alpha 4$ is present on the secondary myotubes.[136] In the adult, neither fiber type expresses the $\alpha 4$ subunit. The $\alpha 4\beta 1$ integrin has two ligands, an alternatively spliced form of fibronectin[137–139] and VCAM-1,[140–142] a cell surface adhesion molecule. Fibronectin is abundant throughout this developmental period,[143] whereas VCAM-1, in contrast, is absent from primary myoblasts and myotubes. Secondary myoblasts and myotubes do, however, express VCAM-1. As seen with the $\alpha 4$ subunit, VCAM-1 is not detected on adult muscle except on satellite cells. Thus, it appears that the $\alpha 4\beta 1$/VCAM-1 system is involved in the organization of the secondary muscle fibers by aligning them along the primary fibers and, perhaps, in fusion. At an earlier developmental stage, ectopic expression of different α isoforms significantly affects activation of $\beta 1$ integrin signaling pathways, which in turn regulate myoblast cell-cycle withdrawal.[144]

The latter possibility was explored using the C2C12 muscle cell line.[136] In accord with in vivo results, the $\alpha 4$ subunit was not detected on mitotic myoblasts but was present on postmitotic myoblasts, with increased expression on myotubes. VCAM-1 was seen on myoblasts and myotubes and localized at sites of cell-cell contact. Antibodies against either VCAM-1 or the $\alpha 4$ subunit inhibited fusion but not differentiation.

During myogenesis in vitro, expression of the $\alpha 5$ subunit undergoes a marked increase.[64] These changes correlate with early events in myofibrillogenesis. The $\alpha 5$ integrin localizes in adhesion plaque–like structures on myoblasts and myotubes, where actin bundles, precursors of myofibrils, and/or nascent myofibrils terminate and where newly synthesized fibrillar fibronectin is deposited.[145,146] These sites are precursors of the MTJ (see "The Myotendinous and Neuromuscular Junctions," above). The observation that integrin and α-actinin interact in vitro, together with the homology between α-actinin and dystrophin,[112,147] suggests a potential direct connection between dystrophin and integrin; however, there is no evidence at present supporting such a direct interaction.

Marked changes in expression and organization of the $\alpha 5$ integrin are seen in cultures growing on fibronectin and may be related to its role in the organization and myofibrillogenesis. In older cultures, the staining intensity of the $\alpha 5$ integrin correlates with registration of myofibrils into defined sarcomeres. Eventually adhesion plaques remain as the only intensely staining structure. The sustained presence of the adhesion plaques raises the possibility that they continue to function, not only in their adhesive capacity to bind to connective tissue fibronectin, but also as a possible template for the continued assembly of myofibrils. The $\alpha 1$, $\alpha 3$, $\alpha 6$, and $\alpha 7$ subunits have different distributions in muscle.[83,86,148,149] In particular, it is interesting to note that the location of alternative $\alpha 7$ isoforms on lateral surfaces and at NMJs and MTJs is developmentally regulated[150–152] in concert with the expression of laminin isoforms (see Chap. 20).[92,153] Indeed, integrins act as the leading element in the hierarchy of protein recruitment during the formation of focal adhesions.[154]

Microtubules

Striated muscle fibers have an extensive and intricate microtubule lattice located in subsarcolemmal, perinuclear, and intermyofibrillar spaces. Intermyofibrillar microtubules have a mostly longitudinal orientation with some oblique or transverse elements; subsarcolemmal regions and the cell ends have the highest density of tubules.[155–158] The density of microtubules is fiber type–dependent, and tubulin levels increase after denervation in both fast- and slow-twitch muscles, while intermediate filaments decrease.[159]

Myotubes grown in paclitaxel (Taxol), which stabilizes microtubules, and in colchemid, which disrupts them, demonstrate an abundance of tubulin and the requirement of microtubules for orderly alignment of myofibrils.[160,161] Interestingly, while under normal conditions microtubules are excluded from the myofibril, paclitaxel-stabilized microtubules interact with myosin filaments[161] and may extensively interdigitate with them to form apparent A bands.[160] Additional evidence for the role of microtubules in myogenesis comes from work on MURF, a protein expressed specifically in skeletal and cardiac muscle. MURF is associated with microtubules and stabilizes them; its presence is required for skeletal myoblast differentiation and fusion.[162]

In muscle as in other cells, microtubules act as pathways for the movement of membrane vesicles and for dispersal of the membrane systems in the cells. Markers involved with the endoplasmic reticulum–to-Golgi transport are found colocalized with microtubules in the interfibrillar spaces. Thus interfibrillar membranes seem to be active in protein export, and trafficking between endoplasmic reticulum and Golgi elements occurs throughout the myofibers.[163] Golgi apparatus and microtubule organizing centers have a unique disposition at multiple sites located circumferentially around nuclei rather than at opposite nuclear poles in both skeletal[164] and cardiac[165] muscle. In addition, thousands of dispersed Golgi elements are also found in the intermyofibrillar spaces, in association with microtubules[166]—a dispersal that is achieved during muscle differentiation, is microtubule-dependent, and is analogous to that observed in other cells after microtubule disruption.[167] This organization is dynamic and dependent on fiber type and activity.[168,169] Microtubule organization is clearly disrupted in dysgenic muscle, which is paralyzed owing to a defect in excitation-contraction coupling (see Chaps. 11 and 12).[170] However, it is not clear whether all intermyofibrillar microtubules are involved in Golgi-related traffic.

Other Structural Connections

The entire architecture of muscle fibers is structurally coordinated in a species- and fiber type–dependent fashion, so that each muscle fiber has a stereotyped and highly specific alignment of cross striations, localization of the internal membrane system (sarcoplasmic reticulum, or SR), and T tubules as well as location of mitochondria. In addition to the cytoskeletal elements described above, other structural connections have come to light. An interesting new discovery is that of obscurin, a giant sarcomeric protein that is connected to titin.[171] In parallel with the discovery of obscurin came the observation that the SR contains a small, alternatively spliced form of ankyrin,[172] one of a family of membrane-to-cytoplasm adapter proteins,[173] and that the SR ankyrin interacts with titin.[174] More specifically, it turns out that the small SR ankyrin most likely binds to obscurin, so that the obscurin-ankyrin bridge, located at the Z and M lines of striated (skeletal and cardiac) muscles,[175,176] may be responsible for the association of SR and myofibrils (see also Chap. 2).[177]

Association of myofibrils at the M line may be mediated by a large protein (skelemin) linking adjacent myofibrils.[178] Such an association may be required to explain the development of fairly well aligned A bands, complete with M lines, in the absence of I-Z-I assemblies in a cell line.[176]

Finally, it is not clear whether myofibrillar actin filaments may be involved in cytoskeletal interactions. I-Z-I bodies may form independently of myosin filaments.[179] Studies of isolated myofibrils have revealed that a number of actin filaments at the fibril's periphery are not involved in interactions with the myosin filaments but may be available for other associations.[180]

Acknowledgments

CFA is grateful to Prof. Eijiro Ozawa for contributing ideas and background for this chapter.

List of Abbreviations

AChR	acetylcholine receptor	NCAM	neural cell adhesion molecule
DAP	dystrophin-associated protein	NMJ	neuromuscular junction
ECM	extracellular matrix	RGD	arginine-glycine-aspartate
MTJ	myotendinous junction	SR	sarcoplasmic reticulum

References

1. Wakayama Y, Shibuya S: Gold-labeled dystrophin molecule in muscle plasmalemma of *mdx* control mice as seen by electron microscopy of deep etching replica. *Acta Neuropathol* 82:178–184, 1991.
2. Pierobon-Bormioli S: Transverse sarcomere filamentous systems: Z- and M-cables. *J Muscle Res Cell Motil* 2:401–413, 1981.
3. Street SF: Lateral transmission of tension in frog myofibers: A myofibrillar network and transverse cytoskeletal connections are possible transmitters. *J Cell Physiol* 114:346–364, 1983.
4. Granger BL, Lazarides E: The existence of an insoluble Z disc scaffold in chicken skeletal muscle. *Cell* 15:1253–1268, 1978.
5. Law DJ, Caputo A, Tidball JG: Site and mechanics of failure in normal and dystrophin-deficient skeletal muscle. *Muscle Nerve* 18:216–223, 1995.
6. Robinson TF, Winegrad S: A variety of intercellular connections in heart muscle. *J Mol Cell Cardiol* 13:185–192, 1981.
7. Pardo JV, Siliciano JD, Craig SW: A vinculin-containing cortical lattice in skeletal muscle: Transverse lattice elements ("costameres") mark sites of attachment between myofibrils and sarcolemma. *Proc Natl Acad Sci USA* 80:1008–1012, 1983.
8. Danowski BA, Imanaka-Yoshida K, Sanger JM, et al: Costameres are sites of force transmission to the substratum in adult rat cardiomyocytes. *J Cell Biol* 118:1411–1420, 1992.
9. Clark KA, McElhinny AS, Beckerle MC, et al: Striated muscle cytoarchitecture. An intricate web of form and function. *Annu Rev Cell Dev Biol* 18:637–706, 2002.
10. Ishikawa H: Plasmalemmal undercoat: The cytoskeleton supporting the plasmalemma. *Arch Histol Cytol* 51:127–145, 1988.
11. Bloch RJ, Capetanaki Y, O'Neill A, et al: Costameres: Repeating structures at the sarcolemma of skeletal muscle. *Clin Orthop* 403:S203–S210, 2002.
12. Masaki T, Endo M, Ebashi S: Localization of 6S component of alpha-actinin at Z-band. *J Biochem (Tokyo)* 62:630–632, 1967.
13. Nakata T, Nishina Y, Yorifuji H: Cytoplasmic gamma actin as a Z-disc protein. *Biochem Biophys Res Commun* 286:156–163, 2001.
14. Poon E, Howman EV, Newey SE, et al: Association of syncoilin and desmin. Linking intermediate filament proteins to the dystrophin-associated protein complex. *J Biol Chem* 277:3433–3439, 2002.
15. Berthier C, Blaineau S: Supramolecular organization of the subsarcolemmal cytoskeleton of adult skeletal muscle fibers. *Biol Cell* 89:413–434, 1997.
16. Ervasti JM: Costameres: Achilles' heel of Herculean muscle. *J Biol Chem* 278:13591–13594, 2003.
17. Tokuyasu KT, Dutton AH, Geiger B, et al: Ultrastructure of chicken cardiac muscle as studied by double immunolabeling in electron microscopy. *Proc Natl Acad Sci USA* 78:7619–7623, 1981.
18. Lazarides E, Hubbard BD: Immunological characterization of the subunit of the 100 A filaments from muscle cells. *Proc Natl Acad Sci USA* 73:4344–4348, 1976.
19. Lazarides E: Intermediate filaments as mechanical integrators of cellular space. *Nature* 283:249–256, 1980.
20. Boriek AM, Capetanaki Y, Hwang W, et al: Desmin integrates the three-dimensional mechanical properties of muscles. *Am J Physiol* 280:C46–C52, 2001.
21. Fuchs E: Intermediate filaments and disease: Mutations that cripple cell strength. *J Cell Biol* 125:511–516, 1994.
22. Schultheiss T, Lin Z, Ishikawa H, et al: Desmin/vimentin intermediate filaments are dispensable for many aspects of myogenesis. *J Cell Biol* 114: 953–966, 1991.
23. Carlsson L, Li ZL, Paulin D, et al: Differences in the distribution of synemin, paranemin, and plectin in skeletal muscles of wild-type and desmin knock-out mice. *Histochem Cell Biol* 114:39–47, 2000.
24. O'Neill A, Williams MW, Resneck WG, et al: Sarcolemmal organization in skeletal muscle lacking desmin: Evidence for cytokeratins associated with the membrane skeleton at costameres. *Mol Biol Cell* 13:2347–2359, 2002.
25. Milner DJ, Weitzer G, Tran D, et al: Disruption of muscle architecture and myocardial degeneration in mice lacking desmin. *J Cell Biol* 134:1255–1270, 1996.
26. Hijikata T, Murakami T, Imamura M, et al: Plectin is a linker of intermediate filaments to Z-discs in skeletal muscle fibers. *J Cell Sci* 112:867–876, 1999.
27. Hijikata T, Murakami T, Ishikawa H, et al: Plectin tethers desmin intermediate filaments onto subsarcolemmal dense plaques containing dystrophin and vinculin. *Histochem Cell Biol* 119:109–123, 2003.
28. Wiche G, Gromov D, Donovan A, et al: Expression of plectin mutant cDNA in cultured cells indicates a role of COOH-terminal domain in intermediate filament association. *J Cell Biol* 121:607–619, 1993.
29. Schroder R, Furst DO, Klasen C, et al: Association of plectin with Z-discs is a prerequisite for the formation of the intermyofibrillar desmin cytoskeleton. *Lab Invest* 80:455–464, 2000.
30. Wiche G: Role of plectin in cytoskeleton organization and dynamics. *J Cell Sci* 3:2477–2486, 1998.
31. McLean WH, Pulkkinen L, Smith FJ, et al: Loss of plectin causes epidermolysis bullosa with muscular dystrophy: cDNA cloning and genomic organization. *Genes Dev* 10:1724–1735, 1996.
32. Uitto J, Pulkkinen L, Smith FJ, et al: Plectin and human genetic disorders of the skin and muscle. The paradigm of epidermolysis bullosa with muscular dystrophy. *Exp Dermatol* 5:237–246, 1996.
33. Newey SE, Howman EV, Ponting CP, et al: Syncoilin, a novel member of the intermediate filament superfamily that interacts with α-dystrobrevin in skeletal muscle. *J Biol Chem* 276:6645–6655, 2001.
34. Mizuno Y, Thompson TG, Guyon JR, et al: Desmuslin, an intermediate filament protein that interacts with α-dystrobrevin and desmin. *Proc Natl Acad Sci USA* 98:6156–6161, 2001.
35. Ozawa E, Nishino I, Nonaka I: Sarcolemmopathy: Muscular dystrophies with cell membrane defects. *Brain Pathol* 11:218–230, 2001.
36. Tinsley JM, Potter AC, Phelps SR, et al: Amelioration of the dystrophic phenotype of mdx mice using a truncated utrophin transgene. *Nature* 384:349–353, 1996.
37. Burkin DJ, Wallace GQ, Nicol KJ, et al: Enhanced expression of the alpha-7 beta-1 integrin reduces muscular dystrophy and restores viability in dystrophic mice. *J Cell Biol* 152:1207–1218, 2001.
38. Abbott BC, Baskin RJ, et al: Volume changes in frog muscle during contraction. *J Physiol (Lond)* 161:379–391, 1962.
39. Elliott GF, Matsubara I: The constant-volume behaviour of the myofilament lattice in frog skeletal muscle: Studies on skinned and intact single fibres by x-ray and light diffraction. *J Physiol* 226:88P–89P, 1972.
40. Dulhunty AF, Franzini-Armstrong C: The relative contributions of folds and caveolae to the surface membrane of frog skeletal muscle fibre to different sarcomere lengths. *J Physiol (Lond)* 250:513–539, 1975.
41. Frigeri A, Nicchia GP, Verbavatz JM, et al: Expression of aquaporin-4 in fast-twitch fibers of mammalian skeletal muscle. *J Clin Invest* 102:695–703, 1998.
42. Ellisman MH, Rash JE, Staehlin LA, et al: Studies of excitable membranes. II. A comparison of specializations at neuromuscular junctions and nonjunctional sarcolemmas of mammalian fast and slow twitch muscle fibers. *J Cell Biol* 68:752–774, 1976.
43. Hatton JD, Ellisman MH: The distribution of orthogonal arrays and their relationship to intercellular junctions in neuroglia of the freeze-fractured hypothalamo-neurohypophysial system. *Cell Tissue Res* 215:309–323, 1981.
44. Yang B, Verbavatz JM, Song Y, et al: Skeletal muscle function and water permeability in aquaporin-4 deficient mice. *Am J Physiol Cell Physiol* 278:1108–1115, 2000.
45. Danowski BA, Imanaka-Yoshida K, Sanger JM, et al: Costameres are sites of force transmission to the substratum in adult rat cardiomyocytes. *J Cell Biol* 118:1411–1420, 1992.
46. Samuelsson SJ, Luther PW, Pumplin DW, et al: Structures linking microfilament bundles to the membrane at focal contacts. *J Cell Biol* 122:485–496, 1993.
47. Mondello MR, Bramanti P, Cutroneo G, et al: Immunolocalization of the costameres in human skeletal muscle fibers: Confocal scanning laser microscope investigations. *Anat Rec* 245:481–487, 1996.
48. Masuda T, Fujimaki N, Ozawa E, et al: Confocal laser microscopy of dystrophin localization in guinea pig skeletal muscle fibers. *J Cell Biol* 119:543–548, 1992.
49. Williams MW, Bloch RJ: Differential distribution of dystrophin and beta-spectrin at the sarcolemma of fast twitch skeletal muscle fibers. *J Muscle Res Cell Motil* 20:383–393, 1999.
50. Porter GA, Dmytrenko GM, Winkelmann JC, et al: Dystrophin colocalizes with β-spectrin in distinct subsarcolemmal domains in mammalian skeletal muscle. *J Cell Biol* 117:997–1005, 1992.
51. Williams MW, Resneck WG, Bloch RJ: Membrane skeleton of innervated and denervated fast- and slow-twitch muscle. *Muscle Nerve* 23:590–599, 2000.
52. Pardo JV, Pittenger MF, Craig SW: Subcellular sorting of isoactins: Selective association of gamma actin with skeletal muscle mitochondria. *Cell* 32:1093–1103, 1983.
53. Pardo JV, Siliciano JD, Craig SW: Vinculin is a component of an extensive network of myofibril-sarcolemma attachment regions in cardiac muscle fibers. *J Cell Biol* 97:1081–1088, 1983.
54. Sharp WW, Simpson DG, Borg TK, et al: Mechanical forces regulate focal adhesion and costamere assembly in cardiac myocytes. *Am J Physiol* 273:546–556, 1997.
55. Craig SW, Pardo JV: Gamma actin, spectrin, and intermediate filament proteins colocalize with vinculin at costameres, myofibril-to-sarcolemma attachment site. *Cell Motil Cytoskeleton* 3:449–462, 1983.
56. Shear CR, Bloch RJ: Vinculin in subsarcolemmal densities in chicken skeletal muscle: Localization and relationship to intracellular and extracellular structures. *J Cell Biol* 101:240–256, 1985.
57. Hijikata T, Fujimaki N, Osawa H, et al: The direct visualization of structural array from laminin to dystrophin in sarcolemmal vesicles prepared from rat skeletal muscles. *Biol Cell* 90:629–639, 1998.
58. McDonald KA, Lakonishok M, Horwitz AF: Alpha v and alpha 3 integrin subunits are associated with myofibrils during myofibrillogenesis. *J Cell Sci* 108:2573–2581, 1995.
59. Brancaccio M, Guazzone S, Menini N, et al: Melusin is a new muscle-specific interactor for beta(1) integrin cytoplasmic domain. *J Biol Chem* 274:29282–29288, 1999.

60. Geiger B, Dutton AH, Tokuyasu KT, et al: Immunoelectron microscope studies of membrane-microfilament interactions: Distributions of alpha-actinin, tropomyosin, and vinculin in intestinal epithelial brush border and chicken gizzard smooth muscle cells. *J Cell Biol* 91:614–628, 1981.
61. Rybakova IN, Patel JR, Ervasti JM: The dystrophin complex forms a mechanically strong link between the sarcolemma and costameric actin. *J Cell Biol* 150:1209–1214, 2000.
62. Sheard P, Paul A, Duxson M: Intramuscular force transmission. *Adv Exp Med Biol* 508:495–499, 2002.
63. Rafael JA, Cox GA, Corrado K, et al: Forced expression of dystrophin deletion constructs reveals structure-function correlations. *J Cell Biol* 134:93–102, 1996.
64. Lakonishok M, Muschler J, Horwitz AF: The alpha 5 beta 1 integrin associates with a dystrophin-containing lattice during muscle development. *Dev Biol* 152:209–220, 1992.
65. Arahata K, Ishiura S, et al: Immunostaining of skeletal and cardiac muscle surface membrane with antibody against Duchenne muscular dystrophy peptide. *Nature* 333:861–863, 1988.
66. Straub V, Bittner RE, Léger JJ, et al: Direct visualization of the dystrophin network on skeletal muscle fiber membrane. *J Cell Biol* 119:1183–1191, 1992.
67. Williams MW, Bloch RJ: Extensive but coordinated reorganization of the membrane skeleton in myofibers of dystrophic (*mdx*) mice. *J Cell Biol* 144:1259–1270, 1999.
68. Watkins SC, Hoffman EP, Slayter HS, et al: Immunoelectron microscopic localization of dystrophin in myofibers. *Nature* 333:863–866, 1988.
69. Harris JB, Cullen MJ: Ultrastructural localization and the possible role of dystrophin, in Kakulas BA, Howell JMcC, Roses AD (eds): *Duchenne Muscular Dystrophy: Animal Models and Gene Manipulation.* New York: Raven Press; 1992, pp 19–40.
70. Klietsch R, Ervasti JM, Arnold W, et al: Dystrophin-glycoprotein complex and laminin colocalize to the sarcolemma and transverse tubules of cardiac muscle. *Circ Res* 72:349–360, 1993.
71. Luther PW, Samuelsson SJ, Bloch RJ, et al: Cytoskeleton-membrane interactions at the postsynaptic density of *Xenopus* neuromuscular junctions. *J Neurocytol* 25:417–427, 1996.
72. Williams MW, Bloch RJ: Differential distribution of dystrophin and beta-spectrin at the sarcolemma of fast twitch skeletal muscle fibers. *J Muscle Res Cell Motil* 20:383–393, 1999.
73. Williams MW, Resneck WG, Bloch RJ: Membrane skeleton of innervated and denervated fast- and slow-twitch muscle. *Muscle Nerve* 23:590–599, 2000.
74. Ojima K, Lin ZX, Zhang ZQ, et al: Initiation and maturation of I-Z-I bodies in the growth tips of transfected myotubes. *J Cell Sci* 112:4101–4112, 1999.
75. Mayer U: Integrins: Redundant or important players in skeletal muscle? *J Biol Chem* 278:14587–14590, 2003.
76. Patton BL: Laminins of the neuromuscular system. *Microsc Res Techn* 51:247–261, 2000.
77. Shimizu T, Matsumura K, Sunada Y, et al: Dense immunostaining on both neuromuscular and myotendon junctions with an anti-dystrophin monoclonal antibody. *Biomed Res* 10:405–409, 1989.
78. Fardeau M, Tomé FM, Collin H, et al: Presence of dystrophine-like protein at the neuromuscular junction in Duchenne muscular dystrophy and in "mdx" mutant mice. *C R Acad Sci Paris Sci Vie* 311:197–204, 1990.
79. Cote PD, Moukhles H, Lindenbaum M, et al: Chimaeric mice deficient in dystroglycans develop muscular dystrophy and have disrupted myoneural synapses. *Nat Genet* 23:338–342, 1999.
80. Bloch RJ, Bezakova G, Ursitti JA, et al: A membrane skeleton that clusters nicotinic acetylcholine receptors in muscle. *Soc Gen Physiol Ser* 52:177–195, 1997.
81. Dmytrenko GM, Pumplin DW, Bloch RJ: Dystrophin in a membrane skeletal network: Localization and comparison to other proteins. *J Neurosci* 13:547–558, 1993.
82. Tidball JG, O'Halloran TBK: Talin at myotendinous junctions. *J Cell Biol* 103:1465–1472, 1986.
83. Tidball JG: Force transmission across muscle cell membranes. *J Biomech* 24:43–52, 1991.
84. Frenette J, Tidball JG: Mechanical loading regulates expression of talin and its mRNA, which are concentrated at myotendinous junctions. *Am J Physiol* 275:C818–C825, 1998.
85. Yang B, Jung D, Rafael JA, et al: Identification of alpha-syntrophin binding to syntrophin triplet, drystophin, and utrophin. *J Biol Chem* 270:4975–4978, 1995.
86. Tidball JG: Assembly of myotendinous junctions in the chick embryo: Deposition of P68 is an early event in myotendinous junction formation. *Dev Biol* 163:447–456, 1994.
87. Nagano Y, Matsuda Y, Desaki J, et al: Morphodifferentiation of skeletal muscle fiber ends at the myotendinous junction in the postnatal Chinese hamster: A scanning electron microscopic study. *Arch Histol Cytol* 61:89–92, 1998.
88. Bao Z, Lakonishok M, Kaufman S, et al: Alpha 7 beta 1 integrin is a component of the myotendinous junction on skeletal muscle. *J Cell Sci* 106:579–589, 1993.
89. Miosge N, Klenczar C, Herken R: Organization of the myotendinous junction is dependent on the presence of alpha7beta1 integrin. *Lab Invest* 79:1591–1599, 1999.
90. Ridge JC, Tidball JG, Ahl K: Modifications in myotendinous junction surface morphology in dystrophin-deficient mouse muscle. *Exp Mol Pathol* 61:58–68, 1986.
90a. Mokri B, Engel AG: Duchenne dystrophy: Electron microscopic findings pointing to a basic or early abnormality in the plasma membrane of the muscle fiber. *Neurology (Minneapolis)* 25:1111–1120, 1975.
91. Mayer U, Saher G, Fassler R, et al: Absence of integrin alpha 7 causes a novel form of muscular dystrophy. *Nat Genet* 17(3):318–323, 1997.
92. Burkin DJ, Kaufman SJ: The alpha7beta1 integrin in muscle development and disease. *Cell Tissue Res* 296:183–190, 1999.
93. Buck CA, Horwitz AP: Cell surface receptors for extracellular matrix molecules. *Annu Rev Cell Biol* 3:179–205, 1987.
94. Ruoslahti E, Pierschbacher MD: New perspectives in cell adhesion: RGD and integrins. *Science* 238:491–497, 1987.
95. Hynes RO: Integrins: A family of cell surface receptors. *Cell* 48:549–554, 1987.
96. Burridge K, Fath K, Kelly T, et al: Focal adhesions: Transmembrane junctions between the extracellular matrix and the cytoskeleton. *Annu Rev Cell Biol* 4:487–525, 1988.
97. Albelda SM, Buck CA: Integrins and other cell adhesion molecules. *FASEB J* 4:2868–2880, 1990.
98. Hynes RO: Integrins: Versatility, modulation, and signaling in cell adhesion. *Cell* 69:11–25, 1992.
99. Belkin AM, Stepp MA: Integrins as receptors for laminins. *Microsc Res Techn* 51:280–301, 2000.
100. van der Flier A, Sonnenberg A: Function and interactions of integrins. *Cell Tissue Res* 305:285–298, 2001.
101. Hynes RO: Integrins: Bidirectional, allosteric signaling machines. *Cell* 110:673–687, 2002.
102. Plow EF, Haas TA, Zhang L, et al: Ligand binding to integrins. *J Biol Chem* 275:21785–21788, 2000.
103. Humphries MJ: The molecular basis and specificity of integrin-ligand interactions. *J Cell Sci* 97:585–592, 1990.
104. Springer TA: Adhesion receptors of the immune system. *Nature* 346:425–434, 1990.
105. Schwartz MA, Ginsberg MH: Networks and crosstalk: Integrin signalling spreads. *Nat Cell Biol* 4:E65–E68, 2002.
106. Schwartz MA: Integrin signaling revisited. *Trends Cell Biol* 11:466–470, 2001.
107. Pierschbacher MD, Ruoslahti E: Cell attachment activity of fibronectin can be duplicated by small synthetic fragments of the molecule. *Nature* 309:30–33, 1984.
108. Pierschbacher MD, Ruoslahti E: Influence of stereochemistry of the sequence Arg-Gly-Asp-Xaa on binding specificity in cell adhesion. *J Biol Chem* 262:17294–17298, 1987.
109. Obara M, Kang MS, Yamada KM: Site-directed mutagenesis of cell-binding domain of human fibronectin: Separable, synergistic sites mediate adhesive function. *Cell* 53:649–657, 1988.
110. Liu S, Calderwood DA, Ginsberg MH: Integrin cytoplasmic domain binding proteins. *J Cell Sci* 113:3563–3571, 2000.
111. Horwitz AF, Duggan K, Buck C, et al: Interaction of plasma membrane fibronectin receptor with talin—A transmembrane linkage. *Nature* 320:531–533, 1986.
112. Otey CA, Pavalko FM, Burridge K: An interaction between alpha-actinin and the beta 1 integrin subunit in vitro. *J Cell Biol* 111:721–729, 1990.
113. Reszka AA, Hayashi Y, Horwitz AF: Identification of amino acid sequences in the integrin B 1 cytoplasmic domain implicated in cytoskeletal interaction. *J Cell Biol* 117:1321–1330, 1992.
114. Menko AS, Boettiger D: Occupation of the extracellular matrix receptor, integrin, is a control point for myogenic differentiation. *Cell* 51:51–57, 1987.
115. Bozyczko D, Decker C, Muschler J, et al: Integrin on developing and adult skeletal muscle. *Exp Cell Res* 183:72–91, 1989.
116. Swasdison S, Mayne R: Location of the integrin complex and extracellular matrix molecules at the chicken myotendinous junction. *Cell Tissue Res* 257:537–543, 1989.
117. Wallace BG: Agrin-induced specializations contain cytoplasmic, membrane, and extracellular matrix-associated components of the postsynaptic apparatus. *J Neurosci* 9:1294–1302, 1989.
118. Song WK, Wang W, Foster R, et al: H36-alpha 7 is a novel integrin chain that is developmentally regulated during skeletal myogenesis. *J Cell Biol* 117:643–657, 1992.
119. Rosen GD, Sanes JR, LaChance R, et al: Roles for the integrin VLA-4 and its counter receptor VCAM-1 in myogenesis. *Cell* 69:1107–1119, 1992.
120. Jaffredo T, Horwitz AF, Buck CA, et al: Myoblast migration specifically inhibited in the chick embryo by grafted CSAT hybridoma cells secreting an anti-integrin antibody. *Development* 103:431–446, 1988.
121. Damsky CH, Knudsen KA, Bradley D, et al: Distribution of the cell substratum attachment (CSAT) antigen on myogenic and fibroblastic cells in culture. *J Cell Biol* 100:1528–1539, 1985.

122. George-Weinstein M, Foster RF, Gerhart JV, et al: In vitro and in vivo expression of alpha 7 integrin and desmin define the primary and secondary myogenic lineages. *Dev Biol* 156:209–229, 1993.
123. Crawley S, Farrell EM, Wang W, et al: The alpha 7 beta 1 integrin mediates adhesion and migration of skeletal myoblasts on laminin. *Exp Cell Res* 235:274–286, 1997.
124. Chatila TA, Geha RS, Arnaut MA: Constitutive and stimulus-induced phosphorylation of CD11/CD18 leukocyte adhesion molecules. *J Cell Biol* 109:3435–3444, 1989.
125. Valmu L, Autero M, Siljander P, et al: Phosphorylation of the beta-subunit of CD11/CD18 integrins by protein kinase C correlates with leukocyte adhesion. *Eur J Immunol* 21:2857–2862, 1991.
126. Wayner EA, Garcia PA, Humphries MJ, et al: Identification and characterization of the T lymphocyte adhesion receptor for alternative cell attachment domain (CS-1) in plasma fibronectin. *J Cell Biol* 109:1321–1330, 1989.
127. Dahl SC, Grabel LB: Integrin phosphorylation is modulated during the differentiation of F-9 teratocarcinoma stem cells. *J Cell Biol* 108:183–190, 1989.
128. Hirst R, Horwitz A, Buck C, et al: Phosphorylation of the fibronectin receptor complex in cells transformed by oncogenes that encode tyrosine kinases. *Proc Natl Acad Sci USA* 83:6470–6474, 1986.
129. Buck CA, Shea E, Duggan K, et al: Integrin (the CSAT antigen): Functionality requires oligomeric integrity. *J Cell Biol* 103:2421–2428, 1986.
130. Damsky CH, Knudsen KA, Bradley D, et al: Distribution of the cell substratum attachment (CSAT) antigen on myogenic and fibroblastic cells in culture. *J Cell Biol* 100:1528–1539, 1985.
131. Kaufman SJ, Foster RF: Replicating myoblasts express a muscle-specific phenotype. *Proc Natl Acad Sci USA* 85:9606–9610, 1988.
132. Kaufman SJ, George-Weinstein MG, Foster RF: In vitro development of precursor cells in the myogenic lineage. *Dev Biol* 156:228–238, 1991.
133. Foster RF, Thompson JM, Kaufman SJ: A laminin substrate promotes myogenesis in rat skeletal muscle cultures: Analysis of replication and development using antidesmin and anti-BrdUrd monoclonal antibodies. *Dev Biol* 122:11–20, 1987.
134. Ocalan M, Goodman SL, Kauhl U, et al: Laminin alters cell shape and stimulates motility and proliferation of murine skeletal myoblasts. *Dev Biol* 125:158–167, 1988.
135. von der Mark K, Ocalan M: Antagonistic effects of laminin and fibronectin on the expression of the myogenic phenotype. *Differentiation* 40:150–157, 1989.
136. Rosen GD, Sanes JR, LaChance R, et al: Roles for the integrin VLA-4 and its counter receptor VCAM-1 in myogenesis. *Cell* 69:1107–1119, 1992.
137. Wayner EA, Garcia PA, Humphries MJ, et al: Identification and characterization of the T lymphocyte adhesion receptor for alternative cell attachment domain (CS-1) in plasma fibronectin. *J Cell Biol* 109:1321–1330, 1989.
138. Guan JL, Hynes RO: Lymphoid cells recognize an alternatively spliced segment of fibronectin via the integrin receptor alpha 4 beta 1. *Cell* 60:53–61, 1990.
139. Mould AP, Wheldon LA, Komorya A, et al: Affinity chromatographic isolation of the melanoma adhesion receptor for the IIICS region of fibronectin and its identification as the integrin alpha 4 beta 1. *J Biol Chem* 265:4020–4024, 1990.
140. Osborn L, Hession C, Tizard R, et al: Direct expression cloning of vascular cell adhesion molecule-1, a cytokine-induced endothelial protein that binds to lymphocytes. *Cell* 59:1203–1211, 1989.
141. Elices MJ, Osborn L, Takada Y, et al: VCAM-1 on activated endothelium interacts with the leukocyte integran VLA-4 at a site distinct from the VLA-4/fibronectin binding site. *Cell* 60:577–584, 1990.
142. Rice GE, Munro JM, Corless C, et al: Vascular and nonvascular expression of INCAM-110: A target for mononuclear leukocyte adhesion in normal and inflamed human tissues. *Am J Pathol* 138:385–393, 1991.
143. Chiu AY, Sanes JR: Differentiation of basal lamina in synaptic and extrasynaptic portions of embryonic rat muscle. *Dev Biol* 103:456–467, 1984.
144. Sastry SK, Lakonishok M, Wu S, et al: Quantitative changes in integrin and focal adhesion signaling regulate myoblast cell cycle withdrawal. *J Cell Biol* 144:1295–1309, 1999.
145. Terai M, Komiyama M, Shimada Y: Myofibril assembly is linked with vinculin, alpha-actinin, and cell-substrate contacts in embryonic cardiac myocytes in vitro. *Cell Motil Cytoskeleton* 12:185–194, 1989.
146. Lin ZX, Holtzer S, Schultheiss T, et al: Polygons and adhesion plaques and the disassembly and assembly of myofibrils in cardiac myocytes. *J Cell Biol* 108:2355–2367, 1989.
147. Koenig M, Monaco AP, Kunkel LM: The complete sequence of dystrophin predicts a rod-shaped cytoskeletal protein. *Cell* 53:219–228, 1988.
148. Bao ZZ, Lakonishok M, Kaufman S, et al: Alpha 7 beta 1 integrin is a component of the myotendinous junction of skeletal muscle. *J Cell Sci* 106:579–589, 1993.
149. Dubank JL, Belkin AM, Syfrig J, et al: Expression of alpha 1 integrin, a laminin-collagen receptor, during myogenesis and neurogenesis in the anion embryo. *Development* 116:585–600, 1992.
150. Song WK, Wang W, Sato H, et al: Expression of alpha 7 integrin cytoplasmic domains during skeletal muscle development: Alternate forms, conformational change, and homologies with serine/threonine kinases and tyrosine phosphatases. *J Cell Sci* 106:1139–1152, 1993.
151. Collo G, Starr L, Quaranta V: A new isoform of the laminin receptor integrin alpha 7 beta 1 is developmentally regulated in skeletal muscle. *J Biol Chem* 268:19019–19024, 1993.
152. Ziober BL, Vu MP, Waleh N: Alternative extracellular and cytoplasmic domains of the integrin alpha 7 subunit are differentially expressed during development. *J Biol Chem* 268:26773–26783, 1993.
153. Martin PT, Kaufman SJ, Kramer RH, et al: Synaptic integrins in developing, adult, and mutant muscle: Selective association of alpha1, alpha7A, and alpha7B integrins with the neuromuscular junction. *Dev Biol* 174:125–139, 1996.
154. Miyamoto S, Teramoto H, Coso OA, et al: Integrin function: Molecular hierarchies of cytoskeletal and signaling molecules. *J Cell Biol* 131:791–805, 1995.
155. Cartwright J Jr, Goldstein MA: Microtubules in the heart muscle of the postnatal and adult rat. *J Mol Cell Cardiol* 17:1–7, 1985.
156. Cartwright J Jr, Goldstein MA: Microtubules in soleus muscles of the postnatal and adult rat. *J Ultrastruct Res* 79:74–84, 1982.
157. Kano Y, Fujimaki N, Ishikawa H: The distribution and arrangement of microtubules in mammalian skeletal muscle fibers. *Cell Struct Funct* 16:251–261, 1991.
158. Boudriau S, Vincent M, Cote CH, et al: Cytoskeletal structure of skeletal muscle: Identification of an intricate exosarcomeric microtubule lattice in slow- and fast-twitch muscle fibers. *J Histochem Cytochem* 41:1013–1021, 1993.
159. Boudriau S, Cote CH, Vincent M, et al: Remodeling of the cytoskeletal lattice in denervated skeletal muscle. *Muscle Nerve* 19:1383–1390, 1996.
160. Toyama Y, Forry-Schaudies S, Hoffman B, et al: Effects of Taxol and colcemid on myofibrillogenesis. *Proc Natl Acad Sci USA* 79:6556–6560, 1982.
161. Fujii T, Suzuki T, Hachimori A, et al: Effect of Taxol on the interaction of tubulin with myosin filaments. *Can J Biochem Cell Biol* 62:878–884, 1984.
162. Spencer JA, Eliazer S, Ilaria RL Jr, et al: Regulation of microtubule dynamics and myogenic differentiation by MURF, a striated muscle RING-finger protein. *J Cell Biol* 150:771–784, 2000.
163. Rahkila P, Vaananen K, Saraste J, et al: Endoplasmic reticulum to Golgi trafficking in multinucleated skeletal muscle fibers. *Exp Cell Res* 234:452–464, 1997.
164. Tassin AM, Paintrand M, Berger EG, et al: The Golgi apparatus remains associated with microtubule organizing centers during myogenesis. *J Cell Biol* 101:630–638, 1985.
165. Kronebusch PJ, Singer SJ: The microtubule-organizing complex and the Golgi apparatus are co-localized around the entire nuclear envelope of interphase cardiac myocytes. *J Cell Sci* 8:25–34, 1987.
166. Ralston E: Changes in architecture of the Golgi complex and other subcellular organelles during myogenesis. *J Cell Biol* 120:399–409, 1993.
167. Lu Z, Joseph D, Bugnard E, et al: Golgi complex reorganization during muscle differentiation: Visualization in living cells and mechanism. *Mol Biol Cell* 12:795–808, 2001.
168. Ralston E, Lu Z, Ploug T: The organization of the Golgi complex and microtubules in skeletal muscle is fiber type-dependent. *J Neurosci* 19:10694–10705, 1999.
169. Ralston E, Ploug T, Kalhovde J, Lomo T: Golgi complex, endoplasmic reticulum exit sites, and microtubules in skeletal muscle fibers are organized by patterned activity. *J Neurosci* 21:875–883, 2001.
170. Tassin AM, Pincon-Raymond M, Paulin D, et al: Unusual organization of desmin intermediate filaments in muscular dysgenesis and TTX-treated myotubes. *Dev Biol* 129:37–47, 1988.
171. Young P, Ehler E, Gautel M: Obscurin, a giant sarcomeric Rho guanine nucleotide exchange factor protein involved in sarcomere assembly. *J Cell Biol* 154:123–136, 2001.
172. Zhou D, Birkenmeier CS, Williams MW, et al: Small, membrane-bound, alternatively spliced forms of ankyrin 1 associated with the sarcoplasmic reticulum of mammalian skeletal muscle. *J Cell Biol* 136:621–631, 1997.
173. Mohler PJ, Gramolini AO, Bennett V: Ankyrins. *J Cell Sci* 115:1565–1566, 2002.
174. Kontrogianni-Konstantopoulos A, Bloch RJ: The hydrophilic domain of small ankyrin-1 interacts with the two N-terminal immunoglobulin domains of titin. *J Biol Chem* 278:3985–3991, 2003.
175. Kontrogianni-Konstantopoulos A, Jones EM, vanRossum DB et al: Obscurin is a ligand for small ankyrin 1 in skeletal muscle. *Mol Biol Cell* 14:1138–1148, 2003.
176. Bagnato P, Barone V, Giacomello E: Binding of an ankyrin-1 isoform to obscurin suggests a molecular link between the sarcoplasmic reticulum and myofibrils in striated muscles. *J Cell Biol* 160:245–253, 2003.
177. Nunzi G, Franzini-Armstrong C: Trabecular network in adult skeletal muscle. *J Ultrastruct Res* 73:21–26, 1980.
178. Price MG: Skelemins: Cytoskeletal proteins located at the periphery of M-discs in mammalian striated muscle. *J Cell Biol* 104:1325–1336, 1987.
179. Holtzer H, Hijikata T, Lin ZX, et al: Independent assembly of 1.6mm long bipolar MHC filaments and I-Z-I bodies. *Cell Struct Funct* 22:83–93, 1997.
180. Bard F, Franzini-Armstrong C: "Extra" actin filaments at the periphery of skeletal muscle myofibrils. *Tissue Cell* 23:191–197, 1991.

Chapter 19b

The Muscle Fiber Cytoskeleton: The Dystrophin System

EIJIRO OZAWA

Dystrophin and Dystrophin-Associated Proteins
　α- AND β-DYSTROGLYCAN AND THE DYSTROGLYCAN COMPLEX
　SARCOGLYCANS AND THE SARCOGLYCAN COMPLEX
　SARCOSPAN
　SYNTROPHINS
　DYSTROBREVIN
　THE STRUCTURE OF THE DYSTROPHIN-DAP COMPLEXES

Biochemical Treatment of the Cell Membrane
　THE GLYCOPROTEIN COMPLEX
　COMPLEXES OBTAINED FROM MUSCLE CELL MEMBRANE FRACTIONS
　IN VITRO BINDING OF THE DYSTROPHIN-ASSOCIATED PROTEINS TO OTHER PROTEINS
　BINDING OF DYSTROPHIN TO THE ACTIN FILAMENT AND β-DYSTROGLYCAN

Interactions within a Dystrophin-Based Fixation Bolt

The Transverse Fixation System: Intermediate Filaments, Costameres, and Fixation Bolts

The Transverse Fixation System Is Composed of Various Proteins Responsible for Muscular Dystrophy
　MUSCULAR DYSTROPHIES CAUSED BY DEFECTS OF THE EXTRACELLULAR MATRIX AND LAMININ RECEPTORS
　MUSCULAR DYSTROPHIES CAUSED BY DEFECTS OF THE DYSTROPHIN BOLT AND ITS RELATED PROTEINS IN COSTAMERES
　MYOPATHIES CAUSED BY DEFECTS OF DESMIN INTERMEDIATE FILAMENTS

The Cellular Location of the Reponsible Proteins and the Severity of the Disorders

Developmental Expression of the Dystrophin-DAP Complex

The Dystrophin-DAP Complex as a Signaling System
　DYSTROPHIN PHOSPHORYLATION REACTIONS
　POSSIBLE SIGNALING BY THE SARCOGLYCAN COMPLEX
　SYNTROPHINS
　nNOS
　CAVEOLIN-3

Defects in dystrophin and some of its associated proteins result in a variety of muscular dystrophies with common features of muscle degeneration and regeneration. Dystrophin was first identified as the responsible gene of Duchenne muscular dystrophy with the positional cloning method. Needless to say, however, dystrophin and dystrophin-associated proteins (DAPs*) are components of the normal cell, mainly

*A list of abbreviations used in this chapter is given at the end of the chapter.

expressed in skeletal, cardiac, and smooth muscle and nerve cells. Dystrophin and transmembraneous β-dystroglycan (DG) and extracellular α-DG form a functional unit, the dystrophin-based connecting bolt (dystrophin bolt),[1,2] that firmly fixes the subsarcolemmal actin network and basal lamina. This is mechanically reinforced by the sarcoglycan (SG) complex. Thus, plasmalemma composed of lipid bilayer is protected, sandwiched by these two layers sewed by the dystrophin bolt. Here, discussions on the dystrophin-DAP complex are made, but to avoid redundancy, most of the details of the dystrophin gene and protein are described in Chap. 34.

Dystrophin and Dystrophin-Associated Proteins

Dystrophin has a molecular mass of 427 kDa composed of 3865 amino acid residues. Its primary structure reveals a molecule composed of four domains, namely, actin-binding, rod, cysteine-rich and C-terminal domains, three of which share many features with the actin-binding membrane cytoskeletal proteins spectrin and α-actinin, and predicts an elongated rod shape.[3] Electron microscopy of isolated and rotary-shadowed dystrophin molecules shows molecules ~175 nm in length.[4] Although dystrophin was once reported to be a homodimer arranged in an antiparallel manner, it is now known to be present as a monomer both in vivo and in vitro. Dystrophin is immunohistochemically detected on the protoplasmic surface of the plasmalemma.[5–7] It has no transmembrane domains or sugar moiety and is released from the membrane fraction by a low-ionic-strength solution at pH 11; hence it is an intracellular and not an integral membrane protein.[3,8]

Following removal of the lipid bilayer with a detergent, digitonin, dystrophin is extracted from a rabbit cell membrane fraction with approximately 10 associated proteins, appropriately designated as dystrophin-associated proteins (DAPs) (Fig. 19b-1, Table 19b-1).[9–12] The dystrophin-DAP complex includes five membrane-integrated glycoproteins, β-DG and four SGs, and one extracellular glycoprotein, α-DG. Other DAPs are nonglycosylated; one is sarcospan, a membrane-integrated protein, and the rest are intracellular peripheral proteins, namely, dystrophin, syntrophins, and dystrobrevin. n-NO synthase (nNOS) and caveolin-3 are not exactly DAPs but are sometimes discussed with DAPs.

α- AND β-DYSTROGLYCAN AND THE DYSTROGLYCAN COMPLEX

The 42-kb DG mRNA consists of 2685 nucleotides in its open reading frame; it encodes a common precursor protein for both α- and β-DG of 895 amino acids with a calculated molecular mass of 97 kDa. The large precursor molecule is split into α-DG and β-DG between residues 653 and 654 and binds soon after posttranslation procession in the endoplasmic reticulum (ER).[13–15]

The molecular mass of the α-DG core protein is about 74 kDa, but owing to its being heavily glycosylated, the acid residues adjacent to its intracellular C-terminus. The intracellular domain is composed of 121 amino acid residues.

SARCOGLYCANS AND THE SARCOGLYCAN COMPLEX

The SG complex is a tetramer composed of one each of four glycosylated subunits, namely, α-, β-, γ- and δ-SG.[12,17] Each gene for each subunit has been cloned (Table 19b-1).[18–22] The β- and δ-SG subunits directly bind to the DG complex, whereas α- and γ-SG subunits seem to bind indirectly for the most part.[15,23,24] α-SG is special in that it is a transmembrane protein with a cytoplasmic C-terminus, whereas the other three SGs are transmembrane proteins that have cytoplasmic N-termini. These SGs carry a cluster of cysteine residues near their extracellular C-termini.

The fifth member of this group, ε-SG, is 44 percent identical and 66 percent similar to α-SG.[25,26] ε-SG seems to replace α-SG in the complex formation. A very small amount of the ε-substituted SG complex can be detected in skeletal muscle.[27] Existence of ζ-SG was recently reported. ζ-SG is weakly homologous to γ-SG but has somewhat larger molecular mass.

SARCOSPAN

Sarcospan (25 kDa) has four predicted transmembrane domains and intracellular N- and C-termini. Over 60 percent of its residues are predicted to be within the membrane.[28] Sarcospan is specifically expressed in skeletal muscle fibers and firmly binds to the SG complex. It is synthesized in the ER. Although it is a membrane-integrated protein, it does not seem to be glycosylated.

SYNTROPHINS

On the basis of their electrical characteristics, syntrophins in muscle fibers are classified into acidic (α-syntrophin; 54 kDa) and basic members; the latter are further divided according to a small difference in their electrophoretic mobility on SDS PAGE (β1- and β2-syntrophins; 58 kDa each).[29–31] α-Syntrophin mRNA is 2.2 kb in size.[30] β-Syntrophin mRNAs range in size from 1.9 to 10 kb.[32] α-Syntrophin is 54 and 50 percent identical in its amino acid composition to β1- and β2-syntrophin, respectively, whereas β-syntrophins are only 57 percent identical to each other.[33] α- and β1-syntrophins are associated with all muscle membranes, whereas β2-syntrophin is confined to the neuromuscular junction and is reported to interact with diacyl glycerol kinase-ζ.[34]

DYSTROBREVIN

α-Dystrobrevin is a member of the dystrophin-DAP complex[11] and also a member of the dystrophin family, together with dystrophin, utrophin, and DRP 2. *Torpedo* dystrobrevin (an 87-kDa protein) shows homology to the C-terminal domain of dystrophin.[35] The human dystrobrevin gene is located at 18q12.1-12.2, and its open reading frame shows 50 percent homology to the cysteine-rich and C-terminal domains of dystrophin.[36,37] Dystrobrevin has two coiled-coil motifs at its C-terminal region that bind to the same motifs

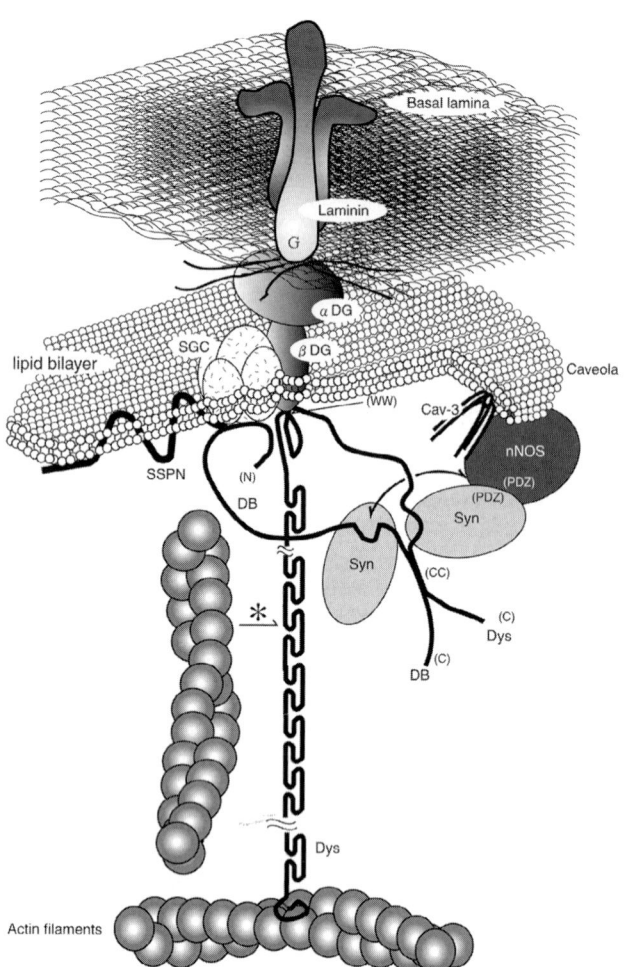

FIGURE 19b-1. Structure of the dystrophin-DAP complex superimposed on the lipid bilayer (plasmalemma) sandwiched by the basal lamina and subsarcolemmal actin network. *(Modified and redrawn from Yoshida et al.[55])* The dystrophin (Dys) bolt composed of β-dystroglycan (DG) and dystrophin connects the g-domain (G) of laminin above and actin filaments below the plasmalemma. (N) and (C) depict the N and C termini, respectively. (WW) shows the WW domain. The sarcoglycan complex (SGC), connected to sarcospan (SSPN), is associated with β-DG. Syntrophin (Syn) molecules, bound to dystrophin and dystrobrevin (DB), additionally bind to nNOS at PDZ domain and caveolin-3 (Cav-3). The mode of association of actin filaments to the rod domain is not known (see text). Asterisk indicates rod domain actin-binding site of dystrophin.

molecular mass of α-DG is difficult to determine because of the broadness of its band in immunoblot analysis, but is usually said to be 156 kDa.[10] Specific O-glycosylation has been reported for α-DG that occurs through serine and threonine residues.[8,16] The glycosyl chains have sequences of Neu5Acα2- or NeuGcα2-3 - 3Galβ1 - 4GlcNAcβ1 - 2Man. This glycosyl chain serves to bind with the G-domain of laminin α1 or α2. The glycosyl chains connecting Man-Ser or Man-Thr have seldom been detected in vertebrates. It is noteworthy that such rare mannose-bearing glycosyl chains play very important roles in cell biology.[16] The molecular mass of glycosylated β-DG is assumed to be 43 kDa. β-DG has a membrane-spanning hydrophobic domain having 24 amino

Table 19b-1. COMPONENTS OF THE CYTOSKELETON AND THEIR RELATION TO MUSCLE DISEASES

Protein	Gene Locus	Molecular Mass (kDa)	Glycosyl Chains	Transmembrane Domains	Presence	Myopathy Due to Mutation in Gene
Dystrophin	Xp21.2	427	—	—	Intracellular	DMD/BMD
Utrophin	6q24	395	—	—	Intracellular	Not known
α-Dystroglycan	3q21	156	+++	—	Extracellular	KO mice: lethal
β-Dystroglycan	3q21	43	+	+	Transmembrane	KO mice: lethal
α-Sarcoglycan	17q21	50	+	+	Transmembrane	α-Sarcoglycanopathy
β-Sarcoglycan	4q12	43	+	+	Transmembrane	β-Sarcoglycanopathy
γ-Sarcoglycan	13q12	35	+	+	Transmembrane	γ-Sarcoglycanopathy
δ-Sarcoglycan	5q33	35	+	+	Transmembrane	δ-Sarcoglycanopathy
Sarcospan	12q11.2	25	—	+++	Largely membrane-integrated	KO mice: normal
α-Dystrobrevin	18q12.1-2	90[a]	—	—	Intracellular	KO mice: dystrophic
α-Syntrophin	20q11.2	60	—	—	Intracellular	KO mice: normal
$β_1$-Syntrophin	8q23-24	60	—	—	Intracellular	Not known
$β_2$-Syntrophin		60	—	—	Intracellular	Not known
nNOS	12q24.2	161	—	—	Intracellular	Not known
Caveolin-3	3p25	22–24	—	+	Partially membrane-integrated, mostly intracellular	LGMD
Dysferlin	2p13	230	—	+	Transmembrane	LGMD and Miyoshi distal myopathy
Plectin	8q24.13-qter	466	—	—	Intracellular	Skin lesion and muscular dystrophy
Desmin	2q35	53	—	—	Intracellular	Desmin-related myopathy
Integrin α7	12q13	130	—	—	Intracellular	Congenital muscular dystrophy
Syncoilin		54	—	—	Intracellular	Not known
Desmuslin	15q26.3	160	—	—	Intracellular	Not known
Laminin α2	6q2	342	—	—	In the basal lamina	Congenital muscular dystrophy
Collagen VI	A1 and A2: 21q22; A3: 2q37	A1 and A2: 140; A3: 200–250	—	—	Outside of the basal lamina	Ullrich CMD and Bethlem myopathy

ABBREVIATIONS: CMD = congenital muscular dystrophy; LGMD = limb-girdle muscular dystrophy; KO = knockout.
[a]Several isoforms are known to be due to alternative splicing.

present in the C-terminal domain of dystrophin.[37] Five dystrobrevin transcripts, 6.5, 5.1, 4, 3.4, and 2.2 kb in size, are expressed in skeletal muscle. At the protein level, there are three major isoforms with molecular masses of 80, 65, and 59 kDa.[38] The β-dystrobrevin gene maps to 2p22-23 and is mainly expressed in nonmuscle tissues.[39,40] Three dystrobrevin-binding proteins are expressed in skeletal muscle: syncoilin,[41] desmuslin,[42] and dysbindin.[43]

THE STRUCTURE OF THE DYSTROPHIN-DAP COMPLEXES

To study how dystrophin is associated with other sarcolemmal proteins, several subcomplexes were prepared from the dystrophin-DAP complex by treatment with different chemical solutions and physical conditions. Some protein complexes made of two DAP were reconstructed in vitro using natural and recombinant proteins. While the solubilization and preparation of subcomplexes of the dystrophin-DAP complexes are straightforward and reflect associations in vivo, they do not indicate binding sites. Probing the complexes with natural and recombinant proteins allows more precise analysis but could be confounded by artifacts. This section reviews studies that have contributed to understanding the subcomplexes of the dystrophin-DAP complex.[1,2,44–46] The architecture of the dystrophin-DAP complex, shown in Fig. 19b-1, is based on these studies.

Biochemical Treatment of the Cell Membrane

THE GLYCOPROTEIN COMPLEX

The glycoprotein complex is a conceptual term coined in the early days of dystrophin research, but such a complex has never been prepared biochemically. Initial biochemical studies focused on muscle membrane preparations.[8,47,48] When muscle membrane fraction was treated at pH 11 to dissociate peripheral proteins from the cytoplasmic membrane surface, dystrophin was in the dissociated fraction. Treatment at pH 12 did not release integral membrane proteins but did release α-DG, a heavily glycosylated protein, suggesting that α-DG is an extracellular protein—a result later confirmed by immunoelectron microscopy[49] and by finding that α-DG binds to α2-laminin, a major component of the basal lamina.[50] Other DAPs known at the time (e.g., β-DG, α-SG, γ-SG, and sarcospan) were not dissociated by alkaline treatments but were bound to 3-(trifluoromethyl)-3-(iodophenyl)diazirine (TID). These are all glycoproteins except sarcospan, suggesting that they are membrane-integrated or transmembrane proteins.[8,29] Subsequently, after their primary sequence became known, these proteins were found to have membrane-spanning domains.

COMPLEXES OBTAINED FROM MUSCLE CELL MEMBRANE FRACTIONS

Subcomplexes of the Dystrophin-DAP Complex

Treatment of the dystrophin-DAP complex with a detergent n-octyl β-D-glucoside yielded three complexes, DG, SG, and peripheral protein complexes, and a separate protein, sarcospan[2,17] (Fig. 19b-2C to F). Biochemical separation of these complexes has been the cornerstone of the classification of DAPs.[51] The following complexes were defined:

1. The DG complex, composed of α- and β-DG.
2. The SG complex. This is a tetramer composed of α-, β-, γ-, and δ-sarcoglycans.[18–22] Initially, it was thought to consist of α-, β-, and γ-SG[17]; the fourth component, δ-SG, was discovered later.[12,52]
3. The peripheral protein complex. This consists of dystrophin, dystrobrevin, and syntrophin.[17]
4. Sarcospan represents a separate entity.

The Binding Site of Dystrophin to the DG and SG Complexes

Calpain digestion of the dystrophin-DAP complex yielded multiple dystrophin fragments,[53] but the glycoproteins remained undigested. A ~32-kDa dystrophin fragment comprising the cysteine-rich domain and the first half of the C-terminal domain remained attached to the DG and SG complexes (Fig. 19b-2A) and thus defined the glycoprotein-binding region of dystrophin.[54]

The SG Complex and Its Attachments

Heat treatment of the dystrophin-DAP complex at various ionic strengths produced three subcomplexes[55]:

1. A large complex composed of the DG complex, the SG complex, and sarcospan (Fig. 19b-2G).
2. The SG complex and sarcospan (Fig. 19b-2H). Sarcospan binds to β- and δ-SG. This complex was also derived by immunoprecipitation.[14,56] Sarcospan binds firmly to the SG complex, but is not a subunit of the SG complex.
3. A large complex composed of syntrophin, dystrobrevin, the SG complex, and sarcospan (Fig. 19b-2I).

The three major dystrobrevin isoforms bind at their N-termini to the intracellular domain of the sarcoglycan com-

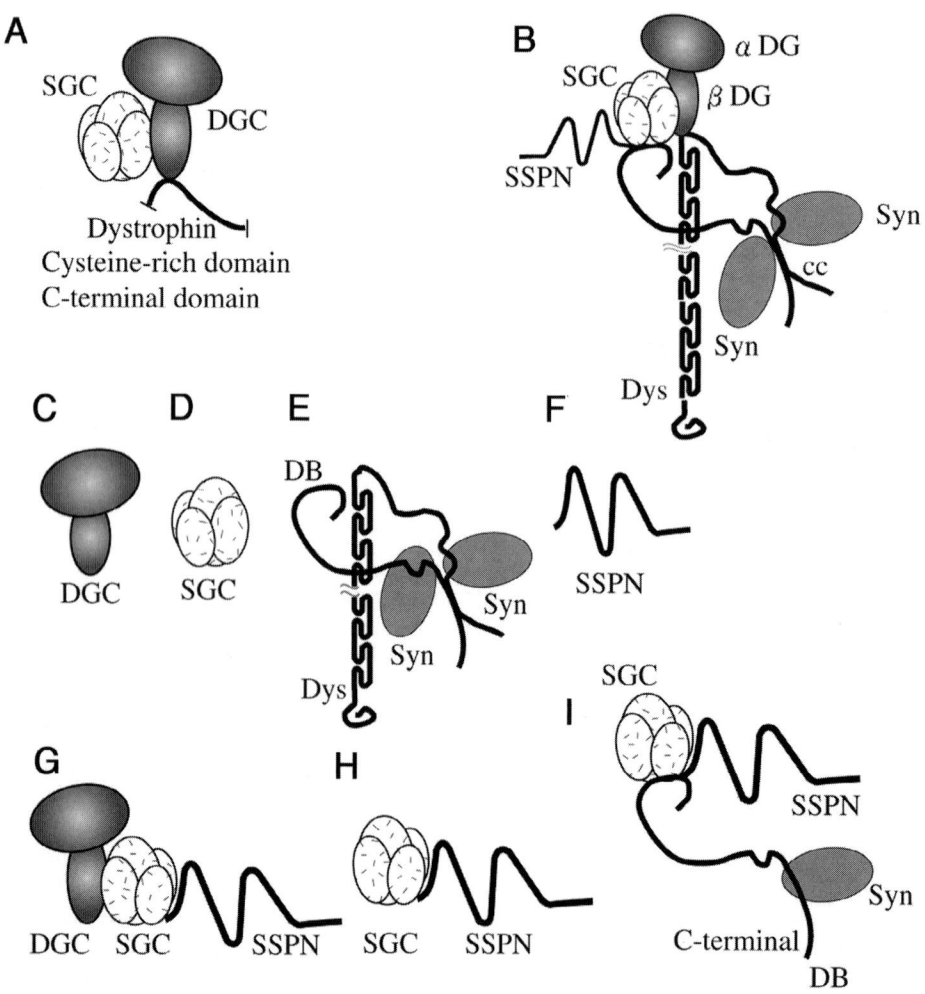

FIGURE 19b-2. The dystrophin-DAP complexes biochemically prepared from muscle. A. Sarcoglycan complex (SGC) and dystroglycan (DGC) bind to a dystrophin fragment containing the cysteine-rich domain and the first half of the C-terminal domain (for the exact binding site of dystrophin to β-DG, see Fig. 19b-4). B. The complete dystrophin-DAP complex model is composed by superimposing the biochemically prepared subcomplexes. C–F. Octyl-glucoside detergent treatment of the dystrophin-DAP complex releases dystroglycan (C); the sarcoglycan complex (D); a peripheral complex composed of dystrophin (Dys), dystrobrevin (DB), and syntrophin (Syn) (E); and sarcospan (SSPN) (F). The binding sites of syntrophin to dystrophin are determined by an in vitro assay (see Fig. 19b-3). G–I. Heat treatment of the dystrophin-DAP complex at different ionic strength releases the DG-SG-SSPN complex (G), the SG-SSPN complex (H), and the SSPN-SG-DB-Syn complex (I).

plex, but the SG subunit that binds to dystrobrevin has not been identified.[55] These studies elucidate the architectural organization of the dystrophin-DAP complex (Fig. 19b-2B).

IN VITRO BINDING OF THE DYSTROPHIN-ASSOCIATED PROTEINS TO OTHER PROTEINS

Binding of α2-Laminin to α-DG

α-DG binds to the laminin on the basal lamina,[50] which in the extrajunctional sarcolemma is laminin 2, composed of α2, β1, and γ1 subunits. The globular (G) domain of the α2 subunit binds to O-linked glycosyl chains of α-DG. (Fig. 19b-3A).[16,57] The glycosyl chains of α-DG bind to G-domain-like sequences of other extracellular matrix molecules, such as agrin[58] and possibly perlecan.[59] This mode of binding is assumed because α-DG binds to the C-terminal G-domain of the laminin α1 subunit.[60] Binding of laminin α1 to α-DG requires calcium ions and is inhibited by heparin,[61,62] but how this occurs is not known.

Binding of α- to β-Dystroglycan

Thirty-six residues (amino acids 550 to 585) close to the C-terminus of α-DG are required for binding α-DG to the extracellular N-terminus of β-DG (amino acids 654 to 750). The N-terminus of β-DG is partially folded in vitro.[63,64]

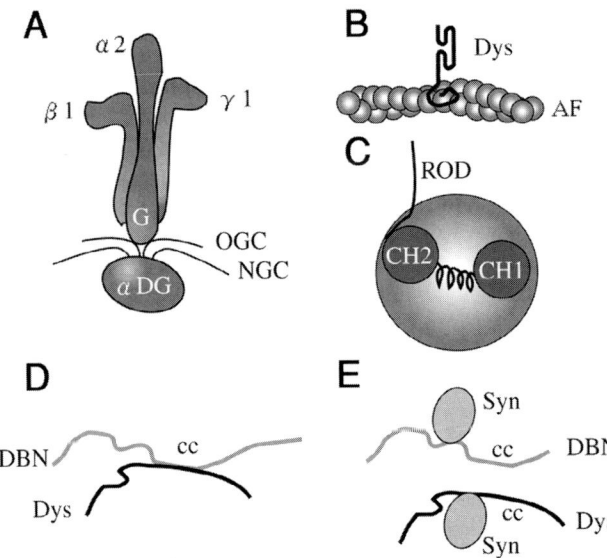

FIGURE 19b-3. Complexes examined by in vitro binding experiments or yeast two-hybrid system. A. The G domain of α2 laminin binds to the O-linked glycosyl chain (OGC) of α-DG in the presence of calcium ions. NGC: N-linked glycosyl chain. B. Three actin-binding sites (ABS) of the dystrophin (Dys) actin-binding domain bind to actin. C. A single g-actin unit in the f-actin filament associates with type-1 and -2 calponin homology domains (CH1 and 2) that include ABS 1-2 and ABS 3, respectively. D. Dystrophin (Dys) and dystrobrevin (DB) bind to each other at their coiled-coil (cc) domains. E. Syntrophin (Syn) binds to both DB and Dys at the N-terminal end of the cc domain.

Binding of Dystrophin to Dystrobrevin

The C-terminal domains of dystrophin, utrophin, and α-dystrobrevin-1 and -2 have two coiled-coil (cc) domains.[65] Dystrophin (residues 3474 to 3603, encoded by exons 74 to 76) and dystrobrevin (residues 399 to 491) bind to each other at their cc domains by hydrophobic bonds[37] (Fig. 19b-3D).

Binding of Dystrophin and Dystrobrevin to Syntrophins

α- and β1-syntrophins are present in the undercoat of the entire sarcolemma, whereas β2-syntrophin is largely restricted to the neuromuscular junction.[30,66] The binding site of dystrophin to syntrophin is located at residues 3444 to 3495 (encoded by exons 73 and 74)[67-69] (Fig. 19b-3E). Syntrophin also binds to the homologous regions of dystrobrevin and utrophin.[70] Recently, a second binding site on dystrobrevin to syntrophin was proposed.[71] Syntrophin associates with utrophin and short dystrophin.[72]

Binding of Syntrophin to nNOS

Syntrophin is a protein containing one PDZ-binding domain composed of ~90 residues, 2 pleckstrin homology domains, and a syntrophin-unique domain responsible for binding to dystrophin/utrophin.[73] Syntrophin binds to nNOS or voltage-gated sodium channel by PDZ-PDZ interactions.[74,75]

Binding of nNOS to Caveolin-3

nNOS binds to the N-terminal scaffolding domain of caveolin-3,[76] which possibly binds with various specified motifs.[77] Synthetic peptides corresponding to caveolin-3 residues 65 to 84 and 109 to 130 inhibit the activity of purified recombinant nNOS.

Binding of Caveolin-3 to β-Dystroglycan and to Dysferlin

Caveolin-3 has a WW-like domain at residues 71 to 105. This domain is predicted to bind directly to the intracellular C-terminal domain of β-DG containing the motif proline-proline-arbitrary amino acid-tyrosine (PPXY). This domain is located between N- and C-membrane-attachment domains and has been shown to bind to the cell membrane.[78] Coimmunoprecipitation studies indicate that caveolin-3 binds to dysferlin, a transmembrane protein responsible for Miyoshi distal myopathy and limb-girdle dystrophy 2B.[79,80]

Other Binding Proteins

Binding of filamin 2 to the SG complex has been reported.[81] Aciculin, a 60- to 63-kDa cytoskeletal protein with high homology to phosphoglucomutase and expressed by myotubes but not myoblasts, binds to dystrophin and utrophin.[82-84]

BINDING OF DYSTROPHIN TO THE ACTIN FILAMENT AND β-DYSTROGLYCAN

Dystrophin is connected (1) to actin filaments at its N-terminal actin-binding domain and probably at the central part of the rod domain and (2) to the intracellular domain of β-DG via its WW-cysteine-rich domain. Absence of either the actin- or the β-DG-binding site results in a dystrophinopathy (see below).[2,54,61,85]

Actin-Binding Sites in the Actin-Binding Domain

The dystrophin-DAP complex prepared from a sarcolemmal preparation binds to actin filaments (F-actin)[61,86,87] but not to single actin molecules (g-actin). However, dystrophin reacts with a single g-actin unit of F-actin (Fig. 19b-3B). The binding involves three actin-binding sites (ABS) at residues 17 to 26 (exon 1), 88 to 116 (exons 4 to 5), and 128 to 156 (exon 6), respectively.[88–91] ABS 1 and 3 bind to residues 83~117 and 350~373 at the C-terminus of actin, respectively.[89] ABS 1 and 2 are in a type 1 calponin homology (CH) domain while actin-binding site 3 is located in a type 2 CH domain (Fig. 19b-3C).[92] By analogy from studies of utrophin, the CH domains are connected with an α-helical polypeptide. When dystrophin is attached to a single g-actin unit of F-actin, the α-helix part is extended.[93]

CH domains are composed of ~100 amino acid residues and are found in signaling and cytoskeletal proteins. Type 1 CH domains have intrinsic ability to interact with F-actin, while type 2 CH domains do not. The type 2 CH domain contributes substantially to the interaction of the complete actin-binding domain, perhaps by acting as a locator or a low-affinity docking site for the actin filament.

The Rod Domain Actin-Binding Site

This site is located at residues 1416 to 1494 (exons 32~40), which span triple-helical segments 11 to 17.[94,95] The dissociation constants of the rod ABS and of N-terminal ABSs 1 to 3 are 14.2 and 13.7 μM, respectively. That the rod-domain ABS is biologically significant is supported by the observation that *mdx* mice can be rescued by a dystrophin transgene that has no N-terminal ABS or by a Dp260 gene that lacks the N-terminal actin-binding domain (see Chap. 34). Both transgenes include the rod ABS, suggesting that the ABS is functional.[96,97] A side-to-side association of the actin filament with the dystrophin rod domain has been proposed,[98] but the mode of binding to the actin filament remains to be clarified experimentally.

Binding of Dystrophin to β-Dystroglycan

The binding site of dystrophin to β-DG was at first determined to fall approximately in the cysteine-rich domain and the first half of the C-terminal domain by analysis of a complex preparation obtained from a natural source and also by an overlay assay.[54,99] Because loss of this region results in dystrophic phenotypes,[100] it became clear that failure of dystrophin to bind β-DG causes DD. Various recombinant dystrophin fragments (Df) were examined for binding to β-DG (Fig. 19b-4A). (1) A Df spanning residues 3026 to 3232 (encoded by exons 62 to 66) did not bind β-DG. (2) A Df spanning residues 3026 to 3257 or 3026 to 3324 (encoded by exons 62 to 67 or 68) and a Df spanning residues 3026 to 3345 (encoded by exons 62 to 69) showed reduced and full binding, respectively.[99,101] The *mdx* mouse with a transgene of various Df genes showed that a full binding site is physiologically required to prevent the dystrophic change.[102]

The WW Domain Binding Motif and Its Ligand PPXY

The WW domain present in some proteins acts as a binding motif to other proteins having the consensus sequence PPXY. The WW domain was defined as a domain composed of approximately 34 residues characteristically having two Ws (tryptophans) at positions 7 and 29 in the WW domain[103,104] (Fig. 19b-4A).

The dystrophin WW domain (residues 3055 to 3088, encoded by exons 62~63, with tryptophan residues at positions 3061 and 3083) is located at the last 25 amino acid residues of the rod domain and the initial part of the cysteine-rich domain (residues 3080~3360).[3] Generally, the WW domain suffices for protein-protein binding. However, in the case of the dystrophin WW domain, the connection of about 270 residues in tandem is required, although the dystrophin WW domain was reported to bind β-DG in vitro under specified conditions.[105]

The PPXY consensus domain is at the C-terminus of β-DG. Dystrophin lacking the WW domain cannot bind to β-DG in overlay assay, although the WW domain alone does not bind to β-DG.[101,106]

X-ray diffraction analysis of the WW-cysteine-rich domain (residues 3046 to 3306), the dystrophin fragment that shows the reduced binding with β-DG, reveals that the domain is composed of four subdomains: WW, WE, EF1, and EF2 (Fig. 19b-4B), each forming blocks of a specified secondary structure. These subdomains are positioned very close to each other in a three-dimensional structure. The long polypeptide composed of about 250 residues associates only with 8 residues of the C-terminus of β-DG (amino acid residues 886~892: PYR-SPPPY) (Fig. 19b-4B and C).[107] For the reduced binding, dystrophin R3246 (encoded at the locus near the 3' terminus of exon 67) has to bind to β-DG Y886. (Note that the ranges of EF1 and EF2 used by the authors of this x-ray diffraction study are different from those defined originally by Koenig et al.[3])

The ZZ Domain of Dystrophin

For the full binding to β-DG, Df 3026 to 3345 is necessary. The last part of the dystrophin fragment, Df 3310 to 3345, which comprises most of the ZZ domain, does not bind to β-DG but to the EF1. Therefore it is possible that Df 3310 to 3345 forms a fifth subdomain working to reinforce the binding to β-DG together with the four subdomains originally defined by x-ray diffraction analysis (Fig. 19b-4A to D).[108]

The cysteine-rich region of dystrophin encompasses a ZZ domain (residues 3307 to 3354), resembling zinc-finger motifs, that is present in many DNA-binding proteins. In dystrophin, the ZZ domain appears to mediate interaction with β-DG.[109] For binding to β-DG, two histidine residues of the ZZ domain are not required, but cysteine residue 3340 is indispensable for binding.[108]

A truncated dystrophin transgene lacking exons 64 to 67, which encodes the full length of the WW domain, and the transgene lacking exons 68 to 70, which encodes the full length of the reduced β-DG-binding domain, including R3246, fail to ameliorate the *mdx* phenotype. Third, a truncated transgene lacking exons 71 to 74 but encoding the whole length of the full β-DG-binding domain does rescue the *mdx* phenotype.[102,110] This suggests that the full binding sequence is required for dystrophin function and, further,

Chapter 19b. The Muscle Fiber Cytoskeleton: The Dystrophin System

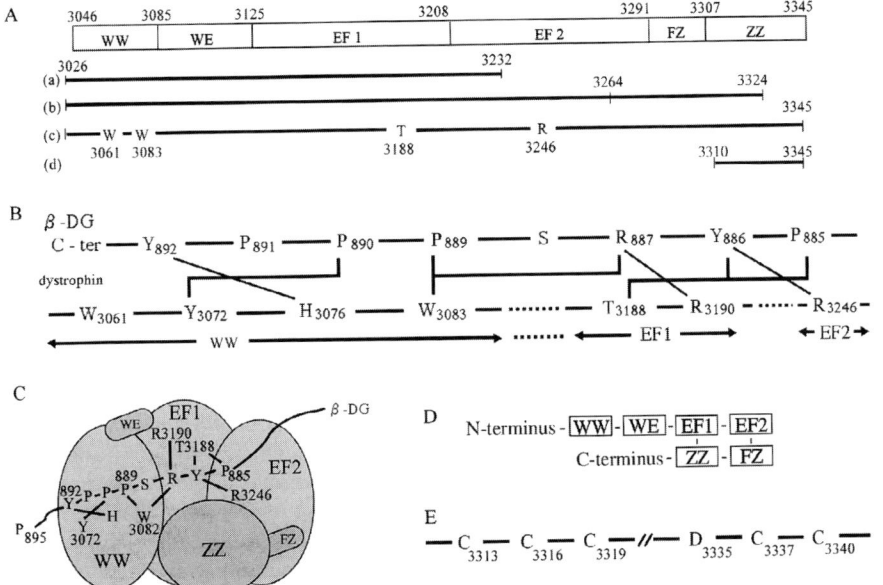

FIGURE 19b-4. Structures and binding functions of the WW-cysteine-rich domain and recombinant dystrophin fragments to β-DG. A. Top: broad bar shows six domains and denominations used in x-ray analysis of the WW-cysteine-rich domain. Sections of the domains figure are named according to Huang et al.[107] The WW domain is slightly shorter than originally defined. EF1 includes both original EF1 and EF2 as defined by Koenig et al.[3] EF2 in this figure does not contain the classic EF hand structure. The ZZ domain is also shorter than that originally defined.[73] The anonymous sites present between WW and EF1 and between EF2 and ZZ domains are tentatively designated as WE and FZ, respectively. Dystrophin fragments show (a) no binding activity, (b) reduced activity, and (c) full activity. Fragment (d) binds to EF1. (Based on Refs. 99, 101, 106, and 107.) B,C. Interaction of dystrophin and β-DG: Interacting amino acid residues of each molecule are picked up from a figure depicted by Huang et al.[107] based on their x-ray analysis of the weak binding domain. D. Interaction of dystrophin subdomains. E. Cysteine (C) and aspartic acid (D) residues in the ZZ domain.

that the ZZ domain is indispensable for the physiologic binding to β-DG. Thus, at least 8 amino acid residues of β-DG, including PPPY, interact with the Df 3026 to 3345.

An in vitro binding assay suggests that β-DG has a second binding site (probably RKKRK) for dystrophin connected in tandem with its membrane-spanning domain.[101]

Utrophin binding to β-DG is similar to that of dystrophin, but with some small differences.[111]

Interactions within a Dystrophin-Based Fixation Bolt

To summarize the dystrophin and DAP interactions (Fig. 19b-1): (1) Extracellular α-DG binds to laminin, with its O-linked glycosyl chains, and associates with transmembrane β-DG at its C-terminus. (2) α-DG binds to the extracellular N-terminal of β-DG. (3) The C-terminus of the intracellular domain of β-DG binds to the WW-cysteine-rich domain of dystrophin (amino acid residues 3026 to 3345). (4) Dystrophin binds to actin filaments via its actin-binding and rod domains, spanning the β-DG and actin networks. (5) The transmembrane SG complex binds side by side to the DG complex, reinforcing the binding of β-DG to dystrophin intracellularly and to α-DG extracellularly. (6) The WW cysteine-rich domain of dystrophin and the N-terminus of dystrobrevin are fixed at intracellular domains of the DG and SG complexes, respectively. The C-terminal regions of dystrophin and dystrobrevin are fixed at coiled-coil domains. In addition, α- and/or β1-syntrophins bind to dystrophin and dystrobrevin close to the coiled-coil domains.

An overview of the dystrophin-DAP interactions suggests a complicated model for the complex (Fig. 19b-1). This model can be conceptually divided into two components. One component consists of the dystrophin-DG complex attached to the SG complex and dystrobrevin. These proteins are mainly concerned with mechanical support. The second component consists of syntrophins, nNOS, and caveolin-3; this component may be related to a sarcolemmal signaling system. Some DAPs, such as the SG complex and dystrobrevin, might also be related to this functional group in addition to the first group.

Other interactions include syntrophin binding to nNOS, which, in turn, binds to caveolin-3 (Figs. 19b-1 and 19b-3). Growth factor receptor 2 (Grb 2), with its SH3 domain, binds to the C-terminal proline-rich domain of β-DG. Dystrobrevin binds to syncoilin, desmuslin, and dysbindin.

The Transverse Fixation System: Intermediate Filaments, Costameres, and Fixation Bolts

The name *costamere* applies to the rib-like appearance of cytoskeketal and adhesion molecule clusters at the plasmalemma, when detected by immunolabeling.[114] Costameres are constituted of two groups of interacting proteins, both anchored on actin filaments: One group comprises dystrophin and DAPs and the other ankyrin, vinculin, talin, vimentin, and velusin, with integrin as the transmembrane link (see Chap. 19a).[114–126] The term *bolt*, with its structural and functional meaning, was initially used to indicate the dystrophin complex. However, it could be extended to the protein complex that includes talin, vinculin, and integrin α1β7, which constitute an additional sarcolemmal "bolt."[1] In the two types of fixation bolts, α-DG and integrin are designated as laminin receptors (see details in the next section below), and the two types of bolts are colocalized within costameres,[118–120,124] but it is not yet clear to what extent the two systems may interact and/or overlap at the molecular level.

Desmin intermediate filaments (DIFs) connect bundles of myofibrils at the Z-disk level and the sarcolemma at the costameres.[112–115] DIFs bind to actin filaments at the costamere via plectin[117,127] and to dystrobrevin via syncoilin and desmuslin. Thus, in addition to the transmembranous connection, the dystrophin bolt and some of the DAPs are fixed via DIFs to myofibrils intracellularly, providing connection from the myofibril to the plasmalemma and mechanical continuity between the myofibrils and the surface membrane (see Chap. 19a for details).[114–127] The complex fixes laminin in the basal lamina to the subsarcolemmal actin network to prevent mechanical injury of the lipid bilayer.[1,2] In this way, DIFs are responsible for constraining the sarcolemma at the level of the Z disks (Fig. 19b-5). There is only small play in the length of the DIF, judging from some electron microscopic (EM) reports; the subsarcolemmal space between the plasmalemma and the myofibrils is not much extended even on strong contraction. This fixation restricts bulging of the sarcolemma in shortened fibers,[128–130] resulting in festooning and possibly preventing T-systems from overstretching. The tubules exist along the DIFs but are not directly associated with them.[131]

Within the dystrophin bolt, dystrophin is incorporated in the meshwork of sarcolemma-associated cytoskeleton[132,133] at sites where the myofibrils are directly or indirectly connected to the extracellular matrix either longitudinally (at the myotendinous junction) or transversely (at costameres).[117–123] Dystrophin is concentrated at costameres, but EM shows dystrophin to be present over the entire fiber surface membrane[6,128,129]; thus dystrophin is also present at the intervening membrane sites, though at a lower density, together with an α5β1 variant of integrin.[135] The molecular significance of this colocalization is also unclear. Dystrophin does not localize to T tubules in skeletal muscle,[6,7] but it is present in the walls of T tubules in cardiac muscle.[136]

The Transverse Fixation System Is Composed of Various Proteins Responsible for Muscular Dystrophies

Defects in a number of proteins composing basal lamina, laminin receptors, costamere proteins, and intermediate filaments connecting costameres and Z disks result in various

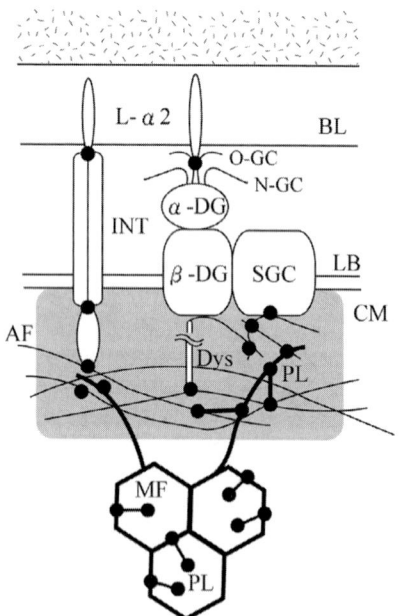

FIGURE 19b-5. The transverse fixation system and myopathy resulting from its defects. *Left*: Dystrophin- and integrin-based bolts are connected to the subplasmalemmal and intermyofibrillar protection systems. Both bolts link laminin-α2 in the basal lamina to the submembranous actin network. An *O*-linked glycosyl chain constitutes the α-DG receptor site. The function of the *N*-glycosyl chain (*N*-GC) is not understood. The actin network is connected to the transverse cytoskeleton composed of plectin linkers and desmin intermediate filaments (DIF). Thus, DIF links the Z disks of myofibrils (shown as hexagons) to the submembranous cytoskeleton. The two protecting systems are structurally linked within the costamere (*shaded area*). (See text for further details.) *Right*: myopathies arising from defects in proteins associated with the two sarcolemmal protection systems. BL = basal lamina, L-α2 = laminin-α2; O-GC = O-linked glycosyl chain; N-GC = N-linked glycosyl chain; DG = dystroglycan; SGC = sarcoglycan; LB = lipid bilayer; CM = costamere; AF = actin filament; MF = myofibril; PL = plectin; DIF = desmin intermediate filament; CMD = congenital muscular dystrophy; FKRP = Fukutin-related protein; MEB = muscle-eye-brain disease; WWS = Walker Warburg syndrome.

types of muscular dystrophies or myopathies (Fig. 19b-5). Their cellular position is closely related to the severity of the disease.

MUSCULAR DYSTROPHIES CAUSED BY DEFECTS OF THE EXTRACELLULAR MATRIX AND LAMININ RECEPTORS

Disorders arising from defects in the extracellular matrix are discussed in Chaps. 39 and 54 and are mentioned here only briefly.

Defects of the Basal Lamina

Mutation of the laminin α2 gene results in merosin-negative congenital muscular dystrophy (CMD).[137] In Fukuyama CMD and Walker Warburg syndrome, the basal lamina is morphologically defective.[138–140] Mutations in the α or β subunit of collagen VI, which is localized on the outer surface of the basal lamina, result in Ullrich's CMD,[141,142] and those of the α, β, or γ subunit cause Bethlem myopathy.[143–145]

Defects of Laminin Receptors: α-Dystroglycan and Integrin

Functional defects of laminin receptors dismantle the basal lamina from the lipid bilayer of the muscle fiber. Defects in glycosylation and a decreased expression of α-DG occur with mutations of the *POMGnT1* and *POMT1* genes and result in the Santavuori type of muscle-eye-brain disease[146] and Walker-Warburg syndrome,[147] respectively. The former gene encodes O-mannose β-1,2-N-acetylglucosaminyl transferase, which catalyzes the transfer GlcNAc to O-linked mannose on brain α-DG,[16] and the latter gene probably encodes the O-mannosyl-transferase gene.

Mutations in the *FUKUTIN* gene cause Fukuyama CMD.[148,149] Mutations of the *FKRP* gene that encodes fukutin-related protein cause limb-girdle muscular dystrophy 2I and a CMD.[150,151] Both genes are assumed to encode glycosylating enzymes because their amino acid sequences show homology to glycosylating enzymes.[152]

Large, a gene encoding a glycosyl transfer enzyme in the mouse, is responsible for murine myodystrophy.[153]

Although these enzymes work in the ER and/or Golgi apparatus, their products work externally on the cell membrane.

Mutations of integrin α7, which is also a laminin receptor, cause a mild congenital muscular dystrophy.[154] Targeted deletion of the homologous gene in the mouse also induces mild dystrophy.[155] Integrin α7β1 is expressed in myotubes and muscle fiber and serves as the laminin receptor.[156]

MUSCULAR DYSTROPHIES CAUSED BY DEFECTS OF THE DYSTROPHIN BOLT AND ITS RELATED PROTEINS IN COSTAMERES

Defects of the Dystroglycan Complex

Muscular dystrophy due to defects of the DG complex has not been reported in humans.

DG-null mice die at embryonic day 6.5, before skeletal or cardiac muscle begins to develop.[157] Skeletal muscles of chimeric mice generated with ES cells targeted for both DG alleles are essentially devoid of the DG complex.[158] Dystrophin, utrophin, and α-SG are not detected immunohistochemically, but laminins 2 and 4, perlecan, β1-integrin, and agrin are normally present. These mice show dystrophic phenotypes as severe as those of dystrophin-utrophin double-deficient mice, consistent with disruption of the connection between the basal lamina and the submembranous actin network[158] (see also Chap. 34).

Transgenic overexpression of the caveolin-3 gene in normal mice causes partial dystrophin deficiency and a dystrophic phenotype.[159] By virtue of its WW domain, wild-type caveolin-3 may bind to β-DG; when expression of caveolin-3 is enhanced, it likely competes with dystrophin for the WW-binding consensus domain of β-DG.[78]

Defects of Dystrophin

In Duchenne dystrophy (DD) and in *mdx* mice, dystrophin is absent. β-DG expression on the lipid bilayer is reduced when dystrophin is absent.[160,161] Some of the remaining β-DG probably binds to utrophin, which is upregulated in DD muscles.[161,162] Expression of the SG complex is reduced in DD muscle, and the decreased availability of the SG complex weakens the connecting bolt that attaches the basal lamina to the subsarcolemmal actin network.[1,2] For further details see Chap. 34.

Experimental Mitigation of the mdx Phenotype by Dystrophin

Absence and partial decrease of dystrophin at the sarcolemma cause DD and Becker dystrophy (BD), respectively.[163] In mice, dogs, and cats, absence of dystrophin results in dystrophic phenotype (see Chap. 34) The severity of the phenotype depends on the amount of dystrophin expressed on the sarcolemma.[164] Patients with very mild BD, who are able to ambulate in their fifties or later, have a 200- to 320-kDa rod-domain deletion owing to various large deletions in the range of exons 13 to 48 but express the truncated dystrophin on the sarcolemma.[165–168] A dystrophin gene lacking exons 17 to 48 used for transgene experiments ameliorates the dystrophic phenotype of *mdx* mice lacking dystrophin.[169]

Functions of various regions of dystrophin and utrophin have been examined by introducing wild-type and mutant dystrophin cDNAs into dystrophin- (and utrophin-) deficient mice. Transgenic *mdx* mice overexpressing full-length dystrophin cDNA have a normal phenotype. Utrophin is not upregulated.[170] Full-length utrophin also prevents muscular dystrophy in *mdx* mice.[171] By contrast, the DNA construct lacking most of the dystrophin C-terminal domain encoded by exons 71 to 78, which includes the syntrophin-binding site and the coiled-coil domain, does not alter the dystrophic phenotype in *mdx* mice.[172]

A cDNA transgene of Dp71, a short dystrophin without the actin-binding and rod domains (see Chap. 34), in *mdx* mice restored the sarcolemmal expression of the DAPs dystrobrevin, α-SG, and β-DG but failed to alleviate the dystrophic phenotype even though sarcolemmal utrophin remained upregulated. The inability of Dp71 to link with the submembranous actin network explains the necessity of the connection between the actin network and basal lamina.[173,174]

Truncated dystrophin that retains actin- and β-DG-binding sites prevents the development of dystrophic changes.

Indeed, most of the dystrophin rod domain can be removed without functional impairment because dystrophin maintains its ability to bolt the extracellular matrix to the subsarcolemmal actin network.[175,176] One type of rod-deleted functional dystrophin, depicted in Fig. 34-2A, is composed of a spacer, followed by the first to third repeats 1 to 3, another spacer, and repeats 19 to 24, followed by a final spacer as well as the actin-binding, cysteine-rich, and C-terminal domains. This construct provides morphologic rescue, but the animals are still weaker than controls. Introduction of utrophin with a large rod-domain deletion into *mdx* mice also improves the phenotype.[177] A utrophin transgene introduced into dystrophin-utrophin double-deficient mice prevents development of the severe phenotype.[178]

Dystrophin lacking N-terminal actin-binding domain[96] or Dp 260[97] introduced into *mdx* mice results in a milder phenotype. In these animals, the rod-domain actin-binding site serves as a bolt to the subplasmalemmal actin network. On the other hand, *mdx* mice transgenic for dystrophins with cysteine-rich domain deletions show a severe phenotype.[112,169,179]

The above examples indicate that functional dystrophin or utrophin that binds to both actin filaments and β-DG is essential for amelioration of the dystrophic phenotype.

Defects of the Sarcoglycan Complex

Mutations in any of the four sarcoglycans can result in autosomal recessive limb-girdle dystrophies termed *sarcoglycanopathies* (see Chap. 37 and Ref. 51). SG-null mice and hamsters similarly show the dystrophic phenotype.[180–186] Absence of the sarcoglycan complex attenuates β-DG binding to α-DG and dystrophin[182,187,188] and likely contributes to the deleterious effects and DD-like features in sarcoglycanopathy.

Defects of Dystrobrevin and Sarcospan

No human disease caused by a mutation in dystrobrevin has been reported to date. α-Dystrobrevin-deficient mice display mild dystrophic alterations in muscle.[189] No human disease due to the absence of sarcospan has been reported. Sarcospan-deficient mice maintain normal muscle function.[190]

Defects of Plectin, an Intermediate Filament Linker

Mutations in the plectin gene are associated with recessive epidermolysis bullosa simplex, absence of plectin from skeletal muscle, myopathic alterations that affect many organelles of the muscle fiber, and sometimes a defect of neuromuscular transmission[191] (see Chap. 66). This disorder is not associated with abnormal ectopic accumulation of multiple proteins. In plectin-deficient mice, the Z bands lose their tight arrangements. Dystrophin expression is diminished, and vinculin expression is dramatically reduced.[192]

MYOPATHIES CAUSED BY DEFECTS OF DESMIN INTERMEDIATE FILAMENTS

Defects of Desmin

Desmin is the intermediate filament composing the transverse network, and αB-crystallin is a chaperon protein for desmin, microtubular proteins, and some soluble enzymes.

Desmin-null mice show myofibrillar disarray beginning at the Z disk associated with accumulation of abnormal degraded myofibrillar material.[193,194] The mice transmit the defect in an autosomal recessive manner. Human desminopathies stem from dominant or sometimes recessive mutations in desmin.[195,196] Myofibrillar degeneration is associated with abnormal or ectopic sarcoplasmic accumulation of a number of proteins (e.g., dystrophin, αB-crystallin, NCAM, Cdc2 kinase).[197] Dominant mutations in αB-crystallin have similar morphologic consequences.[198,199,199a] Desminopathy and αB-crytallinopathy are further discussed in Chap. 43, on myofibrillar myopathies.

The Cellular Location of the Responsible Proteins and the Severity of the Disorders

The following generalizations can be made regarding the transverse fixation system[1] (Fig 19b-5): (1) Defects in the extracellular matrix, especially the basal lamina, and/or laminin receptors result in congenital muscular dystrophies. (2) Defects of molecules located in the costamere result in DD or Duchenne-like dystrophy. (3) Defects in molecules deeper in the cytoplasm cause milder myopathies.

Developmental Expression of the Dystrophin-DAP Complex

Proliferating myoblasts do not express appreciable amounts of dystrophin, DAPs, or desmin; do not contain myofibrils; and have no basal lamina. Myoblasts committed to fusion and small noncontractile myotubes with a few nuclei begin to express desmin,[113] myofibrillar proteins, and utrophin[200] but not dystrophin. Dystrophin and the basal lamina appear about the same time in growing myotubes harboring well-arrayed myofibrils.[201,202] In humans, dystrophin is first detected, and can be identified as a single band in immunoblots, after the ninth week of gestation, when fetal movements commence.[203] This is consistent with the notion that the dystrophin bolt stabilizes the lipid bilayer together with the basal lamina and subsarcolemmal actin network, protecting it from stress imposed by contraction.

De Novo Formation of the Architecture of the Dystrophin-DAP Complex

In the DG precursor protein molecule, the signal sequence is located at the N-terminal. As soon as DG is synthesized as a single molecule, the newly formed molecule is cut in two and they immediately bind each other to form the DG complex (Fig. 19b-6). These processes take place in the ER.[15]

The developmental appearance of four SG mRNAs is not synchronous in cultured muscle cells, but mRNAs of all four SGs are present in myoblasts. Following cell fusion, α- and γ-SG mRNAs increase remarkably, whereas β- and δ-SG mRNAs do not.[204,205] However, the expression of the four SG molecules is almost simultaneous,[15] and SG complex appears as soon as the four SG subunits are synthesized at the ER. The following sequence of events is likely: The δ- or γ-SG binds to β-SG to form a dimer; then γ- or δ-SG is added to form a trimer; finally α-SG is added to form a tetramer.[15]

In the ER, the DG and SG complexes and sarcospan are separate (Fig. 19b-6), but they associate in the Golgi complex or in transport vesicles to form a large complex.[15] When transport vesicles released from the Golgi complex finally fuse with the plasma membrane, the orientation of transmembrane proteins carried by the vesicle is inverted in the plasma membrane. Glycosylation of the DG and SG subunits commences in the ER, but extensive glycosylation of α-DG takes place in the Golgi complex.[15] Since glycosylation occurs inside the vesicles, the glycosyl groups decorate future extracellular domains of the proteins. Peripheral proteins, namely, dystrophin, dystrobrevin, and syntrophin, are synthesized on free ribosomes present in the cytoplasm. They associate with protein domains exposed on the outside of transport vesicles, which will become intracellular when DG and SG complexes are incorporated into the sarcolemma. The exact time when peripheral proteins associate with DG and SG complexes is not known.

The Dystrophin-DAP Complex as a Signaling System

Some sarcolemma-associated signaling molecules are connected to the dystrophin-DAP complex, and these may also be involved in the pathogenesis of DD. The signaling molecules include growth factor receptor 2 (Grb 2), which interacts with β-DG,[206,207] nNOS,[208] and caveolin 3[209] (Fig. 19b-1). On the other hand, signaling processes are usually concerned with rapid cellular responses, whereas the dystrophic changes are inherently slow. Thus it is not necessarily easy to confidently relate altered signaling processes to the pathogenesis of the dystrophinopathies. Below we briefly review the signaling reactions related to the dystrophin complex and their possible effects in dystrophinopathies.

DYSTROPHIN PHOSPHORYLATION REACTIONS

Dystrophin can be phosphorylated at its N-terminal actin-binding domain, rod domain, and C-terminal region.[210–212] Enzymes capable of phosphorylating these sites include a mitogen-activated protein kinase,[213] cyclic AMP- and cyclic GMP-dependent protein kinase, protein kinase C, and casein kinase II,[214] as well as calmodulin-activated protein kinase II.[211] Tyrosine phosphorylation of β-DG inhibits binding to dystrophin[215,216] and utrophin.[217] The cellular significance of the relation of these phosphorylations to the pathogenesis of DD have not been clarified.

POSSIBLE SIGNALING BY THE SARCOGLYCAN COMPLEX

The SG complex serves to strengthen the binding of β-DG to α-DG and dystrophin, but the requirement for four SG subunits has not been rationalized. This raises the question of whether the SG complex may have an as yet undefined signaling function. Related to this notion is the fact that α-SG binds to ATP, and the binding is inhibited by 3′-O-(4-benzoyl) benzoyl ATP and ADP.[218] Immunocytochemical studies indicate that γ- and δ-SG are associated with the sarcoplasmic reticulum as well as the sarcolemma. This, however, suggests that both of these SGs can function independently of the dystrophin complex, and does not assign a signaling function to the sarcolemma-associated sarcoglycans.[219]

SYNTROPHINS

Signaling roles have been ascribed to syntrophin, but the functions of α-, β1-, and β2-syntrophins have not been elucidated. α-Syntrophin binds Ca^{220} and is phosphorylated by

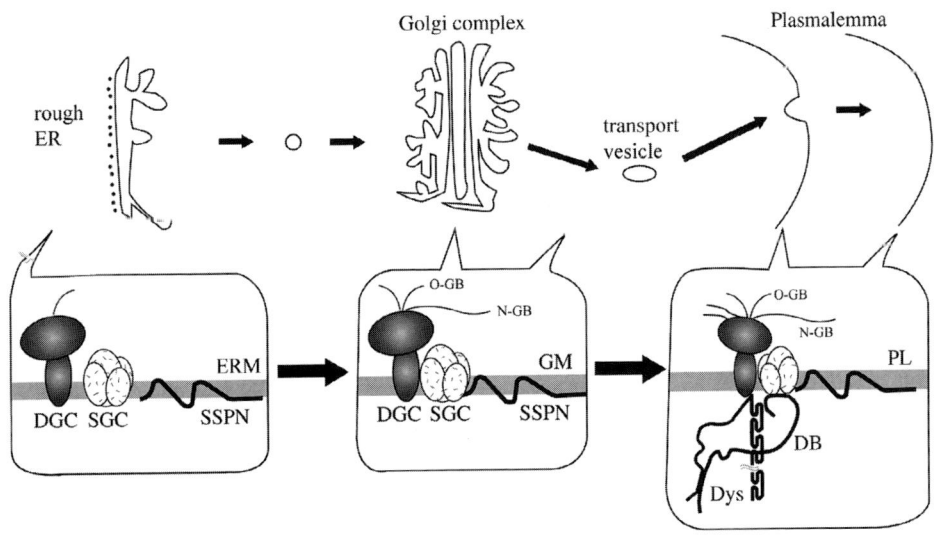

FIGURE 19b-6. Biosynthesis and assembly of the dystrophin-DAP complex. The DG and SG complexes and sarcospan (SSPN) are synthesized and glycosylated but remain unassociated in the ER. The top and bottom of the ER membrane (ERM) correspond to the lumenal and cytoplasmic sides of the ER. DG-SG-SSPN association occurs after translocation to the Golgi or en route to the sarcolemma. During their journey to the cell surface, dystrophin and other molecules become anchored to cytoplasmic extensions of the membrane-integrated DG and SG complexes. O-GB and N-GB = O- and N-glycosyl chains, GM = Golgi complex membrane, PL = plasma membrane. (Revised from Ref. 15.)

calmodulin-dependent protein kinase II.[221] α-Syntrophin forms oligomers by self-association.[222] The marked decrease of α-syntrophin in DD likely results in absence of nNOS from the subsarcolemmal region, but total muscle nNOS activity is unaffected. α-Syntrophin-deficient mice express no nNOS at the sarcolemma and show no structural abnormality at the light microscopic level.[223] However, after cardiotoxin-induced necrosis, the regenerating fibers are hypertrophied. This may be due to increased autocrine release of insulin-like growth factor I by muscle.[224]

nNOS

Nitric oxide (NO) is a gaseous signaling molecule synthesized by NOS present in various tissues.[225,226] NO has vasodilating effects[227] and also mediates satellite cell activation in injured muscle.[228] In DD, BD, and *mdx* muscles, nNOS is absent from the sarcolemma[208,229] but persists in the cytosol, which might contribute to sarcolemmal vulnerability in the dystrophinopathies. nNOS-null mice, however, show neither sarcolemmal damage nor dystrophic changes,[230] and the dystrophin and nNOS double-deficient mice show the expected pathology of the *mdx* mouse.[231] On the other hand, overexpression of nNOS in *mdx* mice ameliorates the dystrophic phenotype, apparently by suppression of macrophage response to fiber necrosis.[232] Both *mdx* and NOS-deficient mice show reduced vasodilator response to exercise.[233] Some reports suggest decreased muscle blood flow in DD patients,[234] but this has not been shown to be due to decreased NO production.

CAVEOLIN-3

Caveolin-3 deficiency causes autosomal dominant limb-girdle dystrophy in humans[235] and autosomal recessive muscular dystrophy in caveolin-3-deficient mice,[236,237] although whether impairment of the signaling functions related to caveolin-3 is responsible for these diseases is not known. As already mentioned, overexpression of caveolin-3 in the mouse induces sarcolemmal dystrophin deficiency, probably by displacing dystrophin from β-DG.[78] Caveolin-3 also associates with dysferlin,[79,80] the protein responsible for Miyoshi distal myopathy and limb-girdle muscular dystrophy.[238] In DD, the expression of caveolin-3 is enhanced, which might contribute to the pathologic process.

Acknowledgment

The author is grateful to Professor Clara Franzini-Armstrong for her expertise and suggestions, which played an important role in the writing of this manuscript.

List of Abbreviations

ABS	actin-binding site	DIF	desmin intermediate filaments
BD	Becker dystrophy	EM	electron microscopy
CH	calponin homology	ER	endoplasmic reticulum
CMD	congenital muscular dystrophy	nNOS	n-NO synthase
DAP	dystrophin-associated protein	NO	nitric oxide
DD	Duchenne dystrophy	PPXY	proline-proline-arbitrary amino acid-tyrosine
Df	dystrophin fragments	SG	sarcoglycan
DG	dystroglycan	TID	3-(trifluoromethyl)-3-(iodophenyl)diazirine

References

1. Ozawa E, Nishino I, Nonaka I: Sarcolemmopathy: Muscular dystrophies with cell membrane defects. *Brain Pathol* 11:218–230, 2001.
2. Ozawa E, Yoshida M, Suzuki A, et al: Dystrophin-associated proteins in muscular dystrophy. *Hum Molec Genet* 4:1711–1716, 1995.
3. Koenig M, Monaco AP, Kunkel LM: The complete sequence of dystrophin predicts a rod-shaped cytoskeletal protein. *Cell* 53:219–228, 1988.
4. Pons F, Augier N, Heilig R, et al: Isolated dystrophin molecules as seen by electron microscopy. *Proc Natl Acad Sci USA* 87:7851–7855, 1990.
5. Sugita H, Arahata K, Ishiguro T, et al: Negative immunostaining of Duchenne muscular dystrophy (DMD) and mdx muscle surface membrane with antibody against synthetic peptide fragment predicted from DMD cDNA. *Proc Jpn Acad* 64:37–39, 1988.
6. Arahata K, Ishiura S, et al: Immunostaining of skeletal and cardiac muscle surface membrane with antibody against Duchenne muscular dystrophy peptide. *Nature* 333:861–863, 1988.
7. Watkins SC, Hoffman EP, Slayter HS, et al: Immunoelectron microscopic localization of dystrophin in myofibers. *Nature* 333:863–866, 1988.
8. Ervasti JM, Campbell KP: Membrane organization of the dystrophin-glycoprotein complex. *Cell* 66:1121–1131, 1991.
9. Campbell KP, Kahl SD: Association of dystrophin and an integral membrane glycoprotein. *Nature* 338:259–262, 1989.
10. Ervasti JM, Ohlendieck K, Kahl SD, et al: Deficiency of a glycoprotein component of the dystrophin complex in dystrophic muscle. *Nature* 345:315–319, 1990.
11. Yoshida M, Ozawa E: Glycoprotein complex anchoring dystrophin to sarcolemma. *J Biochem (Tokyo)* 108:748–752, 1990.
12. Yoshida M, Noguchi S, Wakabayashi E, et al: The fourth component of the sarcoglycan complex. *FEBS Lett* 403:143–148, 1997.
13. Smalheiser NR, Kim E: Purification of cranin, a laminin binding membrane protein. Identity with dystroglycan and reassessment of its carbohydrate moieties. *J Biol Chem* 270:15425–15433, 1995.
14. Holt KH, Crosbie RH, Venzke DP, et al: Biosynthesis of dystroglycan: Processing of a precursor propeptide. *FEBS Lett* 468:79–83, 2000.
15. Noguchi S, Wakabayashi E, Imamura M, et al: Formation of sarcoglycan complex with differentiation in cultured myocytes. *Eur J Biochem* 267:640–648, 2000.
16. Chiba A, Matsumura K, Yamada H, et al: Structures of sialylated O-linked oligosaccharides of bovine peripheral nerve alpha-dystroglycan. The role of a novel O-mannosyl-type oligosaccharide in the binding of alpha-dystroglycan with laminin. *J Biol Chem* 272:2156–2162, 1997.
17. Yoshida M, Suzuki A, Yamamoto H, et al: Dissociation of the complex of dystrophin and its associated proteins into several unique groups by n-octyl beta-D-glucoside. *Eur J Biochem* 222:1055–1061, 1994.
18. Roberds SL, Leturcq F, Allamand V, et al: Missense mutations in the adhalin gene linked to autosomal recessive muscular dystrophy. *Cell* 78:625–633, 1994.

19. Lim LE, Duclos F, Broux O, et al: Beta-sarcoglycan: Characterization and role in limb-girdle muscular dystrophy linked to 4q12. *Nat Genet* 11:257–265, 1995.
20. Bonnemann CG, Modi R, Noguchi S, et al: Beta-sarcoglycan (A3b) mutations cause autosomal recessive muscular dystrophy with loss of the sarcoglycan complex. *Nat Genet* 11:266–273, 1995.
21. Noguchi S, McNally EM, Ben Othmane K, et al: Mutations in the dystrophin-associated protein gamma-sarcoglycan in chromosome 13 muscular dystrophy. *Science* 270:819–822, 1995.
22. Nigro V, de Sa Moreira E, Piluso G, et al: Autosomal recessive limb-girdle muscular dystrophy, LGMD2F, is caused by a mutation in the delta-sarcoglycan gene. *Nat Genet* 14:195–198, 1996.
23. Sakamoto A, Ono K, Abe M, et al: Both hypertrophic and dilated cardiomyopathies are caused by mutation of the same gene, delta-sarcoglycan, in hamster: An animal model of disrupted dystrophin-associated glycoprotein complex. *Proc Natl Acad Sci USA* 94:13873–13878, 1997.
24. Chan YM, Bonnemann CG, Lidov HGW, et al: Molecular organization of sarcoglycan complex in mouse myotubes in culture. *J Cell Biol* 143:2033–2044, 1998.
25. Ettinger A, Feng G, Sanes J: Epsilon-sarcoglycan, a broadly expressed homologue of the gene mutated in limb-girdle muscular dystrophy 2D. *J Biol Chem* 272:32534–32538, 1997.
26. McNally EM, Ly CT, Kunkel LM: Human epsilon-sarcoglycan is highly related to alpha-sarcoglycan (adhalin), the limb girdle muscular dystrophy 2D gene. *FEBS Lett* 422:27–32, 1998.
27. Liu LA, Engvall E: Sarcoglycan isoforms in skeletal muscle. *J Biol Chem* 274:38171–38176, 1999.
28. Crosbie R, Heighway J, Venzke D, et al: Sarcospan, the 25-kDa transmembrane component of the dystrophin-glycoprotein complex. *J Biol Chem* 272:31221–31224, 1997.
29. Yamamoto H, Hagiwara Y, Mizuno Y, et al: Heterogeneity of dystrophin-associated proteins. *J Biochem (Tokyo)* 114:132–139, 1993.
30. Adams ME, Butler MH, Dwyer TM, et al: Two forms of mouse syntrophin, a 58 kd dystrophin-associated protein, differ in primary structure and tissue distribution. *Neuron* 11:531–540, 1993.
31. Yoshida M, Yamamoto H, Noguchi S, et al: Dystrophin-associated protein A0 is a homologue of the Torpedo 87K protein. *FEBS Lett* 367:311–314, 1995.
32. Ahn AH, Yoshida M, et al: Cloning of human basic A1, a distinct 59-kDA dystrophin-associated protein encoded on chromosome 8q23-24. *Proc Natl Acad Sci USA* 91:4446–4450, 1994.
33. Ahn AH, Freener CA, Gussoni E, et al: The three human syntrophin genes are expressed in diverse tissues, have distinct chromosmal localizations, and each bind to dystrophin and its relatives. *J Biol Chem* 271:2724–2730, 1996.
34. Hogan A, Shepherd L, Chabot J, et al: Interaction of gamma1-syntrophin with diacylglycerol kinase-zeta: Regulation of nuclear localization by PDZ interactions. *J Biol Chem* 276:26526–26533, 2001.
35. Wagner KR, Cohen JB, Huganir RL: The 87K postsynaptic membrane protein from Torpedo is a protein-tyrosine kinase substrate homologous to dystrophin. *Neuron* 10:511–522, 1993.
36. Sadoulet-Puccio HM, Khurana TS, Cohen JB, et al: Cloning and characterization of the human homologue of a dystrophin related phosphoprotein found at the Torpedo electric organ post-synaptic membrane. *Hum Mol Genet* 5:489–496, 1996.
37. Sadoulet-Puccio H, Rajala M, Kunkel L: Dystrobrevin and dystrophin: An interaction through coiled-coil motifs. *Proc Natl Acad Sci USA* 94:12413–12418, 1997.
38. Nawrotzki R, Loh NY, Ruegg MA, et al: Characterisation of alpha-dystrobrevin in muscle. *J Cell Sci* 111:2595–2605, 1998.
39. Peters M, O'Brien K, Sadoulet-Puccio HM, et al: Beta-dystrobrevin, a new member of the dystrophin family. Identification, cloning, and protein associations. *J Biol Chem* 272:31561–31569, 1997.
40. Blake DJ, Nawrotzki R, et al: Beta-dystrobrevin, a member of the dystrophin-related protein family. *Proc Natl Acad Sci USA* 95:241–246, 1998.
41. Newey SE, Howman EV, Ponting CP, et al: Syncoilin, a novel member of the intermediate filament superfamily that interacts with alpha-dystrobrevin in skeletal muscle. *J Biol Chem* 276:6645–6655, 2001.
42. Mizuno Y, Thompson TG, Guyon JR, et al: Desmuslin, an intermediate filament protein that interacts with alpha-dystrobrevin and desmin. *Proc Natl Acad Sci USA* 98:6156–6161, 2001.
43. Benson MA, Newey SE, et al: Dysbindin, a novel coiled coil containing protein that interacts with the dystrobrevins in muscle and brain. *J Biol Chem* 276:24232–24241, 2001.
44. Tinsley JM, Blake DJ, Zuellig RA, et al: Increasing complexity of the dystrophin-associated protein complex. *Proc Natl Acad Sci USA* 91:8307–8313, 1994.
45. Campbell KP: Three muscular dystrophies: Loss of cytoskeleton-extracellular matrix linkage. *Cell* 80:675–679, 1995.
46. Blake DJ, Weir A, et al: Function and genetics of dystrophin and dystrophin-related proteins in muscle. *Physiol Rev* 82:291–329, 2002.
47. Ervasti JM, Kahl SD, Campbell KP: Purification of dystrophin from skeletal muscle. *J Biol Chem* 266:9161–9165, 1991.
48. Ohlendieck K, Ervasti JM, Snook JB, et al: Dystrophin-glycoprotein complex is highly enriched in isolated skeletal muscle sarcolemma. *J Cell Biol* 112:135–148, 1991.
49. Watkins SC, Cullen MJ, Hoffman EP, et al: Plasma membrane cytoskeleton of muscle: A fine structural analysis. *Microsc Res Tech* 48:131–141, 2000.
50. Ibraghimov-Beskrovnaya O, Ervasti JM, Leveille CJ, et al: Primary structure of dystrophin-associated glycoproteins linking dystrophin to the extracellular matrix. *Nature* 355:696–702, 1992.
51. Ozawa E, Noguchi S, Mizuno Y, et al: From dystrophinopathy to sarcoglycanopathy: Evolution of a concept of muscular dystrophy. *Muscle Nerve* 21:421–438, 1998.
52. Nigro V, Piluso G, Belsito A, et al: Identification of a novel sarcoglycan gene at 5q33 encoding a sarcolemmal 35 kDa glycoprotein. *Hum Mol Genet* 5:1179–1186, 1996.
53. Yoshida M, Suzuki A, Shimizu T, et al: Proteinase-sensitive sites on isolated rabbit dystrophin. *J Biochem (Tokyo)* 112:433–439, 1992.
54. Suzuki A, Yoshida M, Yamamoto H, et al: Glycoprotein-binding site of dystrophin is confined to the cysteine-rich domain and the first half of the carboxy-terminal domain. *FEBS Lett* 308:154–160, 1992.
55. Yoshida M, Hama H, Ishikawa-Sakurai M, et al: Biochemical evidence for association of dystrobrevin with the sarcoglycan-sarcospan complex as a basis for understanding sarcoglycanopathy. *Hum Mol Genet* 9:1033–1040, 2000.
56. Crosbie RH, Lim LE, Moore SA, et al: Molecular and genetic characterization of sarcospan: Insights into sarcoglycan-sarcospan interactions. *Hum Mol Genet* 9:2019–2027, 2000.
57. Yoshida A, Kobayashi K, Manya H, et al: Muscular dystrophy and neuronal migration disorder caused by mutations in a glycosyltransferase, POMGnT1. *Dev Cell* 1:717–724, 2001.
58. O'Toole JJ, Deyst KA, Bowe MA, et al: Alternative splicing of agrin regulates its binding to heparin, alpha-dystroglycan, and the cell surface. *Proc Natl Acad Sci USA* 93:7369–7374, 1996.
59. Peng HB, Ali AA, Daggett DF, et al: The relationship between perlecan and dystroglycan and its implication in the formation of the neuromuscular junction. *Cell Adhes Commun* 5:475–489, 1998.
60. Gee SH, Blacher RW, Douville PJ, et al: Laminin-binding protein 120 from brain is closely related to the dystrophin-associated glycoprotein, dystroglycan, and binds with high affinity to the major heparin binding domain of laminin. *J Biol Chem* 268:14972–14980, 1993.
61. Ervasti JM, Campbell KP: A role for the dystrophin-glycoprotein complex as a transmembrane linker between laminin and actin. *J Cell Biol* 122:809–823, 1993.
62. Pall EA, Bolton KM, Ervasti JM: Differential heparin inhibition of skeletal muscle alpha-dystroglycan binding to laminins. *J Biol Chem* 271:3817–3821, 1996.
63. Di Stasio E, Sciandra F, Maras B, et al: Structural and functional analysis of the N-terminal extracellular region of beta-dystroglycan. *Biochem Biophys Res Commun* 266:274–278, 1999.
64. Sciandra F, Schneider M, Giardina B, et al: Identification of the beta-dystroglycan binding epitope within the C-terminal region of alpha-dystroglycan. *Eur J Biochem* 268:4590–4597, 2001.
65. Blake DJ, Tinsley JM, Davies KE: Coiled-coil regions in the carboxy-terminal domains of dystrophin and related proteins: Potentials for protein-protein interactions. *Trends Biochem Sci* 20:133–135, 1995.
66. Peters MF, Kramarcy NR, Sealock R, et al: beta2-Syntrophin: Localization at the neuromuscular junction in skeletal muscle. *Neuroreport* 5:1577–1580, 1994.
67. Ahn AH, Kunkel LM: Syntrophin binds to an alternatively spliced exon of dystrophin. *J Biol Chem* 128:363–371, 1995.
68. Suzuki A, Yoshida M, Ozawa E: Mammalian alpha1- and beta1-syntrophin bind to the alternative splice-prone region of the dystrophin COOH terminus. *J Cell Biol* 128:373–381, 1995.
69. Yang B, Jung D, Rafael JA, et al: Identification of alpha-syntrophin binding to syntrophin triplet, dystrophin, and utrophin. *J Biol Chem* 270:4975–4978, 1995.
70. Peters MF, Adams ME, Froehner SC: Differential association of syntrophin pairs with the dystrophin complex. *J Cell Biol* 138:81–93, 1997.
71. Newey SE, Benson MA, Ponting CP, et al: Alternative splicing of dystrobrevin regulates the stoichiometry of syntrophin binding to the dystrophin protein complex. *Curr Biol* 10:1295–1298, 2000.
72. Kramarcy N, Vidal A, Froehner SC, et al: Association of dystrophin and multiple dystrophin short forms with the mammalian M_r 58,000 dystrophin-associated protein (syntrophin). *J Biol Chem* 269:2870–2876, 1994.
73. Ponting CP, Phillips C, Davies KE, et al: PDZ domains: Targeting signalling molecules to sub-membranous sites. *Bioessays* 19:469–479, 1997.
74. Brenman J, Chao D, Gee S, et al: Interaction of nitric-oxide synthase with the postsynaptic density protein psd-95 and alpha-1-syntrophin mediated by PDZ domains. *Cell* 84:757–767, 1996.
75. Adams ME, Mueller HA, Froehner SC: In vivo requirement of the alpha-syntrophin PDZ domain for the sarcolemmal localization of nNOS and aquaporin-4. *J Cell Biol* 155:113–122, 2001.
76. Venema VJ, Ju H, Zou R, et al: Interaction of neuronal nitricoxide synthase with caveolin-3 in skeletal muscle. Identification of a novel caveolin scaffolding/inhibitory domain. *J Biol Chem* 272:28187–28190, 1997.
77. Okamoto T, Schlegel A, Scherer PE, et al: Caveolins, a family of scaffolding proteins for organizing "preassembled signaling complexes" at the plasma membrane. *J Biol Chem* 273:5419–5422, 1998.

78. Sotgia F, Lee JK, Das K, et al: Caveolin-3 directly interacts with the C-terminal tail of beta-dystroglycan. Identification of a central WW-like domain within caveolin family members. *J Biol Chem* 275:38048–38058, 2000.
79. Liu J, Aoki M, Illa I, et al: Dysferlin, a novel skeletal muscle gene, is mutated in Miyoshi myopathy and limb girdle muscular dystrophy. *Nat Genet* 20:31–36, 1998.
80. Bashir R, Britton S, Strachan T, et al: A gene related to *Caenorhabditis elegans* spermatogenesis factor *fer-1* is mutated in limb-girdle muscular dystrophy type 2B. *Nat Genet* 20:37–42, 1998.
81. Thompson TG, Chan YM, Hack AA, et al: Filamin 2 (FLN2): A muscle-specific sarcoglycan interacting protein. *J Cell Biol* 148:115–126, 2000.
82. Belkin A, Burridge B: Localization of utrophin and aciculin at sites of cell-matrix and cell-cell adhesion in cultured cells. *Exp Cell Res* 221:132–140, 1995.
83. Moiseeva EP, Belkin AM, Spurr NK, et al: A novel dystrophin/utrophin-associated protein is an enzymatically inactive member of the phosphoglucomutase superfamily. *Eur J Biochem* 235:103–113, 1996.
84. Wakayama Y, Inoue M, Kojima H, et al: Aciculin and its relation to dystrophin: Immunocytochemical studies in human normal and Duchenne dystrophy quadriceps muscles. *Acta Neuropathol* 99:654–662, 2000.
85. Hoffman EP, Kunkel LM: Dystrophin abnormalities in Duchenne/Becker dystrophy. *Neuron* 2:1019–1029, 1989.
86. Senter L, Luise M, Presotto C, et al: Interaction of dystrophin with cytoskeletal proteins: Binding to talin and actin. *Biochem Biophys Res Commun* 192:899–904, 1993.
87. Ohlendieck K: Towards an understanding of the dystrophin-glycoprotein complex: Linkage between the extracellular matrix and the membrane cytoskeleton in muscle fibers. *Eur J Cell Biol* 69:1–10, 1996.
88. Levine BA, Moir AJG, Patchell VB, et al: The interaction of actin with dystrophin. *FEBS Lett* 263:159–162, 1990.
89. Levine BA, Moir AJ, Patchell VB, et al: Binding sites involved in the interaction of actin with the N-terminal region of dystrophin. *FEBS Lett* 298:44–48, 1992.
90. Way M, Pope B, Cross RA, et al: Expression of the N-terminal domain of dystrophin in *E. coli* and demonstration of binding to F-actin. *FEBS Lett* 301:243–245, 1992.
91. Winder S, Gibson T, Kendrick-Jones J: Dystrophin and utrophin—The missing links. *FEBS Lett* 369:27–33, 1995.
92. Keep NH, Norwood FL, Moores CA, et al: The 2.0 A structure of the second calponin homology domain from the actin-binding region of the dystrophin homologue utrophin. *J Mol Biol* 285:1257–1264, 1999.
93. Moores CA, Keep NH, Kendrick-Jones J: Structure of the utrophin actin-binding domain bound to F-actin reveals binding by an induced fit mechanism. *J Mol Biol* 297:465–480, 2000.
94. Rybakova IN, Amann KJ, Ervasti JM: A new model for the interaction of dystrophin with F-actin. *J Cell Biol* 135:661–672, 1996.
95. Amann KJ, Renley BA, Ervasti JM: A cluster of basic repeats in the dystrophin rod domain binds F-actin through an electrostatic interaction. *J Biol Chem* 273:28419–28423, 1998.
96. Corrado K, Rafael JA, Mills PL, et al: Transgenic *mdx* mice expressing dystrophin with a deletion in the actin-binding domain display a "mild Becker" phenotype. *J Cell Biol* 134:873–884, 1996.
97. Warner LE, DelloRusso C, Crawford RW, et al: Expression of Dp260 in muscle tethers the actin cytoskeleton to the dystrophin-glycoprotein complex and partially prevents dystrophy. *Hum Mol Genet* 11:1095–1105, 2002.
98. Rybakova IN, Ervasti JM: Dystrophin-glycoprotein complex is monomeric and stabilizes actin filaments *in vitro* through a lateral association. *J Biol Chem* 272:28771–28778, 1997.
99. Suzuki A, Yoshida M, Hayashi K, et al: Molecular organization at the glycoprotein-complex-binding site of dystrophin. Three dystrophin-associated proteins bind directly to the carboxy-terminal portion of dystrophin. *Eur J Biochem* 220:283–292, 1994.
100. Beggs A, Hoffman EP, Snyder JR, et al: Exploring the molecular basis for variability among patients with Becker muscular dystrophy: Dystrophin gene and protein studies. *Am J Hum Genet* 49:54–67, 1991.
101. Rentschler S, Linn H, Deininger K, et al: The WW domain of dystrophin required EF-hands region to interact with beta-dystroglycan. *Biol Chem* 380:431–442, 1999.
102. Rafael JA, Cox GA, Corrado K, et al: Forced expression of dystrophin deletion constructs reveals structure-function correlations. *J Cell Biol* 134:93–102, 1996.
103. Andre B, Springael JY: WWP, a new amino acid motif present in single or multiple copies in various proteins including dystrophin and the SH3-binding Yes-associated protein YAP65. *Biochem Biophys Res Commun* 205:1201–1205, 1994.
104. Bork P, Sudol M: The WW domain: A signalling site in dystrophin? *Trends Biochem Sci* 19:531–533, 1994.
105. Chung W, Campanelli JT: WW and EF hand domains of dystrophin-family proteins mediate dystroglycan binding. *Mol Cell Biol Res Commun* 2:162–171, 1999.
106. Jung D, Yang B, Meyer J, et al: Identification and characterization of the dystrophin anchoring site on beta-dystroglycan. *J Biol Chem* 270:27305–27310, 1995.
107. Huang X, Poy F, Zhang R, et al: Structure of a WW domain containing fragment of dystrophin in complex with beta-dystroglycan. *Nat Struct Biol* 7:634–638, 2000.
108. Ishikawa-Sakurai M, Yoshida M, Imamura M, et al: ZZ domain is essentially required for the physiological binding of dystrophin to beta-dystroglycan. *Hum Mol Genet* Feb, 2004.
109. Ponting CP, Blake DJ, Davies KE, et al: ZZ and TAZ: New putative zinc fingers in dystrophin and other proteins. *Trends Biochem Sci* 21:11–13, 1996.
110. Chamberlain JS, Corrodo K, Rafael JA, et al: Interaction between dystrophin and the sarcolemma membrane. *Soc Gen Physiol Ser* 52:19–29, 1997.
111. Tommasi di Vignano A, Di Zenzo G, Sudol M, et al: Contribution of the different modules in the utrophin carboxy-terminal region to the formation and regulation of the DAP complex. *FEBS Lett* 471:229–234, 2000.
112. Lazarides E, Hubbard BD: Immunological characterization of the subunit of the 100 A filaments from muscle cells. *Proc Natl Acad Sci USA* 73:4344–4348, 1976.
113. Gard DL, Lazarides E: The synthesis and distribution of desmin and vimentin during myogenesis in vitro. *Cell* 19:263–275, 1980.
114. Pardo JV, Siliciano JD, Craig SW: A vinculin-containing cortical lattice in skeletal muscle: Transverse lattice elements ("costameres") mark sites of attachment between myofibrils and sarcolemma. *Proc Natl Acad Sci USA* 80:1008–1012, 1983.
115. Hijikata T, Murakami T, Imamura M, et al: Plectin is a linker of intermediate filaments to Z-discs in skeletal muscle fibers. *J Cell Sci* 112:867–876, 1999.
116. Hijikata T, Murakami T, Ishikawa H, et al: Plectin tethers desmin intermediate filaments onto subsarcolemmal dense plaques containing dystrophin and vinculin. *Histochem Cell Biol* 119:109–123, 2003.
117. Mondello MR, Bramanti P, Cutroneo G, et al: Immunolocalization of the costameres in human skeletal muscle fibers: Confocal scanning laser microscope investigations. *Anat Rec* 245:481–487, 1996.
118. Masuda T, Fujimaki N, Ozawa E, et al: Confocal laser microscopy of dystrophin localization in guinea pig skeletal muscle fibers. *J Cell Biol* 119:543–548, 1992.
119. Porter GA, Dmytrenko GM, Winkelmann JC, et al: Dystrophin colocalizes with b-spectrin in distinct subsarcolemmal domains in mammalian skeletal muscle. *J Cell Biol* 117:997–1005, 1992.
120. Straub V, Bittner RE, Leger JJ, et al: Direct visualization of the dystrophin network on skeletal muscle fiber membrane. *J Cell Biol* 119:1183–1191, 1992.
121. Williams MW, Resneck WG, Bloch RJ: Membrane skeleton of innervated and denervated fast- and slow-twitch muscle. *Muscle Nerve* 23:590–599, 2000.
122. Pardo JV, Pittenger MF, Craig SW: Subcellular sorting of isoactins: Selective association of gamma-actin with skeletal muscle mitochondria. *Cell* 32:1093–1103, 1983.
123. Pardo JV, Siliciano JD, Craig SW: Vinculin is a component of an extensive network of myofibril-sarcolemma attachment regions in cardiac muscle fibers. *J Cell Biol* 97:1081–1088, 1983.
124. Rybiakova IN, Patel JR, Ervasti JM: The dystrophin complex forms a mechanically strong link between the sarcolemma and costameric actin. *J Cell Biol* 150:1209–1214, 2000.
125. Berthier C, Blaineau S: Supramolecular organization of the subsarcolemmal cytoskeleton of adult skeletal muscle fibers. A review. *Biol Cell* 89:413–434, 1997.
126. Brancaccio M, Guazzone S, Menini N, et al: Melusin is a new muscle-specific interactor for beta(1) integrin cytoplasmic domain. *J Biol Chem* 274:29282–29288, 1999.
127. Clark KA, McElhinny AS, Beckerle MC, et al: Striated muscle cytoarchitecture. An intricate web of form and function. *Annu Rev Cell Dev Biol* 18:637–706, 2002.
128. Cullen MC, Fulthorpe JJ: Stages in fiber breakdown in Duchenne muscular dystrophy. *J Neurol Sci* 24:179–200, 1975.
129. Pierobon-Bormioli S: Transverse sarcomere filamentous systems: Z- and M-cables. *J Muscle Res Cell Motil* 2:401–413, 1981.
130. Shear CR, Bloch RJ: Vinculin in subsarcolemmal densities in chicken skeletal muscle: Localization and relationship to intracellular and extracellular structures. *J Cell Biol* 101:240–256, 1985.
131. Tokuysu KT, Dutton AH, Singer SJ: Immunoelectron microscopic studies of desmin (skeletin) localization and intermediate filament organization in chicken skeletal muscle. *J Cell Biol* 96:1727–1735, 1983.
132. Harris JB, Cullen MJ: Ultrastructural localization and the possible role of dystrophin, in Kakulas BA, Howell JMcC, Roses AD (eds): *Duchenne Muscular Dystrophy: Animal Models and Gene Manipulation*. New York: Raven Press; 1992, pp 19–40.
133. Wakayama Y, Shibuya S: Gold-labelled dystrophin molecule in muscle plasmalemma of mdx control mice as seen by electron microscopy of deep etching replica. *Acta Neuropathol* 82:178–184, 1991.
134. Lakonishok M, Muschler J, Horwitz AF: The alpha5 beta1 integrin associates with a dystrophin-containing lattice during muscle development. *Dev Biol* 152:209–220, 1992.
135. Klietsch R, Ervasti JM, Arnold W, et al: Dystrophin-glycoprotein complex and laminin colocalize to the sarcolemma and transverse tubules of cardiac muscle. *Circ Res* 72:349–360, 1993.
136. Danofski BA, Imanaka-Yoshida K, Sanger JM, et al: Costameres are sites of force transmission to the substratum in adult rat cardiomyocytes. *J Cell Biol* 118:1411–1420, 1992.
137. Tome FM, Evangelista T, Leclerc A, et al: Congenital muscular dystrophy with merosin deficiency. *C R Acad Sci Paris Sci Vie* 317:351–357, 1994.

138. Osari S, Kobayashi O, Yamashita Y, et al: Basement membrane abnormality in merosin-negative congenital muscular dystrophy. Acta Neuropathol 91:332–336, 1996.
139. Ishii H, Hayashi YK, Nonaka I, et al: Electron microscopic examination of basal lamina in Fukuyama congenital muscular dystrophy. Neuromuscul Disord 7:191–197, 1997.
140. Vajsar J, Ackerley C, Chitayat D, et al: Basal lamina abnormality in the skeletal muscle of Walker-Warburg syndrome. Pediatr Neurol 22:139–143, 2000.
141. Higuchi I, Shiraishi T, Hashiguchi T, et al: Frameshift mutation in the collagen VI gene causes Ullrich's disease. Ann Neurol 50:261–265, 2001.
142. Venegas OC, Bertini E, Zhang RZ, et al: Ullrich scleroatonic muscular dystrophy is caused by recessive mutations in collagen type VI. Proc Natl Acad Sci USA 98:7516–7521, 2001.
143. Jobsis GJ, Keizers H, Vreijling JP, et al: Type VI collagen mutations in Bethlem myopathy, an autosomal dominant myopathy with contractures. Nat Genet 14:113–115, 1996.
144. Pan TC, Zhang RZ, Pericak-Vance MA, et al: Missense mutation in a von Willebrand factor type A domain of the alpha3(VI) collagen gene (COL6A3) in a family with Bethlem myopathy. Hum Mol Genet 7:807–812, 1998.
145. Vanegas OC, Zhang RZ, Sabatelli P, et al: Novel COL6A1 splicing mutation in a family affected by mild Bethlem myopathy. Muscle Nerve 25:513–519, 2002.
146. Yoshida A, Kobayashi K, Manya H: Muscular dystrophy and neuronal migration disorder caused by mutations in a glycosyltransferase, POMGnT1. Dev Cell 1:717–724, 2001.
147. Beltran-Valero de Bernabe D, Currier S, Steinbrecher A, et al: Mutations in the O-mannosyltransferase gene POMT1 give rise to the severe neuronal migration disorder Walker-Warburg syndrome. Am J Hum Genet 71:1033–1043, 2002.
148. Toda T, Segawa M, Nomura Y, et al: Localization of a gene for Fukuyama type congenital muscular dystrophy to chromosome 9q31-33. Nat Genet 5:283–286, 1993.
149. Kobayashi K, Nakahori Y, Miyake M, et al: An ancient retrotransposal insertion causes Fukuyama-type congenital muscular dystrophy. Nature 394:388–392, 1998.
150. Driss A, Amouri R, Ben Hamida C, et al: A new locus for autosomal recessive limb-girdle muscular dystrophy in a large consanguineous Tunisian family maps to chromosome 19q13.3. Neuromuscul Disord 10:240–246, 2000.
151. Brockington M, Blake DJ, Prandini P, et al: Mutations in the fukutin-related protein gene (FKRP) cause a form of congenital muscular dystrophy with secondary laminin alpha2 deficiency and abnormal glycosylation of alpha-dystroglycan. Am J Hum Genet 69:6, 2001.
152. Aravind L, Koonin EV: The fukutin protein family—Predicted enzymes modifying cell-surface molecules. Curr Biol 9:R836–R837, 1999.
153. Grewal PK, Holzfeind PJ, Bittner RE, et al: Mutant glycosyltransferase and altered glycosylation of alpha-dystroglycan in the myodystrophy mouse. Nat Genet 28:151–154, 2001.
154. Hayashi YK, Chou FL, Engvall E, et al: Mutations in the integrin alpha7 gene cause congenital myopathy. Nat Genet 19:94–97, 1998.
155. Mayer U, Saher G, Fässler R, et al: Absence of integrin alpha7 causes a novel form of muscular dystrophy. Nat Genet 17:318–323, 1997.
156. Vachon P, Xu H, Liu L, et al: Integrins (alpha7 beta-1) in muscle function and survival. Disrupted expression in merosin-deficient congenital muscular dystrophy. J Clin Invest 100:1870–1881, 1997.
157. Williamson RA, Henry MD, Daniels KJ, et al: Dystroglycan is essential for early embryonic development: Disruption of Reichert's membrane in Dag1-null mice. Hum Mol Genet 6:831–841, 1997.
158. Cote PD, Moukhles H, Lindenbaum M, et al: Chimaeric mice deficient in dystroglycans develop muscular dystrophy and have disrupted myoneural synapses. Nat Genet 23:338–342, 1999.
159. Galbiati F, Volonte D, Chu JB, et al: Transgenic overexpression of caveolin-3 in skeletal muscle fibers induces a Duchenne like muscular dystrophy phenotype. Proc Natl Acad Sci USA 97:9689–9694, 2000.
160. Ohlendieck K, Matsumura K, Ionasescu VV, et al: Duchenne muscular dystrophy: Deficiency of dystrophin-associated proteins in the sarcolemma. Neurology 43:795–800, 1993.
161. Mizuno Y, Yoshida M, Nonaka I, et al: Expression of utrophin (dystrophin-related protein) and dystrophin-associated glycoproteins in muscles from patients with Duchenne muscular dystrophy. Muscle Nerve 17:206–216, 1994.
162. Tanaka H, Ishiguro T, Eguchi C, et al: Expression of a dystrophin-related protein associated with the skeletal muscle cell membrane. Histochemistry 96:1–5, 1991.
163. Arahata K, Ishihara T, Kamkura K: Mosaic expression of dystrophin in symptomatic carriers of Duchenne muscular dystrophy. N Engl J Med 320:138–142, 1989.
164. Hoffman EP, Fischbeck KH, Brown RH, et al: Characterization of dystrophin in muscle biopsy specimens from patients with Duchenne's or Becker's muscular dystrophy. N Engl J Med 318:1363–1368, 1988.
165. England SB, Nicholson LVB, Johnson MA, et al: Very mild muscular dystrophy associated with the deletion of 46% of dystrophin. Nature 343:180–182, 1990.
166. Passos-Bueno MR, Vainzof M, Marie SK, et al: Half the dystrophin gene is apparently enough for a mild clinical course: Confirmation of its potential use for gene therapy. Hum Mol Genet 3:919–922, 1994.
167. Morandi L, Mora M, Bernasconi P, et al: Very small dystrophin molecule in a family with a mild form of Becker dystrophy. Neuromuscul Disord 3:65–70, 1993.
168. Palmucci L, Doriguzzi C, Mongini T, et al: Unusual expression and very mild course of Xp21 muscular dystrophy (Becker type) in a 60-year-old man with 26 percent deletion of the dystrophin gene. Neurology 44:541–543, 1994.
169. Phelps SF, Hauser MA, Cole NM, et al: Expression of full-length and truncated dystrophin mini-genes in transgenic mdx mice. Hum Mol Genet 4:1251–1258, 1995.
170. Cox GA, Cole NM, Matsumara K, et al: Overexpression of dystrophin in transgenic mdx mice eliminates dystrophic symptoms without toxicity. Nature 364:725–729, 1993.
171. Tinsley J, Deconinck N, Fisher R, et al: Expression of full-length utrophin prevents muscular dystrophy in mdx mice. Nat Med 4:1441–1444, 1998.
172. Crawford GE, Faulkner JA, Crosbie RHCKP, et al: Assembly of the dystrophin-associated protein complex does not require the dystrophin COOH-terminal domain. J Cell Biol 150:1399–1410, 2000.
173. Cox GA, Sunada Y, Campbell KP, et al: Dp71 can restore the dystrophin-associated glycoprotein complex in muscle but fails to prevent dystrophy. Nat Genet 8:333–339, 1994.
174. Greenberg DS, Sunada Y, Campbell KP, et al: Exogenous Dp71 restores the levels of dystrophin associated proteins but does not alleviate muscle damage in mdx mice. Nat Genet 8:340–344, 1994.
175. Harper SQ, Hauser MA, DelloRusso C, et al: Modular flexibility of dystrophin: Implications for gene therapy of Duchenne muscular dystrophy. Nat Med 8:253–261, 2002.
176. Sakamoto M, Yuasa K, Yoshimura M, et al: Micro-dystrophin cDNA ameliorates dystrophic phenotypes when introduced into mdx mice as a transgene. Biochem Biophys Res Commun 293:1265–1272, 2002.
177. Tinsley JM, Potter AC, Phelps SR, et al: Amelioration of the dystrophic phenotype of mdx mice using a truncated utrophin transgene. Nature 384:349–353, 1996.
178. Rafael JA, Tinsley JM, Potter AC, et al: Skeletal muscle-specific expression of a utrophin transgene rescues utrophin-dystrophin deficient mice. Nat Genet 19:79–82, 1998.
179. Rafael JA, Sunada Y, Cole NM, et al: Prevention of dystrophic pathology in mdx mice by a truncated dystrophin isoform. Hum Mol Genet 3:1725–1733, 1994.
180. Duclos F, Straub V, Moore SA, et al: Progressive muscular dystrophy in alpha-sarcoglycan-deficient mice. J Cell Biol 142:1461–1471, 1998.
181. Araishi K, Sasaoka T, et al: Loss of the sarcoglycan complex and sarcospan leads to muscular dystrophy in beta-sarcoglycan-deficient mice. Hum Mol Genet 8:1589–1598, 1999.
182. Hack AA, Ly CT, Jiang F, et al: Gamma–sarcoglycan deficiency leads to muscle membrane defects and apoptosis independent of dystrophin. J Cell Biol 142:1279–1287, 1998.
183. Sasaoka T, Imamura M, Araishi K, et al: Pathological analysis of muscle hypertrophy and degeneration in muscular dystrophy in gamma-sarcoglycan-deficient mice. Neuromuscul Disord 13:193–206, 2003.
184. Coral-Vazquez R, Cohn RD, Moore SA, et al: Disruption of the sarcoglycan-sarcospan complex in vascular smooth muscle: A novel mechanism for cardiomyopathy and muscular dystrophy. Cell 98:465–474, 1999.
185. Okazaki Y, Okuizumi H, Ohsumi T, et al: A genetic linkage map of the Syrian hamster and localization of cardiomyopathy locus on chromosome 9qa2.1-b1 using RLGS spot-mapping. Nat Genet 13:87–90, 1996.
186. Nigro V, Okazaki Y, Belsito A, et al: Identification of the Syrian hamster cardiomyopathy gene. Hum Mol Genet 6:601–607, 1997.
187. Roberds SL, Anderson RD, Ibraghimov-Beskrovnaya O, et al: Primary structure and muscle-specific expression of the 50-kDa dystrophin-associated glycoprotein (adhalin). J Biol Chem 268:23739–23742, 1993.
188. Iwata Y, Nakamura H, Mizuno Y, et al: Defective association of dystrophin with sarcolemmal glycoproteins in the cardiomyopathic hamster. FEBS Lett 329:227–231, 1993.
189. Grady RM, Grange RW, Lau KS, et al: Role for alpha-dystrobrevin in the pathogenesis of dystrophin-dependent muscular dystrophies. Nat Cell Biol 1:215–220, 1999.
190. Lebakken CS, Venzke DP, Hrstka RF, et al: Sarcospan-deficient mice maintain normal muscle function. Mol Cell Biol 20:1669–1677, 2000.
191. Banwell BL, Russel J, Fukudome T, et al: Myopathy, myasthenic syndrome, and epidermolysis bullosa simplex due to plectin deficiency. J Neuropathol Exp Neurol 58:832–846, 1999.
192. Andra K, Lassmann H, et al: Targeted inactivation of plectin reveals essential function in maintaining the integrity of skin, muscle, and heart cytoarchitecture. Genes Dev 11:3143–3156, 1997.
193. Milner DJ, Weitzer G, Tran D, et al: Disruption of muscle architecture and myocardial degeneration in mice lacking desmin. J Cell Biol 134:1255–1270, 1996.
194. Li Z, Mericskay M, Agbulut O, et al: Desmin is essential for the tensile strength and integrity of myofibrils but not for myogenic commitment, differentiation, and fusion of skeletal muscle. J Cell Biol 139:129–144, 1997.
195. Goldfarb LG, Park KY, Cervenáková L, et al: Missense mutations in desmin associated with familial cardiac and skeletal myopathy. Nat Genet 19:402–403, 1998.

196. Munoz-Mármol AN, Strasser G, Isamat M, et al: A dysfunctional desmin mutation in a patient with severe generalized myopathy. *Proc Natl Acad Sci USA* 95:11312–11317, 1998.
197. De Bleecker JL, Engel AG, Ertl BB: Myofibrillar myopathy with abnormal foci of desmin positivity. II. Immunocytochemical analysis reveals accumulation of multiple other proteins. *J Neuropathol Exp Neurol* 55:563–577, 1996.
198. Fardeau M, Godet-Guillain J, Tome FMS, et al: Une nouvelle affection musculaire familiale, définie par l'accumulation inta-sarcoplasmique d'un matériel granulo-filamentaire dense en microscopie électronique. *Rev Neurol* 134:411–425, 1978.
199. Vicart P, Caron A, Guicheney P, et al: A missense mutation in the alphaB-crystallin chaperone gene causes a desmin-related myopathy. *Nat Genet* 20:92–95, 1998.
199a. Selcen D, Engel AG: Myofibrillar myopathy caused by novel dominant negative αB-crystallin mutations. *Ann Neurol* 54:804–810, 2003.
200. Takemitsu M, Ishiura S, Koga R, et al: Dystrophin-related protein in the fetal and denervated skeletal muscles of normal and *mdx* mice. *Biochem Biophys Res Commun* 180:1179–1186, 1991.
201. Hagiwara Y, Yoshida M, Nonaka I, et al: Developmental expression of dystrophin on the plasma membrane of rat muscle cells. *Protoplasma* 151:11–18, 1989.
202. Chiu AY, Sanes JR: Development of basal lamina in synaptic and extrasynaptic portions of embryonic rat muscle. *Dev Biol* 103:456–467, 1984.
203. Clerk A, Strong PN, Sewry CA: Characterisation of dystrophin during development of human skeletal muscle. *Development* 114:395–402, 1992.
204. Noguchi S, Wakabayashi E, Sasaoka T, et al: Analysis of the special, temporal and tissue-specific transcription of *gamma-sarcoglycan* gene using a transgeneic mouse. *FEBS Lett* 495:77–81, 2001.
205. Wakabayashi-Takai E, Noguchi S, Ozawa E: Identification of myogenesis-dependent transcriptional enhancers in promoter region of mouse gamma-sarcoglycan gene. *Eur J Biochem* 268:948–957, 2001.
206. Yang B, Jung D, Motto D, et al: SH3 domain-mediated interaction of dystroglycan and Grb2. *J Biol Chem* 270:11711–11714, 1995.
207. Russo K, Di Stasio E, Macchia G, et al: Characterization of the beta-dystroglycan-growth factor receptor 2 (Grb2) interaction. *Biochem Biophys Res Commun* 274:93–98, 2000.
208. Brenman JE, Chao DS, Xia H, et al: Nitric oxide synthase complexed with dystrophin and absent from skeletal muscle sarcolemma in Duchenne muscular dystrophy. *Cell* 82:743–752, 1995.
209. Song KS, Scherer PE, Tang Z, et al: Expression of caveolin-3 in skeletal, cardiac, and smooth muscle cells. Caveolin-3 is a component of the sarcolemma and co-fractionates with dystrophin and dystrophin-associated glycoproteins. *J Biol Chem* 271:15160–15165, 1996.
210. Senter L, Ceoldo S, Petrusa MM, et al: Phosphorylation of dystrophin: Effects on actin binding. *Biochem Biophys Res Commun* 206:57–63, 1995.
211. Madhavan R, Jarrett HW: Interactions between dystrophin glycoprotein complex proteins. *Biochemistry* 34:12204–12209, 1995.
212. Milner RE, Busaan JL, Holmes CF, et al: Phosphorylation of dystrophin. The carboxyl-terminal region of dystrophin is a substrate for in vitro phosphorylation by p34cdc2 kinase. *J Biol Chem* 268:21901–21905, 1993.
213. Shemanko CS, Sanghera JS, Milner RE, et al: Phosphorylation of the carboxyl terminal region of dystrophin by mitogen-activated protein (MAP) kinase. *Mol Cell Biochem* 152:63–70, 1995.
214. Luise M, Presotto C, Senter L, et al: Dystrophin is phosphorylated by endogenous protein kinases. *Biochem J* 293:243–247, 1993.
215. Ilsley JLSM, Winder SJ: The interaction of dystrophin with beta-dystroglycan is regulated by tyrosine phosphorylation. *Cell Signal* 13:625–632, 2001.
216. Sotgia F, Lee H, Bedford MT, et al: Tyrosine phosphorylation of beta-dystroglycan at its WW domain binding motif, PPxY, recruits SH2 domain containing proteins. *Biochemistry* 40:14585–14592, 2001.
217. James M, Nuttall A, Ilsley JL, et al: Adhesion-dependent tyrosine phosphorylation of beta-dystroglycan regulates its interaction with utrophin. *J Cell Sci* 113:1717–1726, 2000.
218. Betto R, Senter L, et al: Ecto-ATPase activity of alpha-sarcoglycan (adhalin). *J Biol Chem* 274:7907–7912, 1999.
219. Ueda H, Ueda K, Baba T, et al: Delta- and gamma-sarcoglycan localization in the sarcoplasmic reticulum of skeletal muscle. *J Histochem Cytochem* 49:529–538, 2001.
220. Newbell BJ, Anderson JT, Jarrett HW: Ca2+-calmodulin binding to mouse alpha 1 syntrophin: Syntrophin is also a Ca2+-binding protein. *Biochemistry* 36:1295–1305, 1997.
221. Madhavan R, Jarrett HW: Phosphorylation of dystrophin and alpha-syntrophin by Ca(2+)-calmodulin dependent protein kinase II. *Biochim Biophys Acta* 1434:260–274, 1999.
222. Oak SA, Jarrett HW: Oligomerization of mouse alpha1-syntrophin and self-association of its pleckstrin homology domain 1 containing sequences. *Biochemistry* 39:8870–8877, 2000.
223. Kameye S, Miyagoe Y, Nonaka I, et al: Alpha1-syntrophin gene disruption results in the absence of neuronal-type nitric-oxide synthase at the sarcolemma but does not induce muscle degeneration. *J Biol Chem* 274:2193–2200, 1999.
224. Hosaka Y, Yokota T, Miyagoe-Suzuki Y, et al: Alpha1-syntrophin-deficient skeletal muscle exhibits hypertrophy and aberrant formation of muscular junctions during regeneration. *J Cell Biol* 158:1097–1107, 2002.
225. Bredt DS: Endogenous nitric oxide synthesis: Biological functions and pathophysiology. *Free Radic Res* 31:577–596, 1999.
226. Rando TA: Role of nitric oxide in the pathogenesis of muscular dystrophies: A "two hit" hypothesis of the cause of muscle necrosis. *Microsc Res Tech* 55:223–235, 2001.
227. Thomas GD, Sander M, Lau KS, et al: Impaired metabolic modulation of alpha-adrenergic vasoconstriction in dystrophin-deficient skeletal muscle. *Proc Natl Acad Sci USA* 95:15090–15095, 1998.
228. Anderson JE: A role for nitric oxide in muscle repair: Nitric oxide–mediated activation of muscle satellite cells. *Mol Biol Cell* 11:1859–1874, 2000.
229. Chang WJ, Iannaccone ST, Lau KS, et al: Neuronal nitric oxide synthase and dystrophin-deficient muscular dystrophy. *Proc Natl Acad Sci USA* 93:9142–9147, 1996.
230. Bredt DS: Targeting nitric oxide to its targets. *Proc Soc Exp Biol Med* 211:41–48, 1996.
231. Crosbie RH, Straub V, Yun HY, et al: *mdx* muscle pathology is independent of nNOS perturbation. *Hum Mol Genet* 7:823–829, 1998.
232. Wehling M, Spencer MJ, Tidball JG: A nitric oxide synthase transgene ameliorates muscular dystrophy in *mdx* mice. *J Cell Biol* 155:123–132, 2001.
233. Thomas GD, Victor RG: Nitric oxide mediates contraction-induced attenuation of sympathetic vasoconstriction in rat skeletal muscle. *J Physiol (Lond)* 506:817–826, 1998.
234. Sander M, Chavoshan B, Harris SA, et al: Functional muscle ischemia in neuronal nitric oxide synthase-deficient skeletal muscle of children with Duchenne muscular dystrophy. *Proc Natl Acad Sci USA* 97:13818–13823, 2000.
235. Minetti C, Sotgia F, Bruno C, et al: Mutations in the caveolin-3 gene cause autosomal dominant limb-girdle muscular dystrophy. *Nat Genet* 18:365–368, 1998.
236. Hagiwara Y, Sasaoka T, Araishi K, et al: Caveolin-3 deficiency causes muscle degeneration in mice. *Hum Mol Genet* 9:3047–3054, 2000.
237. Galbiati F, Engelman JA, Volone D, et al: Caveolin-3 null mice show a loss of caveolae, changes in the microdomain distribution of the dystrophin-glycoprotein complex, and T-tubule abnormalities. *J Biol Chem* 276:21425–21433, 2001.
238. Matsuda C, Hayashi YK, Ogawa M, et al: The sarcolemmal proteins dysferlin and caveolin-3 interact in skeletal muscle. *Hum Mol Genet* 10:1761–1766, 2001.

Chapter 20
The Extracellular Matrix

JOSHUA R. SANES

Structure
   MORPHOLOGY
   COMPONENTS
   SPECIALIZED REGIONS
   DEVELOPING MUSCLE
   CULTURED MUSCLE

Roles in Muscle Maintenance and Function
   MECHANICAL STRENGTH
   MUSCLE MAINTENANCE
   MYOGENESIS
   MUSCLE REGENERATION

Roles at the Neuromuscular Junction
   NEUROMUSCULAR TRANSMISSION
   SYNAPTIC ADHESION
   REINNERVATION
   PRESYNAPTIC DIFFERENTIATION
   POSTSYNAPTIC DIFFERENTIATION

Pathology

Muscle fibers, like many other cells, are embedded in a protein- and carbohydrate-rich *extracellular matrix* (ECM).* This acellular material, along with a variety of nonmuscle cells, forms the *connective tissue* of skeletal muscle. Components of the extracellular matrix contribute to the mechanical properties of muscle, promote myogenesis, and organize muscle regeneration. One particular structure, the *basal lamina* (BL), is also involved in synaptic interactions at the neuromuscular junction. This chapter reviews the morphology, molecular architecture, functions, and pathology of the ECM of skeletal muscle, with particular emphasis on the BL.

*A list of abbreviations used in this chapter is given at the end of the chapter.

motor and sympathetic nerve branches, fibroblasts, macrophages (histiocytes), and a network of extracellular fibrils. The BL is the endomysial component that lies closest to the muscle fiber surface.

Peripheral nerves also bear connective tissue sheaths, whose structures parallel those of muscle. Individual Schwann cells and the axon or axons they wrap are surrounded by an *endoneurial* BL. Fascicles of axon-Schwann cell units, along with fibroblasts and capillaries, are covered by a *perineurium*, consisting of multiple layers of fibroblast-like cells that assemble a multilamellar BL.[2] Multiple perineurial bundles are then collected by a coarse, fibrous *epineurium*. The endoneurium and the perineurium but not the epineurium extend into the intramuscular course of motor nerves (Fig. 20-2). The perineurium is relatively impermeable and contributes to the "blood-nerve barrier" that protects axons from the environment.[3]

Although we now know that BLs are present in nearly all tissues, their existence was first appreciated in muscle. In 1840, using unstained muscle, Bowman[4] discovered that a delicate, nearly transparent tube surrounds each muscle fiber. This sheath, which he called the *sarcolemma*, was revealed because it survived injuries that caused the muscle cell proper to break and retract (Fig. 20-3). Subsequent light microscopic studies of sectioned and stained muscle revealed three components of the sarcolemma: (1) reticular *fibrils*, composed of small bundles of collagen fibers that stain with silver and follow a roughly spiral course around the muscle fiber[5]; (2) a continuous, amorphous layer of *basement membrane* that stains with the periodic acid–Schiff reagent[6]; and (3) the *plasma membrane*. With the introduction of electron microscopy, it became clear that the basement membrane consists of two discrete layers that had not been resolved by the light microscope: a felt-like BL and a *reticular lamina* of collagen and other fibrils embedded in an amorphous *ground substance*.[7] Further ultrastructural studies, using a variety of electron-dense stains, revealed subdivisions within the BL itself, most notably a 10- to 15-nm-thick *lamina densa* that is separated from the plasma membrane by

Structure

MORPHOLOGY

The connective tissue of muscle is organized into three discrete but interconnected sheaths[1] (Fig. 20-1). A collagenous *epimysium* surrounds each whole muscle. Smaller bundles of coarse collagen fibers extend inward from the epimysium to form the *perimysium*, a system of septa that group muscle fibers into bundles or fascicles. Nerve branches, blood vessels, muscle spindles, and fat cells lie within the perimysium (Fig. 20-2). Finally, individual muscle fibers are invested with a sheath of *endomysium*. The endomysium contains a variety of structures and cells, including capillaries, fine

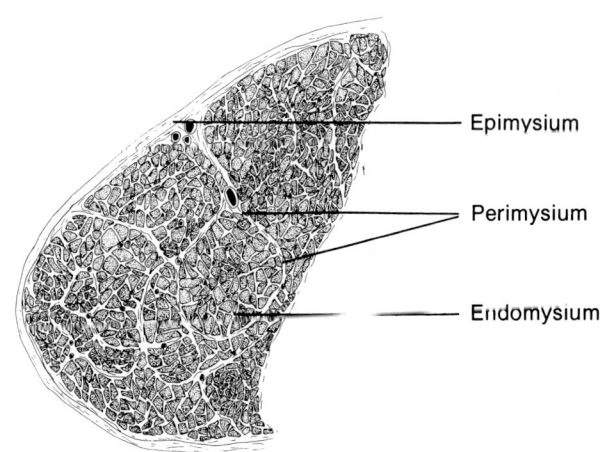

FIGURE 20-1. Sketch of a cross-sectioned whole muscle showing the arrangement of its epimysial, perimysial, and endomysial connective tissue sheaths. (*From Ham AW, Cormack DH: Histology, 8th ed. Philadelphia: Lippinott, 1979, p 54. With permission.*)

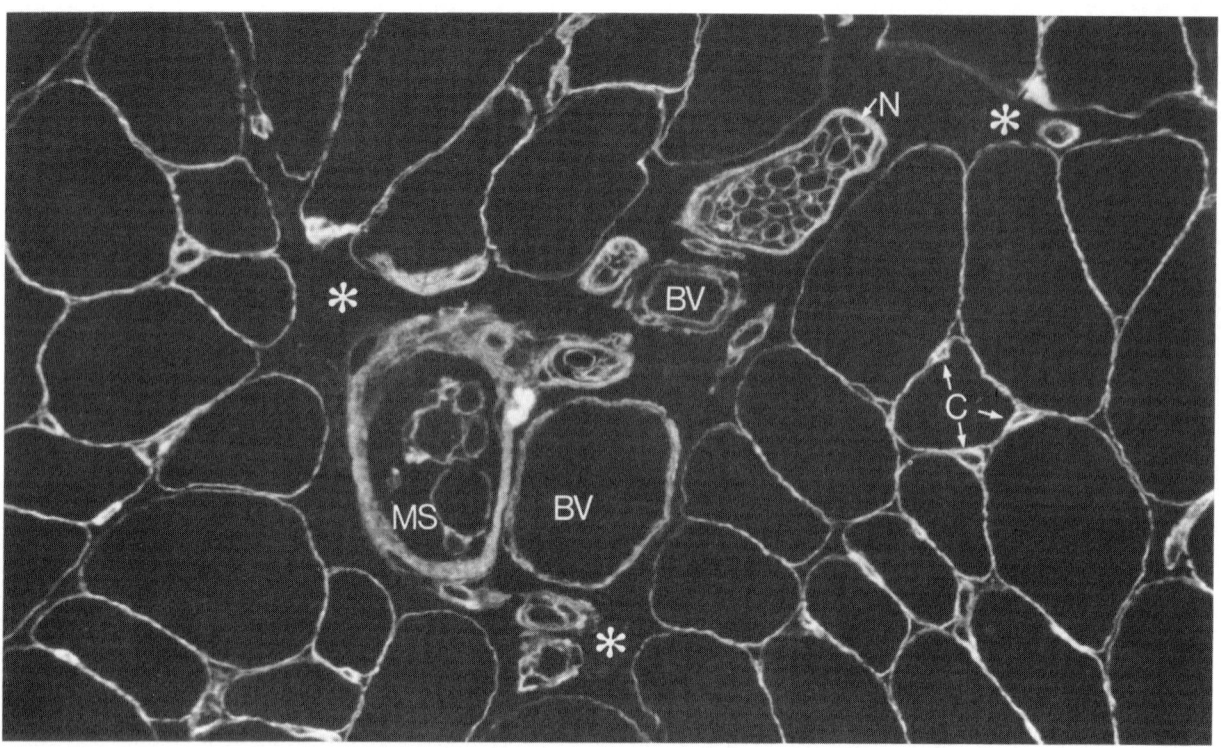

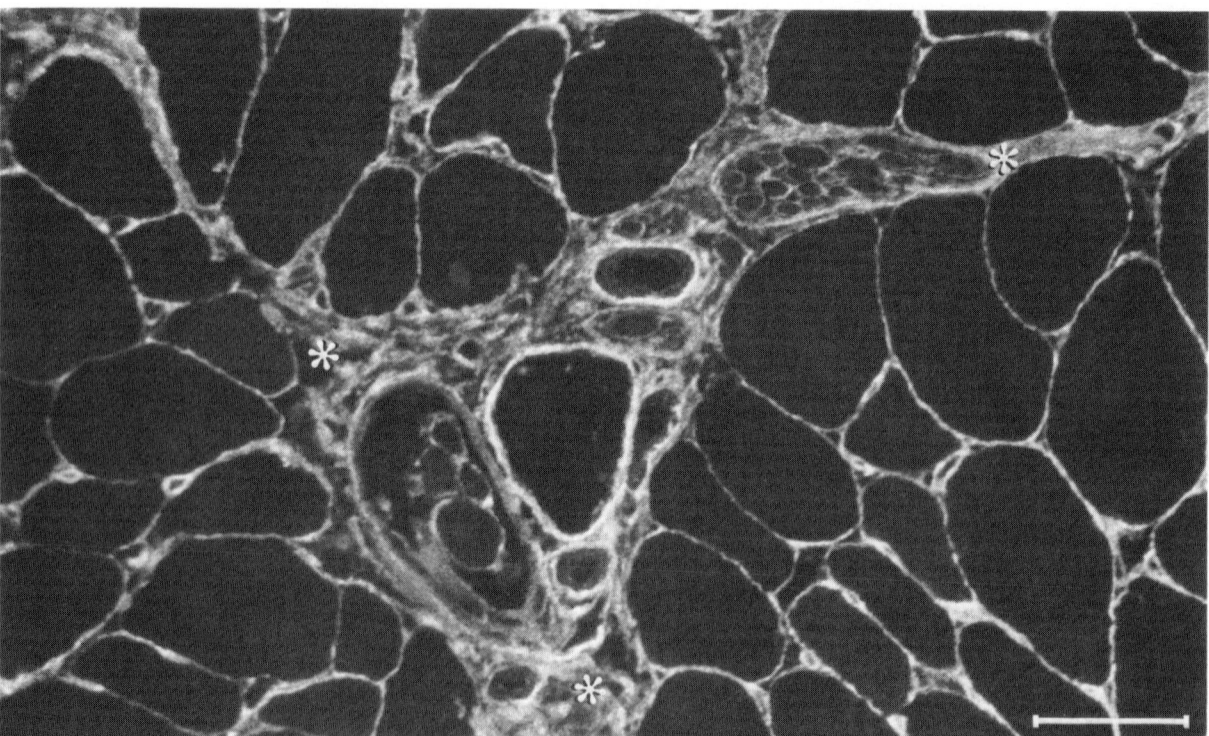

FIGURE 20-2. Cross sections of rat skeletal muscle stained with antibody to laminin (top) or to a collagen (bottom). Both antibodies bind to muscle fiber surfaces and capillaries (C) in the endomysium as well as to the surfaces of structures in the perimysium (asterisk), including intramuscular nerves (N), blood vessels (BV), and muscle spindle (MS) fibers and capsules. Collagen but not laminin is present in the loose connective tissue of the perimysium. Bar is 50 μm.

Chapter 20. The Extracellular Matrix

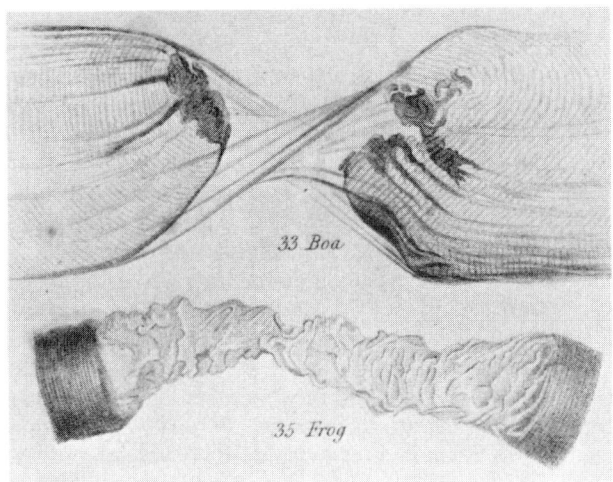

FIGURE 20-3. Bowman's drawings of the sarcolemma of snake and frog muscle fibers as revealed by damage to and retraction of the muscle cell cytoplasm (*From Bowman W: On the minute structure and movements of voluntary muscle. Philos Trans R Soc Lond (Biol)130:457, 1840.*)

a 2- to 5-nm-thick relatively electron-lucent layer, the *lamina rara*[8] (Fig. 20-4). Coating the muscle fiber's plasma membrane and continuous with the lamina rara is a *glycocalyx*, which includes the external domains of integral membrane proteins as well as molecules more loosely adherent to the cell surface. Immunohistochemical studies have now begun to show how individual molecules are arranged within these ultrastructurally defined laminae (Fig. 20-5).

COMPONENTS

For many years, molecular analysis of the ECM lagged behind comparable studies of cytosolic and membrane-bound molecules. In large part this was because extracellular materials in general and BLs in particular are extensively and covalently cross-linked; they are, therefore, insoluble and not susceptible to analysis by conventional biochemical tech-

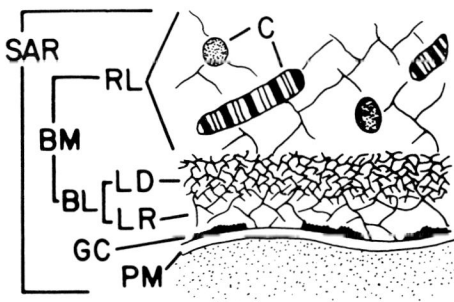

FIGURE 20-4. The surface, or sarcolemma (SAR), of a muscle fiber; drawing from electron micrographs, such as those in Fig. 20-5. Cytoplasm of the muscle cell is surrounded by layers of plasma membrane (PM), glycocalyx (GC), basal lamina (BL), and reticular lamina (RL). RL contains collagen (C) and other fibrils. BL comprises a feltlike lamina densa (LD) and a relatively electron-lucent lamina rara (LR). BL and RL together compose basement membrane (BM).

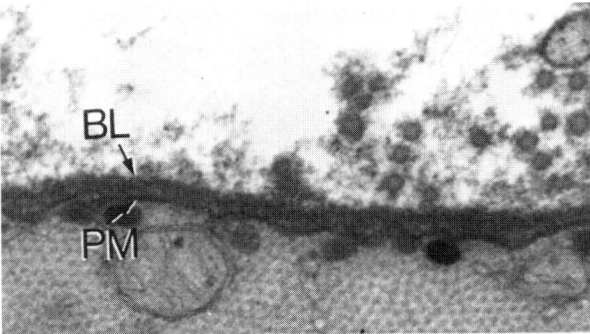
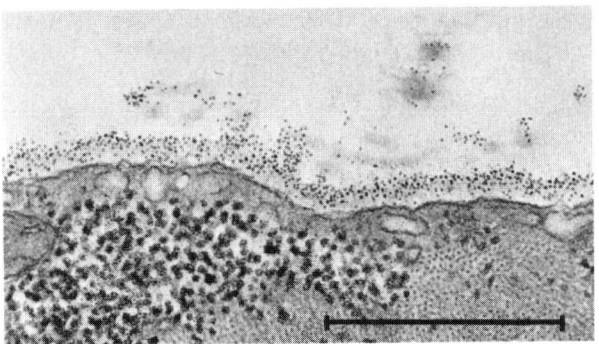

FIGURE 20-5. Muscle fiber basement membrane stained nonselectively with tannic acid (top) or with rabbit antilaminin and ferritin-conjugated goat antirabbit antibody (bottom). PM=plasma membrane, BL=basal lamina. Laminin is concentrated in the BL. Bar is 0.5 μm. (*From Sanes JR: Laminin, fibronectin, and collagen in synaptic and extrasynaptic portions of muscle fiber basement membrane. J Cell Biol 93:442, 1982. With permission.*)

niques, such as chromatography or electrophoresis. Eventually, however, immunohistochemical and molecular genetic methods provided means of circumventing these obstacles, and most major components of the ECM have now been identified. Because most of these components are broadly distributed, a summary of the composition of ECM in general precedes a description of features unique to skeletal muscle.

Major Components of the Extracellular Matrix

ECMs contain protein and carbohydrate but no detectable lipid or nucleic acid. Virtually all the protein is glycosylated, and nearly all the carbohydrate is covalently bound to protein. The three most prevalent classes of molecules in ECMs are *collagens*, *noncollagenous glycoproteins*, and *proteoglycans* (reviewed in Refs. 9 to 16).

The collagens[11] are a large family of proteins distinguished by the presence of triple-helical segments with unusually high contents of glycine, and proline, often in a characteristic repeated "gly-pro-x" sequence. Most collagens also contain the unusual amino acid hydroxyproline. Their triple-helical portions are susceptible to collagenase, a bacterial protease, which spares most proteins, and are resistant to proteolysis by enzymes such as pepsin, which are otherwise fairly indiscriminate. Over 30 proteins that share these features have been enumerated (collagen types I, II, and so on). Several other proteins, including one form of acetylcholinesterase (AChE) (see below), have collagenous sequences or subunits; they are not numbered only because they were initially described in other contexts. Large striated fibers of collagen are usually made of type I collagen, whereas smaller fibrils may contain types II, III, V, or XI, depending on the tissue. Collagens IX, XII, XIV, XVI, and XIX are not themselves fibrillar but are usually associated with fibrils. Collagen IV, described below, is a major component of all BLs.

Many of the noncollagenous glycoproteins that have been isolated so far serve to link cells to the ECM. Well-studied members of this class include fibronectin, the laminins, entactin/nidogen, vitronectin, the thrombospondins, and the tenascins.[12–14] Some, like laminins and entactin, are largely restricted to BLs; others, like tenascins, are present in fibrillar matrix; and still others, like fibronectin and vitronectin, are present both in soluble and matrix-associated forms. Most of these molecules are unusually large. For example, tenascin C is a hexamer of subunits, each of which is >200 kDa. Given their size, it is unsurprising that these glycoproteins contain multiple binding sites for other matrix molecules and for cell surface receptors. For example, laminins and fibronectin bear discrete binding sites for collagen and glycosaminoglycans and also have multiple distinct sites recognized by matrix receptors on cell membranes. What has been surprising is that many of these sites can be mapped to small, discrete domains in the molecule, some as small as three to six amino acids in length. For example, integrins on cell membranes (see Chap. 19) recognize the amino acid sequence arginine-glycine-aspartate in several matrix molecules, including fibronectin, thrombospondin, and some laminins. The current view is that the noncollagenous glycoproteins of the extracellular matrix are assemblies of remarkably independent binding sites, which are repeated, strung together, and separated by other sequences to form large, elongated proteins that are well suited to cross-link cells and matrix and to interact with different cells in different ways.

Proteoglycans are defined by the unique oligosaccharides, called *glycosaminoglycans*, that they bear.[15,16] Glycosaminoglycans are long, unbranched polymers of disaccharide units. Each glycosaminoglycan is defined by the sugars of its disaccharide, one of which is hexosamine and the other a carboxyl or sulfate ester. Abundant glycosaminoglycans include hyaluronic acid, chondroitin sulfate, and heparan sulfate. All glycosaminoglycans in tissue with the possible exception of hyaluronic acid are linked to a core protein to form proteoglycans. Distinct proteoglycans are associated with laminins in BL (see below) and with collagen fibrils in the ground substance; still others are membrane-bound. Molecular cloning has revealed a great diversity in the core proteins that bear glycosaminoglycans; single types of glycosaminoglycans can decorate radically different proteins and individual proteins can bear a variety of types of glycosaminoglycan.

Basal Lamina

Like other structures within the ECM, the BL is composed of collagen, noncollagenous glycoproteins, and proteoglycans.[9,10] The most abundant protein of the BL is collagen IV, a triple-helical collagen whose subunits, called α chains, have prominent terminal noncollagenous domains.[11] The major noncollagenous protein, and the best characterized, is laminin, which is also a heterotrimer of related chains, in this case called α, β, and γ.[12] Both collagens IV and laminins exist in multiple isoforms: there are six collagen IV alpha chains (α_1 to α_6), each encoded by a distinct gene, and laminins are assembled from products of 5α, 4β, and 3γ genes. All basal laminae contain at least one collagen IV trimer and one laminin trimer.[17–19] The most abundant proteoglycan in most BLs is perlecan.[16]

The basic structure of BLs appears to involve distinct networks of collagens IV and laminin, each of which is capable of self-assembly.[10,12] The collagen network becomes cemented by covalent cross-links, and the two separate networks are linked to each other by entactin/nidogen, another noncollagenous glycoprotein.[10] These core components bear a multitude of recognition sites that bind other BL components (including proteoglycans), anchor reticular lamina components (such as collagen VI) to the BL, and serve as ligands for membrane-associated receptors. Among the transmembrane receptors are the integrins and dystroglycans, both of which have cytoplasmic domains that link to components of the cytoskeleton (see Chap. 19). Thus, one can envision a complex series of direct linkages that together span the distance from reticular lamina to BL to plasma membrane to cytoskeleton.

Extracellular Matrix of Muscle

The most thorough analyses of muscle ECM have been immunohistochemical and have used antibodies to molecules prepared from nonmuscle sources.[20–38] Light and electron microscopic methods show that laminin, fibronectin, entactin, perlecan, and collagen I, III, IV, V, VI, and XV are all associated with the muscle fiber surface. Collagens V and VI are concentrated external to the BL; thus, though closely associated with BL, they may not be bona fide components of its lamina densa. Fibronectin is present in both BL and reticular lamina. Collagens I and III have not been localized ultrastructurally but are likely to be in the reticular lamina, perhaps in fibrils. Laminin and collagen IV are present in the lamina densa of the BL, the most abundant trimers being collagen $[\alpha1\ (IV)]_2 [\alpha2(IV)]_1$, and laminin $\alpha2\beta1\gamma1$ (also called laminin 2).

Carbohydrates as well as proteins are prominent constituents of extracellular matrices, and muscle fiber basement membrane binds carbohydrate-selective dyes such as alcian blue, the periodic acid–Schiff reagent, and ruthenium red.[6] Direct sequencing of the carbohydrates remains a formidable technical problem; the most frequently used method for obtaining structural information remains staining with lectins or monoclonal antibodies. Lectins are proteins that bind tightly and specifically to saccharide groups; dozens of lectins have been isolated, each with its own sugar specificity. Fluorescent conjugates of many lectins, including ones that bind to mannose, N-acetylglucosamine, sialic acid, and galactose, all stain rat muscle fiber basement membrane[39,40]; thus, carbohydrates that contain or resemble these sugars are associated with the basement membrane, presumably as sugar moieties of glycoproteins. In addition, antibodies to heparan sulfate and chondroitin glycosaminoglycans stain muscle basement membrane[24,26,40]; these sugars are presumably associated with proteoglycans.

A few molecules have been localized in the perimysium and epimysium.[20,21,37,38] Fibronectin is present in both of these sheaths, as are collagens V and VI. Collagen I is concentrated in the epimysium and collagen III in the perimysium; both these molecules are present at higher concentrations in epi- and perimysium than in endomysium. Laminin and collagen IV are present in the BLs of structures embedded in the perimysium, such as nerves and blood vessels, but are absent from perimysium and epimysium themselves (Fig. 20-2).

Finally, muscle ECM contains four groups of molecules that are not generally thought of as matrix components:

1. The neural cell adhesion molecule, N-CAM, is normally tightly associated with plasma membranes but is sometimes found in BLs, perhaps anchored to heparan sulfate proteoglycans by a specific binding site.[41]
2. Several polypeptide growth factors, originally thought to act in soluble form, are actually matrix-associated in vivo. Some, like fibroblast growth factor (FGF), are associated with the endomysium of embryonic and adult muscle.[42] FGF acts in concert with heparan sulfate proteoglycan sugars and protein and is likely to be bound to them.[43,44]
3. Several proteases are suspected to be involved in remodeling ECM, and some of these have endogenous inhibitors, which may regulate the remodeling. Components of this system are associated with ECM in skeletal muscle.[45,46]
4. Endogenous lectins are thought to mediate cell-cell and cell-matrix interactions in several tissues. Some lectins, including members of the galectin family, are associated with muscle matrix.[47,48]

Together, these observations suggest that "intrinsic" components of matrix not only interact with each other and with cells but also provide binding sites for other bioactive molecules that otherwise occur in soluble or membrane-bound forms.

SPECIALIZED REGIONS

Neuromuscular Junction

The ECM is structurally and functionally specialized in areas where nerves abut muscle fibers. The BL but not the reticular lamina passes between nerve and muscle membranes at the neuromuscular junction and extends into the junctional folds that invaginate the postsynaptic membrane (Fig. 20-6). The BL thus constitutes a sizable fraction of the synaptic cleft material of the neuromuscular junction. The Schwann cell that caps the nerve terminals is also coated with BL; muscle and Schwann cell BLs fuse at the terminal's edge. Although synaptic and extrasynaptic BLs are ultrastructurally similar, they are molecularly distinct.[49,50]

Several molecules have now been described that are concentrated in synaptic BL (Fig. 20-7). These include site-restricted laminin and collagen IV variants, proteoglycans, and growth factors held in place by interactions with proteoglycans. Individual components of synaptic BL are discussed below, in conjunction with specific functions that have been attributed to them. Some other components, such as the collagen IV α_1 and α_2 chains, are excluded from synaptic sites and could, in principle, also contribute to synapse-specific properties. A third class of components, including entactin and perlecan, is present both synaptically and extrasynaptically.[21,34,50]

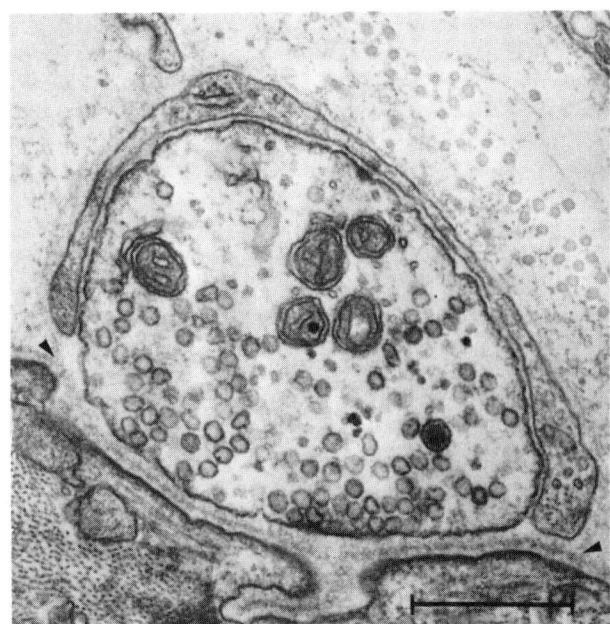

FIGURE 20-6. Frog neuromuscular junction. The nerve terminal, capped by a Schwann cell process, is separated from the muscle fiber by a 50-nm-wide synaptic cleft. Synpatic vesicles in the terminal cluster at an active zone that lies opposite the mouth of a junctional fold in the muscle fiber surface. BL ensheaths muscle fiber and Schwann cell, passes through the synaptic cleft, and extends into junctional folds. Muscle and Schwann cell BL fuse at terminal's edge (arrowheads). Reticular lamina, rich in collagen fibrils, lies outside the BL but does not extend into the synaptic cleft. Bar is 0.5 μm.

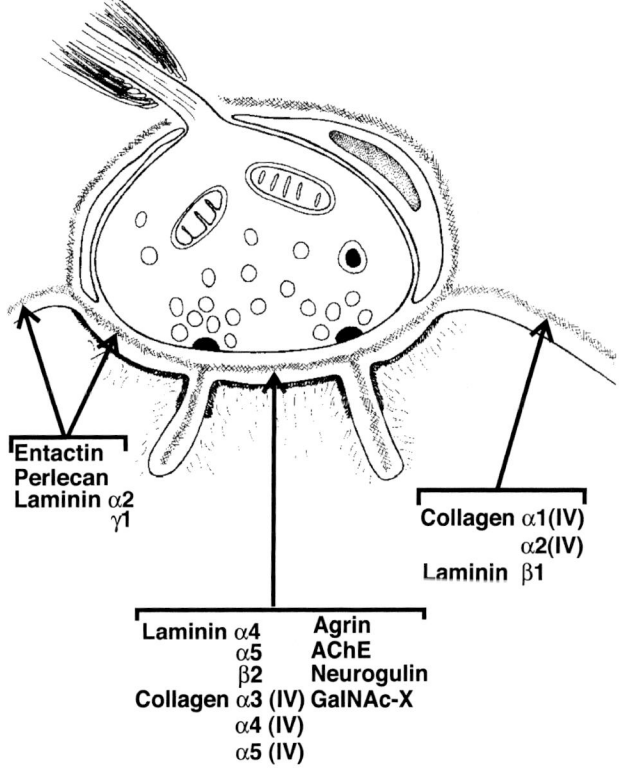

FIGURE 20-7. Molecules concentrated in adult synaptic BL, more abundant in extrasynaptic than synaptic BL, or present throughout adult muscle fiber BL.

Lectins specific for β-N-acetylgalactosamine (GalNAc)-terminated glycoconjugates selectively stain synaptic sites on muscle fibers from many vertebrate species, including humans.[40,51] Several lectins that recognize other sugars stain the muscle fiber surface uniformly. These results argue that β-GalNAc-terminated glycoconjugates rather than carbohydrates in general are selectively associated with the neuromuscular junction. At least some of the lectin-binding material is associated with synaptic BL (Fig. 20-8), and one of the molecules that bears the sugar is the collagen-tailed form of AChE (see Chap. 18), itself selectively associated with synaptic BL (see below). However, other synapse-specific molecules, including both glycoproteins and glycolipids, also appear to bear β-GalNAc terminal sugars,[37,52,53] raising the possibility that β-GalNAc plays some general role in synaptic targeting or differentiation.

Finally, several components of the endomysium have a peculiar distribution that does not correspond to any obvious structure: they are concentrated in areas surrounding synaptic sites.[54–60] Such molecules include thrombospondin 4 and tenascin C. For several, the perisynaptic distribution is most apparent after denervation, apparently because they are produced in part by a population of synapse-associated fibroblasts that proliferate following nerve injury. This distribution and regulation, along with the ability of these molecules to promote axon outgrowth, has suggested that they may be involved in guiding axons to the original synaptic sites that they preferentially innervate (see below).

Myotendinous Junctions

At the myotendinous junction, the surface of the muscle fiber is thrown into elaborate invaginations into which BL and collagen fibrils extend.[61] The BL is thickened in the invaginations and is attached to the plasma membrane by periodically arrayed microfibrils. These fibrils and the increased area of membrane-matrix apposition provided by the invaginations are undoubtedly adaptations for the transmission of force from muscle to tendon. Some molecular differences have been noted between the BL at the myotendinous junction and that coating adjoining regions of the sarcolemma, including high levels of laminin β_2,[34,62,63] but the functional significance of these differences is unknown. Tenascin C is also highly concentrated at the myotendinous junction; indeed, it was originally isolated as a "myotendinous antigen."[64]

DEVELOPING MUSCLE

Several studies have described the development of muscle BL, with emphasis on the appearance of specialized synaptic features. Myoblasts and newly formed myotubes bear little BL. BL then appears in a patchy distribution, with synaptic sites among the first regions to acquire a BL coating (Fig. 20-9). Thus, axons contact myotubes and form synapses before much BL accumulates,[65] but soon thereafter the entire myotube surface acquires a BL coat. Soon after synapses begin to form, laminin β2 and AChE appear at synaptic sites, but laminin β2 is detectable before AChE. Laminin β1 becomes excluded from these sites at a still later stage. A third pattern is observed for the laminin chains α4 and α5 and agrin: these moieties are broadly distributed in embryos and become restricted to synaptic site perinatally, as the muscle matures. Thus, the synaptic BL is not assembled as a unit; rather, components are added, lost, or modified as synaptogenesis proceeds.[31,34,66]

Although each muscle fiber is covered by its own BL in adulthood, there is a transient stage in which several myotubes lie together in a cluster ensheathed by a single BL (Fig. 20-10). The cluster comprises an early-born primary

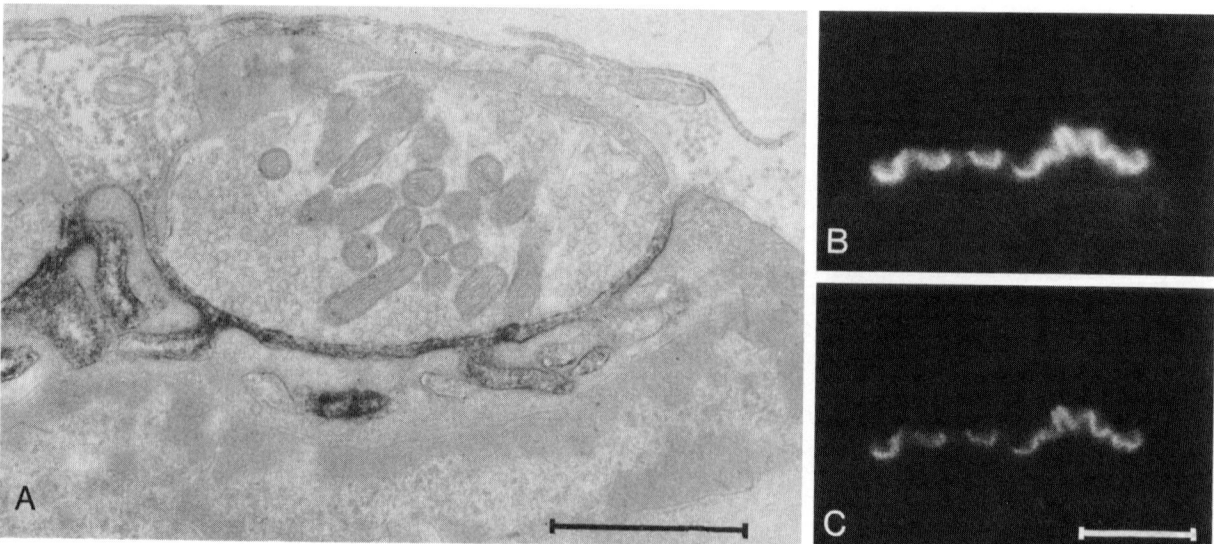

FIGURE 20-8. Immunohistochemical demonstration of a synapse-specific component of muscle fiber BL. *A.* Electron micrograph of a neuromuscular junction from a muscle incubated with a monoclonal antibody to laminin-β_2 (C1) and peroxidase-conjugated second antibody, then fixed and stained for peroxidase. Reaction product is confined to the synaptic cleft and junction folds. *B* and *C.* Light micrographs of cross-sectioned muscle incubated with anti-C1, fluorescein second antibody, and rhodamine bungarotoxin, then photographed with fluorescein optics to show antibody (*B*) or with rhodamine optics to show bungarotoxin and thus synaptic sites. Antibody stains synaptic but not extrasynaptic regions of the muscle fiber surface. Bar is 1 μm in *A*, 10 μm in *C*.

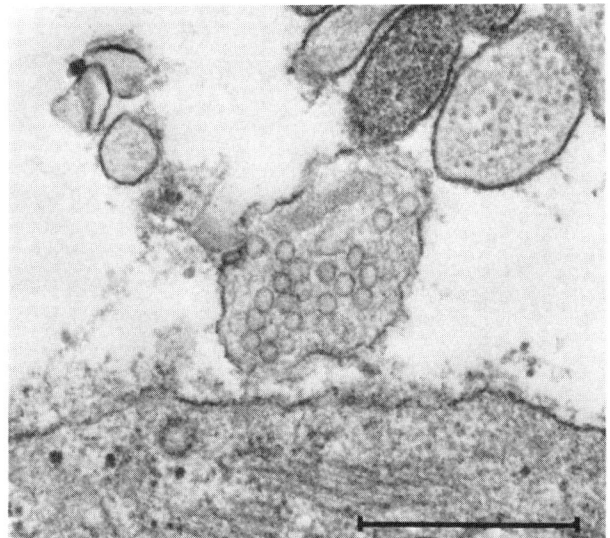

FIGURE 20-9. Neuromuscular junction from a 17-day rat embryo. BL is present in the synaptic cleft and elsewhere on the myotube surface but does not yet form a continuous sheath. Bar is 0.5 μm.

myotube plus one or a few secondary myotubes, which form along the surface of the primary myotube (see Chap. 2). Subsequently (perinatally in rodents), the myotubes in a cluster separate, and each acquires its own BL.

CULTURED MUSCLE

Myotubes grown in culture from embryonic muscle or from cell lines assemble an ECM that includes a BL and a network of extracellular fibrils. These cultures accumulate members of all three categories of ECM molecule: collagen types I, III, IV, and V as well as collagen-tailed AChE, noncollagenous glycoproteins such as fibronectin and laminin, and heparan sulfate proteoglycans including agrin, as well as chondroitin sulfate proteoglycans and hyaluronic acid[67-71] (see Ref. 72 for review of older literature).

Several antigens that are shared by synaptic and extrasynaptic BL in vivo are present throughout the myotube BL, whereas "synaptic" BL antigens—including laminin β2, agrin, and AChE—are concentrated in small patches, many of which coincide with regions of high AChR density. Collagen V and fibronectin, associated with reticular lamina in vivo, are found in reticular fibrils in the cultures. Thus, in the absence of nerves, cultured muscle can form an elaborate ECM and arrange its components in a way that reflects their distribution in vivo (Fig. 20-11).

How might nerves contribute to the matrix? One way is by producing matrix molecules such as agrin (discussed below). Another is by regulating muscle metabolism. Two means by which nerves can influence muscle are by evoking muscle activity and by releasing soluble factors. Both these mechanisms can be studied in vitro: activity by comparing spontaneously active with toxin or anesthetic-paralyzed myotubes, soluble factors by supplementing the medium with neural extracts. Results of such experiments show that activity selectively stimulates accumulation of shared antigens and that neural extracts, including agrin, enhance accumulation of synaptic antigens. These results suggest that nerves regulate BL by both activity-dependent and activity-independent mechanisms.[70]

Roles in Muscle Maintenance and Function

Until about 20 years ago, the ECM was viewed largely as an unspecialized, inert supporting material that filled the space between cells. It is now apparent, however, that ECM subserves many and diverse functions in cellular physiology and development. Several roles of the ECM have been demonstrated in skeletal muscle, and others have been suggested.

MECHANICAL STRENGTH

As the body's motor, muscle must be strong, flexible, and stress-resistant. ECM contributes to these mechanical characteristics in many ways and accounts to some extent for the tensile strength of muscle, the distribution of force within muscle, and the transmission of force from muscle to tendon.[73-76] Formal models of these mechanical properties include contractile, series-elastic, and parallel-elastic elements; this reflects the observation that some of the elasticity that muscle displays when it is stretched acts as if it were in parallel with the contractile apparatus and some in series. The contractile element is, of course, the sarcomere (see Chap. 7). The collagen bundles of the perimysium and possibly also of the endomysium constitute a major fraction of the parallel-elastic element. About half of the series-elastic

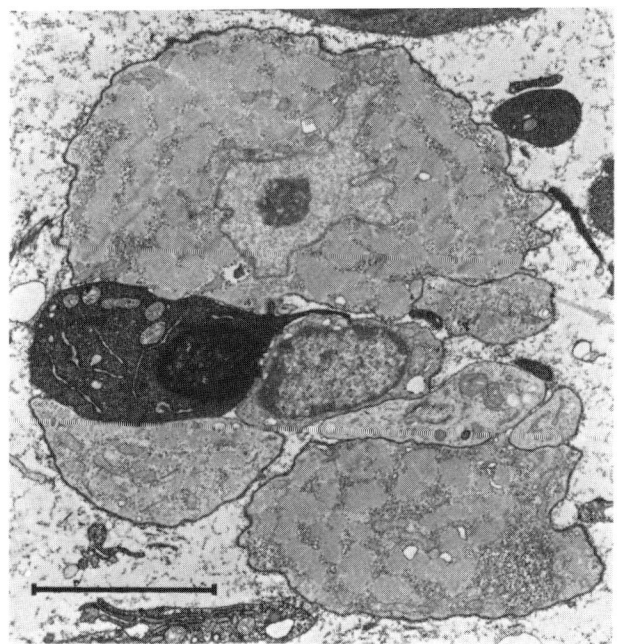

FIGURE 20-10. Developing myotube from a 19-day rat embryo. Several cells share a single BL sheath, which has been stained here with tannic acid. Compare with adult fiber in Fig. 20-12a. Bar is 5 μm.

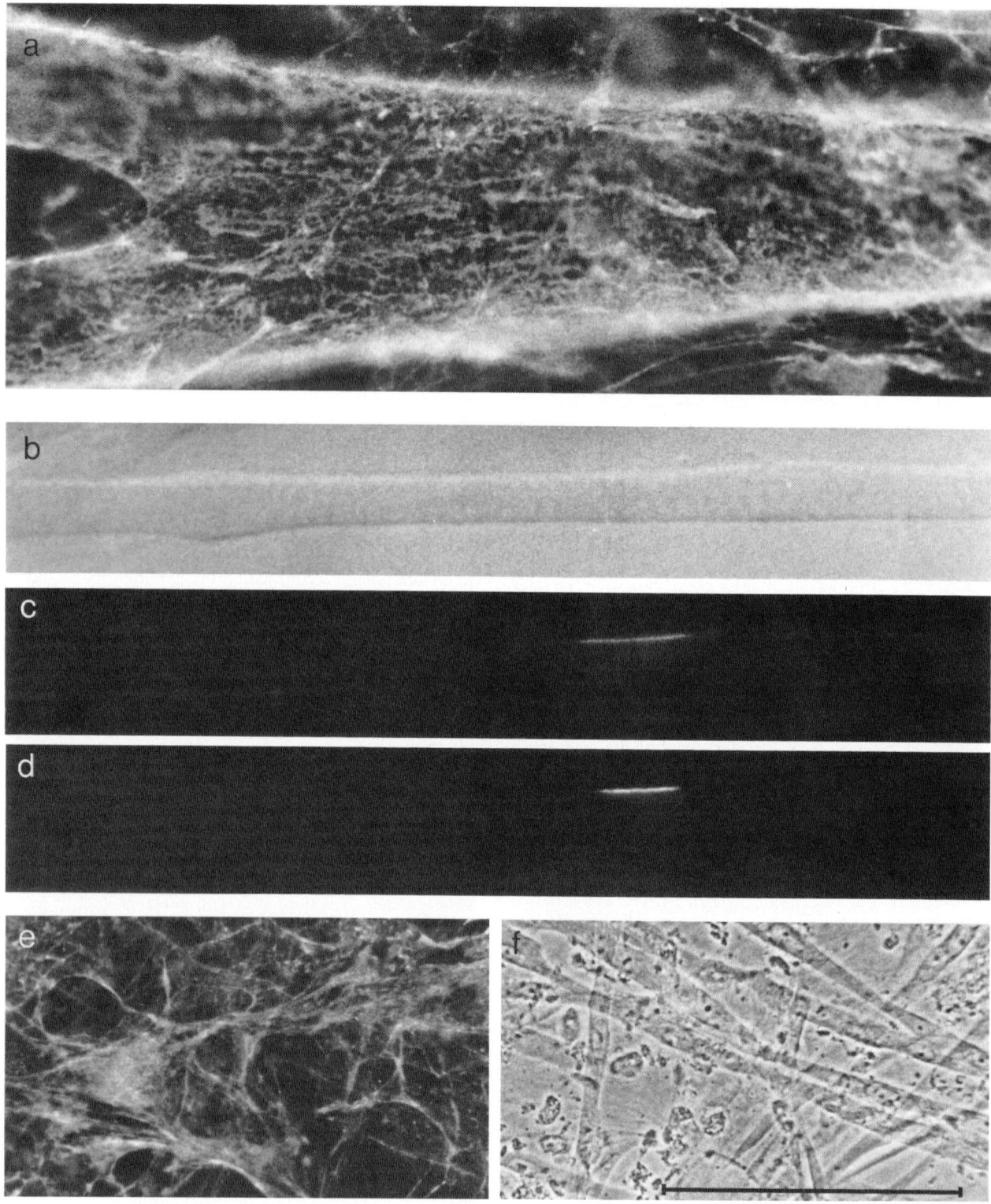

FIGURE 20-11. Cultured rat myotubes stained by an indirect immunofluorescence method with antibodies to muscle fiber basement membrane. *a.* Myotube incubated with an antibody that binds to synaptic and extrasynaptic BL in vivo stains most of the myotube surface and fibrils that run between cells. *b* to *d.* An antibody that binds specifically to synaptic BL in vivo (see Fig. 20-8) stains a small patch on the myotube surface (*c*). The patch occurs at a region of high AChR density, as shown by double staining with rhodamine bungarotoxin (*d*). The fiber is viewed with Nomarski optics in *B.* (*e* to *f*) An antibody that binds to extrasynaptic basement membrane in vivo stains extracellular fibrils but not myotube surfaces. *f.* A phase micrograph of the field shown in *e.* Bar is 50 μm in *a* to *d*, 150 μm in *e* and *f.* (From Sanes JR, Lawrence JC Jr: Activity-dependent accumulation of basal lamina by cultured rat myotubes. Dev Biol 97:123, 1983. With permission.)

element can be accounted for by the tendon, which is itself largely ECM. The other half is distributed along the muscle fiber. Of this fraction, some elasticity is intrinsic to the sarcomeres, but a sizable fraction has been shown to reside in the endomysium.[76] BL could, therefore, take part in the distribution of force along the muscle fiber as well as in the transmission of force from muscle to tendon. Molecules that connect BL to muscle plasma membrane along its length and, more prominently, at the myotendinous junction[77,78] provide possible bases for this mechanical linkage.

Direct biophysical analysis of BL is lacking, but keys to its strength most likely are its major structural components, collagen IV and laminin. As noted above, they form networks that are linked to each other by entactin/nidogen and anchored to reticular lamina and membrane–associated receptors. A key component at the myotendinous junction may be tenascin C. Expression of tenascin C is regulated by mechanical stress, suggesting a means by which the muscle can adjust matrix composition to compensate for changes in loading.[79,80]

MUSCLE MAINTENANCE

Genetic studies of muscle disease show that the BM is critical for the maintenance of muscle integrity. Positional cloning in humans and analysis of naturally occurring and targeted mutants in mice have revealed that muscular dystrophy can arise from loss of any of several components in the reticular lamina-BL-membrane-cytoskeleton linkage. These include laminin $\alpha 2$ (congenital muscular dystrophy); its major transmembrane receptors, integrin $\alpha 7$ and dystroglycan; dystrophin, which links dystroglycan to the cytoskeleton (Duchenne muscular dystrophy); the dystroglycan and dystrophin-associated sarcoglycans (limb-girdle muscular dystrophies 2C-2F); and the α chains of collagen VI, which help connect the BL to the reticular lamina (Bethlem myopathy and Ullrich syndrome).[81–91] Importantly, in all of these diseases, muscles develop normally but then degenerate. Thus, even though the BL does play roles in myogenesis (see below), it is separately required for muscle maintenance. In part, this requirement may be a passive, mechanical one, but more active mechanisms also contribute. The core BL components, laminin and collagen IV, are signaling as well as structural molecules, and their receptors, dystroglycan and integrins, are signal transducers. For example, active signaling from laminin $\alpha 2$ may provide a survival signal for muscle, and its absence in congenital dystrophy is associated with particularly high levels of apoptosis.[92] In short, muscle maintenance requires both the structural and signaling properties of BL.

MYOGENESIS

In one of the first clear demonstrations that ECM influences cellular differentiation, Hauschka and Konigsberg[93] showed that substrate-bound collagen could replace "conditioned medium" factors in promoting the formation of myotubes from cultured myoblasts. Subsequent work showed that several matrix components affect myogenesis. Of these, laminin appears to be particularly critical. Laminin enhances proliferation of myoblasts, stimulates their motility, and leads them to assume the bipolar shape characteristic of fusing cells.[94,95] Myotube formation is decreased although not abolished in the absence of laminin.[96] In contrast, fibronectin selectively promotes adhesion of fibroblasts and may lead to dedifferentiation of myoblasts.[97] The locations of these proteins also differ: laminin adjoins myotubes as soon as the BL begins to form, whereas fibronectin is largely associated with interstitial matrix and is initially excluded from myogenic regions.[98] Therefore, laminin and fibronectin may be involved in sorting myoblasts from fibroblasts as well as in orchestrating their differentiation.

In addition to their direct effects on cells, laminin and collagen IV provide binding sites for less abundant BL components such as proteoglycans, the principal one in muscle being perlecan. The glycosaminoglycan chains of the proteoglycans, in turn, provide an additional set of binding sites that concentrate and present bioactive polypeptides such as FGFs and transforming growth factors, which are critical for myogenesis.[42–44] Indeed, it is increasingly clear that these nominally soluble factors are predominantly matrix-associated in vivo. Thus, major BL components not only promote myogenesis directly but also orchestrate muscle development by presentation of morphogenic, mitogenic, and trophic factors.

Experiments originally designed to elucidate the embryologic origin of limb muscle provided unexpected evidence that ECM may have a profound influence on muscle patterning that extends beyond its role in myogenesis per se.[99–105] Somites were removed from a young chick embryo and replaced by somites from a quail embryo. Later, the limb was examined to see whether its muscle fibers were of quail or chick origin, taking advantage of a characteristic difference in the appearance of chick and quail nuclei under the light microscope. The main result was that myotubes had quail nuclei, which showed that the muscle was derived from cells that migrated to the limb from the somite. However, three other crucial observations were also made. First, muscles developed in the correct positions and patterns even when somites were grafted from an inappropriate level or age; thus, muscle morphogenesis is guided by environmental cues. Second, although myotube nuclei in the chimeric limbs were of graft (somite) origin, most nuclei in the muscle's connective tissue—including epimysium, perimysium, and endomysium—were derived from the host (limb). Third, the innervation of muscles that developed in chimeric limbs was appropriate for the muscle that actually formed rather than for the somite from which it originated. Finally, related experiments have shown that properly shaped muscles form in limbs made aneural before cleavages occur; that properly shaped nerves form in limbs rendered amyogenic by ablation of somites; and even that rudimentary muscle patterning occurs in limbs devoid of myogenic cells. Together, these results lead to the conclusion that developing muscles take account of cues that connective tissue provides. In addition, as discussed further below, the ECM provides cues that promote and guide neurite outgrowth,[106,107] thereby determining the innervation that each muscle receives.

MUSCLE REGENERATION

When skeletal muscle is submitted to ischemic, pharmacologic, thermal, or mechanical insult, muscle fibers degenerate and are phagocytized, but their basement membrane sheaths survive[108–110] (Fig. 20-12). New muscle fibers regenerate from a resident population of stem cells, called *satellite cells*, that are wedged between muscle fiber and BL (see Chap. 3). Although macrophages make their way into the sheaths after injury to remove dead myotubes, satellite cells apparently penetrate the BL poorly unless it is torn or proteolytically digested. New myotubes, therefore, form within the original sheaths. Thus, by constraining the growth and migration of activated satellite cells, BL orients the regeneration of new muscle fibers. In addition, BL acts as a mechanical barrier to prevent migratory loss of satellite cells from normal muscle and could be involved in repressing satellite cell mitosis and differentiation in the absence of damage.

The guidance that BL provides is of considerable functional importance. Muscles do regenerate if the BL is disrupted, but myotubes are not oriented in parallel and the regenerate may develop little net force. Furthermore, because the BLs of nerves and blood vessels also act as scaffolds for regeneration,[106,111] integrity of connective tissue favors rapid revascularization and reinnervation of damaged muscle. In general, recovery of function is good following injuries that minimally disrupt the integrity and orientation of the sheaths and poor following injuries that destroy these scaffolds.

Roles at the Neuromuscular Junction

NEUROMUSCULAR TRANSMISSION

The key events in synaptic transmission at the neuromuscular junction are release of acetylcholine from the nerve terminal and activation of acetylcholine receptors in the postsynaptic membrane. One might imagine that the BL would block movement of acetylcholine across the synaptic cleft, but kinetic studies show that its diffusion to receptors is unimpeded.[112] This result is consistent with conclusions reached from analysis of glomerular BL in kidney, which is an effective filter only for macromolecules.[113] Thus, diffusion of transmitter to receptors and the passive components of its subsequent dispersal are not significantly affected by BL.

On the other hand, the BL is actively involved in the enzymatic hydrolyis of acetylcholine by AChE, which terminates transmitter action faster than would occur by diffusion alone. It was initially believed that AChE was attached to the synaptic membranes, as is the case in cholinergic neuron-neuron synapses. Subsequent studies showed, however, that a major fraction of AChE at the neuromuscular synapse is stably associated with synaptic BL.[114,115] The key to the association is a collagen-like "tail" that is disulfide-bonded to tetramers of catalytic AChE subunits; much of the synaptic enzyme in muscle but little in brain is associated with the tail.[116] The gene encoding the collagenous subunit, named *ColQ* (*queue* is French for "tail") has now been cloned, and its association with the catalytic subunit has been studied in detail.[117–119] Mutation of the *ColQ* gene in mice leads to loss of synaptic AChE, and mutations of *ColQ* in humans have been found to underlie some cases of congenital myasthenia gravis.[120,121] ColQ, in turn, binds to perlecan in the BL.[122,123]

This interaction is critical for the anchoring of AChE to BL, although it is possible that additional interactions account for its *selective* association with synaptic BL.

SYNAPTIC ADHESION

Like pre- to postsynaptic elements at other synapses, nerve terminals adhere tenaciously to muscle fibers at the neuromuscular junction. Several lines of evidence argue that BL is involved in mediating this attachment. First, when muscles are treated with proteases that digest BL but not plasma membrane, nerve terminals lose their firm attachment to the end plate and can easily be pulled away.[124] Second, when muscle is damaged but not denervated, nerve terminals remain at their original sites on the BL for weeks after the muscle fiber has been removed.[110,125] Third, attachment of neuronal somata and processes to BL or components of BL has been documented in many systems.[107,126] The final and most compelling evidence is that nerve and muscle plasma membranes abut the BL of the synaptic cleft but do not directly contact each other. Instead, they are separated by 50 nm, a distance greater than that spanned by membrane-associated adhesion molecules (e.g., cadherins).[127] Based on these considerations, it is evident that the BL must contribute to the tight adhesion of pre- and postsynaptic partners. Adhesion is likely to be mediated in part by integrins on nerve terminals and both integrins and dystroglycan on the postsynaptic membrane. Other potential adhesive systems are mentioned below.

REINNERVATION

Axons that reinnervate denervated muscle fibers show a remarkable preference for original synaptic sites. Although synapses form at completely new sites under some circumstances, preferential reinnervation of patches of original postsynaptic membrane has been documented in mammalian, avian, and amphibian muscles reinnervated by their own or by foreign nerves.[49,110,111,128] In some cases, over 95 percent of the contacts formed by regenerating axons on muscle fibers occur at original sites, even though these sites occupy only about 0.1 percent of the muscle fiber surface.

Experiments on injured muscle have implicated the ECM in the reinnervation of original synaptic sites. Frog muscles were denervated and damaged and then x-irradiated to prevent satellite cell divisions and consequent muscle regeneration (Fig. 20-12). Nerve terminals and muscle fibers degenerated and were removed, but original synaptic sites were identifiable by a histochemical stain for AChE and by the struts of BL that had once lined junctional folds (Fig. 20-13). Axons regenerated to contact BL sheaths and reinnervated original synaptic sites on the BL as precisely in the absence of muscle fibers as they did in their presence (Fig. 20-14). Over 95 percent of the contacts that axons made with BL were at original synaptic sites, and nearly half of the original sites were reinnervated.[110] Thus, the muscle cell itself need not be present for axons to contact target sites selectively. Some of this precision reflects regrowth of axons along the connective tissue pathways that had been associated with the original nerve—a

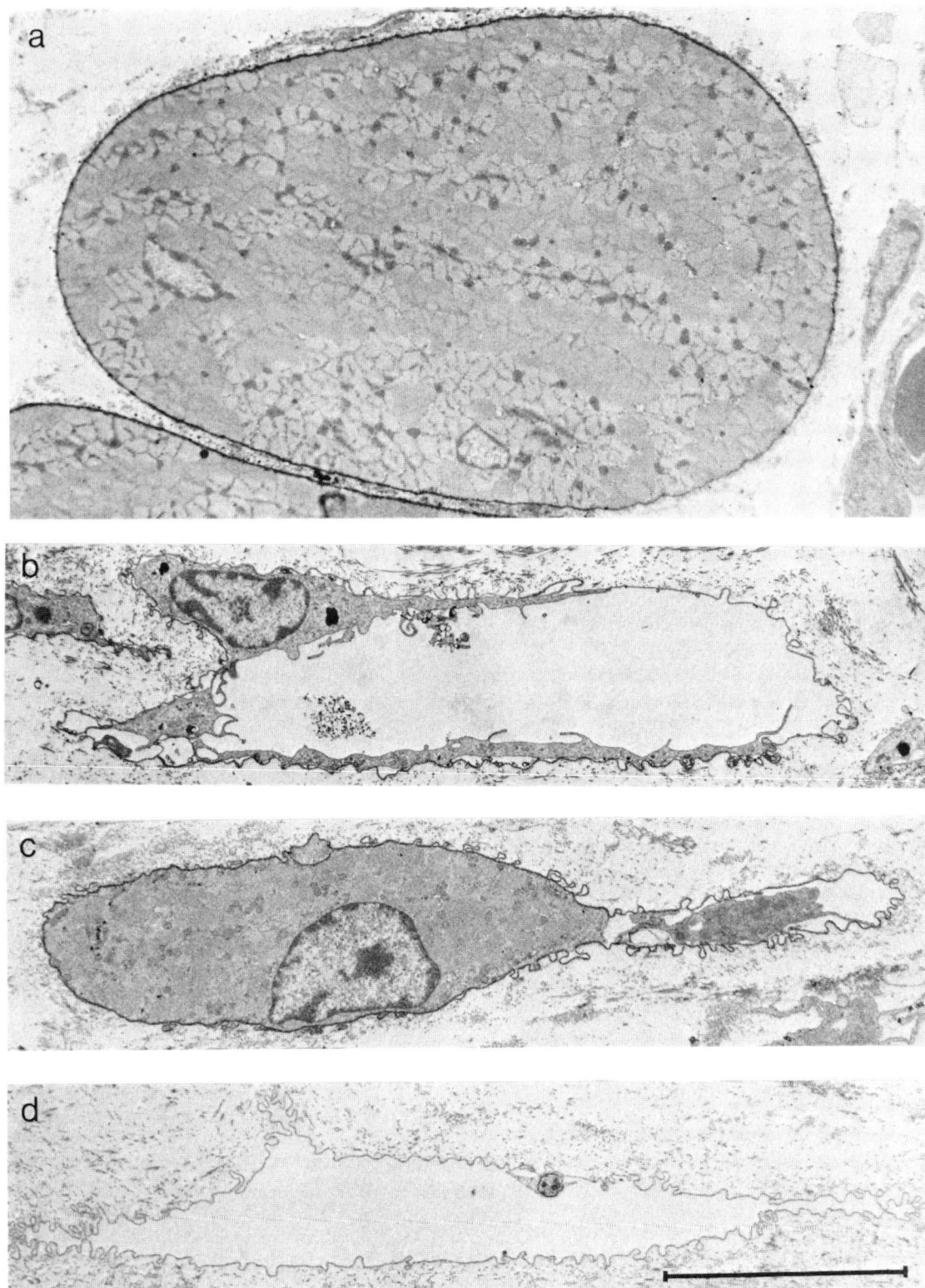

FIGURE 20-12. Damaged muscle degenerates and then regenerates; x-ray irradiation prevents its regeneration. *a.* Normal frog muscle fiber ensheathed in BL, which has been stained here with ruthenium red. *b.* Four days after muscle damage, most of the muscle fiber has been removed but BL persists. A mononucleated cell remains within the BL. *c.* Two weeks after damage, a new muscle fiber has regenerated within the sheath. *d.* Four weeks after damage plus irradiation, the BL sheath remains nearly empty. Bar is 10 μm. (*From Sanes JR, Marshall LM, McMahan VJ: Reinnervation of muscle fiber basal lamina after removal of myofibers. Differentiation of regenerating axons at original synaptic sites. J Cell Biol 78:176, 1978. With permission.*)

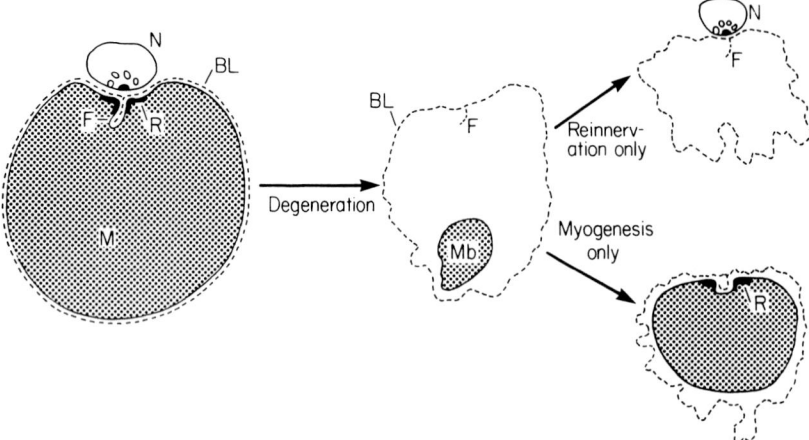

FIGURE 20-13. BL survives damage to nerve (N) and muscle (M). Regeneration of myotubes from myoblastic satellite cells (Mb) can be prevented by x-ray irradiation (top right). Reinnervation can be prevented by repeated nerve damage (bottom right). Axons that regenerate in the absence of muscle fibers contact synaptic BL and form active zones opposite struts of BL that mark sites of junctional folds (F). When myotubes regenerate but axons do not, AChRs (R) accumulate in regions where myotube membrane contacts synaptic BL. (Sanes JR: Roles of extracellular matrix in neural development. Annu Rev Physiol 45:581, 1983. With permission.)

guidance in which the nerve BL plays a prominent role.[111,129] However, neither tubes of perineural connective tissue nor Schwann cells that remain at denervated synaptic sites are required for precise reinnervation of synaptic sites on the BL sheath. Thus, axons might adhere selectively to synapse-specific components of BL or be shielded from contact with nonsynaptic regions by components of BL or reticular lamina that are absent from synaptic sites.

Denervation of skeletal muscle leads to a series of changes in the interstitial spaces that lie between muscle fibers: mononucleated cells proliferate and collagens and fibronectin accumulate. As noted above, some of these changes are concentrated perisynaptically: tenascin, fibronectin (a heparan sulfate proteoglycan), and neural cell adhesion molecule (N-CAM) all accumulate selectively in interstitial spaces surrounding denervated synaptic sites, in part because they are synthesized by a specialized subpopulation of fibroblasts that proliferate in perisynaptic areas following denervation.[58] In light of evidence that axons interact with tenascin, fibronectin, proteoglycans, and N-CAM, this pattern of regulation suggests that perisynaptic matrix could be involved in guiding regenerating axons to the original synaptic sites that they preferentially reinnervate. Evidence favoring this suggestion is that cultured neurons grow longer neurites on fragments of denervated muscle from the earliest steps of synaptic differentiation.[57] However, mutants lacking N-CAM or tenascin C show subtle or no defects in reinnervation.[130–132]

PRESYNAPTIC DIFFERENTIATION

When axons innervate myotubes during embryogenesis or in culture or when they reinnervate muscle fibers in adults, they

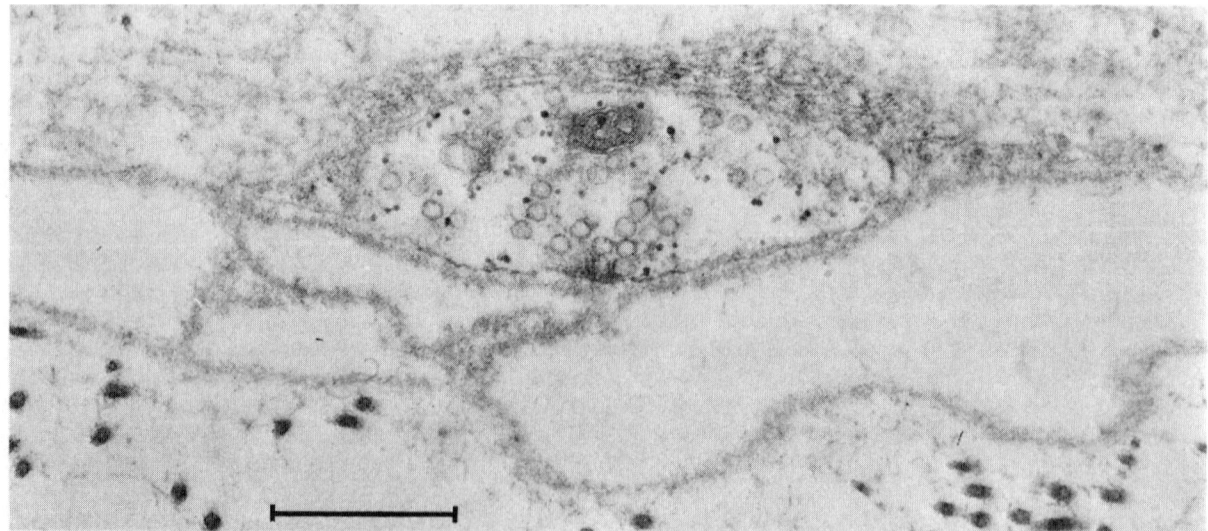

FIGURE 20-14. Regenerated nerve terminal at original synaptic site on a BL sheath, 3 weeks after muscle was denervated, damaged, and irradiated. Some of the vesicles in this terminal are focused on an active zone that lies opposite an intersection of synaptic cleft and junctional fold BL. Compare with Fig. 20-6. Bar is 0.5 μm.

form nerve terminals that contain clusters of neurotransmitter-filled synaptic vesicles and membrane-associated release sites called *active zones*.[49] Importantly, these presynaptic specializations are largely confined to the tiny fraction of the axon that directly contacts the postsynaptic cell, indicating that myotube-derived factors organize presynaptic differentiation. Portions of axons contacting BL sheaths from which muscle fibers had been removed (see above) also acquired active zones and synaptic vesicles as well as the ability to recycle vesicles when electrically stimulated.[110,133] Moreover, new active zones formed in these terminals precisely in register with the struts of BL that marked sites where junctional folds had once been (Fig. 20-14). This association of active zones with folds of BL reconstituted the normal geometry of the synapse, providing strong evidence that some organizers of presynaptic differentiation were contained within the BL.

Among the muscle-derived organizers of presynaptic differentiation are the synaptic laminins. The laminin $\beta 2$ chain was initially identified by virtue of its concentration in synaptic BL.[134] Myotubes are able to target $\beta 2$ to postsynaptic specializations,[68] leading to formation of a BL in which synaptic sites bear primarily if not exclusively $\beta 2$-containing trimers, whereas extrasynaptic regions are enriched in $\beta 1$-containing trimers. Moreover, presentation of $\beta 2$ fragments or $\beta 2$-containing trimers to motor axons in vitro causes them to stop growing and to start differentiating into nerve terminals.[135,136] This behavior contrasts with the robust neurite outgrowth that $\beta 1$-containing trimers promote.[107] Together these results provided one of the first rationales for the existence of multiple laminins: They generate local functional diversity (here, synaptic versus extrasynaptic) in a common structural framework.

In direct support of this model, presynaptic differentiation is aberrant at neuromuscular junctions of $\beta 2$ "knockout" mutant mice: few active zones form, transmitter release is decreased, Schwann cell processes invade the synaptic cleft, and animals die of neuromuscular weakness around the time of weaning (Fig. 20-15).[137,138] Thus, $\beta 2$ laminins qualify as muscle-derived organizers of presynaptic differentiation. On the other hand, the fact that presynaptic differentiation proceeds to a considerable extent in the absence of $\beta 2$ indicates that additional organizers exist.

Additional analysis of muscle laminins revealed the presence of three α chains in synaptic BL (laminin $\alpha 2$, $\alpha 4$, and $\alpha 5$) but only one ($\alpha 2$) extrasynaptically.[31,34] Thus, whereas the predominant extrasynaptic laminin is laminin 2 ($\alpha 2\beta 1\gamma 1$), synaptic BL may contain laminins 4, 9, and 11 ($\alpha 2\beta 1\gamma 1$, $\alpha 4\beta 1\gamma 1$, and $\alpha 5\beta 1\gamma 1$). Any or all of these trimers might be involved in presynaptic differentiation. Genetic studies and analyses in vitro suggest distinct roles for each trimer (Fig. 20-15). Laminin 11 promotes presynaptic differentiation and repels Schwann cell processes in vitro (embryonic lethality of the null mutant from extramuscular defects has hindered analysis in vivo); laminin 9 promotes the precise alignment of pre- and postsynaptic specializations; and laminin 4 appears to have little specifically synaptic role but may be important for structural integrity, as is $\alpha 2$-containing laminin 2 extrasynaptically.[31,139,140] Thus three members of the same gene family collaborate to promote, organize, and maintain presynaptic differentiation.

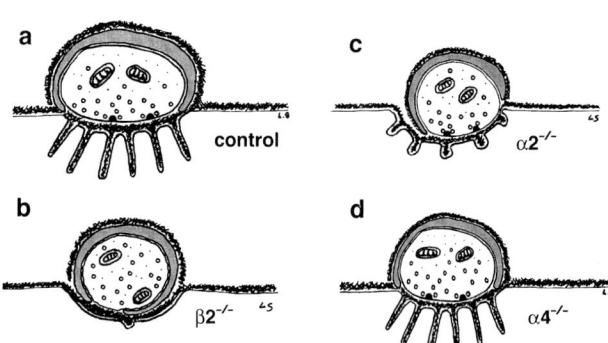

FIGURE 20-15. Neuromuscular junctions in mutants lacking laminin chains normally present in the synaptic cleft. Sketches are from electron micrographs. (*a*) Normal junction.s (*b*) In mice lacking laminin $\beta 2$, presynaptic differentiation is compromised and Schwann cells invade the nerve terminal. (*c*) In mice lacking laminin $\alpha 4$, differentiation is unimpeded but active zones in nerve terminals are not apposed to junctional folds in the postsynaptic membrane. (*d*) Mice lacking laminin $\alpha 2$ have muscular dystrophy but minimal neuromuscular abnormalities. Prenatal lethality prevents assessment of the neuromuscular phenotype in mice lacking laminins $\alpha 5$ or $\gamma 1$. (*Modified by Bruce Patton from his drawings in Ref. 34. With permission.*)

The distinct activities of synaptic laminins suggest that they have multiple receptors on axons and Schwann cells. Receptors presumably include integrins, which major receptors for laminins generally; indeed, integrin $\alpha 3$ is concentrated at active zones.[141] In addition, laminins 9 and 11 copurify with the calcium channels that trigger transmitter release and SV2, the vesicle-associated protein, respectively.[142,143] The biological significance of these associations remains obscure, but they raise the possibility that laminins could organize presynaptic differentiation in part by direct interactions with critical components of the release apparatus.

POSTSYNAPTIC DIFFERENTIATION

Acetylcholine receptors (AChRs) are diffusely distributed in newly formed myotubes but highly concentrated in the postsynaptic membrane of adult muscle ($\sim 10,000/\mu m^2$ synaptically versus $<10/\mu m^2$ extrasynaptically). Myotubes can cluster diffuse AChRs on their own in vitro and may do so to some extent in vivo, but classic studies have demonstrated a striking ability of ingrowing axons to organize postsynaptic specializations, including AChRs, precisely at sites of nerve-muscle contact.[144]

Experiments on BL sheaths suggested that some nerve-derived organizers of AChR clustering are associated with synaptic BL: when myotubes regenerated in these sheaths following damage and denervation (Fig 20-13), new postsynaptic specializations, including AChRs, formed in precise apposition to synaptic BL, even though the axon was absent.[145] These results have demonstrated that components of synaptic BL can promote post- as well as presynaptic differentiation and raised the possibility that some of the nerve-derived organizers of postsynaptic differentiation might be stably maintained in the BL or presented by it. In fact, of numerous candidate postsynaptic organizers, only one has unequivocally been shown to play a role in vivo, and this is z-agrin, a nerve-derived synaptic BL component. Agrin was isolated by McMahan and colleagues in a search for bioactive components of synaptic BL.[146–148] Immunochemical studies showed that agrin is synthesized by motor neurons, transported down axons, and released into the synaptic cleft.[149] Biochemical and, eventually, molecular analysis showed that agrin is a heparan sulfate proteoglycan with a C-terminal domain that interacts with the muscle membrane and an N-terminal domain that mediates binding to laminin in the BL.[150–153] Both loss- and gain-of-function studies have amply supported the idea that agrin is both necessary and sufficient for postsynaptic differentiation: targeted deletion of the agrin gene in mice leads to devastating (and lethal) defects in neuromuscular synaptogenesis, and local expression of agrin in muscle leads to assembly of a complete postsynaptic apparatus.[154–156] A potential complication is that muscles as well as motor neurons synthesize agrin. However, only the latter express an isoform, generated by inclusion of C-terminal exons called "z"; z-containing isoforms are ≥ 1000-fold more active than z-minus isoforms at clustering AChRs in vitro,[157,158] and targeted deletion of just the z exons leads to postsynaptic defects as severe as those seen in the absence of all agrin.[159]

As a large multidomain protein, it is not unexpected that agrin interacts with many cellular receptors, including the neural cell adhesion molecules, N-CAM, dystroglycan, and integrins.[160] Genetic analysis has shown, however, that none of these are required for AChR clustering; instead, agrin's critical receptor, at least for this function, is a receptor tyrosine kinase called MuSK.[161] Activation of MuSK, in turn, leads to association of AChRs with the cytoskeleton via a cytoplasmic protein called rapsyn. Thus, the pathway for postsynaptic differentiation at the neuromuscular junction (NMJ) involves agrin as a signal, MuSK as a receptor, and rapsyn as an effector.

By binding agrin, the BL both localizes the signal and allows it persistence following delivery by the nerve. Once formed, synaptic specializations are stable: aggregates of AChRs—associated with a variety of synaptic cytoskeletal, transmembrane, and BL components—persist at synaptic sites for many weeks following denervation. The stability of BL makes it likely that it plays a role in maintaining postsynaptic integrity. The agrin-binding protein dystroglycan and proteins associated with it appear to be dispensable for initial formation of the postsynaptic membrane but critical for its long-term maintenance.[162,163] Thus, agrin (and laminins) in the BL may use different receptor systems to regulate synapse formation and synapse maintenance.

Pathology

Nerve and muscle regenerate following trauma in human beings as in animals, and new synapses form. The importance of ECM in guiding these processes has been well established in experimental situations, and there is no reason to doubt that similar regulatory interactions occur in people. That preserving BL and endomysium benefits muscle regeneration has been understood for some time. Reinnervation of denervated muscle is also facilitated when original synaptic sites are available, and techniques of muscle transplantation and nerve repair might profitably incorporate measures to maximize the chance that regenerating axons will have access to synaptic BL. In this context, it is worth noting that muscle BL can support and orient the growth of peripheral axons and is now sometimes used as graft material to improve axonal regeneration through damaged areas.[164,165]

A variety of conditions in which muscle function is impaired are characterized by a buildup of connective tissue within muscles. These include conditions such as polymyositis and Duchenne muscular dystrophy, mechanical trauma, and aging. Immunohistochemical studies have documented the accumulation of collagen types I to V, laminin, fibronectin, and several proteoglycans in several of these conditions.[32,33,72] In general, however, such accumulations are not disease-specific and are likely to be secondary to muscle atrophy and/or degeneration.

Finally, when the previous edition of this book was published,[72] no matrix molecules had been implicated in the etiology of any neuromuscular disease. Perhaps the most exciting development in the past decade is the discovery that in some cases, defects in matrix assembly are directly rather than secondarily involved in several such diseases. As mentioned above, mutations in laminin α2 (Chap. 44) and collagen VI (Chap. 39) lead to muscular dystrophies; perlecan defects underlie the Schwartz-Jampel syndrome (Chap. 46) in humans[81–91]; and mutations in ColQ underlie some cases of congenital myasthenia[121] (Chap. 66). Targeted or naturally occurring mutations in mice confirm the phenotypes of the laminin and collagen VI mutations[84,120]; reveal mild myopathies in mice lacking collagens XIII and XV[166–167]; and demonstrate neuromuscular (synaptic) roles for laminins α4, β2, and agrin.[137–139,156,159] Thus, our growing knowledge of matrix biology is now contributing to our understanding of clinical myology, and this understanding, in turn, is suggesting new therapeutic approaches. For example, replacement of mutated matrix components by forced expression or upregulation of other matrix molecules has already shown promising results in genetically valid animal models of muscular dystrophy.[168–170]

List of Abbreviations

AChE	acetylcholinesterase	ECM	extracellular matrix
AChRs	acetylcholine receptors	GalNAc	β-N-acetylgalactosamine
BL	basal lamina	N-CAM	neural cell adhesion molecule
FGF	fibroblast growth factor	NMJ	neuromuscular junction

References

1. Borg TK, Caulfield JB: Morphology of connective tissue in skeletal muscle. *Tissue Cell* 12:197, 1980.
2. Bunge MB, Wood PM, Tynan LB, et al: Perineurium originates from fibroblasts: Demonstration in vitro with a retroviral marker. *Science* 243:229, 1989.
3. Todd BA, Inman C, Sedgwick EM, Abbott NJ: Ionic permeability of the frog sciatic nerve perineurium: Parallel studies of potassium and lanthanum penetration using electrophysiological and electron microscopic techniques. *J Neurocytol* 29:551, 2000.
4. Bowman W: On the minute structure and movements of voluntary muscle. *Philos Trans R Soc Lond (Biol)* 130:457, 1840.
5. Swatland HJ: Morphology and development of endomysial connective tissue in porcine and bovine muscle. *J Anat* 41:78, 1975.
6. Zacks SL, Sheff MP, Saito A: Structure and staining characteristics of myofiber external lamina. *J Histochem Cytochem* 21:703, 1973.
7. Mauro A, Adams WR: The structure of the sarcolemma of the frog skeletal muscle fiber. *J Biophys Biochem Cytol (Suppl)* 10:175, 1961.
8. Inoue S: Ultrastructure of basement membranes. *Int Rev Cytol* 1117:57, 1989.
9. Timpl R, Rohrbach OH (eds): *Molecular and Cellular Aspects of Basement Membranes*. New York: Academic Press, 1993.
10. Timpl R, Brown JC: Supramolecular assembly of basement membranes. *Bioessays* 18:123, 1996.
11. Olsen BR, Ninomya Y: Collagens, in Kreis T, Vale R (eds): *Guidebook to the Extracellular Matrix, Anchor, and Adhesion Proteins*. Oxford, UK: Oxford Univesity Press, 1999, pp 380–407.
12. Colognato H, Yurchenco PD: Form and function: The laminin family of heterotrimers. *Dev Dyn* 218:213, 2000.
13. Jones FS, Jones PL et al: The tenascin family of ECM glycoproteins: structure, function, and regulation during embryonic development and tissue remodeling. *Dev Dyn* 218:235, 2000.
14. Adams JC: Thrombospondins: Multifunctional regulators of cell interactions. *Annu Rev Cell Dev Biol* 17:25, 2001.
15. Iozzo RV: Matrix proteoglycans: from molecular design to cellular function. *Annu Rev Biochem* 67:609, 1998.
16. Erickson AC, Couchman JR: Still more complexity in mammalian basement membranes. *J Histochem Cytochem* 48:1291, 2000.
17. Sanes JR, Engvall E, Butkowski R, Hunter DD: Molecular heterogeneity of basal laminae isoforms of laminin and collagen IV at the neuromuscular junction and elsewhere. *J Cell Biol* 111:1685, 1990.
18. Miner JH, Sanes JR: Collagen IV α3, α4 and α5 chains in rodent basal laminae: Sequence, distribution, association with laminins and developmental switches. *J Cell Biol* 127:879, 1994.
19. Miner JH, Patton BL, Lentz SI, et al: The laminin α chains: Expression, developmental transitions, and chromosomal locations of α1–5, identification of heterotrimeric laminins 8–11, and cloning of a novel α3 isoform. *J Cell Biol* 137:685, 1997.
20. Light N, Champion AE: Characterization of muscle epimysium, perimysium and endomysium collagens. *Biochem J* 219:1017, 1984.
21. Sanes JR: Laminin, fibronectin, and collagen in synaptic and extrasynaptic portions of muscle fiber basement membrane. *J Cell Biol* 93:442, 1982.
22. Kuo HJ, Maslen CL, Keene DR, Glanville RW: Type VI collagen anchors endothelial basement membranes by interacting with type IV collagen. *J Biol Chem* 272:26522, 1997.
23. Eldridge CF, Sanes JR, Chiu AY, et al: Basal lamina-associated heparan sulfate proteoglycan in the rat peripheral nervous system. Characterization and localization using monoclonal antibodies. *J Neurocytol* 15:37, 1986.
24. Bertolotto A, Palmucci L, Mongini T, et al: Chondroitin, chondroitin 6-sulphate, chondroitin 4-sulphate and dermatan sulphate proteoglycans in normal and pathological human muscle. *J Neurol Sc* 81:247, 1987.
25. Vannahme C, Smyth N, Miosge N, et al: Characterization of SMOC-1, a novel modular calcium-binding protein in basement membranes. *J Biol Chem* 277:37977, 2002.
26. Jenniskens GJ, Oosterhof A, Brandwijk R, et al.: Heparan sulfate heterogeneity in skeletal muscle basal lamina: demonstration by phage display-derived antibodies. *J Neurosci* 20:4099, 2000.
27. Sanes JR, Schachner M, Covault J: Expression of several adhesive macromolecules (N-CAM, L1, J1, NILE, uvomorulin, laminin, fibronectin, and a heparan sulfate proteoglycan) in embryonic, adult and denervated adult skeletal muscles. *J Cell Biol* 102:420, 1986.
28. Tomono Y, Naito I, Ando K, et al: Epitope-defined monoclonal antibodies against multiplexin collagens demonstrate that type XV and XVIII collagens are expressed in specialized basement membranes. *Cell Struct Funct* 27:9, 2002.
29. Sewry CA, Chevallay M, Tome FM: Expression of laminin subunits in human fetal skeletal muscle. *Histochem J* 27:497, 1995.
30. Ehrig K, Leivo L, Argraves WS, et al: Merosin, a tissue-specific basement membrane protein, is a laminin-like protein. *Proc Natl Acad Sci USA* 87:3264, 1990.
31. Patton BL, Miner JH, Chiu AY, et al: Distribution and function of laminins in the neuromuscular system of developing, adult and mutant mice. *J Cell Biol* 139:1507, 1997.
32. Patton BL, Connolly AM, Martin PT, et al: Distribution of ten laminin chains in dystrophic, regenerating, and denervated muscles. *Neuromuscul Disord* 9:423, 1999.
33. Ringelmann B, Roder C, Hallmann R, et al: Expression of laminin alpha1, alpha2, alpha4, and alpha5 chains, fibronectin, and tenascin-C in skeletal muscle of dystrophic 129ReJ dy/dy mice. *Exp Cell Res* 246:165, 1999.
34. Patton BL: Laminins of the neuromuscular system. *Microsc Res Tech* 51:247–261, 2000.
35. Cifuentes-Diaz C, Alliel PM, Charbonnier F, et al: Regulated expression of the proteoglycan SPOCK in the neuromuscular system. *Mech Dev* 94:277, 2000.
36. Kannus P, Jozsa L, Jarvinen TA, et al: Location and distribution of non-collagenous matrix proteins in musculoskeletal tissues of rat. *Histochem J* 30:799, 1998.
37. Bertolotto A, Palmucci L, Ooriguzzi C, et al: Laminin and fibronectin distribution in normal and pathological human muscle. *J Neurol Sci* 60:377, 1983.
38. Bowe MA, Mendis DB, Fallon JR: The small leucine-rich repeat proteoglycan biglycan binds to alpha-dystroglycan and is upregulated in dystrophic muscle. *J Cell Biol* 148:801, 2000.
39. Pena SDJ, Gordon BB, Karpati G, et al: Lectin histochemistry of human skeletal muscle *J Histochem Cytochem* 29:542, 1981.
40. Scott LJC, Bacou F, Sanes, JR: A synapse-specific carbohydrate at the neuromuscular junction. Association with both acetylcholinesterase and a glycolipid. *J Neurosci* 8:932, 1988.
41. Booth CM, Brown MC: Localization of neural cell adhesion molecule in denervated muscle to both the plasma membrane and extracellular compartments by immuno-electron microscopy. *Neuroscience* 27:699, 1988.
42. DiMario J, Buffinger N, Yamada S, Strohman RC: Fibroblast growth factor in the extracellular matrix of dystrophic (mdx) mouse muscle. *Science* 244:688, 1989.
43. Baeg GH, Perrimon N: Functional binding of secreted molecules to heparan sulfate proteoglycans in *Drosophila*. *Curr Opin Cell Biol* 12:575, 2001.
44. Pirskanen A, Kiefer JC, Hauschka SD: IGFs, insulin, Shh, bFGF, and TGF-beta1 interact synergistically to promote somite myogenesis in vitro. *Dev. Biol* 224:189, 2000.
45. Festoff BW, Suo Z, Citron BA: Plasticity and stabilization of neuromuscular and CNS synapses: interactions between thrombin protease signaling pathways and tissue transglutaminase. *Int Rev Cytol* 211:153, 2001.
46. Hirohata S, Wang LW, Miyagi M, Yan L, Seldin MF, Keene DR, Crabb JW, Apte SS: Punctin, a novel ADAMTS-like molecule, ADAMTSL-1 in extracellular matrix. *J Biol Chem* 277:12192, 2002.
47. Cooper DN, Massa SM, Barondes SH: Endogenous muscle lectin inhibits myoblast adhesion to laminin. *J Cell Biol* 115:1437, 1991.
48. Cooper DN, Barondes SH: God must love galectins, he made so many of them. *Glycobiology* 9:979, 1999.
49. Sanes JR, Lichtman JW: Development of the vertebrate neuromuscular junction. *Annu Rev Neurosci* 22:389, 1999.
50. Sanes JR:g The synaptic cleft of the neuromuscular junction. *Semin Dev Biol* 6:163, 1995.
51. Kaupmann K, Heimann P, Jockusch H: Dolichos biflorus agglutinin receptors in mouse muscle. 1. Developmental expression in relation to synaptic acetylcholinesterase and to neuromuscular disease. *Eur J Cell Biol* 46:411, 1988.
52. Martin PT, Scott LJ, Porter BE, Sanes JR: Distinct structures and functions of related pre- and postsynaptic carbohydrates at the mammalian neuromuscular junction. *Mol Cell Neurosci* 13:105, 1999.
53. Martin PT: Glycobiology of the synapse. *Glycobiology* 12:1R–7R, 2002.
54. Arber S, Caroni P: Thrombospondin-4, an extracellular matrix protein expressed in the developing and adult nervous system promotes neurite outgrowth. *J Cell Biol.* 131:1083, 1995.
55. Ko CP: A lectin, peanut agglutinin, as a probe for the extracellular matrix in living neuromuscular junctions. *J Neurocytol* 16:567, 1987.
56. Chernousov MA, Carey DJ: Schwann cell extracellular matrix molecules and their receptors. *Histol Histopathol* 15:593, 2000.
57. Covault J, Cunningham JM, Sanes JR: Neurite outgrowth on cryostat sections of innervated and denervated skeletal muscle. *J Cell Biol* 105:2479, 1987.
58. Gatchalian CL, Schachner M, Sanes JR: Fibroblasts that proliferate near denervated synaptic site in skeletal muscle synthesize the adhesive molecules tenasciniJl, NCAM, fibronectin, and a heparan sulfate proteoglycan. *J Cell Biol* 108:1873, 1989.
59. Weis J, Fine SM, David C, et al: Integration site-dependent expression of a transgene reveals specialized features of cells associated with neuromuscular junctions. *J Cell Biol* 113:1385, 1991.
60. Astrow SH, Tyner TR, Nguyen MT, et al: A Schwann cell matrix component of neuromuscular junctions and peripheral nerves. *J Neurocytol* 26:63, 1997.
61. Benjamin M, Ralphs JR: The cell and developmental biology of tendons and ligaments. *Int Rev Cytol* 196:85, 2000.

62. Maier A, Mayne R: Connective-tissue macromolecules in Golgi chicken tendon organs and at their interface with muscle fibers and adjoining tendinous structures. *Am J Anat* 188, 1990.
63. Pedrosa-Domellof F, Tiger CF, Virtanen I, et al: Laminin chains in developing and adult human myotendinous junctions. *J Histochem Cytochem* 48:201, 2000.
64. Chiquet M, Fambrough DM: Chick myotendinous antigen. 1. A monoclonal antibody as a marker for tendon and muscle morphogenesis. *J Cell Biol* 98:1926, 1984.
65. Kelly AM, Zacks ST: The fine structure of motor end-plate morphogenesis. *J Cell Biol* 42:154, 1969.
66. Chiu AY, Sanes JR: Differentiation of basal lamina in synaptic and extra synaptic portions of embryonic rat muscle. *Dev Biol* 103:456, 1984.
67. Anderson MJ, Fambrough DM: Aggregates of acetylcholine receptors are associated with plaques of a basal lamina heparan sulfate proteoglycan on the surface of skeletal muscle fibers. *J Cell Biol* 97:1396, 1983.
68. Martin PT, Ettinger AM, Sanes JR: A synaptic localization domain in the synaptic cleft protein laminin β2 (s-laminin). *Science* 269:413, 1995.
69. Sasse J, von der MH, Kuhl U et al: Origin of collagen types I, III, and V in cultures of avian skeletal muscle. *Dev Biol* 83:79, 1981.
70. Sanes JR, Lawrence JC Jr: Activity-dependent accumulation of basal lamina by cultured rat myotubes. *Dev Biol* 97:123, 1983.
71. Silberstein L, Inestrosa N, Hall ZW: Aneural muscle cell cultures make synaptic basal lamina components. *Nature* 295:143, 1982.
72. Sanes JR: The extracellular matrix, in Engel, AG, Franzini-Armstrong C (eds): *Myology*, 2d ed. New York: McGraw Hill, 1994, pp 242–260.
73. Jewell BR, Wilkie DR: An analysis of the mechanical components in frog's striated muscle. *J Physiol* 143:515, 1958.
74. Fields RW: Mechanical properties of the frog sarcolemma. *Biophys J* 10:462, 1970.
75. Street SF, Ramsey RW: Sarcolemma. Transmitter of active tension in frog skeletal muscle. *Science* 149:1379, 1965.
76. Tidball JG: Energy stored and dissipated in skeletal muscle basement membranes during sinusoidal oscillations. *Biophys J* 50:1127, 1986.
77. Tidball JG, Chan M: Adhesive strength of single muscle cells to basement membrane at myotendinous junction. *J Appl Physiol* 67:1063, 1989.
78. Law DJ, Caputo A, Tidball JG: Site and mechanics of failure in normal and dystrophin-deficient skeletal muscle. *Muscle Nerve* 18:216, 1995.
79. Fluck M, Tunc-Civelek V, Chiquet M: Rapid and reciprocal regulation of tenascin-C and tenascin-Y expression by loading of skeletal muscle. *J Cell Sci* 113(Pt 20):3583, 2000.
80. Chiquet M: Regulation of extracellular matrix gene expression by mechanical stress. *Matrix Biol* 18:417, 1999.
81. Cohn RD, Herrmann R, Sorokin L, et al: Laminin α2 chain-deficient congenital muscular dystrophy. *Neurology* 51:94, 1998.
82. Helbling-Leclerc A, et al: Mutations in the laminin a-chain gene (LAMA2) cause merosin-deficient congenital muscular dystrophy. *Nat Genet* 11:216, 1995.
83. Mayer U, et al: Absence of integrin alpha 7 causes a novel form of muscular dystrophy. *Nat Genet* 17:318, 1997.
84. Xu H, Wu XR, Wewer UM, et al: Murine muscular dystrophy caused by a mutation in the laminin a-2 (LAMA2) gene. *Nat Genet* 8:297, 1994.
85. Scacheri PC, Gillanders EM, Subramony SH, et al: Novel mutations in collagen VI genes: Expansion of the Bethlem myopathy phenotype. *Neurology* 58:593, 2002.
86. Brockington M, Blake DJ, Prandini P, et al: Mutations in the fukutin-related protein gene (FKRP) cause a form of congenital muscular dystrophy with secondary laminin alpha2 deficiency and abnormal glycosylation of alpha-dystroglycan. *Am J Hum Genet* 69:1198, 2001.
87. Ishikawa H, Sugie K, Murayama K, et al: Ullrich disease: Collagen VI deficiency: EM suggests a new basis for muscular weakness. *Neurology* 59:920, 2002.
88. Jobsis GJ, Keizers H, Vreijling JP, et al: Type VI collagen mutations in Bethlem myopathy, an autosomal dominant myopathy with contractures. *Nat Genet* 14:113, 1996.
89. Nicole S, Davoine CS, Topaloglu H, et al: Perlecan, the major proteoglycan of basement membranes, is altered in patients with Schwartz-Jampel syndrome (chondrodystrophic myotonia). *Nat Genet* 26:480, 2000.
90. Arikawa-Hirasawa E, Le AH, Nishino I, et al: Structural and functional mutations of the perlecan gene cause Schwartz-Jampel syndrome, with myotonic myopathy and chondrodysplasia. *Am J Hum Genet* 70:1368, 2002.
91. Miyagoe-Suzuki Y, Nakagawa M, Takeda S: Merosin and congenital muscular dystrophy (review). *Microsc Res Tech* 48:181, 2000.
92. Vachon PH, Loechel F, Xu H, et al: Merosin and laminin in myogenesis; Specific requirement for merosin in myotube stability and survival. *J Cell Biol* 134:1483, 1996.
93. Hauschka SO, Konigsberg IR: The influence of collagen on the development of muscle clones. *Proc Natl Acad Sci USA* 55:119, 1966.
94. Balan M, Goodman SL, Kuhl U, et al. Laminin alters cell shape and stimulates motility and proliferation of murine skeletal myoblasts. *Dev Biol* 125:158, 1988.
95. Goodman S, Oeutzmann R, Nurcombe V: Locomotory competence and laminin-specific cell surface binding sites are lost during myoblast differentiation. *Development* 105:795, 1989.
96. Smyth N, Vatansever HS, Murray P, et al: Absence of basement membranes after targeting the LAMC1 gene results in embryonic lethality due to failure of endoderm differentiation. *J Cell Biol* 144:151, 1999.
97. Kuhl U, Ocalan RT, von der MK: Role of laminin and fibronectin in selecting myogenic versus fibogenic cells from skeletal muscle cells in vitro. *Dev Biol* 117:628, 1986.
98. Godfrey EW, Gradall KS: Basal lamina molecules are concentrated in myogenic regions of the mouse limb bud. *Anat Embryol (Berl)* 198:48, 1998.
99. Christ B, Jacob HJ, Jacob M: Experimental analysis of the origin of the wing musculature in avian embryos. *Anat Embryol* 150.171, 1977.
100. Shellswell GB: The formation of discrete muscles from the chick wing dorsal and ventral muscle masses in the absence of nerves. *J Embryol Exp Morphol* 41:269, 1977.
101. Chevallier A, Kieny M: On the role of the connective tissue in the patterning of the chick limb musculature. *Wilheim Roux Archiv* 191:277, 1982.
102. Lance-Jones C, Dias M: The influence of presumptive limb connective tissue on motoneuron axon guidance. *Dev Biol* 14393, 1991.
103. Wolpert L: Vertebrate limb development and malformations. *Pediatr Res* 46:247, 1999.
104. Kardon G: Muscle and tendon morphogenesis in the avian hind limb. *Development* 125:4019, 1998.
105. Kardon G, Campbell JK, Tabin CJ: Local extrinsic signals determine muscle and endothelial cell fate and patterning in the vertebrate limb. *Dev Cell* 3:533, 2002.
106. Fu SY, Gordon T: The cellular and molecular basis of peripheral nerve regeneration. *Mol Neurobiol* 14:67, 1997.
107. Powell SK, Kleinmann HK: Neuronal laminins and their cellular receptors. *Int J Biochem Cell Biol* 29:401, 1997.
108. Vracko R, Benditt EP: Basal lamina. The scaffold for orderly cell replacement. Observations on regeneration of injured skeletal muscle fibers and capillaries. *J Cell Biol* 55:406, 1972.
109. Kaariainen M, Jarvinen T, Jarvinen M, et al: Relation between myofibers and connective tissue during muscle injury repair. *Scand J Med Sci Sports* 10:332, 2000.
110. Sanes JR, Marshall LM, McMahan VJ: Reinnervation of muscle fiber basal lamina after removal of myofibers. Differentiation of regenerating axons at original synaptic sites. *J Cell Biol* 78:176, 1978.
111. Nguyen QT, Sanes JR, Lichtman JW: Preexisting pathways promote precise projection patterns. *Nat Neurosci* 5:861, 2002.
112. Land BR, Harris WV, Salpeter EE, Salpeter MM: Diffusion and binding constants for acetylcholine derived from the falling phase of minature endplate currents. *Proc Natl Acad Sci USA* 81:1594, 1984.
113. Tryggvason K, Wartiovaara J: Molecular basis of glomerular permselectivity. *Curr Opin Nephrol Hypertens* 10:543, 2001.
114. Hall ZW, Kelly RB: Enzymatic detachment of end-plate acetylcholinesterase from muscle. *Nature New Biol* 232:62, 1971.
115. McMahan VJ, Sanes JR, Marshall LM: Cholinesterase is associated with the basallamina at the neuromuscular junction. *Nature* 271:172, 1978.
116. Massoulie J. et al: Acetylcholinesterase C-terminal domains, molecular forms and functional localization. *J Physiol Paris* 92:183, 1998.
117. Krejci E, Coussen F, Duval N, et al: Primary structure of a collagenic tail peptide of *Torpedo* acetylcholinsterase: Coexpression with catalytic subunit induces the production of collagen-tailed forms in transfected cells *EMBO J* 10:1285, 1991.
118. Bon S, Massoulie J: Quaternary association of acetylcholinesterase. I. Oligomeric associations of T subunits with and without the amino-terminal domain of the collagen tail. *J Biol Chem* 272:3007, 1997.
119. Krejci E, et al: The mammalian gene of acetylcholinesterase-associated collagen. *J Biol Chem* 272:22840, 1997.
120. Feng G, Krejci E, Molgo J, et al: Genetic analysis of Collagen Q: Roles in acetylcholinesterase and butyrylcholinesterase assembly and in synaptic structure and function. *J. Cell Biol.* 144:1349, 1999.
121. Ohno K, Brengman J, Tsujino A, et al: Human endplate acetylcholinesterase deficiency caused by mutations in the collagen-like tail subunit (COLQ) of the asymmetric enzyme. *Proc Natl Acad Sci USA* 95:9654, 1998.
122. Peng HB, Xie H, Rossi SG, et al: Acetylcholinesterase clustering at the neuromuscular junction involves perlecan and dystroglycan. *J Cell Biol* 145:911, 1999.
123. Arikawa-Hirasawa E, Rossi SG, Rotundo RL, et al: Absence of acetylcholinesterase at the neuromuscular junctions of perlecan-null mice. *Nat Neurosci* 5:119, 2002.
124. Betz W, Sakmann B: Effects of proteolytic enzymes on function and structure of frog neuromuscular junctions. *J Physiol (Lond)* 230:673, 1973.
125. Dunaevsky A., Connor EA: Stability of frog motor nerve terminals in the absence of target muscle fibers. *Dev Biol* 194:61, 1998.
126. Perris R, Perissinotto D: Role of the extracellular matrix during neural crest cell migration (review). *Mech Dev* 95:3–21, 2000.
127. Yamagata M, Sanes JR, Weiner JA. Synaptic adhesion molecules. *Curr Opin Cell Biol* 15:621–632, 2003.
128. Ramon y Cajal S: *Degeneration and Regeneration of the Nervous System.* London: Hafner, 1928; new printing, 1968.

129. Ide C: Peripheral nerve regeneration. *Neurosci Res* 25:101, 1996.
130. Moscoso LM, Cremer H, Sanes JR: Organization and reorganization of neuromuscular junctions in mice lacking neural cell adhesion molecule, tenascin-C, or fibroblast growth factor-5. *J Neurosci* 18:1465, 1998.
131. Cifuentes-Diaz C, Velasco E, Meunier FA, et al: The peripheral nerve and the neuromuscular junction are affected in the tenascin-C-deficient mouse. *Cell Mol Biol (Noisy-le-Grand)* 44:357, 1998.
132. Cifuentes-Diaz C, Faille L, Goudou D, et al: Abnormal reinnervation of skeletal muscle in a tenascin-C-deficient mouse. *J Neurosci Res* 67:93, 2002.
133. Glicksman M, Sanes JR: Differentiation of motor nerve terminals formed in the absence of muscle fibers. *J Neurocytol* 12661, 1983.
134. Hunter DD, Shah V, Merlie JP, Sanes JR: A laminin-like adhesive protein concentrated in the synaptic cleft of the neuromuscular junction. *Nature* 338:229, 1989.
135. Porter BE, Weis J, Sanes JR: A motoneuron-selective stop signal in the synaptic protein, s-laminin. *Neuron* 14:549, 1995.
136. Son YJ, Patton BL, Sanes JR: Induction of presynaptic differentiation in cultured neurons by extracellular matrix components. *Eur J Neurosci* 11:3457, 1999.
137. Noakes PG, Gautam M, Mudd J, et al: Aberrant differentiation of neuromuscular junctions in mice lacking s-laminin/laminin β2. *Nature* 374:258, 1995.
138. Patton BL, Chiu AY, Sanes JR: Synaptic laminin prevents glial entry into the synaptic cleft. *Nature* 393:698, 1998.
139. Patton BL, Cunningham JM, Thyboll J, et al: Properly formed but improperly localized synaptic specializations in the absence of laminin α4. *Nature Neurosci* 4:597, 2001.
140. Edwards JP, Hatton PA, Wareham AC: Electrophysiology of the neuromuscular junction of the laminin-2 (merosin) deficient C57 BL/6J dy2J/dy2J dystrophic mouse. *Brain Res* 788:262, 1998.
141. Cohen MW, Hoffstrom BG, DeSimone DW: Active zones on motor nerve terminals contain alpha 3 beta 1 integrin. *J Neurosci* 20:4912, 2000.
142. Son Y-J, Scranton TW, Sunderland WJ, et al: The synaptic vesicle protein SV2 is complexed with an α5-containing laminin on the nerve terminal surface. *J Biol Chem* 275:451, 2000.
143. Sunderland WJ, Son YJ, Miner JH, et al: The presynaptic calcium channel is part of a transmembrane complex linking a synaptic laminin (α4β2γ1) with non-erythroid spectrin. *J Neurosci* 20:1009, 2000.
144. Sanes JR, Lichtman JW: Development induction, assembly, maturation and maintenance of a postsynaptic apparatus. *Nat Rev Neurosci* 2:791, 2001.
145. Burden SJ, Sargent PB, McMahan VJ: Acetylcholine receptors in regenerating muscle accumulate at original synaptic sites in the absence of the nerve. *J Cell Biol* 84:412, 1979.
146. Godfrey EW, Nitkin RM, Wallace BG, et al: Components of *Torpedo* electric organ and muscle that cause aggregation of acetycholine receptors on cultured muscle cells. *J Cell Biol* 99:615, 1984.
147. Nitkin RM, Smith MA, Magill C, et al: Identification of agrin, a synaptic organizing protein from *Torpedo* electric organ. *J Cell Biol* 105:2471, 1987.
148. McMahan UJ: The agrin hypothesis. *Cold Spring Harbor Symp Quant Biol* 4:407, 1990.
149. Reist NE, Magill C, McMahan UJ: Agrin-like molecules at synaptic sites in normal, denervated and damaged skeletal muscles. *J Cell Biol* 105:2457, 1987.
150. Rupp F, Payan DG, Magill-Solc C, et al: Structure and expression of a rat agrin. *Neuron* 68:11, 1991.
151. Tsim KWK, Ruegg MA, Escher G, et al: cDNA that encodes active agrin. *Neuron* 8677, 1992.
152. Denzer AJ, Brandenberger R, Gesemann M, et al: Agrin binds to the nerve-muscle basal lamina via laminin. *J Cell Biol* 137:671, 1997.
153. Burgess RW, Skarnes W, Sanes JR: Agrin isoforms with distinct amino termini: differential expression, localization and function. *J Cell Biol* 151:41, 2000.
154. Jones G, et al: Induction by agrin of ectopic and functional postsynaptic-like membrane in innervated muscle. *Proc Natl Acad Sci USA* 94:2654, 1997.
155. Cohen I, Rimer M, Lomo T, et al: Agrin-induced postsynaptic-like apparatus in skeletal muscle fibers in vivo. *Mol Cell Neurosci* 9:237,1997.
156. Gautam M, Noakes PG, Moscoso L, et al: Defective neuromuscular synaptogenesis in agrin-deficient mutant mice. *Cell* 85:525, 1996.
157. Ruegg MA, Tsim KWK, Horton SE, et al: The agrin gene codes for a family of basal lamina proteins that differ in function and distribution. *Neuron* 8:691, 1992.
158. Ferns M, Hoch W, Campanelli JT, et al: RNA splicing regulates agrin mediated acetylcholine receptor clustering activity on cultured myotubes. *Neuron* 8:1079, 1992.
159. Burgess RW, Nguyen QT, Son Y-J, et al: Alternatively spliced isoforms of nerve- and muscle-derived agrin: Their roles at the neuromuscular junction. *Neuron* 23:33, 1999.
160. Sanes JR, Apel ED, Gautam M, et al: Agrin receptors at the skeletal neuromuscular junction. *Ann N Y Acad Sci* 13:1, 1998.
161. DeChiara TM, et al: The receptor tyrosine kinase MuSK is required for neuromuscular junction formation in vivo. *Cell* 85:501, 1996.
162. Jacobson C, Cote PD, Rossi SG, et al: The dystroglycan complex is necessary for stabilization of acetylcholine receptor clusters at neuromuscular junctions and formation of the synaptic basement membrane. *J Cell Biol* 152:435, 2001.
163. Grady RM, Zhou H, Cunningham JM, et al: Maturation and maintenance of the neuromuscular synapse: genetic evidence for roles of the dystrophin glycoprotein complex. *Neuron* 25:279, 2000.
164. Fansa H, Keilhoff G, Wolf G, et al: Tissue engineering of peripheral nerves: A comparison of venous and acellular muscle grafts with cultured Schwann cells. *Plast Reconstr Surg* 107:485, 2001.
165. Fansa H, Schneider W, Wolf G, Keilhoff G: Influence of insulin-like growth factor-I (IGF-I) on nerve autografts and tissue-engineered nerve grafts. *Muscle Nerve* 26:87, 2002.
166. Kvist AP, Latvanlehto A, Sund M, et al: Lack of cytosolic and transmembrane domains of type XIII collagen results in progressive myopathy. *Am J Pathol* 159:1581, 2001.
167. Eklund L, Piuhola J, Komulainen J, et al: Lack of type XV collagen causes a skeletal myopathy and cardiovascular defects in mice. *Proc Natl Acad Sci USA* 98:1194, 2001.
168. Moll J, Barzaghi P, Lin S, et al: An agrin minigene rescues dystrophic symptoms in a mouse model for congenital muscular dystrophy. *Nature* 413:302, 2001.
169. Nguyen HH, Jayasinha V, Xia B, et al. Overexpression of the cytotoxic T cell GalNAc transferase in skeletal muscle inhibits muscular dystrophy in mdx mice. *Proc Natl Acad Sci USA* 99:5616, 2002.
170. Yang DD, Tarumi YS, Miyagoe-Suzuki Y, et al: Dual mechanisms of action for laminin α5 in preventing muscular dystrophy. *Neurosci Abstr* 699.8, 2002.

Chapter 21
The Muscle Spindle

ROBERT W. BANKS
DAVID BARKER

Introduction
Number and Distribution
  TYPES OF SPINDLE UNIT
  NUMBER
  DISTRIBUTION
Capsule and Vascular Supply
Intrafusal Muscle Fibers
  LENGTH, DIAMETER, AND NUCLEATION
  ULTRASTRUCTURE
  HISTOCHEMISTRY
Sensory Innervation
  PRIMARY ENDINGS
  SECONDARY ENDINGS
  NUMBER OF AFFERENT AXONS
Motor Innervation
  THE γ MOTOR INNERVATION
  THE β MOTOR INNERVATION
  THE PATTERN OF INNERVATION
Autonomic Innervation
The Spindle as a Receptor
  INPUT-OUTPUT PROPERTIES
  INPUT-OUTPUT CONVERSION
  FUNCTIONAL ORGANIZATION OF SENSORY TERMINALS
Development
  ORGANOGENESIS AND INNERVATION
  TROPHIC AND TRANSCRIPTION FACTORS

Introduction

Muscle spindles are mechanoreceptors sensitive to muscle length and changes in muscle length that occur in the somatic muscles of tetrapod vertebrates. They are composed of small (*intrafusal*) muscle fibers that lie as bundles in parallel with ordinary (*extrafusal*) muscle fibers, their ends attached to connective tissue, tendon, or extrafusal endomysium. They receive both a motor and a sensory innervation. The sensory innervation, which responds to active and passive changes in muscle length, is protected by a fusiform, fluid-filled capsule and occupies the *equatorial region* of the intrafusal bundle, whereas the motor innervation is distributed to the *polar regions* that extend on each side. Activation of the motor innervation elicits contractions in the polar regions that modify the sensory discharge.

The nonmammalian spindle is supplied with one sensory ending and receives its motor innervation from branches of axons that also innervate extrafusal muscle fibers.[1] Mammalian spindles are supplied with a *primary* sensory ending (the homologue of the sensory ending in nonmammalian spindles) and may, in addition, be supplied with one or more *secondary* sensory endings. Their motor innervation involves two components: an exclusively intrafusal system provided by specialized *fusimotor* (γ) neurons, and a *skeletofusimotor* (or so-called β) system, in which intrafusal and extrafusal muscle fibers are collaterally innervated, as in nonmammalian spindles. Each system contains two functional types of motor neuron (*dynamic* and *static*) whose activation produces different effects on the response of the primary ending.

This chapter is about mammalian spindles. It is mostly about those of the cat because more is known about them than any others. Such information as there is about spindles of other eutherian mammals, including humans, indicates that they do not differ qualitatively in any radical respect from those in the cat. A typical spindle in a cat's hindlimb muscle (see Fig. 21-1) consists of a 7- to 10-mm-long bundle of six to nine muscle fibers that is richly vascularized, partly encapsulated (generally the middle third), and innervated by a spindle nerve that leaves a nearby intramuscular nerve trunk to enter the equatorial region. Three kinds of muscle fiber can be recognized on the basis of differences in length, diameter, equatorial nucleation, ultrastructure, and histochemistry. Two of these, the longest and thickest, share a similar morphology and were originally called *nuclear-bag fibers* because for a short length in the equatorial region they contain few myofibrils and are full of round vesicular nuclei, thus forming what Barker described as a *nuclear bag*.[2] The distinguishing properties of the two types, now called bag_1 and bag_2 fibers, are described below, but their morphologic similarity should not be allowed to disguise their fundamental differences (see virtually any recent textbook of neuroscience for this error). The shortest and thinnest fibers contain a single central row of nuclei in the equatorial region and are called *nuclear-chain fibers* or simply *chain fibers*[3] (see Fig. 21-1D). There are usually one bag_1 fiber, one bag_2 fiber, and four to seven chain fibers in each spindle.

The site of the equatorial nuclei is occupied by a primary ending, supplied by a group Ia axon. Secondary endings supplied by group II axons may also be present adjacent to the primary. The motor innervation consists of a *trail ending*[4] and two types of plate, designated p_1 and p_2,[5,6] all of which may be variably present. The p_1 *plates* are supplied by β axons, the p_2 *plates* and trail endings by γ axons. Dynamic fusimotor actions are mediated by the bag_1 fiber and static actions by the bag_2 and chain fibers. Apart from this somatic innervation, some spindles also receive autonomic axons that are in neuroeffective association mainly with the intrafusal muscle fibers.[7]

The following sections are restricted to descriptions of the structure, innervation, and development of the mammalian spindle, with some account of how it functions. Recent reviews of work on these topics include those of Poppele,[8] Barker and Banks,[9] Hunt,[10] and Zelená[11]; for reviews that deal also with nonmammalian spindles, see Barker,[1] Hunt,[12] and Maier.[13] The proceedings of international symposia held in Paris (1991),[14] Glasgow (1993),[15] and London (1994)[16] provide useful sources for recent research papers. We have been obliged by limitations of space to remove from consideration the regeneration and reinnervation of spindles that we had included on pages 394 to 395 of our review in the second edi-

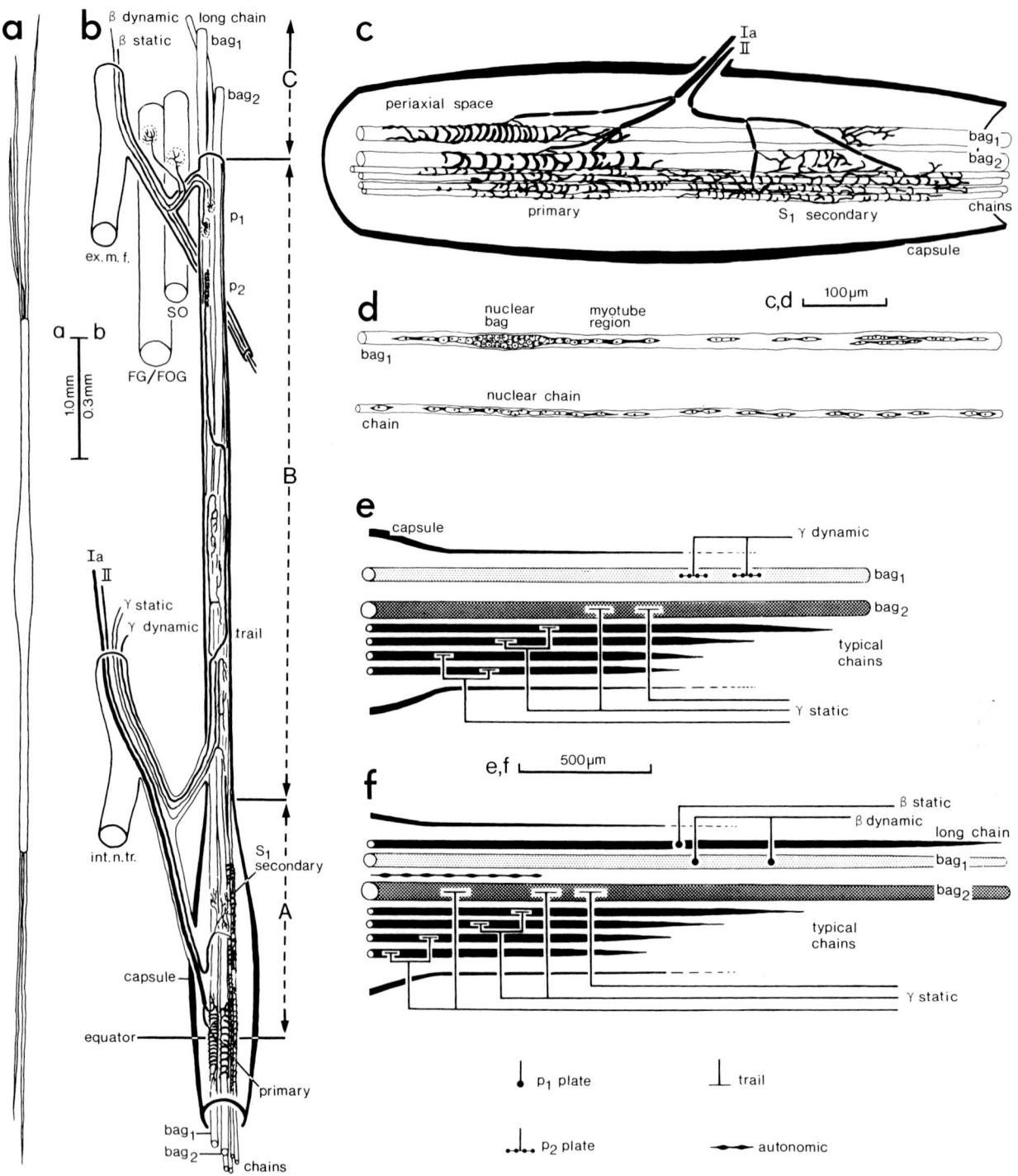

FIGURE 21-1. Schema illustrating the structure and innervation of mammalian muscle spindles, as exemplified by the cat tenuissimus. *a.* The encapsulated bundle of intrafusal muscle fibers that constitutes a spindle. *b.* The equatorial region and part of one pole illustrating the descriptive regions *a, b, c* and innervation by Ia and II sensory and β and γ motor axons. Abbreviations: ex.m.f. = extrafusal muscle fibers; FG/FOG = fast glycolytic or fast oxidative-glycolytic muscle fiber; SO = slow oxidative muscle fiber. *c.* Sensory innervation comprising a primary ending and an S_1 secondary ending, in this instance. The distribution of the total terminal contact area of a primary ending is about 35 percent bag_1, 25 percent bag_2, 40 percent chains; of an S_1 secondary, 10 percent bag_1, 20 percent bag_2, 70 percent chains. *d.* Nuclear-bag and nuclear-chain intrafusal muscle fibers showing nucleation in primary and S_1 secondary regions. *e.* and *f.* Motor innervation of a typical pole (e). The most common variation (f) is for static and dynamic β axons to participate in the motor innervation. Some spindles receive a nonvascular autonomic innervation. *a–d.* Features drawn to the scale of average dimensions. *c* and *d.* Based on reconstructions.[60] *e* and *f.* Schematic diagrams.

tion of *Myology*[9]—topics that have also been reviewed by Zelená.[11] For more recent work on regeneration, see Maier[17] and Soukup and Novotova.[18] The functional role of the spindle as an element of a motor control system is altogether too large a subject to receive any attention here other than to note that the reviews by Whelan[19] and Bosco and Poppele[20] can serve as introductions to it and its extensive literature.

Number and Distribution

TYPES OF SPINDLE UNIT

Spindles occur singly or may be variously combined in groups or intimately associated with tendon organs. The functional significance of the single encapsulated receptor with its sensory and motor innervation is sometimes stressed by using the term *spindle unit.* Spindle units may be linked in series as *tandem spindles*[21] or combined in pairs in which the intrafusal bundles either remain separately encapsulated or equatorially share a common capsule.[22] Richmond and colleagues[23-25] have shown that in cat neck and intervertebral muscles many spindle units are linked together in tandem and compound fashion to form *spindle complexes*. In rat deep masseter, some spindles are crowded together to form *spindle clusters* of up to 40 spindle units, a few of which share a common capsule.[26]

The standard spindle unit is provided with one bag_1 fiber, one bag_2 fiber, and about half a dozen chain fibers, but variations can occur in the complement of any of the three types of intrafusal fiber. For example, absence of the bag_1 fiber may occur, most commonly in certain tandem spindle units.[27]

NUMBER

From the tables published by Voss,[28] it can be estimated that the human body possesses about 50,000 spindles. The total number of axons, both afferent and efferent, involved in their innervation must be far greater. The characteristic numbers of spindles possessed by different muscles have normally been compared using spindle density, which is simply the number of capsules per gram of the adult muscle. On this basis it is often stated (e.g., Cooper,[29] Zelená[11]) that spindles are relatively common in small muscles involved in fine control, such as the intrinsic muscles of the hand.

Spindle density, however, is useful as a relative measure of abundance in muscles of different size only if, on average, the number of capsules tends to scale directly with muscle mass. Banks and Stacey[30] used data from three species (rat, cat, and human) that range in body size over more than two orders of magnitude to show that this was not so. Logarithmic transformations of the number of capsules (n) and the muscle weight in grams (m) yielded a linear regression of the form $y = 0.32x + 1.58$, where $y = \log_{10} n$ and $x = \log_{10} m$. The slope of the regression relationship (0.32) is geometrically significant, since it is virtually identical to that (0.33) which would be expected for a feature scaling isometrically with dimensions of length.

In principle, the relative abundance of spindles in a particular muscle, independent of its size, may be expressed as the amount by which the actual number of capsules deviates from the number expected on the basis of the regression relationship. In the original sample, this varied from 0.13 (or − 0.88 log units) for the infrahyoideus to 5.4 (or + 0.73 log units) for the intertransversarius C2-C3, both from the cat. Furthermore, muscles sharing broadly similar functions within and between species have similar distributions about the regression. Thus there are relatively few spindles in shoulder-girdle muscles and relatively many in dorsal neck muscles, whereas hindlimb muscles often have close to average, or typical, numbers.

Muscles operating synergistically about a joint often differ considerably in size. The combination of high spindle density with low force output in the small as compared with the large muscles of a synergistic group suggested to Peck and coworkers[31] that the small muscles are functionally specialized as "kinesiological monitors." It is now clear, however, that their relatively high spindle densities are a direct consequence of the small size of these muscles and that, in general, they are not specialized in respect of their spindle complement. As a specific example, consider the tenuissimus of the cat, which crosses both hip and knee joints yet weighs a mere 0.28 g. With an average of 16.7 capsules, its spindle density (60 g^{-1}) and lack of any obvious mechanical function have led some authors to suggest a sensory role for the muscle. However, the regression relationship shows that a typical muscle of the same size would be expected to have about 25 capsules, thus contradicting the hypothetical sensory specialization.

In the preliminary analysis by Banks and Stacey,[30] it was tacitly assumed that the function relating number of spindles to muscle mass within a species was the same as that between species. A more recent analysis[32] has shown that this is not so. The human species is the only one for which an almost complete data set is available.[28] In this case the regression relationship derived from a log:log plot of spindle number against muscle mass has the form $y = 0.50x + 1.31$. Although at 0.5 the slope is very different from the isometric relationship seen between species (and confirmed in the new analysis), it is again geometrically very significant as the square-root function. That a similar function exists within other species is indicated by a comparison of a subset of human muscles homologous to those from the cat, for which quantitative data are available, the two samples showing virtually identical regression slopes intermediate between the isometric and square-root values. The relative abundance of spindles in human muscles, based on the square-root relationship and expressed linearly, ranges from 0.13 for digastricus to 8.91 for longissimus capitis (only two muscles, pterygoideus lateralis and mylohyoideus, are recorded by Voss[28] as having no spindles). The intrinsic muscles of the hand, long regarded on the basis of spindle density as the paradigm of an abundant supply of spindles being related to fine control, emerge from the new analysis as quite unexceptional. Lumbricalis manus III (1.64 g, 26 spindles), for example, has a relative abundance of 1.01. Immediately below it in rank order is adductor magnus (487.5 g, 437 spindles), with a relative abundance of 1.00.

DISTRIBUTION

Several detailed maps are available showing the distribution of spindles and other encapsulated receptors in a variety of muscles. Some of the best, together with additional references, are given in van der Wal.[33] Two important features of the distribution of spindles emerge from the maps, as originally described by Gregor[34] and Yellin,[35] respectively: (1) Spindles are concentrated in the region of nerve entry and around the subdivisions of the intramuscular nerves, and (2) they occur preferentially among extrafusal fibers with a high proportion of oxidative [slow oxidative (SO)* and fast oxidative-glycolytic (FOG)] types. It should be noted, however, that these two features are not necessarily independent of each other.

Cameron et al.[36] refer to the differential sensitivity of spindles to surrounding, adjacent, and distant motor units as "sensory partitioning" of the muscle. It is, of course, an inevitable consequence of the mechanical relationships of the spindles and motor units, but it is likely to be of functional importance only if, as Cameron et al. suggest, there are local (intramuscular) reflexes. However, these do not seem to occur,[37] despite evidence for a degree of intramuscular somatotopic organization of both motor neurons and spindles.[38,39] Conversely, in a simply structured muscle whose motor-unit architecture appears to rule out local reflexes, differential distribution of spindles is still present.[40] An extensive discussion of sensory partitioning may be found in the review by Windhorst and colleagues.[41]

It has been argued that it is functionally appropriate for spindles to be particularly associated with oxidative motor units, since these are recruited first and are thought to be especially important in small postural movements.[42] One might, then, reasonably expect spindles to be particularly abundant in muscles with an overall high proportion of oxidative fibers, but there is no evidence for this when the relative abundance of spindles in various cat muscles is compared with the proportion of oxidative fibers in them. It may be, as Richmond and Stuart[43] suggest, that spindles occur among predominantly oxidative (S) fibers because this allows them to sample the activity of all motor units, including the fast, fatigable (glycolytic) type. If so, it is not clear why the spindles are still unevenly distributed in cat soleus, which consists only of S fibers, nor why spindles are so often clumped, as is particularly noticeable in muscles especially rich in them (the spindle complexes of Bakker and Richmond,[25] for example).

Intriguing as are many of the functional speculations concerning the intramuscular distribution of spindles, they remain unconvincing. We are left with the clear association between spindles and subdivisions of the intramuscular nerves. If the total number of spindles in a particular muscle (but not their precise distribution) is a controlled variable of muscle design and if, as seems likely on the evidence from studies on early spindle development (see below), Ia and α axons compete for sites on primary myotubes, the observed distribution of spindles would be expected, especially when it is borne in mind that α axons branch much more freely than Ia axons.

---

*A list of abbreviations used in this chapter is given at the end of the chapter.

Capsule and Vascular Supply

The *outer capsule* is a lamellated structure that encloses the sensory innervation within a fusiform dilation and extends as a sleeve on each side to enclose part of each pole. The lamellae are composed of layers of thin, flat cells arranged in concentric tubular fashion alternating with collagenous and elastic fibrils. Each *capsular sheet cell*[44] is surrounded by a basal lamina and closely interdigitates with its neighbors to form a continuous layer one cell thick. The outermost capsular layer is composed of thick collagenous fibrils and scattered fibrocytes. The innermost layer is composed of a lining of fibrocytes, some of which cross the periaxial space to join other cells of the same type that enclose individual intrafusal muscle fibers (the *inner capsule*). The cells of both the inner and outer capsule express the transcription factor gene *Pax-7* in adult mouse spindles, as shown by in situ hybridization,[45] but the significance of this is unknown.

The capsular sheet cells are continuous with the cells that form the perineurium of the spindle nerve and, according to Low,[46] may confidently be equated with them. Tight junctions between capsular sheet cells[47] act as a barrier to the diffusion of substances into the periaxial space in the same way that the perineurium acts as a diffusion barrier in peripheral nerves. Such junctions are presumably located in the inner layers of the capsule, since horseradish peroxidase (HRP) flooded directly onto the living spindle penetrates the outer layers but fails to enter the periaxial space.[48] After systemic injection of HRP, Dow and coworkers[49] showed that passive flow of the tracer into the periaxial space was prevented by the capsular cell's tight junctions, but there was some leakage into the poles through the open end of each capsule sleeve.

The periaxial space is full of a highly viscous gel containing the glycosaminoglycan hyaluronate.[50,51] Following long-term deafferentation, the space disappears or is greatly diminished.[52] The origin of the periaxial fluid and its functions are uncertain. Fukami[51] has shown that a transcapsular potential of -15 mV is due in part to a relatively high $[K^+]$ in the fluid, which may contribute to the excitability of the endings.

Capillaries course for long distances between capsular layers; they are invariably present in the periaxial space of rabbit spindles[53] but only occasionally so in those of cat. In rabbit tenuissimus spindles, Miyoshi and Kennedy[54] have shown that there is a short direct pathway from the main muscle artery to the spindle capillaries, which are separate from those supplying extrafusal muscle and different from them in being larger and having intercellular tight junctions. The capillaries supplying intramuscular nerves are similar, and HRP injected intraaortically does not leak from either nerve or spindle capillaries, whereas it leaks rapidly from those supplying extrafusal muscle.[48] A blood–nervous system barrier, therefore, obtains in both endoneurial and periaxial spaces.

According to the descriptions of Cooper and Gladden[55] and Gladden,[56] elastic fibers are most numerous around the bag_2 fiber and anchor the spindle at each end to the elastic fiber network among extrafusal muscle fibers. In passing through the spindle, they branch to form smaller fibers that travel alongside muscle fibers or within intercellular spaces in the inner and outer capsules. Observations by Banks[57] have revealed that the bag fibers have peg-like projections on their surface over a length of 300 to 400 μm on either side of the primary region. Each projection slants toward the equator and appears to serve as an anchoring point for an elastic fiber originating from the opposite pole. Such attachments must greatly enhance the elastic properties of the primary region.

Intrafusal Muscle Fibers

LENGTH, DIAMETER, AND NUCLEATION

In most spindles, the bag_2 is the longest intrafusal fiber. Kucera[58] reports mean polar lengths of 2947 μm for bag_2 fibers, 2760 μm for bag_1 fibers, and 1382 μm for chain fibers (tenuissimus, frozen sections). In 77 percent of 313 spindle poles, the bag_2 was the longest fiber, in 14 percent, the bag_1 was the longest; in 3 percent, the bag fibers were of equal length; and in 6 percent, the longest was a chain fiber. Mean juxtaequatorial diameters (inner region B, as defined in Fig. 21-1) given by Boyd[59] are 16.86 ± 2.35 μm for bag fibers and 8.37 ± 1.85 μm for chains (tenuissimus, Susa fixation, paraffin sections). No systematic study of intrafusal muscle-fiber diameters has been made since it was established that there are two types of bag fiber. All types of fiber become thinner as they pass through the equatorial region (once again, contrast this with most textbook representations!), and those that extend well into region C tend to become thickest in this region. This is most notable for the bag_1 fibers of superficial lumbrical (flexores superficialies) muscles of the cat hindfoot, where their diameter can resemble that of a small extrafusal fiber.[22] The presence of a secondary ending adjacent to the primary results in the bag fibers undergoing a marked increase in diameter at the sites where they receive secondary terminals.[60]

The nuclei of intrafusal muscle fibers are located either peripherally underneath the sarcolemma (subsarcolemmal nuclei), as in the polar regions, or internally among the myofibrils (myonuclei), as in the equatorial region. Satellite cells occur mostly in association with bag_2 fibers in region C; they are less frequently associated with the bag_1 fibers and rarely occur on chain fibers.[61]

ULTRASTRUCTURE

Observations on the ultrastructure of intrafusal muscle fibers that were made before the present classification of fiber types was fully established have been reviewed by Barker.[1] It is now apparent that the fibers display two types of myofibrillar ultrastructure, which for convenience have been designated M and dM, according to the appearance of the M line.[62,63] In the M condition, the M line appears as a single prominent line at low power or as five parallel faint lines at high power; the discrete myofibrils are separated by sarcoplasm rich in glycogen, mitochondria, and membranous systems (transverse tubules and sarcoplasmic reticulum). In the dM condition, the M line either cannot be seen or appears as two parallel faint lines,[64] and there is very little interfibrillar sarcoplasm. Chain fibers have the M type of ultrastructure, whereas, remarkably, the bag fibers are a mixture of both M and dM. Unpublished observations by us suggest that the transition from M to dM is from a five- to a four- to a two-line substructure, the middle line being lost first, followed by the two outermost lines. In the bag_1 fiber, the ultrastructure is dM in region A and most of region B; it then changes to the M condition toward the outer end of region B. The sarcomere length is consistently longer than in the bag_2 or chain fibers.[65] In the bag_2 fiber, the condition is dM in region A and changes to M at level A/B,[63,65] though the membranous systems become progressively less developed toward the polar end in region C.[66]

HISTOCHEMISTRY

The histochemical profiles of intrafusal muscle fibers are similar to those of extrafusal fibers in that they vary according to fiber type but are dissimilar in that they are subject to regional variation. The three fiber types—bag_1, bag_2, and chain—differ in their glycogen content and in their profiles of the enzymes adenosine triphosphatase (ATPase), phosphorylase, and nicotinamide adenine dinucleotide tetrazolium reductase (NADH-TR).[65,67–69]

The technique most favored for demonstrating fiber type is that which stains ATPase, as it enables the types to be checked against the different staining reactions that follow alkaline or acid preincubation of the sections. The profiles of the bag fibers but not those of the chains show regional variation; the optimum level for distinguishing between fiber types is midregion B (see Fig. 21-2). In transverse sections cut

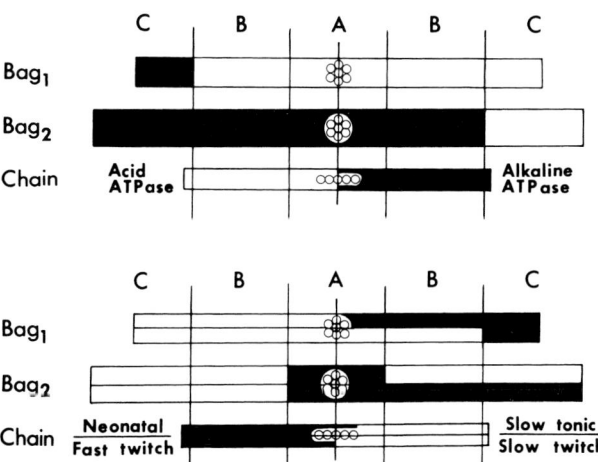

FIGURE 21-2. Schematic summary (top) of the general patterns of ATPase reactivity (black is high) following acid and alkaline preincubation in rat intrafusal fibers; and (bottom) reactivity of the three intrafusal fiber types with antibodies against slow-tonic MHC, slow-twitch MHC, neonatal MHC, and fast-twitch MHC. (*Modified from Pedrosa F, Butler-Browne GS, Dhoot GK, et al: Diversity in expression of myosin heavy chain isoforms and M-band proteins in rat muscle spindles. Histochemistry 92:185–194, 1989. With permission.*)

at this level, the staining intensities for alkali-stable ATPase are low for bag_1, medium or high for bag_2, and high for chains, whereas the staining for acid-stable ATPase is low for bag_1, high for bag_2, and low for chains.

The use of immunohistologic techniques has shown that the differences in ATPase activity between the three types of intrafusal muscle fiber reflect differences in their possession of various isoforms of the myosin heavy chain (MHC). Thus bag fibers have been shown to contain slow-tonic MHC (mostly in bag_1) and slow-twitch MHC (mostly in bag_2), whereas chain fibers are characterized by fast-twitch and neonatal MHC (see Fig. 21-2).[70–74] Slow-tonic MHC, such as is found in the slow-tonic muscles of frogs and birds, does not occur extrafusally in mammalian skeletal muscles, though it is present in the slow-tonic portions of the extraocular muscles.[75] The bag fibers are also unique in mammalian skeletal muscle in that they react positively to anti-α cardiac MHC (mostly bag_2)[74,76] and antiembryonic MHC (mostly bag_1).[77] The fast-twitch MHC (which occurs in bag_2 as well as chain fibers) differs from that of the surrounding type 2 extrafusal fibers but appears to be similar to that of fast-twitch avian muscle.[74] In rat spindles, reactivity to antibodies against M-band proteins and the MM form of creatine kinase[73] is, as might be expected, negative for bag_1 fibers, whose myofibrillar ultrastructure is dM throughout[63]; mixed for bag_2 fibers, which switch from the dM to the M condition; and positive for the chain fibers, which are M throughout. Most of the immunohistologic work has been done on rat spindles. When other species have been used, some species-specific differences have emerged—e.g., embryonic MHC is present in cat chain fibers but absent from rat and rabbit chain fibers.[77]

Sensory Innervation

The first detailed account of spindle sensory innervation in terms of its distribution to the three types of intrafusal muscle fiber was given by Banks and coworkers,[60] who used reconstruction, electron microscopy, and examination of teased silver preparations. In addition to their description of the form of the primary and secondary endings, they noted that the number of secondary endings in individual spindles followed a binomial frequency distribution. The terminals of the primary ending were further studied by Banks,[78] and the numbers of sensory endings by Banks and Stacey.[30,79] The descriptions given under the next three subheadings are based on these studies unless otherwise indicated. An account of recent studies on the functional organization of the sensory terminals, mainly using immunocytochemistry, may be found under "The Spindle as a Receptor," below.

PRIMARY ENDINGS

The primary ending terminates on the densely nucleated equatorial parts of the intrafusal muscle fibers (the nuclear bags, myotubes, and nuclear chains) and occupies a length of about 350 μm. The terminals are annulospiral in form.[80] Spirals are more common and more extensive around chain fibers than around bag fibers; rings are formed by blind-ended terminals that wind once around an intrafusal fiber before abutting against themselves.

In three primary endings reconstructed from serial sections, bag_1 fibers received more terminals (on average, 5.7 separately derived from nonmyelinated preterminal axonal branches) than did bag_2 fibers (2.7 on average), and both received more than chain fibers (average of 0.7 per fiber). Sensory cross terminals[81] occurred frequently in all three endings. They were formed exclusively among chain fibers, a feature that, taken together with regions of close apposition between fibers of this type,[82] may be attributed to the incomplete separation of chain fibers during development (see "Development," below) and correlates with the fact that chain fibers frequently contract as a group on fusimotor stimulation.[83]

Within a primary ending the terminals are not symmetrically distributed, and the form of each one depends on its location in the complete system. On the bag fibers, for example, pure spirals are confined to those parts of the terminals that happen to overlie the nuclear bag. Despite close similarity in the overall form of the three reconstructed endings, the domains of individual terminals varied considerably between the endings (Fig. 21-3). Thus, underlying the constant overall form of the primary ending, there is an independently varying finer level of organization.

Ultrastructural studies of primary axon terminals (reviewed by Barker[1]) have shown that they lie in shallow grooves on the surface of the muscle fibers, forming smooth myoneural junctions. In contrast to the motor myoneural junctions, there is no intervening basal lamina, and the terminals are not covered by Schwann cells but rather by basal lamina continuous with that of the muscle fibers. This separation of the structural components of the sarcolemma is associated with an annulospiral pattern of the deficiency or absence of dystrophin, this being elsewhere associated with the sarcolemma of all three types of intrafusal fiber.[84]

In longitudinal sections of spindles the terminals are typically lenticular in profile, and it is immediately apparent that they are differentially indented into the three types of muscle fiber: most deeply in the chain and least in the bag_1 fibers (Fig. 21-4). The lenticular profile is consistent with the terminals being deformed from a condition of minimum energy and surface area (circular profile) by longitudinal tension in the muscle fibers as well as in the basal laminae that cover the outer surfaces of both the fibers and the terminals. If the basal laminae associated with the different types of intrafusal fiber have similar mechanical properties, the differential indentation of the fibers by the terminals would be due to the mechanical properties of the fibers. Moreover, increased static stretch of the spindle would be expected to increase standing tension in the basal laminae and muscle fibers, thereby also causing the radii of curvature of the outer and inner surfaces of the lenticular terminal profiles to increase. A preliminary study by Banks[79] bears this out (Fig. 21-4), and the proposed mechanism for transduction has been supported by Patten and Ovalle's scanning electron microscope (SEM) study of the terminals and basal laminae.[85]

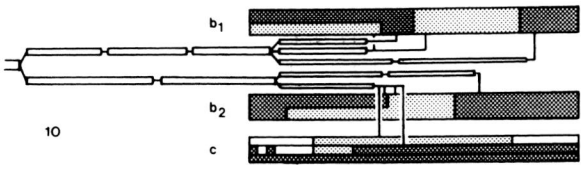
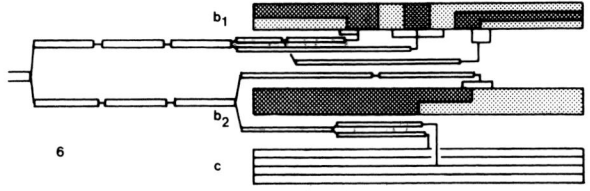
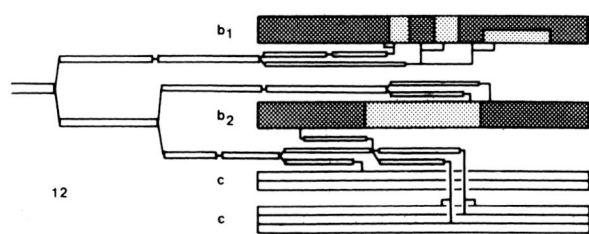

FIGURE 21-3. Diagrams showing the preterminal branches and terminal domains of primary endings innervating cat tenuissimus spindles reconstructed from serial longitudinal (spindle 10) or transverse (spindles 6 and 12) sections. In each case the parent axon (left) divides to form myelinated branches that ultimately give rise to several nonmyelinated branches, each of which distributes terminals within a separate domain. The approximate locations and extents of individual terminal domains are shaded; those belonging to the chain fibers in spindles 6 and 12 could not be determined. Despite close similarity in the overall form of all three endings, details of the preterminal branching patterns and terminal domains vary considerably. (From Banks RW: Observations on the primary sensory ending of tenuissimus muscle spindles in the cat. Cell Tissue Res 246:309–319, 1986. With permission.)

SECONDARY ENDINGS

Secondary endings terminate on one or both sides of the primary. The most we have seen on one side is five and on both sides, six. Each occupies a length of about 350 μm and is designated S_1, S_2, S_3, and so on, according to its position relative to the primary. Most secondaries terminate next to the primary in the S_1 position, though the proportion varies from muscle to muscle depending on the parameters of binomial frequency distributions (see "Number of Afferent Axons," below). Of 1250 secondary endings from a variety of mainly hindlimb muscles, the percentages of secondaries in the different locations were S_1, 71; S_2, 22; S_3, 6; S_4, 1; S_5, 0.3 (Banks and Stacey, unpublished results). The proportion of S_1 endings ranged from 56 percent in the complexus muscle to 100 percent in extensor digitorum lateralis. Chain fibers are innervated in all secondary endings, but few secondaries are restricted to chain fibers only; most are distributed to all three fiber types. Restriction of terminals to one or two fiber types is more prevalent among secondaries terminating in the more polar positions.

NUMBER OF AFFERENT AXONS

The provision of both Ia and II axons to the spindle complement of a muscle varies characteristically among different muscles and is therefore another controlled variable of the functional design of muscles. Since a single Ia axon is required to initiate and maintain a differentiated spindle (see "Development," below), the variability can be described by considering the number (a) of afferent axons supplied to individual spindles, additional to a single Ia. The parameter is expressed in this way, rather than as the number of secondary endings, to take account of those spindles whose primary endings appear to be supplied by two or more Ia axons, and of those II axons that branch within a spindle to

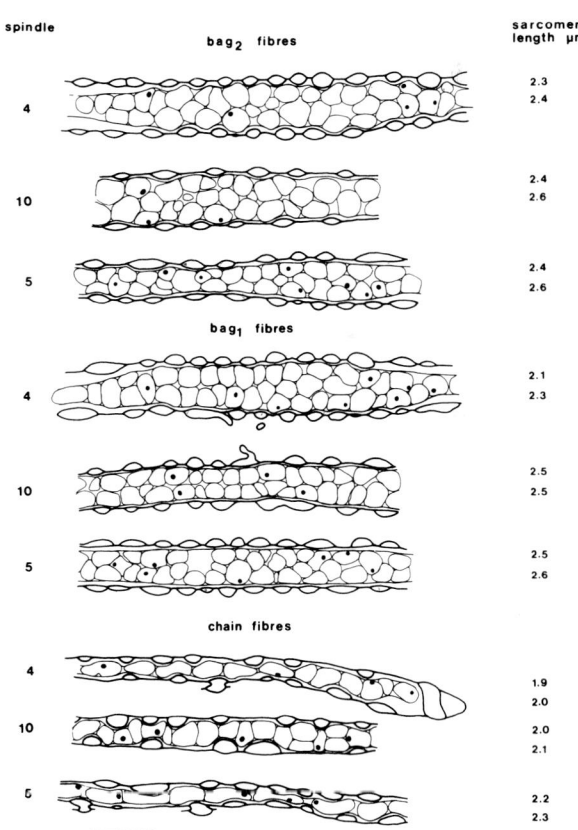

FIGURE 21-4. Tracings of 1-μm-thick longitudinal sections through the equatorial regions of the bag_2 fiber, bag_1 fiber, and one chain fiber from each of three cat tenuissimus spindles. Sections passing closest to the diameter of each fiber were selected. Mean sarcomere lengths of 50 sarcomeres on either side of the primary ending are given for each fiber. They are consistently shortest in spindle 4 and longest in spindle 5, suggesting increasing amounts of static stretch during fixation in the order 4, 10, 5. The terminals are progressively less indented into the bag fibers in the same order, but among the chain fibers only those of spindle 5 are clearly less indented than others. (From Banks RW: Observations on the primary sensory ending of tenuissimus muscle spindles in the cat. Cell Tissue Res 246:309–319, 1986. With permission.)

end in both S_1 positions. These features are rare in most cat muscles so far studied, though in certain muscles the proportion of spindles with primary endings supplied by two Ia axons is quite high (12 percent in EDL and 8 percent in popliteus). In rat masseter multiply-innervated primary endings are the rule (92 percent) rather than the exception and up to 5 axons may be involved[86]; they are also common in rat hindlimb muscles (Banks and Stacey, unpublished data).

In a sample of cat muscles, mainly from the hindlimb, the mean value of a varied from 0.56 in extensor digitorum lateralis to 3.5 in complexus. The greatest number of afferents occurred in a popliteus spindle with a complement of $S_2S_1PPS_1S_2S_3S_4$ (8 afferents). Frequency distributions for a are well described by binomial statistics, and they are also characteristic for different muscles (Fig. 21-5). This suggests that after the initial determinative contact by a Ia axon, the remaining, mostly II, afferents are distributed randomly among the developing spindles. If so, the greater availability of afferents at the point of nerve entry to the muscle might be expected to result in spindles close to this point receiving more afferents than average. This prediction is borne out by a study on tenuissimus, facilitated by its linear spindle arrangement.[79]

These results suggest that any afferent, Ia or II, entering the spindle during development should be able to make an ending capable of persisting into the adult. At first sight, it seems difficult to reconcile this with the observation[87] that transient multiple contacts of the future primary region by several presumed Ia axons occur in the early development of the rat hindlimb spindle. Whereas it is possible that supernumerary Ia afferents may be lost by "programmed" cell death, most of such loss of the dorsal-root ganglion cells occurs before their innervation of the muscle primordium.[88] The explanation may be that individual afferents are also making transient contacts with several presumptive spindles[87] and that the vast majority of them soon withdraw all but one of these contacts.

Motor Innervation

Analysis of the intrafusal distribution of motor axons and their endings has proved to be one of the most difficult problems in studies of the mammalian spindle and has led to much controversy. The interested reader will find accounts of the resolution of this problem in the second edition of *Myology*[9] and in Banks.[89] The following description is a simplified and updated version of the comprehensive review of the intrafusal motor innervation by Banks,[89] which should be consulted for detailed attributions.

THE γ MOTOR INNERVATION

The γ innervation is provided by small motor neurons that have an exclusively fusimotor distribution.[90] Each γ axon is distributed to several spindles, but in a selective manner so as to supply either bag_1 fibers or bag_2 and chain fibers. Exceptions to this dichotomy are rare in the cat but more common in the rat[91] and monkey,[92] though even in these species the overall distribution of the axons concerned may be predominantly of one kind or the other. The functional

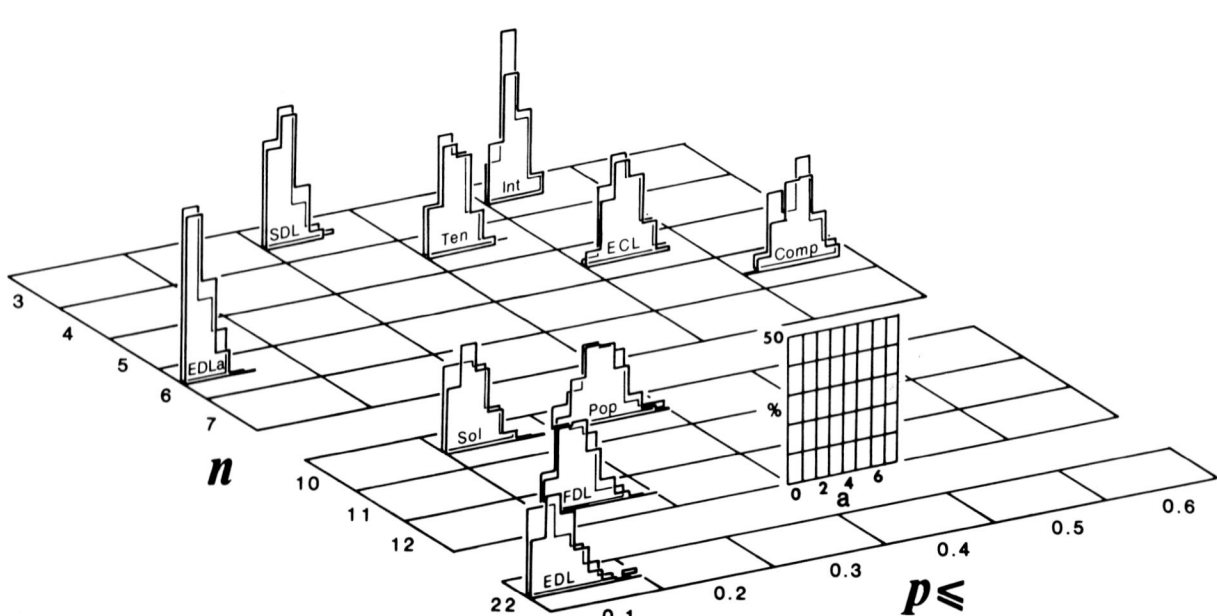

FIGURE 21-5. Pairs of histograms showing the observed distributions (rear of each pair) and best-fitting binomial distributions (front of each pair) of numbers of afferents (a) in excess of a single Ia for various cat muscles. The histograms are positioned on the grid according to their binomial parameters (n, p). Abbreviations: Comp(lexus); ECL, extensor caudae lateralis; EDLa, extensor digitorum lateralis; EDL, extensor digitorum longus; FDL, flexor digitorum longus; Int(erosseus); Pop(liteus); Sol(eus); SDL, superficial and deep lumbrical; Ten(uissimus). (*Modified from Banks R, Stacey M: Quantitative studies on mammalian muscle spindles, in Hník F, Soukup T, Vejsada R, Zelená J (eds): Mechanoreceptors. New York: Plenum Press, 1988; pp 263–269. With permission.*)

classification of γ motor neurons into dynamic and static types[93,94] corresponds with their segregated distribution, those having dynamic effects being distributed to bag$_1$ fibers. There is, however, no distinction between the axonal conduction velocities of the two types; both cover a range from 15 to 55 m s^{-1}.[95] In general, static γ axons seem to outnumber dynamic γ axons by about 3:1,[96] but the ratio may be much higher in tenuissimus.[97]

This muscle has proved to be particularly useful in studying the distribution of static γ axons because of its almost linear arrangement of spindles. Individual primary endings can be located and their responses to fusimotor stimulation correlated with directly observed intrafusal contractions and with the pattern of motor innervation subsequently observed histologically. Boyd[98] showed that different types of static effect could be related to either bag$_2$ or chain fiber activity and went on to use the relationship to infer the distribution of individual static axons in several spindles.[99,100] Some of the spindles were subsequently analyzed by serial section for light and electron microscopy.[101–103] Boyd and colleagues concluded that there are two types of static axon whose neuromuscular junctions display different postjunctional characteristics. According to Boyd,[100] one type always innervates bag$_2$ fibers, whereas the other always innervates chain fibers, but neither is restricted to its characteristic effector. Gladden and Sutherland[104] later suggested that there may, in addition, be a third type that exclusively supplies chain fibers.

Against this, it has been our experience[105] that postjunctional structure is related to muscle fiber type and to location of motor endings with respect to the primary ending rather than to axonal type, and Kucera and Walro[106] have described similar relationships. Furthermore, Banks[97] has used a tenuissimus preparation combined with silver histology to produce an independent correlation of primary responses to static stimulation with motor innervation patterns. He found no evidence for two or more distinct kinds of static γ axon but did find that static γ axons were differentially distributed according to conduction velocity (see Table 21-1). Faster-conducting axons tended to be more widely distributed and less likely to innervate chain fibers alone than slower ones. In the innervation of individual spindles, axons that produced 1:1 driving were likely to be the slowest-conducting static axons supplying the spindles concerned, even though they might not have the slowest conduction velocity of all the static axons supplying the muscle. It could be argued that as the tenuissimus is unusual mechanically, it might be atypical in this respect as well, so it is important to note that entirely consistent results have been obtained by Celichowski et al.[107] in peroneus tertius and by Emonet-Dénand and coworkers[108] in peroneus longus. The results from these larger muscles have necessarily been obtained using exclusively physiologic criteria for identifying the intrafusal distribution of individual static γ axons,[107] the bases of which have recently been critically examined by Petit et al.[109]

Experiments involving cortical, brainstem, or reflex activation of intrafusal muscle fibers have been interpreted as supporting the subdivision of static γ axons into two kinds.[110–112] The existence of a differential distribution of a single population of axons might provide sufficient segregation to account for these observations. Nevertheless, functional segregation of bag$_2$ and chain fiber activation is undoubtedly far from complete; further evidence, presented below (see "The Pattern of Innervation"), raises serious doubts about the existence of functional benefits arising from a segregated bag$_2$/chain system.

Table 21-1. SYMBOLIC REPRESENTATION OF THE EFFECTS OF STIMULATING γ-EFFERENTS ON THE RESPONSES OF PRIMARY ENDINGS IN A CAT TENUISSIMUS MUSCLE[a]

Efferents by cv	D	E	A	J	B	H	C	No. of spindles
41	●	●	●	●	○	—	○	6
40	—	—	●	●	●	●	●	5
33	●	○	●	—	○	▲	▲	6
31	—	—	○	○	—	—	—	2
30	—	▲	—	—	—	—	—	1
28	—	—	—	●	—	—	—	1
27	▲	—	—	—	—	▲	—	2
27	▲	—	●	—	○	—	—	3
24	—	—	—	●	—	—	—	1
23	❑	❑	❑	❑	❑	—	—	5
No. static	4	3	5	5	4	3	3	
No. dynamic	1	1	1	1	1	0	0	
Total	5	4	6	6	5	3	3	

Header for afferent columns: Afferents: proximal → distal

[a]Each row shows the effects of a single efferent on the several primaries activated by it: —, no effect; ●, biasing; ○, indeterminate; ▲, 1:1 driving; ❑, dynamic. The afferents are arranged in the proximal-to-distal sequence of their corresponding spindles and are identified alphabetically according to the order in which they were isolated. Efferents are arranged by conduction velocity (cv, in m/s) as shown in the column at the left; the total number of spindles supplied by each one is given in the column at the right. The numbers of efferents supplying each spindle are summarized at the bottom of the table in the corresponding column.

SOURCE: Banks.[97]

THE β MOTOR INNERVATION

Physiologic evidence for the existence of mammalian skeletofusimotor, later referred to as β,[113] axons was first demonstrated by Bessou and colleagues[114,115] in the first deep lumbrical muscle of the cat. They showed that the repetitive stimulation of such axons not only produced extrafusal contraction but also activated spindles by increasing the dynamic sensitivity of the primary ending. Histologic evidence was provided by Adal and Barker,[116] who traced the intramuscular branching of the motor supply to this muscle in teased osmium tetroxide preparations and showed that it included fibers that had a skeletofusimotor distribution. These had a diameter range of 6.0 to 12.5 μm, which corresponded well with the slow conduction velocities (31 to 61 m s^{-1}) of the skeletofusimotor axons described by Bessou and associates.[115] As osmium tetroxide stains only myelin, no information was obtained on the form and location of the intrafusal β terminals, but Barker and coworkers[117] recognized these as p_1 plates in their teased silver preparations, with a bag/chain fiber distribution of 75/25. The fact that β axons terminated in p_1 plates was later demonstrated in spindles deprived of their γ innervation by degeneration.[118]

Barker and colleagues[117] observed that p_1 innervation was widespread in cat hindlimb muscles and considered it unlikely that the presence of a skeletofusimotor innervation was a vestigial feature, as had been suggested.[115,119] In flexor hallucis longus, they found that 73 percent of spindle poles were innervated by p_1 plates. They argued that this proportion was too high for them all to have been supplied by the collaterals of slow-conducting β axons, and suggested that the deficit was made up by fast β axons.

The use of the glycogen-depletion technique, combined with ATPase staining for muscle fiber type, showed that the intrafusal contraction produced by slow dynamic β (βd) axons was almost exclusively restricted to bag_1 fibers, and that the extrafusal contraction was confined to SO fibers.[120, 121] The predicted existence of fast β axons was confirmed by glycogen-depletion studies on peroneus tertius by Harker et al.[122] and Jami et al.[123] These showed that fast β axons selectively depleted long chain fibers,[122] were static in action, and activated FOG fibers.[124]

Skeletofusimotor axons are now regarded as an integral feature of the somatic neuromuscular system in mammals. Estimates by Jami and associates,[124] based on the physiologic identification of β axons with conduction velocities of 55 m s^{-1} or more (any slower β axons would have been excluded), indicate that at least 50 percent of the spindles in peroneus tertius receive a β innervation and that one-third of the supply is dynamic and two-thirds static. Apart from the occurrence of β axons in cat spindles, there is physiologic evidence for their existence in rabbit,[125] rat,[126] and monkey[127–129] spindles, and histologic evidence in rat,[91] rabbit,[64] monkey,[126,130] and human[131] spindles. Reconstructions of rat[91] and monkey[130] spindles have shown that the β innervation is selectively distributed to the bag_1 and long chain fibers, as in cat spindles. Some distal muscles of the rat's tail contain spindles that lack any γ innervation and are activated entirely by β axons, dynamic and static.[126,132]

In his review of intrafusal motor innervation, Banks[89] concluded that the skeletofusimotor supply is provided by α motor neurons that happen to have encountered spindles during development, and that consequently there is no distinct category of β motor neuron. However, we retain the use of the terms *β innervation* and *β axon* for descriptive convenience.

THE PATTERN OF INNERVATION

It is useful to summarize the present view of how motor axons are "wired up" in cat hindlimb spindles. Inevitably the view is based on tenuissimus, because most is known about spindles in this muscle. The following summary is based largely on teased, silver-impregnated spindles[97,133–135] supplemented by serial-section reconstructions.[133,136–139] On average each spindle, containing one bag_1, one bag_2, and four chain fibers, receives branches of nearly 7 motor axons in a range of 2 to 13. The frequency of occurrence of different numbers of branches follows a binomial distribution, indicating that the branches are randomly distributed with respect to the spindles. It is usually possible to identify the intrafusal branches of β and γ axons by their presynaptic form.[105,135] They number 1 to 6 (mean 3.2) and 1 to 7 (mean 3.8), respectively. In each case they appear to be randomly distributed to their spindles. However, the number of afferent axons additional to a single Ia also follows a binomial frequency distribution (see "Number of Afferent Axons," above), and there is a very clear tendency for spindles with more afferents to receive more γ branches, though there is no relationship between the numbers of β branches and afferents. Banks[135] has suggested that this reflects the different requirements of γ and β branches for guidance during development. Consistent with this view is the observation that in mice carrying a targeted deletion of the gene for neurotrophin-3, both Ia afferents and γ motor neurons (but not α motor neurons) are absent from muscles innervated by spinal segments but are present in some that receive trigeminal innervation[140] (see "Development," below). Also, Tourtellotte et al.[141] have found that survival of γ but not α spinal motor neurons is dependent on glial cell line–derived neurotrophic factor (GDNF) in vivo.

The bag_1 fiber is almost always separately innervated, receiving 38 percent (mean of 3 muscles, range 34 to 41 percent) of the motor branches in cat tenuissimus spindles.[135] Tenuissimus seems to have very few dynamic γ axons, and in some cases they may be absent altogether. Most of the branches to bag_1 fibers in our sample are derived from β axons. Occasionally the bag_1 fiber is coinnervated with a long chain pole, but these account for less than 1 percent of the total motor branches. Static β branches supplied exclusively to long chain poles amount to a further 8 percent of the total, leaving the balance of 53 percent (range 49 to 56 percent) supplied to bag_2 or chain fibers or both. These are almost without exception branches of static γ axons. The proportion that coinnervates both types of fiber in this group is quite variable, ranging in our sample from 17 to 40 percent.

The bag_2 and chain fibers may receive a completely segregated input in each pole, or a completely mixed input, or an input variously segregated—e.g., a branch to bag_2 alone plus another to the bag_2 and chain fibers. Examples are shown in Fig. 21-6. When analyzed without reference to the sensory innervation, poles with different degrees of segregated input appear to be randomly associated in complete spindles; but if account is taken of the occurrence of secondary endings in each pole, then a relationship between the sensory and motor systems again emerges. However, the relationship is not what would be expected if a segregated motor supply to the bag_2 and chain fibers were functionally desirable. Thus the degree of segregation in the motor input increases rapidly, then more slowly, as first one pole and then the other receives secondary endings. Ultimately, as more static γ branches enter, the degree of segregation may actually fall, since complete segregation is most likely to occur when only two branches supply each pole. What is remarkable is that when secondary endings are present in only one pole, it is that pole which normally receives the more segregated static γ input, despite the fact that such segregation is virtually

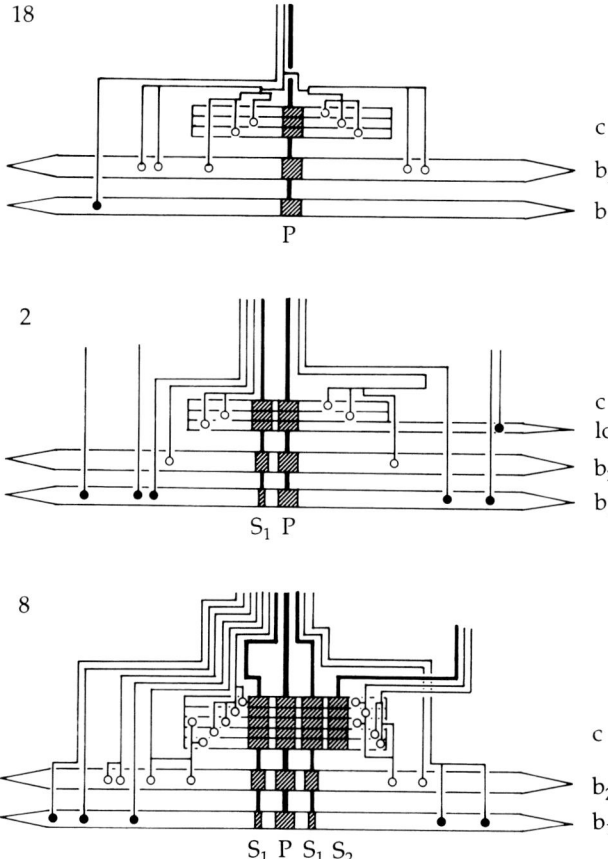

FIGURE 21-6. Schematic representation of the innervation of three cat spindles from a tenuissimus muscle, illustrating the range of complexity. The numbers refer to the order of the spindles in a proximal to distal sequence in the muscle, which contained 20 spindles. Static γ axons end as trail plates (open circles) on bag_2 (b_2) and chain (c) fibers, whereas β axons end as p_1 plates (filled circles) on bag_1 (b_1) and long chain (lc) fibers and are dynamic or static accordingly. Notice the concomitant increase in the number of γ axons and afferents, but not of β axons; and, in spindle 2, note the occurrence of a segregated input to the bag_2 and chain fibers in the same pole as the secondary endings. (Data from Banks [97] experiment C883, in which there was no evidence for any dynamic γ innervation.)

Autonomic Innervation

For many years it was widely held that skeletal muscle fibers are not innervated by sympathetic axons. It was acknowledged that such axons enter muscle spindles, but opinion was divided as to whether they supplied a vascular or nonvascular innervation. In 1981 Barker and Saito[7] demonstrated unequivocally that an autonomic innervation is distributed to some extrafusal muscle fibers and that it also has a nonvascular presence in some spindles. In the muscles sampled (from cat hindlimb), the proportion of spindles receiving autonomic axons was highest in the lumbricals (65 percent) and lowest in peroneus brevis (8 percent). Autonomic axons were absent from 18 tendon organs examined.

On the basis of the vesicle content of varicosities examined by electron microscopy, the extrafusal innervation was identified as noradrenergic (32 axons traced) and the spindle innervation as involving noradrenergic, cholinergic, and nonadrenergic, noncholinergic axons (14 traced). Varicosities were located within the capsule lamellae, inside the periaxial space, and in neuroeffective association with intrafusal muscle fibers (without preference for fiber type) in regions B and C.

The histologic evidence demonstrating the presence of a nonvascular autonomic innervation in some spindles prompted Passatore and Fillipi[143,144] and Hunt and colleagues[145] to study the effects of sympathetic stimulation on the discharge of spindle afferents. The responses were summarized in the second edition of *Myology*; in view of their weak and variable nature, they are not described here. A more marked effect is the long-lasting reduction in the tonic vibration reflex of the rabbit masseter that follows cervical sympathetic nerve stimulation.[146,147] The effect lasts as long as stimulation is continued, but with long (7- to 15-s) latencies of onset and termination. The mechanism remains unclear, though it may be humoral in origin, since it can be mimicked by close arterial injection of phenylephrine.[147] It does, however, appear to be located in the spindles themselves, which become less sensitive to stretch during sympathetic stimulation.[147a]

The Spindle as a Receptor

INPUT-OUTPUT PROPERTIES

When a ramp-and-hold stretch is applied to an adapted, deefferented spindle, the primary ending fires a short, high-frequency burst of impulses at the start of the ramp, and this is followed by a more or less steady increase in the rate of firing until a peak is reached at the end of the ramp. During the held phase there is an initial adaptation, rapid at first, then slower, until a new maintained level of firing is reached. The relation between this static firing level and the extension of the muscle is approximately linear and has been called

irrelevant to the response of the secondary ending.[98] Furthermore, although spindles that possess only a primary ending typically receive two static γ axons, it is the poles rather than the bag_2 and chain fibers that are separately innervated.

Perhaps the most important functional requirement is for a muscle to receive several distributed, exclusively fusimotor static axons that provide both divergence of individual motor neurons to several spindles and convergence of different motor neurons onto individual spindles. The development program may then result in a degree of intrafusal segregation, which is itself of little functional significance. Note that this partial segregation at the level of the individual spindle, which has also been detected in gastrocnemius using physiologic criteria,[142] does not imply the existence of more than one type of static γ motor neuron.

length, or position, sensitivity[148] (see Fig. 21-7). As the velocity of stretch increases, the frequency of the initial burst becomes higher and the slope of the response during the ramp becomes steeper, leading to higher peak rates at the end of the ramp. However, stretch velocity does not affect length sensitivity, so that the difference between the peak rate and the adapted rate at some arbitrary later time (0.5 s in the case of the widely used dynamic index) is some measure of the dynamic response of the ending. Thus for an ending with low dynamic sensitivity, or one in a muscle stretched at a low velocity, the slope of the dynamic response closely corresponds to the length sensitivity (indeed, Boyd[83] uses the term *length sensitivity* to mean the slope of the dynamic response). All these features are recognizable in secondary endings, although the initial burst and dynamic response are usually much less well developed.

Although the effects of dynamic fusimotor axons are mediated through the bag_1 fiber, it does not necessarily follow that the dynamic response of passive spindles is due in whole or part to the bag_1. Several authors have now succeeded in identifying primary afferents from spindle units that lack bag_1 fibers, and all are agreed that they show substantial passive dynamic behavior.[149–155] As in secondary endings, it cannot be selectively increased by dynamic fusimotor stimulation.

The effects of motor stimulation (β or γ) on the primary-ending response depend on the rate of stimulation and the type of muscle fiber activated (see Fig. 21-8). Stimulation of a dynamic axon activates the bag_1 fiber and may produce an increase in the static firing level, though not in the length sensitivity. When a ramp-and-hold stretch is applied in addition, the initial burst is abolished and the slope of the dynamic response is increased. Stimulation of a static axon under these conditions activates the bag_2 fiber or chain fibers or both, and again there is an increase in the static firing level and the initial burst is abolished. In this case, however, the slope of the dynamic response is usually unaffected, so that, although the actual dynamic response remains constant during static stimulation, the dynamic index is usually reduced. The length sensitivity is increased.[128]

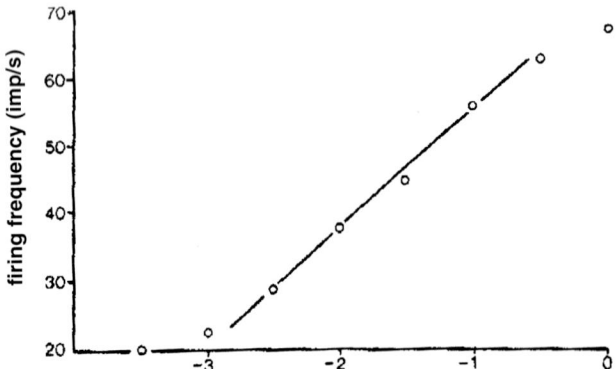

FIGURE 21-7. Length sensitivity of a spindle afferent unit, probably a secondary ending, shown by the slope (18 imp/s/mm) of the adapted firing frequency against muscle length. Maximum physiologic length corresponds to zero on the abscissa. With the muscle completely slack, the ending had a tonic discharge of 20 imp/s. Conduction velocity 63 m/s, cat peroneus brevis.

Some static γ axons elicit 1:1 driving of the primary response over a range of fusimotor stimulus frequencies, typically 50 to 100 Hz, whereas at higher stimulus frequencies very irregular, high-mean-frequency responses are produced. These effects are undoubtedly due to chain fibers,[83,156] probably active alone.[97] Bag_2 activity results in biasing of the primary response, but driving does not occur, even at subharmonic rates.[97,156] According to Banks,[97] bag_2 activity can partially or completely occlude the effect on the primary ending (though not the secondary) of simultaneous chain action in the same pole.

The behavior of the primary ending described above suggests that it is measuring the length (length sensitivity), velocity (dynamic index), and perhaps acceleration (initial burst) of the muscle in which it occurs, and this interpretation is usually found in introductory accounts of the muscle spindle. If this were so, it would be a simple matter to describe the output of the primary ending mathematically by a linear transfer function.[157] However, the sensitivity to velocity declines rapidly with increasing velocity,[158] and for large-amplitude stretches there is no particular response to acceleration.[159] Furthermore, the use of sinusoidal stretches has shown that the primary ending is about twenty times more sensitive to small-amplitude stretches (up to 0.1 mm for cat soleus)[160] than to larger stretches. These complications make the fitting of a linear transfer function more difficult, though various attempts have been made, ranging from power functions[161] to a second-order relation.[162] Nonlinear functions give better fits to the observed behavior,[163] but it seems necessary to suppose that there is more than one site of impulse initiation, such that their individual outputs may be variously summed or occluded. This phenomenon of *pacemaker switching* is to be expected in a branched axonal system.[164] Evidence that it occurs in mammalian spindles was first presented by Crowe and Matthews.[93] Quick et al.[165] provided ultrastructural and cytologic evidence that the sites for impulse generation in Ia axons are the heminodes and some of the penultimate nodes of the final branches. For Ia axons whose first-order branches have a segregated distribution, there would presumably be separate dynamic and static pacemakers. These have been demonstrated by Hulliger and Noth,[166] and the interaction of spiking nodes in a real preterminal tree has been modeled by Otten and colleagues.[167]

Banks et al.[168,169] carried out a correlated physiologic and histologic study in which they observed the responses of tenuissimus primary endings on stimulating pairs of dynamic and static axons, separately or combined, and then reconstructed the preterminal branches of the Ia afferents supplying those endings. When the response to combined stimulation (R_c) was compared with the responses to separate stimulation (R_l and R_h), occlusion of the momentarily lesser response (R_l) by the greater (R_h) tended to be the dominant effect. The amount of summation varied not only from one primary to another but also under different conditions of stretch and fusimotor stimulation. For this reason the quantitative analysis used to compare the different primary endings was restricted to the condition $R_h - R_l < 10$ impulses s^{-1}. Banks et al.[168,169] found that the summation was in part inversely correlated with the shortest distance around the Ia preterminal branches that linked potential dynamic and

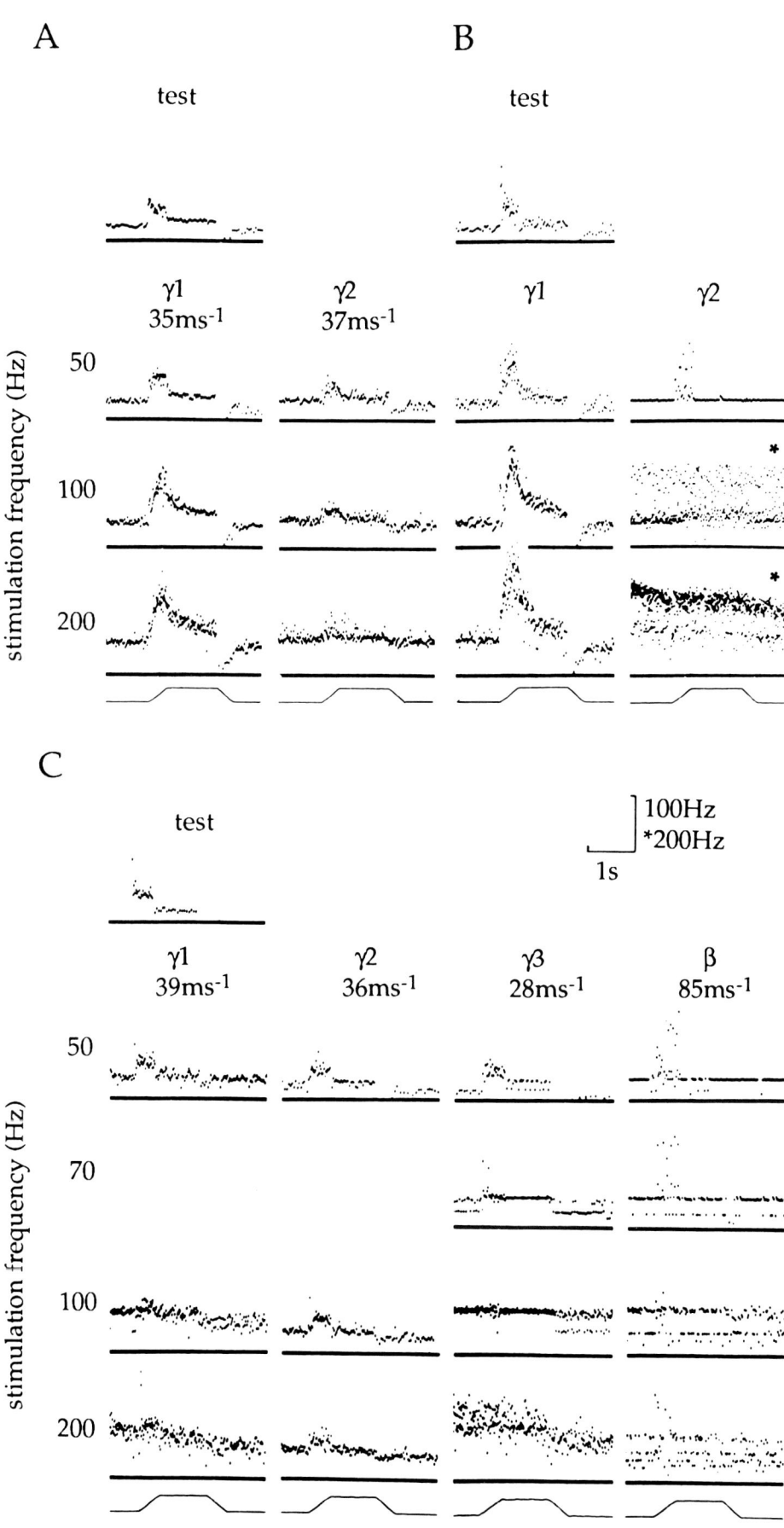

FIGURE 21-8. Responses of primary endings in three cat tenuissimus spindles to ramp-and-hold stretch in the absence (Test) and presence (β, γ) of motor stimulation. Responses are shown as instantaneous frequencies above zero baselines; muscle length is indicated at the bottom of each column. A. The effects of dynamic (γ1) and static (γ2) fusimotor stimulation on a single primary ending. B. The effects of stimulating the same fusimotor axons as in A but acting on a different primary ending: γ1 is again dynamic and γ2 static, but whereas γ2 biases the primary in A, it drives the primary in B at 1:1. Subsequent histological analysis indicated that the static γ supplied the bag_2 and all the chain fibers of one pole in A, but only the chain fibers of one pole in B; the dynamic γ supplied one pole of the bag_1 fiber in each case. C. The effects of stimulating the complete static input to a single spindle, which, on histologic analysis, proved to be segregated to the bag_2 and chain fibers, one of which possessed a long pole. γ1 and γ2 were identified with axons that supplied one pole each of a bag_2 fiber. Note the biasing effect as in A. γ3 was identified with an axon that supplied all the chain fibers in both poles, except for the single long pole; this was supplied by the β axon. Note that both γ3 and the β axon can drive the primary 1:1, and that when only a single chain pole is active, high rates of stimulation lead to preferential primary discharge at a series of subharmonic (1:2, 1:3, 1:4, 1:5) frequencies. (*From Banks RW: The distribution of static γ-axons in the tenuissimus muscle of the cat. J Physiol 442:489–512, 1991. With permission.*)

static pacemakers. They estimated this distance by counting the number of nodes of Ranvier in the linking path. Their conclusion, supported with model simulations, was that this component of summation was most likely due to electrotonic spread of receptor potentials from one sensory terminal to another around the preterminal branches. Fallon et al.[170] have reached similar conclusions using the soleus muscle, while emphasizing the probable additional factor of mechanical interactions. Furthermore, Taylor et al.[171] successfully incorporated the electrotonic model using data from Banks et al.[168] in their analysis of the input-output relationships of tibialis anterior and medial gastrocnemius spindles during treadmill walking in the decerebrate cat.

INPUT-OUTPUT CONVERSION

The spiking activity of the final branches of spindle afferents is generated by receptor potentials produced by their terminals.[172,173] Hunt and Wilkinson[173] analyzed receptor potentials recorded from afferent axons whose impulse activity had been blocked with tetrodotoxin. The contribution of pacemaker switching to the overall input-output properties was therefore absent in these experiments. The responses of primary and secondary endings were essentially similar, the main difference being the greater sensitivity of the primary endings. Moreover, the overall tension of these isolated spindles showed similar nonlinearities in response to sinusoidal amplitude and frequency as did the receptor potentials. It is therefore clear that pacemaker switching cannot account for all of the nonlinearities in the spindle's response to stretch and that there is at least a mechanical contribution as well.

The receptor potentials are generated mainly by an influx of Na^+ into the sensory terminals,[172] though there is also a significant Ca^{2+} current. Reduction in extracellular $[Ca^{2+}]$ increases the firing rate and dynamic response of primary and secondary endings.[174] This effect may be due to a K^+_{Ca} channel, which has also been implicated in Ca^{2+}-dependent modulation of center-frequency dynamics of the primary ending.[175] Nevertheless, as a first approximation we may suppose that the receptor potential is linearly related to the longitudinal tension through the terminals, this being locally modified by such elements as the elastic fibers that insert into the juxtaequatorial regions of bag fibers and thus differing, particularly in phase, from the overall tension (see "Ultrastructure," under "Intrafusal Muscle Fibers," above).

The cause of the mechanical contribution to nonlinearities in the sensory responses may then be sought primarily in the intrafusal muscle fibers, on the basis of the cross-bridge model of muscle activation. Cross-bridges may be regarded as elements of low compliance whose breakage under tension is manifest as viscosity.[176,177] The number of cross-bridges at any one time will be a function of the rate at which they are being formed, the rate at which they spontaneously break, and the rate at which they break under tension. Each of these factors will have an associated time constant, the actual value of which will vary according to muscle fiber type, particularly in the case of the first two. The bag_1 fiber is especially interesting on account of its peculiar properties, which include the presence of tonic myosin, and the discrepancy between the locations of its motor endings and the convergent sarcomere movements seen during the stimulation of dynamic motor axons.[178] If the bag_1 fiber pole normally has a large number of cross-bridges, activation may produce only a modest shortening restricted to the region with M-line sarcomeres, whereas the stiffness will increase. The time course of the shortening[83] may be much longer than that of the activation giving rise to it[179] because of series viscoelastic components.

The prominent dynamic response of the primary is thus seen as a consequence of the stiffness of the bag_1 fiber. Exposure of potential cross-bridge sites by breakage of cross-bridges under tension will automatically lead to an increased rate of cross-bridge formation, recognizable as stretch activation,[180,181] that tends to maintain the muscle fiber stiffness. The importance of stretch activation in the generation of the dynamic response is, however, still debated. At the peak of a ramp stretch the longitudinal tension in the primary terminals on the bag_1 fiber may fall abruptly, perhaps aided by the effectively in-parallel elastic fibers, to be followed by the compensatory length change ("creep"[83,182]) with a longer time course.

The mechanical properties of chain fibers are diametrically opposed to those of the bag_1 fiber in that they show lack of stiffness, low viscosity, and rapid overt contraction. They can be accounted for by assuming that chain fibers have a small number of cross-bridges with a rapid turnover as a result of a high rate of spontaneous breakage. Static fusimotor activation leads to shortening of the chain fiber poles with little, if any, increase in stiffness. Because of the lack of viscosity, small fluctuations in polar length are readily transmitted to the equatorial region and the primary response can be "driven" at the static fusimotor stimulation rate over a wide range of frequencies.[97,98]

FUNCTIONAL ORGANIZATION OF SENSORY TERMINALS

The process of mechanosensory transduction by sensory terminals, such as those of the spindle's primary and secondary endings, has been traditionally seen as entirely passive, but our understanding of it is now undergoing a fundamental revision. We begin with the long-established observation that the terminals contain a population of membrane-bound vesicles, in particular small, clear microvesicles with a mean diameter of 50 nm[81] (also Barker and Saito, unpublished). The apparent similarity of these "synaptic-like vesicles" to the synaptic vesicles of presynaptic terminals, including motor neuromuscular junctions, was greatly increased when De Camilli et al.[183] showed that synapsin 1 and synaptophysin are colocalized in the sensory terminals of muscle spindles and tendon organs.

Use of the fluorescent styryl dye FM1-43 has provided evidence for recycling of the synaptic-like vesicles in rat lumbrical primary endings, the rate being activity-dependent.[184] The possibility that the vesicles may be releasing glutamate is indicated first by elevated levels of glutamate in the sensory terminals (as shown by immunogold labeling for electron microscopy[185]) and second by the enhanced response to stretch in the presence of 0.1 to 1 mM of exogenously applied glutamate.[184] We suggest that this autogenic excitation is a basic feature of the functional organization of at least those mechanoreceptors in which the transduction process occurs in the peripheral terminals of the primary afferent axon. Of course, other functions may also be mediated by the recycling of synaptic-like vesicles—for example, the neurotrophic effect of the afferent innervation on the maintenance of differentiation of the intrafusal muscle fibers.

Activity-dependent recycling of synaptic-like vesicles implies a control mechanism; the central role of Ca^{2+} is indicated by immunocytochemical evidence for the presence of various Ca^{2+}-binding proteins in the spindle. So far, in mammalian spindles, these include calbindin D-28k,[186,187] calretinin,[187,188] and neurocalcin.[189] In addition, frequenin has been described as occurring in the frog spindle.[190] They are all members of the EF-hand superfamily and represent two families of proteins with either 6 EF-hands (calbindin D-28k, calretinin) thought to act as Ca^{2+} buffers[191] or 4 EF-hands (neurocalcin, frequenin) that function as Ca^{2+}-activated switches.[191,192] The distribution of the various proteins differs: All have been found in primary sensory endings, calbindin D-28k also occurs in the intrafusal muscle fibers of rat spindles,[187] and calretinin also occurs in the chain fibers of cat spindles.[188] Duc et al.[187] found calretinin absent from rat spindle secondary endings and tendon organs and used this in part as evidence for a general scheme relating the presence or absence of calretinin in mechanoreceptors to their response properties, respectively phasic or tonic. El-Tarhouni and Banks,[188] however, found calretinin in tendon organs of cat muscle, while confirming its absence from spindle secondaries. Neurocalcin has been reported from a variety of mechanoreceptors in addition to the spindle, including tendon organs,[189,193] Meissner's corpuscles, and perimysial but not cutaneous pacinian corpuscles.[193]

Another aspect of intracellular signaling that probably also involves Ca^{2+} and adds to its complexity in mechanosensory endings is represented in spindle primary endings by immunocytochemical labeling for protein kinase Cβ in rat neck muscle[194] and for protein kinase C α, β, and γ in rat lumbrical muscle.[195]

Development

ORGANOGENESIS AND INNERVATION

The role of innervation in the development of muscle spindles (and other mammalian mechanoreceptors) has recently been fully reviewed by Zelená[11]; consequently, this section focuses on the most salient and recent points.

Electron microscopic (EM) investigations of spindle development in rat,[87,196,197] mouse,[198] and cat[199] have revealed close parallels between intrafusal and extrafusal myogenesis. Both involve the sequential production of myotubes, beginning with a population of primary myotubes that is generated before the innervation of the muscle primordium, and continuing after innervation by the assembly, maturation, and separation of successive series of secondary myotubes forming clusters, each one typically centered on a primary myotube. Thus Milburn[199] demonstrated that the intrafusal muscle fibers in the cat develop in the order bag_2 (primary myotube), bag_1, and chains (successive generations of secondary myotubes). The equatorial position of the bag_1 and chain fibers in the mature spindle reflects the pattern of their assembly and separation[63] (see Fig. 21-9).

An immunohistologic study of developing rat spindles by Pedrosa and Thornell[200] has shown that, whereas all primary myotubes contain neonatal and slow-twitch MHC at E17, there are some that also contain slow-tonic MHC (see Fig. 21-10). These are presumed to be the precursors of the bag_2 fiber, and their positive antitonic staining serves to indicate the sites of future spindles. The bag_1 fiber contains only neonatal MHC when it first appears at E19 and does not stain positively for anti–slow-tonic or anti–slow-twitch MHC until 2 days later. When the first chain fiber appears (E21), it contains only neonatal MHC according to Pedrosa and Thornell,[200] but Kucera and Walro,[201] using a different set of antibodies, find that it also expresses both slow-twitch and fast-twitch MHC. A similar sequence of events occurs in human spindle development, the presumptive bag_2 fibers being identifiable from the 10th week of gestation, though in this case secondary myotubes that differentiate as bag_1 and chain fibers may appear together.[202] For further details and references, see Zelená[11] and the reviews of the developmental expression of MHC isoforms in rat spindles by Soukup et al.[203] and by Walro and Kucera.[204]

Pedrosa and Thornell[200] proposed that the three types of intrafusal fiber arise from three different myoblast lineages already committed to differentiate along specifically intrafusal paths, cells in the bag_2 lineage necessarily being capable of attracting Ia afferent terminals. Kucera and Walro[205] likewise argued for the existence of three lineages of myoblasts, but they proposed that each is pluripotent and may give rise sequentially either to the three types of intrafusal fiber or to successive generations of extrafusal fiber. On this view, the switch to the intrafusal phenotype is signaled by contact by a presumptive Ia afferent. As evidence for this, Kucera and Walro[205] showed that a slow (tonic) MHC is expressed in rat hindlimb muscles from E15 to E17 in all primary myotubes that subsequently differentiate as bag_2 or type I extrafusal fibers. The arrival of the earliest innervation (presumptive Ia and α axons) at E17/E18 results in upregulation of the slow MHC in the presumptive bag_2 fibers and its downregulation and suppression in the presumptive type I extrafusal fibers. The close association between the primary and secondary myotubes does not appear to be necessary for the sequential differentiation of the bag_1 and chain fibers, since neonatal nerve crush and treatment with nerve growth factor (NGF) results in almost 90 percent of spindles that lack bag_2 fibers.[206]

An EM study of the development of spindles in the rat (21 to 23 days gestation) by Kucera et al.[87] has revealed that there is a transient fetal stage of multiple afferent innervation. The first afferent-muscle contacts occur at E17 when en passant contacts are formed between primary myotubes and sensory axons located within intramuscular nerves. Initially, only one primary (Ia) afferent occupies the contact area, but several follow before the capsule begins to form and for a

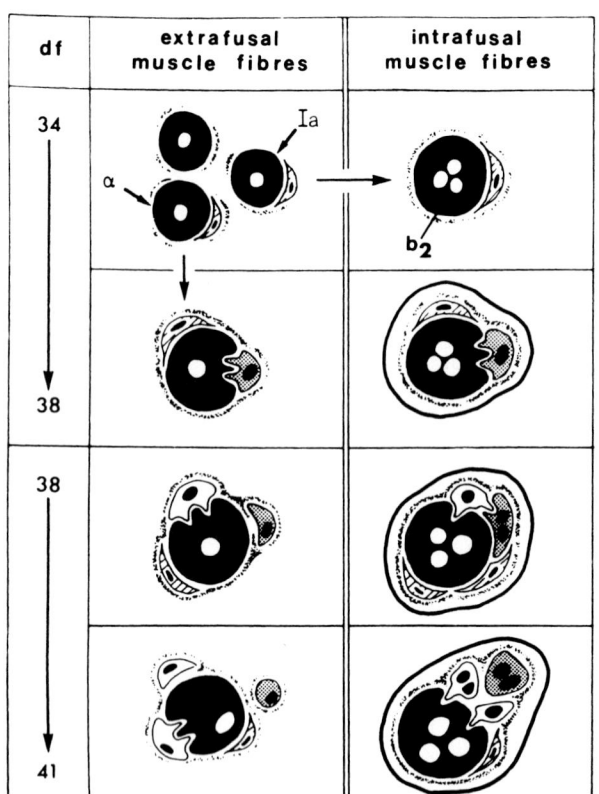 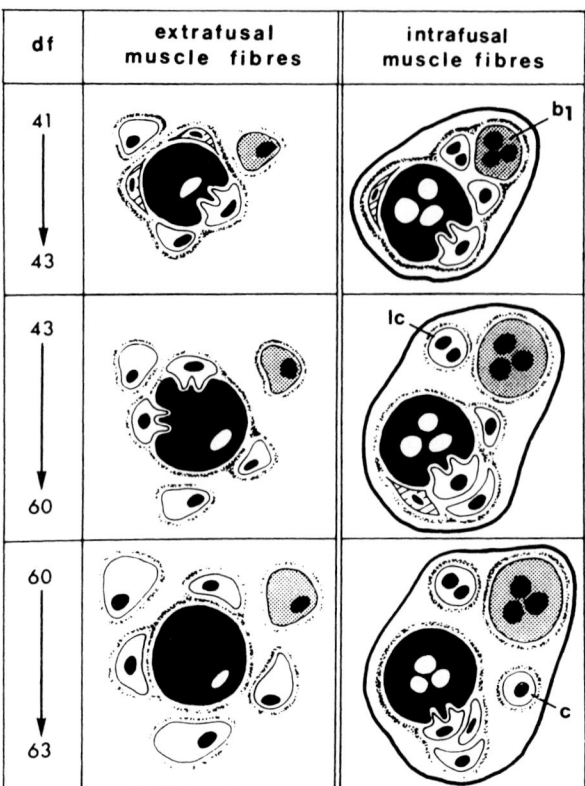

FIGURE 21-9. Schematic diagrams of transverse sections of developing extrafusal and intrafusal muscle fibers in cat peroneal muscles. In the extrafusal fascicle note how the first-series secondary myotube (stippled) separates from the primary myotube (black) and acquires its own basal lamina (stippled halo) before the assembly of subsequent series of secondary myotubes (white). The thin fusiform cells (hatched) are myoblasts. The diagrams of intrafusal muscle fibers illustrate the process of myogenesis as seen at the spindleequator. Abbreviations: α = alpha motor neuron; b_1 = bag_1 fiber; b_2 = bag_2 fiber; lc, c = chain fibers; df = days fetal; Ia = Ia afferent. (*Modified from Milburn A: Stages in the development of the cat muscle spindle. J Embryol Exp Morphol 82:177–216, 1984. With permission.*)

time there is a phase of multiple afferent innervation in which secondary (II) afferents, in some spindles, also take part, arriving on E19. In the soleus spindles studied by Kucera et al.,[87] the supernumerary afferents have withdrawn by E20, but they evidently persist in some muscles, since Banks et al.[86] have described mature spindles in rat deep masseter in which a single primary region may be innervated by up to five Ia afferents. Motor endings appear in developing soleus spindles at E20 on the bag_2 fiber, at E22 on the bag_1 fiber, and 4 days after birth on the first chain fiber.[87,207] These may be regarded as γ endings, since no β innervation occurs in rat soleus.[208] Most of these perinatal motor endings are multiply innervated. It is assumed that a stage of polyneuronal innervation is followed by the loss of some motor axons and connections, but the details of this and of the development of the β innervation are at present unknown. At E18, some of the nonencapsulated primary myotubes that have sensory terminals also receive motor terminals from α axons,[87] as occurs at a similar stage in the development of cat spindles.[199] It is conceivable that in certain muscles some of these motor terminals might persist and represent the first stage in the development of a β innervation. In rat soleus their presence is transitory, since no motor endings occur at E18 and E19 on primary myotubes that are encapsulated.[87]

TROPHIC AND TRANSCRIPTION FACTORS

Within the last decade, molecular biological techniques have begun to shed new light on the interactions between the neural and muscular components of the muscle spindle. A proportion of dorsal-root ganglion cells, including the large muscle afferents, express tyrosine kinase C (trk-C). This is the receptor for NT-3, one of the neurotrophin family of trophic factors. Targeted disruption of the genes encoding trk-C or NT-3 in the mouse results in various deficiencies, among which is the absence of muscle spindles and tendon organs.[88,209] In rat muscles, NT-3 mRNA is expressed only in the bag fibers of muscle spindles, from E19 (bag_2) and E21 (bag_1) through to maturity.[210] In situ hybridization showed it to be especially concentrated in the small amounts of sarcoplasm between the nuclei of the nuclear bags.[210] However, it will be seen that this expression does not begin until after the time of arrival of the afferent innervation and after the bag_2 fiber has begun to differentiate (see above). Moreover,

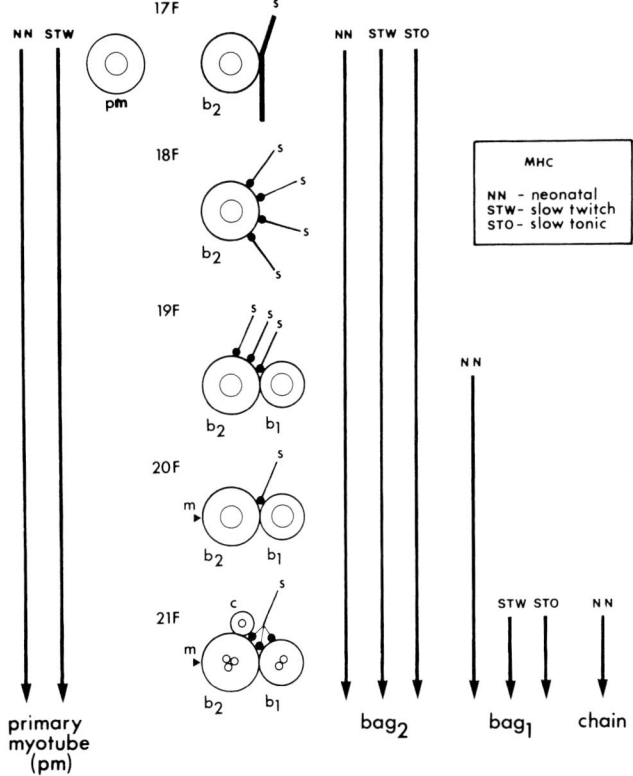

FIGURE 21-10. Simplified illustration of the development of rat soleus spindles showing the acquisition of sensory (s) and motor (m) innervation (based on Kucera et al.[87]) and MHC expression (based on Pedrosa and Thornell[200]). Spindle capsule omitted; intrafusal myotubes/myofibers abbreviated b_1, bag_1; b_2, bag_2; c, chain. (*Modified from Pedrosa F, Soukup T, Thornell L-E: Expression of an alpha cardiac-like myosin heavy chain in muscle spindle fibres. Histochemistry 95:105–113, 1990. With permission.*)

appropriate numbers of muscle afferents may normally depend on NT-3 derived from a source other than the muscle spindle itself.

It should not, of course, surprise us to find that a gene so intimately embedded in a developmental control system as that coding for NT-3 produces nonlinear effects when its spatiotemporal expression is disturbed in any way. Evidence that this might be so may be summarized as follows: (1) A nestin-promoted NT-3 transgene inserted into the NT-3 null mutant rescued NT-3-dependent drg neurons, but nevertheless the mice lacked limb muscle spindles[214]; (2) there is a synergistic interaction between NT-3 and the p75 receptor[215]; and (3) ectopic expression of NT-3 throughout skeletal muscle, produced by a myosin light chain–promoted NT-3 transgene, resulted in progressively worsening locomotor deficits associated with abnormal spindles.[216] Moreover, in NT-3 null mice a proportion of spindles (38 percent in masseter) within the territory of the trigeminal mesencephalic nucleus survive,[217] and in trk-C null mice all of them do,[218] whereas there is some loss of these spindles in brain-derived neurotrophic factor (BDNF) null mutants and to a lesser extent in NT-4 null mutants.[217]

A member (Egr-3) of the early growth response family of zinc-finger transcription factors has been shown to be expressed in intrafusal fibers of the mouse hindlimb from E15.5 onward, but not at all in the surrounding extrafusal fibers.[219] It appears to be another gene that is induced in myotubes by presumptive Ia afferents, and though its function is unknown, its deletion once again results in the absence of spindles in the adult. However, spindles do begin to form in the absence of Egr-3, but the characteristic slow myosin is not induced and the incipient spindles degenerate after withdrawal of their sensory and motor innervation.[220] In this case, however, the afferents are generated and project appropriately into the ventral spinal cord at least up to P7.[219] Expression of Egr-3 and other transcription factors in intrafusal fibers is regulated by immunoglobulin-like neuregulin 1 (Ig-Nrg1); presumptive Ia afferents deficient in neuregulin 1 isoforms make contact with myotubes but fail to initiate spindle development.[221]

the continued intrafusal expression of NT-3 in the adult is itself nerve-dependent.[211] In mice homozygous for a deletion in the gene for NT-3, the NT-3-dependent drg neurons, their peripheral and central processes, seem to be absent or greatly reduced in number from E10.5, which precedes hindlimb innervation[212] but approximately coincides with the onset of "programmed" cell death in normal mice.[88] So, despite the most interesting observation that heterozygotes possess half the normal number of spindles[209] and the rescue of muscle afferents and spindles in NT-3 null mutants by a myogenin-promoted NT-3 transgene,[213] the early survival of

Acknowledgment

We wish to thank Dr. Michael Stacey for his help in preparing the figures.

List of Abbreviations

BDNF	brain–derived neurotrophic factor
EM	electron microscopic
FOG	fast oxidative-glycolytic
GDNF	glial cell line–derived neurotrophic factor
HRP	horseradish peroxidase
Ig-Nrg1	immunoglobulin-like neuregulin 1
MHC	myosin heavy chain
NADH-TR	nicotinamide adenine dinucleotide tetrazolium reductase
NGF	nerve growth factor
NT-3	neurotrophin-3
SEM	scanning electron microscope
SO	slow oxidative
trk-C	tyrosine kinase C

References

1. Barker D: The morphology of muscle receptors, in Hunt CC (ed): *Muscle Receptors: Handbook of Sensory Physiology.* Vol 3, Pt 2. Berlin: Springer-Verlag, 1974; pp 1–190.
2. Barker D: The innervation of the muscle spindle. *Q J Microsc Sci* 89:143–186, 1948.
3. Boyd IA: The diameter and distribution of the nuclear bag and nuclear chain muscle fibres in the muscle spindles of the cat. *J Physiol* 153:23P–24P, 1960.
4. Barker D, Ip MC: The motor innervation of cat and rabbit muscle spindles. *J Physiol* 177:27P–28P, 1965.
5. Barker D: Three types of motor ending in cat spindles. *J Physiol* 186:27P–28P, 1966.
6. Barker D: The innervation of mammalian skeletal muscle, in de Reuck AVS, Knight J (eds): *Myotatic, Kinesthetic and Vestibular Mechanisms* (Ciba Foundation Symposium). London: Churchill, 1967; pp 3–15.
7. Barker D, Saito M: Autonomic innervation of receptors and muscle fibres in cat skeletal muscle. *Proc R Soc Lond Biol Sci* 212:317–332, 1981.
8. Poppele RS: The muscle spindle, in Dyck PJ, Thomas PK, Griffin JW, et al (eds): *Peripheral Neuropathy*, 3d ed. Philadelphia: Saunders, 1993; pp 121–140.
9. Barker D, Banks RW: The muscle spindle, in Engel AC, Franzini-Armstrong C (eds): *Myology* 2d ed. New York: McGraw-Hill, 1994; pp 333–360.
10. Hunt CC: The mammalian muscle spindle: Peripheral mechanisms. *Physiol Rev* 70:643–663, 1990.
11. Zelená J: *Nerves and Mechanoreceptors.* London: Chapman & Hall, 1994.
12. Hunt CC: The physiology of muscle receptors, in Hunt CC (ed): *Muscle Receptors: Handbook of Sensory Physiology.* Vol 3, Pt 2. Berlin: Springer-Verlag, 1974; pp 191–234.
13. Maier A: The avian muscle spindle. *Anat Embryol* 186:1–25, 1992.
14. Jami L, Pierrot-Deseilligny E, Zytnicki D (eds): *Muscle Afferents and Spinal Control of Movement.* Oxford, UK: Pergamon Press, 1992.
15. Ferrell WR, Proske U (eds): *Neural Control of Movement.* New York: Plenum Press, 1995.
16. Taylor A, Gladden MH, Durbaba R (eds): *Alpha and Gamma Motor Systems.* New York: Plenum Press, 1995.
17. Maier A: Development and regeneration of muscle spindles in mammals and birds. *Int J Dev Biol* 41:1–17, 1997.
18. Soukup T, Novotova M: Ultrastructure and innervation of regenerated intrafusal muscle fibres in heterochronous isografts of the fast rat muscle. *Acta Neuropathol* 100:435–444, 2000.
19. Whelan PJ: Control of locomotion in the decerebrate cat. *Prog Neurobiol* 49:481–515, 1996.
20. Bosco G, Poppele RE: Proprioception from a spinocerebellar perspective. *Physiol Rev* 81:539–568, 2001.
21. Cooper S, Daniel PM: Human muscle spindles. *J Physiol* 133:1P–3P, 1956.
22. Banks RW, Emonet-Dénand F: Characteristic properties of superficial lumbrical spindles in the cat hind limb, related to their bag$_1$ fibres. *J Anat* 189:65–71, 1996.
23. Richmond FJR, Abrahams VC: Morphology and distribution of muscle spindles in dorsal muscles of the cat neck. *J Neurophysiol* 38:1322–1339, 1975.
24. Bakker GJ, Richmond FJR: Two types of muscle spindles in cat neck muscles: A histochemical study of intrafusal fiber composition. *J Neurophysiol* 45:973–986, 1981.
25. Bakker GJ, Richmond FJR: Muscle spindle complexes in muscles around upper cervical vertebrae in the cat. *J Neurophysiol* 48:62–74, 1982.
26. Rowlerson A, Mascarello F, Barker D, Saed H: Muscle-spindle distribution in relation to the fibre-type composition of masseter in mammals. *J Anat* 161:37–60, 1988.
27. Barker D, Ip MC: A study of single and tandem types of muscle spindle in the cat. *Proc R Soc Lond Biol Sci* 154:377–397, 1961.
28. Voss H: Tabelle der absoluten und relativen Muskelspindelzahlen der menschlichen Skeletmuskulatur. *Anat Anz* 129:562–572, 1971.
29. Cooper S: Muscle spindles and other muscle receptors, in Bourne GH (ed): *The Structure and Function of Muscle.* New York: Academic Press, 1960; pp 381–420.
30. Banks R, Stacey M: Quantitative studies on mammalian muscle spindles, in Hník F, Soukup T, Vejsada R, Zelená J (eds): *Mechanoreceptors.* New York: Plenum Press, 1988; pp 263–269.
31. Peck D, Buxton DF, Nitz A: A comparison of spindle concentrations in large and small muscles acting in parallel combinations. *J Morphol* 180:243–252, 1984.
32. Banks RW: On the number of spindles in mammalian muscles. *J Physiol* 511:69P, 1998.
33. van der Wal JC: *The Organization of the Substrate of Proprioception in the Elbow Region of the Rat.* Thesis. Maastricht: Rijksuniversiteit Limburg, 1988.
34. Gregor A: Über die Vertheilung der Muskelspindeln in der Musculatur des menschlichen Fötus. *Arch Anat Physiol Anat Abt* 12:191, 1904.
35. Yellin H: A histological study of muscle spindles and their relationship to extrafusal fiber types in the rat. *Am J Anat* 125:31–45, 1969.
36. Cameron WE, Binder M, Botterman BR, et al: "Sensory partitioning" of cat medial gastrocnemius muscle by its muscle spindles and tendon organs. *J Neurophysiol* 46:32–47, 1981.
37. Munson JB, Fleshman JW, Zengel JE, Sypert GW: Synaptic and mechanical coupling between type-identified motor units and individual spindle afferents of medial gastrocnemius muscle of the cat. *J Neurophysiol* 51:1268–1283, 1984.
38. Donselaar Y, Kernell D, Eerbeek O, Verhey BA: Somatotopic relations between spinal motoneurones and muscle fibres of the cat's musculus peroneus longus. *Brain Res* 335:81–88, 1985.
39. Huhle R: Topographic studies relating distribution of Ia- and γ-fibres in spinal cord and position of muscle spindles in cat tibialis anterior muscle. *Brain Res* 333:299–304, 1985.
40. Eldred E, Yung L, Eldred D, Roy RR: Distribution of muscle spindles in a simply structured muscle: Integrated total sensory representation. *Anat Rec* 251:161–172, 1998.
41. Windhorst U, Hamm TM, Stuart DG: On the function of muscle and reflex partitioning. *Behav Brain Sci* 12:629–681, 1989.
42. Botterman BR, Binder MD, Stuart DG: Functional anatomy of the association between motor units and muscle receptors. *Am Zool* 18:135–152, 1978.
43. Richmond FJR, Stuart DG: Distribution of sensory receptors in the flexor carpi radialis muscle of the cat. *J Morphol* 183:1–13, 1985.
44. Merrillees NCR: The fine structure of muscle spindles in the lumbrical muscles of the rat. *J Biophys Biochem Cytol* 7:725–740, 1960.
45. Rodger J, Ziman MR, Papadimitriou JM, Kay PH: Pax7 is expressed in the capsules surrounding adult mouse neuromuscular spindles. *Biochem Cell Biol* 77:153–156, 1999.
46. Low FN: The perineurium and connective tissue of peripheral nerve, in Landon DN (ed): *The Peripheral Nerve.* London: Chapman & Hall, 1976, pp 159–187.
47. Kennedy WR, Quick DC, Reese TR: Freeze-fracture of muscle spindles. *Abstr Soc Neurosci* 5:304, 1979.
48. Kennedy WR, Yoon KS: Permeability of muscle spindle capillaries and capsule. *Muscle Nerve* 2:101–108, 1979.
49. Dow PR, Shinn SL, Ovalle WK: Ultrastructural study of a blood-muscle spindle barrier after systemic administration of horseradish peroxidase. *Am J Anat* 157:375–388, 1980.
50. von Brzezinski DK: Untersuchungen zur Histochemie der Muskelspindeln. II. Mitteilung: Zur Topochemie und Funktion des Spindelraumes und der Spindelkapsel. *Acta Histochem (Jena)* 12:277–288, 1961.
51. Fukami Y: Studies of capsule and capsular space of cat muscle spindles. *J Physiol* 376:281–297, 1986.
52. Kucera J: Myofibrillar ATPase activity of intrafusal fibers in chronically deafferented rat muscle spindles. *Histochemistry* 66:221–228, 1980.
53. Banks RW, James NT: The blood supply of rabbit muscle spindles. *J Anat* 114:7–12, 1973.
54. Miyoshi T, Kennedy WR: Microvasculature of rabbit muscle spindles. *Arch Neurol* 36:471–475, 1979.
55. Cooper S, Gladden MH: Elastic fibres and reticulin of mammalian muscle spindles and their functional significance. *Q J Exp Physiol* 59:367–385, 1974.
56. Gladden MH: Structural features relative to the function of intrafusal muscle fibres in the cat, in Homma S (ed): *Understanding the Stretch Reflex. Progress in Brain Research.* Vol 44. Amsterdam: Excerpta Medica, 1976; pp 51–59.
57. Banks RW: On the attachment of elastic fibres in cat tenuissimus spindles. *J Physiol* 348:16P, 1983.
58. Kucera J: Morphometric studies on tenuissimus muscle spindles in the cat. *J Morphol* 171:137–150, 1982.
59. Boyd IA: The structure and innervation of the nuclear bag muscle fibre system and the nuclear chain muscle fibre system in mammalian muscle spindles. *Philos Trans R Soc Lond [Biol]* 245:81–136, 1962.
60. Banks RW, Barker D, Stacey MJ: Form and distribution of sensory terminals in cat hindlimb muscle spindles. *Philos Trans R Soc Lond [Biol]* 299:329–364, 1982.
61. Banks RW: The number and distribution of satellite cells of intrafusal muscle fibres in a muscle spindle of the cat. *J Anat* 133:694, 1981.
62. Banks RW, Barker D, Harker DW, Stacey MJ: Correlation between ultrastructure and histochemistry of mammalian intrafusal muscle fibres. *J Physiol* 252:16P, 1975.
63. Barker D, Banks RW, Harker DW, et al: Studies of the histochemistry, ultrastructure, motor innervation and regeneration of mammalian intrafusal muscle fibres, in Homma S (ed): *Understanding the Stretch Reflex. Progress in Brain Research.* Vol 44. Amsterdam: Excerpta Medica, 1976; pp 67–88.
64. Barker D, Stacey MJ: Rabbit intrafusal muscle fibres. *J Physiol* 210:70P, 1970.
65. Banks RW, Harker DW, Stacey MJ: A study of mammalian intrafusal muscle fibres using a combined histochemical and ultrastructural technique. *J Anat* 123:783–796, 1977.
66. Adal MN: The transverse tubular system of cat intrafusal muscle fibres. *Cell Tissue Res* 244:197–202, 1986.
67. Ovalle WK, Smith RS: Histochemical identification of three types of intrafusal muscle fibers in the cat and monkey based on the myosin ATPase reaction. *Can J Physiol Pharmacol* 50:195–202, 1972.

68. Soukup T: Intrafusal fiber types in rat limb muscle spindles. Morphological and histochemical characteristics. *Histochemistry* 47:43–57, 1976.
69. Kucera J: Histochemical profiles of cat intrafusal muscle fibers and their motor innervation. *Histochemistry* 73:397–418, 1981.
70. Pierobon-Bormioli S, Sartore S, Vitadello M, Schiaffino S: "Slow" myosins in vertebrate skeletal muscle. An immunofluorescence study. *J Cell Biol* 85:672–681, 1980.
71. Rowlerson A, Gorza L, Schiaffino S: Immunohistochemical identification of spindle fibre types in mammalian muscle using type-specific antibodies to isoforms of myosin, in Boyd IA, Gladden M (eds): *The Muscle Spindle*. London: Macmillan, 1985; pp 29–34.
72. Kucera J, Walro JM: Postnatal expression of myosin heavy chains in muscle spindles of the rat. *Anat Embryol* 179:369–376, 1989.
73. Pedrosa F, Butler-Browne GS, Dhoot GK, et al: Diversity in expression of myosin heavy chain isoforms and M-band proteins in rat muscle spindles. *Histochemistry* 92:185–194, 1989.
74. Kucera J, Walro JM, Gorza L: Expression of type-specific MHC isoforms in rat intrafusal muscle fibers. *J Histochem Cytochem* 40:293–307, 1992.
75. Mascarello F, Rowlerson AM: Myosin isoform transitions during development of extraocular and masticatory muscles in the fetal rat. *Anat Embryol* 185:143–153, 1992.
76. Pedrosa F, Soukup T, Thornell L-E: Expression of an alpha cardiac-like myosin heavy chain in muscle spindle fibres. *Histochemistry* 95:105–113, 1990.
77. Maier A, Gambke B, Pette D: Immunohistochemical demonstration of embryonic myosin heavy chains in adult mammalian intrafusal fibers. *Histochemistry* 88:267–271, 1988.
78. Banks RW: Observations on the primary sensory ending of tenuissimus muscle spindles in the cat. *Cell Tissue Res* 246:309–319, 1986.
79. Banks RW, Stacey MJ: A quantitative analysis of the sensory innervation of cat tenuissimus muscle spindles. *J Physiol* 429:129P, 1990.
80. Ruffini A: On the minute anatomy of the neuromuscular spindles of the cat, and on their physiological significance. *J Physiol* 23:190–208, 1898.
81. Adal MN: The fine structure of the sensory region of cat muscle spindles. *J Ultrastruct Res* 26:332–354, 1969.
82. Corvaja N, Marinozzi V, Pompeiano O: Close opposition and junctions of plasma membranes of intrafusal muscle fibres in mammalian muscle spindles. *Pflügers Arch* 296:337–345, 1967.
83. Boyd IA: The response of fast and slow nuclear bag fibres and nuclear chain fibres in isolated cat muscle spindles to fusimotor stimulation, and the effect of intrafusal contraction on sensory endings. *Q J Exp Physiol* 61:203–254, 1976.
84. Nahirney PC, Ovalle WK: Distribution of dystrophin and neurofilament protein in muscle spindles of normal and mdx-dystrophic mice: An immunocytochemical study. *Anat Rec* 235:501–510, 1993.
85. Patten RM, Ovalle WK: Muscle spindle ultrastructure revealed by conventional and high-resolution scanning electron microscopy. *Anat Rec* 230:183–198, 1991.
86. Banks RW, Barker D, Saed HH, Stacey MJ: Innervation of muscle spindles in rat deep masseter. *J Physiol* 406:16P, 1988.
87. Kucera J, Walro JH, Reichler J: Role of nerve and muscle factors in the development of rat muscle spindles. *Am J Anat* 186:144–160, 1989.
88. Chen H-H, Frank E: Development and specification of muscle sensory neurons. *Curr Opin Neurobiol* 9:405–409, 1999.
89. Banks RW: The motor innervation of mammalian muscle spindles. *Prog Neurobiol* 43:323–362, 1994.
90. Leksell L: The action potential and excitatory effects of the small ventral root fibres to skeletal muscle. *Acta Physiol Scand* 10(Suppl 31):1–84, 1945.
91. Kucera J, Walro JM, Reichler J: Neural organization of spindles in three hindlimb muscles of the rat. *Am J Anat* 190:74–88, 1991.
92. Kucera J: Characteristics of motor innervation of muscle spindles in the monkey. *Am J Anat* 173:113–125, 1985.
93. Matthews PBC: The differentiation of two types of fusimotor fibre by their effects on the dynamic response of muscle spindle primary endings. *Q J Exp Physiol* 47:324–333, 1962.
94. Crowe A, Matthews PBC: The effects of stimulation of static and dynamic fusimotor fibres on the response of stretching of the primary endings of muscle spindles. *J Physiol* 174:109–131, 1964.
95. Brown MC, Crowe A, Matthews PBC: Observations on the fusimotor fibres of the tibialis posterior muscle of the cat. *J Physiol* 177:140–159, 1965.
96. Murthy KSK: Vertebrate fusimotor neurones and their influences on motor behaviour. *Prog Neurobiol* 11:249–307, 1978.
97. Banks RW: The distribution of static γ-axons in the tenuissimus muscle of the cat. *J Physiol* 442:489–512, 1991.
98. Boyd IA: The action of the three types of intrafusal fibre in isolated cat muscle spindles on the dynamic and length sensitivities of primary and secondary endings, in Taylor A, Prochazka A (eds): *Muscle Receptors and Movement*. London: Macmillan, 1981, pp 17–33.
99. Boyd IA, Gladden MH, Ward J: Two types of static γ-axon having a predominantly static bag_2 action or predominantly chain fibre action in the several cat muscle spindles they supply. *J Physiol* 343:110P, 1983.
100. Boyd IA: Two types of static γ-axon in cat muscle spindles. *Q J Exp Physiol* 71:307–327, 1986.
101. Arbuthnott ER, Ballard KJ, Boyd IA, et al: The ultrastructure of cat fusimotor endings and their relationship to foci of sarcomere convergence in intrafusal fibres. *J Physiol* 331:285–309, 1982.
102. Sutherland FI, Arbuthnott ER, Boyd IA, Gladden MH: Two ultrastructural types of fusimotor ending on typical chain fibres in cat muscle spindles, in Boyd IA, Gladden MH (eds): *The Muscle Spindle*. London: Macmillan, 1985; pp 51–56.
103. Arbuthnott ER, Sutherland FI, Boyd IA, Gladden MH: Axon terminal indentation and postsynaptic folding as criteria for classifying fusimotor nerve endings, in Boyd IA, Gladden MH (eds): *The Muscle Spindle*. London: Macmillan, 1985; pp 57–62.
104. Gladden MH, Sutherland FI: Do cats have three types of static gamma axon? *J Physiol* 414:19P, 1989.
105. Banks RW, Barker D, Stacey MJ: Form and classification of motor endings in mammalian muscle spindles. *Proc R Soc Lond Biol Sci* 225:195–212, 1985.
106. Kucera J, Walro JM: Factors that determine the form of neuromuscular junctions of intrafusal fibers in the cat. *Am J Anat* 176:97–117, 1986.
107. Celichowski J, Emonet-Dénand F, Laporte Y, Petit J: Distribution of static γ axons in cat peroneus tertius spindles determined by exclusively physiological criteria. *J Neurophysiol* 71:722–732, 1994.
108. Emonet-Dénand F, Laporte Y, Petit J: Comparison of static fusimotor innervation in cat peroneus tertius and longus muscles. *J Neurophysiol* 80:249–254, 1998.
109. Petit J, Banks RW, Laporte Y: Testing the classification of static γ axons using different patterns of random stimulation. *J Neurophysiol* 81:2823–2832, 1999.
110. Gladden MH, McWilliam PN: The activity of intrafusal muscle fibres during cortical stimulation in the cat. *J Physiol* 273:28P, 1977.
111. Gladden MH, McWilliam PN: The activity of intrafusal muscle fibres in anaesthetized, decerebrate and spinal cats. *J Physiol* 273:49P, 1977.
112. Wand P, Schwarz M: Two types of cat fusimotor neurones under separate central control? *Neurosci Lett* 58:145–149, 1985.
113. Kidd GL: Excitation of primary muscle spindle endings by β-axon stimulation. *Nature* 203:1248–1251, 1964.
114. Bessou P, Emonet-Dénand F, Laporte Y: Occurrence of intrafusal muscle fibres innervated by branches of slow α motor fibres in the cat. *Nature* 198:594–595, 1963.
115. Bessou P, Emonet-Dénand F, Laporte Y: Motor fibres innervating extrafusal and intrafusal muscle fibres in the cat. *J Physiol* 180:649–672, 1965.
116. Adal MN, Barker D: Intramuscular branching of fusimotor fibres. *J Physiol* 177:288–299, 1965.
117. Barker D, Stacey MJ, Adal MN: Fusimotor innervation in the cat. *Philos Trans R Soc Lond [Biol]* 258:315–346, 1970.
118. Barker D, Emonet-Dénand F, Laporte Y, Stacey MJ: Identification of the intrafusal endings of skeletofusimotor axons in the cat. *Brain Res* 185:227–237, 1980.
119. Boyd IA, Davey MR: *Composition of Peripheral Nerves*. Edinburgh: Livingstone, 1968.
120. Barker D, Emonet-Dénand F, Harker DW, et al: Types of intra- and extrafusal muscle fibre innervated by dynamic skeletofusimotor axons in cat peroneus brevis and tenuissimus muscles, as determined by the glycogen-depletion method. *J Physiol* 266:713–726, 1977.
121. Burke RE, Tsairis P: Histochemical and physiological profile of a skeletofusimotor (β) unit in cat soleus muscle. *Brain Res* 129:341–345, 1977.
122. Harker DW, Jami L, Laporte Y, Petit J: Fast conducting skeletofusimotor axons supplying intrafusal chain fibers in the cat peroneus tertius muscle. *J Neurophysiol* 40:791–799, 1977.
123. Jami L, Lan-Couton D, Malmgren K, Petit J: Histophysiological observations on fast skeletofusimotor axons. *Brain Res* 164:53–59, 1979.
124. Jami L, Murthy KSK, Petit J: A quantitative study of skeleto-fusimotor innervation in the cat peroneus tertius muscle. *J Physiol* 325:125–144, 1982.
125. Emonet-Dénand F, Jankowska E, Laporte Y: Skeletofusimotor fibres in the rabbit. *J Physiol* 210:669–680, 1970.
126. Andrew BL, Part NJ, Wait F: Muscle spindles without γ-efferents. *J Physiol* 219:28P, 1971.
127. Cheney PD, Preston JB: Effects of fusimotor stimulation on dynamic and position sensitivities of spindle afferents in the primate. *J Neurophysiol* 39:20–30, 1976.
128. Murthy KSK, Letbetter WD, Eidelberg E, et al: Histochemical evidence for the existence of skeletofusimotor (β) innervation in the primate. *Exp Brain Res* 46:186–190, 1982.
129. Murthy KSK: Physiological identification of static β axons in primate muscle. *Exp Brain Res* 52:6–8, 1983.
130. Kucera J: Distribution of skeletofusimotor axons in lumbrical muscles of the monkey. *Anat Embryol* 173:95–104, 1985.
131. Kennedy WR: Innervation of normal human spindles. *Neurology* 20:463–475, 1970.
132. Andrew BL, Part NJ: The division of control of muscle spindles between fusimotor and mixed skeletofusimotor fibres in a rat caudal muscle. *Q J Exp Physiol* 59:331–349, 1974.
133. Banks RW, Barker D, Stacey MJ: Structural aspects of fusimotor effects on spindle sensitivity, in Taylor A, Prochazka A (eds): *Muscle Receptors and Movement*. London: Macmillan, 1981; pp 5–16.

134. Banks RW: Studies on the motor innervation of the cat's muscle spindle, in Jami L, Pierrot-Deseilligny E, Zytnicki D (eds): *Muscle Afferents and Spinal Control of Movement.* Oxford, UK: Pergamon Press, 1992; pp 31–36.
135. Banks RW: Intrafusal motor innervation: A quantitative histological analysis of tenuissimus muscle spindles in the cat. *J Anat* 185:151–172, 1994.
136. Banks RW: A histological study of the motor innervation of the cat's muscle spindle. *J Anat* 133:571–591, 1981.
137. Kucera J: Ultrastructure of extrafusal and intrafusal terminals of a (dynamic) skeletofusimotor axon in cat tenuissimus muscle. *Brain Res* 298:181–186, 1984.
138. Kucera J, Hammar K, Meek B: Ultrastructure of dynamic and static skeletofusimotor endings in a cat muscle spindle. *Cell Tiss Res* 238:151–158, 1984.
139. Kucera J, Hughes R: Histological study of motor innervation to long nuclear chain intrafusal fibers in the muscle spindle of the cat. *Cell Tiss Res* 228:535–547, 1983.
140. Ringstedt T, Copray S, Walro J, Kucera J: Development of fusimotor innervation correlates with group Ia afferents but is independent of neurotrophin-3. *Dev Brain Res* 111:295–300, 1998.
141. Tourtellotte WG, Keller-Peck CP, Kucera J, et al: Gamma, but not alpha, spinal motor neurons require glial cell line-derived neurotrophic factor (GDNF) for their survival in vivo. *J Neuropathol Exp Neurol* 59:136, 2000.
142. Taylor A, Ellaway PH, Durbaba R: Physiological signs of the activation of bag$_2$ and chain intrafusal muscle fibers of gastrocnemius muscle spindles in the cat. *J Neurophysiol* 80:130–142, 1998.
143. Passatore M, Filippi GM: On whether there is a direct sympathetic influence on jaw muscle spindles. *Brain Res* 225:162–165, 1981.
144. Passatore M, Filippi GM: A dual effect of sympathetic nerve stimulation on jaw muscle spindles. *J Auton Nerv Syst* 6:347–361, 1982.
145. Hunt CC, Jami L, Laporte Y: Effects of stimulating the lumbar sympathetic trunk on cat hindlimb muscle spindles. *Arch Ital Biol* 120:371–384, 1982.
146. Grassi C, Deriu F, Passatore M: Effect of sympathetic nervous-system activation on the tonic vibration reflex in rabbit jaw-closing muscles. *J Physiol* 469:601–613, 1993.
147. Passatore M, Deriu F, Grassi C, Roatta S: A comparative study of changes operated by sympathetic nervous system activation on spindle afferent discharge and on tonic vibration reflex in rabbit jaw muscles. *J Auton Nerv Syst* 57:163–167, 1996.
147a. Routta S, Windhorst U, Ljubisavljevic M, et al. Sympathetic modulation of muscle spindle afferent sensitivity to stretch in rabbit jaw closing muscles. *J Physiol* 540:237–248, 2002.
148. Lennerstrand G: Position and velocity sensitivity of muscle spindles in the cat. I. Primary and secondary endings deprived of fusimotor activation. *Acta Physiol Scand* 73:281–299, 1968.
149. Dutia MB: Activation of cat muscle spindle primary, secondary and intermediate sensory endings by suxamethonium. *J Physiol* 304:314–330, 1980.
150. Price RF, Dutia MB: Properties of neck muscle spindles and their excitation by succinylcholine. *Exp Brain Res* 68:619–630, 1987.
151. Price RF, Dutia MB: Physiological properties of tandem muscle spindles in neck and hindlimb muscles, in Allum JHJ, Hulliger M (eds): *Afferent Control of Posture and Locomotion. Progress in Brain Research.* Vol 80. Amsterdam: Excerpta Medica, 1990; pp 47–56.
152. Taylor A, Durbaba R: Classification of jaw-closer muscle spindle afferents in the anaesthetized cat. *J Physiol* 426:56P, 1990.
153. Taylor A, Rodgers JF, Fowle AJ, Durbaba R: The effect of succinylcholine on cat gastrocnemius muscle spindle afferents of different type. *J Physiol* 456:629–644, 1992.
154. Scott JJA: Responses of Ia afferent axons from muscle spindles lacking a bag$_1$ intrafusal muscle fibre. *Brain Res* 543:97–101, 1991.
155. Gioux M, Petit J, Proske U: Responses of cat muscle spindles which lack a dynamic fusimotor supply. *J Physiol* 432:557–571, 1991.
156. Boyd IA: Intrafusal muscle fibres in the cat and their motor control, in Barnes WJP, Gladden MH (eds): *Feedback and Motor Control in Invertebrates and Vertebrates.* London: Croom Helm, 1985; pp 123–144.
157. Crowe A: A mechanical model of the mammalian muscle spindle. *J Theor Biol* 21:21–41, 1968.
158. Houk JC, Rymer WZ, Crago PE: Dependence of the dynamic response of spindle receptors on muscle length and velocity. *J Neurophysiol* 46:143–166, 1981.
159. Lennerstrand G, Thoden U: Dynamic analysis of muscle spindle endings in the cat using length changes of different length-time relations. *Acta Physiol Scand* 73:234–250, 1968.
160. Matthews PBC, Stein RB: The sensitivity of muscle spindle afferents to small sinusoidal changes of length. *J Physiol* 200:723–743, 1969.
161. Brown MC, Stein RB: Quantitative studies on the slowly adapting stretch receptor of the crayfish. *Kybernetik* 3:175–185, 1966.
162. Rudjord T: A second-order mechanical model of muscle-spindle primary endings. *Kybernetik* 6:205–213, 1970.
163. Schaafsma A, Otten E, van Willigen JD: A muscle spindle model for primary afferent firing based on a simulation of intrafusal mechanical events. *J Neurophysiol* 65:1297–1312, 1991.
164. Eagles JP, Purple RL: Afferent fibers with multiple encoding sites. *Brain Res* 77:187–193, 1974.
165. Quick DC, Kennedy WR, Poppele RE: Anatomical evidence for multiple sources of action potentials in the afferent fibres of muscle spindles. *Neuroscience* 5:109–115, 1980.
166. Hulliger M, Noth J: Static and dynamic fusimotor interaction and the possibility of multiple pacemakers operating in the cat muscle spindles. *Brain Res* 173:21–28, 1979.
167. Otten E, Scheepstra KA, Hulliger M: An integrated model of the mammalian muscle spindle, in Taylor A, Gladden MH, Durbaba R (eds): *Alpha and Gamma Motor Systems.* New York: Plenum Press, 1995; pp 294–301.
168. Banks RW, Hulliger M, Scheepstra KA, Otten E: Pacemaker activity in a sensory ending with multiple encoding sites: The cat muscle spindle primary ending. *J Physiol* 498:177–199, 1997.
169. Banks RW, Hulliger M, Scheepstra KA: Correlated histological and physiological observations on a case of common sensory output and motor input of the bag$_1$ fibre and a chain fibre in a cat tenuissimus spindle. *J Anat* 193:373–381, 1998.
170. Fallon JB, Carr RW, Gregory JE, Proske U: Summing responses of cat soleus muscle spindles to combined static and dynamic fusimotor stimulation. *Brain Res* 888:348–355, 2001.
171. Taylor A, Durbaba R, Ellaway PH, Rawlinson S: Patterns of fusimotor activity during locomotion in the decerebrate cat deduced from recordings from hindlimb muscle spindles. *J Physiol* 522:515–532, 2000.
172. Hunt CC, Wilkinson RS, Fukami Y: Ionic basis of the receptor potential in primary endings of mammalian muscle spindles. *J Gen Physiol* 71:683–698, 1978.
173. Hunt CC, Wilkinson RS: An analysis of receptor potential and tension of isolated cat muscle spindles in response to sinusoidal stretch. *J Physiol* 302:241–262, 1980.
174. Fischer M, Schäffer SS: Effects of calcium on the discharge pattern of primary and secondary endings in isolated cat muscle spindles recorded under a ramp-and-hold stretch. *Brain Res* 875:78–88, 2000.
175. Kruse MN, Poppele RE: Components of the dynamic-response of mammalian muscle spindles that originate in the sensory terminals. *Exp Brain Res* 86:359–366, 1991.
176. Matthews PBC: Muscle spindles and their motor control. *Physiol Rev* 44:219–288, 1964.
177. Baumann TK, Hulliger M: The dependence of the response of cat spindle Ia afferents to sinusoidal stretch on the velocity of concomitant movement. *J Physiol* 439:325–350, 1991.
178. Banks RW, Barker D, Bessou P, et al: Histological analysis of cat muscle spindles following direct observation of the effects of stimulating dynamic and static motor axons. *J Physiol* 283:605–619, 1978.
179. Hulliger M: The responses of primary spindle afferents to fusimotor stimulation at constant and abruptly changing rates. *J Physiol* 294:461–482, 1979.
180. Poppele RE, Quick DC: Stretch-induced contraction of intrafusal muscle in cat muscle spindle. *J Neurosci* 1:1069–1074, 1981.
181. Pringle JWS: Stretch activation of muscle: Function and mechanisms. *Proc R Soc Lond Biol Sci* 201:107–130, 1978.
182. Smith RS: Properties of intrafusal muscle fibres, in Granit R (ed): *Muscular Afferents and Motor Control.* Stockholm: Almqvist & Wiksell, 1966; pp 69–80.
183. De Camilli P, Vitadello M, Canevini MP, et al: The synaptic vesicle proteins synapsin I and synaptophysin (protein p38) are concentrated both in efferent and afferent nerve endings of the skeletal muscles. *J Neurosci* 8:1625–1631, 1988.
184. Bewick GS, Reid B, Banks RW: Investigating the role of small clear vesicles in vertebrate mechanosensory endings using rat muscle spindles. *J Physiol* 528:62P, 2000.
185. Banks RW, Richardson C, Bewick GS: Immunocytochemical demonstration of glutamate in the sensory terminals of rat muscle spindles. *J Physiol* 528:62P, 2000.
186. Hietanen-Peltola M, Pelto-Huikko M, Rechardt L, et al: Calbindin-D-28k-immunoreactivity in rat muscle spindle; a light and electron microscopic study. *Brain Res* 579:327–332, 1992.
187. Duc C, Barakat-Walter I, Droz B: Innervation of putative rapidly adapting mechanoreceptors by calbindin- and calretinin-immunoreactive primary sensory neurons in the rat. *Eur J Neurosci* 6:264–271, 1994.
188. El-Tarhouni A, Banks RW: The distribution of calretinin in muscle receptors of the cat. *J Physiol* 487:77P, 1995.
189. Iino S, Kobayashi S, Hidaka H: Neurocalcin-immunopositive nerve terminals in the muscle spindle, Golgi tendon organ and motor endplate. *Brain Res* 808:294–299, 1998.
190. Werle MJ, Roder J, Jeromin A: Expression of frequenin at the frog (*Rana*) neuromuscular junction, muscle spindle and nerve. *Neurosci Lett* 284:33–36, 2000.
191. Ikura M: Calcium binding and conformational response in EF-hand proteins. *Trends Biochem Sci* 21:14–17, 1996.
192. Burgoyne RD, Weiss JL: The neuronal calcium sensor family of Ca^{2+}-binding proteins. *Biochem J* 353:1–12, 2001.

193. Galeano RM, Germanà A, Vázquez MT, et al: Immunohistochemical localization of neurocalcin in human sensory neurons and mechanoreceptors. *Neurosci Lett* 279:89–92, 2000.
194. Hietanen-Peltola M, Rechardt L, Pelto-Huikko M: Protein kinase C β-subtype-immunoreactive motor and sensory nerves in rat muscle spindle. *Neurosci Lett* 132:65–68, 1991.
195. Masutani M, Mizoguchi A, Arii T, et al: Localization of protein kinase-C-α, kinase-C-β and kinase-C-γ subspecies in sensory axon terminals of the rat muscle spindle. *J Neurocytol* 23:811–819, 1994.
196. Landon DN: The fine structure of the equatorial regions of developing muscle spindles in the rat. *J Neurocytol* 1:189–210, 1972.
197. Milburn A: The early development of muscle spindles in the rat. *J Cell Sci* 12:175–195, 1973.
198. Kozeka K, Ontell M: The three-dimensional cytoarchitecture of developing murine muscle spindles. *Dev Biol* 87:133–147, 1981.
199. Milburn A: Stages in the development of the cat muscle spindle. *J Embryol Exp Morphol* 82:177–216, 1984.
200. Pedrosa F, Thornell L-E: Expression of myosin heavy chain isoforms in developing rat muscle spindles. *Histochemistry* 94:231–244, 1990.
201. Kucera J, Walro JM: Origin of intrafusal muscle fibers in the rat. *Histochemistry* 93:567–580, 1990.
202. Pedrosa-Domellöf F, Thornell L-E: Expression of myosin heavy chain isoforms in developing human muscle spindles. *J Histochem Cytochem* 42:77–88, 1994.
203. Soukup T, Pedrosa-Domellöf F, Thornell L-E: Expression of myosin heavy chain isoforms and myogenesis of intrafusal fibres in rat muscle spindles. *Microsc Res Tech* 30:390–407, 1995.
204. Walro JM, Kucera J: Why adult mammalian intrafusal and extrafusal fibers contain different myosin heavy-chain isoforms. *Trends Neurosci* 22:180–184, 1999.
205. Kucera J, Walro JM: Origin of intrafusal fibers from a subset of primary myotubes in the rat. *Anat Embryol* 192:149–158, 1995.
206. Kucera J, Walro JM, Gao Y: Influence of muscle cell substrates on differentiation of intrafusal fiber types in neonatal rats. *Neurosci* 52:1001–1008, 1993.
207. Kucera J, Walro JM, Reichler J: Innervation of developing intrafusal muscle fibers in the rat. *Am J Anat* 183:344–358, 1988.
208. Andrew BL, Leslie GC, Part NJ: Some observations on the efferent innervation of rat soleus muscle spindles. *Exp Brain Res* 31:433–443, 1978.
209. Ernfors P, Lee KF, Kucera J, Jaenisch R: Lack of neurotrophin-3 leads to deficiencies in the peripheral nervous system and loss of limb proprioceptive afferents. *Cell* 77:503–512, 1994.
210. Copray JCVM, Brouwer N: Selective expression of neurotrophin-3 messenger RNA in muscle spindles of the rat. *Neurosci* 63:1125–1135, 1994.
211. Copray JCVM, Brouwer N: Neurotrophin-3 mRNA expression in rat intrafusal muscle fibres after denervation and reinnervation. *Neurosci Lett* 236:41–44, 1997.
212. Kucera J, Fan GP, Jaenisch R, et al: Dependence of developing group Ia afferents on neurotrophin-3. *J Comp Neurol* 363:307–320, 1995.
213. Wright DE, Zhou L, Kucera J, Snider WD: Introduction of a neurotrophin-3 transgene into muscle selectively rescues proprioceptive neurons in mice lacking endogenous neurotrophin-3. *Neuron* 19:503–517, 1997.
214. Ringstedt T, Kucera J, Lendahl U, et al: Limb proprioceptive deficits without neuronal loss in transgenic mice overexpressing neurotrophin-3 in the developing nervous system. *Development* 124:2603–2613, 1997.
215. Fan G, Jaenisch R, Kucera J: A role for p75 receptor in neurotrophin-3 functioning during the development of limb proprioception. *Neuroscience* 90:259–268, 1999.
216. Taylor MD, Vancura R, Patterson CL, et al: Postnatal regulation of limb proprioception by muscle-derived neurotrophin-3. *J Comp Neurol* 432:244–258, 2001.
217. Fan GP, Copray S, Huang E, et al: Formation of a full complement of cranial proprioceptors requires multiple neurtrophins. *Dev Dyn* 218:359–370, 2000.
218. Matsuo S, Ichikawa H, Silos-Santiago I, et al: Proprioceptive afferents survive in the masseter muscle of trkC knockout mice. *Neuroscience* 95:209–216, 2000.
219. Tourtellotte WG, Milbrandt J: Sensory ataxia and muscle spindle agenesis in mice lacking the transcription factor Egr-3. *Nat Genet* 20:87–91, 1998.
220. Tourtellotte WG, Keller-Peck C, Milbrandt J, Kucera J: The transcription factor Egr3 modulates sensory axon-myotube interactions during muscle spindle morphogenesis. *Dev Biol* 232:388–399, 2001.
221. Chen H-H, Hippenmeyer S, Arber S, et al: Development of the monosynaptic stretch reflex circuit. *Curr Opin Neurobiol* 13:96–102, 2003.

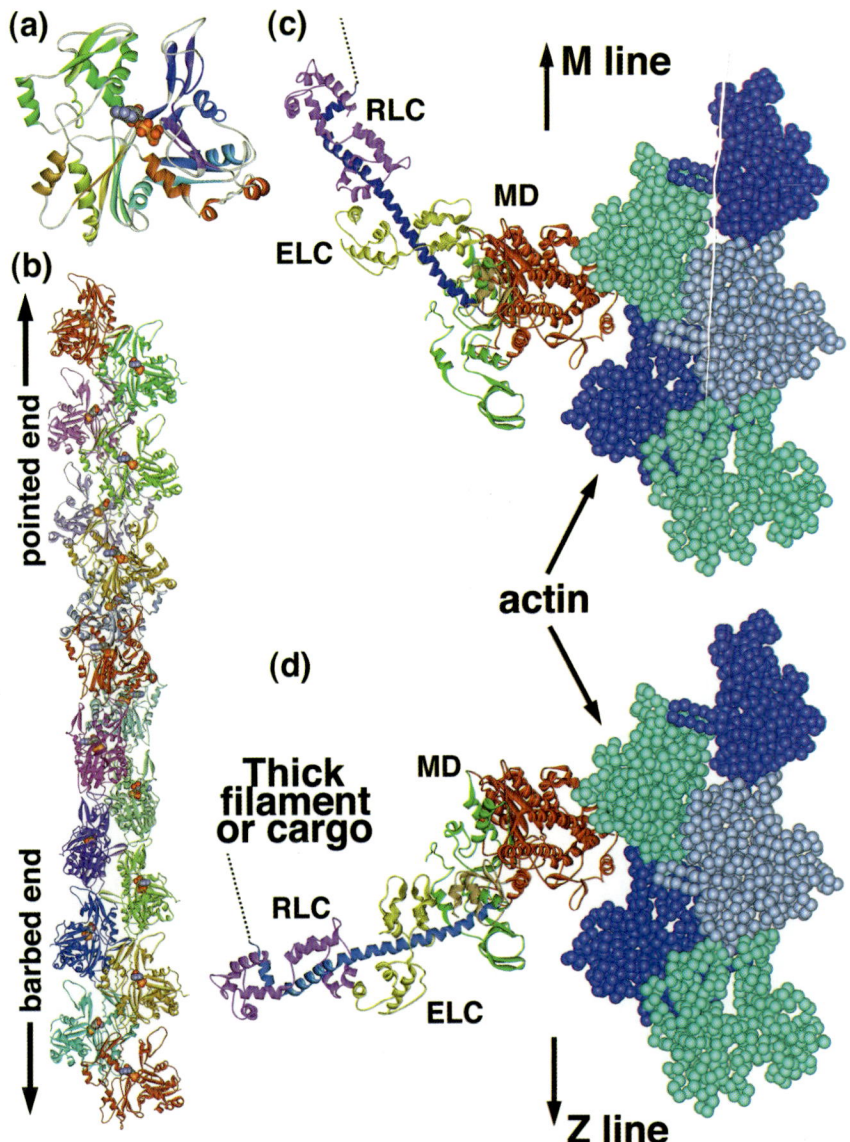

Color Plate 1. Actin and myosin: the architecture of chemomechanical transduction.

Muscle contraction consists of a cyclic interaction between myosin and actin driven by the concomitant hydrolysis of adenosine triphosphate (ATP). The atomic structures of actin and of myosin were defined within a few years of each other and immediately suggested a novel working hypothesis for the mechanism of myosin action. *a* and *b*. A crystal of actin was obtained by combining the molecule with DNase (*a*),[1] and the high-resolution molecules were fitted into filaments (*b*), shown with the pointed end—in the direction of the M line—upward. In the filament (*b*), each monomer is represented by a different color. The individual monomer (*a*) is colored from violet at the N terminus to red at the C terminus. ADP is present as a space-filling model in the center of the molecule. *c* and *d*. The three-dimensional structure of the myosin S1 subfragment or head was independently obtained in the pre-power stroke conformation for a smooth muscle myosin (*c*)[3] and in the "rigor" state, in the absence of ATP, for a skeletal muscle myosin (*d*).[2] These images identify key elements of the motor, or catalytic, domain (MD): the N-terminal region (green), the central 50-kDa region (red), and the converter domain (tan). The C-terminal domain forms a single long α helix (blue), associated with the light chains (yellow and magenta) constituting the lever arm. The two myosin states are distinguished by a large tilt in the orientation of the lever arm around a pivot at its base, where it links to the motor domain. Fitting the high-resolution actin and rigor myosin maps into the low-resolution electron-density maps of decorated actin filaments derived by cryoelectron microscopy resulted in the model presented in *d*.[4] The domain structure suggested that the position of the MD may remain fixed during the power stroke and that the critical movement would be tilting the lever arm. The power stroke would result from the movement of the lever arm between images *c* and *d*, driven by smaller positional shifts of residues at the active site. This hypothesis fits well the x-ray diffraction data during force generation in intact single muscle fibers.[5] The observed positions of active cross-bridges in situ rapidly frozen in action confirm the lever-arm movement but also indicate a tilt and slew of the MD on actin.[6] (See also Chaps. 7 to 9.) (*The coordinates for b were kindly supplied by Dr. Ken Holmes and for c and d by Dr. M. Irving.[5] Molecular models were rendered using WebLab Viewer Pro software. We thank Dr. Yale Goldman for figures and legends on Color Plates 1, 3, and 4.*)

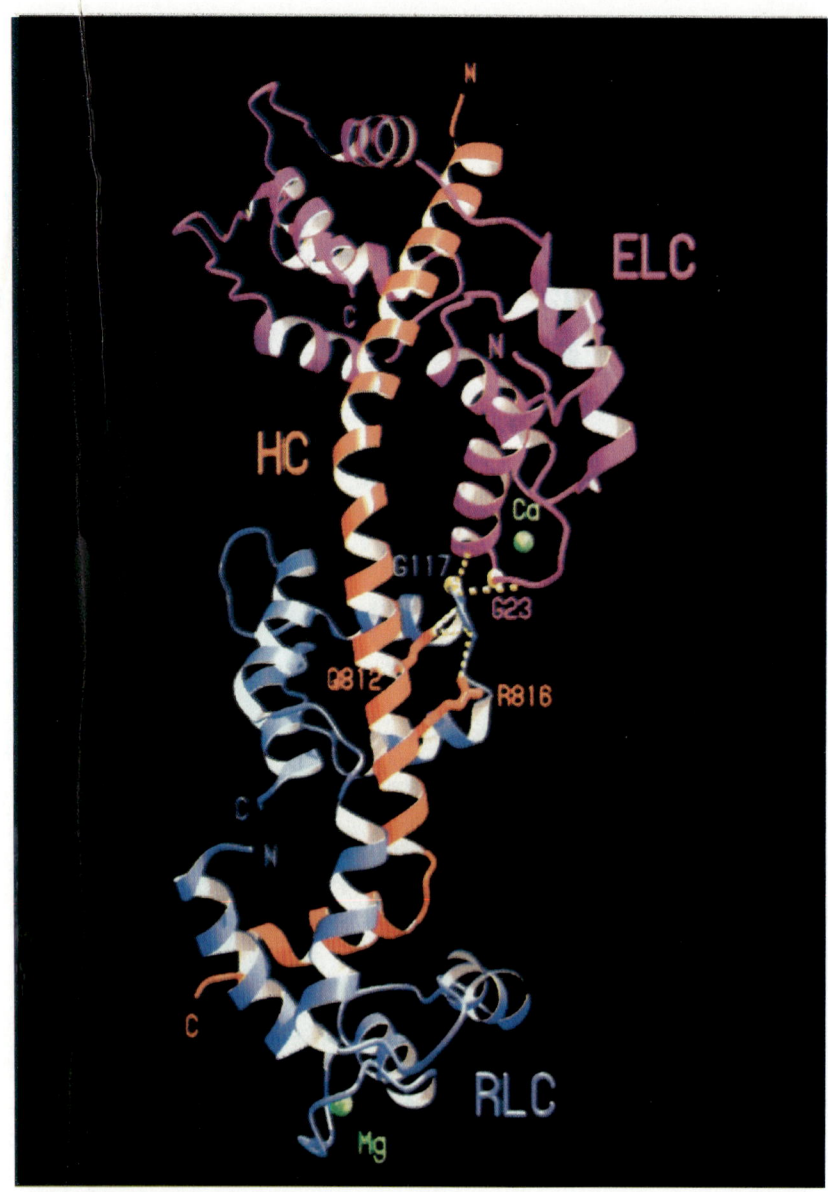

COLOR PLATE 2. The myosin regulatory domain.
The myosin molecule lever arm (see Color Plate 1) is constituted of a single α helix, part of the myosin heavy chain, around which are wrapped the two light chains: the essential light chain, ELC in purple, and the regulatory light chain, RLC in blue. The regulatory domain of scallop myosin is shown here. A Mg^{2+} in green is shown bound to the divalent cation binding site in domain 1 of the RLC. A Ca^{2+} in green is located in the specific Ca^{2+}-binding site of the ELC. The site, which regulates the scallop myosin activity, is surrounded by a loop of nine residues and stabilized by key linkages involving ELC and myosin heavy chain. See Chap. 13 and Fig. 13-14 for details.[1,2] *(Figure kindly provided by C. Cohen and M. Silver, Brandeis University.)*

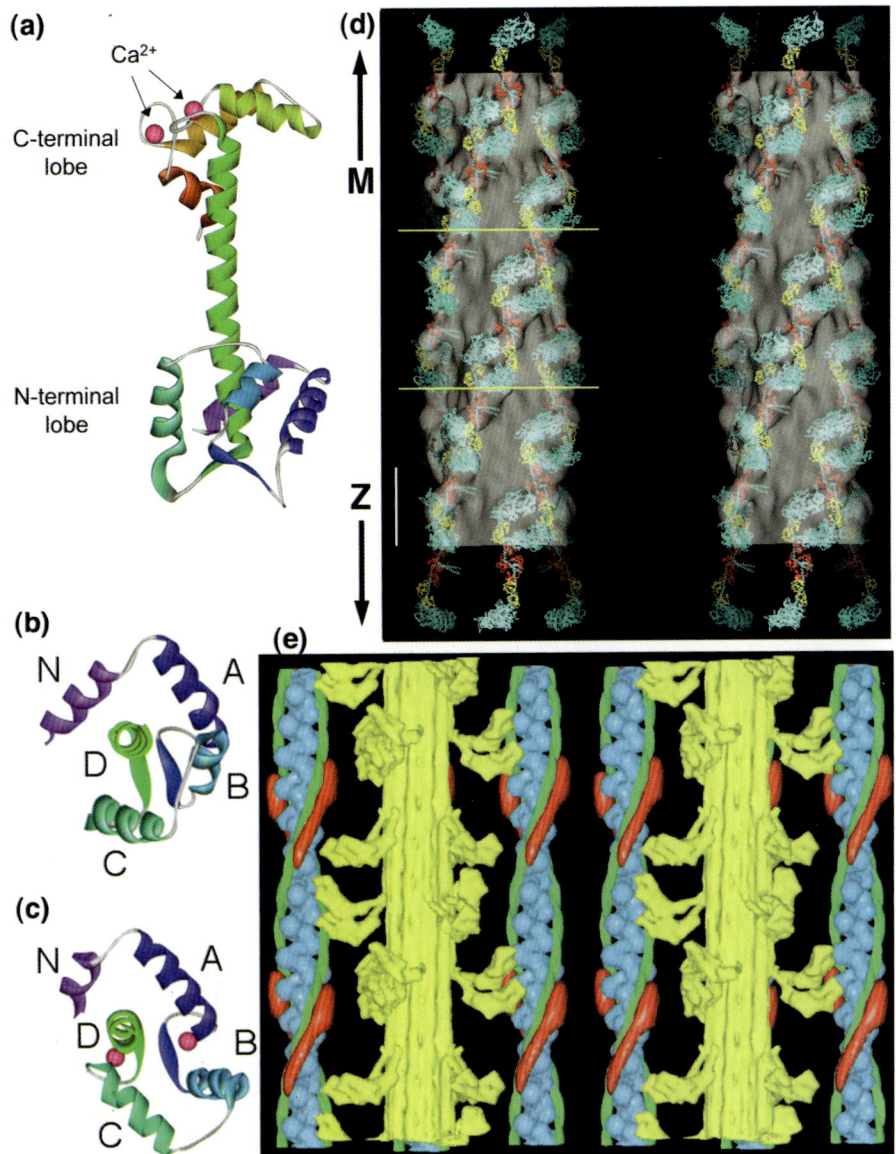

Color Plate 3. Troponin C (TnC), thick filaments, and the sarcomere: a molecular switch and muscle control.

a to *c*. TnC, the regulatory Ca^{2+}-binding component of the sarcomeric thin filaments' troponin complex, has been solved in two states. In one state (*a*),[1] the two high-affinity binding sites in the C-terminal domain are occupied by Ca^{2+}. This is the condition of TnC in relaxed muscle. In the other state (*c*),[2] the two-low affinity sites in the N-terminal domain are also occupied: this is the condition in the contracting muscle. Both domains have two EF hand helix-loop-helix Ca^{2+}-binding motifs approximately related by a twofold rotation. However, H-L-H motifs in the N and C domains have very different conformations, the latter more closely resembling the EF hand domain of parvalbumin. In *b* and *c*, the conformation of the N-terminal domain in the absence and presence of Ca^{2+} is compared. The molecules are colored from violet at the N terminus to orange at the C terminus (see Chap. 13). *d* and *e*. these figures are stereo images: They can be seen either by crossing eyes or by using a stereo viewer. Both images are shown in the same orientation as those in Color Plate 1—that is, the M line upward. *e*. Fitting of the atomic model of myosin on a three-dimensional helical reconstruction of the relaxed myosin filament from tarantula muscle.[3] The myosin heavy chain is turquoise; the light chains are red and yellow. The myosin heads are positioned so that their long axis is oriented approximately along the four strands of the long pitch helix marking the S1-S2 junction on the surface of the filament. This has been shown to be the case for myosin filaments in two arthropods.[3,4] *f*. Model of the disposition of actin (blue), myosin (yellow), tropomyosin (green), and the troponins (red) in the relaxed sarcomere from a fish muscle. The images were modeled from x-ray diffraction data and fitted with the atomic structure of the myosin head. The three actin filaments on the viewer's side of the myosin molecule are not shown in order to reveal the myosin disposition. The crossbridges in this reconstruction reach toward the thin filaments but are not attached to them, as they would be if the muscle were in rigor. The myosin heads in the model are less tightly arranged around the thick filament than in the isolated filament shown in *e*. (See Chaps. 7 to 9.) (*Courtesy of Carlo Knupp and John Squire.*[5–7])

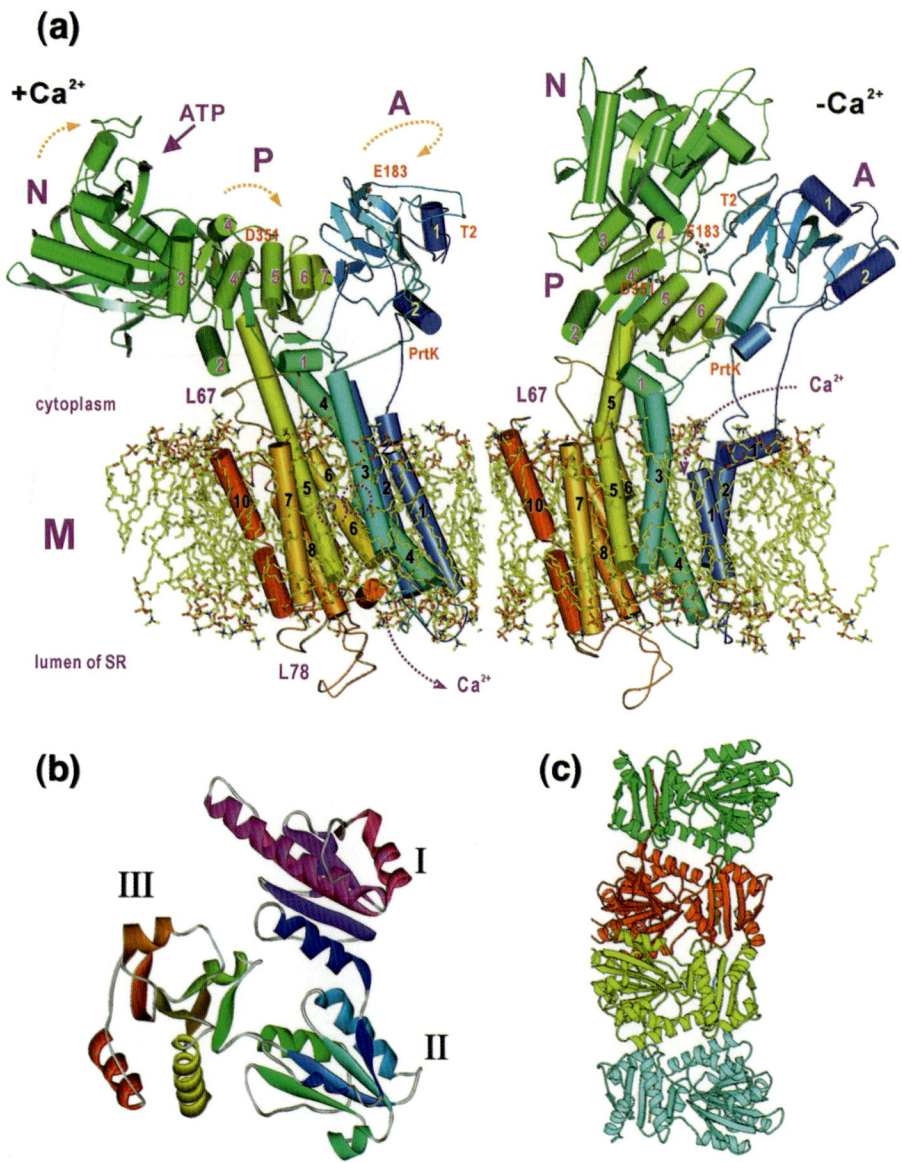

COLOR PLATE 4. **The Ca^{2+}-ATPase: transporting ions against a gradient. Calsequestrin: the anatomy of calcium binding.**
a. The crystal structure of Ca^{2+}-ATPase (SERCA1a) in skeletal muscle sarcoplasmic reticulum (SR) was solved in its Ca^{2+}-bound (E1) state in 2000 (left)[1] and captured in the E^2, Ca^{2+}-free state in 2002 (right).[2,3] Three well-separated domains of the head piece are the phosphorylation (P), nucleotide-binding (N), and actuator (A) domains. The 2.6-Å resolution Ca^{2+}-bound structure, left, shows two Ca^{2+} ions (red spheres) in the transmembrane domain, ready to be released to the SR lumen. Interestingly, no direct connection leading from the cytoplasmic surface to the binding sites is present in this configuration, suggesting that the entry pathway is already closed. The difference between the Ca^{2+}-free and the Ca^{2+}-bound states involves large-scale movements of the N, P, and A domains, which cluster closer together in the absence of Ca^{2+} (right). This is coupled to changes in tilt and position of several intramembrane helices (see Chap. 14). Although the structures of the ATP-bound and phosphorylated states are not yet available, these images provide direct snapshots of the protein in action that fit remarkably well with previous predictions on the basic mechanism of transport by a family of cation pumps (see Chap. 14). The molecules in *a* and *b* are colored from blue at the N terminus to orange at the C terminus. *(Reprinted with permission from Ref. 2.)* *b* and *c*. Calsequestrin releases and binds 40 to 50 Ca^{2+} ions per molecule during a contraction-relaxation cycle. *b*. The crystal structure of calsequestrin, solved in 1998,[4,5] shows three similarly folded domains (I to III). Domain III has the highest electronegative surface potential. *c*. The clever mechanism by which the calsequestrin molecule is compacted and polymer formation is initiated by low concentrations of cations. Each molecule in the polymer has different color. An initial back-to-back dimeric interaction, related by a crystallographic twofold axis, forms a large pocket lined by acidic residues. Calcium occupation of the pocket stabilizes the dimer. A subsequent front-to-front interaction is stabilized by an interaction between two helices of the molecule. Polymerization results in the loose network that fills the luminea of the junctional SR cisternae (see Chaps. 11 and 14). *(From Wang et al.[4] Reproduced by permission.)*

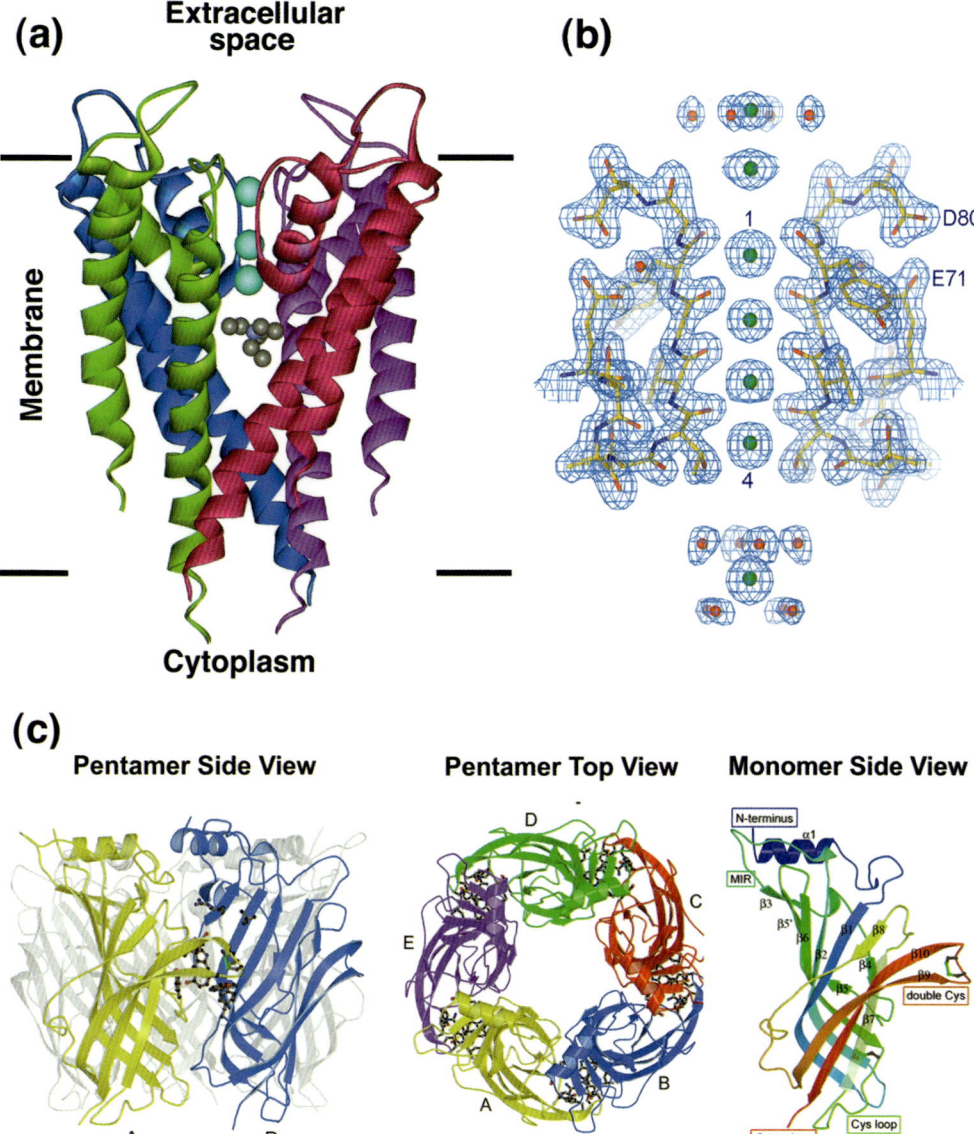

COLOR PLATE 5. Ionic channels: ions in transit.

The K$^+$ ion selective channel a. The first atomic-level-resolution image of an ionic channel (a bacterial K$^+$ selective potassium channel)[1] has provided stunning views of the channel's selectivity filter, surrounded and supported by a tepee of alpha helices. Cations within the selectivity filter are indicated as blue spheres. A TEA molecule (gray spheres) is shown in the hydrophobic central cavity located within the membrane on the cytoplasmic side of the selectivity filter. b. Subsequent refinements following immobilization by cross-linking with FAB fragments[2] illustrate a fully hydrated K$^+$ ion (green) within the central cavity, surrounded by eight ordered water molecules (red), poised to enter the filter. A specific arrangement of carbonyl oxygen atoms protruding into the solution allows the ions to be dehydrated and transferred into the selectivity filter. Several ions can occupy the selectivity filter in a single line, and the conformation of the filter depends on the presence of ions. For the first time, the structural counterparts of selectivity and conductivity are directly seen, deepening our understanding of channel function.[3] Visualization of the K$^+$ ion with its hydration shell hovering at the edges of the selectivity filter is astounding (see Chap. 10). c. The extracellular domain of the pentameric acetylcholine receptor (AChR) channel has been solved by taking advantage of a water-soluble Ach-binding protein that could be used to crystallize portions of a protein closely related to a neuronal AChR.[4] The monomer is colored from blue at the N terminus to orange in at the C terminus. These images account very well for the overall shape of the extracellular domain and for the structure of the ACh binding site (see Chap. 17.)

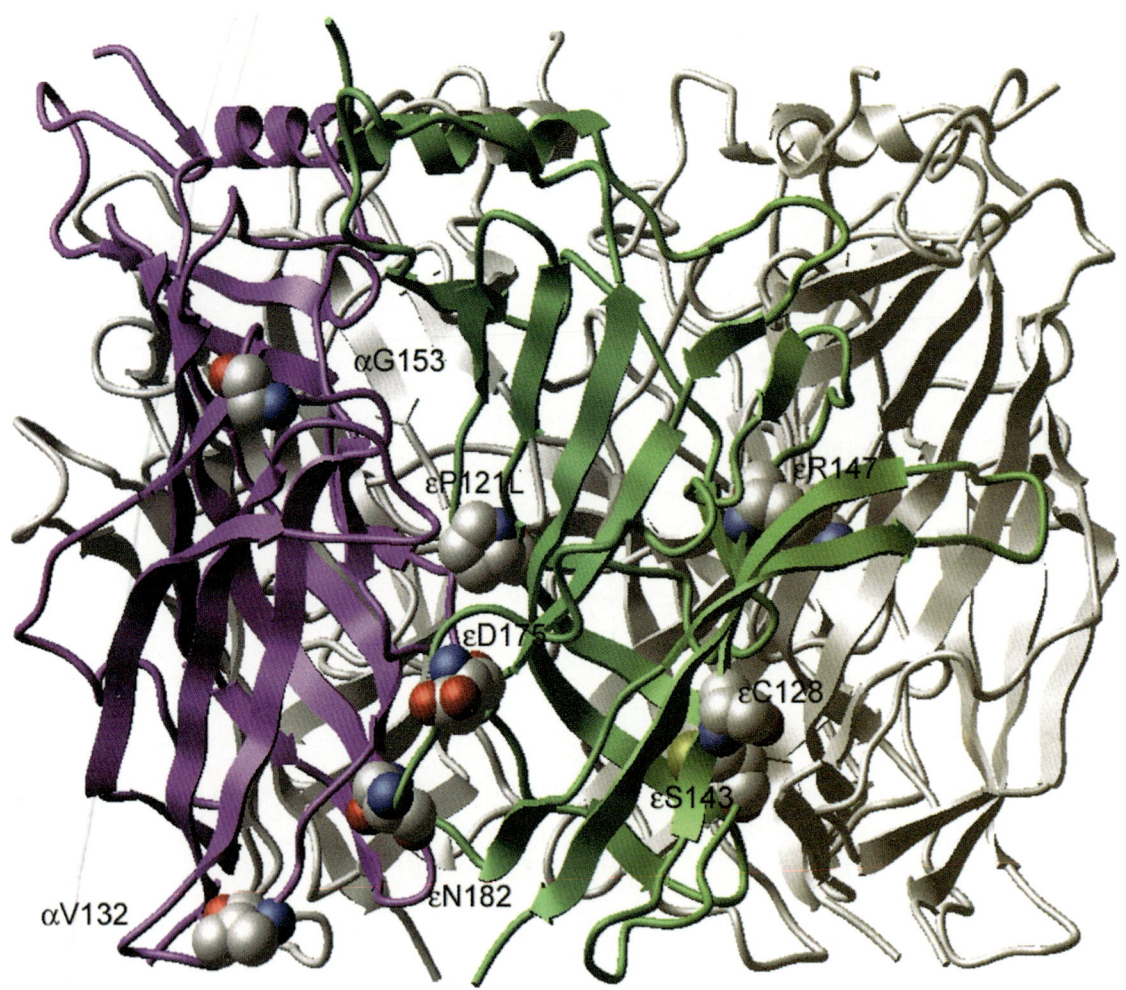

COLOR PLATE 6.   Mutations in the ACh binding site of AChR causing congenital myasthenic syndromes.
Residues found to be mutated are shown on a structural model of the ligand-binding domain formed by α and ε subunits based on lysine scanning and homology modeling. (*From Sine SM et al: J Biol Chem 277:29210-29223, 2002. Reproduced by permission.*) The alpha subunit is highlighted in magenta and the epsilon subunit in green. The three other subunits are depicted in gray. Residues mutated in CMS are shown in space-filling representation on a secondary structural rendering of the subunits. In a slow-channel syndrome, αG153 is mutated; whereas εP121, αV132, εD175, and εN182 are mutated and cause the functional consequences in the fast-channel syndromes. Mutations of εC128, εS143, and εR147 impair assembly and are null mutations in fast-channel patients. (Cited in Chap. 66.)

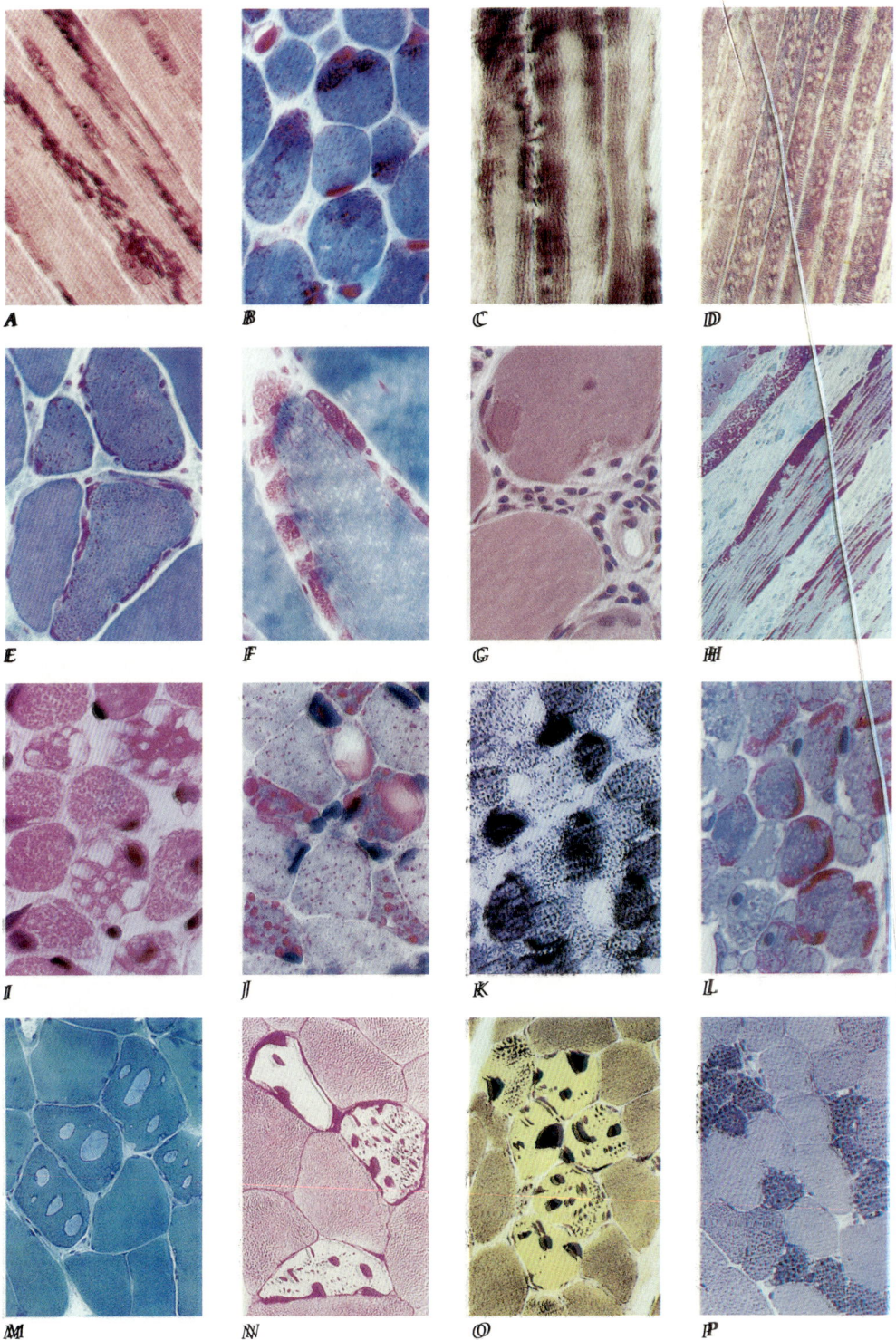

COLOR PLATE 7. *A, B.* Congenital nemaline myopathy. *A.* Phosphotungstic acid hematoxylin stain, paraffin section, ×520. *B.* Trichrome stain, frozen section, ×660. *C.* Central core disease, NADH dehydrogenase, ×210. *D.* Multicore disease, NADH dehydrogenase, ×130. *E, F.* Ragged red fibers in mitochondrial myopathy, trichrome stain, ×210. *G.* Inclusion body myositis. Upper muscle fiber contains eosinophilic nuclear and cytoplasmic inclusions, ×325. *H.* Adult acid maltase deficiency, PAS methylene blue, ×210. *I–L.* Benign infantile cytochrome *c* oxidase deficiency. *I,* hematoxylin and eosin, ×400; *J,* oil red O, ×400; *K,* NADH dehydrogenase, ×260; *L,* PAS methylene blue, ×520. *M–O.* Polyglucosan storage disease. The abnormal polysaccharide in the vacuoles is strongly PAS (*N*) and iodine (*O*) positive. The vacuolated fibers contain decreased intermyofibrillar glycogen (*N*). *M,* trichrome, ×130; *N,* PAS, ×210; *O,* phosphorylase reaction developed with iodine, ×130 *P.* Muscle carnitine deficiency. The lipid deposits are most abundant in type 1 fibers and there is type 1 fiber atrophy. Sudan black B, ×130. (Cited in Chaps. 30 and 31.))

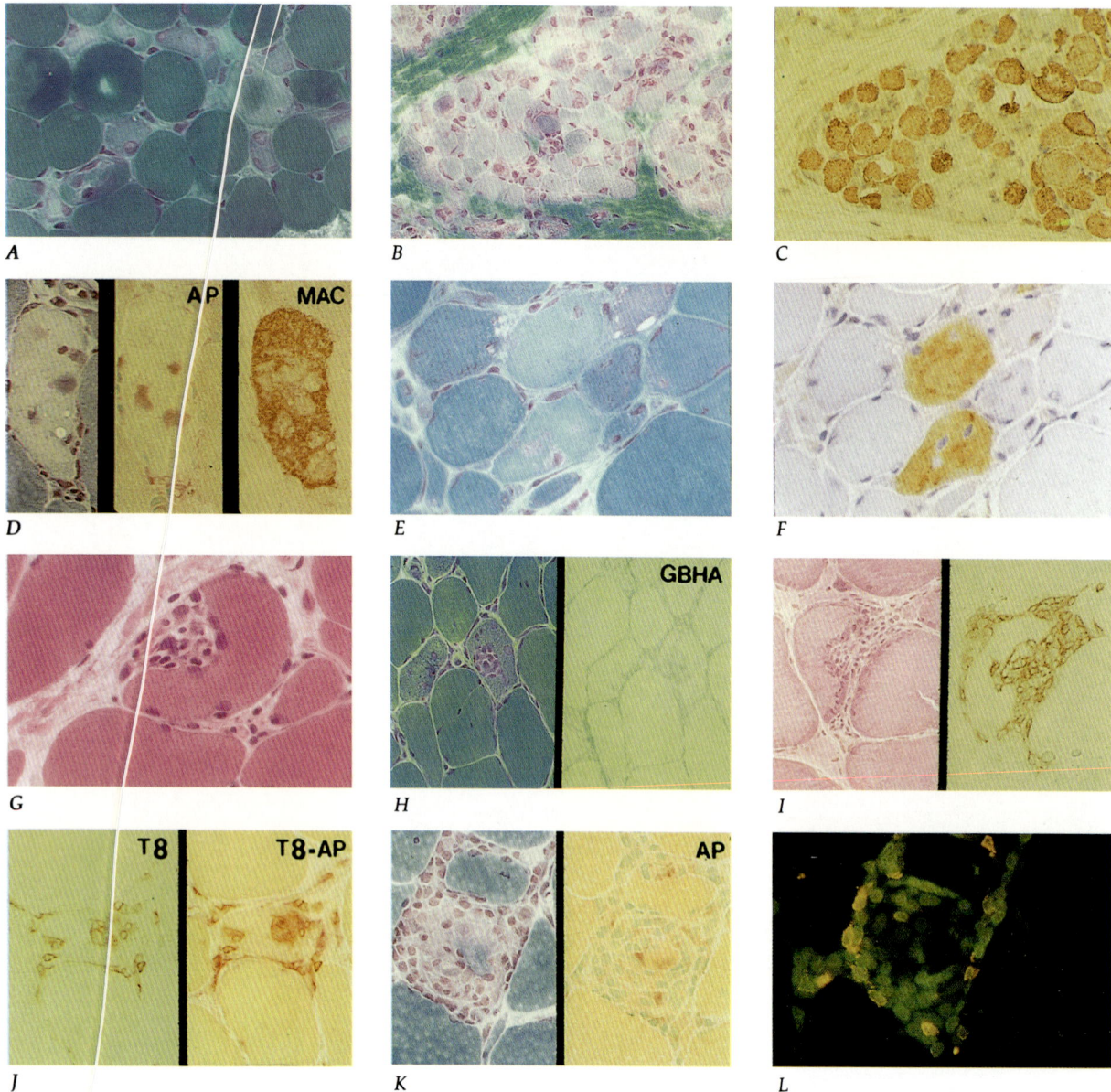

COLOR PLATE 8. *A-F.* Necrotic muscle fibers after an attack of rhabdomyolysis *(A-C)* and in polymyositis *(D-F)*. The sections are stained with trichrome *(A, B,* left panel in *D,* and *E)*, reacted for acid phosphatase (middle panel in *D)*, and reacted for the complement membrane attack complex (MAC) *(C* and *F)*. Pallid necrotic fibers are invaded by acid-phosphatase-positive macrophages and react for MAC. In *A, B,* and *E,* regenerating fibers with large nuclei and red-blue cytoplasm occur near the necrotic fibers. *A, E, F,* × 240; *B, C,* × 150; *D,* × 370. *G-L.* Cell-mediated destruction of nonnecrotic muscle fibers in inclusion body myositis *(G-I)* and polymyositis *(J-L)*. The sections are stained with hematoxylin and eosin *(G,* left panel in *I)*, trichrome (left panels in *H* and *K)*, and with glyoxal-bix-(2-hydroxyanil) (GBHA) (right panel in *H)*. Macrophages are identified by the acid phosphatase (AP) reaction (right panels in *J* and *K)*. The CD8 antigen, found on cytotoxic and suppressor T cells, is localized by the immunoperoxidase method (right panel in *I* and both panels in *J)*. The CD3 antigen, found on all T cells, and the CD57 antigen, found on natural killer (NK) cells, are shown by paired immunofluorescence *(L)*. The invaded fibers do not stain for calcium with GBHA *(H)*. Most invading cells are antigen-specific CD8+ cells *(I, J)*. About one-third of the invading cells are cytotoxic macrophages (right panels in *J* and *K)*. In *K* and *L* serial sections of two invaded fibers show sparse macrophages (right panel in *K)*, many CD3+ T cells (green fluorescence in *L)*, and a few CD3+ CD57+ immature NK cells (yellow fluorescence in *L)*. *H, I, J,* × 150; *G, K, L,* × 375. (Cited in Chaps. 30, 31, and 49.) *(Panels A to D, G to I, and L are reproduced from Selcen and Engel: Brain 127:439-451, 2004, by permission.)*

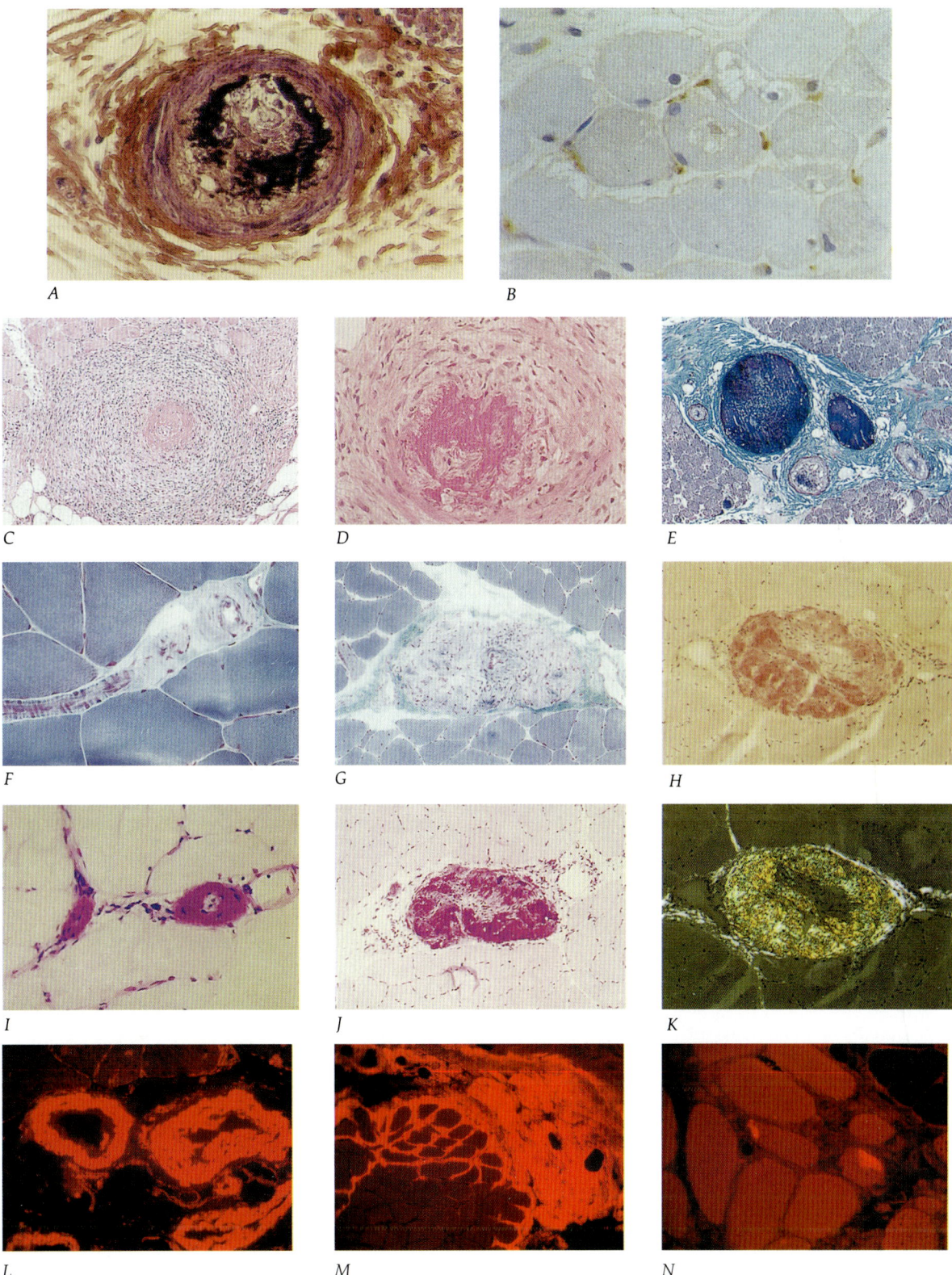

Color Plate 9. *A.* Perimysial artery in dermatomyositis with a fibrin thrombus and early recanalization. Phosphotungstic acid–hematoxylin, ×150. *B.* Necrotic endomysial capillaries in dermatomyositis react for the complement membrane attack complex (MAC). Adjacent muscle fibers show vacuolar change. ×320. *C, D.* Periarteritis nodosa. Perimysial arterioles show fibrinoid necrosis of their mural elements, have occluded lumens, and are surrounded and infiltrated by inflammatory cells. *C,* ×60; *D,* ×150. *E.* Scleroderma. Hyalinization of blood vessel walls and perimysial fibrosis. Trichrome, ×60. *F–N.* Systemic amyloidosis. Amyloid deposits infiltratre the walls of the intramuscular blood vessels and extend into the adjacent interstitial regions. The deposits stain pink-gray with trichrome *(F, G)*, show metachromasia with crystal violet *(I, J)*, and are Congo red-positive *(H).* The Congo red-positive deposits display apple-green birefringence in polarized light *(K)* and strong red fluorescence under rhodamine optics *(L and M). H, J, K,* ×60; *L,* ×90; *M,* ×150. *N.* Fluorescent Congophilic inclusions in inclusions body myositis viewed under rhodamine optics. ×220. (Cited in Chaps. 30, 31, 49, and 53.)

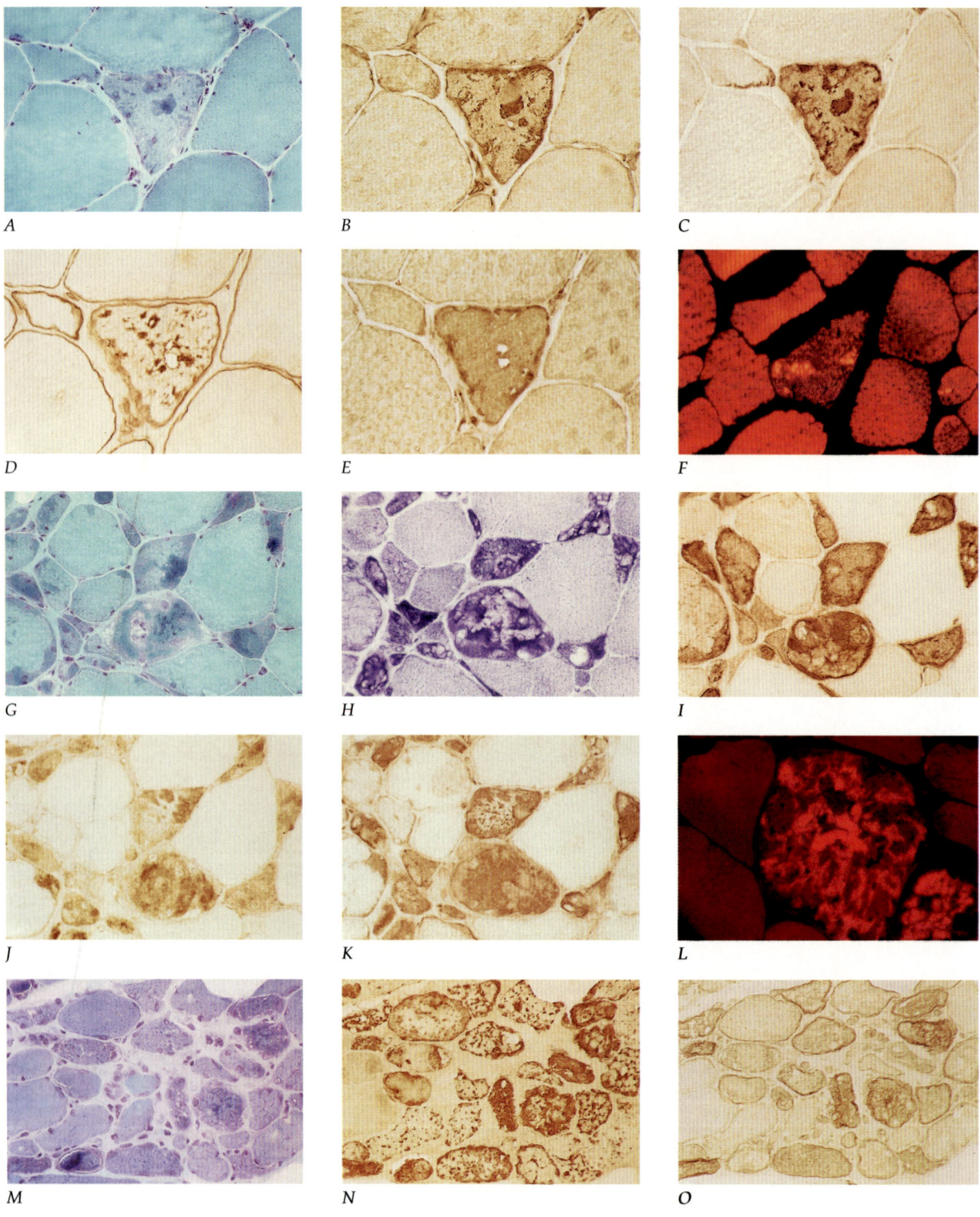

COLOR PLATE 10. *A–O*. Myofibrillar myopathy. Trichromatically stained sections (*A, G,* and *M*) show accumulation of irregularly shaped amorphous, hyaline and granular structures and vacuolar change. Note accumulation of desmin (*B*), αB-crystallin (*C*), dystrophin (*D*), gelsolin (*E*), NCAM (*I*), CDC2 kinase (*J*), prion protein (*K*), myotilin (*N*), and plectin (*O*), and sharply circumscribed decreases of oxidative enzyme activity (*H*) in fiber regions that appear abnormal in serial trichrome-stained sections. Also note intense reaction for actin in some hyaline structures revealed by rhodamine-labeled phalloidin (*F*) and intense congophilia of the hyaline structures (*L*). Panels *A–E, G–K,* and *M–O* image sections from the same series. *A–K,* and *M–O,* ×140; *L* ×220. (Cited in Chaps. 30, 31, and 43.)

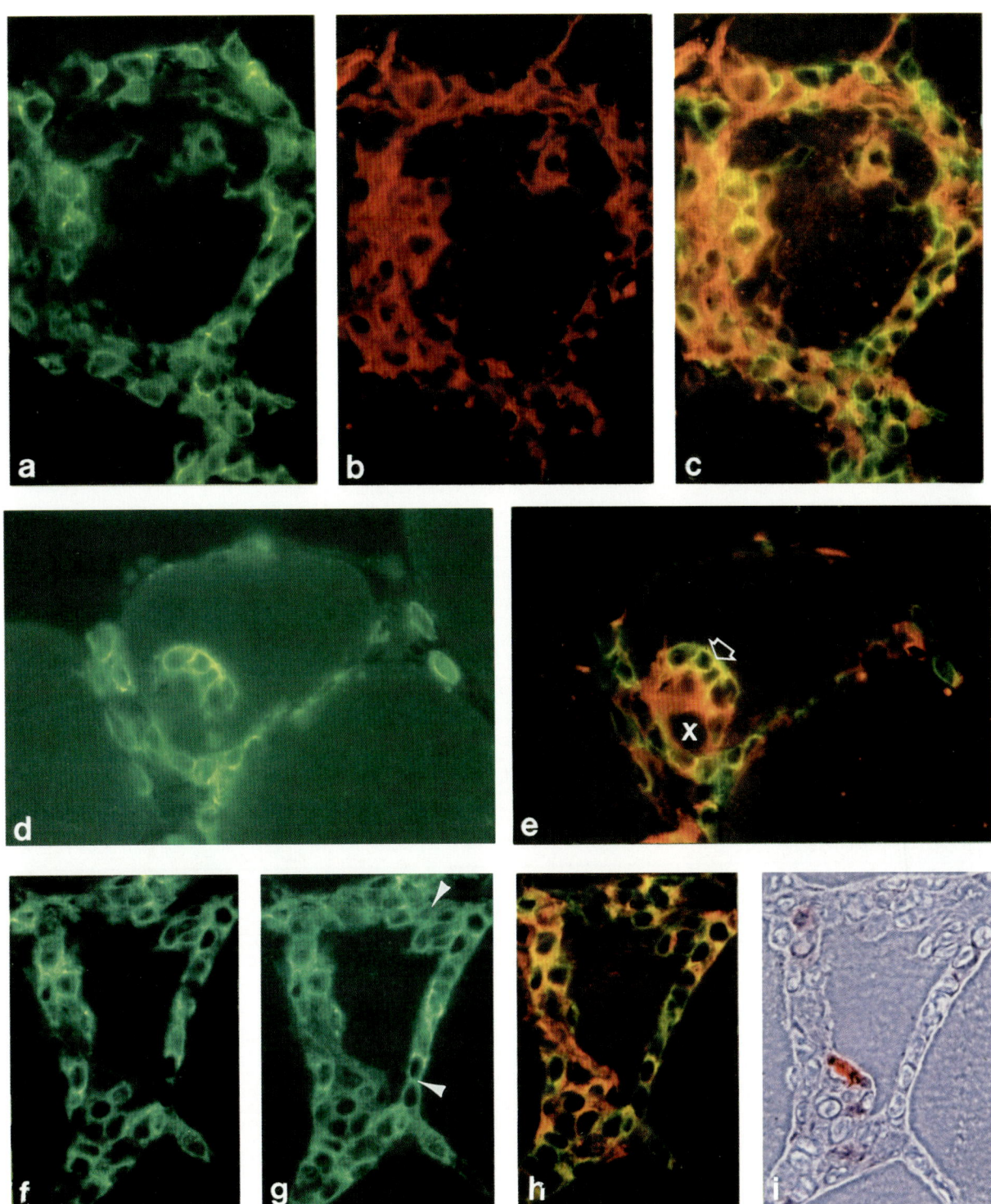

Color Plate 11. Nonnecrotic muscle fibers surrounded and invaded by mononuclear cells in polymyositis *(a-e)* and inclusion body myositis *(f-i)*.

a-c. Multiple rows of cells surround a fiber and invade it in several places. In *a,* CD8+ cells are visualized by green fluorescence; in *b,* the Ia+ cells are demonstrated by red fluorescence; *c* is a double exposure of *a* and *b,* revealing activated CD8+Ia+ cells in yellow. The CD8+Ia- cells remain green, and the CD8-Ia+ cells remain red. × 500. *d, e.* Mononuclear cells partially surround a muscle fiber and invade its lower border at two sites. A small portion of the fiber has been split off (x) by the invading cells. In *d,* the CD8 marker is shown in green; in *e,* a double exposure of the green CD8 and red Ia markers confers a yellow color on the activated CD8+Ia+ cells. Note the four adjacent yellow invading cells (arrow), × 500. f–i. Mononuclear cells surround a fiber and invade it from three sides. The CD8 marker is shown in *f* and the CD8 and CD4 markers in *g; h* is a double exposure of the green T-cell markers and of the red Ia marker; *i* is a phase optic micrograph after staining for acid phosphatase. Most of the surrounding and invading cells are CD8+ and are visualized in *f.* A few cells (some shown by arrowheads) are revealed by the additional reaction for the CD4 marker in *b.* Some of the invading cells are yellow in *h,* indicating that they are activated CD8+Ia+ cells. Note correspondence between the red CD8-CD4-Ia+ cells in *h* and the red- or pink-staining acid-phosphatase-positive macrophages in *i.* × 500. (*Engel AG, Arahata K, Ann Neurol 16:209, 1984. Reproduced by permission.*). (Cited in Chaps. 30, 31, 49, and 50.)

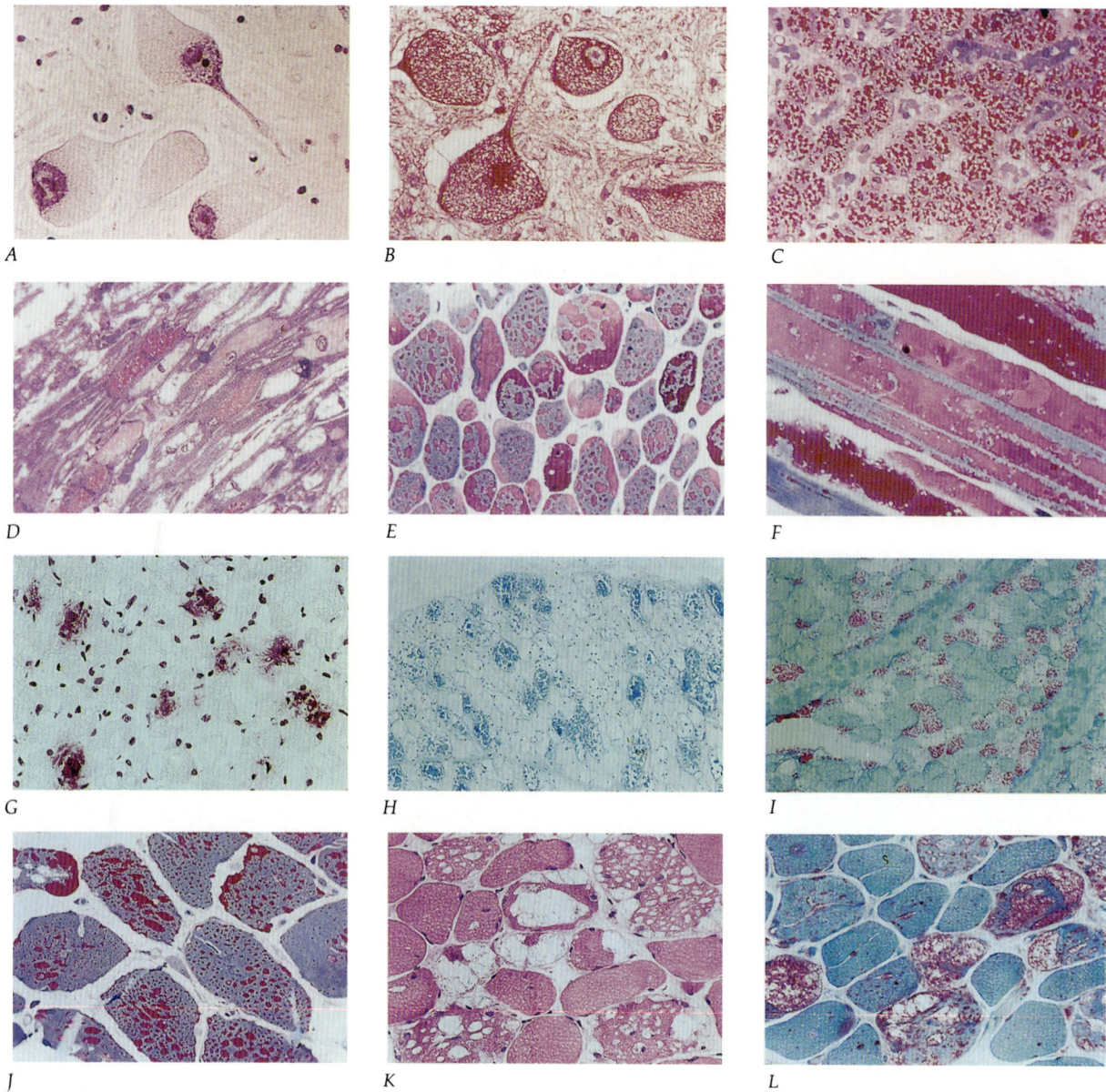

COLOR PLATE 12. *A–F.* Infantile acid maltase deficiency. Distended medullary motor neurons *(A)* are filled with glycogen *(B)*. Glycogen also accumulates in hepatocytes *(C)* and in cardiac *(D)* and skeletal *(E, F)* muscle fibers. *A,* cresyl violet; *B,* periodic acid-Schiff (PAS); *C–E,* PAS-methylene blue. *A–C,* ×240; *D, E,* ×370; *F,* ×600. *G–I.* Acid mucosubstance accumulation in muscle fibers in childhood acid maltase deficiency demonstrated with toluidine blue *(G),* alcian blue *(H),* and basic fuchsion *(I)*. *G,* ×150; *H, I,* × 60. *J–L.* Adult acid maltase deficiency: PAS-methylene blue *(J),* hematoxylin and eosin *(K),* and acid-phosphatase *(L)* stains. From a few to many vacuoles appear in the muscle fibers. The vacuoles are filled with glycogen *(J)* and are highly reactive for acid phosphatase *(L)*. *J, K, L,* ×150. (Cited in Chaps. 31 and 56.)

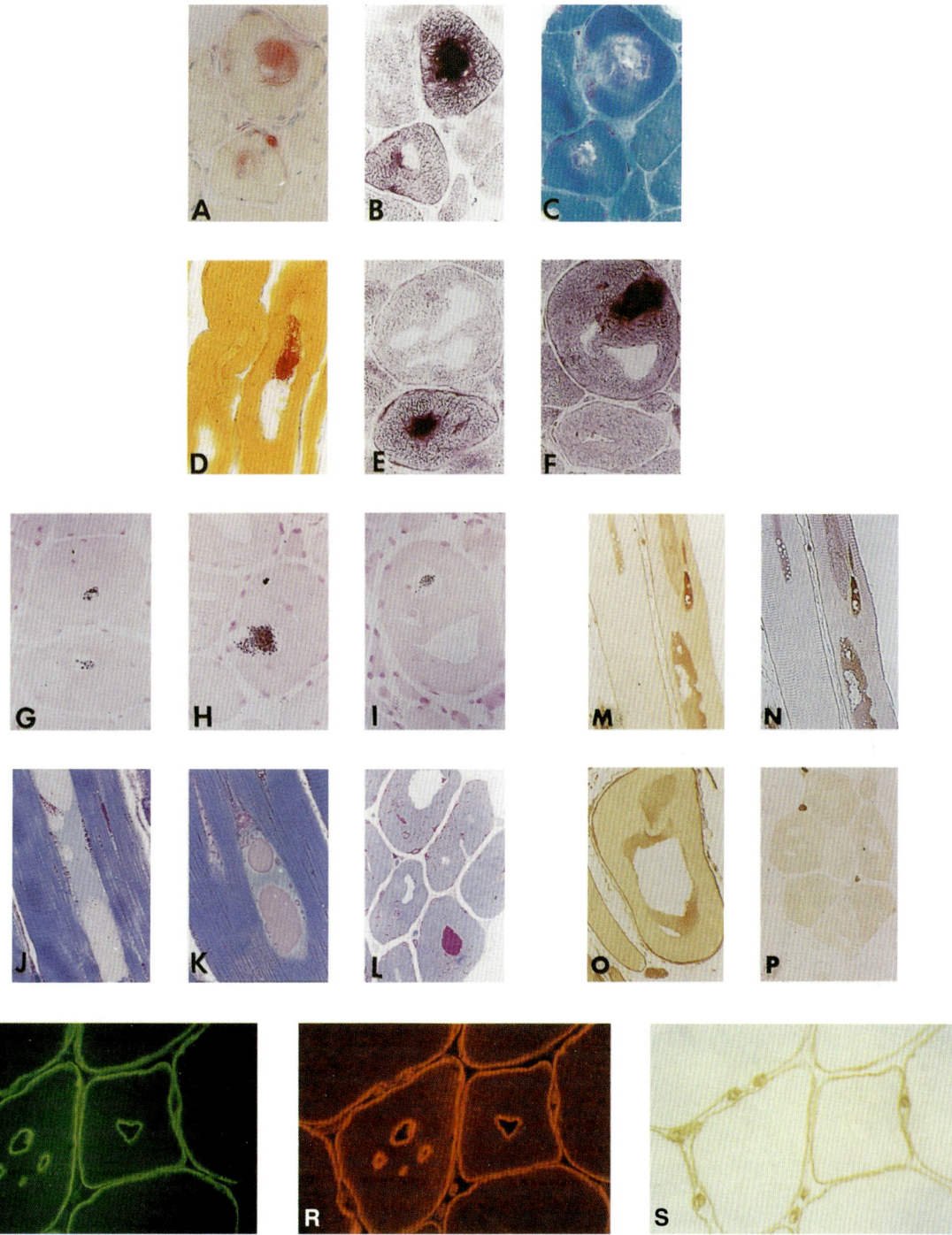

COLOR PLATE 13. The vacuolar myopathy of primary hypokalemic periodic paralysis.

A–C. Serial sections of muscle fibers containing evolving vacuoles. The degenerating material in these abnormal spaces stains dark blue with trichrome *(C)* and reacts strongly for acid phosphatase *(A)* and NADH dehydrogenase *(B)*. ×160. *D–F.* Muscle fibers containing evolving and more mature vacuoles. The evolving vacuoles react strongly for acid phosphatase *(D)* and NADH dehydrogenase *(E, F)*, whereas the mature vacuoles lack enzyme reactivity. *E* and *F* are serial sections separated by a 30-µm interval. Note transition from mature to immature vacuole in the upper fiber. *D*, ×200; *E, F*, ×160. *G–I.* Intravacuolar calcium deposits demonstrated by the von Kossa stain. ×160. *J–L.* Periodic acid Schiff (PAS)-azure II-methylene blue-stained semithin resin sections. Mature vacuoles with sarcoplasmic invaginations. The invaginations contain PAS-positive material *(J, K)*. In *L*, one vacuole is filled with PAS-positive material; here also note fiber splitting. *J, K*, ×400; *L* ×160. *M–P.* Muscle specimens imaged in *M, N*, and *O* were exposed to peroxidase-containing extracellular fluid before fixation. Peroxidase appears in all vacuoles in *M, N*, and *O* but is excluded from lobulated regions of the vacuoles. Parallel ultrastructural studies indicate that peroxidase enters mature vacuoles via the transverse tubules, but it is excluded from sarcoplasmic invaginations into the vacuoles (compare *M* and *N* with *J* and *K*). Specimen imaged in *P* was fixed without exposure to peroxidase. Erythrocytes are intensely peroxidatic; the vacuoles and extracellular space show no reaction. *M, N*, ×160; *O* ×400; *P*, ×200. (*From Engel AG, Mayo Clin Proc 45:774–814, 1970, by permission.*) *Q–S.* Dystrophin *(Q)*, spectrin *(R)* and laminin *(S)* immunolocalization in the same section. The muscle fiber surface membrane and the membranes lining the large mature vacuoles are supported by dystrophin and spectrin. Laminin surrounds the muscle fiber surface membrane and the endomysial capillaries but is not associated with the vacuolar membranes. ×240. (*From De Bleecker I, Engel AG, Am J Pathol 143:1200, 1993, by permission.*) (Cited in Chaps. 31 and 46.)

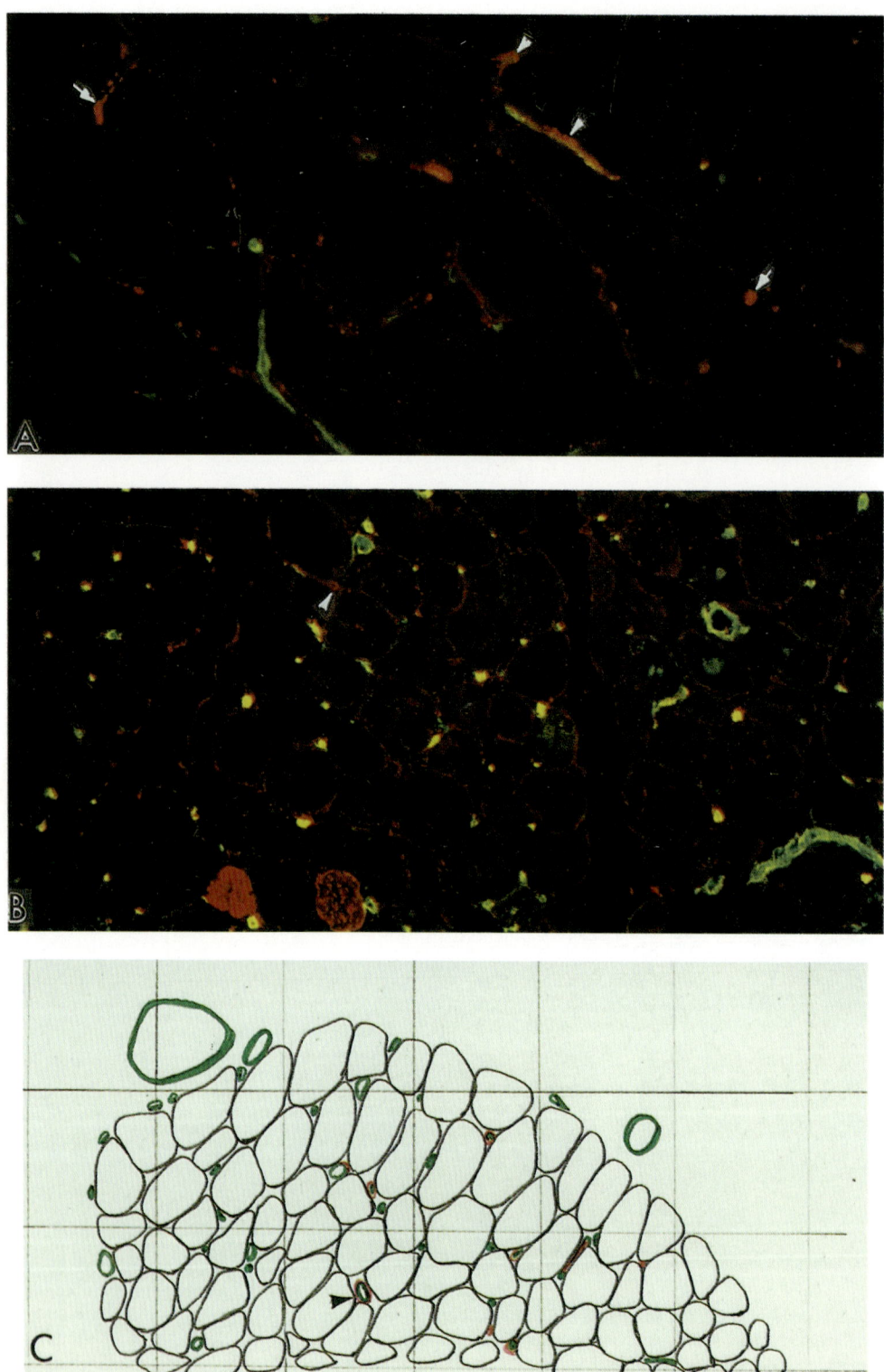

COLOR PLATE 14. *A–C.* Immunolocalization of capillaries and of the complement membrane attack complex (MAC) in dermatomyositis. The capillaries are visualized with the lectin Ulex europaeus agglutinin 1 (green fluorescence); MAC is localized with an anti-MAC antibody (red fluorescence). Green capillaries are MAC-negative and lectin-positive; yellow capillaries are MAC-positive and lectin-positive; red capillaries are MAC-positive and lectin-negative. *A* is from dermatomyositis muscle specimen that showed no apparent pathological change on conventional light microscopy. Note capillary with MAC reactivity exterior to lectin reactivity (arrowheads) and MAC-positive lectin-negative capillaries (arrows). The intensity of the green lectin reaction is attenuated, and the capillary count per unit fiber area is reduced. *B* and *C* are from a dermatomyositis muscle sample that showed advanced structural changes on light microscopy. *C* is a tracing from an immunoreacted section with a superimposed 100 × 100-μm morphometry grid. In *B*, most capillaries display yellow dual fluorescence for lectin and MAC; few capillaries react only for MAC (arrowhead). Two necrotic fibers show intense red MAC reaction. In panel *C*, note several vessels, including a venule (arrowhead) reacting for both lectin and MAC, and two capillaries reacting for MAC only. The capillary count in the grid squares overlying the muscle fibers is markedly reduced. *A* ×290; *B*, ×180; *C*, ×230. (*From Emslie-Smith AM, Engel AG: Ann Neurol 27:343, 1990, by permission.*) (Cited in Chaps. 30, 31, and 49.)

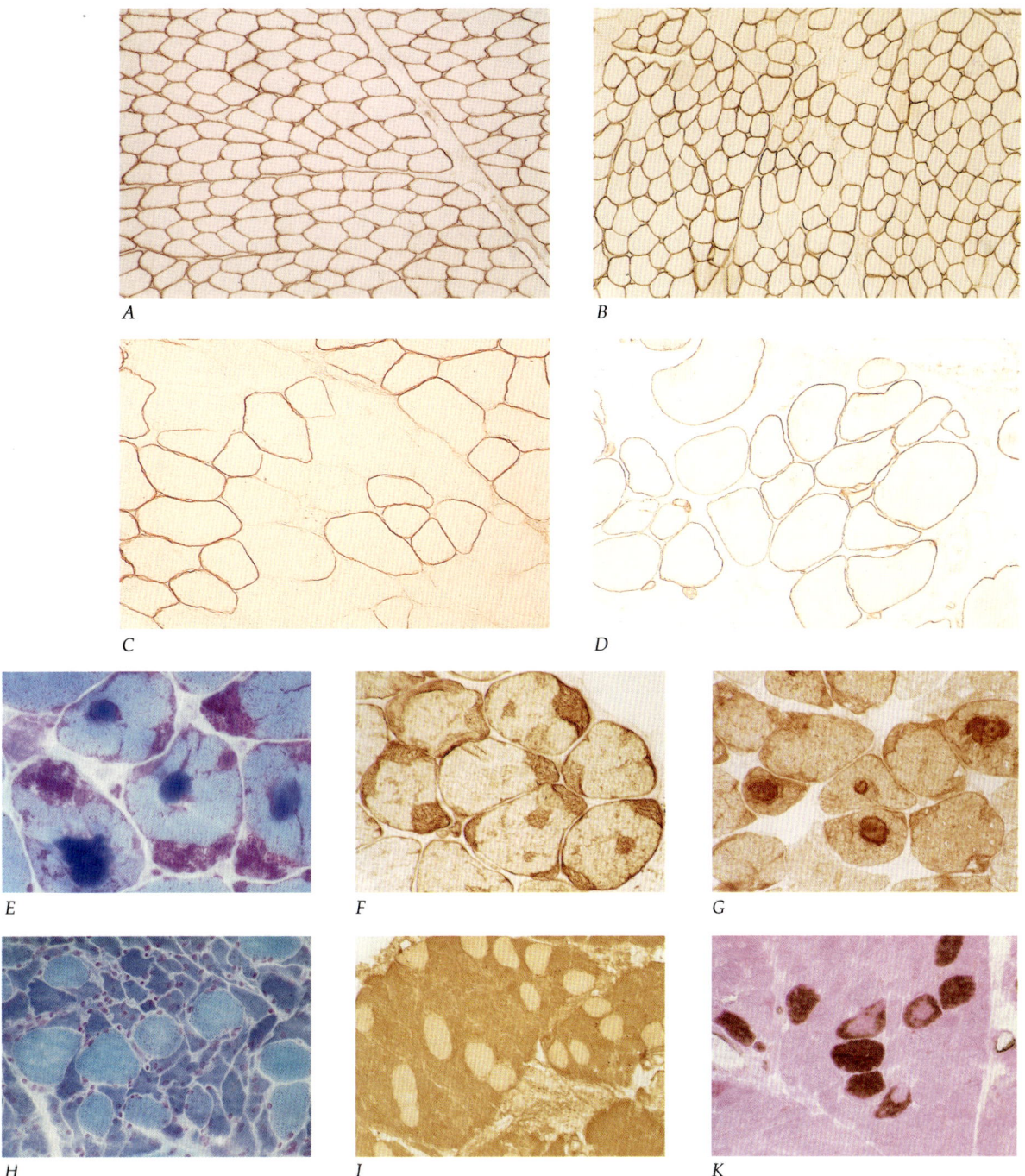

COLOR PLATE 15. *A–D.* Dystrophin immunolocalizations in normal skeletal muscle *(A)*, in asymptomatic carrier of Duchenne dystrophy *(B)*, in symptomatic carrier of Duchenne dystrophy *(C)*, and in patient with Becker dystrophy. (D). *A, B,* ×80; *C, D* ×200. *E–I.* Late onset myopathy associated with central hyaline structures and peripheral nemaline rods observed in trichrome stained *(E)* and desmin *(F)* and αB-crystallin *(G)* immunoreacted sections. The hyaline structures react strongly for desmin and αB crystallin; desmin and αB-crystallin immunoreactivities are also associated with the nemaline rods. *E,* ×300; *F, G* ×200. *H–K.* Acute quadriplegic (critical illness) myopathy. The abnormal fibers are decreased in size (H), immunoreact for calpain (I), and show total or focal loss of ATPase (pH 4.3) reactivity *(K). H–I.* ×150. (Cited in Chaps. 31, 34, 54, 61, and 62.)

References

COLOR PLATE 1.

1. Kabsch W, Mannherz HG, Suck D, et al: Atomic structure of the actin:DNase I complex. *Nature* 347:37–44, 1990.
2. Rayment I, Rypniewski WR, Schmidt-Base K, et al: Three-dimensional structure of myosin subfragment-1: A molecular motor *Science* 261:50–58, 1993.
3. Dominguez R, FreyzonY, Trybus KM, et al: Crystal structure of a vertebrate smooth muscle myosin motor domain and its complex with the essential light chain: Visualization of the pre-power stroke state. *Cell* 94:559–571, 1998.
4. Rayment I, Holden HM, Whittaker M, et al: Structure of the actin-myosin complex and its implications for muscle contraction. *Science* 261:58, 1993.
5. Irving M, Piazzesi G, Lucii L, et al: Conformation of the myosin motor during force generation in skeletal muscle. *Nat Struct Biol* 7:482–485, 2000.
6. Taylor KA, Schmitz, H Reedy MC, et al: Tomographic 3D reconstruction of quick-frozen, Ca^{2+} activated contracting insect flight muscle. *Cell* 99: 421–431, 1999.

COLOR PLATE 2.

1. Xie X, Harrison DH, Schlichting I, et al: Structure of the regulatory domain of scallop myosin at 2.8 Å resolution. *Nature* 368:306–312, 1994.
2. Trybus KM: Role of myosin light chains. *J. Muscle Res. Cell Motil* 15:587–594, 1994.

COLOR PLATE 3.

1. Herzberg O, James MN: Refined crystal structure of troponin C from turkey skeletal muscle at 2.0 Å resolution. *J Mol Biol* 203:761–769, 1988.
2. Strynadka NC, Cherney M, Sielecki AR, et al: Structural details of a calcium-induced molecular switch: X-ray crystallographic analysis of the calcium-saturated N-terminal domain of troponin C at 1.75 Å resolution. *J Mol Biol* 273:238–255, 1997.
3. Offer G, Knight PJ, Burgess SA, et al: A new model for the surface arrangement of myosin molecules in tarantula thick filaments. *J Mol Biol* 298:239–260, 2000
4. Stewart M, Kensler RW, Levine RJC: Structure of *Limulus* telson muscle thick filaments. *J Mol Biol* 153:781–790, 1981.
5. AL-Khayat HA, Yagi N, Squire JM: Structural changes in actin-tropomyosin during muscle regulation: Computer modelling of low-angle x-ray diffraction data. *J Mol Biol* 252:611–632, 1995.
6. Hudson L, Harford JJ, Denny RJ, et al: Myosin head configurations in relaxed fish muscle: Resting state myosin heads swing axially by 150 Å or turn upside down to reach rigor. *J Mol Biol* 273:440–445, 1997.
7. Squire JM, Cantino M, Chew M, et al: Myosin rod packing schemes in vertebrate muscle thick filaments. *J Struct Biol* 122:128–138, 1998.

COLOR PLATE 4.

1. Toyoshima C, Nakasako M, Nomura H, Ogawa H: Crystal structure of the calcium pump of sarcoplasmic reticulum at 2.6 Angstrom resolution. *Nature* 405:647–655, 2000.
2. Toyoshima C, Nomura H: Structural changes in the calcium pump accompanying the dissociation of calcium. *Nature* 418:605–611, 2002.
3. Green NM, Maclennan DH: Calcium calisthenics. *Nature* 418:598–599, 2002.
4. Wang S, Trumble WR, Liao H, et al: Crystal structure of calsequestrin from rabbit skeletal muscle sarcoplasmic reticulum. *Nat Struct Biol* 5:476–483, 1998.
5. MacLennan DH, Reithmeier RA: Ion tamers. *Nat Struct Biol* 5:409–411, 1998.

COLOR PLATE 5.

1. Doyle DD, Cabral JM, Pfuetzner RA, et al: The structure of the potassium channel: Molecular basis of K^+ conduction and selectivity. *Science* 280:69–77, 1988.
2. ZhouY, Morais-Cabral JH, Kaufman et al.: Chemistry of ion coordination and hydration revealed by a K-channel-FAB complex at 2Å of resolution. *Nature* 414:45–48, 2001.
3. Morais-Cabral JH, Zhou Y, Mackinnon R: Energetic optimization of ion conduction rate by the K^+ selectivity filter *Nature* 414:37–40, 2001.
4. Brejc K, van Dijk WJ, Klaasen RV, et al: Crystal structure of an ACh-binding protein reveals the ligand-binding domain of nicotinic receptors. *Nature* 411:269–276, 2001.

Chapter 22
Microcirculation in Muscle

O. HUDLICKA
M. D. BROWN
S. EGGINTON

Introduction
Anatomy of Vascular Supply
   MACROSCOPIC STRUCTURE
   MICROSCOPIC STRUCTURE
   NUTRITIVE AND NONNUTRITIVE FLOW AND FLOW
      HETEROGENEITY
   MUSCLE SPINDLES
Fine Structure of Blood Vessels
   ARTERIES, ARTERIOLES, AND VENULES
   CAPILLARIES
Physiologic Control of the Microcirculation
   SITE OF CONTROL
   CAPILLARY PERFUSION AND RECRUITMENT
   NERVOUS CONTROL
   LOCAL CONTROL
   CONDUCTED RESPONSES AND CELL-CELL INTERACTION
   COORDINATED CONTROL OF FUNCTIONAL HYPEREMIA
   HORMONAL CONTROL
Remodeling of the Microcirculation under Physiologic Conditions
   INCREASED ACTIVITY
   COMPENSATORY HYPERTROPHY
   MUSCLE INACTIVITY
   HYPOXIA
   HORMONES
Remodeling of the Microcirculation under Pathologic Conditions
   DENERVATION AND REGENERATION
   MUSCULAR DYSTROPHIES
   INFLAMMATORY MYOPATHIES
   MUSCLE ISCHEMIA
   REPERFUSION INJURY
   ENDOTHELIAL-LEUKOCYTE INTERACTIONS
Muscle Microcirculation in Other Pathologic States
   HYPERTENSION
   DIABETES
   HEART FAILURE
Conclusions

Introduction

Skeletal muscles comprise about 40 percent of total body weight and require approximately 20 percent of the total cardiac output to meet their basal metabolic needs. This proportion increases dramatically during exercise, particularly if it involves large muscle groups, as in running or swimming. The increased flow is necessary not only to supply oxygen and substrates—e.g., glucose—but also to remove metabolites such as lactate and carbon dioxide. The 10- to 20-fold increase in blood flow to individual muscle groups can be met mostly by local regulation, which ensures dilation of all categories of vessels, with the possible exception of capillaries, and increased perfusion of the microcirculation. When the demand of working muscles exceeds the maximal possible increase in cardiac output, however, systemic neural and hormonal regulation is necessary to enable redistribution of blood toward and within the working muscles. Such regulation can also divert blood from muscles and tissues elsewhere when necessary—for instance, during hemorrhage.

Muscle circulation can adapt structurally to increased levels of contractile activity and/or metabolism or to changes in the environment, such as chronic exposure to cold or hypoxia, by growth of new blood vessels. Conversely, regression of some portions of the vascular bed takes place in response to muscle inactivity or following long-term restriction of blood flow, as, for instance, in arteriosclerosis. Furthermore, diseases such as hypertension, chronic heart failure, and diabetes significantly affect muscle microcirculation both structurally and functionally so as to have a detrimental effect on muscle performance. Endothelial cells can also respond to humoral and mechanical stimuli by release of a number of biologically active molecules involved in the prevention of blood coagulation, transmigration of white blood cells to sites of injury, and regulation of the vascular tone and growth.

Anatomy of Vascular Supply

MACROSCOPIC STRUCTURE

Skeletal muscles are supplied by one or more feed arteries that divide into a network of smaller arteries and arterioles and finally capillaries, which then join into venules and veins. In some muscles these branching networks form arcades with arterioarterial and venovenular anastomoses. In human muscles, the number of supplying arteries varies and is decisive for the formation of collateral circulation. Thus muscles supplied by a single main artery—e.g., medial and lateral head of gastrocnemius, crureus, or gracilis—experience greater damage when this is occluded than muscles supplied by one to three arteries with some anastomoses between regions, such as gluteus maximus, biceps femoris, semitendinosus, and semimembranosus. Muscles such as the deltoid, biceps and triceps brachii, adductor magnus, and gluteus medius and minimus are supplied by vessels from several sources and are hence relatively unaffected by occlusion of one artery, since circulation is maintained by numerous anastomoses between individual regions.[1]

MICROSCOPIC STRUCTURE

Our present knowledge of microcirculation in skeletal muscle is largely based on studies of thin muscles in the musculature of relatively small animals—such as cat and rabbit tenuissimus; rat spinotrapezius and gracilis; and rat, hamster, or mouse cremaster—since these can be transilluminated and exposed for direct observation under the microscope. While the vascular network in spinotrapezius and cremaster forms arcades, other muscles have feed arteries branching into arterioles positioned transversely with respect to muscle fibers. These arterioles are usually classified as first- to fourth-order, according to their location within the branching system, with the smallest terminal arterioles dividing into capillaries oriented in parallel with muscle fibers. Several capillaries then join to form confluent venules and a system of larger venules, classified according to their position and size as V4 (smallest) to V1 (largest) (Fig. 22-1). Direct observations on bulk muscles such as tibialis anterior, extensor digitorum longus, or soleus using epi-illumination have confirmed this branching arrangement. For example, in hamster tibialis anterior muscle, capillaries are arranged in units, with 15 to 20 capillaries branching from a single arteriole and draining typically but not always into one venule with some countercurrent flow between units.[2] This arrangement enables some shunting of oxygen from arterioles to venules and explains the fact that Po_2 is usually higher in the venous blood than in the muscle itself.

The regulation of flow through capillaries, the exchange vessels for oxygen and solutes, is by terminal arterioles and not, as previously thought, by opening or closing of precapillary sphincters, since these are absent in skeletal muscle. Capillaries are 4 to 10 μm in diameter, vary in length between 500 and 1000 μm, and form a rich lattice around muscle fibers, usually with one to four vessels per fiber, depending on its metabolic type. The numbers of capillaries counted in muscle differ between studies largely as a result of their method of detection or because of tissue shrinkage during preparation for histology. Hence capillary densities derived from muscle that has been perfusion-fixed and pre-

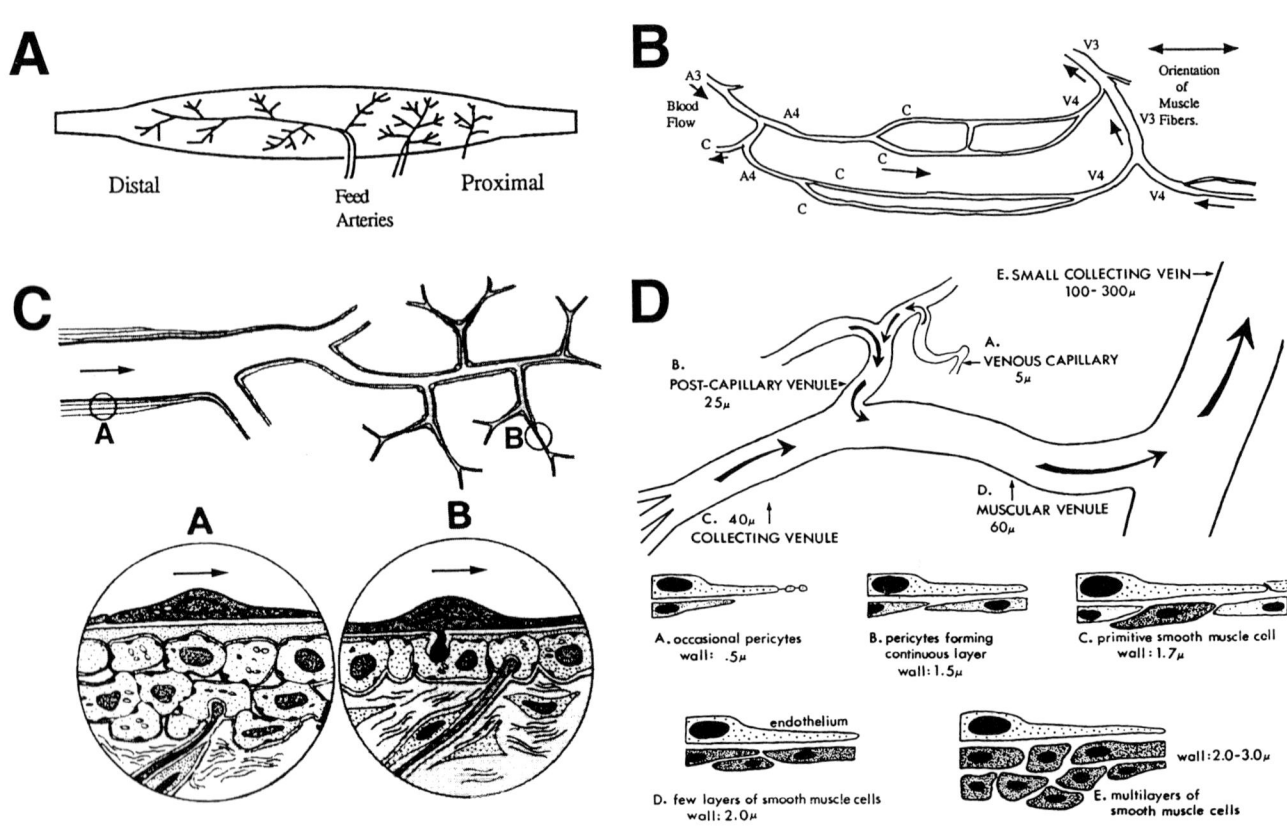

FIGURE 22-1. Scheme of the organization and structure of blood supply to skeletal muscle. A and B. Macroscopic and microscopic arrangement of blood vessels in rat EDL. (*After Williams DA, Segal SS: Feed artery role in blood flow control to rat hindlimb skeletal muscles. J Physiol (Lond) 463:631–646, 1993. With permission.*) Note the multiple feed vessels and the microvascular unit with capillaries running parallel with the orientation of muscle fibers (double-headed arrow). Classification of vessels is given as Strahler branching order: third-order arterioles (A3), terminal arterioles (A4), capillaries (C), postcapillary venules (V4), third-order venules (V3); direction of blood flow is shown by arrows. C. Fine structure of mammalian arterioles, sketched from electron micrographs. (*After Rhodin JAG: The ultrastructure of mammalian arterioles and precapillary sphincters. Ultrastruct Res 18:181–223, 1967. With permission.*) Expanded views of (A) A3 vessels with the smooth muscle cell layer separated from the endothelium by a continuous elastica interna and innervated by nonmyelinated nerves in the outer VSM layer and (B) terminal arterioles, showing the development of myoendothelial junctions as the elastica interna disappears and the sparse innervation by free nerve endings on the single layer of VSMCs; direction of blood flow is shown by arrows. D. Structure of mammalian venules, sketched from electron micrographs. (*After Rhodin JAG: Ultrastructure of mammalian venous capillaries, venules and collecting veins. Ultrastruct Res 25:452–500, 1968. With permission.*) Expanded views of (A) transition between capillary and venular endothelium, (B) V4, (C) V3, (D) V2, and (E) V1 vessels showing the gradual investment of the wall with mural cells (pericytes and smooth muscle cells and increasing wall thickness); direction of blood flow is shown by arrows.

pared for electron microscopy are higher than those obtained from cryostat sections and stained for enzymes (ATPase, PAS amylase, alkaline phosphatase), lectins, or antigens such as factor VIII or CD31 present in the capillary endothelium or basement membrane. The length and tortuosity of the capillary bed varies among muscle types but also with changes in muscle length due to stretch, contraction, and relaxation, while the intercapillary distance varies with fiber size (Fig. 22-2). Capillary supply, whether expressed as capillary density (number of capillaries per square millimeter), capillary:fiber ratio (C:F),* number of capillaries around fibers, or capillary length (millimeters per cubic millimeter),

*A list of abbreviations used in this chapter is given at the end of the chapter.

is related to the size of animal (higher in smaller animals)[3] and muscle fiber size (Table 22-1) and to fiber composition, muscles with a high proportion of oxidative fibers having higher capillary supply[4] (Fig. 22-2).

During postnatal development, the rapid increase in fiber size, which pushes existing capillaries apart, results in a decrease in capillary density; but as the capillaries are still growing, C:F increases. This basic relationship has been established for individual muscles in rodents (see Ref. 4), and humans.[5] Indeed, stretch of the capillary wall as fibers increase in girth may act as a stimulus to endothelial cell growth. Capillarization of skeletal muscles in early postnatal development proceeds much faster in oxidative than in glycolytic muscles.[4,6] Both capillaries and arterioles initially grow by elongation rather than sprouting, while postcapil-

Table 22-1. CAPILLARY SUPPLY TO SKELETAL MUSCLE

Subject	Muscle	Condition	CD, mm^{-2}	C:F	a(f), μm^2	Reference, see legend
Biopsy	Lateral quadriceps	Control	442 ± 52	1.3 ± 0.42	4308 ± 324	1
Endurance exercise	Lateral quadriceps	Control (males)	585 ± 40	1.77 ± 0.10	1870 ± 96^b	2
		Trained	821 ± 28^a	2.49 ± 0.08^a	1893 ± 39^b	2
Endurance exercise	Lateral quadriceps	Control (females)	579 ± 19	1.11 ± 0.07	1201 ± 55^b	3
		Trained	777 ± 45^a	1.69 ± 0.13^a	1432 ± 56^b	3
Endurance exercise	Vastus lateralis	Control	423 ± 30	2.07 ± 0.11	4707 ± 351	4
		Trained	492 ± 14	2.21 ± 0.08^a	4490 ± 337	4
High-resistance exercise	Vastus lateralis	Control	320^b	1.35^b	3886–4927^b	5
		Trained	320	2.64	6800–10,100	5
Rat	Medial gastrocnemius	Control	—	2.53	1199	6
		Swimming	—	2.63	1492^a	6
		Running wheel	—	2.65	1442^a	6
	Lateral gastrocnemius	Control	—	1.22	1959	6
		Swimming	—	1.35	2163^a	6
		Running wheel	—	1.42	2284^a	6
Biopsy	Vastus lateralis?	Control	393 ± 29	—	—	7
		Dermatomyositis	217 ± 24^a	—	—	7
		Polymyositis	372 ± 47	—	—	7
Biopsy	Deltoid	Control	355 ± 148	0.98 ± 0.45	963 ± 81^b	8
		Dermatomyositis	351 ± 121	0.54 ± 0.12^a	594 ± 155^{a,b}	8
		Polymyositis	421 ± 173^a	0.89 ± 0.26^a	698 ± 278^{a,b}	8
Biopsy	Lateral gastrocnemius	NGT	321 ± 59	1.51 ± 0.36	—	9
		IGT, not NIDDM	328 ± 115	1.50 ± 0.38	—	9
		IGT, NIDDM	365 ± 65^a	1.82 ± 0.38^a	—	9
Biopsy	Medial gastrocnemius	IDDM, no neuropathy	374 ± 106	1.3 ± 0.1	—	10
		IDDM with neuropathy	283 ± 67	1.3 ± 0.1	—	10
Rat	Soleus	Control	543 ± 17	2.83 ± 0.05	—	11
		Streptozotocin	601 ± 21	3.00 ± 0.06	—	11
		Streptozotocin and evening primrose oil	655 ± 37^a	3.24 ± 0.09	—	11

^{a}Significantly different from respective controls. ^{b}Calculated from data in the reference.
KEY: NGT, normal glucose tolerance; IGT, impaired glucose tolerance; NIDDM, non-insulin-dependent diabetes mellitus; IDDM; insulin-dependent diabetes mellitus; CD, capillary density; C:F, capillary-to-fiber ratio; a(f), fiber cross-sectional area.

1. Ahmed et al: *Exp Physiol* 82:231–234, 1997.
2. Brodal et al: *Am J Physiol* 232:H705–H712, 1977.
3. Ingjer & Brodal: *Eur J Appl Physiol Occup Physiol* 38:291–299, 1978.
4. Klausen et al: *Acta Physiol Scand* 113:9–16, 1981.
5. Schantz: *Acta Physiol Scand* 114:635–637, 1982.
6. Carrow et al: *Anat Rec* 159:33–39, 1967.
7. Emslie-Smith & Engel: *Ann Neurol* 27:343–356, 1990.
8. Estruch et al: *Hum Pathol* 23:888–895, 1992.
9. Eriksson et al: *Diabetes* 43:805–808, 1994.
10. Matikainen et al: *Eur Neurol* 21:22–28, 1982.
11. Cameron et al: *Diabetes* 40:532–539, 1991.

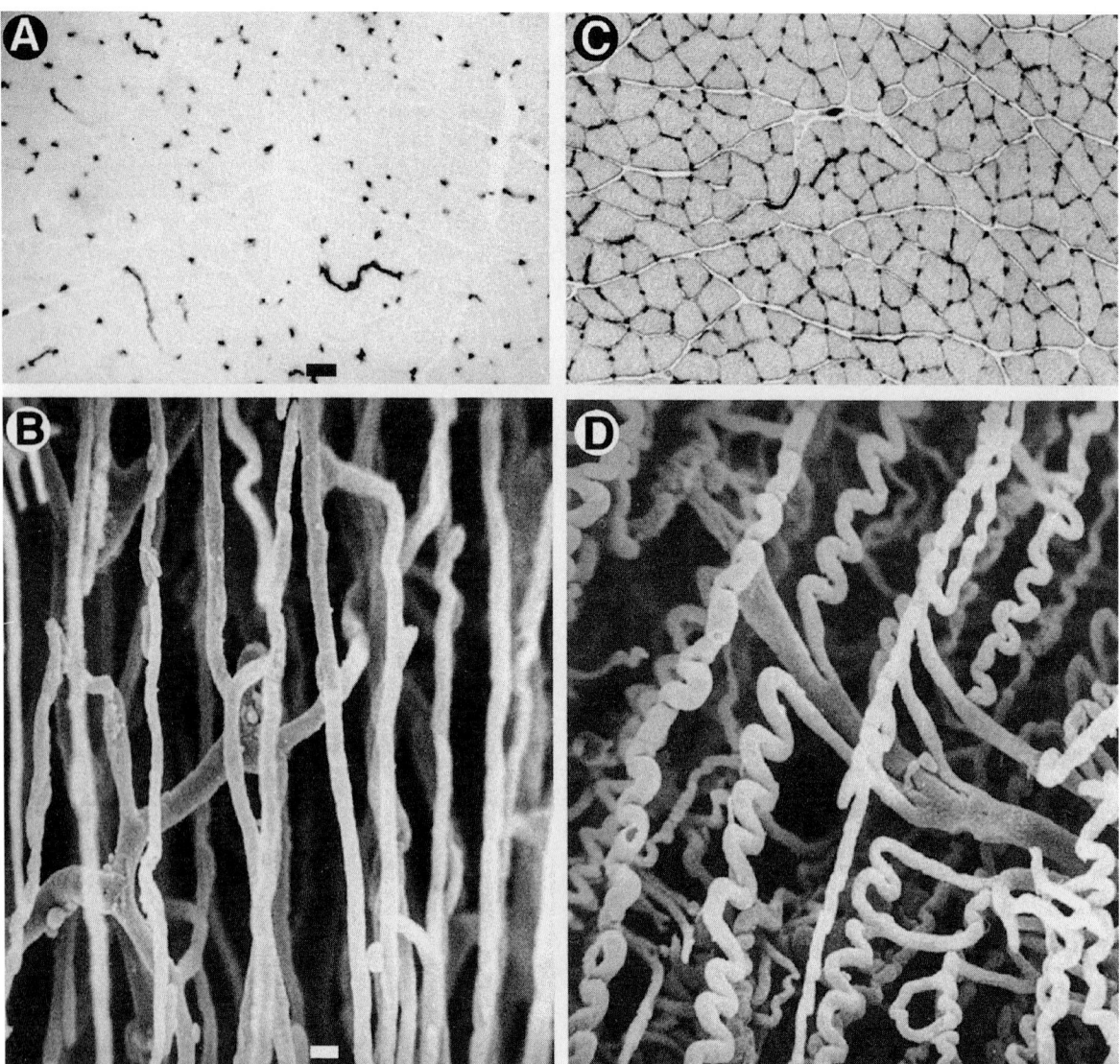

FIGURE 22-2. Comparison of the microcirculation in glycolytic (*A* and *B*, outer cortex of rat tibialis anterior) and oxidative (*C* and *D*, medial portion of rat soleus) skeletal muscles, illustrated by light microscopy (*A* and *C*, alkaline phosphatase staining of frozen sections, scale bar = 50 μm) and scanning electron microscopy (*B* and *D*, acrylic casts with muscle digested by alkaline maceration, scale bar = 10 μm). Contrast the widely spaced and relatively straight capillary bed in glycolytic muscle with the dense and tortuous network found in oxidative muscle.

lary venules increase in numbers. Capillary supply in old animals either is maintained or appears to increase, mainly due to decreased diameter or loss of muscle fibers.[7]

NUTRITIVE AND NONNUTRITIVE FLOW AND FLOW HETEROGENEITY

As in the case of other organs, it has been assumed that blood can bypass some capillaries via arteriovenous shunts. However, direct intravital observation of muscle microcirculation does not confirm the presence of arteriovenous anastomoses, although the possibility of nonnutritive flow supplying connective tissue and tendons rather than muscle fibers has been demonstrated.[8] Another interpretation of "nonnutritive" flow relates to the fact that perfusion of individual capillaries is not uniform. Considerable variability in red cell transit times results from perfusion through capillaries of different lengths.[9] For instance, capillaries supplying the glycolytic part of the tibialis anterior are longer than those supplying oxidative fibers in the soleus,[10] and the time spent by red cells in individual capillaries is longer. Since most muscles are composed of mixed fiber populations, nutritive blood flow will vary with capillary length and diameter, and this spatial heterogeneity has been shown for red cell velocity (V_{rbc}) and red cell flux (0.018 to 0.324 mm·s^{-1} and 0.6 to 16.5 s^{-1}, respectively, in rat gracilis muscle).[11] Temporal heterogeneity of capillary flow depends on cyclic changes in the diameter of the supplying arteriole (vasomotion), occurring usually three times per minute.[11,12] Since vasodilation abolishes vasomotion, temporal and spatial heterogeneity diminish.[13] Uniformity of flow through different parts of a muscle is also affected by physical compression during contractions, whereby stretch or tetanic contraction can result in minimal flow to the central part of calf muscles while blood flow in the periphery is maintained or increased.[14]

MUSCLE SPINDLES

The microcirculation of the muscle spindle originates from two or three precapillary arterioles which extend into a limited number of large capillaries destined exclusively for the spindle. The intrafusal microcirculation includes a longitudinal capillary loop in the region of sensory nerve endings. The capillaries are wider than those supplying extrafusal muscle fibers, but have fewer endothelial cell vesicles and have tight junctions, which would explain the fact that they are relatively impermeable. Pericyte processes cover a greater proportion of the capillary circumference than in nonspindle capillaries, and the basement membrane around endothelial cells and pericytes is thick and often multilayered (Table 22-2).[15]

Fine Structure of Blood Vessels

ARTERIES, ARTERIOLES, AND VENULES

The principal vascular arrangement of microcirculation in skeletal muscle, based on observations in animal muscles, is shown in Fig. 22-1. It is difficult to study in human muscles, in which vessels can be examined only in small biopsies; these do not allow the whole vascular architecture to be visualized. The different categories of vessels have then to be classified approximately, according to the number and arrangement of smooth muscle cells and the ratio of lumen to wall thickness, which is larger in venules than in arterioles.

The feed arteries vary in size according to muscle type and species. They are composed of an inner coat, the tunica intima, formed by endothelial cells; a middle tunica media, composed of several layers of vascular smooth muscle cells (VSMCs); and an outer tunica adventitia, consisting of connective tissue elements. The elastica interna, or internal elastic membrane, separates the tunica intima from the tunica media; likewise, the external elastic membrane separates the tunica media from the tunica adventitia. The adventitia is

Table 22-2. MORPHOMETRIC ANALYSIS OF MUSCLE CAPILLARIES

Muscle	Condition	a(c), μm^2	V_v (endo, cap)	BM thickness, nm	PC area, % capillary	Reference, see legend
Vastus lateralis	Child/control	14.6 ± 1.9	40.0 ± 3.1	84 ± 6^b	6.8 ± 0.8	1
	Duchenne	21.4 ± 1.6^a	37.1 ± 1.6	75 ± 3^b	7.7 ± 0.8^a	1
	Adult/control	12.5 ± 1.3	34.0 ± 2.0	172 ± 13^b	7.1 ± 0.8	2
	Scleroderma	26.4 ± 3.5^a	47.6 ± 4.2^a	$145 \pm 12^{a,b}$	14.5 ± 2.8^a	2
	Polymyositis	12.1 ± 1.5^a	46.4 ± 2.8^a	152 ± 10^b	14.7 ± 2.0	2
	Dermatomyositis	21.1 ± 2.3^a	51.0 ± 3.1^a	$169 \pm 9^{a,b}$	21.0 ± 3.9^a	2
	Lupus erythematosus	17.3 ± 1.4^a	44.6 ± 2.4^a	191 ± 11^b	12.8 ± 2.0^a	2
Vastus lateralis?	Control	—	—	93 ± 18	—	3
	Myotonic dystrophy	—	—	77 ± 26	—	3
	NIDDM	—	—	122 ± 61	—	3
Quadriceps	Control	—	—	126 ± 20	—	4
	IDDM	—	—	186 ± 51	—	4
Medial gastrocnemius	IDDM, no neuropathy	18.5 ± 2.9^b	20.7 ± 4.0	277 ± 27^b	No data	5
	IDDM with neuropathy	19.4 ± 4.5^b	18.9 ± 5.7	$291 \pm 9^{a,b}$	Unchanged	5
Sartorius	Control	15.1 ± 0.5	40.0 ± 1.4	328 ± 32	—	6
	PVD	13.0 ± 0.9	53.0 ± 6.2	320 ± 46	—	6
Gastrocnemius	PVD	13.7 ± 0.6	54.3 ± 3.5^a	427 ± 57^a	—	6
Quadriceps	Control	11.6 ± 1.9	42.1 ± 10.1	246 ± 47	—	7
	Chronic heart failure	13.6 ± 2.8	44.2 ± 11.7	310 ± 77^a	—	7
Rat EDL	Control	12.1 ± 1.3	53.0 ± 1.6	—	—	8
	Chronic ischemia	13.7 ± 0.6^a	60.8 ± 3.3	—	—	8
Rabbit tenuissimus	Intrafusal	37.1 ± 17.7	35.5 ± 16.8^b	78.7 ± 11.6	14.9 ± 15.2^b	9
	Endoneural	32.3 ± 11.2	34.8 ± 16.1^b	60.3 ± 16.2	11.1 ± 8.5^b	9
	Extrafusal	12.2 ± 7.8	32.6 ± 24.8^b	48.0 ± 12.6	5.1 ± 4.7^b	9

[a]Significantly different from respective controls. [b]Calculated from area data.
KEY: NIDDM, non-insulin-dependent diabetes mellitus; IDDM, insulin-dependent diabetes mellitus; PVD, peripheral vascular disease; a(c), capillary cross-sectional area; V_v(endo, cap), volume density of capillary endothelium; BM, basement membrane; PC, pericyte.

1. Jerusalem et al: *Brain* 97:115–122, 1974.
2. Jerusalem et al: *J Neurol Sci* 23:391–402, 1974.
3. Olson et al: *Diabetes* 28:686–689, 1979.
4. Ellis et al: *Diabetes* 35:421–425, 1986.
5. Matikainen et al: *Eur Neurol* 21:22–28, 1982.
6. Thomson et al: *Int J Microcirc Clin Exp* 16:284–290, 1996.
7. Lindsay et al: *Eur Heart J* 15:1470–1476, 1994.
8. Egginton et al: *Int J Microcirc Clin Exp* 12:33–44, 1993.
9. Miyoshi et al: *Arch Neurol* 36:547–552, 1979.

composed of loosely arranged bundles of collagen and occasional spindle-shaped fibroblasts.[15] On branching into arterioles, the number of VSMC layers gradually decreases and the elastica externa disappears. Larger arterioles have smooth muscle cells arranged both helically and circularly in the outer layer, which enables constriction of the vessel lumen on contraction. Terminal arterioles, which vary in size between 6 and 10 μm, typically contain just one layer of smooth muscle cells arranged circularly around the endothelial cells. These two cell types are connected by gap junctions, which are also present between individual smooth muscle cells and are important for communication and signaling in flow regulation. Collecting venules contain only sparse smooth muscle cells, and the three coats present in arterioles are sometimes difficult to distinguish (Fig. 22-1).

Arterioles, but not venules, are supplied by autonomic nerves that pass through the adventitia and terminate in close vicinity of the smooth muscle cells (Fig. 22-3).

CAPILLARIES

The terminal arterioles give rise to a cluster of minute vessels—the capillaries. In skeletal muscle, these are structurally similar to those in other tissues—such as skin, lung, fat, and connective tissue—and are of the continuous phenotype. They therefore lack the fenestrations seen in the more permeable capillary beds of the kidney or the endocrine or exocrine glands and the intercellular gaps of discontinuous or sinusoidal capillaries that allow cellular exchange in bone

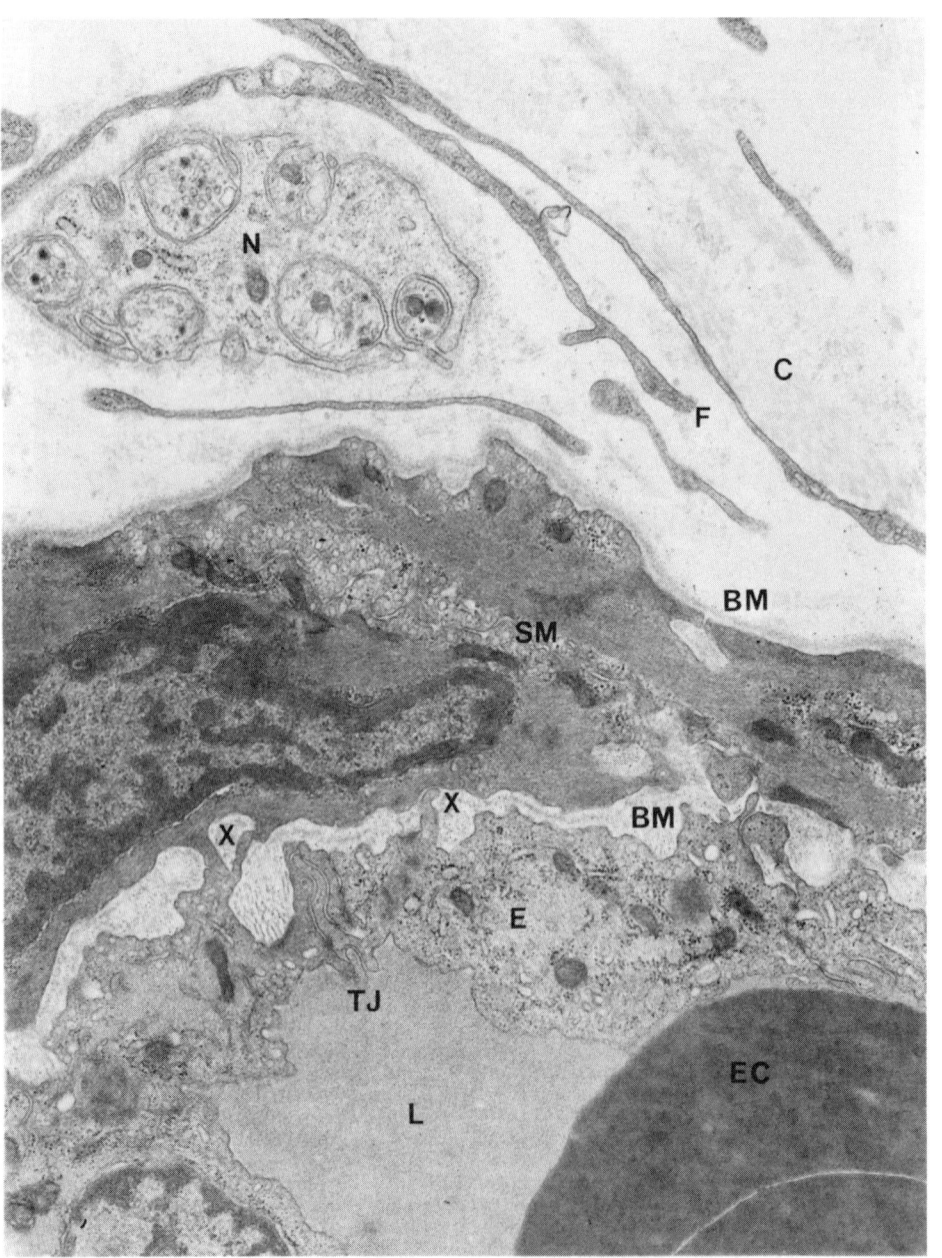

FIGURE 22-3. Transmission electron micrograph of a terminal arteriole shown in cross section. (From Jerusalem F: The microcirculation of muscle, in Engel AG, Franzini-Armstrong C (eds): Myology, 2d ed. Vol I. New York: McGraw-Hill, 1994; pp 361–374. With permission.) Several footlike processes (X) form myoendothelial junctions between a smooth muscle cell (SM) and endothelial cells (E). Adjacent E are connected by tight junctions (TJ) and surrounded by a basement membrane (BM). The lumen (L) contains an erythrocyte (EC), and the adventitial space contains slender fibroblast processes (F) and loose collagen bundles (C). Nerve bundle (N). Magnification ×14,000. (Corrected for shrinkage factor.)

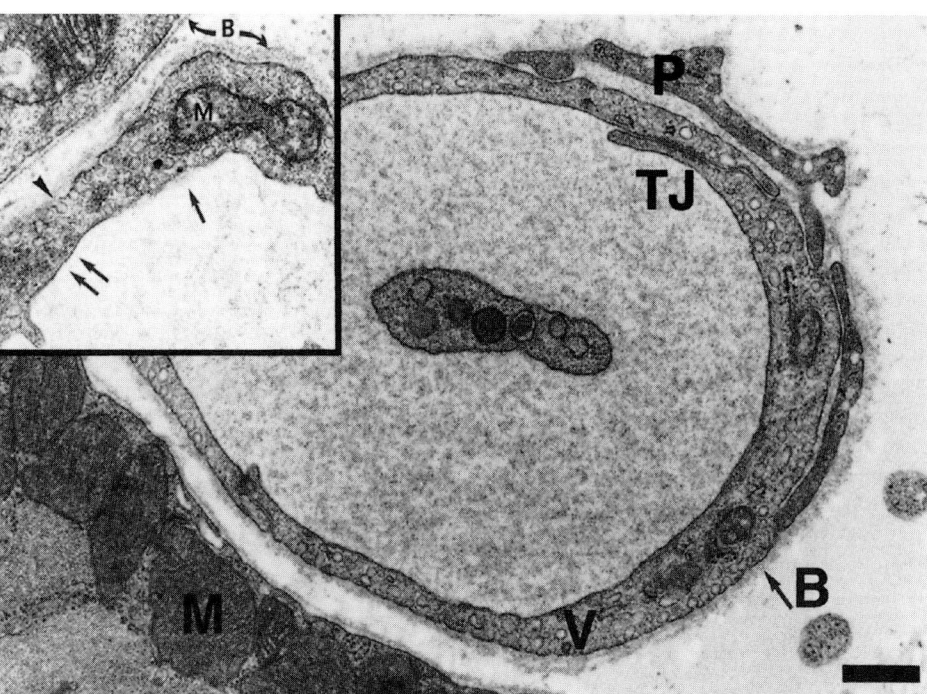

FIGURE 22-4. Transmission electron micrograph of a capillary from rat skeletal muscle, scale bar = 0.5 μm. The role of exchange vessel demands a thin wall made up of a single layer of endothelial cells containing numerous cytoplasmic vesicles (V) and sparse mitochondria (M) joined by tight junctions (TJ) and covered by a distinct basement membrane (B, arrows). The abluminal surface is partially covered with pericyte processes (P) that occasionally make close contact with the endothelium. Inset: Higher-power view showing an intact B, discontinuous glycocalyx (arrows), and erupting vesicles or caveolae (arrowhead).

marrow, spleen, or liver. The endothelial tube is formed from one to three flattened endothelial cells, depending on vessel diameter, elongated along the capillary axis with tapered ends. As the wall is only one cell thick, the diffusion distance is very small (usually < 0.5 μm). Endothelial cells are covered by a basal lamina (or basement membrane) and pericytes on the outer (abluminal) surface and a glycocalyx coat on the inner (luminal) surface. The endothelial cell cytoplasm contains sparse, rough endoplasmic reticulum and mitochondria (around 2 percent by volume) but numerous pinocytic vesicles of ~60 nm diameter, occupying some 25 to 30 percent of cytoplasmic volume. The latter arise from saccular invaginations, or caveolae, of the plasma membrane (Fig. 22-4). These contain cell-surface proteins, the caveolins, involved in mechanotransduction of fluid forces generated by flowing blood. The endothelium bulges in the region of the nucleus, narrowing the vessel lumen and increasing the resistance to passage of erythrocytes. The endothelial cells form tight junctions (zona occludens) around the periphery and occasionally pseudopodia-like structures, which protrude into the lumen. Cytoplasmic filaments of actin, 4 to 6 nm thick, are present, and may form stress fibers. Unlike splenic capillaries, however, those found in skeletal muscle are not thought to be contractile under physiologic conditions.

The thin layer of negatively charged material that forms the glycocalyx lining and covers the intercellular cleft and fenestrae can be identified by labels such as cationic ferritin. This meshwork of fibrous molecules, sialoglycoproteins and glycosaminoglycans, may have narrow enough spaces to act as a macromolecular sieve, increasing hydraulic resistance (the fiber matrix theory of Curry and Michel).[16] Intercellular junctions are parallel-sided clefts of 15 to 20 nm width that form the transcapillary pathway for exchange of most fluid and metabolites—e.g., glucose. The close proximity of adjacent cell membranes in the region of tight junctions is discontinuous around the cell perimeter to allow such exchange, and the permeability may to some extent vary according to the tortuosity of the cleft pathway imposed by these strands of membrane particles.[17]

Endothelial vesicles are thought to be involved in the transport of macromolecules into the cell (endocytosis) and across the cell (transcytosis). The latter process has been a source of controversy for many years. The presence of apparently free-floating vesicles in the cytoplasm is an artifact of the techniques used to visualize them, as their dimensions are similar to the thickness of section used (such that any estimate of dimension or number is subject to very large errors) and appear to connect with adjacent vesicles out of the plane of the section. Thus, they are envisaged to represent more a bunch of grapes than isolated vesicles. Depending on their size, they may play a role in transport by transient fusion and exchange of material, or they may form a continuous channel between the luminal and abluminal surfaces.[17]

The basal lamina varies in width between 50 and 300 nm, averaging around 150 nm in normal human muscle capillaries (Table 22-2). It forms a continuous covering of the abluminal surface with poorly defined dense (lamina densa) and light (lamina rara) regions. The lamina densa contains type IV collagen and heparan sulfate proteoglycan anchored to the endothelial cell by the laminins. The lamina rara includes cablin, a rod-like molecule with integrin-binding properties.[18] Peptide growth factors such as FGF-2, which lacks the leader sequence usually associated with cellular secretion, may also be sequestered within the basement membrane. The physical strength of the basement membrane is important in resisting capillary deformation as a result of hydrostatic pressure and also prevents leakage of macromolecules such as proteins.

The perivascular pericytes, or Rouget cells, are stellate cells with extensive branches that run longitudinally along the capillary for some considerable distance (e.g., up to 150 μm for rat muscle).[19] Although pericytes cover only a relatively small proportion of the capillary surface, around 30 percent, circumferential branches are present along ~90 percent of the capillary length.[20] Pericytes secrete their own basement membrane, such that they are bounded by a common basement membrane with endothelial cells. At a number of points around the circumference there is direct endothelial-pericyte cell contact. The possibility of cellular cross talk is increased by interdigitation of cell processes.[21] Although the presence of actin filaments has led some to conclude that pericytes are contractile and hence regulate microvascular perfusion, there is little direct evidence for this. They may regulate endothelial proliferation by either secreted factors or contact inhibition.[22] Possibly more important is their role in modification of the extracellular matrix and as precursors of smooth muscle cells, supporting endothelial migration and transformation of capillaries into arterioles (arteriolarization) during adaptive growth and remodeling of the microcirculation.

Physiologic Control of the Microcirculation

SITE OF CONTROL

The interactions between nervous, myogenic, hormonal, and metabolic influences that control muscle microcirculation are complex, operating at different levels of the microvascular network. Vascular smooth muscle, which is present in arterioles right down to the smallest precapillary vessels (Fig. 22-1), acts as the final integrator of these regulatory mechanisms, and protein kinase C provides a common signal transduction pathway for modulation of the contractile process.[23] The endothelium is important for the initiation and coordination of signaling throughout the network (Fig. 22-5).

Different control mechanisms operate according to the segmental position of different classes of vessels within the microvascular network. Estimates of the distribution of resistance throughout the microcirculation of muscle have been based on measurements of intravascular pressure profiles along the network, observations of vessel diameters, and assumptions about viscosity obtained mainly from flat,

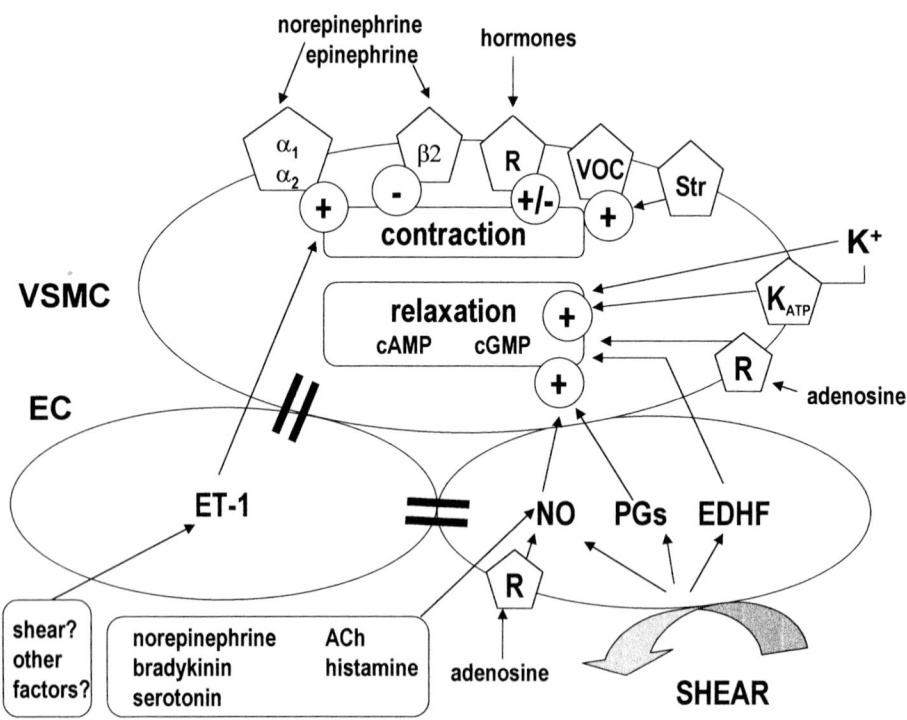

FIGURE 22-5. Schematic representation of vascular smooth muscle cell (VSMC)–endothelial cell (EC) regulatory pathways. The smooth muscle cell receives input via adrenergic receptors from neurally released and circulating catecholamines, from circulating hormones (e.g., vasopressin, angiotensin, insulin), and via voltage-operated Ca^{2+} channels (VOC) and stretch-activated Ca^{2+} channels (myogenic responses). Potassium may vasodilate via different types of K^+ channels, the K_{ATP} channel being important in metabolic control of tone and reactive hyperemia. Cyclic AMP and GMP act as second messengers for several of the VSMC agonists. Communication between smooth muscle and endothelial cells is via gap junctions (indicated by thick, short, parallel lines). Endothelial cells generate both relaxing (nitric oxide, NO; prostaglandins, PGs; endothelial-derived hyperpolarizing factor, EDHF) and contracting (endothelin, ET-1) factors in response to circulating agonists (bradykinin, etc.) and to shear stress resulting from blood flow across the luminal surface.

easily accessible muscles in the rat and cat under anesthesia. They show that the biggest drop in pressure occurs from vessels around 50 μm diameter, in which it is 70 percent of systemic, to those around 10 μm diameter, in which it is approximately 25 percent of systemic (see Ref. 24). Nevertheless, a significant portion of resistance to flow in skeletal muscle resides in large arterioles and arteries with diameters > 100 μm.[25]

CAPILLARY PERFUSION AND RECRUITMENT

Capillary perfusion depends on the pre- to postcapillary resistance, which regulates not only the velocity of flow, red cell flux, and red cell transit time—factors crucial for oxygen delivery—but also transcapillary transport of solutes. In rat cremaster and other muscles, pressure in preterminal arterioles is about 30 to 40 mmHg; in capillaries, 25 mmHg; and in the smallest venules, 15 mmHg.[26] The Vrbc decreases with decreasing vessel diameter: 11 $\mu m \cdot s^{-1}$ in 40-μm-wide arterioles, 4 $\mu m \cdot s^{-1}$ in terminal arterioles (9 μm) in cat tenuissimus, and 0.4 to 1.5 $\mu m \cdot s^{-1}$ in capillaries.[27] Red cell flux (number of red cells per second) also varies with vessel diameter, with values of 43 cells per second in terminal arterioles in hamster cremaster[28] and 7 cells per second in capillaries in hamster tibialis anterior.[29] Capillary transit times, calculated from maximal blood flow and total capillary volume to be between 0.3 and 1.0 s, were shorter in the muscles of small (agouti, fox) than large (steer, horse) animals and showed a negative correlation with oxidative capacity.[30] Direct measurements in the glycolytic cortex of tibialis anterior and the oxidative soleus of rats showed shorter transit times in the latter muscle, 1.5 and 1.1 s, respectively.[10] The short transit times permit adequate oxygen supply, however, because of greater oxygen extraction and the fact that there are multiple capillary pathways available through a dense network. Longer transit time through longer capillaries in glycolytic muscles may ensure adequate washout of metabolites.

While all arterioles, arteries, and the feed artery are capable of dilation or constriction under appropriate stimuli, it has been held that capillary diameters do not change. Recent observations have challenged this assumption, demonstrating that diameter varies along capillary length,[31] that it varies with perfusion pressure[32] or in response to local application of drugs.[33] Such changes can, of course, alter the red cell flux as well as transit times.

During and immediately after muscle contraction or on application of a vasodilator such as adenosine, which increases blood flow to a similar extent as contractions, the diameters of all categories of vessels increase and pressures, velocities, red cell flux, and transit times change accordingly. Thus Vrbc in muscles contracting at 8 Hz can double (cremaster[28]) or treble (extensor digitorum[13]). Pressure measurements are difficult enough to make in muscle microcirculation under resting conditions and impossible during contractions. Data obtained during the administration of vasodilators that caused a 10- to 15-mmHg decrease in systemic blood pressure indicate that the main changes in pressures occur in arterioles > 20 μm, with relatively small changes in capillary and venular pressures.[34]

The enormous increase in muscle blood flow that occurs during contractions, enabled by dilation of supplying arteries and arterioles, has been proposed to involve recruitment of previously unperfused capillaries.[35] However, the majority of direct intravital observations reveal that most capillaries contain red cells under resting conditions, albeit showing temporal and spatial heterogeneity, and that the changes occurring during muscle contractions or vasodilation entail increases in red cell velocity, hematocrit, and flux. Even in bulk locomotor muscles, perfusion with India ink or fluorochromes shows that all capillaries are perfused under resting conditions within 20 s.[36] Conversely, constriction of arterioles would decrease velocity of flow and hematocrit, so that the spacing of red blood cells would become greater and cells may even be stationary.

NERVOUS CONTROL

Adrenergic sympathetic nerve fibers, visualized by catecholamine fluorescence, form a dense network around arterial vessels from large vessels (40 to 70 μm internal diameter) down to terminal precapillary arterioles (7 to 13 μm diameter), while venous microvessels have none.[37] So far, there is no evidence of adrenergic innervation of capillaries. At rest, basal sympathetic constrictor tone in skeletal muscle is relatively high such that pharmacologic adrenergic blockade or denervation leads to significant increases in flow. The response to sympathetic nerve stimulation or application of norepinephrine is constriction of all arterial vessels but greatest in those with diameters less than 25 μm,[38] while venous vessels show little or no response to either. Vessels supplying slow oxidative muscles are also less responsive to sympathetic activation or catecholamines than those to fast muscles, in accord with their lower basal constrictor tone. In larger arterioles and venules, VSMCs possesses both α_1 and α_2 receptors, whereas the small terminal arterioles (~13 μm) contain predominantly α_2 receptors.[39] It has been proposed that low-frequency sympathetic activation would preferentially constrict small arterioles via α_2 receptors, while high-frequency stimulation would act via α_1 receptors on the larger vessels.[40] The importance of sympathetic innervation becomes obvious in situations where it is necessary to divert blood from skeletal muscles to other organs—e.g., during hemorrhage or shock.

Anatomically, cholinergic nerve fibers of sympathetic origin have been described innervating blood vessels in muscles of the cat, dog, and pig, but not rodents or humans. Grasby et al.[41] described a population of nonadrenergic neurons coming from the lumbar sympathetic ganglia and supplying the blood vessels of a number of skeletal muscles in the guinea pig. These were positive for vasoactive intestinal polypeptide (VIP) and neuropeptide Y (NPY), which were found mainly on feed arteries > 80 μm diameter but rarely in small arteriolar vessels of < 20 μm and were more evident in muscles with more type I than type II fibers. Their function was unknown, although it was presumed that they were vasodilator fibers contributing to early increases in muscle blood flow while metabolites acted to vasodilate vessels more distally.

LOCAL CONTROL

Myogenic Control

The intrinsic myogenic response of vascular smooth muscle in the skeletal muscle microcirculation—i.e., vessel constriction in response to increased pressure and dilation in response to decreased pressure—is more apparent in intermediate-sized vessels than in larger or very small arterioles[42] and is relatively strong compared with other vascular beds such as mesentery. It is stimulated by alterations of vessel wall tension and does not require the presence of the endothelium. In response to pressure increases, it is accompanied by membrane depolarization and an increase in intracellular Ca^{2+} concentration (see Ref. 42 for review of mechanisms). In vivo, it serves to generate intrinsic basal tone, maintain normal arterial pressure at rest, and autoregulate perfusion if inflow pressure is altered, as during reactive hyperemia. In arteries > 50 μm, myogenic responses are attenuated by endothelial dilator mechanisms; in microvessels, they can be attenuated by concurrent metabolite accumulation during light exercise, α stimulation by adrenaline, anesthetic (barbiturate), or calcium antagonists (e.g., nifedipine).[43] Myogenic constriction can also be exacerbated in diseases such as diabetes or hypertension,[44] contributing to impaired muscle perfusion and performance.

Metabolic Control

The primary determinant of skeletal muscle blood flow is the metabolic rate of the muscle. The involvement of a host of substances—including decreased tissue and/or blood P_{O_2}, decreased pH, increased P_{CO_2}, increased osmolality, increased adenosine and/or adenosine nucleotides, potassium, phosphates, kinins, and prostaglandins—has been tested (see Refs. 45 to 47 for reviews). Although all of the above can be shown to produce vasodilation in skeletal muscle, and removal of each individually by blockade of synthesis, release, or action on VSMCs attenuates functional hyperemia to some degree, it is clear that none alone can account for the magnitude of blood flow increases.[48]

The site of action of metabolites is presumed to be in all segments of the microvascular network lying within the muscle parenchymal tissue that are exposed to interstitial concentrations. The largest dilation in response to stimulation-evoked contractions occurs in preterminal and terminal arterioles 7 to 13 μm diameter in rat spinotrapezius[49] and cat sartorius.[50] Lash[51] reported that decreases in resistance during contractions occurred in both upstream (including feed arteries) and microvascular segmental resistances of rat spinotrapezius, and it is clear that for muscle blood flow to increase to the magnitude that it does and to provide optimal perfusion, a coordinated dilation of both small and large arterioles has to occur.[52]

To determine whether there is differential regulation of larger versus small arterioles, the direct effects of metabolites on different classes of vessels can best be tested using isolated vessel preparations or intravital observation. Hilton et al.[53] observed that terminal arterioles of the rat spinotrapezius, 7 to 13 μm in diameter, were most sensitive to topical application of potassium and phosphate, the latter producing rapid dilation, whereas Wunsch et al.[54] showed that first-order arterioles from soleus and gastrocnemius of rats, 100 to 200 μm in diameter, also dilated significantly to a variety of substances [potassium, adenosine, acetycholine (ACh), sodium nitroprusside (SNP)]. However, the onset of dilation in these larger, more proximal arterioles was not rapid enough to account for the initiation of exercise hyperemia, although it can contribute significantly to determining the magnitude of perfusion through the microcirculation by both metabolic vasodilation and "ascending dilation" (see below and Ref. 55). Furthermore, feed arteries lying outside the muscle also provide significant resistance to flow and dilate during contractions.[56]

With respect to the time course of metabolic factors in control of muscle microcirculation, factors responsible for the initiation of functional hyperaemia are likely to be different from those that sustain it. The major difficulties in establishing the involvement of specific metabolites as dilators during muscle activity are those of estimating precisely the concentrations to which the vessel wall will be exposed and, as indicated above, showing that their time course of action is appropriate. Even with the use of microdialysis techniques to estimate local adenosine production in skeletal muscle, its source and concentration are still disputed. Marshall[57] argues that during systemic hypoxia, adenosine is released primarily from endothelial rather than muscle cells and acts to cause vasodilation via nitric oxide. Potassium has been measured in the interstitial space using microelectrodes in animal and human muscles; in the latter, microdialysis showed graded increases in concentration with knee extensor exercise[58] and accumulation during static contractions.[59] Joyner and Proctor[60] have recently reiterated the limitations of attempting to "isolate" a potential vasodilator metabolite in view of the multifactorial nature and likely compensatory mechanisms operating in control of muscle blood flow.

Endothelial Control

The endothelium regulates VSMC tone in the muscle microcirculation by releasing relaxing and/or contracting factors in response to chemical and physical signals. Of these factors, nitric oxide (NO), prostaglandins (PGs), endothelial-derived hyperpolarizing factor (EDHF), and endothelin (ET) have been most investigated. In resting muscle, inhibition of NO synthesis by competitive inhibitors increases vascular resistance to a greater degree in larger (> 25 μm) than in smaller (< 25 μm) vessels[61] and decreases blood flow at rest more than 40 percent in cat muscles[62] and human forearm muscles.[63] Likewise, cyclooxygenase inhibitors of prostaglandin synthesis such as indomethacin vasoconstrict arterioles in resting muscle.[64]

The most significant stimulus for release of NO and PGs from the endothelium is shear stress on the luminal vessel surface, although other physical stimuli, such as pulsatile stretching of the vascular wall and low arterial P_{O_2}, are also effective. Increased blood flow through one arteriolar branch following occlusion of flow in a parallel branch induced dilation that was dependent on endothelium, via PGs in rat cremaster[65] and NO in rat spinotrapezius.[64] In isolated arterioles from rat cremaster (85 μm diameter), increasing perfusate flow rate significantly attenuated pressure-induced myogenic constrictions while increasing pressure-reduced flow-induced dilations.[66] Thus if myogenic constriction decreases diameter at constant flow, shear stress would be increased to counteract constriction via enhanced NO release. This mechanism may be more effective in the larger upstream vessels, which are poorly regulated by metabolites and depend more on endothelium.[25] Indeed, endothelial-dependent flow-mediated dilation can even be demonstrated in large conduit arteries such as brachial or femoral in animals and humans, where it contributes to both functional and reactive hyperemia in arms and legs. It can be a sensitive indicator of impairment of endothelial function in diseases such as diabetes, hypertension, and cardiac failure.[67]

Localization of endothelial NO synthase expression by immunoelectron microscopy showed that it is concentrated in the caveolae on the luminal cell surface, where it is activated by increasing vascular flow and pressure.[68] NO synthase and caveolin were found to be coexpressed in the endothelium of feed artery, arterioles, capillaries, and veins of the retractor muscle of the hamster cheek pouch,[69] and it is thought that the caveolae act as flow-sensing organelles involved in the rapid transduction of mechanical stimuli into flow-induced responses. Endothelial NO and PG release may also be agonist-induced—by catecholamines, ACh, histamine, and bradykinin.[70] However, there remains a degree of vasodilation in muscle microcirculation that is resistant to NO or PG synthesis inhibition and is dependent upon VSMC hyperpolarization by EDHF. The characterization of this factor is yet to be fully determined, but it is likely to be a cytochrome-P450 metabolite or K^+. It appears to have greater importance in small than in large vessels and contributes to maintaining vascular responsiveness when other endothelial-dependent dilators are impaired by disease.[71] Endothelin, on the other hand, as a potent endothelial-derived vasoconstrictor, may antagonize dilator mechanisms in skeletal muscle,[72] particularly in disease conditions, such as hypertension.[73]

CONDUCTED RESPONSES AND CELL-CELL COMMUNICATION

The endothelium is important in the transmission of signals between different segments of the microvascular network. Segal and colleagues have shown that if an agonist such as ACh or norepinephrine is applied locally to an arteriole, the vasoactive response is not confined to the site of stimulation but is propagated along the vessel for a distance of several millimeters independently of innervation or flow. This mechanism, termed "conducted" dilation or constriction, appears to depend on direct coupling between endothelial and VSMCs via gap junctions and electrotonic spread of changes in membrane potential,[55,74] and the mechanisms have been reviewed.[75] This ability of specific sections of the microvascular tree to transmit signals up- and downstream is now recognized as very important for the coordination and integration of responses regulating capillary flow, particularly during muscle contractions.

As the microvascular units do not supply distinct motor units, the necessity to match perfusion to dispersed muscle fibers of individual active motor units suggests that dilator signals induced by muscle contractions should originate and be detected at the capillary level and that this should dictate the increase in capillary flow. Indeed, Berg et al.[28] showed that contraction of small groups of muscle fibers caused dilation in arterioles supplying, but lying distant from, the capillaries around active muscle fibers and that capillaries are thus capable of determining their own perfusion, possibly via gap junction communication and/or local paracrine signal such as NO.[76,77] However, since each microvascular unit is positioned to supply fibers that may not all be activated,[74] the perfusion to a specific fiber type will to some degree be dependent on capillary dimension and flow velocity.

COORDINATED CONTROL OF FUNCTIONAL HYPEREMIA

The sites of action of the various control mechanisms with muscle microcirculation are illustrated in Fig. 22-6. As metabolite concentrations take several seconds to accumulate in contracting muscle depending on the intensity of work done, they are in general discounted as the initiators of functional hyperemia. Other mechanisms responsible for the onset of vasodilation in contracting muscle include the muscle pump, whereby rhythmic propulsion of blood out of muscle by mechanical compressive forces facilitates systemic venous return during contraction and venous filling within the muscle during relaxation. Recent reviews[47,78] conclude that this mechanism is likely to contribute significantly to functional hyperemia during voluntary exercise, although whether it can provide sufficient flow in the absence of dilation is not clear.

Another possibility is that of neurally mediated vasodilation. Despite evidence for the presence of sympathetic cholinergic fibers to muscle in some species, albeit not in humans, this mechanism has been discounted, since neither sympathectomy, atropine, nor autonomic blockade alters the rate or magnitude of increase in hyperemia at the onset of exercise (see Refs. 47 and 79). Welsh and Segal[80] proposed that dilation in contracting muscles could be evoked by spillover of ACh released from neuromuscular junctions on the active muscle fibers, a mechanism that could explain the close matching between blood flow and muscle activity. ACh could act indirectly by stimulating release of the vasodilator NO from the endothelium.[81]

On the basis that metabolically driven vasodilation and feedforward flow from elevated cardiac output would increase shear stress on the endothelium, the contribution of dilating factors NO and PGs during exercise has been examined in many studies in animals and humans by the use of appropriate synthesis inhibitors. These studies have failed, however, to show a clear role for either NO[82] or PGs[83] in functional hyperemia in whole muscles or limbs. This may be because the effects of substance elimination are masked by compensatory increases in other vasodilators, but a recent study using microdialysis in contracting human muscles found no effect of NO synthesis blockade on adenosine or prostaglandins.[84]

For the body as a whole, blood flow to skeletal muscle during exercise must be regulated with respect to cardiac output and the maintenance of arterial blood pressure. Sympathetic nerve activity is targeted to both active and inactive muscles

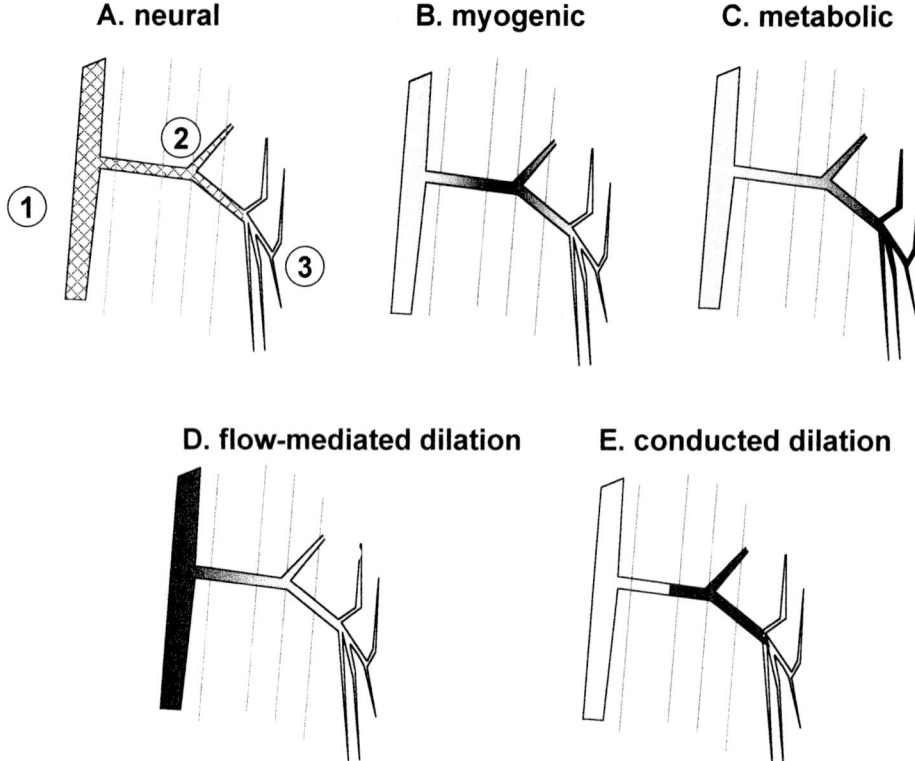

FIGURE 22-6. The location of control mechanisms in different segments of the microcirculation (1 = feed arteries, primary arterioles; 2 = small arterioles < 25 μm in diameter down to terminal precapillary arterioles; 3 = capillaries) is demonstrated. A. Sympathetic vasoconstrictor innervation (crosshatching) is present down to terminal arterioles. B. Myogenic responses are more evident in smaller (darker) than in larger (lighter) arterioles. C. Metabolic dilation can be initiated by capillaries themselves (darker), and although all upstream vessels lying within muscle tissue will be exposed to metabolites during muscle contractions, small arterioles dilate the most. D. Flow-mediated dilation is observed in small arterioles but is probably more important in larger arterioles and arteries (darker shading). E. Conducted responses may spread a few millimeters along the arteriolar network (dark shading).

during exercise. In the former, its constrictor effects are attenuated by metabolites, the so-called functional sympatholysis. In contracting rat hindlimb muscles, NO has been shown to be important in opposing sympathetic constriction[85]; moderate acidic conditions, a consequence of contractions, inhibited α_2 vasoconstriction in small muscle arterioles more than in larger upstream arterioles.[86] Functional sympatholysis has also been studied in human forearms, showing that propagated or local endothelial responses may mediate attenuation of adrenergic vasoconstriction in large conduit arteries remote from metabolites.[87] By contrast, it is well known that during intense steady-state exercise or activation of a large muscle mass, there is effective sympathetic restraint of blood flow even in active muscles in order to maintain arterial pressure. How the switch from functional sympatholysis to sympathetic restraint is regulated remains to be determined.

HORMONAL CONTROL

Hormones other than epinephrine and norepinephrine are less important for short-term vascular regulation than neural or metabolic influences. These catecholamines are released from the adrenal medulla in response to exercise, fight-or-flight situations, hypotension, or hypoglycemia and act on α or β receptors in muscle circulation, resulting in significant β_2-mediated dilation via epinephrine. This occurs in arterioles and results in increased velocity of flow through capillaries (see Ref. 1). Arginine vasopressin (AVP) can vasodilate muscle via V2 receptors; however, during high-stress states such as hemorrhagic hypotension or congestive heart failure, it may have a predominantly vasoconstrictor effect via V1 receptors to support arterial pressure. High levels of circulating angiotensin II, in response to activation of the renin-angiotensin system—by, for example, hemorrhage or cardiac failure—can lead to vasoconstriction by direct action on VSM or by facilitating norepinephrine release and enhancing sympathetic drive. By contrast, atrial natriuretic peptide (ANP) induces dose-dependent dilation in human forearm skeletal muscle[88] and can antagonize α_1-mediated vasoconstriction in large arterioles.[39] Skeletal muscle microcirculation is significantly affected by insulin. Systemic administration of insulin caused arteriolar dilation in rat spinotrapezius[89] and increased velocity of red blood cells in both arterioles and capillaries in rat cremaster.[90] Thyroxine increases both muscle blood flow and metabolism.

Remodeling of the Microcirculation under Physiologic Conditions

INCREASED ACTIVITY

Extensive remodeling of the vascular supply takes place when muscle activity is increased over several weeks, either by training or by chronic electrical stimulation. Repeated muscle biopsies have enabled longitudinal studies on changes in capillary supply in human and animal muscle subjected to different types of training (Table 22-1). Endurance training leads to increased capillary supply in human muscles irrespective of age, predominantly in the particular muscles involved in the training protocol—e.g., the deltoid muscle in rowers and swimmers and the vastus lateralis in cyclists. Capillary growth is related to the intensity of muscle activity. This was clearly shown in cross-country skiers, where electromyographic (EMG) monitoring showed greater activity and greater increase in capillarization in the triceps brachii than in the vastus lateralis. The increase occurs predominantly around oxidative fibers (see Refs. 4 and 91), since these are preferentially recruited and receive increased blood flow during voluntary activity.[92] Fast glycolytic fibers are activated only during supramaximal contractions of short duration, yet capillary growth was observed in the glycolytic parts of gastrocnemius muscle in rats trained by sprint training,[93] again possibly linked with increased blood flow to this region.[94] Duration of training is as important as intensity, since minimal changes were found in muscles of animals trained for only 3 weeks. With heavy resistance training, capillary supply was either not changed (see Ref. 4) or only modestly increased.[95] Capillary growth induced by training is not due to proliferation of endothelial cells[96] but to elongation of existing capillaries and probably capillary splitting.[97] It is usually but not always preceded or accompanied by increased muscle fiber oxidative capacity and is likely due to hemodynamic factors (shear stress, capillary wall tension) associated with increased blood flow. Training also resulted in increased diameter of the feed artery and arterioles[51,98] and increased numbers of terminal arterioles in rats.[99] The size of the whole forearm vascular bed, assessed by maximal vascular conductance, was also increased as a result of several weeks of training in humans,[100] and large conduit arteries increased in diameter.[101]

There is little information about the impact of either a single bout of exercise or short-term training on skeletal muscle microcirculation, in particular in arterioles smaller than 25 μm, which contribute significantly to regulation of flow; hence there is no knowledge of how such changes relate to subsequent structural alterations. However, on an acute basis, muscle activity upregulates endothelial NO synthase activity and NO production in skeletal muscle,[102] while chronic exercise upregulates mRNA for NO synthase in large arteries.[103]

With training, growth of vessels usually appears after many weeks, but increasing muscle activity in selected animal muscle groups (hindlimb ankle flexors) by chronic electrical stimulation induced capillary growth within only 4 days and doubled C:F ratio within a month.[104] The capillaries formed a very complex network, with multiple intercapillary connections and sprouts (Fig. 22-7).[105] The increase in C:F ratio was preceded by intense proliferation of the capillary-linked nuclei and appeared simultaneously with increased numbers of capillaries expressing vascular endothelial growth factor (VEGF), which may be linked to increased capillary shear stress.[106] Capillary growth in stimulated muscles is also accompanied by growth of arterioles,[107] and the size of the whole vascular bed demonstrated by corrosion casts is therefore enlarged.[108]

Growth of vessels induced by increased activity can be initiated by growth factors secreted from muscle, connective tissue, or endothelium or by mechanical factors. Gustafsson and Kraus[109] recently reviewed their involvement, in particular that of VEGF, which appears to be the most important factor stimulating growth of endothelial cells. Although there is some evidence that it may be involved in capillary growth in chronically stimulated muscles,[106,110] direct evidence for its involvement in angiogenesis during exercise is still lacking. VEGF also makes vessels more permeable, so that during development,

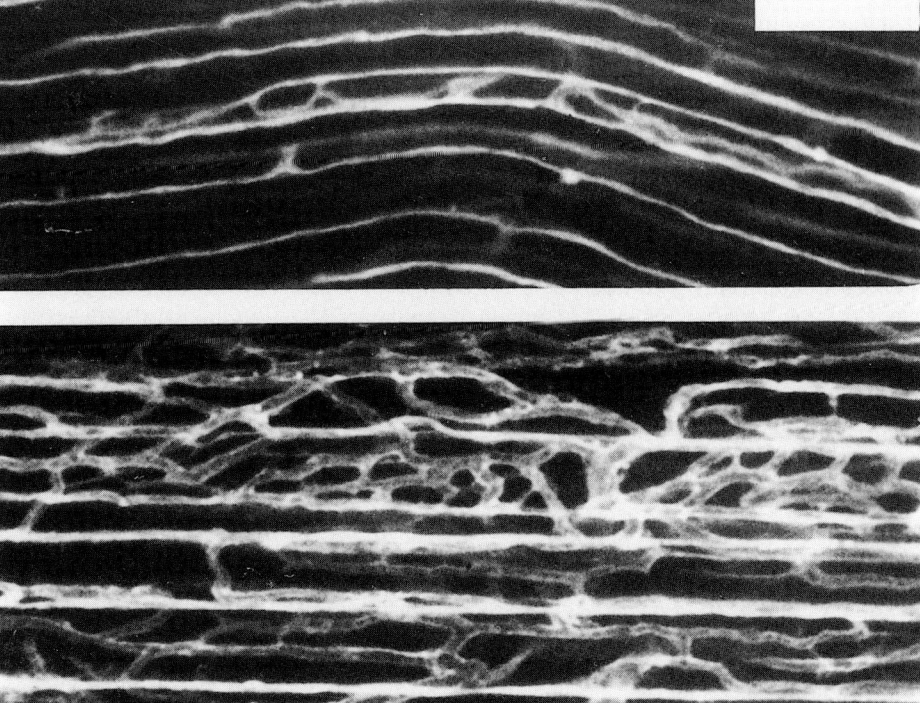

FIGURE 22-7. Laser scanning confocal micrograph of a whole-mount muscle preparation (rat extensor hallucis proprius, fluorescence image of rhodamine-labeled *Griffonia simplicifolia* I lectin). Top panel, control muscle showing some degree of anastomosis between capillaries; bottom panel, appearance following angiogenesis induced by 7 days of indirect electrical stimulation, showing both an increase in microvascular density and a higher frequency of intercapillary anastomoses. (Scale bar = 100 μm.) (*From Hansen-Smith FM, Hudlicka O, Egginton S: In vivo angiogenesis in adult rat skeletal muscle: Early changes in capillary network architecture and ultrastructure. Cell Tissue Res 286: 123–136, 1996. With permission.*)

the factor angiopoietin-1 is required for stabilization of vessels by promoting interaction between endothelium and mesenchymal cells such as fibroblasts or pericytes to make the vessels fully mature, although there is no evidence for its involvement in vessel growth induced by increased activity, whereas angiopoietin-2 is involved in vessel regression. Fibroblast growth factor-2, which is important in angiogenesis in tumors, does not appear to be involved in capillary growth in skeletal muscle, while another factor, endothelial cell–stimulating angiogenic factor (ESAF), which, although not well characterized, can activate metalloproteinases during the angiogenic process, was elevated in muscles where capillary growth was induced by both increased activity and stretch.[111,112] Stretch also activates integrins, which mediate communication between endothelial cells and the extracellular matrix and are involved in angiogenesis in organs other than skeletal muscle. Transforming growth factor-β_1 (TGF-β_1) and platelet-derived growth factor-β (PDGF-β) are not directly involved in capillary growth but may be significant for growth of smooth muscle cells and transformation of capillaries into arterioles. They also have been shown to be upregulated by increased shear stress in vitro, as are many other factors.[113,114]

The role that mechanical factors—namely blood flow, increased shear stress, increased wall tension, and increased stretch—play in capillary growth has been reviewed by Hudlicka[115] and Hudlicka et al.[116] While shear stress results in capillary growth by luminal sprouting and stretch in abluminal sprouting, repeated muscle contractions combine both factors, and capillary growth in stimulated muscles occurs by both mechanisms.[117] Although the signaling pathways in vivo are not fully clarified, increased shear stress can initiate proliferation of endothelial cells via release of NO and/or prostaglandins, or, more directly, by activation of phospholipase C, leading to splitting of phosphatidylinositol to diacylglycerol and IP3; these can initiate the pathway leading to increase of intracellular Ca^{2+}, activation of protein kinase C, mitogen-activated protein kinases, and endothelial cell proliferation.

COMPENSATORY HYPERTROPHY

Most data on hypertrophy derive from muscle overload in mammals and birds, caused by stretch due to extirpation of synergistic muscles, and reveal an almost linear relationship between C:F and fiber area (see Ref. 4). Arteriolar growth may either accompany[118] or precede growth of capillaries.[119] In hypertrophic muscles, growth is mainly due to mechanical forces acting on the outer vessel surface, since blood flow does not increase prior to growth of new vessels[112] and is accomplished only by abluminal sprouting.[120] Capillaries are tethered to muscle fibers and are stretched with increasing sarcomere length.[121] Thus their basement membrane may be disturbed,[117] which would facilitate abluminal endothelial sprouting or release of sequestered growth factors. This process is helped by increased activity of metalloproteinases.[122] Muscle overload also results in upregulation of insulin-like growth factor-1 (IGF-1) production, including a splice variant termed *mechano growth factor*,[123] which may have both paracrine and autocrine influences on angiogenesis.[124]

MUSCLE INACTIVITY

As increased muscle activity is so important for stimulating capillary growth, it could be anticipated that decreased activity would result in capillary loss. However, this is not always the case. It takes a comparatively long time for capillaries to regress if muscle activity is restricted, e.g., 20 months in cats kept caged.[125] In humans, the high capillary supply achieved by training cannot be sustained without continued activity and returns to pretraining values within 4 to 8 weeks (see Ref. 4). Inactivity from hypokinesia (in animals suspended in a position that prevented the limbs from supporting body weight) resulted in muscle atrophy in the antigravitational muscles, which increased capillary density but decreased C:F ratio.[126] Although total blood flow in muscles exposed to the latter type of inactivity was not lower, arteriolar dilation to endothelial-dependent dilators was attenuated[127] and capillary perfusion could thus be decreased. Preservation of capillary supply following unloaded atrophy as a result of unilateral limb suspension in humans[128] or rats following space flight[129] was, presumably, also due to maintenance of normal blood flow.

HYPOXIA

Long-term exposure to hypoxia results in muscle fiber atrophy, and earlier reports of increased capillarization were due to the fact that more capillaries were found per area because of the smaller fibers. More recent studies report no change in C:F ratio (see Ref. 4 for review), total capillary length, tortuosity, or diameters.[130] However, despite low oxygen values in the arterial blood, oxygen supply to muscles is maintained by increased capillary hematocrit, red cell flux, and flow.[131] This is due in the short term to dilatation of feed arteries and arterioles, mediated by adenosine, that produces dilation in an NO-dependent manner.[57] In the long term, adequate oxygen supply is enabled by growth of new arterioles[132] and even capillaries in the vicinity of large muscle fibers, which may experience greater hypoxia because of longer diffusion distances.[133] Growth during hypoxia may be due to enhanced expression of VEGF, which is well known to be upregulated by hypoxia in many tissues.

HORMONES

Aside from their effects on muscle blood flow, a number of hormones also directly or indirectly stimulate capillary proliferation. After administration of insulin, capillary growth reached a maximum after 3 days and was abolished by cortisone.[134] Increased capillary growth after administration of angiotensin II, particularly in combination with angiotensin II AT_2 receptor, was described by Greene.[135] Administration of angiotensin II also caused transformation of capillaries into arterioles.[136] Anabolic steroids increased capillary supply in fast but not slow muscles[137] but did not alter capillarization in trained muscles.[1] Increased C:F ratio has been reported in hyperthyroid animals (see Ref. 4), but was also described in hypothyroid rats, where muscle oxidative capacity was decreased and blood flow was maintained.[138] Thus the effects of thyroid hormones on muscle microcirculation are far from clear.

Remodeling of the Microcirculation under Pathologic Conditions

DENERVATION AND REGENERATION

As capillary density is inversely related to fiber area, muscles undergoing atrophy after denervation (decreased fiber size and number) would be expected to show increases in this parameter. This has indeed been described not only in denervated muscles but also in muscles that atrophy after tenotomy (for review see Refs. 4 and 91). Capillaries degenerated and many disappeared, but only with long-lasting denervation (2 to 18 months), such that some parts of the affected muscles became avascular. Capillaries had endothelial processes protruding into the lumen and collagen deposits externally, which increased diffusion distances and could cause ischemia in the later stages of muscle degeneration.[139] However, blood flow during the first 1 to 2 months after denervation or tenotomy remains similar to that in control muscles after an initial increase due to the section of the sympathetic vasoconstrictor fibers. When referred to muscle weight, flow gradually increased, since the size of the vascular bed remained relatively constant while muscle fibers atrophied.[91] The velocity of red blood cells in capillaries was increased,[127] possibly because metabolites released from the degenerating muscle fibers maintained arteriolar dilation.[1] Thus, although lack of capillary perfusion is not causative at the onset of muscle atrophy after denervation or tenotomy, it may contribute to a progressive atrophy with prolonged periods after these procedures. Degeneration and loss of capillaries in the later stages could be due to lack of perfusion and/or lack of mechanical stretch, as the muscles are not capable of contractions. One explanation, although not proven, for the limited perfusion might lie in dysfunction of arteriolar endothelium, which would render the vessels less responsive to vasodilator stimuli.

In contrast to denervation, there is active vessel growth in regenerating muscles, whether after reinnervation, during wounding, or after transplantation. C:F ratio was lower than in control muscles 7 weeks after nerve crush only in the regions of the largest fibers, and this was corrected by long-term increase in blood flow by α_1 blocker prazosin, indicating the importance of normal perfusion for capillary growth.[140] Growth of vessels in muscles after wounding is characterized by tortuous capillaries, which appear before sprouting. Endothelial cells in the newly formed vessels showed mitoses near the sprout tips and migrated distally, with the remnants of sarcolemma or fibrin acting as contact guidance. Capillary sprouts were fenestrated and showed high permeability, which decreased with maturation. Revascularization of freely grafted muscles (rat extensor digitorum longus) started by vessel growth into the graft from the surrounding tissue, albeit not from the original supplying vessels. These vessels occupied a greater portion of the graft after 5 days, and vascularization was completed by day 10. Revascularization of larger (cat) muscles took longer, 6 to 8 weeks, but even when almost complete, the C:F ratio was lower. It was increased by chronic stimulation, perhaps because this procedure increases muscle blood flow and shear stress and stimulates further capillary growth. Even when the circulation within a relatively small transplant was fully established, the normal reactivity of arterioles to dilators (adenosine) or constrictors (norepinephrine) was not established until 180 days after transplantation (see Ref. 4).

MUSCULAR DYSTROPHIES

Abnormalities in the microcirculation have been considered important in the pathogenesis of Duchenne muscular dystrophy. However, reports on dystrophic muscle blood flow[141,142] or capillary supply indicate either no difference[142a] or higher-than-normal values.[143,144] Nevertheless, venous obliteration,[145] swelling of endothelial cells, and thickening of the basement membrane[146] were observed and could cause impairment of oxygen and solute diffusion (Table 22-2). A decrease in vesicle numerical density[143] may also contribute to limited capillary transport capacity.

INFLAMMATORY MYOPATHIES

Capillary supply is lower in all types of inflammatory myositis,[147] as confirmed by Carry et al.,[5] who described decreased C:F ratio in different types of dystrophy as well as in dermatomyositis, polymyositis, and other inflammatory muscle conditions (Table 22-2). The reduction in C:F in degenerative dermatomyositis[148] is accompanied by capillary necrosis.[149] The proximity of degenerated capillaries and fibers in patients with dermatomyositis, but not in those with polymyositis, suggests that capillary damage may be an early target for the disease process.[150] Capillaries in myopathies of inflammatory origin also have altered ultrastructure, with thicker endothelium in polymyositis and dermatomyositis compared to controls (Table 22-2).[151] The hypertrophic endothelial cells had increased volume density of mitochondria and endoplasmic reticulum. Muscles from patients with polymyositis had significantly thicker and multilaminated capillary basement membrane compared with controls (Table 22-2), and this, together with an increased amount of collagen fibrils in the endomysial space, may represent an advanced stage of vascular regeneration.[147,152] With the exception of an increase in endoplasmic reticulum, pericytes associated with capillaries were relatively unaffected.[147]

Other pathologic myopathies with disturbed capillary supply include necrotizing myopathy with depletion of capillaries due to deposits of the complement membrane attack complex,[153] mitochondrial myopathies with capillaries with swollen endothelium and decreased C:F ratio,[154] and perivascular inflammatory responses in skeletal muscles in patients with rheumatoid arthritis.[155]

MUSCLE ISCHEMIA

In spite of numerous reports published on the changes in muscle blood flow after acute or chronic occlusion of vascular supply, the data on changes in microcirculation are relatively sparse. In rabbit tenuissimus, acute occlusion of large supplying vessels resulted in disappearance of vasomotion;

decreased diameter of terminal arterioles, capillaries, and confluent venules; and decreased capillary Vrbc to such extent that flow in some capillaries stopped. Release of the occlusion was followed by reactive hyperemia with dilation of all microvessels and an almost fourfold increase in capillary Vrbc.[156] Capillary luminal dimensions depended on the transmural pressure (pressure inside the vessels − pressure outside), with partial collapse due to passive recoil[156] and formation of intraluminal pseudopodia at low transmural pressures, which further impeded red blood cell flow.[157] Narrowing of capillaries was also described, with pressure decrease during hemorrhage, but in this case it was due to endothelial cell swelling and could be corrected by infusion of hypertonic solutions.[158]

Chronic ischemia, resulting either from partial or complete occlusion of main supplying arteries in animals or from vessel narrowing by arteriosclerotic changes in patients, leads to impairment of microcirculation with compensatory changes including development of collateral circulation by large vessels and remodeling of arteriolar and capillary vascular bed. This has been recently reviewed.[116,159] The development of collateral circulation seems to be better the further the muscle is from the site of obstruction. Thus, occlusion of the iliac artery has less serious consequences for blood flow, performance, and metabolism in muscles of the lower leg than occlusion of the femoral artery, while ligation of the anterior tibial artery resulted in partial necrosis of the muscles it supplies. Collateral vessels usually develop by enlargement of preexisting vessels with some new growth, particularly of arterioles, close to the site of the occlusion. Diameters of arterioles and venules in muscles such as tibialis anterior, extensor digitorum longus, and soleus, which are remote from the site of iliac artery ligation, were unaffected after this procedure. Diameters of capillaries, however, were diminished and, since capillary Vrbc was slightly higher, capillary shear stress was unchanged, which could help to maintain the integrity of the capillary bed. Maintenance and/or growth of vessels in ischemic areas could also be due to growth factors. Ischemia upregulated VEGF mRNA expression in muscles and in newly developed arteries. mRNA for fibroblast growth factor-1 receptors (FGFR-1), which may mediate signal transduction in proliferating smooth muscle cells and thus contribute to arteriolar growth, was also upregulated, but neither FGF-1 nor FGF-2 mRNA was changed in either muscles or arteries, so that their role in vascular remodeling in chronic ischemia is questionable. Whether chronic ischemia leads to capillary growth in the more remote muscles[159] or not[116] is still unresolved. There are no reports of loss of capillaries, and perfusion of the capillary bed in ischemic muscles at rest is no different from that in normal muscles for up to 5 weeks after ligation of the iliac artery. However, total muscle blood flow, capillary Vrbc, and red cell flux do not increase during contractions, and arterioles do not dilate. This is likely due to endothelial dysfunction, since arteriolar dilation to an endothelium-independent agonist in these ischemic muscles is more or less preserved while responses to endothelium-dependent dilators are either absent or severely attenuated.[160]

The narrowing of capillaries is largely due to capillary endothelial swelling, which has been described in ischemic rat[161,162] and human muscles.[163,164] Endothelial cell swelling may limit microvascular function by increasing the barrier thickness for diffusive exchange of oxygen and metabolites (Table 22-2). The smaller luminal cross-sectional area resulting from endothelial swelling could also restrict flow or in extreme cases impede it. Based on erythrocyte volume and surface area, the lower limit of capillary diameter that will allow erythrocyte passage is about 3 μm. Endothelial cell swelling may result in lumen areas less than the required 7 μm^2 in around 30 percent of capillaries from calf muscles of patients with critical limb ischemia (CLI).[164] This increased microvessel resistance may be accentuated by the bulging endothelial cell nuclei, which can narrow the lumen at some 30 to 40 points along a capillary.[165] At rest the effects may be quite modest, and self-limiting activity patterns may minimize further damage. Making an ischemic muscle perform work in animals[162] or patients with peripheral arterial insufficiency[164] increased the degree of swelling in calf muscle capillaries (Fig. 22-8).

REPERFUSION INJURY

Chronic ischemia, and particularly reperfusion, whether after acute arterial occlusion or in the course of development of the collateral circulation or during permanent limitation of blood supply, alters the quality of both endothelial cells and cells passing through microvessels. The most important changes occur on white blood cells and endothelium in postcapillary venules (see Refs. 166 through 168 for reviews). Exposure of endothelial cells to reoxygenation after ischemia brings about activation of xanthine oxidase and generation of reactive oxygen species. The imbalance between superoxide and nitric oxide formation leads to production and release of inflammatory mediators, such as tumor necrosis factor, and enhanced synthesis of adhesion molecules on the surface of leukocytes (CD11/CD18, L-selectin) and endothelial cells (ICAM-1, P- and E-selectin). This process results in leukocyte rolling and adhesion to the venular endothelium and microvessel plugging, which, together with increased capillary permeability, leads to edema formation, increased interstitial pressure, further narrowing of capillaries, and the no-reflow phenomenon. Generation of reactive oxygen species also inhibits the formation of nitric oxide in arterioles and thus attenuates or eliminates their ability to dilate.

The deleterious effects of chronic ischemia and/or reperfusion can be alleviated or prevented by elimination of oxygen free radicals generation using catalase, superoxide dismutase, oxypurinol, or antioxidants (vitamins C and E). Leukocyte depletion or antibodies against adhesion molecules is also very effective, although less practical for treating reperfusion in humans.[169] However, preconditioning—a short period of ischemia followed by short periods of reperfusion before the onset of longer reperfusion[168]—may be particularly useful in cases of reperfusion after arterial bypass operations in patients with critical limb ischemia. Supplementation of L-arginine, a substrate for NO formation, has also been utilized.[170]

Microcirculation in chronically ischemic muscles can also be improved by exercise. Both treadmill[171] and strength training[172] increased capillary supply in ischemic hindlimb mus-

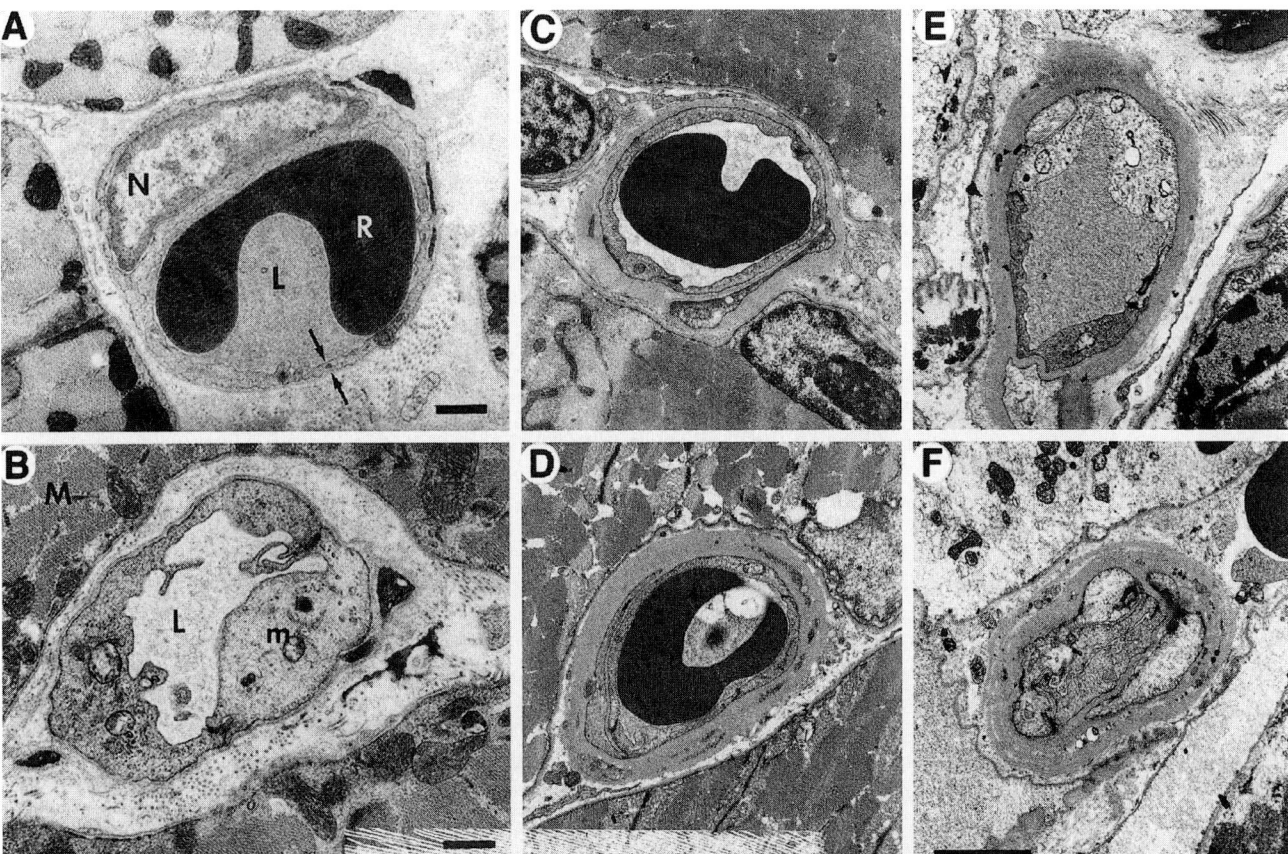

FIGURE 22-8. Transmission electron micrograph of capillaries from rat (*A* and *B*, scale bar = 0.7 μm) and human (*C* to *F*, scale bar = 4.0 μm) skeletal muscle. *A*. Control muscle showing thin capillary wall (arrows), red blood cell (R) in the lumen (L), and endothelial cell nucleus (N). *B*. Capillary from an ischemic muscle following induced activity showing gross edema of endothelial cells and resultant partial occlusion of the capillary lumen. m = mitochondrion. (*From Egginton S, Hudlicka O, Glover M: Fine structure of capillaries in ischaemic and nonischaemic rat striated muscle: Effect of torbafylline. Int J Microcirc Clin Exp 12:33–44, 1993. With permission.*) Appearance of capillaries following femorodistal bypass surgery from muscles proximal (*C, E*) and distal (*D, F*) to the bypass subsequent to infusion of a prostacyclin analogue to reduce endothelial swelling (*C, D*) or placebo (*E, F*). Note the presence of endothelial swelling in capillaries proximal to the site of arterial stenosis, i.e., from nonischemic muscle, demonstrating the systemic effect of local ischemia. (*From Thomson IA, Egginton S, Simms MH, Hudlicka O: Effect of muscle ischaemia and iloprost during femorodistal reconstruction on capillary endothelial swelling. Int J Microcirc Clin Exp 16:284–290, 1996. With permission.*)

cles in rats. Increases in muscle activity by chronic electrical stimulation also increased capillary supply and furthermore restored the ability of arterioles to dilate, also improving total muscle blood flow and performance.[173] In contrast to these beneficial effects of muscle activity were the changes in capillary ultrastructure. Vigorous activity can cause capillary endothelial swelling in human[174] and animal[175] muscles with normal blood supply. In ischemic muscles, contractile activity resulted in an even higher proportion of damaged capillaries[162] and increased the adherence of leukocytes in postcapillary venules.[176] However, the perfusion deficit resulting from lower capillary conductance because of reduced lumen size was ameliorated when arteriolar dilation improved and perfusion pressure increased.[173]

Muscle ischemia and reperfusion result in activation of leukocytes and generation of inflammatory mediators which affect endothelial cells even in sites remote from the intervention. In rats, this included capillaries in muscles contralateral to the ischemic stimulated muscle as well as cardiac muscle and diaphragm.[177,162] In humans, samples from muscles proximal to the site of femorodistal bypass also showed more endothelial swelling than from non-CLI control patients, and this was increased further after distal ischemia and subsequent reperfusion following surgery.[164] Ischemic muscles therefore appear to initiate systemic microvascular damage, which is characteristic of multiple organ dysfunction syndrome (see Ref. 168) and may be accentuated in patients with intermittent claudication by exercise.[178]

ENDOTHELIAL-LEUKOCYTE INTERACTIONS

Any insult to skeletal muscle fibers leads to transmigration of leukocytes. The factors involved in this process have been reviewed.[179] As vessel diameter increases and blood moves from capillaries to venules, red blood cells travel along the center line of the vessel and deflect the larger white blood cells toward the vessel wall, thereby enhancing close contact between the latter and the venular endothelium. In the presence of factors that activate adhesion molecules E- and P-selectin on the endothelium, leukocytes start to roll along the vessel wall, adhere, and eventually transmigrate. L-selectin is expressed on most leukocytes all the time and is necessary for the mediation of rolling and adherence to endothelial cells. It is rapidly shed after contact has been established, and this enables leukocytes to transmigrate. E-selectin synthesis is induced by cytokines, endotoxins, and anoxia and reoxygenation, requiring several hours for maximal expression. P-selectin is expressed within 5 to 10 min due to translocation from the Weibel-Palade bodies, where it is normally stored. It is no longer evident 1 h after exposure to the stimulus but appears again later due to synthesis of new protein. Endothelial cells also constitutively express intercellular adhesion molecule-1 (ICAM-1), a member of the immunoglobulin family that mediates adhesion. This molecule serves as a ligand for leukocyte glycoprotein complexes CD11a/CD18 and CD11b/CD18, the expression of which is rapidly upregulated by inflammatory mediators. Transmigration of leukocytes involves another member of the immunoglobulin family, platelet endothelial adhesion molecule-1 (PECAM-1), which is expressed on most leukocytes and platelets and on intercellular junctions in endothelial cells. PECAM-1 can activate $\beta 1$ and $\beta 2$ integrins, suggesting that it may play an important role in the regulation of leukocyte adhesion to endothelium. Adhesion molecules are also upregulated in inflammatory myopathies. ICAM-1 is strongly expressed on endothelial cells or perimysial arterioles and venules and on some perifasicular capillaries in dermatomyositis, and on capillary endothelium in all other myopathies; and vascular cell adhesion molecule, VCAM-1, was detected in a few arterioles in all inflammatory myositis and in Duchenne dystrophy.[180]

Muscle Microcirculation in Other Pathologic States

HYPERTENSION

Remodeling of the microvascular bed in skeletal muscles in rats with spontaneous hypertension involves an increased arterial media/lumen ratio, due to both hyperplasia and hypertrophy of the smooth muscle cells, and vessel rarefaction (decreased numbers) of arterioles and venules. This is likely due to a combination of high pressure in arterioles and their reduced vasodilator capacity because of impaired NO production and increased vasoconstriction to norepinephrine and endothelin. Consequently, capillary pressure could be lower, which may account for the decreased capillary supply reported by some authors. However, direct measurements of capillary pressures showed no difference with respect to control animals, and an extensive study on a number of muscles did not confirm loss of capillaries (see Ref. 116). Microvessel rarefaction also occurs in hypertension of renal origin, where it has been attributed to occlusion of small vessels by proliferating and hypertrophic endothelial cells under the direct influence of angiotensin II. This would impair perfusion and create conditions for obliteration of arterioles (see Ref. 116). An additional factor is the limited ability of arterioles to dilate in response to both endothelium-dependent and -independent dilators.[181] Administration of angiotensin-converting enzyme inhibitors[182] or an angiotensin II receptor-1 inhibitor[183] reversed changes in the muscle microcirculation of hypertensive animals, as did treatment with the β_2 agonist salbutamol[184] or 13 weeks of treadmill training,[185] conceivably by inducing long-term dilation and improved perfusion.

DIABETES

Muscle blood flow in patients with type I (insulin-dependent) diabetes is higher than normal, with a direct correlation between muscle blood flow and insulin blood levels. Blood flow also increased more during exercise in diabetics, but responses to endothelium-dependent agonists were attenuated.[186] Capillary density and total capillary area in the muscles of patients with diabetes were similar to those of controls, but the diffusion capacity was higher[187] despite thickening of the capillary basement membrane (Table 22-2). In contrast, patients with type II (non-insulin-dependent) diabetes have lower capillary density.[188] Studies in animals with streptozotocin-induced diabetes showed no difference in C:F ratio with short disease duration, but a decrease was observed after 4 months.[189] Capillaries were straighter, wider, and less branching than in control animals, and capillary Vrbc, red cell flux, and the proportion of continuously flowing capillaries were all lower.[190] This, together with the loss of vasomotion and impaired constrictor reactivity of terminal arterioles, would lead to the increased capillary pressure and hyperperfusion implicated in the ultrastructural changes in capillaries and the pathogenesis of microangiopathy.

One of the most commonly reported findings in diabetes, thickening of the capillary basement membrane, was first described 50 years ago.[191] An increase is observed even in normal human capillaries with gravity, from about 100 nm in the neck to 120 nm in the foot, and this is accentuated in diabetic subjects, reaching twice the value of controls in foot capillaries.[192] Thickening of the basement membrane may not lead to any impairment of oxygen transfer, but it may impair glucose transport. Pericyte coverage of capillaries did not vary between diabetic and nondiabetic subjects (about 20 percent in the neck and 30 percent in the foot). However, the incidence of pericyte debris in the basement membrane increased from 3 to 5 percent of capillaries in controls to between 8 and 50 percent of capillaries in diabetics, depending on the site of sampling.[192] These authors also reported an order of magnitude higher occurrence of "acellular" capillaries (up to 12 percent in the foot) of diabetic subjects, which could explain the lower-than-normal capillary density reported in some studies.

Several interventions can improve microcirculation in muscles of diabetic humans or animals. Aerobic training increased C:F ratio in muscles of type I diabetics.[193] Supplementations with evening primrose oil in the diet of diabetic rats increased capillary supply in muscle and, perhaps more importantly, in the sciatic nerve, improving both the nerve conduction velocity and muscle function. A similar effect was achieved by treatment with the angiotensin-converting enzyme inhibitor lisinopril, which was claimed to improve muscle blood flow.[194,195]

HEART FAILURE

Myocardial infarction and congestive heart failure (CHF) both result in increased skeletal muscle fatigue that is largely due to perfusion deficit and endothelial dysfunction in large and small vessels[196] and to alterations in the microcirculation. In animals, even small myocardial infarctions that did not proceed to heart failure led to decreased arteriolar diameters in limb muscles, smaller dilation to adenosine, constriction to ACh, and enhanced constriction to norepinephrine.[197,198] The percentage of capillaries with intermittent flow was increased, and capillary Vrbc and red cell flux were decreased.[199] Muscle C:F ratio in this rat model was unchanged[198]; but in patients with established CHF, it was significantly lower[200] and capillary basement membrane was thickened (Table 22-2). All these changes would impair oxygen delivery and may explain the metabolic changes observed in skeletal muscles as a result of heart failure, although it is still not known to what extent they stem from relative inactivity caused by cardiac limitations or direct effects. Endothelial dysfunction in CHF may be alleviated by interventions such as L-arginine treatment or training.[201] Increasing muscle activity by electrical stimulation prevented the narrowing of arterioles and increased C:F ratio in rats with myocardial infarction.[202] Although physical training can reverse reduced microvascular density in heart failure patients, endothelial NO synthase and VEGF expression were not altered[203]; improvements may be linked instead to the enhanced vasodilator capacity and increased blood flow.

Conclusions

As the primary role of muscle microcirculation is to supply oxygen, nutrients, hormones, and perhaps growth factors to muscle fibers and to remove metabolic products, capillary supply and the size of the microvascular bed would be expected to be more extensive in muscles or regions of muscle with higher metabolic demands. This is mostly but not always true. The microvascular bed undergoes structural and functional adaptation to some, but not all, types of training. It remains comparatively unaffected in the early stages of muscle inactivity or degeneration but is clearly modified in certain diseases, e.g., hypertension, that do not primarily affect skeletal muscle. One reason for this may be the fact that adaptation to metabolic demand is accompanied by general regulation and redistribution of blood flow, and this of itself can alter the capacity of muscle microvascular bed per se without concomitant alterations in metabolism.[115,117] Other physical factors connected with changes in sarcomere length, muscle movements, or increases in fiber girth during growth, immobilization, or denervation also modify the capillary bed and its perfusion. Perfusion of capillaries supplying a group of muscle fibers that may have different metabolic characteristics is dependent on the anatomic dimensions of the vessels. Perfusion of separate microvascular units, which are sited differently from motor units and cannot individually perfuse the entire muscle fiber length, is regulated at the level of small resistance arterioles and larger more proximal arterioles and arteries. Endothelium plays a very important role in this regulation by transmission of metabolic signals upstream to smooth muscle and endothelial cells. It is also crucial in regulation of flow in muscle disease states, particularly in acute and chronic ischemia, where, upon exposure to substances released from muscles, it attracts leukocytes that adhere to venular walls and limit capillary perfusion. Endothelial dysfunction in ischemic and other diseases—such as diabetes, hypertension, or chronic heart failure—can severely limit the vasodilator capacity of arterioles and hence be detrimental to muscle performance. Endothelium is also a target for an assortment of growth factors, and one in particular, VEGF, is currently being utilized for the treatment of peripheral vascular diseases.[204] Thus, structurally, the plasticity of the muscle microcirculation enables it to adapt to acute changes in metabolic demand or to chronic alterations in functional requirements of the muscle fibers by intensive vascular growth or regression.

List of Abbreviations

ACh	acetylcholine	NPY	neuropeptide Y
ANP	atrial natriuretic peptide	PECAM	platelet endothelial adhesion molecule
AVP	arginine vasopressin	PG	prostaglandin
C:F	capillary:fiber ratio	SNP	sodium nitroprusside
CHF	congestive heart failure	TGF	transforming growth factor
EDHF	endothelial-derived hyperpolarizing factor	VCAM	vascular cell adhesion molecule
EMG	electromyography	VEGF	vascular endothelial growth factor
ESAF	endothelial cell–stimulating angiogenic factor	VIP	vasoactive intestinal polypeptide
ET	endothelin	Vrbc	red cell velocity
FGF	fibroblast growth factor	VSM	vascular smooth muscle
IGF-1	insulin-like growth factor-1	VSMC	vascular smooth muscle cell

References

1. Hudlicka O: *Muscle Blood Flow.* Amsterdam: Swets & Zeitlinger, 1973; pp 3–4, 61, 130–138.
2. Lund N, Damon DH, Damon DN, Duling BR: Capillary grouping in hamster tibialis anterior muscles; Flow patterns and physiological significance. *Int J Microcirc Clin Exp* 5:359–372, 1987.
3. Hoppeler H, Weibel ER: Structural and functional limits for oxygen supply to muscle. *Acta Physiol Scand* 168:445–456, 2000.
4. Hudlicka O, Brown MD, Egginton S: Angiogenesis in skeletal and cardiac muscle. *Physiol Rev* 72:369–417, 1992.
5. Carry M, Ringel SP, Starcevich JM: Distribution of capillaries in normal and diseased human skeletal muscles. *Muscle Nerve* 9:445–454, 1986.
6. Stingl J, Hansen-Smith FM: Development of the vascular system in skeletal muscle, in Risau W, Rubanyi GM (eds): *Morphogenesis of the Endothelium.* Amsterdam, The Netherlands: Harwood Academic Publishers, 2000; pp 207–236.
7. Davidson YS, Clague JE, Horan MA, Pendleton N: The effect of aging on skeletal muscle capillarization in a murine model. *J Gerontol Series A* 54:B448–451, 1999.
8. Clark MG, Rattigan S, Clerk LH, et al: Nutritive and non-nutritive blood flow: Rest and exercise. *Acta Physiol Scand* 168:519–530, 2000.
9. Renkin EM: The nutritional shunt-flow hypothesis in skeletal muscle circulation. *Circ Res* 28I:I21–I25, 1971.
10. Dawson JM, Tyler KR, Hudlicka O: A comparison of the microcirculation in rat fast glycolytic and slow oxidative muscles at rest and during contractions. *Microvasc Res* 33:167–182, 1987.
11. Ellis CG, Wrigley SM, Potter RF, Groom AC: Temporal distribution of red cell supply rate to individual capillaries of resting skeletal muscle in frog and rat. *Int J Microcirc Clin Exp* 9:67–84, 1990.
12. Slaaf DW, Bosman J, Tangelder GJ, et al: Oxygen and pressure dependent functional capillary density in rabbit tenuissimus muscle. *Int J Microcirc Clin Exp* 15:271–275, 1995.
13. Tyml K, Cheng L: Heterogeneity of red blood cell velocity in skeletal muscle decreases with increased flow. *Microcirculation* 2:181–193, 1995.
14. Wisnes A, Kirkebo A: Regional distribution of microspheres in calf muscles of rat during stretch and tetanic contraction. *Microvasc Res* 6:256–266, 1973.
15. Jerusalem F: The microcirculation of muscle, in Engel AG, Franzini-Armstrong C (eds): *Myology,* 2d ed. New York: McGraw-Hill, 1994; pp 361–374.
16. Curry FE, Michel CC: A fiber matrix model of capillary permeability. *Microvasc Res* 20:96–99, 1980.
17. Michel CC, Curry FE: Microvascular permeability. *Physiol Rev* 79:703–761, 1999.
18. Charron AJ, Xu W, Bacallao RL, Wandinger-Ness A: Cablin: A novel protein of the capillary basal lamina. *Am J Physiol* 277:H1985–H1996, 1999.
19. Mazanet R, Franzini-Armstrong C: Scanning electron microscopy of pericytes in rat red muscle. *Microvasc Res* 23:361–369, 1982.
20. Egginton S, Hudlicka O, Brown MD, et al: In vivo pericyte-endothelial cell interaction during angiogenesis in adult cardiac and skeletal muscle. *Microvasc Res* 51:213–228, 1996.
21. Tilton RG, Kilo C, Williamson JR: Pericyte-endothelial relationship in cardiac and skeletal muscle capillaries. *Microvasc Res* 18:325–335, 1979.
22. Orlidge A, D'Amore PA: Inhibition of capillary endothelial cell growth by pericyte and smooth muscle cells. *J Cell Biol* 105:1455–1462, 1987.
23. Laughlin MH, Korzick DH: Vascular smooth muscle: Integrator of vasoactive signals during exercise hyperemia. *Med Sci Sports Exerc* 33:81–91, 2001.
24. Christensen KL, Mulvany MJ: Location of resistance arteries. *J Vasc Res* 38:1–12, 2001.
25. Pohl U, de Wit C, Gloe T: Large arterioles in the control of blood flow: Role of endothelium-dependent dilation. *Acta Physiol Scand* 168:505–510, 2000.
26. Zweifach BW: Local regulation of capillary pressure. *Circ Res* 28:I129–I134, 1971.
27. Fronek K, Zweifach B: Microvascular blood flow in cat tenuissimus muscle. *Microvasc Res* 14:181–189, 1977.
28. Berg BR, Cohen KD, Sarelius IH: Direct coupling between blood flow and metabolism at the capillary level in striated muscle. *Am J Physiol* 272:H2693–H2700, 1997.
29. Damon DH, Duling BR: Evidence that capillary perfusion heterogeneity is not controlled in striated muscle. *Am J Physiol* 249:H386–H392, 1985.
30. Kayar SR, Hoppeler H, Jones JH, et al: Capillary blood transit time in muscles in relation to body size and aerobic capacity. *J Exp Biol* 194:69–81, 1994.
31. Cokelet GR, Sarelius IH: Perceived vessel lumen and cell-blood velocity ratio. *Am J Physiol* 262:H1156–H1163, 1992.
32. Schmid-Schoenbein GW, Lee J: Leukocytes in capillary flow. *Int J Microvasc Clin Exp.* 15:255–264, 1995.
33. Bosman J, Tangelder GJ, oude Egbrink MG, et al: Local application of adenosine induces an increase in capillary diameter in skeletal muscle of anesthetized rabbits. *J Vasc Res* 33:111–118, 1996.
34. Fronek K, Zweifach B: Microvascular pressure distribution in skeletal muscle and the effect of vasodilatation. *Am J Physiol* 228:791–796, 1975.
35. Klitzman B, Damon DN, Gorczynski RJ, Duling BR: Augmented tissue oxygen supply during striated muscle contraction in the hamster. *Circ Res* 51:711–721, 1982.
36. Hargreaves D, Egginton S, Hudlicka O: Changes in capillary perfusion induced by different patterns of activity in rat skeletal muscle. *Microvasc Res* 40:14–28, 1990.
37. Marshall JM: The influence of the sympathetic nervous system on individual vessels of the microcirculation of skeletal muscle in the rat. *J Physiol (Lond)* 332:169–186, 1982.
38. Mellander S, Bjornberg J: Regulation of vascular smooth muscle tone and capillary pressure. *NIPS* 7:113–119, 1992.
39. Faber JE: In situ analysis of α-adrenoceptors on arteriolar and venular smooth muscle in rat skeletal muscle microcirculation. *Circ Res* 62:37–50, 1988.
40. Ohyanagi M, Faber J, Nishigaki K: Differential activation of α1- and α2-adrenoceptors on microvascular smooth muscle during sympathetic stimulation. *Circ Res* 68:232–244, 1991.
41. Grasby DJ, Gibbins IL, Morris JL: Projections of sympathetic non-adrenergic neurons to skeletal muscle arteries in guinea-pig limbs vary with the metabolic character of muscles. *J Vasc Res* 34:351–364, 1997.
42. Schubert R, Mulvany MJ: The myogenic response: Established facts and attractive hypotheses. *Clin Sci* 96:313–326, 1999.
43. Grande P-O: Myogenic mechanism in skeletal muscle circulation. *J Hypertens* 7(Suppl 4):S47–S53, 1989.
44. Izzard AS, Heagerty AM: Hypertension and the vasculature: Arterioles and the myogenic response. *J Hypertens* 13:1–4, 1995.
45. Brown MD: Metabolic control of blood flow, with reference to heart, skeletal muscle and brain, in Jordan D, Marshall JM (eds): *Cardiovascular Regulation.* London: Portland Press, 1995; pp 113–126.
46. Lash JM: Regulation of skeletal muscle blood flow during contractions. *Proc Exp Biol Med* 211:218–235, 1996.
47. Delp MD: Control of skeletal muscle perfusion at the onset of exercise. *Med Sci Sports Exerc* 31:1011–1018, 1999.
48. Gorman MW, Sparks HV: The unanswered question. *NIPS* 6:191–193, 1991.
49. Marshall JM, Tandon HC: Direct observations of muscle arterioles and venules following contraction of skeletal muscle fibers in the rat. *J Physiol (Lond)* 350:447–459, 1984.
50. Dodd LR, Johnson PC: Diameter changes in arteriolar networks of contracting skeletal muscle. *Am J Physiol* 260:H662–H670, 1991.
51. Lash JM: Contribution of arterial feed vessels to skeletal muscle functional hyperemia. *J Appl Physiol* 76:1512–1519, 1994.
52. Segal SS: Communication among endothelial and smooth muscle cells coordinates blood flow control during exercise. *NIPS* 7:156, 1992.
53. Hilton SM, Hudlicka O, Marshall JM: Possible mediators of functional hyperaemia in skeletal muscle. *J Physiol (Lond)* 282:131–147, 1978.
54. Wunsch SA, Muller-Delp J, Delp MD: Time course of vasodilatory responses in skeletal muscle arterioles: Role in hyperemia at onset of exercise. *Am J Physiol* 279:H1715–H1723, 2000.
55. Segal SS, Kurjiaka DT: Coordination of blood flow control in the resistance vasculature of skeletal muscle. *Med Sci Sports Exerc* 27:1158–1164, 1995.
56. Williams DA, Segal SS: Feed artery role in blood flow control to rat hindlimb skeletal muscles. *J Physiol (Lond)* 463:631–646, 1993.
57. Marshall JM: Adenosine and muscle vasodilation in acute systemic hypoxia. *Acta Physiol Scand* 168:561–573, 2000.
58. Juel C, Pilegaard H, Nielsen JJ, Bangsbo J: Interstitial K(+) in human skeletal muscle during and after dynamic graded exercise determined by microdialysis. *Am J Physiol* 278:R400–R406, 2000.
59. MacLean DA, Imadojemu VA, Sinoway LI: Interstitial pH, K(+), lactate, and phosphate determined with MSNA during exercise in humans. *Am J Physiol* 278:R563–R571, 2000.
60. Joyner MJ, Proctor DN: Muscle blood flow during exercise: The limits of reductionism. *Med Sci Sports Exerc* 31:1036–1040, 1999.
61. Ekelund U, Bjornberg J, Grande P-O, et al: Myogenic vascular regulation in skeletal muscle in vivo is not dependent of endothelium-derived nitric oxide. *Acta Physiol Scand* 144:199–207, 1992.
62. Poucher SM: The effect of NG-nitro-L-arginine methyl ester upon hindlimb blood flow responses to muscle contraction in the anaesthetized cat. *Exp Physiol* 80:237–247, 1995.
63. Vallance P, Collier J, Moncada S: Nitric oxide synthesised from L-arginine mediates endothelium dependent dilatation in human veins in vivo. *Cardiovasc Res* 23:1053–1057, 1989.
64. Friebel M, Klotz KF, Ley K, et al: Flow dependent regulation of arteriolar diameter in rat skeletal muscle in situ: Role of endothelium-derived relaxing factor and prostanoids. *J Physiol (Lond)* 483:715–726, 1995.
65. Koller A, Kaley G: Endothelial regulation of wall shear stress and blood flow in skeletal muscle microcirculation. *Am J Physiol* 260:H862–H868, 1991.
66. Sun D, Huang A, Koller A, Kaley G: Flow-dependent dilation and myogenic constriction interact to establish the resistance of skeletal muscle arterioles. *Microcirculation* 2:289–295, 1995.
67. Kiowski W, Sutsch G, Schalcher C, et al: Endothelial control of vascular tone in chronic heart failure *J Cardiovasc Pharmacol* 32(Suppl 3): S67–S73, 1998.

68. Rizzo V, Sung A, Schnitzer J: Rapid mechanotransduction in situ at the luminal cell surface of vascular endothelium and its caveolae. *J Biol Chem* 273:26323–26329, 1998.
69. Segal SS, Brett SE, Sessa WC: Codistribution of NOS and caveolin throughout peripheral vasculature and skeletal muscle of hamsters. *Am J Physiol* 277:H1167–H1177, 1999.
70. Mombouli JV, Vanhoutte PM: Endothelial dysfunction: From physiology to therapy. *J Mol Cell Cardiol* 31:61–74, 1999.
71. Feletou M, Vanhoutte PM: The third pathway: Endothelium-dependent hyperpolarization. *J Physiol Pharmacol* 50:525–534, 1999.
72. Bakker EN, van der Linden PJ, Sipkema P: Endothelin-1 induced constriction inhibits nitric-oxide mediated dilation in isolated rat resistance arteries. *J Vasc Res* 34:418–424, 1997.
73. Hergenroder S, Munter K, Kirchengast M: Effects of endothelin and endothelin receptor antagonism on arteriolar and venular microcirculation. *Vasa* 27:216–219, 1998.
74. Segal SS: Dynamics of microvascular control in skeletal muscle, in Saltin B, Boushel R, Secher N, Mitchell JH (eds): *Exercise and Circulation in Health and Disease*. Champaign, IL: Human Kinetics, 2000; pp 141–153.
75. Gustafsson F, Holstein-Rathlou N-H: Conducted vasomotor responses in arterioles: Characteristics, mechanisms and physiological significance. *Acta Physiol Scand* 167:11–21, 1999.
76. Sarelius IH, Cohen KD, Murrant CL: Role for capillaries in coupling blood flow with metabolism. *Clin Exp Pharmacol Physiol* 27:826–829, 2000.
77. Murrant CL, Sarelius IH: Local and remote arteriolar dilations initiated by skeletal muscle contraction. *Am J Physiol* 279:H2285–H2294, 2000.
78. Laughlin MH, Schrage WG: Effects of muscle contraction on skeletal muscle blood flow: When is there a muscle pump? *Med Sci Sports Exerc* 31:1027–1035, 1999.
79. Joyner MJ, Halliwil JR: Neurogenic vasodilation in human skeletal muscle: Possible role in contraction-induced hyperaemia. *Acta Physiol Scand* 168:481–488, 2000.
80. Welsh DG, Segal SS: Endothelial and smooth muscle cell conduction in arterioles controlling muscle blood flow. *Am J Physiol* 274:H178–H186, 1998.
81. Dietz NM, Engelke KA, Samuel TT, et al: Evidence for nitric oxide-mediated sympathetic forearm vasodilatation in humans. *J Physiol (Lond)* 498:531–540, 1997.
82. Radegran G, Hellsten Y: Adenosine and nitric oxide in exercise-induced human skeletal muscle vasodilatation. *Acta Physiol Scand* 168:575–593, 2000.
83. Shoemaker JK, Naylor HL, Prozeg ZI, Hughson RL: Failure of prostaglandins to modulate the time course of blood flow during dynamic forearm exercise in humans. *J Appl Physiol* 81:1516–1521, 1998.
84. Frandsen U, Bangsbo J, Langberg H, et al: Inhibition of nitric oxide synthesis by systemic N(G)-monomethyl-L-arginine administration in humans: Effects on interstitial adenosine, prostacyclin and potassium concentration in resting and contracting skeletal muscle. *J Vasc Res* 37:297–302, 2000.
85. Thomas GD, Victor RG: Nitric oxide mediates contraction-induced attenuation of sympathetic vasoconstriction in rat skeletal muscle. *J Physiol (Lond)* 506:817–826, 1997.
86. McGillivray-Anderson KM, Faber JE: Effect of acidosis on contraction of microvascular smooth muscle by alpha 1- and alpha 2-adrenoceptors: Implications for neural and metabolic regulation. *Circ Res* 66:1643–1657, 1990.
87. Hansen J, Sayad D, Thomas GD, et al: Exercise induced attenuation of alpha-adrenoceptor mediated vasoconstriction in humans. *Cardiovasc Res* 41:220–228, 1999.
88. Branten AJ, Smits P, Jansen TL, et al: Effect of atrial natriuretic factor on skin microcirculation versus skeletal muscle blood flow. *J Cardiovasc Pharmacol* 27:303–306, 1996.
89. Renaudin C, Michoud E, Rapin JR, et al: Hyperglycaemia modifies the reaction of microvessels to insulin in rat skeletal muscle. *Diabetologia* 41:26–33, 1968.
90. Iwashita S, Yanagi K, Ohshima N, Suzuki M: Insulin increases blood flow rate in microvasculature of cremaster muscle of the anesthetized rats. *In Vivo* 15:11–15, 1997.
91. Hudlicka O: The response of muscle to enhanced and reduced activity. *Baillière's Clin Endocrinol Metab* 4:417–439, 1990.
92. Laughlin MH, Armstrong RB: Muscle blood flow during locomotory exercise. *Exerc Sport Sci Rev* 13:95–136, 1985.
93. Gute D, Laughlin MH, Amann JF: Regional changes in capillary supply of interval-sprint and low-intensity endurance trained rats. *Microcirculation* 1:183–193, 1994.
94. Sexton WL, Korthuis RJ, Laughlin MH: High intensity exercise training increases vascular transport capacity in rat hindquarters. *Am J Physiol* 254:H274–H278, 1988.
95. Green H, Goreham C, Ouyang J, et al: Regulation of fiber size, oxidative potential and capillarization in human muscle by resistance exercise. *Am J Physiol* 276:R591–R596, 1999.
96. Ljungqvist A, Unge G: Capillary proliferation activity in myocardium and skeletal muscle of exercised rats. *J Appl Physiol* 43:306–307, 1977.
97. Appell H-J: Morphological studies on skeletal muscle capillaries under conditions of high altitude training. *Int J Sports Med* 1:37–41, 1980.
98. Lash JM, Bohlen VHG: Time and order dependent changes in functional and NO-mediated dilation during exercise training. *J Appl Physiol* 82:460–468, 1997.
99. Lash JM, Bohlen HG: Functional adaptations of rat skeletal muscle arterioles to aerobic exercise training. *J Appl Physiol* 72:2052–2062, 1992.
100. Snell PG, Martin WH, Buckey JC, Blomqviust CG: Maximal vascular leg conductance in trained and untrained men. *J Appl Physiol* 62:606–610, 1987.
101. Dinenno FA, Tanaka H, Monahan KD, et al: Regular endurance exercise induces expansive arterial remodelling in the trained muscle limbs of healthy men. *J Physiol (Lond)* 534:287–295, 2001.
102. Roberts CK, Barnard RJ, Jasman A, Balon TW: Acute exercise increases nitric oxide synthase activity in skeletal muscle. *Am J Physiol* 277:E390–E394, 1999.
103. Woodman CR, Muller JM, Laughlin MH, Price EM: Induction of nitric oxide synthase mRNA in coronary resistance arteries isolated from exercise-trained pigs. *Am J Physiol* 273:H2575–H2579, 1997.
104. Brown MD, Cotter MA, Hudlicka O, Vrbova G: The effect of different patterns of muscle activity on capillary density, mechanical properties and structure of slow and fast rabbit muscles. *Pflügers Archiv* 361:241–250, 1976.
105. Hansen-Smith FM, Hudlicka O, Egginton S: In vivo angiogenesis in adult rat skeletal muscle: Early changes in capillary network architecture and ultrastructure. *Cell Tissue Res* 286:123–136, 1996.
106. Milkiewicz M, Brown MD, Egginton S, Hudlicka O: Shear modulation of angiogenesis and VEGF in skeletal muscles in vivo. *Microcirculation* 8:229–241, 2001.
107. Hansen-Smith FM, Egginton S, Hudlicka O: Growth of arterioles in chronically stimulated adult skeletal muscle. *Microcirculation* 5:49–59, 1998.
108. Dawson JM, Hudlicka O: The effect of long-term activity on the microvasculature of rat glycolytic skeletal muscle. *Int J Microcirc Clin Exp* 8:53–69, 1989.
109. Gustafsson T, Kraus WE: Exercise-induced angiogenesis-related growth and transcription factors in skeletal muscle and their modification by muscle pathology. *Frontiers Biosci* 6:D75–D89, 2001.
110. Skorjanc D, Jaschinski F, Heine G, Pette D: Sequential increases in capillarization and mitochondrial enzymes in low-frequency-stimulated rabbit muscle. *Am J Physiol* 274:C810–C818, 1998.
111. Brown MD, Hudlicka O, Makki RF, Weiss JB: Low-molecular-mass endothelial cell-stimulating angiogenic factor in relation to capillary growth induced in rat skeletal muscle by low-frequency electrical stimulation. *Int J Microcirc Clin Exp* 15:111–116, 1995.
112. Egginton S, Hudlicka O, Brown MD, et al: Capillary proliferation in overloaded rat skeletal muscle: Correlation with blood flow and performance. *J Appl Physiol* 85:2025–2032, 1998.
113. Resnick N, Gimbrone MA Jr: Hemodynamic forces are complex regulators of endothelial gene expression. *FASEB J* 9:874–882, 1995.
114. Chien S, Li S, Shyy YJ: Effects of mechanical forces on signal transduction and gene expression in endothelial cells. *Hypertension* 31:162–169, 1998.
115. Hudlicka O: Is physiological angiogenesis in skeletal muscle regulated by changes in microcirculation? *Microcirculation* 5:7–23, 1998.
116. Hudlicka O, Brown MD, Egginton S: The role of hemodynamic and mechanical factors in vascular growth and remodeling, in Lelkes PI (ed): *Mechanical Forces and the Endothelium*. Amsterdam, The Netherlands: Harwood Academic Publishers, 1999; pp 291–359.
117. Egginton S, Zhou A-L, Brown MD, Hudlicka O: Unorthodox angiogenesis. *Cardiovasc Res* 49:634–646, 2001.
118. Snyder GK, Coelho JR: Microvascular development in chick anterior latissimus dorsi following hypertrophy. *J Anat* 162:215–224, 1989.
119. Hansen-Smith F, Egginton S, Zhou A-L, Hudlicka O: Growth of arterioles precedes that of capillaries in stretch-induced angiogenesis in skeletal muscle. *Microvasc Res* 62:1–14, 2001.
120. Zhou A-L, Egginton S, Brown MD, Hudlicka O: Capillary growth in overloaded hypertrophic adult rat muscles. *Anat Rec* 252:49–63, 1998.
121. Ellis CG, Mathieu-Costello M, Potter RF, et al: Effect of sarcomere length on total capillary length in skeletal muscle: In vivo evidence for longitudinal stretching of capillaries. *Microvasc Res* 40:63–72, 1990.
122. Rivilis I, Milkiewicz M, Boyd P, Goldstein J, et al: Differential involvement of MMP-2 and VEGF during muscle stretch- versus shear-induced angiogenesis. *Am J Physiol* 283:H1430–H1438, 2002.
123. McKoy G, Ashley W, Mander J, et al: Expression of insulin growth factor-1 splice variants and structural genes in rabbit skeletal muscle induced by stretch and stimulation. *J Physiol (Lond)* 516:83–92, 1999.
124. Smith LE, Shen W, Perruzzi C, et al: Regulation of vascular endothelial growth factor-dependent retinal neovascularization by insulin-like growth factor-1 receptor. *Nat Med* 5:1390–1395, 1999.
125. Hernandez N, Torres SH, Rivas M: Inactivity changes fiber proportion and capillary supply in cat muscle. *Comp Biochem Physiol A* 117:2111–2117, 1997.
126. Desplanches D, Kayar SR, Sempore B, et al: Rat soleus muscle ultrastructure after limb suspension. *J Appl Physiol* 69:504–508, 1990.

127. Tyml K, Mathieu-Costello O: Structural and functional changes in the microvasculature of disused skeletal muscle. *Frontiers Biosci* 6:d45–d52, 2001.
128. Hather BM, Adams GR, Tesch PA, Dudley GA: Skeletal muscle responses to lower limb suspension in humans. *J Appl Physiol* 72:1493–1498, 1992.
129. Roy RR, Baldwin KM, Edgerton VR: Response of the neuromuscular unit to spaceflight: What has been learned from the rat model. *Exer Sports Sci Rev* 24:399–425, 1996.
130. Poole DC, Mathieu-Costello O: Skeletal muscle capillary geometry: Adaptation to chronic hypoxia. *Respir Physiol* 77:21–29, 1989.
131. Fisher AJ, Schrader NW, Klitzman B: Effects of chronic hypoxia on capillary flow and hematocrit in rat skeletal muscle. *Am J Physiol* 262: H1877–H1883, 1992.
132. Price RJ, Skalak TC: Arteriolar remodeling in skeletal muscles of rats exposed to chronic hypoxia. *J Vasc Res* 35:238–244, 1998.
133. Deveci D, Marshall JM, Egginton S: Relationship between capillary angiogenesis, fiber type and fiber size in chronic systemic hypoxia. *Am J Physiol* 281:H241–H252, 2001.
134. Holmang A, Jennische E, Bjorntorp P: Rapid formation of capillary endothelial cells in skeletal muscle after exposure to insulin. *Diabetologia* 39:206–211, 1996.
135. Greene AS: Life and death in the microcirculation: A role of angiotensin II. *Microcirculation* 5:101–107, 1998.
136. Le Noble FAC, Kessels van Nylick LCGA, Hacking WJG, et al: The role of angiotensin II and prostaglandins in arcade formation in a developing microvascular network. *J Vasc Res* 33:480–488, 1996.
137. Egginton S: Effects of anabolic hormones on aerobic capacity of rat striated muscle. *Pflügers Arch* 410:356–361, 1987.
138. McAllister RM, Ogilvie RW, Terjung RL: Functional and metabolic consequences of skeletal muscle remodeling in hypothyroidism. *Am J Physiol* 260:E272–E279, 1991.
139. Borisov AB, Huang SK, Carlson BM: Remodeling of the vascular bed and progressive loss of capillaries in denervated skeletal muscle. *Anat Rec* 258:292–304, 2000.
140. Ziada AMAR, Hudlicka O, Tyler KR: The effect of long-term administration of α_1-blocker prazosin on capillary density in cardiac and skeletal muscle. *Pflügers Arch* 415:355–360, 1989.
141. Bradley WG, O'Brien MD, Walder DN, et al: Failure to confirm a vascular cause of muscular dystrophy. *Arch Neurol* 32:466–473, 1975.
142. Leinonen H, Juntunen J, Somer H, Rapola J: Capillary circulation and morphology in Duchenne muscular dystrophy. *Eur Neurol* 18:249–255, 1979.
142a. Burch TG, Prewitt RL, Law PK: In vivo morphometric analysis of muscle microcirculation in dystrophic mice. *Muscle Nerve* 4:420–424, 1981.
143. Jerusalem F, Engel AG, Gomez MR: Duchenne dystrophy: I. Morphometric study of muscle microvasculature. *Brain* 97:115–122, 1974.
144. Atherton GW, Cabric M, James NT: Stereological analysis of capillaries in muscles of dystrophic mice. *Virchows Arch A Pathol Anat Hist* 397:347–352, 1982.
145. Koehler J: Blood vessel structure in Duchenne muscular dystrophy. *Neurology* 27:861–868, 1977.
146. Miike T, Sugino S, Ohtani Y, et al: Vascular endothelial cell injury and platelet embolism in Duchenne muscular dystrophy at the preclinical stage. *J Neurol Sci* 82:67–80, 1987.
147. Jerusalem F, Rakusa M, Engel AG, MacDonald RD: Morphometric analysis of skeletal muscle capillary ultrastructure in inflammatory myopathies. *Neurol Sci* 23:392–402, 1974.
148. Casademont J, Grau JM, Estruch R, et al: Relationship between capillary and muscle damage in dermatomyositis. *Int J Dermatol* 29:117–120, 1990.
149. Banker BQ: Dermatomyositis of childhood, ultrastructural alterations of muscle and intramuscular vessels. *J Neuropathol Exp Neurol* 34:46–75, 1975.
150. Emslie-Smith AM, Engel AG: Microvascular changes in early and advanced dermatomyositis: A quantitative study. *Ann Neurol* 27:343–356, 1990.
151. Estruch R, Grau JM, Fernandez-Sola J, et al: Microvascular changes in skeletal muscle in idiopathic inflammatory myopathy. *Hum Pathol* 23:888–895, 1992.
152. Vlodavsky EA, Ludatscher RM, Sabo E, Kerner H: Evaluation of muscle capillary basement membrane in inflammatory myopathy: A morphometric ultrastructural study. *Virchows Arch* 435:58–61, 1999.
153. Emslie-Smith AM, Engel AG: Necrotizing myopathy with pipestem capillaries, microvascular deposition of the complement membrane attack complex (MAC) and minimal cellular infiltration. *Neurology* 41:936–939, 1991.
154. Scelsi R: Morphometric analysis of skeletal muscle fibers and capillaries in mitochondrial myopathies. *Pathol Res Pract* 188:607–611, 1992.
155. Brooke MH, Kaplan H: Muscle pathology in rheumatoid arthritis, polymyalgia rheumatica and polymyositis. *Arch Pathol Lab Med* 94:101–118, 1972.
156. Bosman J, Tangelder GJ, oude Egbrink MG, et al: Capillary diameter changes during low perfusion pressure and reactive hyperemia in rabbit skeletal muscle. *Am J Physiol* 269:H1048–H1055, 1995.
157. Lee J, Schmid-Schoenbein GW: Biomechanics of skeletal muscle capillaries: Hemodynamic resistance, endothelial distensibility and pseudopod formation. *Ann Biomed Eng* 23:226–246, 1995.
158. Mazzoni MC, Borgstrom P, Warnke KC, et al: Mechanism and implications of capillary endothelial swelling and luminal narrowing in low flow ischemias. *Int J Microcirc Clin Exp* 15:265–270, 1995.
159. Deindl E, Schaper W: Collateral and capillary formation—A comparison, in Dormandy JA, Dole WP, Rubanyi GM (eds): *Therapeutic Angiogenesis*. Berlin, Heidelberg: Springer-Verlag, 1999; pp 67–86.
160. Kelsall CJ, Brown MD, Hudlicka O: Alterations of small arterioles in rat skeletal muscles as a result of chronic ischaemia. *J Vasc Res* 38:212–218, 2001.
161. Strock PE, Majno G: Microvascular changes in acutely ischemic rat muscle. *Surg Gynecol Obstet* 129:1215–1224, 1969.
162. Egginton S, Hudlicka O, Glover M: Fine structure of capillaries in ischaemic and nonischaemic rat striated muscle: Effect of torbafylline. *Int J Microcirc Clin Exp* 12:33–44, 1993.
163. Gidlof A, Lewis DH, Hammersen F: The effect of prolonged total ischemia on the ultrastructure of human skeletal muscle capillaries. *Int J Microcirc Clin Exp* 7:67–86, 1988.
164. Thomson IA, Egginton S, Simms MH, Hudlicka O: Effect of muscle ischaemia and iloprost during femorodistal reconstruction on capillary endothelial swelling. *Int J Microcirc Clin Exp* 16:284–290, 1996.
165. Burns RR, Palade GE: Studies on blood capillaries: I. General organization of blood capillaries in muscle. *J Cell Biol* 37:244–276, 1968.
166. Gute DC, Ishida T, Yarimizu K, Korthuis RJ: Inflammatory responses to ischemia and reperfusion in skeletal muscle. *Moll Cell Biochem* 179:169–187, 1998.
167. Granger DN: Ischemia-reperfusion: Mechanisms of microvascular dysfunction and the influence of risk factors for cardiovascular disease. *Microcirculation* 6:167–178, 1999.
168. Carden DL, Granger DN: Pathophysiology of ischemia-reperfusion injury. *J Pathol* 190:255–266, 2000.
169. Korthuis RJ, Gute DC: Postischemic leukocyte/endothelial cell interaction and microvascular barrier dysfunction in skeletal muscle. *Int J Microcirc Clin Exp* 17(Suppl 1):11–17, 1997.
170. Brevetti G, Corrado S, Martone VD, et al: Microcirculation and tissue metabolism in peripheral arterial disease. *Clin Rheol Microcirc* 21:245–254, 1999.
171. Roberts KC, Nixon C, Unthank JL, Lash JM: Femoral artery ligation stimulates capillary growth and limits training-induced increases in oxidative capacity in rats. *Microcirculation* 4:253–260, 1997.
172. Suzuki J, Kobayashi T, Uruma T, Koyama T: Strength training with partial ischemia stimulates microvascular remodeling in rat calf muscles. *Eur J Appl Physiol* 82:215–222, 2000.
173. Hudlicka O, Brown MD, Egginton S, Dawson JM: Effect of long-term electrical stimulation on vascular supply and fatigue in chronically ischemic muscles. *J Appl Physiol* 77:1317–1324, 1994.
174. Warhol MJ, Siegel AJ, Evans WJ, Silverman LM: Skeletal muscle injury and repair in marathon runners after competition. *Am J Pathol* 118:331–339, 1985.
175. Hoppeler H, Hudlicka O, Uhlmann E, Claasen H: Structural adaptations to ischaemic and severe exercise in rat fast muscle. *J Clin Sports Med* 2:43–51, 1992.
176. Hickey NC, Hudlicka O, Gosling P, et al: Intermittent claudication incites systemic neutrophil activation and increased vascular permeability. *Br J Surg* 80:181–184, 1993.
177. Hickey NC, Hudlicka O, Simms MH: Claudication induces systemic capillary endothelial swelling. *Eur J Vasc Surg* 6:36–40, 1992.
178. Hickey NC, Shearman CP, Gosling P, Simms MH: Assessment of intermittent claudication by quantitation of exercise-induced microalbuminuria. *Eur J Vasc Surg* 4:603–606, 1990.
179. Korthuis RJ, Gute DC: Adhesion molecule expression in postischemic microvascular dysfunction. *J Vasc Res* 36(Suppl 1):15-23, 1999.
180. De Bleecker JL, Engel AG: Expression of cell adhesion molecules in inflammatory myopathies and Duchenne dystrophy. *J Neuropathol Exp Neurol* 53:369–376, 1994.
181. Frisbee JC, Lombard JH: Acute elevations in salt intake and reduced renal mass hypertension compromises arteriolar dilation in cremaster muscle. *Microvasc Res* 57:273–283, 1999.
182. Wang DH, Prewitt RL: Captopril reduces aortic and microvascular growth in hypertensive and normotensive rats. *Hypertension* 15:68–77, 1990.
183. Scheidegger KJ, Wood JM, Van Essen H, et al: Effect of prolonged blockade of the renin angiotensin system on striated muscle microcirculation of spontaneously hypertensive rats. *J Pharmacol Exp Ther* 278:1276–1281, 1996.
184. Dusseau JW, Hutchins DM: Stimulation of arteriolar number by salbutamol in spontaneously hypertensive rats. *Am J Physiol* 236:H134–H140, 1979.
185. Amaral SL, Zorn TM, Michelini LC: Exercise training normalizes wall-lumen ratio of the gracilis muscle arterioles and reduces pressure in spontaneously hypertensive rats. *J Hypertens* 18:1563–1572, 2001.
186. Skyrme-Jones RA, Berry KL, O'Brien RC, Meredith IT: Basal and exercise-induced skeletal muscle blood flow is augmented in type I diabetes mellitus. *Clin Sci* 98:111–120, 2000.

187. Leinonen H, Matikainen E, Juntunen J: Permeability and morphology of skeletal muscle capillaries in type 1 (insulin-dependent) diabetes mellitus. *Diabetologia* 22:158–162, 1982.
188. Marin P, Andersson B, Krotkiewski M, Bjorntorp P: Muscle fiber composition and capillary density in women and men with NIDDM. *Diabetes Care* 17:382–386, 1994.
189. Cotter MA, Cameron NE: Metabolic, neural and vascular influences on muscle function in experimental models of diabetes mellitus and related pathological states. *Basic Appl Myol* 4:293–307, 1994.
190. Kindig CA, Sexton WL, Fedde MR, Poole DC: Skeletal muscle microcirculatory structure and hemodynamics in diabetes. *Respir Physiol* 111:163–176, 1998.
191. Friedenwald JS: Diabetic retinopathy. *Am J Ophthalmol* 33:1187–1199, 1950.
192. Tilton RG, Faller AM, Burkhardt JK, et al: Pericyte degeneration and acellular capillaries are increased in the feet of human diabetic patients. *Diabetologia* 28:895–900, 1985.
193. Wallenberg-Henriksson H, Gunnarsson R, Henriksson J, et al: Influence of physical training on formation of muscle capillaries in type I diabetes. *Diabetes* 33:851–857, 1984.
194. Cameron NE, Cotter MS, Robertson S: Essential fatty acid diet supplementation—effect on peripheral nerve and skeletal muscle function and capillarization in streptozotocin-induced diabetic rats. *Diabetes* 40:532–539, 1991.
195. Cameron NE, Cotter MA, Robertson S: Angiotensin converting enzyme inhibition prevents development of muscle and nerve dysfunction and stimulates angiogenesis in streptozotocin-diabetic rats. *Diabetologia* 35:12–18, 1992.
196. Drexler H, Coats AJS: Explaining fatigue in congestive heart failure. *Annu Rev Med* 47:241–256, 1996.
197. Didion SP, Mayhan WG: Effect of chronic myocardial infarction on in vivo reactivity of skeletal muscle arterioles. *Am J Physiol* 272:H2403–H2408, 1997.
198. Thomas DP, Hudlicka O, Brown MD, Deveci D: Alterations in small arterioles precede structural and functional changes in limb skeletal muscle following myocardial infarction. *Am J Physiol* 275:H1032–H1039, 1998.
199. Kindig CA, Musch TI, Basaraba RJ, Poole DC: Impaired capillary hemodynamics in skeletal muscle of rats in chronic heart failure. *J Appl Physiol* 87:652–660, 1999.
200. Duscha BD, Kraus WE, Keteyian SJ, et al: Capillary density in skeletal muscle: A contributing mechanism of exercise intolerance in class II–III chronic heart failure independent of other peripheral alterations. *J Am Coll Cardiol* 33:1956–1963, 1999.
201. Hambrecht R, Hilbrich L, Erbs S, et al: Correlation of endothelial dysfunction in chronic heart failure: Additional effects of exercise training and oral L-arginine supplementation. *J Am Coll Cardiol* 35:706–713, 2000.
202. Thomas DP, Hudlicka O: Arteriolar reactivity and capillarization in chronically stimulated rat limb skeletal muscle post-MI. *J Appl Physiol* 87:2259–2265, 1999.
203. Testa M, Ennezat PV, Vikstrom KL, et al: Modulation of vascular endothelial gene expression by physical training in patients with chronic heart failure. *Italian Heart J* 1:426–430, 2000.
204. Baumgartner I, Isner JM: Somatic gene therapy in the cardiovascular system. *Annu Rev Physiol* 63:427–450, 2001.

Chapter 23
Protein and Amino Acid Metabolism in Muscle

R. THOMAS JAGOE
NICHOLAS E. TAWA, JR.
ALFRED L. GOLDBERG

Overview
    PROTEIN METABOLISM IN MUSCLE
    METHODS FOR THE STUDY OF PROTEIN METABOLISM IN MUSCLE
    AMINO ACID METABOLISM IN MUSCLE

Amino Acid Metabolism In Muscle
    OXIDATION OF BRANCHED-CHAIN AMINO ACIDS
    CONTRIBUTION OF AMINO ACIDS TO MUSCLE ENERGY
        METABOLISM
    ALANINE PRODUCTION AND RELEASE FROM MUSCLE
    GLUTAMINE PRODUCTION AND RELEASE FROM MUSCLE

Protein Metabolism in Muscle
    PROTEOLYTIC PATHWAYS IN MUSCLE
    REGULATION OF MUSCLE PROTEIN TURNOVER AND GROWTH
        BY NUTRIENTS AND HORMONES
    NUTRITIONAL FACTORS AFFECTING PROTEIN BALANCE IN MUSCLE
    MUSCLE ACTIVITY AND THE CONTROL OF PROTEIN METABOLISM
    CYTOKINES AND THE REGULATION OF PROTEIN METABOLISM
        IN MUSCLE

A General Program for Muscle Atrophy

Overview

PROTEIN METABOLISM IN MUSCLE

Physiologic Significance

The mechanisms of protein synthesis in mammalian cells and bacteria have been extensively investigated and are well understood.[1] Moreover, significant advances have recently occurred in elucidating the fundamental mechanisms of intracellular protein degradation as well as their importance and regulation. Prior to the introduction of isotopic tracers, proteins in mammalian cells were generally believed to be completely stable. The classic experiments by Schoenheimer and coworkers in the 1940s[2] with 15N-labeled amino acids demonstrated the dynamic state of body constituents and showed that cellular proteins are synthesized and degraded continuously. Subsequent work has directly confirmed that all cell proteins are subject to this continued replacement and that different proteins turn over at different rates, having characteristic half-lives that range from a few minutes to many days.[3] By contrast, mammalian cells are often very long-lived (typically with generation times of many days to years); in the case of muscle, the fibers generally last the lifetime of the organism.

There are many reasons for wanting to understand the factors that regulate protein breakdown in skeletal muscle. Rates of proteolysis are an important factor determining the levels of specific muscle proteins. For example, in myasthenia gravis, surface receptors for acetylcholine are broken down very rapidly, and this degradative process contributes to the deficiency of receptors and the failure of neuromuscular transmission.[4] In addition, the overall balance between rates of protein synthesis and degradation determines whether a muscle undergoes normal growth, atrophy, or work-induced hypertrophy.[5] Protein balance in muscle is also important in overall energy homeostasis of the organism, since muscle contains most of the body's protein reserves.[6,7] Net mobilization of muscle protein can provide amino acids for metabolism by other tissues, while net uptake of amino acids by muscle and their incorporation into protein is a form of energy storage. Early in fasting, for example, the mobilization of amino acids stored in muscle protein helps provide the organism with essential precursors for hepatic gluconeogenesis and direct oxidation for energy. Therefore protein breakdown and synthesis in skeletal muscle are subject to precise regulation by a variety of hormones and cytokines as well as contractile activity. Many of the factors that control muscle protein turnover have been identified; this chapter summarizes our knowledge in this area.

Pathways for Protein Degradation

Several pathways for intracellular proteolysis are active in muscle, and each pathway utilizes a unique complement of proteases. These include acid-dependent proteases in lyssomes, calcium-dependent calpains, caspases, and the adenosine triphosphate (ATP)*–ubiquitin-proteasome (Ub-proteasome) pathway (see below).[8] In addition, within mitochondria, there exists an additional ATP-dependent pathway for breakdown of organelle proteins.[9] It is now well established that the proteasome is responsible for the majority of protein degradation in mammalian cells, including skeletal muscle.[9–14] The other soluble pathways may have a variety of specific roles (e.g., caspases in apoptosis) and the importance of the lysosomal pathway varies depending on the cell type, growth rate, and nutritional conditions. For instance, basal proteolysis in rapidly dividing fibroblasts and myoblasts seems primarily to occur by the Ub-proteasome pathway[15]; but if these cells are deprived of serum or insulin, the lysosomal pathway is activated. In contrast, the lysosomal pathway is responsible for a large fraction of proteolysis in the perfused liver, especially in nutrient-deficient states.[16]

METHODS FOR THE STUDY OF PROTEIN METABOLISM IN MUSCLE

In Vivo Methods

A major factor limiting progress in the study of protein metabolism in muscle has been technical problems involving the measurement of degradative rates. A variety of in vivo methods have been used, and all are subject to a number of potential artifacts.[17–19] For example, in early studies, rates of degradation of specific proteins or average rates of protein

---
*A list of abbreviations used in this chapter is given at the end of the chapter.

degradation were estimated from the loss of radioactivity in prelabeled muscle protein. However, such measurements can give artificially low rates of proteolysis because the labeled amino acids released by protein breakdown tend to be reutilized in protein synthesis. Alternatively, overall rates of protein degradation have been estimated by comparing the net gain in muscle protein occurring over several days with the rate of protein synthesis measured during short periods of amino acid infusion. From such data, rates of protein degradation can be calculated, but the values found by this indirect approach are imprecise and necessarily are based on many weak assumptions (e.g., linearity of growth rates). In particular, the validity of using this method seems especially questionable for short-term adaptations or in rapidly progressing diseases, as these processes are not steady states. In addition, urinary urea or total nitrogen excretion is often regarded as an index of muscle protein breakdown, but these measurements actually represent processes of amino acid catabolism and will be influenced by amino acids released from nonmuscle tissues and from the diet.

More recently some investigators have tried to study muscle tissue alone, using selective cannulation techniques in combination with infusions of labeled amino acids or other approaches. In one study protein degradation rates were measured in thigh muscles during exercise by measuring the production of amino acids released, but not metabolized in muscle.[20] Such approaches require accurate measurement of blood flow and become less reliable when flow rates are high and arteriovenous difference is reduced. Though these approaches have yielded valuable insights into aspects of protein metabolism specific to muscle, they are usually subject to the same criticisms noted above. In addition, it is also assumed that the contribution due to protein degradation of other tissues in the limb being studied and associated extracellular proteins is trivial.

One useful method for estimating rates of degradation of certain muscle proteins in vivo is the measurement of urinary N-methylhistidine excretion. This approach has proven valuable in studying muscle protein catabolism in human patients as well as in laboratory animals.[21] This amino acid is found almost exclusively in all types of actin but also in myosin of pale muscles.[22] It is formed by a posttranslational modification of certain histidine residues in these proteins. When generated by proteolysis, it cannot be reincorporated into protein or significantly metabolized; therefore its release in urine must reflect breakdown of these contractile proteins. However, actin and myosin also exist in other tissues; skin, gastrointestinal tract, and possibly other organs besides muscle may contribute significantly to urinary N-methylhistidine excretion.[23] Furthermore, protein and cell turnover in nonmuscle tissues can exceed that in muscle; in addition, these tissues can comprise different proportions of body weight in disease states. Finally, data on N-methylhistidine excretion are influenced by muscle protein mass and are interpretable only if renal function is not impaired and dietary intake of meat is avoided. Thus, in practice, these approaches have proved difficult and have generated some controversy.

In Vitro Methods

In analyzing rates of protein degradation under carefully controlled conditions, simple in vitro techniques offer many advantages.[24] These approaches employ certain thin rodent muscles that can be maintained for many hours in a good physiologic state (e.g., the diaphragm, red soleus, pale extensor digitorum longus, epitrochlearis muscles, and atrial strips). Similar techniques have been applied for measuring rates of protein synthesis and degradation in human muscle biopsies.[25] After correcting for the specific activity of intracellular amino acid pools, rates of protein synthesis are generally determined by measuring rates of incorporation of [^{14}C]-tyrosine or phenylalanine into muscle protein. Rates of protein degradation are measured by following the net release of tyrosine or phenylalanine from cell proteins.[26] Tyrosine is especially useful because it is easily measured fluorometrically and because this amino acid is neither synthesized nor catabolized by muscle. Consequently its production by isolated muscles must reflect net protein breakdown. Absolute rates of protein degradation can be determined by measuring net tyrosine release in the presence of an inhibitor of protein synthesis, such as cycloheximide. Alternatively, absolute rates of protein catabolism can be calculated from simultaneous measurements of net protein balance and rates of protein synthesis.

Similar methods have been used in perfused hearts and hindlimbs (although in the latter experiments, amino acids released from nonmuscle tissues—e.g., skin and adipose tissue—may contribute to the amino acid production and complicate measurements of protein breakdown or amino acid metabolism). Generally, isolated muscle preparations are in a highly catabolic state, in which the overall rate of protein degradation exceeds that of protein synthesis.[27] This property can be advantageous for studying the effects of endocrine factors or pharmacologic agents that suppress proteolysis. Incubating muscles in the presence of glucose, insulin, and amino acids, especially the branched-chain residues,[26] lowers the overall rates of protein degradation and increases overall rates of protein synthesis. If the muscles are maintained near the resting length in situ, protein breakdown is further reduced by 25 to 45 percent.[28] By adding agents to the incubation medium that block a specific proteolytic pathway (for example, nontoxic inhibitors of lysosomal proteases), the contribution of a particular proteolytic process to overall proteolysis can be measured quantitatively as well (see "Protein Metabolism in Muscle," below). These types of analyses have also been adapted to measure proteolysis using homogenates of muscle tissue.[29]

The measurement of tyrosine release reflects the breakdown of all classes of proteins, but does not distinguish between the breakdown of myofibrillar proteins and nonmyofibrillar components. To evaluate the breakdown of myofibrillar proteins, which correspond to 60 to 70 percent of all proteins in skeletal muscle, the rates of release of N-methylhistidine can be measured in vitro.[30] The simultaneous measurements of tyrosine and N-methylhistidine release from the muscle can be particularly informative; in particular, some studies have suggested that the breakdown of myofibrillar and nonmyofibrillar proteins can be regulated independently.[31]

Unfortunately, the various approaches described above measure only the total breakdown of cell proteins over the time period of the study. The data obtained have provided valuable physiologic insights into the overall regulation of protein turnover, but they do not address questions about the fate of individual muscle proteins, which have a wide range of half-lives. Several methods exist for studying the degradation of shorter-lived proteins and for following the fate of individual proteins in muscle and other cells, but they are beyond the scope of this chapter. For example, cells in culture may be "pulse-labeled" during a short exposure to radioactive amino acids, followed by a "chase" of nonradioactive amino acids in a sufficient concentration to block reincorporation of the tracer.[32] By this means, rapidly degraded proteins may be identified, and when this method is combined with electrophoresis or immunoprecipitation, the breakdown of specific proteins can be studied.

AMINO ACID METABOLISM IN MUSCLE

Traditionally, the liver has been thought to be the major site in the body for the degradation and synthesis of amino acids. However, it is now firmly established that skeletal and cardiac muscle are very active in the catabolism of several amino acids—most notably leucine, isoleucine, and valine—and in the synthesis of others, specifically alanine and glutamine.[6,7,33] In fact, muscle appears to be the major site in the body for these processes. These processes are discussed extensively in this chapter because they are important for understanding not only muscle function but also overall energy homeostasis, protein balance, and nitrogen metabolism of the organism.

Amino Acid Metabolism in Muscle

OXIDATION OF BRANCHED-CHAIN AMINO ACIDS

Amino Acids Degraded in Muscle

The first indication that skeletal muscle might be an important site of amino acid catabolism came from the observations of Miller in the early 1960s[34] that [^{14}C]-leucine, isoleucine, and valine were degraded at similar rates by normal and hepatectomized animals. Subsequently Manchester[35] and Odessey and Goldberg[18] demonstrated that isolated rat diaphragms rapidly degrade these three amino acids as well as several nonessential amino acids, including alanine, glutamate, and aspartate. Isolated rat muscles, even those of rapidly growing animals, oxidize branched-chain amino acids at rates comparable to their rates of incorporation into muscle protein. By contrast, muscle does not degrade to any significant extent the carbon skeletons of other amino acids found in plasma—such as lysine, serine, proline, threonine, methionine, cysteine, phenylalanine, histidine, tyrosine, and tryptophan[18,35,36] which can, however, be metabolized by other tissues.

The rate of degradation of the branched-chain amino acids in muscle is greater than in the liver, where these metabolic pathways were first elucidated,[18,36] and given that muscle constitutes up to 40 percent of body mass, it is probably the major site for degradation of branched-chain amino acids. Unlike most ingested amino acids, the branched-chain amino acids are not efficiently extracted from the portal circulation by the liver and pass directly into the systemic circulation, to be taken up by peripheral tissues.[6,7] Though leucine is readily oxidized by muscle, it is also degraded by the kidney,[18] adipose tissue,[37] and brain.[38] The physiologic significance of branched-chain amino acid metabolism in these tissues is probably distinct from that in skeletal muscle. For example, in adipose tissue, leucine degradation serves an anabolic function by providing acetyl-CoA precursors for triglyceride synthesis,[37] while in muscle, leucine is oxidized to CO_2 to provide energy.

Regulation of Branched-Chain Amino Acid Oxidation

In certain catabolic states—including fasting, diabetes, and following traumatic injury—the rates of degradation of the branched-chain amino acids increase markedly in skeletal and cardiac muscle and in the kidney, under conditions when overall protein synthesis falls.[18,33,39,40] Food deprivation leads to a two- to fourfold increase in the capacity of muscle to oxidize leucine, isoleucine, and valine,[18,39] and this adaptation appears to provide an alternative source of energy in the fasting state. The refeeding of animals reduces the muscle's capacity to degrade these amino acids. Liver and brain show no such effects. By contrast, adipose tissue in the fed state rapidly degrades leucine and uses the acetyl groups for synthesis of fatty acids.[37] The capacity of adipose tissue to metabolize branched-chain amino acids falls dramatically in fasting,[41] when lipid synthesis ceases. It is interesting that when animals are fed a protein-deficient diet, leucine oxidation falls in both muscle and adipose tissue.[41,42] This response appears to be a mechanism for conserving essential amino acids.

In muscle, the oxidation of leucine, isoleucine, and valine occurs by an initial transamination to α-ketoacids in the cytosol. The transaminase reaction is reversible and the enzyme is present in large excess in muscle. The α-ketoacids are subsequently decarboxylated by α-ketoacid dehydrogenase, which is localized exclusively in the mitochondria.[43] Thus leucine is converted to isovaleryl-CoA, and this compound is eventually degraded to three acetyl-CoA moieties, which are then oxidized in the tricarboxylic acid cycle. Studies with cell-free extracts clearly indicate that the rate-limiting step in this pathway in muscle (but not in liver) is α-ketoacid decarboxylation.[43,44] As a result, when muscles are incubated or perfused with leucine, this tissue releases significant amounts of the α-ketoisocaproate into the medium. The α-ketoacid decarboxylation reaction is regulated in muscle by glucocorticoids and other stimuli. Thus adrenalectomized rats treated with dexamethasone and made acidotic had increased activity and mRNA levels for muscle branched-chain α-ketoacid dehydrogenase, but the same conditions induced the opposite effects in liver.[45]

The accelerated degradation of branched-chain amino acids in muscles of fasted rats results from stimulation of the α-ketoacid dehydrogenase,[46] with no change in the transaminase.[43] The biochemical mechanism leading to increased dehydrogenase activity in fasting has been elucidated. Normally ATP inhibits the mitochondrial ketoacid dehydrogenase by allowing its specific phosphorylation, which inactivates this enzyme in muscle.[43,47,48] In fasting or diabetes, phosphorylation is reduced, and this change leads to more rapid oxidation of branched-chain amino acids. In muscle[49,50] and adipose tissue,[51] α-ketoacids can autoactivate the dehydrogenase by inhibiting its phosphorylation. The increased blood and tissue levels of leucine and α-ketoacids in fasting may thus directly signal more rapid oxidation in muscle. These mechanisms appear to be important in determining the rate of utilization of amino acids for energy and may also influence rates of protein breakdown in this tissue.

CONTRIBUTION OF AMINO ACIDS TO MUSCLE ENERGY METABOLISM

Leucine as an Energy Source

Since leucine can serve as an alternative energy source for muscle during fasting, it can also reduce glucose utilization in this tissue. In muscles of fasted (but not those of fed) rats, leucine inhibits oxidation of glucose as well as pyruvate by 40 percent. Simultaneously, leucine promotes lactate release from the muscle but does not affect the uptake of glucose or the rate of glycolysis.[52] Studies with transamination inhibitors indicate that leucine degradation is necessary for this inhibition of pyruvate oxidation to occur. While it has long been known that utilization of fatty acids or ketone bodies can also inhibit glucose and pyruvate oxidation, the effects of leucine are demonstrable at much lower concentrations (0.1mM) and seem to involve distinct mechanisms.[53] Therefore, during fasting, when leucine rises in blood and muscle, its degradation in muscle increases and gluconeogenic precursor molecules (pyruvate) are preserved. It is noteworthy that the amount of ATP derived from leucine under these conditions exactly equals the amount of ATP lost by the decrease in glucose oxidation.[52]

It has proved surprisingly difficult to evaluate rigorously the amount of energy obtained from amino acid oxidation in muscle.[33] To determine the contribution of amino acids derived from protein breakdown to the energy requirement of skeletal muscle, the rate of acetyl group formation from leucine and from other amino acids, and the rate of total acetyl group oxidation in the tricarboxylic acid (TCA) cycle were compared.[54] This comparison indicated that for diaphragms of fasted rats incubated with glucose, the net breakdown of proteins provides only 5 percent of all the acetyl groups oxidized, of which leucine provides about 4 percent and the other amino acids accounted for 1 percent, as summarized in Fig. 23-1. Thus leucine appears to be the only amino acid that can provide significant energy for the tissue. When muscles from fasting rats were incubated with physiologic levels of leucine as well as glucose, this amino acid seemed to contribute as much as 20 percent of the energy needs of the muscle. Thus leucine may be an important alternative energy source for skeletal and cardiac muscle in starvation or diabetes, where the levels of the branched-chain amino acids increase and muscle's capacity to degrade them also rises.

Purine Nucleotide Cycle and Effects of Exercise

Amino acid metabolism is altered during exercise; this may occur to help supply the increased energy requirements during muscular contraction.[55,56] The changes include increased muscle protein degradation, increased uptake of branched-chain amino acids and leucine oxidation, and greater net degradation of some other amino acids.[20] NH_3 production is increased during exercise, and one source of NH_3 is the purine-nucleotide pathway described by Lowenstein and coworkers,[57,58] which is activated during exercise.[57] In the purine-nucleotide pathway, amino groups derived from amino acid degradation are transferred to oxaloacetate to form aspartate. Aspartate combines with inosine monophosphate (IMP) to yield adenylsuccinate, which is cleaved to yield fumarate and adenosine monophosphate (AMP). The fumarate can enter the TCA cycle, while the AMP is hydrolyzed by adenylate deaminase to yield free NH_3 and IMP. During muscular work, the NH_3 production occurs directly from AMP and, in accord with the proposed cycle, IMP and adenylosuccinate are also released from muscle. Activation

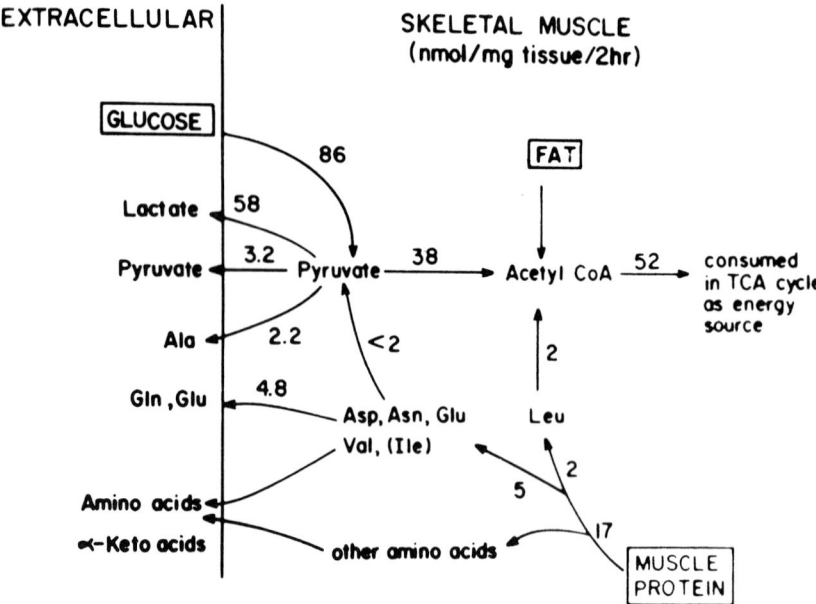

FIGURE 23-1. Utilization of glucose, endogenous fatty acids, and amino acids derived from protein breakdown for energy.[48,55] Values were measured in diaphragms from fasted rats incubated in the presence of glucose (5 mM). These data indicate the absolute fluxes through different pathways and are likely to vary under different conditions which influence net protein breakdown, glycolysis, and ATP demands.

of this cycle during exercise may be mediated by elevated adenosine diphosphate (ADP) levels, which can stimulate adenylate deaminase.

The purine nucleotide cycle may serve important regulatory and metabolic functions in muscle. For example, IMP is a potent stimulator of glycogen phophorylase, and both NH_3 and AMP are activators of phosphofructokinase; therefore the rise in these metabolites may be important in promoting glycogenolysis and glycolysis during exercise. Furthermore, removal of AMP during operation of the cycle will displace the adenylate kinase reaction toward the formation of adenosine triphosphate (ATP) and thus help maintain a high ATP/ADP ratio in the muscle despite rapid ATP hydrolysis. It had been proposed that the purine nucleotide cycle serves an important "anapleurotic" function, replenishing tricarboxylic acid cycle intermediates, the intracellular levels of which actually increase during exercise. However, a more recent study has failed to support this proposal, as those with AMP deaminase deficiency did not have altered exercise tolerance or levels of TCA intermediates.[59,60] The purine nucleotide cycle may also be a source of NH_3 used for glutamine synthesis in muscle as well (see below). In addition, utilization of aspartate by the purine nucleotide cycle may provide an additional energy for muscle contraction.

ALANINE PRODUCTION AND RELEASE FROM MUSCLE

The breakdown of branched-chain amino acids in muscle generates amino groups, whose accumulation in the organism could be toxic. Unlike liver, muscle lacks the enzymes necessary to dispose of ammonia as urea. The initial clue to the fate of these amino groups came from the studies of Cahill and colleagues,[61] who found that the amino acids released from muscle in the postabsorptive state or during starvation do not represent a simple hydrolysate of muscle protein.[6,7] Instead, alanine and glutamine are released in much greater amounts than would be expected simply by the net breakdown of muscle proteins. These two amino acids are synthesized in muscle de novo, using amino groups generated by degradation of branched-chain amino acids and aspartate.[6,33,54,62] In fact, in fasting or following injury, human and rat muscles release leucine, valine, isoleucine, and aspartate in much lower amounts than would be expected from their frequency in muscle protein. These findings reflect the rapid degradation of these residues in muscle.

Alanine production by muscle seems to play an important role in the maintenance of blood glucose, especially in the postabsorptive or fasted state. The liver is very active in extracting alanine from the blood, and alanine is the most important amino acid utilized for gluconeogenesis in the liver.[6,7,61] On this basis, Felig et al.[6,61] and Mallette et al.[63] originally proposed the existence of a "glucose-alanine cycle" in which alanine derived from amino acid metabolism in muscle is carried in the circulation to the liver for conversion into urea and glucose. The glucose synthesized by the liver can then be taken up again by muscle and be converted back to alanine. The flux of alanine between muscle and liver thus appears analogous to that of lactate in the Cori (glucose-lactate) cycle, but in addition alanine helps to ferry potentially toxic amino groups to the liver for disposal as urea. The excretion of urea is increased during exercise[64]; its production is even higher in glycogen-depleted subjects,[65] who also have higher rates of muscle protein degradation and alanine production.[20]

Studies in this laboratory[36,54,62] have established that the production of alanine and glutamine in muscle are coupled to the degradation of the branched-chain and certain other amino acids. Addition of any of the branched-chain amino acids to incubated muscles stimulates the formation of alanine and glutamine, and this effect is most pronounced in the muscle of fasted animals. In starvation, when the capacity of muscle to degrade branched-chain amino acids rises, alanine and glutamine production also increases. Conversely, in protein deficiency, when leucine oxidation in muscle falls, the synthesis of alanine and glutamine is reduced.[42] Thus the original proposal of the glucose-alanine cycle has been modified to incorporate the unique role of the branched-chain amino acids (Fig. 23-2). This cycle also recognizes that the liver tends to release branched-chain amino acids for peripheral use in catabolic states.[53]

A variety of studies by Chang and Goldberg[33,54,62] originally suggested that alanine and glutamine are synthesized in muscle by the pathways summarized in Fig. 23-3. Transamination of the branched-chain amino acids occurs almost exclusively with α-ketoglutarate to form glutamate, which may either donate its amino group to pyruvate to form alanine or incorporate free ammonia to form glutamine. The relative amounts of each amino acid produced depend largely on the concentration of ammonia within the tissue. Increased levels of NH_3 will promote glutamine production and decrease alanine synthesis. Free NH_3 in muscle may arise from extracellular sources or by degradation of purines and amino acids in the purine nucleotide cycle, as discussed above.

The branched-chain amino acids (and possibly glutamate and aspartate) thus appear to contribute only α-amino groups for the synthesis of alanine, while exogenous glucose or muscle glycogen provides the pyruvate.[62] In accord with this idea, exogenous glucose increases alanine production, inhibitors of glycolysis decrease it, and the stimulatory effect of glucose is additive with that of leucine. Since alanine is derived from preexistent glucose, this cycle does not allow the generation of new carbohydrate from muscle proteins, but the oxidation of leucine and the prevention of pyruvate degradation in muscle spares glucose in fasting. Other mod-

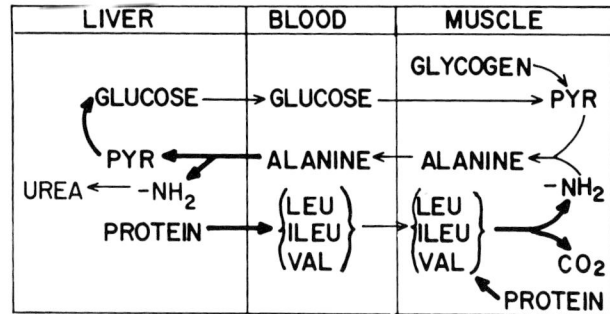

FIGURE 23-2. Relationship between the degradation of branched-chain amino acids and the glucose-alanine cycle. PYR–pyruvate.

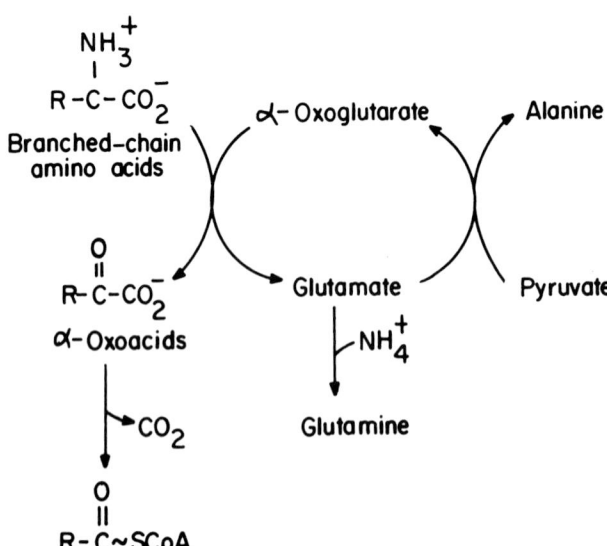

FIGURE 23-3. The linkage between branched-chain amino acid metabolism and the synthesis of alanine and glutamine. In accord with this reaction scheme, the branched chain amino acids stimulate alanine and glutamine production by increasing the transamination of α-ketoglutarate.

els have suggested that alanine is produced from the carbon skeletons of degraded amino acids in muscle.[66,67] However such a mechanism is not consistent with the fact that leucine is degraded to acetyl CoA, which cannot be converted to pyruvate. Also, in vitro experiments have shown that, for example, [^{14}C] from valine was recovered in glutamine but not alanine or pyruvate,[33,54] and in vivo studies have shown that alanine carbon is derived from glucose and muscle glycogen but not protein.[68]

GLUTAMINE PRODUCTION AND RELEASE FROM MUSCLE

Skeletal muscle in vitro and in vivo synthesizes de novo and releases glutamine in similar or even greater amounts than alanine, and in cardiac muscle, glutamine production far exceeds that of alanine.[69] Insight into the origin of the carbon skeleton of glutamine came from studies by Chang and Goldberg,[54] who were attempting to establish the metabolic fates of the amino acids that are generated by muscle protein degradation and then enter the tricarboxylic acid cycle (i.e., valine, isoleucine, aspartate, asparagine, and glutamate). Incubated muscles release these five amino acids in much lower amounts than would be anticipated from the composition of muscle protein. The missing amounts of these five amino acids together equal the amount of glutamine synthesized de novo by the muscle. Similarly, tracer experiments in postabsorptive humans have shown that the carbon atoms in glutamine originate primarily from protein-derived amino acids.[70]

Amino acids generated by protein breakdown in fasting or other catabolic states thus can have several distinct fates in muscle (Table 23-1 and Fig. 23-1). Most residues do not enter the TCA cycle and seem to be released from the tissue intact or as their α-ketoacid derivatives for use by other tissues. By comparison, the branched-chain amino acids, especially leucine, may provide some energy and amino groups for alanine and glutamine synthesis. The carbon skeletons of the five amino acids that can enter the TCA cycle are mainly converted to glutamine, which is then released from muscle. This process should therefore be viewed as an important initial step in gluconeogenesis from muscle protein.

It has been estimated that about 87 percent of the glutamine released from muscle is derived from de novo synthesis, rather than being liberated as a result of proteolysis.[71] As a consequence, glutamine production and release by muscle is a continual drain on intracellular pools of glutamate and therefore on the α-ketoglutarate pool and TCA cycle intermediates. After eating, amino acids taken up from the blood, or, in fasting, those generated by the breakdown of muscle proteins may serve to replenish these pools of TCA cycle intermediates. The glutamine released by muscle is an important energy source for many cells. For example, glutamine is extensively oxidized by leukocytes and fibroblasts.[72] It is taken up from the blood primarily by the kidney, where it serves as a precursor for urinary ammonia, and its carbon skeleton may be used either for gluconeogenesis or energy production, or some of the carbons may be released into the blood as alanine.[73] In addition, the small intestine takes up and metabolizes large amounts of glutamine; it, in turn, releases appreciable amounts of alanine.[74] This complex multiorgan process appears to play an important role in net gluconeogenesis from the five amino acids originating in proteins and converted to glutamine in muscle. Although these patterns of metabolism are firmly established, it remains quite unclear what advantage the organism may gain by carrying out this complex series of reactions or what selective advantage conversion of other amino acids into glutamine in muscle confers to the organism.

The level of glutamine within different tissues is determined by the relative activities of glutamine synthase and glutaminase. The mechanisms underlying the expression and activity of these enzymes have recently been the subject of detailed studies.[75] These have revealed different tissue-specific enzyme isoforms under both transcriptional and posttranscriptional regulation. Thus, for instance, the transcription of glutamine synthase is strongly activated by corticosteroids in lung and muscle tissue. Induction of this enzyme underlies the increased production and release of glutamine from muscle in starvation and disease states such

Table 23-1. AMINO ACIDS CLASSIFIED ACCORDING TO THE PATTERN OF METABOLISM OF THEIR CARBON SKELETONS IN SKELETAL MUSCLE

Amino Acids	Metabolism in Muscle
Ala, Gln	Synthesized de novo and released.
Gly, Cys, Ser, Thr, Met, Pro, Lys, Arg, His, Phe, Tyr, Trp	Not oxidized; released intact or as α-ketoacids upon net proteolysis.
Leu	Utilized as an energy source
Asp, Asn, Glu, Val, Ile	Mainly converted to Gln, some oxidized, some converted to lactate, the remainder released intact or as α-ketoacids.

as sepsis or other critical illness where glucocorticoid levels are high.[76,77] However the increased content of glutamine synthase in these states is dependent on the rapid export of glutamine, because if glutamine accumulates in cells, it induces the accelerated degradation of glutamine synthase in a process involving the proteasome.[75]

It has been proposed that in pathologic conditions, such as following traumatic injury or during infection, energy production from glutamine released from muscle is critical for maintaining the function of gastrointestinal and immune cells.[72,78] Furthermore, it has also been suggested that under these conditions a state of glutamine "deficiency" may exist, and that the administration of supplemental glutamine under such circumstances is beneficial.[78] Glutamine supplementation can raise levels of TCA cycle intermediates, and though this response does not appear to increase energy production or endurance in healthy skeletal muscle, there is some evidence to suggest improved functioning of ischemic heart muscle.[79,80] Also, administration of large amounts of glutamine with parenteral nutrition has been reported to improve patients' recovery rates (e.g., following bone marrow transplantation) and to promote protein accretion in skeletal muscle.[78]

Protein Metabolism in Muscle

PROTEOLYTIC PATHWAYS IN MUSCLE

At least four different cytosolic proteolytic pathways have been identified, each of which uses a unique complement of proteases. The best-characterized proteases include those in the lysosome, such as the cathepsins, the calcium-dependent proteases (calpains), the caspases, and the proteasome. Many studies have attempted to define which of the above pathways is implicated in causing muscle atrophy via accelerated proteolysis. Such studies have been made possible by the use of protease inhibitors, and, as described below, there is considerable evidence that the Ub-proteasome pathway is responsible for the majority of this accelerated proteolysis in many different conditions. However, in reviewing the literature, it is important to remember that some protease inhibitors are neither exclusive nor completely effective in inhibiting their targets (e.g., weak bases such as chloroquine may not block activity of lysosomal proteases, such as cathepsin B, which is active over a broad pH range,[81] and the proteasome inhibitors MG132 and lactacystin also inhibit other proteases, such as cathepsins).[82] Furthermore, effects observed during relatively short-lived experiments in vitro have the potential to give a distorted impression of the critical changes involved in the process of muscle atrophy, which lasts for much longer periods in vivo. Two themes emerging from recent studies are that degradation of individual proteins is highly regulated, and frequently more than one proteolytic pathway is activated during muscle atrophy. Activation of proteolysis via some pathways—e.g., Ca^{2+}-dependent calpains—may contribute relatively little to the increase in proteolysis under most conditions yet still play a vital role in the overall process of atrophy. There is also evidence that certain muscle proteins are degraded by more than one proteolytic pathway,[83,84] but as yet it is unclear how common this is or how the actions of different proteolytic pathways are coordinated.

Lysosomal Proteolytic Process

Lysosomes are membrane-enclosed organelles that contain a large number of proteases (e.g., cathepsins B, D, H, and L) as well as other acid hydrolases. In all cells, these organelles play a critical role in the breakdown of endocytosed extracellular proteins. In muscle, liver, and other cells, the lack of insulin or of essential amino acids stimulates the sequestration of many cytosolic proteins and organelles and their subsequent hydrolysis within enlarged lysosomes called "autophagic vacuoles." This conclusion is based on morphologic evidence[16,85] as well as physiologic data.[13,15,86] Also, in serum-deprived cells, certain proteins are selectively transported into lysosomes prior to their degradation. This "selective autophagy" promotes the degradation of proteins containing specific peptide sequences and involves specific intracellular recognition proteins (members of the hsp 70 family) that facilitate protein entry into the lysosome.[86]

It is possible to measure the contribution of these lysosomal pathways to overall proteolysis in incubated muscles and other cells by using nontoxic agents that block the lysosomal process, such as the weak bases chloroquine or methylamine (which raise lysosomal pH), or with inhibitors of lysosomal cysteine proteases (e.g., leupeptin or E64, both of which inhibit cathepsins B, H, and L).[13] Muscles are incubated under conditions that enhance the lysosomal process (e.g., without insulin or amino acids), and the magnitude of the fall in proteolysis upon addition of the inhibitor represents the lysosomal component of overall proteolysis. Using these approaches in cultured fibroblasts[15] and isolated rat muscles,[13] the lack of insulin or of serum leads to a twofold increase in overall proteolysis, which can be blocked with methylamine. However, when muscles are maintained in vitro under optimal nutritional conditions (with tension, insulin, and amino acids present), the lysosome does not contribute significantly to overall proteolysis.[13] Inhibitors of lysosomal function also have little or no effect on the breakdown of myofibrillar proteins, which make up the majority of the proteins in muscle.[31,87,88]

Many studies have been performed in models of different pathologic conditions to establish what role lysosomal proteolysis may play in muscle atrophy associated with disease. In tissue culture, low insulin or serum starvation stimulates autophagy (see above), but in whole muscle preparations from low insulin states, due, for example, to fasting or untreated diabetes, the increased proteolysis observed was not affected by lysosome inhibitors.[89–91] It seems likely that the explanation for this apparent discrepancy is that in mammals, acidosis and increased circulating glucocorticoids, which are a feature of uncontrolled diabetes, lead to activation of the Ub-proteasome pathway, and that this is responsible for most of the accelerated proteolysis in muscle.[92,93] In rats, burn injury leads to increased lysosomal proteolysis in addition to activating other proteolytic pathways,[94] and this induction of lysosmal proteolysis can be inhibited by insulin.[95] Also, in a rat model of cancer cachexia, up to 30 percent of the accelerated proteolysis in muscle was inhibited by lysosome inhibitors[96]; in other models such as chronic sepsis[97] as well as in atrophy due to disuse,[98] lysosomal proteases were activated in muscle but appeared to have only a minor role in overall proteolysis. Studies in humans with disease-related muscle atrophy are scarce and have largely focused on changes in mRNA levels for components of different proteolytic pathways in muscle. Patients in negative nitrogen balance following head trauma had raised mRNA levels for cathepsin D, and other pathways appeared to be activated simultaneously.[99] By contrast, in subjects with early lung cancer, mRNA levels for cathepsin B but not other proteolytic pathway components were increased in muscle and were inversely related to fat-free mass.[100] Many chronic wasting conditions are characterized by a systemic inflammatory response linked to the development of muscle atrophy. Results from studies of direct trauma to muscle have shown activation of lysosomes in infiltrating macrophages without any similar effects in the surrounding muscle fibers.[101] This finding raises the possibility that, in other wasting conditions, some of the increase proteolysis attributed to muscle fiber lysosomes might be due to effects of circulating inflammatory cells rather than changes in muscle fibers themselves.

Calcium-Dependent Proteases

Calcium-dependent thiol proteases, or calpains, are also present in muscle cytosol. The calpains present in muscle include the ubiquitous calpain 1 (μ or I) and 2 (m or II) and the muscle-specific calpain 3 (p94). The ubiquitous calpains are heterodimers that share a common catalytic subunit but have unique larger regulatory subunits conferring differing affinities for Ca^{2+}.[102–104] Incubation of isolated muscles with a Ca^{2+} ionophore (e.g., A23187) leads to a large activation of overall protein breakdown.[105,106] This response to ionophores presumably reflects the maximal capacity of the muscle to carry out Ca^{2+}-dependent proteolysis. A similar activation of calcium-dependent proteolysis is found in isolated muscle incubated in an unrestrained position. In these muscle preparations, shortening is thought to impair diffusion of oxygen and nutrients from surrounding fluid.[28] The resulting ischemia and loss of membrane integrity appears to allow increased entrance of Ca^{2+} from the medium into the cell and activation of Ca^{2+}-dependent proteases.[28,31] Selective inactivators of thiol proteases (e.g., leupeptin or E64) inhibit the increased proteolysis seen under these conditions. Uncontrolled influx of calcium may also be relevant to the activation of the ubiquitous calpains in the mouse model (mdx) of Duchenne muscular dystrophy. Enhanced proteolytic activity by calpains in mdx myotubes was found to be due to increased Ca^{2+}-influx through Ca^{2+}-leak channels in the plasma membrane,[107] and calpain translocation from the plasma membrane to the cytosol coincides with the occurrence of degeneration/regeneration in muscle fibers of adult mdx mice.[108]

Contractile activity in normal muscle, which is dependent on controlled, rapid Ca^{2+} flux across the plasma membrane and release from the sarcoplasmic reticulum, also leads to increased calpain activity.[109] As a result, exercise-induced muscle injury may involve calpain-dependent proteolysis.[110] Also, changing the pattern of contractile activity of a muscle induces fiber type transition. In one study of the transition from fast fiber to slow fiber, induced by chronic low-frequency stimulation, one of the early changes was increased activity and translocation of calpain 1 from the soluble to the particulate fraction containing myofibrillar proteins and microsomes. This observation may indicate that calpain 1 has a role in adaptation to contractile activity and perhaps aids the removal of fast myosin heavy-chain proteins to allow their replacement by better-adapted slow isoforms.[111] The same authors also examined the effects of regeneration after injection of bupivacaine (Marcaine) and showed that in regenerating muscle fibers a similar early translocation of calpain 2 to the particulate fraction occurs. Similarly, changes in the localization and activity of calpains characterize different phases of muscle cell differentiation, suggesting that these proteases also have additional adaptive roles in muscle cells.[112]

Although the in vivo substrates for calpains are largely unknown, some indication of the role of individual proteases may be gleaned from the substrates that they are able to cleave in vitro. Calpains are implicated in the degradation of proteins containing regions rich in proline, glutamic acid, serine, and threonine amino acids (the PEST sequence), including N-myristoyltransferase, which is highly expressed in cardiac tissue,[113] and Ca^{2+}/calmodulin-dependent cyclic nucleotide phosphodiesterase 1.[114] In addition, calpains cleave cytoskeletal proteins such as talin[115] and ankyrins,[116] myofibrillar components such as actinin and tropomyosin,[109] and the sarcoplasmic reticulum calcium-release channel.[117] The transcription factor YY1 represses expression of certain muscle proteins such as α-actin. During muscle differentiation, degradation of YY1 protein is the primary method of inhibiting its activity, and YY1 is a substrate for both calpains and the Ub-proteasome pathway.[84]

In addition to the effects of Ca^{2+}, the activity of calpains can be modulated by the binding of calpastatin, a naturally occurring inhibitor. The localization and amount of this inhibitor in muscle may determine changes in calpain activity, rather than any alteration in the concentration of the proteases.[111] Thus, during muscle cell differentiation, calpastatin levels are high initially and then drop markedly after myotube fusion, while calpain levels do not change. The associated increase in calpain activity in myotubes may be important for further muscle cell differentiation.[118] A similar increase in the calpain/calpastatin ratio has been described in muscle from rats with cancer cachexia induced by AH-130 tumor, and this change correlated with a fall in the levels of Ca^{2+}-ATPase, a calpain substrate.[119] The calpain/calpastatin ratio is also of interest to the food industry, where a negative correlation between calpastatin activity and meat tenderness has been described. Furthermore, studies suggest that the postmortem degradation of calpastatin is principally performed by calpains.[120]

Despite extensive study and many intriguing observations, there has been no definitive evidence for a functional role for calpains 1 and 2 or calpastatin in muscle protein turnover, and major conceptual issues remain (e.g., are Ca^{2+} levels in muscle sufficient to activate calpains in physiologic or pathologic conditions?). However, in a recent report, transgenic mice with muscle-specific overexpression of calpastatin were found to have no fiber type change and reduced muscle atrophy after unloading.[121] This demonstrates that, at least in this type of muscle atrophy, inhibition of calpain activity can reduce loss of muscle mass, but the molecular basis for this important observation (e.g., which calpain is affected? which proteins are spared and how?) remains to be studied. Though Ca^{2+}-dependent proteolysis appears to have a number of important roles in muscle, it does not contribute significantly to the overall acceleration in proteolysis in any experimental model of muscle wasting studied to date,[12,30,31] and calcium-dependent proteolysis is not increased in muscles atrophying due to uremia[89] or cancer cachexia due to Yoshida hepatoma.[96] Also Ca^{2+}-dependent proteolysis made only a small contribution to the overall increase in proteolysis in sepsis,[97] diabetes,[91] and disuse atrophy.[98] In all these conditions the Ub-proteasome pathway is responsible for the bulk of proteolysis. However, calpains may serve some complementary role. In rats with wasting due to sepsis, Williams et al. described calcium-dependent release of myofibrils and disintegration of the Z band along with increased mRNA levels for calpains 1, 2, and 3. This suggests that, in sepsis, calpains might be important in releasing myofibrils from the contractile apparatus, which presumably then may serve as substrates for ubiquitination and degradation by the proteasome.[122]

Much of the discussion above has concerned the ubiquitous calpains 1 and 2. However, the muscle-specific calpain 3 is of special interest because hereditary loss of function of this protease leads to limb-girdle muscular dystrophy.[123,124] Furthermore, in wasting due to starvation,[125] cancer cachexia,[126] and denervation,[127] levels of mRNA encoding calpain 3 are reduced, though proteolysis increases. Thus this protease, which also has titin- and connectin-binding properties, appears to have an as yet undefined role in maintaining muscle fiber integrity and function, even though it is not implicated in the enhanced proteolysis in many forms of muscle wasting.

ATP-Ubiquitin-Proteasome Proteolytic Pathway

The depletion of ATP leads to a dramatic fall in overall protein breakdown in most cells.[32] However, ATP depletion can have a number of toxic effects, and further investigation into the nature of this ATP requirement defined a soluble ATP-dependent proteolytic process.[128] Subsequent studies designed to elucidate the reasons for this ATP requirement for proteolysis in the cytosol led to the discovery of the Ub-proteasome pathway[10] (see details below). With the advent of proteasome inhibitors in 1994, the dominant role of the proteasome in degrading the majority of intracellular proteins was demonstrated.[14,82] Furthermore, it has become increasingly clear that regulated proteolysis via the Ub-proteasome pathway is a fundamental feature of many constitutive and adaptive processes within cells, and derangements of this proteolytic system underlie many human diseases.[129]

The importance of the Ub-proteasome pathway in muscle atrophy is also now well established. In isolated muscle preparations, blocking of lysosomal and calpain proteases only reduced protein breakdown by 10 to 20 percent and did not inhibit the breakdown of contractile proteins,[13,87] but the majority of basal proteolysis (50 to 70 percent) was blocked by ATP depletion.[11] Furthermore, the majority of the acceleration in proteolysis induced by a variety of catabolic conditions—including diabetes,[130] acidosis,[131] sepsis, thyroid hormone treatment, and denervation atrophy[132]—can be blocked by proteasome inhibitors. Additional confirmation of the activation of the Ub-proteasome pathway in atrophying muscle has come from a variety of studies of muscle under different conditions; these have demonstrated dramatic increases in Ub-protein conjugates, which are key intermediates in this pathway, as well as increases in mRNAs encoding multiple components of the Ub-proteasome pathway.[133]

Table 23-2 summarizes the proteolytic pathways in muscle.

Despite the advances in knowledge of the importance of the Ub-proteasome pathway in muscle, several outstanding questions remain. How are different muscle proteins targeted for proteolysis via the proteasome, and how are the rates of breakdown of different proteins regulated? Some of the answers to these questions are becoming clearer with emerging data about the range and activity of the many components of the Ub-proteasome pathway.

Features of the ATP-ubiquitin-proteasome pathway. Degradation of proteins via the Ub-proteasome pathway is a multistep process and, as highlighted above, requires the hydrolysis of ATP in addition to the 8-kDa protein cofactor Ub and the 26S proteasome (Fig. 23-4). The 26S proteasome is a very large (2-MDa) complex made up of at least 50 subunits.[134] Proteins are digested within the central core, the 20S particle, which is a cylindrical complex containing multiple proteolytic sites with three different specificities. Unlike typical proteases, the proteasome requires ATP for the degradation of proteins; in particular, ATP hydrolysis is needed to drive the unfolding of globular proteins and for protein translocation into the 20S proteolytic compartment.[135]

The majority of protein substrates are marked for degradation by covalent linkage of a chain of Ub molecules to the ε-amino group of an internal lysine of the protein substrate. This process requires at least three enzymes. The Ub-activating enzyme (E1) utilizes ATP to create a highly reactive thiolester form of Ub and then transfers it to a Ub carrier protein (E2). The subsequent transfer of activated Ub to the substrate requires a Ub-protein ligase (E3). The E3 binds both the protein substrate and the E2 carrying the activated Ub and transfers the activated Ub from the E2 to the substrate. When a chain of four or more Ub molecules has been formed on the protein, it is then usually degraded rapidly by the 26S proteasome to yield small peptides.[136] The polyubiquitin chain is also disassembled to release free Ub, which can then be reused. Isopeptidases which remove Ubs from substrate are associated with the 26S proteasome and also found in the cytosol. These deubiquitinating enzymes may also be sites of regulation, and their activation may even block degradation of a polyubiquitinated protein by removing or shortening the polyubiquitin tag.[137]

The E3 Ub-protein ligase can only bind specific protein substrates, and it ubiquitinates these proteins with the aid of a specific E2. Thus which proteins are degraded by the proteasome is critically dependent on which E3s and E2s are present and active in each cell. Numerous E3s from several distinct families have been discovered to date, but there are indications that many other E3s, remain to be identified.[129,138] The binding of an E3 to a protein substrate is determined by the presence of certain structural features within the protein. A number of these degradation signals, which accelerate ubiquitination and thus speed degradation, have been identified. For example, one E3, Ubr1/E3α, ubiquitinates proteins with certain unusual NH_2-terminal residues. This enzyme, and perhaps this form of protein recognition (termed the "N-end rule"), appears to be important in the degradation of muscle proteins[139] (see below). In contrast, a nine–amino acid sequence or "destruction box" motif is required for the ubiquitination and degradation of certain regulatory proteins (e.g., cyclins) during mitosis. This ubiquitination is performed by a large E3 complex called the anaphase-promoting complex.[140] Phosphorylation or dephosphorylation of certain proteins can also trigger their ubiquitination and degradation. This form of destruction signal is involved in the onset of an inflammatory response when IkBα, the inhibitor of the transcription factor NF-kB, is phosphorylated on two serines, and this marking reaction initiates its rapid ubquitination and degradation.[141]

The role of ubiquitin carrier proteins (E2s) and ubiquitin-protein ligases (E3s) in muscle wasting. In most models of muscle wasting so far studied, the rapid loss of muscle protein is largely due to an activation of the Ub-proteasome pathway.[133] However, which E2s and E3s are involved in this acclerated proteolysis is still incompletely understood. One pair of ubiquitinating enzymes, $E2_{14K}$ and E3α, have been identified as possibly being critically involved in muscle wasting. In muscles, mRNA levels for one or both of these proteins increased upon starvation[142] as well as in diabetes,[92,143] sepsis,[144,145] disuse atrophy,[98] and dexamethasone treatment.[146] In addition, in rabbit muscle homogenates, competitive inhibitors of E3α markedly inhibited degradation of muscle proteins.[139] In extracts of rat muscles atrophying due to tumor implantation or sepsis, the conjugation of Ub to endogenous proteins was again markedly reduced by inhibitors of E3α.[139] These results were surprising, because previous experiments in yeast and mammalian cells[147,148] had shown that E3α and $E2_{14K}$ primarily target proteins with abnormal or "destabilizing" NH_2-terminal residues. It remains unclear which muscle proteins were being ubiquitinated by E3α and $E2_{14K}$ in these experiments and how they came to have the requisite N-terminal residues. One possibility is that normal muscle proteins are first modified or even clipped by other proteases to reveal destabilizing N-terminal residues, which then make them substrates for ubiquitination by E3α and $E2_{14K}$. However, the

Table 23-2. PATHWAYS FOR PROTEIN BREAKDOWN IN SKELETAL MUSCLE

Pathway	Summary of Features	Notes
Lysosomes	Lysosomal proteases are optimally active at acid pH. Lysosomal proteolysis (autophagy) is stimulated by low insulin states and lack of amino acids. These proteases can degrade soluble but not myofibrillar muscle proteins. Lysosomal proteolysis increases in muscle during starvation and in muscle wasting due to cancer cachexia, chronic sepsis, and disuse atrophy. Overall, however, lysosomal proteases contribute only a minor proportion of the total increase in proteolysis in these conditions.	Some cathepsins are still active at neutral pH. Muscle lysosomal proteolysis may include a contribution from infiltrating macrophages in some conditions.
Ca^{2+}-dependent	Calpains have varying affinities for Ca^{2+} and are inhibited by calpastatin, a naturally occurring inhibitor. Several muscle protein substrates are known in vitro, but true in vivo substrates are unknown. Calpains are activated by increases in Ca^{2+} induced by Ca^{2+} ionophores. Ca^{2+}-dependent proteolysis is also increased in ischemic conditions and makes a small contribution to increased proteolysis in animal models of sepsis and diabetes. Calpains are also implicated in enhanced proteolysis in Duchenne muscular dystrophy and in development- and exercise- or disuse-induced adaptive change in muscle fibers.	The muscle-specific calpain 3 may have a different role, as loss of function leads to one type of limb-girdle muscular dystrophy, and mRNA levels for this protease are reduced rather than increased in many types of muscle wasting.
Ub-proteasome	Ub-proteasome proteolysis is ATP-dependent and has a central role in the regulated degradation of muscle proteins, including myofibrillar proteins, under catabolic conditions. Activation of this pathway is responsible for the majority of the increase in muscle proteolysis in starvation, diabetes, acidosis, sepsis, thyroid hormone treatment, and denervation or disuse atrophy. Proteins destined for breakdown are bound and ubiquitinated by a series ubiquitination enzymes: E1, E2, and E3.	Two newly discovered muscle-specific E3s—atrogin-1 and MuRF-1—are required for certain forms of muscle wasting and are highly regulated in all wasting conditions studied.
Caspases	Their principal role is in apoptosis, but the role of apoptosis in muscle wasting is unclear. Apoptosis in skeletal muscle is a feature of certain forms of muscular dystrophy and some systemic illnesses; it is also seen after denervation.	Certain muscle cells (e.g., satellite cells) may be more likely to proceed to apoptosis than others.

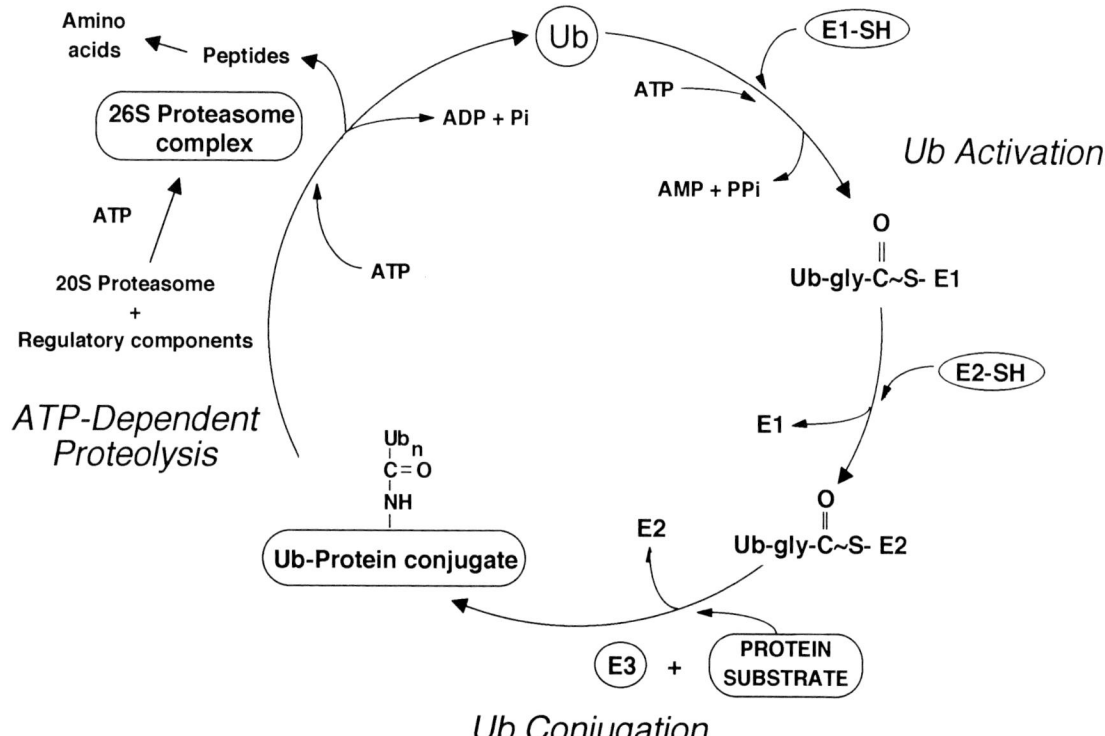

FIGURE 23-4. The ATP-ubiquitin (Ub) dependent pathway for protein degradation. Three enzymes, E1, E2, and E3, are involved in the formation of Ub-protein conjugates.[10] ATP hydrolysis occurs at several sites in this degradative pathway. A single ATP is necessary for the initial activation of the carboxyl terminus of Ub by E1. ATP is used in formation of the 26S proteasome complex from the 20S proteasome and additional regulatory polypeptides. ATP molecules are also consumed in the degradative function of the 26S complex. *Ub activation:* A high energy thiol-ester bond is formed between the C-terminal glycine of Ub and the Ub-activating enzyme E1. Ub is then transferred to the active site thiol group of one of several carrier proteins (E2s). *Ub ligation:* The proteolytic substrate is recognized by a Ub-protein ligase (E3) which mediates transfer of Ub from E2 to the protein. Multiple Ub moities may be covalently bound to each other and to one or more lysines on the protein substrate through isopeptide bonds between the carboxyl terminus of Ub and the ε-amino group of lysine. The addition of Ub to preexisting Ub side chains leads to the formation of high molecular weight Ub-protein conjugates. *ATP-dependent proteolysis:* The protein substrate is degraded by the 26S proteasome complex, which produces short peptides and regenerates free Ub by an associated isopeptidase activity. The released Ub can be reutilized in degradation of other proteins.

experiments by Solomon et al.,[29] followed only degradation of soluble muscle proteins, and thus may give a mistaken impression of the importance of E3α and E2$_{14K}$ in ubiquitination and degradation of muscle proteins generally, or the turnover of specific components (e.g., myofibrillar proteins). Furthermore, other enzymes can ubiquitinate muscle proteins such as actin, troponin T, and the transcription factor MyoD,[149] and there is transcriptional activation of other E2s in addition to E2$_{14K}$ in muscle in response to dexamethasone treatment.[146] These findings suggest that E3α and E2$_{14K}$ do not have an exclusive or dominant role as first thought. Ubiquitination of proteins serves a variety of functions in cells, in addition to marking them for degradation, and recent work has suggested another possible role for E2$_{14K}$. The yeast homologue of E2$_{14K}$, Ubc2/Rad 6, ubiquitinates histone H2B, which leads to methylation of histone H3B and inhibition of gene expression.[150] Whether E2$_{14K}$ has such a role in chromatin remodeling in muscle atrophy remains to be seen.

Our laboratory and others have used genomic approaches (e.g., transcriptional microarray analysis) to identify genes, which we term *atrogins,* whose expression increases or decreases during muscle atrophy. These studies have revealed two novel E3s that appear to be directly involved in accelerated proteolysis in many, perhaps all forms of muscle atrophy. mRNA levels for one of these new E3s, named atrogin-1, increase up to tenfold in muscle atrophying due to fasting, diabetes, cancer cachexia, uremia,[151] immobilization, denervation, and unweighting.[152] The importance of atrogin-1 in determining muscle wasting in response to denervation and disuse was elegantly demonstrated in studies on knockout mice. When muscles from mice lacking a functional atrogin-1 gene were denervated or subjected to unloading (by hindlimb suspension), they lost less mass than muscles in wild-type mice.[152] Atrogin-1 is a member of the large SCF family of Ub ligases, and is expressed exclusively in striated muscle. Another E3, named MuRF1, is also upregulated in these various forms of atrophy, and muscles from MuRF1 knockout mice are also more resistant to denervation atrophy than the wild type.[152] Muscles from animals lacking both these enzymes show very little loss of weight upon denervation. MuRF-1 is a very different type of enzyme and is a member of the ring-finger family of E3s. Atrogin-1 and MuRF-1 are not essential for normal development or function of muscle, though they are essential for atrophy. The protein substrates for these E3s are the subject of current research. Recent data indicate that atrogin-1, which includes a nuclear localization signal, and MuRF-1 may also target nuclear proteins such as transcription factors.

Caspases

Caspases are a family of intracellular proteases that cleave proteins after aspartic acid residues and play a major role in the process of programmed cell death or apoptosis. Caspases are synthesised as proenzymes, and initiator caspases such as caspase 8 and 9 are cleaved and activated in response to either stimulation of a membrane death receptor (extrinsic pathway) or DNA damage by mutagens or ionizing radiation (intrinsic pathway). In most cases, especially for apoptosis via the intrinsic pathway, other proapoptotic proteins translocate to the mitochondrion, causing release of cytochrome c, which contributes to further activation of "executioner" caspases such as caspases 3 and 7. The actions of executioner caspases are then thought to initiate the systematic dismantling of the cell.[153]

The process of apoptosis is vital for normal embryonic development and functioning caspase 3 is essential for normal muscle development.[154] Despite abundant caspase-3 mRNA in rodent muscle, the corresponding protein is undetectable in adult rat and mouse skeletal muscle, and levels of caspase-3 protein increase only transiently in response to injury in regenerating fibers.[155] In humans, certain types of muscular dystrophy are characterized by increased apoptosis in affected muscles,[156] and in denervated muscles features of apoptosis are prominent.[157] Indeed, one reason for impaired recovery after prolonged denervation may be the apoptosis and depletion of muscle satellite cells.[158] Other systemic illnesses are frequently associated with muscle atrophy, and recent studies in heart failure[159] and chronic obstructive pulmonary disease[160] have shown increased apoptosis in the skeletal muscle of affected patients, particularly those with more marked atrophy and reduced exercise capacity.

The role of apoptosis in skeletal muscle is still the subject of debate, but it seems likely that a limited form of apoptosis (e.g., activation of certain caspases) is an adaptive feature of atrophying skeletal muscle that may serve to reduce the number of myonuclei. In addition, caspase activation may cleave proteins, even myofibrillar proteins, and target them for complete degradation by other pathways (e.g., ubiquitination by the N-end pathways E3α and E2$_{14k}$).

REGULATION OF MUSCLE PROTEIN TURNOVER AND GROWTH BY NUTRIENTS AND HORMONES

Great advances have been made in understanding the signaling mechanisms that mediate the effects of various nutrients and anabolic hormones on protein synthesis in eukaryotic cells. In particular, the central role of two protein kinases, Akt and mTOR, in regulating mRNA translation and protein synthesis, is now well established. The lipophilic macrolide rapamycin is an extremely potent inhibitor of yeast cell growth and mammalian cell proliferation. It acts by inhibiting the protein kinase mTOR.[161] In the presence of nutrients, mTOR phosphorylates and activates a protein kinase (S6 kinase), which, in turn, phosphorylates the ribosomal protein S6. Simultaneously, mTOR kinase inactivates a translation-initiation factor binding protein, 4E-BP1. These phosphorylation events promote translation initiation and thus protein synthesis and play an important role in controlling cell size.[162] Upstream of mTOR, Akt, another protein kinase, is activated at the cell membrane by the signaling pathway involving phosphatidylinositol-3-kinase (PI3 kinase). Various growth factors, including insulin and insulin-like growth factors (IGFs), stimulate this pathway. Activated Akt phosphorylates and activates mTOR as well as other kinases not directly regulated by mTOR, which also induce enhanced protein synthesis.[161] Many of the details of the individual steps linking each of these signaling events are still unclear, but it is firmly established that activation of this pathway triggers muscle hypertrophy by enhancing protein synthesis. In addition to its other effects, this pathway also inhibits expression of atrogin-1 and MuRF-1 and suppresses proteolysis in atrophying muscles.[163] Also, identification of this signaling cascade has provided a framework in which to understand the effects of nutrients and amino acids such as leucine and anabolic hormones in promoting muscle growth.

Influence of Leucine on Muscle Protein Turnover

It has been known for some time that branched-chain amino acids in general and leucine in particular have regulatory effects on muscle protein balance. Studies from several laboratories[26,164,165] have shown that branched-chain amino acids stimulate protein synthesis and reduce protein breakdown in isolated skeletal and cardiac muscle. These anabolic effects of leucine can be demonstrated even at physiologic intracellular concentrations of leucine. It has been suggested that leucine's ability to inhibit protein breakdown might be due to increases in leucyl-tRNA, as in bacteria, where the lack of any single species of charged tRNA causes a reduction in protein synthesis and enhanced proteolysis.[32] However, studies of the charging of leucyl-tRNA in muscle extracts have indicated that the charging reaction has a Km of 6 μM or less.[166] Thus the supply of leucyl-tRNA should not vary over the physiologic range of intracellular leucine concentration (0.1 and 0.5 mM) as at these concentrations the tRNA should remain saturated. Some metabolites of leucine, generated by transamination, can also inhibit protein breakdown in muscle,[53,166] and the transamination product, α-ketoisocaproic acid, can reduce proteolysis in isolated muscles as well as urea production in human patients with renal failure and can also improve protein balance.[167]

Leucine and other branched-chain amino acids promote protein synthesis in muscle at the translational level.[165,168] Accordingly, leucine increases polysome formation and reduces the number of free ribosomes in skeletal and cardiac muscle. Furthermore, leucine stimulates synthesis of soluble and contractile proteins to similar extents and thus probably increases production of most (if not all) muscle proteins. Recent studies have shown that an infusion of branched-chain amino acid in humans decreases urinary nitrogen excretion and improves forearm phenylalanine balance; in addition, it leads to increased phosphorylation of S6 kinase and 4E-BP1.[169] Furthermore the effects of leucine on phosphorylation of S6 kinase are additive to those mediated by insulin,[170] but both insulin and leucine are involved in regulation of the translation initiation complex.[171] These and other studies in rats and L6 myoblasts have established that leucine, more than other branched-chain amino acid, stimulates protein synthesis and mRNA translation principally via the nutrient-sensing pathway described above, which involves mTOR.[172,173] However there is also increasing evidence that leucine's stimulation of protein synthesis involves additional rapamycin-insensitive pathways.[174,175] Reduced protein synthesis in muscle is a feature of muscle loss in aging, and one study in old rats suggests that leucine supplementation of meals can restore postprandial stimulation of protein synthesis, raising the possibility that such dietary maneuvers might be useful in aging.[176]

The inhibitory effects of leucine on protein degradation have been less extensively investigated. When the effect of amino acid starvation was tested using cultured C2C12 muscle cells, up to 40 percent of the increase in protein breakdown induced by total amino acid removal was attributable to removal of leucine alone, and the withdrawal of leucine induced enhanced lysosmal proteolysis and autophagy.[175] In addition to lack of nutrients, many other conditions, such as acidosis, can induce accelerated proteolysis. In cultured L6 muscle cells, leucine can reverse the loss of protein and increased protein degradation induced by acidotic conditions. This action of leucine is not related to its role as a metabolic fuel, as other carbon sources such as alanine and pyruvate failed to have the same anabolic effects despite being consumed by the cells.[177]

Insulin and Glucose

Insulin levels in blood have a profound effect on protein balance in muscle and other tissues. Insulin increases rates of transport of many amino acids into muscle tissue, increases rates of protein synthesis, and inhibits muscle protein breakdown.[6,7,178] Thus the rise in insulin after meals promotes net protein accumulation in muscle, while in the postabsorptive state, when insulin is low, there is a net loss of protein and a release of amino acids from muscle. However, the literature contains many apparently conflicting reports about the effects of insulin on protein metabolism, and a number of sources for this confusion can be identified. In particular, the effects of insulin in stimulating protein synthesis are critically dependent on the availability of amino acids, and, as outlined above, leucine alone has similar anabolic effects overlapping those of insulin.

Insulin stimulates amino acid transport into muscle by recruiting specific sodium-dependent amino acid transporters to the plasma membrane.[179] The enhanced uptake of amino acids in a variety of tissues, induced by systemic infusion of insulin, can cause hypoaminoacidemia; in some studies, the resulting reduced availability of amino acids may have actually inhibited the effects of insulin on protein synthesis. However, other studies in postabsoptive human subjects, using leg arteriovenous catheterization and direct measurement of protein fractional synthetic rates, have confirmed that insulin causes increased protein synthesis.[180] Binding of insulin to its receptor on the plasma membrane leads to activation of phophatidylinositol-3 kinase (PI-3 kinase); this initiates a signaling cascade including activation of Akt and S6 kinase[181] and ultimately enhanced initiation of translation. It has been suggested that insulin preferentially stimulates synthesis of myofibrillar proteins. However, in some reports of experiments in pigs, insulin stimulated mitochondrial protein synthesis and had no effect on myosin heavy-chain synthesis,[182] while studies in neonatal animals have suggested an equal effect on the synthesis of myofibrillar and sarcoplasmic protein.[183] Such discrepancies may relate to differences in the sensitivity to insulin during development.[184]

Overall insulin has a permissive role in protein synthesis, and its effects, such as the postprandial stimulation of protein synthesis, are dependent on the presence of a supply of amino acids. The source of amino acids is commonly dietary, but it can include increased protein degradation and release from other tissues. Hence insulin can have a limited role in promoting protein synthesis in some catabolic conditions such as after burns[185] or muscle-damaging exercise.[186]

In addition to its effects on protein sythesis, insulin inhibits protein degradation[13,26,85,187,188]; in isolated muscles, insulin's effects on protein synthesis and degradation appear to be of comparable import in improving nitrogen balance. The effects of insulin in inhibiting protein breakdown in liver center on blocking lysosomal autophagy,[16] although the effects on the Ub-proteasome pathway in liver have not been systematically studied. In skeletal and cardiac muscle, insulin inhibits overall protein breakdown and decreases lysosomal fragility (an indicator of reduced lysosome size) without altering the total content of lysosomal enzymes in this tissue.[85,189] In addition, in the perfused heart, as in liver, insulin withdrawal causes the appearance of autophagic vacoules in electron micrographs.[85] Various observations with inhibitors of lysosomal function also indicate that insulin and amino acids, particularly leucine, inhibit protein degradation in muscle largely by an effect on the lysosomal pathway.[13,175] There is also evidence that the lysosomal proteolysis may be inhibited by insulin in slow-twitch muscle like soleus but not in fast-twitch muscles, where the mechanism of its antiproteolytic effect is still unclear.[188]

Although insulin can rapidly reduce the breakdown of certain cytosolic proteins, this hormone does not inhibit the degradation of myofibrillar proteins in incubated muscles. For example, when added in vitro, insulin failed to reduce N-methylhistidine production by incubated[13,31] or perfused[87,190,191] muscle and heart from starved rats, although it did decrease overall protein breakdown, as shown by a diminished release of tyrosine. Refeeding fasted rats with a complete diet decreased myofibrillar proteolysis[190,192] provided that proteins or amino acids were included in the test meal.[193] In contrast, refeeding with carbohydrate alone raised insulin but did not retard myofibrillar protein degradation.[193] These refeeding studies argue that hormonal and/or nutritional factors other than insulin are involved in the regulation of myofibrillar protein degradation. Lysosomal proteases cannot degrade myofibrillar proteins[87]; thus the lack of an effect of insulin on myofibrillar proteolysis in vitro[31,87,190,191] may be expected. Other studies have confirmed that actin and other myofibrillar components are degraded by the ATP-ubqiuitin-proteasome pathway.[29] Many studies that have examined the effect of insulin on incubated or perfused muscles have involved relatively short periods of incubation—i.e. less than 2 to 4 h. However, insulin treatment for 3 days in insulopenic[92] or burn-injured[95] rats reduced muscle proteolysis, as well as reducing Ub-protein conjugation and mRNA levels for certain components of the Ub-proteasome pathway. Thus sustained treatment with insulin in vivo can inhibit muscle protein breakdown via the Ub-proteasome pathway. In isolated C2C12 cells, insulin and IGF-1 prevent the induction of the Ub-ligases atrogin-1 and MuRF-1, and this effect is associated with a prolonged retardation of proteolysis (evident up to 18 h after treatment). Also, these growth factors and activation of the AKt pathway can reduce atrogin-1 levels in these cells within 2 h.[163] Thus, insulin has coordinated effects on both lysosmal and Ub-proteasome pathways. In addition, in the whole organism, the systemic effects of low insulin states such as fasting or diabetes include muscle wasting, which is principally due to acclerated proteolysis via the Ub-proteasome pathway.[143,194] It is now clear that raised levels of glucocorticoids contribute to the activation of the Ub-proteasome pathway and are required for muscle wasting in fasting[93] and diabetes[92] (see below).

The ability of insulin to reduce net proteolysis is demonstrable when glucose is not in the medium, and thus proteolysis is not dependent on enhanced glucose uptake.[26] In addition, glucose by itself can inhibit protein degradation in isolated muscles[26] and in liver[195] without affecting overall protein synthesis. This effect of glucose in muscle is not simply due to the need to supply energy to the tissue, since fatty acids or ketone bodies do not reduce proteolysis[26] despite their rapid oxidation. Therefore elevated plasma levels of insulin and glucose following food intake together promote the accumulation of amino acids in muscle.

Growth Hormone and Insulin-like Growth Factors

It has long been known that hypophysectomy of young animals prevents normal body growth, including that of skeletal muscle. In muscles from hypophysectomized animals, rates of protein synthesis and tissue RNA content are markedly reduced below levels in normal muscles.[187,196,197] When hypophysectomized animals are treated with growth hormone, overall body growth is reinitiated and rates of protein synthesis in leg muscles increase. This anabolic effect has led to the clinical use of cloned human growth hormone. Pharmacologic levels of this hormone can promote positive nitrogen balance in sepsis and following major injury.[78] However, rates of protein breakdown are also reduced in muscles of hypophysectomized animals, and treatment with growth hormone fails to increase proteolysis.[187,196,197] Subsequent studies have shown that a lack of thyroid hormone is responsible for the decrease in muscle protein breakdown after hypophysectomy (see "Thyroid Hormones," below).

The polypeptide IGFs, IGF-I and IGF-II, are known to have growth-promoting activity when added to cultured cells. Investigations of the effects of IGFs on nonmuscle cells in culture (fibroblasts, myoblasts, chondrocytes, adipocytes) have shown that they stimulate cell division and related processes, including increased amino acid uptake and net protein accumulation.[198,199] The circulating level of IGF-I correlates with body growth, and growth hormone stimulates its synthesis by liver[200]; however, IGF-I production also depends on insulin levels and nutritional status.[201] While IGF-I has a well-defined role as a mediator of growth hormone's actions and has well-documented insulin-like effects, IGF-II appears to be less potent and its in vivo role has been studied less extensively. In hypopituitary dwarfism,[202] starvation,[203] dietary protein deficiency,[202,204] and diabetes,[205] the blood levels of IGFs are low and normal growth of muscle and other tissues ceases. Muscle is a major source of IGF-I and produces two isoforms. The first resembles the liver form of IGF-I, but the second, also known as mechano-growth factor (MGF), has a different 3' exon sequence. MGF is thought to have a paracrine or autocrine action, but in fact mRNA levels for both transcripts are increased in response to mechanical stimuli such as stretch and electrical stimulation.[206] Muscles undergoing work-induced hypertrophy synthesize increased amounts of IGF-I.[207] In addition virally mediated gene transfer of IGF-I in mice led to local hypertrophy due to a combination of increased size of differentiated muscle fibers and proliferation of muscle satellite cells.[208]

The actions of IGFs are modulated by a number of extracellular binding proteins (IGFBPs). A variety of IGFBPs are expressed by different tissues, and these proteins bind both IGF and components of the extracellular matrix.[209] Their role is often unclear but may include inhibiting degradation of IGF in the extracellular space and stabilizing the concentration of IGF near its target receptor on the cell surface. Skeletal muscle secretes primarily IGFBPs 2, 4, and 5,[209] and levels of mRNA for some or all of these are regulated under a variety of conditions. A fall in IGFBP-5 mRNA level is a feature of the response to starvation,[125] overloading muscle causes an increase in IGFBP-4 but a decrease in IGFBP-5 mRNA levels, and unweighting causes an increase in IGFBP-5 mRNA levels.[210] The potential importance of the interaction between the IGFBPs and the extracellular matrix can be seen in experiments such as those using cultured smooth muscle cells, in which the binding of IGFBP-5 to vitronectin in the matrix was shown to enhance the anabolic response to IGF-I; but a mutant IGFBP-5, which did not bind vitronectin, had no such effect.[211] In addition, the potential anabolic effects of infused recombinant IGF in cancer cachexia and starvation can be enhanced by administering IGF with IGFBP-3.[212–214] However, the relative local concentrations of IGF and its binding proteins are likely to be critical in enhancing or blocking the effects of IGF-I. A reduction in IGF-I mRNA levels and an increase in transcription of IGFBP-3 in vascular smooth muscle cells has been shown to be induced by tumor necrosis factor alpha (TNF-α); this has been suggested as an important contributory factor in the pathogenesis of atherosclerotic plaques.[215]

Growth failure of diabetic rats can be overcome by infusion of IGF-I, even though IGF-I, unlike insulin, does not normalize blood glucose levels.[216] In common with insulin, IGFs enhance protein synthesis by activating the PI3 kinase/AKt/mTOR pathway which acclerates the initiation of translation.[217] Previous reports of a central role for calcium/calcineurin–mediated signaling in skeletal muscle hypertophy have not been confirmed,[218] and indeed this signaling pathway is inhibited by IGF-I.[217] It remains possible that the calcium/calcineurin pathway has a more prominent role in hypertophy of cardiac muscle cells, as blocking the L-type calcium channels in these cells completely inhibited IGF-I–induced hypertrophy.[219] In addition to enhancing protein synthesis, IGF-I and IGF-II inhibit protein breakdown in rat myoblasts[220] and reduce the rate of protein breakdown by 20 to 30 percent in isolated mature muscles.[221] The increase in protein degradation in isolated muscles following burn injury can be reversed by IGF-I in a dose-dependent manner.[222] However, this effect was not seen in muscles from septic animals, where IGF-I increased protein synthesis but had no effect on protein degradation rates.[223] The inhibition of protein breakdown by IGF-I is thought to involve a suppression of the lysosomal process, as shown previously for insulin. However, recent evidence suggests that IGF-I, but not growth hormone, can reduce mRNA levels for components of the Ub-proteasome pathway, and this might be an additional mechanism to reduce proteolysis.[146] Evidence against this suggestion comes from one study of incubated muscles from septic rats, where mRNA levels for Ub and $E2_{14K}$ were reduced by administration of IGF-I but no parallel reduction in proteolysis was demonstrated.[224]

Thyroid Hormones

The fall in muscle protein breakdown after hypophysectomy appears to result from the low levels of thyroid hormone in these animals.[187,197] Treatment of hypophysectomized rats with either thyroxine (T_4) or triiodothyronine (T_3) increases rates of protein degradation to levels seen in normal animals. This effect of T_3 requires 2 days, which is similar to the lag time seen in many other responses induced by these hormones. The stimulation of proteolysis in skeletal muscle must be a normal, physiologic action of thyroid hormones, since thyroidectomy also decreases protein breakdown.[196] Protein turnover in liver seems to be regulated in a similar fashion, but no increase in protein degradation in cardiac muscle was found upon thyroid hormone treatment.[225] Though thyroid hormones in large doses are catabolic to skeletal muscle, they increase the workload on the heart and can even induce cardiac hypertrophy. Cardiac hypertrophy induced by thyroid hormones may involve reduced proteolysis, and thus the effects of thyroid hormone on protein turnover in the heart may not be directly comparable to those in skeletal muscle. It is interesting that treatment of rats with T_3 increases protein synthesis in muscle to approximately the same extent as growth hormone. However, treatment of hypophysectomized rats with growth hormone is more effective in inducing growth than T_3 or T_4, probably because growth hormone enhances protein synthesis without also increasing protein breakdown.[187]

One clinically important aspect of thyroid hormone action is that in high and low doses, these agents have opposite effects on body growth. A minimal level of T_3 is essential for the growth of muscle and other tissues, and lack of normal levels of thyroid hormone during early human development leads to dwarfism and mental retardation. By contrast, excessive amounts of the thyroid hormones, as in thyrotoxicosis, lead to a general loss of body weight and severe muscle wasting. Experiments with isolated muscles[187,196] have led to the conclusion that physiologic levels of thyroid hormones induce growth because they stimulate protein synthesis more than they promote breakdown in muscle, whereas high (pharmacologic) doses of T_4 increase rates of protein degradation more than protein synthesis. Thyroid hormones enhance protein breakdown in muscle by activation of both the lysosomal and the nonlysosomal ATP-dependent pathways. Following hypophysectomy, both ATP-dependent and lysosomal proteolysis is reduced, and, for example, the normal activation of lysosomes, induced by lack of insulin and amino acids, is inhibited.[226,227] However, the reduction in both the lysosomal and the ATP-dependent components is eliminated after T_3 treatment of hypophysectomized animals.

Hypophysectomy or thyroidectomy alone cause a 50 percent decrease in the content of the lysosomal proteases cathepsin B and D in skeletal muscle and liver,[228] and the enhancement of protein degradation induced by thyroid hormones is associated with a coincidental two- to threefold increase in the content of these lysosomal proteases in skeletal muscle.[228] In addition, thyroid hormones influence the levels of a variety of lysosomal hydrolases in tissues, including muscle and liver, and these enzymes are implicated in other features of hypothyroidism, such as the accumulation of mucopolysaccharides in the skin (i.e., pretibial myxedema) and the increase in cholesterol esters in the serum.[228,229] The ATP-dependent Ub-proteasome pathway is also regulated by thyroid hormones and is probably responsible for the majority of the increase in proteolysis induced by excess thyroid hormone. This is demonstrated by the dramatic inhibition (up to 70 percent) of the acceleration in proteolysis induced by thyroid hormone due to treatment with proteasome inhibitors.[132] Also, the total proteasome content of skeletal muscle falls 50 percent upon hypophysectomy, and in hypothyroid rats, muscle contains reduced levels of protein-Ub conjugates.[230] However, the levels of Ub conjugates are increased to normal by treating the animals with thyroid hormone.[230]

There is some evidence to suggest that thyroid hormones do not activate Ca^{2+}-dependent proteolysis in muscle, as the capacity of Ca^{2+}-dependent proteases in isolated muscle and muscle homogenates is actually substantially higher after hypophysectomy.[231] Furthermore, T_3 treatment of the hypophysectomized rats promotes overall protein breakdown but does not increase the capacity for the Ca^{2+}-dependent process.[226] However, studies on cultured chick muscle cells exposed to physiologic levels of T_4 or T_3 showed that calpain activity was increased by either treatment.[232] The same experiments also showed that T_3, but not T_4, activates both the proteasome and cathepsin D but not cathepsins B or L.

Newer experimental techniques are now revealing more about the complex actions of thyroid hormone on muscle. A recent study of the transcriptional adaptations induced in muscle in five individuals after treatment with thyroid hormone for 2 weeks showed that mRNAs for 380 genes are increased and are decreased for only 2. The functions of the regulated genes included modulating energy metabolism and protein turnover, and several mRNAs for protesome subunits were significantly increased, consistent with previous evidence that thyroid hormone activates this pathway. In addition, genes involved in many other cellular functions were also increased, including components of the cytoskeleton, which may influence muscle remodeling, and several genes involved in transcriptional control of gene expression.[233]

Glucocorticoids and Nutritional Status

Another class of hormones that markedly influence muscle size are the glucocorticoids. For example, the overproduction of adrenal steroids in Cushing's syndrome or the high levels used clinically often lead to marked muscle weakness and wasting. Glucocorticoids act in several ways to retard growth and to promote the release of amino acids from muscle. These include decreasing DNA[234] and protein synthesis,[235–240] and reducing amino acid uptake by muscle.[236] Such growth-limiting effects on protein and DNA synthesis occur with normal circulating concentrations of glucocorticoids and are reversed in muscle upon adrenalectomy.[187] Experiments to determine the actions of glucortcoids on muscle protein metabolism have often yielded conflicting results and, as detailed below, the effects of glucocorticoids are modified by the influence of hormones such as insulin, nutritional intake, and time course of elevation of glucocorticoids level.

Recent studies have shown that the effects of glucocorticoids on protein degradation in muscle are highly dependent on food intake. In fact, these experiments suggest that in fed animals administered cortisol, a fall in protein synthesis is the primary cause of muscle protein loss, and protein degradation is not necessarily elevated. Early isotopic studies in intact animals suggested that cortisol stimulates breakdown of soluble and contractile proteins in muscle[235]; accordingly, some studies have demonstrated increased N-methylhistidine excretion.[239,241] However, several other groups have failed to observe a significant stimulation of proteolysis in muscle with either in vivo or in vitro approaches, and in some studies, glucocorticoids have appeared to inhibit protein breakdown.[237,238]

By contrast, in the fasted state, glucocorticoids play an important physiologic role in promoting the net breakdown of muscle protein, and this response appears important in the regulation of blood glucose. The classic studies by Long and others[187,242] demonstrated that adrenalectomized animals cannot maintain blood glucose levels in fasting. When fasted, these animals show a dramatic reduction in urea production, which indicates a failure in gluconeogenesis from endogenous protein reserves. The glucocorticoids thus appear to have important actions in facilitating the mobilization of amino acids from peripheral tissue proteins, and this complements the other permissive actions of cortisol in enhancing gluconeogenesis in liver and kidney. In the fed state, rates of protein degradation appear similar in normal and adrenalectomized animals. Although, when normal rats are deprived of food, protein breakdown in muscle rises, no such increase occurs in adrenalectomized rats. In other words, glucocorticoids seem to be required for the acceleration of protein breakdown during fasting. Accordingly, when fasting adrenalectomized rats were treated with cortisol, proteolysis increased in their muscles, as occurs in muscles of normal rats during fasting. By contrast, the reduction in protein synthesis after food deprivation does not require the adrenal hormones and occurs in adrenalectomized animals.[187]

The influence of nutritional intake on the effects of glucocorticoids on muscle protein metabolism suggests that other hormones, such as insulin, present in higher circulating levels in the fed state, might antagonize the effects of glucocorticoids. This was confirmed when experiments with muscles removed from fasted adrenalectomized animals showed that insulin can prevent the increase in proteolysis normally seen with glucocorticoids.[243] These interactions of insulin and cortisol may be useful to the organism in stress in ensuring that the release of steroids does not cause an inappropriate breakdown of muscle protein while on a nutritionally adequate diet.

Very high doses of glucocorticoids can accelerate muscle protein breakdown even in the fed state[187,244]; however, the acute effects of excessive doses of glucocortoids on muscle protein metabolism appear to differ from those of more prolonged exposure. Thus, labeled amino acid infusion studies in humans treated with high-dose prednisolone for 3 days showed raised protein breakdown[245] with no clear effect on protein synthesis. In rats treated with corticosterone for up to 5 days, proteolysis was increased initially in both fast-twitch EDL and slow-twitch soleus, but proteolysis rates declined in soleus and were not elevated after 4 days of treatment,[246] consistent with the observation that, in general, pale (glycolytic) muscle fibers appear more sensitive to the catabolic effects of glucocorticoids than dark (oxidative) fibers.[235] However, in patients with established Cushing's syndrome studied before and after treatment, whole-body leucine oxidation was not elevated, but leucine incorporation into protein was reduced in the untreated state, suggesting that the predominant effect of prolonged glucocorticoids excess is a reduction in protein synthesis.[247]

The accelerated proteolysis due to glucocorticoids is largely due to activation of the Ub-proteasome pathway in muscle. In fasting-related muscle atrophy, accelerated proteolysis is principally due to ATP-dependent proteolysis,[11] and this accelerated ATP-dependent proteolysis is substantially dependent on the presence of glucocorticoids. Thus muscles from fasted adrenalectomized rats exhibited lower levels of ATP-dependent proteolysis and protein-Ub conjugates and polyubiquitin mRNA than control fasted animals.[93,194] Furthermore, the treatment of adrenalectomized rats with dexamethasone rapidly restored both Ub mRNA levels and proteolysis rates to normal.[93] In other studies, treatment of rats with dexamethasone induced loss of muscle mass and substantial increases in mRNAs for polyubiquitin and several Ub-conjugating enzymes.[146] In tissue culture, dexamethasone treatment of C2C12 or L6 myotubes induced increases in mRNA for Ub and other Ub-proteasome pathway components.[241,248] In addition, the transcriptional activation of the Ub-proteasome pathway by dexamethasone can be reversed by treatment with IGF-1.[146] It should be noted that in human studies, no increase in transcripts for proteolytic pathway components have been demonstrated, whether after short exposure to high-dose prednisolone, which induces proteolysis,[245] or in those with untreated Cushing's disease.[249]

There is also evidence for glucocorticoid activation of other proteolytic pathways, but these appear to have a minor role in overall proteolysis. Wang et al. used protease inhibitors to show some increase in calcium-dependent proteolysis,[248] and the same authors also recorded a rise in mRNA for cathepsin B in L6 myotubes treated with dexamethasone. Others have reported increased cathepsin L early after treatment of rats with dexamethasone.[250]

Experiments to define the effects of glucocorticoids on protein synthesis have identified that these hormones impair protein translation and ribosome biogenesis by inhibiting phosphorylation and activation of p70 S6 kinase.[251] Simultaneously, glucocorticoids induce dephosphorylation and increased levels of the translation suppressor protein 4EBP-1.[251] Thus glucocorticoids directly antagonize the effects of insulin and nutrients such as leucine on protein synthesis[169,252] and, in one study, the actions of glucocorticoids on protein synthesis were reversed by oral leucine supplements.[251] Thus insulin and branched-chain amino acids such as leucine have opposing actions to glucocorticoids, with regard to both proteolysis and protein synthesis in muscle. Controlling for these confounding effects is difficult and may explain the inconsistency in the results of experiments attempting to define the true role of glucocorticoids in this tissue.

The sensitivity of tissues to the action of glucocorticoids is dependent on their expression of the glucocorticoid receptor (GR) and the enzyme 11β-hydroxysteroid dehydrogenase (11βHSD), which colocalizes with GR and whose main function is to convert inactive cortisone to active cortisol. Recent studies in muscle demonstrated that glucocorticoids regulate both GR and 11βHSD in opposing ways. Cortisol suppresses expression of the active GR isoform (GRα) but increases expression of the truncated GR (GRβ), which inhibits cortisol binding to GRα. However, in addition, there is glucocorticoid-dependent activation of 11βHSD. In the presence of serum, insulin does not alter expression of GR but does reduce expression and activity of 11βHSD and thus antagonizes the glucocorticoid activation of 11βHSD. However, in the absence of serum, insulin has the opposite effect and downregulates 11βHSD. The active component of serum that alters the effects of insulin has not been identified, but these studies illustrate another level at which the actions of glucocorticoids and insulin interact with opposing effects.[253]

In addition to fasting, glucocorticoids are also important for the increase in proteolysis seen in other physiologic or pathologic states. The increased protein breakdown occurring in the muscles of rats with metabolic acidosis,[254,255] diabetes,[92] and sepsis[256] is dependent on this class of hormone. However, the accelerated proteolysis and atrophy in a denervated muscle is not prevented in adrenalectomized animals.[235]

Table 23-3 summarizes the major endocrine and nutrient factors that can influence protein turnover in skeletal muscle.

Other Hormones Implicated in Regulating Muscle Protein Metabolism

Angiotensin II. Muscle wasting occurs in conditions such as chronic heart failure and chronic renal failure, in which the renin-angiotensin system is activated. Angiotensin II increases cardiac protein synthesis[257] and infusion of angiotensin II causes cardiac muscle hypertrophy.[258] Inhibition of the cardiac hypertrophy induced by elevated circulating levels of angiotensin II in cardiac failure is thought to be one of the major reasons for the protective role of drugs that inhibit angiotensin-converting enzyme or angiotensin II receptor in congestive cardiac failure.[259] However, there is conflicting evidence for the role of angiotensin II in modulating skeletal muscle protein metabolism. In one study, rats infused with angiotensin II suffered muscle weight loss and had significantly elevated muscle protein degradation rates as well as lower circulating levels of IGF-1.[258] However, in another study in rats of similar size, blocking of angiotensin II markedly impaired the skeletal muscle hypertrophy response to overloading, and infusion of angiotensin II rescued this response.[260]

Catecholamines. Catecholamines released from the adrenal medulla or from adrenergic nerve endings can exert an anabolic effect on muscle principally by reducing the Ca^{2+}-dependent proteolysis[261,262] but also by increasing protein synthesis. The anabolic effect of catecholamines is also mimicked by the adrenergic β2 agonist clenbuterol. Treatment of rats with clenbuterol for 10 days induced marked gain in muscle weight,[263] and 20 days' treatment of broiler chickens increased carcass and muscle weights by 6 to 22 percent.[264] Furthermore, clenbuterol can inhibit wasting due to hindlimb suspension[265] or denervation[168] in rats and can also attenuate cachexia after scald injury.[266] Conversely, overactivity of the adrenergic system may contribute to negative energy balance by accelerating metabolic rate and increasing energy demands leading to loss of muscle protein. For this reason β-adrenergic blockade with propranolol was used to reduce protein loss in children after severe burn injury.[267]

Testosterone. The increased secretion of testosterone in males at puberty is thought to determine the increased skeletal muscle mass that occurs at this stage in development and is maintained into adult life. However, in humans, evidence for sustained gender differences in muscle protein metabolism in adulthood is lacking.[268] Nevertheless, suppressing testosterone in healthy young men reduces fat-free mass and fractional muscle protein synthesis, and androgen supplementation to normal physiologic levels in androgen-deficient men leads to increased muscle mass and strength.[269] There is some evidence for the use of testosterone to reverse the loss of muscle mass and strength that occurs in normal aging in males.[269] The potential therapeutic use of testosterone has also been explored in a number of studies. In human immunodeficiency virus (HIV)–infected men with weight loss and low testosterone levels, testosterone supplements led to a 30 percent improvement in strength,[270] and two weekly injections of testosterone after severe burn injury reduced muscle

Table 23-3. THE INFLUENCE OF NUTRIENTS AND HORMONES ON PROTEIN TURNOVER IN SKELETAL MUSCLE

	Protein Synthesis	Protein Degradation	Net Effect
Nutrients			
Leucine	Increase	Decrease	Anabolic
Glucose	No change	Decrease	Anabolic
Hormones			
Insulin	Increase	Decrease	Anabolic
IGF-1	Increase	Decrease	Anabolic
Growth hormone	Increase	No change	Anabolic
Triiodothyronine			
Euthyroid	Increase	Increase	Anabolic
Hyperthyroid	Increase	Increase	Catabolic
Glucocorticoids			
Fed, low dose	Decrease	No change	Catabolic
Fed, high dose	Decrease	Increase	Catabolic
Fasted	Decrease	Increase	Catabolic

loss by improving the efficiency of protein synthesis and reducing degradation rates of muscle protein.[271]

Other hormones. Few studies have been done to establish whether other hormones with a role in control of nutrient metabolism, such as leptin, have a direct effect on muscle protein metabolism. The mRNA and protein levels of leptin increase rapidly in response to increased levels of UDP-N-acetylglucosamine (UDP-GlcNAc) in fat and muscle, and this nutrient-sensing pathway is activated by hyperglycemia or hyperlipidemia.[272] However, circulating leptin induces its own expression in muscle while suppressing further expression in fat tissue.[273] Leptin has many insulin-like effects on muscle glucose metabolism.[274] However, in one study, leptin infusion reduced labeled leucine incorporation into muscle, but muscles incubated with leptin in the medium did not have altered rates of protein synthesis or degradation, suggesting that any effect of circulating leptin may be indirect.[275]

NUTRITIONAL FACTORS AFFECTING PROTEIN BALANCE IN MUSCLE

Short-Term Fasting

As discussed earlier, complete food deprivation leads to a mobilization of body protein reserves to support the energy requirements of animals and humans. However, the changes in muscle protein metabolism in fasting occur in at least two phases. An early event in fasting is increased amino acid release from skeletal muscle, which results from a decrease in protein synthesis and from a marked rise in protein degradation.[26,276–279] However, during prolonged fasting of humans or animals, protein degradation in muscle actually may fall below the rate observed in the fed state (see "Long-Term Fasting," below). Within 24 to 48 h of fasting in humans, urinary nitrogen excretion rises, and net protein degradation in muscle seems to increase substantially when evaluated by forearm arteriovenous differences in amino acid release.[276] Likewise, in young rats, increased protein degradation within the initial period of fasting has been shown in skeletal muscles incubated in vitro[26,277] and by a variety of in vivo approaches.[278, 279] These adaptive changes in muscle protein metabolism seem to result from the low level of circulating insulin, although glucocorticoids also play an essential permissive role for the increased proteolysis (see above).

One expected consequence of the low insulin levels of fasting animals is an increase in intralysosomal proteolysis (i.e., in autophagic vacuole formation) in muscle. There is evidence for changes in lysosomal function accompanying the early rise in muscle protein degradation in fasting. In incubated muscles[13] and in perfused hindlimbs[87] from fasted animals, inhibitors of lysosomal proteases cause a greater absolute reduction in protein breakdown in fasted than fed rats. Under these conditions, the total tissue content of lysosomal proteases does not change.[227] Thus, increased access of substrate proteins to the lysosomal enzymes—in other words, autophagic vacuole formation—seems to be the most likely mechanism. There are excellent morphologic data that the accelerated proteolysis in the liver induced by fasting occurs largely in lysosomes.[16] However, studies reveal that even in the presence of lysosomal inhibitors, a large part of the increase in overall proteolysis in incubated muscles from fasted rats remains unaffected.[12] Addition of agents that inhibit Ca^{2+}-dependent proteases also has no effect on the rise in overall proteolysis induced by fasting. Only depletion of ATP in these muscles with 2,4-dinitrophenol and 2-deoxyglucose eliminates the increased proteolysis due to fasting. Furthermore, refeeding of the animals abolishes this difference in the ATP-dependent process.[11] These data—in conjunction with the finding that fasting leads to a preferential increase in the degradation of myofibrillar proteins,[190,193] which is not blocked by lysosomal inhibitors[87,193,277]—suggest that activation of the ATP-Ub–dependent proteolytic pathway in muscle must be primarily responsible for the increased protein degradation in short-term fasting.

Subsequent studies investigated the nature of the ATP-dependent pathway responsible for most of the accelerated muscle proteolysis during fasting-induced atrophy.[11,93] These experiments have shown that after 48 h of food deprivation, the levels of total Ub mRNA in hindlimb muscles increase fourfold over levels in fed control animals. When the fasted rats are refed, the content of Ub mRNA in their muscles returns to normal levels within 24 h. This rise and fall in the amount of Ub mRNA parallels the changes in overall[192,277] and ATP-dependent[11,12] protein breakdown in the muscle. Expression of other components of the ATP-Ub–dependent pathway also increases during fasting, in parallel with changes in Ub mRNA, and mRNAs for several of the 20- to 30-kDa subunits of the 20S proteasome. More recent microarray studies have confirmed that many but not all 20S proteasome subunits and many subunits of the 19S proteasome regulatory particle are increased coordinately.[125]

In addition to their increased levels of specific mRNAs, muscles from fasted animals contain higher amounts of proteins conjugated to Ub than muscles of fed controls.[11,194] This finding suggested an increased rate of Ub conjugation in muscle during fasting, and it correlated with the activation of the ATP-Ub–dependent pathway in the isolated muscles. It is noteworthy that this rise in Ub-conjugate formation occurs in the myofibrillar fraction of total muscle protein,[194] whose degradation requires the nonlysosomal ATP-dependent pathway,[31,87] but it does not appear in the soluble cytosolic fraction. A rise in the activity of the ATP-dependent proteases in muscle may also occur during fasting. For example, a twofold increase in ATP-Ub–dependent hydrolysis of endogenous muscle proteins and of exogenous radioactive protein substrates (e.g., casein) was demonstrated in soluble extracts of skeletal muscle from fasted rabbits.[243] Presumably this increased proteolytic activity occurs because of an increase in Ub-conjugating activity in the extracts. As indicated previously, many of these responses to fasting require adrenal steroids. Glucocorticoids are necessary for the activation of the ATP-dependent proteolytic process in fasting but not for the rise in the lysosomal process.[93] Glucocorticoids are also necessary for the accompanying increase in Ub mRNA levels and in the muscle content of Ub-protein conjugates.[11,93]

Further detailed analysis of the transcriptional adaptations occuring in muscles of mice fasted for 48 h has recently been performed using cDNA microarrays.[125] This technique makes possible the simultaneous measurement of changes in mRNA levels for several thousand genes and has revealed a number of important new changes of gene expression that had not been noted before. The microarray study confirmed that fasting induces significant increases in mRNAs for polyubiquitin and many proteasome subunit genes. In addition, there were increases in transcript levels for certain other components of the Ub-proteasome pathway, including one new gene that has subsequently proved to be a new Ub-ligase or E3, called atrogin-1.[151,152] However mRNAs for some proteasome subunits were not differentially expressed for reasons still unclear. Other features of the transcriptome in fasting-induced muscle atrophy include reduced transcripts for many of the enzymes involved in later stages of glycolysis but increases in mRNAs for pyruvate dehydrogenase kinase, which inhibits pyruvate dehydrogenase. There was a reduction in mRNA levels for several extracellular matrix proteins and coordinated changes in mRNAs encoding translation initation factors that might favor translation of a subset of stress-related proteins. These and several other transcriptional adaptations in muscle during fasting confirm the wide-ranging and complex nature of the transcriptional response; though the increase in mRNAs for members of the Ub-proteasome pathway is a prominent feature, it is only one component of this response.

Long-Term Fasting

In prolonged fasting in humans and animals, gluconeogenesis from body proteins and loss of muscle mass is gradually reduced, as suggested by a fall in urinary nitrogen excretion and less amino acid release in limb perfusion studies.[24,276,278] Several factors help reduce glucose needs during fasting, the most important being a decrease in the brain's requirement for glucose, as this organ comes to utilize ketone bodies for a large part of its ATP production. As the use of fuels alternative to glucose increases, the need to utilize amino acids for gluconeogenesis is reduced, and muscle protein breakdown appears to fall below the levels seen early in starvation. Eventually net proteolysis is lower than in the fed state, and this adaptation should help preserve muscle protein content and contractile function. For example, both overall and myofibrillar protein degradation fall by up to 30 percent in incubated[24,227] or perfused[192,280] skeletal muscles within several days of fasting, and the excretion of urinary nitrogen and N-methylhistidine is reduced below levels in fed animals.[24,278,281] In humans, 1 week of fasting is necessary before net muscle proteolysis falls, as indicated by a diminished forearm arteriovenous difference of amino acids and by decreased urinary N-methylhistidine excretion.[276,282] In the absence of such mechanisms to conserve protein, the continual rapid loss of muscle protein and the associated loss of muscle function could presumably become life-threatening.

Multiple proteolytic pathways are suppressed in the muscle of rats fasted for prolonged periods.[227] Coordinate reduction in both the lysosomal and nonlysosomal ATP-dependent processes was found in incubated skeletal muscles after 72 h of food deprivation. Furthermore, the contents of the lysosomal thiol protease cathepsin B1 and of the lysosomal hydrolase N-acetyl-β-D-glucosaminidase fell by 40 to 50 percent in muscles of long-term fasted rats, when protein degradation falls. A very similar reduction in muscle proteolysis is found in animals on a protein-deficient diet and may involve similar mechanisms (see "Protein Deficiency," below). These changes in proteolysis and in lysosomal enzyme activity during long-term fasting, as well as related observations (see below), suggest that the muscles of rats fasted for prolonged periods are similar in many ways to those of thyroidectomized animals.[24,227]

Various factors have been proposed to signal the fall in muscle proteolysis during prolonged fasting, including a decrease in thyroid status,[24,227,282] animal adiposity or size,[192,278,280,281] changes in muscle redox state,[278,283] or the elevation of blood ketones.[276] Obesity in animals, as in humans, reduces the extent of whole-body nitrogen loss and prolongs survival during fasting.[192,280,281] Many indicators of thyroid status fall in animals fasted for 72 h or longer: sodium-dependent respiration in muscle, whole body O_2 consumption, and rectal temperature are reduced,[231,284] as are the total and free concentrations of T_4, T_3, and TSH.[285] Similarly, humans fasted for several days have decreased levels of T_3 and a lowered basal metabolic rate.[282,286,287] Accordingly, restoration of the level of T_3 in fasted humans to values seen in the fed state appeared to increase muscle proteolysis.[282,286] Thus the decrease in T_3 levels may be important for the fall in muscle protein breakdown in prolonged fasting. However, certain features of the fasted state differ from those of hypothyroidism and suggest that reduced thyroid status cannot fully explain the adaptations in muscle protein metabolism during prolonged fasting. For example, obese rats have a marked decrease in urinary N-methylhistidine excretion during prolonged fasting, but T_3 levels in these animals do not fall for a sustained period.[278,281]

Protein Deficiency

The physiologic response to complete food deprivation has been extensively studied, but metabolic adaptations to restricted protein intake with adequate caloric intake are poorly understood. Dietary protein deficiency in humans, referred to as kwashiorkor, is a major health problem worldwide, especially for the newborn and growing child. Animal experiments[42,288] have helped to define certain metabolic alterations in skeletal and cardiac muscle that may help the organism preserve amino acids and body protein during protein deprivation rather than utilizing them for energy production or gluconeogenesis, as occurs in starvation, diabetes, and following trauma.

When young rats are fed a protein-free diet, skeletal muscle mass and protein content stop increasing but are remarkably well preserved. By contrast, other organs, such as the liver, undergo a marked reduction in size. Protein synthesis falls in skeletal muscle of protein-deficient animals,[42,289] and this effect by itself should promote muscle atrophy. However, recent experiments have shown that the rates of protein degradation in incubated skeletal and cardiac muscles[42] and urinary N-methylhistidine excretion[290] also fall 30 to 40 percent within 72 h of feeding a protein-deficient diet. This adaptation accounts for the relative constancy of muscle size. Similarly, a fall in N-methylhistidine excretion has been described in children suffering from protein malnutrition.[291]

In addition, under these conditions, rates of branched-chain amino acid oxidation in skeletal muscle and rates of transport of amino acids into the tissue fall, presumably to help reduce the utilization of amino acids.[42] The de novo synthesis of glutamine and alanine are also reduced,[42] and this change conserves amino acids as well, since these processes are coupled to the irreversible degradation of essential amino acids.

In protein deficiency, muscle protein breakdown falls through a reduced contribution of both the lysosomal and nonlysosomal ATP-dependent pathways to overall proteolysis.[288] These changes resemble the effects of hypothyroidism and of prolonged fasting in muscle (see above).[227] Studies of protein-deficient rats also indicate that a decrease in the proteolytic capacity of the lysosomal system accounts for the reduction in the lysosomal process. Accordingly, skeletal and cardiac muscle show a 50 to 70 percent lower activity of cathepsin B1 and H and several other lysosomal proteases and acid hydrolases during protein deficiency.[288] In addition, the fall in overall protein breakdown and lysosomal enzyme content during protein deprivation follow an identical time course, and they return to normal levels simultaneously upon refeeding a diet containing protein. Protein deficiency was also found to reduce the muscle content of proteasomes by 50 percent or more when measured by a sensitive immunoassay for this ATP-dependent protease complex.[292] A similar decrease in proteasome content in muscle was found following hypophysectomy. Thus in each condition, the proteolytic capacity of the ATP-dependent process in muscle appears to be reduced (see "Thyroid Hormones," above). Additional studies have examined the possible contribution of the Ca^{2+}-dependent proteases to changes in muscle protein breakdown in protein deficiency. However, even though overall proteolysis falls in protein deficiency, the stimulation of muscle proteolysis by Ca^{2+} ionophores and the activity of Ca^{2+}-dependent proteases in tissue extracts increase considerably[17,288] and thus do not correlate with overall protein breakdown. These findings in protein deficiency emphasize the uncertain physiologic significance of the calpains and Ca^{2+}-dependent proteolysis in muscle.[17]

The signals that reduce proteolysis during protein deficiency are unclear. Circulating insulin[293] and blood and tissue leucine[42] concentrations are low in protein-deficient animals, but these changes should stimulate net protein catabolism in muscle (not reduce it). By contrast, the fall in proteolysis and protease content during protein deficiency most closely resembles the effects of thyroidectomy described earlier (decreased proteolysis and reduced protease content). It is noteworthy that plasma T_3 and T_4 concentrations, caloric intake, body temperature, and the contribution of sodium transport to total respiration in the diaphragm are reduced in protein-deficient animals,[231] as occurs in hypothyroidism. Thus normal animals in some way seem to become physiologically hypothyroid during protein deficiency. It should be noted that the adaptations to a protein-deficient diet in healthy individuals may not be preserved under other conditions. Thus, in patients with metabolic acidosis due to renal failure, a low-protein diet exacerbated rather than ameliorated muscle protein catabolism as measured by urinary 3-methyl histidine:creatinine ratio.[294]

There are a number of similarities in the changes in lysosomal and nonlysosomal ATP-dependent proteolysis and lysosomal enzyme activity in muscles of long-term starved and protein-deficient animals. It remains likely that these nutritional states share common signals and mechanisms for reducing proteolysis, as through reduced thyroid status.

MUSCLE ACTIVITY AND THE CONTROL OF PROTEIN METABOLISM

Hypertrophy and Atrophy

It is well established that the pattern of contractile activity influences the size of skeletal muscle as well as many of its fundamental biochemical and physiologic properties.[295] Muscle disuse or denervation leads to marked atrophy,[5,296] while increased work of a muscle, especially if it is isometric, can cause very rapid compensatory growth.[5] For example, if the gastrocnemius muscle in a rat is tenotomized, the remaining soleus muscle, which must support body weight on that side, will increase in size and protein content by about 40 percent within 5 days. Unlike normal developmental growth, this work-induced hypertrophy can be induced in hypophysectomized or diabetic animals and also in fasted animals, which undergo generalized muscle wasting.[5,297] As discussed previously, IGF-I, which mediates the effects of growth hormone in normal growth,[200] is also produced locally in muscle, and its production rises in work-induced hypertrophy[206] even in hypophysectomized animals[207] (see "Growth Hormone and Insulin-like Growth Factors," above). However, work-induced growth can occur independently of growth hormone and insulin, even though these agents and other hormones (e.g., testosterone and thyroid hormones)[5] may influence this growth process in vivo. In fact, exercise has been shown to increase the sensitivity of glucose metabolism in muscle to insulin[298] by increasing expression of components of the insulin-signaling pathway.[299] In addition, exercise activates other parallel signaling pathways in muscle, including mitogen-activated protein kinase pathways.[300,301] The central role for activation of the Akt/mTOR pathway (see above) in skeletal muscle growth and hypertrophy was demonstrated recently when rapamycin inhibited 95 percent of the hypertrophy induced in rat or mouse plantaris by removing ipsilateral gastrocnemius and soleus.[302] The same pathway is also vital for the hypertrophy needed to recover from atrophy after hindlimb suspension.[302] A number of humoral factors in addition to insulin and IGF-1 may modulate the response to disuse or increased work including adrenergic receptors agonists such as clenbuterol (see above).

The increase in muscle weight during hypertrophy reflects a rise in protein content, and experiments with incubated muscles have clearly established that this increase results from greater protein synthesis and more rapid uptake of certain amino acids.[295,296] RNA and DNA synthesis also increase in the tissue, but the significance of these changes is difficult to evaluate, since they occur primarily in interstitial and satellite cells. While some in vivo studies have also indicated reduced proteolysis during rapid hypertrophy of muscle,[5] others have reported no change or, in some instances, enhanced protein breakdown.[296] The importance of reduced proteolysis in vivo during work-induced hypertrophy thus remains uncertain, although it is clear that maintaining muscle under tension at or beyond its resting length reduces protein breakdown in vitro.[28] In various in vivo experiments, muscle stretch has also been shown to stimulate protein synthesis,[303] although similar effects in incubated muscles have not been consistently obtained.[5,105,295] These conflicting results may reflect methodologic differences, species differences, or, more importantly, differences in the experimental models used to induce hypertrophy in muscle, as some models used may induce muscle injury as well as increased workload.

Denervation Atrophy

Muscle atrophy induced by denervation or disuse is associated with increased rates of proteolysis, with little or no apparent changes in overall protein synthesis.[5,31,296] Studies by Goldberg and colleagues of rat muscles undergoing denervation atrophy indicated that the marked increase in protein breakdown is due primarily to increased activity of a nonlysosomal pathway,[11,12,31] which requires ATP. These atrophying muscles show a large increase in the breakdown of myofibrillar proteins, which appears to be specifically catalyzed by the ATP-dependent proteolytic process.[31] Following denervation, levels of mRNA for Ub and for several subunits of the proteasome increase several times over levels in the contralateral innervated muscle.[11] Similarly, the content of Ub and Ub-protein conjugates increases in the denervated muscle by 2 days after nerve section.[194] All of these changes occur simultaneously with the rise in the ATP-dependent degradative process.[11]

In addition, other degradative processes also increase in denervated muscles. Under conditions that activate in vitro the lysosomal and Ca^{2+}-dependent proteolytic processes (i.e., insulin deprivation or addition of a Ca^{2+} ionophore), these processes rise more in muscles undergoing denervation atrophy than in normal muscles. Furthermore, the content of lysosomal proteases increases two- to fourfold after nerve section.[31] Levels of the calpains in muscle also appear to increase following denervation.[304] Since the lysosomal and Ca^{2+}-dependent processes do not appear to participate in the degradation of myofibrillar proteins, these pathways presumably contribute to muscle atrophy by degrading different classes of cellular proteins. Thus, multiple degradative pathways are coordinately regulated in muscle during denervation atrophy and contribute to the increased proteolysis.

Though a variety of proteolytic pathways may have a minor role in denervation atrophy, recent studies demonstrated a central role for the Ub-proteasome pathway and, in particular, two Ub-ligases, atrogin-1 (or MAFbx) and MuRF1, whose expression rose four- to eightfold after denervation or inactivation of muscle.[152] When genes for these proteins were inactivated, mice grew normally; but, on denervation, leg muscles from adult mice lacking the active proteins atrophied 56 percent (atrogin-1) or 36 percent (MuRF1) less than controls. Moreover, animals lacking both these E3s are almost totally resistant to denervation-induced loss of weight and strength.[305] These two genes were targeted because they were identified as transcriptionally activated in muscle atrophy due to denervation, disuse, and unweighting[152]; however, atrogin-1 and MuRF-1 are also transcriptionally activated in many other atrophy states.[151] In fact, atrogin-1 was independently discovered as the gene most dramatically induced upon cancer cachexia and fasting, where it rises even before muscle atrophy is demonstrated. These mRNAs also rise dramatically in limb muscles in the first few days after denervation or disuse induced by spinal section and remain high for 1 to 2 weeks when atrophy is rapid. Atrogin-1 and MuRF-1 mRNAs then fall to control levels, when the process of weight loss slows considerably.[306] Thus, there seem to be two phases of the atrophy process, and genes induced or suppressed during atrophy may appear normal in tissues already atrophied. An important challenge now is to identify what muscle proteins are ubiquitinated by atrogin-1 and MuRF1. Aside from helping us understand the process of muscle atrophy, such information may even suggest new approaches to prevent or reverse the muscle atrophy seen in various pathologic states.

Effects of Calcium and Muscle Length

The biochemical mechanisms by which contractile function or passive stretch alter muscle proteolysis remain largely unknown. Many of the changes occurring in muscle hypertrophy (e.g., accelerated uptake of amino acids) can be mimicked by electrical stimulation or passive stretch of incubated muscles.[5,28,206] As these effects of passive tension in vitro occur in isolated muscles, they do not involve stretch receptors, any associated reflex arcs, or any "trophic substance" released from the motor neuron. The effects of passive tension in vitro are particularly interesting, since passive stretch in vivo can promote net growth of muscle, retard muscle wasting induced by endocrine and nutritional treatments, and even cause hypertrophy of denervated muscle.[5] It seems likely that the crucial factor inducing growth and retarding atrophy in vivo is increased tension resulting from passive stretch or resulting from normal contractions. However, the molecular mechanism by which increased muscle tension results in alterations in protein and amino acid metabolism in this tissue is unclear. When cardiac myocytes are maintained at greater than normal lengths in vitro, they undergo hypertrophy. Very quickly, several early growth-related genes, such as c-*fos* and c-*jun*, are induced, followed by increased actin and myosin synthesis.[307] These studies suggest certain gene promoter regions may contain unique "stretch response elements." These new approaches hold great promise for understanding how muscle tension is transduced to signal the biochemical changes accompanying hypertrophy.

Since calcium is also an essential mediator in the normal coupling of excitation and contraction in muscle, changes in the release or uptake of this ion have been an attractive signal for the regulation of proteolysis during muscle contraction or stretch. In vitro, calcium ionophores (e.g., A23187) activate protein breakdown in isolated muscles.[105,106] Increased external calcium in shortened muscles (but not in muscles maintained at resting length)[13] also signals a rise in intracellular proteolysis,[28] probably by raising cytosolic Ca^{2+}. However, this effect of external Ca^{2+} during muscle shortening may result from an anoxia-induced rise in Ca^{2+} permeability (see below) and is thus of uncertain physiologic significance. Furthermore, this activation of proteolysis in skeletal muscle by Ca^{2+} is not prevented by inhibitors of voltage-dependent Ca^{2+} channels, calmodulin, metalloendoproteases, microtubules, or microfilaments.[308]

Injury or anoxia of incubated muscles (as induced by unrestrained muscle shortening) increases proteolysis by a Ca^{2+}-dependent mechanism.[13,28] ATP depletion also causes proteolysis to rise, but only if Ca^{2+} is present in the medium.[12] Thus the calpain-dependent process may be important in damaged or ischemic tissues. However, degradation of most proteins in muscle maintained at normal length, including actin, is independent of Ca^{2+}[30,31,87] and is not affected by inactivation of calpains.[309] Furthermore, although the response to Ca^{2+} ionophores[30,31,87] and the content of Ca^{2+}-dependent proteases[304] increase in denervated muscles, where overall muscle proteolysis rises, inactivation of Ca^{2+}-activated proteases does not block the accelerated proteolysis caused by denervation[30,31,87] or fasting.[12] In addition, in dietary protein deficiency (see above), the muscle content of the calpains and the sensitivity of proteolysis to calcium ionophores increases, even though overall proteolysis in muscle is suppressed when measured in vitro or in vivo.[288] These findings suggest that under physiologic conditions, the Ca^{2+}-dependent degradative process is unlikely to contribute significantly to overall proteolysis in muscle. On the other hand, the Ca^{2+}-dependent process may be very important in muscle injury, e.g., when ATP levels fall or when membrane permeability to Ca^{2+} increases, and perhaps in muscle diseases such as dystrophy. Also, recently the overexpression of calpastatin, the calpain inhibitor, in vivo has been found to retard disease atrophy.[121] Thus, a critical role of some calpains, perhaps in the degradation of specific muscle components, remains likely.

CYTOKINES AND THE REGULATION OF PROTEIN METABOLISM IN MUSCLE

Sepsis

It is well known that patients with fever, sepsis, and also traumatic injury or burns often suffer severe loss of body protein and a generalized muscle wasting.[310] HIV infection is frequently accompanied by profound muscle atrophy, and this is markedly aggravated by concurrent bacterial infection—for example, by *Mycobacterium* species.[311] A number of observations indicate that the nitrogen loss during sepsis results primarily from accelerated degradation of cell proteins, primarily in skeletal muscle, with normal or even enhanced rates of protein synthesis.[25,312–316] However, others have shown that sepsis also leads to reduced protein synthesis, especially in fast-twitch muscles,[317] due to reduced rates of translation initiation.[317,318] Most of the increase in total protein breakdown in muscle in different animal models of bacterial infection appears to result from enhanced hydrolysis of myofibrillar proteins.[319,320] In humans with sepsis, there is clear evidence of increased muscle proteolysis and net release of amino acids from this tissue.[25] Similarly, in experimental animals, the administration of live *Streptococcus pneumoniae*[315] or *Escherichia coli* endotoxin[312] causes a marked loss of muscle mass, and rapid breakdown of muscle proteins.

Many of the systemic manifestations of infection are mediated by cytokines including interleukin-1 (IL-1)[321] and tumor necrosis factor (TNF),[322] raised levels of which circulate in the blood in various natural infections, including HIV[311] and in fevers induced in laboratory animals (e.g., by endotoxin administration). In addition, IL-1 and TNF have been proposed as the primary mediators for cachexia and shock in gram-negative septicemia.[323–326] Some polypeptide(s) circulating in infected animals can stimulate muscle proteolysis,[327] and a number of experiments have suggested that partially purified preparations of human IL-1 ("leukocyte pyrogen") increased proteolysis in isolated muscle preparations.[313,314,328] However, in vitro muscle experiments using recombinant cytokines failed to demonstrate any catabolic effect of IL-1-α or β,[327,329] TNF,[322,327,329–331] epidermal thymocyte activating factors,[332,333] eosinophil cytoxicity enhancing factor,[334] interferon-α, β, or γ,[335] platelet-derived growth factor,[336] or TGF-α or β.[327,337] In addition, combinations between IL-1 and TNF or IL-1, TNF, and phorbol esters, and also TGF-α, all failed to elicit any increase in protein degradation in isolated muscles.[327] Particularly interesting were the negative results with TNF, a macrophage product proposed to play a critical role in the pathogenesis of fever,[331,338] cachexia,[339,340] and shock.[325,326]

The results of several studies where cytokines were administered in vivo, however, suggested that IL-1 alone[319,341,342] or TNF alone[343–345] can induce increased skeletal muscle proteolysis. In contrast, a number of other groups failed to consistently detect or confirm any effect on muscle proteolysis by either IL-1[327,329,343] or TNF[331,346] when administered to intact animals. The effects on protein synthesis, however, appear to be somewhat more consistent. TNF reduced protein synthesis in myofibrillar and sarcoplasmic fractions.[347] TNF reduced translation initiation in the heart and skeletal muscle by reducing EIF-4E availability.[348] Similarly administration of a TNF-binding protein also reduced the effects of sepsis on protein synthesis and corrected some of the changes in peptide translation initiation.[349] Experiments using an IL-1 receptor antagonist showed that it protected against the sepsis-associated inhibition of protein synthesis and normalized peptide chain initiation.[350–352]

Muscles atrophying due to sepsis undergo accelerated proteolysis via the Ub-proteasome pathway. Studies of isolated skeletal muscles have confirmed that endotoxin injection in vivo enhances proteolysis via a nonlysosomal ATP-dependent proteolytic pathway,[353] with little change in lysosomal and Ca^{2+}-activated proteolytic pathways. Furthermore, in endotoxin-treated rats, rates of ATP-dependent proteolysis correlate closely with Ub mRNA levels.[353] Ub mRNA increased by several times in pale EDL muscles, where ATP-dependent proteolysis rose, but it did not change in dark soleus muscles, in which ATP-dependent proteolytic activity was unchanged.[353] mRNAs for other components of the Ub-proteasome pathway were raised in muscle in experimental models of sepsis[144,145,256,354] and in septic patients.[355] Sepsis increased rates of ubiquitination of muscle proteins,[230] and inhibitors of the proteasome dramatically reduced proteolysis in muscle from septic animals.[132] More recently proteasome inhibitors have been used to prevent total and myofibrillar protein breakdown in a rat model of sepsis.[356]

When given together in vivo, IL-1 and TNF were also found to reproduce all of the effects of endotoxin on protein breakdown in muscle (increased Ub mRNA and increased ATP-dependent proteolysis measured in vitro), whereas neither IL-1 nor TNF administration alone was able to signal such changes, as reported earlier.[327,329,331,346] In addition, pretreatment of endotoxin-injected rats with either an anti-TNF antiserum or an IL-1 receptor antagonist partially inhibited the increase in ATP-dependent proteolysis typically observed in endotoxin-treated animals.[353] Treatment of rats with TNF and IL-1 also increases muscle mRNA levels for polyubiquitin,[357] as did treatment with another cytokine, interferon-γ. However, interleukin-6 (IL-6) did not induce changes in muscle mRNA for Ub 357, and this is consistent with evidence from an IL-6–deficient mouse, which demonstrated that this cytokine is not involved in sepsis-related acceleration in proteolysis.[358] Inhibition of TNF production in sepsis and other conditions may be of benefit in inhibiting muscle wasting, and recent experiments with Torbafylline, a xanthine derivative, demonstrated inhibition of proteolysis via the Ub-proteasome pathway and prevented muscle wasting in a rat model of cancer cachexia and in sepsis.[359]

Both IL-1 and/or TNF elicit the release of prostaglandin E2 from muscle.[326,329] Even though prostaglandin E2 had been proposed to be critical for increased muscle proteolysis in septic models,[312,313,315] no decrease in ATP-dependent proteolysis[353] or in Ub mRNA levels[353] occurred in muscles from endotoxin-treated rats that received naproxen, a potent inhibitor of prostaglandin E2 production. Therefore prostaglandins are not necessary for the rise in muscle proteolysis during infection.

Though they contribute little to overall proteolysis, other pathways, in addition to the Ub-proteasome pathway, may still have a role in muscle wasting in sepsis. Increased mRNA levels for cathespin B and m-calpain have been found in muscle after a prolonged septic episode,[97] and others have demonstrated a calcium-dependent release of myofibrillar proteins, possibly due to activity of Ca^{2+}-activated proteases at the Z band, which is disrupted in muscles from septic animals.[122]

Another possible signal for increased proteolysis in muscle during systemic infection is fever. Studies of the influence of temperature on protein degradation and synthesis in isolated muscles demonstrated a linear increase in the rate of proteolysis from 33 to 42°C, whereas protein synthesis was relatively unchanged.[360] In addition, the catabolic effects of leukocyte pyrogen were even larger in muscles treated at 39 than at 37°C.[313] The proteolytic system, which is activated by elevated temperature, is insensitive to lysosomal protease inhibitors[360] and seems to be primarily the ATP-dependent pathway.[353] Therefore, in febrile animals, the rise in body temperature induced by cytokines and their direct catabolic effects on skeletal muscle appear to act synergistically to induce amino acid release and to promote muscle wasting. This increased rate of proteolysis in muscle may account for the worsening of various neuromuscular symptoms (e.g., in myasthenia gravis) during febrile illness.

The discrepancies in the experimental results obtained in relation to muscle metabolism after administration of TNF and other cytokines have been the subject of considerable debate. Differences may arise because of variation in the timing or amount of administered doses, and experimental use of cytokines derived from one species (e.g., human or mouse) may not share the same affinity for receptors in the host (e.g., rat). Studies in sepsis have shown that glucocorticoids are required for full activation of the Ub-proteasome pathway and accelerated proteolysis,[256] and the effects of interaction between different procachexia cytokines and other hormones such as glucocorticoids, insulin, or IGF-1 are difficult to control and may also lead to variation in results. Even in tissue culture, different groups have had conflicting results. Li et al. added TNF to myotubes derived from C2C12 cells and rat primary muscle cultures and demonstrated time- and concentration-dependent loss of protein and reduction in heavy-chain myosin content.[361] However, others showed that though TNF disrupted the normal myocyte differentiation program, it had no effect on more mature myotubes,[362] and coadministration of IFN-γ was required before myosin heavy-chain protein levels were reduced.[363] Another study revealed two distinct effects of TNF on C2C12 myotubes in culture. At low doses TNF caused a reduction in protein content, but at higher doses an anabolic effect was observed, with an increase in protein synthesis and reduction in proteolysis.[364] Although cultured myocytes offer many advantages for studies of growth and development, such cultures can be problematic for studies of atrophy or cytokine actions due to variations in the nature and composition of serum and the fact that most cultures are heterogeneous mixtures of myoblasts and myotubes, which differ in composition and receptor content from each other and from mature muscles.

Cancer Cachexia

Marked muscle wasting and generalized cachexia are common and debilitating features of advanced cancer. There are probably many contributing factors to cachexia in cancer, including reduced food intake, altered metabolic rate, endocrine abnormalities, and the effects of anticancer treatments, but various cytokines and other circulating factors that may play a role have also been identified, including TNF, IL-1, IL-6, and IFN-γ.[365] In rats bearing the Yoshida ascites hepatoma, a model of the tumor-bearing state, severe muscle wasting occurs, mediated by TNF and resulting primarily from an increased rate of proteolysis, as shown in incubated muscles.[366] Furthermore in muscles of rats bearing the Yoshida tumor, an ATP-dependent proteolytic pathway is activated, and there are increased levels of mRNAs for Ub and subunits of the proteasome increase, especially in the pale muscle fibers, which atrophy most profoundly.[96] Most other animal tumors that cause cachexia are also associated with activation of the Ub-proteasome pathway in muscle. However, additional proteolytic pathways may also be activated and different cytokines or other circulating factors are frequently implicated in the genesis of cachexia.[365]

One other factor implicated in some types of cancer cachexia is proteolysis-inducing factor (PIF). This was first identified in mice with the MAC 16 tumor and, when injected into healthy mice, produced profound weight loss.[367] PIF is reported to be a glycoprotein which, when purified, induces catabolism in muscle cells[368] and activates the Ub-proteasome pathway in muscle.[369] PIF has also been found in urine of a large proportion of patients with weight loss due to pancreatic cancer,[370] and treatment with eicosapentaenoic acid, which blocks formation of 15-hydroxyeicosatetraenoic acid by PIF in muscle cells, inhibits weight loss even in those with advanced disease.[371]

A General Program for Muscle Atrophy

Similar cellular mechanisms seem to underly the muscle atrophy seen in fasting, denervation, and a variety of other catabolic states, including cancer, chronic uremia, acquired immunodeficiency syndrome (AIDS), sepsis, diabetes mellitus, and hyperthyroidism.[8,372] In some of these conditions (e.g., in fasting or following cortisol treatment), overall protein synthesis falls, but in all, a clear rise in protein degradation also occurs and is critical to muscle wasting. In fact, after denervation, or in acidotic, tumor-bearing, or endotoxin-treated animals, muscles show a large enhancement of proteolysis with relatively little change in protein synthesis. The acceleration of protein degradation is due largely to activation of the ATP-dependent Ub-proteasome pathway in skeletal muscle. The activity of this proteolytic process appears to be precisely regulated in muscle by hormones (e.g., glucocorticoids), nutritional factors (e.g., caloric and protein intake), and cytokines (e.g., IL-1 and TNF). Common features in atrophying muscles include increased rates of Ub conjugation to muscle proteins and transcriptional regulation of essential components of the Ub-proteasome pathway; in particular, the dramatic transcriptional induction of atrogin-1 and MuRF-1 is essential for rapid atrophy. Genomic approaches to transcription profiling have made possible a systematic and comprehensive analysis of transcriptional adaptations in all forms of muscle atrophy, and this information should lead in coming years to a much better understanding of the final common cellular pathway by which muscle atrophy occurs.

List of Abbreviations

11βHSD	11β-hydroxysteroid dehydrogenase
ADP	adenosine diphosphate
AMP	adenosine monophosphate
ATP	adenosine triphosphate
GR	glucocorticoid receptor
HIV	human immunodeficiency virus
IGF	insulin-like growth factor
IGFBP	insulin-like growth factor binding protein
IMP	inosine monophosphate
MGF	mechano-growth factor
PI-3 kinase	phophatidylinositol-3 kinase
PIF	proteolysis-inducing factor
SCF	S-phase kinase, associated protein 1A (SKP1A), cullin-1, f-box
T_3	triiodothyronine
T_4	thyroxine
TCA	tricarboxylic acid
TNF	tumor necrosis factor
TSH	thyroid-stimulating hormone
Ub	ubiquitin

References

1. Hershey JW: Translational control in mammalian cells. *Annu Rev Biochem* 60:717–755, 1991.
2. Schoenheimer R: *Dynamic State of Body Constituents*. Cambridge, MA: Harvard University Press, 1942.
3. Olson TS, Dice JF: Regulation of protein degradation rates in eukaryotes. *Curr Opin Cell Biol* 1:1194–1200, 1989.
4. Drachman DB: Myasthenia gravis (first of two parts). *N Engl J Med* 298:136–142, 1978.
5. Goldberg AL, Etlinger JD, Goldspink DF, et al: Mechanism of work-induced hypertrophy of skeletal muscle. *Med Sci Sports* 7:185–198, 1975.
6. Felig P: Amino acid metabolism in man. *Annu Rev Biochem* 44:933–955, 1975.
7. Ruderman NB: Muscle amino acid metabolism and gluconeogenesis. *Annu Rev Med* 26:245–258, 1975.
8. Lecker SH, Solomon V, Mitch WE, et al: Muscle protein breakdown and the critical role of the ubiquitin-proteasome pathway in normal and disease states. *J Nutr* 129:227S–237S, 1999.
9. Goldberg AL: The mechanism and functions of ATP-dependent proteases in bacterial and animal cells. *Eur J Biochem* 203:9–23, 1992.
10. Hershko A, Ciechanover A: The ubiquitin system for protein degradation. *Annu Rev Biochem* 61:761–807, 1992.
11. Medina R, Wing SS, Haas A, et al: Activation of the ubiquitin-ATP-dependent proteolytic system in skeletal muscle during fasting and denervation atrophy. *Biomed Biochim Acta* 50:347–356, 1991.
12. Han HQ, Furuno K, Goldberg AL: The activation of the ATP-dependent proteolytic system in skeletal muscle during denervation atrophy and fasting. *Fed Proc* 2:A564, 1988.
13. Furuno K, Goldberg AL: The activation of protein degradation in muscle by Ca2+ or muscle injury does not involve a lysosomal mechanism. *Biochem J* 237:859–864, 1986.
14. Rock KL, Gramm C, Rothstein L, et al: Inhibitors of the proteasome block the degradation of most cell proteins and the generation of peptides presented on MHC class I molecules. *Cell* 78:761–771, 1994.
15. Gronostajski RM, Goldberg AL, Pardee AB: The role of increased proteolysis in the atrophy and arrest of proliferation in serum-deprived fibroblasts. *J Cell Physiol* 121:189–198, 1984.
16. Lardeux BR, Mortimore GE: Amino acid and hormonal control of macromolecular turnover in perfused rat liver. Evidence for selective autophagy. *J Biol Chem* 262:14514–14519, 1987.
17. Kettelhut IC, Wing SS, Goldberg AL: Endocrine regulation of protein breakdown in skeletal muscle. *Diabetes/Metab Rev* 4:751–772, 1988.
18. Goldberg AL, Odessey R: Oxidation of amino acids by diaphragms from fed and fasted rats. *Am J Physiol* 223:1384–1391, 1972.
19. Pisters PWT, Pearlstone DB: Protein and amino acid metabolism in cancer cachexia: Investigative techniques and therapeutic interventions. *Crit Rev Clin Lab Sci* 30:223–272, 1993.

20. Van Hall G, Saltin B, Wagenmakers AJ: Muscle protein degradation and amino acid metabolism during prolonged knee-extensor exercise in humans. *Clin Sci (Lond)* 97: 557–567, 1999.
21. Young VR, Munro HN: Ntau-methylhistidine (3-methylhistidine) and muscle protein turnover: An overview. *Fed Proc* 37:2291–2300, 1978.
22. Huszar G: Developmental changes of the primary structure and histidine methylation in rabbit skeletal muscle myosin. *Nat New Biol* 240:260–264, 1972.
23. Millward DJ, Bates PC: 3-Methylhistidine turnover in the whole body, and the contribution of skeletal muscle and intestine to urinary 3-methylhistidine excretion in the adult rat. *Biochem J* 214:607–615, 1983.
24. Goldberg AL, DeMartino G, Chang TW: Release of gluconeogenic precursors from skeletal muscle, in Essman V (ed): *Regulatory Mechanisms of Carbohydrate Metabolism.* New York: Pergamon Press, 1978, pp 347–358.
25. Clowes GH Jr, George BC, Villee CA Jr, et al: Muscle proteolysis induced by a circulating peptide in patients with sepsis or trauma. *N Engl J Med* 308:545–552, 1983.
26. Fulks RM, Li JB, Goldberg AL: Effects of insulin, glucose, and amino acids on protein turnover in rat diaphragm. *J Biol Chem* 250:290–246, 1975.
27. Goldberg AL, Martel SM, Kushmerick MJ: In vitro preparation of the diaphragm and other muscles. *Methods Enzymol* 39:82–93, 1975.
28. Baracos VE, Goldberg AL: Maintenance of normal length improves protein balance and energy status in isolated rat skeletal muscles. *Am J Physiol* 251:C588–C596, 1986.
29. Solomon V, Goldberg AL: Importance of the ATP-ubiquitin-proteasome pathway in the degradation of soluble and myofibrillar proteins in rabbit muscle extracts. *J Biol Chem* 271: 26690–26697, 1996.
30. Goodman MN: Differential effects of acute changes in cell Ca2+ concentration on myofibrillar and non-myofibrillar protein breakdown in the rat extensor digitorum longus muscle in vitro. Assessment by production of tyrosine and N tau-methylhistidine. *Biochem J* 241:121–127, 1987.
31. Furuno K, Goodman MN, Goldberg AL: Role of different proteolytic systems in the degradation of muscle proteins during denervation atrophy. *J Biol Chem* 265:8550–8557, 1990.
32. Goldberg AL, St John AC: Intracellular protein degradation in mammalian and bacterial cells: Part 2. *Annu Rev Biochem* 45:747–803, 1976.
33. Goldberg AL, Chang TW: Regulation and significance of amino acid metabolism in skeletal muscle. *Fed Proc* 37:2301–2307, 1978.
34. Miller LL: The role of the liver and the non-hepatic tissues in the regulation of free amino acid levels in the blood, in Holden JT (ed): *Amino Acid Pools.* Amsterdam: Elsevier, 1961, pp 708–721.
35. Manchester KL: Oxidation of amino acids by isolated rat diaphragm and the influence of insulin. *Biochim Biophys Acta* 100:295–298, 1965.
36. Odessey R, Khairallah EA, Goldberg AL: Origin and possible significance of alanine production by skeletal muscle. *J Biol Chem* 249:7623–7629, 1974.
37. Goodman HM: Site of action of insulin in promoting leucine utilization in adipose tissue. *Am J Physiol* 233:E97–E103, 1977.
38. Chaplin ER, Goldberg AL, Diamond I: Leucine oxidation in brain slices and nerve endings. *J Neurochem* 26:701–707, 1976.
39. Odessey R, Goldberg AL: Oxidation of leucine by rat skeletal muscle. *Am J Physiol* 223:1376–1383, 1972.
40. Buse MG, Biggers JF, Drier C, et al: The effect of epinephrine, glucagon, and the nutritional state on the oxidation of branched chain amino acids and pyruvate by isolated hearts and diaphragms of the rat. *J Biol Chem* 248:697–706, 1973.
41. Tischler ME, Goldberg AL: Amino acid degradation and effect of leucine on pyruvate oxidation in rat atrial muscle. *Am J Physiol* 238:E480–E486, 1980.
42. Tawa NE Jr, Goldberg AL: Suppression of muscle protein turnover and amino acid degradation by dietary protein deficiency. *Am J Physiol* 263: E317–25, 1992.
43. Odessey R, Goldberg AL: Leucine degradation in cell-free extracts of skeletal muscle. *Biochem J* 178:475–489, 1979.
44. Shinnick FL, Harper AE: Branched-chain amino acid oxidation by isolated rat tissue preparations. *Biochim Biophys Acta* 437: 477–486, 1976.
45. Price SR, Wang X, Bailey JL: Tissue specific responses of branched-chain alpha-ketoacid dehydrogenase activity in metabolic acidosis. *J Am Soc Nephrol* 9:1892–1898, 1998.
46. Holecek M: Effect of starvation on branched-chain alpha-keto acid dehydrogenase activity in rat heart and skeletal muscle. *Physiol Res* 50:19–24, 2001.
47. Odessey R: Reversible ATP-induced inactivation of branched-chain 2-oxo acid dehydrogenase. *Biochem J* 192:155–163, 1980.
48. Parker PJ, Randle PJ: Active and inactive forms of branched-chain 2-oxoacid dehydrogenase complex in rat heart and skeletal muscle. *FEBS Lett* 112:186–190, 1980.
49. Odessey R: Purification and phosphorylation of branched chain oxoacid dehydrogenase, in Walser M, Williamson JR (eds): *Metabolism and Clinical Implications of the Branched Chain Amino and Ketoacids.* New York: Elsevier/North-Holland, 1981, pp 23–28.
50. Randle PJ, Lau KS, Parker PJ: Regulation of branched chain 2-oxoacid dehydrogenase complex, in Walser M, Williamson JR (eds): *Metabolism and Clinical Implications of the Branched Chain Amino And Ketoacids.* New York: Elsevier/North-Holland, 1981, pp 13–22.

51. Frick GP, Goodman HM: Regulation of branched chain a-ketoacid dehydrogenase by insulin and leucine, in Walser M, Williamson JR (eds): *Metabolism and Clinical Implications of the Branched Chain Amino And Ketoacids.* New York: Elsevier/North-Holland, 1981, pp 73–78.
52. Chang TW, Goldberg AL: Leucine inhibits oxidation of glucose and pyruvate in skeletal muscles during fasting. *J Biol Chem* 253:3696–701, 1978.
53. Goldberg AL, Tischler ME: Regulatory effects of leucine on carbohydrate and protein metabolism, in Walser M, Williamson JR (eds): *Metabolism and Clinical Implications of the Branched Chain Amino and Ketoacids.* New York: Elsevier/North-Holland, 1981, pp 205–216.
54. Chang TW, Goldberg AL: The metabolic fates of amino acids and the formation of glutamine in skeletal muscle. *J Biol Chem* 253:3685–3693, 1978.
55. Goodman MN, Ruderman NB: Influence of muscle use on amino acid metabolism. *Exerc Sport Sci Rev* 10:1–26, 1982.
56. Holloszy JO, Booth FW: Biochemical adaptations to endurance exercise in muscle. *Annu Rev Physiol* 38:273–291, 1976.
57. Lowenstein JM, Goodman MN: The purine nucleotide cycle in skeletal muscle. *Fed Proc* 37:2308–2312, 1978.
58. Lowenstein JM: Ammonia production in muscle and other tissues: The purine nucleotide cycle. *Physiol Rev* 52:382, 1972.
59. Tarnopolsky MA, Parise G, Gibala MJ, et al: Myoadenylate deaminase deficiency does not affect muscle anaplerosis during exhaustive exercise in humans. *J Physiol* 533: 881–889, 2001.
60. Gibala MJ, MacLean DA, Graham TE, et al: Anaplerotic processes in human skeletal muscle during brief dynamic exercise. *J Physiol* 502 (Pt 3): 703–713, 1997.
61. Felig P, Pozefsky T, Marliss E, et al: Alanine: Key role in gluconeogenesis. *Science* 167:1003–1004, 1970.
62. Chang TW, Goldberg AL: The origin of alanine produced in skeletal muscle. *J Biol Chem* 253:3677–3684, 1978.
63. Mallette LE, Exton JH, Park: Effects of glucagon on amino acid transport and utilization in the perfused rat liver. *J Biol Chem* 244:5724–5728, 1969.
64. Rennie MJ, Edwards RH, Krywawych S, et al: Effect of exercise on protein turnover in man. *Clin Sci (Lond)* 61:627–639, 1981.
65. Lemon PW, Mullin JP: Effect of initial muscle glycogen levels on protein catabolism during exercise. *J Appl Physiol* 48:624–629, 1980.
66. Garber AJ, Karl IE, Kipnis DM: Alanine and glutamine synthesis and release from skeletal muscle. II. The precursor role of amino acids in alanine and glutamine synthesis. *J Biol Chem* 251:836–843, 1976.
67. Goldstein L, Newsholme EA: The formation of alanine from amino acids in diaphragm muscle of the rat. *Biochem J* 154:555–558, 1976.
68. Perriello G, Jorde R, Nurjhan N, et al: Estimation of glucose-alanine-lactate-glutamine cycles in postabsorptive humans: role of skeletal muscle. *Am J Physiol* 269:E443–E450, 1995.
69. Tischler ME, Goldberg AL: Production of alanine and glutamine by atrial muscle from fed and fasted rats. *Am J Physiol* 238:E487–E493, 1980.
70. Nurjhan N, Bucci A, Perriello G, et al: Glutamine: A major gluconeogenic precursor and vehicle for interorgan carbon transport in man. *J Clin Invest* 95:272–277, 1995.
71. Kuhn KS, Schuhmann K, Stehle P, et al: Determination of glutamine in muscle protein facilitates accurate assessment of proteolysis and de novo synthesis-derived endogenous glutamine production. *Am J Clin Nutr* 70: 484–489, 1999.
72. Parry-Billings M, Newsholme EA: The possible role of glutamine substrate cycles in skeletal muscle. *Biochem J* 279(Pt 1):327–328, 1991.
73. Pitts RF, Pilkington LA, MacLeod MB, et al: Metabolism of glutamine by the intact functioning kidney of the dog. Studies in metabolic acidosis and alkalosis. *J Clin Invest* 51:557–565, 1972.
74. Windmueller HG, Spaeth AE: Respiratory fuels and nitrogen metabolism in vivo in small intestine of fed rats. Quantitative importance of glutamine, glutamate, and aspartate. *J Biol Chem* 255:107–112, 1980.
75. Labow BI, Souba WW, Abcouwer SF: Mechanisms governing the expression of the enzymes of glutamine metabolism—Glutaminase and glutamine synthetase. *J Nutr* 131:2467S–2474S; discussion 2486S–2487S, 2001.
76. Karinch AM, Pan M, Lin CM, et al: Glutamine metabolism in sepsis and infection. *J Nutr* 131:2535S–2538S; discussion 2550S–2551S, 2001.
77. Mittendorfer B, Gore DC, Herndon DN, et al: Accelerated glutamine synthesis in critically ill patients cannot maintain normal intramuscular free glutamine concentration. *J Parenter Enteral Nutr* 23:243–250; discussion 250–252, 1999.
78. Wilmore DW: Catabolic illness. Strategies for enhancing recovery. *N Engl J Med* 325:695–702, 1991.
79. Rennie MJ, Bowtell JL, Bruce M, et al: Interaction between glutamine availability and metabolism of glycogen, tricarboxylic acid cycle intermediates and glutathione. *J Nutr* 131:2488S–2490S; discussion 2496S–2497S, 2001.
80. Bruce M, Constantin-Teodosiu D, Greenhaff PL, et al: Glutamine supplementation promotes anaplerosis but not oxidative energy delivery in human skeletal muscle. *Am J Physiol Endocrinol Metab* 280:E669–E675, 2001.
81. Spiess E, Bruning A, Gack S, et al: Cathepsin B activity in human lung tumor cell lines: Ultrastructural localization, pH sensitivity, and inhibitor status at the cellular level. *J Histochem Cytochem*, 42: 917–29, 1994.

82. Lee DH, Goldberg AL: Proteasome inhibitors: Valuable new tools for cell biologists. *Trends Cell Biol* 8:397–403, 1998.
83. Laing JG, Tadros PN, Westphale EM, et al: Degradation of connexin43 gap junctions involves both the proteasome and the lysosome. *Exp Cell Res* 236:482–492, 1997.
84. Walowitz JL, Bradley ME, Chen S, et al: Proteolytic regulation of the zinc finger transcription factor YY1, a repressor of muscle-restricted gene expression. *J Biol Chem* 273:6656–6661, 1998.
85. Jefferson LS, Rannels DE, Munger BL, et al: Insulin in the regulation of protein turnover in heart and skeletal muscle. *Fed Proc* 33:1098–1104, 1974.
86. Dice JF: Peptide sequences that target cytosolic proteins for lysosomal proteolysis. *Trends Biochem Sci* 15:305–309, 1990.
87. Lowell BB, Ruderman NB, Goodman MN: Evidence that lysosomes are not involved in the degradation of myofibrillar proteins in rat skeletal muscle. *Biochem J* 234:237–240, 1986.
88. Fernandez C, Sainz RD: Pathways of protein degradation in L6 myotubes. *Proc Soc Exp Biol Med* 214:242–247, 1997.
89. Bailey JL, Price SR, England BK, et al: Signals regulating accelerated muscle protein catabolism in uremia. *Miner Electrolyte Metab* 23:198–200, 1997.
90. Kettelhut IC, Pepato MT, Migliorini RH, et al: Regulation of different proteolytic pathways in skeletal muscle in fasting and diabetes mellitus. *Braz J Med Biol Res* 27:981–993, 1994.
91. Pepato MT, Migliorini RH, Goldberg AL, et al: Role of different proteolytic pathways in degradation of muscle protein from streptozotocin-diabetic rats. *Am J Physiol* 271:E340–E347, 1996.
92. Mitch WE, Bailey JL, Wang X, et al: Evaluation of signals activating ubiquitin-proteasome proteolysis in a model of muscle wasting. *Am J Physiol* 276:C1132-C1138, 1999.
93. Wing SS, Goldberg AL: Glucocorticoids activate the ATP-ubiquitin-dependent proteolytic system in skeletal muscle during fasting. *Am J Physiol* 264:E668–E676, 1993.
94. Fang CH, Tiao G, James H, et al: Burn injury stimulates multiple proteolytic pathways in skeletal muscle, including the ubiquitin-energy-dependent pathway. *J Am Coll Surg* 180:161–170, 1995.
95. Solomon V, Madihally S, Yarmush M, et al: Insulin suppresses the increased activities of lysosomal cathepsins and ubiquitin conjugation system in burn-injured rats. *J Surg Res* 93:120–126, 2000.
96. Baracos VE, DeVivo C, Hoyle DHR, et al: Activation of the ATP-ubiquitin-proteasome pathway in skeletal muscle of cachectic rats bearing a hepatoma. *Am J Physiol* 268:E996–E1006, 1995.
97. Voisin L, Breuille D, Combaret L, et al: Muscle wasting in a rat model of long-lasting sepsis results from the activation of lysosomal, Ca2+ -activated, and ubiquitin-proteasome proteolytic pathways. *J Clin Invest* 97:1610–1617, 1996.
98. Taillandier D, Aurousseau E, Meynial-Denis D, et al: Coordinate activation of lysosomal, Ca 2+-activated and ATP-ubiquitin-dependent proteinases in the unweighted rat soleus muscle. *Biochem J* 316(Pt 1):65–72, 1996.
99. Mansoor O, Beaufrere B, Boirie Y, et al: Increased mRNA levels for components of the lysosomal, Ca2+-activated, and ATP-ubiquitin-dependent proteolytic pathways in skeletal muscle from head trauma patients. *Proc Natl Acad Sci USA* 93:2714–2718, 1996.
100. Jagoe RT, Redfern CPF, Roberts RG, et al: Skeletal muscle mRNA levels for cathepsin B, but not components of the ubiquitin-proteasome pathway, are increased in patients with lung cancer referred for thoracotomy.*Clin Sci* 102:353–361, 2002.
101. Farges MC, Balcerzak D, Fisher BD, et al: Increased muscle proteolysis after local trauma mainly reflects macrophage-associated lysosomal proteolysis. *Am J Physiol Endocrinol Metab* 282:E326–E335, 2002.
102. Murachi T, Tanaka K, Hatanaka M, et al: Intracellular Ca2+-dependent protease (calpain) and its high molecular weight inhibitor (calpastatin). *Adv Enzyme Regul* 19:407–424, 1981.
103. Waxman L: Calcium-activated proteases in mammalian tissues. *Methods Enzymol* 80:664–680, 1981.
104. Mellgren R: Calcium-dependent proteases: An enzyme system active at cellular membranes. *FASEB J* 1:110–115, 1987.
105. Kameyama T, Etlinger JD: Calcium-dependent regulation of protein synthesis and degradation in muscle. *Nature* 279:344–346, 1979.
106. Zeman RJ, Kameyama T, Matsumoto K, et al: Regulation of protein degradation in muscle by calcium. Evidence for enhanced nonlysosomal proteolysis associated with elevated cytosolic calcium. *J Biol Chem* 260:13619–24, 1985.
107. Alderton JM, Steinhardt RA: Calcium influx through calcium leak channels is responsible for the elevated levels of calcium-dependent proteolysis in dystrophic myotubes. *J Biol Chem* 275:9452–9460, 2000.
108. Spencer MJ, Tidball JG: Calpain translocation during muscle fiber necrosis and regeneration in dystrophin-deficient mice. *Exp Cell Res* 226:264–272, 1996.
109. Belcastro AN: Skeletal muscle calcium-activated neutral protease (calpain) with exercise. *J Appl Physiol* 74:1381–1386, 1993.
110. Belcastro AN, Shewchuk LD, Raj DA: Exercise-induced muscle injury: A calpain hypothesis. *Mol Cell Biochem* 179:135–145, 1998.
111. Sultan KR, Dittrich BT, Pette D: Calpain activity in fast, slow, transforming, and regenerating skeletal muscles of rat. *Am J Physiol Cell Physiol* 279:C639–C647, 2000.
112. Moraczewski J, Piekarska E, Bonavaud S, et al: Differential intracellular distribution and activities of mu- and m-calpains during the differentiation of human myogenic cells in culture. *C R Acad Sci III* 319:681–686, 1996.
113. Raju RV, Kakkar R, Datla RS, et al: Myristoyl-coA:protein N-myristoyltransferase from bovine cardiac muscle: molecular cloning, kinetic analysis, and in vitro proteolytic cleavage by m-calpain. *Exp Cell Res* 241:23–35, 1998.
114. Kakkar R, Raju RV, Sharma RK: Calmodulin-dependent cyclic nucleotide phosphodiesterase (PDE1). *Cell Mol Life Sci* 55:1164–1186, 1999.
115. Koh TJ, Tidball JG: Nitric oxide inhibits calpain-mediated proteolysis of talin in skeletal muscle cells. *Am J Physiol Cell Physiol* 279:C806–C812, 2000.
116. Yoshida K, Harada K: Proteolysis of erythrocyte-type and brain-type ankyrins in rat heart after postischemic reperfusion. *J Biochem (Tokyo)* 122:279–285, 1997.
117. Gilchrist JS, Wang KK, Katz S, et al: Calcium-activated neutral protease effects upon skeletal muscle sarcoplasmic reticulum protein structure and calcium release. *J Biol Chem* 267:20857–20865, 1992.
118. Barnoy S, Zipser Y, Glaser T, et al: Association of calpain (Ca(2+)-dependent thiol protease) with its endogenous inhibitor calpastatin in myoblasts. *J Cell Biochem* 74:522–531, 1999.
119. Costelli P, Tullio RD, Baccino FM, et al: Activation of Ca(2+)-dependent proteolysis in skeletal muscle and heart in cancer cachexia. *Br J Cancer* 84:946–50, 2001.
120. Doumit ME, Koohmaraie M: Immunoblot analysis of calpastatin degradation: Evidence for cleavage by calpain in postmortem muscle. *J Anim Sci* 77:1467–1473, 1999.
121. Tidball JG, Spencer MJ: Expression of a calpastatin transgene slows muscle wasting and obviates changes in myosin isoform expression during murine muscle disuse. *J Physiol* 545:819–828, 2002.
122. Williams AB, Decourten-Myers GM, Fischer JE, et al: Sepsis stimulates release of myofilaments in skeletal muscle by a calcium-dependent mechanism. *Faseb J* 13:1435–1443, 1999.
123. Richard I, Broux O, Allamand V, et al: Mutations in the proteolytic enzyme calpain 3 cause limb-girdle muscular dystrophy type 2A. *Cell* 81:27–40, 1995.
124. Ono Y, Shimada H, Sorimachi H, et al: Functional defects of a muscle-specific calpain, p94, caused by mutations associated with limb-girdle muscular dystrophy type 2A. *J Biol Chem* 273:17073–17078, 1998.
125. Jagoe RT, Lecker SH, Gomes M, et al: Patterns of gene expression in atrophying skeletal muscles: the response to food deprivation. *FASEB J* 16:1697–1712, 2002.
126. Busquets S, Garcia-Martinez C, Alvarez B, et al: Calpain-3 gene expression is decreased during experimental cancer cachexia. *Biochim Biophys Acta* 1475:5–9, 2000.
127. Stockholm D, Herasse M, Marchand S, et al: Calpain 3 mRNA expression in mice after denervation and during muscle regeneration. *Am J Physiol Cell Physiol* 280:C1561–1569, 2001.
128. Etlinger J, Goldberg AL: A soluble ATP-dependent proteolytic system responsible for the degradation of abnormal proteins in reticulocytes. *Proc Natl Acad Sci USA* 74: 54–58, 1977.
129. Schwartz AL, Ciechanover A: The ubiquitin-proteasome pathway and pathogenesis of human diseases. *Annu Rev Med* 50:57–74, 1999.
130. Price SR, Bailey JL, Wang X, et al: Muscle wasting in insulinopenic rats results from activation of the ATP-dependent, ubiquitin-proteasome proteolytic pathway by a mechanism including gene transcription. *J Clin Invest* 98:1703–1708, 1996.
131. Bailey JL, Wang X, England BK, et al: The acidosis of chronic renal failure activates muscle proteolysis in rats by augmenting transcription of genes encoding proteins of the ATP-dependent ubiquitin-proteasome pathway. *J Clin Invest* 97:1447–1453, 1996.
132. Tawa NE Jr, Odessey R, Goldberg AL: Inhibitors of the proteasome reduce the accelerated proteolysis in atrophying rat skeletal muscles. *J Clin Invest* 100:197–203, 1997.
133. Jagoe RT, Goldberg AL: What do we really know about the ubiquitin-proteasome pathway in muscle atrophy? *Curr Opin Clin Nutr Metab Care* 4:183–190, 2001.
134. Baumeister W, Walz J, Zuhl F, et al: The proteasome: Paradigm of a self-compartmentalizing protease. *Cell* 92:367–380, 1998.
135. Navon A, Goldberg AL: Proteins are unfolded on the surface of the ATPase ring before transport into the proteasome. *Mol Cell* 8:1339–1349, 2001.
136. Pickart CM: Ubiquitin in chains. *Trends Biochem Sci* 25: 544–548, 2000.
137. Lam YA, Xu W, DeMartino GN, et al: Editing of ubiquitin conjugates by an isopeptidase in the 26S proteasome. *Nature* 385:737–740, 1997.
138. Deshaies RJ: SCF and Cullin/Ring H2-based ubiquitin ligases. *Annu Rev Cell Dev Biol* 15:435–467, 1999.
139. Solomon V, Lecker SH, Goldberg AL: The N-end rule pathway catalyzes a major fraction of the protein degradation in skeletal muscle. *J Biol Chem* 273:25216–25222, 1998.

140. Bastians H, Topper LM, Gorbsky GL, et al: Cell cycle-regulated proteolysis of mitotic target proteins. *Mol Biol Cell* 10:3927–3941, 1999.
141. Chen Z, Hagler J, Palombella VJ, et al: Signal-induced site-specific phosphorylation targets I kappa B alpha to the ubiquitin-proteasome pathway. *Genes Dev* 9:1586–1597, 1995.
142. Wing SS, Banville D: 14-kDa ubiquitin-conjugating enzyme: Structure of the rat gene and regulation upon fasting and by insulin. *Am J Physiol* 267:E39–E48, 1994.
143. Lecker SH, Solomon V, Price SR, et al: Ubiquitin conjugation by the N-end rule pathway and mRNAs for its components increase in muscles of diabetic rats. *J Clin Invest* 104:1411–1420, 1999.
144. Hobler SC, Wang JJ, Williams AB, et al: Sepsis is associated with increased ubiquitin-conjugating enzyme $E2_{14k}$ mRNA in skeletal muscle. *Am J Physiol* 276:R468–R473, 1999.
145. Fischer D, Sun X, Gang G, et al: The gene expression of ubiquitin ligase E3alpha is upregulated in skeletal muscle during sepsis in rats: Potential role of glucocorticoids. *Biochem Biophys Res Commun* 267:504–508, 2000.
146. Chrysis D, Underwood LE: Regulation of components of the ubiquitin system by insulin-like growth factor I and growth hormone in skeletal muscle of rats made catabolic with dexamethasone. *Endocrinology* 140:5635–5641, 1999.
147. Varshavsky A: The N-end rule: Functions, mysteries, uses. *Proc Natl Acad Sci USA* 93:12142–12149, 1996.
148. Reiss Y, Kaim D, Hershko A: Specificity of binding of NH_2-terminal residue of proteins to ubiquitin- protein ligase. Use of amino acid derivatives to characterize specific binding sites. *J Biol Chem* 263:2693–2698, 1988.
149. Gonen H, Stancovski I, Shkedy D, et al: Isolation, characterization, and partial purification of a novel ubiquitin-protein ligase, E3. Targeting of protein substrates via multiple and distinct recognition signals and conjugating enzymes. *J Biol Chem* 271:302–310, 1996.
150. Sun ZW, Allis CD: Ubiquitination of histone H2B regulates H3 methylation and gene silencing in yeast. *Nature* 418:104–148, 2002.
151. Gomes MD, Lecker SH, Jagoe RT, et al: Atrogin-1, a muscle-specific F-box protein highly expressed during muscle atrophy. *Proc Natl Acad Sci USA* 98:14440–14445, 2001.
152. Bodine SC, Latres E, Baumhueter S, et al: Identification of ubiquitin ligases required for skeletal muscle atrophy. *Science* 294:1704–1708, 2001.
153. Salvesen GS , Dixit VM: Caspase activation: The induced-proximity model. *Proc Natl Acad Sci USA* 96:10964–10967, 1999.
154. Fernando P, Kelly JF, Balazsi K, et al: Caspase 3 activity is required for skeletal muscle differentiation. *Proc Natl Acad Sci USA* 2002.
155. Ruest LB, Khalyfa A, Wang E: Development-dependent disappearance of caspase-3 in skeletal muscle is post-transcriptionally regulated. *J Cell Biochem* 86:21–28, 2002.
156. Sandri M, El Meslemani AH, Sandri C, et al: Caspase 3 expression correlates with skeletal muscle apoptosis in Duchenne and facioscapulo human muscular dystrophy. A potential target for pharmacological treatment? *J Neuropathol Exp Neurol* 60: 302–312, 2001.
157. Jin H, Wu Z, Tian N, et al: Apoptosis in atrophic skeletal muscle induced by brachial plexus injury in rats. *J Trauma* 50:31–35, 2001.
158. Jejurikar SS, Marcelo CL, Kuzon WM Jr: Skeletal muscle denervation increases satellite cell susceptibility to apoptosis. *Plast Reconstr Surg* 110:160–168, 2002.
159. Vescovo G, Volterrani M, Zennaro R, et al: Apoptosis in the skeletal muscle of patients with heart failure: Investigation of clinical and biochemical changes. *Heart* 84:431–437, 2000.
160. Agusti AG, Sauleda J, Miralles C, et al: Skeletal muscle apoptosis and weight loss in chronic obstructive pulmonary disease. *Am J Respir Crit Care Med* 166:485–489, 2002.
161. Gingras AC, Raught B, Sonenberg N: Regulation of translation initiation by FRAP/mTOR. *Genes Dev* 15: 807–826, 2001.
162. Fingar DC, Salama S, Tsou C, et al: Mammalian cell size is controlled by mTOR and its downstream targets S6K1 and 4EBP1/eIF4E. *Genes Dev* 16:1472–1487, 2002.
163. Ohtsaka A, Sacheck J, Goldberg AL: Unpublished observations.
164. Buse MG, Reid SS: Leucine. A possible regulator of protein turnover in muscle. *J Clin Invest* 56:1250–1261, 1975.
165. Chua BH, Siehl DL, Morgan HE: A role for leucine in regulation of protein turnover in working rat hearts. *Am J Physiol* 239:E510–E514, 1980.
166. Tischler ME, Desautels M, Goldberg AL: Does leucine, leucyl-tRNA, or some metabolite of leucine regulate protein synthesis and degradation in skeletal and cardiac muscle? *J Biol Chem* 257:1613–1621, 1982.
167. Mitch WE, Collier VU, Walser M, Treatment of chronic renal failure with branched chain ketoacids plus the other essential amino acids or their nitrogen free analogues, in Walser M, Williamson JR (eds): *Metabolism and Clinical Implications of the Branched Chain Amino and Ketoacids*. New York: Elsevier/North-Holland, 1981, pp 587–592.
168. Li JB, Jefferson LS: Influence of amino acid availability on protein turnover in perfused skeletal muscle. *Biochem Biophys Acta* 544:351–359, 1978.
169. Liu Z, Jahn LA, Long W, et al: Branched chain amino acids activate messenger ribonucleic acid translation regulatory proteins in human skeletal muscle, and glucocorticoids blunt this action. *J Clin Endocrinol Metab* 86:2136–2143, 2001.

170. Greiwe JS, Kwon G, McDaniel ML, et al: Leucine and insulin activate p70 S6 kinase through different pathways in human skeletal muscle. *Am J Physiol Endocrinol Metab* 281: E466–E471, 2001.
171. Balage M, Sinaud S, Prod'homme M, et al: Amino acids and insulin are both required to regulate assembly of the eIF4E. eIF4G complex in rat skeletal muscle. *Am J Physiol Endocrinol Metab* 281:E565–E574, 2001.
172. Anthony JC, Yoshizawa F, Anthony TG, et al: Leucine stimulates translation initiation in skeletal muscle of postabsorptive rats via a rapamycin-sensitive pathway. *J Nutr* 130:2413–2419, 2000.
173. Kimball SR, Shantz LM, Horetsky RL, et al: Leucine regulates translation of specific mRNAs in L6 myoblasts through mTOR-mediated changes in availability of eIF4E and phosphorylation of ribosomal protein S6. *J Biol Chem* 274:11647–11652, 1999.
174. Anthony JC, Reiter AK, Anthony TG, et al: Orally administered leucine enhances protein synthesis in skeletal muscle of diabetic rats in the absence of increases in 4E-BP1 or S6K1 phosphorylation. *Diabetes* 51:928–936, 2002.
175. Mordier S, Deval C, Bechet D, et al: Leucine limitation induces autophagy and activation of lysosome-dependent proteolysis in C2C12 myotubes through a mammalian target of rapamycin-independent signaling pathway. *J Biol Chem* 275:29900–29906, 2000.
176. Dardevet D, Sornet C, Bayle G, et al: Postprandial stimulation of muscle protein synthesis in old rats can be restored by a leucine-supplemented meal. *J Nutr* 132:95–100, 2002.
177. Bevington A, Brown J, Walls J: Leucine suppresses acid-induced protein wasting in L6 rat muscle cells. *Eur J Clin Invest* 31:497–503, 2001.
178. Newsholme EA, Dimitriadis G: Integration of biochemical and physiologic effects of insulin on glucose metabolism. *Exp Clin Endocrinol Diabetes* 109:S122–S134, 2001.
179. Hyde R, Peyrollier K, Hundal HS: Insulin promotes the cell surface recruitment of the SAT2/ATA2 system A amino acid transporter from an endosomal compartment in skeletal muscle cells. *J Biol Chem* 277: 13628–13634, 2002.
180. Biolo G, Declan Fleming RY, Wolfe RR: Physiologic hyperinsulinemia stimulates protein synthesis and enhances transport of selected amino acids in human skeletal muscle. *J Clin Invest* 95:811–819, 1995.
181. Dardevet D, Sornet C, Vary T, et al: Phosphatidylinositol 3-kinase and p70 s6 kinase participate in the regulation of protein turnover in skeletal muscle by insulin and insulin-like growth factor I. *Endocrinology* 137:4087–4094, 1996.
182. Boirie Y, Short KR, Ahlman B, et al: Tissue-specific regulation of mitochondrial and cytoplasmic protein synthesis rates by insulin. *Diabetes* 50:2652–2658, 2001.
183. Davis TA, Fiorotto ML, Burrin DG, et al: Stimulation of protein synthesis by both insulin and amino acids is unique to skeletal muscle in neonatal pigs. *Am J Physiol Endocrinol Metab* 282:E880–E890, 2002.
184. Suryawan A, Nguyen HV, Bush JA, et al: Developmental changes in the feeding-induced activation of the insulin-signaling pathway in neonatal pigs. *Am J Physiol Endocrinol Metab* 281:E908–E915, 2001.
185. Ferrando AA, Chinkes DL, Wolf SE, et al: A submaximal dose of insulin promotes net skeletal muscle protein synthesis in patients with severe burns. *Ann Surg* 229:11–18, 1999.
186. Fluckey JD, Asp S, Enevoldsen LH, et al: Insulin action on rates of muscle protein synthesis following eccentric, muscle-damaging contractions. *Acta Physiol Scand* 173:379–384, 2001.
187. Goldberg AL, Tischler M, DeMartino G, et al: Hormonal regulation of protein degradation and synthesis in skeletal muscle. *Fed Proc* 39:31–36, 1980.
188. Larbaud D, Balage M, Taillandier D, et al: Differential regulation of the lysosomal, Ca2+-dependent and ubiquitin/proteasome-dependent proteolytic pathways in fast-twitch and slow-twitch rat muscle following hyperinsulinaemia. *Clin Sci (Lond)* 101:551–558, 2001.
189. Rannels SR, Rannels DE, Pegg AE, et al: Glucocorticoid effects on peptide-chain initiation in skeletal muscle and heart. *Am J Physiol* 235: E134–E139, 1978.
190. Li JB, Wassner SJ: Effects of food deprivation and refeeding on total protein and actomyosin degradation. *Am J Physiol* 246:E32–E37, 1984.
191. Smith DM, Sugden PH: Contrasting response of protein degradation to starvation and insulin as measured by release of N tau-methylhistidine or phenylalanine from the perfused rat heart. *Biochem J* 237:391–395, 1986.
192. Lowell BB, Ruderman NB, Goodman MN: Regulation of myofibrillar protein degradation in rat skeletal muscle during brief and prolonged starvation. *Metabolism* 35:1121–1127, 1986.
193. Goodman MN, del Pilar Gomez M: Decreased myofibrillar proteolysis after refeeding requires dietary protein or amino acids. *Am J Physiol* 253: E52–E58, 1987.
194. Wing SS, Haas AL, Goldberg AL: Increase in ubiquitin-protein conjugates concomitant with the increase in proteolysis in rat skeletal muscle during starvation and atrophy denervation. *Biochem J* 307:639–645, 1995.
195. Mortimore GE, Ward WF, Schworer CM: Lysosomal processing of intracellular proteins in rat liver and its general regulation by amino acids and insulin, in Segal HL, Doyle DJ (eds): *Protein Turnover and Lysosome Function*. New York: Academic Press, 1978, pp 67–87.
196. Griffin GE, Goldberg AL: Hormonal control of protein synthesis and degradation in rat skeletal muscle. *J Physiol (Comm)* 54P–55P, 1977.

197. Flaim KE, Li JB, Jefferson LS: Protein turnover in rat skeletal muscle: Effects of hypophysectomy and growth hormone. *Am J Physiol* 234: E38–E43, 1978.
198. Van Wyk JJ, Underwood LE: The somatomedins and their actions, in Litwack G (ed): *Biochemical Actions of Hormones.* New York: Academic Press, 1978, pp 101–148.
199. Uthne K, Reagan CR, Gimpel LP, et al: Effects of human somatomedin preparations on membrane transport and protein synthesis in isolated rat diaphragm. *J Clin Endocrinol Metab* 39:548–554, 1978.
200. D'Ercole AJ, Stiles AD, Underwood LE: Tissue concentrations of somatomedin C: further evidence for multiple sites of synthesis and paracrine or autocrine mechanisms of action. *Proc Natl Acad Sci USA* 81:935–939, 1984.
201. Roberts CT Jr, Brown AL, Graham DE, et al: Growth hormone regulates the abundance of insulin-like growth factor I RNA in adult rat liver. *J Biol Chem* 261:10025–10028, 1986.
202. Underwood LE: Clinical relevance of somatomedin, in Lifshitz F (ed): *Pediatric Endocrinology: A Clinical Guide.* New York: Marcel Dekker, 1985, pp 37–59.
203. Underwood LE, Clemmons DR, Maes M, et al: Regulation of somatomedin-C/insulin-like growth factor I by nutrients. *Horm Res* 24:166–176, 1986.
204. Thissen JP, Triest S, Underwood LE, et al: Divergent responses of serum insulin-like growth factor-I and liver growth hormone (GH) receptors to exogenous GH in protein-restricted rats. *Endocrinology* 126:908–913, 1990.
205. Phillips LS, Young HS: Nutrition and somatomedin. II. Serum somatomedin activity and cartilage growth activity in streptozotocin-diabetic rats. *Diabetes* 25:516–527, 1976.
206. McKoy G, Ashley W, Mander J, et al: Expression of insulin growth factor-1 splice variants and structural genes in rabbit skeletal muscle induced by stretch and stimulation. *J Physiol* 516(Pt 2):583–592, 1999.
207. DeVol DL, Rotwein P, Sadow JL, et al: Activation of insulin-like growth factor gene expression during work-induced skeletal muscle growth. *Am J Physiol* 259:E89–E95, 1990.
208. Barton-Davis ER, Shoturma DI, Sweeney HL: Contribution of satellite cells to IGF-I induced hypertrophy of skeletal muscle. *Acta Physiol Scand* 167:301–305, 1999.
209. Clemmons DR: *Insulin-like growth factor binding proteins,* in Kostoyo JL (ed): *Handbook of Physiology: Section 7. The Endocrine System.* New York: Oxford University Press, 1999, pp 573–602.
210. Awede B, Thissen J, Gailly P, et al: Regulation of IGF-I, IGFBP-4 and IGFBP-5 gene expression by loading in mouse skeletal muscle. *FEBS Lett* 461:263–267, 1999.
211. Nam T, Moralez A, Clemmons D: Vitronectin binding to IGF binding protein-5 (IGFBP-5) alters IGFBP-5 modulation of IGF-I actions. *Endocrinology* 143:30–36, 2002.
212. Debroy MA, Wolf SE, Zhang XJ, et al: Anabolic effects of insulin-like growth factor in combination with insulin-like growth factor binding protein-3 in severely burned adults. *J Trauma* 47: 904–910; discussion 910–911, 1999.
213. Svanberg E, Ohlsson C, Kimball SR, et al: rhIGF-I/IGFBP-3 complex, but not free rhIGF-I, supports muscle protein biosynthesis in rats during semistarvation. *Eur J Clin Invest* 30:438–446, 2000.
214. Wang W, Iresjo BM, Karlsson L, et al: Provision of rhIGF-I/IGFBP-3 complex attenuated development of cancer cachexia in an experimental tumor model. *Clin Nutr* 19: 127–132, 2000.
215. Anwar A, Zahid AA, Scheidegger KJ, et al: Tumor necrosis factor-alpha regulates insulin-like growth factor-1 and insulin-like growth factor binding protein-3 expression in vascular smooth muscle. *Circulation* 105:1220–1225, 2002.
216. Scheiwiller E, Guler HP, Merryweather J, et al: Growth restoration of insulin-deficient diabetic rats by recombinant human insulin-like growth factor I. *Nature* 323:169–171, 1986.
217. Rommel C, Bodine SC, Clarke BA, et al: Mediation of IGF-1-induced skeletal myotube hypertrophy by PI(3)K/Akt/mTOR and PI(3)K/Akt/GSK3 pathways. *Nat Cell Biol* 3:1009–1013, 2001.
218. Musaro A, McCullagh KJ, Naya FJ, et al: IGF-1 induces skeletal myocyte hypertrophy through calcineurin in association with GATA-2 and NF-ATc1. *Nature* 400:581–585, 1999.
219. Huang CY, Hao LY, Buetow DE: Insulin-like growth factor-induced hypertrophy of cultured adult rat cardiomyocytes is L-type calcium-channel-dependent. *Mol Cell Biochem* 231:51–59, 2002.
220. Ballard FJ, Read LC, Francis GL, et al: Binding properties and biological potencies of insulin-like growth factors in L6 myoblasts. *Biochem J* 233: 223–230, 1986.
221. Kettelhut IC, Goldberg AL: Unpublished observations.
222. Fang CH, Li BG, Wang JJ, et al: Insulin-like growth factor 1 stimulates protein synthesis and inhibits protein breakdown in muscle from burned rats. *J Parenter Enteral Nutr* 21: 245–251, 1997.
223. Hobler SC, Williams AB, Fischer JE, et al: IGF-I stimulates protein synthesis but does not inhibit protein breakdown in muscle from septic rats. *Am J Physiol* 274:R571–R576, 1998.
224. Fang CH, Li BG, Sun X, et al: Insulin-like growth factor I reduces ubiquitin and ubiquitin-conjugating enzyme gene expression but does not inhibit muscle proteolysis in septic rats. *Endocrinology* 141:2743–2751, 2000.
225. Hjalmarson AC, Rannels DE, Kao R, et al: Effects of hypophysectomy, growth hormone, and thyroxine on protein turnover in heart. *J Biol Chem* 250:4556–4561, 1975.
226. Kettelhut IC, Leopold B, Tawa NE Jr, et al: Protein deficiency and lack of pituitary hormones reduce both lysosomal and ATP-dependent proteolytic processes in skeletal muscle. *Fed Proc* 2:564, 1988.
227. Tawa NE Jr, Goldberg AL: Prolonged fasting, dietary protein restriction, or lack of thyroid hormones suppress both lysosomal and ATP-dependent proteolytic systems in muscle. *Surg Forum* 42:25–28, 1991.
228. DeMartino GN, Goldberg AL: Thyroid hormones control lysosomal enzyme activities in liver and skeletal muscle. *Proc Natl Acad Sci USA* 75:1369–1373, 1978.
229. DeMartino GN, Goldberg AL: A possible explanation of myxedema and hypercholesterolemia in hypothyroidism: Control of lysosomal hyaluronidase and cholesterol esterase by thyroid hormones. *Enzyme* 26: 1–7, 1981.
230. Solomon V, Baracos V, Sarraf P, et al: Rates of ubiquitin conjugation increase when muscles atrophy, largely through activation of the N-end rule pathway. *Proc Natl Acad Sci USA* 95:12602–12607, 1998.
231. Tawa NE Jr: *Metabolic Consequences of Protein Deficiency and Long-Term Starvation.* Cambridge, MA: Harvard University, 1984.
232. Nakashima K, Ohtsuka A, Hayashi K: Effects of thyroid hormones on myofibrillar proteolysis and activities of calpain, proteasome, and cathepsin in primary cultured chick muscle cells. *J Nutr Sci Vitaminol (Tokyo)* 44:799–807, 1998.
233. Clement K, Viguerie N, Diehn M, et al: In vivo regulation of human skeletal muscle gene expression by thyroid hormone. *Genome Res* 12: 281–291, 2002.
234. Goldberg AL, Goldspink DF: Influence of food deprivation and adrenal steroids on DNA synthesis in various mammalian tissues. *Am J Physiol* 228:310–317, 1975.
235. Goldberg AL: Protein turnover in skeletal muscle: II. Effects of denervation and cortisone on protein catabolism in skeletal muscle. *J Biol Chem* 244:3223–3229, 1969.
236. Kostyo JL, Redmond AF: Role of protein synthesis in the inhibitory action of adrenal steroid hormones on amino acid transport by muscle. *Endocrinology* 79:531–540, 1966.
237. McGrath JA, Goldspink DF: Glucocorticoid action on protein synthesis and protein breakdown in isolated skeletal muscles. *Biochem J* 206: 641–645, 1982.
238. Shoji S, Pennington RJ: The effect of cortisone on protein breakdown and synthesis in rat skeletal muscle. *Mol Cell Endocrinol* 6:159–169, 1977.
239. Tomas FM, Munro HN, Young VR: Effect of glucocorticoid administration on the rate of muscle protein breakdown in vivo in rats, as measured by urinary excretion of N tau-methylhistidine. *Biochem J* 178:139–146, 1979.
240. Odedra BR, Bates PC, Millward DJ: Time course of the effect of catabolic doses of corticosterone on protein turnover in rat skeletal muscle and liver. *Biochem J* 214:617–627, 1983.
241. Thompson MG, Thom A, Partridge K, et al: Stimulation of myofibrillar protein degradation and expression of mRNA encoding the ubiquitin-proteasome system in C(2)C(12) myotubes by dexamethasone: Effect of the proteasome inhibitor MG-132. *J Cell Physiol* 181:455–461, 1999.
242. Long CNH, Katzin B, Fry EG: The adrenal cortex and carbohydrate metabolism. *Endocrinology* 26:209, 1940.
243. Goldberg AL: Unpublished observations.
244. Tischler ME, Goldberg AL: Effect of glucocorticoids on protein and amino acid metabolism in muscle from fasted rats. *Fed Proc* 28:823, 1979.
245. Lofberg E, Gutierrez A, Wernerman J, et al: Effects of high doses of glucocorticoids on free amino acids, ribosomes and protein turnover in human muscle. *Eur J Clin Invest* 32:345–353, 2002.
246. Bowes SB, Jackson NC, Papachristodoulou D, et al: Effect of corticosterone on protein degradation in isolated rat soleus and extensor digitorum longus muscles. *J Endocrinol* 148:501–507, 1996.
247. Bowes SB, Benn JJ, Scobie IN, et al: Leucine metabolism in patients with Cushing's syndrome before and after successful treatment. *Clin Endocrinol (Oxf)* 39:591–598, 1993.
248. Wang L, Luo GJ, Wang JJ, et al: Dexamethasone stimulates proteasome- and calcium-dependent proteolysis in cultured L6 myotubes. *Shock* 10:298–306, 1998.
249. Ralliere C, Tauveron I, Taillandier D, et al: Glucocorticoids do not regulate the expression of proteolytic genes in skeletal muscle from Cushing's syndrome patients. *J Clin Endocrinol Metab* 82:3161–3164, 1997.
250. Deval C, Mordier S, Obled C, et al: Identification of cathepsin L as a differentially expressed message associated with skeletal muscle wasting. *Biochem J* 360:143–150, 2001.
251. Shah OJ, Anthony JC, Kimball SR, et al: Glucocorticoids oppose translational control by leucine in skeletal muscle. *Am J Physiol Endocrinol Metab* 279: E1185–E1190, 2000.
252. Long W, Wei L, Barrett EJ: Dexamethasone inhibits the stimulation of muscle protein synthesis and PHAS-I and p70 S6-kinase phosphorylation. *Am J Physiol Endocrinol Metab* 280:E570–E575, 2001.
253. Whorwood CB, Donovan SJ, Wood PJ, et al: Regulation of glucocorticoid receptor alpha and beta isoforms and type I 11beta-hydroxysteroid dehydrogenase expression in human skeletal muscle cells: A key role

254. May RC, Kelly RA, Mitch WE: Metabolic acidosis stimulates protein degradation in rat muscle by a glucocorticoid-dependent mechanism. *J Clin Invest* 77:614–621, 1986.
255. Price SR, England BK, Bailey JL, et al: Acidosis and glucocorticoids concomitantly increase ubiquitin and proteasome subunit mRNAs in rat muscle. *Am J Physiol* 267:C955–C960, 1994.
256. Tiao G, Fagan J, Roegner V, et al: Energy-ubiquitin-dependent muscle proteolysis during sepsis in rats is regulated by glucocorticoids. *J Clin Invest* 97:339–348, 1996.
257. Geenen DL, Malhotra A, Scheuer J: Angiotensin II increases cardiac protein synthesis in adult rat heart. *Am J Physiol* 265:H238–H243, 1993.
258. Brink M, Price SR, Chrast J, et al: Angiotensin II induces skeletal muscle wasting through enhanced protein degradation and down-regulates autocrine insulin-like growth factor I. *Endocrinology* 142:1489–1496, 2001.
259. Lijnen P, Petrov V: Renin-angiotensin system, hypertrophy and gene expression in cardiac myocytes. *J Mol Cell Cardiol* 31:949–970, 1999.
260. Gordon SE, Davis BS, Carlson CJ, et al: ANG II is required for optimal overload-induced skeletal muscle hypertrophy. *Am J Physiol Endocrinol Metab* 280:E150–E159, 2001.
261. Navegantes LC, Resano NM, Migliorini RH, et al: Catecholamines inhibit Ca(2+)-dependent proteolysis in rat skeletal muscle through beta(2)-adrenoceptors and cAMP. *Am J Physiol Endocrinol Metab* 281:E449–E454, 2001.
262. Navegantes LC, Resano NM, Migliorini RH, et al: Effect of guanethidine-induced adrenergic blockade on the different proteolytic systems in rat skeletal muscle. *Am J Physiol* 277:E883–E889, 1999.
263. Maltin CA, Hay SM, McMillan DN, et al: Tissue specific responses to clenbuterol: Temporal changes in protein metabolism of striated muscle and visceral tissues from rats. *Growth Regul* 2:161–166, 1992.
264. Rehfeldt C, Schadereit R, Weikard R, et al: Effect of clenbuterol on growth, carcase and skeletal muscle characteristics in broiler chickens. *Br Poult Sci* 38:366–373, 1997.
265. Dodd SL, Koesterer TJ: Clenbuterol attenuates muscle atrophy and dysfunction in hindlimb-suspended rats. *Aviat Space Environ Med* 73:635–639, 2002.
266. Martineau L, Little RA, Rothwell NJ, et al: Clenbuterol, a beta 2-adrenergic agonist, reverses muscle wasting due to scald injury in the rat. *Burns* 19:26–34, 1993.
267. Herndon DN, Hart DW, Wolf SE, et al: Reversal of catabolism by beta-blockade after severe burns. *N Engl J Med* 345:1223–1229, 2001.
268. Tipton KD: Gender differences in protein metabolism. *Curr Opin Clin Nutr Metab Care* 4:493–498, 2001.
269. Bhasin S, Woodhouse L, Storer TW: Proof of the effect of testosterone on skeletal muscle. *J Endocrinol* 170:27–38, 2001.
270. Bhasin S, Javanbakht M: Can androgen therapy replete lean body mass and improve muscle function in wasting associated with human immunodeficiency virus infection? *J Parenter Enteral Nutr* 23:S195–S201, 1999.
271. Ferrando AA, Sheffield-Moore M, Wolf SE, et al: Testosterone administration in severe burns ameliorates muscle catabolism. *Crit Care Med* 29:1936–1942, 2001.
272. Wang J, Liu R, Hawkins M, et al: A nutrient-sensing pathway regulates leptin gene expression in muscle and fat. *Nature* 393:684–688, 1998.
273. Wang J, Liu R, Liu L, et al: The effect of leptin on Lep expression is tissue-specific and nutritionally regulated. *Nat Med* 5:895–899, 1999.
274. Ceddia RB, William WN Jr, Curi R: Comparing effects of leptin and insulin on glucose metabolism in skeletal muscle: Evidence for an effect of leptin on glucose uptake and decarboxylation. *Int J Obes Relat Metab Disord* 23:75–82, 1999.
275. Carbo N, Ribas VV, Busquets S, et al: Short-term effects of leptin on skeletal muscle protein metabolism in the rat. *J Nutr Biochem* 11:431–435, 2000.
276. Saudek CD, Felig P: The metabolic events of starvation. *Am J Med* 60:117–126, 1976.
277. Li JB, Goldberg AL: Effects of food deprivation on protein synthesis and degradation in rat skeletal muscles. *Am J Physiol* 231:441–448, 1976.
278. Goodman MN, Larsen PR, Kaplan MM, et al: Starvation in the rat. II. Effect of age and obesity on protein sparing and fuel metabolism. *Am J Physiol* 239:E277–E286, 1980.
279. Li JB, Higgins JE, Jefferson LS: Changes in protein turnover in skeletal muscle in response to fasting. *Am J Physiol* 236:E222–E228, 1979.
280. Goodman MN, McElaney MA, Ruderman NB: Adaptation to prolonged starvation in the rat: Curtailment of skeletal muscle proteolysis. *Am J Physiol* 241: E321–E327, 1981.
281. Goodman MN, Lowell B, Belur E, et al: Sites of protein conservation and loss during starvation: influence of adiposity. *Am J Physiol* 246:E383–E390, 1984.
282. Vignati L, Finley RJ, Hagg S, et al: Protein conservation during prolonged fast: A function of triiodothyronine levels. *Trans Assoc Am Physicians* 91:169–79, 1978.
283. Tischler ME, Fagan JM: Relationship of the reduction-oxidation state to protein degradation in skeletal and atrial muscle. *Arch Biochem Biophys* 217:191–201, 1982.
284. Wimpfheimer C, Saville E, Voirol MJ, et al: Starvation-induced decreased sensitivity of resting metabolic rate to triiodothyronine. *Science* 205:1272–1273, 1979.
285. Kaplan MM, Utiger RD: Iodothyronine metabolism in rat liver homogenates. *J Clin Invest* 61: 459–471, 1978.
286. Gardner DF, Kaplan MM, Stanley CA, et al: Effect of tri-iodothyronine replacement on the metabolic and pituitary responses to starvation. *N Engl J Med* 300:579–584, 1979.
287. Drenick EJ, Dennin HF: Energy expenditure in fasting obese men. *J Lab Clin Med* 81:421–430, 1973.
288. Tawa NE Jr, Kettelhut IC, Goldberg AL: Dietary protein deficiency reduces lysosomal and nonlysosomal ATP-dependent proteolysis in muscle. *Am J Physiol* 263:E326–E334, 1992.
289. Garlick PJ, Millward DJ, James WP, et al: The effect of protein deprivation and starvation on the rate of protein synthesis in tissues of the rat. *Biochim Biophys Acta* 414:71–84, 1975.
290. Haverberg LN, Deckelbaum L, Bilmazes C, et al: Myofibrillar protein turnover and urinary N-tau-methylhistidine output. Response to dietary supply of protein and energy. *Biochem J* 152:503–510, 1975.
291. Narasinga Rao BS, Nagabhushan VS: Urinary excretion of 3-methylhistidine in children suffering from protein-calorie malnutrition. *Life Sci* 12:205–210, 1973.
292. Tawa NE Jr: Unpublished observations.
293. Young VR, Vilaire G, Newberne PM, et al: Plasma insulin and amino acid concentrations in rats given an adequate or low protein diet. *J Nutr* 103:720–729, 1973.
294. Williams B, Hattersley J, Layward E, et al: Metabolic acidosis and skeletal muscle adaptation to low protein diets in chronic uremia. *Kidney Int* 40:779–786, 1991.
295. Pette D: *Plasticity of Muscle*. Berlin: de Gruyter, 1980.
296. Goldspink DF, Garlick PJ, McNurlan MA: Protein turnover measured in vivo and in vitro in muscles undergoing compensatory growth and subsequent denervation atrophy. *Biochem J* 210:89–98, 1983.
297. Goldberg AL: Work-induced growth of skeletal muscle in normal and hypophysectomized rats. *Am J Physiol* 213:1193–1198, 1967.
298. Richter EA, Garetto LP, Goodman MN, et al: Muscle glucose metabolism following exercise in the rat: Increased sensitivity to insulin. *J Clin Invest* 69:785–793, 1982.
299. Chibalin AV, Yu M, Ryder JW, et al: Exercise-induced changes in expression and activity of proteins involved in insulin signal transduction in skeletal muscle: Differential effects on insulin-receptor substrates 1 and 2. *Proc Natl Acad Sci USA* 97:38–43, 2000.
300. Martineau LC, Gardiner PF: Insight into skeletal muscle mechanotransduction: MAPK activation is quantitatively related to tension. *J Appl Physiol* 91:693–702, 2001.
301. Widegren U, Ryder JW, Zierath JR: Mitogen-activated protein kinase signal transduction in skeletal muscle: effects of exercise and muscle contraction. *Acta Physiol Scand* 172:227–238, 2001.
302. Bodine SC, Stitt TN, Gonzalez M, et al: Akt/mTOR pathway is a crucial regulator of skeletal muscle hypertrophy and can prevent muscle atrophy in vivo. *Nat Cell Biol* 3:1014–1019, 2001.
303. Palmer RM, Reeds PJ, Atkinson T, et al: The influence of changes in tension on protein synthesis and prostaglandin release in isolated rabbit muscles. *Biochem J* 214:1011–1014, 1983.
304. Elce JS, Hasspieler R, Boegman RJ: Ca^{2+}-activated protease in denervated rat skeletal muscle measured by an immunoassay. *Exp Neurol* 81:320–329, 1983.
305. Glass DJ: Personal communication, 2003.
306. Sacheck J, Gomes MD, Goldberg AL: Unpublished observations.
307. Sadoshima J, Jahn L, Takahashi T, et al: Molecular characterization of the stretch-induced adaptation of cultured cardiac cells. An in vitro model of load-induced cardiac hypertrophy. *J Biol Chem* 267:10551–10560, 1992.
308. Baracos V, Greenberg RE, Goldberg AL: Influence of calcium and other divalent cations on protein turnover in rat skeletal muscle. *Am J Physiol* 250:E702–E710, 1986.
309. Rodemann HP, Waxman L, Goldberg AL: The stimulation of protein degradation in muscle by Ca^{2+} is mediated by PGE$_2$ and does not require the calcium activated protease. *J Biol Chem* 257:8716–8723, 1982.
310. Beisel WR: Metabolic effects of infection. *Prog Food Nutr Sci* 8:43–75, 1984.
311. Grunfeld C, Feingold KR: Metabolic disturbances and wasting in the acquired immunodeficiency syndrome. *N Engl J Med* 327:329–337, 1992.
312. Fagan JM, Goldberg AL: Muscle protein breakdown, prostaglandin E2 production, and fever following bacterial infection, in Kluger MJ, Oppenheimer JJ, Powanda MC (eds): *The Physiological, Metabolic, and Immunologic Actions of Interleukin-1*. New York: Liss, 1985, pp 202–210.
313. Baracos V, Rodemann HP, Dinarello CA, et al: Stimulation of muscle protein degradation and prostaglandin E2 release by leukocytic pyrogen (interleukin-1). A mechanism for the increased degradation of muscle proteins during fever. *N Engl J Med* 308: 553–558, 1983.
314. Goldberg AL, Baracos V, Rodemann P, et al: Control of protein degradation in muscle by prostaglandins, Ca^{2+}, and leukocytic pyrogen (interleukin 1). *Fed Proc* 43:1301–1306, 1984.
315. Ruff RL, Secrist D: Inhibitors of prostaglandin synthesis or cathepsin B prevent muscle wasting due to sepsis in the rat. *J Clin Invest* 73:1483–1486, 1984.

316. Jepson MM, Pell JM, Bates PC, et al: The effects of endotoxaemia on protein metabolism in skeletal muscle and liver of fed and fasted rats. *Biochem J* 235:329–336, 1986.
317. Vary TC, Kimball SR: Sepsis-induced changes in protein synthesis: Differential effects on fast- and slow-twitch muscles. *Am J Physiol* 262:C1513–C1519, 1992.
318. Voisin L, Gray K, Flowers KM, et al: Altered expression of eukaryotic initiation factor 2B in skeletal muscle during sepsis. *Am J Physiol* 270:E43–E50, 1996.
319. Zamir O, Hasselgren PO, von Allmen D, et al: The effect of interleukin-1 alpha and the glucocorticoid receptor blocker RU 38486 on total and myofibrillar protein breakdown in skeletal muscle. *J Surg Res* 50:579–583, 1991.
320. Hasselgren PO, James JH, Benson DW, et al: Total and myofibrillar protein breakdown in different types of rat skeletal muscle: Effects of sepsis and regulation by insulin. *Metabolism* 38:634–640, 1989.
321. Dinarello CA, Wolff SM: The role of interleukin-1 in disease. *N Engl J Med* 328:106–113, 1993.
322. Beutler B, Cerami A: Cachectin and tumour necrosis factor as two sides of the same biological coin. *Nature* 320:584–588, 1986.
323. Okusawa S, Gelfand JA, Ikejima T, et al: Interleukin-1 induces a shock-like state in rabbits. A synergistic effect with TNF. *J Clin Invest* 81:1162–1172, 1988.
324. Ohlsson K, Bjork P, Bergenfeldt M, et al: Interleukin-1 receptor antagonist reduces mortality from endotoxin shock. *Nature* 348:550–552, 1990.
325. Tracey KJ, Beutler B, Lowry SF, et al: Shock and tissue injury induced by recombinant human cachectin. *Science* 234:470–474, 1986.
326. Kettelhut IC, Fiers W, Goldberg AL: The toxic effects of tumor necrosis factor in vivo and their prevention by cyclooxygenase inhibitors. *Proc Natl Acad Sci USA* 84:4273–4277, 1987.
327. Goldberg AL, Kettelhut IC, Furuno K, et al: Activation of protein breakdown and prostaglandin E2 production in rat skeletal muscle in fever is signaled by a macrophage product distinct from interleukin 1 or other known monokines. *J Clin Invest* 81:1378–1383, 1988.
328. Dinarello CA, Clowes GH Jr, Gordon AH, et al: Cleavage of human interleukin 1: Isolation of a peptide fragment from plasma of febrile humans and activated monocytes. *J Immunol* 133:1332–1338, 1984.
329. Moldawer LL, Svaninger G, Gelin J, et al: Interleukin 1 and tumor necrosis factor do not regulate protein balance in skeletal muscle. *Am J Physiol* 253:C766–C773, 1987.
330. Carswell EA, Old LJ, Kassel RL, et al: An endotoxin-induced serum factor that causes necrosis of tumors. *Proc Natl Acad Sci USA* 72:3666–3670, 1975.
331. Kettelhut IC, Goldberg AL: Tumor necrosis factor can induce fever in rats without activating protein breakdown in muscle or lipolysis in adipose tissue. *J Clin Invest* 81:1384–1389, 1988.
332. Sauder DN: Epidermal cytokines: Properties of epidermal cell thymocyte-activating factor (ETAF). *Lymphokin Res* 3:145–151, 1984.
333. Luger TA, Stadler BM, Luger BM, et al: Characteristics of an epidermal cell thymocyte-activating factor (ETAF) produced by human epidermal cells and a human squamous cell carcinoma cell line. *J Invest Dermatol* 81:187–193, 1983.
334. Silberstein DS, Dessein AJ, Elsas PP, et al: Characterization of a factor from the U937 cell line that enhances the toxicity of human eosinophils to *Schistosoma mansoni* larvae. *J Immunol* 138:3042–3050, 1987.
335. Murray HW: Interferon-gamma, the activated macrophage, and host defense against microbial challenge. *Ann Intern Med* 108:595–608, 1988.
336. Shimokado K, Raines EW, Madtes DK, et al: A significant part of macrophage-derived growth factor consists of at least two forms of PDGF. *Cell* 43:277–286, 1985.
337. Sporn MB, Roberts AB, Wakefield LM, et al: Transforming growth factor-beta: Biological function and chemical structure. *Science* 233:532–534, 1986.
338. Dinarello CA, Cannon JG, Wolff SM, et al: Tumor necrosis factor (cachectin) is an endogenous pyrogen and induces production of interleukin 1. *J Exp Med* 163:1433–1450, 1986.
339. Cerami A, Ykeda Y, LeTrang N, et al: Weight loss associated with an endotoxin-induced mediator from peritoneal macrophages: The role of cachectin (tumor necrosis factor). *Immun Lett* 11:173–177, 1985.
340. Oliff A, Defeo-Jones D, Boyer M, et al: Tumors secreting human TNF/cachectin induce cachexia in mice. *Cell* 50:555–563, 1987.
341. Yang RD, Moldawer LL, Sakamoto A, et al: Leukocyte endogenous mediator alters protein dynamics in rats. *Metabolism* 32:654–660, 1983.
342. Sobrado J, Moldawer LL, Bistrian BR, et al: Effect of ibuprofen on fever and metabolic changes induced by continuous infusion of leukocytic pyrogen (interleukin 1) or endotoxin. *Infect Immun* 42:997–1005, 1983.
343. Goodman MN: Tumor necrosis factor induces skeletal muscle protein breakdown in rats. *Am J Physiol* 260:E727–E730, 1990.
344. Flores EA, Bistrian BR, Pomposelli JJ, et al: Infusion of tumor necrosis factor/cachectin promotes muscle catabolism in the rat. A synergistic effect with interleukin 1. *J Clin Invest* 83:1614–1622, 1989.
345. Zamir O, Hasselgren PO, Kunkel SL, et al: Evidence that tumor necrosis factor participates in the regulation of muscle proteolysis during sepsis. *Arch Surg* 127:170–174, 1992.
346. Hall-Angeras M, Angeras U, Zamir O, et al: Interaction between corticosterone and tumor necrosis factor stimulated protein breakdown in rat skeletal muscle, similar to sepsis. *Surgery* 108:460–466, 1990.
347. Cheema IR, Hermann C, Postell S, et al: Effect of tumour necrosis factor-alpha on total myofibrillar and sarcoplasmic protein synthesis and polysomal aggregation in rat skeletal muscles. *Cytobios* 97:133–139, 1999.
348. Lang CH, Frost RA, Nairn AC, et al: TNF-alpha impairs heart and skeletal muscle protein synthesis by altering translation initiation. *Am J Physiol Endocrinol Metab* 282: E336–E347, 2002.
349. Cooney R, Kimball SR, Eckman R, et al: TNF-binding protein ameliorates inhibition of skeletal muscle protein synthesis during sepsis. *Am J Physiol* 276:E611–E619, 1999.
350. Cooney R, Owens E, Jurasinski C, et al: Interleukin-1 receptor antagonist prevents sepsis-induced inhibition of protein synthesis. *Am J Physiol* 267: E636–E641, 1994.
351. Vary TC, Owens EL, Beers JK, et al: Sepsis inhibits synthesis of myofibrillar and sarcoplasmic proteins: modulation by interleukin-1 receptor antagonist. *Shock* 6:13–18, 1996.
352. Vary TC, Voisin L, Cooney RN: Regulation of peptide-chain initiation in muscle during sepsis by interleukin-1 receptor antagonist. *Am J Physiol* 271:E513–E520, 1996.
353. Attaix DA, Goldberg AL: Unpublished observations.
354. Hobler SC, Williams A, Fischer D, et al: Activity and expression of the 20S proteasome are increased in skeletal muscle during sepsis. *Am J Physiol* 277:R434–R440, 1999.
355. Tiao G, Hobler S, Wang JJ, et al: Sepsis is associated with increased mRNAs of the ubiquitin-proteasome proteolytic pathway in human skeletal muscle. *J Clin Invest* 99:163–168, 1997.
356. Fischer D, Gang G, Pritts T, et al: Sepsis-induced muscle proteolysis is prevented by a proteasome inhibitor in vivo. *Biochem Biophys Res Commun* 270:215–221, 2000.
357. Llovera M, Carbo N, Lopez-Soriano J, et al: Different cytokines modulate ubiquitin gene expression in rat skeletal muscle. *Cancer Lett* 133:83–87, 1998.
358. Williams A, Wang JJ, Wang L, et al: Sepsis in mice stimulates muscle proteolysis in the absence of IL-6. *Am J Physiol* 275:R1983–R1991, 1998.
359. Combaret L, Tilignac T, Claustre A, et al: Torbafylline (HWA 448) inhibits enhanced skeletal muscle ubiquitin-proteasome-dependent proteolysis in cancer and septic rats. *Biochem J* 361:185–192, 2002.
360. Baracos VE, Wilson EJ, Goldberg AL: Effects of temperature on protein turnover in isolated rat skeletal muscle. *Am J Physiol* 246:C125–C130, 1984.
361. Li YP, Schwartz RJ, Waddell ID, et al: Skeletal muscle myocytes undergo protein loss and reactive oxygen-mediated NF-kappaB activation in response to tumor necrosis factor alpha. *FASEB J* 12:871–880, 1998.
362. Langen RC, Schols AM, Kelders MC, et al: Inflammatory cytokines inhibit myogenic differentiation through activation of nuclear factor-kappaB. *FASEB J* 15:1169–1180, 2001.
363. Guttridge DC, Mayo MW, Madrid LV, et al: NF-kappaB-induced loss of MyoD messenger RNA: possible role in muscle decay and cachexia. *Science* 289:2363–1366, 2000.
364. Alvarez B, Quinn LS, Busquets S, et al: Direct effects of tumor necrosis factor alpha (TNF-alpha) on murine skeletal muscle cell lines. Bimodal effects on protein metabolism. *Eur Cytokine Netw* 12:399–410, 2001.
365. Baracos VE: Regulation of skeletal-muscle-protein turnover in cancer-associated cachexia. *Nutrition* 16:1015–1018, 2000.
366. Strelkov AB, Fields AL, Baracos VE: Effects of systemic inhibition of prostaglandin production on protein metabolism in tumor-bearing rats. *Am J Physiol* 257:C261–C269, 1989.
367. Todorov P, Cariuk P, McDevitt T, et al: Characterization of a cancer cachectic factor. *Nature* 379:739–742, 1996.
368. Smith HJ, Lorite MJ, Tisdale MJ: Effect of a cancer cachectic factor on protein synthesis/degradation in murine C2C12 myoblasts: Modulation by eicosapentaenoic acid. *Cancer Res* 59:5507–5513, 1999.
369. Lorite MJ, Smith HJ, Arnold JA, et al: Activation of ATP-ubiquitin-dependent proteolysis in skeletal muscle in vivo and murine myoblasts in vitro by a proteolysis-inducing factor (PIF). *Br J Cancer* 85:297–302, 2001.
370. Wigmore SJ, Todorov PT, Barber MD, et al: Characteristics of patients with pancreatic cancer expressing a novel cancer cachectic factor. *Br J Surg* 87:53–58, 2000.
371. Wigmore SJ, Barber MD, Ross JA, et al: Effect of oral eicosapentaenoic acid on weight loss in patients with pancreatic cancer. *Nutr Cancer* 36: 177–184, 2000.
372. Mitch WE, Goldberg AL: Mechanisms of muscle wasting: The role of the ubiquitin-proteasome pathway. *N Engl J Med* 335:1897–1905, 1996.

Chapter 24
Lysosomal Metabolism and Its Relevance to Skeletal Muscle

JOSEPH ALROY
EDWIN H. KOLODNY

Lysosomal Metabolism
    THE CONCEPT OF LYSOSOMES
Skeletal Muscle Lysosomes
    EFFECTS OF EXERCISE
    PROTEOLYSIS IN SKELETAL MUSCLE
    DENERVATION
    HYPERTROPHY
    FORCED LENGTHENING
    NEUROMUSCULAR DISEASES
    RIMMED VACUOLES
    HEAT-SHOCK PROTEINS
    TRAFFICKING OF LYSOSOMAL ENZYMES IN SKELETAL MUSCLE
Lysosomal Storage Diseases
    PATHOPHYSIOLOGY
    GENETICS
    MUSCLE INVOLVEMENT
    CLINICAL DIAGNOSIS
    LABORATORY DIAGNOSIS
    TREATMENT
    INHERITED DISEASES
    ACQUIRED STORAGE DISEASES
    CONDITIONS THAT MAY SIMULATE LYSOSOMAL STORAGE DISEASES

The lysosome is the primary disposal and recycling apparatus of the cell. It degrades cellular and extracellular macromolecules, providing amino acids, fatty acids, nucleic acids, and carbohydrate residues for reutilization in cellular synthesis. It is present in all cell types including skeletal muscle. This chapter describes how lysosomal enzymes are formed, their intra- and intercellular transport, their involvement in disorders of skeletal muscle, and their effects on skeletal muscle in lysosomal storage diseases.

Lysosomal Metabolism

THE CONCEPT OF LYSOSOMES

DeDuve coined the term *lysosome*, in Greek meaning "lytic body," in 1955 to describe a sedimentable acidified cytoplasmic organelle containing various hydrolases that degrade cellular and extracellular products and foreign materials ingested by the cell (for review, see Ref. 1). The lysosome has a single limiting membrane that contains several highly N-glycosylated proteins. The lysosomal membrane protects the cell from the destructive action of the degradative enzyme within it. It sediments in a density gradient in the light mitochondrial fraction with an isopyknic distribution separate from that of both mitochondria and peroxisomes. Lysosomal enzymes have structure-linked latency; that is, their full catalytic activity is exhibited only after the lysosomal membrane is disrupted by osmotic shock, detergents, freeze-thaw, or sonication.

To begin the process of intracellular digestion, a hydrolase-free vacuole containing macromolecular material coalesces, via the lysosomal associated membrane protein-2 (LAMP-2),* with a primary lysosome to form a complex known as a secondary lysosome (Fig. 24-1). The vacuoles contain intracellular debris (autophagy) or extracellular foreign materials (heterophagy). The heterophagic vacuoles are formed by endocytosis. In the case of extracellular material, a pinocytotic vesicle forms by invagination of the cell membrane, completely surrounding the extracellular or foreign material. Following digestion of the macromolecules, their individual components are transported to the cytosol for reutilization. Any undigested material remaining in the secondary lysosomes after the hydrolytic enzymes have acted coalesces into a residual body. These dense polymorphic bodies are able to leave the cell if an excretory pathway such as bile or urine is available.

Lysosomal enzymes may also be secreted by the cells to be taken up by other cells and for the extracellular digestion of connective tissue and bone. They are also commonly released to the extracellular space in inflammatory reactions and in response to tissue injury.

Lysosomal enzymes

Lysosomal enzymes are glycoproteins that act on lipids, carbohydrates, proteins, and nucleotides to catalyze irreversibly their hydrolysis to their basic structural units. More than 50 such enzymes are known. Most lysosomal hydrolases except glucocerebrosidase and acid phosphatase are soluble proteins associated with the lysosomal membrane.[2] The genes coding for many of these enzymes and those coding lysosomal membrane proteins have been mapped to specific human chromosomes; for most, genomic or cDNA clones have been isolated and sequenced (Table 24-1).

Lysosomal enzymes have a high degree of specificity for one particular linkage, but the structural requirements for the remainder of the molecule are less and less stringent the greater the distance from the point of hydrolysis. For this reason, it is often possible to employ an artificial compound as the substrate for a lysosomal enzyme reaction rather than the more complex natural product. Assays employing this type of substrate usually yield higher levels of more easily detectable activity.

However, different enzymes may act on the same artificial substrate. Examples of such complex isoenzyme systems are the β-N-acetylhexosaminidases, arylsulfatases, α-mannosidases, and α-neuraminidases. Assay of individual

---

*A list of abbreviations used in this chapter is given at the end of the chapter.

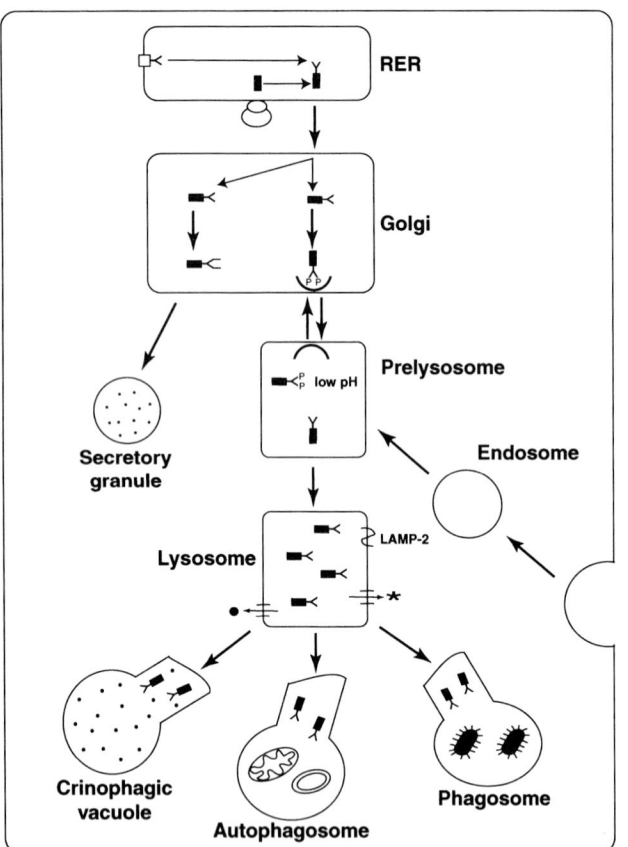

FIGURE 24-1. Schematic illustration of synthesis and targeting of lysosomal hydrolases to lysosomes and mechanisms for transferring substrates to lysosomes for degradation. Nascent lysosomal hydrolase, secretory, and membrane proteins are glycosylated in the RER by transference of preformed oligosaccharide from dolichol-P-P-oligosaccharide. These glycosylated glycoproteins are translocated to the Golgi apparatus, where secretory and membrane glycoproteins are further modified and oligosaccharides of lysosomal hydrolases are phosphorylated (P). All but two lysosomal enzymes bind to M-P receptors and are transported to a prelysosome compartment, where the enzymes are released and the receptor shuttles back to the Golgi apparatus. In the primary lysosome, the prohydrolase is cleaved. The secondary lysosome is formed by fusion of a phagosome with the primary lysosomes via LAMP-2. The catabolic products exit via transporters such as sialin (*) and cystein (.). (Modified from Jones TC, Hunt RD, King NW: Veterinary Pathology, 6th ed. Baltimore: Williams & Wilkins, 1996. With permission from Williams & Wilkins.)

enzymes in a multiple component system requires either that reaction conditions be altered to take advantage of subtle differences in their properties or that the competing activities be physically separated and assayed separately.

Biosynthesis and processing

Lysosomal enzymes are synthesized as preproteins on membrane-bound ribosomes attached to the rough endoplasmic reticulum (RER) (Fig. 24-1); thereafter, they undergo a series of posttranslational modifications involving protein and carbohydrate recognition signals that enable them to reach their final destination in lysosomes.[3] A hydrophobic amino-terminal signal peptide on the nascent protein directs its transport into the lumen of the RER, where it undergoes glycosylation of selected asparagine residues. In this glycosylation step, a large preformed oligosaccharide containing three glucose, nine mannose, and two N-acetylglucosamine residues is transferred in toto from a lipid-linked intermediate to the enzyme polypeptide. The signal peptide is cleaved and the asparagine-linked oligosaccharide modified by the removal of three glucose residues and one mannose residue. It is noteworthy that ingestion of plants such as *Astragalus lentginosus, Oxiftropis serica, Swainsona canescens,* and *Ipomoea carnea* result in acquired lysosomal storage disease. This is due to inhibition of α-mannosidase II with swainsonine and two glycosidase inhibitors, calystegine B_2 and calystegine C_1, at this stage of posttranslational modification.[4]

The lysosomal protein in a vesicular form then enters the Golgi apparatus, a stack of flattened cisternae, where a series of covalent modifications occur to the transported proteins. The cis face is nearer the nucleus and adjacent to the region of the RER that lacks bound ribosomes. There it is acted upon by a phosphotransferase, UDP-N-acetylglucosamine-lysosomal-enzyme N-acetylglucosamine phosphotransferase, that transfers N-acetylglucosamine-1-phosphophate from UDP-N-acetylglucosamine to certain of the mannose residues on the lysosomal enzyme. The N-acetylglucosamine residue is then removed by action of a second enzyme, N-acetylglucosamine-1-phosphodiester-α-N-acetylglucosminidase. A phosphomonoester (Man-6-P) is formed, which later serves as a recognition marker for specific receptors in the trans-Golgi network.

A fraction of the newly synthesized acid hydrolases are glycosylated with high mannose-type oligosaccharide and are not phosphorylated but instead pass on to the trans face of the Golgi stack, where they are processed to complex-type units containing galactose and sialic acid residues. These then exit the trans Golgi as secretory glycoproteins.

The hydrolases containing the Man-6-P marker form a ligand-receptor complex and move to prelysosomal endocytic compartments in coated vesicles. It is here that the biosynthetic and endocytotic pathways converge. The low pH in this endosome facilitates uncoupling of the receptor and its ligand, allowing recycling of the Man-6-P receptor back to the trans Golgi. The acid hydrolase proforms then undergo proteolytic maturation and partial dephosphorylation before entering the lysosome. A small amount is instead secreted and some of this enzyme is subsequently recaptured by binding to Man-6-P receptors on the cell surface. The exogenous acid hydrolase molecules then enter the cell in endosomes and undergo similar modifications en route to the lysosomal compartment.[5]

Man-6-P receptors

Much of our knowledge of lysosomal enzyme trafficking derives from studies of patients with mucolipidosis II (I-cell disease) and mucolipidosis III (pseudo-Hurler polydystrophy). Fibroblasts cultured from the skin of patients with these diseases are deficient in lysosomal enzymes, while the activity of these enzymes in serum and in the extracellular medium of cultured cells is increased severalfold. The primary defect is a deficiency in phosphotransferase. Therefore, the cells are unable to synthesize the phosphomannosyl receptor marker. Consequently, the newly formed lysosomal

Table 24-1. CHROMOSOMAL LOCALIZATION OF LYSOSOMAL ENZYMES AND PROTEINS, THEIR SIZE, AND NUMBER OF KNOWN MUTATIONS

Enzyme or Protein	Chromosomal Location	Gene Size	Exons, n	Mutations, n
di-N-acetylchitobiase	1p22			
Acetyl-CoA: α-glucosaminide acetyltransferase		43 kb	14	1
N-acetylglucosamine 6-sulfatase	12q14			
N-acetylgalactosamine 4-sulfatase	5q13-q14			45+
α-N-acetylgalactosaminidase	22q13.1-q13.2		9	4
α-N-acetylglucosaminidase	17q21.1	9 kb	8	84
N-acetylglucosaminyl-1-phosphotransferase α/β subunit	4q21-q23	80 kb	22	1
N-acetylglucosamine 1-phosphotransferase γ subunit	16p			1
β-N-acetylhexosaminidase α subunit	15q23-q24	35 kb	14	100+
β-N-acetylhexosaminidase β subunit	5q13	45 kb	14	30
Acid ceramidase	8p21.3-22	30 kb	14	10
Acid α-glucosidase	17q25.2-q25.3	20 kb	20	142
Acid lipase	10q23.2-q23.3	38.8 kb	10	25
Arylsulfatase A	22q13.31-qter	3.3 kb	8	100
Aspartylglucosaminidase	4q34-q35	13 kb	9	20
Battenin (JCLN3)	16p12	15 kb	15	31
Cathepsin K	1q21	12 kb	8	15
CLN4				
CLN5	13q22	13 kb	4	4
CLN6	15q21-23	23 kb	7	6
CLN7				
CLN8	8p2.3			1
Cystosin	17p13		12	65
α-L-fucosidase	1p34.1-36.1	23 kb	8	22
Galactosamine 6-sulfatase	16q24.3	40 kb	14	89
β-Galactosidase	3p21.33	62.5 kb	16	46
α-Galactosidase A	Xq22.1	12.5 kb	7	200
Galactosylceramidase	14q31	60 kb	7	70
Glucosylcerebrosidase	1q21	7.5 kb	11	200
β-Glucuronidase	7q21.1-q22	21 kb	12	41
G_{M2}-activator	5q32-q33	16 kb	4	5
Hyaluronidase	3p21.3			2
Iduronate-2-sulfatase	Xq28.3-q28	24 kb	9	286
α-L-iduronidase	4p16.3	9 kb	14	170
Lysosome-associated membrane protein-2 (LAMP-2)	Xq24-25	40 kb	9	8
α-Mannosidase	19p13.1	21.5 kb	24	25
β-Mannosidase	4q22-q25	3.7 kb		2
Mucolipin 1	19p13.2-13.3	14 kb	14	5
α-Neuraminidase	6p21.3		5	26
Niemann-Pick C1	18q11-12	47+kb	25	100
Niemann-Pick C2 (HE1)	14q24.3			5
Palmityl protein thioesterase (CLN 1)	1p32	25 kb	8	39
Prosaposin	10q21	20 kb	13	9
Protective protein/cathepsin A	20q13.1			17
Sialin	6q		11	10
Sphingomyelinase	11p15.1-p15.4		6	57
Sulfaminidase	17q25.3	11 kb	8	62
Tripeptidyl peptidase I (CLN2)	11p15	6.65 kb	13	44
Uridinediphosphate N-acetyl-glucosamine 2 epimerase	6q14-15			6

enzyme is not targeted to the lysosome but instead escapes to the extracellular space and cannot be recaptured by the Man-6-P receptor mechanism. Two distinct Man-6-P receptors have been identified. Both are lysosomal membrane glycoproteins. One is a ≈ 275,000-Da cation-dependent glycoprotein; the other is a ≈ 46,000-Da cation-dependent glycoprotein. Each is composed of four structural domains: a signal sequence, an extracytoplasmic amino-terminal domain, a hydrophobic transmembrane region, and a cytoplasmic domain. The only region of homology in amino acid sequence between the two receptor proteins is the extracytoplasmic domain that contains the ligand binding site.

Interestingly, another receptor, for insulin-like growth factor II (IGF-II), shares 80 percent sequence with the cation-independent Man-6-P receptor. Insulin induces a translocation of the IGF-II/Man-6-P receptor from an intracellular site to the plasma membrane. In this way it competes with the lysosomal enzyme for the Man-6-P receptor and disrupts their intracellular trafficking. This mechanism could explain insulin's ability to decrease intracellular proteolysis.[6]

There is evidence for the existence of alternative mechanisms for the translocation of acid hydrolases to lysosomes that do not involve Man-6-P receptors. I-cell fibroblasts contain normal levels of acid phosphatase and glucocerebrosidase, and other cell types in patients with I-cell disease have near normal levels of lysosomal enzymes. Certain murine cell lines lacking the Man-6-P receptor have also been shown to possess high levels of intracellular acid hydrolase activity. Therefore, intracellular mechanisms independent of the Man-6-P receptor probably exist for the delivery of acid hydrolases to lysosomal organelles.[7]

Lysosomal membrane proteins

The pathway and targeting signal for lysosomal membrane proteins differs from those used by soluble lysosomal hydrolases. These proteins contain a high number of *N*-linked, sialylated oligosaccharides, a single membrane-spanning domain, and relatively short carboxy-terminal cytoplasmic tails of 10 to 11 residues.[8] They contribute to the special properties of the lysosomal membrane—i.e., maintenance of an acidic pH environment, sequestration of acid hydrolases, resistance to degradation by lysosomal enzymes, and the ability to fuse with other membrane organelles. They do not bind to Man-6-P specific receptors but instead are transported to the plasma membrane prior to endocytosis and delivery to the lysosome. Mutations blocking endocytosis cause lysosomal membrane proteins to accumulate in the plasma membrane.[9]

Whereas the molecular signal for targeting of lysosomal enzymes resides in the mannosylphosphate moiety, lysosomal membrane glycoproteins reach the lysosome independently of the attached *N*-glycans. Their transport to the lysosome depends instead on the cytoplasmic tail of the protein, in which a tyrosine residue is essential.[8] The tyrosine plays a critical conformational role in producing a tight turn signal needed for recognition by the putative cytoplasmic receptor.[10] An example is lysosomal acid phosphatase, which undergoes Man-6-P independent targeting to the cell surface, internalization into endosomes, and recycling many times between the cell surface and endosomes before delivery to lysosomes, where it is subjected to limited proteolysis to generate the mature soluble form of the enzyme.[11]

The two best-known lysosomal-associated membrane proteins (LAMP) are LAMP-1 and LAMP-2. These two glycoproteins are structurally similar and evolutionarily related. Expression of LAMP-2 is increased in tissues of mice deficient in LAMP-1.[12] Furthermore, LAMP-2 is a family of membrane proteins, and LAMP-2a was identified as a receptorz in lysosomes known as chaperone-mediated autophagy.[13] Recent studies indicate that LAMP-2 may be involved in the process of fusion of autophagic vacuoles with lysosomes.[14] As a result, deficiency in LAMP-2 results in accumulation of autophagic vacuoles.[14,15]

In addition, there are two other lysosomal associated membrane transporter proteins that participate in efflux of degradation products from the lysosomes. Mutations of the gene coding for cystinosin lead to lysosomal storage of cystein,[16] whereas mutations of the gene coding for sialin lead to storage of free sialic acid.[17]

Skeletal Muscle Lysosomes

The lysosomal system in normal skeletal muscle is poorly developed. One possible reason is that muscle does not normally engage in absorptive, secretory, or excretory activities.[18] Also, with the recurring buildup of lactic acid in muscle, an abundance of lysosomes might conceivably lead to activation of hydrolytic enzymes and autolysis of muscle fibers.

Normal skeletal muscle contains a full complement of acid hydrolases. They are latent and sedimentable, properties normally associated with lysosomal enzymes.[19] There are two populations of lysosomes in skeletal muscle. Those from the muscle itself account for 75 to 95 percent of the enzyme activity. The remainder are derived from connective tissue and macrophages.[18,20] Together they account for less than 1 percent of the protein[21] but contain 5 percent of glycogen in muscle.[22]

That muscle cells possess the potential to form lysosomes can be demonstrated with myoblasts in cell culture. These cells form lysosome-like granules. However, lysosomal activity does not appear to be involved in the digestion of plasma membrane separating fusing myoblasts.[23] Developmentally, lysosomal enzyme activities are higher in fetal muscle and muscle of young animals than in muscle of older animals.[20,22] Histochemical studies demonstrate greater activity in the oxidative than in the glycolytic fibers,[24] and biochemical measurements indicate higher activity in red slow-twitch than white fast-twitch fibers.[25]

The origins and subcellular localization of lysosomes in skeletal muscle can be demonstrated with lysosomotrophic agents. *N*-Dodecyl (C_{12}) imidazole enters lysosomes and disrupts the lysosomal membrane, causing cell death. Its action on skeletal muscle is to cause swelling of the sarcotubular system, leading to rapid myofilament damage. These findings led Duncan and Rudge[26] to postulate that the function of lysosomes in skeletal muscle is subserved by parts of the sarcotubular system. Incubation of mouse skeletal muscle with protamine results in the formation of membrane-limited vacuoles. Their location throughout the muscle fiber and adjacent to the A-I junction suggests that they arise as endocytic vesicles from the transverse tubules. They acquire acid phosphatase activity and become secondary lysosomes, which localize to the longitudinal sarcoplasmic reticulum.[27] Incubation of isolated rat myotubes with horseradish peroxidase reveals a proliferating tubular and vesicular network stained by the peroxidase which has been endocytosed. The network is present in segments that also contain high lysosomal activity, suggesting that the lysosomes are closely associated with the t-tubular system.[28] After ischemic injury to rabbit muscle, histochemical staining for lysosomal enzyme activity discloses granules arranged longitudinally along the muscle fiber.[29] Together, these studies indicate, as first suggested by Pearce,[30] that normal muscle lysosomes exist as part of the sarcotubular system.

EFFECTS OF EXERCISE

Exercise poses a significant metabolic demand on muscle homeostasis. A marked buildup in lactic acid, depletion of energy stores, and rise in temperature can threaten the integrity of muscle. These circumstances could activate the intracellular release of hydrolytic enzymes, degrading cell components and accelerating the breakdown of the muscle tissue itself. To investigate this effect, several researchers have studied acid hydrolase activity in mice or rats after treadmill exercise.

Moderately intense exercise results in a mild increase in lysosomal enzyme activity.[31,32] With more vigorous exercise, fiber necrosis and inflammation may occur due especially to compartmental injury by the accumulation of water, causing increased tissue pressure and ischemic lesions.[33,34] Two to seven days after exertion, an autophagic response occurs in the fibers near the necrotic focus and macrophages move in to remove the debris by heterophagic uptake. The peak response in lysosomal enzyme activity occurs 3 to 5 days after the exercise. While some muscle acid hydrolase activity is induced, the major response is from macrophages. These invading cells secrete lysosomal enzymes that are taken up through the muscle phosphomannosyl-enzyme receptor system. Training confers resistance to the damaging effects of exhaustive exercise.[33]

PROTEOLYSIS IN SKELETAL MUSCLE

Compared to other tissues, skeletal muscle has low proteolytic activity.[20] However, it is important to total body metabolism because skeletal muscle represents the principal store of amino acids in the body, which are the building blocks for protein synthesis and a source of fuel during starvation. Both lysosomal and nonlysosomal degradative pathways have been described.[21] In normal muscle, specific activities of the acidic proteases and the cytosolic (neutral and alkaline) proteases are similar.[21]

DENERVATION

Pathologic states that produce muscle breakdown, such as denervation, provide an opportunity to study proteolysis in skeletal muscle. The degradation of sarcolemmal and myofibrillar proteins is thought to occur differently. Proteolysis of the sarcolemma is attributed to acid hydrolases, whereas nonlysosomal mechanisms cause breakdown of contractile protein.[33] Duncan and Rudge[26] proposed that the calcium concentration rises in injured muscle, producing rapid damage to the myofibrillar apparatus by a mechanism in which lysosomes are not involved. They postulate that the rise in calcium concentration also causes activation of phospholipase A_2, which generates prostaglandins and leukotrienes. These, in turn, damage lysosomal membranes, causing the much slower appearance of acid hydrolases.

Denervation of skeletal muscle leads to rapid loss of muscle bulk and an increase in lysosomal enzyme activities.[35] Very little infiltration of white cells and macrophages occurs, so that nearly all of the increase in enzyme activity would appear to come from the muscle fibers themselves.[36] Drugs that are known to inhibit lysosomal enzyme activity retard the appearance of denervation-derived muscle atrophy, but their effects are transitory.[37] Von Steyern and Josefsson[38] have demonstrated the increased secretion of plasminogen activator and lysosomal β-glucuronidase following muscle denervation. Their studies support the concept that the release of these enzymes may participate in the formation of the neuromuscular synapse and reinnervation of denervated muscle fibers.

Proteolysis in denervated muscle is increased two- to threefold by conditions that activate intralysosomal proteolysis as well as by those that activate calcium-dependent protein breakdown. Similarly, treatments that block both forms of proteolysis do not reduce the increase in protein degradation that occurs in denervated muscle. These results suggest that multiple proteolytic systems increase in parallel in denervated muscle.[39]

Loss of a nerve trophic factor has been suggested to explain the increase in lysosomal enzyme activity that is induced by denervation.[40] Endocytic and lysosomal activities are increased after denervation, especially in the end plate region of the skeletal muscle fiber.[41] Myotubes in culture develop specialized segments with endocytotic activity, high lysosomal enzyme activity, high acetylcholine receptor content, and a proliferating tubular network in communication with the extracellular space.[28] These properties are similar to the characteristics of the denervated end plate region of adult muscle.

HYPERTROPHY

When compensatory hypertrophy is induced in synergistic muscle by experimental tenotomy, it is accompanied by a progressive increase in lysosomal enzyme activity after 3 and 7 days. If the hypertrophied muscle is then denervated, lysosomal activity is greatly enhanced. Bass et al.[42] found the degree of muscle atrophy after the combined procedure to be twice that of denervation alone. Enhanced proteolytic activity in the hypertrophied muscle could explain the alteration in muscle cells after denervation. It has been suggested that the newly synthesized proteins in the hypertrophied muscle are more "labile" and therefore more susceptible to breakdown after denervation.[43]

FORCED LENGTHENING

Injury of muscle induced by forced lengthening causes cellular proliferation, especially near the torn ends of the myofibers. Immunohistochemical staining of these cells indicates that most are myogenic in origin. Lysosomal proteolytic activity indicative of the presence of phagocytic cells is not increased in or between damaged myofibers. However, elevated lysosomal proteolytic activity is present in normal-appearing myofibrils of the injured muscle.[44]

NEUROMUSCULAR DISEASES

Lysosomal enzyme activities in muscle are increased in several neuromuscular diseases of humans. These include amyotrophic lateral sclerosis[45–47] and polymyositis.[46–49] In patients with muscular dystrophy, levels of acid hydrolase activity correlate better with the severity of muscle wasting than with the specific type of muscle disease.[37,39]

RIMMED VACUOLES

Vacuolar degeneration, with rimmed vacuoles containing increased acid phosphatase activity, has been found in acid maltase deficiency, acid lipase deficiency, distal myopathy with rimmed vacuoles, oculopharyngeal muscular dystrophy, and experimental chloroquine myopathy.[50–52] Rimmed vacuoles are also seen in inclusion body myositis. In this disease, autophagic vacuoles containing Congo red–positive amyloid protein are a characteristic feature.[53]

HEAT-SHOCK PROTEINS

Protein degradation in lysosomes is facilitated by cell stress proteins, also known as heat-shock proteins (HSP). These include HSP-70—which acts as molecular chaperone facilitating the folding, assembly, and transport of cellular proteins[54]—and ubiquitin, which conjugates with proteins destined for lysosomal uptake and metabolism.[55] Lysosomal protein degradation also requires the ubiquitin-activating protein E1.[56] Heat-shock proteins are expressed constitutively and are also induced under conditions such as heat shock, nutritional deprivation, and exposure to cytokines or inflammatory mediators.

A 65-kDa HSP has been detected by antibody immunostaining in several inflammatory myopathies on degenerating muscle fibers and on some nonnecrotic muscle fibers invaded by T cells. Hohlfeld and Engel[57] speculate that the expression of the 65-kDa HSP could be a nonspecific response to cellular stress and also an autoantigen recognized by autoreactive T cells.

TRAFFICKING OF LYSOSOMAL ENZYMES IN SKELETAL MUSCLE

Intracellular transfer of lysosomal enzyme activity in muscle occurs via the Man-6-P receptor system as well as through direct cell-to-cell contact. Both the cation-independent and cation-dependent Man-6-P receptors can be detected in muscle cells in culture. The amount of cation-independent receptor mRNA increases tenfold during the first 48 h of culture in C2 myotubes and in primary cultures of fetal muscle. However, there is no change in the amount of cation-independent mRNA, suggesting that the two receptors serve separate functions during development.[58]

The high-molecular-weight cation-independent receptor has also been shown by immunoelectron microscopy to be present in the pericapillary space in human skeletal muscle tissue. Acid α-glucosidase and glucocerebrosidase colocalize with albumin in the pericapillary space, suggesting that these high-molecular-weight proteins can pass the endothelial barrier in the skeletal muscle.[59] Using cultured skeletal muscle cells from a patient with infantile glycogenosis, Van der Ploeg et al.[60] have shown that acid α-glucosidase purified from human urine enters the cells and reverses the glycogen storage. The enzyme, containing phosphorylated high-mannose-type oligosaccharide chains, passed through the cell membrane and was targeted to lysosomes by use of the Man-6-P receptors on the cell surface.

Phosphomannosyl-enzyme receptors can also be shown in the membranes of skeletal muscles.[47,61] Their concentration is one-third that of liver membranes.[61] During repair of exercise-induced muscle injury, the content of receptors rises only slightly, but the occupancy of the receptors by lysosomal enzyme is strikingly increased.[62] In myogenic muscle diseases, such as polymyositis and muscular dystrophy, the specific binding capacity of phosphomannosyl receptors increases significantly. The increase in receptors in neurogenic muscle diseases is much less.[47] Salminen et al.[47] have proposed that the increase in receptors is associated with increased metabolism of connective tissue, thereby accounting for the deposition of collagen in polymyositis and muscular dystrophy.

Uptake of an exogenous lysosomal enzyme into skeletal muscle myoblasts can occur by a pathway independent of Man-6-P receptor-mediated endocytosis. Beauchamp et al.[63] have demonstrated transfer of the lymphocyte form of lysosomal β-glucuronidase by coculture of myoblasts with lymphocytes. Direct cell-to-cell contact with muscle cells was required and was not inhibited by Man-6-P enzyme uptake by the muscle cells.[63]

The existence of these receptor mechanisms suggests that skeletal muscle would be a good target for enzyme replacement therapy in lysosomal storage diseases. They provide a rationale for the use of bone marrow transplantation and direct infusion of purified enzyme. Indeed, as the largest single tissue in the body, skeletal muscle has the greatest potential for the uptake and storage of lysosomal enzymes.

Lysosomal Storage Diseases

Lysosomal storage diseases (LSDs) are a group of more than 45 genetically determined heterogenous metabolic disorders.[64,65] Biochemically, the majority are characterized by deficient activity of specific lysosomal hydrolases and the intralysosomal accumulation of one or more substrates in affected cells. In a few instances, lysosomal storage results from the deficiency of an enzyme coactivator membrane transporter-targeting mechanism for localizing proteins to the lysosomes or for intracellular vesicular trafficking.

The LSDs are often categorized according to the chemical nature of the most prominent storage compounds. They include lipid storage diseases, glycoprotein storage diseases, mucopolysaccharidoses, and mucolipidoses. It is noteworthy that deficient enzyme activity occurs in all cell types of the affected individual. However, the degree of abnormal storage in different cell types and organs is determined by the amount of substrate normally present in these cells. As there is no storage in cardiac and skeletal myocytes in several of the common LSDs, we have chosen to exclude these from this chapter.

PATHOPHYSIOLOGY

Insights concerning the synthetic pathway of lysosomal enzymes, their functions, the role of activator and protective proteins, transporter, and lysosomal associated membrane proteins have led to their classification according to the mechanisms which produce the various disorders.[67] Eleven such mechanisms are recognized and are summarized in Table 24-2. The consequence of the above mechanisms is lysosomal accumulation (i.e., storage) of catabolites, resulting in severe impairment of cellular structure and function. Since it is possible for each of the above mechanisms to occur in all cell types of affected individuals, the degree of abnormal accumulation in each cell type depends on the amount of substrate available in these cells. The substrate load, in turn, is influenced by the cell membrane composition, the rate of membrane recycling and cellular catabolism, the phagocytic ability of affected cells, and the nature of phagocytosed substrates.[66]

Table 24-3 summarizes the lysosomal storage disorders, with a listing of their eponyms, their primary and secondary deficiency, and their clinical manifestations (for reviews, see Refs. 68, 69). These diseases are progressive. Clinically, the initial manifestations begin in childhood and, in many of these disorders, death can occur at an early age. Often they are manifest by generalized neurologic and/or visceral impairment; frequently skeletal abnormalities also occur. In many, the central nervous system (CNS) is particularly affected, because neurons whose function is impaired by lysosomal storage lack the ability to regenerate. When the substrate whose metabolism is blocked is especially abundant in nerve cells, as in the G_{M2} gangliosidoses, there is cognitive decline, loss of motor control, and, ultimately, the destruction of all CNS functions.

Other lysosomal storage diseases affect predominantly the reticuloendothelial system or connective tissue because the substrate whose metabolism is blocked is primarily found in these tissues. These diseases have cumulative effects on various tissues including skeletal muscle, but their impact is partially mitigated by the greater ability of these tissues to store and dispose of the undegradable material and to maintain organ function by cell regeneration.

GENETICS

Nearly all lysosomal storage diseases are inborn errors of metabolism. The majority are inherited as autosomal recessive traits. Exceptions are Hunter disease, Fabry disease, and Danon disease—which are X-linked recessive—and Kuf disease, which has been associated in a few families with autosomal dominant inheritance.

Clinical heterogeneity is common among the lysosomal storage diseases. For many of the diseases, severe infantile, less severe juvenile, and milder chronic or late-onset forms are known. With the availability of cDNA clones for the genes coding for many of the lysosomal enzymes, accurate phenotype-genotype correlations are now possible. In certain instances, no transcription takes place, or the mRNA transcript is sufficiently abnormal that it is destroyed before it can be translated into enzyme protein. Such individuals are totally deficient in the relevant enzyme activity and usually have a severe clinical form of the disease. Other mutations permit transcription and translation to occur,

Table 24-2. CLASSIFICATION OF LYSOSOMAL STORAGE DISORDERS ACCORDING TO THE MECHANISMS THAT CAUSE ABNORMAL STORAGE

Mechanisms	Examples
1. Disorders in which no immunologically detectable enzyme is synthesized. This includes conditions with grossly abnormal structural genes.	Infantile forms of glycoprotein, glycolipid, glycogen, or lipid storage disease and mucopolysaccharidoses
2. Disorders in which catalytically inactive polypeptide is synthesized. The mutation may also affect the stability or transport of the polypeptide.	Juvenile and adult forms of glycoprotein, glycolipid, glycogen, or lipid storage diseases and mucopolysaccharidoses
3. Disorders in which a catalytically active enzyme is synthesized but the enzyme does not segregate into lysosomes.	I-cell disease, pseudo-Hurler polydystrophy
4. Disorder in which catalytically active enzymes are synthesized; however, mutation in protective protein results in unstable enzymes.	Galactosialidosis
5. Disorders in which activator proteins (saposins) of lipid-degrading hydrolases are missing.	AB variant of GM_2 gangliosidosis, variants of Gaucher and Farber diseases, juvenile variant of metachromatic leukodystrophy
6. Disorders in which the structural gene for the hydrolase is normal, but there is a mutation in the gene(s) that code for posttranslation modification of the hydrolase.	Multiple sulfatase deficiencies
7. Disorders due to abnormal transport to lysosomes.	Mucolipidosis IV, Niemann-Pick disease type C
8. Disorders due to a decrease in transport of a degradation end product (i.e., free sialic acid, free cystine) out of lysosomes	Infantile sialidosis, Salla disease, cystinosis
9. Disorder due to deficiency of lysosomal-associated membrane protein-2	X-limited vacuolar cardiomyopathy and myopathy (Danon disease)
10. Disorders due to oversupply of substrate	Some leukemias, and thalassemia that are associated with Gaucher cells
11. Disorders in which lysosomal enzyme deficiencies result from intoxication with natural or synthetic inhibitors of lysosomal enzymes	Indolizidine alkaloid (i.e., swainsonine), cationic amphophilic drugs (i.e., amiodarone, chloroquine, suramin, tilorone, etc.)

Table 24-3. SUMMARY OF LYSOSOMAL STORAGE DISEASES

	Eponym	Primary Deficiency (Secondary Deficiency)	Storage Substrate	Clinical Features
Disorders of sphingolipid degradation				
Fabry disease		α-Galactosidase A	Gal-Gal-Glu-ceramide	Angiokeratoma; corneal and lenticular opacities; cardiac, cerebral, renal, and vascular manifestations
Farber lipogranulomatosis	Farber disease	Ceramidase	Ceramide	Skin nodules; joint, lung, hepatic, and CNS involvement
Glucosylceramide lipidosis	Gaucher disease	Glucocerebrosidase	Glucosylceramide, glycopeptides	
Type 1 (nonneuropathic)				Hepatosplenomegaly and bone marrow involvement
Type 2 (acute neuropathic)				Very severe neurovisceral involvement
Type 3 (subacute neuropathic)				Severe neurovisceral manifestations
G_{M1} gangliosidosis				
Type 1, infantile form		Acid β-galactosidase	G_{M1} gangliosides, galactosyl-oligo-saccharides, keratin sulfate	Extensive neurovisceral and skeletal manifestations
Type 2, juvenile form		"	"	Severe CNS and mild visceral and skeletal involvement
Type 3, adult form		"	"	Moderate CNS impairment, mild skeletal manifestations
G_{M2} gangliosidosis				
Variant B and B1	Tay-Sachs disease	β-Hexosaminidase α-subunit (hexosaminidase A)	G_{M2} ganglioside	Severe CNS manifestations in infantile and juvenile forms; moderate to mild CNS manifestations in adult form
Variant O	Sandhoff disease	β-Hexosaminidase β subunit (hexo-samides A and B)	G_{M2} ganglioside, oligosaccharides, and glycosaminoglycans	Severe CNS manifestations and moderate visceral and skeletal involvement
Variant AB	Activator deficiency	G_{M2} activator	G_{M2} ganglioside	Severe to moderate CNS manifestations
Galactosylceramide lipidosis	Krabbe disease Globoid cell leukodystrophy	Galactosylcerebrosidase galactosylsphinogosine	Galactosylceramide	Severe CNS manifestations in infantile form and moderate symptoms in adult form
Metachromatic leukodystrophy			Galactosylsulfatide, lactosylsulfatide	Severe CNS manifestations in infantile form and moderate manifestations in juvenile and adult forms
Classic type		Arylsulfatase A		
Activator deficiency type		Sulfatide activator/saposin B		
Mucolipidosis IV		Mucolipin	Gangliosides, phospho-lipids, acid muco-polysaccharides	Severe CNS manifestations and corneal clouding
Multiple sulfatase deficiency		Posttranslational modification of sulfatases	Various sulfated-lipids and all mucopolysaccharides	Severe CNS manifestations, hepatosplenomegaly and skeletal involvement
Sphingomyelin-cholesterol lipidosis	Niemann-Pick disease			
Type 1, acute	Niemann-Pick A	Sphingomyelinase	Sphingomyelin	Severe CNS and visceral involvement
Type 1, subacute	Niemann-Pick B	Sphingomyelinase	Sphingomyelin	Mostly moderate visceral organ involvement
Subacute, chronic	Niemann-Pick C, D	Niemann-Pick C protein	Glycolipids, bis(monoglycerol) phosphate	Severe CNS involvement, moderate visceral manifestations
Schindler disease				
Type 1		α-N-Acetylgalacto-saminidase	α-galNAc glycolipids, glycoproteins	Severe neuroaxonal dystrophy
Type II		"	"	Mild CNS involvement, angiokeratoma corporis diffusum

Table 24-3 (Continued). SUMMARY OF LYSOSOMAL STORAGE DISEASES

	Eponym	Primary Deficiency (Secondary Deficiency)	Storage Substrate	Clinical Features
Disorders of glycoprotein degradation				
Aspartylglucosaminuria		Aspartylglucosaminidase	Aspartylglucosamine-oligosaccharides	Moderate to mild neurovisceral, skeletal, and dermal involvement
Fucosidosis		α-L-Fucosidase	Fucosyl-oligosaccharides and glycolipids	
Type I				Severe neurovisceral and skeletal manifestations and angiokeratoma in type I
Type II				Moderate involvement of these sites in type II
Galactosialidosis		Protective protein/cathepsin A (β-galactosidase and sialidase)	Substrates of β-galactosidase and sialidase	Severe neurovisceral, skeletal, and dermal in infantile form; mild involvement in juvenile and adult forms
α-Mannosidosis		α-Mannosidase	α-Mannosyl-oligosaccharides	Severe neurovisceral and skeletal manifestations in infantile form (type I); milder manifestations in juvenile and adult form (type II)
β-Mannosidosis		β-Mannosidase	β-Mannosyl-oligosaccharides	Angiokeratoma and mild to moderate CNS manifestations
Sialidosis	Mucolipidosis I	Sialidase	Sialyl-oligosaccharides	Severe neurovisceral and skeletal manifestations in infantile (type II); mild to moderate involvement in juvenile, adult forms (type I)
Disorders of glycosaminoglycan degradation				
Mucopolysaccharidosis I	Hurler	α-L-iduronidase	Dermatan and heparan sulfate	Severe neurovisceral and skeletal manifestations, corneal clouding
	Scheie	α-L-iduronidase	Dermatan and heparan sulfate	Corneal clouding and skeletal involvement
Mucopolysaccharidosis II	Hunter	Iduronate sulfatase	Dermatan and heparan sulfate	Neurovisceral and skeletal manifestations in infantile form; only skeletal involvement in adult form
Mucopolysaccharidosis IIIA	Sanfilippo A	Sulfaminidase	Heparan sulfate	Mental deterioration, mild to moderate skeletal involvement
Mucopolysaccharidosis IIIB	Sanfilippo B	α-N-acetyl glucosaminidase	Heparan sulfate	Phenotype similar to IIIA
Mucopolysaccharidosis IIIC	Sanfilippo C	Acetyl-CoA: α-glucosaminide acetyltransferase	Heparan sulfate	Phenotype similar to IIIA
Mucopolysaccharidosis IIID	Sanfilippo D	N-acetylglucosamine 6-sulfatase	Heparan sulfate	Phenotype similar to IIIA
Mucopolysaccharidosis IVA	Morquio A	Galactose 6-sulfatase	Keratan sulfate, chondroitin 6-sulfate	Corneal clouding, severe skeletal manifestations
Mucopolysaccharidosis IVB	Morquio B	β-Galactosidase	Keratan sulfate	Phenotype similar to IVA
Mucopolysaccharidosis VI	Maroteaux-Lamy	N-Acetylgalactosamine 4-sulfatase (arylsulfatase B)	Dermatan sulfate	Corneal clouding, severe skeletal involvement
Mucopolysaccharidosis VII	Sly	β-Glucuronidase	Dermatan and heparan sulfate, chondroitin-4-6-sulfates	Severe skeletal involvement, hepatosplenomegaly, moderate mental retardation
Mucopolysaccharidosis IX		Hyaluronidase	Hyaluronan	Mild skeletal involvement, transient periarticular swelling

(Continued)

Table 24-3 (Continued). SUMMARY OF LYSOSOMAL STORAGE DISEASES

	Eponym	Primary Deficiency (Secondary Deficiency)	Storage Substrate	Clinical Features
Disorders of neuronal ceroid lipofuscinosis				
Adult form	Kuf's disease	Unknown	Unknown	Moderate CNS involvement
Classic late infantile form	Jansky-Bielschowsky	Tripeptidyl peptidase (cLINCL)	Mitochondrial subunit c ATPase synthase	Severe neuroocular manifestations and moderate visceral involvement
Disorders of neuronal ceroid lipofuscinosis				
Classic juvenile form	Spielmeyer-Sjögren	Battenin (cJNCL)	Mitochondrial subunit c ATPase synthetase	Severe to moderate neuroocular manifestations and moderate visceral involvement
Infantile form (INCL)	Santavouri-Haltia	Palmityl protein-thioesterase	Saposins A and D	Severe neuroocular manifestations and moderate visceral involvement
Other single-enzyme-deficiency disorders				
Glycogenosis type II	Pompe disease	α-Glucosidase	Glycogen (acid maltase)	Severe neurovisceral involvement with functional impairment of cardiac and skeletal muscle in infantile forms; moderate to mild manifestations in juvenile and adult forms
Acid lipase deficiency	Wolman disease Cholesterol ester storage disease	Acid lipase Acid lipase	Cholesterol esters	Hepatosplenomegaly, anemia, gastrointestinal and adrenal manifestations, liver involvement in cholesterol storage disease
Pycnodysostosis		Cathepsin K	Collagen, osteonectin	Skeletal dysplasia, osteochondrodysplasia, short stature, brachycephalic, osteosclerosis, bone fragility
Abnormal lysosomal membrane transport				
I-cell disease	Mucolipidosis II	6-Phospho-*N*-acetylglucosamine transferase	Complex glycoconjugates	Severe neurovisceral and skeletal involvement, and corneal clouding in I-cell disease; moderate to mild skeletal and corneal involvement in pseudo-Hurler polydystrophy
Pseudo-Hurler polydystrophy	Mucolipidosis III	6-Phospho-*N*-acetylglucosamine transferase	Complex glycoconjugates	
Other disorders of lysosomal membrane transport				
Cystinosis		Cystosin	Free, nonprotein cystine	Severe renal involvement, resulting in mental and growth retardation and ocular manifestations
Free sialic acid storage		Sialin (Impaired feedback inhibition of uridinediphosphate-*N*-acetyl-glucosamine-2-epimerase)	Free sialic acid	Severe neurovisceral and skeletal abnormalities in infantile sialic storage disease
Salla disease			Free sialic acid	Moderate neurological manifestations
Glycogen storage with normal acid maltase	Danon disease	Lysosome-associated membrane protein-2 (LAMP-2)	Glycogen and cytoplasmic debris	Visceral organs, skeletal and cardiac muscles

but—because of their effect on one or another of the steps in lysosomal enzyme processing—the nascent acid hydrolase does not complete its journey to the lysosome. In certain instances of this type, the enzyme proform possesses catalytic activity, but it is severely reduced. Another type of mutation specifically affects the substrate-binding ability or catalytic site of the enzyme. The enzyme protein in these circumstances reaches the lysosome, but it cannot fulfill its catalytic function. Accumulation of undegraded substrate occurs only when the residual activity of the enzyme is below the critical threshold of 10 to 15 percent.[70]

MUSCLE INVOLVEMENT

Tissues with secretory functions such as liver and brain and cells with phagocytic functions such as macrophages have relatively intense lysosomal activity. Therefore, the morphologic manifestations of lysosomal storage disorders in muscle tissue are not as obvious as in neural and visceral tissues. Thus it is not surprising that there are only a few reports in which the involvement of muscle tissue in lysosomal storage disease has been documented.

Most cell types such as neurons and hepatocytes undergo expansion of their cell bodies as a result of lysosomal storage. In contrast, muscle cells in patients with lysosomal diseases tend to shrink because of CNS degeneration, with resulting denervation. Consequently, there is loss of contractile elements and exocytosis of their lysosomal content.[71] Thus, standard light microscopy of muscle is not very useful for the diagnosis of the majority of lysosomal storage diseases because of the relative size, amount, and solubility of the storage material. In some conditions, frozen sections or 1-μm sections of resin-embedded muscle—subjected to special fixation (i.e., with 90% ethanol) and staining with Sudan black, Luxol fast blue (LFB), and periodic acid-Schiff (PAS) after predigestion with diastase, alcian blue, and toluidine blue—may be useful in identifying stored glycogen, acid mucopolysaccharides, nonglycogen carbohydrates, and lipids. Furthermore, lectin histochemistry may contribute to the identification of the sugar residues stored in the affected cells.[72]

The metabolic activity of satellite cells is different from that of contracting muscle cells. These cells are involved in lysosomal storage and are found to be affected in conditions such as I-cell disease[73] and in caprine β-manosidosis.[74]

CLINICAL DIAGNOSIS

Lysosomal storage diseases affect all organ systems, but there is a tendency for involvement of those tissues that normally contain the highest concentration of the stored material. Thus, nerve cells in the central and peripheral nervous system are ballooned in the ganglioside storage diseases, G_{M1} and G_{M2} gangliosidosis. Brain white matter is rich in galactocerebrosides, so that storage of galactosylceramide and sulfatide in Krabbe disease and metachromatic leukodystrophy, respectively, results in leukodystrophy. Turnover of blood cells in the reticuloendothelial system releases glucosylceramide, which, in turn, accumulates in the spleen, liver, and bone marrow of patients with Gaucher disease. Glycosaminoglycans (mucopolysaccharides) are widely dispersed in connective tissues; therefore failure of their degradation causes thickening of the skin, skeletal deformity, tendon contractures, spinal cord compression, and airway obstruction. Blockage of sweat glands and tortuosity of small blood vessels in the skin may suggest Fabry disease or fucosidosis. Glycogen storage in muscle can cause pseudohypertrophy, as seen in acid maltase deficiency and Danon disease. Alternatively, denervation due to the loss of anterior horn cells—as in late-onset G_{M2} gangliosidosis or the peripheral neuropathy of Krabbe disease or metachromatic leukodystrophy—produces neurogenic atrophy.

Therefore, the clinical signs may suggest preferential involvement of specific tissues and their constellation, in turn, can point to the nature of the stored material. For example, involvement of the spleen and liver, as well as the brain gray matter, heightens awareness of Niemann-Pick disease type A or C.

The patient's ethnicity may also help to narrow the diagnostic possibilities. Patients with fucosidosis are often of Italian ancestry; those with a Scandinavian heritage are at a greater risk for aspartylglucosaminuria; and individuals of Ashkenazi Jewish background may have a higher incidence of G_{M2} gangliosidosis, Gaucher disease, Niemann-Pick disease type A, and mucolipidosis IV. Family history is another important component of the workup, especially in the case of the X-linked diseases such as Fabry and Hunter diseases, where other relatives on the maternal side, specifically, are likely to be affected as well.

Age of onset also serves as a guide to diagnosis as well as an indication of the degree of residual enzyme present in the patient's tissues. Many of the lysosomal storage diseases can be grouped according to their age of onset—i.e. neonatal, infancy, childhood, adolescence, or adulthood. In general, the earlier symptoms appear, the more severe the enzyme deficiency—that is, the less residual enzyme present and the more rapid the clinical course. Diseases involving the brain are obviously more handicapping, with gray matter diseases causing greater intellectual impairment.

LABORATORY DIAGNOSIS

The first steps generally involve imaging studies [skeletal x-rays, computed tomography (CT) and magnetic resonance imaging (MRI) of the brain] and clinical neurophysiology [electroencephalography (EEG), electromyography (EMG), evoked potentials]. Readily available fluids such as urine and blood can be especially helpful. Urine, particularly a first morning void, may contain increased amounts of mucopolysaccharides or oligosaccharides that can be separated into their individual components by thin-layer chromatography. Peripheral blood smears are studied for the presence of vacuolated monocytes and lymphocytes, such as may occur in Niemann-Pick disease, mannosidosis, Wolman disease, and sialidosis. Serum and leukocytes can be incubated with artificial substrates to determine whether there is a deficiency of a specific lysosomal enzyme. Blood DNA can also be extracted for molecular diagnosis. In cases where a few common mutations are known, these are looked for. If the disease is found by enzyme analysis and the mutations responsible can be identified, the diagnosis of other family members, including carriers, is facilitated and prenatal diagnosis in future pregnancies can be done with greater confidence. Generally, these types of biochemical and molecular analyses are not part of routine diagnostic laboratory practice but must be performed in specialized laboratories.

Skin biopsy is especially valuable when a storage disease is suspected, but the clinical examination does not provide enough clues to focus the search to a limited number of conditions.[75] This is often the circumstance in a very young child with unexplained developmental delay or a dysmorphic youngster with nonspecific features. It is our practice to take two 3-mm specimens from the axilla. One sample is placed in glutaraldehyde for electron microscopy (EM) and the other, into tissue culture media for fibroblast cell culture. The morphologic appearance of inclusions that might be seen by EM often provides a guide to further biochemical testing. The fibroblasts can be harvested for enzymatic determinations as well as for studies of their DNA. The cultured cells also provide a source of mRNA from which cDNA is prepared, permitting direct sequencing of exons of the relevant gene without interference from introns.

Whenever an enzymatic deficiency is identified, specimens from the parents should also be examined to confirm their carrier status. In the case of those lysosomal diseases with autosomal recessive inheritance, one would expect to find that each parent had a reduced level of activity of the relevant enzyme. However, for certain disorders, such as Krabbe disease and the X-linked disorders, this relationship does not pertain and other types of studies are needed for unequivocal carrier identification. Also, conditions for each type of assay vary. For example, when using peripheral blood for acid maltase determinations, lymphocytes are essential, as mixed leukocytes contain several other enzyme components with acid maltase-like activity that can interfere with the reaction.

TREATMENT

Ongoing treatment for these complex disorders requires a multidisciplinary team. The patient and/or family must understand how the deficient enzyme causes the clinical signs and symptoms that have appeared. The nature of the stored substance, its role in normal cellular metabolism, and its regular catabolic route should be reviewed. From this discussion, the family will come to understand why there is skeletal dysplasia, muscle weakness, or swallowing difficulty and what they can do to ameliorate the situation. In patients with CNS manifestations, adequate nutritional intake and hydration are special concerns. Feeding difficulties can lead to aspiration and pneumonia; dehydration can lead to urinary tract infection. Orthopedic advice is sought for orthotics to prevent contractures. Physical therapy and botulinum toxin injections may also be needed, and medications for spasticity and seizures are also common. The young child especially can benefit from an early intervention program.

For a few disorders, therapeutic approaches are available that specifically address the underlying biochemical disturbance. Bone marrow transplantation (BMT) has stabilized and in some cases reversed the course of illness in children with certain leukodystrophies (metachromatic leukodystrophy, Krabbe disease, and adrenoleukodystrophy)[76,77] and has arrested the progression of certain clinical manifestations in the mucopolysaccharidoses (MPS I and II).[78–80] The best results are obtained when the transplant is done before significant clinical deterioration has occurred. The response in the CNS may be delayed for a year, during which the child can continue to deteriorate. The main deterrents to BMT are the difficulty of finding a suitably matched donor, complications of the conditioning regime, the high likelihood of a graft failure, and graft-versus-host disease (GVHD). GVHD may be reduced in the future by the use of umbilical cord cells, an immunologically privileged source that contains stem cells.

Enzyme replacement therapy (ERT) has been effectively utilized to treat Gaucher disease for more than a decade[81] and was recently introduced for the treatment of Fabry disease.[82,83] Surprisingly, few allergic reactions have occurred and only very rarely have neutralizing antibodies developed. Clinical trials of ERT have also shown promise in MPS I[84] and Pompe disease (acid maltase deficiency). Its utility is presently limited to those diseases with extraneural manifestations, since the blood-brain barrier (BBB) prevents entry of the exogenously derived enzyme into the CNS. Substrate synthesis inhibitors, small molecules that can cross the BBB, provide an alternative approach. One such compound, N-butyldeoxynojirimycin (OGT-918, Zevesca), which blocks the synthesis of glucosylceramide, has been used to treat Gaucher disease[87] and has been shown to reduce G_{M2}-ganglioside storage in the Tay-Sachs mouse.[88]

INHERITED DISEASES

Type II glycogenosis (Pompe disease; acid maltase deficiency). A description of this condition may be found in Chap. 56.

Fabry Disease. This X-linked disorder is due to deficiency of lysosomal α-galactosidase A. It results in lysosomal storage of glycosphingolipids containing terminal α-galactosyl residues.[89] The major storage compounds include mostly globotriaosylceramide (Gb_3Cer) and, to lesser extent, globobiosylceramide (Gb_2Cer) and blood group isoantigen B. Onset is in childhood or adolescence. Affected males have intermittently painful hands and feet, angiokeratoma, corneal opacities, and hypohidrosis. Widespread small vessel disease eventually leads to renal failure, myocardial ischemia, and strokes.

The most severely affected cell types are pericytes and endothelial cells in various tissues as well as renal podocytes; cardiac, skeletal, and smooth muscle; and neurons. It is noteworthy that although this is an X-linked disorder, storage material is found in the cardiac and skeletal muscle of carriers.[90,91] Histopathologic examination of paraffin-embedded skeletal muscle from typical Fabry cases stained with hematoxylin and eosin (H&E) demonstrates light staining of the myocytes, vacuolization of the myocyte periphery (Fig. 24-2), and vacuolization in the center of the myocardial cell (Figs. 24-3 and 24-5D). These vacuoles stained positively with LFB. On 1 μm-thick resin-embedded muscle sections stained with toluidine blue (Fig. 24-4), the storage is infrequently observed as blue-stained granular material beneath the sarcolemma.[92] On frozen sections, the stored compounds stain positively with PAS, Sudan black, and *Griffonia simplicifolia-I* (GS-I), a lectin that specifically binds to terminal α-galactosyl residues,[93] and they are birefringent (Fig. 24-5E). The storage of Gb_3Cer can be demonstrated on frozen and paraffin sections using immunohistochemical methods[94,95] or with chromatography (Fig. 24-6).[96] Ultrastructurally, the storage material appears as lamellated membrane structures (Fig. 24-5C),[92,97] which is characteristic for storage of polar lipids. Atypical cases of Fabry disease have been described[95,96,98] that are characterized primarily by cardiac hypertrophy (Fig. 24-5A) without other clinical signs of any tissue involvement, as seen in more typical cases of Fabry disease.

G_{M1} gangliosidosis. This is an autosomal recessive disorder caused by deficient activity of lysosomal β-galactosidase.[99] It results in lysosomal accumulation of glycolipids and oligosaccharides with a nonreducing terminal β-galactosidic linkage and keratan sulfate in multiple cell types as well as in the abnormal excretion of various oligosaccharide compounds in urine. This disorder is classified into three forms—infantile (type 1), juvenile (type 2), and adult (type 3)—on the basis of age at the onset of symptoms, temporal evolution, clinical and pathologic manifestations, urinary oligosaccharide excretion, and quantities of cholesterol, phospholipids, cerebrosides, and sulfatides in brain. In the majority of cases of the severe type 1 form, the clinical manifestations include mental retardation, hepatomegaly, and skeletal changes without primary cardiomyopathy and skeletal myopathy. Cases with cardiomyopathy and neuropathy have also been described.[100,101] Furthermore, an atypical case with progressive cardiomyopathy, skeletal myopathy, and mental and growth retardation has been described.[102] Histopathologic examination of paraffin-embedded cells stained with H&E revealed vacuolated cells. On paraffin sections, the storage of gangliosides could

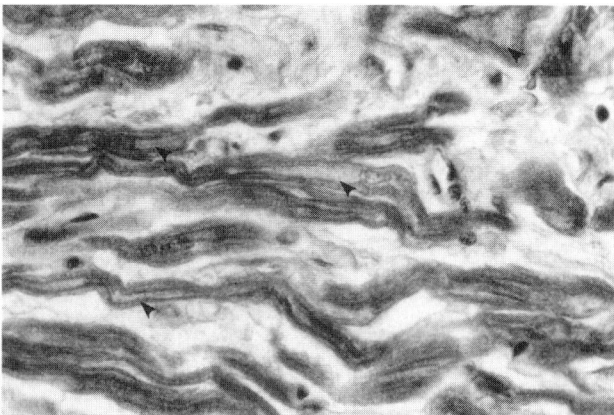

FIGURE 24-3. Formalin-fixed paraffin section of myocardium from the same patient as in Fig. 24-2, who had cardiomegaly with diffuse yellow discoloration of the heart. In the myocardial cells, the contractile filaments are displaced by storage material (arrowheads). (H&E, ×176.)

be demonstrated with LFB[103] and with subunit B of cholera toxin.[104] On frozen sections, it could be identified with *Ricinus communis*-I (RCA-I) lectin—which recognizes nonreducing terminal β-galactosyl residues[72,100]—PAS, Sudan black,[100] and anti G_{M1} antibodies.[105] On paraffin section, the storage of oligosaccharides and keratan sulfate could be demonstrated with PAS, alcian blue,[99] and RCA-I.[103] Ultrastructural changes in endothelial and muscle satellite cells were previously reported.[106] Figure 24-7 demonstrates clear vacuoles, probably indicative of oligosaccharide accumulation, as well as small membrane fragments, which probably represent G_{M1}, in both endothelial cells and myocytes from a 15-month-old infant with G_{M1} gangliosidosis.

G_{M2} gangliosidosis. The G_{M2} gangliosidoses are a group of disorders characterized by primary or secondary deficiency in the activity of lysosomal β-hexosaminidase,

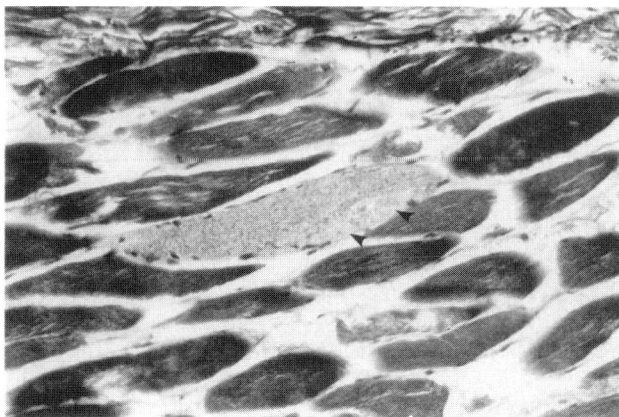

FIGURE 24-2. Formalin-fixed paraffin section of skeletal muscle from a 54-year-old man (Ref. 81, patient 1) with Fabry disease. The cell at the center reveals loss of contractile elements and accumulation of storage material (arrowheads). (H&E, ×176.)

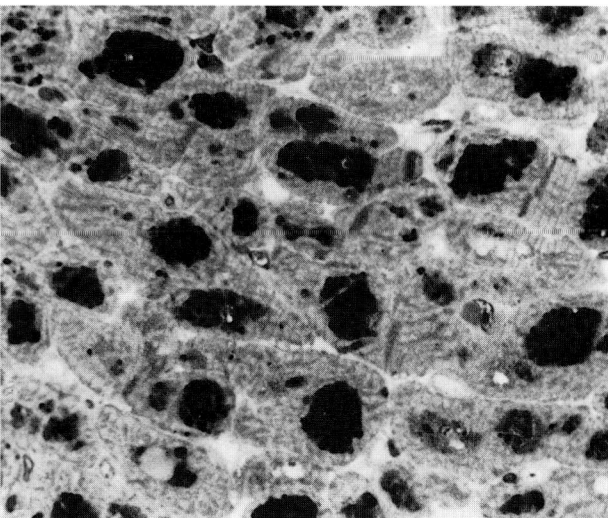

FIGURE 24-4. Glutaraldehyde-fixed resin section of myocardium from an 8-year-old patient illustrating large accumulation of glycolipids in cardiomyocytes. (Toluidine blue, ×480.)

resulting in the accumulation of G_{M2} ganglioside.[107,108] Three genes are required for the lysosomal degradation of this ganglioside. They include the genes that encode the α and β subunits of β-hexosaminidase and the gene encoding the G_{M2} activator protein, required for binding of the lipid (i.e., G_{M2} substrate) to the enzyme.[109] While mutations in the α chain and in the gene coding the activator protein will result mainly in storage of G_{M2} ganglioside, mutation in the β chain will cause additional storage of oligosaccharides and glycosaminoglycans. Mutations on each of the above genes are associated with severe infantile forms as well as an adult form. In cardiac and skeletal muscle from a 3-year-old boy with the infantile form of Tay-Sachs disease, we demonstrated PAS-positive granules in myocytes and nonmuscle cells. Some of the granules were diastase-positive (Fig. 24-8A through C). The positive PAS staining can be in part attrib-

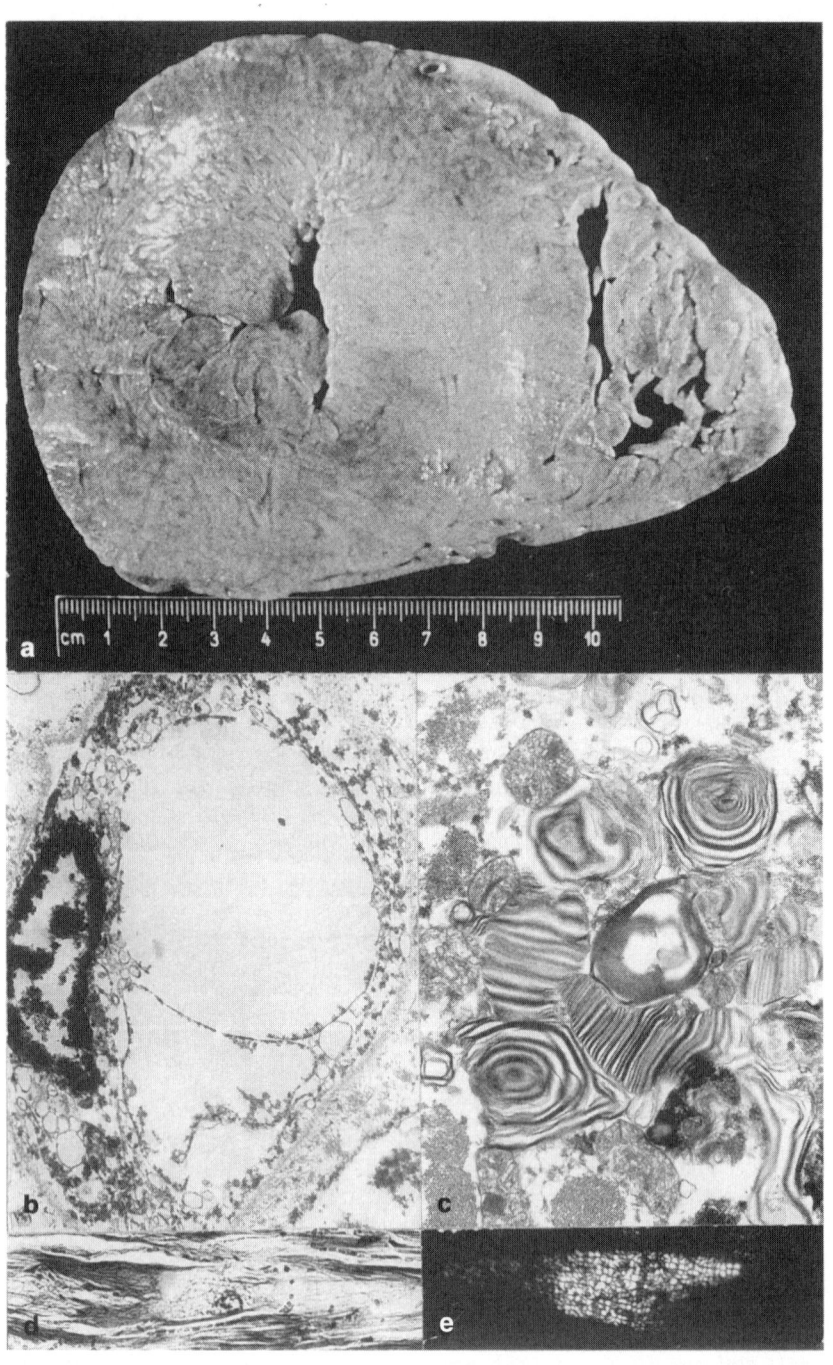

FIGURE 24-5. *a.* Cross section of the heart of a 63-year-old man who had nonobstructive hypertrophic cardiomyopathy due to Fabry disease. *b.* Electron micrograph of an endothelial cell in the heart illustrating the absence of storage material. (×4500.) *c.* Electron micrograph of a myocardial cell illustrating massive storage of lamellated membrane structures. (×15,000.) *d.* Light micrograph of a myocardial cell showing extensive vacuolization. (H&E, ×400.) *(From Elleder M, Bradova V, Smid F, et al: Cardiocyte storage and hypertrophy as a sole manifestation of Fabry's disease: Report on a case simulating hypertrophic non-obstructive cardiomyopathy. Virchows Arch A Pathol Anat A 417:449, 1990. Reproduced with permission from Springer-Verlag.)*

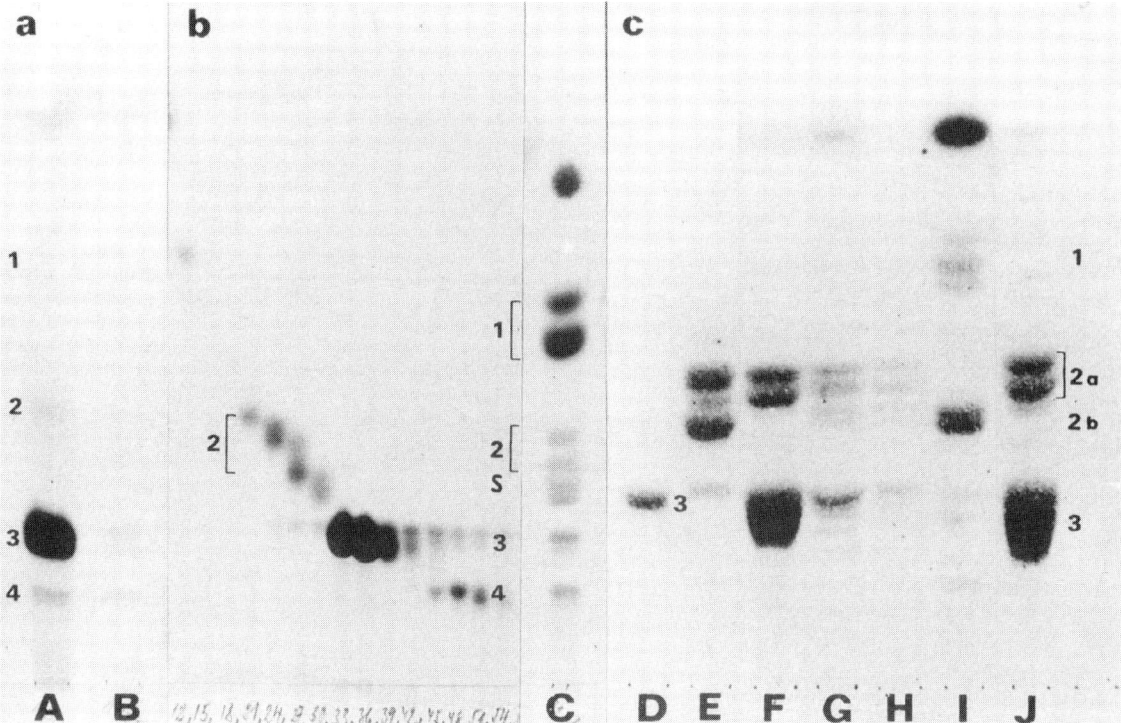

FIGURE 24-6. *a*. Thin-layer chromatography (TLC) of myocardial glycolipid of a patient with Fabry disease (*A*) demonstrating massive accumulation of ceramide trihexoside (globotriasocylceramide), but not in the myocardium. *b*. TLC pattern of myocardial glycolipids, obtained from Fabry patients and separated on silica-gel Separon SGX column (Tessek Ltd., Prague). Fractions 33 to 39 were used for NMR analysis and tissue culture loading tests. Reference glycolipid mixture (*C*). Solvent system and detection used for *A* and *B* include chloroform-methanol-water 65:25:4 by volume and orcinol-H_2SO_4 reagent. *c*. High-performance-TLC separation of lactosylceramide and digalactosylceramide (galabiosylceramide). Marked accumulation of the latter was found in the ceramide dihexoside fraction of the Fabry patient (*E*); it was similarly found in urinary sediments of reference Fabry hemizygotes (*F, J*) and heterozygotes (*G, H*). D. Isolated globotriasocylceramide from the patient's myocardium. *I*. Reference glycolipid mixture with lactosyl ceramide from leukocytes. 1, ceramide monohexoside; 2, ceramide dihexoside; 2a, digalactosylceramide; 2b, lactosylceramide; 3, ceramide trihexoside; 4, ceramide tetrahexosides; S, sulfatide (galactosylceramide I^3-sulfate). Solvent system: isopropanol-28% NH_4OH-water 75:10:15 by vol. Detection by orcinol-H_2SO_4 reaction. *(From Elleder M, Bradova V, Smid F, et al: Cardiocyte storage and hypertrophy as a sole manifestation of Fabry's disease: Report on a case simulating hypertrophic non-obstructive cardiomyopathy. Virchows Arch A Pathol Anat A 417:449, 1990. Reproduced with permission from Springer-Verlag.)*

uted to the "plasma reaction"—i.e., staining of unsaturated lipids that were retained in paraffin section.[110] In Sand-hoff disease, in the nonneuronal cells, the storage of complex carbohydrates with nonreducing terminal β-N-acetylglucosamine can be demonstrated by staining with succinylated wheat germ agglutinin (S-WGA).[111] Lysosomes laden with lamellated membrane structures were noted in myocardial cells from a 2½-year-old boy with Sandhoff disease.[112] Nonspecific secondary changes, such as selective atrophy of type 2 fibers due to disuse or chronic denervation with reinnervation, have been reported in Jewish patients with adult onset of G_{M2} gangliosidosis who are deficient in the activity of lysosomal β-hexosaminidase A.[113,114]

Neuronal ceroid lipofuscinosis (NCL).

This group of progressive neurodegenerative disorders is distinguished from other neurodegenerative diseases by the lysosomal storage of autofluorescent material in multiple tissues.[115,116] The term *ceroid lipofuscinosis* has been given to this class of diseases because the stored substance is stainable with Sudan black and LFB, which stain phospholipids (Fig. 24-9),[117] and is autofluorescent but is not extractable with lipid solvents. It is, however, distinguishable from the aging pigment (i.e., lipofuscin).

The disease is classified into eight different subtypes according to the age of onset, clinical manifestations, biochemical features, and ultrastructure of the storage material. The location of the gene has been identified in six subtypes (Table 24-2), and the gene product in five subtypes[116] (Table 24-3). The onset of the infantile form (NCL1) is at 1 to 2 years of age and is manifest by myoclonus, visual loss with retinopathy, dementia, and extreme cerebral atrophy. Death may occur after 4 to 8 years. It is particularly common among Finnish children. There is deficient activity of palmitoyl protein thioesterase and lysosomal storage of sphingolipid activator proteins (SAPs). Ultrastructurally, the storage material is demonstrated in lysosomes of various cell types including skeletal muscle and is characteristic of granular osmiophilic deposits (GROD).[115]

The onset of the classic late infantile type (NCL2) is at 2 to 5 years of age[118] and of the Finnish late infantile variant (NCL5) at 4½ to 7 years.[119] There are also variant late infan-

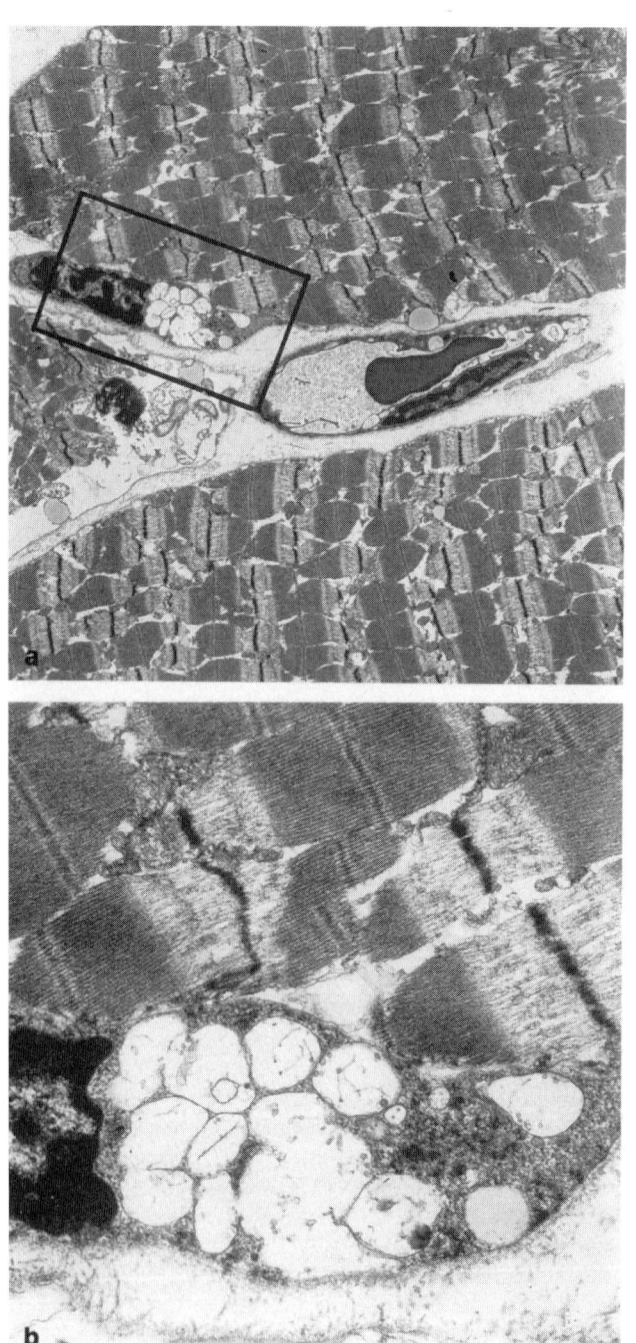

FIGURE 24-7. *A.* Electron micrograph of three myocytes and a capillary from a 15-month-old boy with G_{M1} gangliosidosis. A myocyte and the endothelium contained enlarged secondary lysosomes. (×4000.) *B.* Higher magnification of the myocyte in the rectangle illustrating several lysosomes, some of which are joined together. The lysosomes appear almost empty and contain a few membrane fragments or fine fibrillar material. (×19,000.)

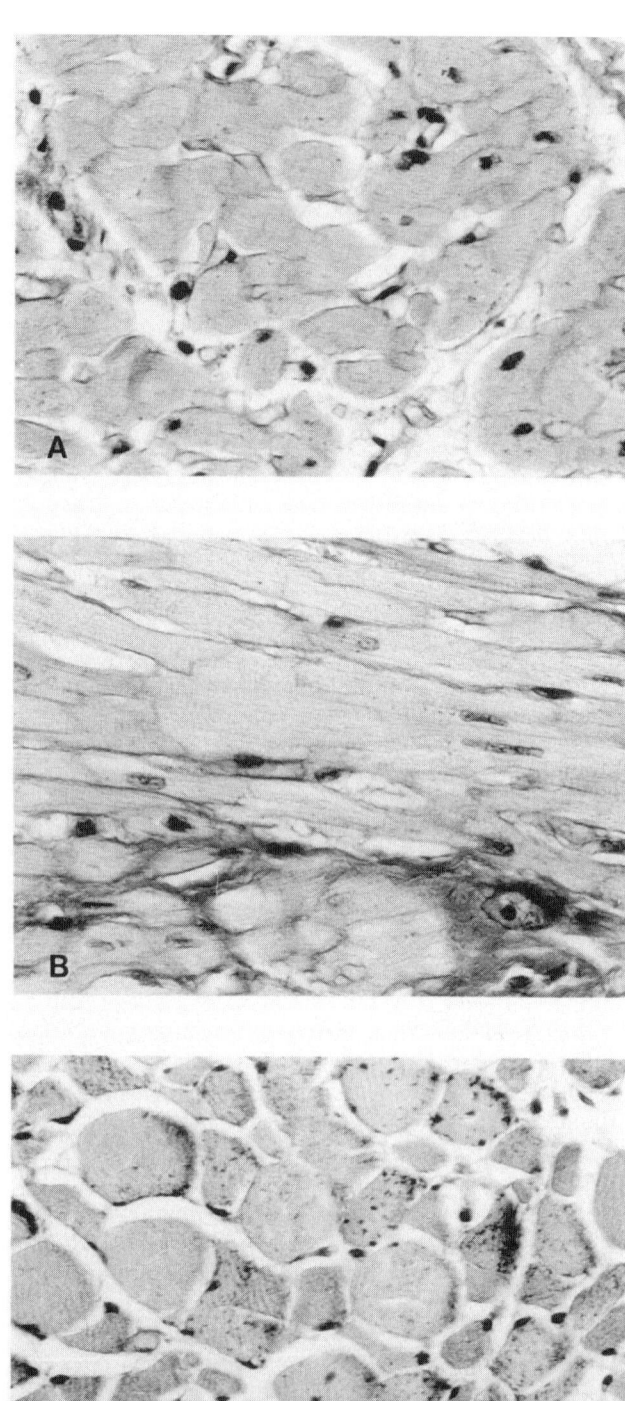

FIGURE 24-8. Formalin-fixed sections of cardiac and skeletal muscle from a 3-year-old boy with the infantile form of Tay-Sachs disease. *A.* Section through cardiac muscle showing the presence of small PAS-positive granules in both myocytes and nonmuscular cells. (PAS, ×440.) *B.* Consecutive section through the same tissue block pretreated with diastase followed by PAS staining reveals fewer PAS-positive granules within myocytes. (D-PAS, ×440.) *C.* Cross section of skeletal muscle demonstrating numerous small, lightly stained granules and larger intensely stained granules. (PAS, ×440.)

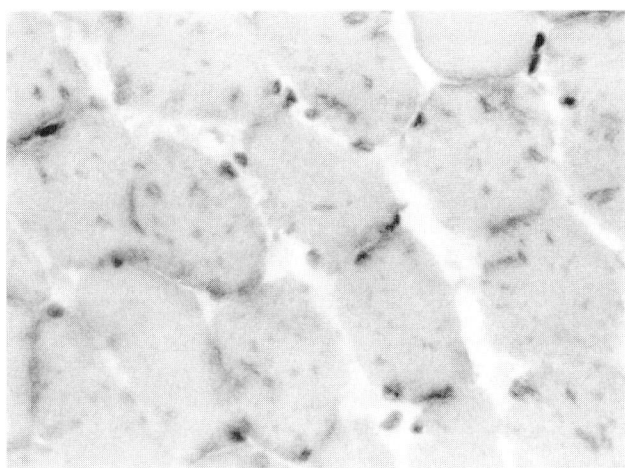

FIGURE 24-9. Frozen section of skeletal muscle from an 8-year-old girl with the juvenile form of neuronal ceroid lipofuscinosis. The section, stained with Luxol fast blue, shows multiple blue cytoplasmic granules, indicating storage of phospholipids. (LFB, ×440.)

However, some patients may have FPP in addition to CVB. Similar LFB-positive granules and CVB (Fig. 24-11) were noted in skeletal and cardiac muscles of an animal model of the juvenile form of NCL.[120] The onset of the adult form, NCL4, is at about 30 years, with death occurring about 10 years later. Patients have normal vision, but they can have either a progressive myoclonic epilepsy or dementia and ataxia. The storage material includes FPP and CVB or GRODs.[121] Northern epilepsy (NCL8) is characterized as an inherited epilepsy. The onset occurs between 5 and 10 years of age and the disease leads to mental retardation by middle age.[122] Ultrastructurally, the storage material includes CVB and GRODs; biochemically, it includes mitochondrial subunit c.[123]

I-cell disease (mucolipidosis II) and pseudo-Hurler polydystrophy (mucolipidosis III). I-cell disease (ML-II) and pseudo-Hurler polydystrophy (ML-III) are biochemically related diseases with an autosomal recessive inheritance. The lysosomal storage is a consequence of a primary deficiency of phospho-N-acetylglucosamine transferase, resulting in failure to transport soluble lysosomal hydrolases from the Golgi apparatus into lysosomes.[124] A characteristic of these conditions is that although all cell types of affected patients are deficient in phosphotransferase activity, not all cell types are deficient in the activity of lysosomal hydrolases. Furthermore, mesenchymal cells are most severely affected.

As a result of a deficiency in the intralysosomal activity of multiple enzymes, the storage material includes both glycolipids and oligosaccharides. Histochemical studies of muscle fibers from an affected 2-year-old girl demonstrated decreased numbers of functioning oxidative (type 1) fibers (Fig. 24-12) and abundant storage of diastase-resistant PAS-positive material within myocytes (Fig. 24-13). Lectin histochemistry of affected cells indicates accumulation of N-linked

tile (NCL6) and Turkish variant late infantile (NCL7) forms.[116] The clinical manifestations of these conditions are similar but not identical. In NCL2, the material that accumulates in numerous cell types, including cardiac[118] and skeletal muscle, has characteristic curvilinear bodies (CVB) (Fig. 24-10). In NCL5, NCL6, and NCL7 the storage material includes both CVB and fingerprint profiles (FPP).[115]

The onset of the juvenile form (NCL3) is at 5 to 10 years of age. Patients present with visual loss and macular degeneration. Seizures, moderate cerebral atrophy, ataxia, and dementia appear several years later. Some patients survive into the third decade. Ultrastructurally, curvilinear bodies are the most commonly observed form of storage material.

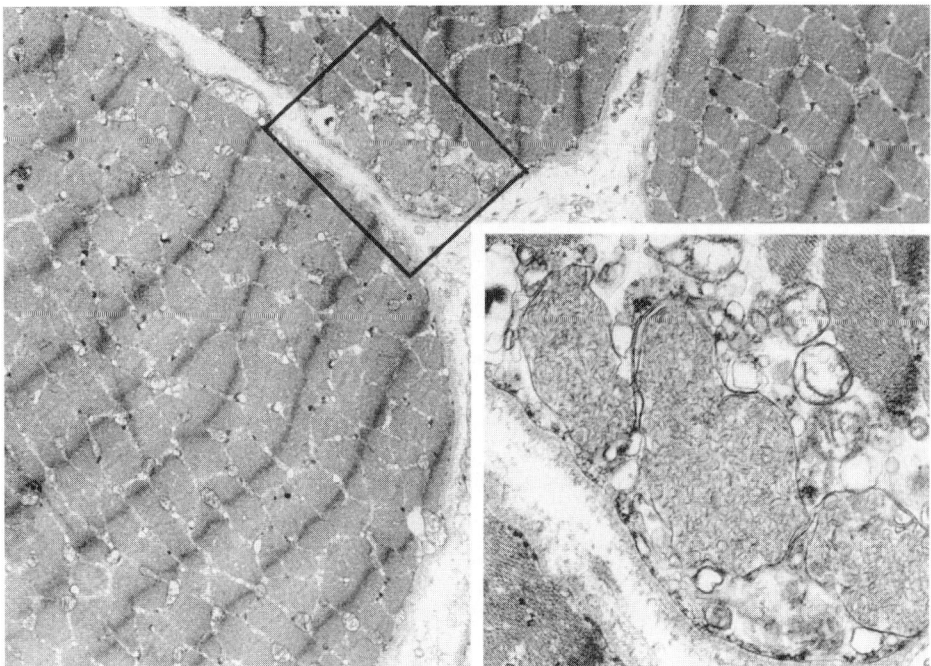

FIGURE 24-10. Low-magnification electron micrograph, from a 4-year-old girl with neuronal ceroid lipofuscinosis, showing three myocytes. The myocyte at the center contains three secondary lysosomes. (×8000.) Inset: The lysosomes in the rectangle are laden with numerous curvilinear bodies. (×18,000.)

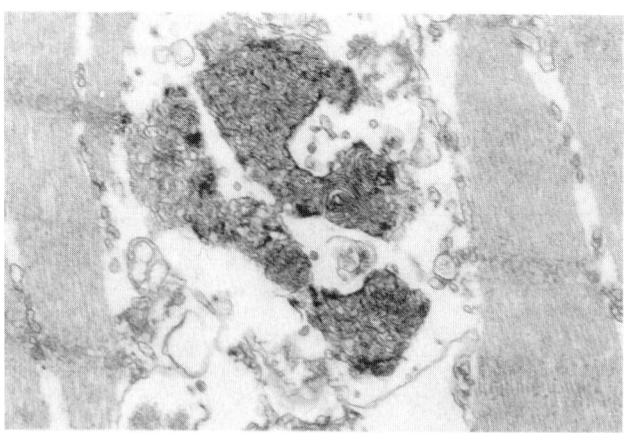

FIGURE 24-11. High-magnification electron micrograph of cardiac muscle from a 2-year-old Australian cattle dog with neuronal ceroid lipofuscinosis[120] showing lysosomes with curvilinear bodies. (×21,000.)

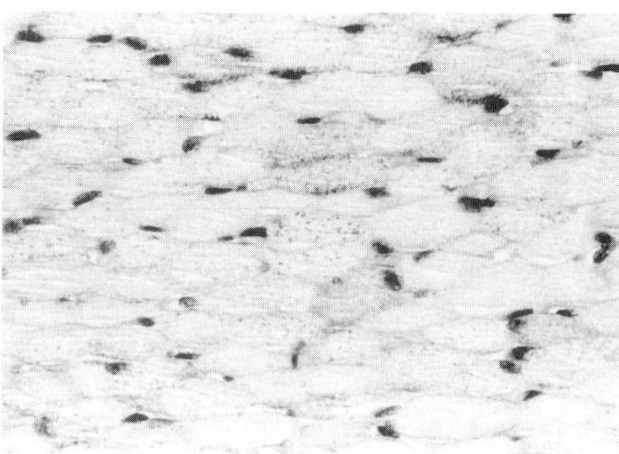

FIGURE 24-13. Formalin-fixed, paraffin-embedded skeletal muscle from a 3-month-old boy affected with I-cell disease. The sarcoplasm of the myocytes contains numerous small PAS-positive granules. (PAS, ×440.)

oligosaccharides containing α-mannosyl, β-N-acetylglucosaminyl, and sialyl residues.[125] Ultrastructural examination revealed numerous lysosomes containing lamellated membrane structures and fibrillar and amorphous material in *satellite cells* (Fig. 24-14), similar to those seen in fibroblasts. Only a few myocytes appear atrophic, with considerable loss of contractile elements. These contained a few enlarged lysosomes with dense particulate material (Fig. 24-15).[72] Similar ultrastructural changes have been noted in myocardial cells.[126] Cultured skeletal muscle of the same patient showed numerous inclusions (i.e., lysosomes) and did not fuse as well as control. However, well-developed myotubes were present, with distinct cross striations, and they did not have inclusions.[127] Both studies indicate that I-cell disease "myopathy" is unique in its characteristic expression in developing but not mature cultured myocytes.

Mucolipidosis IV. This rare lysosomal disorder occurs almost exclusively in Ashkenazi Jews. It is transmitted as an

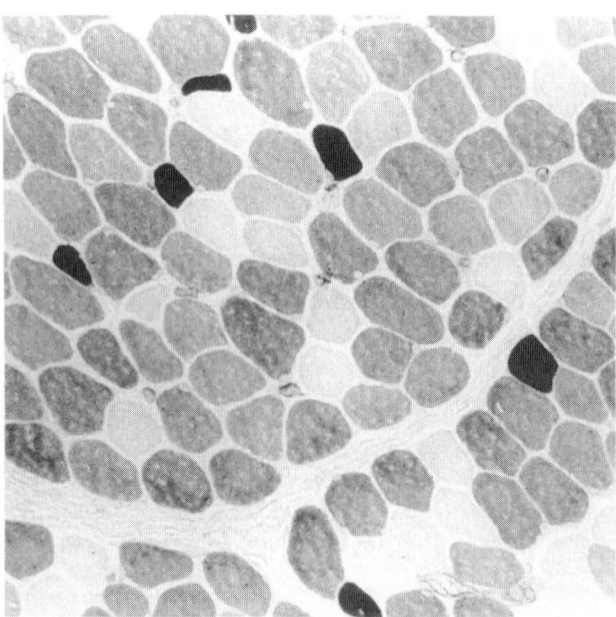

FIGURE 24-12. ATPase reaction (pH 4.6) of a muscle biopsy from a 2-year-old girl with I-cell disease revealing reduction of type I (small dark fibers). (×350.) *(From Kula RW, Shafiq SA, Sher JH, Qazi QH: I-cell disease (mucolipidosis II): Differential expression in satellite cells and mature muscle fibers. J Neurol Sci 63:75, 1984. With permission from Elsevier.)*

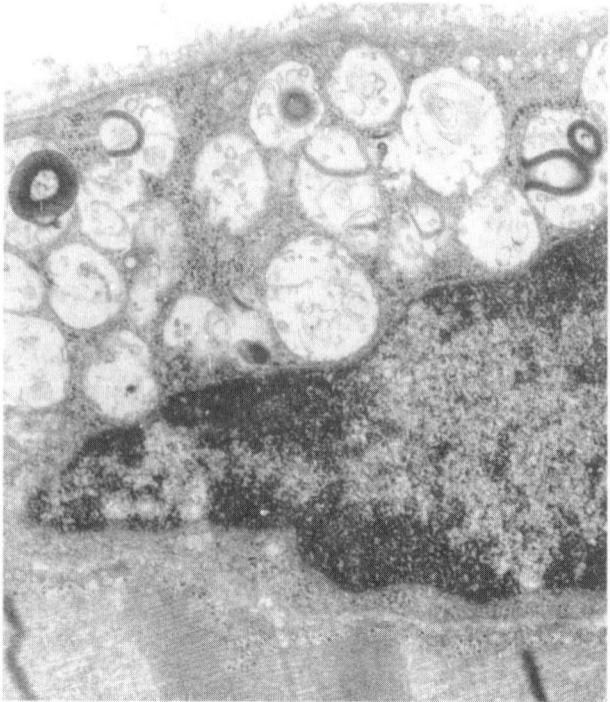

FIGURE 24-14. Electron micrograph of satellite cell and adjacent myocytes. The satellite contains numerous lysosomes laden with lamellated membrane structures as well as fibrillar and amorphous material. (×25,000.) *(From Kula RW, Shafiq SA, Sher JH, Qazi QH: I-cell disease (mucolipidosis II): Differential expression in satellite cells and mature muscle fibers. J Neurol Sci 63:75, 1984. With permission from Elsevier.)*

autosomal recessive trait. Clinically it is characterized by progressive psychomotor retardation and hypotonia beginning within the first year of life, corneal opacities, retinal degeneration, and abnormal gastric function.[128] A milder form with later onset has been described. It is caused by mutations in a gene encoding mucolipin, a protein thought to be a receptor-stimulated cation channel.[129,130] Numerous cell types including muscle are affected. On paraffin sections, the storage material present in myocardiocytes is stained with PAS, LFB, and several different lectins.[128] On frozen sections, almost all muscle fibers contain PAS- and acid phosphatase-positive inclusions, which stain red with the modified trichrome stain. Ultrastructurally, they consist of lysosomes laden with dense lamellated membrane structures[131] (Fig. 24-16). In addition, some of the fibers undergo degenerative changes, such as alterations in Z bands and loss of striation.[132]

α-**Mannosidosis.** α-Mannosidosis is a glycoprotein storage disease caused by deficient activity of lysosomal α-mannosidase. It is inherited as an autosomal recessive trait and results in the accumulation of oligosaccharides containing α-mannosyl residues and 2-acetamido-2-deoxy-D-glucose within lysosomes.[133,134] Since α-mannosidase participates in the catabolism of N-linked glycoproteins, which are major components of intracellular membrane as well as extracellular glycoconjugates, most cell types—including cardiac, smooth, and skeletal muscle—are affected. It is manifested by progressive neurologic impairment and visceral, ocular, and skeletal involvement. In addition, there is compromise of humoral and cellular immune systems.[135]

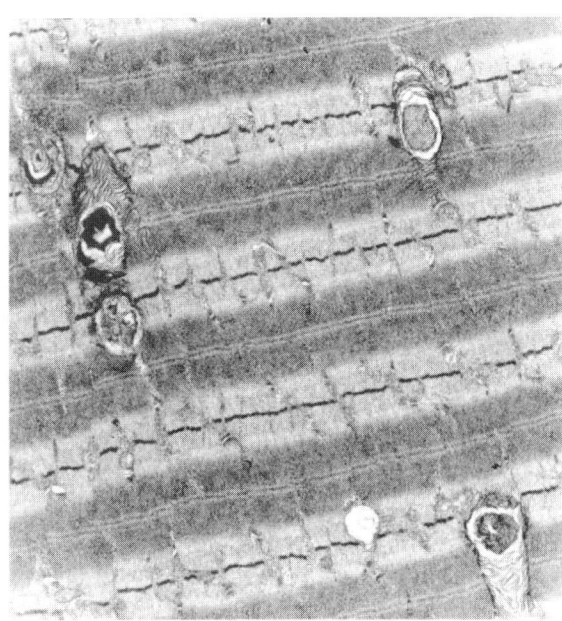

FIGURE 24-16. Electron micrograph of the quadriceps muscle from a 14-year-old boy with mucolipidosis IV, illustrating several secondary lysosomes laden with lamellated membrane structures. (×9000.) *(Courtesy of Dr. Hans Goebel.)*

Light microscopic examination of paraffin sections stained with H&E or PAS and fresh-frozen sections stained with or reacted for NADH-tetrazolium reductase, ATPase (pH 9.4, 4.2, and 4.6), acid phosphatase, modified Gomori trichrome, and PAS do not reveal evidence of lysosomal storage disease. However, toluidine blue-stained semithin sections show many subsarcolemmal vacuoles and some vacuoles in the intermyofibrillar space.[136] The storage material stains with concanavalin ensiformis (ConA), wheat germ agglutinin (WGA) and succinyl-WGA (S-WGA).[137] Ultrastructural examinations demonstrate enlarged lysosomes containing fine fibrillar or granular material, which is occasionally accompanied by lamellated membrane structures, electron-dense bodies, and lipofuscin (Fig. 24-17).[136,138]

β-**Mannosidosis.** Deficient activity of lysosomal β-mannosidase has been described in humans,[139] goats,[74] and cattle.[140] It is associated with lysosomal storage of partially degraded N-linked oligosaccharides with terminal β-mannosyl residues. In the few patients reported, clinical manifestations have varied but included seizures, mental retardation, and angiokeratoma. Comprehensive morphologic studies of different organs including skeletal muscle have been reported in goats. While vacuoles are absent in myofibers, the satellite cells contain coarse vacuoles.[74]

Fucosidosis. This disorder is due to deficient activity of lysosomal α-fucosidase, resulting in the lysosomal storage of fucosylated oligosaccharides, glycopeptides, glycolipids, and mucopolysaccharides. It is inherited as an autosomal recessive trait and is manifest in a severe infantile form as well as in a milder late-onset form. Psychomotor retardation, mild facial coarsening, hepatomegaly, excessive sweating, and angiokeratoma are part of the clinical presentation.

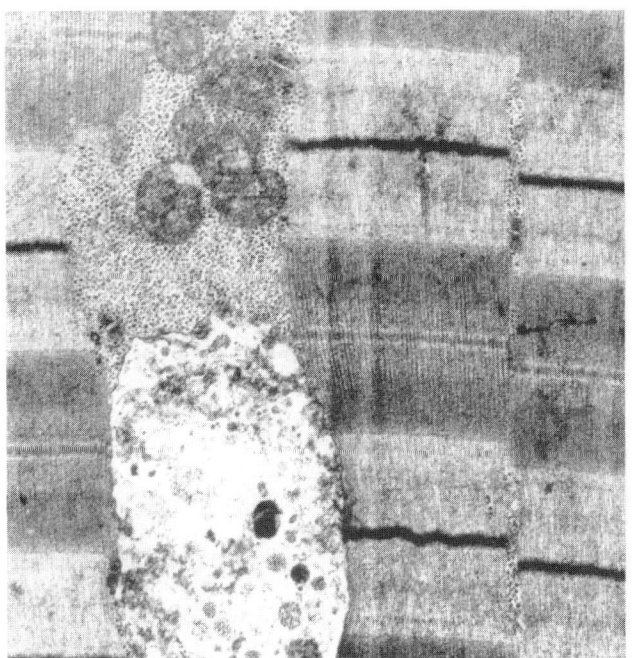

FIGURE 24-15. Electron micrograph of myocyte from the same patient as in Figs. 24-12 and 24-14 demonstrates large lysosome containing dense particulate material. (×25,000.) *(From Kula RW, Shafiq SA, Sher JH, Qazi QH: I-cell disease (mucolipidosis II): Differential expression in satellite cells and mature muscle fibers. J Neurol Sci 63:75, 1984. With permission from Elsevier.)*

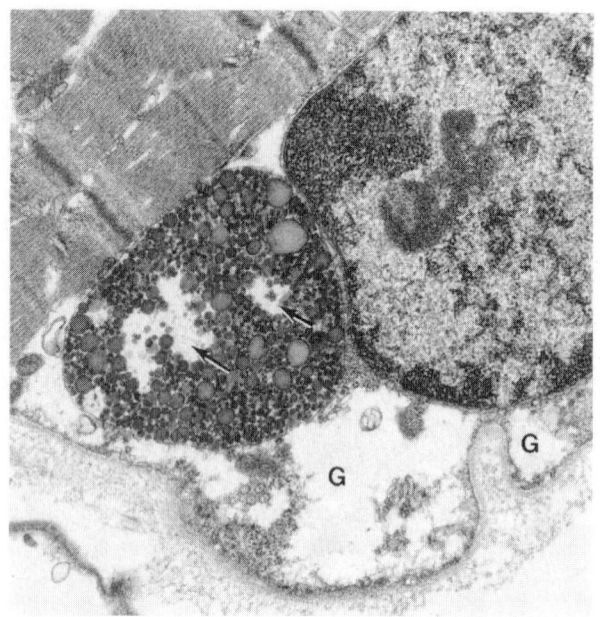

FIGURE 24-17. Electron micrograph of skeletal muscle from a 32-year-old patient with α-mannosidosis (Ref. 137). It illustrates myocytes containing glycogen (G), which was extracted during tissue processing, and a secondary lysosome which contains both electron-dense lipofuscin granules and fine fibrillar material (arrows) representing the storage material. (×24,000.) (*Courtesy of Dr. John Halperin.*)

In the severe infantile form, frozen sections of muscle revealed acid phosphatase-positive sites in the vascular wall and rarely in myocytes.[71] Paraffin sections of skeletal muscle have shown mildly increased variation in fiber size and fine cytoplasmic vacuolization.[141] Paraffin sections of heart demonstrate enlarged endothelium, which is intensely stained with *Ulex europaeus* agglutinin-I (UEA-I),[142] a lectin that specifically binds to nonreducing terminal fucosyl residues (Fig. 24-18). In semithin resin-embedded muscle sections, prominent clear vacuoles are observed in vacuolar endothelium, and there is secondary muscle atrophy.[71]

Sialic acid storage disease. In this condition, free sialic acid accumulates in lysosomes due to mutations in sialin, an anion/cation symporter.[17] There is impairment in the transport of sialic acid and glucuronic acids across the lysosomal membrane into the cytosol, where it would ordinarily be further utilized or degraded.[143] This disease is inherited as an autosomal recessive trait and manifests itself in a severe infantile form, a milder form (i.e., Salla disease), and an intermediate form. Cardiomegaly and vacuolization of myocardial cells have been reported in the infantile form.[144] Muscle biopsies in Salla disease disclose an increase in subsarcolemmal glycogen and lysosomes containing granular and fine filamentous material and small droplets. The vacuoles are present in fibroblasts, vascular endothelium, myocytes, and satellite cells of muscle.[145]

Cystinosis. Cystinosis, an autosomal recessive disorder,[143] is due to mutations of cystinosin, an integral membrane protein with features of a lysosomal membrane protein.[146] This results in lysosomal storage of the disulfide amino acid cysteine. Cysteine crystals form in parenchymal organs such as liver and kidney but have also been observed in ocular, endocrine, neural, and muscular tissues.[143] Among the consequences are renal tubular dysfunction, stunted growth, and progressive photophobia. Oral cysteamine, dialysis, and renal transplantation improve the outcome.

The cystine content of skeletal muscle is increased more than 1000-fold. Muscle specimens show a myopathy characterized by mild increase of connective tissue, variation in the size of fibers, atrophy of type 1 fibers, and numerous ring fibers. Under polarized light, intracellular cystine crystals are noted in the perimysial and endomysial spaces adjacent to the myocytes. Ultrastructural studies have revealed intralysosomal accumulation of rectangular and hexagonal crystals in various mesenchymal cells (i.e., fibroblasts, etc.) but not within myocytes.[147] These findings indicate that the myopathy is secondary to the long-standing cystinosis. It is noteworthy that, as in I-cell disease,[127] cultured myotube cells store cystine.[148]

Mucopolysaccharidosis (MPS). The mucopolysaccharidoses are a group of lysosomal storage diseases that result from deficient activity of specific lysosomal enzymes involved in the degradation of dermatan, heparan, keratan, and chondroitin sulfates, singly or in combination,[149,150] and hyaluronan.[151] In all of these conditions except for mucopolysaccharidosis IIIC, the deficient enzymes are hydrolases. The inheritance in all but mucopolysaccharidosis II (MPS-II) is autosomal recessive. MPS-II is an X-linked syndrome. While multiple tissues and organs are involved in these diseases, mesenchymal cells, which actively participate in proteoglycan catabolism, are more severely affected.

Mucopolysaccharidosis type I (Hurler, Scheie, and Hurler-Scheie syndromes). Deficient activity of α-L-iduronidase results primarily in storage of dermatan and heparan sulfate. Depending on the mutation, it has a wide range of clinical manifestations. Hurler syndrome, the severe form, is associated with progressive facial and skeletal dysmorphism, deafness, and mental retardation, leading to death before the age of 10 years. The mildest form is Scheie

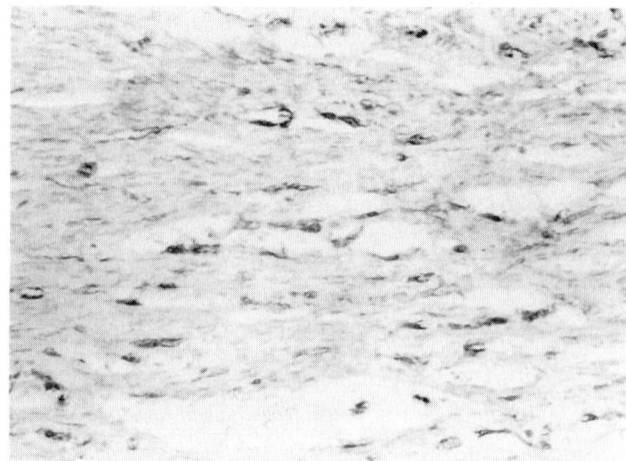

FIGURE 24-18. Formalin-fixed, paraffin-embedded section through the myocardium of a 4-year-old girl with fucosidosis (Ref. 190) stained with UEA-I and counterstained with methyl green. It illustrates enlarged endothelial cells containing cytoplasm intensely stained with UEA-I, indicating the storage of fucosylated oligosaccharides. (×176.)

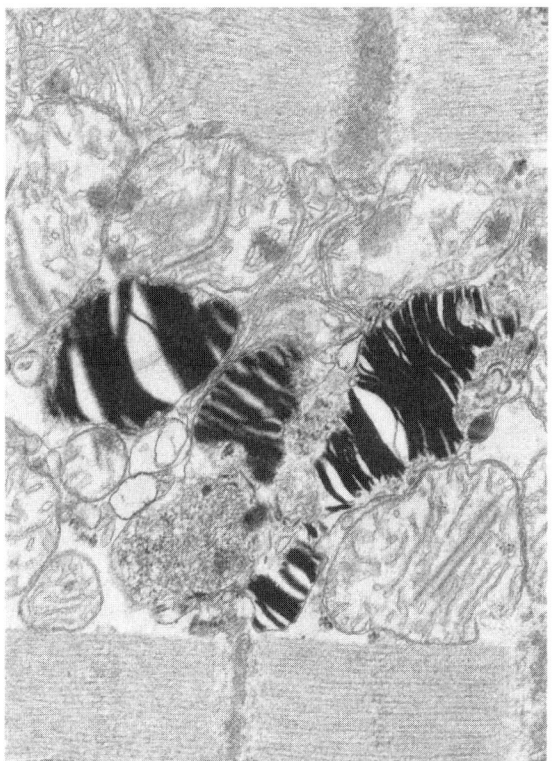

FIGURE 24-19. Myocardial section from an 11-year-old boy (Ref. 151, patient 3) with Hurler disease, showing membrane-bound electron-dense lamellae within the myocyte. (×35,000.) *(From Renteria GS, Ferrans VJ, Roberts WC: The heart in the Hurler syndrome: Gross, histologic and ultrastructural observations in five necropsy cases. Am J Cardiol 38:487, 1976. With permission from the American Journal of Cardiology.)*

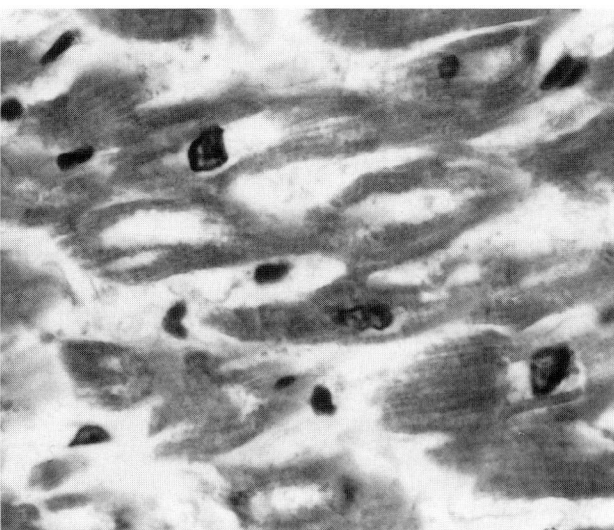

FIGURE 24-20. Formalin-fixed, paraffin-embedded section through the myocardium of a 10-year-old with Hunter disease, demonstrating enlarged, vacuolated cardiomyocytes. (H&E, ×480.)

found in lysosomes of aortic smooth muscle and those of interstitial fibroblast-like cells among the cardiomyocytes.[154]

Mucopolysaccharidosis type III (Sanfilippo disease) type A.
Sanfilippo disease type A is associated with the storage of heparan sulfate, due to deficiency in the activity of heparan N-sulfatase (i.e., sulfaminidase). As in other types of Sanfilippo syndrome, it is characterized clinically by severe progressive mental retardation; but unlike most other mucopolysaccharidoses, these patients have relatively mild somatic changes. On paraffin-embedded H&E-stained heart sections, small vacuoles are noted in a juxtanuclear position (Fig. 24-21).

Mucopolysaccharidosis type III (Sanfilippo disease) type C.
In this disease heparan sulfate storage is due to deficient activity of acetyl CoA: α-glucosaminidase-N-acetyltransferase. Clinically, it is not distinguishable from

syndrome, which features joint contractures without mental retardation; an intermediate form (Hurler-Scheie syndrome) also exists.

The myocardium is mildly hypertrophied in the severe form (i.e., Hurler disease), and small vacuoles can be seen adjacent to myocardial cell nuclei on formalin-fixed, paraffin-embedded H&E-stained sections. In resin-embedded semithin sections stained with toluidine blue, few clear vacuoles can be seen in myocardial cells. Electron microscopic examination of these myocardial cells has revealed, in addition to clear vacuoles,[152] lamellated membrane structures (Fig. 24-19) measuring 1 to 3 μm in diameter and occupying less than 5 percent of the cell volume, indicating the storage of both mucopolysaccharides and lipids. The storage of diverse compounds (i.e., lipids) may be due to the inhibition of multiple lysosomal hydrolases by glyco-saminoglycans that are stored in the mucopolysaccharidoses.[153]

Mucopolysaccharidosis type II (Hunter disease).
Patients with Hunter disease are deficient in the activity of iduronate sulfatase, which results in lysosomal storage of dermatan and heparan sulfate. Clinically, nodular white skin lesions, coarse facial features, stiff joints, and hepatosplenomegaly occur but the corneas are clear. Both severe and mild forms are found. Enlarged, vacuolated cardiomyocytes have recently been observed in a 10-year-old boy with the severe form (Fig. 24-20). Flocculent storage material has been

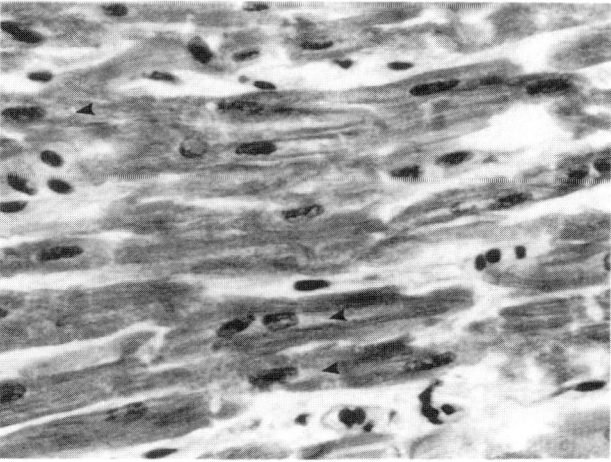

FIGURE 24-21. Formalin-fixed, paraffin-embedded section through the heart of a 4-year-old child who had cardiomegaly and mucopolysaccharidosis IIIA. It reveals cardiomyocyte hypertrophy and cytoplasmic vacuoles (arrowheads) at a juxtanuclear position. (H&E, ×440.)

MPS III type A. Light microscopy has revealed involvement of the nervous system and visceral organs, with storage in mesenchymal cells. Vacuolization and degeneration of cardiomyocytes and myocardial fibrosis distinct from that seen in myocardial infarction have been noted.[155] Affected myocardial cells contained "zebra bodies," membranogranulovacuolar inclusions, and lipofuscin.[156]

Mucopolysaccharidosis type III (Sanfilippo disease) type D. In this condition the storage of heparan sulfate is due to deficient activity of N-acetylglucosamine-6-sulfatase. The onset of variable clinical features becomes apparent in early childhood. The progressive CNS symptoms are more severe than those in the other MPS III syndromes.[157] Storage material is present in both cardiac and skeletal muscle. In both types of muscle, the storage material is stained with toluidine blue and PAS, is diastase resistant, and stains weakly with alcian blue. Human myocardial cells contain both lamellated membrane structures and lipofuscin granules,[157] whereas the myocardial cells of goats with MPS-IIID contain a few fine fibrils.[158]

Mucopolysaccharidosis type VI (Maroteaux-Lamy syndrome). Arylsulfatase B (i.e., N-acetylgalactosamine-4-sulfatase) is deficient in this disease of dermatan sulfate storage. It manifests itself clinically by severe osseous and corneal lesions, contractures, and valvular heart disease. Mesenchymal cells—including fibroblasts, chondrocytes, macrophages, and smooth muscle cells—are most commonly affected. There are no reports on the involvement of skeletal or cardiac muscles. An acute infantile cardiomyopathy without endocardial fibrosis is described. There is vacuolization of interstitial macrophages as the most prominent change, but not of cardiomyocytes.[159]

Galactosialidosis. In galactosialidosis, mutation occurs in the gene for a protective protein/cathepsin A, which forms a multienzyme complex with β-galactosidase and neuraminidase and is required for the intralysosomal activity and stability of these two hydrolases.[160] This leads to rapid degradation of monomeric β-galactosidase by cathepsins within the cell and absence of a subunit essential for neuraminidase activity. As a consequence, there is deficient activity of both β-galactosidase and neuraminidase.[161] Clinically, it manifests itself in severe early-infantile, late-infantile, and juvenile/adult forms. All three forms include mental retardation, visceral organ involvement, and skeletal abnormalities.[162] In skeletal muscle, only prominent vacuolization of interstitial fibroblasts has been noted.[70]

Acid lipase deficiency: Wolman disease and cholesterol ester storage disease. Wolman disease and cholesterol ester storage disease differ in their clinical expression, but both are due to deficient activity of lysosomal acid lipase and have in common the accumulation of cholesterol esters and triglycerides in tissues.[163,164] The infant with Wolman disease develops abdominal distention from massive hepatosplenomegaly. There is vomiting and diarrhea, persistent low-grade fever, and wasting. Death supervenes before 1 year of age. Intracytoplasmic vacuoles are present in lymphocytes and there is vacuolization of macrophages within the bone marrow.

The child with cholesterol ester storage disease is less severely affected. Fatty infiltration of the liver progresses to hepatic fibrosis. The spleen, gastrointestinal tract, lymph nodes, and large arteries are involved. Most patients with this variant grow to adulthood without CNS involvement.

Histopathologic examinations have revealed mild degenerative changes without inflammatory response or myophagia. Oil red O (ORO) staining of a frozen muscle biopsy demonstrated a moderate increase in the number and size of lipid droplets. Under polarized light, the cytoplasm of some muscle fibers contained birefringent, elongated, or ir-regularly shaped crystalline material. Ultrastructural studies exhibited lipid droplets and cholesterol ester crystals in endomysial fibroblasts and muscle fibers.[165] Degenerated and necrotic fibers are observed in the skeletal muscle of rats deficient in lysosomal acid lipase. On H&E, some of the cells had basophilic cytoplasm that revealed reddish granular changes in Gomori-trichrome staining. Others showed vacuolar degeneration that resembled "rimmed vacuoles." Frozen sections demonstrated high acid phosphatase activity in endomysial and perimysial cells and in 5 to 6 percent of the myocytes, whereas ORO staining showed lipid storage in the interstitial cells and in subsarcolemmal spaces of a few fibers. Membrane-bound lipid droplets were noted in fibroblasts, endothelial cells, and the subsarcolemmal space of muscle fibers.

Primary LAMP-2 deficiency (Danon disease). Since 1981, cases have been reported of infantile and adult onset with mental retardation, myopathy, and cardiomyopathy demonstrating autophagic vacuoles with variable storage of glycogen and degraded organelles but normal acid maltase activity.[166–169] This disease is due to a primary deficiency in LAMP-2.[14,15] The gene that encodes LAMP-2 is localized on the X chromosome, and in most familial cases there is no male-to-male transmission; males are affected predominantly and their mothers have milder and later-onset cardiac symptoms.[15,169] It has been proposed that LAMP-2 protects the lysosomal membrane from proteolytic enzymes within lysosomes and that the vacuoles with undegraded substrate seen in primary LAMP-2 deficiency are lysosomal in origin.[14] This hypothesis is supported by the fact that LAMP-2 is a receptor for selective uptake of cytosolic proteins by lysosomes.[170]

Male patients develop hypertrophic cardiomyopathy and female patients manifest dilated cardiomyopathy. The electrocardiogram (ECG) is abnormal, often with the Wolff-Parkinson-White syndrome. Several patients have required a permanent pacemaker and one male patient has received a heart transplant. The myopathy is mild, with proximal limb and neck muscle weakness, and the serum creatine kinase is elevated. Hepatomegaly and an increase in liver enzymes may also be observed. Mild mental retardation occurs in more than half of the male patients.[169]

Exon 9 of LAMP-2 is alternatively spliced with the LAMP-2a isoform, present ubiquitously, whereas the LAMP-2b isoform is expressed predominantly in heart and skeletal muscle. No mental retardation was present in one family with a mutation in the LAMP-2b isoform.[169] A few asymptomatic mothers lack a LAMP-2 mutation in their blood DNA, suggesting that the disease in their affected sons was due either to a spontaneous mutation or to germline mosaicism.[171]

In humans, the vacuolar membranes are reinforced by dystrophin and react strongly for nonspecific esterase. Acid phosphatase reactivity is accentuated around but only infrequently within the vacuoles. Most vacuoles are smaller than 5 μm in diameter and are best observed in 1- to 2-μm-thick resin sections. There is also frequent fiber splitting, giving rise to nonautophagic vacuoles lined by dystrophin, laminin,[172,173] and basal lamina (Fig 24-22).[173] The diagnosis is readily confirmed by failure of an anti-LAMP-2 antibody to immunostain the muscle fibers.[15] Lectin histochemistry of unfixed frozen sections of skeletal muscle is also useful in distinguishing between a patient with primary LAMP-2[15,168] and those patients who have deficient activity of acid maltase.[174] The membrane and content of the vacuoles in the patient with normal acid maltase activity stained intensely with the following lectins: UEA-I, Limas flavus agglutinin (LFA), and WGA; whereas in patients with deficient activity of acid maltase, the lectin stains were negative or only very slightly positive.[174]

There are species differences in organ involvement. In mice, morphologic changes have been described in liver, pancreas, spleen, kidney, and skeletal and cardiac muscles[14]; in humans, they were seen only in cardiac and skeletal muscles.[15] In mice, resin-embedded myocardial sections 1 μm

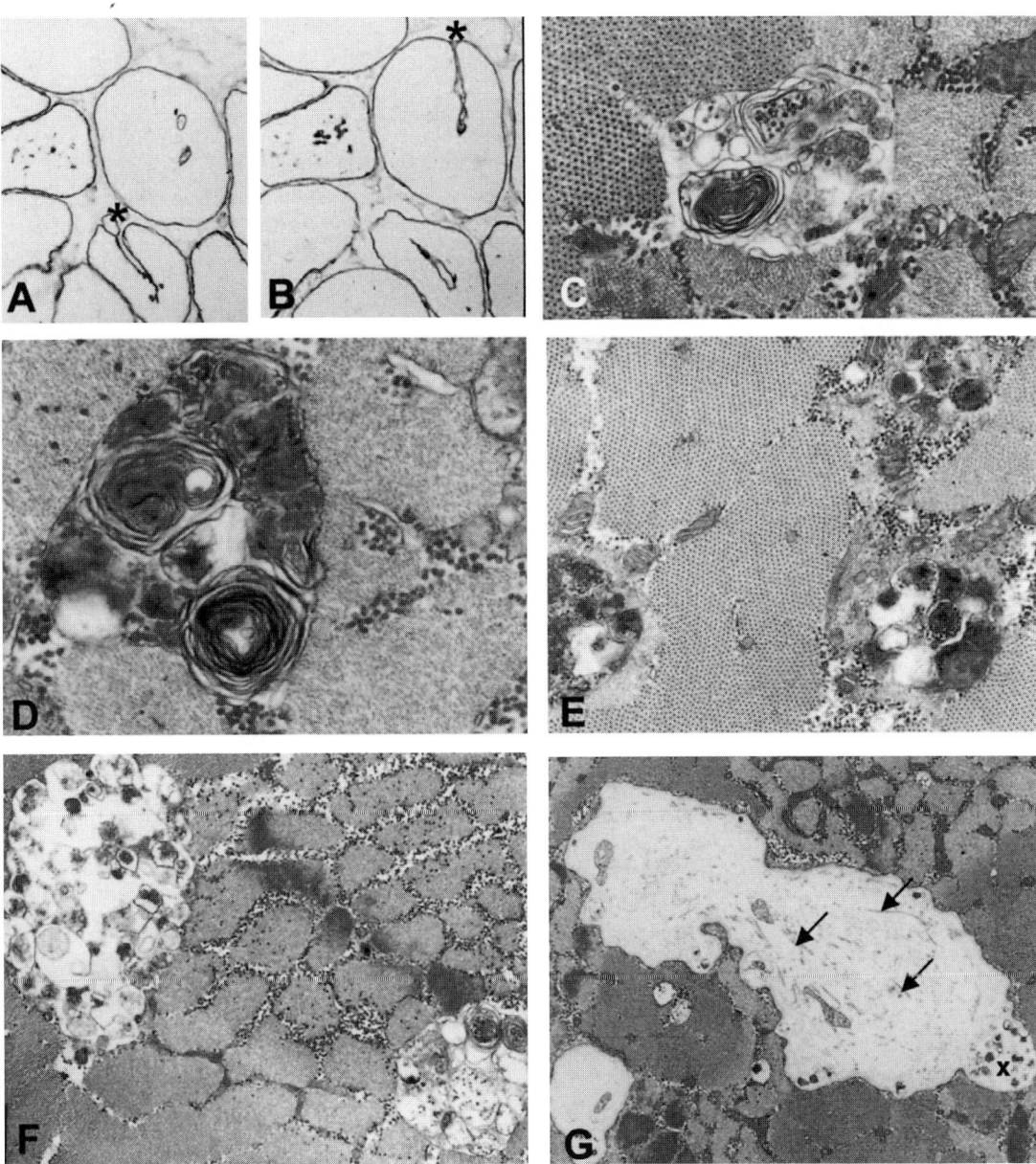

FIGURE 24-22. Danon disease. A and B. Three μm–thick nonconsecutive frozen sections immunostained for α2-laminin reveal sarcolemmal invaginations (fiber splitting,*) that extend to and merge with small vacuoles. C–E. Electron micrographs show that the smallest abnormal spaces contain lamellar structures, amorphous material, and sparse glycogen granules, but are not fully membrane bound and are not lined by basal lamina. F. Classical membrane-bound lobulated autophagic vacuoles not lined by basal lamina. G. Vacuole lined by basal lamina contains collagen fibrils (arrows) and degraded contents of an autophagic vacuole (x). Vacuoles of this type likely arise when the invaginating sarcolemma merges with an autophagic vacuole allowing the contents of the vacuole to leave the fiber. A and B, ×300; C, ×35,300; D, ×46,600; E, ×21,400; F, ×13,700; G, ×9,700. (Courtesy of Dr. Andrew Engel.)

thick stained with toluidine blue reveal the storage of light granular material in cardiomyocytes (Fig. 24-22). Electron microscopic examination of mice deficient in LAMP-2 revealed the presence of membrane-bound vacuoles in various organs and cell types,[14] including endothelial cells, pericytes, and cardiomyocytes (Fig. 24-23A and B). The vacuoles contain pleomorphic fibrillar and lamellated structures.

ACQUIRED STORAGE DISEASES

This group of diseases includes conditions in which there is oversupply of substrate (Table 24-2, mechanism 10), as seen in chronic myelogenous leukemia[175] and conditions in which there is inhibition of lysosomal hydrolases (Table 24-2, mechanism 11). Inhibition of lysosomal storage can be induced experimentally by amphophilic drugs, such as aminoglycoside antibiotics[176] or amiodarone and chloroquine (for an extensive review, see Ref. 177), which results in phospholipidosis. A mucopolysaccharidosis-like condition is induced by the drug suramin[178] and the immunomodulator tilorone.[179] Recent studies indicate that the drug-induced mucopolysaccharidosis is due to the formation of intralysosomal nondegradable dermatan sulfate-drug complexes, which are slow to dissociate.[179]

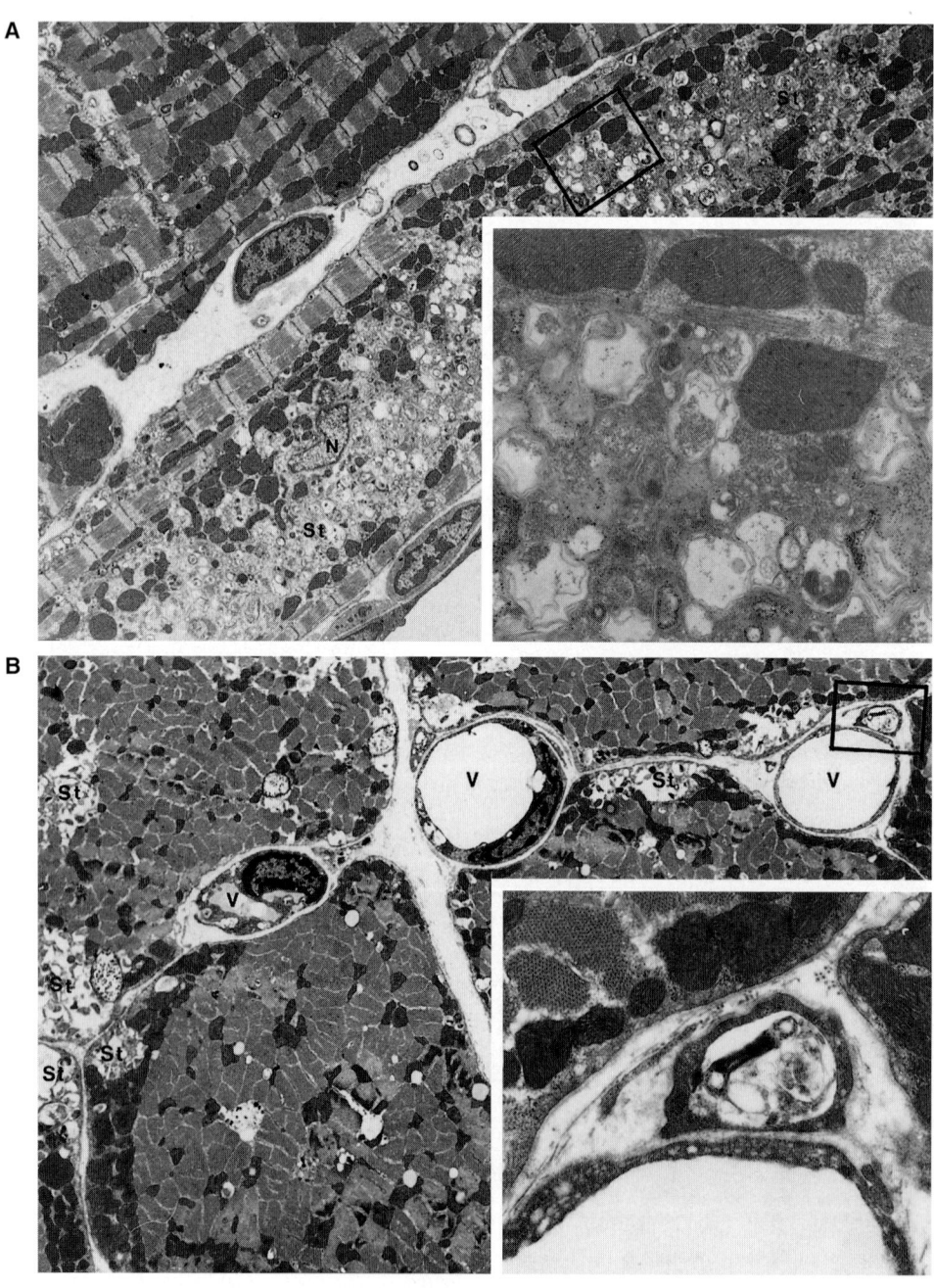

FIGURE 24-23. A. Low-magnification electron micrograph of heart from the same mouse as in Fig. 24-22, showing accumulation of storage (St) material at the center of a cardiomyocyte. (×3,800.) Inset: Higher magnification reveals numerous vacuoles; some are empty, others contain granular and/or fibrillar material. (×18,900.) B. Cross section reveals storage (St) in myocardial cells and in vascular (V) endothelium. (×3800.) Inset: Higher magnification demonstrates storage in pericyte. (×18,900.)

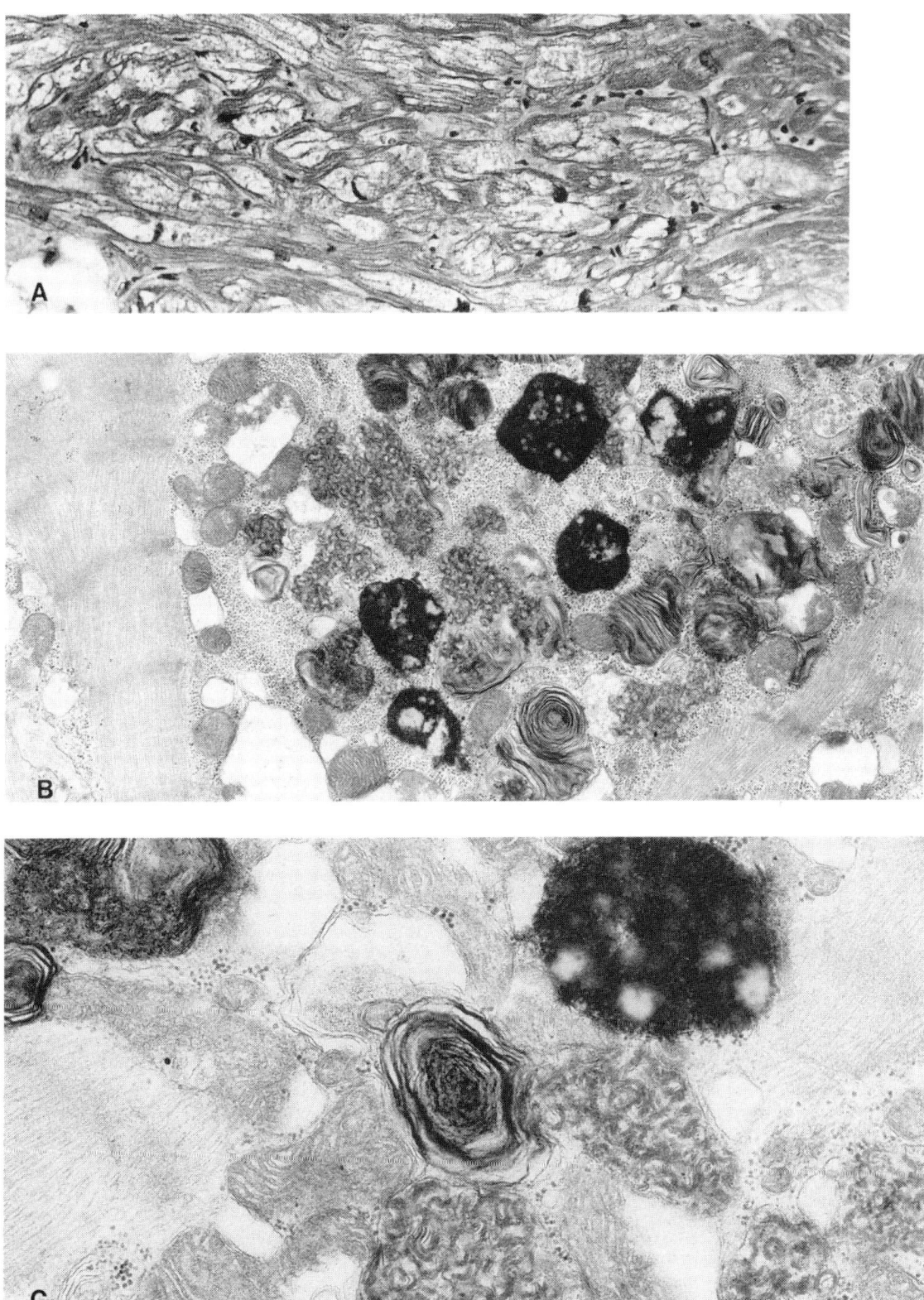

FIGURE 24-24. Light (*A*) and electron (*B* and *C*) micrographs of sections of the right ventricular endomyocardial biopsy from a patient who developed cardiomyopathy after receiving prolonged treatment with chloroquine. *A*. Paraffin section showing enlarged, vacuolated myocytes. (H&E, ×400.) *(Courtesy of Dr. Victor Ferrans.)* *B*. Electron micrograph of a myocyte, showing part of a nucleus, myofilaments, glycogen, lipofuscin granules, and lysosomes laden with lamellated membrane structures and curvilinear bodies. (×16,000.) *(Courtesy of Dr. Victor Ferrans.)* *C*. Higher magnification of electron-dense lipofuscin, lamellated membrane structures, and curvilinear bodies. (×40,000.) *(Courtesy of Dr. Victor Ferrans.)*

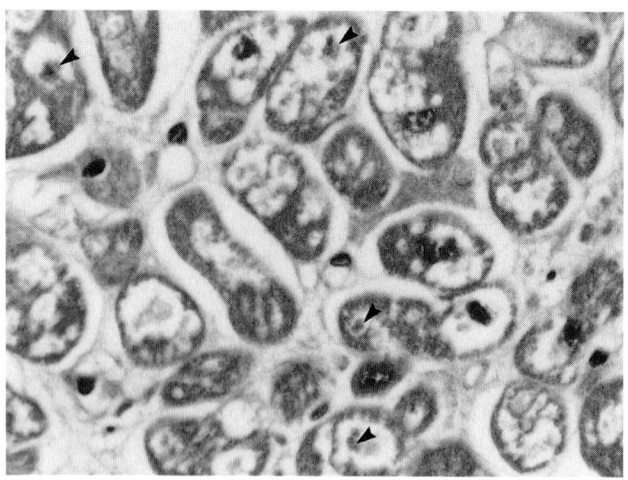

FIGURE 24-25. Formalin-fixed, paraffin section of a heart from a 60-year-old patient[191] with chloroquine-associated cardiomyopathy stained with luxol fast blue, illustrating enlarged vacuolated cardiomyocytes containing some blue granules (arrowheads). (LFB, ×480.)

Swainsonine, an indolizide alkaloid, inhibits the activity of lysosomal α-mannosidase, causing an α-mannosidase-like condition in animals[180] and, in addition, interfering with glycoprotein synthesis.[181] Numerous cell types and various tissues, including cardiac and skeletal muscle,[52,182–184] are affected by the above compounds.

In patients treated with chloroquine, involvement of both skeletal and cardiac muscle has been described. Paraffin sections stained with H&E reveal severe vacuolization of muscle fibers[183] (Fig. 24-24A), which contain LFB-positive granules (Fig. 24-25), indicating the presence of polar lipids.[185] Electron micrographs of affected muscle fibers have demonstrated lamellated membrane structures and curvilinear bodies[182,183] (Fig. 24-24B and C). The storage material gradually disappears after discontinuation of the therapy.

CONDITIONS THAT MAY SIMULATE LYSOSOMAL STORAGE DISEASES

Inclusion body myositis is an idiopathic progressive inflammatory myopathy. Frozen sections stained with H&E revealed basophilic granular inclusions around the edges of slit-like vacuoles, which often stain positively with acid phosphatase. These granules are removed by lipid solvents and are absent from corresponding paraffin sections.[186] EM of skeletal muscle from patients with inclusion body myositis demonstrates numerous enlarged secondary lysosomes laden with coarse membrane structures and amorphous electron-dense material displacing sarcomeres in skeletal muscle (Fig. 24-26).

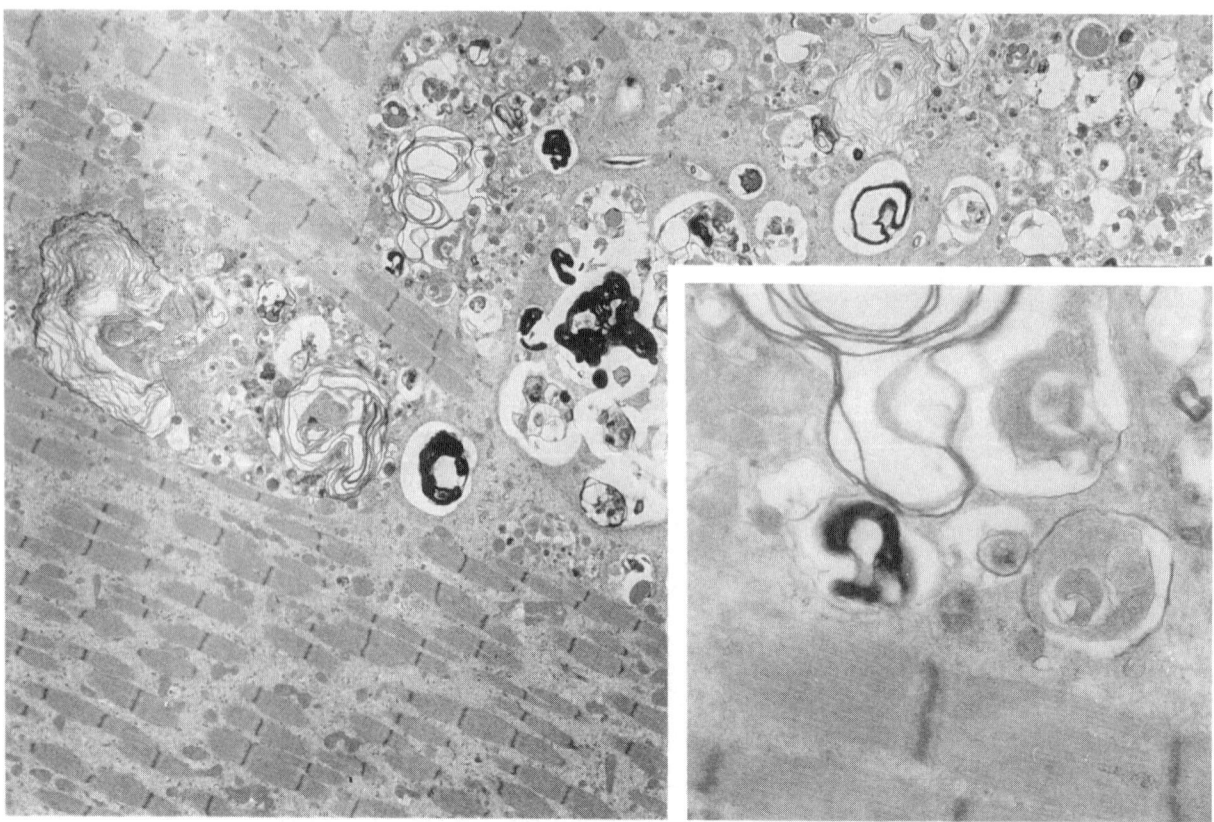

FIGURE 24-26. Electron micrograph of skeletal muscle from a 54-year-old male with inclusion body myositis who presented with a 10-year history of progressive generalized muscle weakness. The levels of his serum CK were 2797 IU/L as compared with 235 in control samples. The micrograph demonstrates fewer sarcomers and displacement of sarcomeres by enlarged secondary lysosomes laden with coarse lamellated membrane structures. ×3500. Inset: Closeup of membrane-bound secondary lysosomes and adjacent sarcomeres. ×19,500.

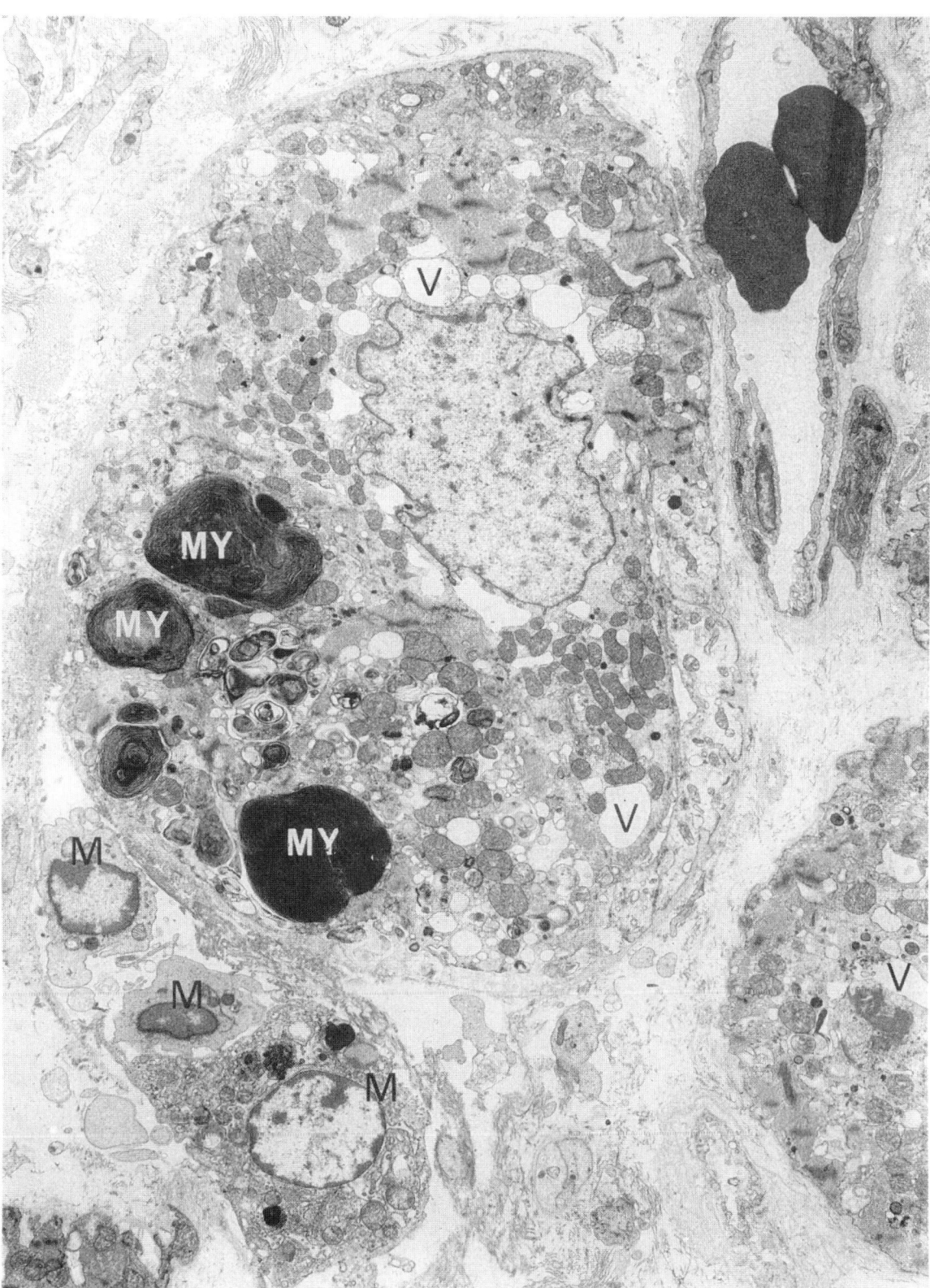

FIGURE 24-27. Electron micrograph of cardiac myocytes, several macrophages (M), and capillary from a rabbit with severe cardiomyopathy after being treated with Adriamycin. The sarcoplasm contains several large myelin figures (MY), small lamellated membrane structures, and vacuoles (V). (×6000.) *(From Van Vleet JF, Greenwood L, Ferrans VJ, Rebar AH: Effect of selenium-vitamin E on Adriamycin-induced cardiomyopathy in rabbits. Am J Vet Res 39:997, 1978. With permission from the American Journal of Veterinary Research.)*

Cardiac and skeletal muscle injury in rabbits treated with doxorubicin (Adriamycin), an antineoplastic chemotherapeutic drug, has resulted in extensive vacuolar degeneration and accumulation of lamellated membrane structures (i.e., myelin figures) (Fig. 24-27).[187] Chronic cases of cardiac and skeletal myopathy have been observed in animals on a diet poor in vitamin E and selenium. This condition is characterized by an accumulation of autofluorescent lipopigments.[188] Similar muscular lesions are seen in patients with abetalipoproteinemia (Bassen-Kornzweig syndrome) They have also been attributed to vitamin E deficiency.[189]

Acknowledgments

The authors are grateful to Dr. L. S. Adelman, Dr. M. W. Ambler, Dr. M. Ellder, Dr. V. J. Ferrans, Dr. R. D. Folkerth, Dr. H. H. Goebel, Dr. J. J. Halpern, Dr. R. Jaffe, Dr. R. W. Kula, Dr. R. Matalon, Dr. P. O'Shea, Dr. A. E. Rosenberg, Dr. P. Saftig, Dr. G. Sahagian, Dr. T. J. Schuetz, Dr. J. F. Van Vleet, Dr. J. P. Veinot, and Dr. D. Zagzag for identifying or providing tissue specimens or illustrations for this chapter. We thank Mrs. V. Goyal for her technical assistance and Mss. C. Welch and P. Stewart for their assistance with the chapter.

List of Abbreviations

BBB	blood-brain barrier	IGF	insulin-like growth factor
BMT	bone marrow transplant	LAMP	lysosomal-associated membrane protein
CNS	central nervous system	LFA	*Limas flavus* agglutinin
CT	computed tomography	LFB	Luxol fast blue
CVB	curvilinear bodies	LSD	lysosomal storage disease
ECG	electrocardiography	Man-6-P	mannose-6 phosphate
EEG	electroencephalography	ML	mucolipidosis
EM	electron microscopy	MPS	mucopolysaccharidosis
EMG	electromyography	MRI	magnetic resonance imaging
ERT	enzyme replacement therapy	NCL	neuronal ceroid lipofuscinosis
FPP	fingerprint profiles	ORO	oil red O
Gb_2Cer	globobiosylceramide	PAS	periodic acid–Schiff
Gb_3Cer	globotriaosylceramide	RCA-I	*Ricinus communis*-I
GROD	granular osmiophilic deposits	RER	rough endoplasmic reticulum
GS-I	*Griffonia simplicifolia*-I	SAP	sphingolipid activator protein
GVHD	graft-versus-host disease	S-WGA	succinylated wheat germ agglutinin
H&E	hematoxylin and eosin	UEA-I	*Ulex europaeus agglutinin*-I
HSP	heat-shock protein	WGA	wheat germ agglutinin

References

1. de Duve C, Wattiaux R: Function of lysosomes. *Annu Rev Physiol* 28:435, 1966.
2. Neufeld EF: Lysosomal storage diseases. *Annu Rev Biochem* 60:275, 1991.
3. Sabatini DD, Adesnik MB: The biogenesis of membrane and organelles, in Scriver CR, Beaudet AL, Sly WS, et al (eds): *The Metabolic and Molecular Bases of Inherited Disease*, 8th ed. New York: McGraw-Hill, 2001; pp 433–517.
4. de Balogh KKIM, Dimande AP, van der Lugt JJ, et al: A lysosomal storage disease induced by *Ipomoea caronea* in goats in Mozambique. *J Vet Diagn Invest* 11:266, 1999.
5. Gabel CA, Foster SA: Postendocytic maturation of acid hydrolases: Evidence of prelysosomal processing. *J Cell Biol* 105:1561, 1987.
6. Roth RA: Structure of the receptor for insulin-like growth factor II: The puzzle amplified. *Science* 239:1269, 1988.
7. Gabel CA, Goldberg DE, Kornfeld S: Identification and characterization of cell deficient in the mannose-6-phosphate receptor: Evidence for an alternative pathway for lysosomal enzyme targeting. *Proc Natl Acad Sci USA* 80:775, 1983.
8. Fukuda M: Lysosomal membrane glycoproteins: Structure, biosynthesis, and intracellular trafficking. *J Biol Chem* 266:21327, 1991.
9. Mathews PM, Martinie JB, Fainbrough DM: The pathway and targeting signal for delivery of the integral membrane glycoprotein LEP100 to lysosomes. *J Cell Biol* 118:1027, 1992.
10. Eberle W, Sander C, Klaus W, et al: The essential tyrosine of the internalization signal in lysosomal acid phosphatase is part of a β turn. *Cell* 67:1203, 1991.
11. Peters C, Braun M, Weber B, et al: Targeting of a lysosomal membrane protein: A tyrosine-containing endocytosis signal in the cytoplasmic stain of the lysosomal acid phosphatase is necessary and sufficient for targeting of lysosomes. *EMBO J* 9:3497, 1990.
12. Andrejewski N, Punnonen E-L, Guhde G, et al: Normal lysosomal morphology and function in LAMP-1-deficient mice. *J Biol Chem* 274:12692, 1999.
13. Cuervo AM, Dice JF: Regulation of Lamp2a levels in the lysosomal membrane. *Traffic* 1:570, 2000.
14. Tanaka Y, Guhde G, Suter A, et al: Accumulation of autophagic vacuoles and cardiomyopathy in LAMP-2-deficient mice. *Nature* 406:902, 2000.
15. Nishino I, Fu J, Tanji K, et al: Primary LAMP-2 deficiency causes X-linked vacuolar cardiomyopathy and myopathy (Danon disease). *Nature* 406:906, 2000.
16. Town M, Jean G, Cherqui S, et al: A novel gene encoding an integral membrane protein is mutated in nephrotic cystinosis. *Nature Genet* 18:319, 1998.
17. Verheijen F, Verbeek E, Aula N, et al: A new gene, encoding an anion transporter is mutated in sialic acid storage diseases. *Nature Genet* 23:462, 1999.
18. Canonico PG, Bird JWC: Lysosomes in skeletal muscle tissue: Zonal centrifugation evidence for multiple cellular sources. *J Cell Biol* 45:321, 1970.
19. Bird JWC: Skeletal muscle lysosomes. *Front Biol* 43:75, 1975.
20. Etherington DJ, Wardale RJ: The mononuclear cell population in rat leg muscle: Its contribution to the lysosomal enzyme activities of whole muscle extracts. *J Cell Sci* 58:139, 1982.
21. Gerard KW, Hipkiss AR, Schneider DL: Degradation of intracellular protein in muscle: Lysosomal response to modified proteins and chloroquine. *J Biol Chem* 263:18886, 1988.

22. Oron U: Proteolytic enzyme activity in rat hindlimb muscles in fetus and during post-natal development. *Int J Dev Biol* 34:457, 1990.
23. Norris G, Reporter M: Hydrolysis of phospholipid esters localized in lysosomes and related structures of rat muscle cells in culture. *Nature* 225:1246, 1970.
24. Vihko V, Rantamaki J, Salminen A: Exhaustive physical exercise and acid hydrolase activity in skeletal muscle: A histochemical study. *Histochemistry* 57:237, 1978.
25. Vihko V, Salminen A, Rantimaki J: Acid hydrolase activity in red and white skeletal muscle of mice during a two-week period following exhausting exercise. *Pflugers Arch* 378:99, 1978.
26. Duncan CJ, Rudge MF: Are lysosomal enzymes involved in rapid damage in vertebrate muscle cells? A study of the separate pathways leading to cellular damage. *Cell Tissue Res* 253:447, 1988.
27. Libelius R, Lundquist I: Lysosomal activation in mouse skeletal muscle induced by protamine in vitro. *Cell Tissue Res* 186:1, 1978.
28. Tagerud S, Libelius R, Shainberg A: High endocytic and lysosomal activities in segments of rat myotubes differentiated in vitro. *Cell Tissue Res* 259:225, 1990.
29. Shannon AD, Courtice FC: The lysosomal enzyme N-acetyl-β-glucosaminidase in rabbit muscle following a period of ischemia. *Pathology* 7:25, 1975.
30. Pearce GW: The sarcolemma and sarcotubular systems in normal and dystrophic muscle. *Res Musc Proc 3rd Symp*, p 146, 1965.
31. Schott LH, Terjung RL: The influence of exercise on muscle lysosomal enzymes. *Eur J Appl Physiol* 42:175, 1979.
32. Rusko H, Bosco C, Komulainen J, et al: Muscle ezyme adaptations to added load during training and nontraining hours in rats. *J Appl Physiol* 70:764, 1991.
33. Vihko V, Salminen A, Rantamaki J: Exhaustive exercise, endurance training, and acid hydrolase activity in skeletal muscle. *J Appl Physiol Respir Environ Exerc Physiol* 47:43, 1979.
34. Salminen A: Lysosomal changes in skeletal muscle during the repair of exercise injuries in muscle fibers. *Acta Physiol Scand* 124(suppl 539):1, 1985.
35. Wallace RR, Lewis MHR: Glycosidase in normal and atrophic skeletal muscle. *Biochem Soc Trans* 3:1027, 1975.
36. Maskrey P, Pluskal MG, Harris JB, Pennington RJT: Studies on increased acid hydrolase activities in denervated muscle. *J Neurochem* 28:403, 1977.
37. Schwartz J, Rath-Wolfson L, Varon D, et al: Effects of various drugs on denervation changes in rat muscles. *Clin Neuropathol* 9:305, 1990.
38. von Steyern FV, Josefsson J-O: Secretion of plasminogen activator and lysosomal enzymes from mouse skeletal muscle: Effect of denervation. *J Cell Physiol* 164:555, 1995.
39. Furuno K, Goodman MN, Goldberg AL: Role of different proteolytic systems in degradation of muscle proteins during denervation atrophy. *J Biol Chem* 265:8550, 1990.
40. Elmquist S, Libelius R, Lawoko G, Tagerud S: Dextrans as markers for endocytosis in innervated and denervated skeletal muscle. *Muscle Nerve* 15:876, 1992.
41. Lawoko G, Tagerud S, Libelius R: Increased endocytic and lysosomal activities in denervated type I and type II muscle fibers. *Histochemistry* 97:221, 1992.
42. Bass A, Teisinger J, Hnik P, et al: Lysosomal and enzyme activities in hypertrophied rat soleus muscle after deneravation. *Pfugers Arch* 400:188, 1984.
43. Hink P, Mackova EV, Syrovy I, et al: Contractile properties of muscle undergoing "compensatory" hypertrophy and its increased susceptibility to denervation and reflex atrophy. *Pflugers Arch* 349.171, 1974.
44. Strauber WT, Fritz VK, Vogelbach DW, Dahlmann B: Characterization of muscles injured by forced lengthening: I. Cellular infiltrates. *Med Sci Sports Exerc* 20:345, 1988.
45. Antel JP, Chelmicka-Schorr E, Sportiello M, et al: Muscle acid protease activity in amyotrophic lateral sclerosis: Correlation with clinical and pathological features. *Neurology* 32:901, 1982.
46. Takala TES, Myllyla VV, Salminen A, et al: Lysosomal and nonlysosomal hydrolases of skeletal muscle in neuromuscular diseases. *Arch Neurol* 40:541, 1983.
47. Salminen A, Marjomaki V, Tolonen U, Myllyla VV: Phosphomannosyl receptor of lysosomal enzymes of skeletal muscle in neuromuscular diseases. *Acta Neurol Scand* 77:461, 1988.
48. Kar NC, Pearson CM: Dipeptidyl peptidases in human muscle disease. *Clin Chim Acta* 82:185, 1978.
49. Pearson CM, Kar NC: Muscle breakdown and lysosomal activation (biochemistry), in Harris JB (ed): *Muscular Dystrophy and Other Inherited Diseases of Skeletal Muscle in Animals*. New York: Academic Press, 1979; pp 338–348.
50. Honda Y, Kuriyawa M, Higuschi I, et al: Muscular involvement in lysosomal acid lipase deficiency in rats. *J Neurol Sci* 108:198, 1992.
51. Neville HE, Baumbach LL, Ringel SP, et al: Familial inclusion body myositis: Evidence for autosomal dominant inheritance. *Neurology* 42:897, 1992.
52. Sano MN, Ishiura S, Nonaka I, et al: Chloroquine myopathy in rat soleus muscle: An experimental model for hyman distal myopathy with rimmed vacuoles. *Biomed Res* 7:301, 1986.
53. Mendell JR, Sahenk Z, Gales T, Paul L: Amyloid filaments in inclusion body myositis: Novel findings provide insight into nature of filaments. *Arch Neurol* 48:1229, 1991.
54. Chiang H-L, Terlecky SR, Plant CP, Dice JF: A role for a 70-kilodalton heat shock protein in lysosomal degradation of intracellular proteins. *Science* 246:382, 1989.
55. Laszlo L, Doherty FJ, Osborn NU, Mayer RJ: Ubiquitinated protein conjugates are specifically enriched in lysosomal system of fibroblasts. *FEBS Lett* 261:365, 1990.
56. Gropper R, Brandt AR, Elias S, et al: The ubiquitin-activated enzyme E1 is required for stress-induced lysosomal degradation of cellular proteins. *J Biol Chem* 266:3602, 1991.
57. Hohlfeld R, Engel AG: Expression of 65-kD heat shock proteins in the inflammatory myopathies. *Ann Neurol* 32:821, 1992.
58. Szebenyi G, Rotwein P: Differential regulation of mannose-6-phosphate receptors and their ligands during the myogenic development of C2 cells. *J Biol Chem* 266:5534, 1991.
59. Willemsen R, Wisselaar HA, van der Ploeg AT: Plasmalemmal vesicles are involved in transepithelial transport of albumin, lysosomal enzymes and mannose-6-phosphate receptor fragments in capillary endothelium. *Eur J Cell Biol* 51:235, 1990.
60. Van der Ploeg AT, Loonen MC, Bolhuis PA, et al: Receptor mediated uptake of acid α-glucosidase corrects lysosomal glycogen storage in cultured skeletal muscle. *Pediatr Res* 24:90, 1988.
61. Fischer HD, Gonzalez-Noriega A, Sly WS, Morre DJ: Phosphomannosyl-enzyme-receptors in rat liver: Subcellular distribution and role in intracellular transport of lysosomal enzymes. *J Biol Chem* 255:9608, 1980.
62. Salminen A: Latencies and phosphomannosyl-enzyme receptors of lysosomal enzymes during the appearance and repair of exercise injuries in mouse skeletal muscles. *Exp Mol Pathol* 41:409, 1984.
63. Beauchamp JR, Partridge TA, Olsen I: Acquisition of lysosomal enzyme by myoblasts in tissue culture. *J Cell Physiol* 144:166, 1990.
64. Kornfeld S, Sly WS: Lysosomal storage defects. *Hosp Pract* 20:71, 1985.
65. Reuser AJJ, Kroos MA, Visser R, Willemsen R: Lysosomal storage diseases: Cellular pathology, clinical and genetic heterogeneity, therapy. *Ann Biol Clin* 52:721, 1994.
66. Castagnaro M, Alroy J, Ucci AA, Glew RH: Lectin histochemistry and ultrastructure of feline kidneys from six different storage diseases. *Virchows Arch B* 54:16, 1987.
67. Warren CD, Alroy J: Morphological, biochemical and molecular biology approaches for the diagnosis of lysosomal storage diseases. *J Vet Diagn Invest* 12:483, 2000.
68. Samuels MA, Feske, SK (eds): *Office Practice of Neurology*, 2nd ed. Philadelphia: Churchill Livingstone, 2003; pp 1254–1263.
69. Scriver CR, Beaudet AL, Sly WS, Valle D (eds): *The Metabolic and Molecular Bases of Inherited Disease*, 8th ed. New York: McGraw-Hill, 2001; pp 3371–3894.
70. Leinekugel P, Michel S, Conzelmann E, Sandhoff K: Quantitative correlation between the residual activity of β-hexosaminidase A and arylsulfatase A and the severity of the resulting lysosomal storage disease. *Hum Genet* 88:513, 1992.
71. Carpenter S, Karpati G: Lysosomal storage in human skeletal muscle. *Hum Pathol* 17:683, 1986.
72. Alroy J, DeGaspari R, Warren CD: Application of lectin histochemistry and carbohydrate analysis to the characterization of lysosomal storage diseases. *Carbohydr Res* 213:213, 1991.
73. Kula RW, Shafiq SA, Sher JH, Qazi QH: I-cell disease (mucolipidosis II): Differential expression in satellite cells and mature muscle fibers. *J Neurol Sci* 63:75, 1984.
74. Jones MZ, Cunningham JG, Dade AW, et al: Caprine β-mannosidosis: Clinical and pathological features. *J Neuropathol Exp Neurol* 42:268, 1983.
75. Prasad A, Kaye EM, Alroy J: Electron microscopic examination of skin biopsy as a cost effective tool in the diagnosis of lysosomal storage diseases. *J Child Neurol* 11:301, 1996.
76. Krivit W, Shapiro EG, Peters C, et al: Hematopoietic stem-cell transplantation in globoid-cell leukodystrophy. *N Engl J Med* 338:1119, 1998.
77. Krivit W, Aubourg P, Shapiro E, Peters C: Bone marrow transplantation for globoid cell leukodystrophy, adrenoleukodystrophy, metachromatic leukodystrophy, and Hurler syndrome. *Curr Opin Hematol* 6:377, 1999.
78. Guffon N, Souillet G, Maire I, et al: Follow-up of nine patients with Hurler syndrome after bone-marrow transplantation. *J Pediatr* 133:119, 1998.
79. Vellodi A, Young E, Cooper A, et al: Long-term follow-up following bone marrow transplantation for Hunter disease. *J Inherit Metab Dis* 22:638, 1999.
80. Peters C, Krivit W: Hematopoietic cell transplantation for mucopolysaccharidosis IIB (Hunter syndrome) *Bone Marrow Transplant* 25:1097, 2000.
81. Grabowski GA, Leslie N, Weinstrup R: Enzyme therapy for Gaucher disease: The first five years. *Blood Rev* 12:115, 1998.
82. Schiffman R, Koop JB, Austia HA III, et al: Enzyme replacement therapy in Fabry disease: A randomized controlled trial. *JAMA* 285:2743, 2001.
83. Eng CM, Guffon N, Wilcox WR, et al: Safety and efficacy of recombinant human alpha-galactosidase A-replacement therapy in Fabry's disease. *N Engl J Med* 345:9, 2001.

84. Kakkis ED, Muenzer J, Tiller GE, et al: Enzyme replacement therapy in mucopolysaccharidosis I. *N Engl J Med.* 344:182, 2001.
85. Van den Hout JM, Reuser AJ, de Klerk JB, et al: Enzyme therapy for Pompe disease with recombinant human alpha-glucosidase from rabbit milk. *J Inherit Metab Dis* 24:266, 2001.
86. Amalfitano A, Bengur AR, Morse RP, et al: Recombinant human acid alpha-glucosidase enzyme therapy for infantile glycogen storage disease type II: Results of a phase I/II clinical trial. *Genet Med* 3:132, 2001.
87. Cox T, Lachmann R, Hollak C, et al: Novel oral treatment of Gaucher's disease with N-butyldeoxynojirimycin (OGT 918) to decrease substrate biosynthesis. *Lancet* 355:1481, 2000.
88. Platt FM, Neises GR, Reinkensmeier G, et al: Prevention of lysosomal storage in Tay-Sachs mice treated with N-butyldeoxynojirimycin. *Science* 276:428, 1997.
89. Desnick RJ, Ioannou YA, Eng CM: α-Galactosidase A deficiency : Fabry disease, in Scriver CR, Beaudet AL, Sly WS, Valle D (eds): *The Metabolic and Molecular Bases of Inherited Disease*, 8th ed. New York: McGraw-Hill, 2001; pp 3733-3774.
90. Koitabashi N, Utsugi T, Seki R, et al: Biopsy-proven cardiomyopathy in heterozygous Fabry's disease. *Jpn Cir J* 63:572, 1999.
91. Uchino M, Uyama E, Kawano H, et al: A histochemical and electron microscopy study of skeletal and cardiac muscle from a Fabry disease patient and carrier. *Acta Neuropathol* 90:334, 1995.
92. Sima AA, Robertson DM: Involvement of peripheral nerve and muscle in Fabry's disease: Histologic, ultrastructural, and morphometric studies. *Arch Neurol* 35:291, 1978.
93. Faraggiana T, Churg J, Grishman E, et al: Light- and electron-microscopic histochemistry of Fabry's disease. *Am J Pathol* 103:247, 1981.
94. deVeber GA, Schwarting GA, Kolodny EH, Kowall NW: Fabry disease: Immunocytochemical characterization of neuronal involvement. *Ann Neurol* 31:409, 1992.
95. Ogawa K, Sugamata K, Funamoto N, et al: Restricted accumulation of globotriaosylceramide in hearts of atypical cases of Fabry's disease. *Hum Pathol* 21:1067, 1990.
96. Elleder M, Bradova V, Smid F, et al: Cardiocyte storage and hypertrophy as a sole manifestation of Fabry's disease: Report on a case simulating hypertrophic non-obstructive cardiomyopathy. *Virchows Arch A Pathol Anat A* 417:449, 1990.
97. Pellissier JF, Van Hoof F, Bourdet D, et al: Morphological and biochemical changes in muscle and peripheral nerve in Fabry's disease. *Muscle Nerve* 4:381, 1981.
98. Nagao Y, Nakashima H, Fukuhara Y, et al: Hypertrophic cardiomyopathy in late-onset variant of Fabry disease with high residual activity of α-galactosidase A. *Clin Genet* 39:233, 1991.
99. Suzuki Y, Oshima A, Namba E: β-Galactosidase deficiency (β-galactosidosis): G_{M1} gangliosidosis and Morquio B disease, in Scriver CR, Beaudet AL, Sly WS, Valle D (eds): *The Metabolic and Molecular Bases of Inherited Disease*, 8th ed. New York: McGraw-Hill, 2001; pp 3775-3809.
100. Kohlschutter A, Sieg K, Schulte FJ, et al: Infantile cardiomyopathy and neuromyopathy with β-galactosidase deficiency. *Eur J Pediatr* 139:75, 1982.
101. Lin H-C, Tsai F-J, Shen W-C, et al: Infantile form G_{M1} gangliosidosis with dilated cardiomyopathy: A case report. *Acta Paediatr* 89:878, 2000.
102. Charrow J, Hvizd MG: Cardiomyopathy and skeletal myopathy in an unusual variant of G_{M1} gangliosidosis. *J Pediatr* 108:729, 1986.
103. Alroy J, Orgad U, DeGasperi R, et al: Canine G_{M1}-gangliosidosis: A clinical, morphologic, histochemical, and biochemical comparison of two different models. *Am J Pathol* 140:675, 1992.
104. Iwamasa T, Ohshita T, Nashiro K, et al: Demonstration of G_{M1}-ganglioside in nervous system in generalized G_{M1}-gangliosidosis using cholera toxin B subunit. *Acta Neuropathol* 73:357–360, 1987.
105. Yoshida K, Ikeda S-I, Kawaguchi K, et al: Adult G_{M1} gangliosidosis: Immunohistochemical and ultrastructural findings in an autopsy case. *Neurology* 44:2376, 1994.
106. Tome FMS, Fardeau M: Ultrastructural study of muscle biopsy in a case of G_{M1} gangliosidosis type 1. *Pathol Eur* 11:15, 1976.
107. Gravel RA, Clarke JTR, Kaback MM, et al: The GM2 gangliosidoses, in Scriver CR, Beaudet AL, Sly WS, Valle D (eds): *The Metabolic Basis of Inherited Disease*, 7th ed. New York: McGraw-Hill, 1995; pp 2839–2879.
108. Kolodny EH: The G_{M2} gangliosidoses, in Rosenberg RN, Prusiner S, DiMauro S, Barchi R (eds): *The Molecular and Genetic Basis of Neurological Disease*, 2nd ed. Stoneham, MA: Butterworth-Heinemann, 1997; pp 473–490.
109. Sandhoff K, Harzer K, Furst W: Sphingolipid activator proteins, in Scriver CR, Beaudet AL, Sly WS, Valle D (eds): *The Metabolic Basis of Inherited Disease*, 7th ed. New York: McGraw-Hill, 1995; pp 2427–2441.
110. Pearse AGE: The plasmal reaction, in *Histochemistry, Theoretical and Applied*, 2nd ed. Boston: Little, Brown, 1961; pp 347–355.
111. Alroy J, Adelman L, Warren CD: Lectin histochemistry of gangliosidosis. II. Neurovisceral tissues from patients with Sandhoff's disease. *Acta Neuropathol* 76:359, 1988.
112. Dolman CL, Chang E, Duke RJ: Pathologic findings in Sandhoff disease. *Arch Pathol* 96:272, 1973.
113. Willner JP, Grabowski GA, Gordon RE, et al: Chronic G_{M2} gangliosidosis masquerading as atypical Friedreich ataxia: Clinical, morphologic, and biochemical studies of nine cases. *Neurology* 31:787, 1981.
114. Navon R, Argov Z, Brand N, Sandbank U: Adult G_{M2} gangliosidosis in association with Tay-Sachs disease: A new phenotype. *Neurology* 31:1397, 1981.
115. Goebel HH, Sharp JD: The neuronal ceroid-lipofuscinosis. *Brain Pathol* 8:151, 1998.
116. Peltonen L, Savukoski M, Vesa J: Genetics of the neuronal ceroid lipofuscinosis. *Curr Opion Genet Dev* 10:299, 2000.
117. Pearse AGE: The plasmal reaction, in *Histochemistry, Theoretical and Applied*, 2nd ed. Boston: Little, Brown, 1961; pp 347–355.
118. Dolman CL, Chang E: Visceral lesions in amaurotic idiocy with curvilinear bodies. *Arch Pathol* 94:425, 1972.
119. Tyynela J, Suopanki J, Santavuori P, et al: Variant late infantile neuronal ceroid-lipofuscinosis: Pathology and biochemistry. *J Neuropathol Exp Neurol* 56:369, 1997.
120. Alroy J, Castagnaro M, McCoy JP, et al: Neuronal ceroid lipofuscinosis diseases in Australian Blue Heelers: Clinical morphological and histochemical studies. *Eur J Vet Pathol* 1:61, 1995.
121. Berkovic SF, Carpenter S, Anderman F, et al: Kuf's disease: A critical reappraisal. *Brain* 111:27, 1988.
122. Hirvasniemi A, Lang H, Lehesjoki A-E, Leisti J: Northern epilepsy syndrome: An inherited childhood onset epilepsy with associated mental deterioration. *J Med Genet* 31:177, 1994.
123. Haltia M, Tyynela J, Hirvasniemi A, et al: Northern epilepsy, in Goebel HH, Mole SE, Lake BD (eds): *The Neuronal Ceroid-Lipofuscinosis (Batten's Disease)*. Amsterdam: IOS Press, 1998; pp 117–124.
124. Kornfeld S, Sly WS: I-cell disease and pseudo-Hurler polydystrophy: Disorders of lysosomal enzyme phosphorylation and localization, in Scriver CR, Beaudet AL, Sly WS, Valle D (eds): *The Metabolic Basis of Inherited Disease*, 7th ed. New York: McGraw-Hill, 1995; pp 2495–2508.
125. Castagnaro M, Alroy J, Ucci AA, Jaffe R: Lectin histochemistry and ultrastructure of kidneys from patients with I-cell disease. *Arch Pathol* 11:285, 1987.
126. Martin JJ, Leroy JG, Farriaux JP, et al: I cell disease (mucolipidosis II): A report on its pathology. *Acta Neuropathol* 33:285, 1975.
127. Shanske S, Miranda AF, Penn AS, DiMauro S: Mucolipidosis II (I-cell disease): Studies of muscle biopsy and muscle cultures. *Pediatr Res* 15:1334, 1981.
128. Folkerth RD, Alroy J, Lomakina I, et al: Mucolipidosis IV: Morphology and histochemistry of an autopsy case. *J Neuropathol Exp Neurol* 54:154, 1995.
129. Sun M, Goldin E, Stahl S, et al: Mucolipidosis type IV is caused by mutations in a gene encoding a novel transient receptor potential channel. *Hum Mol Genet* 9:2471, 2000.
130. Alterescu G, Sun M, Moore DF, et al: The neurogenetics of mucolipidosis type IV. *Neurology* 9:306, 2002.
131. Goebel HH, Kohlschutter A, Lenard HG: Morphologic and chemical biopsy findings in mucolipidosis IV. *Clin Neuropathol* 1:73, 1982.
132. Weitz R, Kramer I, Nissenkorn I, et al: Muscle involvement in mucolipidosis IV. *Brain Dev* 12:524, 1990.
133. Thomas GH: Disorders of glycoprotein degradation: α-mannosidosis, β-mannosidosis, fucosidosis, and sialidosis, in Scriver CR, Beaudet AL, Sly WS, Valle D (eds): *The Metabolic and Moleculaar Bases of Inherited Disease*, 8th ed. New York: McGraw-Hill, 2001; pp 3507–3533.
134. Johnson WG: Disorders of glycoprotein degradation: Sialidosis, fucosidosis, alpha-mannosidosis, beta-mannosidosis, and aspartyl-glycosaminuria, in Rosenberg RN, Prusiner S, DiMauro S, et al (eds): *The Molecular and Genetic Basis of Neurological Disease*, 2nd ed. Stoneham, MA: Butterworth-Heinemann, 1997; pp 355–369.
135. Malm D, Halvorsen DS, Tranebjaeg L, Sjursen H: Immunodeficiency in alpha-mannosidosis: A matched case-control study on immunoglobulin, complement factors, receptor density, phagocytosis and intracellular killing in leucocytes. *Eur J Pediatr* 159:699, 2000.
136. Kawai H, Nishino H, Nishida Y, et al: Skeletal muscle pathology of mannosidosis in two siblings with spastic paraplegia. *Acta Neuropathol* 68:201, 1985.
137. Halperin JJ, Landis DMD, Weinstein LA, et al: Communicating hydrocephalus and lysosomal inclusions in mannosidosis. *Arch Neurol* 41:777, 1984.
138. Alroy J, Orgad U, Ucci AA, Pereira MEA: Identification of glycoprotein storage diseases by lectins: A new diagnostic method. *J Histochem Cytochem* 32:1280, 1984
139. Wenger DA, Sujansky E, Fennessey PV, Thompson JN: Human β-mannosidase deficiency. *N Engl J Med* 315:1201, 1986.
140. Patterson JS, Jones MZ, Lovell KL, Abbitt B: Neuropathology of bovine β-mannosidosis. *J Neuropathol Exp Neurol* 50:538, 1991.
141. Landing BH, Donnell GN, Alfi OS, et al: Fucosidosis: Clinical pathologic, and biochemical studies of five patients. *Adv Exp Med Biol* 68:147, 1975.
142. Alroy J, Ucci AA, Warren CD: Human and canine fucosidosis: A comparative lectin histochemistry study. *Acta Neuropathol* 67:265, 1985.
143. Gahl WA, Schneider JA, Aula PP: Lysosomal transport disorders: Cystinosis and sialic acid storage disorders, in Scriver CR, Beaudet AC, Sly WS, Valle D (eds): *The Metabolic Basis of Inherited Disease*, 7th ed. New York: McGraw-Hill, 1995; pp 3763–3797.

144. Pueschel SM, O'Shea PA, Alroy J, et al: Infantile sialic storage disease associated with renal disease. *Pediatr Neurol* 4:207, 1986.
145. Wolburg-Bucholz K, Scholte W, Baumkotter J, et al: Familial lysosomal storage disease with generalized vacuolization and sialic aciduria: Sporadic Salla disease. *Neuropediatrics* 16:67, 1985.
146. Gahl WA, Dalakas MC, Charnas L, et al: Myopathy and cystine storage in muscles in a patient with nephropathic cystinosis. *N Engl J Med* 319:1461, 1988.
147. Harper GS, Bernardini I, Hurko O, et al: Cystine storage in cultured myotubes from patients with nephropathic cystinosis. *Biochem J* 243:841, 1987.
148. Neufeld EF, Muenzer J: The mucopolysaccharidoses, in Scriver CR, Beaudet AL, Sly WS, Valle D (eds): *The Metabolic Basis of Inherited Disease*, 7th ed. New York: McGraw-Hill, 1995; pp 2465–2494.
149. Matalon R, Kaul R, Michals K: The mucopolysaccharidoses and the mucolipidoses, in Rosenberg RN, Pruisner S, DiMauro S, Barchi ET (eds): *The Molecular and Genetic Basis of Neurological Disease*, 2nd ed. Stoneham, MA: Butterworth-Heinemann, 1997; pp 333–354.
150. Triggs-Raine B, Salo TJ, Zhang H, et al: Mutations in HYAL1, a member of a tandemly distributed multigene family encoding disparate hyaluronidase activities, cause a newly described lysosomal disorder, mucopolysaccharidosis IX. *Proc Natl Acad Sci USA* 96:6296, 1999.
151. Renteria GS, Ferrans VJ, Roberts WC: The heart in the Hurler syndrome: Gross, histologic and ultrastructural observations in five necropsy cases. *Am J Cardiol* 38:487, 1976.
152. Avila JL, Convit J: Inhibition of leucocytic enzymes by glycosaminoglycans in vitro. *Biochem J* 152:57, 1975.
153. Oda H, Sasaki Y, Nakatani Y, et al: Hunter syndrome: An ultrastructural study of an autopsy case. *Acta Pathol Jpn* 38:1175, 1990.
154. Kurihara M, Kumagai K, Yagishita S: Sanfilippo syndrome type C: A clinicopathological autopsy study of a long-term survivor. *Pediatr Neurol* 14:317, 1996.
155. Martin JJ, Ceuterick C, Van Dessel G, et al: Two cases of mucopolysaccharidosis type III (Sanfilippo): An anatomopathological study. *Acta Neuropathol* 46:185, 1979.
156. Jones MZ, Alroy J, Rutledge J, et al: Human mucopolysaccharidosis IIID: Clinical, biochemical and immunohistochemical characteristics. *J Neuropathol Exp Neurol* 56:1158, 1997.
157. Jones MZ, Alroy J, Boyer PJ, et al: Caprine mucopolysaccharidosis IIID: Clinical, biochemical and immunohistochemical characteristics. *J Neuropathol Exp Neurol* 57:148, 1998.
158. Hayflick S, Rowe S, Kavanaugh-McHugh A, et al: Acute infantile cardiomyopathy as a presenting feature of mucopolysaccharidosis VI. *J Pediatr* 38:132, 1987.
159. Rudenko G, Bonten E, Hol WGJ, d'Azzo A: The atomic model of the human protective protein/cathepsin A suggests a structural basis for galactosialidosis. *Proc Natl Acad Sci USA* 95:621, 1998.
160. Galjaard H, Willemsen R, Hoogeven AT, et al: Molecular heterogeneity in human β-galactosidase and neuraminidase deficiency. *Enzyme* 38:132, 1987.
161. d'Azzo A, Andria G, Strisciuglio P, Galjaard H: Galactosialidosis, in Scriver CR, Beaudet AL, Sly WS, Valle D (eds): *The Metabolic and Molecular Bases of Inherited Disease*, 8th ed. New York: McGraw-Hill, 2001; pp 3811–3826.
162. Assmann G, Seedorf U: Acid lipase deficiency: Wolman diseases and cholesteryl ester storage disease, in Scriver CR, Beaudet AL, Sly WS, Valle D (eds): *The Metabolic and Molecular Bases of Inherited Disease*, 8th ed. New York: McGraw-Hill, 2001; pp 3551–3572.
163. Yatsu F, Alam R: Wolman disease, in Rosenberg RN, Pruisner S, DiMauro S, Barchi et al (eds): *The Molecular and Genetic Basis of Neurological Disease*, 2nd ed. Stoneham, MA: Butterworth-Heinemann, 1997; pp 371–378.
164. Navarro C, Fernandez JM, Dominguez C, et al: Muscle involvement in cholesterol ester storage disease. *Neurology* 42:1120, 1992.
165. Honda Y, Kuriyama M, Higuchi I, et al: Muscular involvement in lysosomal acid lipase deficiency in rats. *J Neurol Sci* 108:189, 1992.
166. Danon MJ, Oh SJ, DiMauro S, et al. Lysosomal glycogen storage disease with normal acid maltase. *Neurology* 31:51, 1981.
167. Hart ZH, Servidie S, Peterson PL, et al: Cardiomyopathy, mental retardation, autophagic vacuolar myopathy. *Neurology* 37:1065, 1987.
168. Kashio N, Usuki F, Akamine T, et al: Cardiomyopathy, mental retardation, and autophagic vacuolar myopathy: Abnormal MRI findings in the head. *J Neurol Sci* 105:1, 1991.
169. Sugie K, Yamamoto A, Murayama K, et al: Clinicopathological features of genetically confirmed Danon disease. *Neurology*. 58:1773, 2002.
170. Cuervo AM, Dice JF: A receptor for the selective uptake and degradation of proteins by lysosomes. *Science* 273:501, 1996.
171. Takahashi M, Yamamoto A, Takamo K, et al: Germline mosaicism of a novel mutation in lysosome-associated membrane protein-2 deficiency (Danon disease). *Ann Neurol* 52:122, 2002.
172. Muntoni F, Catani G, Mateddu A, et al: Familial cardiomyopathy, mental retardation, and myopathy associated with desmine-type intermediate filaments. *Neuromuscul Disord* 4:233, 1994.
173. Murakami N, Goto Y, Itoh M, et al: Sarcolemmal indentation in cardiomyopathy with mental retardation and vacuolar myopathy. *Neuromuscul Disord* 5:149, 1995.
174. Kashio N, Usuki F, Higuchi I, et al: Lysosomal glycogen storage disease without acid maltase deficiency-A lectin-histochemical study of an unusual type of glycogen storage disease. *Acta Histochem Cytochem* 23:603, 1991.
175. Lee RE: Histiocytic diseases of bone marrow. *Hematol Oncol Clin North Am* 2:657, 1988.
176. Hashino E, Shero M, Salvi RJ: Lysosomal augmentation during aminoglycoside uptake in cochlear hair cells. *Brain Res* 887:90, 2000.
177. Hurban Z: Pulmonary and generalized lysosomal storage induced by amphophilic drugs. *Environ Heath Perspect* 55:53, 1984.
178. Christensen B, Lullmann-Rauch R: On the alcianophilia of the drug suramin used as a tool for inducing experimental mucopolysaccharidosis. *Histochemistry* 89:365, 1988.
179. Bispinck F, Fischer J, Lullmann-Rauch R, von Witzendorf B: Lysosomal glycosaminoglycan storage as induced by dicationic amphophilic drugs: Investigation into the mechanisms underlying the slow reversibility. *Toxicology* 128:91, 1998.
180. Molyneux RJ, James LF: Loco intoxication: Indolizidine alkaloids of spotted locoweed *(Astragalus lentiginosus)*. *Science* 216:190, 1983.
181. Tulsiani DRP, Touster O: Swainsonine causes the production of hybrid glycoproteins by human skin fibroblasts and rat liver hepatocyte preparations. *J Biol Chem* 258:7578, 1983.
182. McAllister HA Jr, Ferrans VJ, Hall RJ, et al: Chloroquine-induced cardiomyopathy. *Arch Pathol Lab Med* 111:953, 1987.
183. Pearse AGE: Lipid, lipoproteins and proteolipids, in *Histochemistry, Theoretical and Applied*, 3rd ed. Boston: Little, Brown, 1968; pp 398–466.
184. Ratliff NB, Estes ML, Myles JL, et al: Diagnosis of chloroquine cardiomyopathy by endomyocardial biopsy. *N Engl J Med* 316:191, 1987.
185. Snyder VL, Bandyopadhyay S, Collins J, et al: Subcellular changes of rat myocardium after treatment with amiodarone or desethylamiodarone, studied with electron microscopy. *J Submicrosc Cytol Pathol* 22:71, 1990.
186. Mastaglia FL, Walton JN: Inflammatory myopathy, in Mastaglia FL, Walton J (eds): *Skeletal Muscle Pathology*. Edinburgh: Churchill Livingstone, 1982; pp 360–392.
187. Van Vleet JF, Greenwood L, Ferrans VJ, et al: Effect of selenium-vitamin E on Adriamycin-induced cardiomyopathy in rabbits. *Am J Vet Res* 39:997, 1978.
188. Howes EL, Price HM, Blumberg JM: The effects of diet producing lipochrome pigment (ceroid) on the ultrastructure of skeletal muscle in the rat. *Am J Pathol* 45:599, 1964.
189. Kott E, Delre G, Kadish U, et al: Abetalipoproteinemia (Bassen-Kornzweig syndrome): Muscle involvement. *Acta Neuropathol* 37:255, 1977.
190. Kolodny EH, Cable W, Daniel P, et al: Fucosidosis presenting as a leukodystrophy. *Trans Am Neurol Assoc* 105:1, 1980.
191. Veinot JP, Mai KT, Zarychanski R: Chloroquine related cardiac toxicity. *J Rheumatol* 25:1221–1225, 1998.

2
General Approaches to Neuromuscular Diseases

Chapter 25
The Clinical Examination

BRENDA L. BANWELL
MANUEL R. GOMEZ

The Clinical History
    PRESENTING SYMPTOMS
    HISTORY OF THE ILLNESS
    FAMILY HISTORY
    THE SYMPTOMS

The Clinical Examination
    SIMPLE INSPECTION AT REST
    WEAKNESS AND ATROPHY
    INSPECTION OF GAIT
    TESTING OF THE CRANIAL MUSCLES
    MANUAL MUSCLE TESTING
    PALPATION OF MUSCLES AND NERVES
    PERCUSSION OF MUSCLES
    REACTIONS AND REFLEXES
    SENSATION

The Clinical Features
    WEAKNESS
    ARTHROGRYPOSIS AND OTHER TENDON CONTRACTURES
    SKELETAL ANOMALIES
    FATIGABILITY
    FASCICULATIONS
    MYOKYMIA
    MYOTONIA

This chapter focuses on the clinical history and examination of adults and children with neuromuscular diseases. The data obtained are essential for defining the clinical problem, but they must be correlated with appropriate ancillary investigations such as electromyographic studies, muscle imaging, muscle biopsy, or DNA analysis.

The Clinical History

PRESENTING SYMPTOMS

Although there are many neuromuscular diseases, they present with relatively few symptoms. Adults complain of weakness, increased fatigability, loss of muscle bulk, or cramps, pain, and stiffness of muscles. Parents note that their affected child is floppy; cannot support his or her head; cannot sit, stand, walk, or run normally; fatigues easily; or has skeletal deformities.

HISTORY OF THE ILLNESS

The history of the illness must be recorded chronologically from its onset. It should include the rate of progression and any symptoms referable to other systems. An abrupt onset of symptoms suggests a toxic or metabolic disturbance, a subacute onset of days to weeks is most commonly associated with an inflammatory or infective process, and weakness that evolves slowly over months to years often has a hereditary, degenerative, or endocrinologic basis.[1] Episodic generalized weakness occurs in patients with electrolyte disturbances, neuromuscular junction disorders, channelopathies, or cataplexy, and in those with metabolic defects of muscle.[2]

It is particularly important to inquire about symptoms of cardiac muscle involvement, either irregularities in cardiac rate or rhythm (palpitations, syncope) or features of cardiac failure (paroxysmal nocturnal dyspnea, orthopnea, fatigue, exercise intolerance, peripheral edema). Direct inquiry should be made as to the effects of diet, medications, exercise, and ambient temperature on muscle symptoms and about ingestion of improperly prepared and potentially poisonous foods, inadvertent intoxication with pharmaceuticals, exposure to oral polio vaccine, or accidental exposure to toxic substances or venomous animals. An insidious onset of weakness often obscures the duration of the illness. Patients with static or slowly progressive myopathies or spinal muscular atrophy (SMA)* type III may show an apparent sudden decompensation during periods of rapid somatic growth, either due to increased body mass or due to progressive worsening of scoliosis. Many patients underreport symptoms, either due to unconscious denial or due to a tendency to disregard symptoms such as cramps that have been present for many years. A direct inquiry into the symptoms mentioned in this chapter could thus be rewarding.

In children, the prenatal and perinatal events are often relevant. A delay in the onset or an impairment of the quality and strength of fetal movements; a history of polyhydramnios (which may suggest impaired fetal swallowing); and a breech presentation at birth are common features of infants with congenital neuromuscular disease. The rate of acquisition of developmental motor milestones (the age when the infant first lifted his or her head from a prone decubitus position, sat alone, pulled himself or herself up to a standing position, stood without assistance, walked unsupported, climbed onto furniture, and climbed one step at a time or with alternating feet, and when the child could run), the speed and agility of the child relative to age-matched peers, and any regression in previously acquired skills should be documented.

FAMILY HISTORY

Many neuromuscular diseases have a heritable basis, and an increasing array of molecular diagnostic tests is available. A pattern of inheritance revealed by the family history can be an important clue leading to diagnosis. If genetic counseling is indicated, a detailed genealogical tree is also required. This must include the sex of all members, age of onset and rate of evolution of symptoms (if known) of affected rela-

---

*A list of abbreviations used in this chapter is given at the end of the chapter.

tives, miscarriages and stillbirths, consanguineous marriages, cause of death of direct relatives of each proband's parents, and the state of health of all living siblings. If possible, the proband's parents and siblings should be examined whenever an inherited neuromuscular disease is considered. For instance, the diagnosis of myotonic dystrophy in a newborn with severe hypotonia is strongly supported by the presence of action and/or percussion myotonia in the mother. In myotonic dystrophy, as in other selected neuromuscular diseases, reliable and confirmatory DNA studies are now available and obviate the need for further invasive studies.

THE SYMPTOMS

Pain at Rest

Acute and subacute inflammatory neuromuscular diseases (acute inflammatory polyradiculoneuropathy, acute anterior poliomyelitis, polymyositis, or dermatomyositis) may be associated with pain at rest and with muscle tenderness as well. Polymyositis is more frequently associated with muscle tenderness than with pain. Children with dermatomyositis or those with acute inflammatory demyelinating polyneuropathy (Guillain-Barré syndrome) often experience significant muscle pain or aching, are noted to be irritable or miserable, and will often refuse to move or bear weight. Painful muscle spasms can occur in acute poliomyelitis or with inflammation of an adjacent joint—e.g., an intervertebral disk space infection. Rheumatoid arthritis, generalized lupus erythematosus, periarteritis nodosa, Sjögren syndrome, and other collagen-vascular diseases and acute viral infections such as influenza are often associated with muscle pain. Viral myositis, and notably epidemic pleurodynia stemming from Coxsackie B infection, is associated with thoracic, upper abdominal, subcostal, and parasternal muscle pain. Polymyalgia rheumatica, a steroid-responsive disease in older patients, is associated with severe pain of the shoulder and the hip girdle muscles and a high sedimentation rate. Acute trichinosis is associated with muscle pain, stiffness, malaise, fever, periorbital edema, skin rash, and petechiae, but the sedimentation rate is normal.

Familial neuralgic amyotrophy with brachial predilection represents a painful, recurrent neuropathy. The onset follows heavy exercise of the upper extremities or appears spontaneously. Pain is the first symptom; unilateral or bilateral weakness of shoulder and upper arm muscles appears a few days later. The pain lasts only a few weeks, but weakness persists for months or years and is associated with atrophy. The condition has now been linked to chromosome 17q24.[3]

Diabetic femoral mononeuropathy causes pain, weakness, and atrophy of the quadriceps muscle. Mononeuropathies and polyneuropathies—and especially those associated with necrotizing vasculitis, porphyria, alcoholism, vitamin B_1 or B_{12} deficiencies, and arsenic intoxication—can cause muscle pain or sensory allodynia that often has a burning quality.

Exertional Pain

This is often the result of muscle ischemia secondary to occlusive arterial disease (intermittent claudication) but may also occur when the energy supply to muscle is restricted, as with deficits in glycolysis, or fatty acid oxidation or in AMP deaminase deficiency. In the latter entity, exercise may be followed by burning muscle pain and stiffness.

Cramps

Muscle cramps are powerful, involuntary, painful contractions lasting from seconds to minutes.[2,4] They may be either spontaneous or provoked by ischemia. When severe, they may be followed by residual muscle tenderness and elevated serum muscle enzymes.[2] They are to be differentiated from muscle contractures induced by exertion, which are also painful but last up to several hours and are electrically silent. With cramps, the electromyogram (EMG) shows high-voltage, high-frequency, irregular bursts of motor unit potentials.

Cramps can occur in normal individuals and are frequent in some children and in the elderly, even at rest. They can also occur with dehydration, uremia, hemodialysis, pregnancy, tetanus, and after exposure to phenothiazines, vincristine, cimetidine, lithium, and other substances. Cramps also occur in partially denervated muscles in motor neuron disease, in peripheral neuropathies, and in myasthenic patients overmedicated with acetylcholinesterase inhibitors. Recurrent cramps that are localized to one muscle group may indicate nerve root disease.[2]

Electrically Silent Muscle Contractures

These occur with strenuous or ischemic exercise in metabolic myopathies associated with defects of glycolysis or glycogenolysis. They are painful, last from a few minutes to more than half an hour, and lead to myoglobinuria if severe or widespread. They are considered in detail in other chapters in this book.

Another type of electrically silent contracture is associated with an exercise-induced defect of muscle relaxation. Relaxation is delayed, and the delay increases relative to the amount of exercise. The patient complains of muscle stiffness or pain. Superficially, the phenomenon resembles myotonia, but it differs in that continued exercise worsens the defect and the contracted muscles are electrically silent.[5,6] The condition is autosomal recessive and is due to mutations in the sarcoplasmic reticulum calcium ATPase encoded on chromosome 16p12.[7]

Tetany

Tetany is a sustained muscle contraction that resembles cramps but affects chiefly the distal segments of the extremities (carpopedal spasms) and the facial and laryngeal muscles. It is associated with irritability to percussion of the facial nerve (Chvostek's sign) and can occur in patients with hypocalcemia, hypomagnesemia, or alkalosis.

Stiffness

There is no precise and generally accepted definition of muscle stiffness. However, the term is often used to describe spontaneously occurring muscle contractions that may be accompanied by painful cramps. These can occur in infants with hypothyroidism and muscle hypertrophy (Hoffman's syndrome)[8] and in disorders associated with continuous muscle fiber activity, such as the "stiff-man" syndrome, Isaacs-Merten syndrome or neuromyotonia, tetanus, strychnine poisoning, the early phase of the bite of the American black widow spider, and the Schwartz-Jampel syndrome. Myotonia is often described by patients as muscle stiffness. Patients with autosomal dominant or recessive myotonia congenita complain of muscle stiffness that is worsened by cold, is most prominent at the onset of movement, and is reduced with activity. Patients with paramyotonia congenita often note worsening of their stiffness with exertion (paradoxical myotonia).[2]

The Clinical Examination

It is best to follow a predetermined sequence so that the entire examination is consistently performed. A practical format includes inspection, palpation of muscles and nerves, manual muscle testing, passive motion of joints, percussion of muscles and tendons, and sensory testing. In young children, a more flexible approach to the examination is often required.

SIMPLE INSPECTION AT REST

One can readily observe muscle wasting or enlargement, spontaneous muscle activity in the form of fasciculations or myokymia, or tremulousness of the fingers and hands. One can also note palpebral ptosis; strabismus; the expressionless face of facial diplegia; the myasthenic snarl; the drooping jaw or drooling caused by weak masticatory muscles; atrophy of the cranial, cervical, torso, and limb muscles; the high-arched palate; tongue fasciculations; weakness of the soft palate on phonation; the shape and size of the chest wall; and scoliosis, kyphosis, or exaggerated lumbar lordosis. The patient must be partially disrobed to allow proper inspection. Hospital gowns are often impractical for this purpose, especially in children, and many patients are uncomfortable being examined in underclothes. For this reason, it is most helpful to tell all patients visiting the neuromuscular clinic to bring a pair of shorts and a sleeveless shirt to the clinic appointment. The patient will then be more comfortable during examination of the limb muscles and during assessment of gait (often performed in the hallway). The shirt can be briefly removed for inspection of the spine and torso muscles.

It is also important to inspect the patient for the presence of dysmorphic features, which might suggest a genetically distinct syndrome associated with hypotonia (such as the Prader-Willi or Beckwith-Wiedemann syndromes) or a congenital muscular dystrophy associated with central nervous system (CNS) involvement. The spine should be inspected for the presence of a sacral dimple. Examination of the skin may reveal the heliotrope rash, Gottron's papules, dystrophic calcification of dermatomyositis, or ulcers and distal limb hair loss seen in chronic diabetic neuropathy. Signs of endocrinopathy, such as frontal balding and testicular atrophy (myotonic dystrophy) or gynecomastia (Kennedy disease) should also be noted.

WEAKNESS AND ATROPHY

Weakness of axial muscles can sometimes be detected by simple inspection. For instance, a newborn infant with weak neck extensor muscles is unable to lift its head when in the prone decubitus position or, if held horizontally and face down, resting on the examiner's hands, is unable to lift its head sufficiently to maintain the cephalic and truncal axes in line. Infants with significant truncal weakness will assume a C-shaped posture when placed in the seated position. In older children and adults, inability to sit up from the supine position or to rise from squatting or sitting indicates weakness of the torso and pelvic girdle muscles, respectively. Weak serratus anterior muscles cause displacement of the scapulas from the trunk, resulting in a wing-like appearance. Weakness of the chest wall muscles results in a bell-shaped thorax and recruitment of accessory muscles of respiration.

As infants have sparse subcutaneous fat in the cervical region, muscle atrophy in this distribution is readily detected. Wasting of periscapular muscle displays the scapular contours. Displacement of the scapula and humerus is common in patients with severe shoulder girdle weakness and atrophy. Deltoid atrophy displays the bony prominences of the scapulohumeral joint. Greater weakness of the lateral than the medial humeral rotators results in internal rotation of the entire upper limb, so that in the standing position the limb dangles with the palm facing backward.

Wasting of arm muscles is easier to recognize during contraction. The patient extends the elbow for demonstrating the triceps and semiflexes at the elbow and supinates the forearm for the biceps. Similarly, flexion-extension of the wrist and pronation-supination of the forearm reveal atrophy of the forearm muscles. Atrophy of the intrinsic hand muscle causes deep grooves between the metacarpal bones. On the dorsum of the hand, this is best seen with the fingers hyperextended and abducted. In the supinated hand, the hypothenar and thenar eminences become flattened. With paralysis of the opponens pollicis, the thumb becomes rotated so that it faces in the same direction as the remaining fingers. This is known as the "simian hand." Selective paralysis of intrinsic hand muscles including the lumbricals with relative sparing of long finger flexors and extensors results in flexed interphalangeal and extended metacarpophalangeal joints, giving a characteristic "claw hand."

Weakness of the paraspinal muscles results in lumbar lordosis, thoracic kyphosis, and scoliosis. Weakness of the hip extensors may cause a "compensatory" lumbar lordosis and a protuberant abdomen.

Atrophy of the gluteal muscles causes flattening of the buttocks and horizontal wrinkling of the overlying skin. Atrophy of the quadriceps muscles produces flattening or depression of the anterior thigh. The medial thigh becomes concave when the hip adductors are wasted. With atrophy of the anterior tibial and peroneal muscles, the anterior edge of the tibia becomes a prominent sharp ridge ("saber's edge"). Atrophy of the lower leg muscles and preservation of the femoral muscles give the extremity the appearance of an "inverted bottle of champagne." With atrophy of the extensor digitorum brevis, its belly does not appear when the patient dorsiflexes the ankle and toes and medially rotates the foot.

Fasciculations

In adults, fasciculating shoulder and thigh muscles are readily observed with oblique illumination. Fasciculations in infants are concealed by subcutaneous fat; but in chronic spinal muscular atrophy, the fasciculations of the chest wall are occasionally seen. Fasciculations of the tongue are seen in approximately 30 to 50 percent of infants with SMA type I. True tongue fasciculations are noted when the infant is calm and the tongue is resting within the mouth. Fasciculation-like movements of the tongue can be seen in healthy infants when crying. Fasciculations are normal if observed in incompletely relaxed muscle, particularly in the calves.[2] A rapid low-amplitude tremor of the fingers and hand is a characteristic of the later-onset forms of SMA. This is related to asynchronous contractions of relatively few and large motor units and does not indicate fasciculations. Fasciculations are further considered below, under "The Clinical Features."

Hypertrophy

Increased muscle bulk of a clinically strong muscle is termed *hypertrophy*. This is a common feature of healthy, athletic individuals but is also seen in patients with myotonia congenita. *Pseudohypertrophy* refers to the enlargement of a clinically weak muscle and is a common finding in the calf muscles of boys with the Duchenne and Becker types of muscular dystrophy, in dystrophies caused by mutations in caveolin-3 or calpain, in some patients with SMA type III, and in the childhood form of acid maltase deficiency.

INSPECTION OF GAIT

Gait disturbances require keen observation. Ambulation is accomplished by the hip extensors and plantarflexors, with the sole pushing against the ground, generating friction between the sole and the ground. Simultaneously, the opposite limb swings forward. The principal ambulatory muscles are the iliopsoas, hip adductors, gluteus maximus, gluteus medius, hamstrings, quadriceps, tibialis anterior, peroneals, gastrocnemius, and soleus. An abnormal gait will result from weakness of any of these muscles or from structural abnormalities of articular surfaces, joint capsules, or ligaments. A normal gait also requires coordination of the gait cycle by the CNS, which stimulates or inhibits flexors, extensors, adductors, and abductors for counteracting gravity.

In general, gait abnormalities result from (1) pain, (2) muscle weakness, (3) reduced range of joint motion, (4) weakness of upper or lower motor neuron origin, (5) spasticity, (6) dystonia, (7) rigidity, (8) ataxia, and, rarely, (9) somatoform disorder (hysteria).

The gait is observed from each side as well as from the front and back, with the patient appropriately disrobed as discussed earlier. The ambulating space should be ample. There are four gait phases for each extremity: heel strike, midstance, pushoff, and midswing. The examiner should notice the cadence, symmetry, and length of strides; trunk lurches; changes in pelvic tilt; base width; and duration of phases. The base width is the distance between the heels at midstance of one leg and midswing of the other.[9] The normal range is between 10 and 20 cm. Vertical foot clearance during midswing should be viewed from the side or the front. Exaggerated pelvic tilts are called *fixed* when they do not change in any gait phases. Lurching of the trunk is best seen from the side. This can be caused by fixed kyphosis or lordosis or by anterior or posterior pelvic rotations.[9]

Young children unable to complain may refuse to walk altogether when they suffer from limb or back pain. This occurs, for instance, with intravertebral disk space infection, epidural abscess, osteomyelitis, benign long-bone tumors irritating the femoral periosteum (osteoid osteoma) or pelvis, or infiltrating tumors of the lumbosacral spinal cord or cauda equina. If the child is compelled to walk, he or she fixes the lumbosacral spine and pelvis to prevent pain while ambulating. When standing on one limb causes pain, the ipsilateral stance phase and the contralateral swing phase are shortened and the heel strike may be absent.[9]

Spasticity of the hip adductors, knee extensors, and plantarflexors produces a characteristic scissoring gait. Sensory gait ataxia, resulting from impairment of position sense, causes a broad-based gait and requires the patient to use visual assistance to compensate for the proprioceptive loss. An asymmetrical paralytic gait caused by weakness of one lower limb was frequently seen when acute anterior poliomyelitis was prevalent. Different types of limp, slow locomotion, and flapping of one foot on the floor are still seen in older patients with weakness caused by poliomyelitis.

Weakness of hip muscles—particularly of the iliopsoas, abductors, and adductors—produces a characteristic gait abnormality. As one leg advances and the heel strikes the floor, the weak abductor muscles cannot prevent the pelvis from tilting more deeply to the opposite side than the normal 5 degrees and the torso lurches laterally as the foot contacts the floor. With bilateral pelvic abductor weakness, the torso lurches laterally from one side to the other, with each leg swing causing a characteristic waddle, as seen in patients with Duchenne dystrophy or any myopathy with significant proximal weakness. With minimal abductor weakness, the torso may not lurch, but there is an excessive pelvic tilt toward the swinging leg ("waddling gait").[9]

With severe weakness of the hip and back extensor muscles, the patient develops a compensatory lumbar lordosis. The upper trunk and shoulders become hyperextended to displace the center of gravity posteriorly. This way, the line of gravity falls on the base formed by the feet, and this prevents falling forward. The gait is now markedly lordotic. With each step there is hyperextension of the trunk, so that the shoulders are thrown backward and the trunk lurches toward the advancing leg. This is the characteristic gait of a youngster with advanced Duchenne dystrophy.

Unilateral weakness of the hip flexor muscles causes lurching of the trunk backward and toward the sound side and reduces the acceleration of the swing phase and the stride length of the affected side.

With paralysis of the hip extensors, a backward trunk lurch appears when the heel strikes at the end of the swing phase, locking the hip in extension to maintain the line of gravity behind the hip axis.[9]

Weakness of the knee extensors may not be recognized during observation of the gait. Normally, as the lower limb advances, the quadriceps relaxes; but when the quadriceps is weak, it paradoxically contracts and the knee flexes slightly when the heel strikes. Paralysis of the quadriceps may be compensated by the gluteus maximus, which pulls on the iliotibial band as the plantarflexors contract to stabilize the knee in extension during stance. Absent quadriceps action produces excessive knee flexion and heel evaluation during the swing phase.[9]

Weakness of the knee flexors causes increased knee extension at the end of the swing phase, with an overshoot of the advancing leg and a hard heel strike. During stance, the knee remains in exaggerated extension (genu recurvatum).[9]

Weakness of the ankle dorsiflexors produces excessive plantarflexion during the swing phase, requiring excessive hip and knee flexion for the foot to clear the floor and causing "foot drop." The patient with proprioceptive loss of the lower limbs who is not looking clears the floor by raising each foot excessively without knowing where it is, and the height to which either foot is raised varies from step to step.

Weakness of the plantarflexors of the foot prevents the propulsion at the end of the stance phase before the leg is advanced. This is partly compensated by knee extension and hip flexion to get the foot off the floor.[9] When the foot dorsiflexors are weak but the peronei and the posterior tibial muscles are relatively strong, as can occur in Duchenne dystrophy, the foot assumes the equinovarus position. The reverse happens when the weakness predominantly involves the posterior tibial muscle: The foot is everted in a valgus position. Early recognition of these foot positions allows for proper physiotherapy and bracing, which may prevent fixed joint deformities.

TESTING OF THE CRANIAL MUSCLES

Extraocular Muscles

Isolated or combined extraocular muscle palsies are common in myasthenia gravis, congenital myasthenic syndromes, botulism and other intoxications, some myopathies, and diseases of the lower motor neuron. Particular attention should be given to diplopia, as it may be the presenting symptom of myasthenia gravis or botulism.

The examiner should note head tilt or rotation, eyelid ptosis, hyperactive frontalis muscle to compensate for the ptosis, eyelid retraction, and the position of the globes relative to each other. Each eye should be observed as it moves fully toward all six cardinal positions of gaze. Infranuclear disorders of eye movements dissociate the conjugate action of the so-called yoke muscles—lateral rectus and contralateral medial rectus, superior rectus and contralateral inferior oblique, inferior rectus and contralateral superior oblique. In a primary position and with the healthy eye fixating, the weak eye deviates opposite to the direction of action of the paralytic muscle because of the unopposed action of the antagonist muscle. During the cover test, the paretic eye is fixating and the healthy eye undergoes secondary deviation in the direction of action of the contralateral paralytic muscle.

Tests for diplopia can be performed with the Maddox rod or the Lancaster red-green projection test. Both tests allow the examiner (usually an ophthalmologist) to distinguish the degree of deviation of the affected eye.

Fluctuating palpebral ptosis and/or ophthalmoplegia are often signs of myasthenia gravis. They can be further investigated with the edrophonium test, which is described below.

Palatal Muscles

The tensor veli palatini is innervated by the trigeminal nerve. Its action is to tense the soft palate. Weakness of this muscle results in a flaccid soft palate. If this flaccidity is unilateral, the affected side sinks below the level of the other side. The levator veli palatini, or palatal levator, is innervated by the cranial nerves IX, X, and XI by way of the pharyngeal plexus. The two levators elevate the palate symmetrically during phonation or gagging.

Pharyngeal Muscles

The superior, middle, and inferior constrictors are innervated by the pharyngeal plexus, and their function is to sequentially constrict the nasopharynx, oropharynx, and hypopharynx by acting as a sphincter. Direct examination of their action is not possible. Fluoroscopic or radiocinematographic examinations can be performed, but these are seldom needed for the diagnosis of neuromuscular diseases. Selectively severe involvement of the pharyngeal muscles is noted in oculopharyngeal muscular dystrophy. In these patients cricopharyngeal myotomy (surgical release of the pharyngeal constrictors) facilitates nutrition and greatly improves quality of life.[10]

Laryngeal Muscles

The many small laryngeal muscles receive their innervation directly from cranial nerve X or through the cranial accessory branch of cranial nerve XI. Some close the inlet of the larynx (aryepiglottic and thyroepiglottic), while others shorten, adduct, or elongate the vocal cords or widen the glottis.

Tongue Muscles

All intrinsic and extrinsic tongue muscles are innervated by cranial nerve XII except the palatoglossus, which is supplied by the pharyngeal plexus (cranial nerves IX, X, and XI). The tongue muscles induce lateral and vertical movements or protrude, retract, shorten, lengthen and narrow, or flatten and broaden the tongue or raise and lower its tip. Atrophy and fasciculations of the tongue occur in patients with bulbar lesions affecting the motor nucleus or intra- and extracranial course of the cranial nerve XII. For facial and mandibular muscles, see Table 25-1.

MANUAL MUSCLE TESTING

Several publications detail this part of the examination.[11–14] Even when the strength is graded as normal, there is a great variation from person to person and according to age. In cooperative patients, an experienced examiner can detect minor degrees of weakness. The muscle grading systems quantitate muscle strength subjectively. The grading of the British Medical Research Council is as follows: 0, no contraction; 1, flicker or trace of contraction; 2, active movement

Table 25-1. INNERVATION AND TESTING OF MUSCLES

Location of Motor Nucleus	Nerve Supply	Muscle Tested	Action Requested of Patient; Examiner's Action
Pons	V	*Mandibular*	
		Masseter, temporal and medial pterygoid[a]	Clench teeth
		Medial and lateral pterygoids[a]	Protrude lower jaw
		Lateral pterygoid	Move lower jaw sideways
Pons	VII	*Facial*	
		Frontalis[a]	Raise eyebrows; lower eyebrows
		Corrugator	Frown
		Orbicularis oculi[a]	Close eyes tightly; spread eyelids open
		Procerus	Pull up skin of nose
		Levator angularis	Draw angle of mouth toward cheek
		Zygomatic	Draw angles of mouth up and out in forced smile
		Orbicularis oris[a]	Protrude closed lips as in whistling
		Buccinator	Press cheeks inward as to blow
		Mentalis	Evert lower lip as in pouting
		Depressor angularis	Draw down angles of mouth
		Depressor labiae inferioris and platysma	Draw angles of mouth downward and pull up skin of neck
Medulla	IX, X, XI	See "Tongue Muscles"	(Palate, pharynx, larynx, tongue)
		Cervical	
C1–3	Cervical	Infrahyoid	Draw chin in and downward
C1–8		Neck flexors[a]	Flex head; rostrodorsal pressure on forehead
C1–8		Neck extensors[a]	Extend head; forward pressure
C2	Spinal accessory	Sternocleidomastoid[a]:	
		Sternal head	Rotate head in opposite direction to muscle tested; resist rotation
		Lateral head	Lateral flexion of head toward muscle tested; resist lateral flexion
		Upper extremity	
C3,4	Spinal accessory	Trapezius (Fig. 25-1)[a]	
		Upper	Shrug shoulder; press shoulder caudally and head away from shoulder
		Middle	Brace shoulder backward and adduct scapula
		Lower	Abduct arm fully and pronate forearm; press on forearm caudally to lower arm
C3–5	Dorsal scapular	Levator scapulae	With elbow flexed, adduct and retract upper arm; force elbow laterally and forward Rhomboids hold scapula in adduction
C4–5	Dorsal scapular	Rhomboids[a]	
C5–8	Long thoracic	Serratus anterior[a]	Thrust outstretched upper limb forward against wall. In paralysis there is winging and medial shift of the scapula
		Lateral shoulder rotators (Fig. 25-2)[a]	
C5,6	Suprascapular	Infraspinatus	Rotate arm laterally, elbow flexed 90°; while placing one hand on
C5,6	Axillary	Teres minor	

[a]Muscles that are commonly examined.

Table 25-1 (Continued). INNERVATION AND TESTING OF MUSCLES

Location of Motor Nucleus	Nerve Supply	Muscle Tested	Action Requested of Patient; Examiner's Action
C5,6	Axillary	Posterior deltoid	medial side of elbow, press on forearm medially toward chest
		Medial shoulder rotators[a]	
C5–7	Lower subscapular	Teres major	Extend and adduct upper arm with dorsum of wrist resting on iliac crest; press against elbow to abduct and flex humerus
C5–7	Upper subscapular	Subscapularis	
C6–8	Thoracodorsal	Latissimus dorsi[a]	With arm in adduction, rotate medially and extend; press against forearm to abduct and flex humerus
		Pectoralis major	With elbow extended, flex arm 90° and slightly rotate medially; press against forearm to abduct humerus horizontally
C5–7	Lateral pectoral	Clavicular head[a]	
C5–8, T1	Lateral and medial pectorals	Sternocostal	Start as for clavicular and try to adduct arm obliquely toward opposite iliac crest; press in a lateral and cephalad direction
C5,6	Subclavian	Supraspinatus (Fig. 25-3)[a]	Abduct arm from full adducted position; press against forearm
C5,6	Axillary	Deltoid[a] (lateral portion)	Abduct arm to horizontal in neutral rotation with elbow flexed; press to adduct humerus
C5,6	Musculocutaneous	Biceps[a]	Flex elbow 100° and supinate forearm; pull forearm to extend elbow
C5,6	Musculocutaneous	Brachialis[a]	
C6–8, T1	Radial	Triceps[a]	Extend elbow from a 90° angle; resistance against forearm to prevent extension
C7,8	Radial	Anconeus[a]	
C5,6	Radial	Brachioradialis[a]	Flex elbow, semipronate forearm; pull forearm to extend elbow
		Wrist extensors[a]	
C5–8	Radial	Extensor carpi radialis longus	Extend wrist; press on dorsum of hand to flex it
			Pronate forearm, extend wrist toward radial side with fingers flexed
C5–8	Radial	Extensor carpi radialis brevis	Press on 2nd metacarpal area to flex hand toward ulnar side
C6–8	Radial	Extensor carpi ulnaris	Extend wrist toward ulnar side; press on 5th metacarpal to flex wrist toward radial side
C5,6	Radial	Supinator	With elbow fully extended and supinated, force forearm to a pronated position
C6–8	Radial	Extensor digitorum[a]	Extend proximal phalanges of fingers with other phalanges relaxed; press on dorsum of proximal phalanges
C6–8	Radial	Abductor pollicis longus	With hand semipronated, thumb radially abducted, press against lateral surface of distal end of 1st metacarpal
C6–8	Radial	Extensor pollicis brevis	With hand semipronated, proximal thumb phalanx extended, press against dorsal surface of proximal phalanx to flex it
C6–8	Radial	Extensor pollicis longus	With hand semipronated, distal thumb phalanx extended, press against dorsal surface of distal phalanx to flex it

[a] Muscles that are commonly examined.

(Continued)

Table 25-1 *(Continued).* INNERVATION AND TESTING OF MUSCLES

Location of Motor Nucleus	Nerve Supply	Muscle Tested	Action Requested of Patient; Examiner's Action
C6–8	Radial	Extensor indicis	Extend index finger; press on proximal phalanx
C6–8	Radial	Extensor digiti minimi	Extend little finger; press on proximal phalanx
C6,7	Median	Pronator teres (Fig. 25-4)	Pronate forearm with elbow flexed 70°; press on forearm above wrist to supinate it
		Wrist flexors (Fig. 25-5)[a]	
C6–8	Median	Flexor carpi radialis (See below for *Flexor carpi ulnaris*)	Flex wrist; press against palm to extend it Flex wrist toward radial side; press against thenar eminence to extend it in ulnar direction
C7,8, T1	Median	Palmaris longus	Flex wrist and cup hand with forearm resting on table; press against thenar and hypothenar eminences to flatten hand
C7,8, T1	Median	Flexor digitorum sublimis[a]	Flex proximal interphalangeal joint with distal IP joint extended; press palmar surface of middle phalanges to extend them
C7,8, T1	Median	Flexor digitorum profundus 1 and 2[a]	Flex distal interphalangeal joints of all fingers; press against palmar surface of distal phalanges to extend them
C7,8, T1	Median	Flexor pollicis longus	Flex distal phalanx of thumb; press against palmar surface of distal phalanx to extend it
C7,8, T1	Median	Pronator quadratus	Pronate forearm with elbow fully flexed; pressure on forearm above wrist
C6–8, T1	Median	Abductor pollicis brevis[a]	Abduct thumb perpendicularly to palm and away from it; press against proximal phalanx toward palm
C6–8, T1	Median	Flexor pollicis brevis (superficial head)	Flex proximal phalanx of thumb; press against palmar surface of proximal phalanx to extend it
C6–8, T1	Median	Opponens pollicis[a]	Oppose thumb; press on thenar eminence to place thumb in a neutral position
C8, T1	Median	Lumbricals 1 and 2	Extend interphalangeal joints and simultaneously flex metacarpophalangeal joints; (a) press against dorsal surface of middle and distal phalanges of 1 and 2, or (b) press against palmar surface of proximal phalanges 1 and 2 (the two fingers are tested individually)
C8, T1	Ulnar	Flexor carpi ulnaris (Fig. 25-5)	See *Flexor carpi radialis*, above. Flex wrist toward ulnar side; press against hypothenar eminence to extend wrist toward radial side
C8, T1	Ulnar	Flexor digitorum profundus 3 and 4[a]	See *Flexor digitorum profundus 1 and 2*, above
C8, T1	Ulnar	Abductor digiti quinti[a]	Abduct little finger; press against ulnar side of little finger to abduct it

[a] Muscles that are commonly examined.

Table 25-1 (Continued). INNERVATION AND TESTING OF MUSCLES

Location of Motor Nucleus	Nerve Supply	Muscle Tested	Action Requested of Patient; Examiner's Action
C8, T1	Ulnar	Flexor digiti quinti	Flex proximal phalanx of little finger; press against palmar surface of first phalanx to extend it
C8, T1	Ulnar	Opponens digiti quinti	Oppose little finger toward thumb; press on palmar surface of 5th metacarpal to flatten hand
C8, T1	Ulnar	Adductor pollicis[a]	Adduct thumb toward palm; press against medial side of thumb to abduct it
C8, T1	Ulnar	Flexor pollicis brevis (deep head)	See *Flexor pollicis brevis* (superficial head), above
C8, T1	Ulnar	Lumbricals 3 and 4	See *Lumbricals* 1 and 2, above
C8, T1	Ulnar	Dorsal interossei[a]: 1 or 2	Abduct index or middle finger toward radial side
		3 or 4	Abduct middle or fourth finger toward ulnar side; for each muscle, press in opposite direction to adduct finger
C8, T1	Ulnar	Palmar interossei[a]	Adduct thumb and fingers toward axis of hand; press to abduct individually, thumb, index, third or fourth fingers
		Trunk muscles	
T1, S3		Trunk extensors	Intrinsic extensors are assisted by trapezius, neck extensors, latissimus dorsi, and quadratus lumborum. To test the trunk extensors, the hip extensors must fixate the pelvis. As the examiner stabilizes the lower extremities of the patient in prone decubitus and with hands clasped behind buttocks, the patient lifts upper trunk from table
L1–4	Lumbar plexus	Quadratus lumborum	To test this hip extensor, the patient is placed in prone decubitus. The lower extremity is slightly abducted and extended. Pressure in ventral and caudal direction is applied against the iliac crest if hip muscles are weak; otherwise, the lower extremity is pulled by the ankle in a direction away from the muscle
		Trunk flexors	The anterior abdominal muscles are tested with the patient in supine position and flexing the neck against resistance applied to the forehead. Also, with hands on occiput, the patient flexes successively trunk and then pelvis by action of hip flexors. The examiner must fixate the patient's legs on the table

[a]Muscles that are commonly examined.

(Continued)

Table 25-1 *(Continued).* INNERVATION AND TESTING OF MUSCLES

Location of Motor Nucleus	Nerve Supply	Muscle Tested	Action Requested of Patient; Examiner's Action
		Lower extremity	
		Thigh flexors[a]:	
L1–4	Lumbar plexus	Psoas (Fig. 25-6)	Sitting with knees flexed, flex thigh; press against thigh to extend it
L2–4	Femoral	Iliacus	
L2,3	Femoral	Sartorius	Supine with thigh flexed, abduct and rotate laterally; press against anterolateral surface of thigh to extend, adduct, and medially rotate it
L2–4	Femoral	Quadriceps femoris[a]	Sitting with knees flexed, extend lower leg; press against leg above ankle to flex it
L2–4	Obturator	Adductors[a]	Supine with knee extended, adduct leg; apply resistance against medial surface of thigh to abduct it
L4,5, S1	Superior gluteus	Gluteus medius (Fig. 25-7)[a]	In lateral decubitus, abduct lower limb; press against region of lateral malleolus to adduct and slightly flex the limb
L4,5, S1	Superior gluteus	Tensor fascia lata	Supine with knee extended, slightly flex and medially rotate abducted limb; press to abduct and extend limb
L5, S1,2	Inferior gluteus	Gluteus maximus (Fig. 25-8)[a]	Prone flex knee and extend thigh; press against lower dorsal aspect of thigh to flex it
L4,5, S1	Superior gluteus	Medial rotators of hip[a] (tensor fascia lata, gluteus minimus, and gluteus medius)	Sitting with knees flexed, rotate thigh medially; fixing knee with hand medially, press above lateral malleolus inward to rotate thigh laterally
		Lateral rotators of hips[a] (gluteus medius obturators, piriformis, gemelli, quadratus femoris, and gluteus maximus)	Sitting with knees flexed, rotate thigh laterally; fixing knee with hand laterally press above medial malleolus outward to rotate thigh medially
L4,5, S1,2	Sciatic	Hamstrings (Fig. 25-9)[a]	Prone, flex knee 45°; press on leg proximal to ankle to extend knee
L4,5, S1	Deep peroneal	Tibialis anterior[a]	Sitting with knees flexed, dorsiflex and invert foot; press on medial side of dorsal foot's surface to plantar flex and evert foot
		Toe extensors[a]:	Extend all joints of four last toes; press on dorsal surface of toes to flex them
L4,5, S1	Deep peroneal	Extensor digitorum longus	
L4,5, S1	Deep peroneal	Extensor digitorum brevis	
L4,5, S1	Deep peroneal	Extensor hallucis longus	Extend metatarsophalangeal joint of great toe; press on dorsal surface of great toe to flex it
		Foot evertors[a]:	Plantarflex and evert foot; press against lateral border of foot to invert it
L4,5, S1	Superficial peroneal	Peroneus longus	
L4,5, S1	Superficial peroneal	Peroneus brevis	
S1,2	Tibial	Gastrocnemius, soleus and other plantar flexors	With knee extended, plantarflex foot; press against plantar surface of forefoot to dorsiflex it
L5, S1	Tibial	Tibialis posterior	Plantarflex and invert foot; press against medial border of foot to evert it and slightly dorsiflex it

[a] Muscles that are commonly examined.

Table 25-1 (Continued). INNERVATION AND TESTING OF MUSCLES

Location of Motor Nucleus	Nerve Supply	Muscle Tested	Action Requested of Patient; Examiner's Action
L5, S1,2	Tibial	Flexor hallucis longus	Flex distal phalanx of great toe; press against plantar surface of distal phalanx to extend it
		Toe flexors:	
L5, S1	Tibial	Flexor digitorum longus	Flex distal phalanx of last four toes; press against plantar surface of distal phalanx to extend them
S1,2	Lat. plantar	Quadratus plantar	
L4,5, S1	Medial plantar	Flexor digitorum brevis	
			Flex middle phalanx of last four toes; press against plantar surface of middle phalanx to extend them
L4,5, S1	Medial plantar	Flexor hallucis brevis	Flex proximal phalanx of big toe; press against plantar surface of proximal phalanx to extend it
L4,5, S1	Medial plantar	Abductor hallucis	Abduct big toe; press against medial side of big toe to adduct it
		Perineal	
S3,4	Pudendal	Rectal sphincter[a]	Squeeze with sphincter; introduce finger in rectum to feel strength of contraction as well as muscle tone during relaxation

[a] Muscles that are commonly examined.

with gravity eliminated; 3, active movement against gravity; 4, active movement against gravity and resistance; 5, normal power. At the Mayo Clinic, the symbols have a different connotation: 0, normal; 0 to −1, questionable weakness; −1, slight weakness; −2, moderate weakness; −3, severe weakness, which can be further graded as +g or −g, indicating ability or failure to move the extremity through full range against gravity alone; and −4, complete paralysis.

To facilitate manual muscle testing, it is convenient to follow a certain order, either by regions or according to muscle innervation, as it is done for the cranial nerves, or according to the sequence of the positions the patient is asked to assume during the examination (standing, sitting, supine, or prone decubitus). Certain key muscles that are involved early and more severely in some diseases should always be examined.

Muscle strength testing in infants depends chiefly on observation of spontaneous movements and adopted postures. In response to tactile stimulation of the feet, a weak infant will be unable to flex the hips to withdraw the legs toward the abdomen and will demonstrate a paucity of limb movements against gravity. The strength of the hand grip can be evaluated by placing the examiner's hand in the infant's palm, while upper limb strength can be evaluated by the degree of flexion and resistance of the infant's biceps muscles when the child is pulled forward into the seated position. Failure of the infant to flex the neck forward during this maneuver implies weakness of the neck flexors, but this can also be seen in neurologically impaired children with increased neck extensor tone.

Muscle strength testing in the young or cognitively impaired child requires ingenuity, patience, and careful observation. Observing the child at play, preferably wearing a diaper only, may yield more information than formal examination. Placing the child on a blanket on the floor with toys allows assessment of the child's ability to sit, to crawl, to grip objects, and, if a chair is placed nearby, to pull itself up to stand. Watching the child jump, run, and climb onto the examination table (or parent's lap if the child is apprehensive) reveals a great deal about proximal muscle strength. Individual muscle testing can be reliably performed in a cooperative child as early as 3 years of age if the examination has a game-like quality. Examples of phrases useful in manual muscle examination are provided in Table 25-2.

Table 25-1 lists the muscles that can be tested, their innervation, and actions by patient and examiner during the test. Asterisks in the table indicate the muscles commonly examined. Other muscles are tested in selected patients. The actions of some muscles are best understood by inspection of Figs. 25-1 through 25-9. It is important to remember that the muscle to be tested must be optimally positioned and that the force produced by the examiner must be exerted gradually.

PALPATION OF MUSCLES AND NERVES

Weak and hypotonic muscles are usually soft to palpation. This is always the case in diseases affecting primarily the anterior horn cell. The muscles in Becker and Duchenne muscular dystrophy, particularly the enlarged gastrocne-

Table 25-2. PHRASES FOR MANUAL MUSCLE STRENGTH TESTING OF SELECTED MUSCLES IN THE YOUNG CHILD

Muscle Tested	Phrase
Deltoid	"Hold your arms up like chicken wings."
Biceps	Place the child's arm at 90° and then ask him or her to "Bring your thumb to your shoulder."
Triceps	Place the child's arm at 90° and then ask the child to "Reach toward my (the examiner's) shoulder."
Wrist extensors	Extend the child's wrist and ask him or her to "Hold your hands up like a stop sign."
Wrist flexors	Flex the child's wrist and say "Your stop sign fell down; don't let me pull it back up."
Interossei	"Open your fingers wide, like a large spider."
Flexor digitorum	"Make your hand look like a squished spider."
Opponens	Have the child make a circle with the thumb opposed across to the fifth digit and say "Make a circle and don't let me pull it apart."
Iliopsoas	Have the child sit on the parent's lap and say "Lift your knee toward your nose."
Quadriceps	Have the child straighten his or her leg until it is almost but not completely extended. "Now try to make your leg straight, like a board."
Hamstrings	"Keep your leg bent and don't let me pull it out."
Tibialis anterior	"Lift your foot up like a stop sign."
Gastrocnemius/soleus	"Step on the gas pedal."

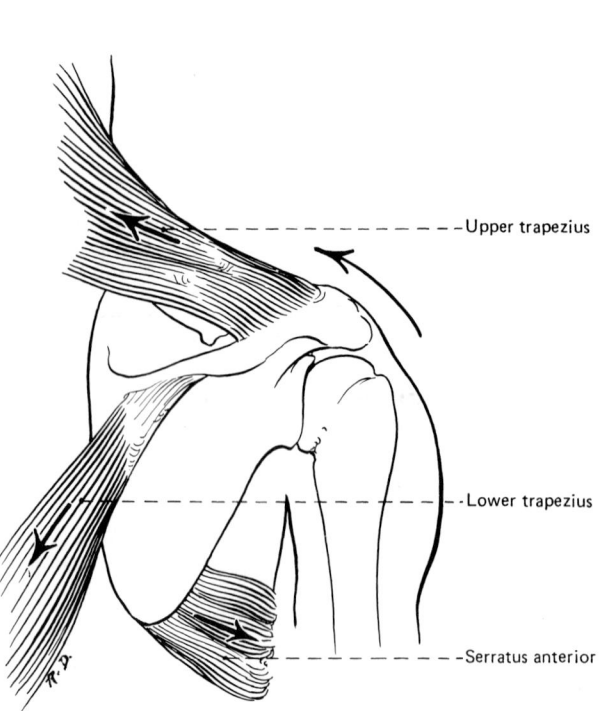

FIGURE 25-1. Upper and lower trapezius and serratus anterior, upward rotators of the scapula. (Redrawn, with permission, from Hollinshead WH: Textbook of Anatomy, 3rd ed. Hagerstown, MD: Harper & Row, 1974.)

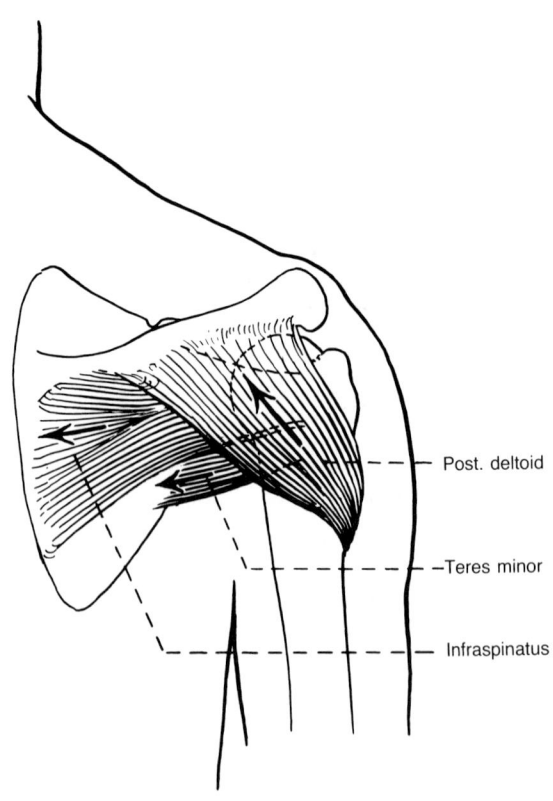

FIGURE 25-2. The external rotators of the humerus. (Redrawn, with permission, from Hollinshead WH: Textbook of Anatomy, 3rd ed. Hagerstown, MD: Harper & Row, 1974.)

Chapter 25. The Clinical Examination

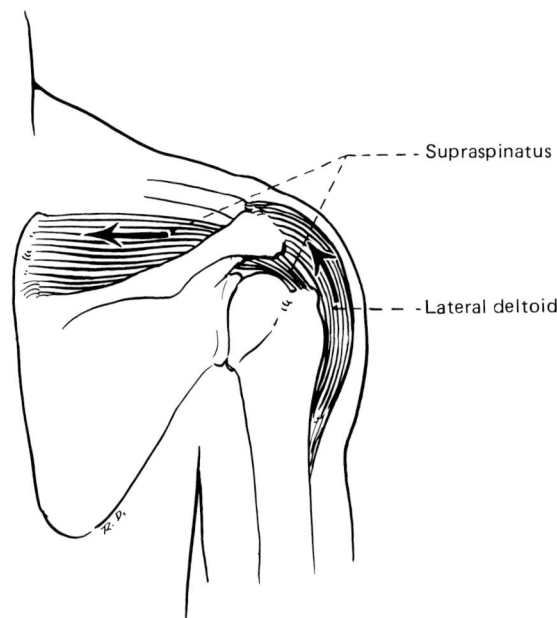

FIGURE 25-3. Abductors of the humerus. *(Redrawn, with permission, from Hollinshead WH: Textbook of Anatomy, 3rd ed. Hagerstown, MD: Harper & Row, 1974.)*

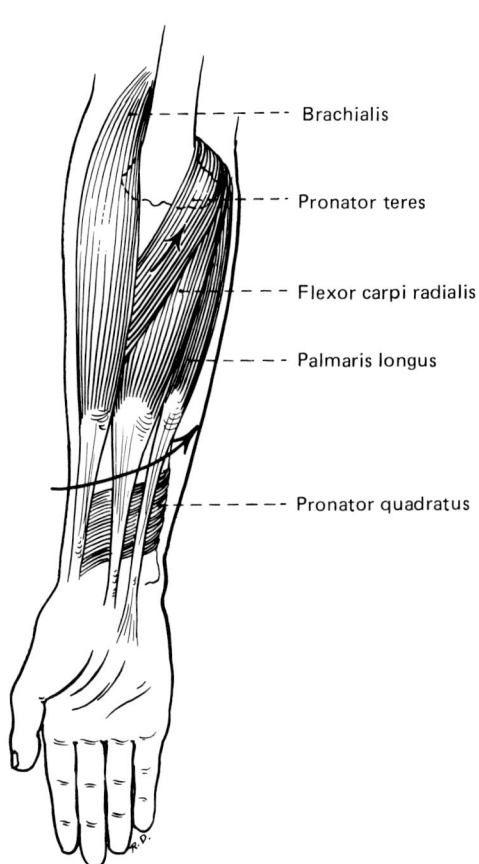

FIGURE 25-4. Pronators of the forearm. *(Redrawn, with permission, from Hollinshead WH: Textbook of Anatomy, 3rd ed. Hagerstown, MD: Harper & Row, 1974.)*

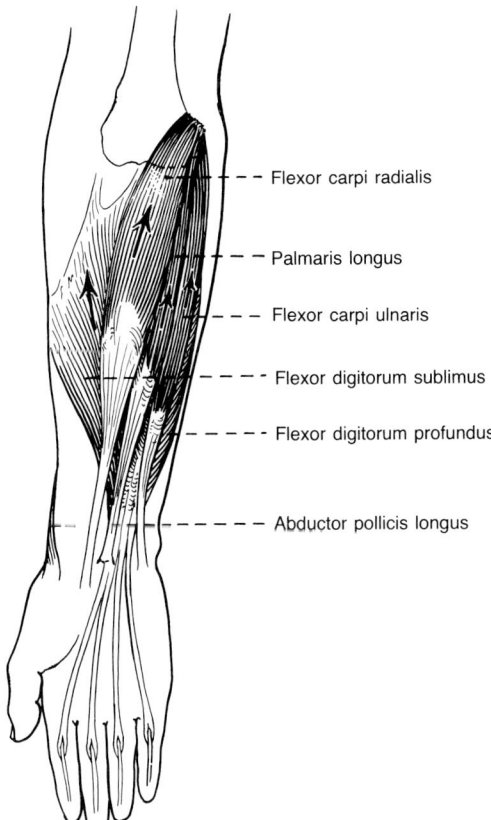

FIGURE 25-5. The flexors of the wrist. *(Redrawn, with permission, from Hollinshead WH: Textbook of Anatomy, 3rd ed. Hagerstown, MD: Harper & Row, 1974.*

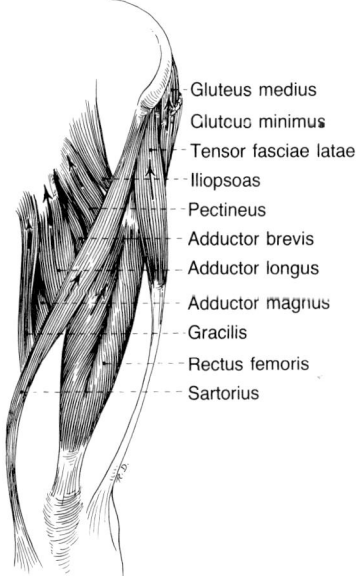

FIGURE 25-6. Flexors of the thigh. *(Redrawn, with permission, from Hollinshead WH: Textbook of Anatomy, 3rd ed. Hagerstown, MD: Harper & Row, 1974.*

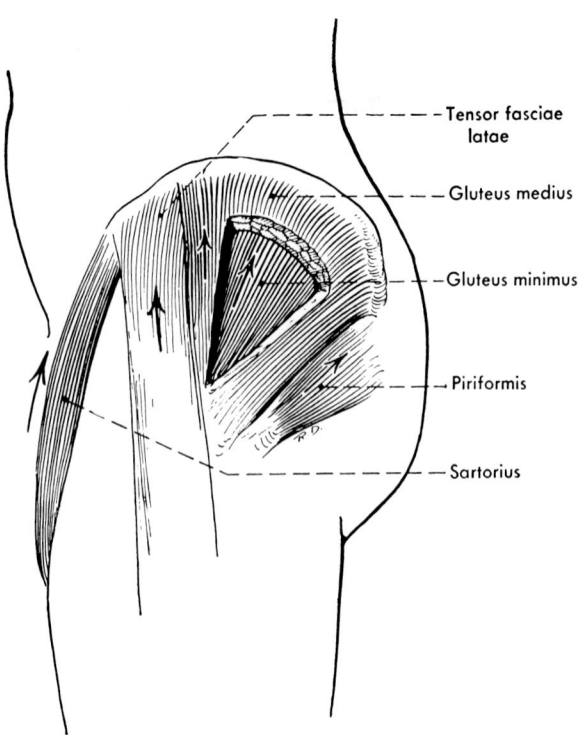

FIGURE 25-7. Abductors of the thigh. *(Redrawn, with permission, from Hollinshead WH: Textbook of Anatomy, 3rd ed. Hagerstown, MD: Harper & Row, 1974.)*

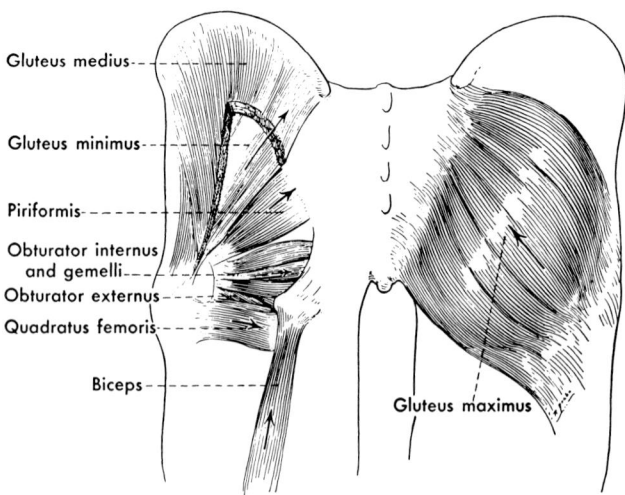

FIGURE 25-8. The external rotators and extensor of the thigh. *(Redrawn, with permission, from Hollinshead WH: Textbook of Anatomy, 3rd ed. Hagerstown, MD: Harper & Row, 1974.)*

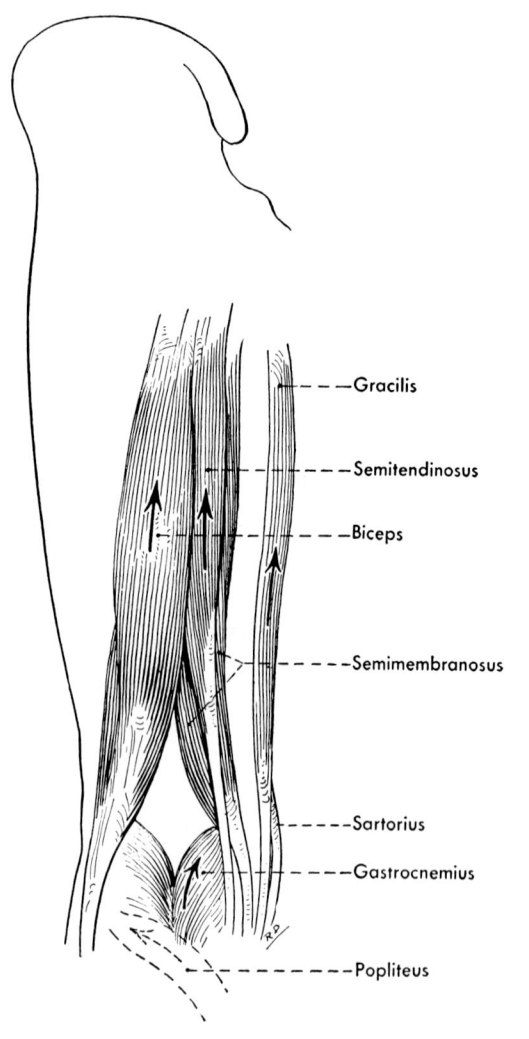

FIGURE 25-9. Flexors of the knee. *(Redrawn, with permission, from Hollinshead WH: Textbook of Anatomy, 3rd ed. Hagerstown, MD: Harper & Row, 1974.)*

mius/soleus muscles, have a rubbery or firm consistency. In infantile acid maltase deficiency, the weak muscles are firmer than normal as a result of glycogen storage.

Palpable enlargement of peripheral nerves is found in hereditary sensorimotor neuropathies type 1 and 3, amyloidosis, Refsum syndrome, acquired demyelinating neuropathies, acromegaly, neurofibromatosis, and leprosy. In the two latter diseases, the nerves have nodular enlargements.

Muscle tone can be assessed by inspection (resting tone), by passively moving a limb segment distal to a joint to feel the resistance encountered, and by shaking the extremity to transmit movements to its distal segments. Hypotonia is often suggested by posture. Rounding of the back in the sitting position is caused by hypotonia of the spine erectors. Droopy shoulders, winged scapulae, hyperextended elbows, and genu recurvatum are also signs of hypotonia but can also be seen in patients with joint laxity due to genetic diseases associated with mutations in connective tissue proteins.

In healthy infants, the resting muscle tone leads to flexion of the elbows, hips, and knees.[15] Limb tone is influenced by the tonic neck reflex; thus it is important to examine the infant with the head in the midline.[15] The scarf sign, or the ability to gently pull the arm across the chest such that the elbow crosses the midline, indicates upper limb hypotonia. The "frog-leg" posture, abduction of the lower limbs when the child is lying supine, indicates lower limb hypotonia. Truncal hypotonia is demonstrated during the Landau reflex. The examiner lifts the supine infant with one hand under the trunk. A normal child will elevate the head, resulting in a convex upward curvature of the spine. The hypotonic infant hangs over the examiner's hand in an inverted U-shaped posture.[15] Infants with shoulder muscle hypotonia slip between the examiner's hands when lifted under the arms.

Hypotonia is a common nonspecific sign of neurologic disease in infants and children. When associated with weakness, it can indicate a disease of the lower motor neuron, neuromuscular junction, peripheral nerve, or muscle. Hypotonia not associated with weakness may occur in disorders of the cerebrum or cerebellum, or it may be an intermittent or persistent finding in children with inborn errors of metabolism. Hypotonia without muscle weakness occurs in premature infants and in infants with progressive or nonprogressive encephalopathies in which the CNS was injured by perinatal trauma, hyperbilirubinemia, ischemia-hypoxia, infection, or congenital malformations. Hypotonia is prominent in Prader-Willi syndrome (obesity, mental retardation, and hypogonadism) and may be seen in other chromosomal disorders, in endocrinopathies (cretinism), or in nutritional deficiencies. Finally, it can also be idiopathic (benign congenital hypotonia).

PERCUSSION OF MUSCLES

Percussion Myotonia

The sign is positive when percussion of a muscle belly elicits a depression of the overlying soft tissues for several seconds (Fig. 25-10). The phenomenon is caused by abnormal mechanical irritability and sustained contraction of the percussed fibers. Percussion of the thenar eminence produces sustained adduction of the thumb. Percussion of extensor digitorum communis muscle about 2 cm below its origin elicits extension of one or more fingers that then slowly return to the resting, slightly flexed position. Percussion of larger muscles, such as the deltoid, may cause contraction of a strip of muscle. Myotonia of the tongue can be elicited by percussing the tongue as it is stretched over a tongue depressor. The examiner then places a second tongue depressor across the tongue, which is then percussed using a reflex hammer. Percussion myotonia of the tongue will manifest as a deep groove along the line of the tongue depressor, pulling the tongue into an hourglass shape.

Myoedema

This consists of mounding of part of a muscle at a percussed site (Fig. 25-11). The mound may move slightly and then flatten until it disappears over a few seconds. Myoedema appears in cachexia, in myxedema, and occasionally in otherwise normal individuals. Myoedema is not associated with electrical activity of the muscle fibers.

Rippling Muscle Disease

This is a benign and dominantly inherited condition, caused in some families by mutations in caveolin-3 on chromosome 1q41. During rippling, a longitudinal indentation parallel to the long axis of the muscle moves to the periphery of the muscle in 10 to 20 s in a wave that resembles the plucking of

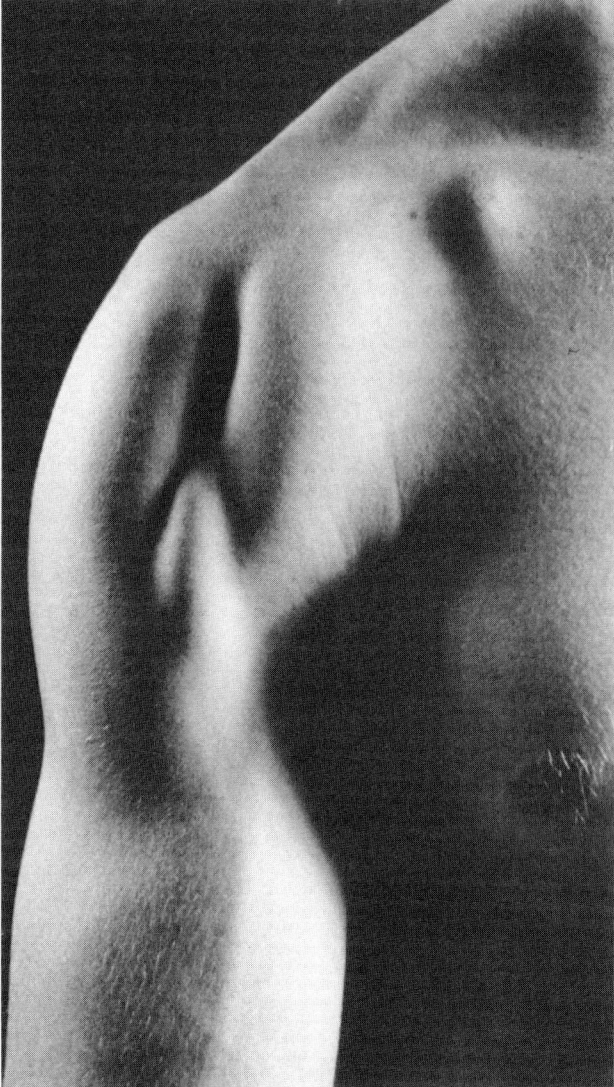

FIGURE 25-10. Percussion myotonia.

a chromatic scale on a harp.[16,17] This phenomenon occurs either spontaneously or after local mechanical stimulation. The rippling muscles are electrically silent.

REACTIONS AND REFLEXES

While the examination of muscle stretch and cutaneous reflexes in the adult is usually straightforward, examination in neonates and young children can be more challenging.

In neonates and small infants, the integrity of the CNS at different levels can be assessed by eliciting reflexes at different segmental levels: blink to light or to noise, vestibuloocular responses, rooting, sucking, righting of the head and trunk, plantar and palmar grasp reflexes, and Moro reaction.

Muscle stretch reflexes can be obtained from relaxed infants and cooperative young children. The triceps and ankle reflexes may not be present in normal infants, but the biceps and quadriceps are always present. Perseverance and patience are needed to elicit deep reflexes in the uncoopera-

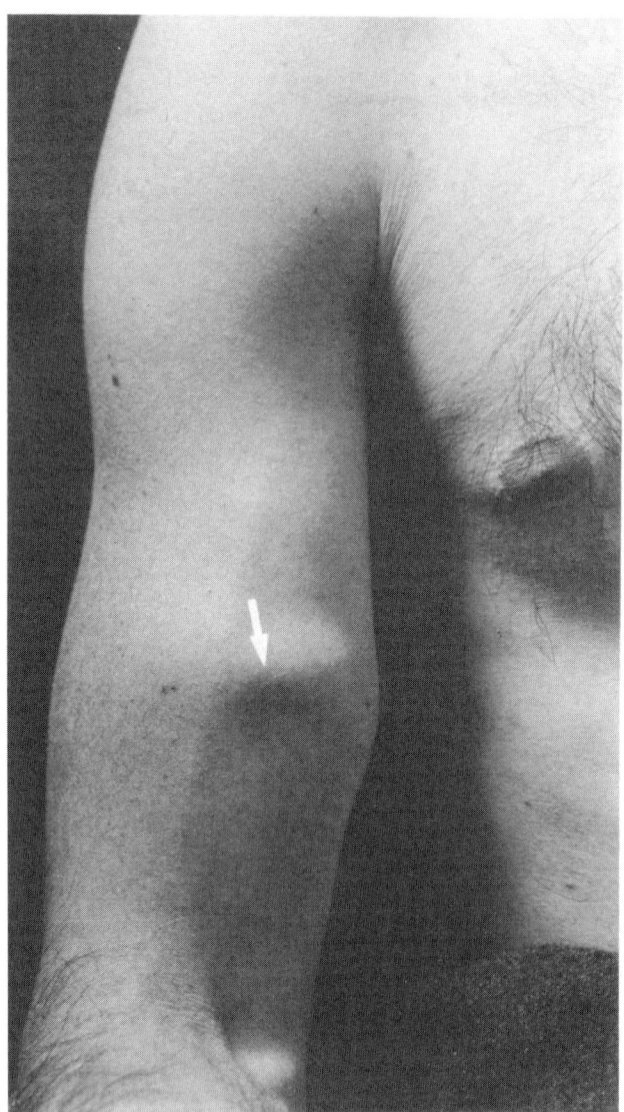

FIGURE 25-11. Myoedema.

flexor in normal children after they have begun to walk. Neuromuscular disorders associated with corticospinal tract involvement are characterized by increased muscle stretch reflexes, loss of cutaneous reflexes, and an extensor plantar reflex or Babinski sign.

SENSATION

Sensory testing is described in Chap. 69, "Diseases of Peripheral Nerves."

The Clinical Features

The following clinical features may be related by the patient or parents or observed during the course of the examination.

WEAKNESS

The clinical history should provide the necessary information to answer four basic questions: Is the patient weak? When did the weakness begin? Is the weakness intermittent? Is the weakness progressive? The examination should determine which muscle groups are affected and whether the weakness is diffuse or focal. Does it affect all limbs? Is it proximal or distal? Is the weakness equal in upper and lower extremities, or is it more severe in the upper or in the lower extremities? Are the muscles innervated by cranial nerves affected? Is there weakness of the respiratory muscles?

A few simple tests may reveal weakness of particular muscle groups.

1. Having the patient sit on a flat surface with no back support may reveal weakness of the spine erectors. If there is mild weakness, the patient supports the torso by placing his or her hands on the sitting surface. With more severe weakness, the ability to sit up is lost. The inability to flex the torso from the supine to the seated position without the use of the arms indicates weakness of the abdominal musculature.
2. Rising from the sitting or from the supine decubitus requires strong hip extensors. With weakness of the gluteus maximus, thigh extension is impossible unless the trunk is pushed up with the aid of both upper extremities. In Duchenne dystrophy, in myopathies with proximal weakness, and in the chronic form of spinal muscular atrophy, the patient attempting to stand up from the supine decubitus position will often demonstrate a Gowers' maneuver (Fig. 25-12).
3. Climbing stairs is difficult to impossible for patients with hip muscle weakness. Patients with mild to moderate weakness are able to negotiate stairs, but only with the use of the banister.
4. Climbing up the examining table requires enough strength in one lower limb to be able to push the entire weight of the body up while the other limb flexes at the knee to reach the surface of the table.

tive or frightened child. The stretch reflexes nearly always disappear in diseases of the anterior horn cells but are present in early muscular dystrophy and are always preserved in myasthenia gravis. They can be reduced or absent in the Lambert-Eaton myasthenic syndrome, botulism, and some congenital myasthenic syndromes. The stretch reflexes are lost during acute attacks of periodic paralysis. They may be preserved or reduced in polymyositis and are often reduced or absent in some of the congenital myopathies. In myxedema, the reflexes, particularly the ankle reflex, are delayed in the relaxation phase.

The superficial reflexes obtained by stimulation of the cornea, skin, or mucous membranes are of little value in assessing patients with neuromuscular disease. In the newborn, flexor or extensor responses may be obtained according to the type of stimulation: light, sustained touch at the base of the toes elicits plantarflexion, but light scratching of the sole produces an extensor response. The extensor response disappears before ambulation. The plantar reflex is

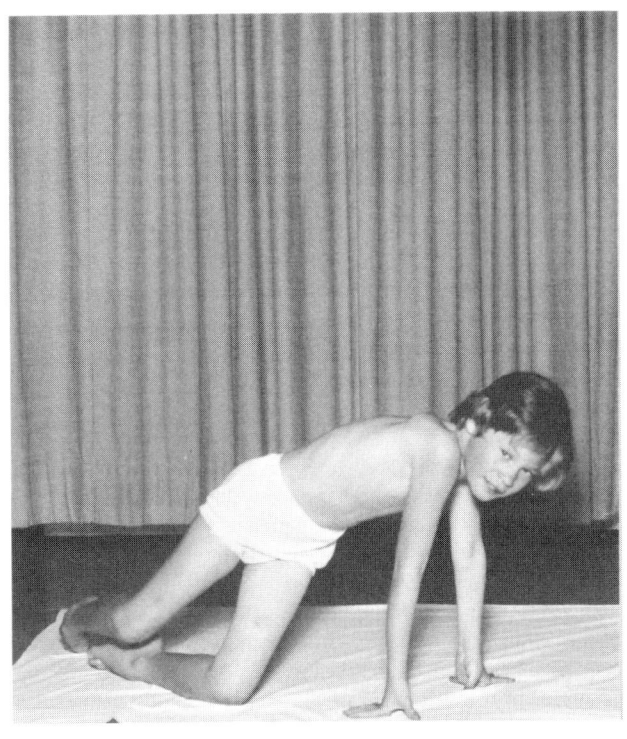
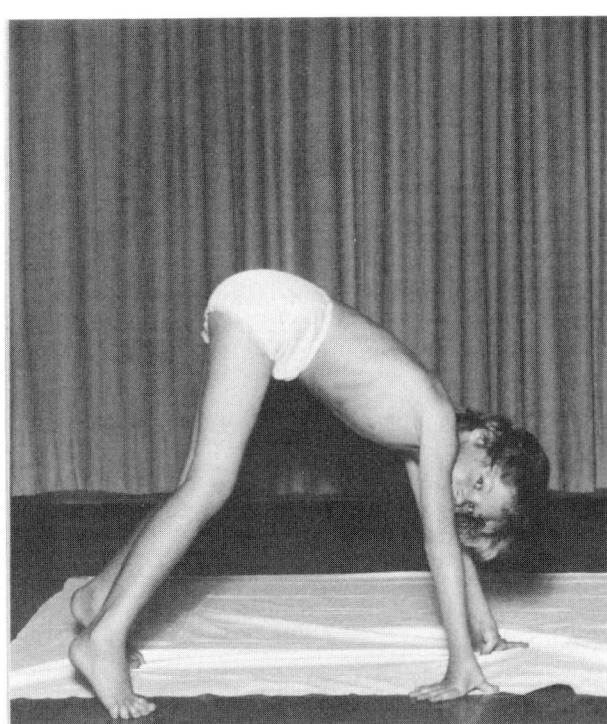
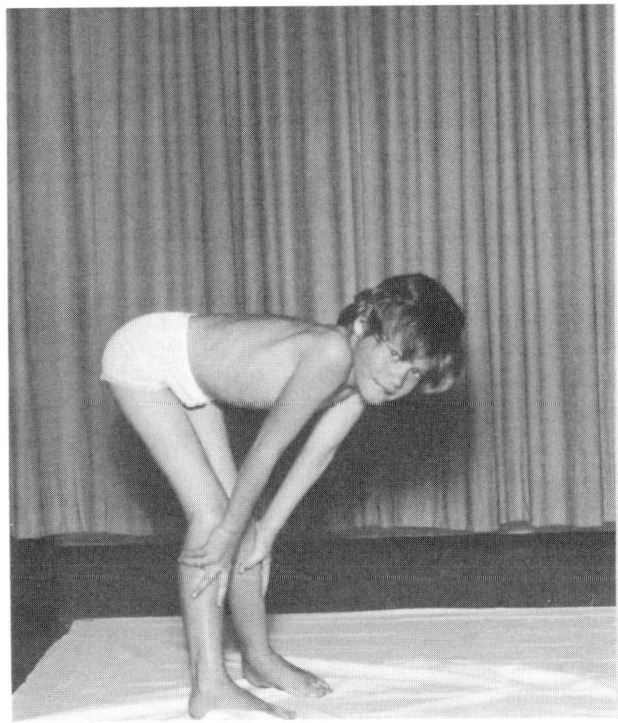
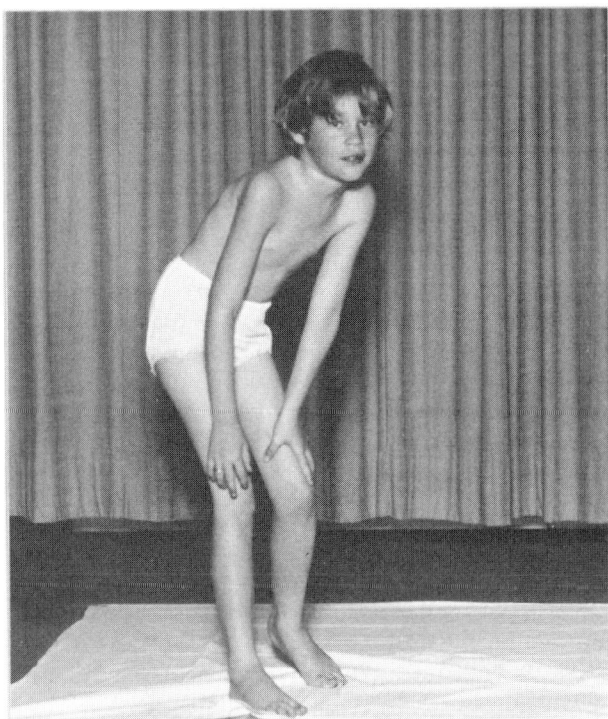

FIGURE 25-12. The Gowers' maneuver: The patient first sits up, then changes from a sitting position to a four-point standing position on the knees and hands. When the upper limbs support the upper trunk, the knees extend and push the lower trunk upward. The hands then move to the knees and gradually extend the trunk until an erect position is attained. A variation of this maneuver consists of rolling from a sitting position to rest on only one knee. As the opposite knee is extended, the weight is shifted to that side and the hand on the same side pushes on the knee to raise the trunk until the erect position is attained. In another variant of Gowers' maneuver, both hands are placed on the floor in line with the center of gravity. Extension of the arms then produces enough momentum to completely extend the hips to adopt the upright position.

5. Walking on the heels or on the toes tests the distal lower limb muscles.
6. Reaching with the arms above the head to get an object is a simple way to elicit flexion and abduction of the upper limb. This maneuver requires fixation of the scapula by the trapezius, rhomboids, and serratus anterior and strong supraspinatus and deltoid muscles. With mild weakness of the proximal upper limb muscles, the patient may be able to raise the hands to face level by rapidly flexing the arm at the shoulder in a throwing motion, which causes the elbow to flex by inertia. Children with upper limb weakness will be unable to support their weight when playing on monkey bars.

ARTHROGRYPOSIS AND OTHER TENDON CONTRACTURES

Arthrogryposis is a malformation of the extremities characterized by contractures of muscles and tendons and limitation of movement of the affected joints without primary joint involvement. In arthrogryposis multiplex congenita, the primary cause may be a disease of the neuromuscular unit: an anomaly of the spinal cord such as myelodysplasia with spina bifida, a congenital myopathy, or a disease of the lower motor neuron. Arthrogryposis may also be caused by an abnormal position of the fetus, in association with oligohydramnios or amniotic bands around the limbs.

Muscle and tendon contractures may also develop after birth from immobilization, usually the result of weakness. Mechanical immobilization of the joints by casts or prolonged bed rest from any cause accelerates the development of contractures. The Achilles tendons, iliotibial bands, and the paraspinal, posterior tibial, hamstring, and pectoral muscles are most often affected.

Contractures develop early in the course of dermatomyositis and juvenile polymyositis. Patients with Duchenne or Becker dystrophy are often referred to the orthopedist because of toe-walking. Examination shows short Achilles tendons and weak anterior tibial muscles. Achilles tendon contracture also occurs in distal motor neuropathy, in spastic diplegia, in patients with a tethered spinal cord, in juvenile dystonia musculorum deformans, and in Hallervorden-Spatz disease. Some normal children also toe-walk for a brief period of time when they first ambulate; other children remain toe-walkers, yet neuromuscular and orthopedic examinations demonstrate no abnormality other than the short Achilles tendons.[18] Joint contractures are particularly prominent in X-linked or autosomal recessive Emery-Dreifuss muscular dystrophy and in myopathies associated with mutations in collagen genes. Arthrogryposis is discussed further in Chap. 70.

SKELETAL ANOMALIES

A number of skeletal anomalies found in the congenital myopathies give a clue to the diagnosis. Patients with central core disease, nemaline myopathy, centronuclear myopathy, congenital fiber type disproportion, and congenital myotonic dystrophy often have an elongated head in the anteroposterior direction, a long and narrow face, high-arched palate, and dental malocclusion. Dislocation of the hips occurs with central core disease. Congenital scoliosis and kyphosis can be associated with congenital anomalies of the vertebral column, such as agenesis or hypoplasia of vertebrae and adjacent muscles, and in infantile spinal muscular atrophy with prenatal onset of symptoms. Progressive scoliosis and other spinal deformities occur in patients with spinal muscular atrophy, some congenital myopathies, spinocerebellar degeneration, or advanced Duchenne dystrophy. Rigidity of the spine occurs in the rigid spine syndrome and in Emery-Dreifuss muscular dystrophy.

FATIGABILITY

Fluctuating weakness and abnormal fatigability that usually worsens by the end of the day or after exercise point to a disorder of neuromuscular transmission. Patients with the Lambert-Eaton myasthenic syndrome may notice an improvement in strength after repeated muscle contractions. Generalized fatigue and limited exercise tolerance is also a feature of metabolic disorders affecting energy production in muscle, such as mitochondrial myopathies.

In children, evaluation of fatigable weakness can be limited by a lack of cooperation or attention to the task. For lid elevation testing, having the child count the numbers on a clock placed high on the wall or asking him or her to identify pictures in a book held at an appropriate height will often allow assessment of lid elevation for 1 to 2 min. Similarly, arm elevation time can be assessed by having the child keep the arms elevated while pointing to objects in a book held at an appropriate height. Children with fatigable weakness of the limbs may develop a compensatory lumbar lordosis in an effort to maintain arm elevation.

In patients with classic myasthenia gravis and in some congenital myasthenic syndromes, the intravenous injection of edrophonium, an acetylcholinesterase inhibitor, will produce a prompt but evanescent increase in strength. It is necessary to assess the strength of selected weak muscles before and after the administration of the drug. The effect appears about 30 s after the injection, peaks in 1 min, and wears off in a few minutes. A test dose (one-tenth of the total dose) is administered intravenously over 10 to 15 s. If there is no response, the remaining dose is injected. In adults, the test dose is 0.1 mL (1 mg) and the maximal dose is 1.0 mL (10 mg). For infants and children, the maximal dose of edrophonium is 0.15 mg/kg and 0.2 mg/kg, respectively. The response must be evaluated immediately, looking for a change in the severity of the ptosis, the range of ocular ductions, or the strength of other skeletal muscles.

FASCICULATIONS

Fasciculations are brief fine twitches of resting muscles caused by spontaneous activation of motor units. They are visible as transient longitudinal depressions of the skin overlying muscle. Fasciculations may be precipitated by gentle tapping of the muscle, fatigue, or exposure to cold or anticholinesterase drugs. They occur in patients with active anterior horn cell degeneration and in neuromyotonia (see Chap. 47), but even normal individuals may fasciculate after receiving anticholinesterase drugs. Benign fasciculations occur in healthy individuals without muscle weakness. These are increased by fatigue, smoking, or drinking coffee. Tongue fasciculations are found in progressive bulbar atrophy, advanced spinal muscular atrophy, and syringobulbia.

Contraction fasciculations are rhythmic fascicular twitches during weak muscle contractions. They occur in patients with chronic poliomyelitis, nerve root compression, and motor neuron disease. They differ from the usual spontaneous fasciculations in that they disappear when the muscle relaxes.

MYOKYMIA

Myokymia is caused by successive spontaneous contractions of motor units, or groups of muscle fibers, and results in a continuous undulation of the overlying body surface. The movements are slower and more prolonged than fasciculations. Myokymia of the hand muscles causes stiffness of the hands. Facial myokymia may be associated with facial spasms and appears as a fine rippling of the facial skin. It can be associated with multiple sclerosis or with brainstem compression by tumors and with episodic ataxia type 1.

MYOTONIA

Myotonia is a painless, sustained muscle contraction associated with abnormal repetitive depolarization of the muscle fibers, which causes tetanic contraction of the muscle fibers. The responding fibers are not neurally linked. Clinical myotonia consists of percussion myotonia (described above) and action myotonia. The following are examples of action myotonia. Myotonia of the upper eyelid can be elicited by having the patient look up and down rapidly: The upper eyelid will descend slowly, exposing the sclera. Myotonia of the orbicularis oculi can be demonstrated by having the patient squeeze the lids for a second and then relax them. There will be a delay of a few seconds before the patient can open his or her eyes. Myotonia of the hand muscles is demonstrated simply by having the patient squeeze the examiner's fingers and then attempt to let go quickly. In congenital myotonia, the onset of myotonia is in infancy or early childhood; but in myotonic dystrophy, it does not appear until late childhood or adult life. In some mildly affected patients with myotonic dystrophy, clinical myotonia cannot be elicited. Myotonia can also occur in some patients with primary hyperkalemic periodic paralysis. Acquired myotonia may occur after exposure to the insecticide dichlorphenoxyacetic acid or to monocarboxylic aromatic acids. Myotonia is further described in Chap. 36, "Myotonic Dystrophy," and Chap. 46, "Nondystrophic Channelopathies: Myotonias and Periodic Paralyses."

List of Abbreviations

| AMP | adenosine monophosphate | EMG | electromyogram |
| CNS | central nervous system | SMA | spinal muscular atrophy |

References

1. Motor deficits, in Simon RP, Aminoff MJ, Greenberg DA (eds): *Clinical Neurology.* Stamford, CT: Appleton & Lange, 1999; pp 159–169.
2. Griggs RC: Episodic muscle spasms, cramps, and weakness, in Fauci AS, Braunwald E, Isselbacher KJ, et al (eds): *Harrison's Principles of Internal Medicine.* New York: McGraw-Hill, 1998; pp 118–122.
3. Pellegrino JE, Rebbeck TR, Brown MJ, et al: Mapping of hereditary neuralgic amyotrophy (familial brachial plexus neuropathy) to distal chromosome 17q. *Neurology* 46(4):1128–1132, 1996.
4. Layzer RB, Rowland LP: Cramps. *N Engl J Med* 285(1):31–40, 1971.
5. Lambert EH, Goldstein NP: An unusual form of "myotonia." *Physiologist* 1:51, 1957.
6. Brody IA: Muscle contracture induced by exercise. A syndrome attributable to decreased relaxing factor. *N Engl J Med* 281(4):187–192, 1969.
7. Odermatt A, Taschner PE, Khanna VK, et al: Mutations in the gene-encoding SERCA1, the fast-twitch skeletal muscle sarcoplasmic reticulum Ca2+ ATPase, are associated with Brody disease. *Nat Genet* 14(2):191–194, 1996.
8. Klein I, Parker M, Shebert R, et al: Hypothyroidism presenting as muscle stiffness and pseudohypertrophy: Hoffmann's syndrome. *Am J Med* 70(4):891–894, 1981.
9. Stolor WC: Normal and pathologic ambulation, in Rosse C, Clawson D (eds): *The Musculoskeletal System in Health and Disease.* New York: Harper & Row, 1980; pp 315–334.
10. Cook IJ, Kahrilas PJ: AGA technical review on management of oropharyngeal dysphagia. *Gastroenterology* 116: 455–478, 1999.
11. Members of the Department of Neurology and the Department of Physiology and Biophysics, Mayo Clinic and Mayo Foundation: *Clinical Examinations in Neurology,* 6th ed. St. Louis: Mosby–Year Book, 1990.
12. Medical Research Council of the United Kingdom: *Aids to the Examination of the Peripheral Nervous System.* United Kingdom: Pendragon House, 1978.
13. Kendall HO, Kendall KP, Wadsworth GE: *Muscle Testing and Function,* 2nd ed. Baltimore: Williams & Wilkins, 1971.
14. Walton JN: Clinical examination, differential diagnosis, and classification of neuromuscular diseases, in Walton JN (ed): *Disorders of Voluntary Muscle,* 5th ed. London: Churchill Livingstone, 1981.
15. Menkes JH, Sarnat HB, Moser FG: Introduction: Neurologic examination of the child and infant, in Menkes JH, Sarnat HB (eds): *Child Neurology.* Philadelphia: Lippincott Williams & Wilkins, 2000; pp 1–32.
16. Betz RC, Shoser BGH, Kasper D, et al. Mutations in *CAV3* cause mechanical hyperirritability of skeletal muscle in rippling muscle disease. *Nature Genet* 28:218–219, 2001.
17. Alberca R, Rafel E, Castilla JM, et al: Increased mechanical muscle irritability syndrome. *Acta Neurol Scand* 62(4):250–254, 1980.
18. Ringel SP: Clinical presentations in neuromuscular disease, in Vinken PJ, Bruyn GW (eds): *Handbook of Clinical Neurology.* Part I: *Diseases of Muscle.* Amsterdam: North-Holland, 1979; pp 295–348.
19. Eunson LH, Rea R, Zuberi SM, et al: Clinical, genetic, and expression studies of mutations in potassium channel gene KCNA1 reveal new phenotypic variability. *Ann Neurol* 48:647–656, 2000.

Chapter 26
Electrodiagnosis of Muscle Disorders

JASPER R. DAUBE
DEVON I. RUBIN

Introduction
Electrodiagnostic Methods
 NEEDLE ELECTROMYOGRAPHY
 SINGLE-FIBER ELECTROMYOGRAPHY
 OTHER ELECTROMYOGRAPHIC RECORDINGS
 NERVE AND MUSCLE STIMULATION
Findings in Muscle Diseases
 INFLAMMATORY MYOPATHIES
 INFILTRATIVE MYOPATHIES
 DISORDERS OF ALTERED CELL MEMBRANE EXCITABILITY
 MUSCULAR DYSTROPHIES
 CONGENITAL MYOPATHIES
 METABOLIC DISORDERS OF MUSCLE
 CRITICAL ILLNESS MYOPATHY
 DISTURBANCES OF NEUROMUSCULAR TRANSMISSION
 MUSCLE SPASMS AND RELATED PHENOMENA
Findings in Neural Diseases
 PERIPHERAL NERVE DISORDERS
 MOTOR NEURON DISEASES
 INTERPRETATION OF EMG AND NCSS
Neuromyopathies

Introduction

Disorders of muscle are characterized and identified most efficiently with the combined application of clinical, histologic, biochemical, and electrophysiologic studies. The clinical features of these disorders are weakness, increase or decrease of muscle bulk, and sometimes cramps.[1] Clinical distinctions are based on age at onset; the distribution, severity, rate of progression, and fluctuation of weakness; and associated clinical findings. This chapter reviews the application of clinical electrodiagnostic studies to the evaluation of muscle disease. First, the types of recordings and the abnormalities detected with each type are considered; second, the patterns of alteration that occur in the major groups of muscle diseases are surveyed; and third, the interpretation of electrodiagnostic studies is discussed.

Analysis of the different kinds of potentials recorded in electrodiagnostic studies can help to identify a disease, assess its severity, or understand its pathophysiologic mechanism. Because electrical recordings are made in a volume conductor, potentials can be recorded at a distance from the generator, just as the electrocardiogram can be recorded from the limbs. However, the amplitude of a potential decreases exponentially with the distance from the generator. Thus, nerve and muscle potentials cannot be recorded reliably at more than a few centimeters from the generator.

Individual potentials have different sites of origin and may display different alterations. The description and naming of these potentials have been standardized.[2]

Electrodiagnostic studies record spontaneous, voluntarily generated and evoked potentials from nerve or muscle with electrodes positioned on the surface of the skin or in the muscle. The multiple generators and the variety of their interactions result in a complex array of electrical waveforms in different disorders. The potentials recorded in electrodiagnosis are derived from either muscle fibers or nerve fibers. Individual fibers of either type generate small potentials that are a few microvolts or less in amplitude. Single-fiber potentials are too difficult to record routinely but can be measured by inserting small needle electrodes into the nerve or muscle.[3] Groups of nerve or muscle fibers that fire in synchrony generate much larger and more readily recorded potentials. Electrical stimulation of a nerve elicits compound nerve action potentials (NAPs),* the summated activity of all axons activated in the nerve, or compound muscle fiber action potentials (CMAPs), the summated activity of all muscle fibers activated in the muscle. The synchronous activation of groups of muscle fibers during voluntary activation of motor units produces motor unit potentials (MUPs).

Disorders of nerve or muscle will alter any or all these potentials. An increase or decrease in the size of muscle fibers will increase or decrease the spontaneous and voluntary potentials generated by the muscle fibers. Changes in the number, distribution, and density of muscle fibers will alter the size and configuration of MUPs and CMAPs, as will alterations in the location of end plate regions and muscle fiber conduction velocity. Alterations in neuromuscular transmission can also alter the MUP and CMAP, especially if the potentials are activated sequentially. The distribution of the abnormalities and the fluctuation of the changes with exercise are also valuable testing methods. The loss of axons or motor neurons will decrease the number of MUPs that can be activated and the size of CMAPs. If there is collateral sprouting of the remaining axons and successful reinnervation of previously denervated muscle fibers, the size and configuration of MUPs are modified. These patterns of abnormality have distinctive features that allow the site and type of change that has occurred in disease to be determined.

The electromyographer provides four kinds of information: (1) classification of a disease into broad categories—in a few instances, disorders can be identified by specific types of electrical potentials or patterns of abnormality; (2) description of the distribution, severity, and progression of disease by the extent and type of change; (3) insight into the pathophysiologic mechanism of the disease; and (4) for a few disorders, identification of subclinical disease.[4] Specialized electrical recording techniques can add to the structural information provided by standard histologic studies.[5,6] The recognition and reliable interpretation of the waveforms and their association with particular diseases requires a trained physician-electromyographer.

---

*A list of abbreviations used in this chapter is given at the end of the chapter.

Electrodiagnostic studies of peripheral neuromuscular disease are grouped into three types: (1) Electromyography (EMG) records spontaneous and voluntary potentials with a needle electrode in muscle. (2) Nerve conduction studies (NCS) measure evoked potentials from peripheral nerve stimulation. (3) Repetitive stimulation tests assess the neuromuscular junction.

Electrodiagnostic Methods

NEEDLE ELECTROMYOGRAPHY

Technique Overview

Electrodes. Experience has shown that the most valuable electrodiagnostic information about muscle disease is obtained with needle electrodes that sample voluntary and spontaneous potentials of muscle fibers in an area a few millimeters in diameter.[7] The two types of electrodes most commonly used are *standard concentric electrodes* and *monopolar electrodes*. Each has advantages and disadvantages, but both record similar potentials and demonstrate similar alterations in disease. The monopolar electrode is a stainless steel needle that is insulated except at its tip. Potential differences are recorded between the needle tip and a large electrode on the surface of the skin. The standard concentric electrode is a bare needle shaft containing within it a fine insulated wire that is exposed at the tip of the needle. The electrical potentials are recorded between this electrode tip and the shaft of the needle. Both electrodes record potentials of comparable size, but the potentials recorded with a monopolar electrode have a slightly longer duration and higher amplitude than those recorded with a concentric electrode. In either case, the MUPs are summated potentials of the muscle fibers in a motor unit located within a few millimeters of the electrode. In most muscles, this area does not include all the muscle fibers in the motor unit; consequently, the electrode must be moved to another area to record the activity of other fibers of the same motor unit or the fibers of other motor units (Fig. 26-1). Single-fiber electrodes and macroelectrodes are specialized electrodes, described below.

Summary of Normal Activity

Most of the activity recorded from normal muscles is the result of voluntary activation of MUPs. However, muscle disease is often associated with spontaneous electrical discharges generated by single muscle fibers, which can be invaluable in identifying the type of disease.[8] Although diseased muscle may show various kinds of spontaneous activity, normal muscle fibers are activated only by lower motor neurons. Therefore, normal muscle is electrically silent at rest except for insertion activity and end plate activity.

Normal spontaneous potentials. Although muscle fibers typically are activated by nerve impulses, they can also be activated mechanically. As a needle electrode passes through a muscle, it mechanically stimulates or damages muscle fibers and, by depolarizing them, initiates brief potentials of varied sizes and shapes. This *insertion activity* occurs as a burst of potentials in response to needle movement (Fig. 26-2, panel 1). A single muscle fiber potential is usually recorded as a triphasic potential as it passes the recording electrode.[9] Mechanical activation usually occurs at the needle tip; thus, the insertion potentials are generally biphasic potentials, which are initially negative. Some muscle fibers may be damaged by the needle tip and thus cannot

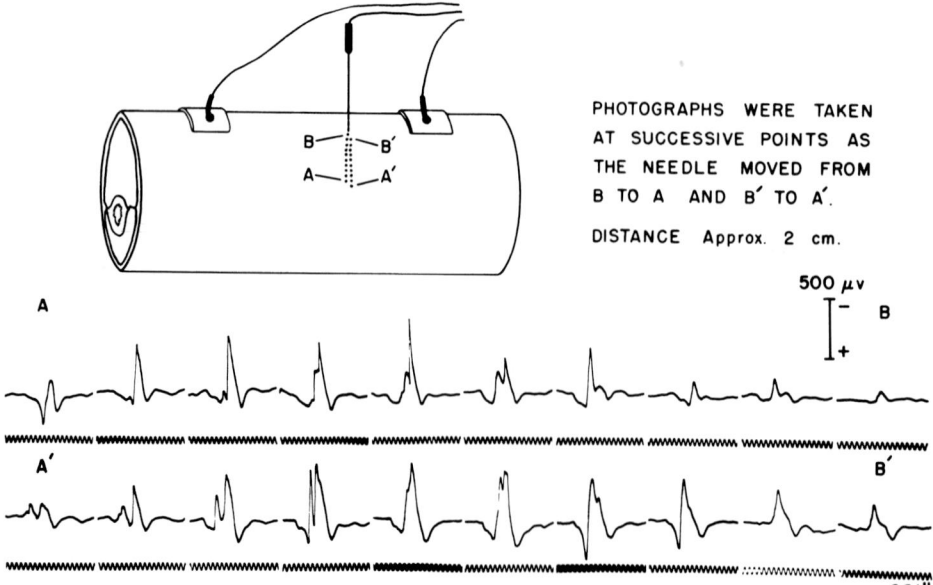

FIGURE 26-1. Recording of different size and shape MUPs from a single motor unit by moving the electrode through the muscle. *(Courtesy of EH Lambert.)*

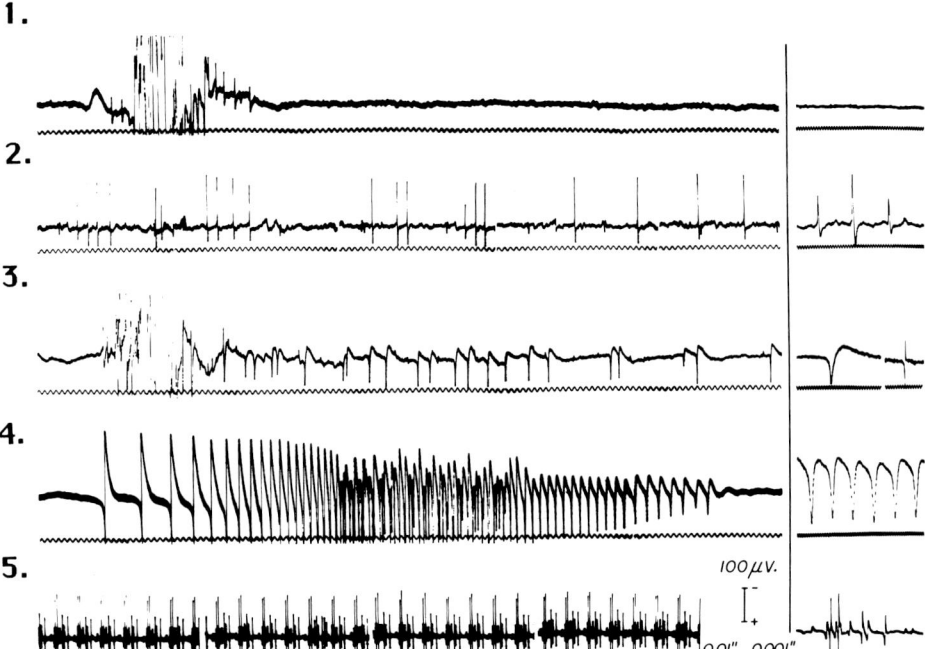

FIGURE 26-2. EMG insertion activity with standard concentric needle electrodes. (From Members of the Department of Neurology and the Department of Physiology and Biophysics, Mayo Clinic and Mayo Foundation for Medical Education and Research: Clinical Examinations in Neurology, 6th ed. St. Louis: Mosby–Year Book, 1991; p 404. With permission from Mayo Foundation.)

generate a depolarization in the region of the electrode; the action potential from the distant intact area is recorded as a positive waveform. Thus, normal insertion activity is typically a mixture of spikes of varying sizes that may be monophasic or biphasic, positive or negative.[10] The number of spikes in a burst depends on the amount of needle movement. The most consistent characteristic of these bursts is that they do not outlast needle movement. Two normal variants can occur. One of these, seen especially in muscular young men, is a rapid, brief, irregular discharge that "snaps, crackles, and pops." The other is familial and consists of short trains of waning, rapid positive waves; it may represent a subclinical form of myotonia. Both of these variants must be recognized so that they are not misinterpreted as signs of disease.

Another normal discharge that may be mistaken for abnormal spontaneous activity occurs in the end plate region. Nerve terminals at the neuromuscular junction continuously and randomly release single packets, or quanta, of acetylcholine (ACh). These quanta produce small, localized depolarization of the postsynaptic membrane called *miniature end plate potentials* (MEPPs). MEPP amplitudes are low and well below the threshold for activation of muscle fibers. MEPPs can be recorded with a standard needle electrode in the end plate region.[11] The relatively large recording surface of the standard electrode records MEPPs from several muscle fibers as low-amplitude, monophasic negative potentials. This *end plate noise* is often not much greater than baseline noise. End plate noise has a characteristic seashell sound.

Another form of normal electrical activity, *end plate spikes*, can also be recorded in the end plate region. End plate spikes are the potentials of single muscle fibers activated indirectly by the mechanical stimulation of the innervating nerve terminal. The nerve terminal, like the muscle fiber, can be mechanically activated, but its small size precludes the potential it generates from being recorded with a standard needle electrode. The indirect effect of this mechanical activation, a muscle fiber action potential, can readily be recorded; it has the features typical of a single fiber potential. End plate spikes are 20 to 100 μV in amplitude and 1 to 3 ms in duration; they are usually biphasic and initially negative because the potential is recorded at the site of its initiation (Fig. 26-2, panel 2). An end plate spike may be a positive waveform if the electrode has damaged the muscle fiber.[10] The most characteristic feature of end plate spikes is their pattern of firing: irregular, high-frequency discharges with interpotential intervals as short as 15 ms. Interpotential intervals this short are seen only with activity generated in nerve.

End plate noise and end plate spikes are of no diagnostic significance, but it is extremely important to recognize them so they are not confused with abnormal spontaneous activity. In infants, the end plate region comprises a larger proportion of the total muscle length than in adults; therefore end plate activity is encountered more frequently in infants and can be particularly confusing.

Insertion activity, end plate noise, and end plate spikes are not recorded with surface or macroelectrodes because of their low amplitude. They are also rarely seen in single-fiber EMG (SFEMG) recordings, because the recording surface of the SFEMG needle is not at the needle tip, where the mechanical activation occurs.

Normal voluntary potentials. Voluntary muscle activity is mediated by the lower motor neuron acting on the muscle fibers that it innervates (motor units). Motor units represent the final common pathway of motor activity. Individual muscles contain 50 to 800 motor units, each unit comprising 50 to 2000 muscle fibers. The number of motor units activated and their rate of discharge determine the

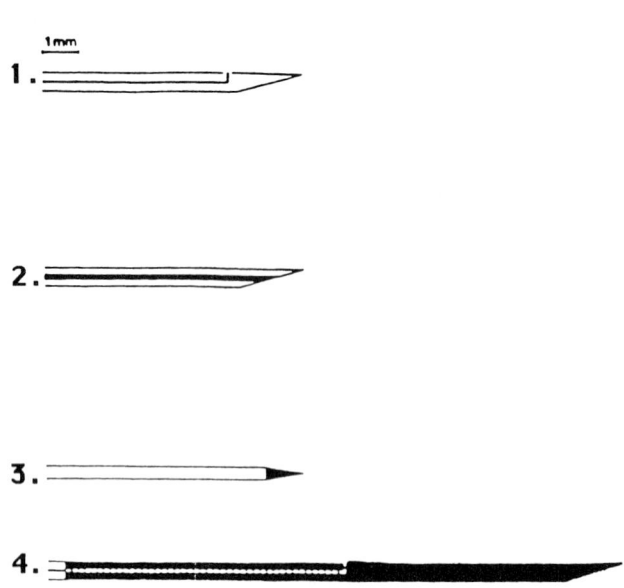

FIGURE 26-3. Recording electrodes for clinical electromyography. (1) Single fiber. (2) Standard concentric. (3) Monopolar. (4) Macro. Shaded areas represent active electrode; unshaded areas represent reference electrode.

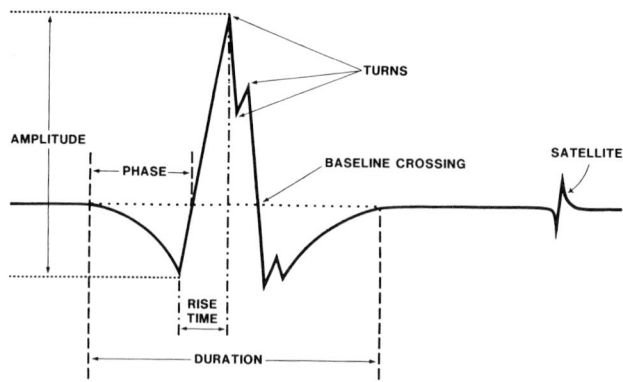

FIGURE 26-4. Diagram of the characteristics of a MUP. Each of the major variables is indicated.

movement and force generated by a muscle. The action potential of an anterior horn cell is transmitted to each muscle fiber in the motor unit through nerve fiber branches. The nearly synchronous discharge of the muscle fibers in the motor unit can be recorded electrically during voluntary activation. The size and shape of the recording electrode determine the number of muscle fibers sampled from a motor unit.[12] Standard clinical recordings are made with electrodes with recording surfaces 100 to 500 μm in diameter (Fig. 26-3). The electrical activity recorded with these electrodes is predominantly from muscle fibers within 0.5 mm of the electrode. Action potentials from single muscle fibers can be recorded with 25-μm electrodes in SFEMG studies. Larger electrodes, either within the muscle (macroelectrode) or on its surface, sample a much larger proportion of muscle fibers or all the muscle fibers in the motor unit.

The *size and shape of a MUP* depend on the number, density, size, conduction velocity, and synchrony of firing of muscle fibers within the recording area and on the intervening inactive tissue, such as connective tissue.[13,14] The firing synchrony varies with the conduction velocity of the muscle fiber (which increases with muscle fiber diameter), the location of the end plates, the length of the nerve terminals, and the conduction velocity of action potentials in the nerve terminals. Variation in muscle fiber diameter and scattered end plates are the primary causes of loss of synchrony.

Single fiber potentials of muscle are recorded as triphasic (positive-negative-positive) spikes. Generally, MUPs are also triphasic because they are the sum of single-fiber potentials (Fig. 26-4). The initial positivity of the potential reflects the recording of current flow from depolarization at a distance; in contrast, recordings made at the site of initiation of the potential are initially negative. Recordings made from damaged areas of the muscle fiber or at a distance from the fiber where no negativity is generated are recorded as entirely positive potentials. The sizes and shapes of MUPs in normal muscle vary markedly from area to area, from muscle to muscle, and with age and muscle temperature.[15]

Normal muscle contains many motor units. Because the needle electrode primarily records from muscle fibers within a millimeter of the needle, different MUPs will be recorded from a single motor unit as the needle is moved through the muscle. Each of these MUPs has different amplitudes and durations. The description of the amplitude and duration of normal MUPs in a muscle is best based on the measurement of at least 20 different MUPs from different areas in the muscle (Fig. 26-5); in most muscles, these will be recorded from 5 to 10 different motor units. Abnormal duration or amplitude is identified by a significant difference of either the mean value or the distributions from normal.

Normal MUPs usually range from 100 to 2000 μV in amplitude and from 3 to 15 ms in duration. They have two to four phases, although up to 15 percent of normal MUPs may have more than four phases. The rise time from the positive to the negative peak depends primarily on the distance

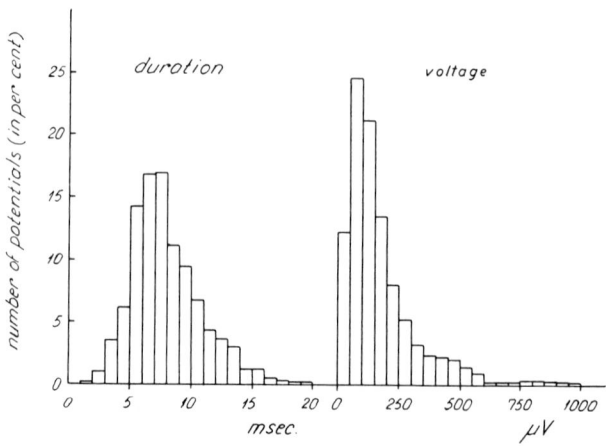

FIGURE 26-5. Distribution of durations and voltages of 1268 MUPs recorded with concentric electrodes in different points of the brachial biceps of a normal subject. *(From Buchthal F: An Introduction to Electromyography. Oslo: Scandinavian University Books, 1957. With permission from the publisher.)*

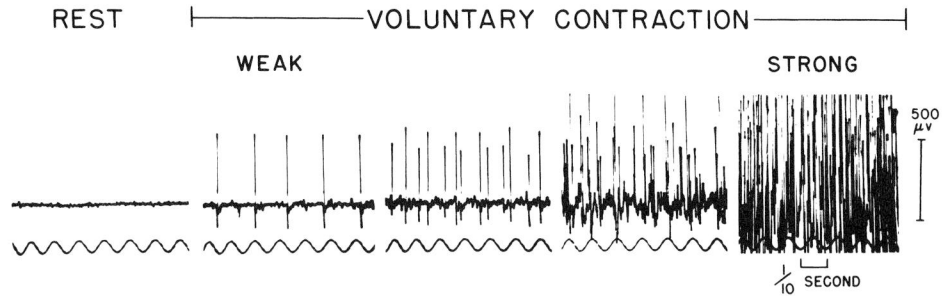

FIGURE 26-6. Recording of MUPs at slow sweep speeds during increasing effort of voluntary contraction illustrating recruitment of MUPs. Note the increased rate of firing of the first recruited MUP as the second MUP is recruited. *(From Members of the Department of Neurology and the Department of Physiology and Biophysics, Mayo Clinic and Mayo Foundation for Medical Education and Research: Clinical Examinations in Neurology, 6th ed. St. Louis: Mosby–Year Book, 1991; p 400. With permission from Mayo Foundation.)*

of the electrode from the muscle fibers, although small differences between slowly contracting and rapidly contracting fibers have been reported. The turns, or peaks, in a MUP represent individual muscle fiber potentials that are not precisely synchronous in activation with the other fibers in that recording area (Fig. 26-4). Each of the muscle fibers in a motor unit is activated every time the motor unit is activated, so that the size and shape of a MUP in normal muscle remain stable at any one location with repeated firing.

During normal muscle activation, one or more motor units are activated at different levels of voluntary effort. Individual anterior horn cells fire at faster rates as the input to the anterior horn cell pool in the ventral horn of the spinal cord increases with effort. Concurrent with this, additional anterior horn cells are activated (Fig. 26-6). The activation of additional anterior horn cells with increasing rates of firing, called *recruitment*, occurs in direct relation to the size of the anterior horn cell. Smaller anterior horn cells are activated first, followed by cells of increasing size. Later-activated cells generally fire at higher rates. An irregular firing rate occurs at the lower and upper ranges of normal firing rates (5 to 25 Hz).[16]

Thus, with increased force of contraction, additional motor units are recruited. This is seen on needle EMG as the progressive activation of additional MUPs as the firing rate of individual MUPs increases. The number of MUPs activated and their rates of firing are determined by the characteristics of their anterior horn cells and change with voluntary effort. Most motor units begin firing at rates of 5 to 10 Hz. With increasing effort, the previously activated MUPs increase their firing frequency and additional MUPs are recruited at higher frequencies. The ratio of the number of different, active MUPs to the rate of firing of an individual MUP varies somewhat in different regions of a muscle and among muscles, but it is constant in an area of the muscle. The ratio is generally less than five. For example, at firing rates of 10 Hz or higher, at least two MUPs are usually active, and at 20 Hz or higher, at least four are active.

Abnormal Spontaneous Activity

In muscle disease, when the muscle is at rest and the needle is not moving, spontaneous electrical discharges produce various patterns in muscle disease. These discharges are recognized most readily by their pattern of firing rather than by their configuration. Insertion activity may be increased in disorders in which there is irritability of the muscle fiber membrane, or it may be decreased if muscle fibers have been replaced by connective tissue or fat or if the muscle fiber membrane has become inactivated. Increased insertion activity is seen as short trains of spikes or positive waves after the initial burst when needle movement stops. Increased insertion activity is a nonspecific finding encountered in many disorders of muscle or nerve. Among the varieties of abnormal spontaneous activity, only myotonic discharges and fibrillation potentials are of help in diagnosis.

Fibrillation potentials. Of the different forms of abnormal spontaneous activity in muscle disease, fibrillation potentials are the most frequent and of the greatest diagnostic importance. *Fibrillation potentials* are regularly firing, spontaneous discharges of single muscle fibers that are not innervated (Fig. 26-7). Their interpotential intervals are longer than 80 ms, in contrast to the shorter intervals of end

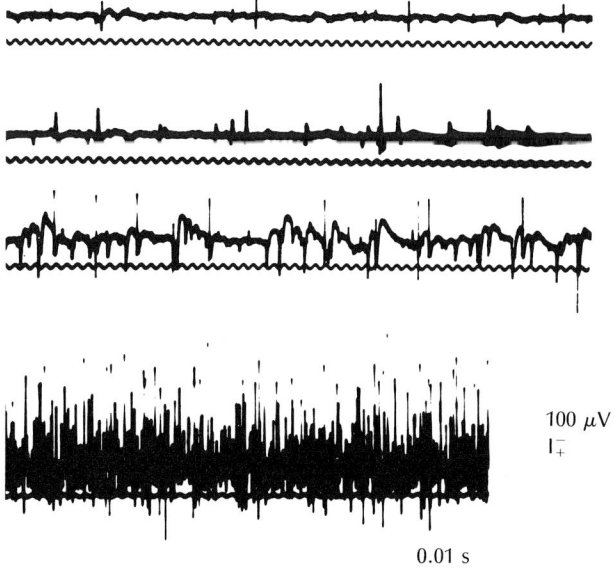

FIGURE 26-7. Fibrillation potentials in denervated muscle. Increasing grades of severity are illustrated (top to bottom). Both spike form and positive waveforms of the fibrillation potentials are present. Different amplitude fibrillation potentials are recorded from different size muscle fibers. *(Courtesy of EH Lambert.)*

plate spikes.[17] They occur in muscle fibers that either have not been innervated or have been denervated for 10 or more days. Thus, split muscle fibers and regenerating muscle fibers fibrillate until nerve terminals innervate them. If reinnervation does not occur, muscle fibers may fibrillate indefinitely. Fibrillation potentials are associated with contractions of individual muscle fibers, but these are not sufficient to produce visible movement.

Muscle fibers may lose their innervation and produce fibrillation potentials by various mechanisms. The most common is damage to or loss of the axon or lower motor neuron innervating the muscle fibers. The death of anterior horn cells; the destruction of nerve roots, plexuses, or peripheral nerves; and the destruction of nerve terminals all result in fibrillation potentials. In each of these, muscle fibers lose their connection with the motor neuron. Blocked conduction of NAPs to muscle fibers alone does not result in fi-brillation.

Fibrillation potentials can also occur with disease of the neuromuscular junction or muscle (Table 26-1). The blocking of neuromuscular transmission by botulinum toxin[18] and the destruction of the postsynaptic elements of the neuromuscular junction can isolate the muscle fiber and result in fibrillation. Direct damage to the muscle fiber, which isolates some portion of the fiber from the remaining innervated portion, may also result in fibrillation.[19]

Fibrillation potentials are usually triphasic (unless initiated at the site of recording), 50 to 300 μV in amplitude, and 1 to 5 ms in duration. Rarely, they may be quite large, up to 1000 μV, or very small, less than 10 μV, if the fibers that generate them are hypertrophied or atrophied, respectively. Rare fibrillation potentials have shapes that are more complex than a triphasic potential. These complex potentials likely arise from time-locked discharges of two fibers or a double discharge of one fiber. The firing pattern is commonly regular, often with a slow increase or decrease in frequency at rates of 0.5 to 10 Hz, but usually at the low end of the range. Some fibrillation potentials have an irregular firing pattern, but usually not until several weeks after the

Table 26-1. MUSCLE DISEASES IN WHICH SPONTANEOUS ACTIVITY CAN OCCUR

Fibrillation potentials	Myotonic discharges	Complex repetitive discharges
Inflammatory myopathies	Inflammatory myopathies	Chronic myositis
Dystrophies	Dystrophies	Duchenne dystrophy
Duchenne	Limb-girdle	Limb-girdle dystrophy
Becker	Distal atrophy	Myxedema
Myotonic	Congenital	Chloroquine myopathy
Congenital	Becker	Local trauma
Distal	Myotonic	Hypothyroid myopathy
Limb-girdle	Altered membrane excitability	
Facioscapulohumeral	Proximal myotonic myopathy	
Altered membrane excitability	Myotonia congenita	
Paramyotonia	Hyperkalemic periodic paralysis	
Hyperkalemic periodic paralysis	Paramyotonia	
Myotonia congenita	Acid maltase deficiency	
Neuromuscular junction disorders	Sarcoid myopathy	
Myasthenia gravis	Centronuclear myopathy	
Botulism	Schwartz-Jampel syndrome	
Metabolic myopathies	Cholesterol-lowering drugs	
Acid maltase deficiency	Traumatic myopathy	
McArdle disease	Myofibrillar myopathy	
Hypothyroid		
Parathyroid		
Carnitine deficiency		
Congenital myopathies		
Centronuclear		
Nemaline		
Desmin storage		
Myotubular		
Mitochondrial		
Other myopathies		
Toxic myopathy		
Cholesterol-lowering agents		
Colchicine		
AZT		
Trichinosis		
Muscle trauma		
Rhabdomyolysis		
Amyloid myopathy		
Sarcoid myopathy		
Late-onset rod myopathy		

onset of fibrillation. In contrast to end plate spikes, even irregular fibrillation potentials do not have interpotential intervals shorter than 70 ms.

Fibrillation potentials occur spontaneously in a muscle fiber that has been denervated for more than 3 weeks, but the rate and amount of fibrillation can be increased by temperature, caffeine, or epinephrine. The shorter the segment of axon attached to the muscle, the shorter the interval from denervation to the appearance of fibrillation potentials, which have been reported as early as 5 days after injury. With the mechanical stimulation of a needle electrode, trains of fibrillation potentials lasting a few seconds can often be initiated in muscle fibers denervated for shorter periods that do not show spontaneous discharges. The duration and number of these mechanically initiated fibrillation potentials increase with time after the loss of innervation. As this irritability of the muscle fibers first appears, many fibers that are mechanically activated are unable to generate a local negative depolarization and produce a positive waveform with the same firing pattern as the spike form of fibrillation potentials. These have been called *positive waves* (Fig. 26-7, *third panel from top*).[20]

Fibrillation potentials with a positive waveform are often seen in muscle diseases in which the muscle fiber membrane is damaged. Positive waves were originally thought to be distinct from the spike form of fibrillation potentials, but they have been shown to be a function of the site of recording and damage to the muscle fiber. Potentials recorded from a damaged area of a muscle fiber have a positive waveform, but those recorded from the undamaged area of the same muscle fiber have a typical triphasic waveform. Thus, positive waves with the firing pattern of fibrillation potentials represent fibrillation potentials recorded from damaged muscle fibers.

Because of the small size of fibrillation potentials, they cannot be recorded with large surface electrodes or macroelectrodes. When recorded with a single-fiber electrode, they have the size and shape of single-fiber potentials from intact motor units. Fibrillation potentials are recorded less commonly with SFEMG than with conventional electrodes because the recording surface of the SFEMG needle is far from its tip, where mechanical activation occurs.

Myotonic discharges. Myotonic discharges, another important form of spontaneous activity in muscle disease, are also generated by single muscle fibers and, like fibrillation potentials, have two waveforms (Fig. 26-2, *panel 4*). If they are recorded from a damaged area of the muscle fiber, the potentials are positive, but if recorded elsewhere, they are triphasic and generally have the same amplitude and duration as fibrillation potentials. They differ from fibrillation potentials in their rate and pattern of firing. The rate is more rapid, ranging from 2 to 100 Hz, and is more variable than that of fibrillation potentials. Most commonly, the discharge rate decelerates, often from more than 50 Hz to less than 10 Hz. However, it may also increase from 10 to 20 Hz up to 40 to 50 Hz.[21] Occasionally, a single potential increases and then decreases its rate (or vice versa).

Concomitant with the change in firing rate, the myotonic discharges often simultaneously change in amplitude, increasing or decreasing up to tenfold. Some potentials show sequential increases and decreases, usually not in direct relation to the change in firing rate. Such discharges, like fibrillation potentials, are recorded most readily with standard needle electrodes, but they can also be recorded with single-fiber electrodes.

Myotonic discharges can result from alterations in the ion channels of the muscle fiber membrane, and they can be produced by changes in more than one ion channel. Like fibrillation potentials, they can also occur after denervation of a muscle fiber, usually many months after denervation. They also occur in a number of other disorders and hence are not specific for any single disease (Table 26-1).[22]

Complex repetitive discharges. These are the third major type of spontaneous discharge that occurs in muscle disease. In the past, they were called "pseudomyotonic discharges," "bizarre high-frequency discharges," and "bizarre repetitive potentials" (Fig. 26-2, *panel 5*).[23] Currently, the accepted term is *complex repetitive discharge* (CRD). CRDs are made up of the discharges of a group of muscle fibers firing together through ephaptic activation. CRDs fire regularly at rates of 2 to 60 Hz, but most commonly at 30 to 40 Hz.[23] CRD rates are more constant than myotonic discharges and show only a slight increase or decrease in frequency before ending abruptly. The configuration depends on the firing synchrony of the individual muscle fibers that contribute to the discharge. Occasionally, individual muscle fibers are not activated, resulting in intermittent loss of single spikes from the CRD. SFEMG of CRDs (see below) shows an absence of jitter between individual components. CRDs are nonspecific, but they are seen most commonly in chronic disorders. Rarely are CRDs present in chronic inflammatory myopathy in sufficient number to produce dystonic postures.[24]

Other spontaneous discharges. Several other spontaneous discharges generated in the lower motor neuron are seen only rarely in primary muscle disease. *Fasciculation potentials* are spontaneous discharges of single motor neurons. They occur because of irritability anywhere along the neuron or its axon. They are most common in amyotrophic lateral sclerosis, but some frequently occur in normal persons and can occur in muscle disease. *Myokymic discharges* are bursts of 2 to 10 MUPs firing at 5 to 60 Hz, which recur regularly at 0.2- to 10-s intervals (Fig. 26-8). They arise in the peripheral part of an axon of a chronically damaged nerve and are associated with clinical myokymia or syndromes of continuous muscle fiber contraction. Myokymia occurs in several brainstem diseases, especially radiation damage and multiple sclerosis, and in chronic peripheral nerve disorders.[25–27] *Neuromyotonic discharges* are trains or bursts of high-frequency discharges at 150 to 300 Hz, which occur in disorders of nerve fibers, especially the nerve terminals, such as tetany and Isaac syndrome (Fig. 26-9).[28–31] *Neurotonic discharges* are similar to neuromyotonic discharges due to mechanical stimulation of axons during surgery. Various other spontaneous, repetitive discharges with a multiplicity of waveforms and firing patterns can occur. They are classified in the broad category of *iterative discharges*; they may be found in several chronic neurogenic processes and some inherited disorders (Fig. 26-10).[32]

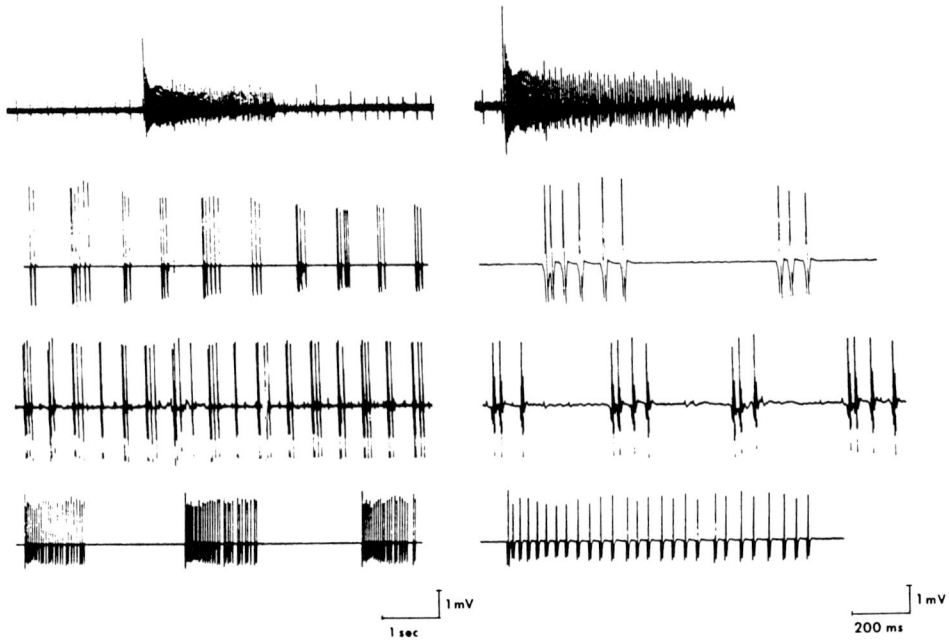

FIGURE 26-8. Myokymic discharges. Various patterns of discharge are illustrated.

Abnormal Motor Unit Potentials

Altered MUP size. Diseases can affect either the appearance or the recruitment of MUPs. Changes in size or shape (or both) of MUPs are the most common findings in myopathy. If the action potentials of individual muscle fibers become smaller because of atrophy or if there are fewer muscle fibers from a motor unit within the recording area of the electrode due to inactivation or destruction of individual fibers, the MUP will become smaller in both amplitude and duration.[33] The *MUP amplitude* reflects primarily the potentials of the nearby muscle fibers, whereas the *MUP duration* depends on both those near the recording electrode and those at some distance. Generally, both amplitude and duration decrease together. Hypertrophied muscle fibers or an increase in the number of muscle fibers in a motor unit within the recording area result in a large MUP. Decomposition analysis of the EMG waveforms may provide a more efficient and reliable method to identify abnormalities,[34] but direct comparisons of automated systems with manual/auditory testing have not borne out this promise.[35] Duration may increase without an increase in amplitude if there is loss of synchrony of muscle fiber activation. Automated computer analysis of MUPs suggests that the ratio

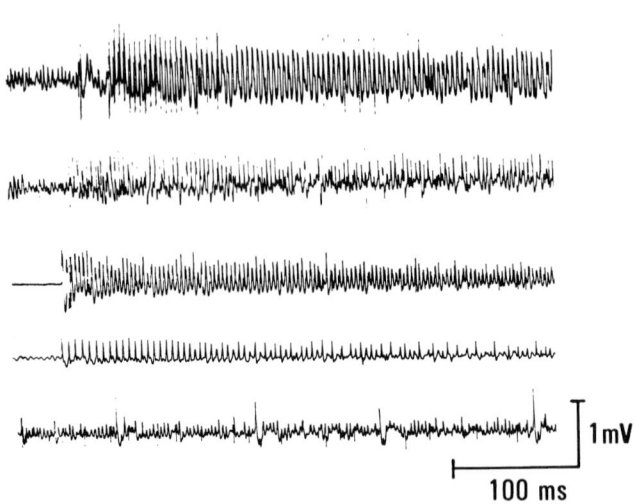

FIGURE 26-9. Neurotonic discharges recorded from spinal muscular atrophy and syndromes of continuous muscle fiber activity. Discharge rates of individual spikes are 200 to 300 Hz.

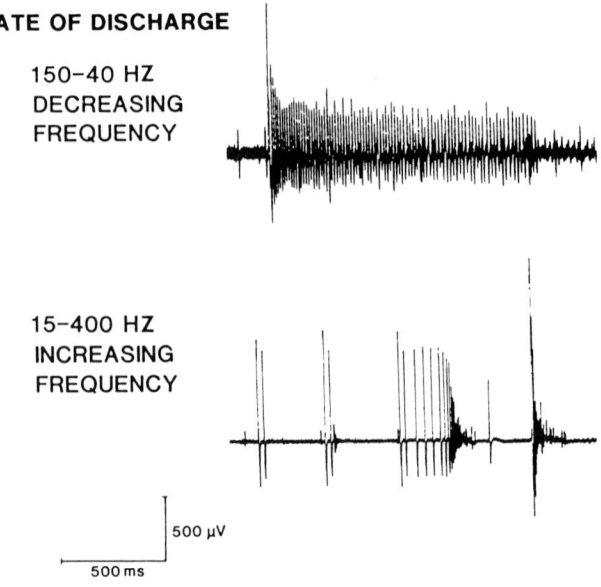

FIGURE 26-10. Iterative discharges with decreasing (top) and increasing (bottom) frequency of firing during the discharge.

of MUP area to amplitude may be a more reliable indicator of muscle disease.

In many disorders of muscle, the major MUP abnormalities are decreases in amplitude and duration. Such potentials have been referred to as "myopathic" but should not be, because similar potentials can occur with neurogenic disorders and disturbances and neuromuscular transmission.[36] For instance, after severe denervation, only a few denervated muscle fibers may become reinnervated. These will generate short-duration or low-amplitude (or both) MUPs. Another example is peripheral nerve disease that selectively involves the distal nerve terminals; this results in a smaller number of fibers contributing to the MUP, thus decreasing the duration and amplitude of the MUP.[36-38] Therefore it is better to describe the type of alteration in the MUP and to interpret the finding in the context of the associated clinical and electrodiagnostic findings. This is especially important because long-duration MUPs occur in some muscle diseases.

The MUP amplitude or duration (or both) is usually decreased in muscle disease, but in some instances amplitude and duration are increased.[39,40] The size of the MUP depends primarily on the number of muscle fibers in the recording area of the electrode and their firing synchrony. If fiber density increases through fiber splitting or regeneration and firing synchrony is maintained, the MUP increases in amplitude and duration. Usually, the firing synchrony of fibers is poor after regeneration and only an increase in polyphasic MUPs occurs. Long-duration MUPs are more likely to occur in chronic disorders. Because various mechanisms can produce both large and small MUPs in either muscle or nerve disease, it is not unexpected that both of these changes can occur in some disorders. In such cases, it becomes doubly important to evaluate the statistical distribution of amplitudes and durations. The mean values may show little change, but the range of distribution of the values will be much wider. Rarely, the amplitudes or durations of MUPs have a bimodal distribution. The MUP "territory" is the area in a muscle over which the MUP can be recorded with a short rise time. This is determined by measuring the distance of needle movement over which a MUP can be recorded. Changes in territory are caused primarily by alterations in the size of the potentials rather than by a change in the anatomic area in which the fibers of the motor unit are distributed.[3]

Altered recruitment. *Reduction in recruitment* is a hallmark of neurogenic disorders.[41] However, it can occur in a severe myopathy if all the muscle fibers of some motor units are lost. In this case, the ratio of the rate of firing of an individual MUP to the number of active MUPs increases. A more common pattern of MUP firing detected in myopathy is "rapid recruitment," in which the ratio remains unchanged but the number of MUPs relative to the effort is increased. Thus, minimal effort in a myopathy is often associated with the firing of many MUPs. Another pattern of firing is called *poor activation*, in which the rate of MUP firing is less than 10 Hz with maximal effort. Poor activation is typical of central disorders.

Altered MUP configuration. Changes in the shape of the MUP are the most common MUP change in muscle diseases. If the muscle fibers in a motor unit do not fire synchronously because of fiber atrophy or other abnormality, the potentials from individual muscle fibers are spread out in time to produce a MUP with multiple phases. A MUP with more than four phases is *polyphasic*, in which a phase is defined as the portion of the potential between baseline crossings. There is always one more phase than there are baseline crossings. Occasional polyphasic MUPs occur in normal muscle; thus, an excess of polyphasic MUPs must be defined in relation to the percentage of polyphasic MUPs in a comparable normal muscle. Polyphasic MUPs may result from several pathophysiologic mechanisms that produce loss of synchrony of muscle fiber potentials. With the destruction and regeneration of muscle fibers in a myopathy, the end plate sites may become more dispersed than normal. If the terminal nerve branches innervating the muscle fibers were of sufficiently different lengths or different conduction velocities, synchrony of activation would be lost and polyphasic potentials would occur. Because muscle fiber conduction velocity is normally slow (3 to 5 m/s) and this velocity is proportional to fiber diameter, the loss of synchrony of firing of muscle fibers and polyphasic MUPs are more likely to occur with an alteration in muscle fiber diameter than with a change in the axon.[36] Polyphasic MUPs may also occur with an increase in the number of muscle fibers in the region of the recording electrode, as could occur with segmental fiber destruction, longitudinal fiber splitting, or regeneration of muscle fibers.

A MUP characteristic closely related to the number of phases is the number of *turns*, or reversals of polarity of the potential. Each phase has at least one turn, but there may be many turns in a phase if a reversal does not cross the baseline (Fig. 26-4). Turns, like phases, are generated by the potentials of single muscle fibers and occur for the same reasons as increased phases. Smaller losses of synchrony of firing result in the generation of a phase rather than a turn. Turns are a normal finding; an increased proportion of turns is necessary to identify an abnormality.

Muscle fiber potentials time-locked to MUPs but completely separated from them have been called *parasite, linked*, or *satellite potentials* (the last is the accepted term). They result from either a very slow muscle fiber conduction velocity or an end plate far from other end plates in the motor unit. These potentials are rare in normal muscle and are evidence of disease only if they occur with a higher-than-normal incidence. The duration of a MUP is usually measured from the point at which the potential first leaves the baseline to the point at which it returns to the baseline. For this reason, measurements of the duration usually exclude satellite potentials.[42] Because it would be equally valid to include satellite potentials in these measurements, the electromyographer must specify the method used when reporting measurements of MUP duration.

MUP Variation. Each characteristic discussed above can be measured in a single MUP; stability cannot. In normal muscle, each muscle fiber in a motor unit is activated each time a motor neuron fires. The size and shape of MUPs remain constant during the repeated firing of normal voluntary activity. In some diseases, MUP variation is seen if not all of the muscle fibers are activated each time. This occurs if there is intermittent block of conduction in the nerve termi-

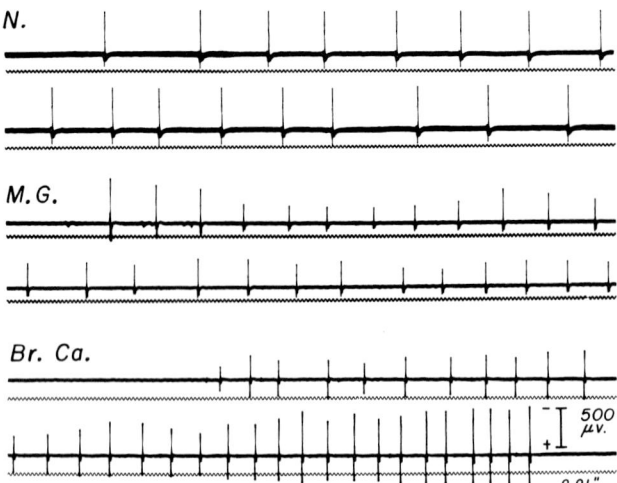

FIGURE 26-11. Variation in MUP amplitude during voluntary activation in myasthenia gravis (M.G.) and Lambert-Eaton myasthenic syndrome (Br. Ca.). N = normal subject. Note the gradual MUP decline in myasthenia gravis and gradual MUP increase in bronchogenic carcinoma (Br. Ca.) after initiation of activity. *(From Lambert EH: Defects of neuromuscular transmission in syndromes other than myasthenia gravis. Ann N Y Acad Sci 135:367–384, 1966. With permission from the New York Academy of Sciences.)*

nal or at the neuromuscular junction. The MUP then varies from moment to moment as the number of muscle fibers contributing to it change (Fig. 26-11). The variation in MUP shape has been termed "jiggle" and can be quantified.[34,43] A block in the transmission of the action potential along the muscle fiber occurs in muscle membrane disorders such as the periodic paralyses or myotonic disorders. This is seen as a gradual change in MUP configuration rather than a moment-to-moment variation.

Other firing pattern abnormalities. Alterations in MUP firing pattern are much less significant than changes in MUP configuration or recruitment. MUPs under voluntary control are activated semirhythmically, in which changes in activation rate (or interpotential interval) occur in a regular fashion. At the onset of voluntary contraction, MUPs may discharge twice, with a short (20- to 30-ms) interpotential interval, a *double discharge*.[16] MUPs with short interpotential intervals (less than 20 ms), *doublets* or *multiplets*, are caused by abnormal irritability of the lower motor neuron, most commonly in the distal axon. Either the spikes in a doublet are identical or the second one is slightly smaller if it occurs when some fibers in the motor unit are still refractory. Doublets and multiplets occur in a semirhythmic pattern under voluntary control. They rarely occur in muscle disease, but they must be differentiated from polyphasic MUPs. Tremor stemming from central nervous system disorders, such as Parkinson disease, may produce MUPs that resemble polyphasic MUPs. Tremor occurs with the synchrony of firing of two or more motor units, resulting in summation of their MUPs and an apparently abnormal polyphasic potential. Tremor potentials can be distinguished from polyphasic MUPs by the variable appearance of the former.

In clinical studies, MUP variables are reliably assessed subjectively at low levels of effort, producing single MUPs. Low levels of effort activate primarily type 1 motor units, which generate smaller MUPs than type 2 motor units. Automated methods are improving the accuracy of the procedure but still provide only a 50 percent concordance with visual assessment.

Stronger contractions activate multiple motor units, unpredictably summating MUPs that cannot be analyzed individually (Fig. 26-6). This complex *interference pattern* can be measured by a turns-amplitude analysis[44] or by frequency analysis. Recently developed computer methods of fast Fourier transform have provided rapid frequency analyses that may become of clinical value. Well-defined changes have been shown to occur in the *frequency distribution* of the EMG signal with both muscle and nerve disease. In primary muscle diseases, the high-frequency components are increased. Mixed myopathies and neurogenic changes, alterations with disease duration, or mild disease cannot be demonstrated with frequency analysis. Comparison of interference analysis with single MUP measurements shows comparable and complementary accuracy up to 80 percent in simply identifying the presence of a myopathy. Simpler methods of interference pattern analysis that provide similar information have also been described.

SINGLE FIBER ELECTROMYOGRAPHY

Standard needle EMG records the potentials within 0.5 mm of the electrode, an area that includes a number of individual muscle fibers. SFEMG is designed to isolate the potentials from individual muscle fibers. For most myopathies, the electrical characteristics of individual muscle fibers have not been found to be of clinical diagnostic value, but they are important in helping to characterize abnormalities of the neuromuscular junction, as described below.[45-47]

In SFEMG recordings, action potentials of individual muscle fibers are isolated by using a small recording surface 25 μm in diameter and filtering frequency components less than 500 Hz generated by distant muscle fibers.[3] SFEMG samples the same activity as EMG with standard needle electrodes, but isolation of single-fiber potentials permits precise measurement of variables unique to the neuromuscular junction. These include jitter or interpotential interval variation, blocking, and fiber density. *Jitter* is defined as the mean consecutive difference (MCD) of a series of 50 or more interpotential intervals. MCD is equal to the standard deviation of a series of interpotential intervals multiplied by 1.13.[48]

A muscle fiber action potential is triggered by the end plate potential (EPP) generated by ACh released from the nerve terminal. Changes in the rates of ACh synthesis and release that occur with activity normally result in EPPs of varying amplitude. Because all EPPs in normal muscle are well above threshold for activation of the muscle fiber (safety factor), each EPP always activates a muscle fiber potential. The summated single muscle fiber potentials in a MUP thus remain unchanged during continued firing and the MUPs do not vary in size or shape.

The variation in EPP amplitude in both normal and abnormal muscle does produce a change that can be measured with SFEMG.[49] Because the rate of rise of the EPP is proportional to its size, a small EPP reaches threshold later than a larger one. Thus, the latency of individual muscle fiber potentials varies slightly with changes in EPP amplitude.

This variation in latency can be measured as a change in the time interval between the potentials of two muscle fibers in a motor unit and is called *jitter* (Fig. 26-12). In normal muscle, jitter is very small, ranging from 15 to 60 μs, with a mean of approximately 30 μs. Jitter varies with age, muscle, and temperature and increases in any disorder of the neuromuscular junction that decreases EPP amplitude.

When the EPP of a muscle fiber becomes subthreshold, the fiber action potential is blocked and the MUP changes in size. This intermittent firing of single-fiber potentials is called *blocking*. In normal muscle, blocking does not occur except, rarely, in elderly persons. If blocking is present, it (like jitter) can be measured quantitatively with SFEMG. Jitter is not seen with standard needle EMG; blocking is the SFEMG concomitant of variation in MUPs referred to as *jiggle*.

Recordings made with a single-fiber electrode sample a much smaller area than those made with standard needle electrodes. It has been estimated that SFEMG effectively records the potentials from fibers within 200 μm of the electrode. In normal muscle, most areas of this size contain only one muscle fiber innervated by a single motor unit. Approximately 30 percent of the areas contain two muscle fibers, and 5 to 10 percent contain three muscle fibers (Fig 26-12A). The number of fibers within the recording area of a single-fiber electrode can be counted in multiple areas and a mean calculated. This is called the *fiber density*. Normal fiber density ranges from 1.5 to 2.0 but varies with age and muscle. Fiber density is related most directly to the turns of a MUP recorded with standard EMG electrodes, but it also is proportional to the number of phases. Increases in fiber density occur by the same mechanisms that result in polyphasic MUPs. Increased fiber density has been reported in several myopathies, including type I hypertrophy, acid maltase deficiency, limb-girdle dystrophy, and polymyositis with normal findings in the central core disease, phosphorylase deficiency, myotonia congenita, and hypokalemic periodic paralysis.[50]

Standard SFEMG measures jitter in pairs of voluntarily activated muscle fibers. Jitter can also be measured from single muscle fibers activated by nerve stimulation, *stimulated SFEMG*.[49] Stimulated SFEMG has different technical problems and lower normal values than standard SFEMG, but it can be particularly useful in the presence of tremor, in children, and in patients in an intensive care unit.[51–53]

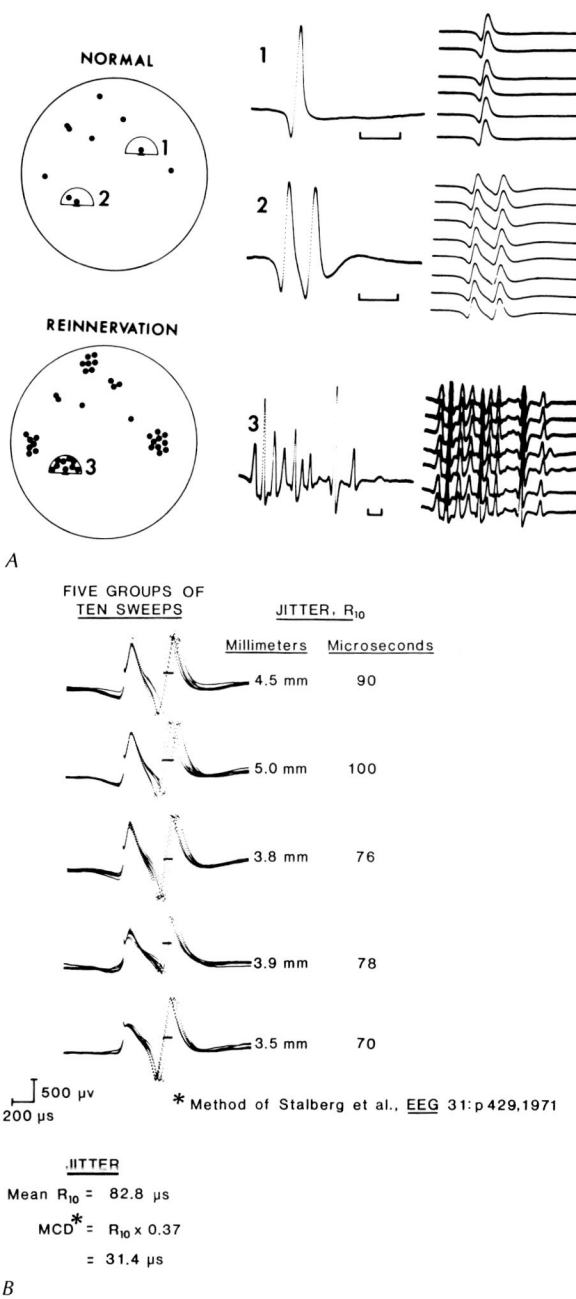

FIGURE 26-12. A. SFEMG recordings with single pairs and multiple single fiber potentials recorded from one motor unit at one site. Tracings at the right show repetitive sweeps of the same potentials. B. Manual method of jitter measurement. R_{10} = range of 10; MCD = mean consecutive difference. (A. from Stålberg E, Trontelj JV: Single Fibre Electromyography, Old Woking, Surrey, UK: Miravalle Press, 1979. With permission from the publisher. B. from Members of the Department of Neurology and the Department of Physiology and Biophysics, Mayo Clinic and Mayo Foundation for Medical Education and Research: Clinical Examinations in Neurology, 5th ed. Philadelphia: Saunders, 1981; p 325. With permission from Mayo Foundation.)

OTHER ELECTROMYOGRAPHIC RECORDINGS

The electrical activity of muscles has been recorded with several varieties of other electrodes, both needle and surface electrodes, that sample larger areas of the muscle. A *macro-EMG* needle electrode records the averaged activity along 15 mm of a needle electrode shaft in a muscle. The activity from a single motor unit is obtained by averaging shaft activity that occurs time-locked with a single fiber potential recorded with an SFEMG electrode located on the macroelectrode.[54] Because MUPs recorded with macroelectrodes are from a much larger proportion of the muscle fibers in the motor unit, they better depict changes in the whole motor unit. Macro-EMG needles record lower-amplitude MUPs if there are fewer muscle fibers in the motor unit, as in muscle disease, and higher-amplitude MUPs if there are more muscle fibers in the motor unit, as in neurogenic disorders. MUP amplitude also increases or decreases with muscle fiber diameter and the size of single muscle fiber potentials. MUP configuration varies with scatter of the end plate region, as do turns and phases in standard recordings. Standard electrodes and macroelectrodes demonstrate different types of changes in disease not seen with either technique alone. For instance, in disorders with prominent local regeneration and reinnervation but with loss of fibers elsewhere, standard electrodes may show polyphasic, long-duration MUPs, whereas macroelectrodes would reflect the overall loss of fibers as small MUPs.[55] Although macroelectrodes and standard concentric electrode recordings show different aspects of motor unit physiology, they have similar sensitivity in identifying myopathies.[56]

Surface recordings summate the activity not only from multiple muscle fibers but also from multiple motor units and multiple muscles in a fashion that precludes the assessment of individual components. Frequency analysis of surface EMG signals has demonstrated differences between myopathic and neurogenic processes, but with less precision than interference pattern studies with needle electrodes.[57] Thus, the application of surface electrode recordings has been limited to kinesiologic studies that gauge the presence and amount of EMG activity with movement. Turns-amplitude analysis of needle EMG recordings is a simplified form of frequency analysis that has been shown to differentiate a myopathy from a neurogenic process.[58,59]

Less commonly used methods have shown central inhibitory changes in motor control in myopathies that can serve to compensate for loss of muscle power.[60] Recently developed multielectrode surface recordings have recorded MUPs from the skin surface and have demonstrated their spread from the end plate region to the tendon. The clinical applications remain to be proven, but some remarkable new information has already been obtained for cramps and disorders of muscle membrane (see below).

NERVE AND MUSCLE STIMULATION

Neuromuscular diseases can also be assessed by their responses to electrical and magnetic stimulation. Peripheral nerve stimulation evokes motor and sensory nerve action potentials that are altered in diseases of nerve and muscle. Nerve conduction studies (NCSs) measure motor and sensory amplitudes, latencies, and velocities to identify and describe neuropathies and occasionally show changes in muscle diseases. Responses to repetitive motor nerve stimulation help to distinguish disorders of neuromuscular transmission. Motor nerve stimulation is also applied in measurements of the number of motor units in a muscle. Direct stimulation of muscle evokes potentials in groups of muscle fibers or in single muscle fibers that are altered in some muscle diseases.

Nerve Conduction Studies

NCSs apply electrical stimuli to a motor or sensory nerve to activate the axons in the nerve.[61] With a supramaximal stimulus that activates all motor axons, all the fibers in the innervated muscles generate nearly synchronous action potentials that summate to produce a CMAP. The CMAP recorded with an electrode in or over the muscle is 2 to 25 mV in amplitude. It is the most readily recordable potential in electrodiagnosis.

The size and shape of the CMAP depend on the number of muscle fibers activated, the size of the muscle fibers, their synchrony of firing, the distance of the muscle fibers from the recording electrode, and the temperature of the muscle. Because most muscles innervated by a single nerve are adjacent to one another, the CMAP recorded over a muscle usually includes contributions from adjacent muscles. This increases the CMAP amplitude and adds irregularities to its waveform. Low temperature *slows* the ionic flow through membrane channels, prolongs the potentials of individual nerve and muscle fibers, and increases the duration and amplitude and, hence, the area of the CMAP.

The CMAP gauges the number of muscle fibers in a muscle. If the location of the recording electrode, the age of the subject, and the temperature of the muscle are constant, the *area* and *amplitude* of the CMAP reflect the number, size, density, and synchrony of firing of the muscle fibers. The area of the CMAP is more directly proportional to the number of muscle fibers than its amplitude, whereas the amplitude of the CMAP more directly reflects the synchrony of firing of the muscle fibers. Loss of synchrony of firing by spread of the end plate regions, differences in conduction velocity of individual muscle fibers, or disease in the nerve fibers disperses the response and decreases the amplitude but not the area of the CMAP (Fig. 26-13, *line 2*). The destruction of axons or muscle fibers and impairment of activation of nerve or muscle fibers decreases the amplitude and area of the CMAP (Fig. 26-13, *line 3*).

The range of normal CMAP amplitudes is so broad that an individual muscle may lose up to half of its fibers before an abnormality of the CMAP can be recognized. Nonetheless, measurement of CMAP amplitudes should be a standard part of the electrodiagnostic testing of a patient with muscle disease. As long as it is recalled that diseases of the motor neuron, nerve, and neuromuscular junction as well as of muscle can reduce the CMAP amplitude, this measurement can be a useful index of the amount of functioning muscle. Measurement of the amount of functioning muscle independent of nerve is not possible, because direct stimulation of muscle cannot reliably activate the whole muscle. Direct stimulation of muscle, as used in strength-duration curve testing, however, can provide an example of the relative amounts of innervated and denervated muscle.

The electrical activation of a muscle results in a contraction that produces the force needed for strength and movement. The force of muscle contraction is not usually measured in electrodiagnostic studies, and muscle diseases that impair the generation of force but spare the electrical response are not detected with standard electrodiagnostic testing.[62] Thus, complete physiologic assessment of the neuromuscular system requires simultaneous measurement of the force and the electrical potentials generated.

The *configuration* of the CMAP can change with several technical and physiologic factors. If electrodes move at the site of stimulation or recording, the CMAP will be altered. A change in conduction velocity of the nerve or muscle fiber can affect the latency and the shape of the potential. Repetitive discharges of the CMAP can occur if there is irritability of the nerve, neuromuscular junction, or muscle. Such spontaneous, repetitive discharges are usually separated by short (3- to 15-ms) intervals.

Chapter 26. Electrodiagnosis of Muscle Disorders

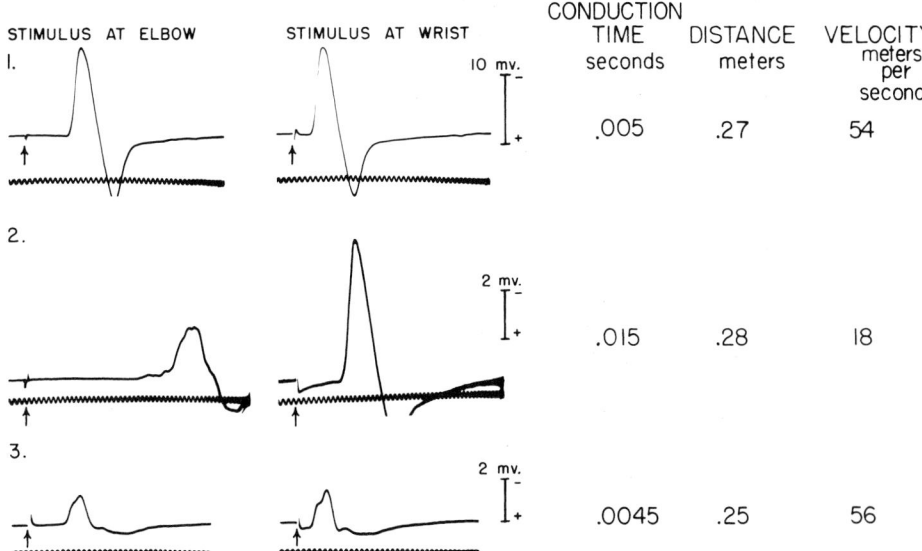

FIGURE 26-13. Measurement of CMAP amplitude and nerve conduction velocity by ulnar nerve stimulation and hypothenar muscle recording. (1) Normal. (2) Neuropathy. (3) Dermatomyositis. Note the dispersion and reduction in CMAP with proximal stimulation in neuropathy and the low-amplitude responses at both sites of stimulation in myositis. *(From Members of the Department of Neurology and the Department of Physiology and Biophysics, Mayo Clinic and Mayo Foundation for Medical Education and Research: Clinical Examinations in Neurology, 6th ed. St. Louis, Mosby–Year Book, 1991; p 428. With permission from Mayo Foundation.)*

The CMAP latency, the time from stimulus to potential, is typically measured in NCSs. This is designated *distal latency* if the stimulus is distal and *proximal latency* if the stimulus is proximal. The latency includes the times required for (1) nerve activation (a very small fraction of the total), (2) conduction of the action potentials along the axons to the muscle, (3) neuromuscular transmission (fraction of a millisecond), and (4) muscle activation (less than one-tenth of a millisecond). Most of the latency is required for conduction of the action potential along the nerve (nerve latency). Nerve latency depends on nerve function and is not altered in pure muscle disease. Compound NAPs have many of the same characteristics as CMAPs but are not altered with muscle damage.

The major application of nerve stimulation and CMAP recording in NCSs is the assessment of peripheral nerve function. Because most of the latency of a CMAP is the time required for the action potential to travel from the site of stimulation to the neuromuscular junction, latency is prolonged in many diseases of peripheral nerve.[63] The rate of action potential conduction along the nerve, *conduction velocity*, is calculated from the distance traversed and the time to traverse it. The calculation is valid only if the times of activation, neuromuscular transmission, and distal latency are not included. Thus, the usual conduction velocity measurement is over a segment of nerve between two sites of stimulation. Conduction velocity calculated from the latency difference between proximal and distal stimulation sites provides an excellent estimate of motor or sensory axon function in peripheral nerve. Conduction velocity measurement has proved useful for the identification of many localized or generalized peripheral nerve diseases and is useful in excluding the presence of certain types of neurogenic process in the evaluation of myopathies.

Repetitive Stimulation Testing

Repetitive stimulation is used to assess the integrity of neuromuscular transmission.[45,64] An increase or decrease in the area of a CMAP with repetitive stimulation identifies activation of more or fewer muscle fibers. Depending on the frequency of stimulation, the amplitude normal EPPs decreases during repetitive stimulation because the immediately available store of ACh is decreased. The amplitude of the normal EPP is well above the muscle fiber threshold, thereby providing a safety factor that prevents the decreasing EPP from becoming subthreshold and causing a decrement in CMAP during repetitive stimulation. If the amplitude of the EPP in rested muscle fibers is decreased to near threshold by disease, the further decrease with repetitive activation results in a block of neuromuscular transmission in an increasing proportion of the fibers and a progressive decrement in the amplitude of the CMAP (Fig. 26-14). The reduction of EPP

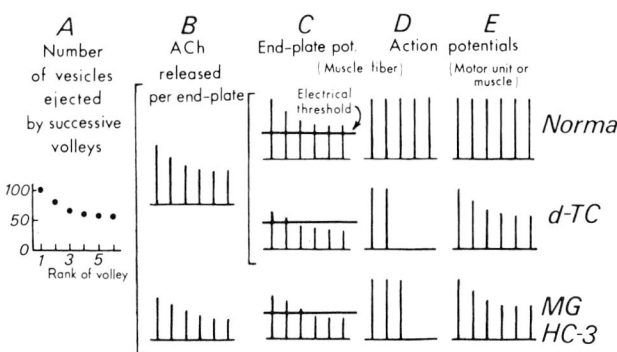

FIGURE 26-14. Scheme of the decrement in EPPs and CMAP that occurs with presynaptic (d-TC = d-tubocurare) and postsynaptic disorders (MG = magnesium, HC-3 = hemicholinium). Note that in normal muscle the EPPs have a decrement but remain above threshold, so that no decrement in CMAP occurs (safety factor). *(From Desmedt JE: The neuromuscular disorder in myasthenia gravis: II. Presynaptic cholinergic metabolism, myasthenic-like syndromes and a hypothesis, in Desmedt JE (ed): New Developments in Electromyography and Clinical Neurophysiology. Vol 1. Basel: Karger, 1973; p 321. With permission from the publisher.)*

amplitude is maximal at stimulation rates of 2 to 5 Hz. At these rates, the CMAP area and amplitude generally do not change in normal muscle, but a decrement occurs with presynaptic or postsynaptic disorders of neuromuscular transmission. The maximal reduction typically occurs between the first two potentials of a train, with smaller reductions between subsequent potentials and stabilization by the fourth or fifth potential. If mobilization of ACh in the nerve terminal is sufficient, the amplitude may increase after the fifth potential. In normal subjects, stimulation greater than 20 Hz causes an increase of up to 20 percent in amplitude, a decrease in duration, but no change in the area of the CMAP.

With disease, stimulation at 20 to 50 Hz may either decrease or increase CMAP amplitude. If neuromuscular transmission is partially blocked, facilitation of ACh release may increase the EPP and CMAP amplitudes. Rapid rates of stimulation may block axonal conduction, which will decrease CMAP amplitude. Nerve and muscle fibers become refractory at rates of stimulation faster than 50 and 300 Hz, respectively; they either do not respond or produce lower-amplitude responses. Disease of nerve, especially of the terminal axon, can increase the refractory period, so that stimulation at even 10 to 40 Hz decreases the CMAP. Infrequently, primary muscle disease may result in an abnormality of membrane activation that is reflected in a decrement on repetitive stimulation.

Exercise, ischemia, and curare have been used in conjunction with repetitive stimulation to identify mild abnormalities of neuromuscular transmission. Exercise enhances the release of ACh from a nerve terminal for a few seconds and depletes presynaptic ACh stores for a few minutes. Thus, the amplitude of the EPP and CMAP is increased during the first 2 min after exercise (*postactivation facilitation*) but decreases between 2 and 15 min after exercise (*postactivation exhaustion*). A decrement is less prominent or is repaired during postactivation facilitation and is increased during postactivation exhaustion (Fig. 26-15). Postsynaptic disorders may show either phenomenon, with postactivation exhaustion usually more prominent. In presynaptic disorders with normal stores but impaired release of ACh, there is marked facilitation of the CMAP amplitude immediately after exercise. In the congenital myasthenic disorder associated with impaired acetylcholine resynthesis, the CMAP amplitude falls abnormally during sustained exercise or subtetanic stimulation for 5 to 10 min and then remains decreased for 5 to 15 min.

Ischemia and *curare* both reduce the safety factor for neuromuscular transmission. Curare partially blocks postsynaptic acetylcholine receptors, and ischemia may reduce the release of ACh from the nerve terminal. A greater-than-normal decrease in the amplitude of the first evoked CMAP or a greater-than-normal CMAP decrement during repetitive stimulation under these conditions indicates a defect of neuromuscular transmission but does not localize it to the presynaptic or postsynaptic site. Both tests require careful definition of normal values and are more time-consuming than standard tests.

The response of a CMAP to *prolonged exercise* can provide information about total stores of ACh in the nerve terminal and the functional integrity of the muscle fiber membrane. More specific testing for disorders of the muscle fiber membrane can be obtained with an *epinephrine test*.[65,66] The intraarterial injection of epinephrine increases glucose metabolism, produces potassium shifts, and secondarily decreases the amplitude of CMAPs in primary hypokalemic periodic paralysis.

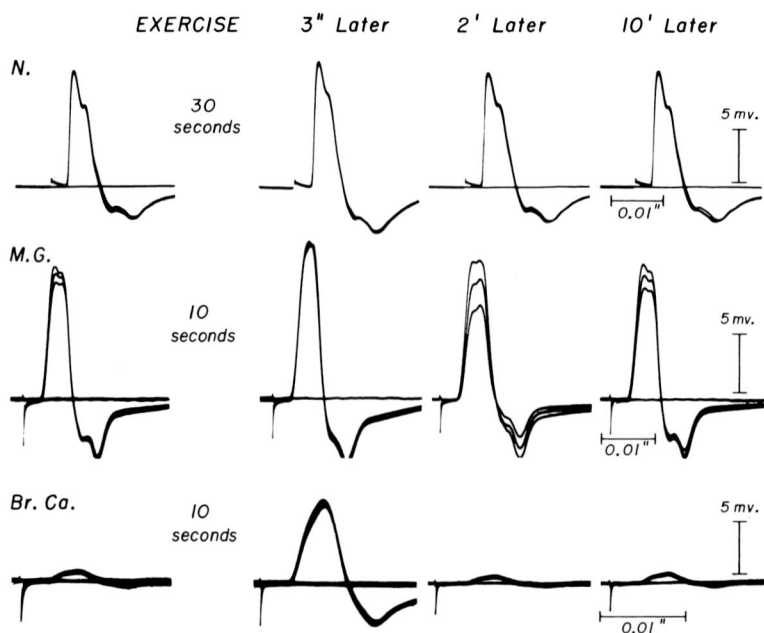

FIGURE 26-15. Examples of the repair of CMAP decrement immediately after exercise (postactivation facilitation) and enhancement of a decrement later after exercise (postactivation exhaustion) in myasthenia gravis and amyotrophic lateral sclerosis. N = normal muscle; M. G., myasthenia gravis; Br. Ca., bronchogenic carcinoma. *(From Lambert EH: Neurophysiologic techniques useful in the study of neuromuscular disorders, in Adams R (ed): Neuromuscular Disorders. Baltimore: Williams & Wilkins, 1960. With permission from the publisher.)*

A decrement of the CMAP during repetitive stimulation or in the course of special tests indicates that some of the muscle fibers are not activated. This could be caused by a defect in the sarcolemmal membrane, the neuromuscular junction, or the nerve terminal.

Motor Unit Number Estimates

A single anterior horn cell innervates from 50 to 2000 muscle fibers via a peripheral nerve axon and its terminal branches. The synchronous activation of the muscle fibers produces a MUP, which usually is activated voluntarily but can be activated by selective stimulation of single motor axons. Carefully graded stimulation and high amplification permits the recording of all-or-none responses of single motor units.[67] The ratio of the amplitude of the maximal CMAP to the mean amplitude of single motor units provides a reproducible estimate of the number of motor units in a muscle.[68-70] Motor unit number estimates (MUNE) may show a loss of lower motor neurons in a neurogenic process when the amplitude of the CMAP remains normal because of reinnervation of muscle fibers through collateral sprouting of intramuscular nerves. MUNE can demonstrate a normal number of motor units in a myopathy when CMAPs are low because of loss of muscle fibers. Small MUPs in a myopathy can make MUNE more technically difficult.

Various methods have been reported for selectively activating single motor units, including incremental stimulation, multipoint stimulation, F-wave recording, and statistical estimates.[71] Activation of single surface motor unit potentials (SMUPs) with intramuscular needle electrodes near the nerve terminals allows simultaneous measurement of SMUPs and the force generated by a motor unit.[72] The twitch duration in the force recording allows the fiber type of the motor unit to be identified.

Other Stimulation Methods

Direct muscle stimulation. Small groups of fibers can be activated directly with an intramuscular electrode to measure the muscle fiber conduction velocity of the muscle fibers, recorded at a fixed distance along the fibers. This is usually in the range of 3 to 5 m/s.[3,73] These velocity measurements are nonspecific because they are abnormal in most myopathies.[74] Direct muscle stimulation has been helpful in distinguishing quadriplegic myopathy from critical illness neuropathy[75] and identifying unsuspected myopathies.[76]

Nerve accommodation testing. Recently developed methods of testing peripheral nerve excitability, threshold, and accommodation have shown differences among some disorders, but none of these methods has demonstrated any clinical usefulness.[77]

Findings in Muscle Diseases

Each of the abnormal electrical potentials described in the preceding section is a nonspecific finding that may occur in multiple disorders. However, the patterns and combinations of these findings provide the electromyographer with a basis for a clinical diagnosis. Both the types of abnormal potentials and their distribution in the patient are important for the electromyographic diagnosis. The EMG and NCS data usually are not sufficient to identify a specific disease, but the pattern of findings in a patient can be associated with groups of disorders that can be listed. The overlap between muscle diseases in children and adults is extensive, with many disorders of childhood onset persisting into adulthood and some disorders that are subclinical in childhood becoming manifest in adulthood. Other reviews have defined the electrodiagnostic features of childhood muscle diseases, and this chapter does not review them separately.[78]

Although EMG and NCS may provide nonspecific data, they still are the most common screening procedures for myopathies and important techniques for assessing the course of myopathy over time.[79] EMG/NCS can confirm an impression based on other clinical and laboratory findings, can suggest disorders that had not been considered in the differential diagnosis, and can characterize the severity and distribution of the disorder. The accessibility of multiple muscles and nerves to EMG examination provides advantages over biochemical studies that sample sera and histologic studies that usually sample single selected sites. EMG is an aid to the clinical, biochemical, and histologic approaches to diagnosis. EMG can not only complement and extend other laboratory studies of muscle disease[80-82] but in some instances can identify abnormalities that cannot be defined by other means—for example, physiologic defects of neuromuscular transmission, myotonia, and inactivation of the action potential mechanism in periodic paralysis.

The characterization of diseases by EMG and NCS has often been limited to two broad groups: muscle disease and nerve disease. In primary muscle disease, the typical findings are a decrease in the average duration and amplitude of individual MUPs, an increased incidence of polyphasic potentials, a full recruitment pattern during effort in spite of weakness and wasting, decreased amplitude and increased density of the interference pattern, and a decrease in the CMAP amplitude. These occur with or without spontaneous electrical activity. However, more specific interpretations can be made than merely identifying the presence of muscle disease. The description of the different patterns of abnormalities in different muscle diseases and the different abnormalities that can occur in a given disease during its evolution make this evident. The general terms *myopathic MUP*, *myopathic EMG*, and *BSAP* (brief duration, short amplitude, abundant, polyphasic) potentials are inadequate descriptions of the wide range of abnormal EMG findings and may obscure clinically relevant information. These terms are not used in this discussion.

The following sections present the EMG findings in specific clinical entities and review applications of EMG in the diagnosis and differential diagnosis of these entities. The disorders presented, and the order in which they are presented, are according to the clinical value of the EMG in their assessment and their frequency in clinical practice.

INFLAMMATORY MYOPATHIES

Inflammatory myopathies are the most common myopathies encountered by electromyographers. The identification of

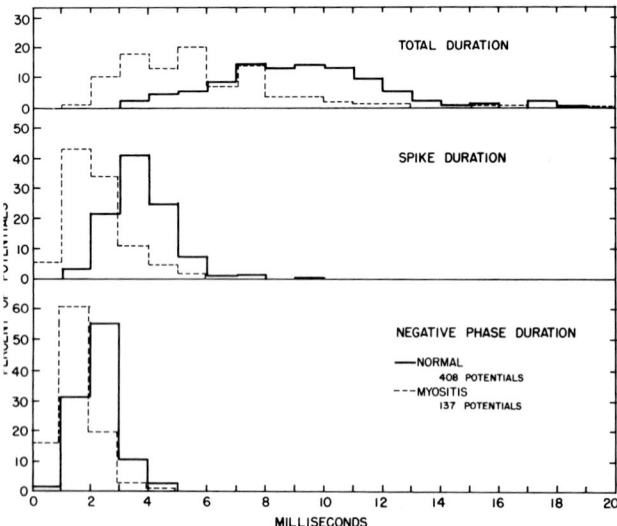

FIGURE 26-16. Duration of MUPs in normal and myositic biceps brachii muscle. *(Courtesy of EH Lambert.)*

tion and low in amplitude, with the amount of this change increasing with the severity of the disease (Fig. 26-16).[81–83] As muscle fibers are lost from individual motor units, the force exerted during activation is reduced. To produce the same force, more motor units must be activated. Therefore, activation of muscle results in an increased number of MUPs for a given force, whereas the pattern of recruitment remains normal. When the disease is severe, all fibers in some motor units are lost, resulting in reduced recruitment. The scattered, spotty character of these changes is striking, especially in comparison with other forms of myopathy. Some areas of muscle may show an entirely normal population of MUPs, whereas others show marked MUP changes. The findings are most marked in proximal muscles, especially the paraspinal muscles. Some muscles, such as the anterior tibial, may show greater involvement than adjacent ones. These changes occur without other EMG findings and are nonspecific, but the scattered distribution of abnormalities in a given muscle suggests an inflammatory process.

If segmental necrosis or regeneration produces fibers that are not innervated, fibrillation potentials occur in addition to the MUP changes (Fig. 26-17).[84] The fibrillation potentials tend to fire at slower rates than those in neurogenic disorders; scattered, slowly recurring fibrillation potentials are typical of myositis. These potentials are found most readily in the paraspinal muscles and are often more prominent in the superficial layers of the muscle, where the pathologic changes are more prominent.[85] An EMG examination of a patient who may have myositis is incomplete if the paraspinal muscles are not examined.

Prominent spontaneous activity is characteristic of most active inflammatory myopathies and distinguishes them from most other myopathies. A higher proportion of the fibrillation potentials occur as positive waves than in neurogenic processes. This is attributed to the fragility of the muscle fiber membrane in myositis and to the relative abundance of recently denervated fibers. If the fibrillating fibers are small because of atrophy or regeneration, the amplitude of the fibrillation potentials will be very low and the dura-

inflammatory myopathy as the cause of proximal muscle weakness and its differentiation from other myopathies, neurogenic processes, or disorders of neuromuscular transmission is an important application of EMG in the study of muscle disease. In most inflammatory myopathies (described in Chaps. 49 through 53), there is destruction of muscle fibers that results in the typical EMG findings. EMG patterns vary enormously with the severity, distribution, and duration of the disease. Some differences can also be identified between subgroups of inflammatory myopathies.

Polymyositis and Dermatomyositis

In polymyositis and dermatomyositis, the major inflammatory myopathies, segmental muscle fiber damage and loss of muscle fibers from the motor unit cause EMG changes in scattered areas of the muscle. MUPs become short in dura-

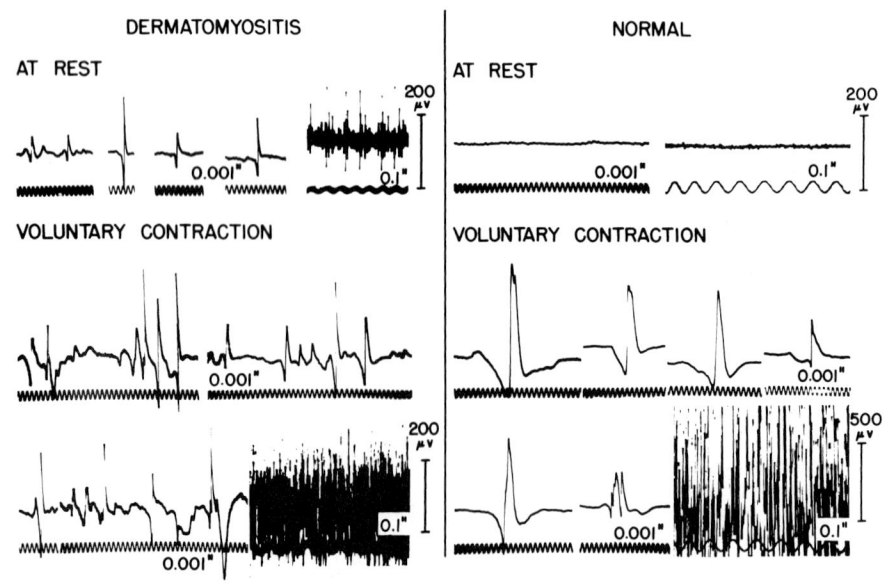

FIGURE 26-17. Electrical activity recorded from normal and myositic biceps brachii muscles. Fibrillation potentials are present in the resting myositic muscle. Polyphasic and short-duration MUPs are present during voluntary contraction. *(From Members of the Department of Neurology and the Department of Physiology and Biophysics, Mayo Clinic and Mayo Foundation for Medical Education and Research: Clinical Examinations in Neurology, 5th ed. Philadelphia: Saunders, 1981. With permission from Mayo Foundation.)*

tion short. These may be difficult to distinguish in the baseline noise. The frequency of fibrillations and the severity of MUP changes increase with the severity of the myositis and are further modified by the duration of the disease. Fibrillation potentials become less prominent as the disease improves with treatment.

Chronic myositis shows more extensive MUP changes and fibrillation potentials. In some patients, MUPs become markedly polyphasic with time; this is associated with an increase in fiber density, suggesting that fibers become reinnervated by axonal sprouting within the motor unit (Fig. 26-17). At the same time, the irritable muscle fiber membranes may produce scattered myotonic discharges and CRDs. These can occur in any muscle but are most prominent in the weakest muscles and the paraspinal muscles. The results of frequency analysis change as patients recover. High-frequency components increase because of the development of polyphasic MUPs; later still, an excess of low-frequency components develops because of the occurrence of long-duration MUPs.[86] However, these changes are not specific for inflammatory myopathies but also occur in other myopathies, e.g., in muscular dystrophies, glycogen storage diseases, the periodic paralyses, and even in autoimmune myasthenia gravis. Thus, the electromyographic interpretation of an inflammatory myopathy must always include the comment that a limited group of other myopathies may be associated with similar findings, and those that are most appropriate clinically should be named.

Inclusion Body Myositis and Chronic Myositis

Chronic myositis can present still another picture as the underlying muscle damage evolves. The progressive reinnervation of regenerated fibers produces a significant number of long-duration MUPs, a few MUPs higher than normal in amplitude, some MUPs with satellite potentials, plus many polyphasic potentials.[39] Inclusion body myositis is a more chronic and severe disease that commonly shows these changes.[87] Inclusion body myositis has prominent small polyphasic potentials, some long-duration potentials, and more involvement of distal muscles.[88,89] Quantitative EMG testing may miss the long-duration potentials by focusing on mean duration rather than on the range and standard deviation of the durations, which are needed when a mixture of some long with many short-duration, which are potentials is present.

This pattern of abnormalities occurring with the chronic course of disease has led to misdiagnoses of amyotrophic lateral sclerosis (ALS). This pattern should always suggest the possibility of inclusion body myositis. The pattern of distribution of abnormalities can help identify inclusion body myositis. Some muscles show more change than others, particularly the long finger flexors and the vastus and medial gastrocnemius muscles. Macro-EMG studies can help distinguish between ALS and chronic myositis when necessary.[90] The duration of the groups of potentials recorded in chronic myositis with SFEMG increases concomitantly with the increase in MUP duration (Fig. 26-18). Damage to a large number of fibers in some motor units produces a reduction in recruitment, so that the distinction from chronic neurogenic atrophy becomes less clear. Along with these electrical

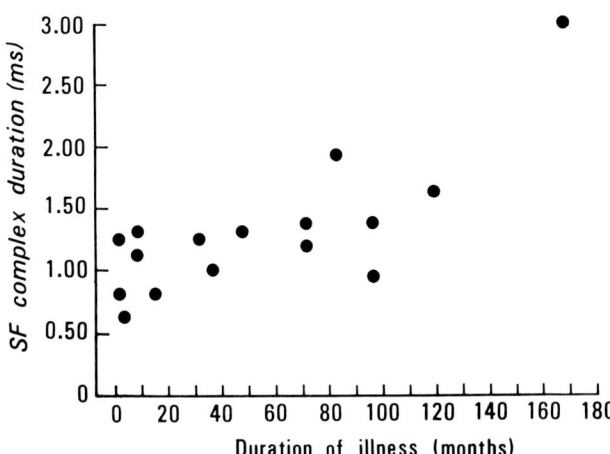

FIGURE 26-18. Increase in the duration of single-fiber potential groups in the quadriceps muscle with duration of disease in 16 subjects with myositis. Each point represents the mean of 20 measurements in individual patients.

changes, an increase in the resistance to needle movement and eventually a decrease in insertion activity develops because of the increase in connective tissue.

NCSs usually show little change in myositis, although the amplitude of the CMAP may be decreased in the muscles that have a sufficient loss of muscle fibers. This occurs rarely in hand and foot muscles but can be seen in the anterior tibial or biceps muscle. Some of the inflammatory myopathies are accompanied by vasculitis or perineural inflammation that also can cause peripheral neuropathy or mononeuritis multiplex. When this occurs, a needle examination of muscles innervated by damaged nerves shows mixed changes, including impaired recruitment and large MUPs caused by nerve damage. Findings on repetitive stimulation are virtually always normal; a decremental response at slow or rapid rates of stimulation has rarely been reported. Most likely, this stems from abnormal properties of the nerve terminals reinnervating regenerating muscle fibers.

SFEMG shows a marked increase in fiber density that is proportional to the duration and severity of the disease. With active disease, jitter is increased and blocking may occur. Blocking has been attributed to the presence of newly formed nerve sprouts, to reinnervated fibers, or to disease of the nerve terminal. Reduced jitter values, attributed to fiber splitting, can also occur. The mean interspike interval is increased, but it decreases with recovery.[91]

Other Inflammatory Myopathies

The EMG/NCS findings in subcategories of inflammatory myopathies show little difference, but some comments may be helpful. The EMG changes in myositis that occur with rheumatoid arthritis, systemic lupus erythematosus, scleroderma, and mixed collagen-vascular disorders can be mild, with few fibrillation potentials, usually only in the paraspinal muscles.[92–94] Some have reported no increase in the incidence of EMG changes of myopathy.[95] Eosinophilic fasciitis and other forms of fascial inflammation may not show any EMG abnormalities.[96] However, MUP abnormalities have been reported.[97,98] Myofascial pain syndromes show no EMG abnormalities.[99]

Except for one report of SFEMG changes,[100] an acute viral myositis rarely shows any EMG changes, perhaps because there is little destruction of muscle fibers. In parasitic myositis, such as trichinosis, and in sarcoid myopathy, the abnormalities are more scattered but may be focally severe; fibrillation potentials and distal changes can be more prominent than in polymyositis.[101–104]

Electrodiagnosis of Inflammatory Myopathy

The major diseases that must be distinguished in identifying myositis are ALS and muscular dystrophy. Early in the course of the disease, the distinction is readily made. In ALS, recruitment is impaired early, with a marked increase in the duration and amplitude of MUPs, in contrast to the opposite changes in myositis. In muscular dystrophy, except for myotonic dystrophy, fibrillation potentials or myotonic discharges are minimal and the MUPs are less polyphasic.

As ALS progresses, MUPs that are of short duration, low amplitude, polyphasic, and varying in amplitude and duration appear and may resemble the potentials of myositis. However, these MUPs are always accompanied by the large potentials typical of ALS. Therefore, multiple MUPs must be studied to determine the relative abundance of large and small potentials. The spontaneous activity in myositis consists of myotonic discharges, CRDs, and slow fibrillation potentials. These are rarely seen in ALS. In ALS but not in myositis, prominent changes are present distally. In the late stages of myositis, when some large potentials may appear, the fibrillation potentials are less prominent, and highly polyphasic potentials are more common than in ALS.

In late polymyositis, EMG/NCS changes become more diffuse and are more difficult to distinguish from those of chronic muscular dystrophy. However, selective muscles are involved in most dystrophies, and associated involvement of the peripheral nervous system in some inflammatory myopathies may help make a distinction. The EMG findings in severe subacute or chronic inflammatory myopathy and childhood muscular dystrophy may be similar, but prominent spontaneous activity is a clue to myositis.

Occasionally, EMG can help to define the activity of myositis. Active fiber injury and hence disease activity are reflected by fibrillations, with the amount of fibrillation correlated partly with the severity of disease progression. In contrast, the MUP changes may persist even after the process subsides. In a patient who has myositis treated with corticosteroids, progressive weakness without continued fibrillation suggests steroid-induced weakness rather than continued disease activity.

INFILTRATIVE MYOPATHIES

Amyloid Myopathy

Myopathy is an uncommon manifestation in patients with primary systemic amyloidosis. Clinical manifestations can include proximal weakness, dysphagia, pseudohypertrophy of muscles, and macroglossia. Electrodiagnostic studies often demonstrate abnormalities on NCS that indicate an underlying peripheral neuropathy or mononeuropathy, such as carpal tunnel syndrome. Needle examination has demonstrated fibrillation potentials and positive waves, and short-duration, low-amplitude, polyphasic MUPs in proximal muscles, such as the paraspinal muscles and gluteus medius, more than distal muscles.[105,106] These findings may be similar in severity and distribution to those that occur in polymyositis and dermatomyositis.

Sarcoid Myopathy

Myopathy may rarely be a manifestation of systemic sarcoidosis and may occur as asymptomatic infiltration of noncaseating granulomas, palpable nodules or pseudohypertrophy within the muscles, or as slowly progressive weakness.[107] Weakness may involve proximal or distal muscles. NCSs are usually normal. Needle EMG may be normal or may show fibrillation potentials and short-duration, polyphasic MUPs in proximal and distal muscles.[104,108] According to one report, prominent myotonic discharges were recorded.[109]

DISORDERS OF ALTERED CELL MEMBRANE EXCITABILITY

Many myopathies have associated excess muscle fiber activation due to disorders of ion channel function.[110] Channelopathies typically show intermittent symptoms. The abnormalities due to the channel deficit may be a "gain of function," in which there is excessive membrane irritability and firing of action potentials, or a loss of function, in which the response to stimuli is decreased. Patients with myotonic disorders are often referred for electrodiagnosis. Clinical myotonia is a finding of prolonged muscle contraction (see Chaps. 36 and 46) associated with specific electrical potentials (myotonic discharges) due to unique alterations in membrane physiology.[111,112] Myotonic discharges may also occur in disorders not associated with clinical myotonia (see discussion of inflammatory and metabolic myopathies). This section focuses on disorders with a primary abnormality in the muscle fiber membrane that is associated with myotonic discharges, a readily recognizable EMG discharge.

Myotonic Dystrophy

Myotonic dystrophy is an inherited disorder that may manifest itself shortly after birth or many years later. The typical EMG findings in clinical myotonia are myotonic discharges and abnormal MUPs, but significant variations from these findings occur among patients and in different muscles of individual patients.[112] An accurate EMG assessment of a patient with suspected myotonic dystrophy requires knowledge of these variations. For instance, in infants, weakness and hypotonia caused by myotonic dystrophy often are not recognized clinically, and the electromyographer called upon to test the infant for hypotonic disease may be the first to recognize the myotonia. To do so requires awareness of differences in the EMG findings in adults and infants.

The myotonic discharges in a symptomatic adult are readily recognizable. They are most common in distal muscles but can be recorded in any muscle, even those without clinical myotonia. These discharges are enhanced with cooling and reduced with warming. They also are reduced after activity, so that a patient who is warm and has walked or exercised just before the EMG examination may show no myotonic discharges until well rested. The myotonic discharges can be elicited with either mechanical or electrical stimulation. The usual method for activating them during EMG is by needle movement. This produces a burst of myotonic discharges composed of positive waves. A tap on the muscle also produces a myotonic burst. Voluntary contractions also induce discharges, called an *afterdischarge*, but because many of the activated fibers are at a distance from the needle tip, the discharges are not well recorded. The myotonic discharges activated with voluntary contraction and tapping are mainly spike forms, because the muscle fiber has not been damaged. The spikes fire rapidly and regularly, but some may discharge at the slower rates seen with fibrillation potentials. Myotonic discharges in myotonic dystrophy last slightly longer (up to 10 s), fire more slowly, and have less frequency increment than the myotonic discharges in myotonia congenita (see below). Slow myotonic discharges cannot be differentiated readily from fibrillation potentials and must be identified by associated findings. The slowly firing myotonic spikes make it difficult to identify a possible superimposed neurogenic lesion that may cause fibrillation potentials in a patient with myotonic dystrophy. Myotonic discharges can be used for early recognition of asymptomatic or mildly affected individuals of families at risk for the disease.[113] The discharge may not be present in subjects carrying the gene who have only a partial syndrome.[114]

Complex or small MUPs (or both) are the other abnormalities in myotonic dystrophy, and these increase as the disease progresses. Regenerating fibers result in polyphasic potentials, often the first indication of a dystrophic process. The MUP amplitude can also change as a result of the sarcolemmal membrane abnormality. A single MUP in a normal muscle remains unchanged as it discharges repeatedly. In myotonic dystrophy, myotonia congenita, and some other myotonic disorders, the MUP amplitude may gradually decrease and finally disappear because the muscle fibers contributing to it become inactivated despite continued firing of the anterior horn cell and axon.[21] With continued activity or rest, the MUP can recover, and the original amplitude is regained over many seconds to a few minutes. The variation in MUP sizes is gradual rather than from moment to moment, as in disorders of neuromuscular transmission (see "Disturbances of Neuromuscular Transmission," below).

Myotonic discharges may be identified in myotonic dystrophy as early as the first week of life. They occur in infants with facial diplegia and hypotonia who may show no clinical evidence of myotonia.[115] Infants normally have smaller MUPs than adults and end plate regions that occupy a larger proportion of the total muscle area. Thus, end plate noise and spikes are more widely distributed, even in most of the area of a small muscle. The end plate activity is of lower amplitude than in adults and must be distinguished from abnormal discharges. In myotonic dystrophy, the myotonic discharges during the first few weeks of life are much less clearly defined than in adults and may be mistaken for the widespread end plate noise.[115–117] The abnormal potentials are low in amplitude and often do not appear in well-defined, recurrent patterns. The duration of the discharge may be shorter, with less waxing and waning. With persistent, careful study of spontaneous activity in these infants, it is possible to record bursts of discharges that are clearly myotonic. Often, these are found more readily in larger muscles and paraspinal muscles. The MUPs usually are normal in size or shape for the age, although some have been reported to be of low amplitude and polyphasic.[117] NCSs are normal in these infants.[112] It is not known whether initially asymptomatic infants who develop myotonia in later life have similar myotonic discharges in infancy.

The inactivation of the muscle fiber membrane with activity is also demonstrated by repetitive stimulation. The initial CMAP is usually normal in amplitude unless atrophy has developed. Repetitive stimulation, especially at more than 5 Hz, often produces an irregular decrement.[118] The amplitude of the response is decreased, and the decrement is usually greater during rest after exercise or with prolonged stimulation, in contrast to neuromuscular junction disorders.[119] The decrease in CMAP amplitude develops rapidly with exercise but may develop over many minutes with stimulation and persist for 30 min after exercise.

Myotonic dystrophy is a systemic disorder with manifestations in many organ systems. Reports of abnormal peripheral nerve conduction, a decreased number of motor units, and abnormal H reflexes have suggested neural involvement.[120–122] Some observers have found little change; others have reported mononeuropathies or diffuse neuropathies. The neuropathy may represent a greater than normal decrease in nerve conduction with age: Younger persons have little or no abnormality of nerve conduction; the older ones have mild impairment. Other reports have suggested that the abnormality is related primarily to associated disorders, such as diabetes mellitus.[123]

Proximal Myotonic Myopathy

Proximal myotonic myopathy (PROMM) is a proximal myopathy that is autosomal dominant and genetically distinct from myotonic dystrophy, although PROMM also has an abundance of myotonic discharges and small motor unit potentials.[124] On routine clinical EMG testing, the myotonic discharges do not appear to be different from those of myotonic dystrophy, but the small MUPs are more prominent in distal muscles. Even more distinctive is the response to exercise. In contrast to the decrease in CMAP amplitude that occurs in myotonic dystrophy and myotonia congenita after 10 to 60 s of exercise, 10 s of exercise can distinguish the lack of amplitude reduction in PROMM.[125]

Myotonia Congenita

Myotonia congenita occurs as an autosomal dominant form (Thompsen disease) or autosomal recessive form (Becker disease). Both forms result from a mutation in the voltage-gated chloride channel and are associated with myotonic discharges, especially in the dominant form.[126] The myotonic discharges in dominant and recessive forms of myotonia congenita and paramyotonia generally are similar to those in myotonic dystrophy, but the trains are shorter and there is more variation in their frequency and amplitude. By contrast, the MUPs and NCSs are normal.[127] The myotonic discharges are often distributed more widely in these disorders and may be detected in infancy.[128] Spike and positive waveforms, MUP variation, and afterdischarges are all similar to those that can occur in myotonic dystrophy. Transient muscle weakness and reduced EMG activity after exercise frequently occur in recessive but not in dominant myotonia congenita.[21,129] The decrement during prolonged repetitive stimulation appears at lower frequency than in myotonic dystrophy[112] and may be delayed.[126] The short-duration, polyphasic MUPs of myotonic dystrophy are the most reliable EMG criterion for differentiating this disorder from myotonia congenita. Major changes in MUPs are not seen in myotonia congenita, but the MUP amplitude may gradually decrease with repeated firing. Multichannel surface EMG recording has shown both a slowing of muscle fiber conduction velocity and a progressive decrease in MUP amplitude as the action potential travels from the end plate to the tendon.[130]

The electrical features of myotonia congenita and paramyotonia are similar at room temperature but can be distinguished by brief exercise or cooling.[131] Cooling the muscle below 20°C inhibits electrical and clinical myotonia in paramyotonia but not in myotonia congenita.[132] During moderate cooling, intense fibrillation potentials may occur in paramyotonia before all activity ceases. Some electrical features of paramyotonia are similar to those of hyperkalemic periodic paralysis.[133,134] Recessive forms of generalized myotonia may be difficult to distinguish from sporadic myotonia congenita.[135] In severe recessive forms, transient weakness occurs because of muscle fiber depolarization with activity, as in myotonic dystrophy (Fig. 26-19A).[129] The EMG may identify myotonic discharges in heterozygotes when no clinical myotonia is present.[136]

Periodic Paralysis

There are characteristic EMG findings in periodic paralysis. Different clinical forms of periodic paralysis have been described (see Chap. 46). The two major types of primary periodic paralysis have distinct EMG features. In the hyperkalemic form due to impaired sodium channel inactivation, there is spontaneous activity; an aberrant depolarization shift inactivates the muscle fiber. In the hypokalemic form there is no spontaneous activity, but there is susceptibility to intraarterially administered epinephrine.

The paralysis during an episode of weakness in both of these forms of periodic paralysis is manifested on EMG as a striking loss of electrical activity.[65] When a muscle is completely paralyzed during an attack, the EMG shows total electrical silence. Insertion activity and voluntary MUPs are both lost. Nerve stimulation produces no CMAPs. With lesser degrees of paralysis, the CMAP is reduced in proportion to the weakness and the MUPs range from short duration and low amplitude to normal. If weakness persists between attacks, the MUPs are generally of short duration and low amplitude.[65,137,138] Although both forms of periodic paralysis produce transient weakness, they differ in their underlying pathophysiologic mechanism. Hyperkalemic periodic paralysis is a sodium channelopathy, like paramyotonia congenita.[139]

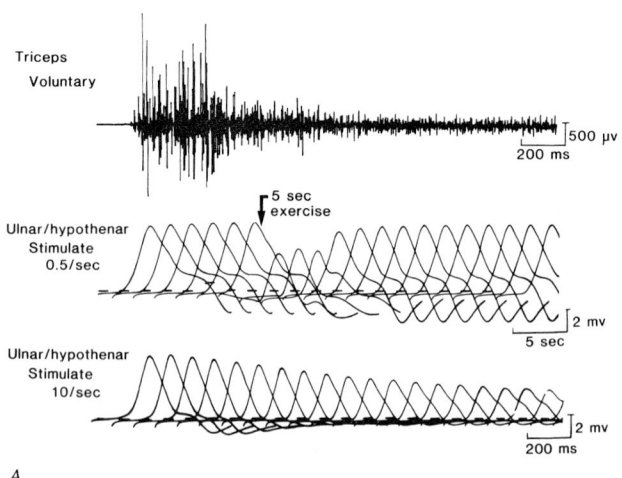

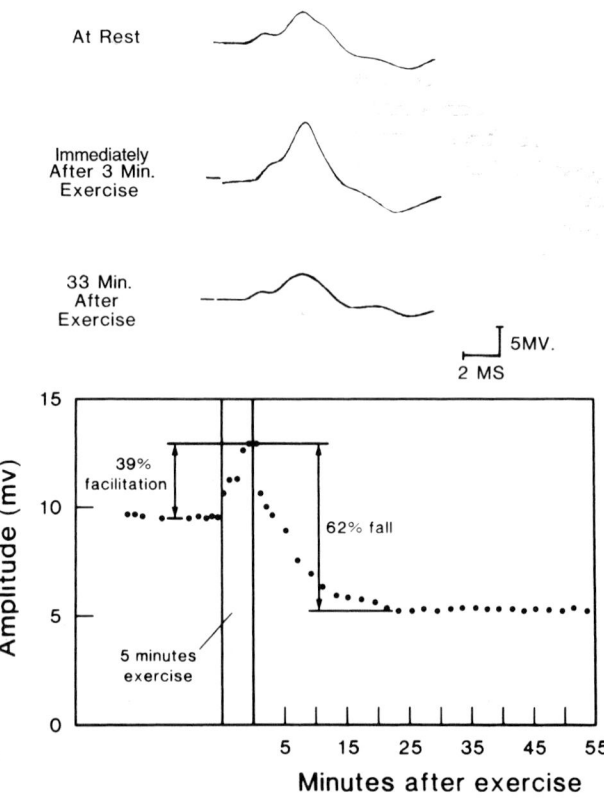

FIGURE 26-19. Compound muscle action potential amplitude reduction after exercise. A. Recessive myotonia congenita. B. Hypokalemic periodic paralysis.

Primary hyperkalemic periodic paralysis. In addition to the changes described above during an attack, spontaneous activity occurs between attacks in hyperkalemic periodic paralysis. In addition, typical myotonic discharges and fibrillation potentials have been reported in this disorder in many muscles, especially the paraspinal muscles.[137,140,141] The abnormal activity increases with cooling, decreases with activity, and subsides completely during paralysis. Nerve conduction studies show no abnormalities, but variable decrements may be seen rarely with repetitive stimulation. After exercise, there is variation in the CMAP but no consistent, major loss of amplitude.[142]

In several muscle diseases with no clinical myotonia, such as myositis and acid maltase deficiency, or with limited or fleeting clinical myotonia, as in hyperkalemic periodic paralysis, electrical myotonia can be prominent and provide an important clue to the correct diagnosis. Occasionally, myotonic discharges also occur in neurogenic disorders; thus, these discharges are not absolute evidence for a primary muscle disease.[22]

Primary hypokalemic periodic paralysis. In contrast to the hyperkalemic form, no spontaneous activity occurs between attacks and the changes in the CMAP are more consistent after exercise (Fig. 26-19B). Prolonged exercise (3 to 5 min) often results in a gradual reduction in the CMAP amplitude 15 to 40 min after exercise (Fig. 26-19B).[65,138] This phenomenon can be used as a screening test for periodic paralysis, but the CMAP must decrease to less than 50 percent of the resting value, because in a few normal subjects the CMAP also decreases after exercise.[65] If a prolonged exercise test does not produce a significant change, epinephrine injected intraarterially into the arm may still produce a significant decrease of the CMAP and twitch tension in primary hypokalemic periodic paralysis.[65] Muscle fiber conduction velocity may be slowed.[73] SFEMG shows little change between attacks but demonstrates decreased fiber density and blocking during attacks caused by failure of the muscle fiber membrane to propagate an action potential.[143]

MUSCULAR DYSTROPHIES

A third major group of muscle disease in which EMG/NCSs can be of particular value is muscular dystrophy. The changes depend on the underlying pathologic process. Small motor unit potentials could result from loss of muscle fibers, atrophy of muscle fibers, or inactivation of muscle fibers due to a membrane channel abnormality.[1] Although the anatomy of the motor unit is altered in a dystrophy, the standard EMG findings are nonspecific in nonmyotonic dystrophies and are of value primarily in defining the distribution and severity of the abnormality.[144]

Dystrophinopathies

Among the nonmyotonic dystrophinopathies, Duchenne dystrophy has the most consistent and abnormal EMG findings. The extent of EMG abnormality is proportional to the severity and rate of progression of the ongoing muscle fiber destruction and the extent of fiber regeneration.[145] The fiber loss results in low-amplitude, short-duration MUPs, most prominent in the weak muscles. Fiber regeneration or splitting (or both) results in polyphasic MUPs that are generally low in amplitude but of long or short duration, depending on the number of fibers and their firing synchrony within the motor unit. MUP changes can also be detected as changes in the interference pattern by change in the frequency, size, and number of spikes.[146] The ongoing segmental necrosis of muscle fibers in a scattered distribution results in a small to moderate number of fibrillation potentials that are generally of low amplitude and short duration because they arise from small muscle fibers. If there has been marked replacement of muscle fibers by fibrous or fatty connective tissue, there will be areas of decreased insertion activity and increased resistance to needle movement. In the late stages of the disease, when a large number of muscle fibers have been lost, whole motor units are missing and recruitment is impaired. The original reports of a loss of motor units[147,148] early in Duchenne dystrophy have not been confirmed.

The changes recorded with standard needle EMG are also reflected in SFEMG recordings by the increase in fiber density and occasional increase in jitter and blocking. NCS findings are generally normal; however, the CMAP amplitude may be mildly reduced. Somatosensory evoked potentials may show abnormal central conduction.[149] Specialized electrophysiologic measurements have shown some abnormalities of muscle fiber conduction velocity: There is (1) faster than normal recovery of conduction velocity after action potential propagation, (2) slowing of conduction in muscle fibers,[111] and (3) an abnormal, immature pattern of muscle fiber action potential activation, implying an abnormality of the muscle fiber membrane.[150] Repetitive stimulation shows little or no abnormality. Abnormal muscle fiber contractility may precede the electrical changes.

The EMG not only can characterize the severity and distribution of abnormality in dystrophy but also is useful in the differential diagnosis. The most common disease that must be distinguished from dystrophy is chronic spinal muscular atrophy, such as Kugelberg-Welander syndrome, which can simulate dystrophy clinically.[151] On EMG, however, the abnormalities are strikingly different. In spinal muscular atrophies, an early, severe loss of motor units reduces recruitment and the MUNE. The MUPs become progressively longer in duration and higher in amplitude. There is little increase in the number of phases because the process is slowly progressive and firing synchrony is maintained. Fibrillation potentials can be scanty and may be less prominent than in some dystrophies; these potentials are less reliable than MUP changes for distinguishing between dystrophy and chronic spinal muscular atrophy.

Milder forms of dystrophinopathies may demonstrate little or no change on EMG.[152]

Limb-Girdle Dystrophies

Less severe forms of dystrophy—such as the Becker form, limb-girdle dystrophy, and facioscapulohumeral dystrophy—show similar but less marked changes and usually few or no fibrillation potentials. Muscular dystrophies caused by dysferlin deficiency can show marked heterogeneity in EMG findings.[153,154] Some of the sarcoglycan-related dystrophies have minimal EMG changes.[155] Some patients with Becker type of muscular dystrophy have more severe EMG changes, including fibrillation potentials, myotonic discharges, and CRDs.[156] Mild EMG changes have been reported in Duchenne dystrophy carriers.[157] This may help in detecting carriers, but immunostains of muscle for dystrophin, measurements of creatine kinase, or specific genetic markers are more efficient and reliable.

Facioscapulohumeral Muscular Dystrophy

Large MUPs have been reported occasionally in cases of facioscapulohumeral muscular dystrophy (FSHD). A loss of motor units has also been reported in limb-girdle dystrophy and FSHD. FSHD is generally identified by the distribution of weakness and the specific genetic defect.[158] EMG findings are nonspecific, with short-duration MUPs in proportion to the severity of deficit, rapid recruitment, and occasional scattered fibrillation potentials. Recent studies have shown considerable clinical heterogeneity, with variation in the severity of the EMG findings.[158] Some FSHD patients have marked involvement of the tongue.[159]

Congenital Dystrophies

The definition of congenital dystrophies not due to α2-laminin (merosin) deficiency is not fully agreed upon, making it difficult to define electrodiagnostic characteristics.[160] The findings consist mainly of short-duration, low-amplitude MUPs. Occasionally, large MUPs have been described, suggesting that this entity is heterogeneous.[161] In the reported congenital dystrophies, the EMG findings consist of short-duration MUPs, with some increase in polyphasic MUPs but few fibrillation potentials. The number of motor units is not decreased.

Oculopharyngeal Dystrophy

Small MUPs or mixtures of small and large MUPs with fibrillation potentials have been reported rarely in oculopharyngeal dystrophy.[162,163]

Distal Dystrophies

Several myopathies may present with distal weakness (e.g., inclusion body myositis, myotonic dystrophy, myofibrillar myopathy) and EMG findings that can be confusing for electromyographers (Table 26-2). The distal dystrophies (Welander, Markesberry-Griggs, Miyoshi, and other types) with a predominantly distal distribution generally have short-duration MUPs, but some have fibrillation potentials and a disturbed motor unit recruitment order consistent with loss of type 1 muscle fibers.[164,165] However, several forms can also have myotonic discharges, CRDs, and some long-duration MUPs with reduced recruitment. Thus, a distal myopathy can resemble a neuropathy clinically, an impression reinforced by the occurrence of fibrillation potentials.[166,167] The small MUPs help in distinguishing the disorder on EMG. In some types of distal dystrophies (such as Welander), the anterior compartment muscles of the legs are affected most, whereas in others (Miyoshi), the calf muscles are affected more. In some cases of oculopharyngeal dystrophy, short-duration MUPs may be seen in distal muscles in addition to facial muscles.[167a] In the localized forms of dystrophy, the EMG changes occur primarily in the areas of clinical weakness, the sites that should be tested first.

CONGENITAL MYOPATHIES

The EMG changes in some of the congenital myopathies (centronuclear, nemaline, myotubular, mitochondrial) are

Table 26-2. MYOPATHIES WITH DISTAL INVOLVEMENT

Myotonic dystrophy
Facioscapulohumeral dystrophy
Scapuloperoneal myopathy
Oculopharyngeal dystrophy
Emery-Dreifuss humeroperoneal dystrophy
Inflammatory myopathy
   Inclusion body myositis
   Sarcoid
Metabolic myopathy
   Debrancher enzyme deficiency
   Acid maltase deficiency
Congenital myopathy
   Nemaline
   Central core
   Centronuclear
Distal myopathies
   Welander
   Markesberry-Griggs
   Nonaka
   Miyoshi
   Laing
   Distal with pharyngeal involvement
   Myofibrillar
   Infantile-onset

mild. MUP amplitude and duration are decreased in proportion to the amount of fiber loss, and there is some increase in the proportion of polyphasic potentials. The major exception to this is myotubular (centronuclear) myopathy, in which a large number of fibrillation potentials occur with occasional myotonic discharges (Table 26-3).[168–181] These changes usually are distributed widely, but they may be more prominent in the paraspinal muscles. Scattered fibrillation potentials and SFEMG abnormalities occur infrequently in congenital and late-onset nemaline myopathy[173–176] and have been noted in two patients with central core disease. Satellite potentials on MUPs and increased fiber density on SFEMG have been reported in central core disease. Mitochondrial myopathy may show neurogenic as well as myopathic abnormalities on EMG, SFEMG, and NCS.[179,180]

Congenital myopathies with an alteration in the proportion of fiber types and multicores have generally been reported to have normal EMG findings.[181] Standard EMG usually assesses only the early recruited type 1 motor units firing at a low level and might be expected to show less change. The congenital myopathies are discussed further in Chap. 54.

METABOLIC DISORDERS OF MUSCLE

Metabolic myopathies arise from enzyme deficiencies in the biochemical pathway of glycogen or lipid metabolism or from a defect in the pathway of energy production within the mitochondria. Among those muscle diseases currently identified as stemming from a specific enzyme deficiency (see Chaps. 55 through 58, on metabolic disorders affecting muscle), most—with some exceptions—show relatively little or no EMG change or only a mild decrease in the amplitude and duration of the MUP (Table 26-4).

Table 26-3. EMG FINDINGS IN CONGENITAL MYOPATHIES

Myopathy	MUP abnormalities		Spontaneous activity		
	Short duration	Polyphasic	Fibrillation potentials	Myotonic discharges	Complex repetitive discharges
Myotubular	++	++	0 to ++	+	0
Nemaline (rod)	++	++	0 or +	0	0
Central core	+	+	0 or +	0	0
Fiber type disproportion	(+)	(+)	0	0	0

KEY: 0 = Not present; (+) = rare reports of abnormality; + to ++++ = severity of abnormality from mild to severe.

Disorders of Glycogen Metabolism

There are several disorders of glycogen metabolism; however, electrophysiologic findings have been described in detail for only the more common ones, including myophosphorylase (McArdle disease) and phosphofructokinase deficiencies. In McArdle disease, routine motor and sensory nerve conduction studies are normal, although repetitive stimulation at high rates has been reported to demonstrate a marked decrement in CMAP amplitude; a smaller decrement has been reported with low rates of stimulation.[182,183] Often, needle EMG does not demonstrate abnormal spontaneous activity, although in some cases a small number of scattered fibrillation potentials may be detected in proximal and paraspinal muscles.[184–189] Often MUP configuration is normal, but the potential may be of short duration and polyphasic. During the period of muscle cramping and weakness following physical exercise or ischemic exercise testing, there may be an alteration in evoked mechanical and electrical responses with electrical silence and, rarely, scattered fibrillation potentials in the paraspinal muscles.[185,187]

In contrast to the rest of the glycogen storage myopathies, the infantile, childhood, and adult forms of *acid maltase deficiency*[190] and *debrancher enzyme deficiency*[191] show prominent changes on needle EMG (Table 26-4). These entities are also discussed in Chaps. 55 and 56. In acid maltase deficiency, the MUPs are often of short duration, and there may be an increase in polyphasic potentials, especially in proximal muscles. The proximal muscles are also the site of striking spontaneous activity, similar to that seen in myositis, with many fibrillation potentials and occasional CRDs.[190,192–195] Myotonic discharges without clinical myotonia are not infrequent in proximal muscles, especially paraspinal muscles.[193,196] These potentials may be prominent in respiratory muscles in patients presenting primarily with respiratory weakness. The abnormalities are more pronounced and widespread in younger patients than in older ones. Also, SFEMG shows a mild increase in fiber density, likely due to local muscle regeneration.[50]

In debranching enzyme myopathy (glycogen storage disease type III), fibrillation potentials, positive sharp waves with short duration, and low-amplitude MUPs in proximal muscles more than distal muscles have been reported in 16 patients. Mild prolongation of ulnar and median sensory distal latencies and slowed motor conduction velocities were also reported in these patients.[197]

Disorders of Lipid Metabolism

EMG findings in disorders of lipid metabolism have not been widely reported. In carnitine palmitoyltransferase type II (CPT II) deficiency and carnitine deficiency, fibrillation potentials may be absent or present in mild degree, and short-duration MUPs may occur.[198–202] NCSs are usually

Table 26-4. EMG FINDINGS IN MUSCLE ENZYME DEFICIENCIES

Deficiency	MUP abnormalities	Fibrillation potentials	Myotonic discharges	Complex repetitive discharges
Glycolytic enzyme deficiencies				
Acid maltase	+++	+++	++	++
Debrancher	++	+++	+	+
Brancher	0	0	0	0
Phosphorylase	(+)	(+)	0	0
Phosphofructokinase	0	0	0	0
Disorders of lipid metabolism				
Muscle carnitine deficiency	+	+	0	0
Systemic carnitine deficiency	0	0	0	0
Palmityltransferase deficiency	0	0	0	0
Other				
Primary adenylate deaminase	0	0	0	0
Mitochondrial myopathies	(+)	(+)	0	0

KEY: 0 = Not present; (+) = rare reports of abnormality; + to ++++ = severity of abnormality from mild to severe.

normal, although there is one report of a decrement in the CMAP amplitude with slow rates of repetitive stimulation in carnitine deficiency.[203]

Disorders of Mitochondrial Function

Defects in the pathway of energy production within mitochondria often produce muscle dysfunction as part of a spectrum of neurologic disease. In several disorders, such as MERRF (myoclonic epilepsy with ragged red fibers), NARP (neuropathy, ataxia, and retinitis pigmentosa), MNGIE (mitochondrial neurogastrointestinal encephalomyopathy), MELAS (mitochondrial myopathy, encephalopathy, lactic acidosis, strokes), and Kearns-Sayre syndrome, various degrees of abnormalities may be found on electrophysiologic testing. Motor and sensory nerve conduction studies may show a decrease in amplitudes and slowing of conduction velocities, indicating a superimposed peripheral neuropathy, in up to 50 percent of patients, including some without clinical findings of neuropathy.[204] On needle EMG, a mild degree of fibrillation potentials and short-duration, low-amplitude MUPs may be detected, even without clinical signs of neuromuscular disease.[205] In a large study of 51 patients with an unspecified type of mitochondrial myopathy, the EMG was normal in 6, demonstrated findings of myopathy in 38, and showed findings suggestive of a peripheral neuropathy in 7.[206] Multiple electrophysiologic techniques—including NCS, concentric needle EMG with interference pattern analysis, quantitative EMG, SFEMG, and macro-EMG—have been used to study large kindreds with mitochondrial myopathies; they have shown variable findings in individual members.[207,208] Many patients had a mild decrease in sensory or motor (or both) amplitudes on NCS, with mild slowing of conduction velocities, indicative of a peripheral neuropathy. Needle EMG findings were normal in some patients, whereas other patients had short-duration, polyphasic MUPs of mild to moderate degree, and a few had increased jitter on SFEMG. Macro-EMG showed increased amplitude in the tibialis anterior muscles of a few patients. These findings indicate that many patients with mitochondrial cytopathy commonly have a combination of myopathy and neuropathy.

Schwartz-Jampel Syndrome

This disorder is now known to be caused by mutations in perlecan, a large heparan sulfate proteoglycan present in basement membrane and other extracellular matrices.[208a] The disease is associated with skeletal abnormalities and continuous muscle contraction. Although the discharges in this disorder have been called myotonic discharges and some of the clinical features resemble myotonia, true myotonic discharges are not present. When the potentials in Schwartz-Jampel syndrome have been isolated, they have consisted, with one exception, of an abundance of CRDs that occurred spontaneously and with voluntary activation. The MUPs are of long duration and complex, resembling the recurring components of the CRDs, and, in some cases, can be seen to be the voluntary activation of potentials that also are active spontaneously.[209–214]

Endocrine Disorders of Muscle

Thyroid disorders. EMG changes may be mild or prominent in thyroid disorders. In *hypothyroid* myopathy, fibrillation potentials or other abnormal spontaneous discharges are usually absent, although in some cases irritability of the muscle fiber membrane may appear as increased insertion activity, complex repetitive potentials, or short myotonic discharges.[215–217] Voluntary MUPs may be normal but in up to 70 percent of patients are short in duration.[218,219] One study demonstrated EMG findings consistent with myopathy in 7 percent of patients with clinical hypothyroidism.[220] Myopathies associated with *hyperthyroidism* may be associated with a normal EMG, without fibrillation potentials or motor unit changes. However, some studies have demonstrated a mild decrease in the size of MUPs and increased polyphasic MUPs in most persons with thyrotoxicosis, even without clinical weakness.[221–223] The myoedema following local percussion has been described by some as "myotonia," but it is associated with electrical silence rather than myotonic discharges on EMG.

Parathyroid disorders. In hypoparathyroidism with hypocalcemia, striking irritability with increased insertion activity, doublet and multiplet MUPs, single or complex fasciculation potentials, and various ill-defined, irregular, spontaneous discharges may be present.[224] In severe cases of primary hyperparathyroidism, with or without osteomalacia, the EMG may be normal, but short-duration, polyphasic MUPs have been reported. Fibrillation potentials and other spontaneous discharges are absent.[225–228] With earlier detection and treatment of hyperparathyroidism, clinical and EMG findings of myopathy have become less common.[229]

Adrenal disorders. Cushing disease, characterized by excess glucocorticoid production, is commonly manifest as progressive muscle weakness. An identical myopathy occurs with chronic exogenous administration of corticosteroids. In these disorders, the EMG findings are almost invariably normal, reflecting the pathologic alteration of type II muscle fiber atrophy.[230,231] With severe involvement, the MUPs may be of short duration and low amplitude.[232] In a single report, three of six patients with endogenous Cushing syndrome had fibrillation potentials or positive waves in addition to short-duration MUPs.[233] NCSs and repetitive stimulation studies are normal.

Acromegaly. Several neuromuscular complications may occur in acromegaly.[234] Most commonly, focal entrapment mononeuropathies, such as median or ulnar neuropathy, or a generalized peripheral neuropathy is present. In rare instances, progressive proximal muscle weakness may occur. NCSs may demonstrate findings consistent with mononeuropathies. In patients with proximal weakness, short-duration MUPs without fibrillation potentials have been reported.[235]

Toxic Myopathies

Many drugs and toxins can have a profound effect on muscle fibers by causing diffuse inflammatory cell infiltration, abnormal functioning of mitochondria, lysosomal dysfunction with autophagic vacuole production, or selective atrophy of muscle fibers (see Chap. 61). EMG abnormalities often occur with these pathologic alterations. The development of drug-induced myopathies is related to the type of medication, the duration and dose administered, the presence of underlying liver or renal failure, and the number of myotoxic medications that have been taken. With each of these drugs, clinical and electrophysiologic manifestations are reversible after discontinuation of the offending agent.

The list of medications that may produce clinical weakness or myalgias and increased serum levels of creatine kinase is extensive; however, EMG findings have been described only in limited series. The best-described toxic myopathies are due to cholesterol-lowering agents, zidovudine (AZT), colchicine, emetine, chloroquine, and penicillamine, although EMG changes have also been found in myopathies due to cardiovascular drugs such as amiodarone, labetalol, and procainamide.[236–241]

Drugs that produced generalized muscle fiber necrosis include cholesterol-lowering agents, such as clofibrate and HMG-CoA reductase inhibitors, AZT, colchicine, and emetine. The EMG may be normal in mild or early disease, but short-duration, low-amplitude, polyphasic MUPs with or without fibrillation potentials may be detected in more severe disease.[242,243] The findings are more prominent in proximal muscles. Experimental myotonia has been produced with the administration of clofibrate, and myotonic discharges may occur in myopathies due to other cholesterol-lowering agents.[243–246]

Mitochondrial dysfunction, as evident by prominent ragged red fibers, is the major pathologic effect of AZT myopathy. On EMG, a mild to moderate degree of fibrillation potentials and rapidly recruited, short-duration, low-amplitude MUPs are present.[237,247]

Chloroquine and hydroxychloroquine cause muscle dysfunction, with the unique feature of vacuole production. NCSs may show mild slowing of motor and sensory conduction velocities, indicating concomitant peripheral nerve dysfunction. Needle EMG demonstrates fibrillation potentials in distal and proximal muscles, occasional CRDs, and short-duration, low-amplitude MUPs.[248–252]

The *eosinophilia-myalgia syndrome*, characterized by the insidious onset of rash, fatigue, myalgias, and peripheral blood eosinophilia, has occurred after ingestion of impure batches of L-tryptophan. The EMG findings may be normal or show fibrillation potentials and mildly short-duration MUPs.

Alcohol is well known to have a toxic effect on muscle. Alcoholic myopathy occurs in two forms: acute and chronic. The characteristics of acute alcoholic myopathy are abrupt onset of muscle pain, swelling, and weakness. This myopathy is often associated with rhabdomyolysis and myoglobinuria. Needle EMG may show fibrillation potentials and short-duration MUPs in affected muscles. Chronic alcoholic myopathy is characterized by the insidious onset and progression of muscle weakness (proximal more than distal), with less muscle pain than in acute alcoholic myopathy. These patients often have an associated alcoholic peripheral neuropathy.[253] NCSs may show slowed motor and sensory conduction velocities, and needle EMG demonstrates short-duration MUPs in proximal muscles, often with a small degree of fibrillation potentials.

Focal and Traumatic Myopathies

Focal myopathies. Focal weakness with hypertrophy or atrophy has been reported in many different muscles. It is due to a wide variety of disorders, including focal myositis, sarcoidosis, local infection, heroin injections, and Becker and other dystrophies.[254,255] Some examples in the calf muscles have been due to localized S1 radiculopathies. One form, called the *dropped head syndrome*, has no defined cause, but the EMG and biopsy findings are those of myopathy. There may be some scattered fibrillation potentials.[256]

Marked focal myopathic changes may occur with repeated intramuscular injections of medications or illicit drugs, such as anesthetic agents, pentazocine, or heroin.[257] Progressive muscle weakness, induration, and fibrosis may lead to severe contractures. Because of fibrous replacement of muscle, a needle examination of the affected muscles demonstrates an absence of or a reduction of insertion activity associated with resistance during manual needle movement. Minimal scattered fibrillation potentials may occur, and occasional CRDs and myotonic discharges have been reported. Voluntary MUPs may be normal or of short duration. Severe local damage and fibrosis result in the loss of all EMG activity.[258]

Less severe forms of focal muscle damage with single injections, lacerations, or surgical procedures cause similar changes that are less severe and more localized.[259] For instance, fibrillation potentials and polyphasic or small MUPs in the paraspinal muscles result less commonly from an underlying myopathy than from the aftereffects of a laminectomy. Thus, surgical and other scars should always be avoided in needle EMG studies. Occasionally, patients are referred for EMG because of localized atrophy due to lipodystrophy.[260,261] Usually, no abnormality is found in the underlying muscle.

Traumatic myopathies. Widespread muscle injury may occur after crush injuries, heat damage, excessive exercise, or prolonged coma. In the severe syndromes, rhabdomyolysis with myoglobinuria and acute renal failure may occur (see Chap. 60). Myoglobinuria may also occur in many other disorders, including glycogen storage myopathies, neuroleptic malignant syndrome, infectious myopathies, toxic myopathies, and medication-induced myopathies and with some environmental toxins.[262] These syndromes almost always are associated with marked changes on needle EMG. In each of these, the destruction of muscle fibers can result in an early decrease in the amplitude and duration of MUPs, followed by fibrillation potentials in the remaining viable but noninnervated segments of muscle fibers.[263] As regeneration occurs, fibrillations decrease and complex long-duration, low-amplitude MUPs appear. These gradually increase in amplitude and duration as the nerve terminals and muscle fibers mature.

CRITICAL ILLNESS MYOPATHY

Critical illness neuropathy is well known, but similar severe weakness from primary muscle damage is less well recognized. Up to 84 percent of patients in an intensive care unit for longer than 1 week have neuromuscular disorders on electrical testing, and most of them have a combination of motor and sensory abnormalities.[264] The identification of critical illness myopathy has relied heavily on electrodiagnostic testing, with confirmation by muscle biopsy.[265] Recent reports have highlighted the importance and frequency of occurrence of primary muscle damage in patients with severe weakness while in an intensive care unit.[266] Sensory NCSs are normal, but CMAPs are of low amplitude and often long duration.[266] Direct muscle stimulation demonstrates an absence of response in this disorder, in contrast to severe nerve damage, in which the response is intact. On needle examination, MUPs have a short duration, with an excess of phases, and recruitment and MUNE are normal.[76]

DISTURBANCES OF NEUROMUSCULAR TRANSMISSION

Disturbances of neuromuscular transmission occur in many disorders of nerve and muscle. The reinnervated muscle fibers in motor neuron disease, muscle fibers damaged in the region of the neuromuscular junction in myositis, or recently reinnervated and regenerated muscle fibers all may show an impairment of neuromuscular transmission. This section focuses only on disorders that primarily affect the neuromuscular junction. Variability of MUPs on standard EMG, abnormal SFEMG, and a decrement on repetitive stimulation are the electrodiagnostic hallmarks of these disorders. Often, these measurements distinguish presynaptic from postsynaptic disorders of the neuromuscular junction.[267,268] The EMG findings in these disorders are among the most specific ones in clinical electrodiagnostic testing. Four major categories of diseases are reviewed: autoimmune myasthenia gravis, Lambert-Eaton myasthenic syndrome, congenital myasthenic syndromes, and botulism. The definitive identification of the electrophysiologic abnormality in these disorders requires intracellular microelectrode recordings from single muscle fibers. These can reveal the size and number of ACh quanta released at rest and with activation and can provide important information about the site of the defect.[269] The pathophysiologic basis defects of neuromuscular transmission is discussed in Chaps. 15, 16, and 64–66.

Acquired Myasthenia Gravis

Autoimmune myasthenia gravis. This is caused by a loss of postsynaptic ACh receptors, which results in low-amplitude EPPs and instability of neuromuscular transmission (see Chap. 64). The latter can be reflected in abnormal CMAP responses to repetitive nerve stimulation, MUPs of varying duration and amplitude during needle EMG, and abnormal jitter and blocking during SFEMG. When a muscle is weak, standard needle EMG is equal in sensitivity to SFEMG. Jitter is not detected on standard EMG, so that SFEMG has a greater overall capacity to show MUP alterations in myasthenia gravis. Standard needle electrode recordings, however, can quickly sample larger areas in many muscles. Therefore, if quantitation of the defect is not needed or if the abnormality is apparent, standard needle recording is sufficient to identify MUP variability.

A decrement of CMAPs on repetitive stimulation is the classic finding in patients with myasthenia gravis (Fig. 26-15). It is most likely to be found in a weak muscle at slow (2 to 3 Hz) stimulation rates. The amplitude of the initial CMAP is usually normal, but subsequent CMAPs decrease in amplitude until the fourth to sixth response. After this, the amplitude transiently increases, followed by a second and more slowly progressive decrease. In some instances, the amplitude may increase after the initial decrement and exceed the initial value by 10 to 20 percent after several seconds. Not infrequently, high rates of stimulation in mild myasthenia gravis increase the CMAP amplitude without an initial decrement, even though at low rates an initial decrement does occur. The increment is usually less than 40 percent. Thus, the optimal frequency of stimulation for observing the characteristic initial decrement is 2 to 3 Hz.

The defect of neuromuscular transmission is characteristically altered after a brief tetanic contraction of the muscle. In myasthenia gravis, after a brief, strong voluntary muscle contraction (10 s is sufficient), the amplitude of the evoked response is increased and the decrement at a low stimulation rate is diminished or absent. This represents postactivation facilitation. From 2 to 4 min after the exercise, the defect of neuromuscular transmission becomes more marked than it had been in the well-rested muscle. This represents postactivation exhaustion. In some instances, when no decrement is present in rested muscle, a decrement may occur during the period of postactivation exhaustion.

The yield of positive tests (i.e., a decrement in CMAPs at slow rates of stimulation) among patients with myasthenia gravis varies from laboratory to laboratory. In general, about 65 percent of patients show a decrement in the hand muscles, the easiest muscles to test. About 85 percent display decrement in proximal muscles, which are more difficult to test. When several distal and proximal muscles and the facial muscles are tested, a decrement may be found in up to 95 percent of patients.[270]

Patients with minimal or only ocular weakness rarely show an abnormal response except in proximal muscles or during selective stimulation of single axons.[271] Depending on the severity and distribution of the weakness, from 30 to 70 percent of cases are abnormal on repetitive stimulation. Repetitive stimulation is easy to apply, causes little discomfort to the patient, and can be quantitated for follow-up. The yield of positive tests can be increased with regional curare testing, but SFEMG is more readily applied. Thus, repetitive stimulation is generally used initially in the assessment of a patient with suspected myasthenia gravis. Only if repetitive stimulation and standard EMG findings are normal or equivocal is SFEMG necessary.[49,52]

Two other standard EMG changes can occur in myasthenia gravis: (1) If there is persistent blocking or if fibers have been lost from the motor unit, the MUPs will be of short duration and low amplitude.[272,273] This generally is not seen unless the disease is particularly severe or of long duration. (2) A more valuable finding clinically is fibrillation potentials,[274] which occur in up to 35 percent of patients with myasthenia gravis, particularly the elderly with mainly bulbar involvement. The fibrillation potentials are genuine, but they must be differentiated carefully from the small MUPs that may also be present. Fibrillations occur most commonly in paraspinal and bulbar muscles, especially the masseter. If fibrillations are present, the patient is less likely to respond well to acetylcholinesterase (AChE) medication.[274] A less obvious change is the decrease in end plate noise in myasthenia gravis because the MEPPs are reduced in amplitude.

The neuromuscular junction impairment is seen best with SFEMG, in which any abnormality of transmission produces an increase in jitter (Fig. 26-12).[3,271,275] Muscles with no decrement of CMAPs on repetitive stimulation have up to 50 percent blocking on SFEMG.[276] Patients with mild myasthenia gravis localized to eye muscles or even those in remission have increased jitter in clinically uninvolved muscles.[277] In ocular myasthenia, SFEMG was 100% sensitive and ACh receptor antibodies were 100 percent specific in one study.[278] Stimulated SFEMG of the frontalis muscle can reliably assess facial muscle involvement when a patient is unable to satisfactorily activate the muscles voluntarily.[279] Asymptomatic relatives of patients with myasthenia gravis have been shown to have higher-than-normal jitter values, although some of the patients may have had congenital myasthenia. Jitter values vary widely between end plates in a given motor unit, with some values normal and others markedly increased, reflecting the spotty distribution of the disease process. In ocular myasthenia gravis, up to 50 percent of jitter values for individual muscle fiber pairs in extensor digitorum communis are abnormal; mean values for jitter in the whole muscle are up to 50 μs (normal mean, less than 35 μs). Normal SFEMG findings in a limb make it more likely that the disease will remain localized to the ocular muscles.[280] The values are lower in patients in remission and higher in those with mild generalized myasthenia gravis.[270,281]

In clinically affected (weak) muscles, the jitter values become markedly prolonged and blocking begins to occur as transmission fails intermittently. The clinical weakness is a function of the number of failures. In normal subjects, there is no blocking. In a weak muscle in myasthenia gravis, blocking may be seen in as many as 90 percent of the fibers; the amount of blocking in individual fibers varies from none to complete blocking. Both jitter and blocking vary with activity, and they are decreased during postactivation facilitation and increased with postactivation exhaustion. They also are decreased by edrophonium and neostigmine. Both jitter and blocking are most prominent in the weakest or most clinically involved muscles. Thus, a higher percentage of abnormality is found in the facial muscles of patients with ocular or bulbar myasthenia. Percentages of abnormality range from 100 percent in patients with clinical weakness to 90 percent in those with focal or no demonstrable weakness. Comparison of the accuracy of SFEMG studies and ACh receptor antibody assay in the diagnosis of myasthenia gravis shows that they have comparable sensitivity. They have complementary roles in diagnosis.[270] SFEMG can identify abnormalities when none are found on immunologic testing and vice versa. The specificity of the immunologic test is much greater. Fiber density shows little change in myasthenia gravis.

Transient neonatal myasthenia gravis. From 10 to 15 percent of infants born to mothers who have generalized myasthenia gravis have neonatal myasthenia as a result of transplacental transfer of ACh receptor antibodies from mother to fetus. During repetitive stimulation of a motor nerve at 2 to 3 Hz in these infants, a progressive decrement occurs in the amplitude of the muscle action potential, reaching a minimum after four to six stimuli. Postactivation facilitation and exhaustion phenomena occur after tetanic stimulation. Edrophonium chloride decreases the decrement. In some infants, the decrement is more severe in distal hand muscles than in the deltoid or quadriceps, in contrast to the greater decrement in proximal muscles in mothers. An abnormal EMG may persist for as long as 2 to 4 months.[282]

As in adults, the CMAP in neonates is well maintained, with protracted stimulation at slow rates. However, in contrast to adults, it is poorly maintained at high rates of stimulation (50 Hz).[283]

Lambert-Eaton Myasthenic Syndrome

The Lambert-Eaton myasthenic syndrome (LEMS), sometimes associated with small cell carcinoma of the lung, also decreases the EPP amplitude.[269] Standard repetitive stimulation provides the most ready electrophysiologic means for distinguishing LEMS from myasthenia gravis. In more than 90 percent of the patients, the CMAP amplitude is low at rest, often less than 10 percent of normal,[284] even in muscles that are not clinically weak or atrophied. A decrement occurs on repetitive stimulation at slow rates, but it may be difficult to recognize because the CMAP amplitude is very low. Characteristically, the CMAP amplitude quickly increases with muscle activation, particularly with rapid rates of stimulation or vigorous exercise (Fig. 26-15). An increment of more than 50 percent is strong evidence for LEMS; the range of increase is usually from 200 to 1,000 percent. No differences in the responses are seen in patients with and in those without a tumor.[285]

SFEMG findings are similar to those in myasthenia gravis, with increased jitter and blocking in proportion to the involvement of the muscle.[286] The abnormalities in jitter and blocking are greater than in myasthenia gravis, with up to 90 percent blocking in rested muscle in the presence of only mild weakness. Both jitter and blocking improve with activation, particularly at rapid rates, because ACh release is facilitated.[51]

Comparable phenomena are found with standard needle EMG. MUPs vary in amplitude and configuration, becoming more stable and of higher amplitude with continued firing, especially at faster rates. MUPs may be of short duration and low amplitude if blocking is extensive. Fibrillation potentials are not seen.

Congenital Myasthenic Syndromes (CMS)

Several congenital defects of neuromuscular transmission have been described (see Chap. 66). These CMS manifest various clinical and EMG findings, depending on whether the defect is presynaptic, synaptic, or postsynaptic.[287–289] As in myasthenia gravis and LEMS, decrement on repetitive stimulation, variation in MUPs on standard needle examination, and abnormal jitter and blocking on SFEMG can occur. Some CMS have unique findings that can help identify the disorder.[267] Some electrodiagnostic changes resemble those of autoimmune disorders, and some suggest a specific CMS. In congenital end plate AChE deficiency and in the slow-channel syndromes, the EPP is prolonged, resulting in repetitive muscle action potential discharges.[289a,289b] This is best seen, after a single stimulus is applied to nerve, as a small second component of the CMAP. The second response may decrease or disappear with exercise or repetitive stimulation. Although repetitive CMAPs can occur from excess ACh drugs or in tetany, its presence should suggest a CMS.[290]

In another CMS, there is a presynaptic abnormality of ACh resynthesis caused by mutations in choline acetyltransferase.[290a] This disorder is typically associated with episodes of acute respiratory embarrassment culminating in apnea. The decrement in evoked response may occur only after prolonged 10-Hz stimulation or exercise and disappears slowly over several minutes after stimulation. Therefore, prolonged exercise followed by monitoring of the decremental response over several minutes should be considered in the evaluation of a patient with myasthenic symptoms associated with episodes of apnea.

Although technically difficult, spectral analysis of end plate activity has been reported to be useful in identifying congenital myasthenic syndromes associated with kinetic abnormalities of the acetylcholine receptor.[291]

Other Disorders of Neuromuscular Transmission

Clostridium botulinum, an anaerobic bacillus, releases a neurotoxin that paralyzes muscle by blocking ACh release from the motor nerve terminals at the neuromuscular junction. The EMG changes are typical.[18,292] The block of ACh release results in low-amplitude CMAPs that may show a small decrement at slow rates of stimulation and an increment with tetanic stimulation. Prolonged posttetanic facilitation of CMAPs has been described as a unique feature of botulism.[285] NCSs are normal. Needle EMG presents striking abnormalities, with prominent fibrillation potentials and MUPs of very short duration (less than 5 ms) and low amplitude (less than 500 μV). Variation in MUP configuration is seldom seen. Stimulated SFEMG may demonstrate the abnormality more clearly, including improvement with higher rates of stimulation.[293,294] The severity of the changes is proportional to the amount of transmission block and slowly subsides over several weeks after toxic exposure. Botulism can occur at any age, but it is particularly difficult to identify in infants, in whom it is less likely to be considered and testing is more difficult. EMG can be particularly helpful in these cases.[295–297]

MUSCLE SPASMS AND RELATED PHENOMENA

Muscle spasm is an inability of muscle to extend fully. It can result from an abnormality anywhere from the central nervous system to the muscle. For most of these disorders, the EMG can readily distinguish the mechanism underlying the inability to extend the muscle fully. Central disorders, such as spasticity, rigidity, dystonia, and other disorders of central motor control, are associated with normal MUPs and normal patterns of recruitment and activation of agonist and antagonist. The contraction is due solely to continued bombardment of the anterior horn cell pool by activity in descending pathways and, thus, is often more prominent in certain muscle groups, such as the leg extensors or arm flexors in spasticity.

Incomplete muscle relaxation also occurs with spinal cord diseases that impair the normal inhibitory mechanisms of motor unit firing. Patients with strychnine poisoning, tetanus, and "stiff-man" syndrome are in this group. The configuration and firing pattern of MUPs are normal,[298] but normal agonist-antagonist interactions are impaired and the normal silent period on nerve stimulation during the persistent MUP discharge may be lost.

The commonest peripheral cause of muscle spasm is a *muscle cramp*. This usually arises from abnormal discharges of nerve terminals in a muscle. Cramps can occur in normal persons and can be familial without known associated disease.[299,300] They also can be symptomatic of neurogenic processes, such as neuropathies, and ALS. Cramps occur in some systemic disorders, such as uremia and hypomagnesemia, but only rarely in myopathies, such as those associated with thyroid disease.[301,302] A cramp is recorded electrically as simple triphasic potentials firing irregularly at rates of 40 to 60 Hz, first in increasing numbers and then, as the cramp subsides, in decreasing numbers. High-density surface EMG suggests that cramps may arise in small groups of nerve terminals or muscle fibers.[303]

Disorders with *continuous muscle fiber activity* caused by primary nerve disease have been described.[29] These can be separated into broad categories by the rate of discharge (interpotential interval) of individual axons and motor units. Those with rates of discharge of 200 Hz and higher are usually due to a channel disorder. *Neuromyotonia* is an autoimmune disorder of voltage-gated potassium channels with characteristics of neuromyotonic discharges of varying length and recurrence.[304] *Tetany* with carpopedal spasm has been attributed to an abnormality of the calcium control of the sodium channel, with spontaneous axonal discharges at high rates of up to 300 Hz. Both the CMAPs and MUPs under voluntary control display repetitive discharges as doublets or multiplets. Tetany is aggravated by hyperventilation or ischemia. The rapid discharges in tetany are like neuromyotonic discharges. Isaac syndrome and other syndromes of continuous muscle fiber activity are also associated with 150- to 300-Hz neurotonic discharges, which have the characteristic sound of a speeding race car.[28] Similar disorders have been reported with some chronic neuropathies. In some hereditary peripheral neuropathies, discharges similar to neuromyotonic discharges can occur but last for shorter periods and recur regularly.[32] On inspection, the involved muscles are in a state of contraction, but with some myokymia-like quivering.

Myokymia is a rippling of muscles that looks like a "can of worms." It is due to various disorders, including radiation damage to nerves, multiple sclerosis, and tumors. EMG shows characteristic recurring bursts of MUPs firing at 30 to 80 Hz. Some forms of muscle contractions are not associated with any EMG activity. Rippling muscle disease involves ongoing spontaneous muscle movement as well as prolonged contraction in response to percussion that is not accompanied by any EMG activity.[305]

Primary muscle diseases can also produce persistent muscle contraction resembling spasms. These occur with or without an associated electrical discharge. Those in myotonia congenita and myotonic dystrophy, described below, are associated with myotonic discharges. Involuntary muscle contraction produced by exercise also occurs with glycolytic enzyme deficiencies, such as phosphorylase deficiency. These are caused by altered contractile mechanisms within the muscle fibers and are not associated with electrical activity. The term *contracture* is applied to this phenomenon. Contractions also can be due to connective tissue proliferation, which prevents muscle extension without involving electrical or contractile mechanisms. These can be due to several neurogenic, myopathic, and orthopedic disorders.

Primary muscle disease with excessive muscle contraction must be distinguished from central disorders with excess muscle contraction, like "stiff-man" syndrome, an immune-mediated disorder with glutamate decarboxylase antibodies. EMG recordings show normal MUPs and patterns of activation that are abnormal only in their persistence and lack of inhibition by antagonist contraction.[306]

One form of contracture in newborn infants is called *arthrogryposis* (see Chap. XX).[307] It may result from intrauterine muscle disease, lower motor neuron disease, or orthopedic disorders. The EMG can be helpful in distinguishing disorders with excess muscle contraction by demonstrating changes typical of one or the other.[308] The most common cause is motor neuron disease, which is associated with poor recruitment and long-duration, high-amplitude MUPs.

Findings in Neural Diseases

PERIPHERAL NERVE DISORDERS

A few peripheral nerve disorders result in proximal weakness, particularly polyradiculopathies. The acute Guillain-Barré syndrome is unlikely to be mistaken for myopathy, but the more slowly progressive, chronic inflammatory demyelinating polyradiculoneuropathy occasionally is. NCSs are of critical importance in making this distinction because they typically show marked slowing of the velocity and dispersion of the CMAPs. In addition, needle examination shows reduced recruitment with large MUPs. Fibrillation potentials may not be prominent.

MOTOR NEURON DISEASES

ALS, the most common adult motor neuron disease, typically has asymmetrical weakness with no sensory loss. Therefore, only infrequently is it mistaken for myopathy, especially if the upper motor neuron signs are not yet evident. In contrast, Kugelberg-Welander disease, a slowly progressive spinal muscular atrophy of childhood that commonly extends into early adulthood, has symmetrical weakness without sensory loss or upper motor neuron signs and may be mistaken for myopathy.[151] The EMG can be extremely helpful in making an accurate diagnosis of spinal muscular atrophy (SMA).[309–311] The EMG findings are those of a chronic neurogenic process with poor recruitment and large MUPs. The severity of findings increases with the duration of the disease. Early in the disease, muscle cramps and minimal EMG abnormalities may be the only findings. If the duration of clinical disease is more than 1 year, impairment of recruitment and large MUPs are widespread and prominent. Fibrillation potentials in SMA are infrequent and scattered, in contrast to their prominence in ALS. The fibrillation potentials may be of such low amplitude and short duration that they are difficult to distinguish from baseline noise. True fasciculation potentials are usually infrequent, but they must be distinguished from contraction fasciculation, the potentials (or twitches) of large motor units in muscles that are not completely relaxed. This differentiation can be made only by recognizing the irregular firing pattern of true fasciculations, as opposed to the semirhythmic pattern of MUP firing. Many forms of iterative discharge can occur in SMA. Complex repetitive discharges are more common than in ALS. Neurotonic discharges (rapidly waning potentials firing at 150 to 300 Hz) are recorded from some patients with long-standing SMA.

Motor unit potentials in SMA are usually long duration and high amplitude.[312] Polyphasic MUPs, although less common than in ALS, may include satellite potentials with the MUP. These late components are the action potentials of atrophic single muscle fibers, of split fibers, or of muscle fibers innervated by a long, thin nerve terminal. In the late stages of SMA, short-duration, low-amplitude MUPs may be found, especially in weight-bearing muscles such as the anterior tibial and gastrocnemius muscles.[33] These small MUPs are typically associated with histologic changes of the type seen in a myopathy.[151] NCSs of motor and sensory fibers in SMA are normal. CMAP amplitudes are not as low as those in ALS and are often normal.[313] MUNE is often markedly reduced.[314] Responses to repetitive stimulation are usually normal.

The EMG diagnosis of SMA usually is not difficult in a patient with atrophic muscles, normal conduction, poor MUP recruitment, and large MUPs. The major distinction is usually a chronic myopathy, which would have small, rather than large, MUPs.[315] However, in the late stages of SMA and some myopathies, severe degeneration of muscle can result in MUP similarities that may make it difficult to distinguish them by EMG. Chronic inflammatory myopathies may show large, long-duration MUPs, suggesting a neurogenic process. Atrophic muscle in neurogenic disease that has been chronically overworked may show the changes of a myopathy, both on EMG and on histologic studies. In these patients, it is better to study less severely involved muscles, which are less likely to have changes resembling those of myopathy. In patients with widespread, chronic, wasting disease, EMG findings that are not clear-cut must be interpreted cautiously.

INTERPRETATION OF EMG AND NCSs

The limited repertoire of EMG changes compared with the large number of muscle diseases implies that the EMG usually can categorize only groups of muscle disorders and not identify specific entities.[38] Therefore, the electromyographer must associate patterns of EMG change with groups of disorders. The summary in Tables 26-3 and 26-4 may help in analyzing and interpreting these observed changes.

Table 26-5. SUMMARY OF CHARACTERISTIC ELECTRODIAGNOSTIC FINDINGS IN SEVERAL DISORDERS CAUSING INFANTILE HYPOTONIA

Disorder	Conduction velocity	CMAP amplitude	CMAP decrement	Fibrillation potentials	Myotonic discharges	MUP recruitment	MUP duration
Motor neuron disease	(Slow)	Low	(+)	+	0	Reduced	Long
Demyelinating neuropathy	Slow	Low	0	(+)	0	Reduced	(Long)
Axonal neuropathy	(Slow)	Low	0	++	0	Reduced	Long
Myasthenia gravis	Normal	Normal	+	0	0	Normal	Vary
Botulism	Normal	Low	(+)	+	0	Reduced	Short
Lambert-Eaton myasthenic syndrome	Normal	Low	+	0	0	Normal	Short
Acid maltase deficiency	Normal	Normal	0	+	+	Normal	Short
Congenital dystrophy	Normal	Normal	0	(+)	0	Normal	Short
Neonatal myotonia	Normal	Normal	0	(+)	+	Normal	Normal

KEY: 0 = Not present; (+) = rare reports of abnormality; + = abnormality present.

The high degree of accuracy of EMG in identifying the type of neuromuscular disease has been confirmed in several studies. In one study in which muscle biopsy and EMG findings were compared, muscle biopsy and EMG were necessary to make a diagnosis in 60 percent of the patients; of these patients, only 6 percent had EMG and biopsy findings that were inconsistent, and all these patients had Kugelberg-Welander disease.[80] In another quantitative analysis of MUPs and recruitment, the EMG findings agreed with the clinical diagnosis in 87 percent of the patients with myopathy and in 91 percent of those with neurogenic disorders, compared with 79 and 92 percent, respectively, for muscle biopsy findings.[316] Among 32 patients in this study with myopathy for whom there was a discordance with clinical classification, 28 were identified by EMG to have myopathy and 2 by biopsy, but the biopsy findings were able to provide a more specific diagnosis. EMG/NCS can be equally effective in diagnosis of infantile hypotonia (Table 26-5).[317,318] The divergence in electrophysiologic and histologic findings in some patients need not imply methodologic error, because some physiologic changes may not be reflected in the biopsy specimen, and histologic changes within muscle fibers may not be expressed electrophysiologically.[319]

Neuromyopathies

Myopathies and neuropathies are not always readily distinguished with electrodiagnostic testing for two reasons. A few myopathies have findings of a neurogenic process, and some neurogenic disorders have findings suggesting a myopathy. The neurogenic changes in myopathy may appear either as clearly defined abnormalities on NCS or as large MUPs of the type usually seen in peripheral nerve disease.

Abnormalities on NCSs are sometimes due to a clearly unrelated disorder, such as diabetes mellitus. If NCSs are abnormal in a case of myopathy, the electromyographer needs to search for evidence of such disorders. If they are not evident, myopathies due to disorders that involve both nerve and muscle must be considered. Among disorders in which the primary disease results in both myopathy and neuropathy, connective tissue disorders, particularly vasculitis, are the most common. Sarcoidoisis and amyloidosis have been shown to involve both muscle and nerve in a patient.[107,320] Some toxic agents may produce changes in nerve and muscle, in particular chloroquine,[239] omeprazole,[321] and amiodarone.

Mixtures of large and small MUPs may be seen in both primary myopathies and primary neurogenic disorders (Table 26-6). The findings of both small and large MUPs are most common in chronic myositis and inclusion body myositis. Infantile acid maltase deficiency, debrancher and brancher enzyme deficiencies, and mitochondrial myopathies may all show some large MUPs. A dominantly inherited, progressive myopathy with clear clinical and EMG features of neuropathy linked to chromosome 19p13 has features similar to those of inclusion body myositis.[322]

Small MUPs are sometimes seen in rapidly progressing motor neuron diseases and in recovery from a severe polyradiculopathy. The sprouting nerve terminals may innervate only a few muscle fibers and produce small MUPs.[310] Such potentials that are polyphasic and vary in size or shape from moment to moment have been called *nascent potentials*.

Table 26-6. DISORDERS WITH LONG- AND SHORT-DURATION MUPS

Chronic myopathy
    Polymyositis and dermatomyositis
    Inclusion body myositis
    Muscular dystrophy
Nerve and muscle involvement
    Connective tissue disorders, especially vasculitis
    Sarcoidosis
    Amyloidosis
    Toxic myopathies
        Chloroquine
        Amiodarone
        Omeprazole
    Infantile acid maltase
    Debrancher enzyme deficiency
    Mitochondrial myopathy
Neurogenic disorders
    Rapidly progressing, e.g., motor neuron disease
    Early reinnervation

List of Abbreviations

ACh	acetylcholine	MELAS	mitochondrial myopathy, encephalopathy, lactic acidosis, strokes
AChE	acetylcholinesterase		
ALS	amyotrophic lateral sclerosis	MEPP	miniature end plate potential
BSAP	brief duration, short amplitude, abundant, polyphasic	MERRF	myoclonic epilepsy with ragged red fibers
		MNGIE	mitochondrial neurogastrointestinal encephalomyopathy
CMAP	compound muscle action potential		
CMS	congenital myasthenic syndrome	MUNE	motor unit number estimate
CRD	complex repetitive discharge	MUP	motor unit potential
EMG	electromyography	NAP	nerve action potential
EPP	end plate potential	NARP	neuropathy, ataxia, and retinitis pigmentosa
FSHD	facioscapulohumeral muscular dystrophy	NCS	nerve conduction study
LEMS	Lambert-Eaton myasthenic syndrome	PROMM	proximal myotonic myopathy
		SFEMG	single-fiber electromyography
MCD	mean consecutive difference	SMA	spinal muscular atrophy

References

1. Cohn RD, Campbell KP: Molecular basis of muscular dystrophies. *Muscle Nerve* 23:1456–1471, 2000.
2. Phillips LH: Chair, AAEM Nomenclature Committee, 1994–2001. AAEM glossary of terms in electrodiagnostic medicine. *Muscle Nerve Suppl* 10:S1–S50, 2001.
3. Stålberg E, Trontelj JV: *Single Fiber Electromyography: Studies in Healthy and Diseased Muscle*, 2nd ed. New York: Raven Press, 1994.
4. Caforio AL, Rossi B, Risaliti R, et al: Type 1 fiber abnormalities in skeletal muscle of patients with hypertrophic and dilated cardiomyopathy: Evidence of subclinical myogenic myopathy. *J Am Coll Cardiol* 14:1464–1473, 1989.
5. Stålberg E: Invited review: Electrodiagnostic assessment and monitoring of motor unit changes in disease. *Muscle Nerve* 14:293–303, 1991.
6. Stålberg E, Antoni L: Electrophysiological cross section of the motor unit. *J Neurol Neurosurg Psychiatry* 43:469–474, 1980.
7. Daube JR: Assessing the motor unit with needle electromyography, in Daube JR (ed): *Clinical Neurophysiology*, 2d ed. New York: Oxford University Press, 2002; pp 293–323.
8. Daube JR: AAEM minimonograph #11: Needle examination in clinical electromyography. *Muscle Nerve* 14:685–700, 1991.
9. Lorente de Nó R: *A Study of Nerve Physiology*. Vol 2. New York: Rockefeller Institute for Medical Research, 1947; p 466.
10. Dumitru D, King JC: Varied morphology of spontaneous single muscle fiber discharges. *Am J Phys Med Rehabil* 77:128–139, 1998.
11. Wiederholt WC: "End-plate noise" in electromyography. *Neurology* 20:214–224, 1970.
12. Dumitru D: Physiologic basis of potentials recorded in electromyography. *Muscle Nerve* 23:1667–1685, 2000.
13. Gath I, Stålberg E: On the volume conduction in human skeletal muscle: In situ measurements. *Electroencephalogr Clin Neurophysiol* 43:106–110, 1977.
14. Lateva ZC, McGill KC: Estimating motor-unit architectural properties by analyzing motor-unit action potential morphology. *Clin Neurophysiol* 112:127–135, 2001.
15. Buchthal F, Pinelli P, Rosenfalck P: Action potential parameters in normal human muscle and their physiological determinants. *Acta Physiol Scand* 32:219–229, 1954.
16. Andreassen S, Rosenfalck A: Regulation of the firing pattern of single motor units. *J Neurol Neurosurg Psychiatry* 43:897–906, 1980.
17. Schulte-Mattler WJ, Georgiadis D, Zierz S: Discharge patterns of spontaneous activity and motor units on concentric needle electromyography. *Muscle Nerve* 24:123–126, 2001.
18. Gutmann L, Pratt L: Pathophysiologic aspects of human botulism. *Arch Neurol* 33:175–179, 1976.
19. Desmedt JE: Muscular dystrophy contrasted with denervation: Different mechanisms underlying spontaneous fibrillations. *Electroencephalogr Clin Neurophysiol Suppl* 34:531–146, 1978.
20. Dumitru D, King JC, Rogers WE, et al: Positive sharp wave and fibrillation potential modeling. *Muscle Nerve* 22:242–251, 1999.
21. Brown JC: Muscle weakness after rest in myotonic disorders; an electrophysiological study. *J Neurol Neurosurg Psychiatry* 37:1336–1342, 1974.
22. Durelli L, Mutani R, Piredda S, et al: The quantification of myotonia. A problem in the evaluation of new antimyotonic drugs. *J Neurol Sci* 59:167–173, 1983.
23. Stoehr M: Low frequency bizarre discharges. A particular type of electromyographical spontaneous activity in paretic skeletal muscle. *Electromyogr Clin Neurophysiol* 18:147–156, 1978.
24. Preston DC, Finkleman RS, Munsat TL: Dystonic postures generated from complex repetitive discharges. *Neurology* 46:257–258, 1996.
25. Albers JW, Allen AA II, Bastron JA, et al: Limb myokymia. *Muscle Nerve* 4:494–504, 1981.
26. Daube JR, Kelly JJ Jr, Martin RA: Facial myokymia with polyradiculoneuropathy. *Neurology* 29:662–669, 1979.
27. Trontelj J, Stålberg E: Bizarre repetitive discharges recorded with single fibre EMG. *J Neurol Neurosurg Psychiatry* 46:310–316, 1983.
28. Subramony SH, Parker CC, Evans OB, et al: Mistaken diagnoses in continuous muscle fiber activity of peripheral nerve origin. *Pediatr Neurol* 6:257–259, 1990.
29. Warmolts JR, Mendell JR: Neurotonia: Impulse-induced repetitive discharges in motor nerves in peripheral neuropathy. *Ann Neurol* 7:245–250, 1980.
30. Coers C, Telerman-Toppet N, Durdu J: Neurogenic benign fasciculations, pseudomyotonia, and pseudotetany. A disease in search of a name. *Arch Neurol* 38:282–287, 1981.
31. Torbergsen T, Stålberg E, Brautaset NJ: Generator sites for spontaneous activity in neuromyotonia. An EMG study. *Electroencephalogr Clin Neurophysiol* 101:69–78, 1996.
32. Auger RG, Daube JR, Gomez MR, et al: Hereditary form of sustained muscle activity of peripheral nerve origin causing generalized myokymia and muscle stiffness. *Ann Neurol* 15:13–21, 1984.
33. Stålberg E, Karlsson L: Simulation of the normal concentric needle electromyogram by using a muscle model. *Clin Neurophysiol* 112:464–471, 2001.
34. Stålberg E, Falck B, Sonoo M, et al: Multi-MUP EMG analysis—a two year experience in daily clinical work. *Electroencephalogr Clin Neurophysiol* 97:145–154, 1995.
35. Jongen PJ, Vingerhoets HM, Roeleveld K, et al: Automatic decomposition electromyography in idiopathic inflammatory myopathies. *J Neurol* 243:79–85, 1996.
36. Gath I, Sjaastad O, Loken AC: Myopathic electromyographic changes correlated with histopathology in Wohlfart-Kugelberg-Welander disease. *Neurology* 19:344–352, 1969.
37. Warmolts JR, Mendell JR: Open-biopsy electromyography. Direct correlation of a pattern of excessively recruited, pathologically small motor unit potentials with histologic evidence of neuropathy. *Arch Neurol* 36:406–409, 1979.
38. Takahashi K, Kameyama M: Electromyography and histopathology of muscle and spinal cord. Analysis of 105 skeletal muscles from 31 autopsy cases. *J Neurol Sci* 16:465–479, 1972.
39. Uncini A, Lange DJ, Lovelace RE, et al: Long-duration polyphasic motor unit potentials in myopathies: A quantitative study with pathological correlation. *Muscle Nerve* 13:263–267, 1990.
40. Nakashima K, Tabuchi Y, Takahashi K: The diagnostic significance of large action potentials in myopathy. *J Neurol Sci* 61:161–170, 1983.
41. Dorfman LJ, Howard JE, McGill KC: Motor unit firing rates and firing rate variability in the detection of neuromuscular disorders. *Electroencephalogr Clin Neurophysiol* 73:215–224, 1989.
42. Lang AH, Partanen VS: "Satellite potentials" and the duration of motor unit potentials in normal, neuropathic and myopathic muscles. *J Neurol Sci* 27:513–524, 1976.
43. Campos C, Malanda A, Gila L, et al: Quantification of jiggle in real electromyographic signals. *Muscle Nerve* 23:1022–1034, 2000.
44. Finsterer J, Mamoli B: Turn/amplitude-analysis in subclinical myogenic lesions. *Acta Neurol Scand* 96:46–51, 1997.

45. AAEM Quality Assurance Committee: Literature review of the usefulness of repetitive nerve stimulation and single fiber EMG in the electrodiagnostic evaluation of patients with suspected myasthenia gravis or Lambert-Eaton myasthenic syndrome. *Muscle Nerve* 24:1239–1247, 2001.
46. Harper CM Jr: Single fiber electromyography, in Daube JR (ed): *Clinical Neurophysiology*, 2d ed. New York: Oxford University Press, 2002; pp 343–347.
47. Stålberg E, Trontelj JV: The study of normal and abnormal neuromuscular transmission with single fibre electromyography. *J Neurosci Methods* 74:145–154, 1997.
48. Ekstedt J, Nilsson G, Stålberg E: Calculation of the electromyographic jitter. *J Neurol Neurosurg Psychiatry* 37:526–539, 1974.
49. Stålberg E, Trontelj JV: *Single Fiber Electromyography: Studies in Healthy and Diseased Muscle*, 2d ed. New York: Raven Press, 1994; pp 31–40.
50. Bertorini TE, Stålberg E, Yuson CP, et al: Single-fiber electromyography in neuromuscular disorders: Correlation of muscle histochemistry, single-fiber electromyography, and clinical findings. *Muscle Nerve* 17:345–353, 1994.
51. Chaudhry V, Watson DF, Bird SJ, et al: Stimulated single-fiber electromyography in Lambert-Eaton myasthenic syndrome. *Muscle Nerve* 14:1227–1230, 1991.
52. Oey PL, Wieneke GH, Hoogenraad TU, et al: Ocular myasthenia gravis: The diagnostic yield of repetitive nerve stimulation and stimulated single fiber EMG of orbicularis oculi muscle and infrared reflection oculography. *Muscle Nerve* 16:142–149, 1993.
53. Schwarz J, Planck J, Briegel J, et al: Single-fiber electromyography, nerve conduction studies, and conventional electromyography in patients with critical-illness polyneuropathy: Evidence for a lesion of terminal motor axons. *Muscle Nerve* 20:696–701, 1997.
54. Stålberg E, Fawcett PR: Macro EMG in healthy subjects of different ages. *J Neurol Neurosurg Psychiatry* 45:870–878, 1982.
55. Roeleveld K, Stegeman DF, Falck B, et al: Motor unit size estimation: Confrontation of surface EMG with macro EMG. *Electroencephalogr Clin Neurophysiol* 105:181–188, 1997.
56. Finsterer J, Fuglsang-Frederiksen A: Concentric-needle versus macro EMG. II. Detection of neuromuscular disorders. *Clin Neurophysiol* 112:853–860, 2001.
57. Fuglsang-Frederiksen A, Ronager J: EMG power spectrum, turns-amplitude analysis and motor unit potential duration in neuromuscular disorders. *J Neurol Sci* 97:81–91, 1990.
58. Fuglsang-Frederiksen A: The utility of interference pattern analysis. *Muscle Nerve* 23:18–36, 2000.
59. Liguori R, Dahl K, Vingtoft S, et al: Determination of peak-ratio by digital turns-amplitude analysis on line. *Electromyogr Clin Neurophysiol* 30:371–378, 1990.
60. Priori A, Cinnante C, Pesenti A, et al: Decreased EMG inhibition following electrical stimulation over muscle tendons in myopathies. *Clin Neurophysiol* 112:1931–1935, 2001.
61. Daube JR: Compound muscle action potentials, in Daube JR (ed): *Clinical Neurophysiology*, 2d ed. New York: Oxford University Press, 2002; pp 231–267.
62. Quinlan JG, Iaizzo PA, Gronert GA, et al: Twitch response in a myopathy with impaired relaxation but no myotonia. *Muscle Nerve* 13:326–329, 1990.
63. Daube JR: Nerve conduction studies, in Aminoff MJ (ed): *Electrodiagnosis in Clinical Neurology*, 4th ed. New York: Churchill Livingstone, 1999; pp 253–289.
64. Hermann RC Jr: Assessing the neuromuscular junction with repetitive stimulation studies, in Daube JR (ed): *Clinical Neurophysiology*, 2d ed. New York: Oxford University Press, 2002; pp 268–281.
65. McManis PG, Lambert EH, Daube JR: The exercise test in periodic paralysis. *Muscle Nerve* 9:704–710, 1986.
66. Engel AG, Lambert EH, Rosevear JW, et al: Clinical and electromyographic studies in a patient with primary hypokalemic periodic paralysis. *Am J Med* 38:626–640, 1965.
67. McComas AJ: Motor-unit estimation: The beginning. *J Clin Neurophysiol* 12:560–564, 1995.
68. Daube JR: Estimating the number of motor units in a muscle, in Daube JR (ed): *Clinical Neurophysiology*, 2d ed. New York: Oxford University Press, 2002; pp 358–369.
69. Shefner JM: Motor unit number estimation in human neurological diseases and animal models. *Clin Neurophysiol* 112:955–964, 2001.
70. Daube JR: Estimating the number of motor units in a muscle. *J Clin Neurophysiol* 12:585–594, 1995.
71. Gooch CL, Harati Y: Motor unit number estimation, ALS and clinical trials. *Amyotroph Lateral Scler Other Motor Neuron Disord* 1:71–82, 2000.
72. Jabre JF, Chirico-Post J, Weiner M: Stimulation SFEMG in myasthenia gravis. *Muscle Nerve* 12:38–42, 1989.
73. Zwarts MJ: Evaluation of the estimation of muscle fiber conduction velocity. Surface versus needle method. *Electroencephalogr Clin Neurophysiol* 73:544–548, 1989.
74. Naumann M, Reiners K: Diagnostic value of in situ muscle fiber conduction velocity measurements in myopathies. *Acta Neurol Scand* 93:193–197, 1996.
75. Rich MM, Bird SJ, Raps EC, et al: Direct muscle stimulation in acute quadriplegic myopathy. *Muscle Nerve* 20:665–673, 1997.
76. Trojaborg W, Weimer LH, Hays AP: Electrophysiologic studies in critical illness associated weakness: Myopathy or neuropathy—a reappraisal. *Clin Neurophysiol* 112:1586–1593, 2001.
77. Kiernan MC, Hart IK, Bostock H: Excitability properties of motor axons in patients with spontaneous motor unit activity. *J Neurol Neurosurg Psychiatry* 70:56–64, 2001.
78. Harper CM Jr: Myopathies, in Jones HR Jr, Bolton CF, Harper CM Jr (eds): *Pediatric Clinical Electromyography*. New York: Lippincott-Raven Publishers, 1996; pp 387–444.
79. Liguori R, Fuglsang-Frederiksen A, Nix W, et al: Electromyography in myopathy. *Neurophysiol Clin* 27:200–203, 1997.
80. Black JT, Bhatt GP, Dejesus PV, et al: Diagnostic accuracy of clinical data, quantitative electromyography and histochemistry in neuromuscular disease. A study of 105 cases. *J Neurol Sci* 21:59–70, 1974.
81. Tymms KE, Beller EM, Webb J, et al: Correlation between tests of muscle involvement and clinical muscle weakness in polymyositis and dermatomyositis. *Clin Rheumatol* 9:523–529, 1990.
82. Barkhaus PE, Nandedkar SD, Sanders DB: Quantitative EMG in inflammatory myopathy. *Muscle Nerve* 13:247–253, 1990.
83. Roddy SM, Ashwal S, Peckham N, et al: Infantile myositis: A case diagnosed in the neonatal period. *Pediatr Neurol* 2:241–244, 1986.
84. Swash M, Schwartz MS: Implications of longitudinal muscle fibre splitting in neurogenic and myopathic disorders. *J Neurol Neurosurg Psychiatry* 40:1152–1159, 1977.
85. Streib EW, Wilbourn AJ, Mitsumoto H: Spontaneous electrical muscle fiber activity in polymyositis and dermatomyositis. *Muscle Nerve* 2:14–18, 1979.
86. Sandstedt PE, Henriksson KG, Larrsson LE: Quantitative electromyography in polymyositis and dermatomyositis. *Acta Neurol Scand* 65:110–121, 1982.
87. Griggs RC, Askanas V, DiMauro S, et al: Inclusion body myositis and myopathies. *Ann Neurol* 38:705–713, 1995.
88. Lotz BP, Engel AG, Nishino H, et al: Inclusion body myositis. Observations in 40 patients. *Brain* 112:727–747, 1989.
89. Julien J, Vital C, Vallat JM, et al: Inclusion body myositis. Clinical, biological and ultrastructural study. *J Neurol Sci* 55:15–24, 1982.
90. Luciano CA, Dalakas MC: Inclusion body myositis: No evidence for a neurogenic component. *Neurology* 48:29–33, 1997.
91. Henriksson KG, Stålberg E: The terminal innervation pattern in polymyositis: A histochemical and SFEMG study. *Muscle Nerve* 1:3–13, 1978.
92. Foote RA, Kimbrough SM, Stevens JC: Lupus myositis. *Muscle Nerve* 5:65–68, 1982.
93. Ringel RA, Brick JE, Brick JF, et al: Muscle involvement in the scleroderma syndromes. *Arch Intern Med* 150:2550–2552, 1990.
94. Bromberg MB, Donofrio PD, Segal BM: Steroid-responsive electromyographic abnormalities in polymyalgia rheumatica. *Muscle Nerve* 13:138–141, 1990.
95. Bekkelund SI, Torbergsen T, Husby G, et al: Myopathy and neuropathy in rheumatoid arthritis. A quantitative controlled electromyographic study. *J Rheumatol* 26:2348–2351, 1999.
96. Simon DB, Ringel SP, Sufit RL: Clinical spectrum of fascial inflammation. *Muscle Nerve* 5:525–537, 1982.
97. Helfrich DJ, Walker ER, Martinez AJ, et al: Scleromyxedema myopathy: Case report and review of the literature. *Arthritis Rheum* 31:1437–1441, 1988.
98. Hens L, Bulcke JA, De Meirsman J, et al: [Shulman's syndrome. Diffuse fasciitis with eosinophilia. A differential diagnosis from polymyositis.] (English translation by the authors.) *Rev Neurol* 137:203–210, 1981.
99. Durette MR, Rodriquez AA, Agre JC, et al: Needle electromyographic evaluation of patients with myofascial or fibromyalgic pain. *Am J Phys Med Rehabil* 70:154–156, 1991.
100. Jamal GA, Hansen S: Electrophysiological studies in the post-viral fatigue syndrome. *J Neurol Neurosurg Psychiatry* 48:691–694, 1985.
101. Herrera R, Varela E, Morales G, et al: Dermatomyositis-like syndrome caused by trichinae. Report of two cases. *J Rheumatol* 12:782–784, 1985.
102. Gross B, Ochoa J: Trichinosis: Clinical report and histochemistry of muscle. *Muscle Nerve* 2:394–398, 1979.
103. Schimrigk K, Uldall B: The disease of Besnier-Boeck-Schaumann and granulomatous polymyositis. *Eur Neurol* 1:137–157, 1968.
104. Gardner-Thorpe C: Muscle weakness due to sarcoid myopathy. Six case reports and an evaluation of steroid therapy. *Neurology* 22:917–928, 1972.
105. Prayson RA: Amyloid myopathy: Clinicopathologic study of 16 cases. *Hum Pathol* 29:463–468, 1998.
106. Rubin DI, Hermann RC: Electrophysiologic findings in amyloid myopathy. *Muscle Nerve* 22:355–359, 1999.
107. Gemignani F, Bellanova MF, Salih S, et al: Sarcoid neuromyopathy with selective involvement of the intramuscular nerves. *Acta Neuropathol (Berl)* 95:437–441, 1998.
108. Robberecht W, Theys P, Lammens M, et al: Distal myopathy as the presenting manifestation of sarcoidosis. *J Neurol Neurosurg Psychiatry* 59:642–643, 1995.
109. Dewberry RG, Schneider BF, Cale WF, et al: Sarcoid myopathy presenting with diaphragm weakness. *Muscle Nerve* 16:832–835, 1993.

110. Celesia GG: Disorders of membrane channels or channelopathies. *Clin Neurophysiol* 112:2–18, 2001.
111. Gruener R, Stern LZ, Weisz RR: Conduction velocities in single fibers of diseased human muscle. *Neurology* 29:1293–1297, 1979.
112. Streib EW: AAEE minimonograph #27: Differential diagnosis of myotonic syndromes. *Muscle Nerve* 10:603–615, 1987.
113. Bundey S, Carter CO, Soothill JF: Early recognition of heterozygotes for the gene for dystrophia myotonica. *J Neurol Neurosurg Psychiatry* 33:279–293, 1970.
114. Pryse-Phillips W, Johnson GJ, Larsen B: Incomplete manifestations of myotonic dystrophy in a large kinship in Labrador. *Ann Neurol* 11:582–591, 1982.
115. Swift TR, Ignacio OJ, Dyken PR: Neonatal dystrophia myotonica. Electrophysiologic studies. *Am J Dis Child* 129:734–737, 1975.
116. Watters GV, Williams TW: Early onset myotonic dystrophy. Clinical and laboratory findings in five families and a review of the literature. *Arch Neurol* 17:137–152, 1967.
117. Zellweger H, Ionasescu V: Early onset of myotonic dystrophy in infants. *Am J Dis Child* 125:601–604, 1973.
118. Aminoff MJ, Layzer RB, Satya-Murti S, et al: The declining electrical response of muscle to repetitive nerve stimulation in myotonia. *Neurology* 27:812–816, 1977.
119. Streib EW, Sun SF, Yarkowsky T: Transient paresis in myotonic syndromes: A simplified electrophysiologic approach. *Muscle Nerve* 5:719–723, 1982.
120. Jamal GA, Weir AI, Hansen S, et al: Myotonic dystrophy. A reassessment by conventional and more recently introduced neurophysiological techniques. *Brain* 109:1279–1296, 1986.
121. Bartel P, Lotz B, Robinson E, et al: Posterior tibial and sural nerve somatosensory evoked potentials in dystrophia myotonica. *J Neurol Sci* 70:55–65, 1985.
122. Panayiotopoulos CP: F-wave conduction velocity in the deep peroneal nerve: Charcot-Marie-Tooth disease and dystrophia myotonica. *Muscle Nerve* 1:37–44, 1978.
123. Roohi F, List T, Lovelace RE: Slow motor nerve conduction in myotonic dystrophy. *Electromyogr Clin Neurophysiol* 21:97–105, 1981.
124. Kohler A, Burkhard P, Hefft S, et al: Proximal myotonic myopathy: Clinical, electrophysiological and pathological findings in a family. *Eur Neurol* 43:50–53, 2000.
125. Sander HW, Scelsa SN, Conigliari MF, et al: The short exercise test is normal in proximal myotonic myopathy. *Clin Neurophysiol* 111:362–366, 2000.
126. Sasaki R, Ito N, Shimamura M, et al: A novel CLCN1 mutation: P480T in a Japanese family with Thomsen's myotonia congenita. *Muscle Nerve* 24:357–363, 2001.
127. Wegmuller E, Ludin HP, Mumenthaler M: Paramyotonia congenita. A clinical, electrophysiological and histological study of 12 patients. *J Neurol* 220:251–257, 1979.
128. Harel S, Chui LA, Shapira Y: Myotonia congenita (Thomsen's disease). Early diagnosis in infancy. *Acta Paediatr Scand* 68:225–227, 1979.
129. Ricker K, Haass A, Hertel G, et al: Transient muscular weakness in severe recessive myotonia congenita. Improvement of isometric muscle force by drugs relieving myotonic stiffness. *J Neurol* 218:253–262, 1978.
130. Drost G, Blok JH, Stegeman DF, et al: Propagation disturbance of motor unit action potentials during transient paresis in generalized myotonia: A high-density surface EMG study. *Brain* 124:352–360, 2001.
131. Gutmann L, Riggs JE, Brick JF: Exercise-induced membrane failure in paramyotonia congenita. *Neurology* 36:130–132, 1986.
132. Nielsen VK, Friis ML, Johnsen T: Electromyographic distinction between paramyotonia congenita and myotonia congenita: Effect of cold. *Neurology* 32:827–832, 1982.
133. de Silva SM, Kuncl RW, Griffin JW, et al: Paramyotonia congenita or hyperkalemic periodic paralysis? Clinical and electrophysiological features of each entity in one family. *Muscle Nerve* 13:21–26, 1990.
134. Ricker K, Rohkamm R, Bohlen R: Adynamia episodica and paralysis periodica paramyotonica. *Neurology* 36:682–686, 1986.
135. Kuhn E, Fiehn W, Seiler D, et al: The autosomal recessive (Becker) form of myotonia congenita. *Muscle Nerve* 2:109–117, 1979.
136. Zellweger H, Pavone L, Biondi A, et al: Autosomal recessive generalized myotonia. *Muscle Nerve* 3:176–180, 1980.
137. Brooks JE: Hyperkalemic periodic paralysis. Intracellular electromyographic studies. *Arch Neurol* 20:13–18, 1969.
138. Campa JF, Sanders DB: Familial hypokalemic periodic paralysis. *Arch Neurol* 31:110–115, 1974.
139. England JD: Mutant sodium channels, myotonia, and propofol. *Muscle Nerve* 24:713–715, 2001.
140. Engel AG, Gomez MR, Groover RV: Multicore disease. A recently recognized congenital myopathy associated with multifocal degeneration of muscle fibers. *Mayo Clin Proc* 46:666–681, 1971.
141. Riggs JE, Moxley RT III, Griggs RC, et al: Hyperkalemic periodic paralysis: An apparent sporadic case. *Neurology* 31:1157–1159, 1981.
142. Subramony SH, Wee AS: Exercise and rest in hyperkalemic periodic paralysis. *Neurology* 36:173–177, 1986.
143. De Grandis D, Fiaschi A, Tomelleri G, et al: Hypokalemic periodic paralysis. A single fiber electromyographic study. *J Neurol Sci* 37:107–112, 1978.
144. Hilton-Brown P, Stålberg E: The motor unit in muscular dystrophy, a single fibre EMG and scanning EMG study. *J Neurol Neurosurg Psychiatry* 46:981–995, 1983.
145. Desmedt JE, Borenstein S: Regeneration in Duchenne muscular dystrophy. Electromyographic evidence. *Arch Neurol* 33:642–650, 1976.
146. Willison RG: Analysis of electrical activity in healthy and dystrophic muscle in man. *J Neurol Neurosurg Psychiatry* 27:386–394, 1964.
147. McComas AJ, Sica RE, Currie S: An electrophysiological study of Duchenne dystrophy. *J Neurol Neurosurg Psychiatry* 34:461–468, 1971.
148. McComas AJ, Sica RE, Brandstater ME: Further motor unit studies in Duchenne muscular dystrophy. *J Neurol Neurosurg Psychiatry* 40:1147–1151, 1977.
149. Sugimoto S, Tsuruta K, Kurihara T, et al: Posterior tibial somatosensory evoked potentials in Duchenne-type progressive muscular dystrophy. *Electroencephalogr Clin Neurophysiol* 64:525–527, 1986.
150. Takagi A, Nonaka I: Duchenne muscular dystrophy: Unusual activation of single fibers in vitro. *Muscle Nerve* 4:10–15, 1981.
151. Meadows JC, Marsden CD, Harriman DG: Chronic spinal muscular atrophy in adults. 1. The Kugelberg-Welander syndrome. *J Neurol Sci* 9:527–550, 1969.
152. Samaha FJ, Quinlan JG: Myalgia and cramps: Dystrophinopathy with wide-ranging laboratory findings. *J Child Neurol* 11:21–24, 1996.
153. Schmalbruch H, Kamieniecka Z, Fuglsang-Frederiksen A, et al: Benign congenital muscular dystrophy with autosomal dominant heredity: Problems of classification. *J Neurol* 234:146–151, 1987.
154. Argov Z, Sadeh M, Mazor K, et al: Muscular dystrophy due to dysferlin deficiency in Libyan Jews. Clinical and genetic features. *Brain* 123:1229–1237, 2000.
155. van der Kooi AJ, de Visser M, van Meegen M, et al: A novel gamma-sarcoglycan mutation causing childhood onset, slowly progressive limb girdle muscular dystrophy. *Neuromuscul Disord* 8:305–308, 1998.
156. Bradley WG, Jones MZ, Mussini JM, et al: Becker-type muscular dystrophy. *Muscle Nerve* 1:111–132, 1978.
157. Toulouse P, Coatrieux JL, LeMarec B: An attempt to differentiate female relatives of Duchenne type dystrophy from healthy subjects using an automatic EMG analysis. *J Neurol Sci* 67:45–55, 1985.
158. Felice KJ, Moore SA: Unusual clinical presentations in patients harboring the facioscapulohumeral dystrophy 4q35 deletion. *Muscle Nerve* 24:352–356, 2001.
159. Yamanaka G, Goto K, Matsumura T, et al: Tongue atrophy in facioscapulohumeral muscular dystrophy. *Neurology* 57:733–735, 2001.
160. Mendell JR: Congenital muscular dystrophy: Searching for a definition after 98 years. *Neurology* 56:993–994, 2001.
161. Lazaro RP, Fenichel GM, Kilroy AW: Congenital muscular dystrophy: Case reports and reappraisal. *Muscle Nerve* 2:349–355, 1979.
162. Schmitt HP, Krause KH: An autopsy study of a familial oculopharyngeal muscular dystrophy (OPMD) with distal spread and neurogenic involvement. *Muscle Nerve* 4:296–305, 1981.
163. Bouchard JP, Brais B, Brunet D, et al: Recent studies on oculopharyngeal muscular dystrophy in Quebec. *Neuromuscul Disord* 7(Suppl 1):S22–S29, 1997.
164. Edstrom L: Histochemical and histopathological changes in skeletal muscle in late-onset hereditary distal myopathy (Welander). *J Neurol Sci* 26:147–157, 1975.
165. Scoppetta C, Vaccario ML, Casali C, et al: Distal muscular dystrophy with autosomal recessive inheritance. *Muscle Nerve* 7:478–481, 1984.
166. Borg K, Ahlberg G, Borg J, et al: Welander's distal myopathy: Clinical, neurophysiological and muscle biopsy observations in young and middle aged adults with early symptoms. *J Neurol Neurosurg Psychiatry* 54:494–498, 1991.
167. Saperstein DS, Amato AA, Barohn RJ: Clinical and genetic aspects of distal myopathies. *Muscle Nerve* 24:1440–1450, 2001.
167a. Goto I, Kanazawa Y, Kobayashi T: Oculopharyngeal myopathy with distal involvement and cardiomyopathy. *J Neurol Neurosurg Psychiatry* 40:600–607, 1977.
168. Hawkes CH, Absolon MJ: Myotubular myopathy associated with cataract and electrical myotonia. *J Neurol Neurosurg Psychiatry* 38:761–764, 1975.
169. Gil-Peralta A, Rafel E, Bautista J, et al: Myotonia in centronuclear myopathy. *J Neurol Neurosurg Psychiatry* 41:1102–1108, 1978.
170. Elder GB, Dean D, McComas AJ, et al: Infantile centronuclear myopathy. Evidence suggesting incomplete innervation. *J Neurol Sci* 60:79–88, 1983.
171. Baradello A, Vita G, Girlanda P, et al: Adult-onset centronuclear myopathy: Evidence against a neurogenic pathology. *Acta Neurol Scand* 80:162–166, 1989.
172. Bill PL, Cole G, Proctor NS: Centronuclear myopathy. *J Neurol Neurosurg Psychiatry* 42:548–556, 1979.
173. Hopkins IJ, Lindsey JR, Ford FR: Nemaline myopathy. A long-term clinicopathologic study of affected mother and daughter. *Brain* 89:299–310, 1966.
174. Radu H, Ionescu V: Nemaline (neuro) myopathy. Rod-like bodies and type I fibre atrophy in a case of congenital hypotonia with denervation. *J Neurol Sci* 17:53–60, 1972.

175. McComb RD, Markesbery WR, O'Connor WN: Fatal neonatal nemaline myopathy with multiple congenital anomalies. *J Pediatr* 94:47–51, 1979.
176. Brownell AK, Gilbert JJ, Shaw DT, et al: Adult onset nemaline myopathy. *Neurology* 28:1306–1309, 1978.
177. Lopez-Terradas JM, Lopez MC: Late components of motor unit potentials in central core disease. *J Neurol Neurosurg Psychiatry* 42:461–464, 1979.
178. Cruz Martinez A, Ferrer MT, Lopez-Terradas JM, et al: Single fibre electromyography in central core disease. *J Neurol Neurosurg Psychiatry* 42:662–667, 1979.
179. Peyronnard JM, Charron L, Bellavance A, et al: Neuropathy and mitochondrial myopathy. *Ann Neurol* 7:262–268, 1980.
180. Jinnai K, Yamada H, Kanda F, et al: A case of mitochondrial myopathy, encephalopathy and lactic acidosis due to cytochrome c oxidase deficiency with neurogenic muscular changes. *Eur Neurol* 30:56–60, 1990.
181. Rowinska-Marcinska K, Strugalska MH, Hausmanowa-Petrusewicz I: Fiber density in congenital muscle fiber type disproportion: II. Congenital muscle hypotonia and hip dislocation. *Electromyogr Clin Neurophysiol* 31:5–8, 1991.
182. Dyken ML, Smith DM, Peake RL: An electromyographic diagnostic screening test in McArdle's disease and a case report. *Neurology* 17:45–50, 1967.
183. Pourmand R, Sanders DB, Corwin HM: Late-onset McArdle's disease with unusual electromyographic findings. *Arch Neurol* 40:374–377, 1983.
184. Cornelio F, Di Donato S, Peluchetti D, et al: Fatal cases of lipid storage myopathy with carnitine deficiency. *J Neurol Neurosurg Psychiatry* 40:170–178, 1977.
185. Brandt NJ, Buchthal F, Ebbesen F, et al: Post-tetanic mechanical tension and evoked action potentials in McArdle's disease. *J Neurol Neurosurg Psychiatry* 40:920–925, 1977.
186. Danon MJ, Servidei S, DiMauro S, et al: Late-onset muscle phosphofructokinase deficiency. *Neurology* 38:956–960, 1988.
187. Hains AD, Pannall PR, Bourne AJ, et al: McArdle's disease presenting with rhabdomyolysis. *Aust N Z J Med* 14:681–684, 1984.
188. Felice KJ, Schneebaum AB, Jones HR Jr: McArdle's disease with late-onset symptoms: Case report and review of the literature. *J Neurol Neurosurg Psychiatry* 55:407–408, 1992.
189. Hays AP, Hallett M, Delfs J, et al: Muscle phosphofructokinase deficiency: Abnormal polysaccharide in a case of late-onset myopathy. *Neurology* 31:1077–1086, 1981.
190. Engel AG, Gomez MR, Seybold ME, et al: The spectrum and diagnosis of acid maltase deficiency. *Neurology* 23:95–106, 1973.
191. DiMauro S, Hartwig GB, Hays A, et al: Debrancher deficiency: Neuromuscular disorder in 5 adults. *Ann Neurol* 5:422–436, 1979.
192. Barohn RJ, McVey AL, DiMauro S: Adult acid maltase deficiency. *Muscle Nerve* 16:672–676, 1993.
193. Engel AG: Acid maltase deficiency in adults: Studies in four cases of a syndrome which may mimic muscular dystrophy or other myopathies. *Brain* 93:599–616, 1970.
194. Karpati G, Carpenter S, Eisen A, et al: The adult form of acid maltase (alpha-1,4-glucosidase) deficiency. *Ann Neurol* 1:276–280, 1977.
195. Rosenow EC III, Engel AG: Acid maltase deficiency in adults presenting as respiratory failure. *Am J Med* 64:485–491, 1978.
196. Bordiuk JM, Legato MJ, Lovelace RE, et al: Pompe's disease. Electromyographic, electron microscopic, and cardiovascular aspects. *Arch Neurol* 23:113–119, 1970.
197. Moses SW, Gadoth N, Bashan N, et al: Neuromuscular involvement in glycogen storage disease type III. *Acta Paediatr Scand* 75:289–296, 1986.
198. Engel AG, Banker BQ, Eiben RM: Carnitine deficiency: Clinical, morphological, and biochemical observations in a fatal case. *J Neurol Neurosurg Psychiatry* 40:313–322, 1977.
199. Karpati G, Carpenter S, Engel AG, et al: The syndrome of systemic carnitine deficiency. Clinical, morphologic, biochemical, and pathophysiologic features. *Neurology* 25:16–24, 1975.
200. Markesbery WR, McQuillen MP, Procopis PG, et al: Muscle carnitine deficiency. Association with lipid myopathy, vacuolar neuropathy, and vacuolated leukocytes. *Arch Neurol* 31:320–324, 1974.
201. VanDyke DH, Griggs RC, Markesbery W, et al: Hereditary carnitine deficiency of muscle. *Neurology* 25:154–159, 1975.
202. Angelini C, Lucke S, Cantarutti F: Carnitine deficiency of skeletal muscle: Report of a treated case. *Neurology* 26:633–637, 1976.
203. Scarlato G, Albizzati MG, Bassi S, et al: A case of lipid storage myopathy with carnitine deficiency. Biochemical and electromyographic correlations. *Eur Neurol* 16:222–229, 1977.
204. Yiannikas C, McLeod JG, Pollard JD, et al: Peripheral neuropathy associated with mitochondrial myopathy. *Ann Neurol* 20:249–257, 1986.
205. Girlanda P, Toscano A, Nicolosi C, et al: Electrophysiological study of neuromuscular system involvement in mitochondrial cytopathy. *Clin Neurophysiol* 110:1284–1289, 1999.
206. Petty RK, Harding AE, Morgan-Hughes JA: The clinical features of mitochrondrial myopathy. *Brain* 109:915–938, 1986.
207. Fawcett PR, Mastaglia FL, Mechler F: Electrophysiological findings including single fibre EMG in a family with mitochondrial myopathy. *J Neurol Sci* 53:397–410, 1982.
208. Torbergsen T, Stålberg E, Bless JK: Nerve-muscle involvement in a large family with mitochondrial cytopathy: Electrophysiological studies. *Muscle Nerve* 14:35–41, 1991.
208a. Arikawa-Hirasawa E, Le AH, Nishino I, et al: Structural and functional mutations of the perlecan gene cause Schwartz-Jampel syndrome, with myotonic myopathy and chondrodysplasia. *Am J Hum Genet* 70:1368–1375, 2002.
209. Pascuzzi RM, Gratianne R, Azzarelli B, et al: Schwartz-Jampell syndrome with dominant inheritance. *Muscle Nerve* 13:1152–1163, 1990.
210. Ferrannini E, Perniola T, Krajewska G, et al: Schwartz-Jampel syndrome with autosomal-dominant inheritance. *Eur Neurol* 21:137–146, 1982.
211. Cadilhac J, Baldet P, Greze J, et al: EMG studies of two family cases of the Schwartz and Jampel syndrome (osteo-chondro-muscular dystrophy with myotonia). *Electromyogr Clin Neurophysiol* 15:5–12, 1975.
212. Cao A, Cianchetti C, Calisti L, et al: Schwartz-Jampel syndrome. Clinical, electrophysiological and histopathological study of a severe variant. *J Neurol Sci* 35:175–187, 1978.
213. Jablecki C, Schultz P: Single muscle fiber recordings in the Schwartz-Jampel syndrome. *Muscle Nerve* 5:S64–S69, 1982.
214. Spaans F, Theunissen P, Reekers AD, et al: Schwartz-Jampel syndrome: I. Clinical, electromyographic, and histologic studies. *Muscle Nerve* 13:516–527, 1990.
215. Venables GS, Bates D, Shaw DA: Hypothyroidism with true myotonia. *J Neurol Neurosurg Psychiatry* 41:1013–1015, 1978.
216. Astrom KE, Kugelberg E, Muller R: Hypothyroid myopathy. *Arch Neurol* 5:472–482, 1961.
217. Salick AI, Colachis SC Jr, Pearson CM: Myxedema myopathy: Clinical, electrodiagnostic, and pathologic findings in advanced case. *Arch Phys Med Rehabil* 49:230–237, 1968.
218. Torres CF, Moxley RT: Hypothyroid neuropathy and myopathy: Clinical and electrodiagnostic longitudinal findings. *J Neurol* 237:271–274, 1990.
219. Rao SN, Katiyar BC, Nair KR, et al: Neuromuscular status in hypothyroidism. *Acta Neurol Scand* 61:167–177, 1980.
220. Scarpalezos S, Lygidakis C, Papageorgiou C, et al: Neural and muscular manifestations of hypothyroidism. *Arch Neurol* 29:140–144, 1973.
221. Verhagen WI, Schimsheimer RJ: Neurologic disease and thyrotoxic storm. A clinical and electrophysiological study. *Electromyogr Clin Neurophysiol* 26:27–32, 1986.
222. Ramsay ID: Electromyography in thyrotoxicosis. *Q J Med* 34:255–267, 1965.
223. Puvanendran K, Cheah JS, Naganathan N, et al: Thyrotoxic myopathy: A clinical and quantitative analytic electromyographic study. *J Neurol Sci* 42:441–451, 1979.
224. Snowdon JA, Macfie AC, Pearce JB: Hypocalcaemic myopathy with paranoid psychosis. *J Neurol Neurosurg Psychiatry* 39:48–52, 1976.
225. Skaria J, Katiyar BC, Srivastava TP, et al: Myopathy and neuropathy associated with osteomalacia. *Acta Neurol Scand* 51:37–58, 1975.
226. Irani PF: Electromyography in nutritional osteomalacic myopathy. *J Neurol Neurosurg Psychiatry* 39:686–693, 1976.
227. Frame B, Heinze EG Jr, Block MA, et al: Myopathy in primary hyperparathyroidism. Observations in three patients. *Ann Intern Med* 68:1022–1027, 1968.
228. Prineas JW, Mason AS, Henson RA: Myopathy in metabolic bone disease. *Br Med J* 1:1034–1036, 1965.
229. Turken SA, Cafferty M, Silverberg SJ, et al: Neuromuscular involvement in mild, asymptomatic primary hyperparathyroidism. *Am J Med* 87:553–557, 1989.
230. Muller R, Kugelberg E: Myopathy in Cushing's syndrome. *J Neurol Neurosurg Psychiatry* 22:314–319, 1959.
231. Kaplan PW, Rocha W, Sanders DB, et al: Acute steroid-induced tetraplegia following status asthmaticus. *Pediatrics* 78:121–123, 1986.
232. Khaleeli AA, Levy RD, Edwards RH, et al: The neuromuscular features of acromegaly: A clinical and pathological study. *J Neurol Neurosurg Psychiatry* 47:1009–1015, 1984.
233. Olafsson E, Jones HR Jr, Guay AT, et al: Myopathy of endogenous Cushing's syndrome: A review of the clinical and electromyographic features in 8 patients. *Muscle Nerve* 17:692–693, 1994.
234. Pickett JB, Layzer RB, Levin SR, et al: Neuromuscular complications of acromegaly. *Neurology* 25:638–645, 1975.
235. Lewis PD: Neuromuscular involvement in pituitary gigantism. *Br Med J* 2:499–500, 1972.
236. Willis JK, Tilton AH, Harkin JC, et al: Reversible myopathy due to labetalol. *Pediatr Neurol* 6:275–276, 1990.
237. Chalmers AC, Greco CM, Miller RG: Prognosis in AZT myopathy. *Neurology* 41:1181–1184, 1991.
238. Chappel R, Willems J: D-penicillamine-induced myositis in rheumatoid arthritis. *Clin Rheumatol* 15:86–87, 1996.
239. Nucci A, Queiroz LS, Samara AM: Chloroquine neuromyopathy. *Clin Neuropathol* 15:256–258, 1996.
240. Kuncl RW, Cornblath DR, Avila O, et al: Electrodiagnosis of human colchicine myoneuropathy. *Muscle Nerve* 12:360–364, 1989.
241. Abourizk N, Khalil BA, Bahuth N, et al: Clofibrate-induced muscular syndrome. Report of a case with clinical, electromyographic and pathologic observations. *J Neurol Sci* 42:1–9, 1979.

242. Rush P, Baron M, Kapusta M: Clofibrate myopathy: A case report and a review of the literature. *Semin Arthritis Rheum* 15:226–229, 1986.
243. London SF, Gross KF, Ringel SP: Cholesterol-lowering agent myopathy (CLAM). *Neurology* 41:1159–1160, 1991.
244. Geltner D, Shapiro M, Chaco M: Reversible myopathy induced by clofibrate. *Postgrad Med J* 51:184–185, 1975.
245. Meriggioli MN, Barboi AC, Rowin J, et al: HMG-CoA reductase inhibitor myopathy: Clinical, electrophysiological, and pathologic data in five patients. *J Clin Neuromusc Dis* 2:129–134, 2001.
246. Schalke BB, Schmidt B, Toyka K, et al: Pravastatin-associated inflammatory myopathy. *N Engl J Med* 327:649–650, 1992.
247. Gertner E, Thurn JR, Williams DN, et al: Zidovudine-associated myopathy. *Am J Med* 86:814–818, 1989.
248. Whisnant JP, Espinosa RE, Kierland RR, et al: Chloroquine neuromyopathy. *Proc Mayo Clin* 38:501–513, 1963.
249. Eadie MJ, Ferrier TM: Chloroquine myopathy. *J Neurol Neurosurg Psychiatry* 29:331–337, 1966.
250. Estes ML, Ewing-Wilson D, Chou SM, et al: Chloroquine neuromyotoxicity. Clinical and pathologic perspective. *Am J Med* 82:447–455, 1987.
251. Hughes JT, Esiri M, Oxbury JM, et al: Chloroquine myopathy. *Q J Med* 40:85–93, 1971.
252. Mastaglia FL, Papadimitriou JM, Dawkins RL, et al: Vacuolar myopathy associated with chloroquine, lupus erythematosus and thymoma. Report of a case with unusual mitochondrial changes and lipid accumulation in muscle. *J Neurol Sci* 34:315–328, 1977.
253. Mills KR, Ward K, Martin F, et al: Peripheral neuropathy and myopathy in chronic alcoholism. *Alcohol Alcohol* 21:357–362, 1986.
254. Lederman RJ, Salanga VD, Wilbourn AJ, et al: Focal inflammatory myopathy. *Muscle Nerve* 7:142–146, 1984.
255. Takuma H, Murayama S, Watanabe M, et al: A severe case of subacute sarcoid myositis. *J Neurol Sci* 175:140–144, 2000.
256. Suarez GA, Kelly JJ Jr: The dropped head syndrome. *Neurology* 42:1625–1627, 1992.
257. Oh SJ, Rollins JL, Lewis I: Pentazocine-induced fibrous myopathy. *JAMA* 231:271–273, 1975.
258. Johnson KR, Hsueh WA, Glusman SM, et al: Fibrous myopathy. A rheumatic complication of drug abuse. *Arthritis Rheum* 19:923–926, 1976.
259. Johnson EW, Braddom R, Watson R: Electromyographic abnormalities after intramuscular injections. *Arch Phys Med Rehabil* 52:250–252, 1971.
260. Orrell RW, Peatfield RC, Collins CE, et al: Myopathy in acquired partial lipodystrophy. *Clin Neurol Neurosurg* 97:181–186, 1995.
261. Afifi AK, Bergman RA, Zaynoun ST, et al: Partial (localized) lipodystrophy. Report of a case with muscle and skin abnormalities. *J Am Acad Dermatol* 12:198–203, 1985.
262. Bertorini TE: Myoglobinuria, malignant hyperthermia, neuroleptic malignant syndrome and serotonin syndrome. *Neurol Clin* 15:649–671, 1997.
263. Penn AS, Rowland LP, Fraser DW: Drugs, coma, and myoglobinuria. *Arch Neurol* 26:336–343, 1972.
264. Coakley JH, Nagendran K, Yarwood GD, et al: Patterns of neurophysiological abnormality in prolonged critical illness. *Intensive Care Med* 24:801–807, 1998.
265. Hoke A, Rewcastle NB, Zochodne DW: Acute quadriplegic myopathy unrelated to steroids or paralyzing agents: Quantitative EMG studies. *Can J Neurol Sci* 26:325–329, 1999.
266. Lacomis D, Zochodne DW, Bird SJ: Critical illness myopathy. *Muscle Nerve* 23:1785–1788, 2000.
267. Harper CM Jr: Electrodiagnosis of endplate disease, in Engel AG (ed): *Myasthenia Gravis and Myasthenic Disorders*. New York: Oxford University Press, 1999; pp 65–84.
268. Maselli RA: Electrodiagnosis of disorders of neuromuscular transmission. *Ann N Y Acad Sci* 841:696–711, 1998.
269. Lambert EH, Elmqvist D: Quantal components of end-plate potentials in the myasthenic syndrome. *Ann N Y Acad Sci* 183:183–199, 1971.
270. Kelly JJ Jr, Daube JR, Lennon VA, et al: The laboratory diagnosis of mild myasthenia gravis. *Ann Neurol* 12:238–242, 1982.
271. Schwartz MS, Stålberg E: Single fibre electromyographic studies in myasthenia gravis with repetitive nerve stimulation. *J Neurol Neurosurg Psychiatry* 38:678–682, 1975.
272. Odabasi Z, Kuruoglu R, Oh SJ: Turns-amplitude analysis and motor unit potential analysis in myasthenia gravis. *Acta Neurol Scand* 101:315–320, 2000.
273. Oosterhuis HJ, Hootsmans WJ, Veenhuyzen HB, et al: The mean duration of motor unit action potentials in patients with myasthenia gravis. *Electroencephalogr Clin Neurophysiol* 32:697–700, 1972.
274. Barbieri S, Weiss GM, Daube JR: Fibrillation potentials in myasthenia gravis (abstract). *Muscle Nerve* 5:S163–S164-A, 1982.
275. Blom S, Ringqvist I: Neurophysiological findings in myasthenia gravis. Single muscle fibre activity in relation to muscular fatiguability and response to anticholinesterase. *Electroencephalogr Clin Neurophysiol* 30:477–487, 1971.
276. Sonoo M, Uesugi H, Mochizuki A, et al: Single fiber EMG and repetitive nerve stimulation of the same extensor digitorum communis muscle in myasthenia gravis. *Clin Neurophysiol* 112:300–303, 2001.
277. Hokkanen E, Emeryk-Szajewska B, Rowinska-Marcinska K: Evaluation of the jitter phenomenon in myasthenic patients and their relatives. *J Neurol* 219:73–82, 1978.
278. Padua L, Stålberg E, LoMonaco M, et al: SFEMG in ocular myasthenia gravis diagnosis. *Clin Neurophysiol* 111:1203–1207, 2000.
279. Valls-Canals J, Montero J, Pradas J: Stimulated single fiber EMG of the frontalis muscle in the diagnosis of ocular myasthenia. *Muscle Nerve* 23:779–783, 2000.
280. Weinberg DH, Rizzo JF III, Hayes MT, et al: Ocular myasthenia gravis: Predictive value of single-fiber electromyography. *Muscle Nerve* 22:1222–1227, 1999.
281. Sanders DB, Howard JF Jr, Johns TR: Single-fiber electromyography in myasthenia gravis. *Neurology* 29:68–76, 1979.
282. Ahlsten G, Lefvert AK, Osterman PO, et al: Follow-up study of muscle function in children of mothers with myasthenia gravis during pregnancy. *J Child Neurol* 7:264–269, 1992.
283. Branch CE Jr, Swift TR, Dyken PR: Prolonged neonatal myasthenia gravis: Electrophysiological studies. *Ann Neurol* 3:416–418, 1978.
284. Lambert EH, Rooke ED, Eaton LM, et al: Myasthenic syndrome occasionally associated with bronchial neoplasm: Neurophysiologic studies, in Viets HR (ed.): *Myasthenia Gravis: The Second International Symposium Proceedings*. Springfield, IL: Charles C Thomas, 1961; pp 362–410.
285. Fakadej AV, Gutmann L: Prolongation of post-tetanic facilitation in infant botulism. *Muscle Nerve* 5:727–729, 1982.
286. Sadeh M, River Y, Argov Z: Stimulated single-fiber electromyography in Lambert-Eaton myasthenic syndrome before and after 3,4-diaminopyridine. *Muscle Nerve* 20:735–739, 1997.
287. Engel AG: Congenital myasthenic syndromes, in Engel AG (ed.): *Myasthenia Gravis and Myasthenic Disorders*. New York: Oxford University Press, 1999; pp 251–297.
288. Ohno K, Engel AG: Congenital myasthenic syndromes: Genetic defects at the neuromuscular junction. *Curr Neurol Neurosci Rep* 2:78–88, 2002.
289. Ohno K, Brengman J, Tsujino A, et al: Human endplate acetylcholinesterase deficiency caused by mutations in the collagen-like tail subunit (ColQ) of the asymmetric enzyme. *Proc Natl Acad Sci USA* 95:9654–9659, 1998.
289a. Engel AG, Lambert EH, Gomez MR: A new myasthenic syndrome with end-plate acetylcholinesterase deficiency, small nerve terminals, and reduced acetylcholine release. *Ann Neurol* 1:315–330, 1977.
289b. Engel AG, Lambert EH, Mulder DM, et al: A newly recognized congenital myasthenic syndrome attributed to prolonged open time of the acetylcholine induced ion channel. *Ann Neurol* 11:553–569, 1982.
290. van Dijk JG, Lammers GJ, Wintzen AR, et al: Repetitive CMAPs: Mechanisms of neural and synaptic genesis. *Muscle Nerve* 19:1127–1133, 1996.
290a. Ohno K, Tsujino A, Brengman J, et al: Choline acetyltransferase mutations cause myasthenic syndrome associated with episodic apnea in humans. *Proc Natl Acad Sci USA* 98:2017–2022, 2001.
291. Maselli RA: End-plate electromyography: Use of spectral analysis of end-plate noise. *Muscle Nerve* 20:52–58, 1997.
292. Maselli RA, Bakshi N: AAEM case report 16. Botulism. American Association of Electrodiagnostic Medicine. *Muscle Nerve* 23:1137–1144, 2000.
293. Chaudhry V, Crawford TO: Stimulation single-fiber EMG in infant botulism. *Muscle Nerve* 22:1698–1703, 1999.
294. Padua L, Aprile I, Monaco ML, et al: Neurophysiological assessment in the diagnosis of botulism: Usefulness of single-fiber EMG. *Muscle Nerve* 22:1388–1392, 1999.
295. Pickett J, Berg B, Chaplin E, et al: Syndrome of botulism in infancy: Clinical and electrophysiologic study. *N Engl J Med* 295:770–772, 1976.
296. Johnson RO, Clay SA, Arnon SS: Diagnosis and management of infant botulism. *Am J Dis Child* 133:586–593, 1979.
297. Pickett JB: Infant botulism—the first five years. *Muscle Nerve* 5:S26–S27, 1982.
298. Rossi B, Massetani R, Guidi M, et al: Electrophysiological findings in a case of stiff-man syndrome. *Electromyogr Clin Neurophysiol* 28:137–140, 1988.
299. Van den Bergh P, Bulcke JA, Dom R: Familial muscle cramps with autosomal dominant transmission. *Eur Neurol* 19:207–212, 1980.
300. Lazaro RP, Rollinson RD, Fenichel GM: Familial cramps and muscle pain. *Arch Neurol* 38:22–24, 1981.
301. Jansen PH, Joosten EM, Vingerhoets HM: Muscle cramp: Main theories as to aetiology. *Eur Arch Psychiatry Neurol Sci* 239:337–342, 1990.
302. de Waal M, Bertelsmann FW, Strijers RL: Syndrome of continuous muscle fibre activity confined to the legs. *Clin Neurol Neurosurg* 92:283–286, 1990.
303. Roeleveld K, van Engelen BG, Stegeman DF: Possible mechanisms of muscle cramp from temporal and spatial surface EMG characteristics. *J Appl Physiol* 88:1698–1706, 2000.
304. Hart IK: Acquired neuromyotonia: A new autoantibody-mediated neuronal potassium channelopathy. *Am J Med Sci* 319:209–216, 2000.
305. So YT, Zu L, Barraza C, et al: Rippling muscle disease: Evidence for phenotypic and genetic heterogeneity. *Muscle Nerve* 24:340–344, 2001.

306. Dalakas MC, Li M, Fujii M, et al: Stiff person syndrome: Quantification, specificity, and intrathecal synthesis of GAD65 antibodies. *Neurology* 57:780–784, 2001.
307. Brownlow S, Webster R, Croxen R, et al: Acetylcholine receptor delta subunit mutations underlie a fast-channel myasthenic syndrome and arthrogryposis multiplex congenita. *J Clin Invest* 108:125–130, 2001.
308. Fleury P, Hageman G: A dominantly inherited lower motor neuron disorder presenting at birth with associated arthrogryposis. *J Neurol Neurosurg Psychiatry* 48:1037–1048, 1985.
309. Buchthal F, Olsen PZ: Electromyography and muscle biopsy in infantile spinal muscular atrophy. *Brain* 93:15–30, 1970.
310. Daube JR: Electrodiagnostic studies in amyotrophic lateral sclerosis and other motor neuron disorders. *Muscle Nerve* 23:1488–1502, 2000.
311. Jones HR Jr, Darras BT: Acute care pediatric electromyography. *Muscle Nerve* Suppl 9:S53–S62, 2000.
312. McLeod JG, Prineas JW: Distal type of chronic spinal muscular atrophy. Clinical, electrophysiological and pathological studies. *Brain* 94:703–714, 1971.
313. Moosa A, Dubowitz V: Motor nerve conduction velocity in spinal muscular atrophy of childhood. *Arch Dis Child* 51:974–977, 1976.
314. Galea V, Fehlings D, Kirsch S, et al: Depletion and sizes of motor units in spinal muscular atrophy. *Muscle Nerve* 24:1168–1172, 2001.
315. Coers C, Telerman-Toppet N: Differential diagnosis of limb-girdle muscular dystrophy and spinal muscular atrophy. *Neurology* 29:957–972, 1979.
316. Buchthal F, Kamieniecka Z: The diagnostic yield of quantified electromyography and quantified muscle biopsy in neuromuscular disorders. *Muscle Nerve* 5:265–280, 1982.
317. Packer RJ, Brown MJ, Berman PH: The diagnostic value of electromyography in infantile hypotonia. *Am J Dis Child* 136:1057–1059, 1982.
318. Jones HR Jr: EMG evaluation of the floppy infant: Differential diagnosis and technical aspects. *Muscle Nerve* 13:338–347, 1990.
319. Werneck LC, Lima JG: Muscle biopsy correlated with electromyography. Study of 100 cases. *Arq Neuropsiquiatr* 46:156–165, 1988.
320. Sobh M, Refaie A, El-Tantawy AE, et al: Study of neuromyopathy in amyloid kidney transplant patients. *Am J Nephrol* 16:114–117, 1996.
321. Faucheux JM, Tournebize P, Viguier A, et al: Neuromyopathy secondary to omeprazole treatment. *Muscle Nerve* 21:261–262, 1998.
322. Servidei S, Capon F, Spinazzola A, et al: A distinctive autosomal dominant vacuolar neuromyopathy linked to 19p13. *Neurology* 53:830–837, 1999.

Chapter 27
Muscle Imaging

MARIANNE DE VISSER
CARL D. REIMERS

Introduction
General Pathologic Features
Common Neuromuscular Disorders
    MUSCULAR DYSTROPHIES
    INFLAMMATORY MYOPATHIES
    METABOLIC MYOPATHIES AND MITOCHONDRIAL DISORDERS
    NEUROGENIC DISORDERS
The Added Value of Muscle Imaging

Introduction

Since O'Doherty et al.[1] first described the usefulness of computed tomography as a noninvasive diagnostic tool for neuromuscular diseases, muscle imaging has been accepted as an important adjunct to the clinical examination. Muscle wasting in deep-seated muscles or in parts of compound muscles may easily escape the attention of the clinician. Replacement of muscle tissue by fibrosis or fat and the presence of edema and even intramuscular calcifications cannot be diagnosed clinically but can readily be visualized by muscle imaging techniques. Myosonography (real-time ultrasound scanning, or US) and computed tomography (CT)* have over the years proven to be of added value in depicting the extent and distribution of muscle changes in neuromuscular diseases, including replacement of skeletal muscle by fat, increase or decrease in size (atrophy or hypertrophy), and calcifications (Table 27-1). However, CT and US have gradually lost their significance and have to a great extent been replaced by magnetic resonance imaging (MRI). Nevertheless, due to its portability, low cost, and freedom from ionizing radiation, muscle US in experienced hands can still be considered a useful tool, particularly for studies involving children.[2] MRI has obvious advantages. First and foremost, as with US, the absence of ionizing radiation allows repeated MRI investigations to document the progression of a disease or, even more importantly, to assess the effect of an intervention. Second, the excellent soft tissue resolution is superior to that of both US and CT. MRI enables the accurate quantification of variations in the relative fat and water content within the muscle. Edema is the predominant imaging finding in inflammatory myopathies. It is observed in metabolic myopathies during rhabdomyolysis, and edema is also considered a characteristic imaging feature in subacute denervation. Third, MRI does not show bone artifacts that often hamper the interpretation of CT images. Fourth, assessment of MRI and CT images is quite easy, whereas the investigator must be skilled in the interpretation of myosonographic images. MRI presents disadvantages for patients with claustrophobia, those with indwelling metallic objects such as pacemakers and other foreign bodies, very obese individuals, and children who have great difficulty lying still in the magnet and thus must undergo some form of sedation.

The relatively new technique of spin-lock imaging, in which—unlike conventional MRI—changes in tissue microstructure may be apparent, makes it possible to screen asymptomatic patients, closely monitor progressive muscle diseases, and follow the patients' responses to therapy.[3]

Another technique that has elicited much interest in recent years is magnetic resonance spectroscopy (MRS). The clinical application of muscle phosphorus (P)-MRS is useful as a diagnostic tool in patients suspected of a disorder associated with impairment of energy metabolism, such as metabolic myopathies and mitochondrial disorders (for review, see Ref. 4). As it is noninvasive, it allows serial monitoring of oxidative glycolytic metabolism of muscle at rest, exercise, and recovery from exercise. Proton nuclear magnetic resonance spectroscopy (^{1}H MRS) can also be used to study skeletal muscle metabolism—e.g., changes in fatty acid chains, membrane lipid fluidity, and amino acid residues.[5]

MRI and MRS are applied not only in humans but increasingly in animal studies on myopathies in which sarcolemmal breakdown is implicated in the degeneration of the skeletal muscle. Identification of dystrophic foci in the muscles of *mdx* mice and investigation of membrane integrity in vivo in animal models of muscular dystrophy has been shown to be feasible by using either MRS[5] or MRI, the latter in combination with a gadolinium-based, albumin-targeted contrast agent.[6,7]

Table 27-1. CHARACTERISTIC FEATURES OF MUSCLE IMAGING IN VARIOUS NEUROMUSCULAR DISEASES

Asymmetrical muscle changes (i.e., fatty infiltration, atrophy)
Anterior horn cell diseases (postpolio syndrome, amyotrophic lateral sclerosis, focal spinal muscular atrophies, Hopkins syndrome)
Radiculopathies
Plexopathies
Mononeuropathies
Myopathies
    Facioscapulohumeral muscular dystrophy
    Inclusion body myositis
Edema (see Table 27-3)
Muscle hypertrophy
    Muscular dystrophies (in particular dystrophinopathies and limb-girdle muscular dystrophy)
    Congenital myotonias
    Hypothyroid myopathy
    Glycogenoses types 2 and 5
    Cysticercosis
    Muscle amyloidosis
    Denervation hypertrophy
Calcifications
    Myositis ossificans
    Childhood dermatomyositis
    Fibrodysplasia ossificans progressiva

---

*A list of abbreviations used in this chapter is given at the end of the chapter.

Table 27-2. PATHOLOGIC FEATURES IN SKELETAL MUSCLE REVEALED BY NONINVASIVE MUSCLE IMAGING TECHNIQUES

Substrate	Computed tomography	Myosonography	Magnetic resonance imaging
Edema	Normal density	Homogeneous increase in echo intensity	Normal T1-weighted signal intensity, increased T2-weighted signal intensity
Replacement of muscle by fat	Decreased attenuation	Nonhomogeneous increase in echo intensity	Increase in T1- and T2-weighted signal intensities
Edema in the initial stage of fatty replacement	Only decreased attenuation	Nonhomogeneous increase in echo intensity	Increased T1- and T2-weighted signal intensities, increase in signal intensity on STIR[a] sequences
Intramuscular fibrosis	Normal density	Normal or slightly increased/decreased echo intensity	Decreased T1- and T2-weighted signal intensities
Calcifications	Markedly increased attenuation	Markedly increased echo intensity	Markedly decreased T1- and T2-weighted signal intensities
Blood	Markedly increased attenuation	Markedly increased echo intensity	Markedly decreased T1- and T2-weighted signal intensities

[a]Short tau inversion recovery.

This chapter does not deal with the basic and technical principles of the various techniques; it is limited to the general pathology found in various neuromuscular conditions and diseases.

General Pathologic Features

All three techniques (CT, US, and MRI) allow the identification of structural changes in skeletal muscle tissue (Table 27-2). MRI is the only tool that can visualize an increase in water content—in terms of true edema or a relative increase due to a shift of water between the intracellular and the extracellular space—in association with fatty changes in the muscle. The edematous changes are seen as elevations in muscle signal intensity on T2-weighted and on short tau inversion recovery (STIR) images, which suppress the fat signal. True edema or edema-like changes can appear as a nonspecific finding in various neuromuscular conditions and diseases[8] (Table 27-3), but also in physiologic conditions in the gastrocnemius muscle and as the muscle's response to exercise.[9]

Replacement of skeletal muscle by fat can be readily visualized by all three techniques and is observed in a large variety of mostly chronic neuromuscular diseases, both myopathic and neuropathic (Figs. 27-1 through 27-4). Fibrosis of muscle tissue is recognizable only on MRI.

Real-time US scanning enables the observation of fasciculations and myoclonus (Fig. 27-5). In motor neuron disease, US appeared to be more sensitive than clinical and electromyographic examination in visualizing fasciculations.[10]

For detection of focal abnormalities—including calcifications (Figs. 27-6 and 27-7), hematomas, cysts, and space-occupying processes such as tumors and abscesses—both CT and US can be applied.

The assessment of muscle wasting or hypertrophy is dependent on parameters related to the individual, including gender, age, height, body weight, and condition,[11] but also on technical aspects of the applied imaging techniques. In particular, standardization of the imaging procedure with regard to the levels of imaging is important. Since the difference between normality and pathology (e.g., atrophy and hypertrophy) may not always be straightforward, the use of reference values either derived from the literature or self-collected is highly recommended. Measurement of cross-sectional areas is more sensitive than that of muscle diameters in the assessment of atrophy or hypertrophy.

Pseudohypertrophy can easily be recognized on US and CT if fat infiltration is prominent (Figs. 27-8 and 27-9). However, in cases of incipient fatty replacement of hypertrophic muscles, MRI is superior in distinguishing between true and pseudohypertrophy.[12]

Quantification of the muscle volume is feasible by application of the stereologic method named after Cavalieri[13,14] and may be helpful in assessing the effects of potential therapeutic interventions aimed at increasing viable muscle mass in muscular dystrophies or other degenerative neuromuscular disorders.[15]

Table 27-3. NEUROMUSCULAR CONDITIONS AND DISEASES INCLUDING EDEMA

Physiologic condition
  M. gastrocnemius (slightly)
  Muscle exercise
Pathologic conditions
  Acute inflammatory myopathy
  Muscular dystrophies (in particular facioscapulohumeral muscular dystrophy)
  Myotonic dystrophy
  Rhabdomyolysis
  Dyskalemic periodic paralyses
  Muscle infarction
  Muscle trauma
  Muscle tumor (at the periphery)
  Postradiation
  Subacute denervation

Common Neuromuscular Disorders

MUSCULAR DYSTROPHIES

Muscular dystrophies are characterized by chronic degeneration and hence muscle wasting and replacement of muscle tissue by connective tissue and fat. Even more than on clinical examination, muscle imaging shows preferential involvement of muscles or of selected parts of compound muscles (Figs. 27-2, 27-10, and 27-11). Although a pattern of muscle involvement may be recognized, this is seldom pathognomonic, since there is clear overlap between various muscular dystrophies.

Characteristically, there is compensatory hypertrophy or pseudohypertrophy in muscular dystrophies (Figs. 27-4, 27-8, 27-9, and 27-10), which seems to be limited to the following muscles: gastrocnemius and in particular the medial head, sartorius, gracilis, adductor longus, rectus femoris, and semitendinosus. Muscle hypertrophy may also be found in various other myopathies and even in chronic neurogenic diseases such as poliomyelitis[11] (Fig. 27-3).

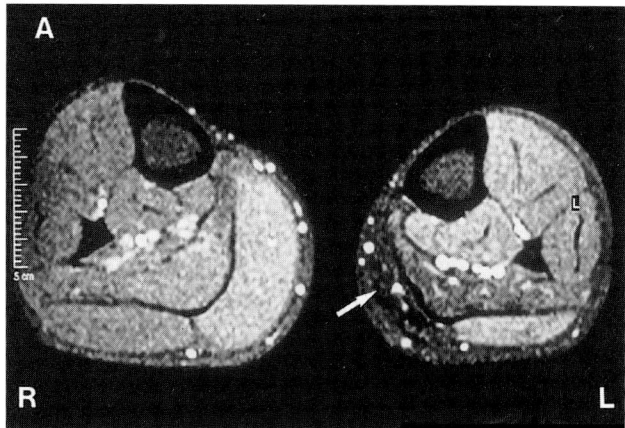

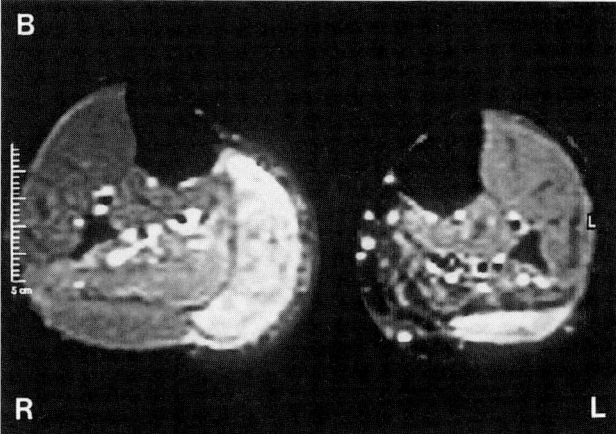

FIGURE 27-2. Magnetic resonance tomography in genetically proven facioscapulohumeral muscular dystrophy. *A.* T1-weighted fat-saturated short tau inversion recovery image: atrophy of the foot flexors of the left lower leg. *B.* Proton-weighted images demonstrate high signal intensities of the medial head of the right and of the lateral head of the left gastrocnemius muscle (indicating edema), whereas the medial head of the left gastrocnemius presents with very low signal intensity, indicating fat tissue. L = left; R = right.

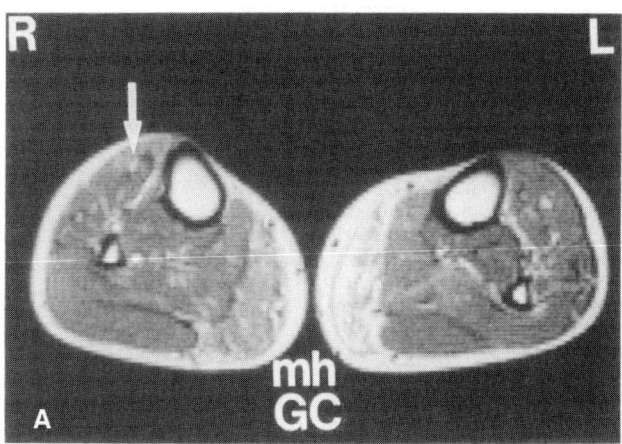

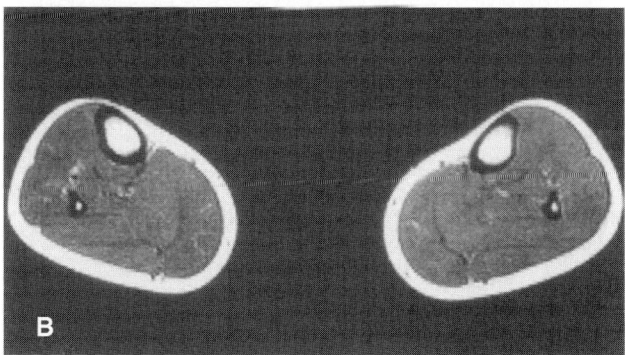

FIGURE 27-1. *A.* Myotonic dystrophy. Proton-weighted magnetic resonance image (1.0 tesla; TR 1600 ms/TE 30 ms) of the lower legs. Note marked increase of signal intensity from medial head of gastrocnemius (mhGC) and slight increase of the signal intensity from right tibialis anterior (arrow). *B.* Proton-weighted image of leg muscle from a normal subject, shown for comparison. R = right; L = left. *(Courtesy of Dr. Thomas Vogl, Department of Radiology, University of Munich, Germany.)*

Edema-like changes are rare and can be detected focally in patients with facioscapulohumeral muscular dystrophy (FSHD) (Fig. 27-2) and myotonic dystrophy. FSHD is also unique in the sense that muscle involvement can be predominantly asymmetrical (Fig. 27-12), whereas most muscular dystrophies show symmetrical involvement.

INFLAMMATORY MYOPATHIES

Active inflammatory diseases such as dermatomyositis and myositis associated with connective tissue disorders manifest with muscle edema,[16–18] whereas inclusion body myositis (IBM), which is a chronic process, instead shows predominantly fatty infiltration (Fig. 27-13). Edema, easily detected by STIR rather than T2-weighted images,[17] can be located not only within the muscle but also in the fascia and the subcutaneous fat even without clinically overt dermatitis or panniculitis (Fig. 27-14).[17,18] T1-weighted images of muscles in dermatomyositis, in contrast to IBM, are mostly normal, since fatty infiltration is lacking.[19]

Another important difference between the active idiopathic inflammatory disorders and IBM is the distribution of muscle changes. In the former, there is predominantly proximal and symmetrical involvement, whereas in IBM muscle changes are often asymmetrical and often located in predominantly distal muscles of the limbs. In particular, the tibialis anterior muscles and the flexors of the forearms are selectively affected at an early stage.[20]

MRI is especially useful in those cases of dermatomyositis in which muscle strength is (near) normal and serum creatine kinase activity within normal limits, so-called amyopathic dermatomyositis.[21,22] Not uncommonly, blind muscle biopsies in inflammatory myopathies yield negative results. However, MRI-guided muscle biopsy greatly reduces the number of false-negative results,[23] which suggests that MRI may be a cost-effective method for diagnosing inflammatory myopathies. Some even claim that MRI suffices for establishing the diagnosis, considering the cost and invasiveness of a muscle biopsy.[19,24] However, given the sensitivity of 80 percent of MRI studies in detecting abnormalities,[25] we and others conclude that a muscle biopsy is still required for the diagnosis.

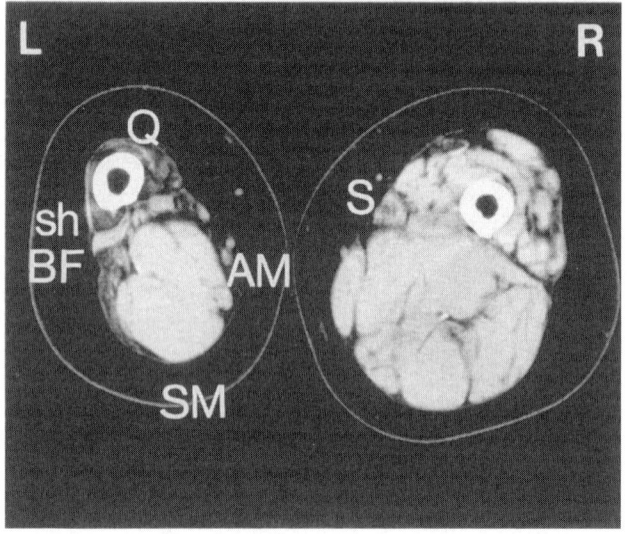

FIGURE 27-3. Late sequelae of acute poliomyelitis. Severe wasting of left thigh muscles and especially of quadriceps femoris (Q). The adductor magnus (AM) and the short head of the biceps femoris (shBF) muscle are preserved, whereas the semimembranosus (SM) is clearly hypertrophic. On the right side, both the quadriceps femoris and sartorius (S) muscles show areas of decreased attenuation. L = left; R = right.

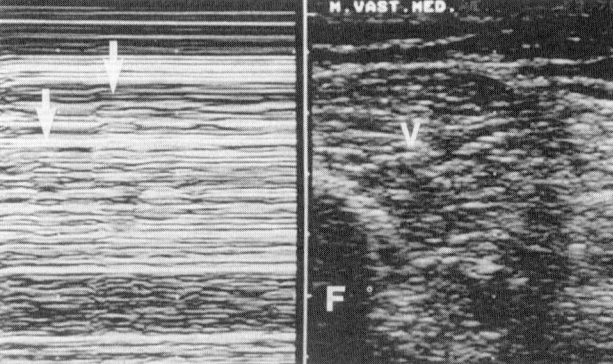

FIGURE 27-5. Adult-onset spinal muscular atrophy. M-mode (left panel) and transverse B-mode (right panel) ultrasound images of the right vastus medialis muscle. No significant abnormality is present in the B-mode image. The M-mode image reveals fasciculations (arrows). F = femur; V = vastus medialis.

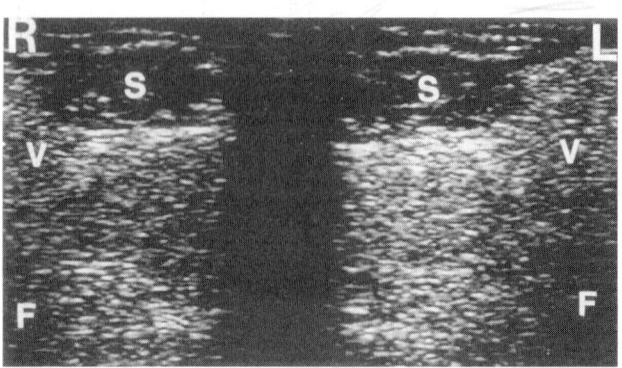

FIGURE 27-4. Duchenne muscular dystrophy. Transverse ultrasound scan of the vastus medialis (V) and sartorius (S) muscles. Note hypertrophy of the sartorius muscle and atrophy and high echo intensities in the vastus medialis muscles. F = femur; R = right; L = left.

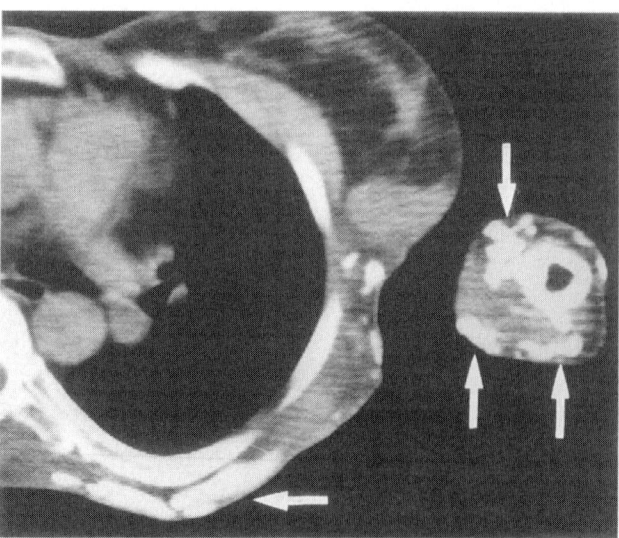

FIGURE 27-6. Childhood dermatomyositis. Note multiple areas of increased attenuation (arrows), indicating calcifications in the upper arm and adjacent to the scapula. (*Courtesy of Dr. Thomas Vogl, Department of Radiology, University of Munich, Germany.*)

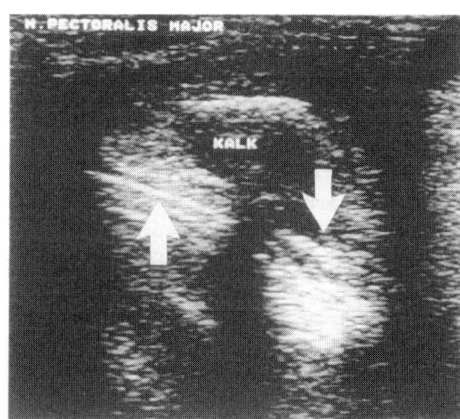

FIGURE 27-7. Progressive ossifying fibrodysplasia of Münchmeyer. Longitudinal ultrasound scan of the left pectoralis major muscle. Note streak of high echo intensity with low echo intensity beneath it, indicating an intramuscular calcification ("Kalk"). Arrows indicate a rib.

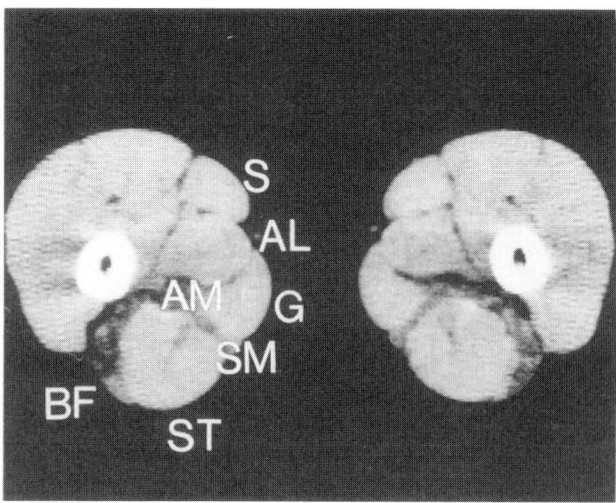

FIGURE 27-10. Becker muscular dystrophy. Hypertrophy of the sartorius (S), adductor longus (AL), gracilis (G), and semitendinosus (ST) muscles. Areas of decreased attenuation are present in the adductor magnus (AM), semimembranosus (SM), and biceps femoris (BF) muscles. (From de Visser M: The diagnosis of neuromuscular diseases using computerized tomography. Ned Tijdschr Geneesk 132:1061, 1988. With permission.)

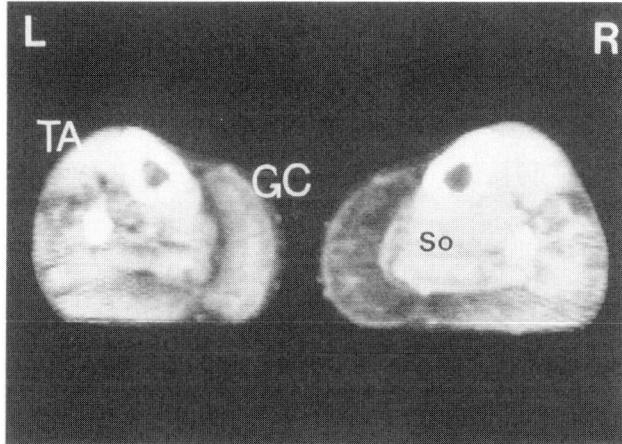

FIGURE 27-8. Becker muscular dystrophy. Pseudohypertrophy of the gastrocnemius muscles (GC). Areas of decreased attenuation are present in all lower leg muscles with the exception of both tibialis anterior muscles (TA) and the right soleus (So) muscle. R = right; L = left.

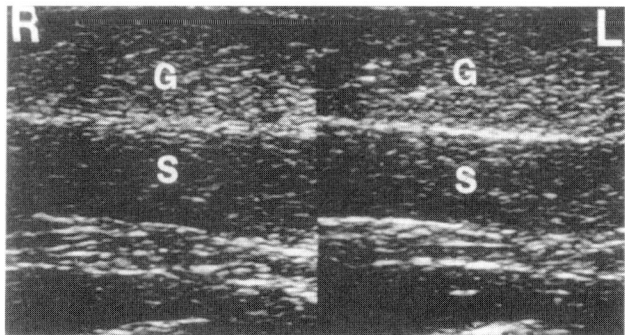

FIGURE 27-9. Becker muscular dystrophy. Longitudinal ultrasound scans of the gastrocnemius (G) and soleus (S) muscles. Note large muscle bulk and increased echo intensities of the gastrocnemius muscles (pseudohypertrophy). R = right; L = left.

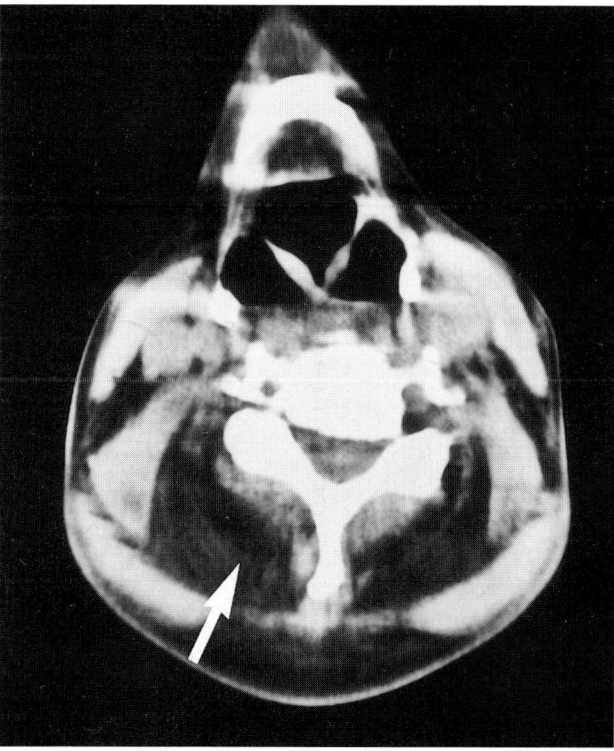

FIGURE 27-11. Oculopharyngeal muscular dystrophy. Paraspinal muscles are completely replaced by fat (arrow).

Another application of MRI in inflammatory myopathies is the evaluation of treatment by monitoring signal intensities.[22] For the same purpose, antimyosin scintigraphy can be used, which seems to reflect disease activity even better than do the T2-weighted images of MRI.[26]

METABOLIC MYOPATHIES AND MITOCHONDRIAL DISORDERS

Disorders that manifest clinically with rhabdomyolysis, such as McArdle disease and carnitine palmityltransferase deficiency, usually produce normal muscle imaging findings between the attacks. However, during the exacerbation, the muscles are edematous, which is readily visible on MRI.[27] In chronic metabolic myopathies such as acid maltase deficiency, there is fatty infiltration and muscle wasting, as in other chronic muscle diseases such as muscular dystrophies (Fig. 27-15).[28]

If a patient with exercise intolerance is suspected of a metabolic myopathy, P-MRS is a useful diagnostic tool. The height of the peak of phosphomonoesters is crucial in determining whether there is a defect in glycogenolysis or glycolysis.[29]

A P-MRS spectrum of resting muscle from a patient with mitochondrial myopathy shows an increase in inorganic phosphates. During exercise, the most sensitive variable is the change in phosphocreatine, showing a more rapid fall in energy state as compared to that in normal individuals.[30] P-MRS has been used as a surrogate outcome parameter in several therapeutic clinical trials, since its noninvasive nature allows repeated measurements.[4]

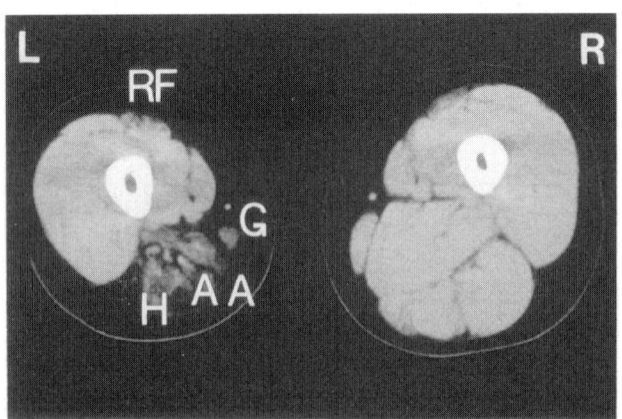

FIGURE 27-12. Facioscapulohumeral dystrophy. The left hamstrings (H), adductors (AA), and gracilis (G) muscle show severe atrophy and fat infiltration. The rectus femoris muscle (RF) is affected on both sides. L = left; R = right. (From de Visser M: The diagnosis of neuromuscular diseases using computerized tomography. Ned Tijdschr Geneesk 132:1061, 1988. With permission.)

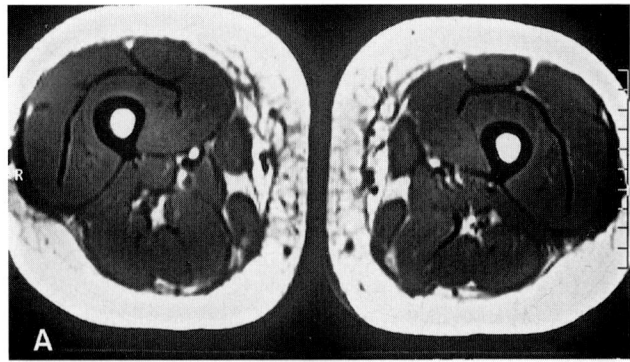

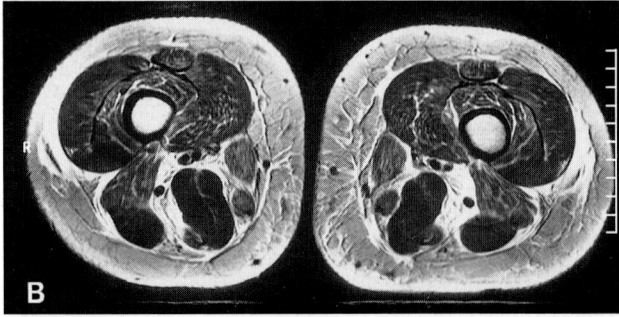

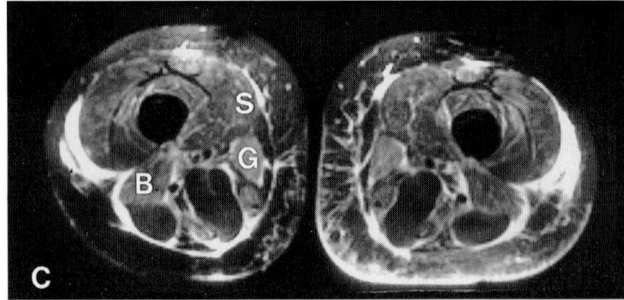

FIGURE 27-14. Magnetic resonance tomography of the thighs in acute polymyositis without clinically overt involvement of the skin and subcutaneous fat tissue. A. T1-weighted image without any abnormality. B. T2-weighted image showing high signal intensities of several fascias and epimysia, indicating fasciitis; slightly increased signal intensities predominantly of the sartorius (S), gracilis (G), and biceps femoris (B) muscles, indicating edema; and normal signal intensity of the semitendinosus muscles. C. T2-weighted, fat-saturated images showing the same abnormalities as non-fat-saturated images, but even more clearly.

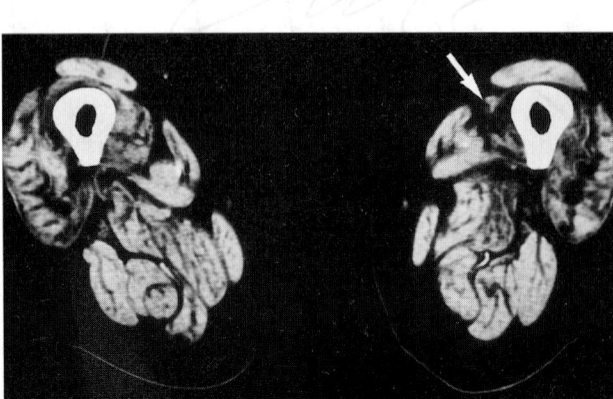

FIGURE 27-13. Inclusion body myositis. There is atrophy of all thigh muscles and especially of the quadriceps femoris muscles (arrows), which also show areas of decreased attenuation.

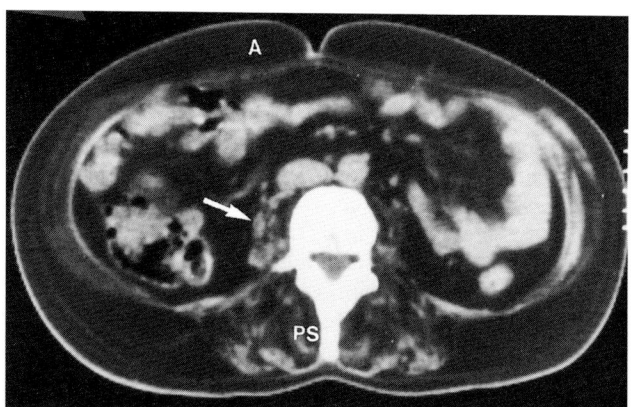

FIGURE 27-15. Adult Pompe disease. Note the wasting of the psoas muscles (arrows), which are also almost completely replaced by fat. The same holds true for the paraspinal (PS) and abdominal (A) muscles.

NEUROGENIC DISORDERS

Subacutely and chronically denervated muscles have increased signal intensities on MR images. In subacute denervation, there is first an edema-like phase in which both T1 and T2 relaxation times are prolonged. If denervation progresses, as is the case in amyotrophic lateral sclerosis, T1 relaxation time is decreased and T2 relaxation time increased. Bryan et al.[31] showed that T2 relaxation time could be a promising tool in evaluating motor dysfunction, based on the observed strong negative correlation with muscle strength and the amplitude of the compound muscle action potential. Gadolinium-enhanced MRI is a new and sensitive technique for visualizing denervated muscle and perhaps even preceding electromyographic changes.[32] Ultrasound is as sensitive as electromyography (EMG) in depicting acute denervation (Fig. 27-16).[33–35]

In slowly progressive neurogenic conditions—e.g., "benign monomelic amyotrophy," a variant of segmental spinal muscular atrophy, Charcot-Marie-Tooth disease, and postpolio syndrome—there is not only marked and selective fatty infiltration[36,37] but sometimes also compensatory hypertrophy (Figs. 27-3 and 27-17). Hypertrophy can also be observed in patients with radiculopathy and is then considered to be stretch- and work-induced.[38,39]

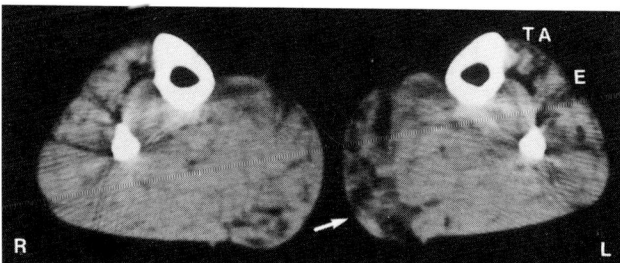

FIGURE 27-16. Charcot-Marie-Tooth disease. Areas of low attenuation in both medial heads of the gastronemius (mhGC) muscles, left more than right, tibialis anterior (TA) muscles, and extensors of the toes (E). Note the increased size (pseudohypertrophy) of the medial heads of the gastrocnemius muscles (arrow). L = left; R = right.

In the past, muscle imaging was used to demonstrate differences between hereditary myopathies and neurogenic disorders,[40,41] showing the preferential involvement of specific muscles and preservation of others in the hereditary conditions (Duchenne/Becker muscular dystrophy) (Fig. 27-10). In neurogenic disorders (spinal muscular atrophy, Kugelberg-Welander type), more diffuse involvement is observed (Fig. 27-18). In addition, the affected muscles showed different patterns: homogeneously infiltrated by fat in Duchenne/Becker muscular dystrophy in contrast to an irregular pattern in spinal muscular atrophy. Today, molecular genetic analysis at either the DNA or the protein level has entirely overshadowed the use of muscle imaging for these diagnostic purposes.

Since MRI is much more sensitive than CT or US in detecting mesenchymal changes, this tool can also be used in

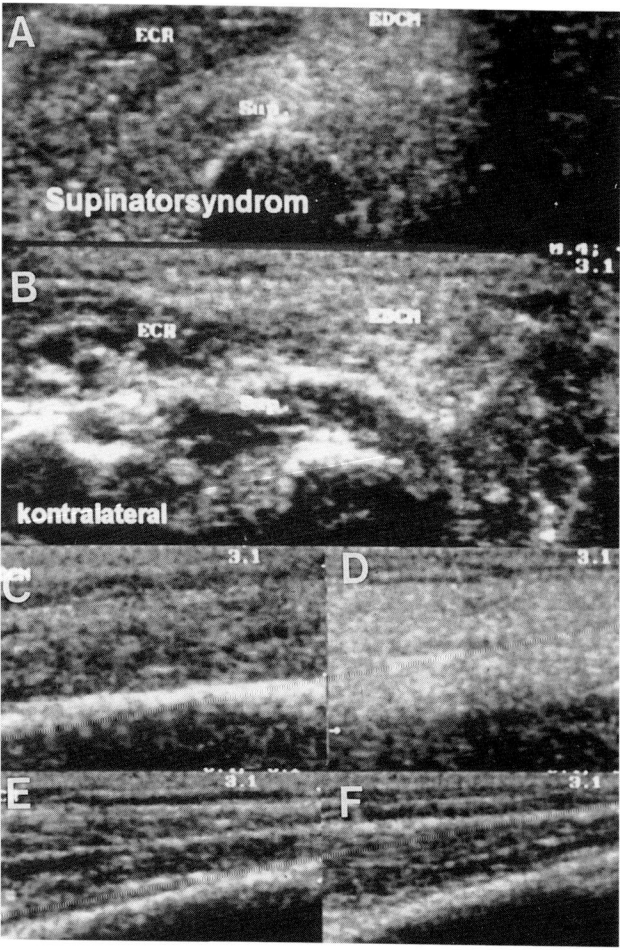

FIGURE 27-17. Transverse ultrasonography of both forearms in radial tunnel syndrome. A. Normal echointensity of the extensor carpi radialis muscle (ECR), whereas the extensor digitorum communis manus (EDCM) and supinator (Sup) muscles show homogeneously increased echointensities. On the contralateral side (B), the extensor digitorum communis manus muscle also presents slightly increased echointensity, indicating incipient disease. On the longitudinal scans, the diseased extensor digitorum communis manus muscle also presents with homogenously increased echointensity (D), whereas the contralateral muscle (C) and both extensor carpi radialis muscles have a normal appearance (E and F).

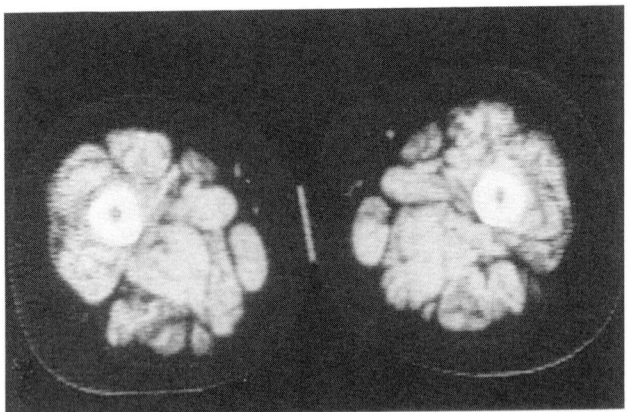

FIGURE 27-18. Spinal muscular atrophy, Kugelberg-Welander type. Diffuse wasting of the thigh muscles is seen. Punctate areas of decreased attenuation are scattered throughout the muscles.

preoperative planning for orthopedic interventions in Charcot-Marie-Tooth disease, where early muscle atrophy and fatty infiltration are easier to discern than with manual examination.[42]

Fasciculations are a feature of lower motor neuron involvement of various kinds. Although these are often not recognized clinically, US can be helpful in detecting this spontaneous muscle activity at the subclinical level[10] (Fig. 27-5).

The Added Value of Muscle Imaging

Muscle imaging is much more accurate in estimating the size of a muscle than is external measurement of the circumference of limbs, since this measurement also includes "nonmuscular tissues" such as the bone and subcutaneous tissue.[43,44]

The same holds true for the localization of structural abnormalities in muscle, most commonly fat infiltration. In particular, if parts of compound muscles are infiltrated by fat, the muscle may have a normal appearance and strength, especially if there is compensatory hypertrophy. Detection of abnormalities on muscle imaging may be helpful in tailoring subsequent invasive investigations—e.g., in directing the needle in EMG, especially in children, or in selecting an appropriate muscle biopsy site. In contrast to the above abnormalities, which may be detected by CT, US, or MRI in (sub)acute diseases such as dermatomyositis or metabolic myopathies manifesting with rhabdomyolysis, edematous changes can be visualized only by MRI. This is important not only in establishing a diagnosis as early as possible but also in maximizing cost-effectiveness, as MRI-guided muscle biopsies also contribute this.[23]

Both US and MRI can be used to monitor the progression of a neuromuscular disease or to document response to treatment in idiopathic inflammatory myopathies.

List of Abbreviations

1H MRS	proton nuclear magnetic resonance spectroscopy
CT	computed tomography
EMG	electromyography
FSHD	facioscapulohumeral muscular dystrophy
IBM	inclusion body myositis
MRI	magnetic resonance imaging
MRS	magnetic resonance spectroscopy
P-MRS	Phosphorus magnetic resonance spectroscopy
STIR	short tau inversion recovery
US	ultrasound

References

1. O'Doherty DS, Schellinger D, Raptopoulos V: Computed tomographic patterns of pseudohypertrophic muscular dystrophy: Preliminary results. J Comput Assist Tomogr 1:482, 1977.
2. Zuberi SM, Matta N, Nawaz S, et al: Muscle ultrasound in the assessment of suspected neuromuscular disease in childhood. Neuromuscul Disord 9:203, 1999.
3. Franczak MB, Ulmer JL, Jaradeh S, et al: Spin-lock magnetic resonance imaging of muscle in patients with autosomal recessive limb girdle muscular dystrophy. J Neuroimaging 10:73, 2000.
4. Argov Z, Lofberg M, Arnold DL: Insights into muscle diseases gained by phosphorus magnetic resonance spectroscopy. Muscle Nerve 23:1316, 2000.
5. McIntosh LM, Baker RE, Anderson JE: Magnetic resonance imaging of regenerating and dystrophic mouse muscle. Biochem Cell Biol 76:532, 1998.
6. Allamand V, Donahue KM, Straub V, et al: Early adenovirus-mediated gene transfer effectively prevents muscular dystrophy in alpha-sarcoglycan-deficient mice. Gene Ther 7:1385, 2000.
7. Straub V, Donahue KM, Allamand V, et al: Contrast agent-enhanced magnetic resonance imaging of skeletal muscle damage in animal models of muscular dystrophy. Magn Reson Med 44:655, 2000.
8. Schedel H, Reimers CD, Vogl T, et al: Muscle edema in MR imaging of neuromuscular diseases. Acta Radiol 36:228, 1995.
9. Fleckenstein JL, Canby RC, Parkey RW, et al: Acute effects of exercise on MR imaging of skeletal muscle in normal volunteers. Am J Roentgenol 151:231, 1988.
10. Reimers CD, Ziemann U, Scheel A, et al: Fasciculations: Clinical, electromyographic, and ultrasonographic assessment. J Neurol 243:579, 1996.
11. Reimers CD, Schlotter B, Eicke BM, et al: Calf enlargement in neuromuscular diseases: A quantitative ultrasound study in 350 patients and review of the literature. J Neurol Sci 143:46, 1996.
12. Fleckenstein JL, Weatherall PT, Bertocci LA, et al: Locomotor system assessment by muscle magnetic resonance imaging. Magn Reson Q 7:79, 1991.
13. Roberts N, Puddephat MJ, McNulty V: The benefit of stereology for quantitative radiology. Br J Radiol 73:679, 2000.
14. Roberts N, Cruz-Orive LM, Reid NM, et al: Unbiased estimation of human body composition by the Cavalieri method using magnetic resonance imaging. J Microsc 171:239, 1993.
15. Gong QY, Phoenix J, Kemp GJ, et al: Estimation of body composition in muscular dystrophy by MRI and stereology. J Magn Reson Imaging 12:467, 2000.
16. Fleckenstein JL, Reimers CD: Inflammatory myopathies: Radiologic evaluation. Radiol Clin North Am 34:427, xii, 1996.
17. Fraser DD, Frank JA, Dalakas M, et al: Magnetic resonance imaging in the idiopathic inflammatory myopathies. J Rheumatol 18:1693, 1991.
18. Adams EM, Chow CK, Premkumar A, et al: The idiopathic inflammatory myopathies: Spectrum of MR imaging findings. Radiographics 15:563, 1995.

19. Park JH, Olsen NJ: Utility of magnetic resonance imaging in the evaluation of patients with inflammatory myopathies. *Curr Rheumatol Rep* 3:334, 2001.
20. Sekul EA, Chow C, Dalakas MC: Magnetic resonance imaging of the forearm as a diagnostic aid in patients with sporadic inclusion body myositis. *Neurology* 48:863, 1997.
21. Stonecipher MR, Jorizzo JL, Monu J, et al: Dermatomyositis with normal muscle enzyme concentrations. A single-blind study of the diagnostic value of magnetic resonance imaging and ultrasound. *Arch Dermatol* 130:1294, 1994.
22. Park JH, Vital TL, Ryder NM, et al: Magnetic resonance imaging and P-31 magnetic resonance spectroscopy provide unique quantitative data useful in the longitudinal management of patients with dermatomyositis. *Arthritis Rheum* 37:736, 1994.
23. Schweitzer ME, Fort J: Cost-effectiveness of MR imaging in evaluating polymyositis. *Am J Roentgenol* 165:1469, 1995.
24. Olsen NJ, Park JH: Inflammatory myopathies: Issues in diagnosis and management. *Arthritis Care Res* 10:200, 1997.
25. Reimers CD, Schedel H, Fleckenstein JL, et al: Magnetic resonance imaging of skeletal muscles in idiopathic inflammatory myopathies of adults. *J Neurol* 241:306, 1994.
26. Lofberg M, Liewendahl K, Lamminen A, et al: Antimyosin scintigraphy compared with magnetic resonance imaging in inflammatory myopathies. *Arch Neurol* 55:987, 1998.
27. Fleckenstein JL, Peshock RM, Lewis SF, Haller RG: Magnetic resonance imaging of muscle injury and atrophy in glycolytic myopathies. *Muscle Nerve* 12:849, 1989.
28. de Jager AE, van der Vliet TM, van der Ree TC, et al: Muscle computed tomography in adult-onset acid maltase deficiency. *Muscle Nerve* 21:398, 1998.
29. Ross BD, Radda GK, Gadian DG, et al: Examination of a case of suspected McArdle's syndrome by 31P nuclear magnetic resonance. *N Engl J Med* 304:1338, 1981.
30. Radda GK, Bore PJ, Gadian DG, et al: 31P NMR examination of two patients with NADH-CoQ reductase deficiency. *Nature* 295:608, 1982.
31. Bryan WW, Reisch JS, McDonald G, et al: Magnetic resonance imaging of muscle in amyotrophic lateral sclerosis. *Neurology* 51:110, 1998.
32. Bendszus M, Koltzenburg M: Visualization of denervated muscle by gadolinium-enhanced MRI. *Neurology* 57:1709, 2001.
33. McDonald CM, Carter GT, Fritz RC, et al: Magnetic resonance imaging of denervated muscle: Comparison to electromyography. *Muscle Nerve* 23:1431, 2000.
34. Kullmer K, Sievers KW, Reimers CD, et al: Changes of sonographic, magnetic resonance tomographic, electromyographic, and histopathologic findings within a 2-month period of examinations after experimental muscle denervation. *Arch Orthop Trauma Surg* 117:228, 1998.
35. Fleckenstein JL, Watumull D, Conner KE, et al: Denervated human skeletal muscle: MR imaging evaluation. *Radiology* 187:213, 1993.
36. de Visser M, Ongerboer de Visser BW, Verbeeten B Jr: Electromyographic and computed tomographic findings in five patients with monomelic spinal muscular atrophy. *Eur Neurol* 28:135, 1988.
37. Di Muzio A, Delli PC, Lugaresi A, et al: Benign monomelic amyotrophy of lower limb: A rare entity with a characteristic muscular CT. *J Neurol Sci* 126:153, 1994.
38. de Visser M, Verbeeten B Jr, Lyppens KC: Pseudohypertrophy of the calf following S1 radiculopathy. *Neuroradiology* 28:279, 1986.
39. Heuss D, Schober S, Eberhardt K, et al: Muscle hypertrophy due to scarring of the S1 nerve root. *Neurol Res* 22:469, 2000.
40. de Visser M, Verbeeten B Jr: Computed tomography of the skeletal musculature in Becker-type muscular dystrophy and benign infantile spinal muscular atrophy. *Muscle Nerve* 8:435, 1985.
41. Suput D, Zupan A, Sepe A, et al: Discrimination between neuropathy and myopathy by use of magnetic resonance imaging. *Acta Neurol Scand* 87:118, 1993.
42. Stilwell G, Kilcoyne RF, Sherman JL: Patterns of muscle atrophy in the lower limbs in patients with Charcot-Marie-Tooth disease as measured by magnetic resonance imaging. *J Foot Ankle Surg* 34:583, 1995.
43. Knapik JJ, Staab JS, Harman EA: Validity of an anthropometric estimate of thigh muscle cross-sectional area. *Med Sci Sports Exerc* 28:1523, 1996.
44. Andersen H, Gadeberg PC, Brock B, Jakobsen J: Muscular atrophy in diabetic neuropathy: A stereological magnetic resonance imaging study. *Diabetologia* 40:1062, 1997.

Chapter 28

Functional Evaluation of Metabolic Myopathies

RONALD G. HALLER
JOHN VISSING

Functional Evaluation of Muscle Disease—Rationale
Energy Utilization in Exercise
Muscle Metabolism in Exercise
   MONITORING GLYCOGENOLYSIS AND AMMONIA PRODUCTION IN FOREARM EXERCISE
   MAGNETIC RESONANCE SPECTROSCOPY
   OTHER METHODS OF MONITORING INTRACELLULAR METABOLITES
   METHODS OF MONITORING OXIDATIVE METABOLISM
Exercise Pathophysiology in Muscle Energy Defects
   RESPIRATORY CHAIN AND RELATED DISORDERS
   DISORDERS OF MUSCLE GLYCOGENOLYSIS—IMPLICATIONS FOR ANAEROBIC AND AEROBIC METABOLISM
   FATTY ACID OXIDATION DEFECTS

Functional Evaluation of Muscle Disease—Rationale

Metabolic myopathies due to inborn errors of muscle energy metabolism often elude diagnosis because symptoms occur predominantly or exclusively during exercise. Premature muscle fatigue and related exercise-induced symptoms often are ascribed to being "out of shape" or to indicate poor effort. Exercise testing provides an objective means to assess the mechanism of exercise limitations by evaluating the metabolic pathways that power muscular work and physiologic responses that support muscle oxidative metabolism. Exercise testing also plays an important role in evaluating treatment efficacy in metabolic myopathies.[1-4]

Symptoms in muscle energy defects are directly linked to a mismatch between the rate of adenosine triphosphate (ATP)* utilization (energy demand) relative to the capacity of muscle metabolic pathways to regenerate ATP (energy supply). This energy supply/demand mismatch impairs energy-dependent processes that power muscle contraction (exertional fatigue, weakness), mediate muscle relaxation (muscle tightness, cramping), and/or maintain membrane ion gradients necessary for normal membrane excitability (fatigue, weakness) and muscle cell integrity (muscle pain, injury, myoglobinuria). The specific metabolic mediators of premature fatigue, cramping, pain, and muscle injury in metabolic myopathies are complex and vary among different metabolic disorders. ATP levels are usually only modestly lower than at rest with fatiguing exercise, implying that frank ATP depletion is not responsible for premature fatigue. Accumulation of end products of ATP hydrolysis (ADP, inorganic phosphate) and H$^+$ ions alone or in combination slows the rate of muscle energy turnover by inhibiting the activity of the ATPases that link the hydrolysis of ATP to cellular work.[5] Substrate-level phosphorylation in glycolysis is closely linked to membrane sodium pump function,[6] and glycolytic defects may promote the increase in extracellular potassium accompanying repetitive muscle activation.[7,8] In McArdle disease, low levels of muscle sodium-potassium ATPase further promote the extracellular potassium accumulation[8] and may account for a characteristic decline in sarcolemmal excitability with rapid stimulation.[9,10]

Energy Utilization in Exercise

The limits of energy utilization in skeletal muscle are set by the ATPases, which couple muscle contraction (myosin ATPase) and ion transport (calcium and sodium, potassium ATPases) to the hydrolysis of ATP to adenosine diphosphate (ADP) and inorganic phosphate (Pi).[11] ADP and Pi, in turn, activate energy-producing reactions which regenerate ATP, without which ATP stores would be exhausted in seconds. The substrates used to replenish ATP are determined by the intrinsic properties of these fuels (Fig. 28-1, Table 28-1) as well as by the intensity and duration of exercise, which modulate fuel selection.[12,13] The major anaerobic sources of ADP phosphorylation are the creatine kinase reaction and anaerobic glycogenolysis. The coupled adenylate kinase (myokinase) and adenylate deaminase (myoadenylate deaminase) reactions serve primarily to buffer the increases in ADP and AMP that accompany heavy exercise. Phosphocreatine hydrolysis and anaerobic glycogenolysis support rates of muscle energy production (power output) that are two- to fourfold higher than those supported by oxidative metabolism.[14] Thus these metabolic pathways are required to support maximal-effort exercise and are engaged whenever the rate of oxidative ATP production fails to meet energy demand. Acceleration to high rates of energy production occurs instantly for ATP, in less than a second for phosphocreatine, and within seconds for anaerobic glycogenolysis, whereas achieving maximal oxidative power requires from 3 (with glycogen as the oxidative substrate) to 30 min (for peak fat oxidation). Thus, anaerobic energy is critical for rapid bursts of exercise and to fuel the transition from rest to exercise. However, anaerobic fuels both are rapidly depleted and cause accumulation of metabolic end products (e.g., protons and inorganic phosphate) that promote muscle fatigue.

Oxidative phosphorylation is the most abundant source of ATP synthesis and is necessary for exercise to be sustained for more than a few minutes. The major *endogenous* oxidative fuel of skeletal muscle is glycogen, while blood glucose and free fatty acids (FFA) are the primary *exogenous* fuels. Amino acids, predominantly branched-chain amino acids, are oxidized to a limited extent and can supply only a small percentage of muscle energy needs. The energetic advantage of oxidative metabolism is indicated by the fact that the yield

---

*A list of abbreviations used in this chapter is given at the end of the chapter.

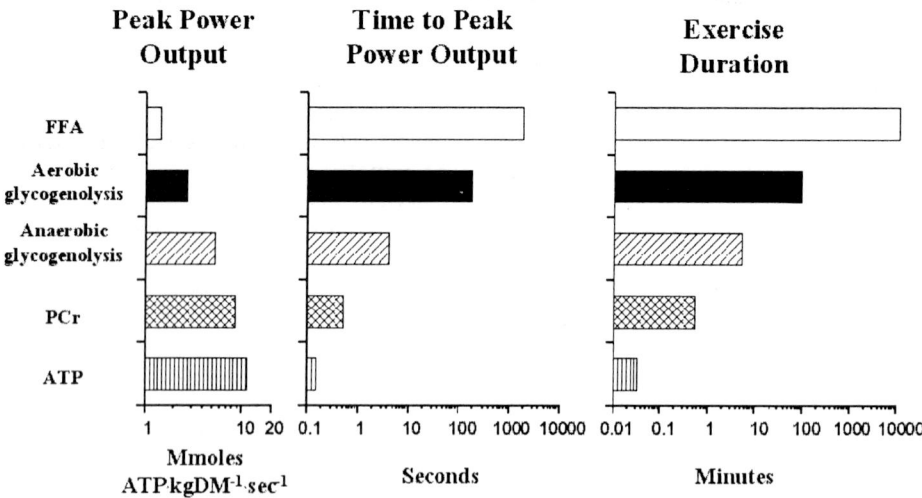

Figure 28-1. Attributes of muscle fuels in terms of peak power output, time to achieve peak power output, and duration of exercise that can be supported by major anaerobic and oxidative fuels in skeletal muscle. The x axis is in a log scale for millimoles of ATP per kilogram per second, seconds, and minutes, respectively. (*Modified from Sahlin K: Metabolic changes limiting muscle performance, in Saltin B (ed): Biochemistry of Exercise VI. Champaign, IL: Human Kinetics, 1986; pp 323–343. With permission.*)

of ATP per mole of substrate rises from 2 to 36 for glucose and from 3 to 37 per glycosyl unit of glycogen metabolized anaerobically versus oxidatively; it is 129 for palmitate. Also, the metabolic end products of oxidative metabolism, CO_2 and water, are readily removed from working muscle and do not promote fatigue. Lipid is by far the most abundant fuel and is critical for supporting prolonged, moderate exercise. Stores of carbohydrate in the form of muscle and hepatic glycogen and blood glucose (derived primarily from hepatic glycogenolysis) are far more limited and can support high-intensity exercise for only 1 to 2 h. However, carbohydrate, and in particular muscle glycogen, is critical for normal oxidative metabolism in several ways. First, glycogen supports a peak rate of oxidative phosphorylation (power output) that is approximately twofold greater than that of fat. The biochemical basis of this enhanced power output is incompletely understood but may involve a requirement for glycogen-derived pyruvate to support optimal function of the tricarboxylic acid cycle.[15–17] The proportion of carbohydrate relative to lipid oxidation progressively rises as the intensity of aerobic exercise increases, and carbohydrate is the exclusive fuel of maximal oxidative metabolism.[14,18] A second critical attribute of glycogen is its capacity to accelerate to maximal oxidative power output rapidly compared to other fuels.[14,19] Finally, the molar ratio of ATP produced to O_2 consumed is higher for glycogen (6.17) and glucose (5.98) than for fatty acids (5.61).[20] This is important because peak O_2 utilization in healthy humans is limited by O_2 delivery.[21] The major disadvantage of carbohydrate fuels is their limited supply. The consequence of muscle glycogen depletion is fatigue.[14,22]

Combustion of fuels in oxidative metabolism involves the generation of reducing equivalents in glycolysis, β-oxidation, and the tricarboxylic acid cycle that are oxidized via the respiratory chain, where the phosphorylation of ADP is coupled to the reduction of molecular oxygen to water. Normal

Table 28-1. ANAEROBIC AND OXIDATIVE REACTIONS SUPPLYING ENERGY TO WORKING MUSCLE

Anaerobic Glycolysis

$$3ATP \rightarrow 3ADP + Pi$$
$$Glycogen_{(n)} + 3Pi + 3ADP \rightarrow Glycogen_{(n-1)} + 2\ \mathbf{lactate} + 2H_2O + 3ATP$$

net
$$Glycogen_{(n)} \rightarrow Glycogen_{(n-1)} + 2\ \mathbf{lactate} + 2H_2O$$

Creatine Kinase

$$ATP \rightarrow ADP + Pi$$
$$ADP + PCr + H^+ \leftrightarrow ATP + Cr$$

net
$$PCr + H^+ \rightarrow \mathbf{Cr + Pi}$$

Adenylate Kinase/Deaminase

$$2ATP \rightarrow 2ADP + 2Pi$$
$$2ADP \leftrightarrow ATP + AMP$$
$$AMP + H_2O \rightarrow NH_3 + IMP$$

net
$$ATP + H_2O \rightarrow NH_3 + IMP + 2Pi$$

Oxidative Phosphorylation

$$Glycogen_{(n)} + 6O_2 + 37Pi + 37ADP \rightarrow Glycogen_{(n-1)} + 6CO_2 + 42H_2O + 37ATP$$
$$Glucose + 6O_2 + 36Pi + 36ADP \rightarrow 6CO_2 + 42H_2O + 36ATP$$
$$palmitate + 23O_2 + 129Pi + 129ADP \rightarrow 16CO_2 + 145H_2O + 129ATP$$

oxidative metabolism necessitates both functional mitochondria to efficiently extract available O_2 from blood and a highly integrated physiologic support system to regulate the flow of oxygen from the lungs to respiring muscle mitochondria. From rest to peak exercise, muscle oxygen utilization in oxidative phosphorylation may increase 50-fold or greater. This is achieved by increases in both the level of O_2 extraction from oxyhemoglobin in red blood cells and the rate of delivery of oxygenated blood to working muscle by the circulation. These variables in oxygen utilization are expressed in the Fick equation: Oxygen utilization ($\dot{V}_{O_2}$) = [arteriovenous (a–v) O_2 difference] × [blood flow ($\dot{Q}$)].

Assuming normal hemoglobin levels and function, arterial blood contains about 20 mL O_2 per 100 mL (~1.34 mL O_2/g of hemoglobin), and mixed venous (right heart) blood 15 mL/dL, so that the resting systemic a–v O_2 difference is about 5 mL O_2/dL of blood (Fig. 28-2). With exercise, levels of O_2 in muscle and in venous effluent blood decrease due to increased mitochondrial O_2 utilization; from rest to peak exercise, the systemic arteriovenous O_2 difference increases threefold, to about 15 mL/dL. Oxygen delivery by the circulation (cardiac output) in exercise increases as a function of increasing heart rate and cardiac stroke volume and is directed primarily to working muscle (Fig. 28-2). Peak levels of O_2 delivery are determined by the level of physical conditioning. Exercise cardiac output and muscle blood flow increase 5 to 6 L per liter of increased O_2 utilization in healthy subjects. Since 5 L of arterial blood contain about 1 L of oxygen, this represents a virtual 1:1 relationship between the increase in O_2 delivery and muscle O_2 utilization. The regulatory mechanisms by which such tight coupling of muscle O_2 delivery/utilization is achieved are poorly understood. Skeletal muscle metabolism participates by stimulating group III and IV neural afferents in muscle, which activate cardiovascular centers in the midbrain to increase sympathetic neural outflow to the heart and blood vessels, and by mediating local vasodilation to direct the resulting increase in cardiac output to working muscle. Available evidence supports the view that intact muscle oxidative phosphorylation is necessary for normal coupling of O_2 delivery and utilization in exercise. This implies that metabolites that reflect the state of oxidative phosphorylation, such as muscle [ADP] or [ATP]/[ADP], may be involved.[23]

Muscle Metabolism in Exercise

Changes in levels of metabolites in muscle cells, within the muscle interstitium, and in blood accompany exercise and provide indices of the integrity of muscle energy pathways (Table 28-2). Although absolute exercise capacity among individuals varies widely due to differences in muscle mass and levels of physical conditioning, work performed at a similar relative workload—i.e., at a similar percentage of one's maximal exercise capacity—elicits comparable metabolic responses in normal subjects. Thus, exercise performed at a similar percentage of maximal voluntary contraction or of $\dot{V}_{O_2max}$ will elicit comparable changes in muscle phosphocreatine, inorganic phosphate, and pH and in blood levels of lactate, pyruvate, and ammonia.

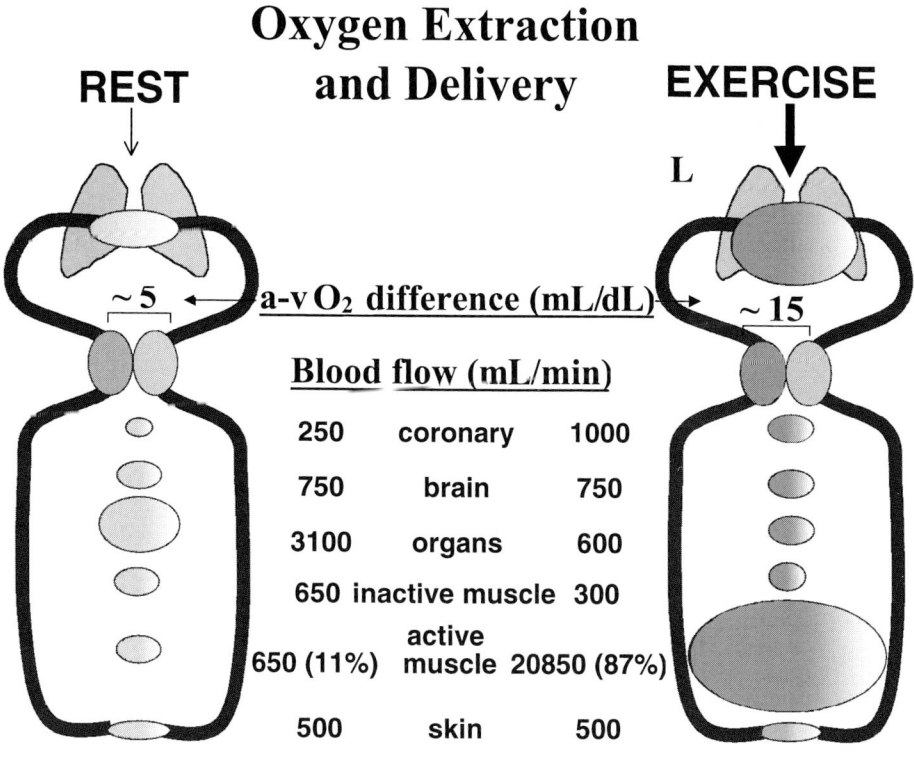

Figure 28-2. Illustration of the physiologic components of oxygen utilization—i.e., oxygen delivery (cardiac output or blood flow) and oxygen extraction from blood (arteriovenous O_2 difference)—at rest and during peak exercise in a healthy human. Note that during peak exercise there is a marked increase in oxygen delivery (blood flow), with approximately 90 percent of total blood flow (and more than 95 percent of the *increase* in blood flow) directed to working muscle. In addition, from rest to exercise, there is a threefold increase in the level of extraction of available oxygen from blood, so that the a–v O_2 difference increases from 5 to about 15 mL O_2/dL blood. (Modified from Mitchell J, Blomqvist CG: Maximal oxygen uptake. N Engl J Med 284:1018–1022, 1971. With permission.)

Table 28-2. MONITORS OF ENERGY METABOLISM IN EXERCISE

Metabolic pathway	Monitor	Method
Oxidative phosphorylation	Oxygen uptake ($\dot{V}_{O_2}$)	Douglas bags, mass spectrometry
	Carbon dioxide production ($\dot{V}_{CO_2}$)	Douglas bags, mass spectrometry
	Fuel mix (lipid vs. carbohydrate)	Gas exchange (RER)
	Oxygen delivery	
	Systemic (cardiac output, $\dot{Q}$)	Acetylene rebreathing
	Local (muscle blood flow)	Dye dilution studies
	Muscle oxygen extraction	Systemic a-v O_2 difference $[=\dot{V}_{O_2}(mL)/\dot{Q}(dL)]$
	Muscle phosphorylation potential	Estimate from PCr/Pi (^{31}P NMR)
	Muscle oxidative metabolites: acetylcarnitine, NADH, etc.	Needle biopsy studies
Anaerobic glycogenolysis	Venous lactate, pyruvate, L/P ratio, pH, alanine, other glycolytic intermediates	Blood chemistry
	Intracellular pH, phosphomonoesters (sugar phosphates)	^{31}P NMR
	Glycolytic end products, intermediates	Needle biopsy studies
Creatine kinase reaction	Phosphocreatine, ATP, H$^+$	^{31}P NMR or needle biopsy
Adenylate kinase/deaminase	Venous NH$_3$, inosine, hypoxanthine, xanthine	Blood chemistry
	ADP (calculated from creatine kinase equilibrium)	^{31}P NMR
	ADP, AMP, IMP	Needle biopsy studies

MONITORING GLYCOGENOLYSIS AND AMMONIA PRODUCTION IN FOREARM EXERCISE

Monitoring levels of lactate and related diffusible metabolites in venous effluent blood before and after forearm exercise is the paradigm most often used to evaluate the integrity of muscle glycogenolysis and glycolysis as well as to assess ammonia production to provide an indication of the integrity of myoadenylate deaminase. Peak rates of ATP hydrolysis produced by intense forearm exercise result in high rates of phosphocreatine hydrolysis, glycogenolysis, and ammonia production (Fig. 28-3). High rates of glycolytic flux produce high levels of cytoplasmic NADH/NAD, favoring the metabolism of pyruvate to lactate as the end product of anaerobic glycogenolysis. The accumulation of [H$^+$] is reflected in a fall in muscle pH that parallels lactate production and, along with increased cytoplasmic ADP, shifts the creatine kinase equilibrium to phosphocreatine hydrolysis. High ADP levels shift the myokinase equilibrium to the production of AMP; and the combination of increased ADP and AMP promotes AMP deamination via myoadenylate deaminase with the production of ammonia and inosine monophosphate (IMP).[24] The formation of other metabolites of purine catabolism—including inosine, hypoxanthine and xanthine—accompanies increased ammonia production. The regulation of these metabolic pathways is complex and beyond the scope of this review, but key interrelationships exist. For example, Pi, which accumulates as a net product of the creatine kinase reaction, activates glycogenolysis at the level of glycogen phosphorylase.[25] Increased [H$^+$] accompanying anaerobic glycogenolysis shifts the equilibrium of the proton-consuming creatine kinase reaction toward phosphocreatine hydrolysis and promotes AMP deamination.[26] Also AMP, IMP, and Pi produced by the myokinase/myoadenylate deaminase reactions activate anaerobic glycogenolysis at the level of muscle phosphorylase and phosphofructokinase. It follows that defects in any of these energy pathways, by altering levels of key regulatory metabolites, may have secondary effects upon remaining mechanisms of ATP production.

As originally described by McArdle a half century ago,[27] the forearm exercise test has traditionally employed ischemia induced by the inflation of a cuff above arterial pressure in combination with high-intensity exercise, commonly 30 maximal-effort hand-grip contractions performed in 1 min. An invariable complication of such testing in patients with defects of muscle glycogenolysis/glycolysis is a painful muscle contracture, which may result in myoglobinuria and/or a compartment syndrome.[28,29] Accordingly, alternatives to the traditional ischemic forearm test (IFT) have been sought. Sustained, intense [70 percent of maximal voluntary contraction (MVC)] isometric handgrip exercise has been reported as an alternative, "nonischemic" forearm test.[30] In fact, such testing is as ischemic as employing a blood pressure cuff, since the intramuscular pressure in isometric contractions of ≥ 50 percent MVC completely occlude muscle blood flow. Thus, any reduction in the incidence of muscle contractures depends on shortening the duration of the test—a method that is also effective in minimizing contractures in the traditional IFT. We have described a nonischemic forearm test (NIFT) consisting of 30 maximal handgrip contractions in 1 min without a blood pressure cuff.[31] The level of increase in lactate and ammonia in control subjects and the diagnostic accuracy in patients were similar to those from ischemic exercise. In contrast to

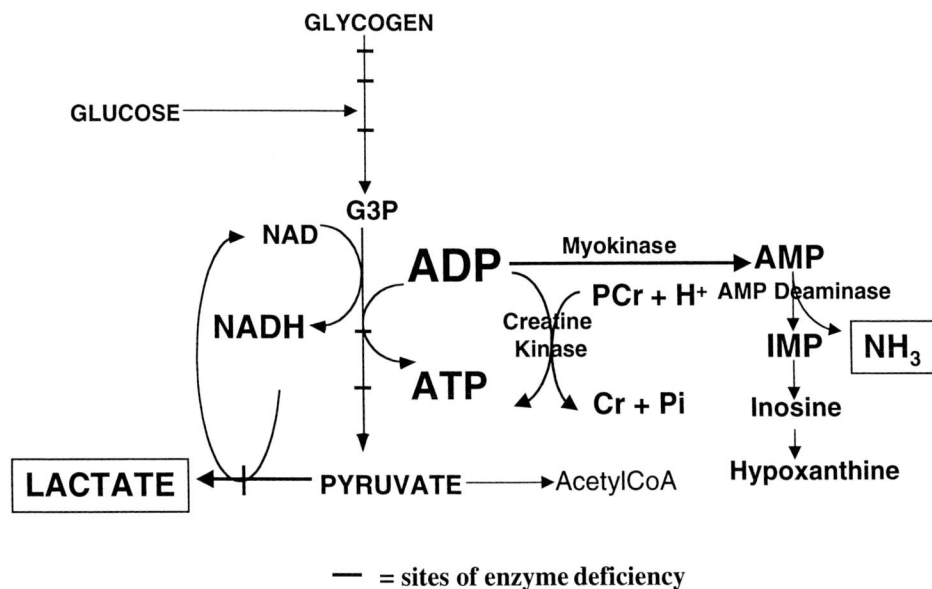

FIGURE 28-3. Metabolic consequences of intense forearm exercise. The accumulation of ADP produced by ATP hydrolysis activates *glycogenolysis*, with cytoplasmic NADH reoxidized via the LDH-mediated reduction of pyruvate to lactate. The accumulation of ADP and of H+ also activates the hydrolysis of phosphocreatine (PCr) and phosphorylation of ADP via *creatine kinase*. Increased cellular ADP also results in the production of ATP and AMP via the *myokinase* reaction, with AMP subsequently deaminated via *myoadenylate deaminase* with the production of ammonia (NH_3) and inosine monophosphate (IMP).

ischemic tests, retained oxidative capacity protects patients from contractures and significant pain.[31]

To perform the test, a catheter is placed in a median antecubital vein proximal to the deep veins of the forearm. After a resting sample has been collected, repetitive maximal hand-gripping at a rate of 30/min for a total duration of 1 min is performed. Recording of the initial maximal voluntary contraction and the strength of successive muscle contractions permits monitoring of the pattern of muscle fatigue and is helpful in identifying blunted metabolic responses that are due to poor and inconsistent effort. Typical responses to forearm exercise are illustrated in Fig. 28-4. Blood lactate normally increases four- to sixfold over baseline (~1 mM), with the peak occurring 1 to 2 min postexercise. In subjects with normal myoadenylate deaminase levels, ammonia typically increases fivefold or more, with levels generally peaking at 2 to 5 min after exercise. In healthy subjects, venous ammonia and lactate are linearly related.[32,33] Thus patients in whom lactate levels are low due to poor effort or to placement of the venous line other than in the median cubital vein show proportionally blunted ammonia responses. In contrast, patients with impaired glycogenolysis have a characteristic exaggerated rise in ammonia (Fig. 28-4), attributable to high cellular levels of ADP resulting from a combination of blocked glycogenolysis/glycolysis and absent cellular acidosis.

MAGNETIC RESONANCE SPECTROSCOPY

Phosphorus-31 magnetic resonance spectroscopy (^{31}P MRS) identifies five major phosphorus peaks involved in energy metabolism: inorganic phosphate (Pi), phosphocreatine (PCr), and three peaks corresponding to the α, β, and γ phosphates of ATP (Fig. 28-5). Additional small spectral signals may arise from phosphomonoesters (PME, representing phosphorylated intermediates of glycolysis) and phosphodiesters (PDE, representing membrane phospholipids), which do not play a direct role in energy metabolism. The separation of different phosphorus peaks relates to differences in resonance frequency of the individual phosphate atoms due to the specific chemical environment of phosphorus. For phosphorus atoms to be "visible" with ^{31}P MRS, they must be freely mobile and present in sufficient concentrations

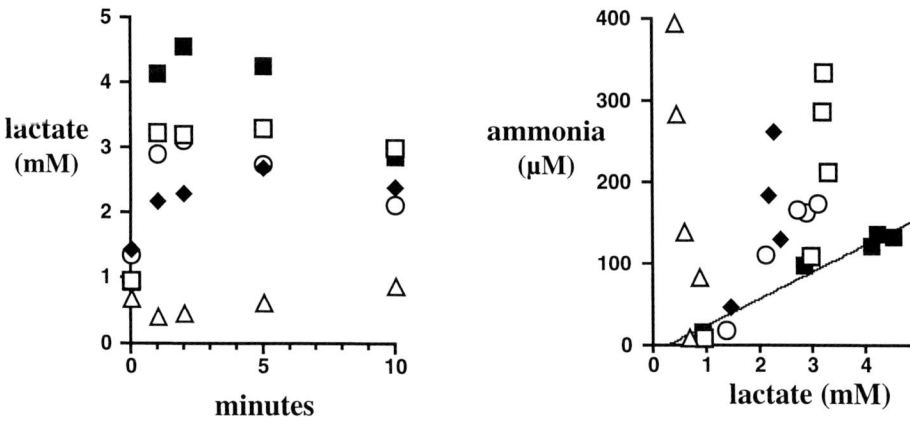

FIGURE 28-4. Venous effluent lactate and levels of ammonia (NH_3) in relation to lactate after forearm exercise in control subjects (closed squares); for patients with complete glycolytic blocks due to myophosphorylase deficiency (McArdle's disease) and PFK deficiency (open triangles); and for patients with partial defects of muscle glycolysis, phosphoglycerate mutase deficiency (closed diamonds), phosphoglycerate kinase deficiency (open squares), and lactate dehydrogenase (open circles).

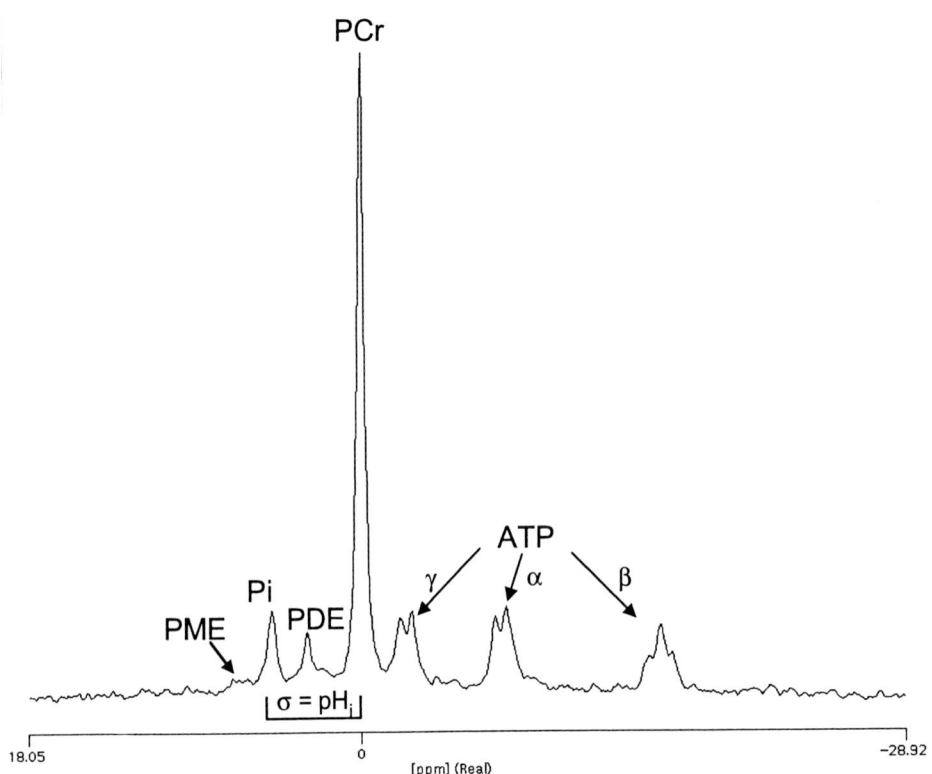

FIGURE 28-5. ^{31}P MRS spectra obtained from vastus lateralis of a healthy subject at rest. The labeled phosphorus peaks are the α, β, and γ phosphates of ATP, phosphocreatine (PCr), and inorganic phosphate (Pi). In addition, a small phosphomonoester (PME) peak corresponding to phosphorylated glycolytic intermediates and a phosphodiester (PDE) peak attributable to membrane phospholipids are indicated.

[~ 0.5 mM or greater in a 1.9-tesla (T) magnetic field]. Peak intensity (or area) is proportional to the concentration of each respective metabolite. Metabolite intensities are converted to concentrations relative to ATP, an internal standard believed to remain constant in normal working muscle; by convention, this is assumed to be 7.97 mM. Direct measures of the relative amounts of ATP, Pi, and PCr provide indirect measurements of intracellular pH and cytosolic free ADP. Free ADP, which is present in micromolar concentrations, is calculated assuming a normal equilibrium of the creatine kinase reaction.[34] The PCr/Pi ratio in normal subjects reflects the phosphorylation potential [ATP]/[ADP][Pi] as an indicator of the integrity of muscle oxidative phosphorylation.

Different paradigms of forearm and leg exercise have been employed to evaluate the effect of increased energy demand on ^{31}P MRS spectra.[35–39] The major ^{31}P MRS features of exercise are (1) a fall in the PCr peak and corresponding rise in the Pi peak attributable to the net phosphorylation of ADP by creatine phosphate via the creatine kinase reaction; and (2) a shift in the Pi resonance frequency toward PCr, attributable to the fall in muscle pH and a consequent increase in the proportion of the $H_2PO_4^-$ relative to the HPO_4^{-2} ion.[40] The separation of the Pi and PCr peaks therefore correlates with muscle pH and can be used to estimate it. Since muscle pH correlates closely with lactate and pyruvate accumulation in exercise, ^{31}P MRS can directly monitor the integrity of muscle glycogenolysis.

^{31}P MRS spectral acquisition during recovery from exercise is particularly informative in assessing the integrity of muscle oxidative phosphorylation. As the recovery period is considered primarily a function of oxidative ATP synthesis, PCr resynthesis and the initial rate of PCr recovery have been used as markers of muscle capacity for oxidative phosphorylation[41] (Fig. 28-6). PCr recovery is pH-dependent, with lower pH associated with slower rates of PCr synthesis, so correction for differences in end-exercise pH is necessary. The rate of postexercise decline in muscle [ADP] has also been employed as a monitor of the peak rate of oxidative phosphorylation.[42,43] Although ^{31}P MRS is noninvasive, it is costly and available in only a few centers. Technical limitations include possible signal inhomogeneity attributable to nonmuscle tissue or, in exercise studies, to inactive muscle within the volume of tissue sampled by the MRS coil.

OTHER METHODS OF MONITORING INTRACELLULAR METABOLITES

The proton (^{1}H) is the standard atom used in imaging. Although proton spectroscopy has increasingly been applied to the evaluation of brain metabolism, the technique has had limited application to skeletal muscle.[44] Separation of intracellular and extracellular lipid with ^{1}H MRS has been achieved in some studies, suggesting utility in identifying metabolic defects associated with excessive intramuscular lipid.[45] In addition, lactate and creatine peaks can be monitored using ^{1}H MRS. ^{13}C is present in low (approximately 1 percent) abundance, so its detection has required high field magnets. Using such devices, measurement of muscle and liver glycogen levels has been possible.[46] Direct needle biopsy of skeletal muscle at rest and during exercise can provide additional information about muscle cellular metabolism. Advantages of the needle biopsy include the capacity to assess levels of metabolites not visible by MRS and to differentiate phosphorus compounds that have the same reso-

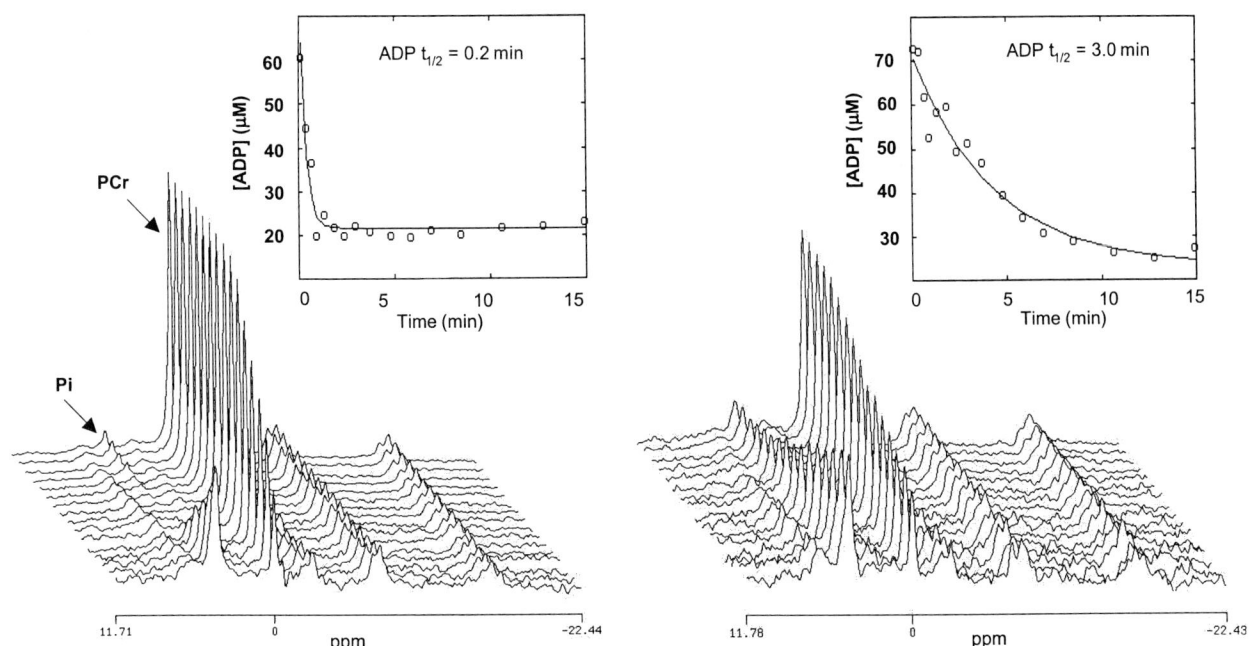

FIGURE 28-6. ^{31}P MRS spectra during recovery of PCr and ADP after quadriceps exercise in a healthy subject (left) and in a patient with a mitochondrial myopathy (right). Note (1) the rapid increase in PCr and fall in calculated ADP (inset) in the healthy subject and (2) delayed recovery of PCr and ADP consistent with impaired oxidative phosphorylation in the patient with mitochondrial myopathy.

nance frequency on MRS. For example, the increase in muscle NADH that accompanies heavy exercise reflects net NADH production [primarily via the tricarboxylic acid (TCA) cycle] relative to oxidation (electron transport). NADH is not detectable by ^{31}P MRS due to its low concentration and primarily intramitochondrial distribution, but it is measurable in needle biopsy samples of working muscle.[47] Laser fluorimetry of the muscle surface has also been used to monitor net production of NADH during exercise.[48] Microdialysis has been employed to sample the interstitial/extracellular milieu in skeletal muscle and other tissues in some research studies.[49,50]

METHODS OF MONITORING OXIDATIVE METABOLISM

Oxidative metabolism can be assessed by determining peak oxygen utilization during cycle or treadmill exercise; by measuring O_2 levels in venous effluent blood from working forearm; by assessing arteriovenous O_2 differences utilizing the Fick equation ($\dot{V}_{O_2} = \dot{Q} \times a{-}v\ O_2$ difference); by monitoring tissue oxygen levels by means of near infrared spectroscopy (NIRS); and by means of ^{31}P MRS measurements of postexercise rates of PCr recovery and ADP phosphorylation. More indirect determinations of oxidative capacity involve measurement of blood lactate levels during submaximal exercise as a surrogate marker of limited oxidative capacity.[51]

Near infrared spectroscopy (NIRS). Tissue O_2 levels and rates of O_2 utilization can be estimated using near infrared spectroscopy.[52,53] The technique depends upon the ability of light in the near infrared spectrum (700 to 1000 nm) to penetrate tissue to a depth of several centimeters and upon the differential absorbance of light at discrete wavelengths in the near infrared (NIR) spectrum by oxygenated versus deoxygenated hemoglobin and myoglobin. Differential absorbance at the sampled wavelengths (including ~760 and ~850 nm) provides outputs corresponding to oxyhemoglobin (+ myoglobin) and deoxyhemoglobin (+ myoglobin).[54] Since the absorbance characteristics of hemoglobin and myoglobin are identical, definitive assessment of the contributions of each to NIRS results is not possible. However, the majority of the NIR signal is generally considered to derive from hemoglobin, and results are often referred to simply as oxy/deoxyhemoglobin.[55] The sum of oxy and deoxy signals provides an estimate of blood volume. Changes in tissue O_2 levels accompany ischemia, exercise, and postexercise recovery. Exercise results in a fall in oxyhemoglobin and a reciprocal rise in deoxyhemoglobin, indicating a net increase in O_2 extraction relative to increased O_2 delivery by the circulation (Fig. 28-7). Results are usually referenced to maximal changes in oxy/deoxyhemoglobin levels during resting ischemia.[54] Postexercise, NIRS detects an increase in oxyhemoglobin that transiently exceeds preexercise resting levels and corresponds to postexercise hyperemia. NIRS has also been used to estimate rates of O_2 utilization at rest and in exercise using estimates of optical

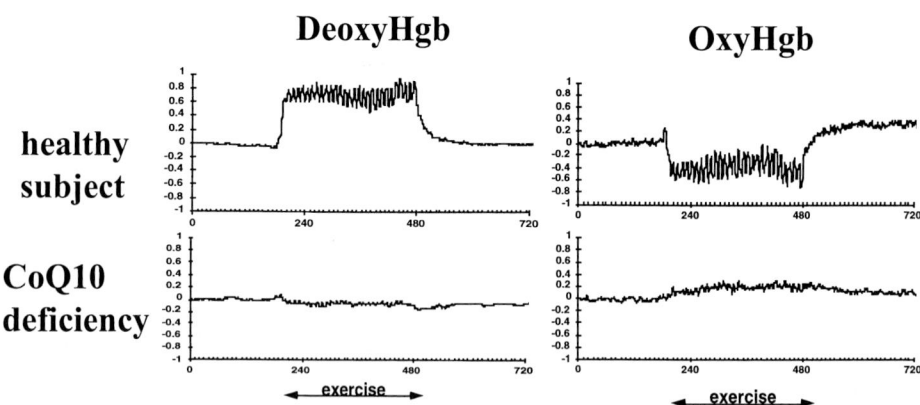

FIGURE 28-7. Near infrared spectra corresponding to oxyhemoglobin (+ myoglobin) and deoxyhemoglobin (+ myoglobin) at rest, during exercise, and after recovery in healthy subjects and a patient with a mitochondrial myopathy. Note the prompt increase in tissue deoxyhemoglobin and corresponding decrease in oxyhemoglobin with exercise in healthy subjects. In contrast, a patient with a severe oxidative defect due to deficiency of coenzyme Q10 shows no ability to increase oxygen extraction during exercise. (*From Sobreira C, Hirano M, Shanske S, et al: Mitochondrial encephalomyopathy with coenzyme Q10 deficiency. Neurology 48:1238–1243, 1997. With permission.*)

path length to determine O_2 concentrations.[52,56] Transient arterial occlusion is used to estimate rates of O_2 uptake. Transient venous occlusion has been used to estimate blood flow. Like MRS, NIRS is subject to technical limitations attributable to sampling nonmuscle tissue or inactive muscle. Considerable subject-to-subject variation exists in healthy subjects. One important variable in the NIR response is the thickness of subcutaneous tissue overlying the sampled muscle. A recent report indicates that low resting rates of oxygen utilization in forearms of patients with mitochondrial myopathy and progressive external ophthalmoplegia can be accounted for by greater subcutaneous tissue thickness in patients compared to control subjects.[56,57]

Venous effluent oxygen levels. From rest to exercise, O_2 levels in venous effluent blood fall due to a net increase in mitochondrial O_2 utilization relative to the increase in O_2 delivery by the circulation, paralleling the decline in tissue oxygen levels monitored with tissue oximetry. This response has been exploited to screen for impaired oxidative phosphorylation in patients with mitochondrial myopathies where impaired respiratory chain function limits the capacity for extraction of available O_2 from blood.[58,59] The forearm testing protocol involves the collection of a resting sample using a blood-gas syringe, followed by rhythmic forearm exercise consisting of repeated brief isometric contractions at low to moderate intensity (30 to 50 percent of maximal voluntary contraction). After 3 min of exercise, and as exercise continues, venous effluent blood is collected. In healthy subjects and in patients with a variety of nonmitochondrial muscle disorders, venous Po_2 and O_2 saturation falls. In contrast, in most patients with mitochondrial myopathies, venous O_2 levels do not decline but increase, indicating impaired oxygen utilization relative to O_2 delivery (Fig. 28-8). More severely restricted respiratory chain function results in larger exercise increases in venous O_2.[58,59]

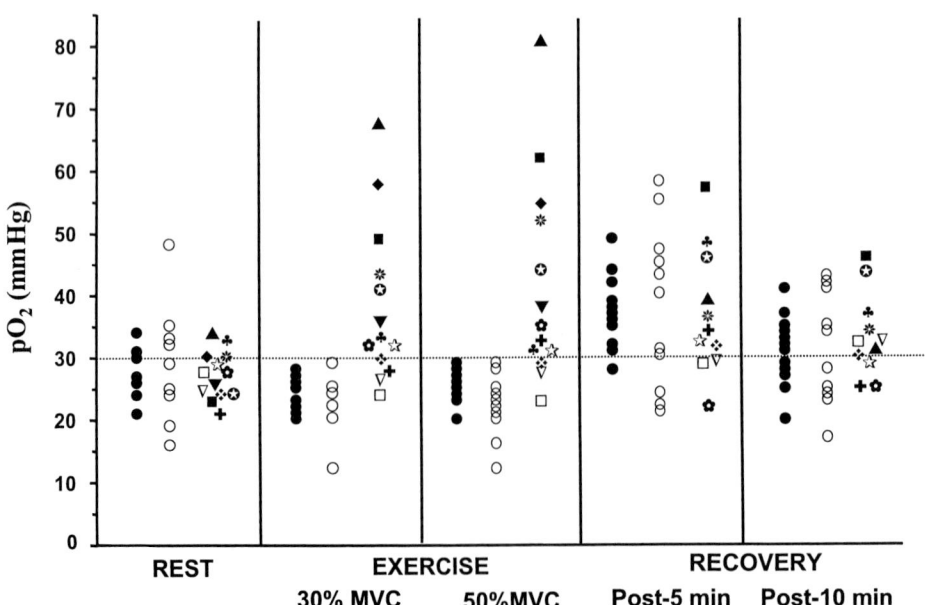

FIGURE 28-8. Venous Po_2 at rest, during exercise at 30 and 50 percent of MVC, and during recovery in control subjects (closed circles), control myopathy patients (open circles), and patients with mitochondrial myopathies. Note the elevated O_2 levels in most mitochondrial myopathy patients during exercise. (*From Taivassalo T, Abbott A, Wyrick P, Haller RG: Venous oxygen levels during aerobic forearm exercise: An index of impaired oxidative metabolism in mitochondrial myopathy. Ann Neurol 51:38–44, 2002. With permission.*)

Cycle ergometry assessment of oxidative metabolism.
The most common paradigm for assessing muscle oxidative capacity is treadmill or cycle exercise in which the workload is increased at regular intervals (ramp test). Oxygen utilization ($\dot{V}_{O_2}$) is determined at rest and during submaximal and peak exercise. Resting oxygen utilization is elevated in hypermetabolic states such as Luft disease[60] and was reported elevated in patients with complex I deficiency[61] but is normal in other metabolic myopathies. During cycle exercise, oxygen uptake is linearly related to work rate. This $\dot{V}_{O_2}$-work relationship is an index of ADP/O coupling. Thus, poorly coupled oxidative phosphorylation would result in high $\dot{V}_{O_2}$ relative to work rate. In some muscle oxidative defects, the O_2 cost of exercise is high due to exaggerated increases in cardiac output and pulmonary ventilation, resulting in increased O_2 utilization by cardiac and ventilatory muscles.[62]

The measurement of maximal oxygen utilization during peak exercise is an important index of the integrity of muscle oxidative phosphorylation.[12] In some patients, symptoms of exertional pain or cramping preclude determining $\dot{V}_{O_2max}$ (defined as a plateau of $\dot{V}_{O_2}$ with increasing exercise workload). Since heart rate is linearly related to relative workload, $\dot{V}_{O_2max}$ can be estimated using the heart rate at which the patient ceased exercise and extrapolating to the $\dot{V}_{O_2}$ that would correspond to the subject's predicted maximal heart rate (220 minus patient age in years). Patients with metabolic defects affecting muscle oxidative phosphorylation typically have a peak $\dot{V}_{O_2}$ of less than 20 mL/kg/min when corrected for ideal weight.

Evaluation of the components of oxygen utilization, i.e., cardiac output and a–v O_2 difference, enhances the diagnostic sensitivity of cycle ergometry. Cardiac output can be measured noninvasively utilizing acetylene rebreathing, in which the rate of disappearance of acetylene from the lungs is directly proportional to lung blood flow and systemic cardiac output.[63] The maximal capacity for O_2 delivery is the limiting factor for peak $\dot{V}_{O_2}$ in healthy subjects, and an increased capacity for O_2 delivery, indicated by a higher peak cardiac output, is a fundamental adaptation to aerobic training.[12] Measurement of maximal cardiac output thus provides an independent measure of aerobic fitness. Determination of $\dot{V}_{O_2}$ and cardiac output permits calculation of systemic arteriovenous O_2 difference from the Fick equation: $\dot{V}_{O_2}$ = cardiac output × a–v O_2 difference. The maximal a-v O_2 difference is increased only slightly by physical conditioning[64]; therefore, in normal subjects of widely differing aerobic capacity, the maximal systemic a-v O_2 difference is similar, i.e., ~15 mL/dL. In contrast, patients with impaired muscle mitochondrial function typically have peak a–v O_2 difference of less than 10 mL/dL[62]; in the most severe oxidative defects, exercise a–v O_2 difference may actually fall from resting levels of 5 mL/dL.[58,65] When defects in the function of the muscle respiratory chain limit oxygen extraction, blood flow and cardiac output are exaggerated relative to oxygen utilization.[23] The normal tight coupling between oxygen delivery and utilization is indicated by an increase in blood flow and cardiac output of 5 to 6 L of arterial blood (containing approximately 1 L of oxygen) for every liter of increase in oxygen utilization (i.e., $\Delta\dot{Q}/\Delta\dot{V}_{O_2}$ ~5 to 6).

Gas-exchange measurements provide information about fuel utilization and ventilatory regulation. At rest and with exercise below the ventilatory threshold, the respiratory exchange ratio (RER = $\dot{V}_{CO_2}/\dot{V}_{O_2}$) provides an indication of the mix of oxidized fuels. Characteristically, the proportion of carbohydrate oxidized increases with increasing exercise intensity, as indicated by a rise in the RER from approximately 0.7 at rest (reflecting virtually exclusive lipid oxidation) to approach 1.0 with near maximal exercise, reflecting exclusive oxidation of carbohydrate.[14,66] The RER also is high during the transition from rest to exercise due to the slower increase in oxidation of fat than carbohydrate. With sustained submaximal exercise, the proportion of lipid oxidized progressively increases, peaking at approximately 30 min of exercise.[14] Limited availability of oxidizable carbohydrate blunts the increase in RER in myophosphorylase deficiency and muscle phosphofructokinase (PFK) deficiency. Conversely, fat oxidation defects may be associated with higher than normal RER at rest and during prolonged exercise.

During submaximal exercise, ventilation is linearly related to oxygen utilization and the ratio of ventilation to oxygen utilization (i.e., the ventilatory equivalent for oxygen, $\dot{V}_E/\dot{V}_{O_2}$) is relatively constant at approximately 30 to 35.[67] At exercise above approximately 70 percent of $\dot{V}_{O_2max}$, ventilation increases more than oxygen utilization, resulting in a progressive increase in $\dot{V}_E/\dot{V}_{O_2}$ to approximately 45. This inflection point is termed the ventilatory or "anaerobic" threshold. Above this threshold, the blood lactate level and lactate/pyruvate ratio increase steeply with exercise. In patients with respiratory chain defects, the anaerobic threshold is exceeded at trivial levels of exertion, and $\dot{V}_E/\dot{V}_{O_2}$ and RER are anomalously high.[62,68]

Neurohumoral responses to exercise govern levels of lipolysis in adipose tissue and of glycogenolysis in liver to increase the availability of fatty acids and of glucose for working muscle. The mismatch between energy supply and demand in metabolic myopathies accelerates rates of production and uptake of these fuels.[69–71] Correspondingly, the neurohumoral responses to exercise, including the increase in cortisol and growth hormone and the decrease in circulating insulin, are exaggerated in these patients compared to control subjects exercising at either the same absolute or relative workload.[69–71]

Exercise Pathophysiology in Muscle Energy Defects

Abnormal muscle metabolism in metabolic myopathies is associated with (1) a lack of increase or decrease in metabolites distal to the site of the metabolic block; (2) an accumulation of metabolic intermediates proximal to the metabolic block; and (3) altered activity of preserved energy pathways and of physiologic responses that normally are modulated by the affected metabolic pathway.

RESPIRATORY CHAIN AND RELATED DISORDERS

Larsson-Linderholm syndrome. The classic physiologic features of a severe defect in muscle oxidative metabolism were described in the 1960s in studies of patients living in the vicinity of Umeå in northern Sweden with an apparently recessively inherited disorder marked by disabling exercise intolerance and episodic myoglobinuria.[72,73] Utilizing exercise testing and cardiac and peripheral vessel catheterization, peak O_2 utilization in exercise was found to be low (one-third to one-fourth of normal) and limited by the level of O_2 extraction from circulating blood. Systemic a–v O_2 difference and femoral venous O_2 saturation remained at essentially resting levels with peak exercise (Fig. 28-9). In contrast to the severe limitation in O_2 extraction, peak O_2 delivery (cardiac output and blood flow) was similar to healthy subjects; and, in relation to oxygen utilization, O_2 delivery was three- to sixfold normal.[72] The molecular defect involves deficiency of multiple iron-sulfur proteins of the tricarboxylic acid cycle (succinate dehydrogenase and aconitase)[65,74,75] and respiratory chain (iron sulfur proteins in complexes I and III) in skeletal muscle.[76]

Extraction of available oxygen from blood. The level of extraction of available oxygen from blood during exercise, as marked by systemic a–v O_2 difference, is now recognized to be a surrogate marker of the integrity of muscle oxidative phosphorylation. A blunted capacity to increase the level of extraction of available O_2 from blood is the hallmark of disorders of muscle oxidative phosphorylation.[62,71,77] In patients with mitochondrial myopathy, the peak a–v O_2 difference correlates directly with the capacity for aerobic exercise, consistent with the view that respiratory chain function governs aerobic capacity in this patient population.[62] This contrasts with the situation in healthy subjects, in whom mitochondrial capacity for O_2 uptake, as reflected in peak a–v O_2 difference, does not limit aerobic exercise and demonstrates no direct correlation with $\dot{V}_{O_2max}$. Low capacity for oxygen extraction from blood in mitochondrial myopathy patients is also detected by NIRS as anomalously high tissue O_2 levels during exercise[53,56,78,79] (Fig. 28-7) and as high levels of O_2 in venous effluent blood during aerobic forearm exercise[58,59] (Fig. 28-8).

Exaggerated oxygen transport and ventilation. A corollary of impaired O_2 extraction in mitochondrial myopathies is exaggerated O_2 delivery in relation to the rate of O_2 utilization. In a large series of patients, we found that the level of increase in systemic O_2 delivery (cardiac output) was, on average, about threefold normal.[62] Furthermore, the degree of exaggerated increase in cardiac output in relation to oxygen utilization correlated with the degree of impaired respiratory chain function (Fig. 28-10). Thus patients with the lowest capacity to extract oxygen from blood had cardiac output responses that were as high as tenfold normal.[4,62] This accounts for the prominent tachycardia with trivial exertion in severe respiratory chain defects. Ventilation is also exaggerated in patients with severe respiratory chain

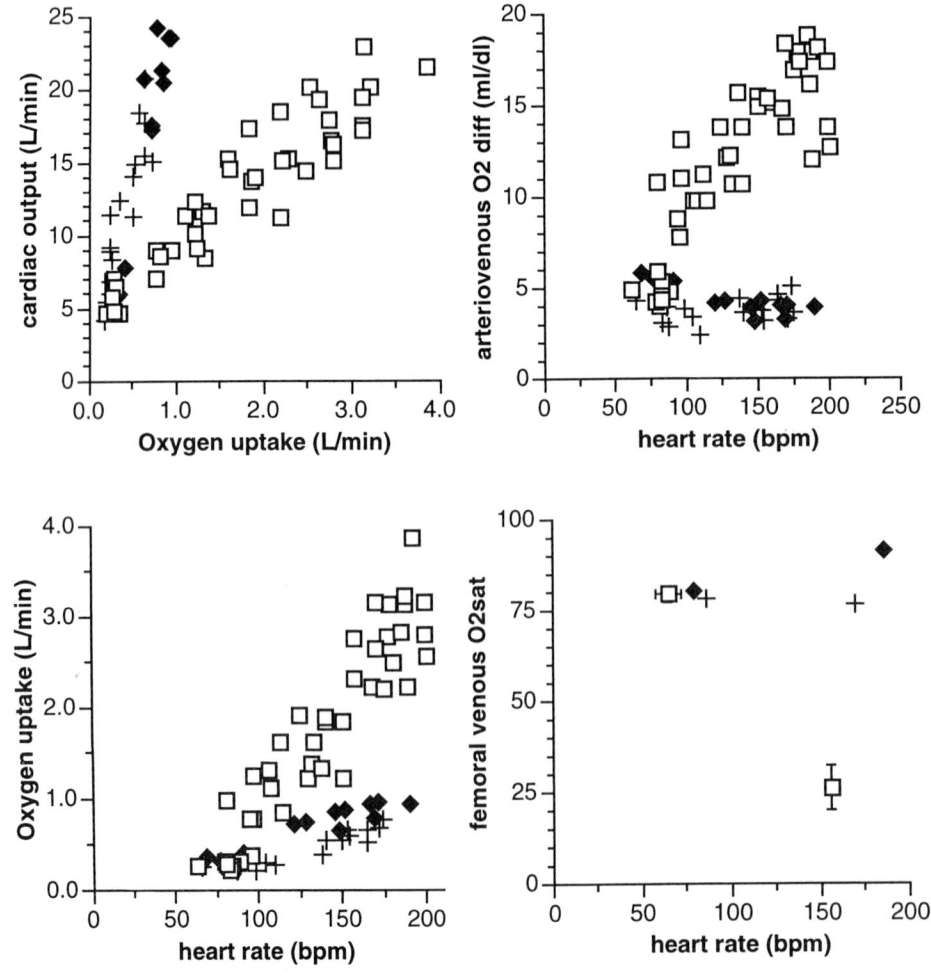

FIGURE 28-9. Cycle exercise responses from patients studied by Larsson, Linderholm and coworkers (pluses), a patient with the same syndrome studied more recently (closed diamonds) and healthy control subjects (open squares). In comparison with healthy control subjects, during cycle exercise, patients demonstrate an absence of the normal increase in systemic a–v O_2 difference (upper right panel) and decrease in femoral venous O_2 saturation (lower right panel); blunted increase in oxygen uptake relative to increased heart rate (lower left panel), and an exaggerated increase in cardiac output relative to O_2 uptake (upper left panel). (From Haller RG, Vissing J: Circulatory regulation in muscle disease, in Saltin B, Boushel R, Seckel N, Mitchell JH (eds): Exercise and Circulation in Health and Disease. Champaign, IL: Human Kinetics, 1999; pp 263–273. With permission.)

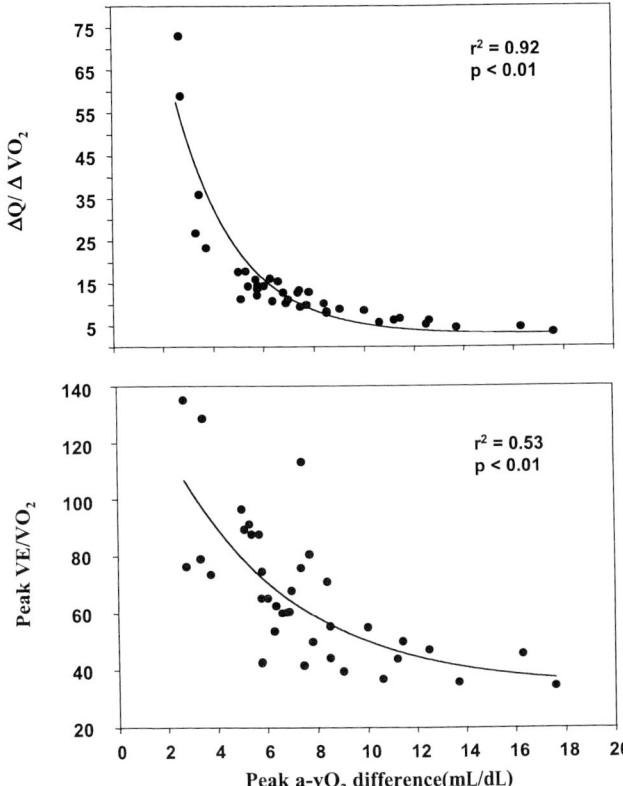

FIGURE 28-10. Relationship between peak a–v O_2 difference and $\Delta\dot{Q}/\Delta\dot{V}_{O_2}$ (the level of increase in cardiac output relative to increased oxygen utilization from rest to exercise) (upper panel) and in peak levels of ventilation relative to oxygen uptake ($\dot{V}_E/\dot{V}_{O_2}$). More severely impaired muscle oxidative phosphorylation as indicated by low peak levels of a–v O_2 difference is linked to progressively exaggerated circulatory and ventilatory responses to exercise as indicated by significant negative exponential relationship between the two variables. Note normal $\Delta\dot{Q}/\Delta\dot{V}_{O_2}$ = ~5; normal peak $\dot{V}_E/\dot{V}_{O_2}$ = ~45; normal peak a–v O_2 difference ≥ 10 mL O_2/dL blood.

defects. We found that the average ventilatory equivalent for oxygen ($\dot{V}_E/\dot{V}_{O_2}$) in peak exercise was 65 in patients compared to 41 in control subjects. Also indicative of hyperventilation in exercise was the observation that the respiratory exchange ratio in peak exercise was 1.31 in patients versus 1.14 in control subjects. As in the circulatory response, more severely impaired respiratory chain function (lower peak levels of a–v O_2 difference) was associated with more severe hyperventilation in exercise (Fig 28-10). In the most extreme cases, a $\dot{V}_E/\dot{V}_{O_2}$ of more than 100 and an RER of more than 2 were recorded during peak exercise.[62] These observations explain the prominence of exertional dyspnea in some mitochondrial myopathies.

Blood lactate and pyruvate levels at rest and during exercise. Respiratory chain defects are associated with elevated levels of lactate at rest in a minority of patients with established mitochondrial myopathy.[62,80,81] However, high lactate levels in relation to work performed and level of O_2 utilization are present in most affected patients.[62,82,83] The lactate/pyruvate ratio similarly rises steeply relative to exercise workload, consistent with high levels of cytoplasmic NADH/NAD mirroring high levels of mitochondrial reducing equivalents. Defects of pyruvate metabolism are associated with high levels of pyruvate relative to lactate and anomalously low lactate/pyruvate ratios in exercise.

^{31}P MRS manifestations of muscle oxidative defects.

Phosphorus MRS has identified a number of abnormalities in patients with respiratory chain defects. At rest, the ^{31}P MRS spectrum may exhibit one or more of the following: low [PCr], high [Pi], high calculated free [ADP], and/or low PP, suggesting that oxidative phosphorylation is deficient even at rest.[84–87] However, the ^{31}P MRS spectrum can also be normal in patients with identified mitochondrial defects, suggesting that the resting state is often not sensitive enough to detect abnormalities in energy metabolism. With exercise, there is typically an exaggerated fall in PCr and rise in Pi relative to work performed, consistent with impaired oxidative phosphorylation. After exercise, recovery of PCr typically is greatly delayed, consistent with the oxidative deficit (Fig. 28-6). Curiously, the fall in muscle pH during exercise as monitored by the chemical shift of Pi relative to PCr is normal or even subnormal and the recovery of pH is rapid despite high and prolonged elevations of venous lactate. Accelerated extrusion of lactic acid from active muscle and/or increased buffering capacity of the muscle may be responsible.[44,84,87]

DISORDERS OF MUSCLE GLYCOGENOLYSIS — IMPLICATIONS FOR ANAEROBIC AND AEROBIC METABOLISM

Forearm exercise. The hallmark of defects in muscle glycogenolysis is failure of lactate to rise normally in blood flowing from exercised muscles.[27] In complete blocks in muscle glycogenolysis due to myophosphorylase or PFK deficiency, lactate levels fall with exercise. Patients with a small residual capacity for glycogenolysis—as with glycogen debrancher enzyme, phosphoglycerate kinase (PGK), phosphoglycerate mutase (PGM), or lactate dehydrogenase (LDH) deficiencies—usually demonstrate a 1.5- to 3-fold rise in lactate (Fig. 28-4). The level of reduction in glycolytic enzymes necessary to result in a clinically significant reduction in glycolytic energy and lactate production is unknown. In our experience, persons who are heterozygous for mutations in enzymes that are rate-limiting for glycogenolysis (myophosphorylase) and glycolysis (PFK), and thus have approximately 50 percent of normal enzyme levels, produce lactate normally during forearm exercise. Changes in venous pH after forearm exercise parallel lactate production, so a lack of normal decline in pH accompanies defects in glycogenolysis.[31,88,89] The normal increase in blood pyruvate is also attenuated or absent, as is the normal, roughly fivefold rise in the lactate/pyruvate (L/P) ratio. A virtually unchanged L/P ratio with exercise typifies myophosphorylase and muscle PFK deficiency. A disproportionate increase in pyruvate relative to lactate occurs in muscle LDH deficiency and is due to the buildup of pyruvate behind the metabolic block[90]; consequently the L/P ratio in this disorder actually *falls* with exercise. A disproportionate increase in ammonia relative to lactate or a low peak lactate/ammonia ratio is characteristic of glycolytic defects. An exception is the occasional patient with combined deficiency of glycolysis or glycogenolysis and myoadenylate deaminase.[91]

^{31}P MRS. The ^{31}P MRS hallmark of defective muscle glycogenolysis is failure of the Pi peak to shift towards the PCr peak, reflecting the absence of the normal fall in muscle pH due to impaired production of lactic acid during exercise.[37,92,93] Muscle pH actually increases when the block in glycogenolysis is complete, as in myophosphorylase and muscle PFK deficiency, due to the proton-utilizing creatine kinase reaction. The decline in pH is blunted with a partial glycolytic defect, as with PGK, PGM, or LDH deficiency. The site of glycolytic block may also be identified from the presence or absence of a phosphomonoester (PME) peak during exercise. Muscle phosphorylase and debrancher deficiencies produce no accumulation of sugar phosphates during exercise, whereas distal glycolytic blocks result in accumulation of sugar phosphates upstream of the metabolic block, as shown by a large phosphomonoester peak on MRS.[38,93,94] Correspondingly, the increase in Pi is attenuated relative to the decrease in PCr attributable to "phosphate trapping" in sugar phosphates (Fig. 28-5). PME accumulation may not be apparent at low levels of exercise with distal glycolytic defects that typically retain some enzyme activity.

Oxidative metabolism. In patients with muscle phosphorylase and PFK deficiency, the capacity for oxidative phosphorylation is substrate-limited. The major elements of this oxidative limitation are as follows: (1) absence of glycogen-derived pyruvate for the production of acetyl-CoA and for pyruvate-dependent anaplerotic reactions (e.g., alanine aminotransferase and pyruvate carboxylase), which, by increasing TCA cycle levels of malate and oxaloacetate, may "spark" the combustion of lipid and carbohydrate fuels[16,95,96]; (2) limited rates of flux through the TCA cycle that restrict the generation of reducing equivalents (NADH, FADH) for oxidation via the respiratory chain, thus restraining peak rates of oxidative phosphorylation[96]; and (3) fluctuations in exercise and oxidative capacity owing to changing availability of extramuscular fuels in response to exercise and diet.[19,97] In McArdle disease and PFK deficiency, impaired oxidative metabolism has been demonstrated using cycle exercise, NIRS, and ^{31}P MRS.[53,98–100] In contrast to complete blocks of glycogenolysis, virtually normal $\dot{V}_{O_2max}$ has been found in a rare patient with McArdle disease with a small amount of preserved myophosphorylase[19] as well as in other glycolytic defects in which some residual glycolytic enzyme activity is preserved.[101,102] These findings are consistent with the view that a relatively small amount of glycolytic flux is sufficient to meet the oxidative requirements of glycogenolysis/glycolysis.

Second wind, "out of wind" phenomena. The clinical manifestations of impaired aerobic glycogenolysis in McArdle disease are epitomized by the spontaneous second wind (Fig. 28-11). This is a stereotyped response that, in our experience, is an invariable feature of complete myophosphorylase deficiency, i.e., typical McArdle disease. The char-

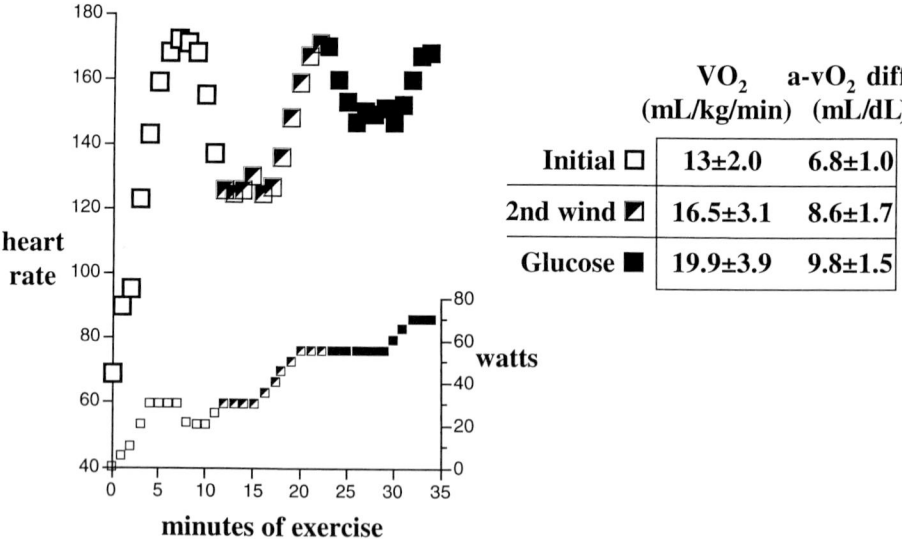

FIGURE 28-11. Spontaneous second wind in McArdle disease. The graph at the left shows peak exercise and exercise heart rate in a 29-year-old woman with McArdle disease as determined in the first 6 to 8 min of cycle exercise (initial, open squares); after the onset of a spontaneous second wind (2nd wind, partially closed squares); and after glucose infusion (glucose, closed squares). Mean (±SD) peak $\dot{V}_{O_2}$ and a–v O_2 difference under each condition for eight McArdle patients undergoing similar testing are shown at the right. The data indicate that improved exercise capacity and fall in exercise heart rate that denotes the onset of a spontaneous second wind is attributable to an approximately 25 percent increase in oxidative capacity that is marked by a 25 percent increase in peak a–v O_2 difference, a surrogate marker of mitochondrial oxidative phosphorylation. Infusion of glucose after a spontaneous second wind induced a second "second wind" that is due to a further increase in mitochondrial oxygen utilization attributable to increased availability of oxidative substrate. (*Modified from Haller RG, Vissing J: Spontaneous second wind and glucose-induced second, "second wind" in McArdle disease: Oxidative mechanisms. Arch Neurol 59:1395–1402, 2002. With permission.*)

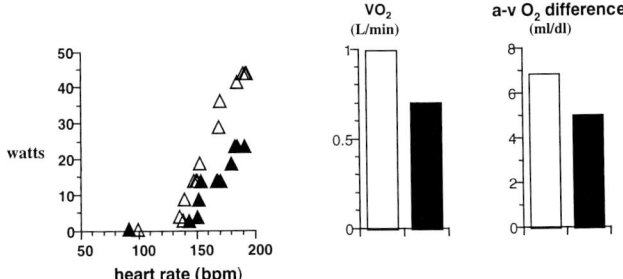

FIGURE 28-12. Carbohydrate-induced "out of wind" phenomenon in muscle PFK deficiency. Heart rate relative to workload in cycle exercise in a 13-year-old boy with previously undiagnosed PFK deficiency (left graph). Exercise was performed after an overnight fast (open triangles) and, the following day, after a carbohydrate meal (closed triangles). The patient displayed a characteristic fall in work capacity (from 45 to 25 W) that corresponded to an approximately 30 percent drop in peak $\dot{V}_{O_2}$ and a–v O_2 difference after a carbohydrate meal (closed bars) compared to fasting (open bars). This decreased oxidative capacity correlates with a carbohydrate/insulin-mediated drop in the availability of free fatty acids, on which oxidative capacity in PFK deficiency depends.

acteristic features are: (1) low capacity for oxidative phosphorylation marked by low peak levels of systemic a–v O_2 difference in the first 5 to 8 min of sustained exercise that is due to low availability of blood-borne fuels; and (2) an abrupt improvement in exercise tolerance between minutes 8 and 12 of sustained exercise due to an approximately 25 percent increase in the rate of oxidative phosphorylation related to increased availability of blood glucose and free fatty acids. Braakhekke et al. concluded that muscle oxidative capacity was normal and comparable to healthy subjects after the onset of a second wind[103]; but we have found that oxidative metabolism remains substrate-limited: Infusion of glucose after a spontaneous second wind resulted in a second "second wind" attributable to a further increase in oxidative capacity consistent with enhanced mitochondrial oxidative phosphorylation.[19]

Muscle PFK deficiency closely resembles McArdle disease clinically, and the degree of oxidative impairment, as assessed in the first 5 to 8 min of exercise, is virtually identical. However, there are important differences in exercise responses, because PFK deficiency blocks the metabolism of glucose as well as of muscle glycogen. Glucose administration improves oxidative capacity in McArdle disease but lowers oxidative capacity in PFK deficiency (Fig. 28-12). Carbohydrate-induced exertional fatigue, which we have termed the "out of wind" phenomenon, is attributable to a carbohydrate-induced reduction in availability of the major oxidative fuel of PFK-deficient muscle, free fatty acids.[97] PFK-deficient patients also do not develop the spontaneous second wind that is characteristic of McArdle disease.[104] Available evidence suggests that enzyme defects that preserve some residual capacity for glycogenolysis are not subject to fluctuations in exercise capacity as a result of changing levels of extramuscular substrates.

FATTY ACID OXIDATION DEFECTS

The oxidation of long-chain fatty acids can be limited by deficiency of carnitine palmitoyl transferase II, very long chain acyl-CoA dehydrogenase (VLCAD), and the trifunctional protein. These deficiencies predispose to the accumulation of potentially toxic intermediates of fat oxidation, and increase dependence upon carbohydrate fuels. Increased dependence upon carbohydrate relative to fat oxidation may be suggested by a higher than normal RER at rest and during exercise.[105–107] As long as carbohydrate availability is preserved, peak rates of oxidative phosphorylation and cardiopulmonary responses to exercise are normal.[83,102,107] Thus in a patient with a history compatible with a disorder of fatty acid oxidation, normal oxygen utilization and delivery during exercise would strongly support the diagnosis.

List of Abbreviations

ADP	adenosine diphosphate	NIRS	near infrared spectroscopy
ATPase	adenosine triphosphatase	PCr	phosphocreatine
FADH	flavine adenine dinucleotide	PDE	phosphodiester
FFA	free fatty acids	PFK	phosphofructokinase
IFT	ischemic forearm test	PGK	phosphoglycerate kinase
IMP	inosine monophosphate	PGM	phosphoglycerate mutase
L/P	lactate/pyruvate	Pi	inorganic phosphate
MVC	maximal voluntary contraction	PME	phosphomonoester
NAD	oxidized nicotinamide adenine dinucleotide	RER	respiratory exchange ratio
NADH	reduced nicotinamide adenine dinucleotide	TCA	tricarboxylic acid
NIFT	nonischemic forearm test	VLCAD	very long chain acyl-CoA dehydrogenase

References

1. Abe K, Matsuo Y, Kadekawa J, et al: Effect of coenzyme Q10 in patients with mitochondrial myopathy, encephalopathy, lactic acidosis, and stroke-like episodes (MELAS): Evaluation by noninvasive tissue oximetry. J Neurol Sci 162:65–68, 1999.
2. MacLean D, Vissing J, Vissing SF, Haller RG: Oral branched-chain amino acids do not improve exercise capacity in McArdle's disease. Neurology 51:1456–1459, 1998.
3. Vissing J, Gansted U, Quistorff B: Exercise intolerance in mitochondrial myopathy is not related to lactic acidosis. Ann Neurol 49:672–676, 2001.
4. Taivassalo T, Shoubridge EA, Chen JEC, et al: Aerobic conditioning in patients with mitochondrial myopathies: Physiological, biochemical and genetic effects. Ann Neurol 50:133–141, 2001.
5. Fitts RH: Cellular mechanisms of muscle fatigue. Physiol Rev 74:49–94, 1994.
6. James JH, Fang CH, Schrantz SJ, et al: Linkage of aerobic glycolysis to sodium-potassium transport in rat skeletal muscle. J Clin Invest 98:2388–2397, 1996.
7. Sejersted OM, Sjøgaard G: Dynamics and consequences of potassium shifts in skeletal muscle and heart during exercise. Physiol Rev 80:1411–1481, 2000.
8. Haller RG, Clausen T, Vissing J: Reduced levels of skeletal muscle Na$^+$K$^+$-ATPase in McArdle disease. Neurology 50:37–40, 1998.
9. Dyken M, Smith D, Peake R: An electromyographic diagnostic screening test in McArdle's disease and a case report. Neurology 17:45–50, 1967.
10. Wiles CM, Jones DA, Edwards RHT: Fatigue in human metabolic myopathy, in Human Muscle Fatigue: Physiological Mechanisms. London: Pitman Medical, 1981; pp 264–282.
11. Kushmerick MJ: Skeletal muscle: A paradigm for testing principles of bioenergetics. J Bioenerg Biomembr 27:555–569, 1995.
12. Åstrand PO, Rodahl K: Textbook of Work Physiology: Physiological Basis of Exercise. New York: McGraw-Hill, 1986.
13. Gollnick PD: Metabolism of substrates: Energy substrate metabolism during exercise and as modified by training. Fed Proc 44:353–357, 1985.
14. Sahlin K: Metabolic changes limiting muscle performance, in Saltin B (ed): Biochemistry of Exercise VI. Champaign, IL: Human Kinetics, 1986; pp 323–343.
15. Sahlin K, Katz A, Broberg S: Tricarboxylic acid cycle intermediates in human muscle during prolonged exercise. Am J Physiol 259:C834–C841, 1990.
16. Sahlin K, Jorfeldt L, Henriksson K-G, et al: Tricarboxylic acid cycle intermediates during incremental exercise: Attenuated increase in McArdle's disease. Clin Sci 88:687–693, 1995.
17. Gibala MJ, MacLean DA, Graham TE, Saltin B: Anaplerotic processes in human skeletal muscle during brief dynamic exercise. J Physiol 502:703–713, 1997.
18. van Loon LJ, Greenhaff PL, Constantin-Teodosiu D, et al: The effects of increasing exercise intensity on muscle fuel utilization in humans. J Physiol 536:295–304, 2001.
19. Haller RG, Vissing J: Spontaneous second wind and glucose-induced second, "second wind" in McArdle disease: Oxidative mechanisms. Arch Neurol 59:1395–1402, 2002.
20. Rennie MJ, Edwards RHT: Carbohydrate metabolism of skeletal muscle and its disorders, in Randle P (ed): Carbohydrate Metabolism and Its Disorders. New York: Academic Press, 1981; pp 1–118.
21. Saltin B: Capacity of blood flow delivery to exercising skeletal muscle in humans. Am J Cardiol 62:30E–35E, 1988.
22. Bergström J, Hultman E, Saltin B: Diet, muscle glycogen and physical performance. Acta Physiol Scand 71:170–176, 1967.
23. Haller RG, Vissing J: Circulatory regulation in muscle disease, in Saltin B, Boushel R, Secker N, Mitchell JH (eds): Exercise and Circulation in Health and Disease. Champaign, IL: Human Kinetics, 1999; pp 263–273.
24. Lowenstein JM: Ammonia production in muscle and other tissues: The purine nucleotide cycle. Physiol Rev 52:382–414, 1972.
25. Chasiotis D: The regulation of glycogen phosphorylase and glycogen breakdown in human skeletal muscle. Acta Physiol Scand (Suppl) 518:1–68, 1983.
26. Dudley GA, Terjung RL: Influence of acidosis on AMP deaminase activity in contracting fast-twitch muscle. Am J Physiol 248:C43–C50, 1985.
27. McArdle B: Myopathy due to a defect in muscle glycogen breakdown. Clin Sci 10:13–33, 1951.
28. Meinck H, Goebel H, Rumpf K, et al: The forearm ischaemic work test—Hazardous to McArdle patients? J Neurol 45:1144–1146, 1982.
29. Lindner N, Reichert M, Eichorn M, et al: Acute compartment syndrome after forearm ischemic work test in a patient with McArdle's disease. Neurology 56:1779–1780, 2001.
30. Hogrel JY, Laforet P, Yaou RB, et al: A non-ischemic forearm exercise test for the screening of patients with exercise intolerance. Neurology 56:1733–1738, 2001.
31. Kazemi-Esfarjani P, Skomorowska E, et al: A nonischemic forearm exercise test for McArdle disease. Ann Neurol 52:153–159, 2002.
32. Coleman RA, Stajich JM, Pact VW, et al: The ischemic exercise test in normal adults and in patients with weakness and cramps. Muscle Nerve 9:216–221, 1986.
33. Sinkeler SPT, Daanen HAM, Wevers RA, et al: The relation between blood lactate and ammonia in ischemic handgrip exercise. Muscle Nerve 8:523–527, 1985.
34. Arnold DL, Matthews PM, Radda GK: Metabolic recovery after exercise and the assessment of mitochondrial function in human skeletal muscle in vivo by means of 31P NMR. Magn Reson Med 1:307–315, 1984.
35. Edwards RHT, Wiles CM, Gohil D, et al: Energy metabolism in human myopathy, in Schotland DL (ed): Disorders of the Motor Unit. New York: Wiley, 1982; pp 715–735.
36. Radda GK, Bore PJ, Gadian DG, et al: 31P NMR examination of two patients with NADH-CoQ reductase deficiency. Nature 295:608–609, 1982.
37. Argov Z, Bank WJ: Phosphorus magnetic resonance spectroscopy in neuromuscular disorders. Ann Neurol 30:90–97, 1991.
38. Bertocci LA, Haller RG, Lewis SF, et al: Altered high energy phosphate metabolism during exercise in muscle phosphofructokinase deficiency. J Appl Physiol 70:1201–1207, 1991.
39. Taivassalo T, De Stefano N, Argov Z, et al: Effects of aerobic training in patients with mitochondrial myopathies. Neurology 50:1055–1060, 1988.
40. Lundberg P, Harmsen E, Ho C, Vogel HJ: Nuclear magnetic resonance studies of cellular metabolism. Anal Biochem 191:193–222, 1990.
41. Harris RC, Edwards RHT, Hultman E, et al: The time course of phosphorylcreatine resynthesis during recovery of the quadriceps muscle in man. Pflügers Arch 367:137–142, 1976.
42. Argov Z, De Stefano N, Arnold DL: ADP recovery after a brief ischemic exercise in normal and diseased human muscle—A 31 MRS study. NMR Biomed 9:165–172, 1996.
43. Chen JT, Argov Z, Kearney RE, Arnold DL: Fitting cytosolic ADP recovery after exercise with a step response function. Magn Reson Med 41:926–932, 1999.
44. Kemp GJ, Radda GK: Quantitative interpretation of bioenergetic data from 31P and 1H magnetic resonance spectroscopic studies of skeletal muscle on analytical review. Magn Reson Q 10:43–63, 1994.
45. Szczepaniak LS, Babcock EE, Schick F, et al: Measurement of intracellular triglyceride stores by 1H spectroscopy: Validation in vivo. Am J Physiol 276:E977–E989, 1999.
46. Shulman RG, Rothman DL: ^{13}C NMR in intermediary metabolism: Implications for systemic physiology. Annu Rev Physiol 63:15–48, 2001.
47. Sahlin K: NADH and NADPH in human skeletal muscle at rest and during ischaemia. Clin Physiol 3:477–485, 1983.
48. Duboc D, Renault G, Polianski J, et al: NADH measured by laser fluorimetry in McArdle's disease. N Engl J Med 316:1664–1665, 1987.
49. MacLean DA, Bangsbo J, Saltin B: Skeletal muscle interstitial glucose and lactate levels during dynamic exercise in humans determined by microdialysis. J Appl Physiol 87:1483–1490, 1999.
50. Vissing J, MacLean D, Vissing S, et al: The exercise metaboreflex is maintained in the absence of muscle acidosis: Insights from McArdle's disease. J Physiol 537:641–649, 2001.
51. Siciliano C, Rossi B, Manca L, et al: Residual muscle cytochrome c oxidase activity accounts for submaximal exercise lactate threshold in chronic progressive external ophthalmoplegia. Muscle Nerve 19:342–349, 1996.
52. Sato T, Hamaoka R, Higuchi H, et al: Validity of NIR spectroscopy for quantitatively measuring muscle oxidative metabolic rate in exercise. J Appl Physiol 90:338–344, 2001.
53. Bank W, Chance B: An oxidative defect in metabolic myopathies: Diagnosis by non-invasive tissue oximetry. Ann Neurol 36:830–837, 1994.
54. Wariar R, Gaffke JN, Haller RG, Bertocci LA: A modular system for clinical measurement of impaired skeletal muscle oxygenation. J Appl Physiol 88:315–325, 2000.
55. Ferrari M, Binzoni T, Quaresima V: Oxidative metabolism in muscle. Phil Trans R Soc Lond 352:677–683, 1997.
56. van Beekvelt MCP, van Engelen BGM, Wevers RA, Colier WNJM: Quantitative near-infrared spectroscopy discriminates mitochondrial myopathies and normal muscle. Ann Neurol 46:667–670, 1999.
57. van Beekvelt MCP, van Engelen BGM, Wevers RA, Colier WNJM: Near-infrared spectroscopy in chronic progressive external ophthalmoplegia: Adipose tissue thickness confounds decreased muscle oxygen consumption. Ann Neurol 51:272–273, 2002.
58. Taivassalo T, Abbott A, Wyrick P, Haller RG: Venous oxygen levels during aerobic forearm exercise: An index of impaired oxidative metabolism in mitochondrial myopathy. Ann Neurol 51:38–44, 2002.
59. Jensen TD, Kazemi-Esfarjani P, Skomorowska E, Vissing J: A forearm exercise screening test for mitochondrial myopathy. Neurology 58:1533–1538, 2002.
60. Luft R, Ikkos D, Palmieri G, et al: A case of severe hypermetabolism of nonthyroid origin with a defect in the maintenance of mitochondrial respiratory control: A correlated clinical, biochemical, and morphological study. J Clin Invest 41:1776–1801, 1962.
61. Roef MJ, Rejingoud DJ, Jeneson JA, et al: Resting oxygen consumption and in vivo ADP are increased in myopathy due to complex I deficiency. Neurology 58:1088–1093, 2002.

62. Taivassalo T, Jensen TD, Kennaway N, et al: The spectrum of exercise tolerance in mitochondrial myopathy—A study of 40 patients. *Brain* 126:413–423, 2003.
63. Triebwasser JH, Johnson RLJ, Burpo RP, et al: Non-invasive determination of cardiac output by a modified acetylene rebreathing procedure utilizing mass spectrometer. *Aviat Space Environ Med* 48:203–209, 1977.
64. Mitchell J, Blomqvist CG: Maximal oxygen uptake. *N Engl J Med* 284:1018–1022, 1971.
65. Haller RG, Henriksson KG, Jorfeldt L, et al: Deficiency of skeletal muscle succinate dehydrogenase and aconitase: Pathophysiology of exercise in a novel human muscle oxidative defect. *J Clin Invest* 88:1197–1206, 1991.
66. Rosell S, Saltin B: Energy need, delivery and utilization in muscular exercise, in Bourne GH (ed): *The Structure and Function of Muscle*. Vol 3. New York: Academic Press, 1973; pp 185–221.
67. Wasserman K, Whipp BJ: Exercise physiology in health and disease. *Am Rev Respir Dis* 112:219–249, 1975.
68. Flaherty KR, Wald J, Weisman IM, et al: Unexplained exertional limitation: Characterization of patients with a mitochondrial myopathy. *Am J Respir Crit Care Med* 164:425–432, 2001.
69. Vissing J, Lewis SF, Galbo H, Haller RG: Effect of deficient muscular glycogenolysis on extramuscular fuel production in exercise. *J Appl Physiol* 72:1773–1779, 1992.
70. Vissing J, Galbo H, Haller RG: Paradoxically enhanced glucose production during exercise in humans with blocked glycolysis due to muscle phosphofructokinase deficiency. *Neurology* 47:766–771, 1996.
71. Vissing J, Galbo H, Haller RG: Exercise fuel mobilization in mitochondrial myopathy: A metabolic dilemma. *Ann Neurol* 40:655–662, 1996.
72. Larsson L-E, Linderholm H, Muller R, et al: Hereditary metabolic myopathy with paroxysmal myoglobinuria due to abnormal glycolysis. *J Neurol Neurosurg Psychiatry* 27:361–380, 1964.
73. Linderholm H, Muller R, Ringqvist R, Sornas R: Hereditary abnormal muscle metabolism with hyperkinetic circulation during exercise. *Acta Med Scand* 185:153–166, 1969.
74. Linderholm H, Essén-Gustavsson B, Thornell L-E: Low succinate dehydrogenase (SDH) activity in a patient with a hereditary myopathy with paroxysmal myoglobinuria. *J Inter Med* 228:43–52, 1990.
75. Drugge U, Holmberg M, Holmgren G, et al: Hereditary myopathy with lactic acidosis, succinate dehydrogenase and aconitase deficiency in northern Sweden. *J Med Genet* 32:344–347, 1995.
76. Hall RE, Henriksson KG, Lewis SF, et al: Mitochondrial myopathy with succinate dehydrogenase and aconitase deficiency: Abnormalities of several iron-sulfur proteins. *J Clin Invest* 92:2660–2666, 1993.
77. Haller RG, Lewis SF, Estabrook RW, et al: Exercise intolerance, lactic acidosis, and abnormal cardiopulmonary regulation in exercise associated with adult skeletal muscle cytochrome c oxidase deficiency. *J Clin Invest* 84:155–161, 1989.
78. Abe K, Matsuo Y, Kadekawa J, et al: Measurement of tissue oxygen consumption in patients with mitochondrial myopathy by noninvasive tissue oximetry. *Neurology* 49:837–841, 1997.
79. Sobreira C, Hirano M, Shanske S, et al: Mitochondrial encephalomyopathy with coenzyme Q10 deficiency. *Neurology* 48:1238–1243, 1997.
80. Petty RKH, Harding AE, Morgan-Hughes JA: The clinical features of mitochondrial myopathy. *Brain* 109:915–938, 1986.
81. Jackson MJ, Schaefer JA, Johnson MA, et al: Presentation and clinical investigation of mitochondrial respiratory chain disease: A study of 51 patients. *Brain* 118:339–357, 1995.
82. Bogaasser M, Busch HFM, Scholte HR, et al: Exercise responses in patients with an enzyme deficiency in the mitochondrial respiratory chain. *Eur Respir J* 1:445–452, 1988.
83. Elliot DL, Buist NRM, Goldberg L, et al: Metabolic myopathies: Evaluation by graded exercise testing. *Medicine* 68:163–172, 1989.
84. Arnold DL, Taylor DJ, Radda GK: Investigation of human mitochondrial myopathies by phosphorus nuclear magnetic resonance spectroscopy. *Ann Neurol* 18:189–195, 1985.
85. Argov A, Bank WJ, Maris J, et al: Bioenergetic heterogeneity of human mitochondrial myopathies as demonstrated by in vivo phosphorus magnetic resonance spectroscopy (31P NMR). *Neurology* 37:257–262, 1987.
86. Matthews PM, Allaire C, Shoubridge EA, et al: In vivo muscle magnetic resonance spectroscopy in the clinical investigation of mitochondrial disease. *Neurology* 41:114–120, 1991.
87. Taylor DJ, Kemp GJ, Radda GK: Bioenergetics of skeletal muscle in mitochondrial myopathy. *J Neurol Sci* 127:198–206, 1994.
88. Barcroft H, Greenwood B, McArdle B, et al: The effect of exercise on forearm blood flow and on venous blood pH, P_{CO_2} and lactate in a subject with phosphorylase deficiency in skeletal muscle. *J Physiol* 189:44P–46P, 1966.
89. Benoit F, Watten R: Observations on venous pH alterations after ischemic exercise in myopathic disorders. *Am J Med Sci* 251:532–534, 1966.
90. Kanno T, Sudo K, Takeuchi I, et al: Hereditary deficiency of lactate dehydrogenase M-subunit. *Clin Chim Acta* 108:267–276, 1980.
91. Tsujino S, Shanske S, Carroll JE, et al: Double trouble: Combined myophosphorylase and AMP deaminase deficiency in a child homozygous for nonsense mutations at both loci. *Neuromuscul Disord* 5:263–266, 1995.
92. Ross BD, Radda GK, Gadian DG, et al: Examination of a case of suspected McArdle's syndrome by 31P nuclear magnetic resonance. *N Engl J Med* 304:1338–1342, 1981.
93. Duboc D, Jehenson P, Dinh S, et al: Phosphorus NMR spectroscopy study of muscular enzyme deficiencies involving glycogenolysis and glycolysis. *Neurology* 37:663–674, 1987.
94. Argov A, Bank WJ, Maris J, Leigh JSJ, Chance B: Muscle energy metabolism in human phosphofructokinase deficiency as recorded by 31P NMR. *Ann Neurol* 22:46–51, 1987.
95. Lewis SF, Haller RG: The pathophysiology of McArdle's disease: Clues to regulation in exercise and fatigue. *J Appl Physiol* 61:391–401, 1986.
96. Sahlin K, Areskog N-H, Haller RG, et al: Impaired oxidative metabolism increases adenine nucleotide breakdown in McArdle's disease. *J Appl Physiol* 69:1231–1235, 1990.
97. Haller RG, Lewis SF: Glucose-induced exertional fatigue in muscle phosphofructokinase deficiency. *N Engl J Med* 324:364–369, 1991.
98. Haller RG, Lewis SF, Cook JD, Blomqvist CG: Myophosphorylase deficiency impairs muscle oxidative metabolism. *Ann Neurol* 17:196–199, 1985.
99. De Stefano N, Argov Z, Matthews PM, et al: Impairment of muscle mitochondrial oxidative metabolism in McArdle's disease. *Muscle Nerve* 19:764–769, 1996.
100. Lewis SF, Haller RG, Cook JD, Nunnally RL: Muscle fatigue in McArdle's disease studied by 31P NMR: Effect of glucose infusion. *J Appl Physiol* 59:1991–1994.
101. Kissel JT, Beam W, Bresolin N, et al: Physiologic assessment of phosphoglycerate mutase deficiency. *Neurology* 35:828–833, 1985.
102. Lewis SF, Haller RG: Skeletal muscle disorders and associated factors that limit exercise performance. *Exerc Sport Sci Rev* 17:67–113, 1989.
103. Braakhekke JP, deBruin MI, Stegeman DF, et al: The second wind phenomenon in McArdle's disease. *Brain* 109:1087–1101, 1986.
104. Haller RG, Vissing J: Lack of a spontaneous second wind in muscle phosphofructokinase deficiency. *Neurology* 56:A231, 2001.
105. Carroll JE, Brooke MH, DeVivo DC, et al: Biochemical and physiologic consequences of carnitine palmitoyl transferase deficiency. *Muscle Nerve* 1:103–110, 1979.
106. Layzer RB, Havel RJ, McIlroy MB: Partial deficiency of carnitine palmityltransferase: Physiologic and biochemical consequences. *Neurology* 30:627–633, 1980.
107. Lewis SF, Vora S, Haller RG: Abnormal oxidative metabolism and O_2 transport in muscle phosphofructokinase deficiency. *J Appl Physiol* 70:391–398, 1991.

Chapter 29
The Muscle Biopsy

ANDREW G. ENGEL

Selection of an Appropriate Muscle
The Biopsy Procedure
Processing the Specimens
    PARAFFIN SECTIONS
    CRYOSTAT SECTIONS
    SEMITHIN RESIN SECTIONS
    ELECTRON MICROSCOPY
    BIOCHEMICAL STUDIES
    IMMUNOBLOT ANALYSIS
    MOLECULAR GENETIC STUDIES

The diagnosis of most neuromuscular diseases rests on careful clinical evaluation of the patient, electromyography, the muscle biopsy, and, in some instances, molecular genetic studies. The information ultimately derived from the biopsy depends on the choice of the muscle, the biopsy technique, and the subsequent studies performed on the biopsy specimens.

The muscle biopsy should be done only after the clinical evaluation, including detailed manual muscle testing, has been completed; after usual tests of blood and urine have been obtained; and after a preliminary diagnosis has been formulated. The risks associated with a muscle biopsy are usually minimal. However, the physician must explain to the patient the need for the muscle biopsy, the discomfort during the postoperative period, the possible complications of the surgical procedure, and what it is hoped will be learned from the biopsy. If the procedure is for research instead of diagnosis—as, for example, in a patient whose diagnosis has been established by a recent biopsy—the biopsy is done only with the patient's informed consent to participate in a research procedure.

Selection of an Appropriate Muscle

The muscle to be biopsied is selected on the basis of the following principles:

1. The muscle should show mild to moderate weakness upon manual muscle testing. This implies a rating of −1 to −2 on the Mayo Clinic examination scale (0 = normal; −4 = no visible contraction) or strength rated at 3 to 4 on the scale adopted by the British Medical Research Council (5 = normal; 0 = no visible contraction). Severely affected muscles are not biopsied because the contractile elements may be so extensively replaced by fibrous and/or fatty connective tissue that a meaningful diagnosis cannot be made. Clinically unaffected muscles are not biopsied, for these may show no pathologic change.

2. The muscle should be free from previous trauma that could confuse the histologic findings. For example, the muscle should not be one that had been previously biopsied, injected with medications, or recently (i.e., within 4 to 6 weeks of the biopsy) subjected to an electromyographic examination by needle electrodes.

3. The muscle should be free from an unrelated disease process. For example, a patient with a myopathy may also have a concurrent cervical lumbar radiculopathy or a compression or entrapment neuropathy. Clearly, a muscle that may be partially denervated or reinnervated because of an unrelated neurogenic disorder should not be biopsied.

4. Muscles subject to a heavy workload may show secondary myopathic changes in the course of denervation atrophy. For example, myopathic alterations are common in the partially denervated gastrocnemius muscle. Further, this muscle in older patients often shows evidence of a previous neurogenic process stemming from an ancient S1 radiculopathy. For this reason, the author prefers to avoid biopsy of this muscle except when a sural nerve biopsy is also done and the underlying gastrocnemius muscle can be readily sampled through the existing skin incision.

5. In some instances a muscle is selected because it is thought to be involved by a contiguous disease process. For example, in fasciitis with eosinophilia, a muscle underlying the indurated fascial zone is biopsied together with the overlying fascia and skin.

6. Facial, cervical, or intrinsic hand muscles are usually not biopsied because of their functional significance or for cosmetic reasons.

7. For a routine diagnostic study, the triceps or biceps muscle in the upper extremity or the vastus lateralis muscle in the lower extremity is often suitable for biopsy. When proximal muscles are severely affected or only distal muscles are involved, the extensor carpi radialis or anterior tibial muscles may prove to be useful for diagnostic studies. However, one must be aware of possible variations in the distribution of fiber types in different muscles.[1] For example, in the tibialis anterior, type 1 fibers are typically more abundant than type 2 fibers.[1]

8. When special diagnostic or research studies of the neuromuscular junction (NMJ*) are planned, the biopsy sample must include the muscle region containing the NMJs (the "motor point"). In biceps or deltoid muscles, this region is usually along the middle third of the muscle. For some in vitro electrophysiologic and immunocytochemical studies of the NMJ, the muscle fibers must be maintained under physiologic conditions in an oxygenated bath for many hours. For these studies, a short muscle or portion of a short muscle is removed from origin to insertion. The peroneus tertius muscle in the lower extremity, the anconeus muscle near the elbow, and the external intercostal muscle in the fifth or sixth intercostal space near the anterior axillary line have been used for this purpose.

*A list of abbreviations used in this chapter is given at the end of the chapter.

The Biopsy Procedure

In all patients over the age of 12, the routine muscle biopsy is done under local anesthesia. After it has been ascertained that the patient has not had an allergic reaction to the anesthetic, the skin and subcutaneous tissues are infiltrated with the anesthetic, such as 2% lidocaine, but the muscle itself is never injected. In children under the age of 12, surgical procedures under local anesthesia are often psychologically traumatizing even after heavy sedation. In these patients, the biopsy is done under light general anesthesia unless this is contraindicated by the patient's general medical condition. Major inhalation anesthetics or succinylcholine, which may precipitate a hyperthermic reaction in susceptible patients and may also cause adverse reactions in Duchenne dystrophy, are avoided in patients at risk.

General anesthesia is preferred for intercostal biopsies for two reasons: (1) Removal of a segment of the external intercostal muscle from origin to insertion requires stripping the periosteum from the adjacent ribs, and the pain associated with this is difficult to control with local anesthesia. (2) Endotracheal intubation is desired so that positive pressure ventilation can be instituted if the pleural cavity is inadvertently entered.

The biopsy should be done by a physician who understands the need for the careful and gentle handling of the tissue and is willing to take the required samples in a manner optimal for the subsequent handling of the specimens. The intercostal muscle biopsy should be done only by a surgeon experienced in thoracic surgery.

Either the technician, pathologist, or investigator who will subsequently work with the muscle specimens should be present in the operating room. This is important so that specimens for histochemical or biochemical studies can be promptly frozen, specimens for electron microscopy fixed without delay, and the surgeon informed of any special requirements regarding the specimens.

Meticulous hemostasis must be maintained during the entire surgical procedure. The fascia overlying muscle is incised in the direction of the underlying muscle fibers and gently retracted. After this, only sponges moistened with physiologic saline are used, and bleeding vessels are ligated rather than electrocoagulated to avoid cautery artifact to the nearby muscle fibers.

In routine biopsies, the muscle strips are removed with small sharp scissors, so that the long axis of the strips is parallel to the long axis of the muscle fibers. The size of these strips and the sequence in which they are excised may vary with the clinical diagnosis, the patient's age, the source of the muscle, and the studies that are planned. For example, the samples removed from an infant's muscle or from muscles that control delicate movements, such as extensor digitorum communis, should be as small as possible. Only a few milligrams of muscle are required for electron microscopy, but relatively large specimens may be needed for biochemical or in vitro physiologic studies.

In a routine biopsy of a relatively large muscle of an adult (e.g., biceps or triceps brachii or vastus lateralis), the following specimens are taken: (1) an optional 2- to 3-cm-long and approximately 0.5-cm-wide strip or cylinder of muscle

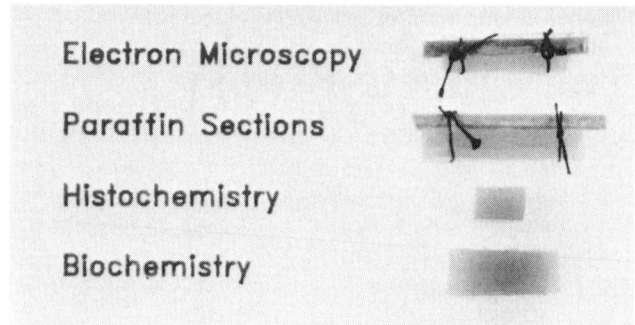

FIGURE 29-1. Wax models of muscle samples obtained in routine biopsy.

for paraffin sections; (2) a 1- to 2-cm-long and approximately 0.1- to 0.2-cm-wide strip or cylinder of muscle for electron microscopy; (3) a 0.6- by 0.6-cm specimen for light microscopic histochemistry; and (4) a specimen of suitable dimensions for biochemical, genetic, immunoblot, tissue culture, or further histologic studies (Fig. 29-1). Specimens 1 and 2 are tied to segments of an applicator stick or toothpick in situ with 3-0 silk ligatures before being excised to hold them at constant length during fixation (Figs. 29-1 and 29-2). This prevents objectionable contraction artifacts and facilitates subsequent orientation for longitudinal and transverse sectioning. Alternatively, specimens 1 and 2 are removed after they are

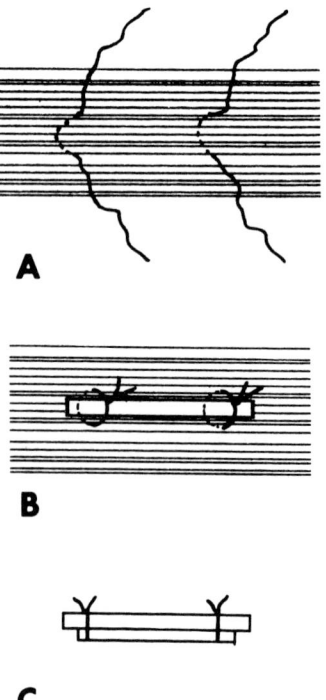

FIGURE 29-2. Schematic diagram of removal of muscle sample at rest length. *A.* Two 3-0 silk ligatures are placed under the strip of muscle to be excised. *B.* Segment of an applicator stick is positioned over the ligatures and is tied into place. Following this, one end of the stick is gently elevated and the strip of muscle held by the ligatures is carefully excised. *C.* Excised muscle strip tied to the stick. A specimen of this size is fixed for electron microscopy.

clamped in situ by a muscle biopsy clamp. However, the clamp is difficult to apply in small children or obese subjects, and the author finds its use more cumbersome than tying a strip of muscle to a stick in situ.

Percutaneous needle biopsy specimens of muscle also can be useful for selected diagnostic or research studies.[2] However, some muscles cannot be biopsied in this manner, the specimens cannot be held at rest length before removal, and the total amount of tissue that can be obtained may not be sufficiently large to detect focally distributed histologic changes or provide enough material for subsequent studies. For these reasons the author prefers the open biopsy in most instances.

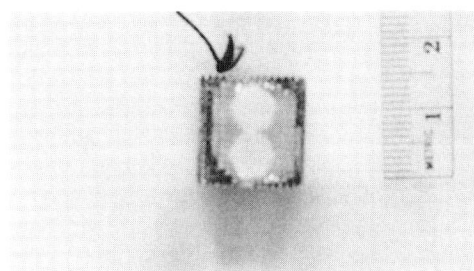

FIGURE 29-3. A wax model of a fresh muscle specimen mounted on a brass microtome chuck.

Processing the Specimens

PARAFFIN SECTIONS

The optional specimen taken for paraffin sections is fixed for 24 h in Bouin's fluid. This fixative is preferable to formalin because trichrome staining can be done without further mordanting. The fixed muscle is trimmed, and those parts not held at rest length or crushed by the ligature are discarded. The remainder is divided into a number of slabs for embedding in paraffin in transverse and longitudinal orientations. The paraffin sections are cut at 5 μm and are routinely stained with hematoxylin and eosin (H&E) and trichrome. The information yielded by these sections is limited by variable shrinkage of the muscle fibers, the appearance of slit-like spaces in the fibers, the loss or displacement of cytoplasmic constituents that are soluble in the dehydrating and clearing media, and the unsuitability for enzyme histochemical and most types of immunocytochemical studies. For these reasons even marked structural, histochemical, and immunocytochemical abnormalities go undetected in paraffin sections. On the other hand, a larger block of tissue can be sampled than in frozen sections; longitudinally oriented paraffin sections stained with H&E and viewed in polarized light or trichrome-stained paraffin sections viewed in bright field optics readily reveal loss of cross striations, whereas transversely oriented frozen sections do not; and inflammatory infiltrates and alterations in blood vessel walls can be seen in paraffin sections as well as in frozen sections. The formalin-fixed specimen can also serve as a backup for the frozen specimen if the latter is inadvertently disfigured by freezing artifact or becomes permeated by quenching fluid. Finally, paraffin blocks are easier and less expensive to store than frozen muscle specimens, which must be kept in a freezer at −70°C or in a liquid nitrogen refrigerator. The author presently obtains specimens for paraffin sections only in selected instances. Without paraffin sections, he relies on resin-embedded semithin sections for detecting loss of cross striations in the muscle fibers.

CRYOSTAT SECTIONS

The specimen collected for cryostat sections is subdivided with a razor blade into two slabs that are then mounted on a brass chuck in transverse orientation (Fig. 29-3). The mounting medium is a paste made up of 1.5 g gum tragacanth, 0.6 mL glycerol, and 15 mL distilled water and contains a crystal of thymol preservative. Other cryostat mounting media are commercially available. Infiltration of the upper surface of the specimen with the mounting medium is avoided because this can cause undesired artifacts in the trichrome stain. The chuck with the tissue facing up is held by a forceps and plunged into a beaker containing isopentane chilled to about −150°C by liquid nitrogen. (Direct immersion into liquid nitrogen is avoided because this causes nitrogen to boil and the gas bubbles insulate the specimen and slow its quenching.) Near −150°C isopentane is a highly viscous transparent fluid just beginning to freeze. At a slightly lower temperature, it freezes solidly but melts readily on contact with the specimen to be frozen. During quenching, the specimen turns milky white. The chuck is kept under isopentane for a further 10 to 20 s while the beaker is vigorously swirled to equalize the temperature of isopentane in the beaker. The frozen specimen is then stored under liquid nitrogen except when it is transferred to the cryostat for the preparation of frozen sections.

If isopentane and liquid nitrogen are unavailable, the specimen can be frozen in a thick slurry of dry ice and acetone at −70°C and then stored under dry ice or in a freezer at −70°C until it is sectioned. However, the quenching is slower and the chances of ice crystal growth are greater at −70°C than at −150°C.

The most important artifact that degrades the quality of the frozen section is ice crystal growth in the tissue. This varies with the speed of freezing and the temperature at which the tissue is stored. Slow freezing over minutes or hours at relatively high temperatures, overnight storage in the cryostat at −15°C to −20°C, or repeated freezing and thawing produce marked ice crystal artifact. Ice crystal growth occurs relatively slowly below −40°C, is very slow at −70°C, and does not occur at liquid nitrogen temperatures.

If an adequately frozen specimen is allowed to thaw completely, the muscle fibers become rounded and swollen and lose their close apposition to each other within the fascicles. This phenomenon occurs during the last moments of thawing and can be readily observed under the dissecting microscope. Therefore, if a frozen specimen must be divided or remounted, this should be done without allowing the specimen to thaw by cutting it in the cryostat or on a block of dry ice, at a temperature at which frozen muscle is no longer too brittle to be cut with a razor blade.

Most specimens can be sectioned at a cryostat temperature of –20°C, but those with abundant fatty or fibrous connective tissue are easier to section at –22°C. For routine studies, 10-μm sections are used because they are easier to cut than thinner ones and because small ice crystal artifacts remain hidden in the depth of the section. Thinner sections reveal even very small vacuoles produced by ice crystal growth but provide better resolution of structures smaller than 10 μm. For cytochemical studies of small structures in serial sections (e.g., inflammatory cells or NMJs), 2-μm sections are preferable.

The cryostat section is obtained by a smooth and even knife stroke and is allowed to slip between the knife and a well-fitting antiroll plate positioned above the knife. The antiroll plate is then lifted and a glass coverslip placed on the section. Next, the coverslip is lifted, the section is rapidly thawed by touching the opposite coverslip surface, and the section is then allowed to dry at room temperature for 20 to 30 min. The quality of the section can be degraded by sectioning artifacts and by failure of the section to adhere to the glass coverslip. A dull microtome knife produces knife marks of varying width and depth and torn or scraped sections. To avoid these, the first complete section obtained from the block is inspected for knife marks in the microscope with a low-power (× 6) objective and with the condenser lowered. If knife marks are noted, an adjacent section of the knife is tested or a new knife is tried.

Failure of the section to adhere to the coverslip may cause loss of part of the section during staining, elevation of the rims of muscle fibers from the coverslip, and uneven staining. Adhesion of the section to the coverslip is improved by the use of meticulously clean coverslips, picking up wrinkle-free sections, and allowing adequate time for the section to dry on the coverslip. Despite these precautions, relatively thin (e.g., 2 μm) sections or cryostat sections of prefixed muscle often fail to adhere to glass coverslips. However, even these sections will adhere to coverslips lightly coated with a solution of 1% gelatin and 0.1% chromium potassium sulfate dodecahydrate (chrome alum) or with L-polylysine.

For routine studies in the author's laboratory, 28 successive cryostat sections are picked up on 28 coverslips. To assure identical orientation of the sections on the coverslips, care is taken that the upper border of each section faces the upper edge of each coverslip. After the appropriate stains or reactions are performed, the 28 coverslips are mounted on 14 glass slides, with 2 coverslips per slide. Table 29-1 shows the routine stains and reactions and the sequence in which the coverslips are mounted on the slides. Tables 29-2 and 29-3 list some of the additional stains or localizations that can be useful in the study of cryostat sections. Selected references for the stains and localizations are indicated in the tables. For the theory and practice of histochemical and cytochemical techniques, the reader is referred to standard texts (see Refs. 3, 13, 14, and 69).

Because the interpretation of frozen sections is considered in Chap. 30, only the following need be mentioned here. In high-quality frozen sections, the dimensions of the muscle fibers are close to those in the native state. The trichrome-

Table 29-1. ROUTINE PROCESSING OF CRYOSTAT SECTIONS

Slide Number	Section Number	Stain or Reaction	Reference
1	1, 14	Hematoxylin and eosin (H&E)[a]	
2	2, 15	Modified Gomori trichrome	3
3	3, 16	NADH dehydrogenase (NADHD)	4
4	4, 17	Succinate dehydrogenase (SDH)	5
5	5, 18	Cytochrome-c oxidase (CCO)	6
6	6	ATPase after preincubation at pH 4.3[b]	7
6	7	ATPase after preincubation at pH 4.5[c]	7
7	9, 20	ATPase after preincubation at pH 9.4 [d]	7
8	8, 21	Toluidine blue–ATPase after preincubation at pH 4.5[c,e]	8
9	9, 22	Acid phosphatase[f]	9, 10
10	10, 23	Phosphorylase	11
11	11, 24	Periodic acid-Schiff (PAS)[g]	12
12	12, 25	Oil red O[a]	13
13	13	Cholinesterase[h]	13
13	27	Nonspecific esterase[i]	13
14	14, 28	Congo red	13a

[a]Fixed with 10% formalin before staining.
[b] Types 1 and 2C fibers react; section is lightly counterstained with eosin.
[c]Types 1, 2B, and 2C fibers react.
[d]Type 2 fibers react; section no. 19 is lightly counterstained with eosin.
[e]Types 1, 2A, and 2B fibers appear dark blue, intermediate blue, and light blue, respectively.
[f]Naphthol AS-BI phosphate substrate.
[g]Fixed with 10% formalin or Newcomer's fluid before staining.
[h]α-Naphthyl phosphate substrate; 0.01 mM iso-OMPA added to inhibit nonspecific cholinesterase; 5 to 10 min incubation at 23°C; light hematoxylin counterstain.
[i]α-Naphthyl phosphate substrate; 1 h incubation at 37°C.

Table 29-2. SELECTED STAINS FOR ADDITIONAL STUDIES OF CRYOSTAT SECTIONS

Substance or Structure Visualized	Stain or Reaction	Reference
Glycolipids, mucins, amylopectins	PAS after diastase digestion	12, 14
Acid mucins	Alcian blue at pH 2.6	14
	Basic fuchsin at pH 1.7	15
	Alcian blue (pH 0.5) plus Alcian yellow (pH 2.5)	16
	Cresyl violet (pH 2.9)	17
Amyloid	Crystal violet, toluidine blue	13
	Congo red, sirius red	13, 13a, 13b
	Thioflavin T (pH 1.4)	13
Lipid material:		
Neutral fats and phospholipids	Sudan black B	13
Phospholipids, neutral fats, cholesterol	OTAN[a]	18
Acidic lipids	Nile blue sulfate	13
Plasmalogen phospholipids	Plasmal reaction	13
Phospholipids containing choline	Acid hematin	13
Cholesterol esters	Perchloric acid–naphthoquinone	13
Free cholesterol	Digitonin method	13
Calcium:		
Calcific minerals	von Kossa stain	14, 19
	Alizarin red	14, 19
Ionized calcium	Glyoxal-bis-(2-hydroxyanil)	19, 20

[a]Osmium tetroxide-α-naphthylamine reaction: phospholipids, orange red; neutral fats and cholesterol, black.

stained sections reveal an intermyofibrillar membranous network composed of mitochondria and sarcoplasmic reticulum. The lipid and glycogen content of the fibers can be estimated by Oil-red-O and PAS stains. The distribution of mitochondria in the individual fibers can be inferred from the oxidative enzyme reactions. Increased lysosomal enzyme activity is detected by the acid phosphatase reaction. Myofibrillar integrity can be evaluated from the ATPase-reacted sections. The presence or absence of selected enzymes (e.g., phosphorylase, phosphofructokinase, cytochrome oxidase, lactate dehydrogenase, AMP deaminase) can be demonstrated enzyme-cytochemically. Each muscle fiber has a distinct histochemical profile determined by its innervation. This allows fiber typing, detection of pathologic changes that selectively affect a given fiber type, and observation of signs of denervation and reinnervation. A number of disease-related muscle fiber or interstitial components (e.g., dystrophin, α-, β-, δ-, and γ-sarcoglycans, β-dystroglycan, dysferlin, caveolin-3, emerin, α2-chain of laminin-2 (merosin), β1-chain of different laminins, collagen VI, LAMP-2, desmin, plectin, αB-crystallin, NCAM, CDC2-kinase, prion protein, and 80 kDa common subunit of μ-calpain) can be shown by appropriate immunostains. Immunolocalization of selected end plate–associated proteins, T- and B-cell and macrophage markers, and different components of the complement cascade are useful in special studies (Table 29-3).

SEMITHIN RESIN SECTIONS

The specimen taken for electron microscopy is also used for the preparation of 0.5- to 1.5-μm-thick resin sections. These sections can be studied under phase optics without further staining or in bright-field optics after staining with toluidine blue, azure B-methylene blue, or other dyes.[50,51] Semithin resin sections provide better resolution and tissue preservation than paraffin sections but are unsuitable for histochemical studies except for localizing PAS-reactive material. In this respect, however, they are superior to fresh-frozen sections. If immunolocalization studies are done with a peroxidase-labeled reagent before embedding, reactive regions large enough to be resolved by the light microscope can be detected in semithin resin sections. In general, the main use of semithin resin sections is selection of areas for further study by electron microscopy. When an area of interest is localized in a semithin section, the corresponding block is trimmed around this area and thin-sectioned for electron microscopy.

ELECTRON MICROSCOPY

The specimen taken for electron microscopy studies is fixed in glutaraldehyde buffered with 0.1 M cacodylate or phosphate buffer (pH 7.3). The concentration of glutaraldehyde, the type of buffer, and the duration and temperature of fixation that provide optimal preservation of muscle fine structure have never been rigorously established. However, the following generalizations can be made: (1) The higher the concentration of glutaraldehyde, the more rapidly it penetrates the specimen; 5% glutaraldehyde penetrates at the rate of about 1 mm/h. (2) Concentrations above 5% glutaraldehyde may cause undue osmotic shrinkage of organelles. (3) Glutaraldehyde concentrations below 0.1% may not preserve muscle fine structure adequately. (4) Fixation at 4°C is

Table 29-3. SELECTED LOCALIZATIONS FOR ADDITIONAL STUDIES OF CRYOSTAT SECTIONS

Procedure	Reference
Enzyme cytochemical localization	
α-Glycerophosphate dehydrogenase	21
Lactate dehydrogenase	13
Catalase	22
Phosphofructokinase	23
AMP deaminase	24
Alkaline phosphatase	13
Carbonic anhydrase	25
Acetylcholinesterase	26,[a] 27[b]
Immunolocalization	
IgG	28, 29
Complement component 3 (C3)	28, 29
Complement component 9 (C9)	29, 30
Complement membrane attack complex (MAC)	29, 31, 32
Mononuclear cell surface antigens	33–36
Class I MHC antigens	37
Class II MHC antigens	38
Heat shock protein 65	39
Cathepsins B, D, and L	40–42
Ubiquitin	42, 43
β-Amyloid precursor protein	42, 44
β-Amyloid	42, 45
Myosin isoforms	46, 47
β-Actin	48
α-Actinin	49
Vinculin	49
Filamin	49
Desmin	50–53
Vimentin	50–53
Myotilin	53a
Plectin	49a
αB-Crystallin	49b
CDC-2 kinase	49c
Prion protein	49d
μ-Calpain	49e
β-Spectrin, muscle-specific isoform	54, 55
Dystrophin[c]	56, 57
Utrophin	58, 59
α-Sarcoglycan	14
β-Sarcoglycan	14
δ-Sarcoglycan	14
γ-Sarcoglycan	14
α-Dystroglycan	60a
β-Dystroglycan	14
Dysferlin	60a
Caveolin-3	14
Emerin	14
α2-Chain of laminin-2 (merosin)	14
β1-Chain of different laminins	14, 62
Collagen VI	61, 62
LAMP-2	63
Neural cell adhesion molecule (NCAM)	64, 65
Acetylcholine receptor	66, 67
Acetylcholinesterase	68

[a]Acetylcholine iodide substrate in the presence of 0.01 mM iso-OMPA.
[b]Dithio-bis-acetic acid substrate in the presence of 0.01 mM iso-OMPA.
[c]Antibodies recognizing the N-terminal, rodlike central, and C-terminal domains of dystrophin.

preferable to fixation at room temperature because the lower temperature retards autolytic and anoxic changes that may occur before fixation in deeper portions of the specimen. (5) Sodium phosphate buffer has a strong buffering capacity around pH 7.3 and enhances subsequent electron staining of glycogen particles by lead salts. However, uranyl phosphate and lead phosphate are highly insoluble; therefore, the use of a phosphate buffer precludes the subsequent use of a lead cytochemical procedure, and en bloc staining with uranyl acetate must be avoided unless the specimen is thoroughly rinsed with another buffer before exposure to the uranyl salt. For these reasons, the author uses ice-cold 5% glutaraldehyde buffered with 0.1 M cacodylate buffer. After fixation for 2 h, the specimen surrounded by the fixative is examined in the dissecting microscope. Muscle strands not held at rest length or compressed by the ligature are trimmed away. The rest is subdivided into numerous smaller blocks that are fixed for an additional 30 min. Alternatively, the specimen held at rest length is immediately injected with a small volume of the ice-cold fixative through a 30-gauge needle. This assures prompt and nearly simultaneous fixation of the entire specimen and uniform and excellent preservation of fine structure. The injected tissue is fixed for an additional hour on ice in the same fixative and is then trimmed and subdivided under the dissecting microscope as described above. The author avoids prolonged (i.e., overnight) fixation with glutaraldehyde, as he finds that this results in less than optimal preservation of membranous organelles.

After an overnight rinse with buffer, the specimens are refixed with 2% ice-cold osmium tetroxide buffered with 0.1 M cacodylate for 3 h, dehydrated with graded alcohols, and embedded in Epon or Spurr's resin. At least 20 blocks are embedded for longitudinal and 10 for transverse sectioning. The remaining blocks are flat-embedded in a small aluminum weighing dish and serve as a reservoir of material that can be reembedded for thick and thin sectioning (Fig. 29-4). For details of dehydration, embedding, thick and thin sectioning, and staining, the reader is referred to standard texts on basic electron microscopic techniques (see Refs. 70 to 73).

Electron microscopy is time-consuming and not required for routine clinical diagnosis. However, it clearly demonstrates pathologic reactions of muscle fiber organelles, the boundaries and contents of vacuoles, and different types of abnormal inclusions (such as fingerprint bodies, nemaline rods, concentric laminar bodies, and so forth). Pathologic alterations in the surface membrane of the muscle fiber, the NMJ, intramuscular nerves, or small blood vessels and events occurring during cell-mediated muscle fiber injury are best detected by electron microscopy. Immunoelectron microscopic and electron-cytochemical studies have applications in the investigation of autoimmune myasthenia gravis, congenital myasthenic syndromes, myofibrillar myopathies, and inflammatory myopathies. The recognition and characterization of a number of neuromuscular disorders have become possible with the added use of the electron microscope in the study of the muscle biopsy.

A description of the numerous preparatory techniques and special methods that have been used in investigating ultrastructural aspects of different neuromuscular disorders is beyond the scope of this chapter; however, approaches to

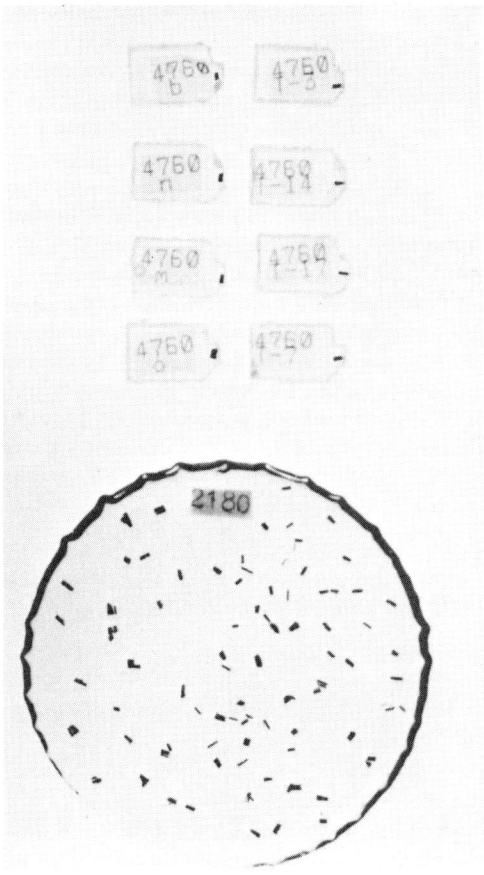

FIGURE 29-4. Specimens for electron microscopy embedded for longitudinal (left upper column) and transverse (right upper column) sectioning and flat-embedded (lower panel) for possible reembedding. At least 20 blocks are embedded for longitudinal and 10 for transverse sectioning. Specimen orientation is again adjusted during trimming and when the specimens are aligned for sectioning in the microtome.

two particularly challenging and interesting problems are considered here.

Localization of the NMJ in the Electron Microscope

For many years, thorough ultrastructural studies of the NMJ have been hindered by the fact that the NMJ, which occupies but a small segment of the muscle fiber, is seldom observed in thin sections of biopsy specimens. To locate the NMJ in the electron microscope, the specimen must include the motor point and those blocks embedded for electron microscopy must be enriched in NMJs. Inclusion of the NMJs in the biopsy was discussed above. To enrich the embedded blocks in NMJs, the following procedure is useful.[66] A thin strip of aldehyde-fixed muscle is put on a glass slide, covered with buffer, and observed in the dissecting microscope. The author uses a Bausch & Lomb stereozoom microscope with a × 0.7 to 3 power pod mounted on a transilluminating base and equipped with an adjustable substage mirror and diffusing reflector. The semitransparent specimen is back-lighted by a horizontally positioned external illuminator directed against the diffusing reflector, which is set at a 45-degree angle in the light path. The intramuscular nerve and its preterminal branches now appear as opaque strands that traverse the specimen more or less perpendicularly to the long axis of the muscle fibers. Next, small blocks of muscle (about 0.3 to 0.5 mm in length and width) are excised from the muscle strip so that a nerve branch traverses the center of each excised block. The NMJs are invariably adjacent to the nerve branches in these blocks. The dissection is done with two 27-gauge needles mounted on tuberculin syringes, the bevels of the needles providing the cutting edge. A small piece of muscle (about 2 cm long and 0.2 cm in diameter) yields 30 to 40 blocks enriched in NMJs. After further cytochemical or immunocytochemical procedures, the blocks are osmicated, dehydrated, infiltrated with resin, and embedded in suitable embedding molds. Semithin (1 to 1.5 μm) sections are cut from the blocks and inspected for the presence of NMJs in the phase microscope. Blocks that yield no NMJs after the first sectioning are resectioned 10 μm below the level of the initial section. About one-half of the initial semithin sections contain one or more NMJ(s), and about one-half of those blocks that show no NMJs after the first sectioning yield NMJs after the second or third sectioning. When a NMJ is encountered in a semithin section, the corresponding block is further trimmed and thin-sectioned for electron microscopy.

Electron Cytochemical and Immunoelectron Microscopic Studies

Electron cytochemical and immunoelectron microscopic studies require adequate preservation of fine structure and reactivity of the substance of interest (e.g., enzyme, antigen, receptor) in the reaction system designed to localize it. Fixation with glutaraldehyde preserves fine structure optimally. However, this cross-links free amino groups, which often inhibits enzyme activity, eliminates affinity for specific ligands, or may so alter epitopes that they lose their immunoreactivity. Paraformaldehyde, which has a low cross-linking potential, and hydroxyadipaldehyde or glyoxal, dialdehyde fixatives that cross-link free amino groups less than glutaraldehyde, provide greater reactivity in cytochemical[71,74] and immunocytochemical[73] studies than glutaraldehyde, but the preservation of fine structure is suboptimal. A fixative consisting of 1 to 2% paraformaldehyde, 10 mM sodium periodate, and 75 mM lysine in 37 mM phosphate buffer (pH adjusted to 7.3) introduced by McLean and Nakane[76] improves preservation of fine structure and reduces loss of immunoreactivity but still does not preserve skeletal muscle fine structure optimally.

Extracellular localizations. If an antigen or a receptor to be localized is on the extracellular surface of the muscle fiber, localization in the unfixed specimen followed by glutaraldehyde fixation provides both optimal sensitivity and preservation of fine structure.[28, 66] A fresh biopsy specimen consisting of a thin strip of muscle intact from origin to insertion is pinned out on a perforated wax plate and maintained in a bath of mammalian Ringer's solution equilibrated with 95% O_2 and 5% CO_2. The reagents are added to the bath in the required concentrations, the reaction is allowed to proceed at room temperature for the required length of time, and the muscle strips are then rinsed with ice-cold oxygenated mammalian Ringer's solution; the procedure is next repeated with a second reagent if a second reagent is required for the localization. The incubations are done at room temperature to prevent patching, capping, and internalization of surface determinants cross-linked by antibody or other ligands and are rinsed on ice to reduce the dissociation of the antigen-antibody or receptor-ligand complex. Pilot studies are required to establish optimal reagent concentrations and incubation and rinsing times. After the last rinse, the specimen is fixed in 2 to 5% glutaraldehyde. If the localization involves the use of a peroxidase-labeled reagent, the specimen is next incubated in Karnovsky's medium containing 0.05% 3,3′-diaminobenzidine, 0.01% H_2O_2, and 50 mM Tris buffer, pH 7.4,[77] again rinsed, osmicated, and then further processed for electron microscopy. This approach has provided optimal sensitivity and preservation of fine structure in the localization at the normal and abnormal NMJ of the acetylcholine receptor with α-bungarotoxin,[66] and of IgG, C3,[28] and C9[30] with peroxidase-labeled reagents.

Restoration of immunoreactivity after glutaraldehyde fixation. The approach described in the preceding section cannot be applied if muscle strips intact from origin to insertion are not available or if an intracellular substance needs to be localized. To obtain maximal sensitivity plus optimal fixation in immunolocalization studies, these specimens are fixed in glutaraldehyde, but the loss of immunoreactivity caused by the fixative is reversed with sodium borohydride before the immunoreagents are applied.[78,79] Sodium borohydride reduces the carbon-nitrogen double bonds in Schiff bases formed between the aldehyde functional groups of glutaraldehyde and the free amino groups of tissue antigens. This decreases the conformational change imposed on the antigen's tertiary structure by the fixative and probably accounts for the restoration of immunoreactivity.[78]

To localize intracellular antigens, the appropriate immunoreagents are applied to glutaraldehyde-fixed, borohydride-treated cryostat sections. This procedure has yielded excellent results in the immunoelectron microscopic localization of surface antigens on lymphoid cells infiltrating muscle with the appropriate monoclonal antibody, a biotinylated second antibody, and the ABC (avidin-biotin-peroxidase complex) reagent.[80,81]

It is very likely that borohydride treatment can restore immunoreactivity of many antigens whose epitopes are altered by glutaraldehyde fixation, but this will have to be evaluated for each individual antigen. It is also possible that borohydride can reactivate enzymes or receptors inactivated by glutaraldehyde and may thus facilitate the electron cytochemical localization of enzymes and receptors in well-fixed tissues.

For additional reading and a survey of well-defined immunolocalization procedures, the reader is referred to Refs. 82 and 83.

Immunogold localizations. These are feasible with the use of appropriate second or third immunoreagents labeled with colloidal gold particles of known size. The immunoreagents are applied either before or after embedding. The preembedding immunogold technique can localize surface-associated antigens on teased muscle fibers, suspended cells, or tissue sections. Its use is limited by the penetration of the gold particles into the tissue, but the method has been successful in localizing β-amyloid protein in muscle.[45] The problem of tissue penetration is avoided with the use of prefixed ultrathin cryosections thawed before labeling, but the efficiency of the labeling is reduced and the preparations lack contrast. The postembedding immunogold technique is applied to ultrathin resin sections. It is also less efficient than the preembedding technique but is well suited for detecting intracellular antigens. For detailed protocols, the reader is referred to relevant reviews.[84,84a,84b]

BIOCHEMICAL STUDIES

Because the biochemical basis of most neuromuscular diseases is still unknown, biochemical studies are applicable only in selected instances. Direct measurement of muscle lipid or glycogen content, structural analysis of glycogen, assay of glycolytic enzymes or substrates, determination of rates and other parameters of mitochondrial respiration, assays of respiratory chain complexes, determination of coenzyme Q levels and cytochrome spectra, assays of carnitine, acylcarnitines, carnitine palmitoyltransferase, and β-oxidation enzymes are examples of biochemical procedures used in the diagnosis of metabolic myopathies.

IMMUNOBLOT ANALYSIS

Extracts of small amounts of tissue (20 to 30 mg) prepared under denaturing conditions in the presence of protease inhibitors can be electrophoresed on minigels, transferred to nitrocellulose membranes, and then immunostained with appropriate antibodies. This approach has been particularly useful in detecting altered amounts or molecular weights of dystrophin and decreased expression of dysferlin, calpain-3, telethonin, and LAMP-2.[84c]

MOLECULAR GENETIC STUDIES

Cryopreserved fresh muscle is a perpetual resource for molecular genetic studies. A small amount of muscle (25 mg) is an excellent source of nuclear DNA, a very rich source of mitochondrial DNA, and an essential source of mRNA for those gene products expressed only in muscle. Deparaffinized paraffin sections of formalin-fixed muscle or cryosections of fresh muscle postfixed with formalin can be used for in situ hybridization studies (for example, see Refs. 85, 86, and 86a). Recent studies have explored the feasibility of combining the extreme sensitivity of the polymerase chain reaction with the cell localizing ability of in situ hybridization.[87] Although a number of protocols and applications have been published,[87] none has been used in studies of muscle specimens to date.

List of Abbreviations

AMP	adenosine monophosphate		NMJ	neuromuscular junction
ATPase	adenosine triphosphatase		OMPA	octamethyl pyrophosphoramide
DMSO	dimethyl sulfoxide		PAS	periodic acid-Schiff
H&E	hematoxylin and eosin			

References

1. Johnson MA, Polgar J, Weightman D, Appleton D: Data on the distribution of fibre types in thirty-six human muscles: An autopsy study. *J Neurol Sci* 18:111, 1973.
2. Edwards RHT, Young A, Wiles CM: Needle biopsy of skeletal muscle in the diagnosis of myopathy and the clinical study of muscle function and repair. *N Engl J Med* 302:261, 1980.
3. Engel WK, Cunningham GC: Rapid examination of muscle tissue: An improved trichrome method for fresh-frozen biopsy sections. *Neurology* 13:919, 1963.
3a. Sewry CA, Lu Q: Immunological reagents and amplification systems, in Bushby KMD, Anderson LVB (eds): *Muscular Dystrophy: Methods and Protocols.* Totowa, NJ: Humana Press, 2001; pp 325–338.
4. Nachlas MM, Walker DG, Seligman AM: A histochemical method for the demonstration of diphosphopyridine nucleotide diaphorase. *J Biophys Biochem Cytol* 4:29, 1958.
5. Nachlas MM, Tsou K-C, de Souza E, et al: Cytochemical demonstration of succinic dehydrogenase by the use of a new p-nitrophenyl substituted ditetrazole. *J Histochem Cytochem* 5:420, 1957.
6. Seligman AM, Karnovsky MJ, Wasserkrug HL, Hanker JS: Non-droplet ultrastructural demonstration of cytochrome oxidase activity with a polymerising osmiophilic reagent, diaminobenzidine (DAB). *J Cell Biol* 38:1, 1968.
7. Round JM, Matthews Y, Jones DA: A quick, simple and reliable histochemical method for ATPase in human muscle preparations. *Histochem J* 12:707, 1980.
8. Ogilvie RW, Feeback DL: A metachromatic dye ATPase method for the simultaneous identification of skeletal muscle fiber types I, IIA, IIB and IIC. *Stain Technol* 65:231, 1990.
9. Barka T: A simple azo dye method for histochemical demonstration of acid phosphatase. *Nature* 187:248, 1960.
10. Barka T, Anderson PJ: Histochemical methods for acid phosphatase using hexazonium pararosanilin as coupler. *J Histochem Cytochem* 10:741, 1962.
11. Takeuchi T: Histochemical demonstration of branching enzyme (amylo-1,4-1,6-transglucosidase) in animal tissues. *J Histochem Cytochem* 6:208, 1958.
12. Lillie RD: *Histopathologic Technique and Practical Histochemistry,* 3d ed. New York: McGraw-Hill, 1965, pp 198, 496.
13. Bancroft JD, Gamble N: *Theory and Practice of Histologic Techniques,* 5th ed. Edinburgh; Churchill Livingstone, 2002.
13a. Mendell JR, Sahenk Z, Gales T, et al: Amyloid filaments in inclusion body myositis. *Arch Neurol* 48:1229, 1991.
13b. Askanas V, Engel WK, Alvarez RB: Enhanced detection of Congo-red-positive amyloid deposits in muscle fibers of inclusion body myositis and brain of Alzheimer's disease using fluorescence techniques. *Neurology* 43:1265, 1993.
14. Johnson MA: Immunocytochemical analysis, in Bushby KMD, Anderson LVB (eds): *Muscular Dystrophy: Methods and Protocols.* Totowa, NJ: Humana Press, 2001; pp 339–368.
15. Stempien MF Jr: Localization of acid mucopolysaccharides with basic fuchsin. *J Histochem Cytochem* 10:766, 1962.
16. Carlo B: Alcian blue-alcian yellow: A new method for the identification of different acidic groups. *J Histochem Cytochem* 12:44, 1964.
17. Hirsch TV, Peiffer J: A histochemical study of pre-lipid and metachromatic degenerative products in leucodystrophy, in Cumings JN (ed): *Cerebral Lipidoses: A Symposium.* Springfield, IL: Charles C Thomas, 1957; pp 68–73.
18. Adams CWM: A histochemical method for the simultaneous demonstration of normal and degenerating myelin. *J Pathol Bact* 77:648, 1959.
19. Bodensteiner J, Engel A: Intracellular calcium accumulation in Duchenne dystrophy and other myopathies: A study of 567,000 muscle fibers in 114 biopsies. *Neurology* 28:439, 1978.
20. Kashiwa HK, Atkinson WB: The applicability of a new Schiff base, glyoxalbis-(2-hydroxyanil), for the cytochemical localization of ionic calcium. *J Histochem Cytochem* 11:248, 1963.
21. Wattenberg LW, Leong LJ: Effects of coenzyme Q_{10} and menadione on succinic dehydrogenase activity as measured by tetrazolium salt reduction. *J Histochem Cytochem* 8:296, 1960.
22. LeHir M, Herzog V, Fahimi HD: Cytochemical detection of catalase with 3,3'-diaminobenzidine. *Histochemistry* 64:51, 1979.
23. Bonilla E, Schotland DL: Histochemical diagnosis of muscle phosphofructokinase deficiency. *Arch Neurol* 22:8, 1970.
24. Fishbein WN, Griffin JL, Armbrustmacher VW: Stain for skeletal muscle adenylate deaminase: An effective tetrazolium stain for frozen biopsy specimens. *Arch Pathol Lab Med* 104:462, 1980.
25. Riley DA, Ellis S, Bain J: Carbonic anhydrase activity in skeletal muscle fiber types, axons, spindles, and capillaries of rat soleus and extensor digitorum longus muscles. *J Histochem Cytochem* 30:1275, 1982.
26. Gomori G: *Microscopic Histochemistry: Principles and Practice.* Chicago: University of Chicago Press, 1952.
27. Gautron J: Cytochimie ultrastructurale des acétylcholinestérases. *Microscopie* 21:259, 1974.
28. Engel AG, Lambert EH, Howard FM: Immune complexes (IgG and C3) at the motor end-plate in myasthenia gravis. Ultrastructural and light microscopic localization and electrophysiologic correlations. *Mayo Clinic Proc* 52:267, 1977.
29. Engel AG, Biesecker G: Complement activation in muscle fiber necrosis: Demonstration of the membrane attack complex of complement in necrotic fibers. *Ann Neurol* 12:289, 1982.
30. Sahashi K, Engel AG, Lambert EH, Howard FM: Ultrastructural localization of the terminal and lytic ninth complement component (C9) at the motor end-plate in myasthenia gravis. *J Neuropathol Exp Neurol* 39:160, 1980.
31. Emslie-Smith AM, Engel AG: Microvascular changes in early and advanced dermatomyositis: A quantitative study. *Ann Neurol* 27:343, 1990.
32. Nakano S, Engel AG: Myasthenia gravis: Quantitative immunocytochemical analysis of inflammatory cells and detection of complement membrane attack complex at the end-plate in 30 patients. *Neurology* 43:1167, 1993.
33. Arahata K, Engel AG: Monoclonal antibody analysis of mononuclear cells in myopathies: I. Quantitation of subsets according to diagnosis and sites of accumulation and demonstration and counts of muscle fibers invaded by T cells. *Ann Neurol* 16:193, 1984.
34. Engel AG, Arahata K: Monoclonal antibody analysis of mononuclear cells in myopathies: II. Phenotypes of autoinvasive cells in polymyositis and inclusion body myositis. *Ann Neurol* 16:209, 1984.
35. Engel AG, Arahata K, Emslie-Smith AM: Immune effector mechanisms in myopathies. *Res Publ Assoc Res Nerv Ment Dis* 68:141, 1990.
36. Hohlfeld R, Engel AG: Polymyositis mediated by T lymphocytes that express the γ/δ receptor. *N Engl J Med* 324:877, 1991.
37. Emslie-Smith AM, Arahata K, Engel AG: Major histocompatibility complex class I antigen expression, immunolocalization of interferon subtypes, and T-cell-mediated cytotoxicity in myopathies. *Hum Pathol* 20:224, 1989.
38. Cifuentes-Diaz C, Delaporte C, Dautréaux B, et al: Class II MHC antigens in normal human skeletal muscle. *Muscle Nerve* 15:295, 1992.
39. Hohlfeld R, Engel AG: Expression of 65 kilodalton heat-shock proteins in the inflammatory myopathies. *Ann Neurol* 32:821, 1992.
40. Whitaker JN, Bertorini TE, Mendell JR: Immunocytochemical studies of cathepsin D in human skeletal muscle. *Ann Neurol* 13:133, 1983.
41. Jimi T, Satoh Y, Takeda A, et al: Strong immunoreactivity of cathepsin L at the site of rimmed vacuoles in diseased muscles. *Brain* 115:249, 1992.
42. Villanova M, Kawai M, Lübke U, et al: Rimmed vacuoles of inclusion body myositis and oculopharyngeal dystrophy contain amyloid precursor protein and lysosomal markers. *Brain Res* 603:343, 1993.
43. Askanas V, Serdaroglu P, Engel WK, et al: Immunolocalization of ubiquitin in muscle biopsies of patients with inclusion body myositis and oculopharyngeal dystrophy. *Neurosci Lett* 130:73, 1991.
44. Askanas V, Engel WK, Alvarez RB: Strong immunoreactivity of β-amyloid precursor protein, including the β-amyloid protein sequence, at human neuromuscular junctions. *Neurosci Lett* 143:96, 1992.
45. Askanas V, Engel WK, Alvarez RB: Light and electron microscopic localization of β-amyloid protein in muscle biopsies of patients with inclusion body myositis. *Am J Pathol* 141:31, 1992.

46. Gauthier GF, Lowey S, Benfield PA, Hobbs AW: Distribution and properties of myosin isozymes in developing avian and mammalian skeletal muscle fibers. *J Cell Biol* 92:471, 1982.
47. Gauthier GF, Burke RE, Lowey S, Hobbs AW: Myosin isozymes in normal and cross-reinnervated cat skeletal muscle fibers. *J Cell Biol* 97:756, 1983.
48. Hall ZW, Lubit BW, Schwartz JH: Cytoplasmic actin in postsynaptic structure at the neuromuscular junction. *J Cell Biol* 90:789, 1981.
49. Showalter CJ, Engel AG: Acute quadriplegic myopathy: Analysis of myosin isoforms and evidence for calpain-mediated proteolysis. *Muscle Nerve* 20:316–322, 1997.
49a. Banwell BL, Russel J, Fukudome T, et al: Myopathy, myasthenic syndrome, and epidermolysis bullosa simplex due to plectin deficiency. *J Neuropathol Exp Neurol* 58:832–846, 1999.
49b. Banwell BL, Engel AG: αB-crystallin immunolocalization yields new insights into inclusion body myositis. *Neurology* 54:1033–1041, 2000.
49c. Nakano S, Engel AG, Akiguchi I, et al: Myofibrillar myopathy: III. Abnormal expression of cyclin-dependent kinases and nuclear proteins. *J Neuropathol Exp Neurol* 56:850–856, 1997.
49d. Askanas V, Bilak M, Leclerc A, et al: Prion protein is strongly immunolocalized at the postsynaptic domain of human normal neuromuscular junctions. *Neurosci Lett* 159:111–114, 1993.
50. Gallanti A, Prelle A, Moggio PM, et al: Desmin and vimentin as markers of regeneration in muscle diseases. *Acta Neuropathol* 85:88, 1992.
51. De Bleecker JL, Ertl BB, Engel AG: Patterns of abnormal protein expression in target formations and unstructured cores. *Neuromuscul Disord* 6:255–260, 1996.
52. De Bleecker JL, Engel AG, Ertl BB: Myofibrillar myopathy with abnormal foci of desmin positivity: II. Immunocytochemical analysis reveals accumulation of multiple other proteins. *J Neuropathol Exp Neurol* 55:563–577, 1996.
53. Bornemann A, Schmalbruch H: Desmin and vimentin in regenerating muscle. *Muscle Nerve* 15:14, 1992.
53a. Schröder R, Reimann J, Salmikangas P, et al: Bayond LDMDIA: Myotilin is a component of central core lesions and nemaline rods. *Neuromuscul Disord* 13:451–455, 2003.
54. Vybiral T, Winkelmann JC, Roberts R, et al: Human cardiac and skeletal muscle spectrins: Differential expression and localization. *Cell Motil Cytoskel* 21:293, 1992.
55. De Bleecker JL, Engel AG, Winkelmann JC: Localization of dystrophin and β-spectrin in vacuolar myopathies. *Am J Pathol.* 143:1200, 1993.
56. Muntoni F, Mateddu A, Cianchetti C, et al: Dystrophin analysis using a panel of anti-dystrophin antibodies in Duchenne and Becker muscular dystrophy. *J Neurol Neurosurg Psychiatry* 56:26, 1993.
57. Nguyen TM, Ginjaar IB, van Ommen G-J B, et al: Monoclonal antibodies for, dystrophin analysis: Epitope mapping and improved binding to SDS treated muscle sections. *Biochem J* 288:663, 1992.
58. Helliwell TR, Nguyen TM, Morris GE, et al: The dystrophin related protein, utrophin, is expressed on the sarcolemma of regenerating human skeletal muscle fibres in dystrophies and inflammatory myopathies. *Neuromusc Disord* 2:177, 1992.
59. Karpati G, Carpenter S, Morris G, et al: Localization and quantitation of the chromosome 6-encoded dystrophin-related protein in normal and pathological human muscle. *J Neuropathol Exp Neurol* 52:119, 1993.
60. Michele DE, Barresi R, Kanagawa M, et al: Post-translational disruption of dystroglycan-ligand interactions in congenital muscular dystrophies. *Nature* 418:417–422, 2002.
60a. Selcen D, Stilling G, Engel AG: The earliest pathologic alterations in dysferlinopathy. *Neurology* 56:1472–1481, 2001.
61. Vanegas OC, Bertini E, Zhang R-Z, et al: Ullrich scleratonic muscular dystrophy is caused by recessive mutations in collagen type VI. *Proc Natl Acad Sci USA* 98:7516–7521, 2001.
62. Merlini L, Villanova M, Sabatelli P, et al: Decreased expression of laminin-β1 in chromosome 21-linked Bethlem myopathy. *Neuromuscul Disord* 9:326–329, 1999.
63. Nishino I, Fu J, Tanji K, et al: Primary LAMP-2 deficiency causes X-linked vacuolar cardiomyopathy and myopathy (Danon disease). *Nature* 406:906–910, 2000.
64. Schubert W, Zimmerman K, Cramer M, et al: Lymphocyte antigen Leu-19 as a molecular marker of regeneration in human skeletal muscle. *Proc Natl Acad Sci USA* 86:307, 1989.
65. Illa I, Leon-Monzon M, Dalakas M: Regenerating and denervated human muscle fibers and satellite cells express neural cell adhesion molecule recognized by monoclonal antibodies to natural killer cells. *Ann Neurol* 31:46, 1992.
66. Engel AG, Lindstrom JM, Lambert EH, et al: Ultrastructural localization of the acetylcholine receptor in myasthenia gravis and in its experimental autoimmune model. *Neurology* 27:307, 1977.
67. Engel AG, Hutchinson DO, Nakano S, et al: Myasthenic syndromes attributed to mutations affecting the epsilon subunit of the acetylcholine receptor. *Ann NY Acad Sci.* 681:496, 1993.
68. Fambrough DM, Engel AG, Rosenberry TL: Acetylcholinesterase of human erythrocytes and neuromuscular junctions: Homologies revealed by monoclonal antibodies. *Proc Natl Acad Sci USA.* 79:1078, 1982.
69. Pearse AGE: *Histochemistry. Theoretical and Applied*, 4th ed. New York: Churchill Livingstone, 1980.
70. Bozzola JJ, Russell LD: *Electron Microscopy: Principles and Techniques for Biologists*. Boston: Jones and Bartlett, 1992.
71. Glauert AM, Lewis PR: *Biological Specimen Preparation for Electron Microscopy*. Princeton, NJ: Princeton University Press, 2002.
72. Hajibagheri MAN (ed): *Electron Microscopy: Methods and Protocols*. Totowa, NJ: Humana Press, 1999.
73. Harris JR, Adrian M: The production of cryosections through fixed and cryoprotected biological material for cryoelectron microscopy, in Hajibagheri MAN (ed): *Electron Microscopy: Methods and Protocols*. Totowa, NJ: Humana Press, 1999; pp 49–75.
74. Sabatini DD, Bensch K, Barrnett RJ: Cytochemistry and electron microscopy: The preservation of cellular ultrastructure and enzymatic activity by aldehyde fixation. *J Cell Biol* 17:19, 1963.
75. Cuello AC: *Immunohistochemistry*. New York: Wiley, 1993.
76. McLean IW, Nakane PK: Periodate-lysine-paraformaldehyde fixative. A new fixative for immunoelectron microscopy. *J Histochem Cytochem* 22:1077, 1974.
77. Karnovsky MJ: The ultrastructural basis of capillary permeability studies with peroxidase as a tracer. *J Cell Biol* 35:213, 1967.
78. Eldred WD, Zucker C, Karten HJ, Yazulla S: Comparison of fixation and penetration enhancement techniques for use in ultrastructural immunocytochemistry. *J Histochem Cytochem* 31:285, 1983.
79. Weber K, Rathke PC, Osborn M: Cytoplasmic microtubular images in glutaraldehyde-fixed tissue culture cells by electron microscopy and by immunofluorescence microscopy. *Proc Natl Acad Sci USA* 75:1820, 1978.
80. Arahata K, Engel AG: Monoclonal antibody analysis of mononuclear cells in myopathies: II. Immunoelectron microscopic aspects of cell mediated muscle fiber injury. *Ann Neurol* 19:112, 1986.
81. Hsu S-M, Raine L, Fanger H: Use of avidin-biotin-peroxidase complex (ABC) in immunoperoxidase techniques: A comparison between ABC and unlabeled antibody (PAP) procedures. *J Histochem Cytochem* 29:577, 1981.
82. Ribeiro-da-Silva A, Priestley JV, Cuello AC: Preembedding ultrastructural immunocytochemistry, in Cuello AC (ed): *Immunohistochemistry*. New York: Wiley, 1993; pp 181–228.
83. Larsson L-I: Antibody specificity in immunocytochemistry, in Cuello AC (ed): *Immunohistochemistry*. New York: Wiley, 1993; pp 79–106.
84. Merighi A, Polak JM: Postembedding immunogold staining, in Cuello AC (ed): *Immunohistochemistry*. New York: Wiley, 1993; pp 229–264.
84a. Hayat MA (ed): *Colloidal Gold: Principles, Methods and Protocol*. Vols 1–3. San Diego, CA: Academic Press, 1991.
84b. Thorpe JR: The application of LR gold resin for immunogold labeling, in Hajibagheri MAN (ed): *Electron Microscopy: Methods and Protocols*. Totowa, NJ: Humana Press, 1999; pp 99–109.
84c. Bushby KMD, Anderson LVB: *Muscular Dystrophy: Methods and Protocols*. Totowa, NJ: Humana Press, 2001.
85. Mita S, Schmidt B, Schon E, et al: Detection of "deleted" mitochondrial genomes in cytochrome-c oxidase-deficient muscle fibers of a patient with Kearns-Sayre syndrome. *Proc Natl Acad Sci USA* 86:9509, 1989.
86. Nishino H, Engel AG, Rima BK: Inclusion body myositis—The mumps virus hypothesis. *Ann Neurol* 25:260, 1989.
86a. Fournier J-G, Escaig-Haye F: In situ molecular hybridization techniques, in Hajibagheri MAN (ed): *Electron Microscopy: Methods and Protocols*. Totowa, NJ: Humana Press, 1999; pp 167–181.
87. Nuovo GJ: *PCR in Situ Hybridization: Protocols and Applications*. New York: Raven Press, 1992.

Chapter 30
Basic Reactions of Muscle

BETTY Q. BANKER
ANDREW G. ENGEL

Histopathologic Study of the Muscle Biopsy
Histochemical Analysis of Muscle Fibers
   PATTERN OF FIBER TYPES
   ANALYSIS OF MUSCLE FIBER DIAMETERS
Alterations in the Muscle Fiber
   CENTRAL MIGRATION OF SUBSARCOLEMMAL NUCLEI
   CHANGE IN CONTOUR
Alterations in Muscle
   DYSTROPHIN DEFICIENCY
Enzymatic Deficiencies
   GLYCOGEN STORAGE DISORDERS
   NEURONAL CEROID LIPOFUSCINOSES
   MUCOPOLYSACCHARIDOSES
   NIEMANN-PICK GROUP OF DISEASES
   G_{M1} GANGLIOSIDOSIS
   FABRY DISEASE
   LAFORA DISEASE
   METACHROMATIC LEUKODYSTROPHY
   GLOBOID CELL LEUKODYSTROPHY
   INFANTILE NEUROAXONAL DYSTROPHY
   CYTOCHROME OXIDASE DEFICIENCY
   MYOADENYLATE DEAMINASE DEFICIENCY
Alterations of the Muscle Spindle

Histopathologic Study of the Muscle Biopsy

The clinical and electromyographic examinations of the patient and the light microscopic study of the muscle biopsy specimen are three essential requirements for the diagnosis of most neuromuscular diseases. At the simplest level, the histopathologic study is likely to provide information as to whether the basic disease process is primarily a myopathy or a neurogenic process. In addition, the muscle biopsy may provide clues for the diagnosis of a specific disorder (such as Duchenne dystrophy or dermatomyositis) or categories of disorders (such as storage diseases or metabolic myopathies) and may yield insights as to the time of onset or rate of evolution of the disease (e.g., a recent attack of rhabdomyolysis or acute versus chronic neurogenic atrophy). Finally, unexpected or unusual histopathologic findings may provide hints for further biochemical, ultrastructural, or genetic studies. A careful and systematic study of the muscle biopsy specimens by currently available histologic techniques may also yield valuable insights into the pathogenesis of selected neuromuscular disorders.

A number of basic pathologic reactions of muscle can be recognized in paraffin sections of fixed biopsy specimens. These alterations include muscle fiber necrosis, regeneration, loss of myofibrillar markings or of cross striations, abnormalities of the muscle fiber diameter (atrophy, hypertrophy, abnormal variation in fiber size), increased number of central nuclei, fiber splitting, vacuolar change, storage of abnormal material, inflammatory infiltrates, and proliferation of connective tissue elements. Small or large groups of atrophic fibers with or without target fibers or hypertrophy of the nonatrophic fibers can indicate a neurogenic process. On the other hand, there are numerous pathologic alterations in muscle that cannot be detected or adequately defined in paraffin sections but can be clearly visualized by histochemical analysis of cryostat sections of unfixed muscle. The present chapter reviews those reactions of muscle that can be observed by light microscopic analysis. The ultrastructural reactions of muscle are considered in Chap. 31 and other chapters dealing with specific disorders.

Histochemical Analysis of Muscle Fibers

There are three approaches to the histochemical analysis of the muscle fiber: (1) the survey of the pattern established by the muscle fibers, (2) the measurement and recording of the diameters of each fiber type (histogram), and (3) the analysis of the various changes within individual fibers. In many muscle biopsies in which the diagnosis is obvious, e.g., inflammatory myopathy, it is not always necessary to analyze fiber types or relative diameters. In others, the muscle fibers must be evaluated very carefully in order to determine the presence of denervation atrophy, atrophy or hypertrophy of a given histochemical fiber type, fiber-type predominance, and altered fibers. Measurements of the fiber diameters and determination of the patterns of muscle fiber types are of particular importance in understanding the muscle disorders of children who present with hypotonia and muscle weakness and are slow to pass their motor milestones (see Chap. 54).

PATTERN OF FIBER TYPES

The pattern of fiber types can be studied accurately only by subjecting cryostat-sectioned unfixed, frozen muscle to myofibrillar adenosine triphosphatase (ATP)* reactions at pHs 4.3, 4.6, and 9.4. The pH lability of this reaction allows the differentiation of the fibers into four types (Figs. 30-1 and 30-2). Such a distinction is possible because type 1 fibers are base-labile and acid-stabile, whereas type 2 fibers possess the reverse properties. Type 2B and 2C fibers display activity in solutions containing a wider pH range than the 2A fibers and thus can be differentiated. Type 2C fibers are infrequent in human muscle (see Table 30-1).

A few basic concepts are important for the understanding of the normal and the altered state. Muscle fibers of a single motor unit are not congregated into a group but are ran-

---

*A list of the abbreviations used in this chapter is given at the end of the chapter.

domly dispersed among fibers of other motor units.[1] All muscle fibers of a single motor unit are of the same fiber type.[1,2] The typical checkerboard or mosaic pattern of normal human muscle is the result of the intermingling of types 1, 2A, 2B, and, infrequently, type 2C fibers of different motor units. The normal pattern is characteristically altered in several situations, which are discussed below.

Differentiation into a Mosaic Pattern

The differentiation into a mosaic of fiber types begins gradually in human muscle after 22 weeks of fetal life, a time when polyneuronal innervation has disappeared and a mature pattern of innervation has been established. Definition of the distribution of fiber types before 30 fetal weeks is not possible because the differentiation into a mosaic of fiber types is not complete until after that time. When the myofibrillar ATPase technique at either alkaline or acid pH is applied before the 30th week of gestation, all fibers stain darkly regardless of the pH of the preincubation medium.[3] These fibers are called undifferentiated, or 2C, fibers. In human muscle, differentiation into the three major fiber types occurs in the last 3 months of fetal life and continues throughout the first year of life and even until early childhood. Between 30 and 40 weeks of fetal life, a small proportion of the type 1 fibers have a large diameter; the remainder are similar to the other fibers. The larger type 1 fiber has been referred to as the B fiber of Wohlfart.[4–6] These larger type 1 fibers are significantly larger than the undifferentiated fibers and the other type 1 fibers that are observed during the last 3 months of fetal life. These large type 1 fibers are not detected in all muscles at any one stage of development; after the 20th week of fetal life, they were found only in three of four muscles studied by Colling-Saltin.[3] Furthermore, these large fibers never constitute more than 4 to 5 percent of all the fibers, and by 40 weeks of gestation they are rarely observed. Not until after the 30th week of gestation are some type 2A fibers detected.[3]

The fiber-type distribution at birth is similar to but not identical with that of adult muscle, the major difference being that up to 20 percent of the fibers are undifferentiated in the newborn compared with 1 to 2 percent in the adult.[3] The decrease in undifferentiated fibers occurs mainly during the first year of life. By 1 year of age, the percentage of fiber types differs very little from the adult. As the percentage of undifferentiated fibers decreases, that of type 1 fibers

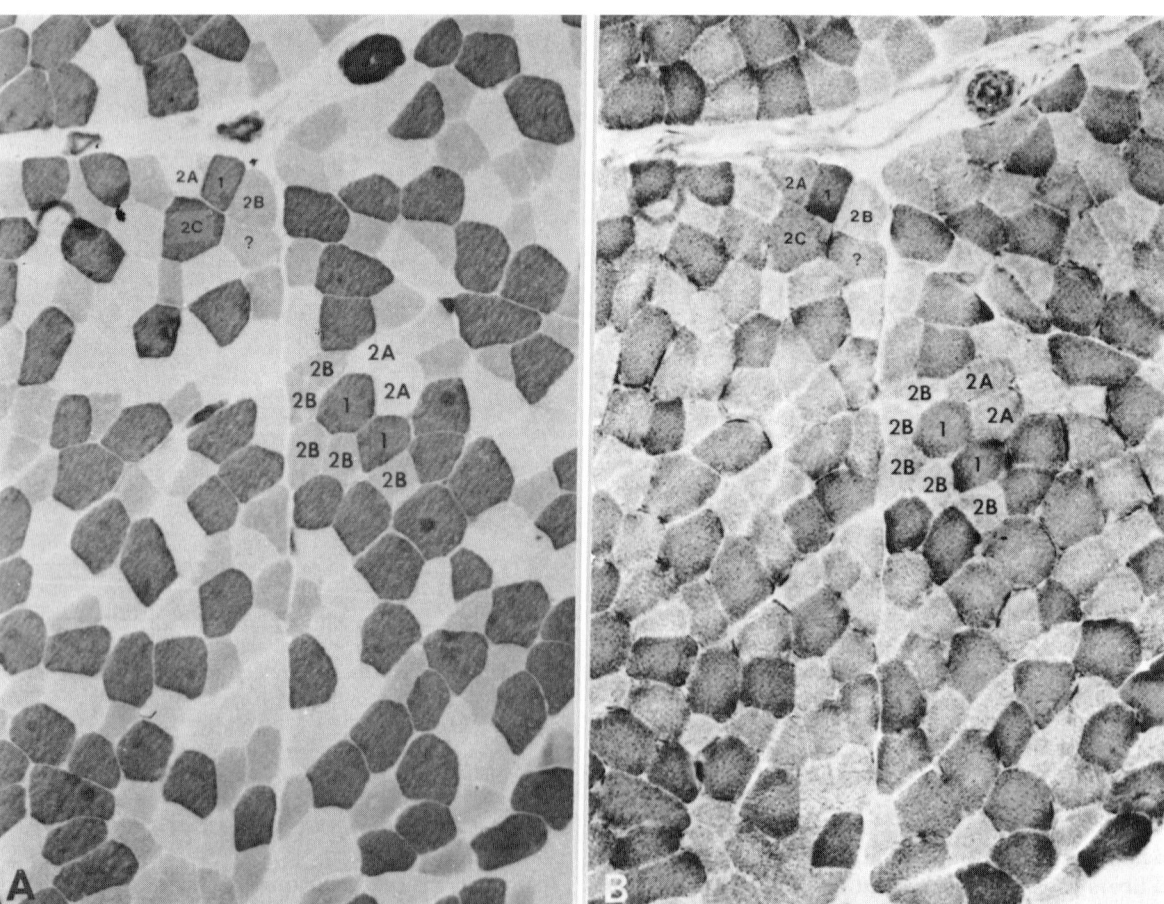

FIGURE 30-1. Normal checkerboard distribution of histochemical fiber types demonstrated by the ATPase (after preincubation at pH 4.6) *(A)* and NADH dehydrogenase *(B)* reactions in lateral vastus muscle of a 6-year-old boy. In *A*, type 1 fibers appear dark, 2B fibers are less dark, and 2A fibers are light. In *B*, type 1 fibers are dark, 2B fibers are light, and 2A fibers are intermediate in reactivity. Few type 2C fibers are present. These are dark with ATPase at pH 4.6 and are of intermediate reactivity for NADH dehydrogenase. Few fibers (indicated by question mark) are of intermediate reactivity with ATPase at pH 4.6 and with NADH dehydrogenase and do not fall into any of the previous fiber types. In this biopsy specimen the type 2B fibers have a smaller mean diameter than the other fiber types. ×160.

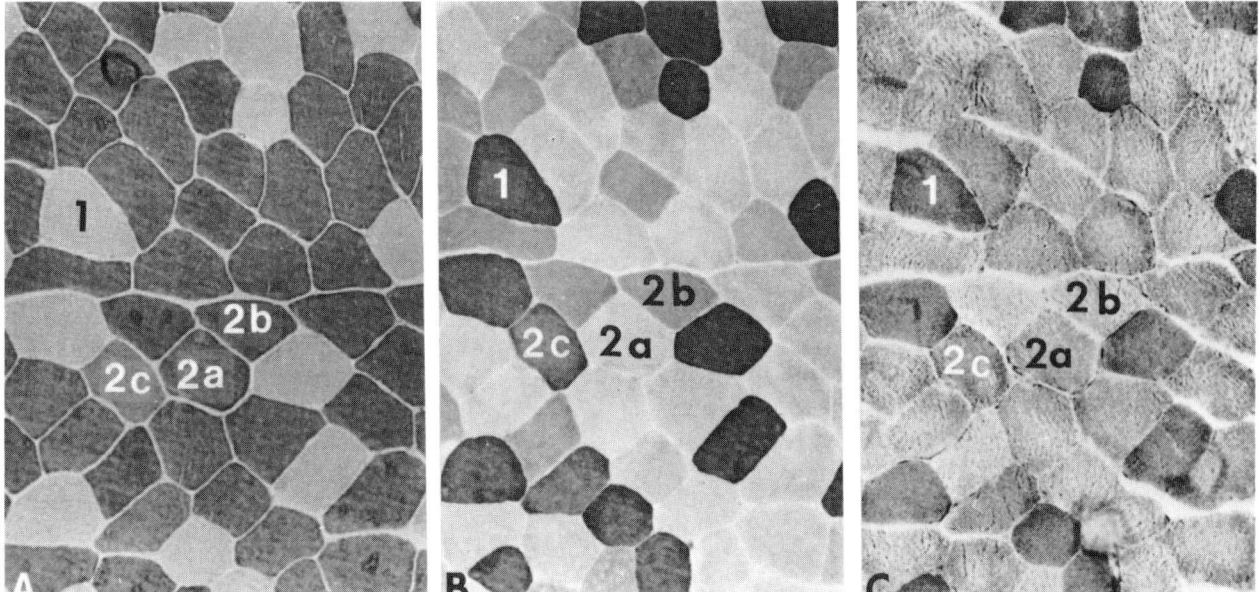

FIGURE 30-2. Normal checkerboard distribution of histochemical fiber types in lateral vastus muscle of a 26-year-old woman demonstrated by the ATPase reaction at pH 9.4 (A) and after preincubation at pH 4.6 (B), and by the NADH dehydrogenase reaction (C). In A, type 2 fibers are more abundant than type 1 fibers; B and C further differentiate the type 2 fibers as 2A, 2B, and 2C and reveal a random distribution of these subtypes. Only rare type 2C fibers are present. ×160.

increases.[3] The total number of type 2 fibers is the same at birth and at 1 year of age; however, the proportions of 2A and 2B fibers change in this period. During the first year of life, 2B fibers constitute only about 2 percent. From 1 year until 5 years of age, the percentage of 2A fibers decreases and that of 2B increases. As there are very few undifferentiated fibers during this period, it appears that the 2A fibers have been converted into 2B fibers.[3]

Normal Predominance of a Fiber Type

In animals the predominance of a fiber type is characteristic of a particular muscle. In the soleus, for example, type 1 fibers predominate; in the medial head of the gastrocnemius muscle, type 2 fibers predominate. In the anterior tibial muscle, two-thirds of the fibers are type 2. By contrast, in human muscle the three fiber types occur in roughly equal proportions in a pattern that rarely varies. Nevertheless, there are certain muscles in humans that have relatively specific characteristics. For example, in anterior tibial and deltoid muscles the type 1 fibers are more numerous than the type 2 fibers; type 1 fiber predominance could be incorrectly assumed if the normal pattern of fiber types for that muscle were not known.[7] Further, in some muscles (e.g., vastus medialis, triceps) type 2 fibers can be more abundant in the superficial than in the deeper regions of muscle.[7] Therefore, in any study that assesses the distribution of fiber types, it is necessary to compare identical muscles and identical areas (superficial versus deep) in a given muscle.

Fiber-Type Predominance

In certain congenital myopathies, the differentiation into fiber types may be delayed or never appear during development. This alteration in pattern is called *fiber-type predominance* (Fig. 30-3A, B, and C). The normal ratio of type 1 to type 2 fibers in some commonly biopsied human muscles (superficial triceps, biceps, vastus lateralis) is approximately 1:2. For these muscles, if the type 2 fibers are further subdivided, types 1, 2A, and 2B each constitute about one-third of the fibers (Fig. 30-3A, B, and C). The term *fiber-type predominance*, a very nonspecific alteration, designates an excess of one fiber type (Figs. 30-1 and 30-2). In most other muscles the normal distribution of type 1 and 2 fibers can vary,[7] and this fact must be taken into account in the evaluation of type predominance.

Table 30-1. INTENSITY OF STAINING REACTION OF THE MUSCLE FIBER TYPES

	Fiber Type			
Stain	1	2A	2B	2C
Hematoxylin and eosin (H&E)	++	+	+	+
Periodic–acid Schiff (PA)	+	+++	++	++
Gomori trichrome	+++	++	++	++
NADH dehydrdogenase	+++	++	+	++
Succinic dehydrogenase	+++	++	+	+1
Cytochrome oxidase	+++	++	+	+
ATPase pH 9.4	+	+++	+++	+++
ATPase pH 4.6	+++	0	++	++
ATPase pH 4.3	+++	0	0	++
Phosphorylase	+	+++	+++	+++
Phosphofructokinase	++	+	+	+
Myoadenylate deaminase	++	++	++	++
Esterase	+++	+	+	+
Acid phosphatase	0	0	0	0
Alkaline phosphatase	0	0	0	0
Menadione-linked α-glycerophosphate dyhydrogenase	+	+++	+++	++

KEY: + = weakly positive; ++ = moderately positive; +++ = strongly positive.

Selective Fiber-Type Involvement

Fibers of one histochemical type may become involved or degenerate when a disease selectively or predominantly affects the muscle fibers of that type. Involvement of both fiber types may also interfere with the normal differentiation into the mosaic pattern. Certain fiber types may be specifically affected in certain disorders. For example, in lipid storage myopathies, the type 1 muscle fibers are particularly affected (see Chap. 57). In a myopathy with tubular aggregates, the type 2 fibers in particular contain large collections of tubules (see Chap. 54). Their specific vulnerability usually relates to the function of the particular fiber involved, as is indicated in the discussion of these disorders.

Reinnervation and Fiber-Type Grouping

The checkerboard pattern of fiber types is altered when denervated muscle is reinnervated.[8] Following the denervation of muscle, sprouts of adjacent intact motor axons reinnervate the muscle fibers. With enlargement of individual motor units during reinnervation, the random distribution of fiber types is so altered that an increased number of fibers of a single type appear immediately adjacent to each other. Such a histochemical change following reinnervation is termed *fiber-type grouping* and provides a means of early recognition of the disorders that result from the denervation of muscle (Fig. 30-4). This change often precedes the more obvious features of denervation atrophy.

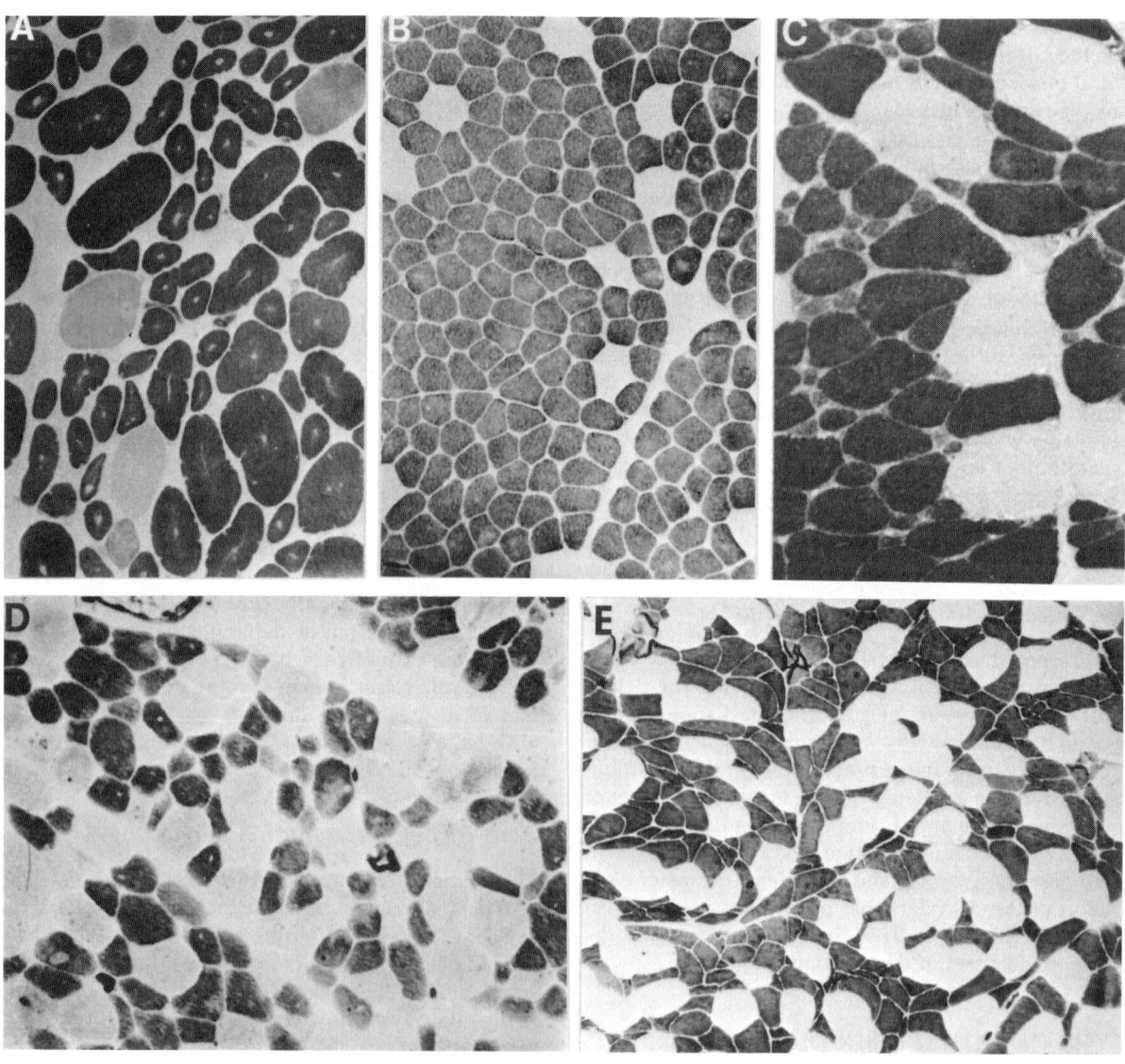

FIGURE 30-3. Fiber–type predominance and atrophy demonstrated by the ATPase reaction after preincubation at pH 4.6 (*A, B*) or pH 4.3 (*C*) and by the regular ATPase reaction at pH 9.4 (*E*). The panels show type 1 fiber predominance and atrophy in myotubular myopathy (*A*), multicore disease (*B*), and fingerprint body myopathy (*C*); type 1 fiber atrophy in myotonic dystrophy (*D*); and type 2 fiber atrophy secondary to disuse (*E*). In *A* and *C* only some of the type 1 fibers are atrophic, and in *C* the type 2 fibers are hypertrophied. *A*, ×120; *B*, ×120; *C*, ×210; *D*, ×120; *E*, ×75.

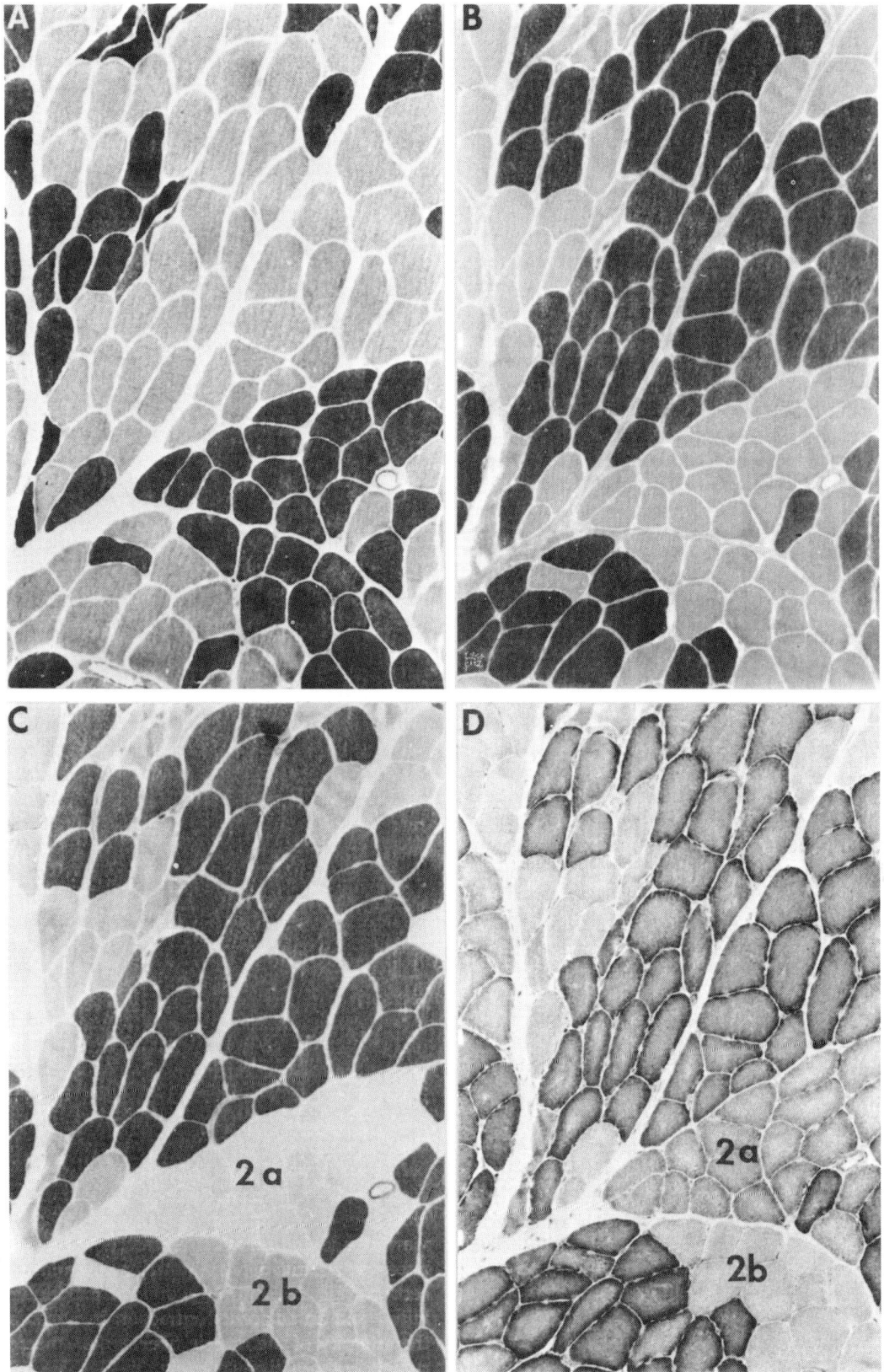

FIGURE 30-4. Grouping of histochemical fiber types demonstrated in chronic neurogenic atrophy; serial sections reacted for ATPase at pH 9.4 (A), for ATPase after preincubation at pH 4.3 (B) and at pH 4.6 (C), and for NADH dehydrogenase. Grouping of types 1 and 2 fibers can be observed in A and B; and C and D also reveal grouping of type 2A and 2B fibers. Two small groups of atrophic fibers and isolated atrophic fibers are present in the left upper quadrant of each panel. As only a small portion of the fibers are atrophic, reinnervation appears to be keeping abreast with denervation. The extensive type grouping indicates that the process is chronic. ×80.

ANALYSIS OF MUSCLE FIBER DIAMETERS

In a series of papers, Brooke and Engel[9–12] introduced the histographic analysis of the diameters of the various muscle fibers in both normal and abnormal muscle. This approach has proved to be important in the definition of certain alterations of muscle. In establishing a histogram, it is necessary to follow a number of basic rules.[9–12] The measurements must be made in one muscle. All comparisons must be established between the same muscles taken from persons of similar age and sex. All muscle used for comparison must be prepared in the same way; there is a 30 percent reduction of diameters of muscle fibers that are embedded in paraffin compared with cryostat-sectioned unfixed, frozen material. In order to measure the diameters of the three types of muscle fibers, the application of the myofibrillar ATPase technique at the varying pH is essential. Histograms are constructed from measurements of photomicrographs, projections, or direct microscopic visualization. Muscle is always studied in cross section when fiber diameters are being determined. The diameter chosen is the shortest dimension bisecting the muscle fiber in a plane through the center of the fiber. The mean fiber diameter is determined for the three principal fiber types. In normal muscle from the age of 40 gestational weeks, the mean fiber diameters of the three principal fiber types do not differ by more than 12 percent of the largest mean diameter,[9–12] and the variability coefficient (standard deviation of the fiber diameters multiplied by 1000 and divided by the mean diameter of all the fibers) is less than 250.[9–12]

Histogram of Normal Muscle Fibers

In the course of development, the diameters of muscle fibers gradually enlarge from 6 to 7 μm in the 20-week fetus[13] to 15 to 17 μm at 1 year of age. After that the measurements increase by about 2 μm each year to 5 years of age.[12] From the age of 5 to 9 years, the diameters increase by about 3 μm. At the age of 10 years, the diameters range from 38 to 42 μm. Adult values are reached between the ages of 12 and 15 years. In infancy and childhood, the average diameters of type 1 and 2 fibers are equal and the variability is small. The type 2 fibers in the adult male are usually larger than the type 1; in women, on the other hand, the type 1 fibers are slightly larger.[11] Although the diameters of type 1 fibers vary very little, those of the type 2 fibers vary over a narrow range. In comparisons of identical muscles in healthy active adults, the diameters of both type 1 and 2 fibers are significantly larger in men than in women. The difference may be as great as 10 μm.

There are a number of categories of deviation from the normal described, as follows.

Type 1 Fiber Disproportion or Atrophy

This change is characterized by a reduction in the diameter of type 1 fibers. The mean diameter of the type 1 fiber is smaller than the mean diameter of the type 2 fiber by more than 12 percent.[14] Type 2 fibers have a variability coefficient less than 250.[14] This selective atrophy of type 1 fibers occurs in myotonic dystrophy (Fig. 30-3D),[11] in children with various types of congenital myopathy (Fig. 30-3A, B, and C) (Chap. 54), in muscle of the lower leg in children with club feet (Chap. 70), and in many other disorders. In the involved muscles, the fibers are not only smaller (disproportion) but are also frequently increased in number (predominance) (Fig. 30-3A, B, and C).

Type 2 Fiber Disproportion or Atrophy

This alteration is characterized by a reduction in the diameter of the type 2 fibers. The mean diameter of the type 2 fibers is at least 12 percent less than the mean diameter of the type 1 fibers. The larger type 1 fibers have a normal variability. This change is often encountered in muscle of patients with involvement of corticospinal tracts.[15] There is also selective type 2 fiber atrophy with disuse from any cause (Fig. 30-3E), malnutrition or cachexia, corticosteroid excess, and sometimes with collagen vascular disease.

Increased Variability

When there is a moderate or conspicuous variation in fiber diameter, the distribution curve of a histogram is widened and the variability coefficient is increased (Fig. 30-5). This alteration is found in primary myopathies and is particularly prominent in muscular dystrophy.

Denervation Atrophy

When a histogram of the various diameters of denervated muscle is plotted, the atrophic and nonatrophic fibers provide at least two peaks. In comparison with the histogram from a myopathy, the range of diameters in the denervated muscle is usually narrower. The small fibers are usually of both types 1 and 2.[14]

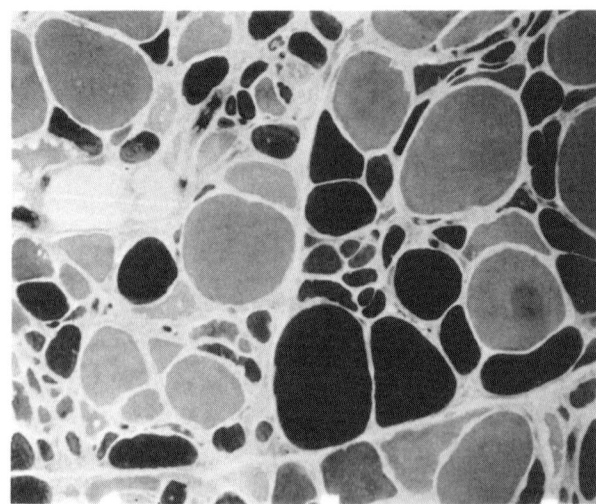

FIGURE 30-5. Fibers of either histochemical type vary abnormally in diameter and show abnormal contours. Some fibers are splitting. Inclusion body myositis, ATPase reaction, pH 9.4. ×120.

Alterations in the Muscle Fiber

CENTRAL MIGRATION OF SUBSARCOLEMMAL NUCLEI

In the normal mature muscle fiber, the nuclei are located at the periphery of the fiber in a subsarcolemmal position. Migration of nuclei to a central position in the mature muscle fiber represents an abnormal but nonspecific, response. In muscular dystrophy, centrally placed nuclei are frequently observed; in myotonic dystrophy, they are particularly prominent (Fig. 30-6). The congenital myopathy called centronuclear myopathy is characterized by a high percentage of muscle fibers displaying centrally positioned nuclei.

CHANGE IN CONTOUR

In cross section, the normal muscle fiber is polygonal in shape. Rounding of the muscle fiber in cross section represents a nonspecific but consistent feature in the myopathies (Fig. 30-5). In addition, rounding as well as angulation are features that often accompany denervation of the fiber.

Necrosis

Muscle fiber necrosis is a stereotyped response to a variety of pathogenic stimuli. It represents an injury to all organelles of the fiber or to a segment or circumscribed region of the fiber (Fig. 30-7). Segmental necrosis affects several sarcomeres of a muscle fiber. Within such fibers the contractile substance appears homogenized, resulting in the obliteration of striations. The sarcolemma is disrupted and disappears, and the contents of the fiber are usually removed by phagocytes (Figs. 30-7 and 30-8). The major portions of the affected fibers may survive and appear quite normal except for the regenerative changes in the vicinity of the damaged segment.

Segmental necrosis must be differentiated from artifactual change. Muscle is a highly irritable tissue, and if it is allowed to contract during removal or before fixation, violent contraction results in irregular banding and deformation of the fibers. Highly concentrated segments of such fibers appear swollen; the fiber contour is rounded and in hematoxylin and eosin (H&E)–stained sections the fiber contents have a homogeneous or vitreous appearance. However, closely spaced striations can still be discerned on viewing a longitudinally oriented contracted segment with phase or polarization optics or in trichromatically stained sections (Fig. 30-9). On the other hand, focal muscle fiber injury and an adjacent contraction band can also occur if the integrity of the muscle fiber surface membrane is disrupted in the native state (Fig. 30-10). This alteration may represent an early stage in muscle fiber destruction. Artifactual contraction bands can be readily distinguished from necrotic fiber segments when the latter are invaded by macrophages.

In the muscle fiber stained by the Gomori trichrome technique, the zone of necrosis appears pale gray or green-blue in color, while the normal fiber stains a deep blue or green (Figs. 30-7 and 30-8; Color Plate 8A and B). The fine inter-

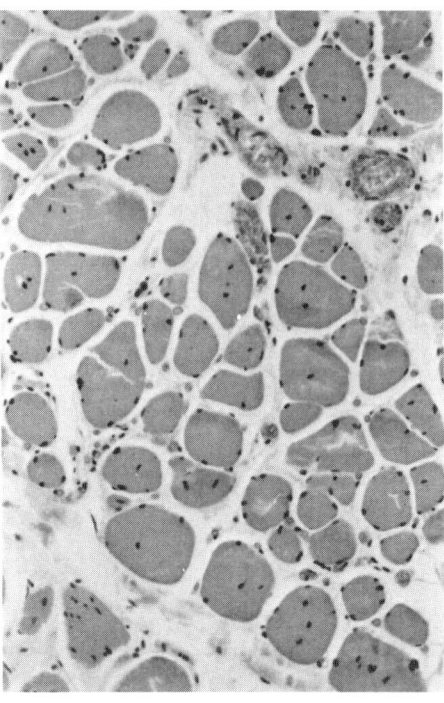

FIGURE 30-6. Many muscle nuclei have migrated centrally from a subsarcolemmal position. Myotonic dystrophy. H&E stain. ×180.

myofibrillar membranous network is absent, attenuated, or clumped. The zone of necrosis may or may not be invaded by macrophages (Color Plate 8E). Necrosis of the entire longitudinal extent of the fiber is referred to as single-fiber necrosis and is particularly prominent in the active stage of polymyositis. The muscle fiber is swollen and homogeneous throughout its length (Fig. 30-7). Histiocytes invade the cytoplasm (Figs. 30-7 and 30-8A and B). The subsarcolemmal nuclei are usually pyknotic and the plasma membrane disappears. The term *acidophilic hyalinization* has been applied to these large swollen muscle fibers; they stain intensely with acidophilic dyes, and the loss of internal structural detail is often described as *hyalinization*. The hyalinized contents retract, leaving large areas partially filled with a loose granular material. Fibroblastic processes circumscribe the degenerating muscle fiber.

Engel and Biesecker[16,17] have shown that complement activation is an invariant concomitant of muscle fiber necrosis. Complement proteins enter the muscle fiber through the damaged surface membrane and become fixed to intracellular organelles. This is followed by assembly of the C5b-9 membrane attack complex (MAC) that lyses membranous organelles. MAC appears only in necrotic fibers and is a reliable marker for such fibers[16,17] (Fig. 30-11; Color Plate 8C–F). Complement activation is also associated with the release of factors that chemotactically attract and immobilize macrophages and opsonize fiber components for destruction by the macrophages. The mechanism that triggers complement activation during fiber necrosis is not known.[16,17]

Delta or Wedge-Shaped Lesions

Regional defects in the plasma membrane are observed in the electron microscope in a proportion of nonnecrotic muscle fibers in Duchenne dystrophy. The light microscopic concomitant of some of these abnormal areas is a wedge-shaped area of rarefaction in the fiber, the base of which rests on the surface of the fiber. These are observed in about 5 percent of the nonnecrotic fibers in resin-embedded sections of fixed tissue viewed by phase microscopy (Fig. 30-12A), but they cannot be seen in fresh-frozen sections.[18,19] The membranous defects allow the penetration of extracellular fluid into the fiber and the accumulation of calcium in fiber zones that abut on the plasma membrane. Zones of calcium accumulation

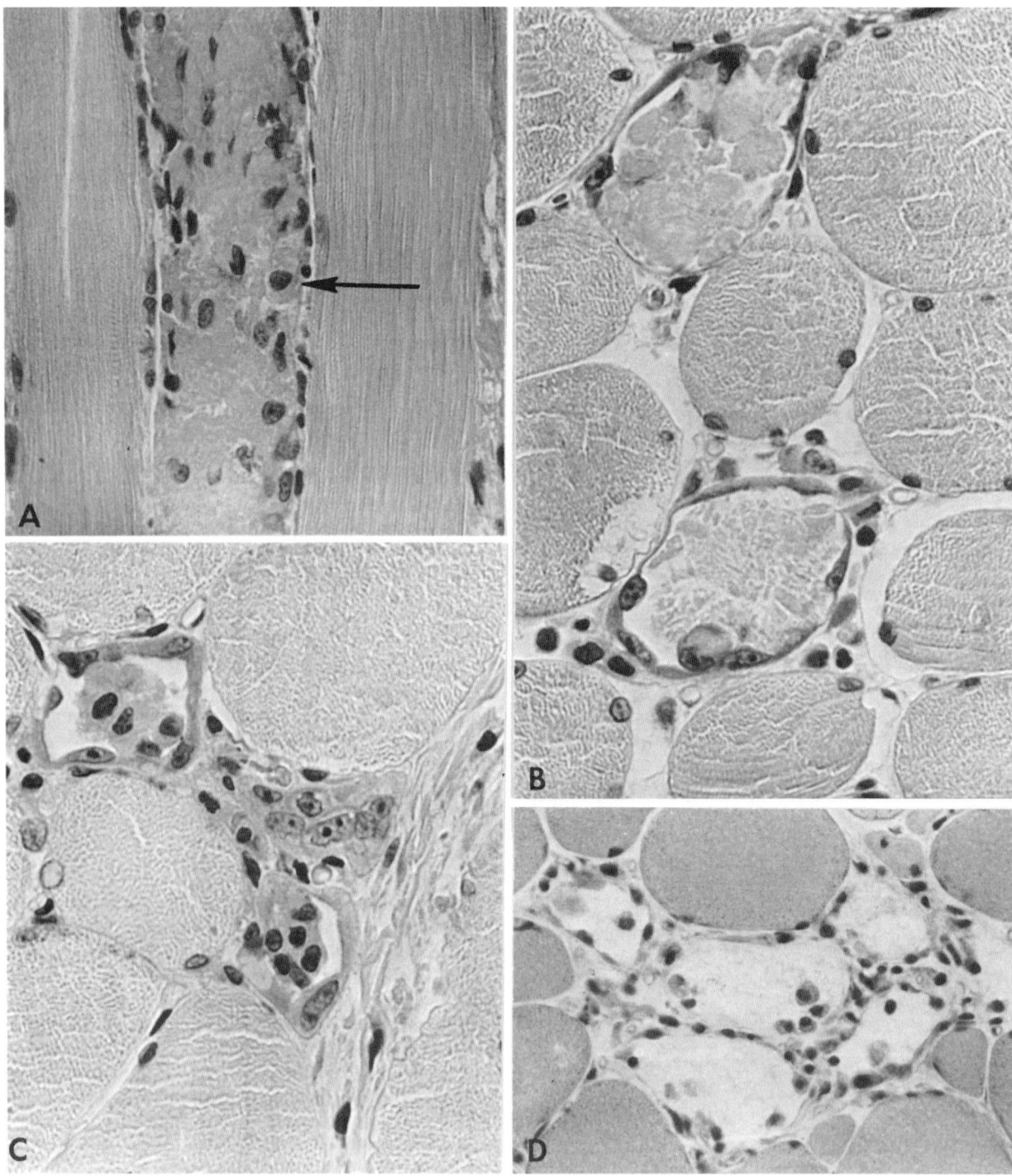

FIGURE 30-7. Muscle fiber necrosis. A. Longitudinal section of a necrotic muscle fiber in which the homogenized contractile substance has been invaded by macrophages (arrow). ×570. B, C, and D. The cytoplasmic components of these necrotic muscle fibers are being phagocytized by macrophages. Each necrotic fiber is encircled by the cytoplasmic extensions of mononuclear cells. H&E stain. B, C, ×665; D, ×319.

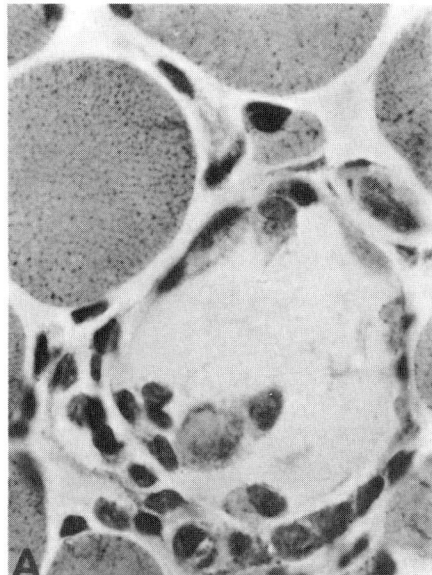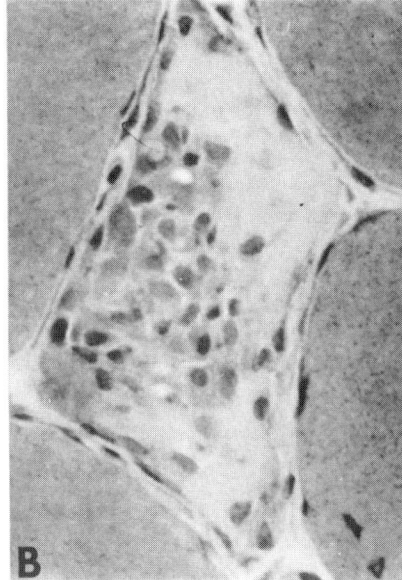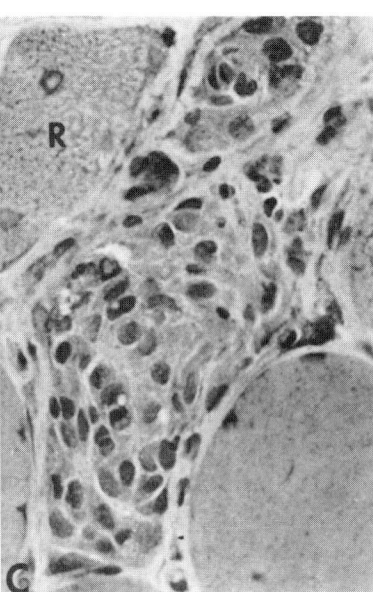

FIGURE 30-8. Muscle fiber necrosis, trichrome-stained frozen sections. In A and B the necrotic fiber can be identified by its pallid cytoplasm. The normal intermyofibrillar membranous network, readily seen in the adjacent nonnecrotic fibers, has disappeared from the necrotic fibers. In A, the necrotic fiber is invaded by few mononuclear cells; in B, a large proportion of the necrotic fiber; and in C, the entire necrotic fiber had been replaced by the invading cells. Most of the invading cells are macrophages, but a few are other lymphoid cells. R = regenerating fiber. A, ×700; B, C, ×420.

can be demonstrated in fresh-frozen sections[20] (Fig. 30-12B and C). In the electron microscope, in many lesions the myofibrils appear rarefied and the myofilaments are sparse; in some lesions the sarcotubular profiles are dilated, and some lesions contain degenerating mitochondria. In bordering regions the myofibrils are contracted.[18] When biopsied muscle is maintained at constant length and rapidly immersed in buffered horseradish peroxidase, the labeled extracellular fluid enters the wedge.[18] These findings indicate that the altered plasma membrane fails to maintain an effective cellular barrier.[18,19] (see also Chap. 34).

Splitting or Branching

When two muscle fibers are in close apposition and occupy the space of one, it can usually be assumed that they have undergone splitting or branching (Fig. 30-13). This is a frequent alteration in primary diseases of muscle, and it is particularly conspicuous in dystrophy.[21,22] This process is best observed in cross section, where the muscle fibers are seen in close proximity and nestled within the same endomysial connective tissue enclosure, like the pieces of a jigsaw puzzle (Fig. 30-14). In longitudinal section, the two fibers fork from the single master fiber, leaving only a small space between the two. The consistent finding of membranous debris and capillaries in the cleavage space suggests that focal damage has occurred at the point of branching. The splitting of muscle fibers that occurs in dystrophic muscle is associated with increased lysosomal activity, also prominent in the vacuolar myopathies such as periodic paralysis, chloroquine myopathy, LAMP2 deficiency, and type 2 glycogenosis (Fig. 30-14). In chloroquine myopathy, the myriad of vacuoles and myeloid bodies in muscle fibers together with extensive fiber splitting have a characteristic appearance.[23] Also in this situation, the split portions are often abnormal.

Regeneration

Muscle tissue is regarded as having an excellent capacity to repair itself. The ability of any striated muscle to regenerate is related to the extent of the tissue necrosis, the preservation of the innervation and the blood supply to the area, and the degree of intactness of the architecture of the muscle (Fig. 30-10). Probably a very important additional factor is the nature of the initiating disease process. Several forms of regeneration are recognized by light microscopy, depending upon whether the architecture of muscle is interrupted or whether the necrosis has been confined to single muscle fibers or portions of those fibers, as indicated below.

The regenerating muscle fiber displays a number of features. When stained with H&E, the cytoplasm of the relatively intact, regenerating muscle fiber is basophilic; the subsar-

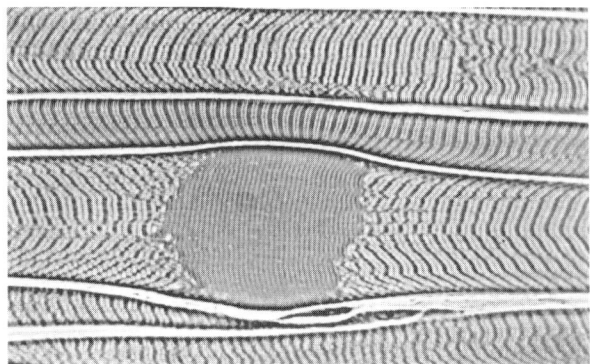

FIGURE 30-9. Phase micrograph of a segmentally contracted muscle fiber. The contracted fiber is swollen but retains its cross-striations. With the H&E stain, the contracted region would have a homogeneous appearance, suggesting segmental fiber necrosis. ×333.

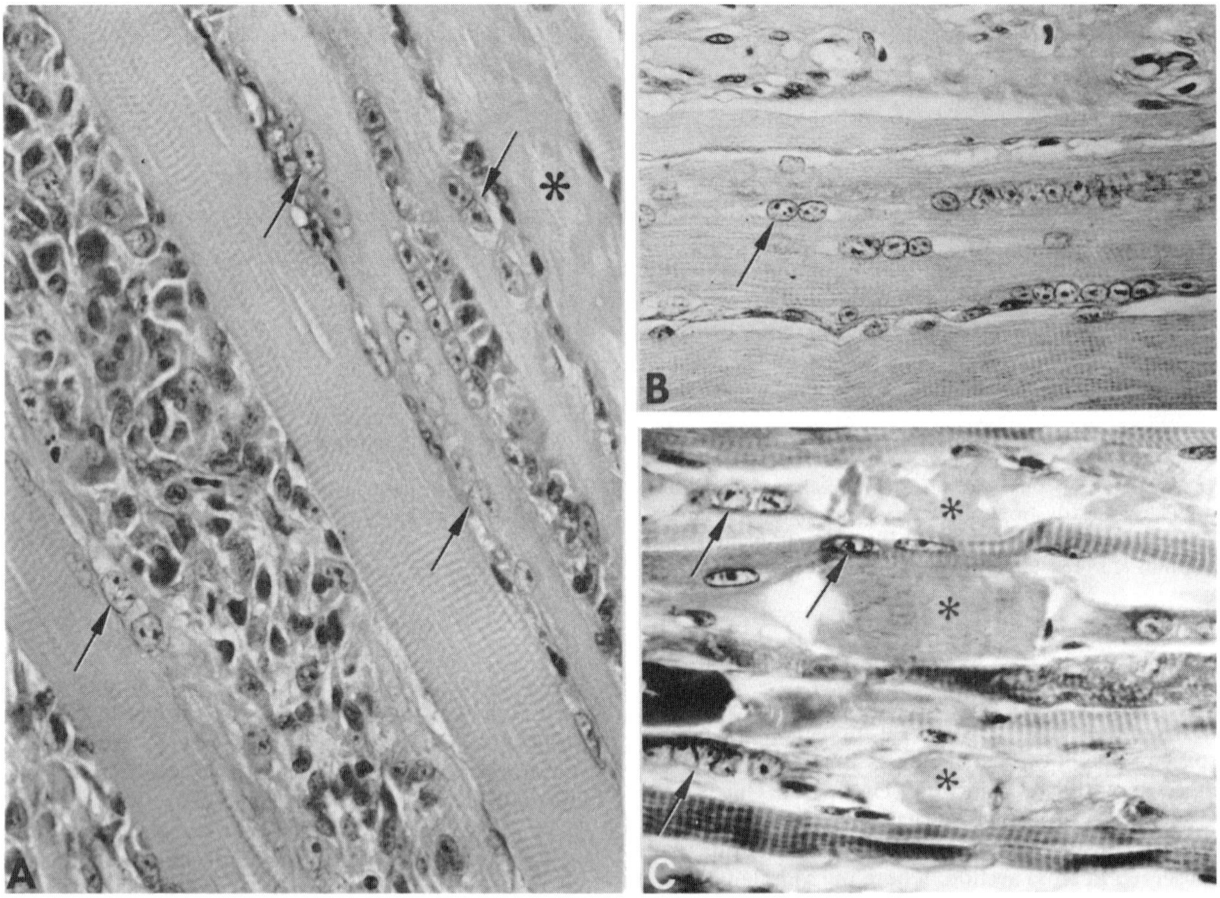

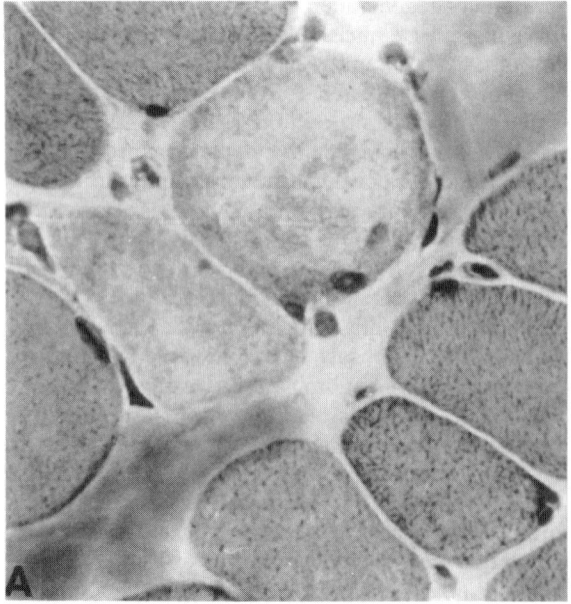
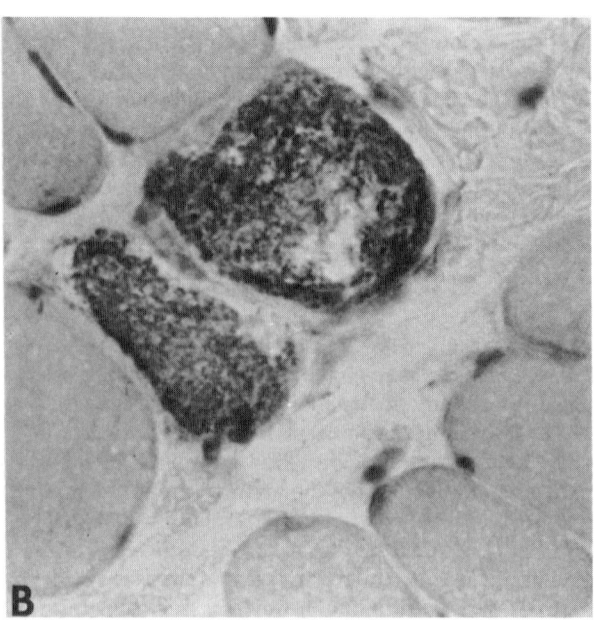

FIGURE 30-10. Regenerating muscle fibers after paroxysmal rhabdomyolysis *(A,B)* and in limb girdle dystrophy *(B)*. H&E *(A, B)* and trichrome *(C)* stained paraffin sections. The regenerating fibers display rows of large vesicular nuclei with prominent nucleoli (arrows). In *A*, two necrotic fibers have been replaced by macrophages; another necrotic fiber in *A* and necrotic fiber regions in *C* (asterisks) are not invaded by macrophages. ×400.

FIGURE 30-11. Duchenne dystrophy: serial cryostat sections stained with trichrome *(A)* and reacted for the neoantigenic determinants of the complement C5b-9 MAC *(B)*. The necrotic fibers, readily recognized in *A*, show intense reactivity for MAC in *B*. ×400. *(Engel AG, Biesecker G: Ann Neurol 12:289, 1982. Reproduced by permission.)*

colemmal nuclei are numerous, and the nucleoli are unusually large, dark, and prominent (Figs. 30-10 and 30-15). Regenerating muscle fibers are also distinguished by the expression of vimentin and desmin, both intermediate filament proteins, neural cell adhesion molecule (NCAM) isoforms, thrombomodulin, midkine, class I MHC molecules, and fetal myosin isoforms. As the fiber matures, vimentin expression disappears, desmin expression becomes attenuated, NCAM expression becomes confined to the region of the neuromuscular junction, class I MHC expression disappears, and adult myosin isoforms are expressed.[23a–f]

Extensive regeneration can occur by proliferation of the surviving muscle nuclei, by extensions from the intact portion of the fiber (muscle budding), and by rebuilding and reorganization of the contractile substance within a framework of a chain of surrounding cells (Fig. 30-15). The characteristic basophilia of the cytoplasm corresponds to the concentration of polysomes and ribosomes in these fibers. These ribonucleoprotein granules represent the precursor building materials of the contractile filaments. The most effective regeneration of muscle occurs when there are supporting cells surrounding the muscle cell to serve as guides to preserve the configuration and the direction of the muscle fiber growth. In such a circumscribed lesion, the extensive proliferation of fibroblasts is lacking.

It appears that the size of the area to be repaired and the degree to which muscle architecture is destroyed are the most important factors governing collagen proliferation. The new growth of fibrous tissue in muscle following injury forms a major obstacle to its reorganization. The larger the devastated area, the more massive the proliferation of collagen. In the course of muscle regeneration, when portions of muscle fibers are separated from each other, the budding and sprouting of myofibrils extend from the ends of existing muscle fibers in an attempt to bridge the gap (Fig. 30-15). The proliferation of collagen across their path inhibits the formation of muscle bridges and prevents the growth to maturity of the young muscle fibers. Muscle sprouts attempt to circumvent the barrier of fibrosis by means of abortive regeneration, but their activity is not effective in large lesions. A small lesion in muscle will usually undergo repair without leaving scar tissue, whereas a large lesion will result in repair by connective tissue replacement. Not infrequently an embryonal form of regeneration is detected in which mononuclear stellate cells with basophilic cytoplasm (myoblasts) form clusters, along with thin fibers containing small amounts of contractile substance, large nuclei, and prominent nucleoli (myotubes). The presence of the mononuclear muscle cells and the myotubes represents a form of regeneration that is referred to as *embryonal*. This particular process of repair and rebuilding of muscle by the fusion of myoblasts and myotubes in an attempt to form more mature muscle fibers is identical to the process by which the muscle fiber develops in early fetal life. The term *satellite cell* is used synonymously for myoblast, presumptive myoblast, or myoblast stem cell. It is usually assumed that the resting satellite cell of muscle is activated when the muscle fiber is damaged and that it plays a major role in the regeneration of the muscle fiber.

Current interest in muscle regeneration has been kindled by the discovery of the basic defect in Duchenne muscular dystrophy and the expectation that the transfer of normal myogenic cells or the grafting of normal muscle tissue into dystrophic muscle might restore the protein dystrophin. Early studies of myoblast implantation, both in mdx mice and in young boys with Duchenne dystrophy, have identified small clusters of dystrophin-positive muscle fibers in the myoblast-injected muscle but not in the contralateral sham-injected muscle.[24,25,26] However, there were obvious practical problems with this approach (Reviewed in Chap. 34). It is now known that satellite cells are heterogeneous and that a small subpopulation of these cells display stem cell characteristics.[27] The possible relevance of this finding to the treatment of muscular dystrophy is considered in Chaps. 3 and 34 as well as in recent publications.[28,28a]

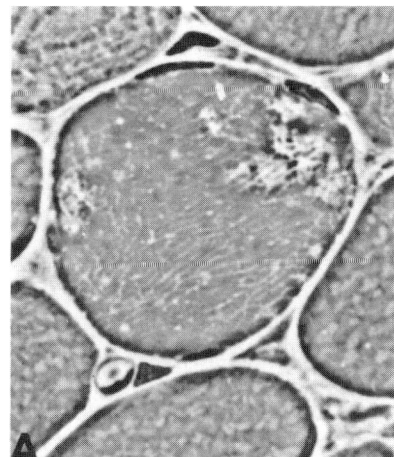
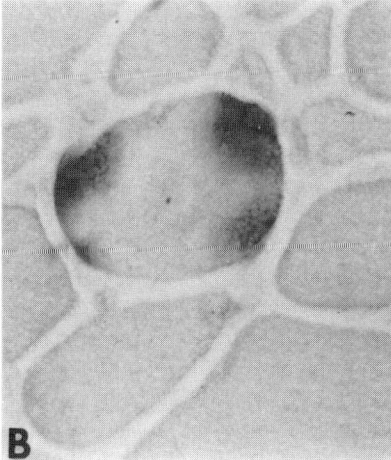
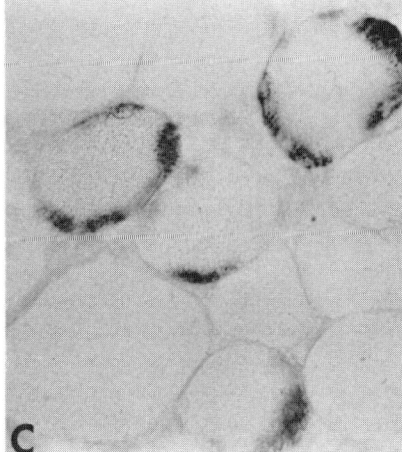

FIGURE 30-12. Focal subsarcolemmal abnormalities in muscle fibers in Duchenne dystrophy. *A.* Phase micrograph. *B* and *C.* Stained for calcium with alizarin red *(B)* and with glyoxal-bis-(o-hydroxyanil) *(C)*. The abnormal regions are crescent or wedge-shaped with their base nesting on the fiber surface. These regions appear rarified in A and show calcium overloading in B and C. A, ×980; B, ×475; C, ×300. *(B and C from Bodensteiner J, Engel A: Neurology 28:439, 1978. Reproduced by permission.)*

Variation in Diameter of Muscle Fibers within Each Fasciculus

The degree of intrafascicular variation in muscle fiber diameter depends upon the type of disorder and the stage of the disease (Figs. 30-5 and 30-6). This variation is a major feature of all dystrophies and is greatest in degree in the Duchenne type, with fibers ranging from 3 to 100 μm within a single fasciculus. In the various congenital myopathies and endocrine myopathies, this feature is much less prominent.

The mechanism of formation of the large and small fibers is really not well understood. Some small fibers represent the products of degeneration of muscle fibers as well as ineffective attempts at regeneration. Numerous small fibers appear in various stages of development. Others are quite mature yet small. Still others, when followed in serial section, represent branches of a larger master fiber. Occasional large fibers, on the other hand, can be observed in lateral apposition to more primitive fibers, their plasma membranes being in various stages of union. This process, by which muscle fibers fuse at their lateral margins, is the same as that by which fetal fibers increase in girth. Other fibers are enlarged yet have a normal architecture.

Accumulation of Lipofuscin and Ceroid

The terms *lipofuscin* and *ceroid* are used synonymously to describe certain yellow-brown pigments that accumulate within various tissues. These pigments are derived from lipid or lipoprotein sources and represent the end products of peroxidation of unsaturated fatty acids present in organelles, primarily lysosomes. Ceroid represents an intermediate stage between the auto-oxidizing lipid and the lipofuscin. In normal muscle, the pigment granules are often found in a paranuclear location or under the sarcolemma. The collections of pigment are irregular in outline and heterogeneous in content, consisting of extremely dense bodies of varying sizes embedded in a matrix of somewhat lower density. They are bounded by a single membrane. The collections are acid-fast and insoluble in acid, alkali, and fat solvents. They fluoresce a golden brown in ultraviolet light, stain with fat-soluble dyes, and are strongly positive with the periodic acid–Schiff (PAS) stain. Acid phosphatase activity is present in the region of the deposits. The collections occur more frequently in type 1 than in type 2 fibers.[29]

The current concept is that lipofuscin-ceroid pigments represent deposits of insoluble residues that are derived

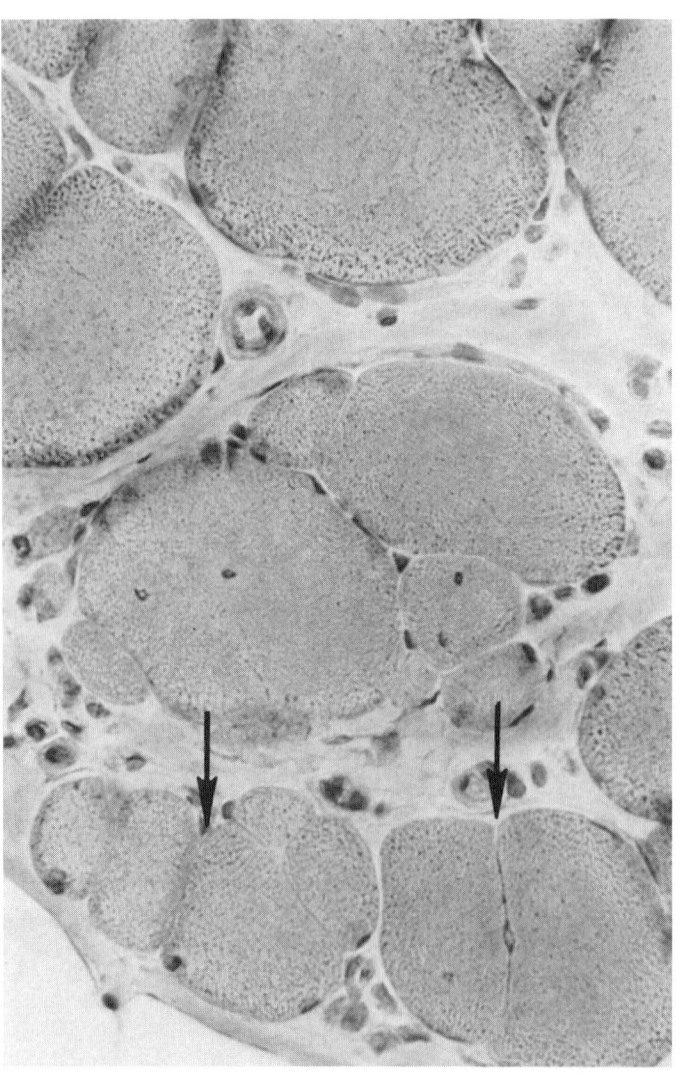

FIGURE 30-13. Many muscle fibers have undergone longitudinal splitting (arrows). Variation in muscle fiber diameter is also a conspicuous feature. Duchenne muscular dystrophy. Gomori trichrome stain. ×390.

from the intracellular degradation of waste products. These accumulations are quite nonspecific. Such deposits are found in normal muscle, increase with age, and are accentuated in vitamin E deficiency and in practically all primary and secondary disorders of muscle. It is not known whether the process leading to lipofuscin collections adversely affects the functional capacity of the muscle fiber.

Ringbinden (Ring Fibers or Spiral Annulets)

The term *ringbinden* designates a peripheral band of myofibrils that encircle a central longitudinal core of normally oriented fibrils (Fig. 30-16). These circumferentially oriented fibers are found in all types of muscular dystrophy, in various myopathies, as well as in muscle undergoing regeneration. Ringbinden are observed most frequently in myotonic dystrophy[30,31] and are detected readily by light or phase microscopy. The abnormal arrangement of myofibrils is best visualized in transverse sections as a circular or concentric striated coil ringing the periphery at right angles to the cross-sectional plane of the muscle fiber. Sections reacted for oxidative enzymes display the ring formations clearly. The presence of ring formations signals a preceding fiber injury followed by reorganization of the fiber architecture and failure of the cytoskeleton to align the myofibrils correctly.

Sarcoplasmic Masses

Sarcoplasmic masses can be detected by phase or light microscopy. The muscle fibers when viewed in cross section display a concentration of sarcoplasm in the subsarcolemmal area (Fig. 30-17). The masses border the more central myofibrils or completely circumscribe the muscle fibers and are relatively free of myofibrils (Fig. 30-17). When frozen tissue is sectioned by cryostat technique, the sarcoplasmic mass has a homogeneous, faintly fibrillar appearance (Fig. 30-17). The lighter-staining mass can be distinguished from the darker staining of the bordering and intact myofibrils. When studied by histochemical techniques,[32,33] the sarcoplasmic mass shows increased oxidative and glycolytic enzyme activity. Bundles of myofilaments that are trapped in these areas are disorganized and in complete disarray. Tubular structures and accumulations of lysosomes and lipofuscin are noted in the mass as well. Although sarcoplasmic masses have been observed in muscular dystrophies such as limb girdle dystrophy and in hypothyroid myopathy, they occur most frequently in myotonic dystrophy.

Lobulated Fibers

These fibers represent a nonspecific change in muscle. In the facioscapulohumeral and limb girdle forms of muscular dystrophy, and especially in calpainopathies, lobulated fibers are often conspicuous[34]; they are also present in myotonic muscular dystrophy and in other chronic myopathies. The lobulated fibers are usually type 1 muscle fibers. Their diameter is often smaller than the average diameter of the fibers in the biopsied muscle. The characteristics of the lobulated fiber are best appreciated by studying muscle in cross section (Fig. 30-18). Lakes of oxidative enzyme activity in the sarcoplasm under the sarcolemma and in sarcoplasmic seams that extend into the interior of the muscle fiber impart a lobulated appearance to the muscle fiber. In longitudinal

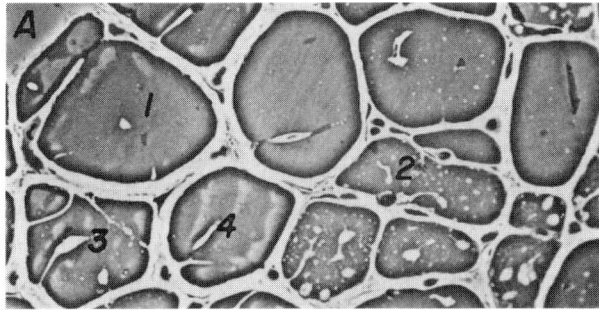
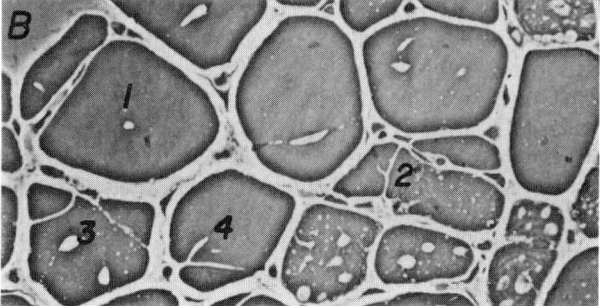

FIGURE 30-14. Fiber splitting in adult acid maltase deficiency; *A* and *B* are nonconsecutive serial sections. Fibers 1 and 2 are incompletely split in *A* and completely split in *B*. Fibers 3 and 4 containing slitlike spaces are partially split in both *A* and *B*. ×390. (Engel AG, Dale AJ; Mayo Clin Proc 43:233, 1968. Reproduced by permission.)

section, bundles of myofibrils are observed to run an aberrant course and the bundles constitute the boundaries of the lobules. The changes persist throughout the length of the muscle fiber. These alterations, like the ring formations, signal antecedent muscle fiber injury followed by incorrect alignment of the myofibrils with the cytoskeleton.

Moth-Eaten Fibers

The term *moth-eaten* has been applied to muscle fibers that show multiple patches of decreased oxidative enzyme activity (Fig. 30-19). The abnormal areas are pleomorphic in shape and size and extend for varying, but relatively short, distances along the long axis of the muscle fiber. They are detected in such diverse disorders as facioscapulohumeral dystrophy, limb girdle dystrophy, oculopharyngeal dystrophy, and malignant hyperthermia. The zones of decreased enzyme activity lack mitochondria and often display disorganization of contractile substance. The individual lesions in such fibers are essentially identical to multicores (see Multicores, below).

Cytoplasmic Bodies

Cytoplasmic bodies represent an alteration in the cytoplasm of the muscle fiber.[35,36] They are located under the plasma membrane or within the more central myofibrils (Fig. 30-20). There are varying degrees of Z-band streaming within the muscle fibers that contain the bodies. The structural continuity of cytoplasmic bodies to Z bands has been well documented.[36] Three distinct zones can be appreciated in the cytoplasmic body by light microscopy.[36,37] The central portion, or the core, is homogeneous, dense, and accentuated by hematoxylin stains. A halo of relatively decreased density, observed as a clear zone, circumscribes the core. The outer zone consists of distorted fibrils (Fig. 30-20B). Cytoplasmic bodies are observed in all fiber types. No enzymatic activity is displayed within the central zone. In the surrounding area, the myofibrillar ATPase activity is accentuated. By phase microscopy, the dense core is surrounded by a zone of decreased lucency (Fig. 30-20B).

These bodies have been observed in such diverse disorders as denervation atrophy, inflammatory myopathy, myotonic dystrophy and other forms of progressive muscular dystrophy, periodic paralysis, Menkes kinky hair disease, and mitochondrial myopathies. Because of their predominance in a particular myopathy, the term *cytoplasmic body myopathy* has been applied to that disorder (see Chap. 43).

Z-Band Streaming

The Z disk, or Z line, is a dense structure that divides each I band transversely at its midpoint and marks the boundary between contiguous sarcomeres. Z-band streaming is one of the commonest pathologic reactions of the muscle fiber. It is a sign of focal myofibrillar degeneration and is frequently associated with a focal loss of mitochondria.[37] It can be recognized in longitudinally oriented muscle fibers by polarization optics in H&E–stained paraffin sections, in bright field optics in trichrome, or phosphotungstic acid hematoxylin (PTAH)–stained paraffin sections and by phase microscopy in resin-embedded sections (Fig. 30-21). The abnormality appears as

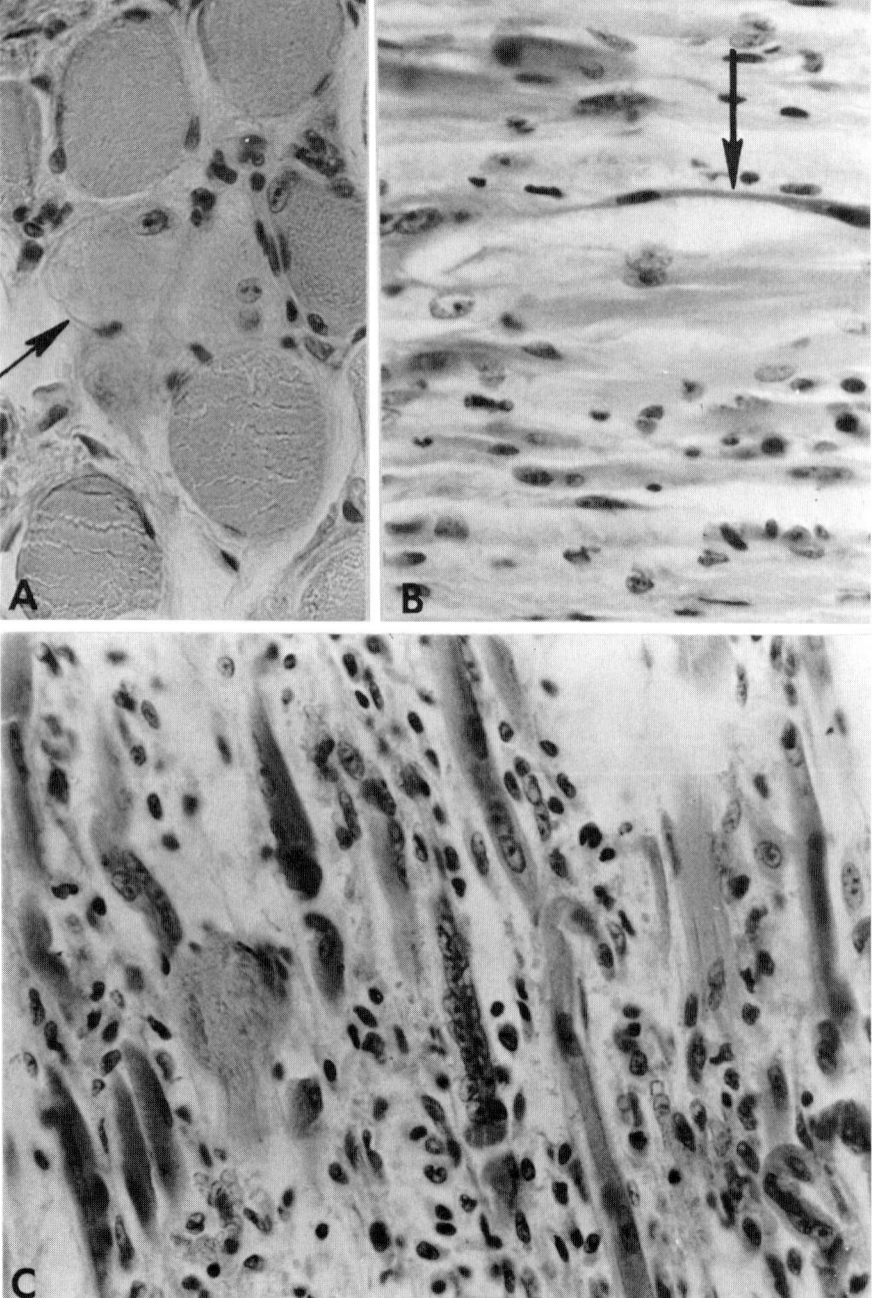

FIGURE 30-15. *A*. Early regenerative changes can be observed in two muscle fibers (arrow). The nuclei are large and the nucleoli prominent. ×350 *B*. A thin extension of regenerating muscle projects across an area of destruction (arrow). ×330. *C*. Muscle nuclei are numerous and nucleoli are prominent in these young fibers that are attempting to transverse a damaged region of muscle. ×370. H&E stain.

an extension of dense Z-disk material into one or both contiguous I band(s). In more advanced lesions the abnormal material spreads through the entire sarcomere; I and Z disks in multiple adjacent sarcomeres in the same and adjacent myofibrils are affected. The nonspecificity of Z-band streaming has been emphasized,[37,38] and the alteration may also appear in normal muscle.[38]

Inclusions in Myofibrillar Myopathy

The light microscopic features consist of multiple abnormal fiber regions of varying shape and size within which normal myofibrillar markings are replaced by amorphous or granular material or pleomorphic hyaline deposits. The majority of the abnormal fiber regions react positively for myotilin, desmin, αB-crystallin, dystrophin, NCAM, β-amyloid precursor protein, prion protein, CDC2 kinase, gelsolin, and ubiquitin, and many are strikingly congophilic (Color Plate 10). Other frequently associated features consist of rimmed vacuoles and signs of denervation atrophy.[38a] Ultrastructural features and the associated clinical and genetic features are discussed further in Chaps. 31 and 43.

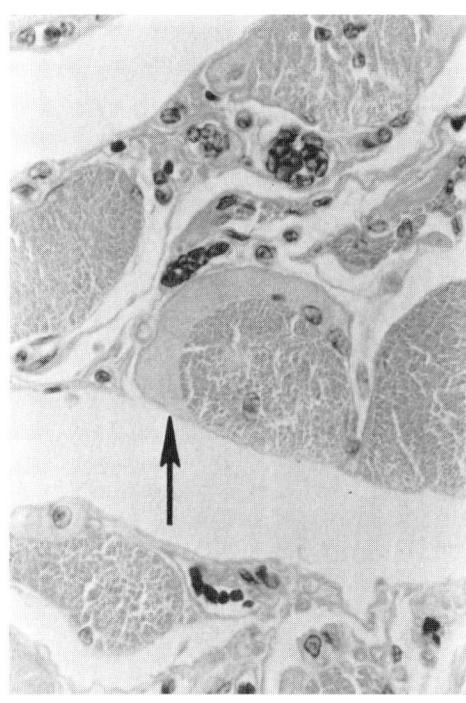

FIGURE 30-17. A sarcoplasmic mass (arrow) consisting of a pad of homogeneous substance that separates the contractile substance from the sarcolemma. Myotonic dystrophy. H&E stain. ×450.

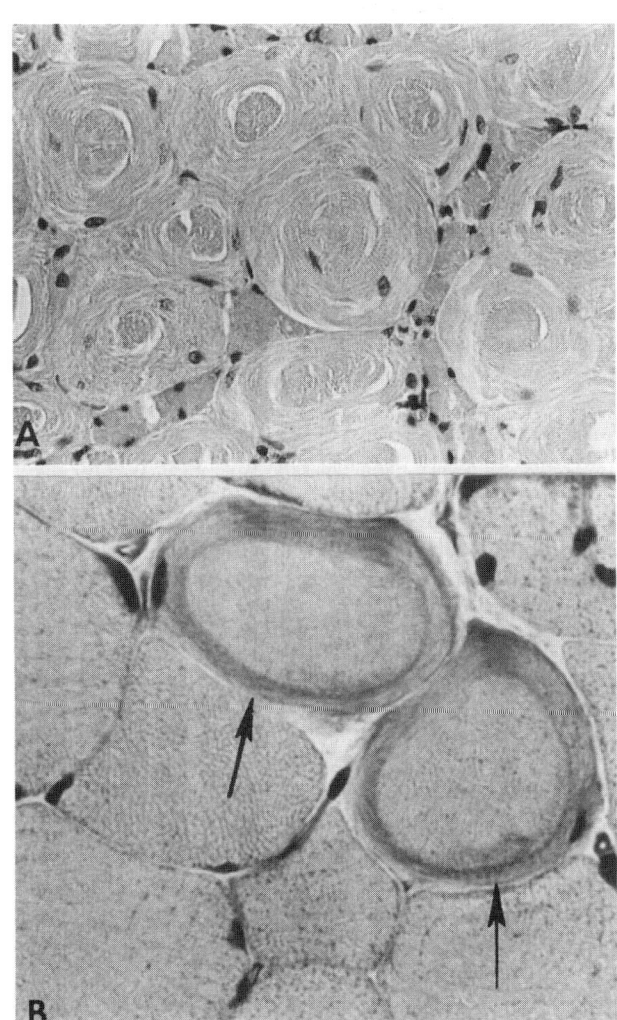

FIGURE 30-16. Peripheral bands of myofibrils (arrows) ring a central core of longitudinally oriented fibrils (ringbinden). Myotonic dystrophy. H&E stain. *A*, ×380; *B*, ×630.

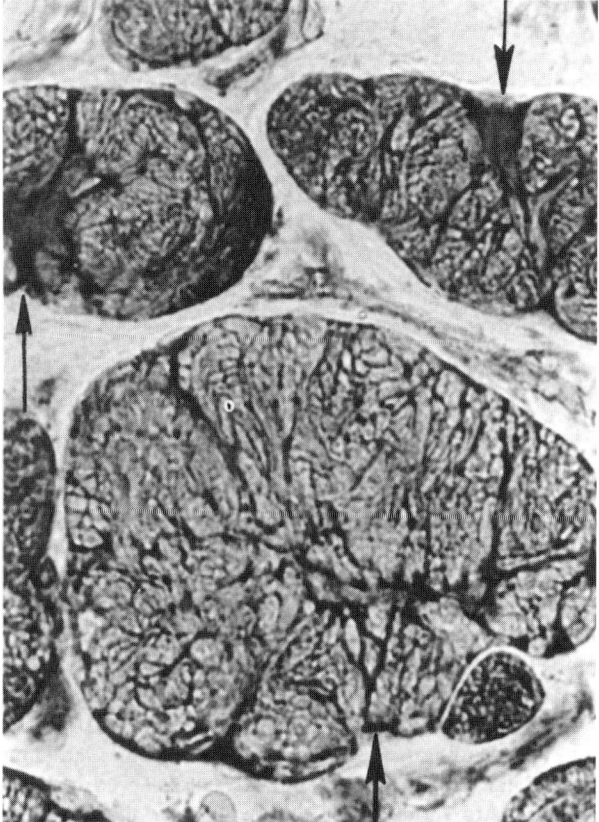

FIGURE 30-18. There are three lobulated fibers in this field (arrows). Seams consisting of lakes of oxidative enzyme activity penetrate the fibers and distort their contours. NADH dehydrogenase. ×720.

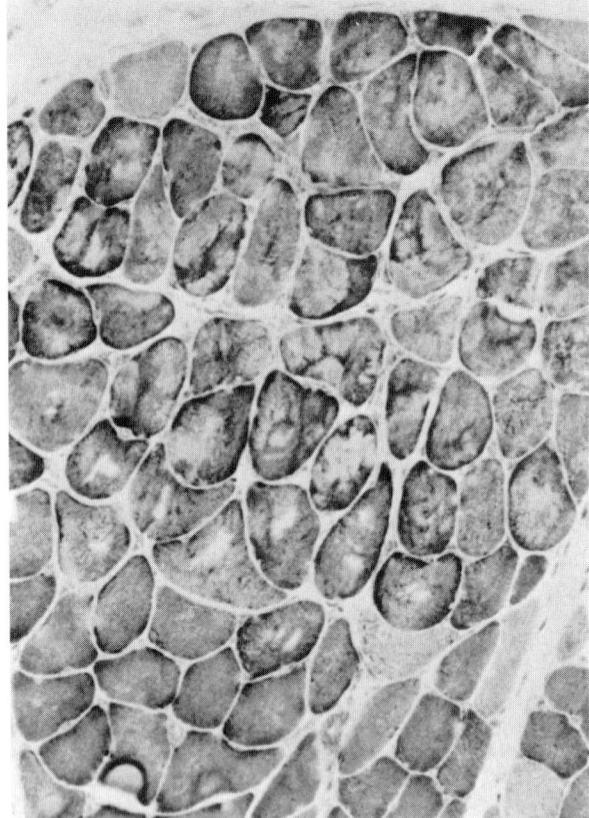

FIGURE 30-19. Multiple small focal decreases of NADH dehydrogenase activity occur in numerous muscle fibers. The affected fibers have a moth-eaten appearance. Dermatomyositis. ×120.

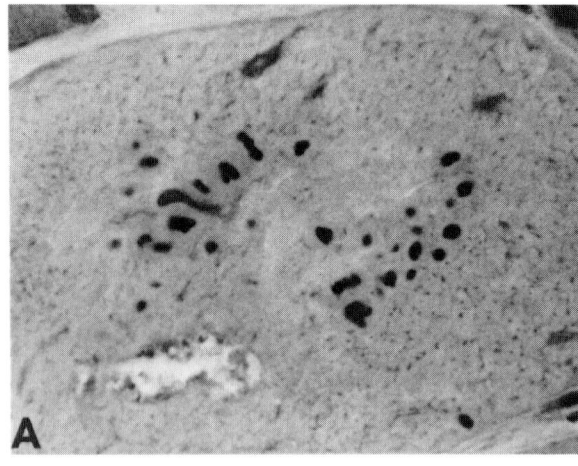

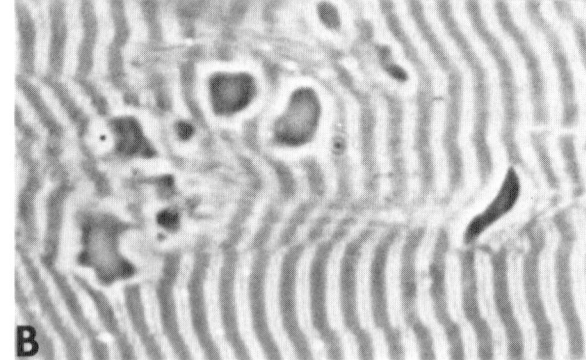

FIGURE 30-20. Cytoplasmic bodies in a trichrome-stained frozen section (A) and in a resin section viewed in phase optics (B). The affected fiber in A also contains a rimmed vacuole. The cytoplasmic bodies are pleomorphic in shape and size and are surrounded by a clear halo. A, ×700; B, ×1300.

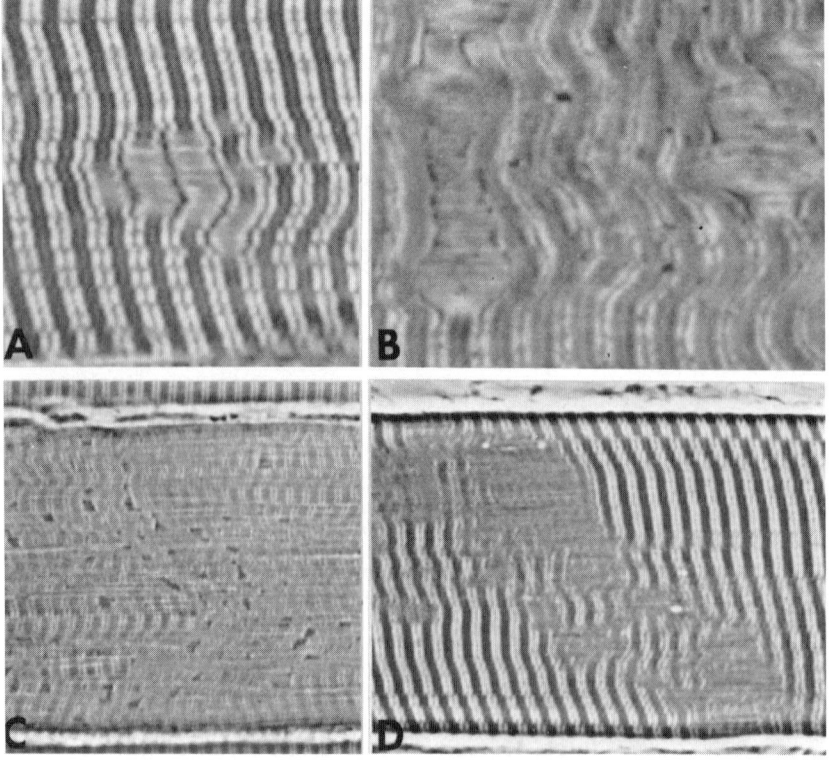

FIGURE 30-21. Focal Z-disk streaming and focal myofibrillar degeneration seen in phase-contrast micrographs. In the abnormal fiber regions the sarcomeres are obscured by optically dense material of Z-disk origin. A. A small lesion involves adjacent sarcomeres in several myofibrils. ×1300. B. Two separate narrow lesions involve several sarcomeres between adjacent Z disks. The affected sarcomeres are stretched and irregularly widened. Where the lesions are widest, the Z disks have completely disintegrated. ×2300. C. A muscle fiber shows numerous early lesions. Narrow bands of optically dense abnormal material simulate nemaline rods. ×940. D. A fiber contains a large lesion. The lesion has irregular outlines and may have arisen by the coalescence of adjacent smaller lesions. (Engel AG: Excerpta Medica International Congress Series 147:398, 1967. Reproduced by permission.)

Rod Body Formation

Rods or rod bodies were first described as the characteristic muscle alteration in nemaline or rod body myopathy[39,40] (Fig. 30-22B and C). Rod bodies also occur as a nonspecific alteration of the myofibril in a number of other unrelated disorders. The rods measure 0.5 to 3 μm in width and up to 7 μm in length and arise in the Z disk (Fig. 30-22D). They are more clearly defined than the irregular components of Z–band streaming. The rods cluster in subsarcolemmal (Fig. 30-23) and paranuclear locations within the muscle fiber (Fig. 30-22A and B). They are usually oriented with their long axis perpendicular to the Z band (Fig. 30-22C, D, and E). In the trichrome-stained cryostat sections, the rods appear a darker blue-green than the normal myofibrils. When the sections are as thin as 5 μm, the rods appear red while the myofibrils remain green to blue. When subjected to polarized light, the rods and the myofibrils are anisotropic. They are clearly seen in resin sections viewed by phase optics (Fig. 30-22D and E). The rod bodies can also be demonstrated in Zenker- or Bouin-fixed muscle that has been embedded in paraffin and stained by PTAH (Fig. 30-22C; Color Plate 7A and B) or a trichrome. The H&E stain fails to outline the rod bodies, nor are they detailed by ATPase, phosphorylase, or oxidative enzyme techniques.

Central Cores

These alterations are characterized by circular zones or cores and are limited to type 1 fibers (Fig. 30-24). Within the cores there is neither oxidative enzyme (Color Plate 7C; Fig. 30-24A and B) nor phophorylase activity and the myofibrillar ATPase activity (pH 9.4) is normal or decreased. The trichrome technique applied to unfixed frozen muscle outlines the cores and separates them from the normal contractile substance (Fig. 30-24C). In Zenker- or Bouin-fixed muscle embedded in paraffin and stained with PTAH or trichrome techniques, the cores are accentuated. The cores are often central in position and extend the length of the muscle fiber (Color Plate 7C). There may be one or, less often, several cores in a single fiber.

The most consistent feature of the cores is a sharply circumscribed decrease in oxidative enzyme activity that extends for at least the length of the fiber represented in the biopsy specimen. For a given core formation, the area of mitochondrial loss is always as large as or larger than the area in which other organelles are affected. The cores are either structured

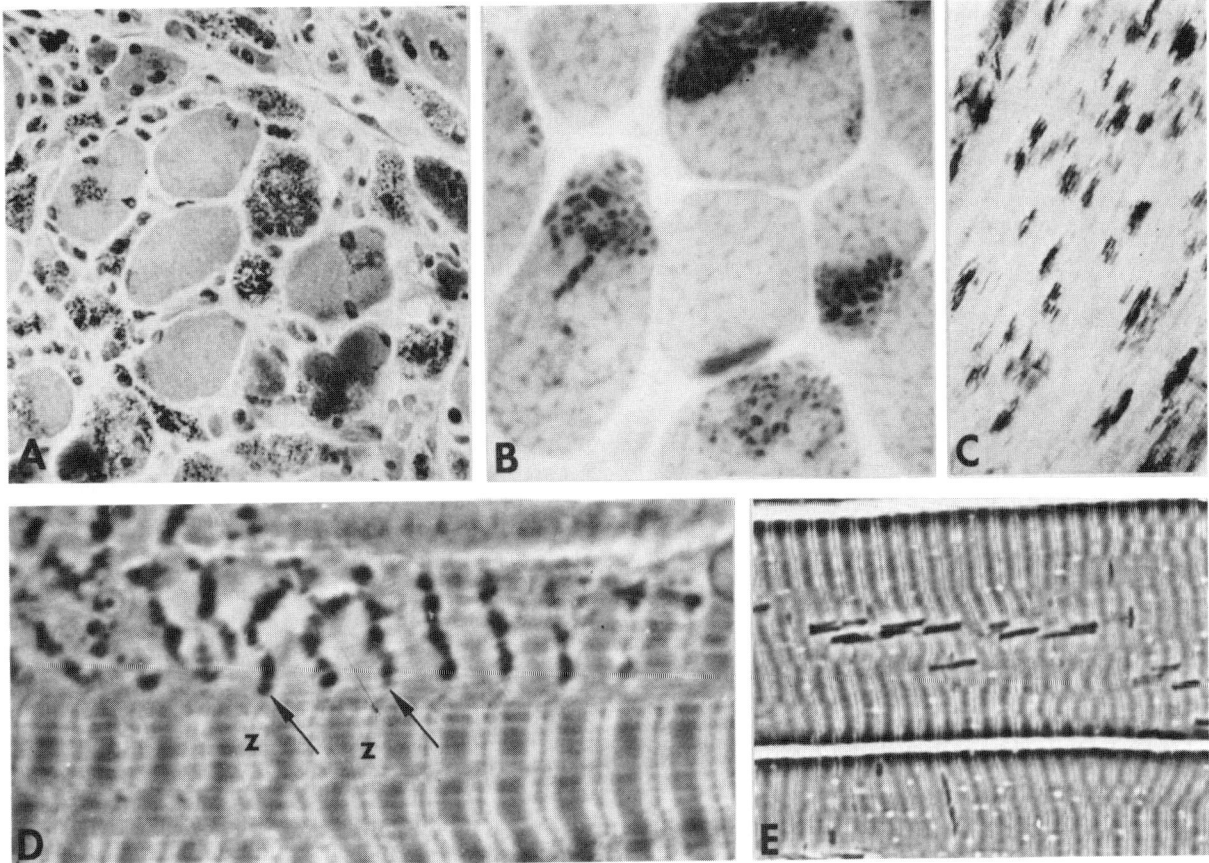

FIGURE 30-22. Nemaline rods demonstrated in trichrome-stained frozen sections (A, B), in phosphotungstic acid–hematoxylin–stained paraffin section (C), and in resin sections viewed in phase optics (D, E). A and D are from patients with late-onset nemaline myopathy; B, C, and E are from patients with congenital nemaline myopathy. In transverse sections (A, B) the long axis of most rods is perpendicular to the plane of the section and, therefore, the rods have circular or irregularly polygonal profiles. In longitudinal sections (C, D, E) the long axis of most rods is parallel to the plane of the section. The origin of the rods from the Z disk is clearly shown in D. Arrows indicate the regions where rod-bearing portions of the Z disk are continuous with normal Z disks. In E, numerous rods extend as many as three sarcomeres. A, ×300; B, ×1500; C, ×300; D, ×2400; E, ×1100. (D is reprinted from Engel AG: Mayo Clinic Proc 47:713, 1966. Reproduced by permission. E is reprinted from Engel AG, Gomez MR: J Neuropathol Exp Neurol 25:601 1967. Reproduced by permission.)

or nonstructured. In the structured core, the pattern of cross striations is quite normal except for the Z band, which appears slightly widened and irregular, and the sarcomeres within the core are usually increased in number in comparison with the adjacent myofibrils. Glycogen and mitochondria are usually decreased or absent in the altered zone. In the unstructured core, the pattern of cross striations is obliterated and mitochondria and glycogen are lacking in the central zone; in the non core areas, all cytochemical reactions are normal.

The unstructured cores, like central zones of target formations, react positively for desmin, dystrophin, and αB-crystallin, and show enhanced reactivity for actin and α-actinin.[40a,b]

Multicores

Multicores consist of numerous small areas of decreased oxidative enzyme activity, some of which also show myofibrillar degeneration. (Fig. 30-25; Color Plate 7D). The latter, when present, is always within the confines of, and usually smaller than, the area of decreased oxidative enzyme activity. The small cores can be observed in both types 1 and 2 fibers.[41] The long axis of the lesion is perpendicular or parallel to the long axis of the muscle fiber. Oxidative enzyme activity as demonstrated by succinic or NADH dehydrogenase is depleted within the cores (Figs. 30-25 and 30-26). Myofibrillar ATPase activity is frequently decreased in the affected zones. Glycogen as demonstrated by PAS or Best carmine technique or phosphorylase activity are reduced in the altered zones.

Paraffin sections stained with H&E reveal only small foci of pallor within muscle fiber (Fig. 30-27); the pale areas may be difficult to differentiate from a staining artifact. However,

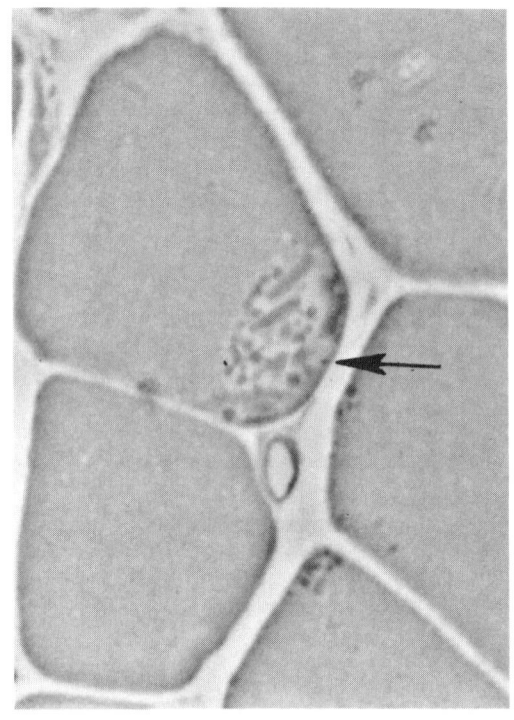

FIGURE 30-23. A subsarcolemmal collection of rod bodies is clearly defined (arrow). Other fibers contain smaller collections of rods. Nemaline myopathy. Phase-contrast microscopy. ×1800.

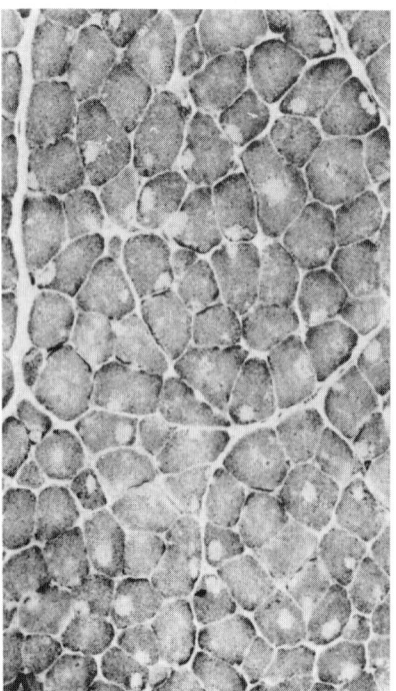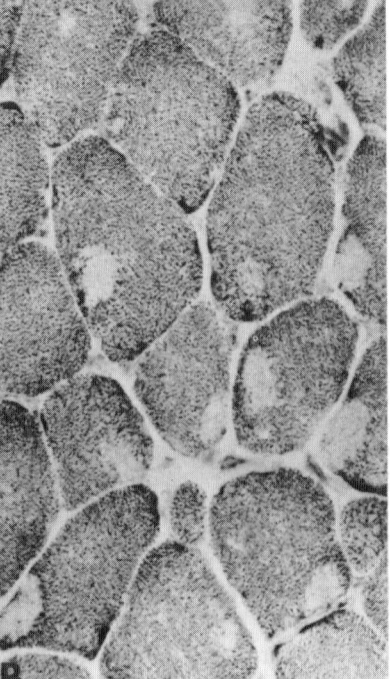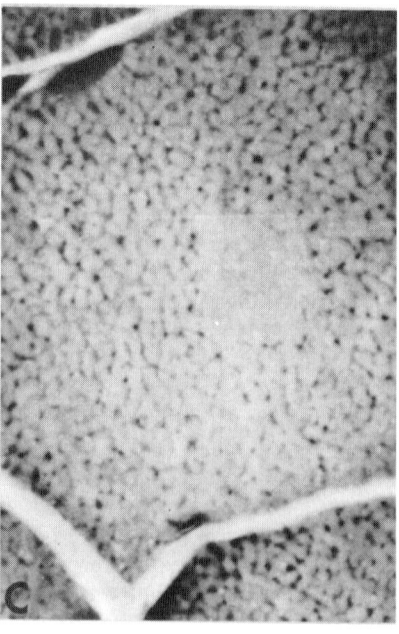

FIGURE 30-24. Central core disease. Frozen sections stained with NADH dehydrogenase (A, B) and trichrome (C). All muscle fibers in these structures react uniformly for NADH dehydrogenase; nearly all fibers contain a core, and enzyme activity is absent from all cores (A, B). Intermyofibrillar membranous material is markedly attenuated in the core (C). A, ×110; B, ×280; C, ×1100.

if the paraffin-embedded material is studied in longitudinal sections by polarization microscopy (Fig. 30-27B, C, and D), the foci are accentuated and the loss of cross striations in these regions can be appreciated.[41] These zones usually measure 5 to 7 μm in length; those 75 μm long or even longer occur but are exceptions. The majority of the cores are 20 μm in diameter or less, but some are as large as those in central core disease. The multicores share one feature with central cores and targets (see "Target Fibers," below): the mitochondria are depleted and the oxidative enzyme activity is abolished within the multiple small cores (Fig. 30-25). The multicores are smaller and more numerous than central cores and extend only a short distance along the long axis of the fiber.[41] Unlike central cores and targets, multicores can be oriented with their long axis perpendicular to the long axis of the muscle fiber (Fig. 30-25B).

The multicores (like moth-eaten fibers) represent a nonspecific change in that they can be observed in various unrelated muscle disorders.[41] Multicores can be detected in the various types of muscular dystrophy as well as in the inflammatory myopathies and at various stages of denervation atrophy. Multicores have been produced in the muscle of rats given emetine or glucocorticoids.[42,43] Multicores have been observed in certain endocrine myopathies and other primary myopathies and represent the predominant alteration in a cogenital myopathy described by Engel et al.[41]

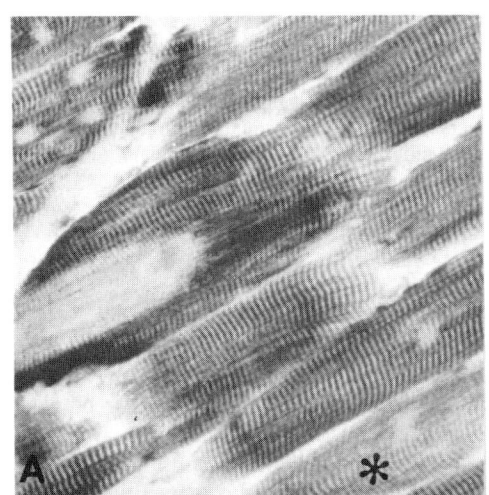
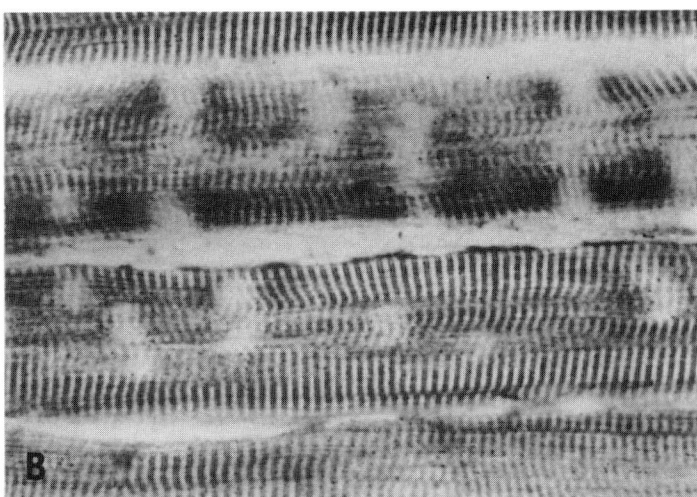
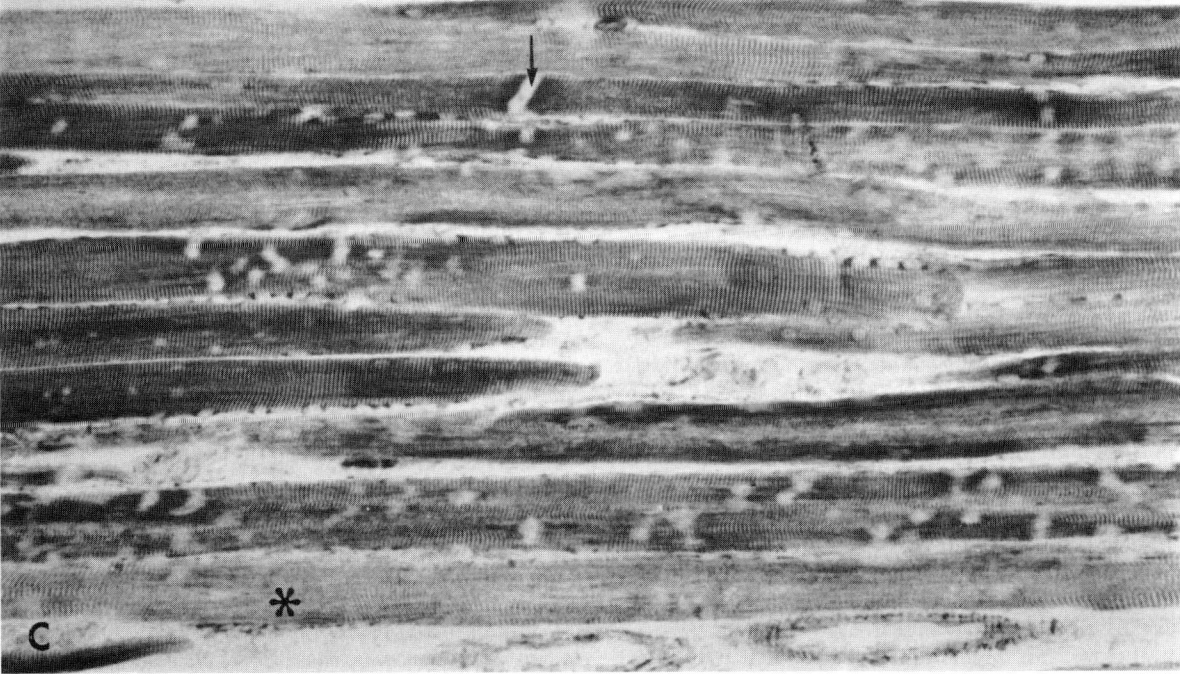

FIGURE 30-25. Multicore disease. Hydroxyadipaldehyde-fixed longitudinal sections processed for oxidative enzyme activity. Innumerable areas of decreased enzyme activity can be seen. Most abnormal areas are small. Large central lesion in fiber in A resembles central core. Some lesions are bandlike and extend across width of fiber (arrow). According to the intensity of the reaction, two histochemical fiber types can be seen. Less intensely reacting fibers (asterisks) are fewer but are also affected. A, ×340; B, ×520; C, ×230. (From Engel AG, Gomez MR, Groover RV: Mayo Clinic Proc 46:666, 1971. Reproduced by permission.)

Target Fibers

A change in the architecture of the muscle fiber occurs frequently in the course of reinnervation[44] (Fig. 30-28). The area of alteration, which usually occupies the center of the muscle fiber, is called a *target* and consists of three concentric zones. The innermost zone displays no mitochondrial (Fig. 30-28A), phosphorylase or ATPase (Fig. 30-28B) enzymatic activity. The activity is increased in the intermediate zone and is normal peripherally (Fig. 30-28A and B). The term *targetoid* has been applied to target fibers in which the intermediate zone is indistinct; the targetoid fibers are often observed together with target formations in reinnervated muscle.[44] Target fibers can also be detected by the Gomori trichrome technique (Fig. 30-28C). The central zones of the target formations react positively for desmin, dystrophin, and αB-crystallin, and show enhanced reactivity for actin and α-actinin.[40a,40b] Thus, their histochemical profile is similar to that of the unstructured cores and even in paraffin-embedded PTAH-stained sections.

Central cores and targets are also similar in that both affect the type 1 fiber and are elongated along the long axis of the fiber. A number of differences have been proposed between core and target formations. In a single muscle fiber there may be one to several cores but usually only one target. Target formations generally do not extend for the whole length of the muscle fiber, whereas core formations probably do. In the central core, the myofibrillar structures are in varying stages of disarray, yet the architecture is not totally abolished as it is in the central zone of the target fiber. The central cores contain only two major concentric zones, whereas the targets contain three. Although a small rim of increased oxidative enzyme reaction often rings the core, this concentric layer lacks the well-formed intermediate zone that characterizes the target fiber. Because targetoid fibers contain only two concentric zones instead of the three of the target fibers, they resemble the central cores.

The central zones of the target formations react positively for desmin, dystrophin, and αB-crystallin, and show enhanced reactivity for actin and α-actinin[40a,40b] Thus, their histochemical profile is similar to that of the unstructured cores. The basic alteration in cores, multicores, targets and targetoid fibers is a decrease in mitochondria within a circumscribed fiber region.(compare Figs. 30-24, 30-25, and 30-28)

However, the three-dimensional configuration of cores, targets/targetoids, and multicores is different, and it is this feature that is most useful in distinguishing between the different formations. Although it has been suggested that the extent of mitochondrial and myofibrillar alterations differs in each formation, strict and consistently reliable criteria based on these features have not been established.

Target and targetoid fibers are usually observed in the course of reinnervation but also have been produced experimentally by tenotomy.[45-48] They can also occur in such diverse conditions as the Lambert-Eaton myasthenic syndrome, myotonic dystrophy, and dermatomyositis.

Angulated Fibers

An angulated fiber is small in diameter and has concave sides. Fibers such as these may occur singly or in groups in certain stages of denervation atrophy (Fig. 30-29A and B). Some stain deeply with the oxidative enzyme techniques and lack phosphorylase activity and thus appear to be type 1 fibers. However, when subjected to the menadione-linked α-glycerophosphate dehydrogenase technique, they stain positively and do not show the expected reciprocal staining pattern for type 1 fibers. In addition, with the basic ATPase technique, they also display enzymatic activity. The angulated fibers usually display a strong nonspecific esterase activity.

Although the presence of small angulated fibers suggests a neurogenic process, these fibers are also detected in polymyositis, facioscapulohumeral dystrophy, myotonic dystrophy, oculopharyngeal dystrophy, Becker dystrophy, distal myopathy, and other myopathies (Fig. 30-5). In these primary disorders of muscle, the angulated fibers are randomly scattered within the fasciculi. Angulated fibers in the myopathies usually display the normal reciprocal staining pattern with menadione-linked α-glycerophosphate dehydrogenase and the oxidative enzyme techniques, in contrast to angulated fibers caused by denervation.

Fingerprint Bodies

Fingerprint bodies are inclusions not recognized in paraffin sections or by histochemical staining. They appear under the sarcolemma as dense foci when viewed by phase microscopy (Fig. 30-30). Frequently they are located in paranuclear position.[49] Fingerprint bodies measure 1 to 10 μm in length and 0.5 to 4 μm in width. They were recognized in about 50 percent of the muscle fibers in the fingerprint myopathy described by Engel at al.[49] These inclusions have also been detected in other myopathies,[50-53] where their presence has not constituted the predominant pathologic change that

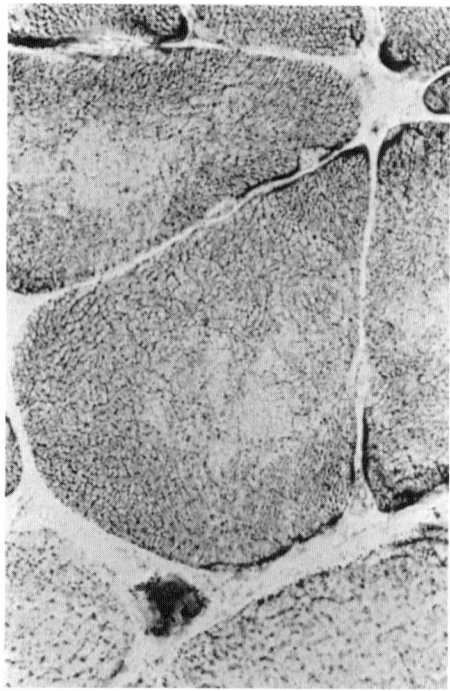

FIGURE 30-26. Multiple foci of decreased oxidative enzyme activity can be seen in three muscle fibers. Oculopharyngeal muscular dystrophy. NADH dehydrogenase. ×450.

characterizes the fingerprint myopathy.[49] Even though the presence of these bodies can be suspected by phase microscopy (Fig. 30-30), electron microscopic studies are essential for their identification.

Reducing Bodies

These inclusions characterize an uncommon myopathy appearing in infancy (see Chap. 54). H&E-stained sections of muscle reveal flocculent eosinophilic bodies under the sarcolemma of many muscle fibers. These bodies are round or oval in shape and many form caps at the outer edge of the muscle fiber. They are sharply demarcated from the normal muscle fiber. Occasional inclusions of this type are detected within muscle fibers undergoing degeneration.

The reducing bodies or inclusions stain strongly for glycogen and ribonucleic acid.[54] There is an intense reaction for α-glycerophosphate dehydrogenase (menadione-linked). Even when this latter reaction is carried out without substrate, the bodies are well outlined. Thus the inclusions contain a substance that is capable of reducing nitro-blue tetrazolium when mediated by menadione.[54] In addition, sulfhydryl groups can also be demonstrated within the inclusions.

Trilaminar Configurations

Fibers containing trilaminar configurations have been observed in a congenital myopathy. The abnormal fibers are enlarged and contain three distinct concentric zones.[55] Each zone stains uniformly and differently. When the central zone is stained with the trichrome technique, it is red; by oxidative enzyme techniques, it is dark. The central zone stains positively for lipid, glycogen, and phosphorylase and acid-phosphatase activity. The intermediate zone is green with

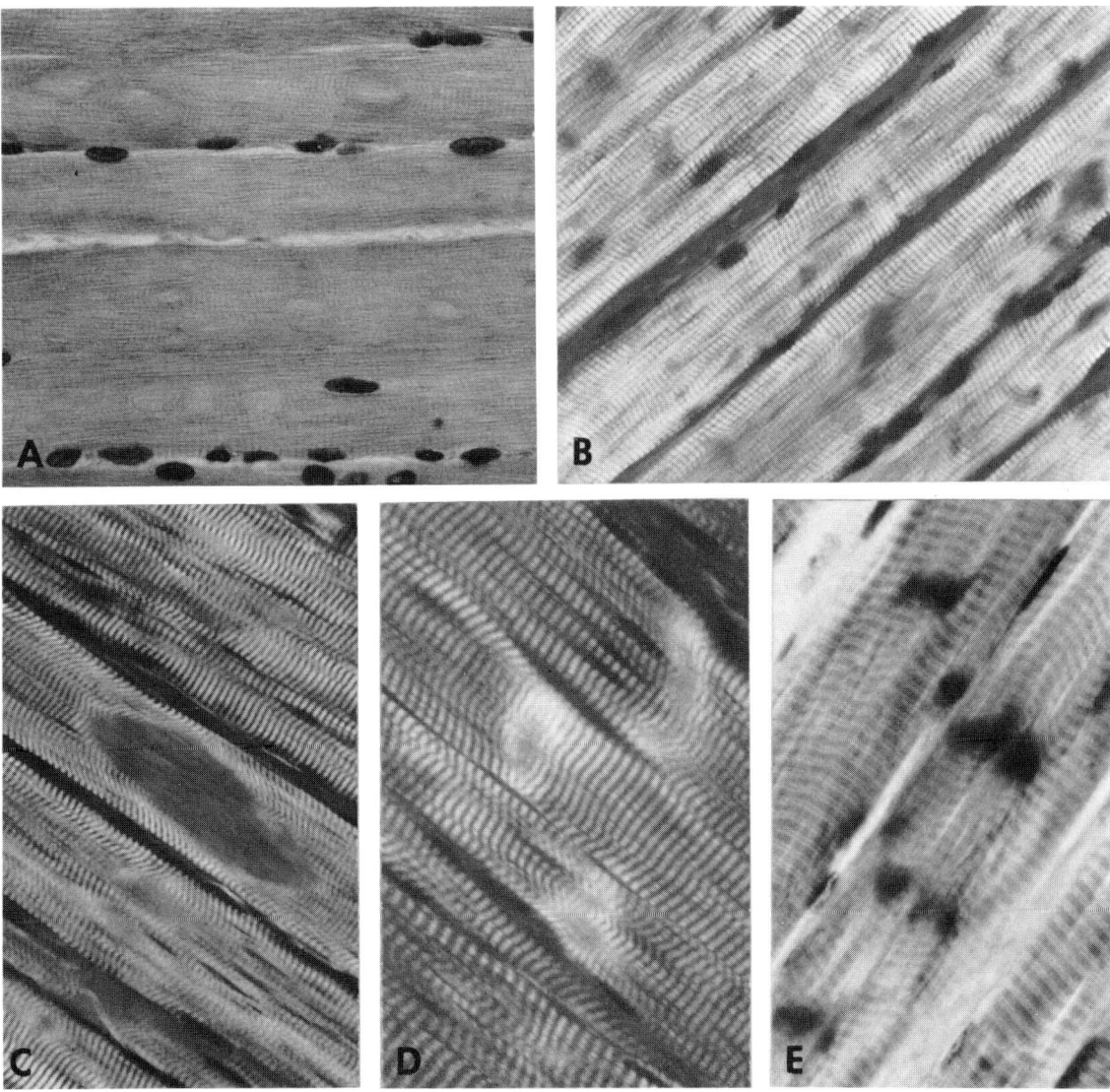

FIGURE 30-27. Focal loss of cross-striations observed in paraffin sections in multicore disease. The lesions are pallid and barely recognizable in section stained with H&E (A) but are seen as nonrefrigent areas in polarized light (B, C, and D). Fuchsinophilic material covers lesions after trichromatic staining (E). Most lesions are small and randomly distributed in the fibers. Large, centrally located lesion is seen in one fiber in C. A, ×44; B, ×510; C, ×370; D, ×600; E, ×750. (Engel AG et al: Mayo Clinic Proc 46:666, 1971. Reproduced by permission.)

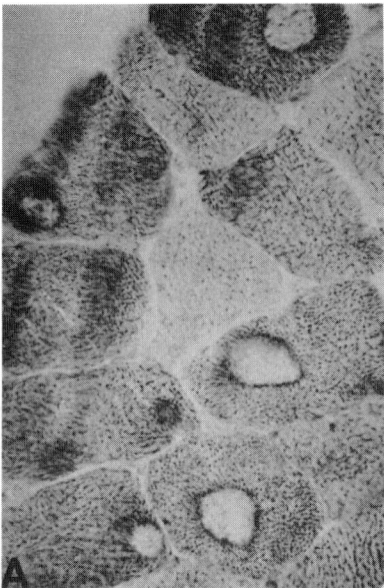 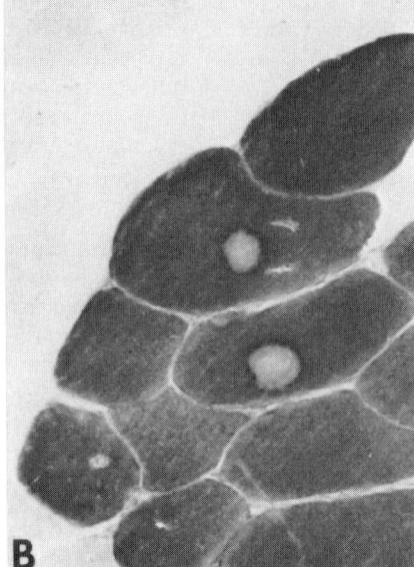 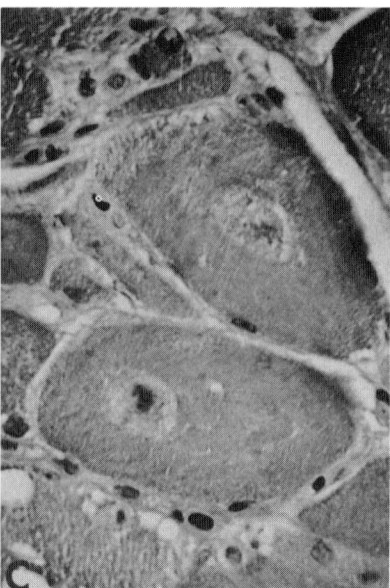

FIGURE 30-28. Target formations in cryostat sections reacted for NADH dehydrogenase (A) and for ATPase after preincubation at pH 4.3 (B) and in a trichrome-stained paraffin section (C). The target formations appear in the type 1 fibers and are surrounded by a rim of increased enzyme activity (A, B). Degenerating myofibrils in the center of the target appear dark in the trichrome stain. A, x250; B, x360; C, x480.

the trichrome stain, deep brown with the ATPase reaction at varying pH, and unreactive with all other enzyme techniques. The outer zone, which resembles a sarcoplasmic mass, stains purple with the trichrome, H&E, and methyl green-pyronin techniques. In this peripheral region, there are lipid bodies and glycogen granules as well as phosphorylase, esterase, and acid phosphatase activities. The array of colors elicited by light microscopy correlates well with the ultrastructural features.[55]

Tubular Aggregates

Tubular aggregates within muscle are found in a variety of disorders such as periodic paralysis, congenital myasthenic syndromes, muscle disorders associated with cramps, pain or stiffness, subacute alcoholic myopathy, or after exposure to various drugs.[56–58] The structural features of the aggregates are identical from case to case. Routinely embedded paraffin material stained by H&E reveal only subsarcolemmal areas devoid of stain. Such zones are easily overlooked or regarded as artifact. When cryostat-sectioned unfixed, frozen muscle is stained by H&E there are conspicuous basophilic zones under the sarcolemma of many fibers, and in some, similar zones occupy the more central portions of the fiber. These zones stain red with the trichrome technique. (Fig. 30-31A) and black with Sudan black. The aggregates react strongly for the NADH tetrazolium reductase (Fig. 30-31B) as well as by the myoadenylate deaminase, phosphofructokinase, and the nonspecific esterase techniques. The tubular aggregates also display activity for lactic dehydrogenase and cytochrome oxidase but not for succinic dehydrogenase or menadione-linked α-glycerophosphate dehydrogenase. The abundant enzymatic activity appears as a deeply stained mass that caps the muscle fibers and extends as threads into the interior (Fig. 30-31). These zones lack myofibrillar structures and thus do not react for the myofibrillar ATPase. Phosphorylase activity is absent from these areas and the aggregates cannot be demonstrated with the PAS stain. The aggregates are confined to the type 2 fibers in many myopathies,[56,57] whereas in others[58] they are observed in both type 1 and type 2 fibers.

Ragged Red Fibers

Ragged red fibers are best demonstrated in cryostat sections of unfixed, frozen muscle. The fibers are randomly distributed, irregular in outline, and display prominent subsarcolemmal and intermyofibrillar deposits of membranous material that stains red with the trichrome stain. The sarcoplasm appears fragmented as if there were artifactual cracking. The membranous material represents the accumulation of mitochondria beneath the sarcolemma and between the myofibrils (Fig. 30-32A and B; Color Plate 7E and F). Collections of glycogen and lipid are also conspicuous under the sarcolemma and between the myofibrils. Ragged red fibers are typically encountered in mitochondrial myopathies caused either by nuclear or mitochondrial DNA mutations involving the respiratory chain. However, they can also occur in adult acid maltase deficiency, in older patients with inflammatory myopathies, and especially in those with inclusion body myositis, as a nonspecific isolated finding in various myopathies, and in normal muscle where their frequency increases with age and reaches a maximum of about 0.4 percent by the eighth decade.[59] This probably reflects the accumulation of the deleted mitochondrial DNA with age.[60] In mitochondrial myopathies, the frequency of ragged red fibers varies widely, ranging from 1 to more than 30 percent of all fibers.

The mitochondria accumulating in ragged red fibers are frequently morphologically abnormal (i.e. abnormally large or harboring crystalloid or amorphous inclusions) and biochemically defective. In the case of heteroplastic mitochondrial DNA mutations, the mitochondrial DNA in the ragged red fibers is composed of an excess of mutant DNA and of variable amounts of wild-type DNA.[61,62] The enzyme cytochemical profile of the ragged red fiber depends on the underlying abnormality. Nuclear DNA mutations involving subunits coding for complex I, II, or IV of the respiratory chain may, respectively, result in reduced reactivity for NADH dehydrogenase, succinate dehydrogenase, or cytochrome c oxydase; but intense reactivity is detected for those respiratory enzymes whose translation is not affected by the mutation. In the case of heteroplastic mitochondrial DNA mutations (as in the Kearns-Sayre syndrome), the ragged red change in the fiber is segmental[62,62a] and the ragged-red-fiber segment can lose its reactivity for a given respiratory enzyme whether or not the mutation encompasses DNA encoding a subunit of the enzyme. Succinate dehydrogenase reactivity is typically preserved and conspicuous. Loss of enzyme reactivity is explained by the observation that the mutant DNA is globally incompetent for translation[63] and by the assumption that the mutant DNA is functionally dominant over the remaining wild-type mitochondrial genome.[62] For these reasons, the ragged red fibers may fail to react for cytochrome c oxydase in mitochondrial cytopathies (Fig. 30-32C and D), and are frequently cyto-

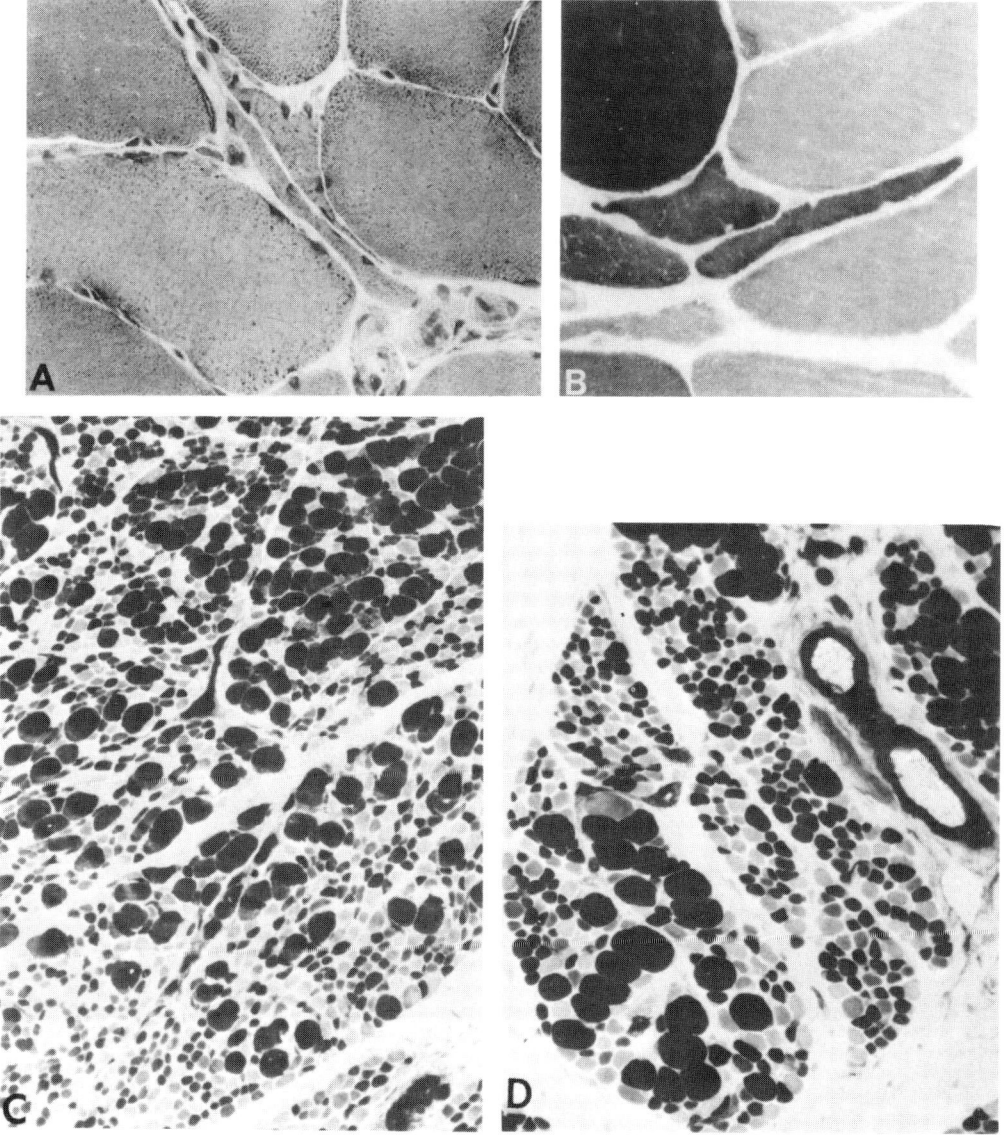

FIGURE 30-29. Neurogenic atrophy in early diabetic neuropathy. Trichrome-stained (A) and ATpase (pH 9.3)-reacted (B) cryostat sections. The small angulated fibers are of either histochemical type and are molded by the adjacent larger fibers. Denervation atrophy in Werdnig-Hoffman disease, ATPase (ph 4.2) (C and D). The small and often angular fibers predominate and contrast sharply with the hypertrophied fibers. The checkerboard pattern of histochemical activity is maintained in the small fibers; the large fibers are primarily type 1. A and B, ×284; C and D, ×205.

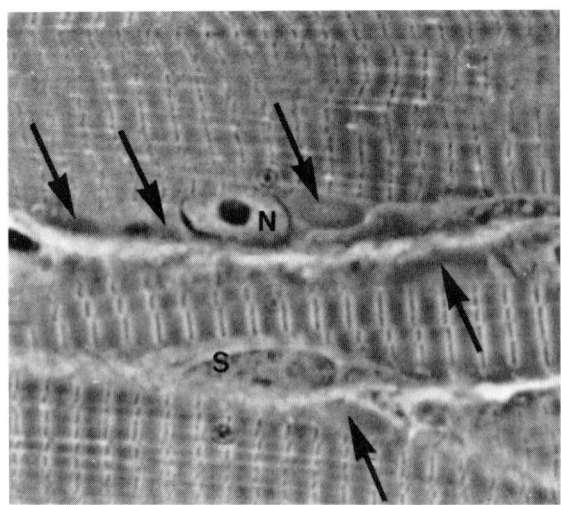

FIGURE 30-30. Five subsarcolemmal fingerprint bodies (arrow) appear in three muscle fibers. S = satellite cell; N = nucleus. Resin section viewed in phase optics. ×1800. (Engel AG et al: Mayo Clinic Proc 47:377, 1972. Reproduced by permission.)

chrome c oxidase-negative in those cytopathies associated with large-scale mitochondrial DNA deletions (Fig. 30-32E and F). Loss of cytochrome c oxidase reactivity also can occur without mitochondrial excess, i.e., in fibers that are not ragged red (Fig. 30-32E and F), indicating a more widespread distribution of abnormal mitochondria than suggested by the frequency of the ragged red fibers.[64]

Vacuoles

A vacuole is defined as an abnormal space or cavity within the muscle fiber that appears empty by at least one method of staining or examination. It is either a membrane limited space, the contents of which vary, or nonmembrane limited space that contains an excess of normal or abnormal cell components. Depending upon the method of fixation and staining, the vacuoles appear empty or partially empty when viewed by bright field (Figs. 30-33 through 30-38), phase, or even electron microscopy. The term *vacuolar myopathy* is applied when vacuoles represent the predominant pathologic feature, as in hypokalemic periodic paralysis.[65–67] On the other hand, vacuoles may be present but inconspicuous, as in oculopharyngeal muscular dystrophy. For this reason the term *vacuolar myopathy* is applied to hypokalemic periodic paralysis and not to oculopharyngeal dystrophy.

Vacuoles in muscle represent a common alteration and are found in a variety of nonrelated disorders. Any morphologic classification of vacuoles must take into account their size, shape, number, and location within the muscle fiber.[67] Also, it is important to note whether the space is enclosed by a membrane or rimmed by a basophilic substance. A determination of the contents of the vacuoles provides important information insofar as the vacuoles may serve as a repository for fat, glycogen, or other storage materials. Vacuoles may also harbor collections of degenerated cytoplasmic material, as in inclusion body myositis (Fig. 30-34), myofibrillar myopathy,[67a] acid maltase deficiency, periodic paralysis (Fig. 30-38B), and oculopharyngeal muscular dystrophy.

No one specific type of vacuole is diagnostic of a particular disease but particular types are associated with certain disorders. The characteristics of the vacuole may change as other pathologic alterations in the muscle fiber develop. The significance of the vacuole is determined by its morphology, its histochemical characteristics, and the overall pathologic changes in the muscle.

Autophagic vacuoles are membrane-bound vacuoles that contain cytoplasmic degradation products and display acid phosphatase activity (Figs. 30-34B, 30-36B, 30-38A). Membranes of autophagic vacuoles are derived in part from the transverse tubules and, in some myopathies, from Golgi membranes.[63] Such vacuoles are observed in a large number of primary or secondary neuromuscular disorders in which there is a degeneration of cytoplasmic components: polymyositis,[68] systemic lupus erythematosus,[69] myotonic dystrophy,[31] muscular dystrophy,[70] distal myopathy,[71] inclusion body myositis

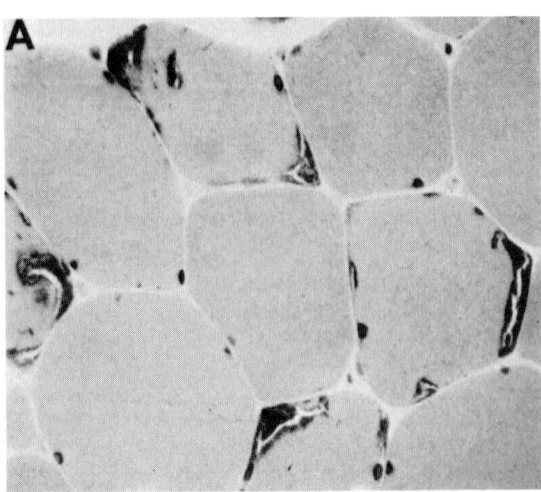 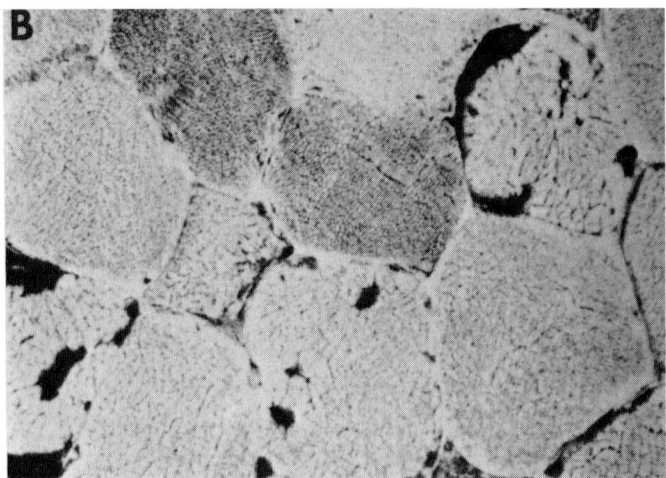

FIGURE 30-31. Tubular aggregates are visualized in trichrome-stained (A) and NADH dehydrogenase-reacted (B) frozen sections. The aggregates appear in type 2 fibers. ×300.

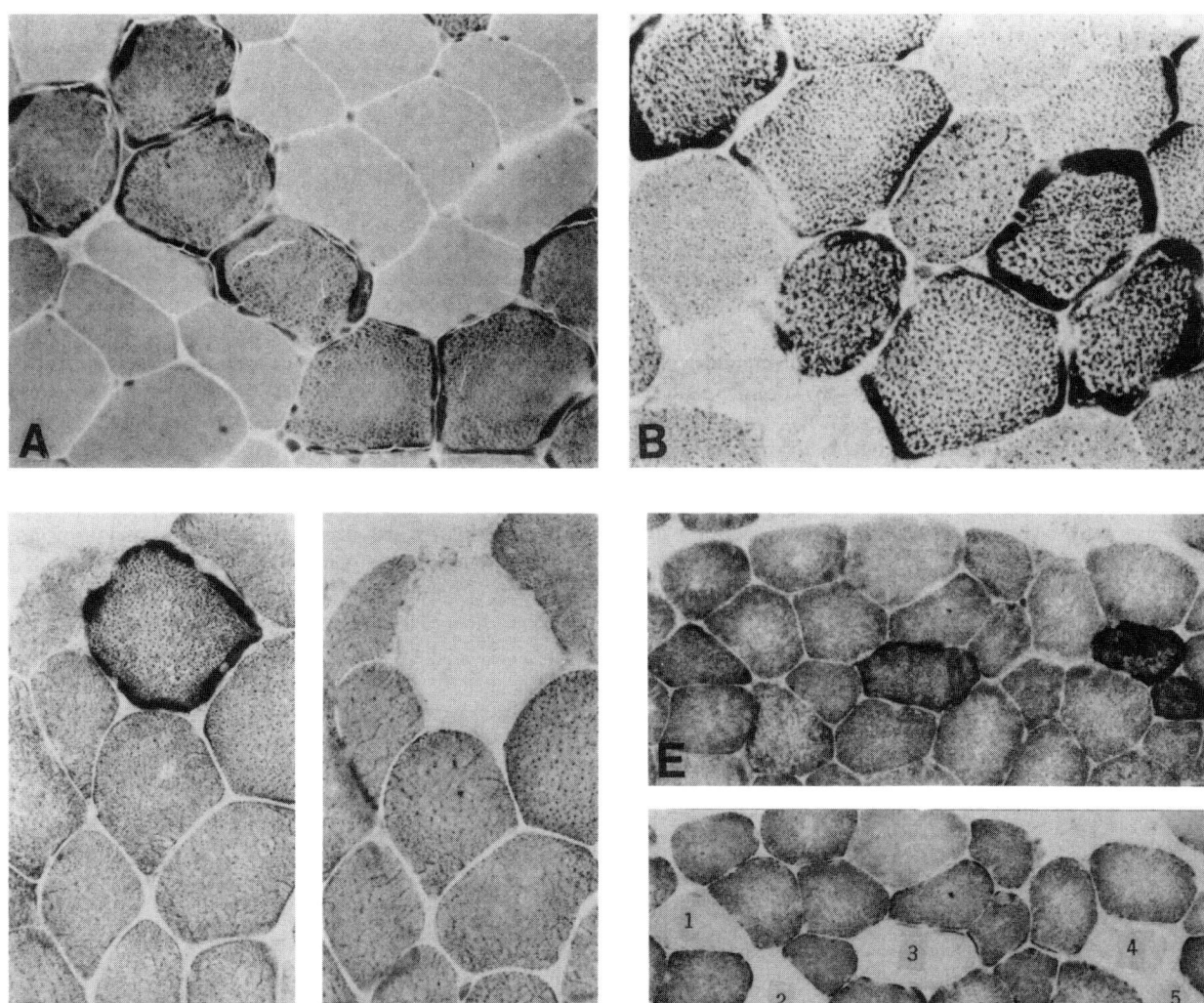

FIGURE 30-32. Mitochondrial abnormalities. A. Trichrome-stained section; several muscle fibers display increased subsarcolemmal and intermyofibrillar membranous material (ragged red fibers). B. Several ragged red fibers show intense subsarcolemmal and intermyofibrillar reactivity for NADH dehydrogenase. C, D, E, and F. Serial sections reacted for succinate dehydrogenase (C, E) and cytochrome c oxidase (D, F). In C, a single ragged red fiber reacts strongly for succinate dehydrogenase, but in D this fiber fails to react for cytochrome c oxidase. In E, three ragged red fibers react strongly for succinate dehydrogenase. In F, the same fibers (fibers 3, 4, and 5) and also two other fibers (fibers 1 and 2) are cytochrome c oxidase–negative. This demonstrates that the distribution of cytochrome c oxidase-negative fibers can be more widespread than that of the ragged red fibers. A, B. Familial coenzyme Q deficiency. C and D. Cerebellar syndrome with peripheral neuropathy and mitochondrial myopathy. E, F. Kearns-Sayre syndrome. A, ×300; B, ×480; C, D, ×215; E, F, ×145.

(Fig. 30-34),[72] oculopharyngeal muscular dystrophy,[73] periodic paralyses (Fig. 30-38),[65,67] vincristine myopathy,[74] chloroquine myopathy,[23] the type 2 glycogenoses (Fig. 30-35),[75,76] and many other disorders.

Rimmed vacuoles are also autophagic in character[77] (Figs. 30-34 and 30-36). These vacuoles are irregular or round in shape. In order to identify them and to appreciate their staining properties, cryostat-sectioned unfixed muscle must be studied, but even under these conditions various degrees of loss of contents occur. The margins of the vacuoles are blue with H&E and red with Gomori trichrome stain. They contain multilaminated, membranous structures accompanied by glycogen granules, dense bodies, and amorphous granular and fibrillar material. These vacuoles are found in inclusion body myositis,[72] myofibrillar myopathy,[67a] and in oculopharyngeal muscular dystrophy.[73,78] They have also been observed in denervated muscle[79] and distal myopathy.[71,77] The vacuoles or their borders are stained by Sudan black B and by osmium tetroxide; they exhibit acid phosphatase activity (Fig. 30-34B). By phase microscopy, the granular lining of the vacuole is readily recognized.

A vacuolar myopathy occurs in both primary and secondary types of periodic paralysis[65–67] (Figs. 30-37 and 30-38). In paraffin sections, a varying proportion of fibers display vacuoles that range from less than 10 μm in diameter to a width that nearly encompasses the entire fiber (Fig. 30-37). In any given section, the vacuoles are usually centrally placed and solitary, but as many as five vacuoles can be seen in one fiber. Most vacuoles appear empty, although some contain varying amounts of granular material. With high magnification by light microscopy, some vacuoles are observed to be compartmentalized (Fig. 30-37C and D). In Epon-embedded material studied by phase-contrast microscopy, it can be appreciated that their interiors are lobulated and their contents heterogeneous (Fig. 30-38B). In zones adjacent to or within some vacuoles, histochemical studies reveal acid phosphatase (Fig. 30-38A) or NADH dehydrogenase reactions. Clusters of calcific deposits and PAS positive material can also be detected within the cavities. (see Color Plate 13 and Chap. 46).

Although not a prominent change in muscle, vacuoles are encountered in the various lysosomal storage disorders. Their contents provide information regarding the substances that have accumulated, and from histochemical and ultrastructural studies of such material it is possible to identify the type of metabolic defect (see "Enzymatic Deficiencies," below).

The most common inclusions in muscle are *lipid bodies* consisting of triglycerides of fatty acids (Color Plate 7I, J, and P). These lipid collections, more conspicuous in type 1 fibers than in type 2, are found in varying amounts in normal muscle. However, in the lipid myopathies the amount of lipid is increased in the muscle fiber and the lipid bodies are large and numerous (Fig. 30-39). If the tissue is embedded in paraffin, the area of lipid loss appears as a vacuole. The type 1 fibers are more severely affected than the type 2. Lipid bodies are best detected with fat stains of cryostat sections. The vacuoles in lipid storage myopathy differ from autophagic vacuoles in that the accumulated material is not enclosed by membranes and autophagy is absent.[67] The vacuoles and their lipid content are quite stereotyped in structure except that some coalesce.

Recent studies indicate that the boundaries of many but not all membrane-bound vacuoles are reinforced by the cytoskeletal proteins dystrophin and β-spectrin. Vacuoles of this type are commonly observed in adult acid maltase deficiency, chloroquine myopathy, and periodic paralysis (Color Plate 13Q, R, and S).[79a]

Inclusion Bodies

The majority of inclusions that are found in muscle, such as rod bodies, reducing bodies, fingerprint bodies, etc., have

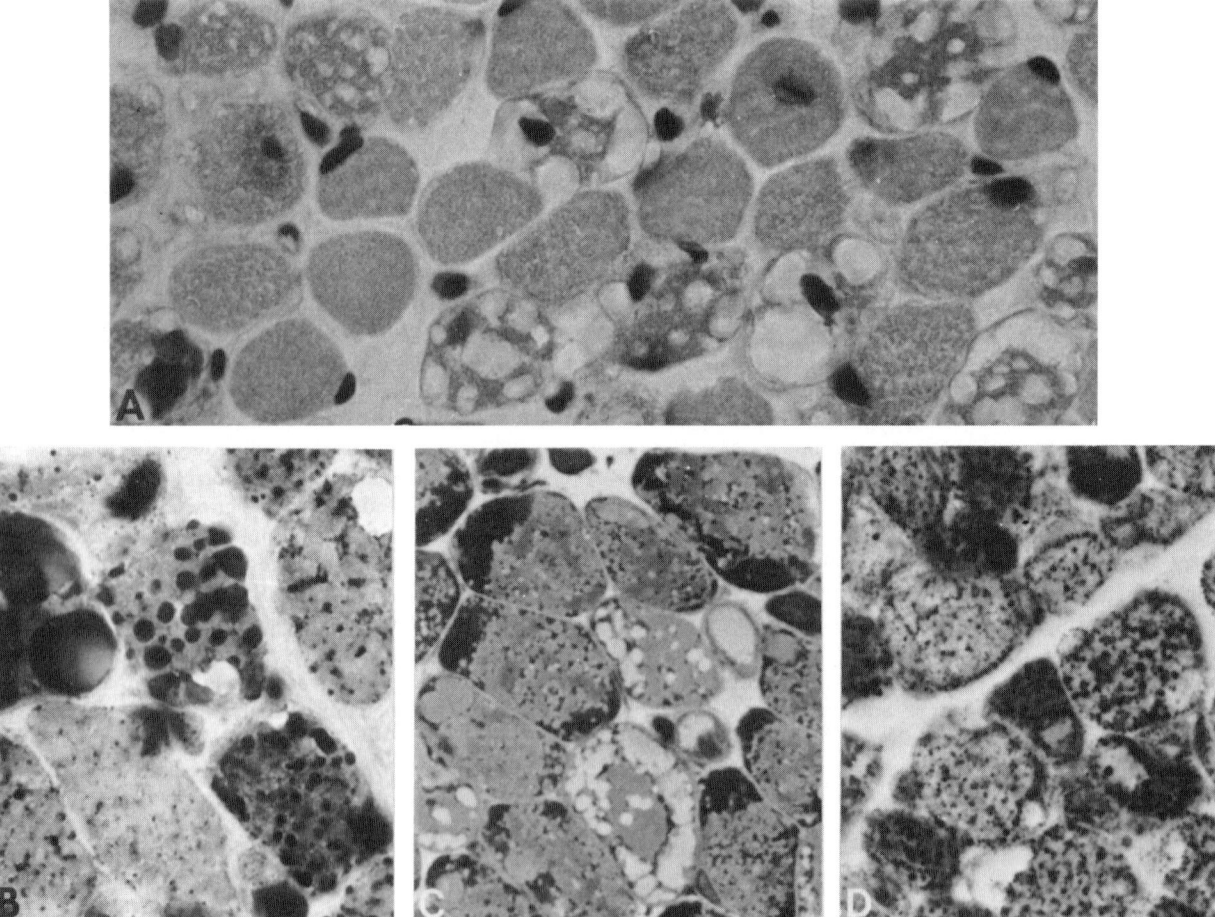

FIGURE 30-33. Cytochemical analysis of vacuolar contents: H&E-stained (A), oil red 0-stained (B), PAS-stained (C), and NADH dehydrogenase-reacted (D) sections from a case of mitochondria-lipid-glycogen disease of muscle. Nearly all fibers contain abnormal empty spaces in A. Lipid material (B), PAS positive material (C), and accumulations of mitochondria (D) account for varying fractions of the vacuolar volume in the individual fibers. Definitive identification of glycogen requires digestion with diastase or observation by electron microscopy. A, ×740; B, C, ×1200; D, ×800. (Jerusalem et al: Arch Neurol 29: 162, 1973. Reproduced by permission.)

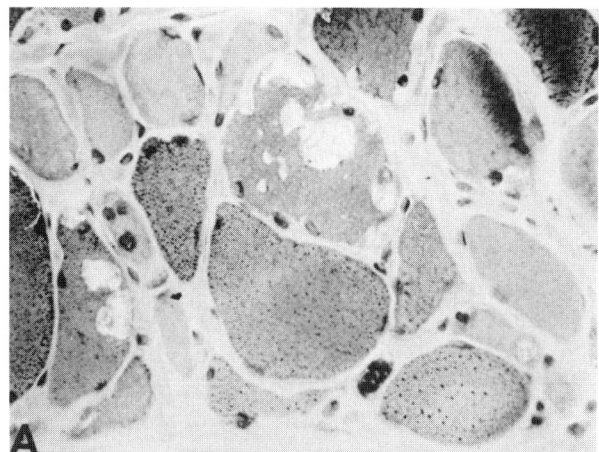
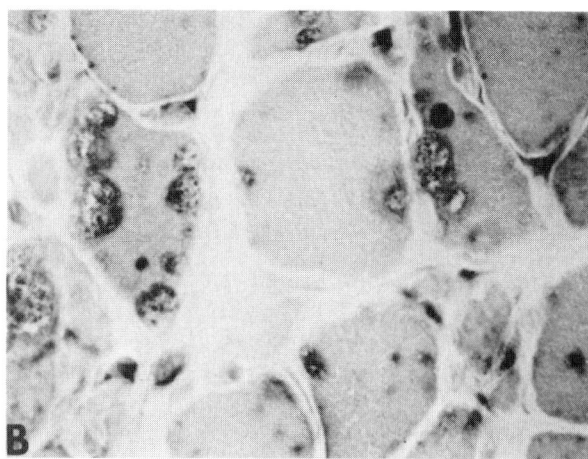

FIGURE 30-34. Vacuoles in inclusion body myositis visualized in trichrome-stained (A) and acid phosphatase–reacted (B) sections. In A, the vacuoles appear nearly empty; in B, the vacuoles react intensely for acid phosphatase, indicating that they are autophagic in character. A, ×300; B, ×480.

already been discussed. In *inclusion body myositis* (Chap. 50), uniform hyaline eosinophilic inclusions are observed by light microscopy within the cytoplasm (Fig. 30-40; Color Plate 7G) and occasionally within the nucleus of some muscle fibers. The inclusions vary in size, are homogeneous, and are rounded or oval and often multiple. They are best seen with Congo red stains of fresh-frozen material sectioned by cryostat. These inclusions can also be recognized by phase microscopy. The filaments that make up the inclusions can be demonstrated only by electron microscopy (Chaps. 31 and 48). These filamentous collections in association with the inflammation and the basophilic granules that line the vacuoles set apart this form of myositis from dermatomyositis and polymyositis. The inclusions or deposits of some associated material stain red with Congo red dye at pH 10.5 to 11[79b] (Color plate 9N) and are associated with material that is immunoreactive for β-amyloid protein[79c] and ubiquitin[79d] (also in Chap. 50).

In *oculopharyngeal muscular dystrophy*, other intranuclear inclusions of muscle can be detected by phase microscopy. These inclusions consist of tubular filaments that also are best defined by electron microscopy (see Chap. 40).

Alterations in Muscle

DYSTROPHIN DEFICIENCY

This section considers the tissue localization of dystrophin. A deficiency of dystrophin, a 420-kDA subsarcolemmal cytoskeletal protein, is the molecular basis of Duchenne and Becker dystrophies.[80] In Duchenne dystrophy, the mutation usually disrupts the codon triplet reading frame of the dystrophin gene and causes severe dystrophin deficiency.

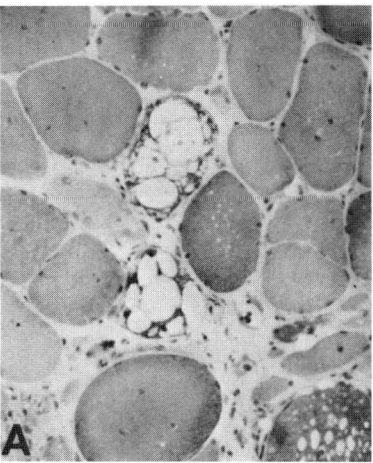
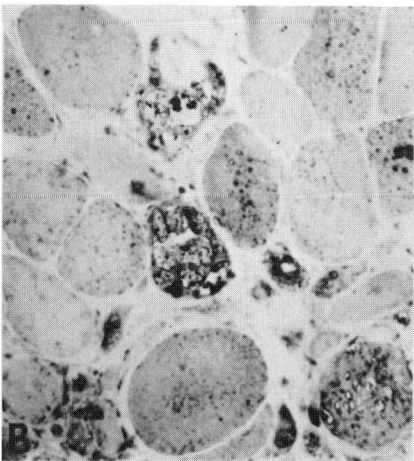
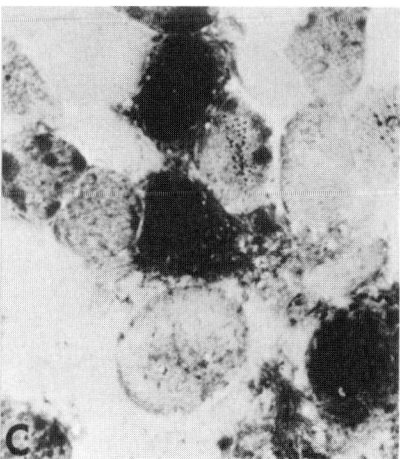

FIGURE 30-35. Vacuolar myopathy of adult acid maltase deficiency. Trichrome-stained (A), acid phosphatase–reacted (B), and PAS-stained (C) serial cryostat sections. The vacuoles react intensely for acid phosphatase and are filled with PAS-positive material. Even those fibers that do not display vacuoles in A contain multiple small regions of acid phosphatase reactivity. ×280.

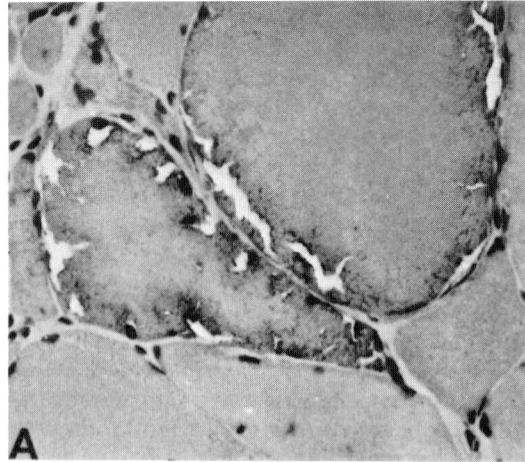
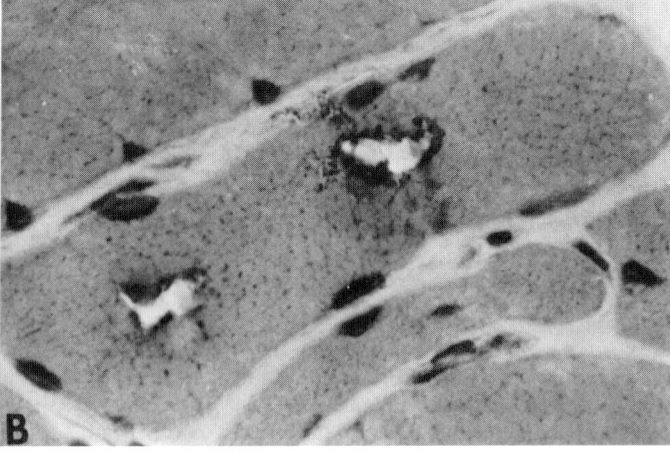

FIGURE 30-36. Rimmed vacuoles in inclusion body myositis; trichrome-stained fresh-frozen sections. The vacuoles vary in shape, size, number, and location and are bordered by dark-staining material that also extends into the nearby fiber regions. A, ×270; B, × 690.

Muscle dystrophin levels generally fall below 25 percent of normal.[81,82] The residual dystrophin, if detectable, is truncated and lacks the carboxy terminus of the wild-type dystophin. In Becker dystrophy, the mutation usually does not disrupt the codon triplet reading frame, the mutant dystrophin retains the carboxy terminus of wild-type dystrophin, and the dystrophin deficiency is less severe than in Duchenne dystrophy.[83] Antibodies useful in the detection of dystrophin in muscle must recognize a segment of the dystrophin molecule and must not cross-react with utrophin,[84] α-actinin,[85,86] or spectrin.[87] Carboxy terminus-specific antibodies are particularly useful in distinguishing between some cases of Duchenne and Becker dystrophy.[83,88] In cryostat

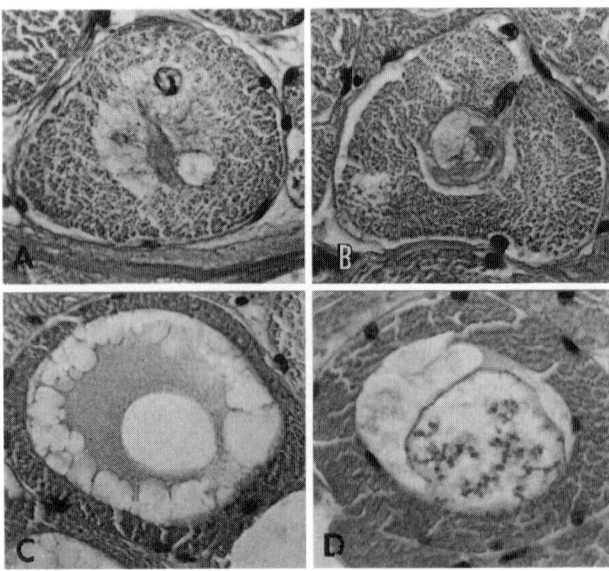

FIGURE 30-37. Vacuoles in periodic paralysis. A, B. Abnormal fiber regions with rarefied or absent myofibrillar markings. C. Numerous round or dome-shaped membrane-limited spaces, many abutting on rim of vacuole. D. Large dome-shaped space containing coarse granules in vacuole. H&E-stained paraffin sections. ×450 (Engel AG; Mayo Clinic Proc 45:774, 1970. Reproduced by permission.)

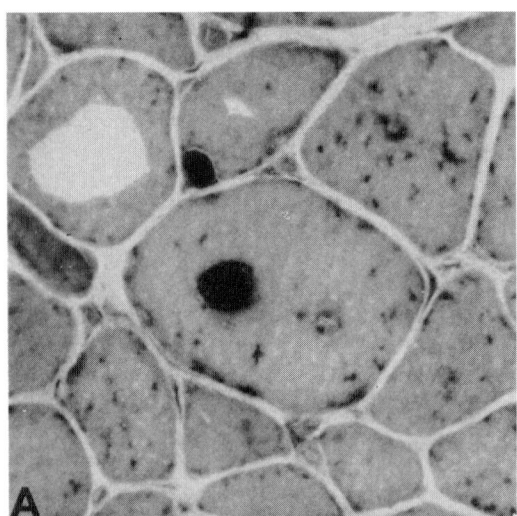
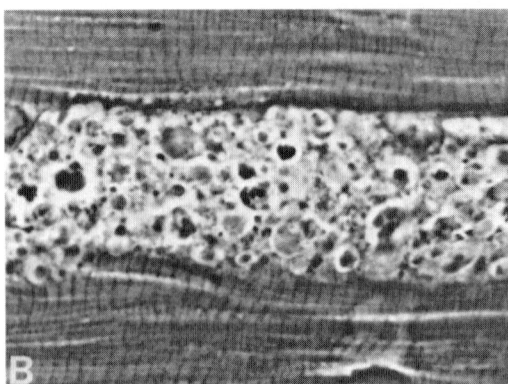

FIGURE 30-38. Vacuoles in period paralysis. A. Acid phosphatase–reacted frozen section. ×340. B. Resin-embedded section viewed in phase optics. ×1200. In A, some vacuoles are intensely reactive for acid phosphatase, indicating that they are secondary lysosomes. Multiple small areas of acid phosphatase reactivity are also present in nonvacuolated fiber regions. In B, the abnormal space contains small collections of abnormal material of varying optical density. Definitive identification of the vacuolar contents requires electron microscopy. (A is from Engel AG: Mayo Clinic Proc 45:774, 1970. Reproduced by permission.)

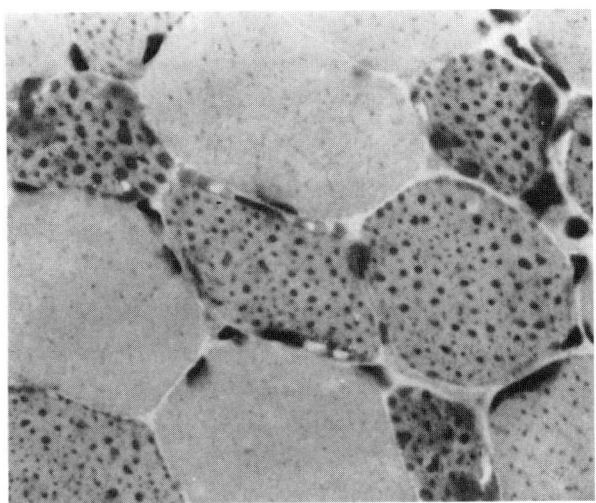

FIGURE 30-39. Vacuolar myopathy of carnitine deficiency. Type 1 fibers contain multiple small, round abnormal spaces filled with Sudan black B-positive lipid material. ×400.

ments may not affect the mutant protein's immunoreactivity. (2) A genetic defect in a given protein may result in a secondary deficiency of other proteins. For example, in Fukuyama muscular dystrophy, mutations in fukutin result in secondary decreases of immunoreactivity for α-dystroglycan and α2-laminin; mutation in one sarcoglycan can attenuate the expression of one or more other sarcoglycans. (3) Some monoclonal antibodies, such as those directed against calpain and telethonin, recognize their target in immunoblots but not in tissue sections. (4) More than one monoclonal antibody, recognizing different regions of a given protein, may be required for diagnosis. (5) Suitable monoclonal antibodies are not available for the diagnosis of several forms of muscular dystrophy. Despite these limitations, a number of immunostains have been useful in the histologic diagnosis of different types of dystrophies (Table 30-2). For a detailed discussion of immunohistochemical methods for the diagnosis of muscular dystrophies the reader is referred to a recent monograph.[100a]

sections of normal muscle and in myopathies without dystrophin deficiency, dystrophin is localized to the sarcolemma without intra- or interfiber-variation of staining intensity[82,89–94] (Fig. 30-41A). In patients with dystrophin deficiency, the immunolocalization is affected by the titer and epitope specificity of the antibody and by the degree of dystrophin deficiency.

In some but not all Duchenne dystrophy carriers, a small proportion of muscle fibers show no, attenuated, or uneven circumferential staining for dystrophin (Fig. 30-41D and E, and Color Plate 15A–D).[95–97] Because the overall dystrophin deficiency in carriers is typically mild, immunocytochemistry is more sensitive for carrier detection than Western blot analysis; but even immunocytochemistry may not be diagnostic.[98,99]

In Becker dystrophy, dystrophin immunoreactivity is preserved but attenuated, and there is both intra- and interfiber variability of immunostaining.[82,88,89] In some instances, when the antidystrophin antibody is directed against a deleted epitope, no immunostaining is detected. This finding might suggest the diagnosis of Duchenne dystrophy; a carboxy terminus–specific antibody, however, will immunostain the fibers.[88,100] Becker specimens with relatively low overall dystrophin content may be immunocytochemically indistinguishable from Duchenne specimens with weak dystrophin immunoreactivity.[82] Neither immunocytochemistry nor Western blot analysis is consistently reliable for detecting carriers of Becker dystrophy.

For a more complete discussion of various aspects of the diagnosis of dystrophin deficiency, the reader is referred to Chap. 34.

Histochemical Diagnosis of Other Dystrophies with Monoclonal Antibodies

Monoclonal antibodies have proved useful in the diagnosis of a number of other muscular dystrophies. This approach, however, has clear limitations: (1) Small DNA rearrange-

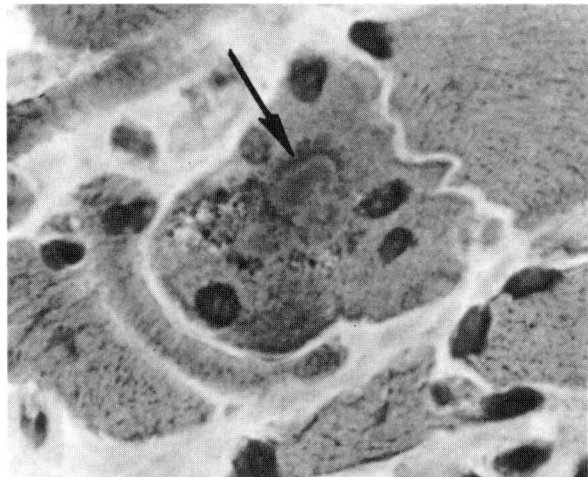

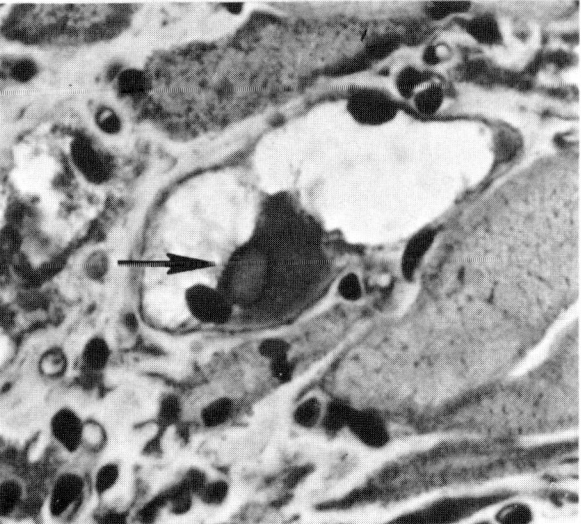

FIGURE 30-40. Well-defined inclusion bodies within the cytoplasm of muscle fibers (arrows). Inclusion body myositis. Cryostat sections stained with H&E. ×800.

Loss of Muscle Fibers

A varying percentage of muscle fibers in certain myopathies disappears as a result of necrosis and ineffective regeneration. This loss of muscle fiber is particularly severe in Duchenne dystrophy (Fig. 30-42C). A slow, gradual disappearance of muscle fibers is a major feature of the pathologic reaction in each of the muscular dystrophies. Equally characteristic is the topography of the fiber loss affecting particularly the proximal muscles. In the most advanced stage of dystrophy, a severely involved muscle contains virtually no muscle fibers.

Increased Connective Tissue

As the muscle fibers disappear, they are replaced by connective tissue. Both endomysial fibrous connective tissue and perimysial fibrous and fatty connective tissue are increased (Figs. 30-42 and 30-43). The more severely affected the muscle, the more conspicuous the connective tissue proliferation. In myopathic disorders associated with fiber destruction, endomysial fibrous connective tissue increases from the onset of the disorder. Increase in endomysial fatty connective tissue is observed only after there has been an extensive loss of muscle fibers from a fascicle (Fig. 30-42C). In denervation atrophy, perimysial connective tissue proliferates at first, followed by endomysial connective tissue when the total number of fibers in a fascicle is reduced.

Table 30-2. IMMUNOHISTOCHEMICAL STUDIES USEFUL IN THE DIAGNOSIS OF SELECTED MUSCULAR DYSTROPHIES

Antigen Localized by Immunostain	Application
α-, β-, δ- and γ-Sarcoglycan	Sarcoglycanopathies
Dysferlin	Dysferlinopathy (LGD2B/Miyoshi myopathy)
Caveolin 3	LGD1C
α2-Laminin (merosin)	Merosin-deficient congenital muscular dystrophy
Emerin	X-linked Emery-Dreifuss muscular dystrophy
Collagen VI	Bethlem myopathy; Ullrich myopathy
β1-Laminin	Bethlem myopathy
Plectin	Myopathy associated with epidermolyis bullosa simplex

Infarction

Muscle infarcts are uncommon, probably because muscle contains a rich collateral vascular supply. The four circumstances in which muscle infarction occurs are atherosclerotic occlusive vascular disease of an extremity, acute compartment syndrome, diabetes, polyarteritis nodosa, and dermatomyositis. The largest infarcts are found in the first three groups.

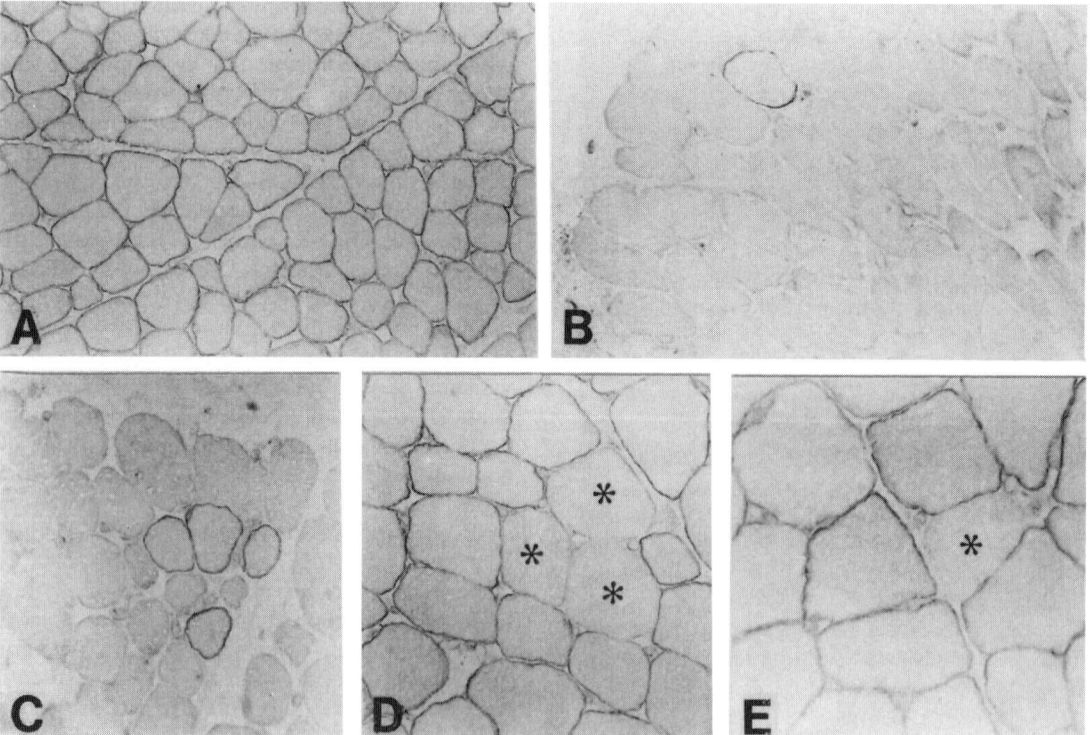

FIGURE 30-41. Dystrophin immunolocalization in a young boy with limb-girdle dystrophy *(A)*, in Duchenne dystrophy *(B, C)* and in an obligate carrier of Duchenne dystrophy *(D, E)*. In limb-girdle dystrophy, all muscle fibers show sarcolemmal dystrophin immunoreactivity. In Duchenne dystrophy, nearly all fibers are dystrophin-negative, but a single fiber in *B* and a small group of fibers in *C* express dystrophin. In the Duchenne carrier, a small proportion of the fibers (asterisks) show attenuated *(D)* or no *(E)* reaction for dystrophin. *A–D*, ×210; *E*, ×330.

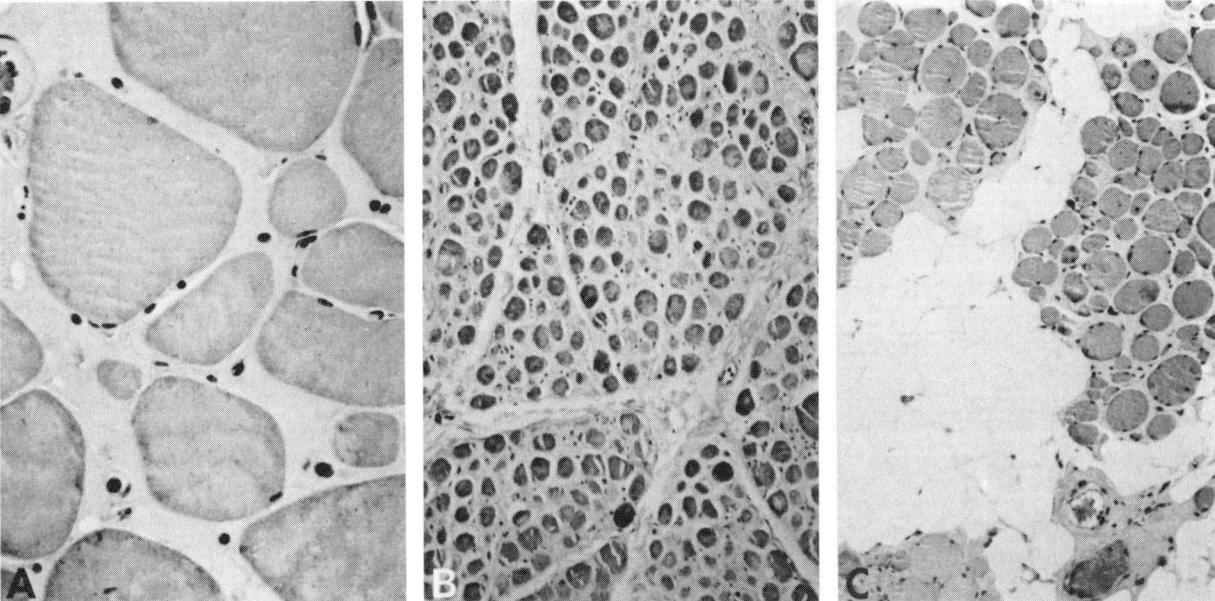

FIGURE 30-42. Increased connective tissue in muscle in muscular dystrophy (A, C) and in chronic polymyositis (B). Endomysial fibrous connective tissue separates muscle fibers in A, B, and C. Perimysial fibrous connective tissue is increased in B, and perimysial fatty connective tissue is markedly increased in C. The increased connective tissue in C indicates that significant loss of muscle fibers has occurred. A, ×283; B, ×70; C, ×100.

Infarction of muscle is a rare but well-documented complication of diabetes mellitus.[101] The thigh muscles are preferentially involved. The course of the illness has been uniform in six patients followed by one of us.[102] The onset is heralded by pain in the thigh muscle accompanied by swelling and tenderness. All these patients have been women in renal failure and with other complications of diabetes. The pathological changes in muscle have also been similar in each patient. The muscle is grossly pale and firm to palpation and contains both pale and hemorrhagic zones (Fig. 30-44). Microscopic examination reveals extensive infarction involving an area 5 to 10 cm in diameter. In the center of the infarct the architecture of muscle is destroyed, while at the periphery the outline of acutely necrotic fibers can be discerned (Fig. 30-44). Many small arteries, arterioles, and capillaries are occluded by fibrin and calcium. Small peripheral nerves are degenerated, and denervation atrophy is evident in the fasciculi bordering the zones of infarction. The walls of many capillaries and small arteries are thickened and homogenized (Fig. 30-45). Calcification of the media is observed in many medium-sized arteries. In the more chronic lesions, recanalization is often observed (Fig. 30-45). At the periphery of the totally ischemic zones, there are attempts at regeneration of muscle fibers as indicated by basophilia of fibers and the prominence of subsarcolemmal nuclei and nucleoli (Fig. 30-46C). The infarcted tissue is infiltrated by small muscle cells that can be identified as myocytes by their lack of syncytial formation, the presence of large nuclei and nucleoli, and the small amount of contractile substance. These cells along with the more mature but still primitive muscle fibers (the myotubes) are aligned in parallel in an attempt to form more mature muscle. The infiltration by collagen is so conspicuous in these areas that the primitive muscle cells represent only a very small portion of the tissue. The infiltration by massive amounts of collagen and the paucity of regeneration prevent the effective repair of infarcted tissue. More effective regenerative activity, such as muscle budding from the peripheral segments of intact muscle fibers or even abortive regeneration, are not evident. Groups of fasciculi, in which the remaining muscle fibers appear small and denervated, intermingle with and

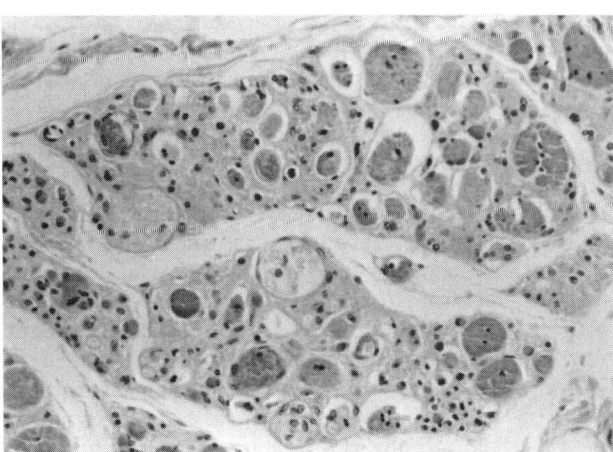

FIGURE 30-43. Muscle fibers are reduced in number. The endomysial connective tissue is increased and collagen replaces the area previously occupied by muscle fibers. Myotonic dystrophy. H&E stain. ×260.

surround the areas of attempted repair. Hemorrhages in various stages of absorption are often found in the infarct (Fig. 30-46). At least three factors appear to prevent effective regeneration in muscle infarcts of diabetics: proliferation of connective tissue, which replaces the necrotic muscle fibers and forms a barrier to regenerative attempts; denervation of muscle within the infarcted area; and failure of collateral blood supply.

In dermatomyositis, the zones of infarction are small and often overlooked microscopically in biopsy material. Portions of two or three fasciculi contain acutely necrotic muscle fibers, all in the same stage of degeneration (Fig. 30-47). When various staining techniques are applied to cryostat sections of fresh-frozen muscle, the zones are accentuated (Fig. 30-47). The altered muscle fibers are strongly eosinophilic. Reactivity for myofibrillar ATPase and other enzymes are markedly attenuated or lost. Numerous large lipid bodies fill the degenerated fibers in the zone of infarction. The PAS–orange G stain outlines the ischemic area; red-staining necrotic fibers are surrounded by the orange-staining normal fibers. Regenerative efforts are minimal in these zones and the changes in small blood vessels are subtle. Nevertheless, even by light microscopy varying degrees of endothelial hyperplasia can be recognized. Fibrin thrombi and recanalized

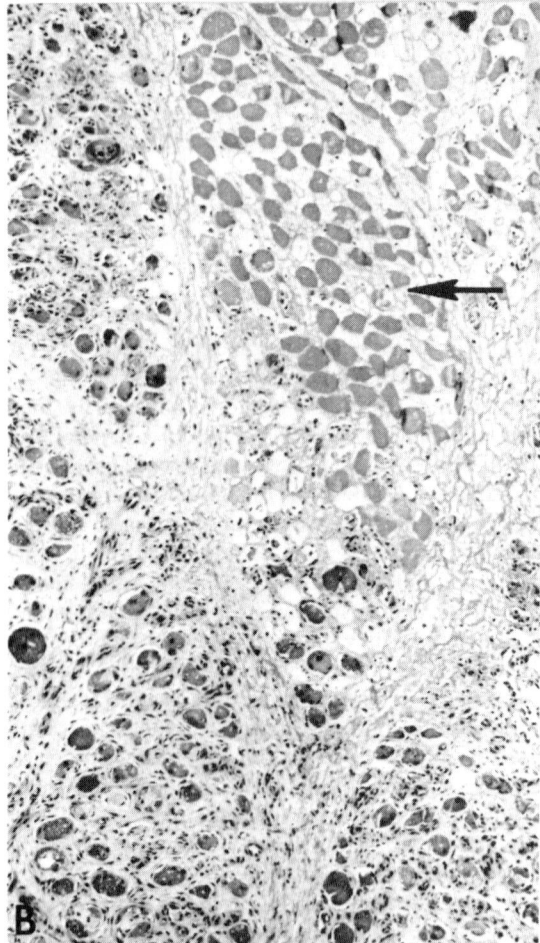

FIGURE 30-44. *A.* Gross specimen of infarcted thigh muscle from a diabetic woman. A zone of pallor is bordered by hemorrhage. ×2.6 *B.* Necrotic fibers (arrow) constitute a large portion of the infarcted tissue. Fasciculi containing muscle fibers in various stages of regeneration surround a large zone of necrosis. Perimysial and endomysial connective tissue is increased in these border regions. H&E stain. ×75.

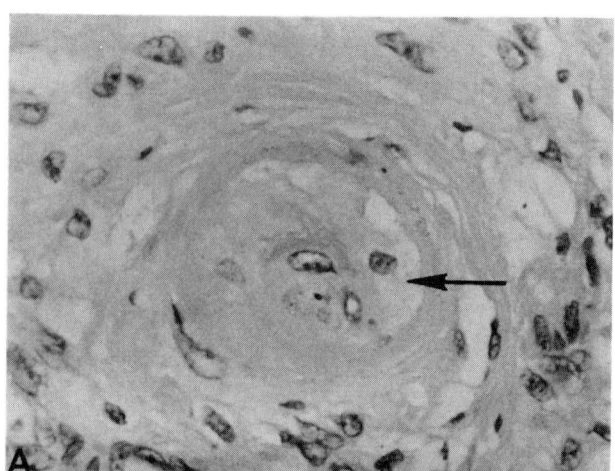

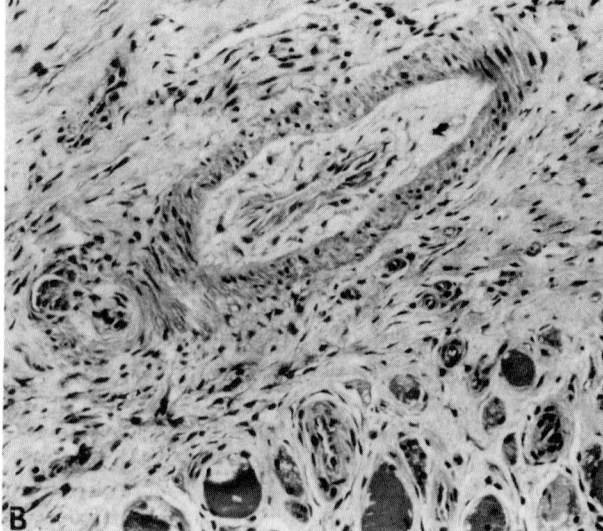

FIGURE 30-45. Muscle infarcts in diabetes. *A.* In acutely infarcted muscle, intimal hyperplasia of small arteries is conspicuous (arrow). ×600. *B.* Later, medium-sized arteries are observed in varying stages of recanalization. ×170. H&E stain.

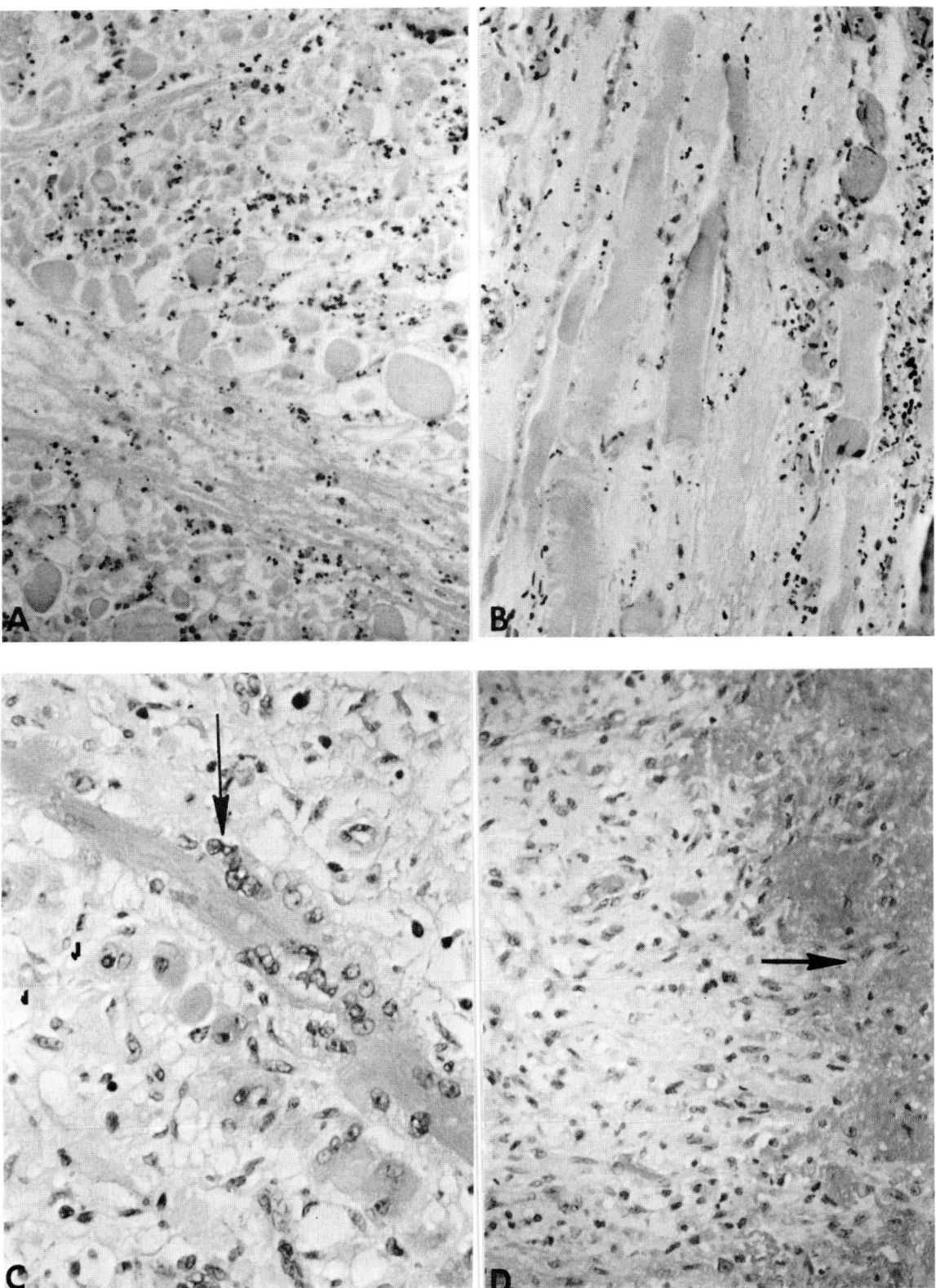

FIGURE 30-46. Muscle infarcts in diabetes A. Zones of acutely infarcted thigh muscle are infiltrated by polymorphonuclear leukocytes. ×230. B. In the more chronic infarct, there is a mixture of necrotic muscle fibers, proliferated connective tissue, and acute and chronic inflammation. ×370. C. Muscle fibers are attempting to regenerate (arrow) but increased connective tissue forms a barrier. ×590. D. a hemorrhagic zone (arrow) is bordered by granulation tissue. ×370. H&E stain.

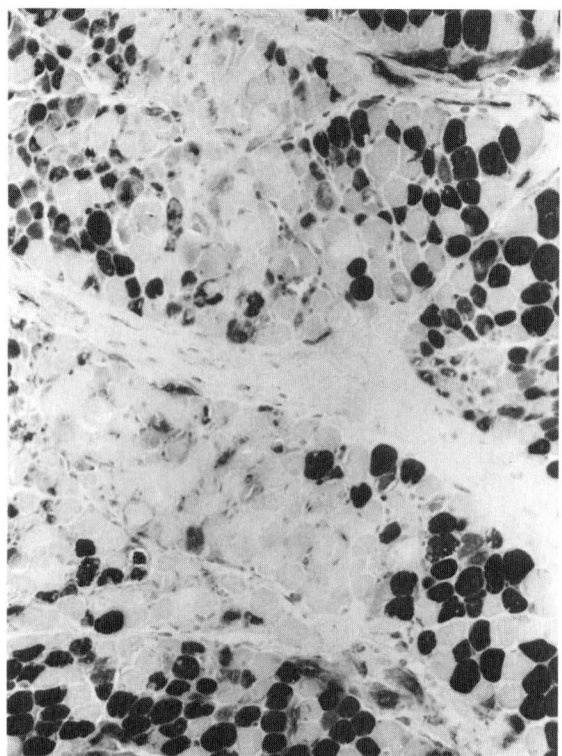

FIGURE 30-47. Dermatomyositis of childhood. An infarct in muscle (zone of pallor) extends from the periphery of several fasciculi toward the more central portion of the muscle. ATPase reacton (pH 9.4). ×240.

blood vessels are more easily identified in autopsy material than in small biopsy blocks (Fig. 30-48). A vasculitis is often detected in the small arteries and veins in perimysial connective tissue.

Perifascicular Atrophy

When the peripheral muscle fibers of a fasciculus are all in one stage of atrophy, the alteration is called perifascicular atrophy. This change is quite conspicuous when the perifascicular fibers are compared with the centrofascicular ones (Fig. 30-49). This alteration can be appreciated by light microscopic study of paraffin-embedded muscle stained by H&E or plastic-embedded muscle viewed by phase-contrast microscopy or studied by histochemical techniques alone.

Perifascicular atrophy is found in a large proportion of muscle biopsies in children and adults with dermatomyositis. The pathogenesis of this form of atrophy is unknown. Some investigators have suggested that the loss or destruction of the perifascicular capillaries results in an ischemic change in the peripheral regions.[103,104] Others have proposed that ischemic changes result in an extensive transverse tubule–sarcoplasmic reticular anastomosis in the affected perifascicular muscle fibers;[105] But these anastomoses would not in and of themselves explain the muscle fiber atrophy. Ultrastructural studies suggest that fiber atrophy results from degeneration of organelles followed by incomplete repair.

Denervation Atrophy

Denervated muscle fibers atrophy. Type grouping and target formations are associated with reinnervation of previously denervated fibers (Figs. 30-4 and 30-28). Hypertrophy of the nondenervated fibers and secondary myopathic changes in these fibers can also occur. The latter include central nuclei, fiber splitting, necrosis and phagocytosis, and the appearance of regenerating fibers. The frequency, grouping, and size distribution of the atrophic fibers, the frequency of target formations, and the extent of type grouping are affected by several variables. These include the fraction of motor nerve fibers that is interrupted (or the proportion of motor units that is denervated), the duration and rate of progression of the denervating process, and the ability of those nerve fibers that remain in muscle to sprout and reinnervate the denervated muscle fibers. Hypertrophy of the nondenervated fibers and the secondary myopathic changes are probably related to the workload imposed on these fibers (Fig. 30-29).

Two extreme types of denervation are considered here first. If a muscle is totally denervated, as by cutting its motor nerve, all fibers in that muscle atrophy. In experimental studies of total muscle denervation, fiber size decreases rapidly. In the rat, sciatic nerve section at the mid-thigh level results in an 80 percent decrease in fiber size in gastrocnemius and soleus muscles during the first 3 weeks after denervation, and a further reduction in fiber size occurs more slowly thereafter.[106]

If a single motor nerve fiber is disrupted or a single anterior horn cell destroyed, only the muscle fibers of the denervated motor unit atrophy. The atrophic fibers occur singly, or in small groups (with two to three fibers per group), corresponding to the arrangement of muscle fibers within the territory of the motor unit.[1] The atrophic fibers are separated by fibers of normal size belonging to intact motor units whose territory overlaps with that of the denervated motor unit. The extent of muscle fiber atrophy will depend on how soon after denervation, reinnervation occurs by collateral sprouts derived from adjacent normal nerve fibers. Reinnervation by collateral sprouting is confined to a given fascicle. Thus muscle fibers in one fascicle are not reinnervated by nerve sprouts arising in an adjacent fascicle.

In naturally occurring illnesses of the anterior horn cell or of peripheral nerves, a variable number of motor units may become denervated within a given period of time and the denervating event recurs at a variable rate (Fig. 30-29). With repeated cycles of denervation and reinnervation, the territory of those motor units from which the reinnervating nerve sprouts arise enlarges and the random distribution of the histochemical fiber types decreases, so that an increasing number of fibers of the same histochemical type appear immediately adjacent to each other (type grouping). The extent of type grouping is thus a measure of reinnervation of previously denervated muscle fibers. When an anterior horn cell or nerve fiber that supplies an enlarged motor unit is destroyed, a relatively large number of adjacent fibers, or even an entire fascicle, of the same histochemical type become atrophic. Target fibers are a sign of relatively recent reinnervation; therefore, their presence suggests that the neurogenic process is active, and their relative abundance reflects on the rate of reinnervation.

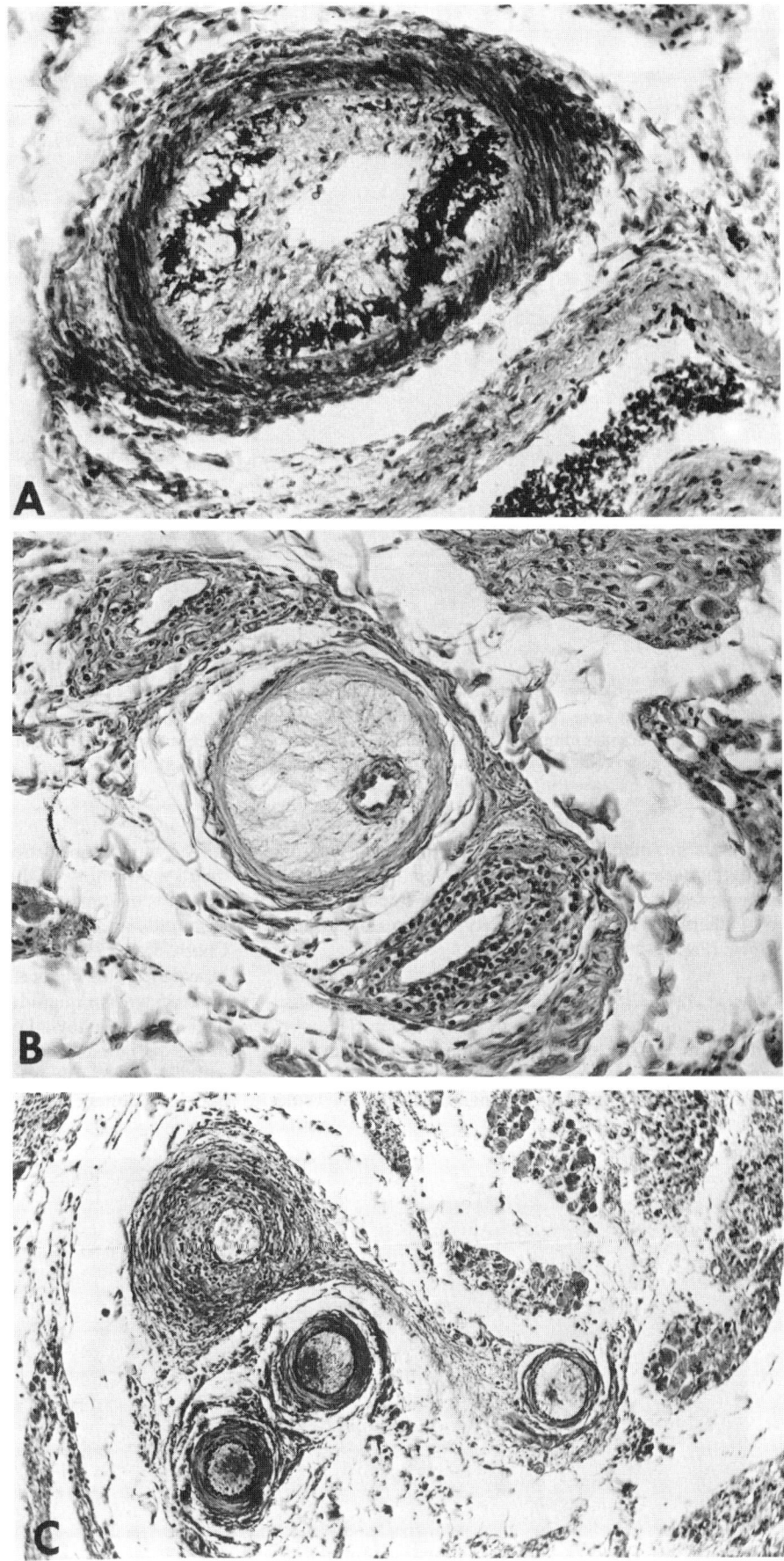

FIGURE 30-48. Dermatomyositis of childhood. *A.* A perimysial artery is partially occluded by a fibrin thrombus which is in the process of resolution PTAH stain. ×260. *B.* Recanalization in a perimysial artery. The wall of the adjacent vein is infiltrated by inflammatory cells. H&E stain. ×190. *C.* The lumina of three perimysial arteries are occluded and the wall of the vein is thickened and infiltrated by inflammatory cells. Weigert's elastic tissue stain. ×160. *(Banker BQ, Victor M: Medicine 45:251, 1966. Reproduced by permission.)*

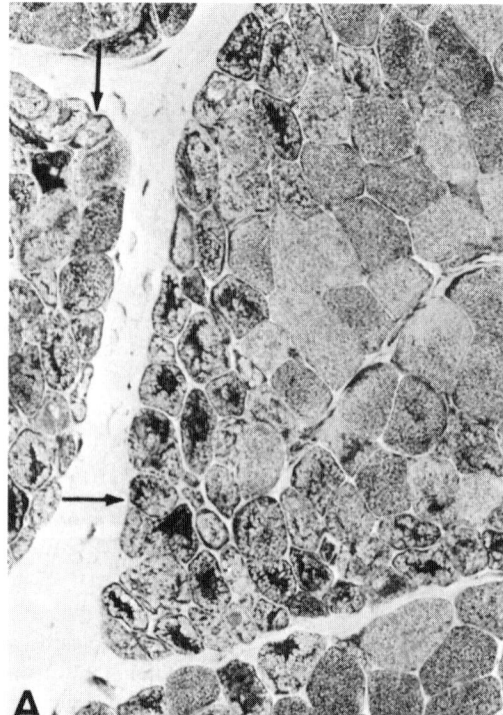
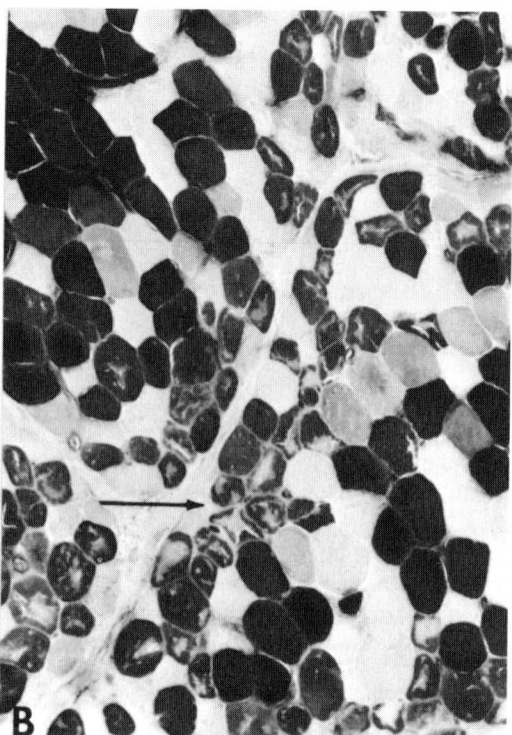

FIGURE 30-49. Muscle from a child with dermatomyositis showing conspicuous perifascicular atrophy. The fibers at the periphery of the fasciculi are undergoing degeneration (arrows). A. Oxidative enzyme activity is increased in many of these peripheral fibers. B. ATPase reaction is decreased in similar zones. The more central fibers are relatively normal. A. NADH dehydrogenase. B. ATPase (pH 9.4). ×350.

Type grouping without atrophic fibers indicates that denervation is keeping up with reinnervation or that the neurogenic process is no longer active. Type grouping plus highly atrophic fibers in groups of varying sizes suggest an ancient neurogenic process. Type grouping and the presence of atrophic fibers of varying sizes appearing in groups of varying sizes and/or target formation indicate an ongoing neurogenic process. Numerous small groups of atrophic fibers of varying sizes but only slight type grouping suggest an active neurogenic process but a limited ability of the surviving motor neurons to reinnervate the denervated fibers (Fig. 30-29C and D).

The workload imposed on nondenervated muscle fibers is a function of the number of surviving nondenervated fibers and the physical activity of the muscle. Those muscles that normally carry a heavy workload, especially the gastrocnemius in ambulatory patients, are particularly prone to show hypertrophy and secondary myopathic changes in nondenervated muscle fibers. Selective hypertrophy of type 1 fibers is a feature of acute (type 1) spinal muscular atrophy (Fig. 30-29C and D).[107]

Myogenic Atrophy

In the course of any myopathy, some muscle fibers may become reduced in size. Decrease in fiber size can result from disuse or fiber splitting, as mentioned before. Widespread muscle fiber atrophy and selective loss of thick filaments are features of the acute quadriplegic myopathy (critical illness myopathy) that develops in some patients treated with high doses of corticosteroids and nondepolarizing muscle relaxants (see also Chaps. 31, 61, and 62).[107a,b] Other causes of myogenic atrophy include repeated cycles of focal cytoplasmic degradation followed by exocytosis of degraded fiber contents; repeated cycles of degeneration followed by incomplete regeneration or repair of the degraded fiber elements; proliferation of a single organelle accompanied by extensive disappearance of other fiber components (as in late-onset nemaline myopathy) (Fig. 30-23A); and compression, replacement, or focal destruction of nonnecrotic muscle fibers by cytotoxic mononuclear cells (Fig. 30-50).

Inflammation

The distribution and type of inflammatory response in muscle help to define the category of the muscle disorder.

In various types of myositis, inflammatory cells collect in the perimysium and endomysium and around blood vessels (Fig. 30-51). The inflammatory exudate may be limited to certain muscles or it may be diffuse. In muscles adjacent to burns or destructive foci, inflammatory cells parade directly into the muscle tissue. In muscle abscesses, large collections of inflammatory cells occupy and replace the destroyed parenchyma (Fig. 30-52). In a vasculitis, inflammatory cells are particularly conspicuous within the walls of the blood vessels. In polyarteritis nodosa, for example, there is necrosis of the media of medium-sized arteries and chronic inflammation of the walls of the arteries as well as nodules of histiocytes and lymphocytes in a perivascular distribution (Fig. 30-53).

Inflammatory cells are detected within and around necrotic or even nonnecrotic muscle fibers. The predominant cell type invading and surrounding the *necrotic fiber* is a macrophage (Figs. 30-8 and 30-10). *Nonnecrotic fibers* are focally surrounded and invaded by lymphoid cells and a smaller number of macrophages (Fig. 30-50 and Color Plates 8G–L and 11). This feature is particularly conspicuous in polymyositis and inclusion body myositis, but even in noninflammatory myopathies, such as Duchenne dystrophy, occasional nonnecrotic muscle fibers are invaded by lymphocytes and macrophages.[108]

When muscle is altered by trauma, infarction, burns, or abscesses, the cellular response is acute and consists mainly of polymorphonuclear leukocytes. When eosinophils are present in conspicuous numbers, attention is directed to parasitic infestations (Chap. 52) and to eosinophilic polymyositis and fasciitis (Chap. 53). A granulomatous response consisting of lymphocytes, histiocytes, and giant cells characterizes Boeck's sarcoid (Fig. 30-54), Wegener's granulomatosis, polyarteritis nodosa, tuberculosis, and rheumatic fever (Chap. 53). In polymyositis and dermatomyositis, the cellular response consists essentially of lymphocytes and macrophages. Even in the various types of muscular dystrophy or metabolic myopathies, occasional perivascular collections of mononuclear cells and histiocytes can be detected. In the muscle of the newborn infant, foci of extramedullary hematopoiesis may be misinterpreted as perivascular collections of inflammatory cells.

In order to determine the distribution of mononuclear cells within muscle among the different inflammatory myopathies, Giorno et al.[109] and Arahata and Engel[108,110] applied monoclonal antibody techniques to biopsy samples. Giorno et al. found no significant differences in the type of lymphocytic response in polymyositis, dermatomyositis, and polymyositis with other connective tissue disorders. Arahata and Engel[110] determined the types of cells that constitute the inflammatory changes in muscle from 76 biopsies. Inflammatory cell subsets were analyzed according to diagnosis and site of accumulation (e.g., perivascular, perimysial, or endomysial). The monoclonal antibodies employed were reactive for B cells, T cells, T-cell subsets, killer (K) or natural killer (NK) cells, and the class 2 HLA antigen; macrophages were identified by the acid phosphatase reaction. In the inflammatory myopathies, the exudates consisted of T cells, B cells, and macrophages. There were more T cells, CD8$^+$ cells, and activated T cells in the endomysium than in perivascular distribution. B cells and CD4$^+$ cells were more numerous in perivascular distribution than in the endomysium. Scleroderma differed in that the conspicuous perimysial collections consisted of mainly T cells and macrophages (Figs. 30-55 and 30-56). In dermatomyositis, the percentage of B cells was increased at all sites and the CD4$^+$/T cell ratio in the endomysium was significantly higher than in the other forms of inflammatory myopathy[110] (Fig. 30-57). In contrast there were large numbers of T cells, CD8$^+$ cells, and activated T cells, whereas B cells were sparse in the endomysium, both in polymyositis and inclusion body myositis.[110] T cells and macrophages surrounded and invaded a significant number of muscle fibers in polymyositis and inclusion body myositis (Fig. 30-58). This T cell-mediated muscle fiber injury was observed only rarely in dermatomyositis and scleroderma. For this reason the authors suggest that a local humoral response predominates in dermatomyositis, whereas cell-mediated immune effector mechanisms are more conspicuous in polymyositis and inclusion body myositis.[110]

In addition, Engel and Arahata[108] found, both in polymyositis and inclusion body myositis, that the cells invading the nonnecrotic fibers were selectively enriched in CD8$^+$ phenotype. One-half of the invading CD8$^+$ cells were activated. The significance of this observation relates to the cytotoxic properties of CD8$^+$ cells and their ability to recognize antigens on the muscle fiber. As only sensitized CD8$^+$ cells can recognize an antigen on the muscle fiber surface, the presence of activated autoinvasive CD8$^+$ cells is evidence for sensitization, and suggests clonal expansion, of these cells to an antigen associated with the muscle fiber surface membrane. In contrast, CD4$^+$ cells were more abundant among the surrounding cells than the invading cells, and only a small proportion of CD4$^+$ cells was activated. Macrophages formed 21 to 31 percent of the cells invading or surrounding nonnecrotic fibers and the remainder were T cells; contrariwise, 80 percent of the mononuclear cells within necrotic muscle fibers

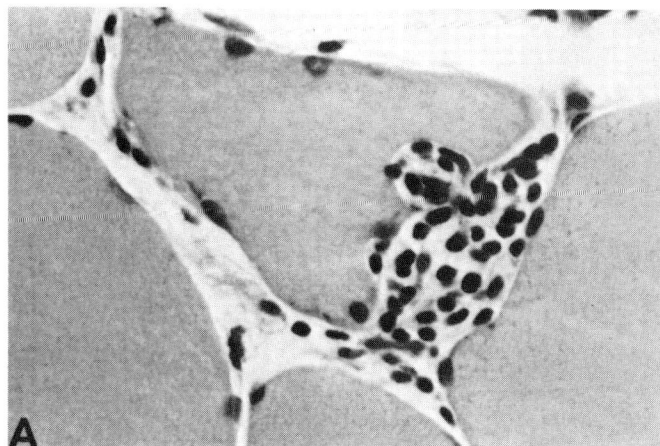
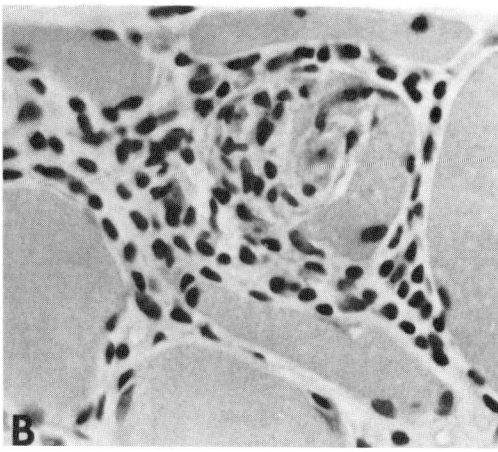

FIGURE 30-50. Nonnecrotic muscle fibers focally invaded and surrounded by mononuclear cells. In *A,* the invading cells have indented and partially replaced two small zones of the muscle fiber. In *B,* the invading cells subdivide and replace a large portion of the affected fiber. H&E–stained cryostat sections. ×450.

were macrophages and only 20 percent were T cells.[108] In polymyositis and inclusion body myositis the autoinvasive CD8+ cells appeared to act in conjunction with macrophages in injuring nonnecrotic muscle fibers. Similarly, occasionally nonnecrotic muscle fibers in Duchenne dystrophy were invaded by T cells and some macrophages.[108]

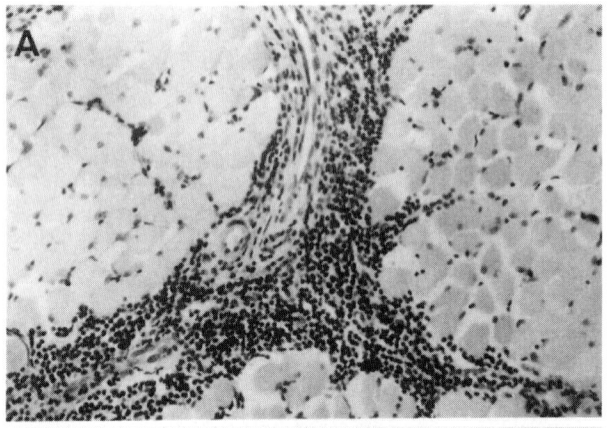
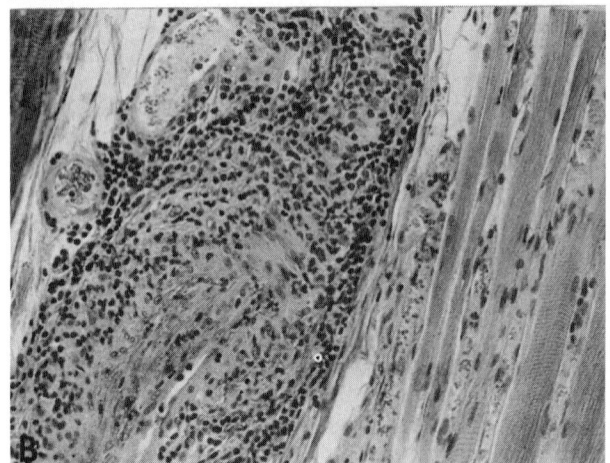
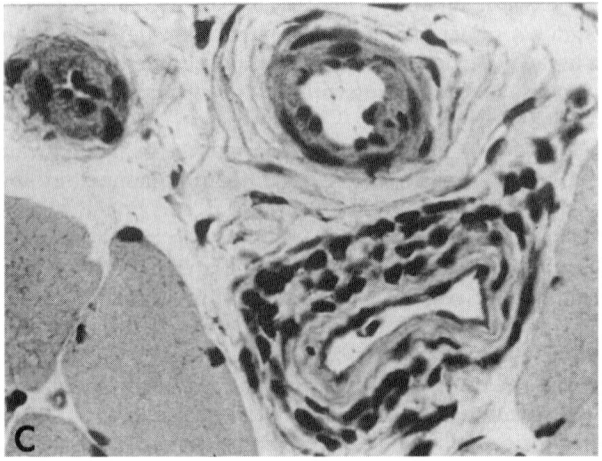

FIGURE 30-51. A. Prominence of inflammatory cells in the perimysial connective tissue. Dermatomyositis of childhood. ×150. B. The wall of this artery is thickened and infiltrated by mononuclear cells. Rheumatoid arthritis. ×292. C. Collection of lymphocytes around and within a perimysial vein. H&E stain. Lupus erythematosus. ×420.

Certain inflammatory changes in muscle are readily recognized because of unusual features of the reaction. In Whipple disease, for example, the diagnosis is established by demonstrating, in the gastrointestinal mucosa, macrophages containing large cytoplasmic granules that give a brilliant magenta stain with periodic acid-Schiff reagent (PAS). Such macrophages may also be detected in other tissues, notably muscle,[111] lymph nodes, spleen, and liver. The presence of PAS-positive granules in macrophages of the lamina propria is not specific for Whipple disease; however, the virtual replacement of most cellular elements in the lamina propria by these macrophages has been seen only in this disorder.

Bacilliform bodies have been detected by electron microscopy within and adjacent to the macrophages. These bodies measure 0.3×1.5 to 2.5 μm and they contain a trilaminar plasma membrane. The bodies have also been observed within epithelial cells and polymorphonuclear leukocytes. With antibiotic therapy, the bacilliform bodies decrease in number or disappear. The PAS-positive granules within macrophages probably represent lysosomes that contain bacilliform bodies in various stages of degradation. In muscle, macrophages containing PAS-positive granules infiltrate the endomysium.[111] The prominence of these cells in muscle as well as their inclusions constitute unique alterations (Figs. 30-59 and 30-60).

Deposition of Amyloid

Amyloidosis. In the course of the various types of amyloidosis, deposition of amyloid in muscle is a common occurrence but is usually clinically silent. Exceptionally, the patient may present with generalized weakness, pseudohypertrophy of muscles, macroglossia, dysphagia, and hoarseness.[112] In the familial form of amyloidosis a slow progression of a proximal weakness may appear in young adults.[113]

Microscopically, amyloid in muscle appears as deposits of amorphous material around and within the walls of blood vessels (Fig 30-61; Color Plate 9F–N) as well as within the perimysial and endomysial connective tissue (Fig. 30-62 and Color Plate 9M and N). The deposits of amyloid blend with contiguous structures and impart an appearance of thickening of the blood vessel wall. Large collections of amyloid are completely devoid of nuclear elements. Amyloid takes the eosin stain and displays metachromasia with crystal violet or methyl violet stains (Color Plate 9I and J). The amyloid deposits outlined by the alkaline Congo red stain manifest as green birefringence when the same sections are studied under polarized light (Color Plate 9K) and show red fluorescence when viewed under rhodamine optics (Color Plate 9L and M). Collections of amyloid stained by thioflavine T also fluoresce.

Although collections of amyloid compress and distort the muscle fibers, they do not penetrate the sarcolemma.[112,114] The muscle fiber changes are subtle and nonspecific. The varying degrees of atrophy that may be detected in fiber types 1 and 2 are often secondary to the peripheral neuropathy that also occurs in the various forms of amyloidosis.[115] Also see Chap. 31

β-Amyloid deposits within muscle fibers. Deposits of β-amyloid[79b–d] and its precursor protein[115a] are associated with the inclusions of inclusion body myositis (Color Plate 9N), the deposits occurring near the rimmed vacuoles.

Similar amyloid deposits also occur in or near rimmed vacuoles in oculopharyngeal dystrophy,[115a,b] in distal myopathies with rimmed vacuoles,[115b] and occasionally in acid maltase deficiency, limb-girdle dystrophy, and Becker dystrophy.[115b] Massive congophilic deposits not consistently associated with accumulation of β-amyloid precursor protein components or gelsolin were observed in myofibrillar myopathy[115c] (Color Plate 10L; see also Chap. 43).

Enzymatic Deficiencies

It has become increasingly apparent that the majority of storage diseases involve most tissues of the body to a greater or lesser extent even though certain organs may be disproportionately affected. In some storage disorders in which the central nervous system is primarily affected, biopsies of muscle and skin have yielded important diagnostic information. It should be stressed that in many of these disorders the standard paraffin-embedded materials are usually of no help. The application of special stains and histochemical techniques to cryostat sections of unfixed material is almost always necessary, and even then the granules that accumulate in the autophagic vacuoles are often so small that they may escape detection. Usually a combination of histochemical and electron microscopic studies are required to detect and define the substances that accumulate in muscle.

The following discussion refers only to the morphologic alterations of intramuscular structures. The clinical, genetic, and laboratory features of these diseases are discussed fully in the monograph by Childs et al.[116]

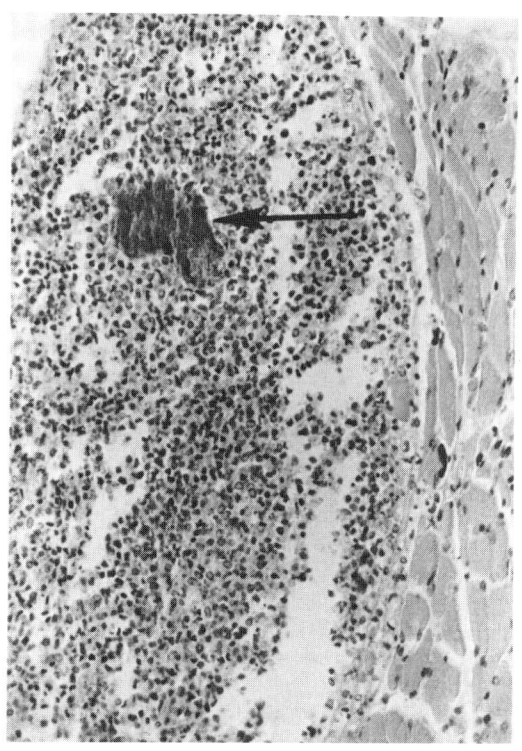

FIGURE 30-52. An abscess within muscle, consisting of neutrophils, fibrin, and bacteria (arrow). The muscle fibers at the periphery are compressed. H&E stain. ×200.

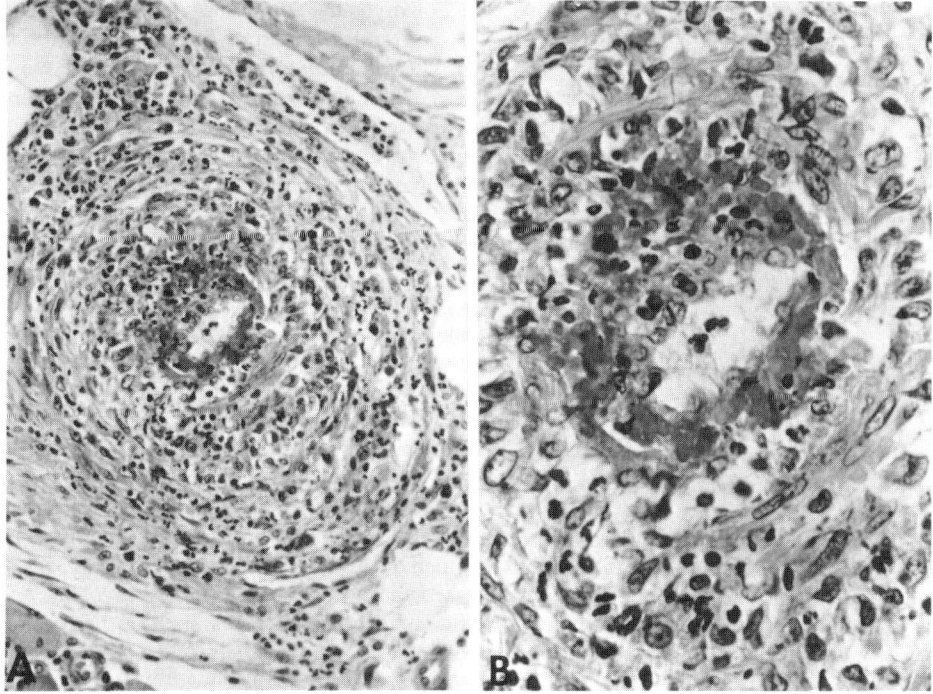

FIGURE 30-53. Polyarteritis nodosa, involving intramuscular blood vessels. Inflammatory cells infiltrate the intima, media, and adventitia of a medium-sized artery. Fibrin is present within the necrotic wall. H&E stain. A, ×180; B, ×450.

GLYCOGEN STORAGE DISORDERS

The glycogen storage diseases (types 2, 3, 4, 5, and 7 and also phosphoglycerate mutase, phosphoglycerate kinase, and beta-enolase deficiencies) that affect muscle all involve defects in glycogen degradation. The myopathologic change common to all of them is the presence of vacuoles containing glycogen.[117] Each of these disorders shows varying degrees of this structural change. In all of them, biochemical studies reveal an increase in muscle glycogen and a deficiency or absence of a specific enzyme. In two of these disorders, myophosphorylase deficiency and phosphofructokinase deficiency, a specific histochemical technique allows a tissue identification of the enzymatic defect. Beta-enolase deficiency can be detected immunohistochemically.[117a]

Acid Maltase Deficiency (Type 2)

Here the fundamental deficiency is in lysosomal acid α-glucosidase. The predominant alteration detected by light microscopic study is the presence of vacuoles containing glycogen within individual muscle fibers (Figs. 30-35 and 30-63). When cryostat-sectioned fresh-frozen muscle is stained by H&E, the majority of the vacuoles contain basophilic granules. PAS and Best Carmine techniques (before and after diastase) identify glycogen collections within the vacuoles (Color Plates 7H and 12E and F). These vacuoles are also strongly reactive for acid phosphatase (Fig. 30-35B; Color Plate 12L). In occasional vacuoles, small amounts of acid mucopolysaccharides can be demonstrated by metachromasia and a positive Alcian blue reaction (Color Plate 12G–I).[117] Similarly, collections of lipid are localized to an occasional vacuole. The vacuoles are found in both types 1 and 2 muscle fibers. In addition, glycogen can be detected in increased amounts between the myofibrils and under the sarcolemma. Many of the muscle fibers appear distended and even distorted. Muscle fibers undergoing regeneration are rarely observed. Occasional necrotic fibers can be seen undergoing phagocytosis. Collections of glycogen granules under the sarcolemma and between the myofibrils are best appreciated by phase-contrast microscopy. Many of the larger vacuoles are subdivided into compartments by complete or incomplete septa.

In the infantile form of this disorder, virtually all muscle fibers contain large vacuoles; in children, the vacuoles tend to be less conspicuous and some muscle fibers or entire muscles may be spared. In adults, almost all fibers of severely weakened muscles contain vacuoles (Fig. 30-63). In less severely affected muscles the vacuolation involves 25 to 75 percent of the fibers, and in clinically unaffected muscles there are only a few vacuolated fibers.[67]

Debranching Enzyme Deficiency (Type 3)

This glycogenosis, also called limit dextrinosis, is due to a deficiency of amylo-1,6-glucosidase. This disorder is also characterized by a vacuolar myopathy (Fig. 30-64). Collections of glycogen are detected within the vacuoles.[67,118] The degree of vacuolar change in muscle appears to correlate closely with the degree of weakness of that muscle. Glycogen is increased between the myofibrils and under the sarcolemma.

Branching Enzyme Deficiency (Type 4)

This disease is also called *amylopectinosis*. A structurally abnormal polysaccharide (amylopectin) with longer outer chains and fewer branch points than normal glycogen is deposited in many tissues and organs. Muscle involvement is variable; not all muscles are equally affected, but the tongue usually is severely involved. The abnormal polysaccharide accumulates in vacuoles. It is PAS-positive but diastase-fast and stains with Alcian blue, colloidal iron, and iodine.[119]

Myophosphorylase Deficiency (McArdle's Disease) (Type 5)

Here the vacuoles are smaller and appear under the sarcolemma as blebs. In many of the vacuoles, glycogen can be detected by PAS and Best Carmine techniques. Empty-appearing subsarcolemmal spaces are well demonstrated in sections reacted for NADH tetrazolium reductase. Cryostat sections of unfixed, frozen muscle lack phosphorylase activity (Fig. 30-65), yet enzyme activity is well demonstrated in

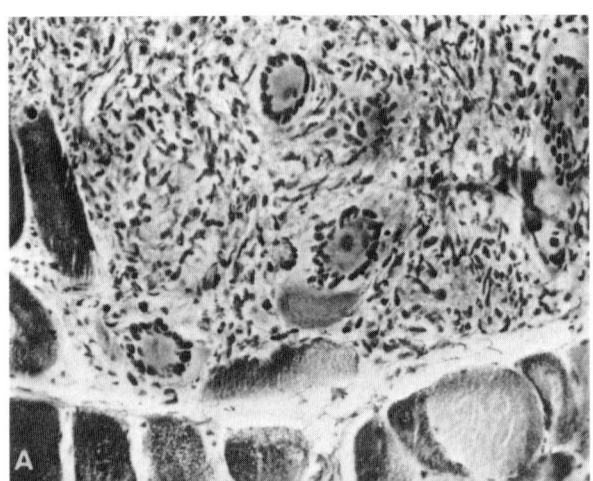

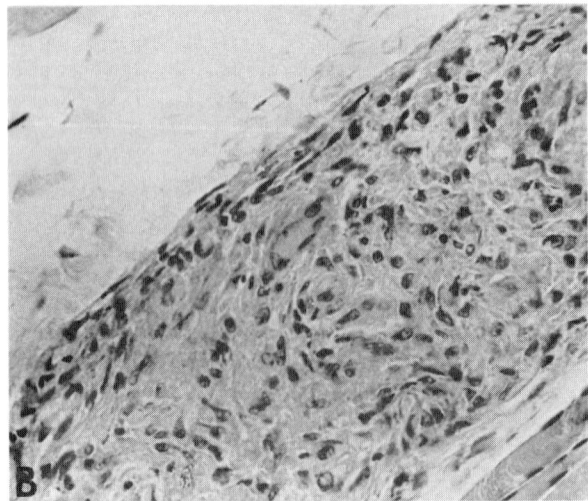

FIGURE 30-54. Conspicuous granulomatous reaction, consisting of giant cells, histiocytes, and lymphocytes within perimysium and adventitia of blood vessels. The infiltrated structures are thickened by connective tissue proliferation. Boeck sarcoid. H&E stain. ×200.

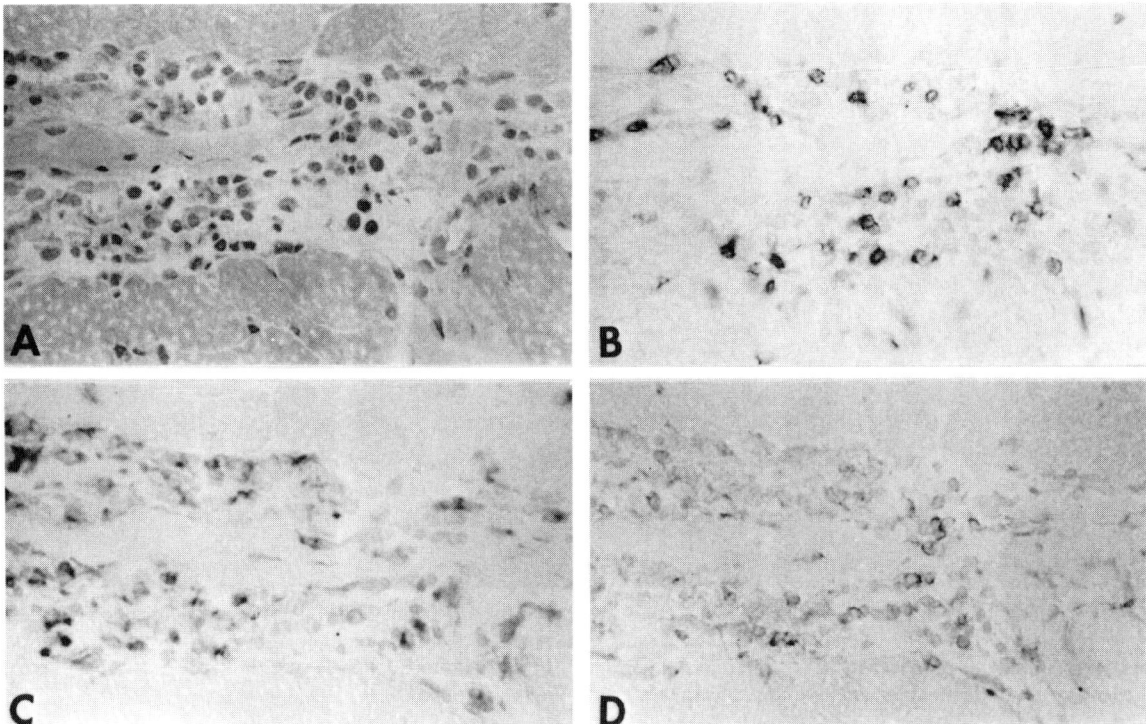

FIGURE 30-55. Perimysial inflammatory cells in scleroderma: 2-μm-thick serial sections stained trichromatically *(A)* and reacted for CD8 *(B)*, acid phosphatase, *(C)* and CD4 *(D)* markers. Nearly all mononuclear cells are accounted for by T cells and macrophages. More CD8⁺ cells and CD4⁺ cells, and more T cells than macrophages, are present. ×260. *(Arahata K, Engel AG: Ann Neurol 16:193, 1984. Reproduced by permission.)*

the muscular layer of the blood vessels. Phase-contrast microscopy of Epon-embedded materials demonstrates the alterations in muscle more clearly. Accumulations of glycogen granules are pocketed particularly in a subsarcolemmal distribution as well as between the myofibrils and between the filaments of the I band.

Phosphofructokinase Deficiency (Tarui's Disease) (Type 7)

This disorder is characterized by the same changes as myophosphorylase deficiency, described above. Histochemical studies reveal the presence of phosphorylase activity and the depletion of phosphofructokinase activity.[120]

NEURONAL CEROID LIPOFUSCINOSES

In the neuronal ceroid lipofuscinoses, the central nervous system is primarily affected. The main alteration is an accumulation within neuronal cytoplasm of substances that possess the staining properties of lipopigments of the ceroid-lipofuscin type. The involvement of tissues other than central nervous system is well appreciated.[121–126] Although storage material can be identified in all organs, the distension and distortion of cells is confined to the central nervous system and the peripheral ganglia.

By light microscopy, two types of vacuoles can be detected in the muscle fiber. In frozen sections stained by H&E, small vacuoles containing coarse basophilic granules are located under the sarcolemma and in the paranuclear zones. In addition, even smaller vacuoles containing fine dustlike basophilic particles are frequently observed within the more central portions of the muscle fiber (Fig. 30-66A). Acid phosphatase activity outlines these vacuoles. The granular collections at the margins of the vacuoles stain red with the trichrome technique and can often be accentuated by the PAS and Sudan black stains. A nitroblue tetrazolium technique such as NADH brings out a deeply colored pigment at the borders of the vacuoles. Both types of vacuoles, ranging in diameter from 1 to 4 μm, are most often detected in the type 1 muscle fiber. They can even be found within intrafusal muscle fibers. In unstained sections, the glycolipid collections within the vacuoles display a yellow-green autofluorescence of lipofuscin.

Electron microscopy shows the vacuoles to be lined by the membranes and to be located within the cytoplasm of muscle fibers, endothelium, fibroblasts, smooth muscle, and Schwann cells.[125] These vacuoles contain membranous structures in the shape of crescents and semicircles called curvilinear or fingerprint profiles (Fig. 30-66B). Each curvilinear body consists of a stack of lamellae in which there are alternating dense and pale lines of equal width. The groups of clusters of curvilinear or fingerprint profiles are usually surrounded by a single membrane. Still other inclusions contain stacks of alternate dark and pale membranes that are straight, wavy, or occasionally circular. Glycogen particles are also observed within the inclusions.[125]

The inclusions containing predominantly the curvilinear profiles are most numerous and conspicuous in the late infan-

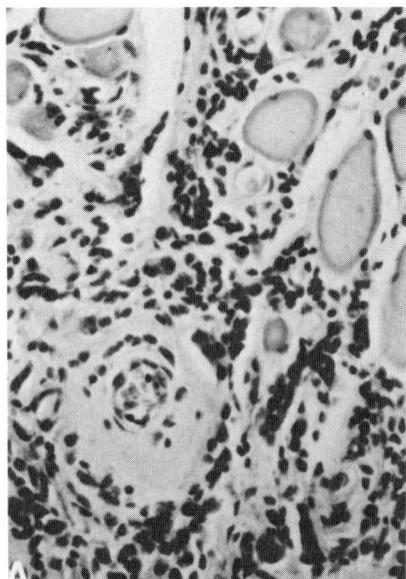 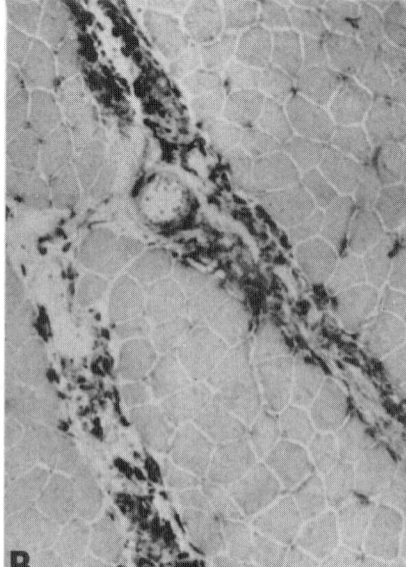 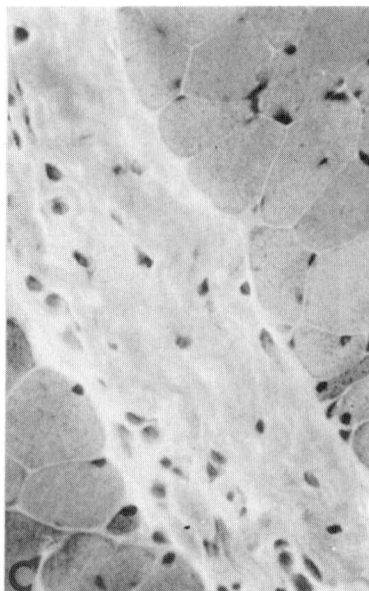

FIGURE 30-56. Inflammatory cells in scleroderma. H&E-(A), acid phosphatase-(B), and trichrome-(C) stained sections. The cells accumulate predominantly at perivascular (A) and perimysial (A, B, C) sites. Many of the inflammatory cells are acid phosphatase— positive macrophages (B). Also note hyalinization of the mural elements of a small blood vessel in A and proliferation of perimysial fibrous connective tissue in C. ×300.

tile group. In the juvenile group an additional type of cytosome with rectilinear profiles is encountered in muscle.[122] These profiles consist of short stacks of alternate dark and pale lines that are straight, wavy, or occasionally circular. The number of lines varies within a stack from 2 to 10 or more, and the fusion of the lines then appears as a thick, dense line. Groups of stacks are enclosed by a membrane. In addition to the profiles within the vacuoles, there are collections of glycogen granules.

Even though these intracytoplasmic inclusions can be detected within muscle, biopsies of skin provide a richer source and are a simpler diagnostic procedure. In skin, the cytosomes are prominent in the endothelial cells of small blood vessels in the dermis. They are also numerous in smooth muscle cells, eccrine sweat glands, Schwann cells, perineurial cells, pericytes, and fibroblasts of the dermis.[124,126]

MUCOPOLYSACCHARIDOSES

The mucopolysaccharidoses (MPS) constitute a group of disorders that are caused by the deficiencies of lysosomal enzymes essential for the stepwise degradation of glycosaminoglycans (mucopolysaccharides). Such deficiencies result in the storage of glycosaminoglycan molecules in lysosomes. At least ten such enzyme deficiencies have been identified. In these disorders the major pathological alterations consist of accumulations of mucopolysaccharides in the viscera and the central nervous system. Accumulations in skin, muscle, and the peripheral nervous system occur as well, but electron microscopic studies are necessary to detect them. The cytoplasm of fibroblasts, Schwann cells, and endothelium of the endomysium, perimysium, endoneurium, and perineurium contain many small intracytoplasmic vacuoles measuring 1 μm at most and enclosed by single membranes. Acid phosphatase activity can be demonstrated within the vacuoles. The mucopolysaccharides within the inclusions frequently disappear when subjected to glutaraldehyde fixation. The inclusions consist of membranous bodies in concentric (membranous cytoplasmic bodies) and parallel configurations (zebra bodies). Many of the lined vacuoles are empty.[127]

Although the vacuoles can be detected within intramuscular structures by electron microscopic techniques, they are more numerous and more easily identified in the dermal layer of skin. Skin biopsy, therefore, is the diagnostic approach of choice.

NIEMANN-PICK GROUP OF DISEASES

These disorders are sphingomyelin-cholesterol lipidoses characterized by an accumulation of sphingomyelin, cholesterol, glycosphingolipids or bis (monoacylglycero)-phosphate, particularly in the viscera. The basic deficiency is that of sphingomyelinase; in the type 2 form, there is a defect in cholesterol esterification as well. The histologic study of skin, muscle, and peripheral nerve reveals large macrophages within the nerve fibers displaying the same characteristics as those of liver, spleen, bone marrow, and lymph nodes.[127,128] Ultrastructural studies reveal numerous dense cytoplasmic bodies in the Schwann cells, macrophages, and fibroblasts of endoneurium and perineurium. The cytoplasmic bodies are also detected in the endothelium, pericytes, smooth muscle cells of blood vessels, and satellite cells of skeletal muscle. The cytoplasmic bodies consist of vacuoles containing membranous structures arranged as parallel dense lines or lamellated inclusions as well as collections of electron-dense confluent materials. Small electron-dense bodies measuring 40 nm in diameter are distributed between the myofibrils.

G_{M1} GANGLIOSIDOSIS

G_{M1} gangliosidosis (generalized gangliosidosis) is characterized by the accumulation of G_{M1} ganglioside and a keratan sulfate–like polysaccharide. A lack of activity of β-galactosidase results in an accumulation of both lipid and mucopolysaccharide, particularly in viscera and the central nervous system. The G_{M1} ganglioside is found in excess in the cytoplasm of the neurons throughout the central and peripheral nervous systems. A keratan sulfate–like mucopolysaccharide accumulates in the viscera. In muscle, abnormalities are observed in blood vessel, nerves, and muscle fibers.[129,130] In the endomysium and perimysium, the cytoplasm of fibroblasts contains material that is outlined by acid phosphatase and mucopolysaccharide techniques. The further identification of the storage material requires electron microscopic study. Two kinds of cytoplasmic inclusions are observed. In the Schwann cells of the intramuscular nerves, the inclusions are filled either with a moderately electron-dense and polymorphous material that corresponds to the

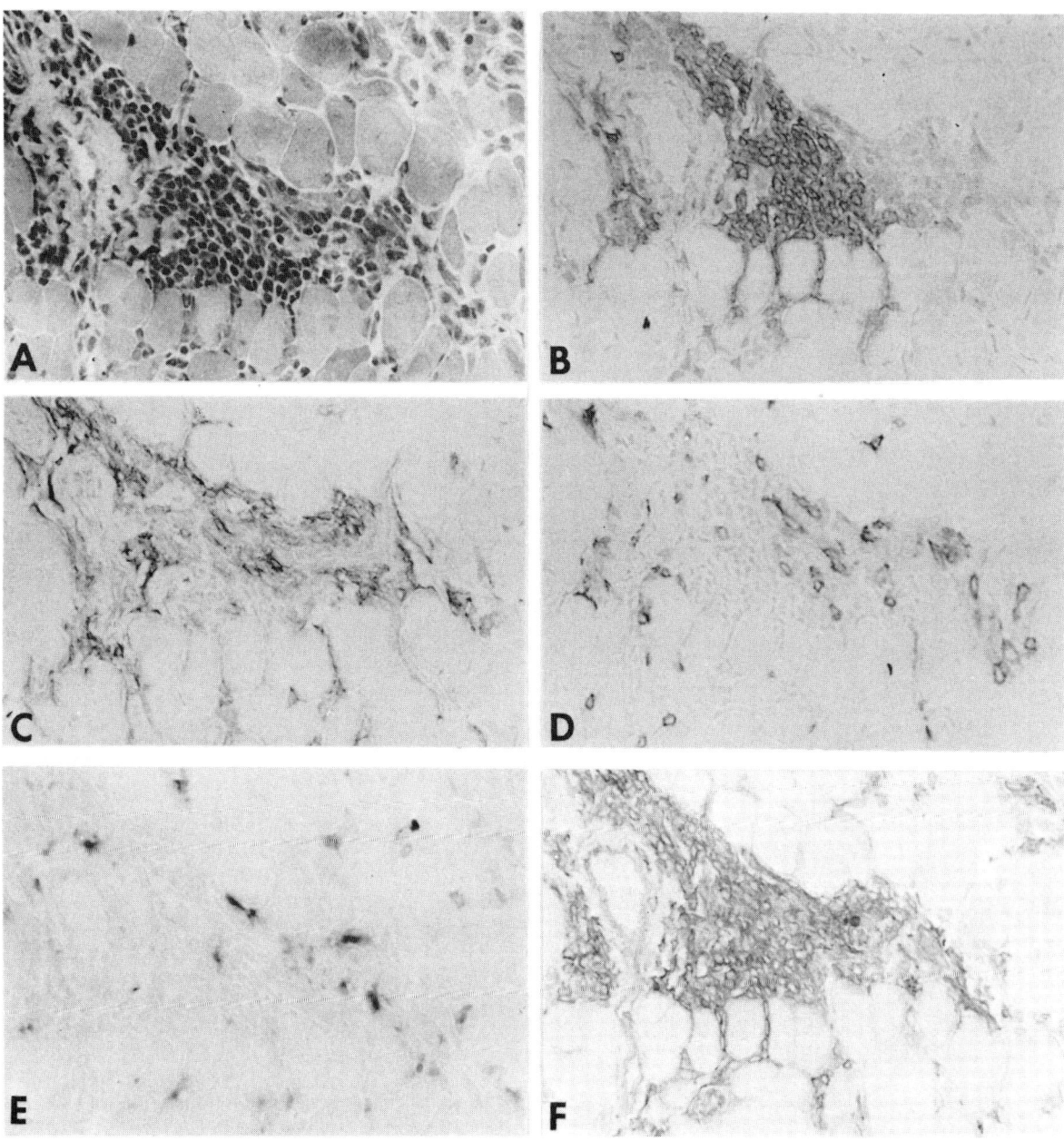

FIGURE 30-57. Inflammatory cells in dermatomyositis: 2-μm-thick serial sections stained trichromatically *(A)* and reacted for B cell *(B)*, CD4 *(C)*, CD8 *(D)*, acid phosphatase *(E)*, and Ia *(F)* markers. A blood vessel at the upper left is surrounded by a compact collection of mononuclear cells. Most of the perivascular cells are B cells. CD8+ cells and macrophages are relatively sparse and have migrated farther from the blood vessels than have B cells. CD4+ cells intermingle with B cells and CD8+ cells Ia+ cells (which include B cells, macrophages, and activated T cells) are more numerous than cells in any subset. Relatively few endomysial mononuclear cells appear in this field. *A–F.* 260. (Arahata K, Engel AG: Ann Neurol 16:193, 1984. Reproduced by permission.)

ganglioside accumulation[130] or with electron-lucent collections containing fibrillar material.[129] In the perineurial fibroblasts, endothelium, pericytes and satellite cells of muscle, the inclusions are bounded by a single membrane and contain a finely granular material that corresponds to the keratan sulfate–like mucopolysaccharide. The nature of the accumulated substances appears to be related to the particular metabolism of the cell involved.[130]

FABRY DISEASE

Fabry disease (angiokeratoma corporis diffusum) is an inborn error of glycosphingolipid metabolism caused by the defective activity of the lysosomal enzyme α-galactosidase A. Neutral glycosphingolipids with terminal galactosyl moieties accumulate in tissues and fluids throughout the body. This material can be detected by light microscopy in cryostat-

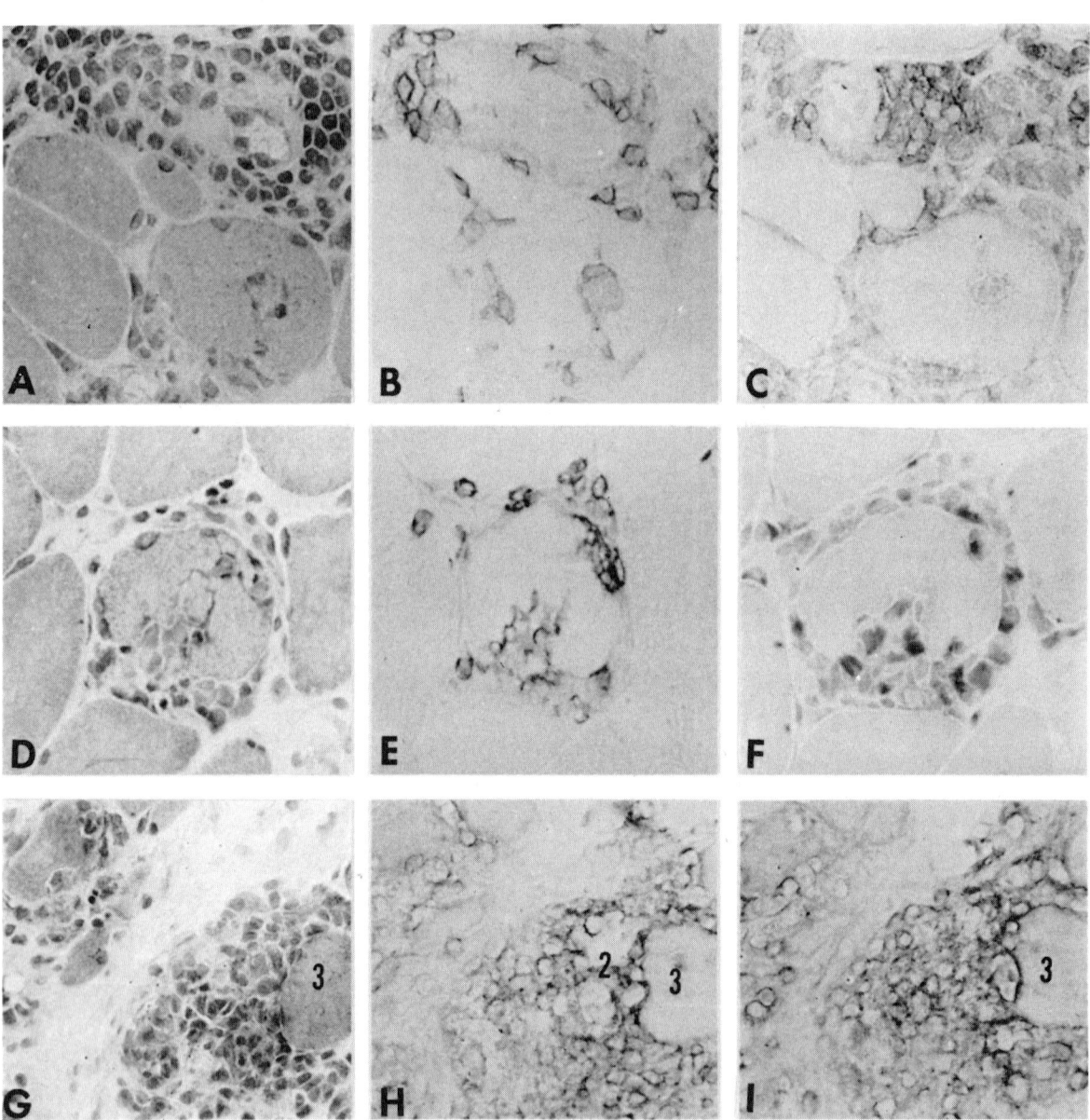

FIGURE 30-58. Inflammatory cells in polymyositis. *A–C.* Nonconsecutive 2-μm-thick sections stained trichromatically (*A*) and reacted for the CD8 (*B*) and CD4 (*C*) antigens. A small perimysial blood vessel is surrounded by numerous CD8+ and CD4+ cells. A muscle fiber at the lower right is focally surrounded and deeply invaded by mononuclear cells (*A*). Some of the invading cells are CD8+ (*B*), but none are CD4+ (*C*). All ×360. *D–F.* Nonconsecutive 2-μm-thick sections stained trichromatically (*D*), reacted for the CD4 antigen (*E*), and stained for acid phosphatase (*F*). The muscle fiber in the center is focally surrounded by mononuclear cells, which invade it at the 2 and 7 o'clock positions. A large fraction of the fiber area is replaced, and the fiber is nearly divided by the invading cells (*D*). Many of the invading cells are CD8+ and are applied directly against the scalloped margins of the fiber (*E*). A proportion of the invading cells are acid phosphatase–positive macrophages (*F*). All ×360. *G–I.* Nonconsecutive 10-μm-thick sections stained trichromatically (*G*) and reacted for Lyt 3 (*H*) and CD4 (*I*) antigens. Three muscle fibers are invaded by mononuclear cells. Fibers 1 and 3, present in each section, are partially replaced by the invading cells. Fiber 2 is represented only in *H*; this fiber has been completely replaced by the invading cells in *G* and *I*. Nearly all the invading cells are Lyt 3+ (*H*) and therefore represent T cells. Most of these cells are also CD8+ (*I*). All ×300. (Arahata K, Engel AG: Ann Neurol 16:193, 1984. Reproduced by permission.)

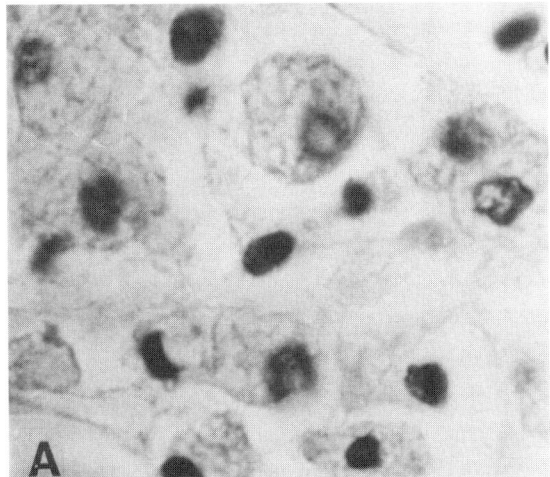

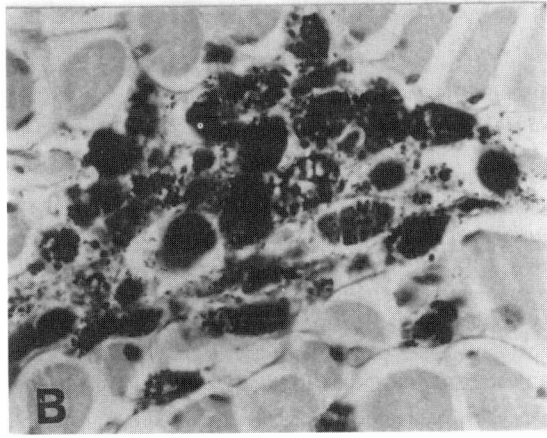

FIGURE 30-59. Whipple disease. Psoas muscle. *A*. Large macrophages form conspicuous clusters in the perimysium. Small intracellular granules are visible. H&E stain. ×1300. *B*. The macrophages are accentuated when stained with PAS. ×536. The slides were supplied by Dr. Ann C. McKee.

LAFORA DISEASE

This is a disorder of the nervous system in children and adolescents; it is characterized by an accumulation of polysaccharide inclusions in neurons as well as in viscera, peripheral nerves, sweat glands, and muscle. In some kinships the metabolic defect is in a tyrosine phosphatase (laforin).[131a] The muscle biopsy can be of value in establishing the diagnosis.[132–134] In many relatively normal-appearing muscle fibers there are numerous scattered, round inclusions (polyglucosans) that stain red with PAS and purple with H&E, modified trichrome stain, and the NADH-TR oxidative enzyme technique. The polyglucosans demonstrate strong diaminobenzidine peroxidase acitivity. This feature and the ultrastructural appearance support the concept that the inclusions have features in common with those in nerve cells in this disorder.[132,135] Ultrastructural studies reveal that in neurons, the polyglucosan accumulations are free in the cytoplasm, while in skeletal muscle they are inside membrane-bound spaces.[132,135] Sheets of glycogen particles and fine granular filamentous materials are observed between myofibrils. Numerous membrane-lined vesicles measuring 3 to 10 μm are seen within the muscle fiber. The vesicles contain small amounts of dense granular material, glycogen particles, fine particles, and filamentous aggregates. Some vesicles also contain lipid droplets. Nishimura et al.[136] have stressed the value of the liver biopsy in establishing the diagnosis of Lafora disease. Busard et al.[137,138] have found axillary skin biopsy of diagnostic value, the polyglucosan bodies being concentrated in the myoepithelial cells of apocrine glands.

sectioned fresh-frozen muscle (Fig. 30-67*A*). The deposits of glycosphingolipid are birefringent in polarized light, often displaying the "Maltese cross" configuration, and are also outlined by lipid, PAS, and acid phosphatase techniques. Within muscle, the material accumulates in the endothelium, pericytes, and smooth muscle of blood vessels. Inclusions are also observed in the histiocytes and in perineurial and endoneurial cells as well as within the muscle fiber.

Ultrastructural study discloses lamellar bodies in the cytoplasm of the various cells listed above. In muscle there are numerous bodies of this type ranging from 0.6 to 1.6 μm in diameter, situated either between the myofibrils or under the plasma membrane.[131] These bodies are round or ovoid and are sparsely distributed singly or in groups (Fig. 30-67*B*). A single membrane encloses electron-dense parallel lamellae. Identical lamellar bodies are observed within capillary endothelium and pericytes, perineurium, and occasional phagocytes.

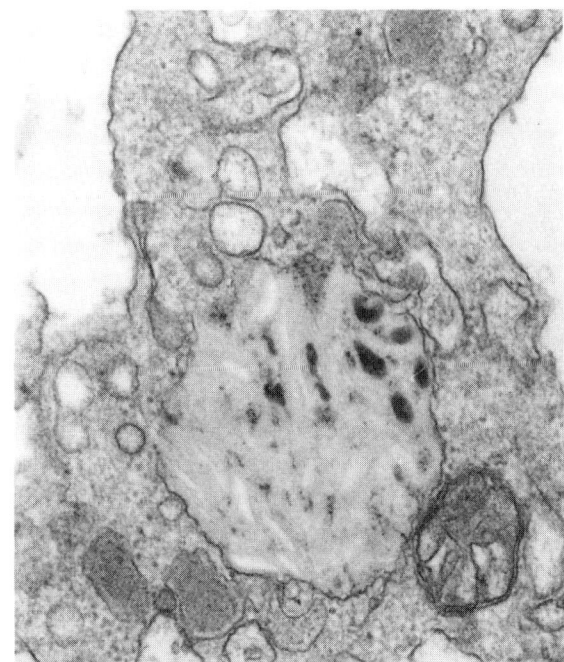

FIGURE 30-60. Whipple disease. Electron micrograph of a macrophage in the perimysium. Electron-dense elongated structures represent the bacilliform bodies. ×44000.

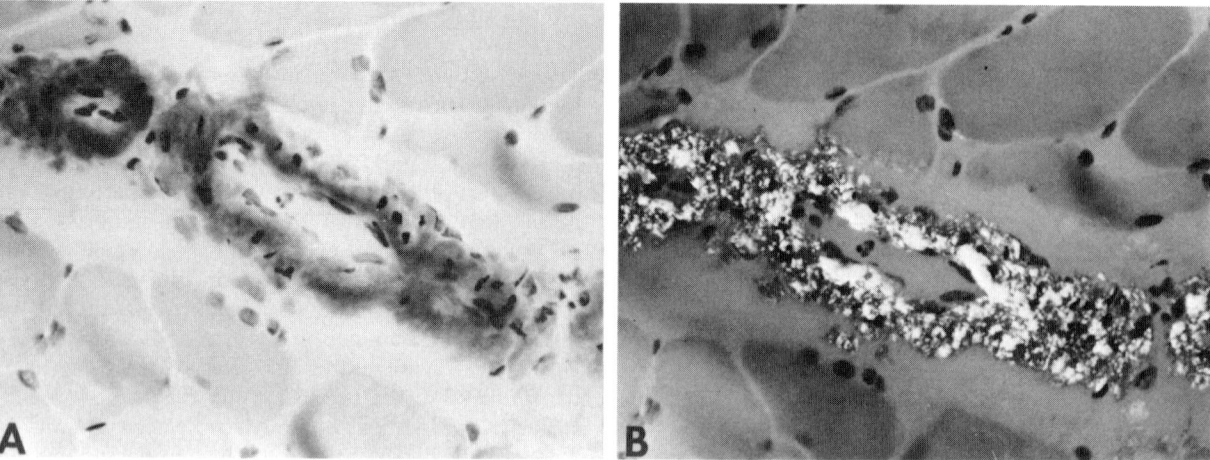

FIGURE 30-61. Amyloid deposition in muscle. The mural elements of a perimysial blood vessel are infiltrated with amorphous Congo red-positive material (A) that displays positive birefringence in polarized light (B). ×270.

METACHROMATIC LEUKODYSTROPHY

The biochemical defect in metachromatic leukodystrophy (MLD) is a deficiency of arylsulfatase A (cerebroside sulfatase) that results in the accumulation of galactosyl sulfatide (cerebroside sulfate) within the white matter of the central nervous system. In addition, metachromatic substances are observed within the neuronal cytoplasm as well as within the peripheral and autonomic nervous systems and certain viscera, particularly kidney and liver. When frozen sections of fresh or formalin-fixed muscle containing intramuscular nerves are subjected to acetic cresyl violet stain at a pH of 3.6, a golden brown metachromasia appears within the intramuscular nerves. This is in contrast to the purple-blue color of the normal myelinated nerves. In addition, it has been shown that when these same sections are viewed by polarized light with the polarizer and analyzer 90° out of phase, the metachromatic granules display a specific lime-green to yellow-green dichroism.[139] The PAS stain of the metachromatic granules is strongly positive as is the alcian blue reaction. The granules are also outlined by Sudan black.

Ultrastructural studies reveal two major types of membrane-enclosed inclusion material within the intramuscular nerves.[140,141] The configurations are located within the endoneurial macrophages, Schwann cytoplasm, and endothelial cells of small blood vessels. The first group of inclusions consists of osmiophilic bodies that contain concentrically arranged lamellar material. These configurations are made up of major dense lines separated by an 8-nm space. These inclusions are particularly conspicuous in the Schwann cytoplasm of myelinated axons and may therefore represent products of myelin breakdown.[140] The second type of inclu-

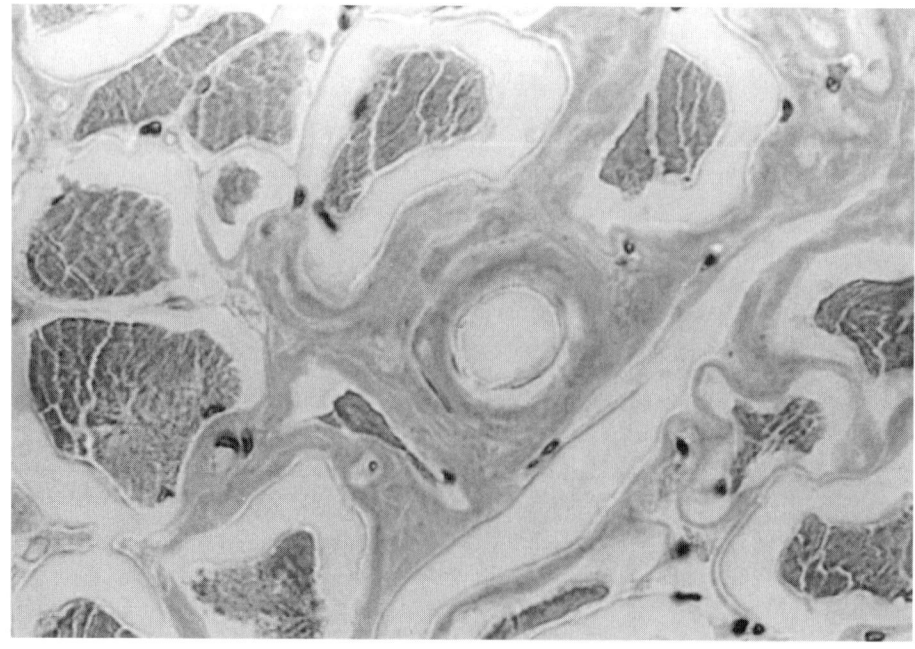

FIGURE 30-62. Deposition of amyloid in perimysial and endomysial spaces as well as within the walls of blood vessels. H&E stain. ×674.

sion is more elaborate and similar to the inclusions within the central nervous system. This second type of inclusion corresponds to the metachromatic material detected by light microscopy. The accumulations in this latter group have the same basic lamellar structure of alternating dark and light bands, with a regular periodicity of 5.8 nm.[140] Zebra bodies, which display parallel lamellae, are observed within Schwann cells and macrophages. Tuffstone bodies, as the name implies, exhibit a pattern that resembles volcanic limestone; these configurations are electron-dense and the lamellae are irregularly oriented. Prismatic inclusions consist of closely packed stacked disks that are composed of the lamellar lipid leaflets. Depending upon the plane in which the prisms are visualized, some appear honeycombed.[142] Although the histologic diagnosis may be suggested by the study of biopsied nerve, conjunctiva, skin, or urinary sediment, the diagnosis is established by the biochemical studies of arylsulfatase A activity in peripheral leukocytes and cultured skin fibroblasts.[143] Prenatal diagnosis is made by measuring the activity of arylsulfatase A in amniotic fluid cells.[143]

GLOBOID CELL LEUKODYSTROPHY

Globoid cell leukodystrophy (Krabbe disease) affects primarily the white matter of the central nervous system. A genetic deficiency of the lysosomal enzyme galoctosylceramidase (galactosyl ceramide β-galactosidase) results in the accumulation of galactosyl ceramide in globoid cells. The peripheral nervous system also is commonly affected.[144,145] Alterations can even be appreciated within intramuscular nerves. However, typical globoid cells are not found in the peripheral nerves, whereas they predominate in the central nervous system. In the peripheral nerves inclusion material is not detected by light microscopy; the distinct alterations are appreciated only by electron microscopy. The inclusions, which are shaped like needles, splinters, or prisms, are found within the histiocytes in the endoneurial connective tissue and around small blood vessels as well as within Schwann cells.[144] The inclusions of Krabbe disease are usually but not always membrane-bound within the cytoplasm of the cell; the endoplasmic reticulum of the cell is often dilated. The inclusions lack the highly structured arrangement of those of metachromatic leukodystrophy, and because the inclusions in Krabbe disease differ from all others, they are considered to represent specific changes.

INFANTILE NEUROAXONAL DYSTROPHY

Infantile neuroaxonal dystrophy is one of the few degenerative neurological disorders that can be diagnosed by skin, conjunctival, nerve, or muscle biopsies,[146-148] even though the major site of the disease is the central nervous system. The basic defect in this disease is not known, unlike most of the storage disorders discussed above. However, a deficient activity of lysosomal alpha-N-acetylgalactosaminidase has been described in two brothers with the clinical and pathologic features of neuroaxonal dystrophy.[149-151] The parents, who were distantly related, had an intermediate degree of activity of this enzyme, while eight unrelated patients with infantile neuroaxonal dystrophy had normal activity. Whether the neuroaxonal dystrophies are genetically heterogeneous and this metabolic defect is directly related to neuroaxonal dystrophy in this particular family or whether the enzymatic defect represents an additional defect remains to be defined.

When peripheral nerve is carefully scrutinized by light or phase microscopy, spheroids or focal swellings of the axons can occasionally be found.[152] These spheroids, like the ones in the central nervous system, are eosinophilc and argyrophilic and stain strongly with PAS. However, by light and phase microscopy they are not readily distinguishable from other types of axonal enlargement. In muscle, zones of denervation atrophy are usually evident.

The ultrastructural alterations are characteristic in that inclusions can be identified within the terminal portion of axons. The alterations in the peripheral axons are identical to those in the central nervous system. The distended axons (spheroids) of the peripheral nerve are filled with smooth membranous tubular and wedge-shaped profiles that are

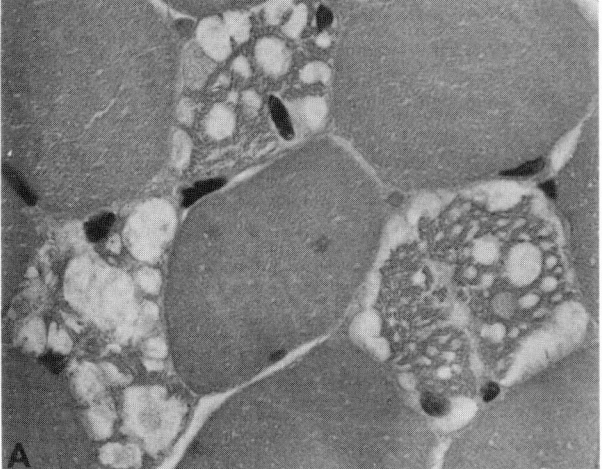

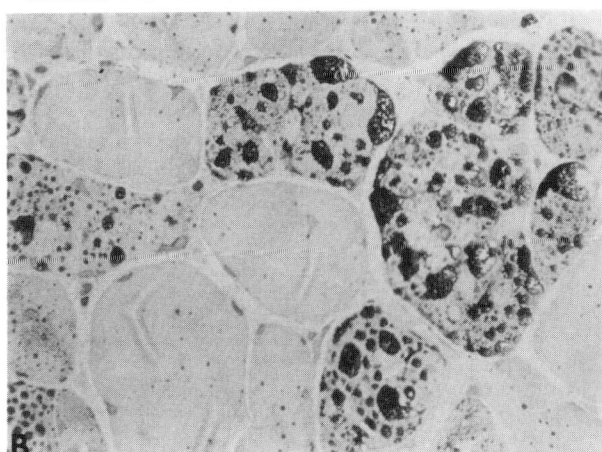

FIGURE 30-63. Adult acid maltase deficiency. H&E-stained paraffin (*A*) and PAS-stained (*B*) resin sections. Multiple vacuoles of varying sizes are present in the abnormal fibers. The vacuoles appear empty or contain finely granular material in *A* but are nearly completely filled with PAS-positive material in *B*. *A*, ×633; *B*, ×460. (*Engel AG, Dale AJ: Mayo Clin Proc 43:233, 1968. Reproduced by permission.*)

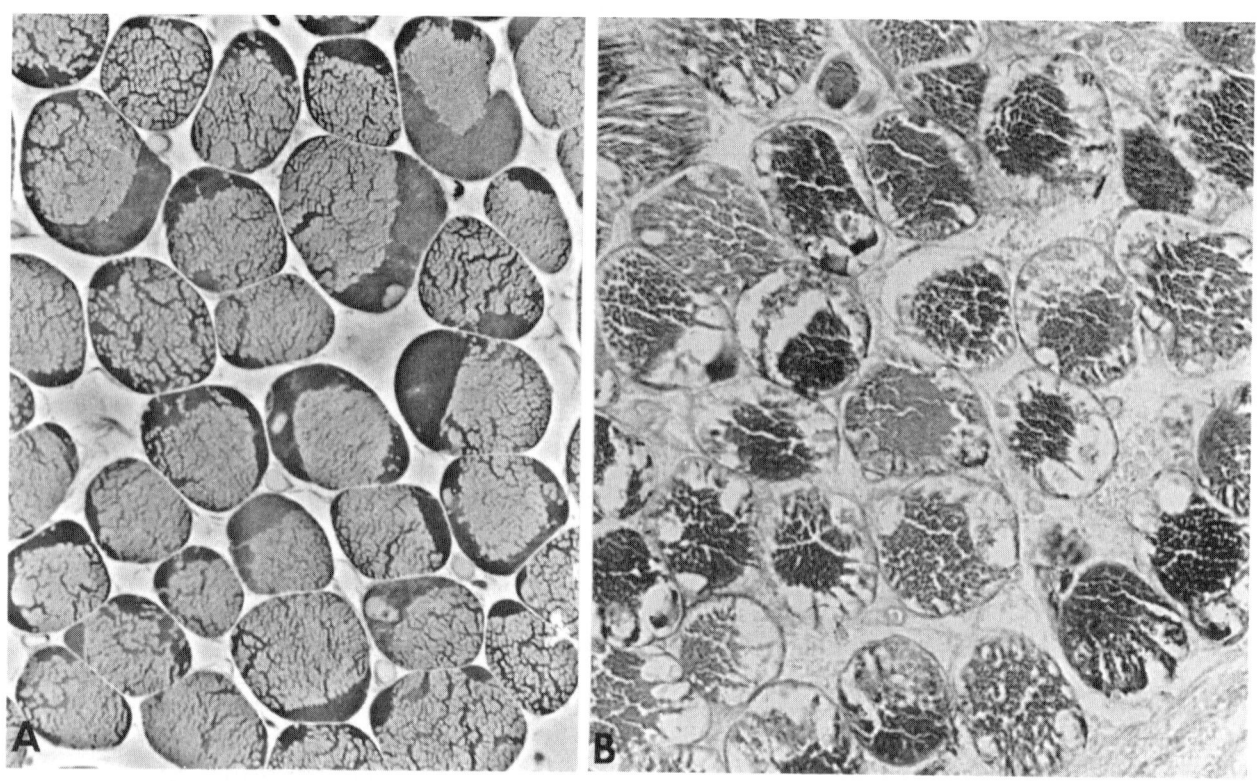

FIGURE 30-64. *A.* Epon-embedded sections stained with PAS, showing collections of glycogen in a subsarcolemmal distribution. *B.* A portion of the same muscle embedded in paraffin and stained with PAS; much of the stored glycogen has been lost by processing. ×600.

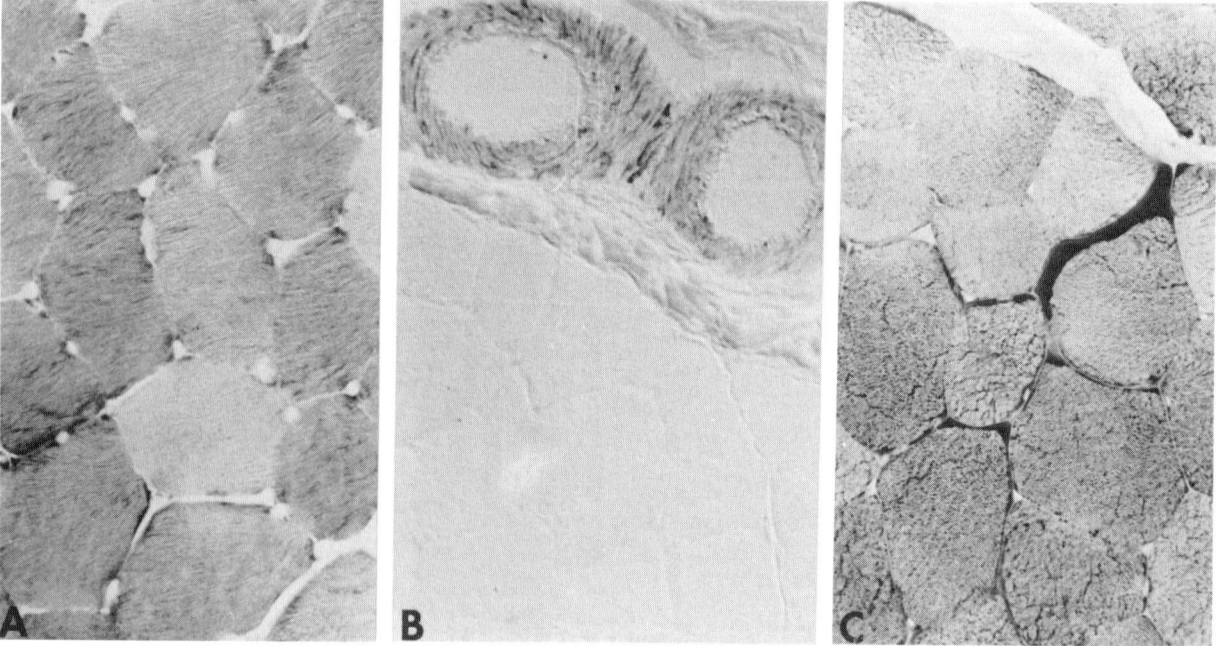

FIGURE 30-65. Normal *(A)* and phosphorylase-deficient *(B, C)* muscle reacted for phosphorylase *(A, B)* and stained with PAS *(C)*. In the patient's muscle, enzyme activity is absent from the muscle fibers but is preserved in vascular smooth muscle *(B)*. In this disorder relatively small amounts of glycogen accumulate in the muscle fibers and the glycogen deposits are often subsarcolemmal *(C)*. *A, C,* ×320; *B,* ×200.

often divided by lamellar arrays into compartments. In the distended axons the neurofilaments are severely depleted; the mitochondria are large but their cristae are normal. The structure of the spheroid is often complex and imparts a density to the axoplasm; cisternae are frequently distended. In skin and conjuctiva, spheroids are detected in the distal portions of both myelinated and unmyelinated axons, particularly in the presynaptic endings. Occasionally they can be observed in the cytoplasm of an endoneurial fibroblast and Schwann cell.[148,153] In muscle, the collections of packed membranous and tubular structures have been found at the motor end plate in the axoplasm of the presynaptic portion of the nerve terminal.[153–156]

It must be stressed that these unique morphological features are primarily located in the axoplasm of both the central and peripheral nervous systems. For muscle to provide diagnostic information, the motor end plate region and/or small intramuscular nerves must be included in the biopsied area. Because of the concentration of small terminal axons and their accessibility, skin and conjuctival biopsies are a more practical means of establishing the diagnosis than is muscle biopsy.

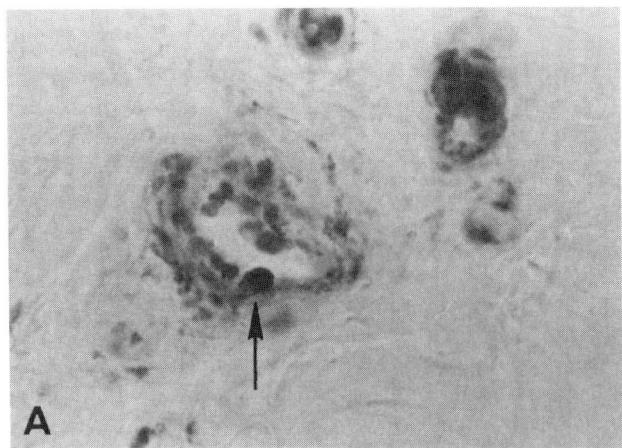

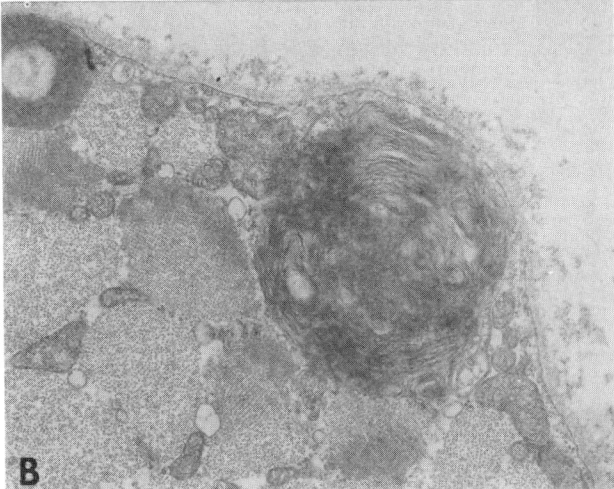

FIGURE 30-67. Fabry disease. *A*. A substance accentuated by PAS and lipid stains collects within the endothelial cytoplasm of small intramuscular blood vessels (arrow). Sudan black stain. ×506. *B*. By electron microscopy, lamellar bodies are found under the sarcolemma of muscle fibers. ×13,000.

CYTOCHROME OXIDASE DEFICIENCY

A defect in cytochrome *c* oxidase has been demonstrated in muscle biopsies from infants and children with severe generalized weakness, lactic acidosis, abnormal muscle mitochondria, and the de Toni-Fanconi-Debré syndrome.[157–160] Muscle studies reveal excessive mitochondria, lipid, and glycogen. The trichrome stain accentuates the sarcoplasmic granules in many muscle fibers. There is often increased succinic dehydrogenase or NADH-tetrazolium reductase activity occurring in a large proportion of the fibers. Histochemically, cytochrome *c* oxidase activity is markedly reduced or absent in the muscle fibers[157–160] (Fig. 30-68). Biochemical studies have confirmed an isolated defect of cytochrome oxidase activity (see Chap. 58). The fatal and benign infantile forms of cytochrome oxidase deficiency myopathies can be differentiated immunohistochemically[161] (see also "Ragged Red Fibers," above).

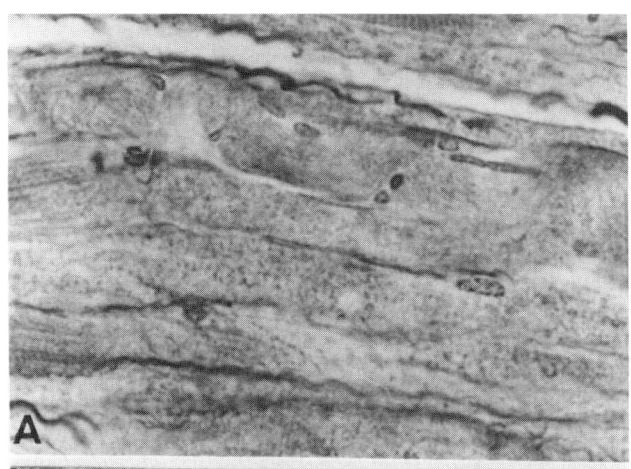

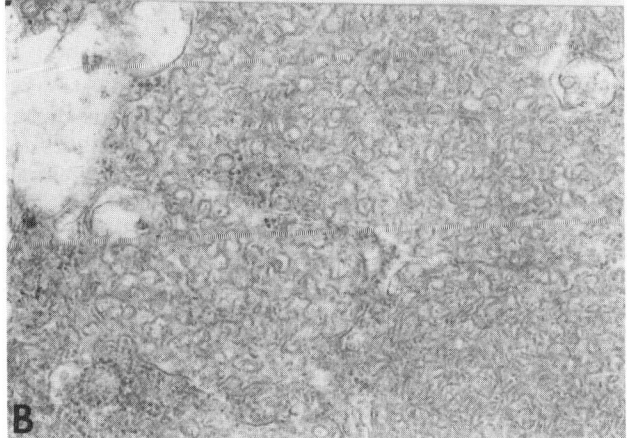

FIGURE 30-66. *A*. The muscle fibers contain a fine granular material that stains as a glycolipid. H&E stain. ×628. *B*. By electron microscopy there are many membranous structures or curvilinear profiles within the muscle fiber. Neuronal lipofuscinosis. ×17,386.

MYOADENYLATE DEAMINASE DEFICIENCY

Fishbein et al.[162] have described a tetrazolium-based histochemical technique for the detection of adenylate deaminase in cryostat sections of unfixed muscle. This method is based on the elaboration of ammonia by adenylate deaminase as the enzyme deaminates 5AMP. Application of this stain allows the screening of muscle biopsies for deficiencies of adenylate deaminase (Fig. 30-69). Although the clinical features are quite diverse, the diagnosis should be suspected when easy fatigue, muscle cramps, and myalgia follow exercise and the ratio of blood ammonia to lactate is abnormal following ischemic exercise.[163,164] In the majority, the serum creatine kinase is elevated.[165] Most patients lacking this enzyme in muscle are identified by the reduced or absent histochemical reaction product for adenylate deaminase. The incidence of the histochemically proved deficiency is as high as 1.5 percent,[162] although not all are of the primary type. In the secondary type, it is not clear what relationship the deficiency of the myoadenylate deaminase activity bears to the presenting disorder. The deficiency state can be confirmed by biochemical assay of muscle.[162] There are no specific structural changes in muscle.

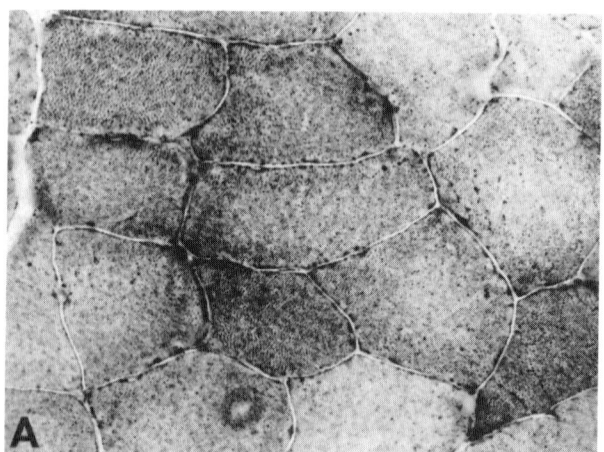

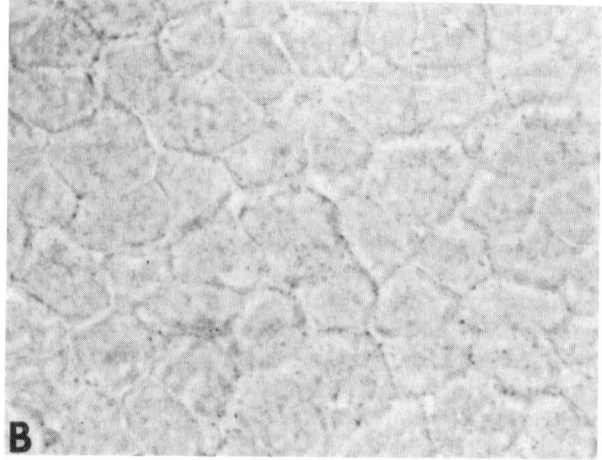

FIGURE 30-68. Cytochrome oxidase activity in normal muscle (A) and in muscle of an infant suffering from mitochondria-lipid-glycogen disease associated with cytochrome oxidase deficiency. A, ×280; B, ×690.

Alterations of the Muscle Spindle

The muscle spindle is a highly complex structure, and recognition of its alterations requires a knowledge of its normal structure and topography (Chap. 21). The alterations of extrafusal fibers and surrounding structures are often identical to changes that occur within the muscle spindle. For example, in the various storage disorders, the abnormal accumulations can be detected in the capsule, endothelial cells, and intrafusal fibers of the spindle as well as the extrafusal fibers. In dermatomyositis of childhood, the microtubular inclusions are found within the endothelium of blood vessels of the spindle as well as within endothelium of the endomysial and perimysial vessels. Certain tumors originating in muscle, e.g., hemangioma, extend directly along nerve to invade the intraaxial space (Fig 30-70). The changes that are confined to the muscle spindle are summarized below.

Denervation. A large number of denervation experiments carried out over a period of more than 100 years have defined the morphologic and physiologic attributes of the neuromuscular spindle apparatus and its role in skeletal muscle function. The first recorded experiment was by Sachs,[166] who severed the anterior roots in frogs and then observed a nerve entering muscle and twisting around a spindle-shaped body, even though the extrafusal muscle fibers were completely degenerated. Onanoff in 1890[167] first studied the specific effects of selective denervation of the muscle spindle. After deafferentation of the spindle by removing the dorsal root ganglia and the dorsal roots, he found a degenration of the spiral endings and of nearly all the nerve fibers within the spindle. On the other hand, after deefferentation only a few nerve fibers had degenerated. From these experiments he concluded that the spindle was a sensory organ that was dependent upon motor control from the anterior horn cells. Sherrington's study in 1894[168] was based on selective denervation techniques in both the cat and monkey. From deefferentation experiments, he concluded that muscle and spindle contained a rich afferent supply. In the muscle spindles subjected to both deefferentation and deafferentation he found no myelinated nerve fibers and concluded that the sympathetic nervous system did not innervate the muscle spindle. Moreover, he observed no atrophy of the intrafusal fibers as long as 5 months after the interruption of the sciatic nerve. On the basis of all these observations he stressed that muscle spindles were elaborately organized sensory organs that were supplied with nerve fibers arising in the dorsal root ganglion cells. In 1897 and 1898, two important contributions to this subject were made by Batten.[169,170] He severed the sciatic nerves in a group of cats and allowed them to survive for 3 weeks to 3 months; although the extrafusal fibers had atrophied and the nerves to the spindles had degenerated, there was no definite change in the intrafusal fibers. A year before, in human autopsy material, Batten had demonstrated that the intrafusal fibers degenerated in peripheral neuropathy provided that there was a sufficiently long period of denervation.[170] He correctly concluded[169,170] that intrafusal fibers atrophy following motor denervation, that muscle spindle is the organ from which muscular afferents are derived, that tendon

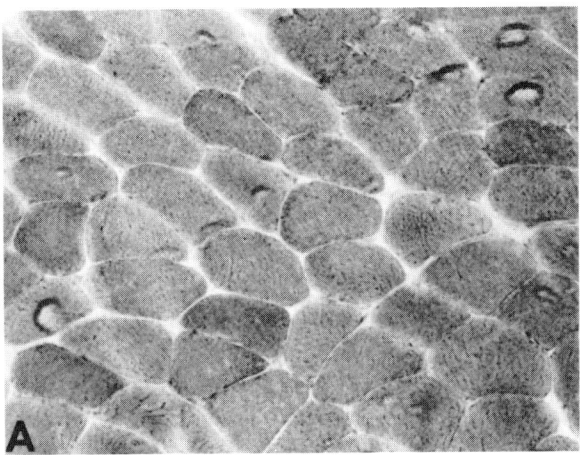
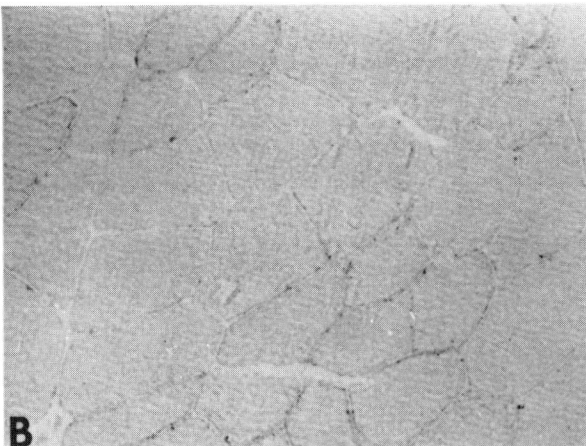

FIGURE 30-69. Reaction for adenylate deaminase in normal subject *(A)* and in patient with adenylate deaminase deficiency *(B)*. ×130.

organs and muscle spindles are closely allied, and that muscle spindles are responsible for position sense.

In another early experiment, Cippolone[171] temporarily compressed the abdominal aorta of rabbits and sacrificed the animals 5 to 10 days later. In the muscle spindles he found a degeneration of the plate endings but not of the equatorial endings and concluded that the ischemia had damaged the spinal cord but not the dorsal root ganglia. He therefore postulated that the plate endings were motor and the more central endings were sensory. Tello[172] studied the muscle spindle after sectioning peripheral nerve and found that the plate endings and the more central endings degenerated at different rates; he also postulated that the two endings had different functions. Investigators followed these leads and carefully defined the motor and sensory endings of the intrafusal fibers through a series of selective denervation experiments.[173–179] A number of more recent reports has added to the descriptions of the innervation of the normal muscle spindle as well as to its ultrastructural features (Chap. 21).

Kennedy[180] has studied the intrafusal innervation in muscle biopsies from patients with amyotrophic lateral sclerosis (ALS). He found that the gamma efferent fibers were reduced in number and altered in their intrafusal course; the gamma endings were altered as well. The changes in the muscle spindle in ALS differed from those in peripheral neuropathy in that the sensory innervation was spared in the former and altered in the latter.[180]

The effect of denervation in the developing spindle is quite different from that in the mature spindle. Zelena et al.[181–183] found that muscle spindle development is highly dependent upon innervation; in the newborn rat, the intrafusal fibers degenerated within a few days after nerve section. McArdle and Sansone[184] were able to prevent the development of muscle spindles in the rat by ablating their innervation at birth.

Regeneration. Although extrafusal muscle fibers have a high potential for regeneration, intrafusal fibers have been thought to lack this capacity.[185] The evidence that supports this concept is derived from the studies of Zelena and Sobotkova.[185] In adult female albino rats they removed that portion of the extensor digitorum longus muscle between its distal third below the entrance of the distal nerve and 2 mm above the distal tendon. The proximal segment of the muscle with blood vessels and innervation and the small remaining distal portion of muscle were left in situ. The intervening gap was filled with minced muscle tissue from the distal part of the ipsilateral anterior tibial muscle, a zone that usually does not contain muscle spindles. The wound was then covered with fascia so that the minced tissue remained in position between the two stumps. In 14

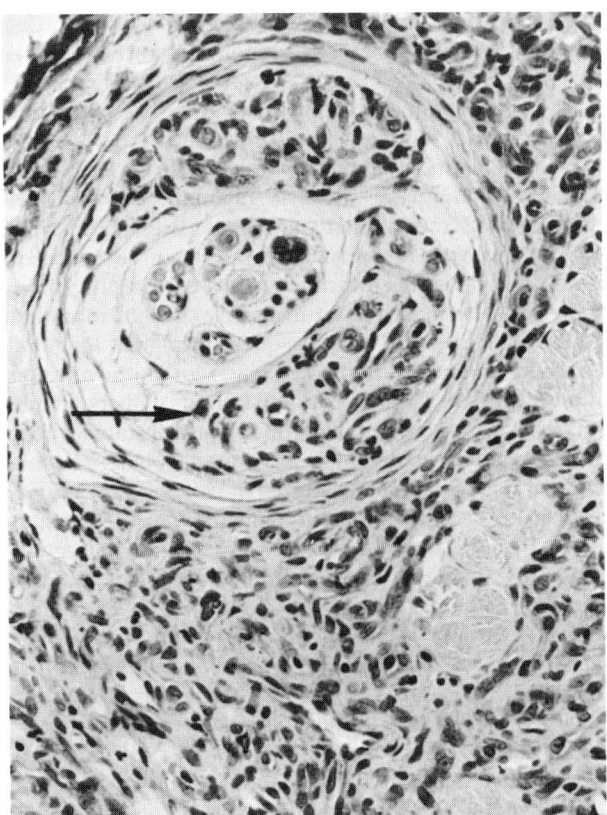

FIGURE 30-70. A hemangioma has infiltrated and destroyed portions of muscle. The tumor appears to have penetrated the periaxial space of a muscle spindle by traveling along nerves (arrow). The spindle capsule is intact. H&E stain. ×450.

animals the operative procedures were the same, but in addition to the original nerve supply the lateral branch of the plantar nerve was joined to the proximal stump of the extensor digitorum longus muscle. The animals were sacrificed either 4 months or 1 year after the operation. Neither muscle spindles nor intrafusal fibers were identified within the regenerated muscle segments after serial sections of the newly formed muscle were studied. These observations confirmed the previous studies of Zhenevskaya[186] and Zhenevskaya and Umnova.[187]

In Schmalbruch's model[188] in which soleus muscle was shifted from the right to the left leg of the rat, regeneration of the extrafusal and intrafusal fibers was observed from 7 to 250 days following the graft procedure. In these grafts, almost all the muscle spindles contained noninnervated intrafusal muscle fibers.[189] In another group of experiments, pigeon muscle that lacked spindles was grafted into a site that had contained muscle with spindles.[189] Contrariwise, muscle that contained spindles was transplanted into the bed of a muscle that lacked spindles. After 2 to 8 months, the graft of the first donor muscle (without spindles) had regenerated and formed a muscle that contained spindles. The muscle that originally contained spindles and that was transplanted to a site lacking spindles regenerated into muscle that contained no spindles. These experiments indicated that a specific type of innervation is required for the formation and regeneration of muscle spindles. These studies also suggested that an intact spindle capsule is not essential for muscle spindle regeneration. In mature rats, Rogers[190] produced three types of extensor digitorum longus grafts in order to vary the extent to which regenerating spindles might be reinnervated: (1) grafts that were reinnervated following the severance of their nerve supply, (2) grafts to facilitate reinnervation through intact nerve sheaths, and (3) grafts in which reinnervation was prevented. In all three types of grafts, complete degeneration of the extrafusal and intrafusal muscle fibers occurred before their regeneration, while the spindle capsules remained intact. The regeneration of the intrafusal muscle fibers followed the patterns that have been associated with regeneration of extrafusal fibers. However, even the reinnervation of regenerating muscle grafts did not result in fully differentiated muscle spindles. Although intrafusal fibers had the ability to regenerate without sensory innervation, there were major histochemical and structural alterations. Even the reinnervation of regenerating muscle grafts did not correct these changes.

Congenital myopathies. Although certain changes in the extrafusal fibers characterize the various congenital myopathies (see Chap. 54), the intrafusal fiber alterations are never conspicuous. Nevertheless, occasional abnormalities of the spindle have been found. In congenital nemaline myopathy, the intrafusal fibers differentiate into types 1 and 2 even though they are located within muscles in which the type 1 extrafusal fibers predominate. Even when type 2 extrafusal fibers are totally lacking, the intrafusal fibers maintain their histochemical differentiation. Although rods are not conspicuous within the intrafusal fibers, they have been observed by light and phase microscopy.[191-194]

Myotonic dystrophy. Daniel and Strich[195] first described the alterations in the muscle spindle of five patients with

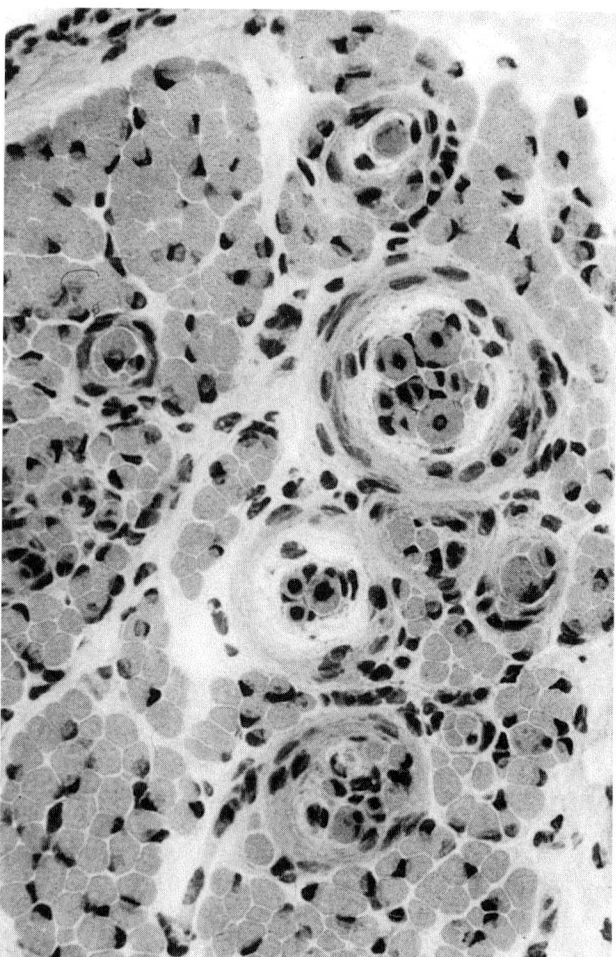

FIGURE 30-71. Myopathy with muscle spindle excess. Biopsy specimen from vastus lateralis muscle. The imaged field displays 6 muscle spindles that harbor a variable number of intrafusal fibers. ×360.

dystrophia myotonica. They observed abnormal spindles in the majority of muscles sampled although the changes were most conspicuous in the small muscles of the hand. The most striking abnormalities were an increase in the number of intrafusal fibers and a reduction in their diameters. In identical muscles of normal controls the average number of intrafusal fibers was 5 (maximum, 14), whereas in myotonic dystrophy they found as many as 60 intrafusal fibers in some muscle spindles.

It has been suggested that the abnormally large number of small intrafusal fibers in myotonic dystrophy results from the longitudinal splitting of parent fibers.[195,196] This abnormality is particularly prominent in polar regions.[197,198] It has been further suggested that the split fibers extend for only a short distance and then recombine into a master fiber. Even in the equatorial region, longitudinal fragmentation is observed.[199] However, in the most distal portion of the polar region, the intrafusal fibers are normal. In the zones of focal abnormality, the intrafusal fibers display a fragmentation in the longitudinal plane. The multitude of fragments are recognized in cross section as small intrafusal fibers.[197,198] The fragments cluster in many groups that are circumscribed by a single layer of basement membrane. Some of the small fragments lack innervation,[196–200] whereas others are innervated.[200] The pathogenesis of the aforementioned changes, which occur even in muscles that contain a large proportion of normal extrafusal muscle fibers, is not understood. It has been postulated that the fragmentation in the polar regions results from the mechanical stresses of myotonic discharges.[197,198] Heene[201] has demonstrated that in the abnormal zones all intrafusal fibers are of histochemical type 1 instead of the normal mixture of three muscle fiber types. He has suggested that this histochemical change expresses either a fiber type grouping flowing gamma denervation or an increased oxidative metabolism from the overloading of spindle activity by the myotonia. Maynard et al.[200] proposed an alternative explanation. They found that the muscle spindle in myotonic dystrophy resembled that of the normal mammalian fetus (the opossum) during development and postulated that there had been an arrest in the development of the intrafusal fibers in myotonic dystrophy.

Agenesis. Krugliak et al.[202] have reported an absence of spindles in 10 skeletal muscles of a newborn infant with arthrogryposis multiplex congenita. A total of 36 blocks of muscle were serially sectioned. All sections displayed varying degrees of denervation of extrafusal muscle fibers. No muscle spindles were detected in any of the material sampled, although no entire muscle was studied from its origin to its insertion. It was suggested that the aplasia of muscle spindles resulted from early intrauterine denervation.[202] The early differentiation of muscle spindles in the rat has been shown to be dependent upon innervation,[181–183] and denervation of muscle in the newborn rat prevents the differentiation of the muscle spindles.[183–184] Although it is conceivable that denervation or lack of innervation of human muscle early enough in intrauterine development could prevent muscle spindle formation, more evidence is necessary in the human to substantiate this concept.

Muscle spindle excess. A marked increase of muscle spindles in skeletal muscle has been observed in two infants with the Noonan phenotype,[203] a disorder assosiated with dysmorphic facial features and cardiac anomalies. Selcen et al. have described increased numbers of muscle spindles in a hypotonic weak infant with congenital neuroblastoma, hypertrophic cardiomyopathy, organomegaly, and arthrogryposis.[204] In this latter child, as many as 12 muscle spindles harboring a variable number of intrafusal fibers were observed in a single fascicle; some fascicles contained predominantly spindle structures (Fig. 30-71). Major sympathetic nerve innervation to muscle spindles has been demonstrated unequivocally in the normal dog by Banker and Girvin.[205,206] It is conceivable, therefore, that the early development of the muscle spindle is stimulated by increased catecholamines, as in the infant reported by Selcen et al., resulting in the development of an excess of muscle spindles in normal positions within muscle.

Inflammation. Inflammatory cells enter the periaxial space along the walls of blood vessels and nerves. In the eosinophil-myalgia syndrome, inflammatory cells display a predilection for the external capsule of the muscle spindle.[207]

List of Abbreviations

ALS	amyotrophic lateral sclerosis	MHC	myosin heavy chain
AMP	adenosine monophosphate	MLD	metachromatic leukodystrophy
ATPase	adenosine triphosphatase	NADH	reduced nicotinamide adenine dinucleotide
DNA	deoxyribonucleic acid	NCAM	neural cell adhesion molecule
H&E	hematoxylin and eosin	PAS	periodic acid–Schiff
MAC	membrane attack complex	PTAH	phosphotungstic acid–hematoxylin

References

1. Edström L, Kugelberg E: Histochemical composition, distribution of fibers and fatigability of single motor units. Anterior tibial muscle of the rat. *J Neurol Neurosurg Psychiatry* 31:424, 1968.
2. Engel WK: Selective and nonselective susceptibility of muscle fiber types. A new approach to human neuromuscular diseases. *Arch Neurol* 22:97,1970.
3. Colling-Saltin A-S:Enzyme histochemistry on skeletal muscle of the human foetus. *J Neurol Sci* 39:169, 1978.
4. Wohlfart G: Uber das Vorkommen verschiedener Arten von Muskelfasern in der Skelettmuskulatur des Menschen und einiger Säugetier. *Acta Psychiatr Neurol Scand* [suppl] 12:1, 1937.
5. Fenichel GM: The B fibre of human fetal skeletal muscle. *Neurology* 13:219, 1963.
6. Fenichel GM: A histochemical study of developing human skeletal muscle. *Neurology* 16:741, 1966.
7. Johnson MA, Polgar J, Leightman D, Pippelton D: Data on the distribution of fiber types in thirty-six human muscles: An autopsy study. *J Neurol Sci* 18:111, 1973.
8. Karpati G, Engel WK: "Type grouping" in skeletal muscles after experimental reinnervation. *Neurology* 18:447, 1968.
9. Brooke MH, Engel WK: The histographic analysis of human muscle biopsies with regard to fiber types. 1. Adult male and female. *Neurology* 19:221, 1969.
10. Brooke MH, Engel WK: The histographic analysis of human muscle biopsies with regard to fiber types: 2. Diseases of the upper and lower motor neuron. *Neurology* 19:378, 1969.
11. Brooke MH, Engel WK: The histographic analysis of human muscle biopsies with regard to fiber types: 3. Myotonias, myasthenia gravis and hypokalemic periodic paralysis. *Neurology* 19:469, 1969.
12. Brooke MH, Engel WK: The histographic analysis of human muscle biopsies with regard to fiber types: 4. Children's biopsies. *Neurology* 19:591, 1969.
13. Mahoney MJ, Haseltine FP, Hobbins JC et al: Prenatal diagnosis of Duchenne's muscular dystrophy. *N Engl J Med* 297:968, 1977.
14. Brooke MH: Congenital fiber type disproportion, in Kakulas BA (ed): *Clinical Studies in Myology*. Amsterdam, Excerpta Medica 1973, pp 147–159.
15. Brooke MH: The pathologic interpretation of muscle histochemistry, in Pearson CM, Mostofi FK (eds): *The Striated Muscle*. Baltimore, Williams & Wilkins, 1973, pp 86–122.

16. Engel AG, Biesecker G: Universal involvement of complement in muscle fiber necrosis, in Schotland DL (ed): *Disorders of the Motor Unit*. New York, Wiley, 1982, pp 535–546.
17. Engel AG, Biesecker G: Complement activation in muscle fiber necrosis: Demonstration of the membrane attack complex of complement in necrotic fibers. *Ann Neurol* 12:289, 1982.
18. Mokri B, Engel AG: Duchenne dystrophy: Electron microscopic findings pointing to a basic or early abnormality in the plasma membrane of the muscle fiber. *Neurology* 25:1111, 1975.
19. Engel AG, Mokri B, Jerusalem F et al: Ultrastructural clues in Duchenne dystrophy, in Rowland LP (ed): *Pathogenesis of Human Muscular Dystrophies*. Amsterdam, Excerpta Medica, 1977, pp 310–324.
20. Bodensteiner J, Engel A: Intracellular calcium accumulaion in Duchenne dystrophy and other myopathies: A study of 567,000 muscle fibers in 114 biopsies. *Neurology* 28:439, 1978.
21. Wohlfart G: Aktuelle Probleme der Muskelpathologie. *Dtsch Z Nervenheilk* 173:426, 1955.
22. Bray GM, Banker BQ: An ultrastructural study of degeneration and necrosis of muscle in the dystrophic mouse. *Acta Neuropathol* 15:34, 1970.
23. MacDonald RD, Engel AG: Experimental cholorquine myopathy. *J Neuropathol Exp Neurol* 29:479, 1970.
23a. Gallanti A, Prelle A, Moggio M et al: Desmin and vimentin as markers of regeneration in muscle diseases. *Acta Neuropathol* 85:88, 1992.
23b. Sarnat HB: Vimentin and desmin in maturing skeletal muscle and developmental myopathies. *Neurology* 42:1616, 1992.
23c. Figarella-Branger D, Calore EE, Boucraut J et al: Expression of cell surface and cytoskeleton developmentally regulated proteins in adult centronuclear myopathies. *J Neurol Sci* 109:69, 1992.
23d. Bornemann A, Schmalbruch H: Desmin and vimentin in regenerating muscles. *Muscle Nerve* 15:14, 1992.
23e. Niiyama T, Higuchi I, Osame M: Expression of thrombomodulin, caveolin-3, and desmin on muscle fibers in neuromuscular diseases. *Muscle Nerve* 22:1713–1716, 1999.
23f. Hu J, Higuchi I, Yoshida Y et al: Expression of midkine in regenerating skeletal muscle fibers and cultured myoblasts of human skeletal muscle. *Eur Neurol* 47:20–25, 2002.
24. Law PK, Fang Q, Goodwin TG et al: First clinical trial of myoblast transfer therapy. *J Neurol Sci* 98:32S, 1990.
25. Miller RG, Blau H, Almada A, Steinman L: Myoblast implantation in Duchenne muscular dystrophy. *J Neurol Sci* 98:32S, 1990.
26. Partridge TA: Invited review: Myoblast transfer: A possible therapy for inherited myopathies? *Muscle Nerve* 14:197, 1991.
27. Qu-Peterson Z, Deasy B, Jankowsky R, et al: Identification of a novel population of stem cells in mice: potential for muscle regeneration. *J Cell Biol* 157:851–864, 2002.
28. O'Brien K, Muskiewicz K, Gussoni E: Recent advances in and therapeutic potential of muscle-derived stem cells. *J Cell Biochem* 38 (suppl): 80–87, 2002.
28a. Ferrari G, Stornaiuolo A, Mavilio F: Bone marrow transplantation. Failure to correct murine muscular dystrophy. *Nature* 411:1014–1015, 2001.
29. Örlander J, Kiessling K-H, Larsson L et al: Skeletal muscle metabolism and ultrastructure in relation to age in sedentary men. *Acta Physiol Scand* 104:249, 1978.
30. Wohlfart G: Dystrophia myotonica and myotonia congenita: Histopathologic studies with special reference to changes in the muscles. *J Neuropathol Exp Neurol* 10:109, 1951.
31. Schröder JM, Adams RD: The ultrastructural morphology of the muscle fiber in myotonic dystrophy. *Acta Neuropathol (Berl)* 10:218, 1968.
32. Engel WK: Chemocytology of striated annulets and sarcoplasmic masses in myotonic dystrophy. *Histochem Cytochem* 10:229, 1962.
33. den Hartog Jager WA, Meijer AEFH, de Jong JMBV: Sarcoplasmic masses: Enzyme histochemistry and autoradiography. *Arch Neurol* 32:247, 1975.
33a. Sabatelli M, Bertini E, Ricci E et al: Peripheral neuropathy with giant axons and cardiomyopathy associated with desmin type intermediate filaments in skeletal muscle. *J Neurol Sci* 109:1, 1992.
34. Bethlem J, Van Wijngaarden GK, de Jong J:The incidence of lobulated fibres in the facioscapulohumeral type of muscular dystrophy and the limb-girdle syndrome. *J Neurol Sci* 18:351, 1973.
35. Engel WK: The essentiality of histo- and cytochemical studies of skeletal muscle in the investigation of neuromuscular disease. *Neurology* 12:778, 1962.
36. MacDonald RD, Engel AG: The cytoplasmic body: Another structural anomaly of the Z disk. *Acta Neuropathol* 14:99, 1969.
37. Engel AG: Pathological reactions of the Z disk. *Excerpta Medica*, International Congress Series 147:398, 1967.
38. Fischman DA, Meltzer HY, Poppei RW: The ultra-structure of human skeletal muscle: Variations from archetypal morphology, in Pearson CM, Mostofi FK (eds): *The Striated Muscle*. Baltimore, Williams & Wilkins, 1973, p 58.

38a. Selcen D, Ohno K, Engel AG: Myofibrillar myopathy. Clinical, morphological and genetic studies in 63 patients. *Brain* 127:439, 2004.
39. Shy GM, EngelWK, Somers JE, Wanko T: Nemaline myopathy. A new congenital myopathy. *Brain* 86:793, 1963.
40. Conen PE, Murphy EG, Donohue WL: Light and electron microscopic studies of "myogranules" in a child with hypotonia and muscle weakness. *Can Med Asoc J* 89:793, 1963.
40a. De Bleecker JL, Ertl BB, Engel AG: Patterns of abnormal protein expression in target formations and unstructured cores. *Neuromuscul Disord* 6:339, 1996.
40b. Banwell BL, Engel AG: AlphaB crystallin immunolocalization yields new insights into inclusion body myositis . *Neurology* 54:1033, 2000.
41. Engel AG, Gomez MR, Groover RV: Multicore disease. A recently recognized congenital myopathy associated with multifocal degeneration of muscle fibers. *Mayo Clinic Proc* 46:666, 1971.
42. Duane DD, Engel AG: Emetine myopathy. *Neurology* 20:733, 1970.
43. Tice LW, Engel AG: The effects of glucocorticoids on red and white muscles in the rat. *Am J Pathol* 50:311,1967.
44. Dubowitz V: Pathology of experimentally re-innervated skeletal muscle. *J Neurol Neurosurg Psychiatry* 30:99, 1967.
45. Shafiq SA, Gorycki MA, Asiedu SA, Milhorat AT: Tenotomy effect on the fine structure of the soleus of the rat. *Arch Neurol* 20:625, 1969.
46. Engel WK, Brooke MH, Nelson PG: Histochemical studies of denervated or tenotomized cat muscle. *Ann NY Acad Sci* 138:160, 1966.
47. Karpati G, Carpenter S, Eisen AA: Experimental core-like lesions and nemaline rods: A correlative morphological and physiological study. *Arch Neurol* 27:237, 1972.
48. Resnick JS, Engel WK, Nelson PG: Changes in the Z disc of skeletal muscle induced by tenotomy. *Neurology* 18:737, 1968.
49. Engel AG, Angelini C, Gomez MR: Fingerprint body myopathy. *Mayo Clin Proc* 47:377, 1972.
50. Tomé FMS, Fardeau M: "Fingerprint inclusions" in muscle fibres in dystrophia myotonica. *Acta Neuropathol* 24:62, 1973.
51. Radnot M: "Fingerprint" Einschlusse im M orbicularis oculi. *Ophthalmologica* 168:282, 1974.
52. Julien J, Vital CL, Vallat J-M et al: Oculopharyngeal muscular dystrophy—A case with abnormal mitochondria and "fingerprint" inclusions. *J Neurol Sci* 21:165, 1974.
53. Sengel A, Stoebner P: Une inclusion musculaire atypique rare: Les "corps en empreintes digitales" ou fingerprint bodies. *Acta Neuropathol* 27:61, 1974.
54. Brooke MH, Neville HE: Reducing body myopathy. *Neurology* 22:829, 1972.
55. Ringel SP, Neville HE, Duster MC, Carroll JE: A new congenital neuromuscular disease with trilaminar muscle fibers. *Neurology* 28:282, 1978.
56. Morgan-Hughes JA, Mair WGP, Lascelles PT: A disorder of skeletal muscle associated with tubular aggregates. *Brain* 93:873, 1970.
57. Brumback RA, Staton RD, Susag ME: Exercise-induced pain, stiffness and tubular aggregation in skeletal muscle. *J Neurol Neurosurg Psychiatry* 44:250, 1981.
58. Johns TR, Campa JF, Adelman LS: Familial myasthenia with "tubular aggregates" treated with prednisone. *Neurology* 23:426, 1973.
59. Müller-Höcher J: Cytochrome c oxidase deficient fibers in the the limb muscle and diaphragm of man without muscular disease: An age-related alteration. *J Neurol Sci* 100:14, 1990.
60. Cortopassi GA, Arnheim N: Detection of a specific mitochondrial DNA deletion in tissues of older humans. *Nucleic Acids Res* 18:6297, 1990.
61. Mita S, Schmidt B, Schon EA et al: Detection of "deleted" mitochondrial genomes in cytochrome-c-oxidase-deficient muscle fibers of a patient with Kearns-Sayre syndrome. *Proc Natl Acad Sci USA* 86:9509, 1989.
62. Shoubridge EA, Karpati G, Hastings KE: Deletion mutants are functionally dominant over wild-type mitochondrial genomes in skeletal muscle fiber segments in mitochondrial disease. *Cell* 62:43, 1990.
62a. Johnson MA, Bindoff LA, Turnbull DM: Cytochrome c oxidase activity in single muscle fibers: Assay techniques and diagnostic approaches. *Ann Neurol* 33:28, 1993.
63. Nakase H, Moraes CT, Rizzuto R et al: Transcription and translation of deleted mitochondrial genomes in Kearns-Sayre syndrome: Implications for pathogenesis. *Am J Hum Genet* 46:418, 1990.
64. Yamamoto M, Clemens PR, Engel AG: Mitochondrial DNA deletions in mitochondrial cytopathies: Observations in 19 patients. *Neurology* 41: 1822, 1991.
65. Engel AG: Electron microscopic observations in primary hypokalemic and thyrotoxic periodic paralyses. *Mayo Clin Proc* 41:797, 1966.
66. Engel AG: Evolution and content of vacuoles in primary hypokalemic periodic paralysis. *Mayo Clin Proc* 45:774, 1970.
67. Engel AG: Vacuolar myopathies: Multiple etiologies and sequential structural studies, in Pearson CM, Mostofi FK (eds): *The Striated Muscle*. Baltimore, Williams & Wilkins, 1973, pp 301–341.
67a. Nakanos, Engel AG, Waclawik AJ et al: Myofibrillar myopathy with abnormal foci of desmin positivity. I. Light and electron microscopy analysis. *J Neuropathol Exp Neurol* 55:549–562, 1996.

68. Shafiq SA, Milhorat AT, Gorycki MA: An electron microscope study of muscle degeneration and vascular changes in polymyositis. *J Pathol Bact* 94:139, 1967.
69. Pearson CM, Yamazaki JN: Vacuolar myopathy in systemic lupus erythematosus. *Am J Clin Pathol* 29:455, 1958.
70. Milhorat AT, Shafiq SA, Goldstone L: Changes in muscle structure in dystrophic patients, carriers and normal siblings seen by electron microscopy: Correlation with levels of serum creatine phosphokinase (CPK). *Ann NY Acad Sci* 138:246, 1966.
71. Markesbery WR, Griggs RC, Herr B: Distal myopathy: Electron microscopic and histochemical studies. *Neurology* 27:727, 1977.
72. Mikol J, Felten-Papaiconomou, Ferchal F et al: Inclusion body myositis: Clinicopathological studies and isolation of an adenovirus type II from muscle biopsy specimen. *Ann Neurol* 11:576, 1982.
73. Tomé FMS, Fardeau M: Nuclear inclusions in oculopharyngeal dystrophy. *Acta Neuropathol* 49:85, 1980.
74. Anderson PJ, Song SK, Slotwinner P: The fine structure of spheromembranous degeneration of skeletal muscle induced by vincristine. *J Neuropathol Exp Neurol* 26:15, 1967.
75. Engel AG, Dale AJD: Autophagic glycogenosis of late onset with mitochondrial abnormalities: Light and electron microscopic observations. *Mayo Clin Proc* 43:233, 1968.
76. Engel AG, Gomez MR, Seybold ME, Lambert EH: The spectrum and diagnosis of acid maltase deficiency. *Neurology* 23:95, 1973.
77. Nonaka I, Sunohara N, Ishiura S, Satoyoshi E: Familial distal myopathy with rimmed vacuole and lamellar (myeloid) body formation. *J Neurol Sci* 51:141, 1981.
78. Dubowitz V, Brooke MH: *Muscle Biopsy: A Modern Approach.* Philadelphia, Saunders, 1973.
79. Fukuhara N, Kumamoto T, Tsubaki T: Rimmed vacuoles. *Acta Neuropathol* 51:229, 1980.
79a. De Bleecker JL, Engel AG, Winkelmann JC: Localization of dystrophin and β-spectrin in vacuolar myopathies. *Am J Pathol* 143:1200, 1993.
79b. Mendell JR, Sahenk Z, Paul L: Amyloid filaments in inclusion body myositis; Novel findings provide insight into nature of filaments. *Arch Neurol* 48:1229, 1991.
79c. Askanas V, Engel WK, Alvarez RB: Light and electron microscopic localization of beta-amyloid protein in muscle biopsies of patients with inclusion-body myositis. *Am J Pathol* 141:31, 1992.
79d. Askanas V, Serdaroglu P, Engel WK et al: Immunolocalization of ubiquitin in muscle biopsies of patients with inclusion body myositis and oculopharyngeal muscular dystrophy. *Neurosci Lett* 130:73, 1991.
80. Kunkel LM, Hoffman EP: Duchenne/Becker muscular dystrophy: A short overview of the gene, the protein, and current diagnostics. *Br Med Bull* 45:630, 1989.
81. Bullman DE, Murphy EG, Zubrzycka-Gaarn EE et al: Differentiation of Duchenne and Becker muscular dystrophy with amino- and carboxy-terminal antisera specific for dystrophin. *Am J Hum Genet* 48:295, 1991.
82. Nicholson LVB, Johnson MA, Gardner-Medwin D et al: Heterogeneity of dystrophin expression in patients with Duchenne and Becker muscular dystrophy. *Acta Neuropathol (Berl)* 80:239, 1990.
83. Hoffman EP: Molecular diagnostics of Duchenne/Becker dystrophy: New additions to a rapidly expanding field. *J Neurol Sci* 101:129, 1991.
84. Khurana TS, Hoffman EP, Kunkel LM: Identification of a chromosome-6 encoded dystrophin-related protein. *J Biol Chem* 265:16717, 1990.
85. Hoffman EP, Watkins SC, Slater HS, Kunkel LM: Detection of a specific isoform of alpha-actinin with antisera directed against dystrophin. *J Cell Biol* 108:503, 1989.
86. Man TN, Ellis JM, Ginjaar IB et al: Monoclonal antibody evidence for structural similarities between the central rod regions of actinin and dystrophin. *FEBS Lett* 272:109, 1990.
87. Cross RA, Stewart M, Kendrick-Jones J: Structural predictions for the central domain of dystrophin. *FEBS Lett* 262:87, 1990.
88. Arahata K, Beggs AH, Honda H et al: Preservation of the C-terminus of dystrophin molecule in the skeletal muscle from Becker muscular dystrophy. *J Neurol Sci* 101:148, 1991.
89. Zubrzycka-Gaarn EE, Bulman DE, Karpati G et al: The Duchenne muscular dystrophy gene product is localized in sarcolemma of human skeletal muscle. *Nature* 333:466, 1988.
90. Arahata K, Ishiura S, Ishiguro T et al: Immunostaining of skeletal and cardiac muscle surface membrane with antibody against Duchenne muscular dystrophy peptide. *Nature* 333:861, 1988.
91. Bonilla E, Samitt CE, Miranda AF et al: Duchenne muscular dystrophy: Deficiency of dystrophin at the muscle surface. *Cell* 54:447, 1988.
92. Shimizu T, Matsumura K, Hashimoto K et al: A monoclonal antibody against a synthetic polypeptide fragment of dystrophin (amino acid sequence from position 215 to 264). *Proc Japan Acad* 64 (ser B):205, 1988.
93. Gold R, Meurers B, Reichmann H et al: Duchenne muscular dystrophy: Evidence for somatic reversion of the mutation in man. *J Neurol* 237:494, 1990.
94. Burrow KL, Coovert DD, Klein CJ et al: Dystrophin expression and somatic reversion in prednisone-treated and untreated Duchenne dystrophy. *Neurology* 41:661, 1991.
95. Bonilla E, Schmidt B, Sammitt CE et al: Normal and dystrophin-deficient muscle fibers in carriers of the gene for Duchenne muscular dystrophy. *Am J Pathol* 133:440, 1988.
96. Arahata K, Ishihara T, Kamakura K et al: Mosiac expression of dystrophin in symptomatic carriers of Duchenne's muscular dystrophy. *N Engl J Med* 320:138, 1989.
97. Morandi L, Mora M, Gussoni E et al: Dystrophin analysis in Duchenne and Becker muscular dystrophy carriers: correlation with intracellular calcium and albumin. *Ann Neurol* 28:674, 1990.
98. Beggs AH, Kunkel LM: Improved diagnosis of Duchenne/Becker muscular dystrophy. *J Clin Invest* 85:613, 1990.
99. Arahata K, Hoffman EP, Kunkel LM et al: Dystrophin diagnosis: Comparison of dystrophin abnormalities by immunofluorescence and immunoblot analysis. *Proc Natl Acad Sci USA* 86:7154, 1989.
100. England SB, Nicholson LVB, Johnson MA et al: Very mild muscular dystrophy associated with the deletion of 46% of dystrophin. *Nature* 343:180, 1990.
100a. Bushby KMD, Anderson LVB: *Muscular Dystrophy. Methods and Protocols.* Totowa, NJ, Humana Press, 2001.
101. Banker BQ, Chester CS: Infarction of thigh muscle in the diabetic. *Neurology* 23:667, 1975.
102. Chester CS, Banker BQ: Focal infarction of muscle in diabetics. *Diabetes Care* 9:623, 1986.
103. Banker BQ: The ultrastructural alterations of the intramuscular blood vessels in dermatomyositis of childhood, in Milhorat AT (ed): *Exploratory Concepts in Muscular Dystrophy II.* Amsterdam, Excerpta Medica, 1974, pp 564–584.
104. Banker BQ: Dermatomyositis of childhood. Ultrastructural alterations of muscle and intramuscular blood vessels. *J Neuropathol Exp Neurol* 34:46, 1975.
105. Chou SM, Miike T: Ultrastructural abnormalities and perifascicular atrophy in childhood dermatomyositis. With special reference to transverse tubular system—sarcoplasmic reticulum junctions. *Arch Pathol Lab Med* 105:76, 1981.
106. Engel AG, Stonnington H: Morphological effects of denervation of muscle: A quantitative ultrastructural study. *Ann NY Acad Sci* 228:68, 1974.
107. Fenichel GM, Engel WK: Histochemistry of muscle in infantile spinal muscular atrophy. *Neurology* 13:1059, 1963.
107a. Waclawick A, Sufit RL, Beinlich BR et al: Acute myopathy with selective degeneration of myosin filaments following status asthmaticus treated with methylprednisolone and vecuronium. *Neuromusc Disord* 2:19, 1992.
107b. Hirano M, Ott BR, Raps EC et al: Acute quadriplegic myopathy: A complication of treatment with steroids, nondepolarizing blocking agents, or both. *Neurology* 42:2082, 1992.
108. Engel AG, Arahata K: Monoclonal antibody analysis of mononuclear cells in myopathies: II. Phenotypes of autoinvasive cells in polymyositis and inclusion body myositis. *Ann Neurol* 16:209, 1984.
109. Giorno R, Barden MT, Kohler PF, Ringel SP: Immunohistochemical characterization of the mononuclear cells infiltrating muscle of patients with inflammatory and noninflammatory myopathies. *Clin Immunol Immunopathol* 30:405, 1984.
110. Arahata K, Engel AG: Monoclonal antibody analysis of mononuclear cells in myopathies: I. Quantitation of subsets according to diagnosis and sites of accumulation and demonstration and counts of muscle fibers invaded by T cells. *Ann Neurol* 16:193, 1984.
111. Swash, M, Schwartz MS, Vandenburg MJ, Pollock DJ: Myopathy in Whipple's disease. *Gut* 18:800, 1977.
112. Whitaker JN, Hashimoto K, Quinones M: Skeletal muscle pseudohypertrophy in primary amyloidosis. *Neurology* 27:47, 1977.
113. Bruni J, Bilbao JM, Pritzker KPH: Myopathy associated with amyloid angiopathy. *Can J Neurol Sci* 4:77, 1977.
114. Lange RK: Primary amyloidosis of muscle. *South Med J* 63:321, 1970.
115. Cohen AS, Rubinow A: Amyloid neuropathy, in Dyck PJ, Thomas PK, Lambert EH, Bunge R (eds): *Peripheral Neuropathy.* Philadelphia, Saunders, 1984, vol 2, pp 1866–1898.
115a. Villanova M, Kawai M, Lübke U et al: Rimmed vacuoles of inclusion body myositis and oculopharyngeal dystrophy contain amyloid precursor protein and lysosomal markers. *Brain Res* 603:343, 1993.
115b. Satayoshi E, Murakami N, Takemitu M, Nonaka I: Significance of "rimmed vacuoles" in various neuromuscular disorders, in Serratrice G, Pellissier J-F, Pouget J et al: (eds): Système nerveux, muscles et maladies sytémiques: Acquisitions récentes. Paris, Expansion Scientifique Francaise, 1993, pp 83–92.
115c. DeBleecker JL, Engel AG: Myopathy with desmin excess. II. Ectopic overexpression of multiple proteins (including dystrophin, gelsolin, NCAM, and serine protease inhibitors) and congophilia. *Neurology* 44(suppl), April 1994.
116. Childs B, Kinzler K et al. (eds): *The Metabolic and Molecular Bases of Inherited Disease,* New York, McGraw-Hill, 2001
117. Engel AG, Gomez MA, Seybold M, Lambert EM: The spectrum and diagnosis of acid maltase deficiency. *Neurology* 23:95, 1973.
117a. Comi GP, Fortunato F, Lucchiari S et al: Beta-enolase deficiency: A new metabolic myopathy of distal glycolysis. *Ann Neurol* 50:202–207, 2001.

118. DiMauro S, Hartwig GB, Hays A et al: Debrancher deficiency: Neuromuscular disorder in 5 adults. *Ann Neurol* 5:422, 1979.
119. Schochet SS Jr, McCormick WF, Zellweger H: Type IV glycogenosis (amylopectinosis). Light and electron microscopic observations. *Arch Pathol* 90:354, 1970
120. Bonilla E, Schotland DL: Histochemical diagnosis of muscle phosphofructokinase deficiency. *Arch Neurol* 22:8, 1970.
121. Kristensson K, Olsson Y, Sourander P: Peripheral nerve changes in Tay-Sachs and Batten-Spielmeyer-Vogt disease. *Acta Pathol Microbiol Scand* 70:630, 1967.
122. Carpenter S, Karpati G, Andermann F: Specific involvement of muscle, nerve, and skin in late infantile and juvenile amaurotic idiocy. *Neurology* 22:170, 1972.
123. Dolman CL, Chang E: Visceral lesions in amaurotic familial idiocy with curvilinear bodies. *Arch Pathol* 94:425, 1972.
124. Martin JJ, Jacobs K: Skin biopsy as a contribution to diagnosis in late infantile amaurotic idiocy with curvilinear bodies. *Eur Neurol* 10:281, 1973.
125. Rapola J, Haltia M: Cytoplasmic inclusions in the vermiform appendix and skeletal muscle in two types of so-called neuronal ceroid-lipofuscinosis. *Brain* 96:833, 1973.
126. Carpenter S, Karpati G, Andermann F et al: The ultrastructural characteristics of the abnormal cytosomes in Batten-Kufs' disease. *Brain* 100:137, 1977.
127. O'Brien JS, Bernett J, Veath ML, Paa D: Lysosomal storage disorders: Diagnosis by ultrastructural examination of skin biopsy specimens. *Arch Neurol* 32:592, 1975.
128. Gumbinas M, Larsen M, Mei Liu H: Peripheral neuropathy in classic Niemann-Pick disease: Ultrastructure of nerves and skeletal muscles. *Neurology* 25:107, 1975.
129. Carpenter S, Karpati G, Andermann FA, Watters G: Muscle, skin and nerve abnormalities in ganglioside storage diseases. *Neurology* 22:446, 1972.
130. Tomé FMS, Fardeau M: Ultrastructural study of a muscle biopsy in a case of GMI gangliosidosis type I. *Pathol Eur* 11:15, 1976.
131. Tomé FMS, Fardeau M, Lenoir G: Ultrastructure of muscle and sensory nerve in Fabry's disease. *Acta Neuropathol* 38:187, 1977.
131a. Serratosa JM, Gomez-Garre P, Gallardo ME et al: A novel protein tyrosine phosphatase gene in progressive myoclonus epilepsy of the Lafora type (EPM2). *Hum Mol Genet* 8:345–352, 1999.
132. Neville HE, Brooke MH, Austin JH: Studies in myoclonus epilepsy. (Lafora body form). IV Skeletal muscle abnormalities. *Arch Neurol* 30:466-74, 1974
133. Carpenter S, Karpati G, Andermann F et al: Lafora's disease: Peroxisomal storage in skeletal muscle. *Neurology* 24:531, 1974.
134. Carpenter S, Karpati G: Ultrastructural findings in Lafora disease. *Ann Neurol* 10:63, 1981.
135. Gambetti P, Di Mauro S, Hirt L et al: Myoclonic epilepsy with Lafora bodies. Some ultrastructural, histochemical, and biochemical aspects. *Arch Neurol* 25:483, 1971.
136. Nishimura RN, Ishak KG, Reddick R et al: Lafora disease: Diagnosis by liver biopsy. *Ann Neurol* 8:409, 1980.
137. Busard HLSM, Gabreels-Festen AAWM, Renier WO et al: Axilla skin biopsy: A reliable test for the diagnosis of Lafora's disease. *Ann Neurol* 21:599, 1987.
138. Busard HLSM, Gabreels-Festen AAWM, Renier WO et al: Adult polyglucosan body disease: The diagnostic value of axilla skin biopsy. *Ann Neurol* 29:448, 1991.
139. Dayan AD: Dichroism of cresyl violet-stained cerebroside sulfate ("sulfatide"). *J Histochem Cytochem* 15:421, 1967.
140. Thomas PK, King RHM, Kocen RS, Brett EM: Comparative ultrastructural observations on peripheral nerve abnormalities in the late infantile, juvenile and late onset forms of metachromatic leukodystrophy. *Acta Neuropathol* 39:237, 1977.
141. Joosten E, Hoes M, Gabreëls-Festen A, Hommes O et al: Electron microscopic investigation of inclusion material in a case of adult metachromatic leukodystrophy: Observations on kidney biopsy, peripheral nerve and cerebral white matter. *Acta Neuropathol* 33:165, 1975.
142. Gregoire A, Périer O, Dustin P: Metachromatic leukodystrophy, an electron microscope study. *J Neuropathol Exp Neurol* 25:617, 1966.
143. Kolodny EH: Metachromatic leukodystrophy and multiple sulfatase deficiency: Sulfatide lipidosis, in Scriver CR, Beaudet AL, Sly WS, Valle D (eds): *The Metabolic Basis of Inherited Disease*, 6th ed. New York, McGraw-Hill, 1989, pp 1721–1750.
144. Bischoff A, Ulrich J: Peripheral neuropathy in globoid cell leukodystrophy (Krabbe's disease): Ultrastructure and histochemical findings. *Brain* 92:861, 1969.
145. Dunn HG, Lake BD, Dolman CL, Wilson J: The neuropathy of Krabbe's infantile cerebral sclerosis (globoid cell leukodystrophy). *Brain* 92:329, 1969.
146. Martin JJ, Leory JG, Libert J et al: Skin and conjunctival biopsies in infantile neuroaxonal dystrophy. *Acta Neuropathol* 45:247, 1979.
147. Arsénio-Nunes ML, Goutières F: Diagnosis of infantile neuroxonal dystrophy by conjunctival biopsy. *J Neurol Neurosurg Psychiatry* 41:5111, 1978.
148. Wisniewski K, Wisniewski HM: Diagnosis of infantile neuroaxonal dystrophy by skin biopsy. *Ann Neurol* 7:377, 1980.
149. Schindler D, Bishop DF, Wolfe DE et al: Neuroaxonal dystrophy due to lysosomal α-N-acetylgalactosaminidase deficiency. *N Engl J Med* 320:1735, 1989.
150. Wang AM, Schindler D, Desnick RJ: Schindler disease: The molecular lesion in the α-N-acetylgalactosaminidase gene that causes an infantile neuroaxonal dystrophy. *J Clin Invest* 86:1752, 1990.
151. Desnick RJ, Wang AM: Schindler disease: An inherited neuroaxonal dystrophy due to α-N-acetylgalactosaminidase deficiency. *J Inher Metab Dis* 13:549, 1990.
152. Duncan C, Strub R, McGarry P, Duncan D: Peripheral nerve biopsy as an aid to diagnosis in infantile neuroaxonal dystrophy. *Neurology* 20:1024, 1970.
153. Yagishita S, Itoh Y, Nakano T et al: Infantile neuroaxonal dystrophy: Schwann cell inclusion in the peripheral nerve. *Acta Neuropathol* 41:257, 1978.
154. Berard-Badier M, Gambarelli D, Pinsard N et al: Infantile neuroaxonal dystrophy or Seitelberger's disease: II. Peripheral nerve involvement; electron microscopic study in one case. *Acta Neuropathol* (suppl V):30, 1971.
155. Sengel A, Stoebner P: Intérêt de la biopsie neuromusculaire dans le diagnostic de la dystrophie neuro-axonale infantile. Étude ultrastructurale de trois cas dont deux familiaux. *Acta Neuropathol* 21:109, 1972.
156. Martin JJ, Martin L: Infantile neuroaxonal dystrophy. Ultrastructural study of the peripheral nerves and of motor end plates. *Eur Neurol* 8:239, 1972.
157. DiMauro S, Mendell JR, Sahenk Z et al: Fatal infantile mitochondrial myopathy and renal dysfunction due to cytochrome-c-coxidase deficiency. *Neurology* 30:795, 1980.
158. Heiman-Patterson TD, Bonilla E, DiMauro S et al: Cytochrome-c-oxidase deficiency in a floppy infant. *Neurology* 32:898, 1982.
159. DiMauro S, Nicholson JF, Hays AP et al: Benign infantile mitochondrial myopathy due to reversible cytochrome-c-oxidase deficiency. *Ann Neurol* 14:226, 1983.
160. Zeviani M, Van Dyke DH, Servidei S et al: Myopathy and fatal cardiopathy due to cytochrome c oxidase deficiency. *Arch Neurol* 43:1198, 1986.
161. Tritschler HJ, Bonilla E, Lombes A et al: Differential diagnosis of fatal and benign cytochrome c oxidase–deficient myopathies of infancy: An immunohistochemical approach. *Neurology* 41:300, 1991.
162. Fishbein WN, Griffin JL, Armbrustmacher VW: Stain for skeletal muscle adenylate deaminase: An effective tetrazolium stain for frozen biopsy specimens. *Arch Pathol Lab Med* 104:462, 1980.
163. Fishbein WN, Armbrustmacher VW, Griffin JL: Myoadenylate deaminase deficiency: A new disease of muscle. *Science* 200:545, 1978.
164. Fishbein WN, Armbrustmacher VM, Griffin JL et al: Levels of adenylate deaminase, adenylate kinase, and creatine kinase in frozen human muscle biopsy specimens relative to type 1/type 2 fiber distribution: Evidence for a carrier state of myoadenylate deaminase deficiency. *Ann Neurol* 15:271, 1984.
165. Sabina RL, Holmes EW. Myoadenylate deficiency, in Server CR, Beavdet Al, Sly WS, et al (eds): *The Metabolic and Molecular Bases of Inherited Disease*, 7th ed. New York, McGraw-Hill, 1995, pp 1769-1780.
166. Sachs, C: Physiologische und anatomische Untersuchungen uber die sensiblen Nerven der Muskeln. *Arch Anat Phys Wissen Med* S175:491, 645, 1874.
167. Onanoff MI: Sur la nature des faisceux neuromusculaires. *Compt Rend Soc Biol* 42:432, 1890.
168. Sherrington CS: On the anatomical constitution of nerves of skeletal muscles; with remarks on recurrent fibers in the ventral spinal nerve root. *J Physiol Lond* 17:211, 1894.
169. Batten FE: Experimental observations on early degenerative changes in the sensory end organs of muscles. *Brain* 21:388, 1898.
170. Batten FE: The muscle-spindle under pathological conditions. *Brain* 20:138, 1897.
171. Cippolone LT: Nuove ricerche sul fuso neuromuscolare. *Ann Med Navale Coloniale* 4:461, 1898.
172. Tello JF: Genesis de las terminaciones nerviosas motrices y sensitivas: I. En el sistema locomotor de los vertebrados superiores. Histogenesis Muscular. *Trab Lab Invest Biol* 15:227, 1917.
173. Boeke J: Die Morphologische Grundlage der Sympathischen Innervation der Quergestreiften Muskelfasern. *Z Mikrosk Anat Forsch* 8:561, 1927.
174. Hinsey JC: Some observations on the innervation of skeletal muscle of the cat. *J Comp Neurol* 44:87, 1927.
175. Hines M, Tower SS: Studies on the innervation of skeletal muscles: II. Of muscle spindles in certain muscles of the kitten. *Bull Johns Hopkins Hosp* 42:264, 1928.
176. Hines M: The innervation of the muscle spindle. *Res Publ Assoc Res Nerv Ment Dis* 9:124, 1930.
177. Tower SS: Atrophy and degeneration in the muscle spindle. *Brain* 55:77, 1932.

178. Cuajunco F: The plurisegmental innervation of neuromuscular spindles. *J Comp Neurol* 54:205, 1932.
179. Boyd IA: The structure and innervation of the nuclear bag muscle fiber system and the nuclear chain muscle fiber system in mammalian muscle spindles. *Philos Trans R Soc Lond [Biol]* 245:81, 1962.
180. Kennedy WR: Innervation of muscle spindles in amyotrophic lateral sclerosis. *Mayo Clin Proc* 46:245, 1971.
181. Zelená J: The morphogenetic influence of innervation on the autogenetic development of muscle spindles. *J Embryol Exp Morphol* 5:283, 1957.
182. Zelená J, Hnik P: Absence of spindles in muscles of rats re-innervated during development. *Physiol Bohemoslov* 9:373, 1960.
183. Zelená J, Hnik P: Effect of innervation on the development of muscle receptors, in Gutman E, Hnik P (eds): *The Effect of Use and Disuse of Neuromuscular Function*. Amsterdam, Elsevier, 1962.
184. McArdle J, Sansone FM: Re-innervation of fast and slow twitch muscle following nerve crush at birth. *J Physiol* 271:567, 1977.
185. Zelená J, Sobotkova M: Absence of muscle spindles in regenerated muscles of the rat. *Physiol Bohemoslov* 20:433, 1971.
186. Zhenevskaya RP: Experimental histologic investigation of striated muscle tissue. *Rev Can Biol* 21:457, 1962.
187. Zhenevskaya RP, Umnova MM: Degeneration and restoration of sensory nerve endings in skeletal muscle (in Russian). *Arkh Anat Gist Embriol* 159:3, 1965.
188. Schmalbruch H: Regeneration of soleus muscle of rat autografted in toto as studied by electron microscopy. *Cell Tissue Res* 177:159, 1977.
189. Mackenson-Dean CA, Hikida RS, Frangowlakis TM: Formation of muscle spindles in regenerated avian muscle grafts. *Cell Tissue Res* 217:37, 1981.
190. Rogers SL: Muscle spindle formation and differentiation in regenerating rat muscle grafts. *Dev Biol* 94:265, 1982.
191. Fardeau M: Etude d'une nouvelle observation de "nemaline myopathy": II. Donnes ultrastructurales. *Acta Neuropathol* 13:250, 1969.
192. Gilles C, Raze J, Vasam V: Nemaline (rod) myopathy: A possible cause of rapidly fatal infantile hypotonia. *Arch Pathol Lab Med* 103:1, 1979.
193. Kolin IS: Nemaline myopathy. A fatal case. *Am J Dis Child* 114:95, 1967.
194. Konda K, Yuasa T: Genetics of congenital nemaline myopathy. *Muscle Nerve* 3:308, 1980.
195. Daniel PM, Strich SJ: Abnormalities in the muscle spindles in dystrophia myotonica. *Neurology* 14:310, 1964.
196. Swash M: The morphology and innervation of the muscle spindle in dystrophia myotonica. *Brain* 95:357, 1972.
197. Swash M, Fox KP: The fine structure of the spindle abnormality in myotonic dystrophy. *Neuropathol App Neurobiol* 1:171, 1975.
198. Swash M, Fox KP: Abnormal intrafusal muscle fibres in myotonic dystrophy: A study using serial sections. *J Neurol Neurosurg Psychiatry* 38:91, 1975.
199. Stranock SD, Newsom Davis J: Ultrastructure of the muscle spindle in dystrophia myotonica: II. The sensory and motor nerve terminals. *Neuropathol App Neurobiol* 4:407, 1978.
200. Maynard JA, Cooper JR, Ionasescu VV: An ultrastructure investigation of intrafusal muscle fibers in myotonic dystrophy. *Virchows Arch [Pathol Anat]* 373:1, 1977.
201. Heene R: Histological and histochemical findings in muscle spindles in dystrophia myotonica. *J Neurol Sci* 18:369, 1973.
202. Krugliak I, Gadoth N, Behar AJ: Neuropathic form of arthrogryposis multiplex congenita: Report of 3 cases with complete necropsy, including the first reported case of agenesis of muscle spindles. *J Neurol Sci* 37:174, 1978.
203. De Boode WP, Semmekrot BA, Ter Laak HJ et al: Myopathology in patients with a Noonan phenotype. *Acta Neuropathol (Berl)* 92:597, 1996.
204. Selcen D, Kupsky WJ, Benjamins D et al: Myopathy with muscle spindle excess: A new congenital neuromuscular syndrome? *Muscle Nerve* 24:138, 2001.
205. Banker BQ, Girvin JP: The ultra-structural features of the normal and de-efferented mammalian muscle spindle. In Banker BQ, Przbylski R, Van Der Meulen J, Victor M (eds): *Research in Muscle Development and the Muscle Spindle*. Excerpta Medica International Congress series No. 240 (ISBN 90 219 01730), Amsterdam, Excerpta Medica, 1972, pp 267–298.
206. Banker BQ, Girvin JP: The ultra-structural features of the mammalian muscle spindle. *J Neuropathol Exp Neurol* 30:155, 1971.
207. Winkelmann RK, Connolly SM, Quimby SR et al: Histopathologic features of the L-tryptophan-related eosinophilia-myalgia (fasciitis) syndrome. *Mayo Clin Proc* 66:457, 1991.

Chapter 31
Ultrastructural Changes in Diseased Muscle

ANDREW G. ENGEL
BETTY Q. BANKER

Patterns of Ultrastructural Changes
Ultrastructural Reactions of Muscle Fiber
  Organelles or Components
    ALTERATIONS OF THE SURFACE MEMBRANE
    ALTERATIONS OF THE NUCLEUS
    ALTERATIONS OF THE T TUBULES
    ALTERATIONS OF THE SARCOPLASMIC RETICULUM
    ALTERATIONS OF THE ENDOPLASMIC RETICULUM
    ALTERATIONS OF THE GOLGI APPARATUS
    ALTERATIONS OF MITOCHONDRIA
    ALTERATIONS OF THE Z DISK
    OTHER MYOFIBRILLAR ALTERATIONS
    MISCELLANEOUS INCLUSIONS

Ultrastructural Alterations in the Muscle Fiber
    CORE, MULTICORE, AND TARGET FORMATIONS
    SARCOPLASMIC MASSES
    DENERVATION ATROPHY
    MYOGENIC MUSCLE FIBER ATROPHY
    FOCAL CYTOPLASMIC DEGRADATION
      AND AUTOPHAGIC MECHANISMS
    LIPID ACCUMULATION IN MUSCLE FIBERS
    GLYCOGEN ACCUMULATION IN MUSCLE FIBERS
    MUSCLE FIBER INVASION AND DESTRUCTION BY T CELLS
      AND MACROPHAGES
    MUSCLE FIBER NECROSIS
    SATELLITE CELLS
    MUSCLE FIBER REGENERATION

Alterations at the Neuromuscular Junction
    PRESYNAPTIC ALTERATIONS
    POSTSYNAPTIC ALTERATIONS

Alterations of the Muscle Microvasculature

Ultrastructural studies provide insights into pathologic cellular mechanisms and suggest etiologic clues in different neuromuscular disorders. For example, such studies suggest that involvement of the muscle fiber surface membrane occurs early in the course of muscle fiber destruction in Duchenne dystrophy[1] and in dysferlinopathy[1a]; that injury of the intramuscular capillaries plays an important role in the pathogenesis of dermatomyositis[2]; that tubulofilamentous inclusions occur in inclusion body myositis [3,4]; and that nonnecrotic muscle fibers are injured by cytotoxic T cells and macrophages in polymyositis and inclusion body myositis.[5,5a] In a late-onset myopathy, electron microscopy revealed sequestration of glycogen in membrane-bound spaces, and this correctly suggested that the myopathy was caused by acid maltase deficiency.[6] Ultrastructural studies have also helped to understand mechanisms that impair neuromuscular transmission in various myasthenic disorders (see Chaps. 64 to 66). Electron cytochemical[7,8] and immunoelectron microscopic methods[5,9,9a,b,c,d] and the correlation of ultrastructural with biochemical or physiologic data[8,10,11] have further enhanced the usefulness of ultrastructural studies.

Patterns of Ultrastructural Changes

Similar ultrastructural changes can occur in individual muscle fibers or fiber regions in diverse neuromuscular diseases. *Consequently, morphologic similarity does not imply etiologic identity.* However, the ultrastructural abnormalities can be resolved into reaction patterns involving muscle fiber, and these reactions, in turn, appear in different sequences and combinations in various diseases.[12]

This chapter describes the ultrastructural changes that involve the various organelles or components of the muscle fiber or the entire fiber, the neuromuscular junction, and the intramuscular capillaries. These alterations are best understood when they are correlated with the corresponding light microscopic changes described in Chap. 30. To avoid needless repetition, only brief light microscopic descriptions are included in this chapter.

The fine structure of normal skeletal muscle is considered in Part I of this volume (Chaps. 2, 3, 6, 7, 11, and 15); therefore only selected electron micrographs of normal muscle are shown in this chapter (Figs. 31-1 to 31-3, 31-15A, 31-35A, 31-39, 31-41, and 31-47A).

Ultrastructural Reactions of Muscle Fiber Organelles or Components

ALTERATIONS OF THE SURFACE MEMBRANE

The normal muscle fiber surface displays straight or faintly undulating plasma and basement membranes with only a few associated caveolae or endocytotic vesicles (Fig. 31-3). The pathologic reactions of the surface membrane include the *formation of papillary projections; increased numbers of endocytotic vesicles; infolding during longitudinal or concentric fiber splitting; focal structural defects of the plasma membrane; disappearance of the plasma membrane* (1) during exocytosis, (2) from circumscribed regions of nonnecrotic fibers, and (3) from large regions of necrotic fibers; and *alterations of the basal lamina.*

Papillary projections. Numerous papillary projections may appear on the surface of abnormal fibers (Figs. 31-4 and 31-5) that may or may not be atrophic. The entire fiber circumference (Fig. 31-4A) or only a segment of it (Fig. 31-86A) is covered by the projections. The projections may be studded by numerous caveolae or endocytotic vesicles (Figs. 31-4A and B, 31-5B) and are always covered by basal lamina. Occasionally, loops of basal lamina surround empty spaces,

---

A list of abbreviations used in this chapter is given at the end of the chapter.

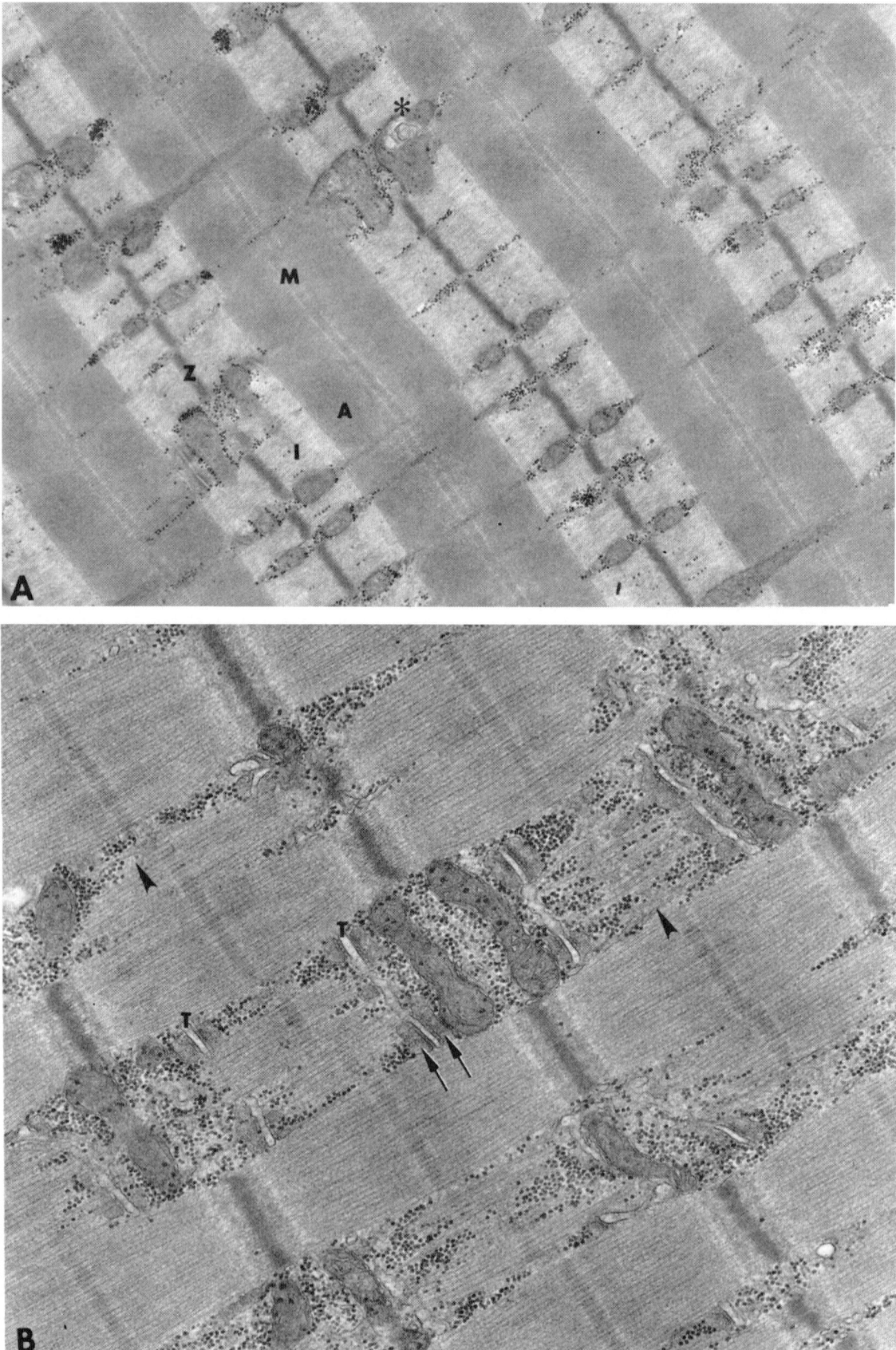

FIGURE 31-1. Longitudinal sections of normal human muscle fibers. A, A band; I, I band; Z, Z disk; M, M band; T, transverse tubule. Arrows indicate junctional SR. Only a few tubular SR profiles are imaged (arrowheads). Note small myeloid structure in one mitochondrion (asterisk). Most glycogen granules are adjacent to I bands and mitochondria. A, ×15,500; B, ×30,800.

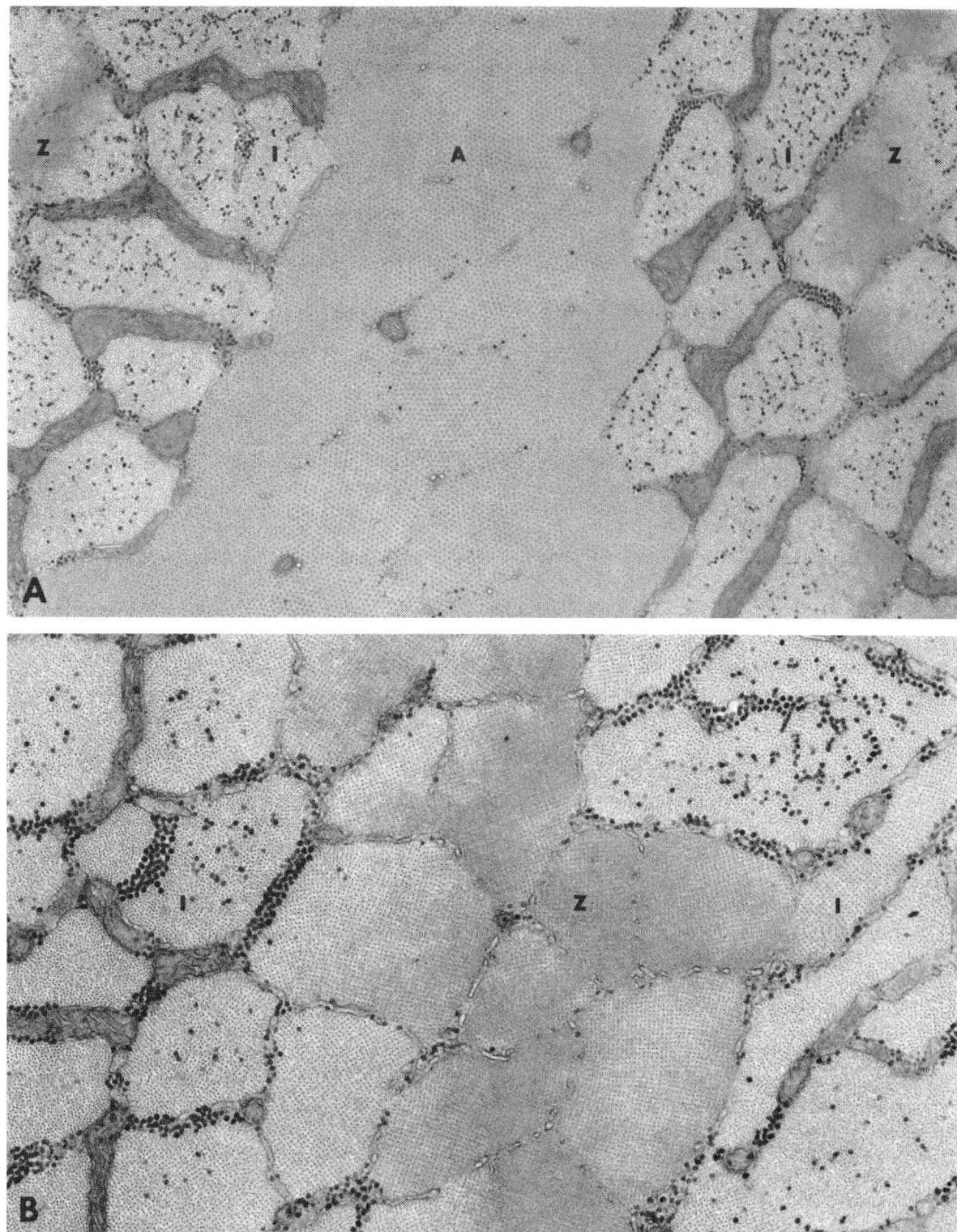

FIGURE 31-2. Transverse sections of normal human muscle fibers. In *A*, the section traverses two Z disks (Z), two I bands (I), and an A band (A); in *B*, it traverses two I bands and a Z disk. Mitochondria form bracelets around myofibrils in the I band and seldom appear in the A band. Most glycogen granules are adjacent to the I band, but a few also occur within the I band. The square filamentous array of the Z disk is apparent in *B*. *A*, ×30,800; *B*, ×39,300.

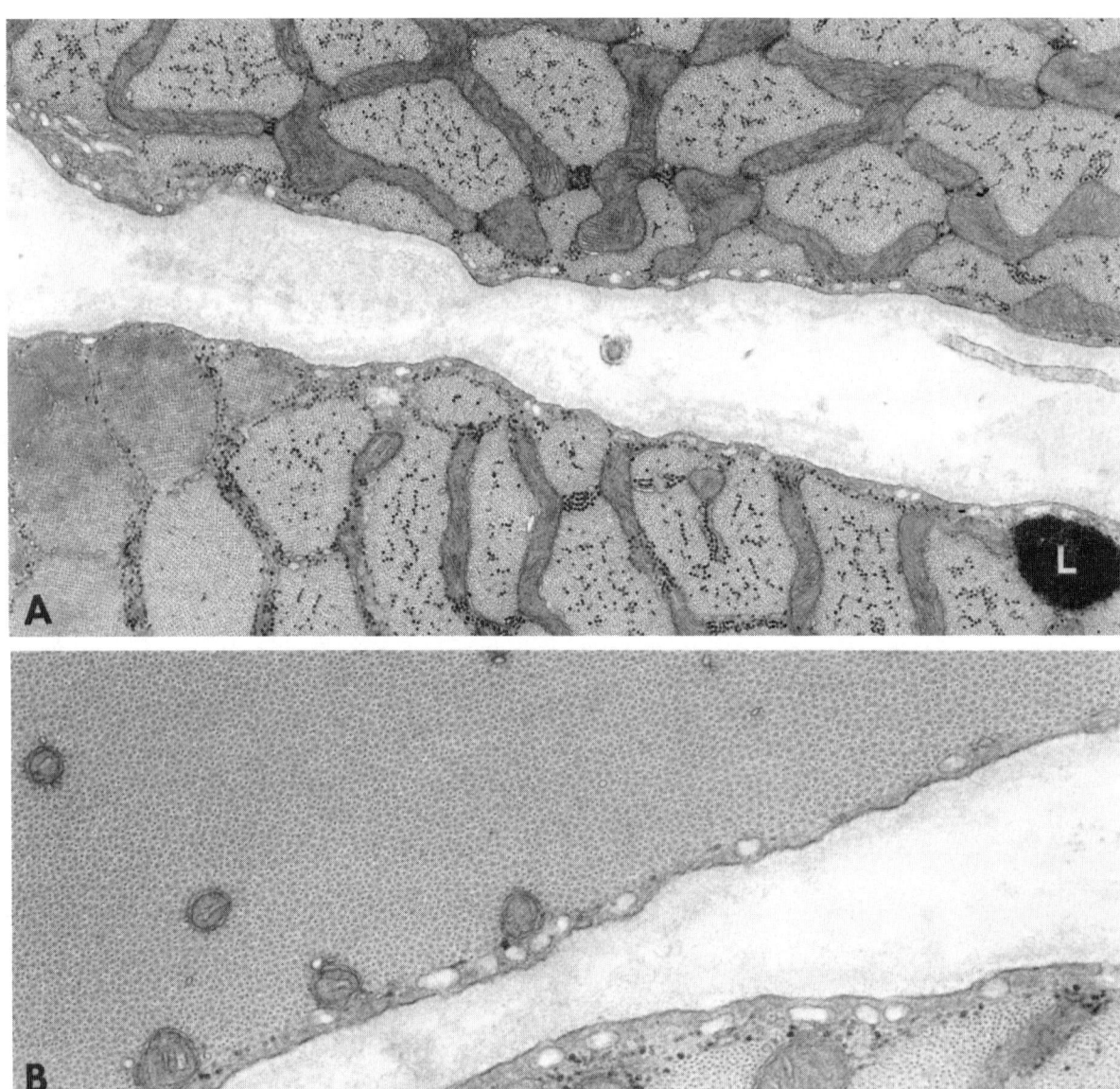

FIGURE 31-3. Transverse sections of peripheral regions of normal human muscle fibers. The muscle fiber surface membrane is smooth or slightly undulating and is associated with a number of caveolae. A thin layer of basal lamina covers the plasma membrane. Endomysial collagen fibrils are unstained. L, lipofuscin granule. A, ×24,800; B, ×49,600.

suggesting disappearance of preexisting folds (Figs. 31-4C, 31-5A). The folds could arise by: (1) Loss of bulk from the fiber interior throwing the surface into folds. (2) Sculpturing of the fiber surface when cytoplasmic degradation products are extruded from the fiber by exocytosis (Fig. 31-5A)—this mechanism may underlie the appearance of numerous papillary projections on muscle fibers in dysferlinopathy. Where frequent disintegration of the papillary folds is associated with activation of the C5b9 complement membrane attack complex.[1a] (3) Sculpting of the fiber surface by spike-like projections of cytotoxic mononuclear cells or by the cytotoxic cells themselves (Fig. 31-5B).

Infolding during fiber splitting. Infolding of the surface and basement membrane can subdivide the fiber into smaller fibers or fiber fragments (Figs. 31-6 to 31-8). The split-off fiber segments remain connected with the parent fiber by one or more anastomoses. Two types of fiber splitting can be distinguished.

In *longitudinal fiber splitting,* the long axis of the pocket formed by the infolding surface membrane is parallel to the fiber axis, and relatively large segments of the fiber are split off. The invaginating plasma and basement membranes are accompanied by collagen fibrils and sometimes by capillaries and fibroblasts. Thus a transverse section of the pocket

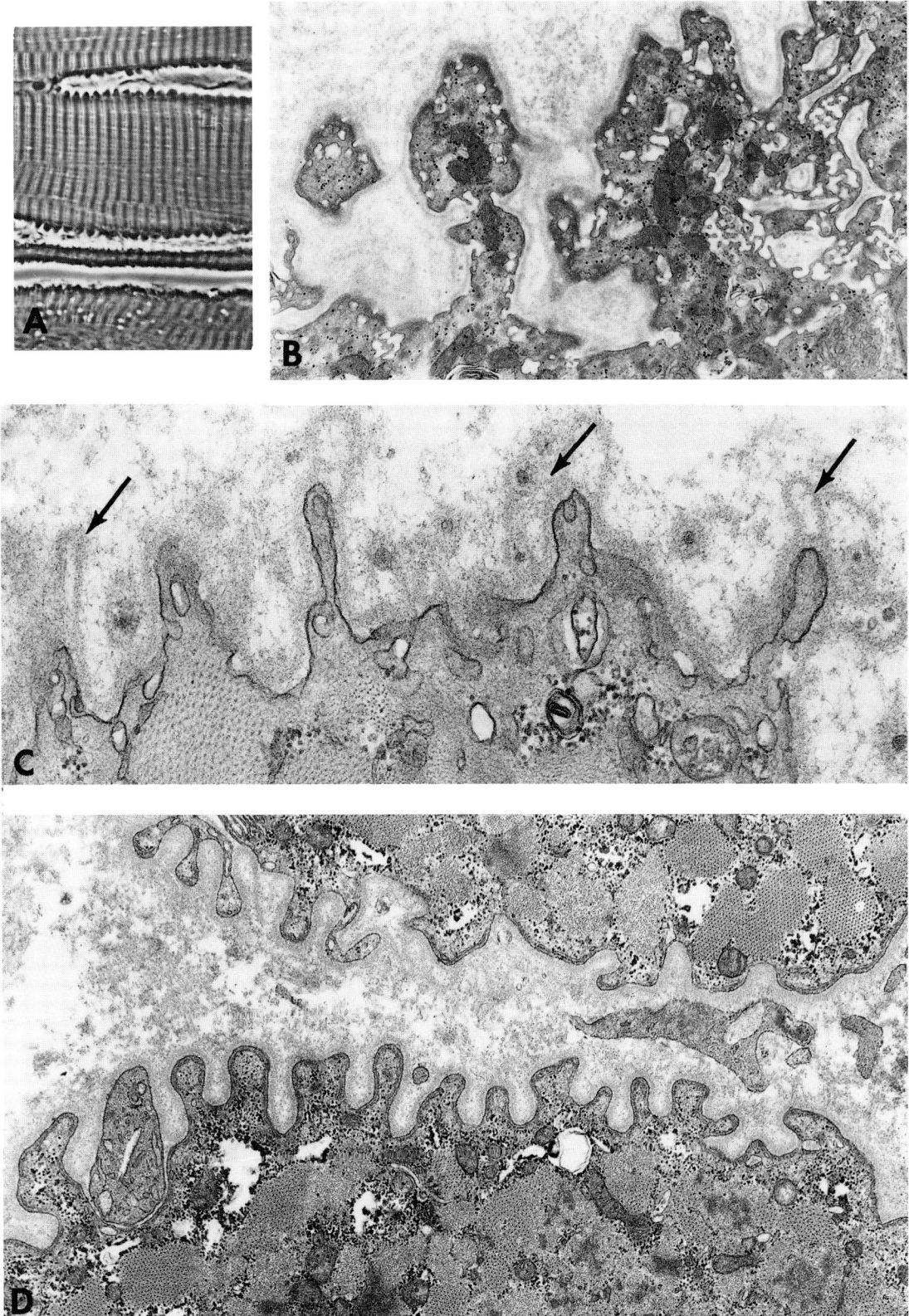

FIGURE 31-4. Papillary projections of the muscle fiber surface membrane in Welander's distal myopathy *(A and B)*, dysferlinopathy *(C)*, and dermatomyositis *(D)*. *A* is a phase micrograph and also demonstrates longitudinal fiber splitting. In *B*, myriad caveolae and caveolar inpocketings are associated with the surface projections. In *C*, collapsed layers of basal lamina indicate sites from which papillary projections have disappeared (arrows). *A*, ×640; *B*, ×19,200; *C*, ×43,000; *D*, ×16,000. *(A and B are reproduced by permission from Engel AG, Macdonald RD, Excerpta Medica ICS 199:71, 1970.)*

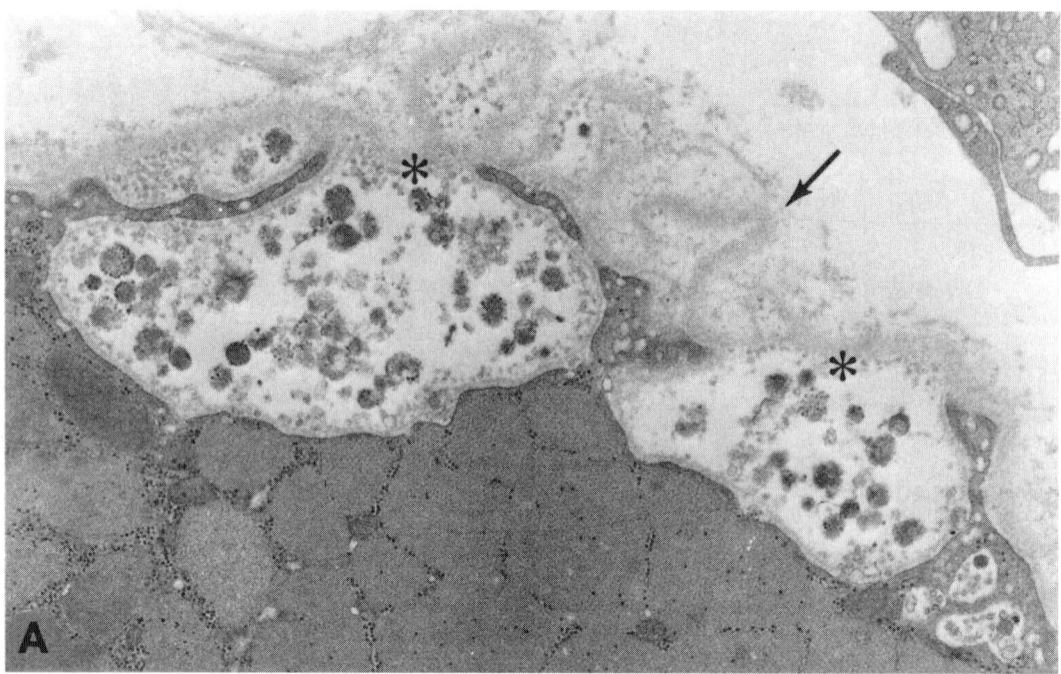
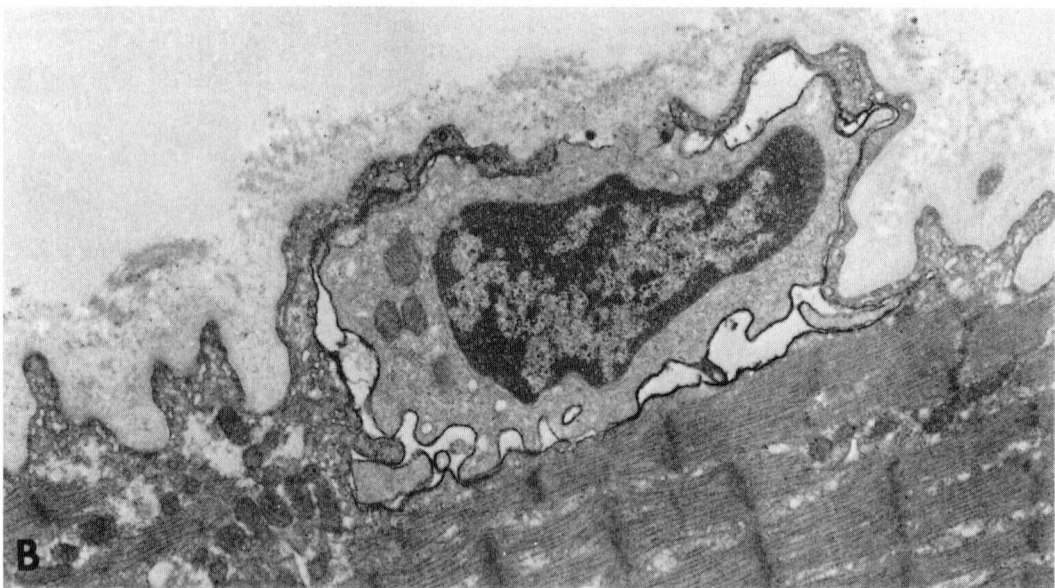

FIGURE 31-5. Sculpturing of the fiber surface by exocytosis (A) and by cytotoxic lymphocyte (B). In A, the plasma membrane has disappeared from the region through which the autophagic vacuole extrudes its content. In B, numerous caveolae occur on the papillary projections of the fiber. In this section, the CD8 antigen is localized by the immunoperoxidase method; the electron-dense reaction product appears on the surface of the autoinvasive lymphocyte. Reciprocal staining of the adjacent muscle fiber surface membrane is due to diffusion of the reaction product. A. Myopathy associated with chronic hypokalemia, ×18,400. B. Polymyositis, ×17,200.

formed by the infolding surface of a splitting fiber may display a capillary surrounded on all sides by the same muscle fiber (Fig. 31-113). The infolding portion of the plasma membrane often displays caveolae, and small membranous networks arising from caveolar inpocketings may abut on or may be continuous with the infolded plasma membrane (Figs. 31-6A, 31-113). Longitudinal fiber splitting is frequently observed in vacuolar myopathies.[6,7] In these disorders, splitting often occurs near abnormal fiber areas, and the split-off part is often diseased. Longitudinal splitting frequently also involves hypertrophied muscle fibers, possibly so as to restore to normal the surface/volume ratio of the hypertrophied fiber.

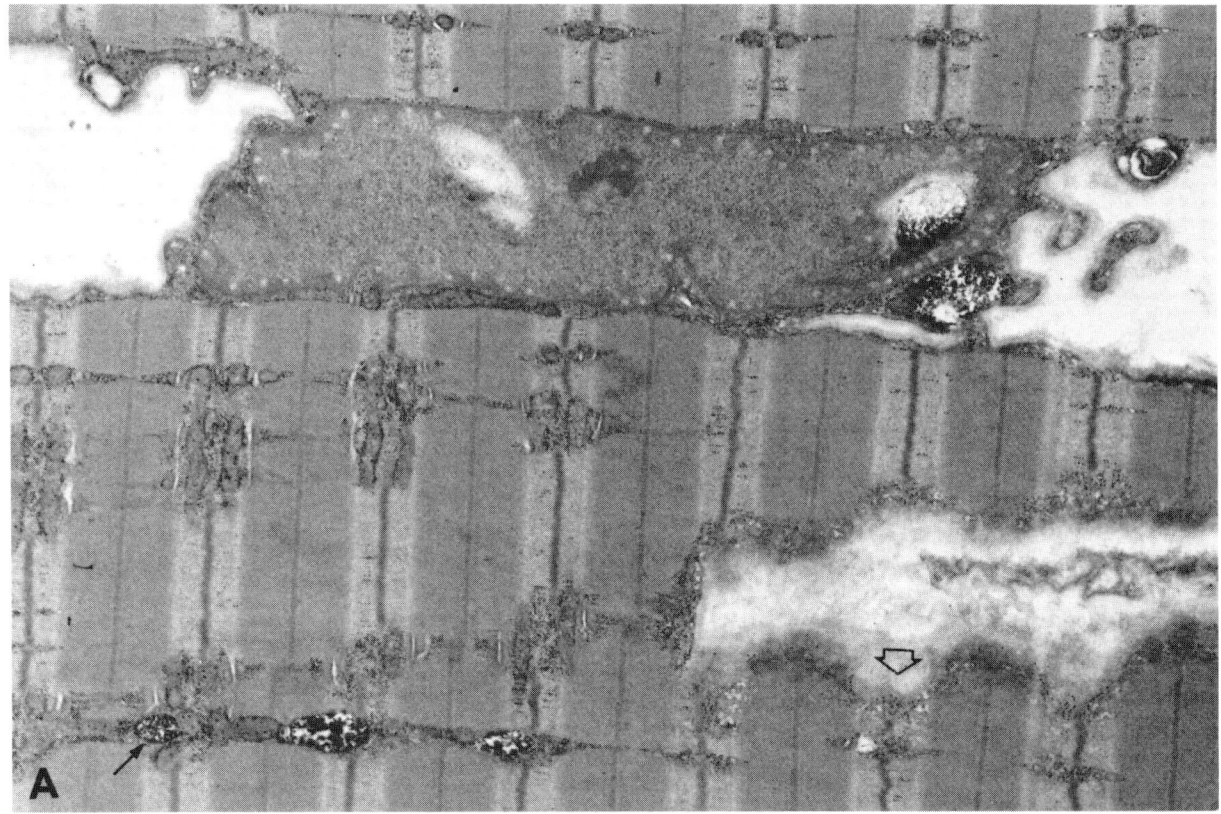
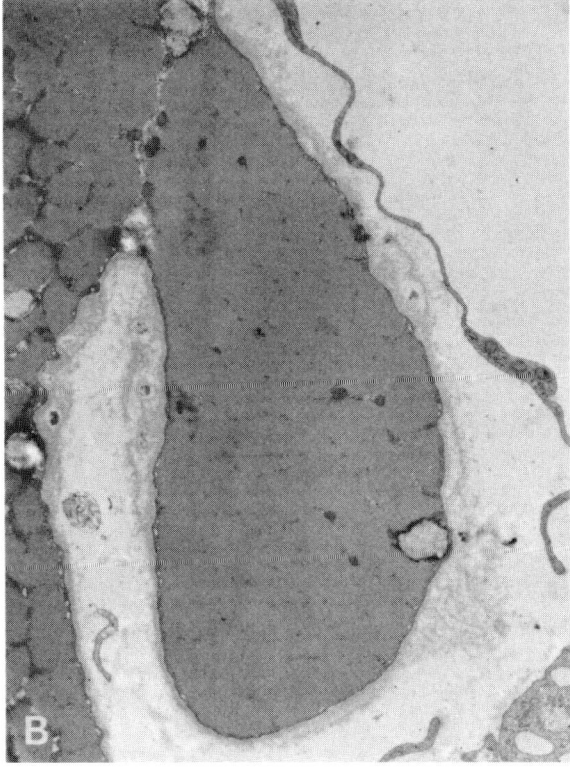
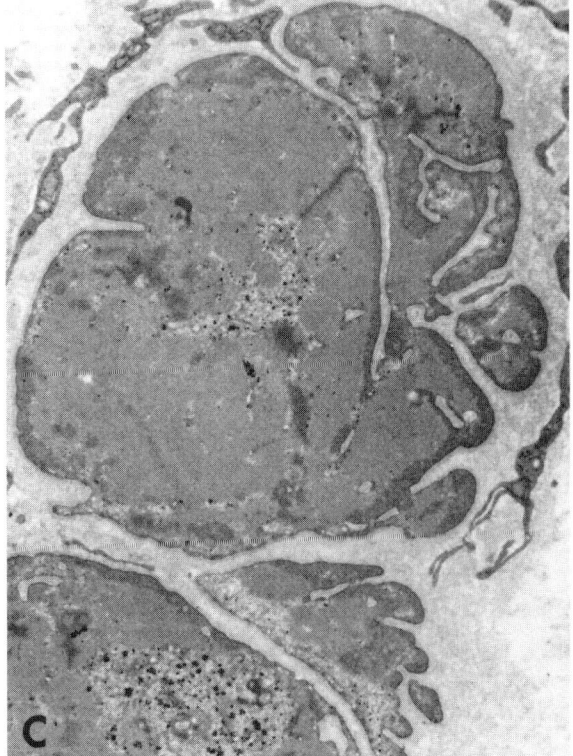

FIGURE 31-6. Longitudinal fiber splitting in acid maltase deficiency (A and B) and limb-girdle dystrophy (C). In A, the subdividing fiber contains three slit-like spaces lined by plasma and basement membrane. Nucleus separates two of these spaces. Numerous caveolar inpocketings line one of these spaces, and these project more deeply into I bands (open arrow) than into A bands. The fiber also contains small lysosomal glycogen sacks (arrow). In C, interdigitating muscle fiber processes of a myomuscular junction are subdividing by splitting. A, ×10,000; B and C, ×9400. (A is reproduced by permission from Engel AG, Dale AJD, Mayo Clin Proc 43:233, 1968.)

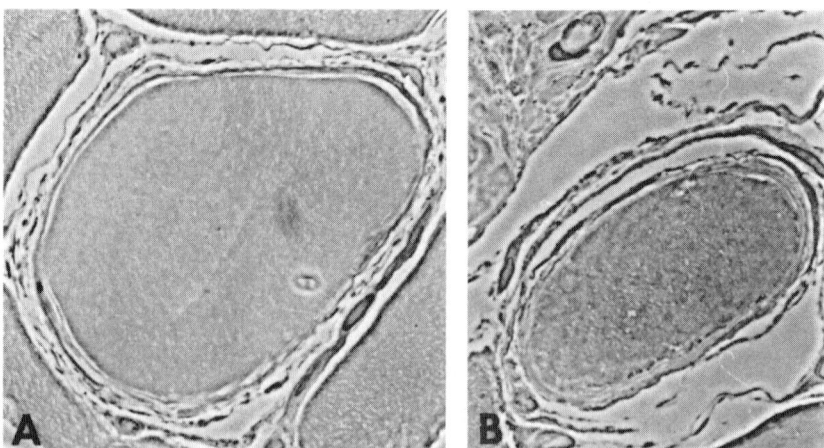

FIGURE 31-7. Semithin resin sections demonstrating concentric fiber splitting in amyloid myopathy. A, ×940; B, ×730.

The incomplete lateral fusion of newly formed myotubes during regeneration produces anastomosing fibers closely molded to each other within the confines of the preexisting fiber that had undergone necrosis.[12a] The incompletely fused fibers resemble a split fiber, and it has been argued that "fiber splitting" is always a sign of preexisting fiber necrosis.

However, there is no rigorous proof that the "split fibers" in diverse myopathies or in hypertrophied muscles always arise from the incomplete fusion of regenerating fibers.

Marked splitting of fiber elements occurs in myomuscular junctions in which processes of two adjacent fibers of the same histochemical type interdigitate (Fig. 31-6C). These formations

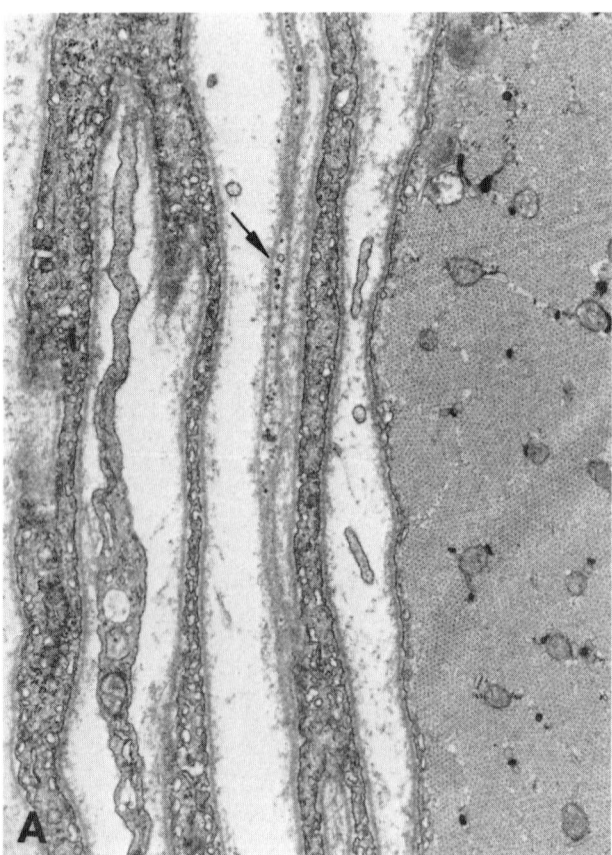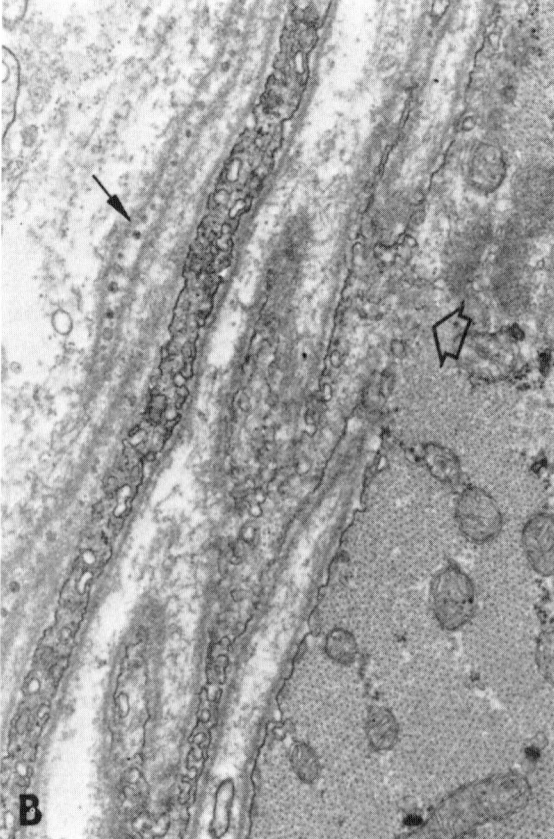

FIGURE 31-8. Concentric fiber splitting in amyloid myopathy. The split-off segments are continuous with the parent fiber (open arrow) and contain myriad caveolae. Degenerate remnants of split-off segments remain sandwiched between adjacent layers of basal lamina (arrows). Electron-dense material in transverse tubules in parent fibers is due to combined fixation with osmium and potassium ferrocyanide. A, ×15,500; B, ×25,900.

are rare in normal and abnormal muscle except in reinnervated rat muscles, in which they are relatively abundant.[13a]

In *concentric fiber splitting*, the pocket formed by the infolding surface membrane forms concentric rings around the entire fiber, splitting off concentric laminae from the superficial regions of the fiber (Figs. 31-7, 31-8). The split-off fiber segments surround the parent fiber like onionskin, anastomose frequently, and are studded by myriad endocytotic vesicles (Fig. 31-8). Some of the split-off segments degenerate into globular fragments that remain sandwiched between adjacent layers of basal lamina (Fig. 31-8A and B). Concentric fiber splitting is an uncommon phenomenon and has been observed by us only in a single case of amyloid neuromyopathy.

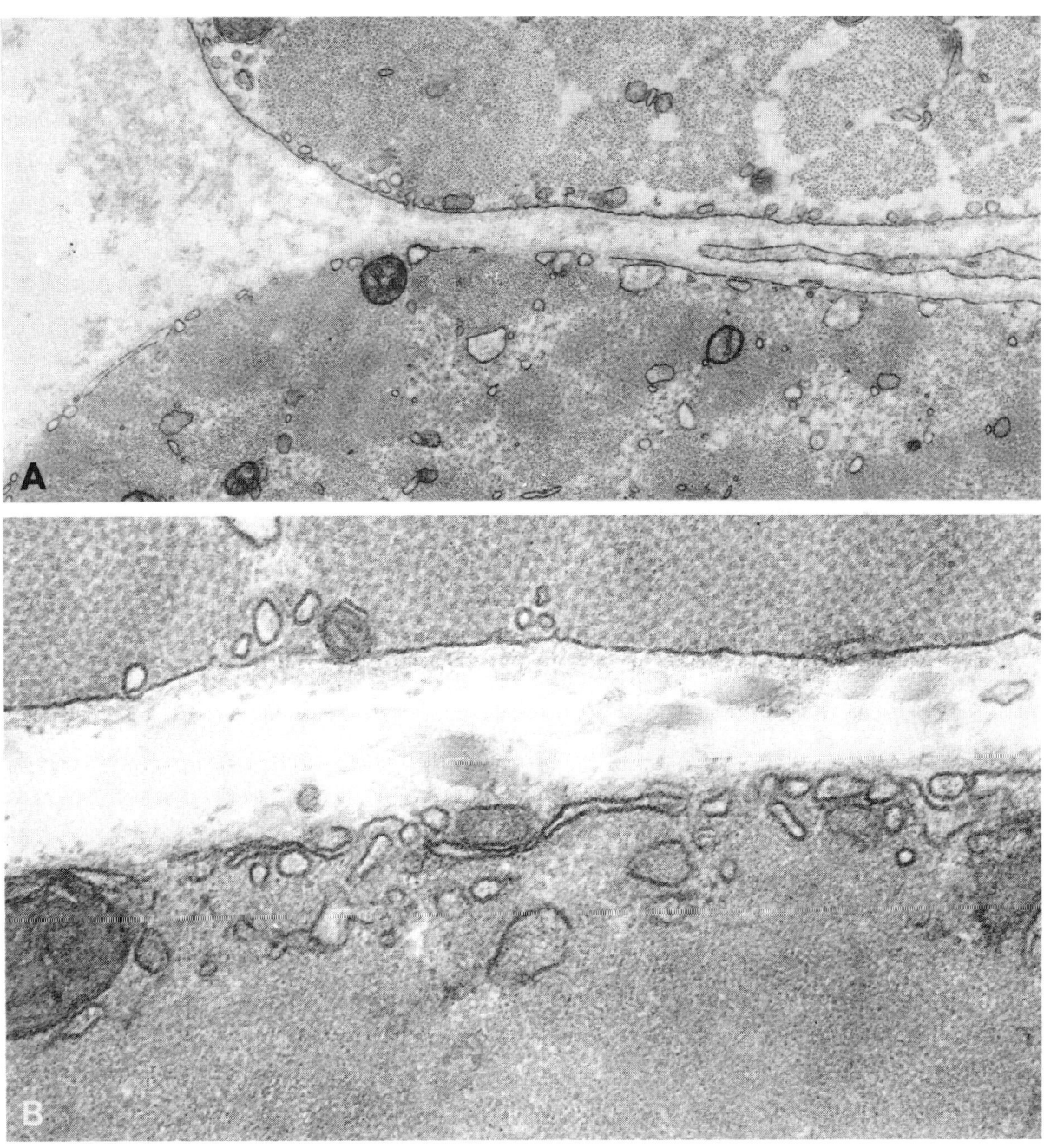

FIGURE 31-9. Focal plasma membrane defects in nonnecrotic fibers in Duchenne dystrophy. The fiber regions under the defect display dilated SR vesicles and rarefied (A) or contracted (B) myofibrils. In B, tubules and vesicles partially cover the fiber surface denuded of its plasma membrane. A, ×29,000; B, ×72,900.

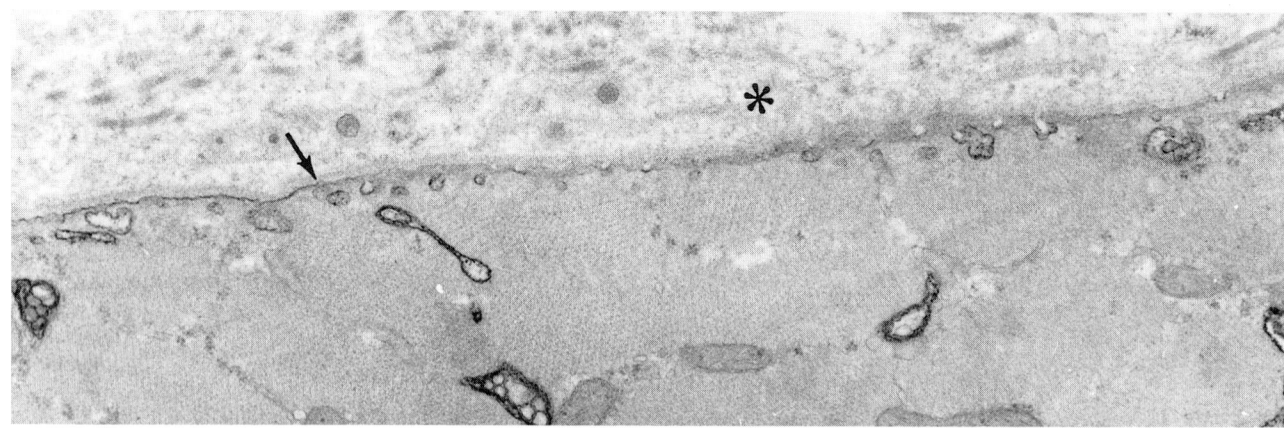

FIGURE 31-10. Extensive plasmalemmal defect in a case of dysferlinopathy. Arrow indicates transition between intact and defective plasmalemma. The basal lamina is focally duplicated (asterisk) and contains small globules of dense material. ×23,000. (From Selcen et al., Neurology 56:1472–1481, 2001. Reproduced by permission.)

Focal structural defects and disappearance of the plasma membrane. Plasma membrane loss during exocytosis occurs when autophagic vacuoles discharge their contents into the extracellular space (Fig. 31-5). The interior of the fiber is not exposed to the extracellular environment, however, because that segment of the vacuolar membrane which does not disappear during exocytosis fuses with the adjacent edges of the muscle fiber plasma membrane.

Focal structural defects of the plasma membrane of nonnecrotic muscle fibers have been observed by electron microscopy in Duchenne dystrophy[1] (Fig. 31-9), in the *mdx* strain of dystrophic mice,[13b] and in dysferlinopathies[1a] (Fig. 31-10). Similar plasmalemmal defects have been detected in α- and γ-sarcoglycanopathies.[13c,d] Permeation studies with Evans blue dye indicate that plasmalemmal integrity is breached in γ sarcoglycan–null mice,[13e] δ sarcoglycan–deficient hamsters,[13f] and calpain 3–deficient mice[13g] but not in the α2 laminin–deficient *dy/dy* mice.[13h] Both in Duchenne dystrophy and in the *mdx* mouse, the plasma membrane defects are due to dystrophin deficiency (see also Chaps. 30 and 34). In either transverse or longitudinal sections, the membrane defects extend over a distance of 0.1 μm to several microns. Tubules and vesicles may become aligned with short segments (Fig. 31-9A) or nearly the entire length (Fig. 31-9B) of the denuded fiber surface, possibly to repair the defect[14] or to seal off the fiber from the extracellular environment. The fiber regions underlying the membrane defect may appear normal.[14] More frequently, either the fiber region under the defect or the adjacent fiber regions are in a contracted state and a wedge- or delta-shaped fiber region under the defect contains dilated vesicles (Fig. 31-9A), scattered myeloid structures, and sometimes small autophagic vacuoles.[1] In some lesions there is also loss of myofilaments. This could be due to pulling apart of the sarcomeres by contractures occurring in the adjacent fiber regions, to proteolytic digestion of the myofibrils, or to both. The basal lamina overlying the plasma membrane defect is either unremarkable (Fig. 31-9), replicated, or thickened.

Extensive loss of the plasma membrane from necrotic fibers (Figs. 31-103, 31-104, 31-111B) is described under "Muscle Fiber Necrosis," later in this chapter.

Alterations of the basal lamina. Replication of the basal lamina commonly occurs around degenerating, regenerating, or necrotic fibers and over focal defects of the muscle fiber plasma membrane. Thickening of the basal lamina over plasma membrane defects was described in the preceding section. The basal lamina often persists when the structures surrounded by it disappear (Figs. 31-4, 31-8, 31-122, 31-131B). Thus basal lamina shells that surround empty spaces or debris represent "tombstones" of preexisting structures.

Thinning and focal discontinuities of the basal lamina are present in α2 laminin (merosin)–deficient muscular dystrophy[14a,b] and its experimental models.[14c,d] Thinning and derangements of the basal lamina have also been observed in the Walker-Warburg syndrome[14e] and in Fukuyama congenital muscular dystrophy.[14f] The basal lamina is preserved, but the overlying collagen network is devoid of microfibrils, with mutations in collagen VI (Ullrich's disease).[14g]

ALTERATIONS OF THE NUCLEUS

Despite the important role of the nucleus in the cell, alterations in the nucleus in muscle diseases are poorly understood. Reactions involving the nucleus include *central migration, regenerative changes in the hof region, extensive infolding of the nuclear membrane, nuclear degeneration and apoptosis, miscellaneous nuclear structures, and nuclear abnormalities.*

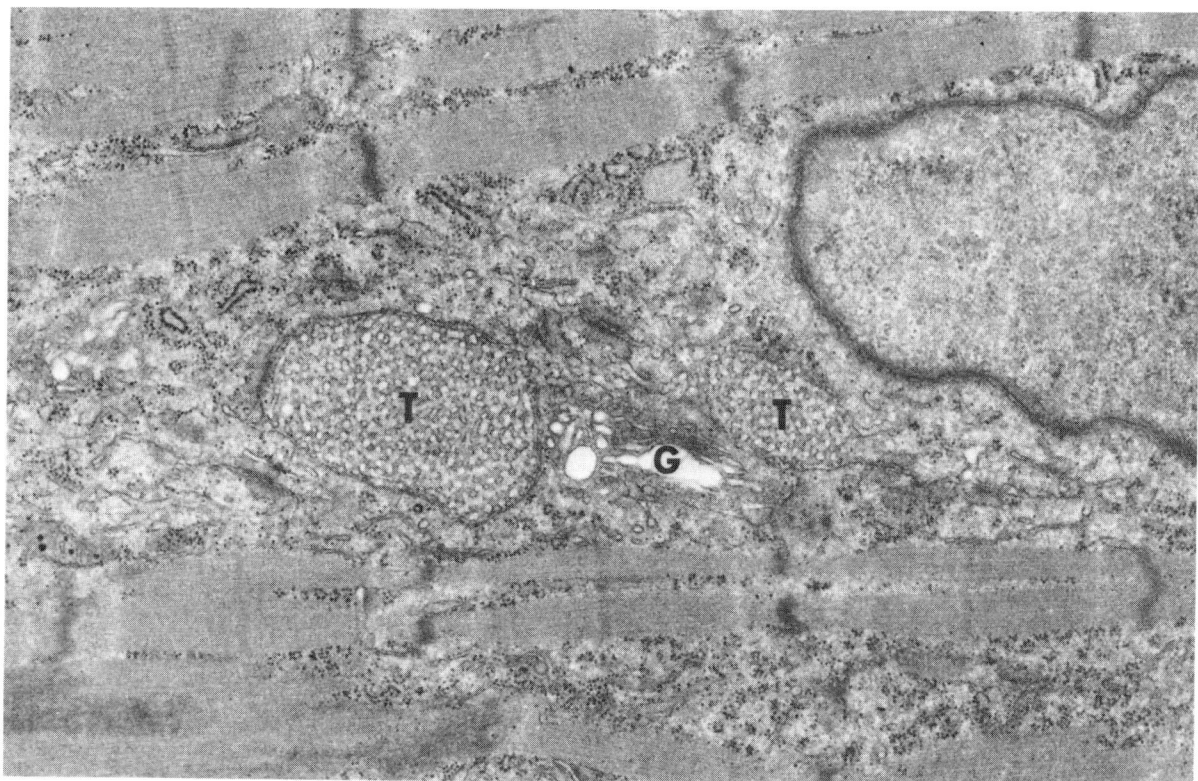

FIGURE 31-11. Regenerative activity in hof region of nucleus. T, T-system network; G, Golgi. Polymyositis, ×22,700. (*Reproduced by permission from Engel AG, Macdonald RD, Excerpta Medica ICS 199:71, 1970.*)

Central migration and regenerative changes in the hof region. Central migration of the nucleus from its normal subsarcolemmal position is common in any myopathy and also occurs in denervation atrophy (Figs. 31-11, 31-12, 31-13A). The hof region of the internal nucleus often shows signs of regenerative activity consisting of abundant rough endoplasmic reticulum, free ribosomes, prominent Golgi networks, transverse (T) tubular networks, and a few too many dilated vesicles of the sarcoplasmic reticulum (SR) (Figs. 31-11, 31-12B and C).

Centrally located nuclei represent the predominant pathological alteration in centronuclear (myotubular) myopathy. Here the centrally positioned nuclei are often surrounded by mitochondria (Fig. 31-12A), glycogen deposits, rough endoplasmic reticulum, and Golgi networks (Fig. 31-12B and C).

Myotubes and immature regenerating fibers in different species typically have central nuclei. In rodents, regenerated muscle fibers bear central nuclei indefinitely. Thus, in *mdx* mice, the proportion of fibers with central nuclei is an index of the number of fibers that had undergone necrosis.[14h]

Extensive infolding of the nuclear membrane. Infolding of the membrane of a subsarcolemmal or central nucleus can incompletely subdivide the nucleus (Fig. 31-13A). It has never been established, however, that this results in amitotic division of the nucleus.

Nuclear degeneration and apoptosis. Invagination of cytoplasmic organelles is an early sign of nuclear degeneration.[15] The invaginated organelles are surrounded by an inwardly displaced nuclear double membrane (Fig. 31-13B). This may occur in the course of apoptosis or independent of apoptosis.

Apoptosis is formally defined by morphologic criteria, and only electron microscopy provides definitive evidence of its occurrence. The sequence of ultrastructural changes during apoptosis is well characterized.[15a] During early apoptosis, chromatin material becomes compacted and segregated into sharply circumscribed masses that abut on the surface of the inner nuclear membrane. This is followed by increased convolution of the entire nucleus, further compaction and enhanced osmophilia of chromatin, loss of all nuclear details, and finally fragmentation of the nucleus. In cells with single nuclei, there is associated blebbing of the plasma membrane and formation of apoptotic bodies that rapidly disappear. This, however, is not true for the multi-

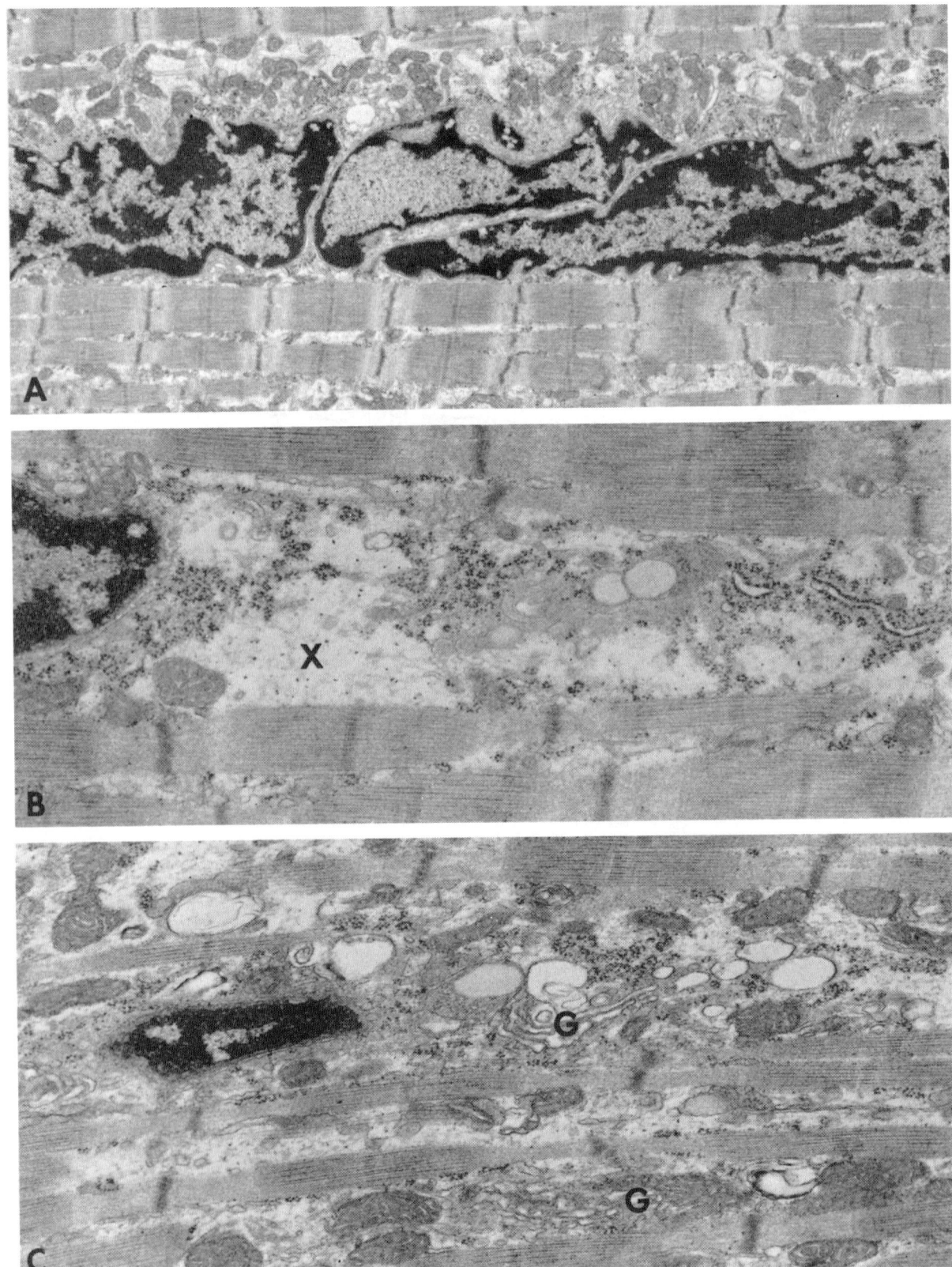

FIGURE 31-12. Central nuclei in centronuclear (myotubular) myopathy surrounded by mitochondria (*A*), rough endoplasmic reticulum (*B* and *C*), and numerous Golgi networks. Empty spaces in *B* (X) are sites from which glycogen was lost during fixation. G, Golgi complex. *A*, ×9300; *B*, ×15,500; *C*, ×25,900.

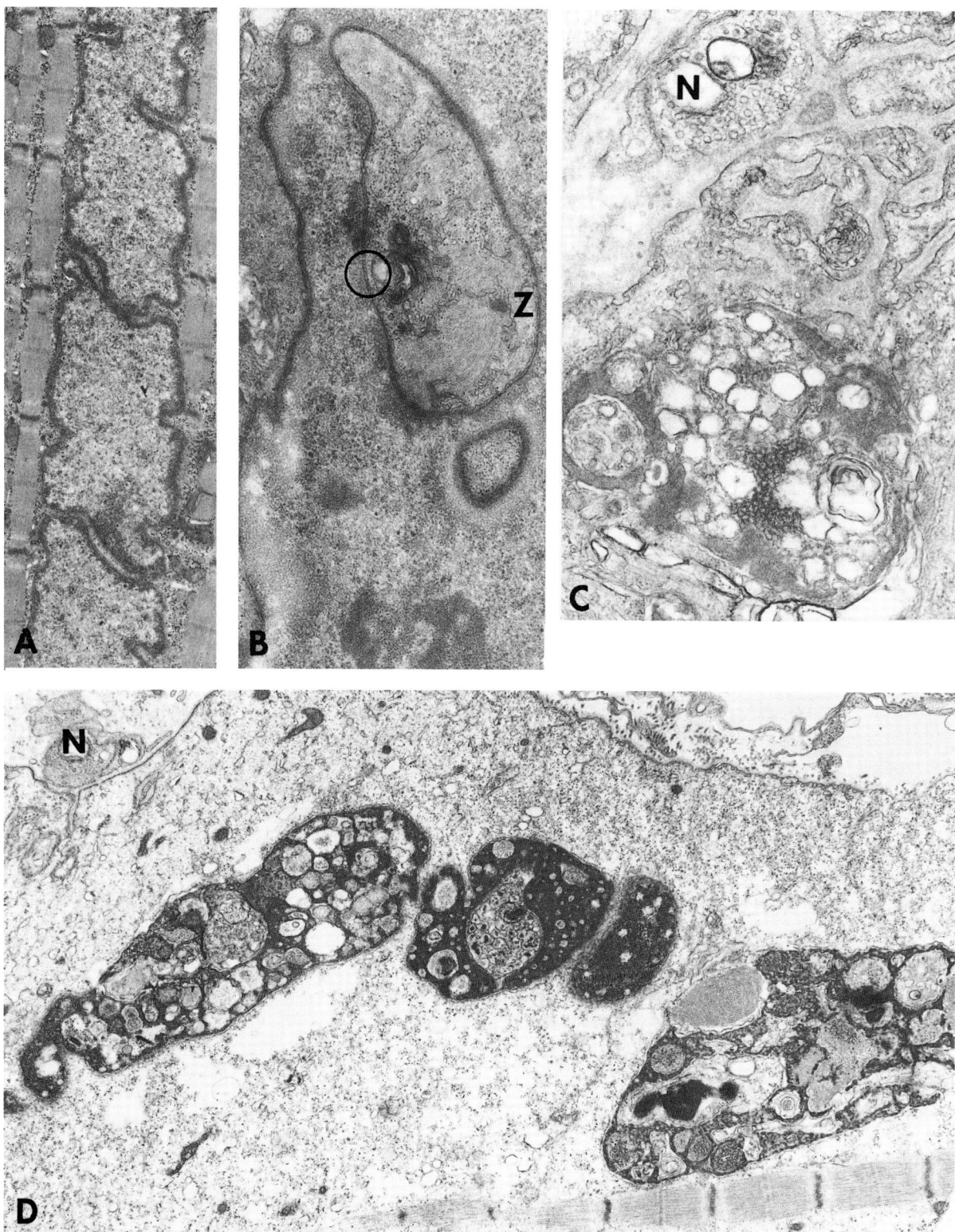

FIGURE 31-13. Nuclear alterations. *A.* Lobulated, centrally migrated nucleus in muscular dystrophy. *B.* Degenerating nucleus with cytoplasmic invaginations in experimental chloroquine myopathy. Circle indicates infolded two-layered sarcolemma. Z, Z disk. *C* and *D.* Apoptotic nuclei at the neuromuscular junction in the slow-channel congenital myasthenic syndrome. Apoptosis in this disease is attributed to calcium overloading of the postsynaptic region. N, nerve terminal. *A,* ×13,300; *B,* ×16,000; *C,* ×26,000; *D,* ×10,000. *(A and B reproduced by permission from Engel AG, Macdonald RD, Excerpta Medica ICS 199:71, 1970.)*

nucleated mature muscle fiber, where apoptotic and non-apoptotic nuclei may appear side by side. The presence of even numerous apoptotic nuclei in the mature muscle fiber has never been convincingly shown to progress to blebbing of the sarcolemma and dissolution of the fiber or to initiate conventional fiber necrosis followed by phagocytosis (see "Muscle Fiber Necrosis," below).

The occurrence of nuclear apoptosis in muscle diseases is often inferred not from electron microscopy studies but by ancillary methods that include detection of nuclei harboring fragmented DNA by the TUNEL method or finding enhanced expression of proapoptotic proteins such as bax and caspase 3 in the muscle fibers. Nuclear apoptosis has been demonstrated by combined electron microscopy and ancillary methods in mitochondrial myopathies,[15b,c] calpain 3–deficient limb-girdle dystrophy 2A,[15d,e] a novel congenital myopathy,[15f] and the Marinesco-Sjögren syndrome.[15g] Striking apoptosis is also seen at the neuromuscular junction in the slow-channel myasthenic syndrome (Fig. 31-13C and D) and in end plate acetylcholinesterase deficiency. In both diseases there is cationic and especially calcium overloading of the junctional sarcoplasm.

Nuclear apoptosis detected by ancillary methods has been reported in spinal muscular atrophy,[15h] myotonic dystrophy,[15i] Duchenne and facioscapulohumeral muscular dystrophies,[15j] and peripheral neuropathies.[15k] Other studies find no evidence for apoptosis in myotonic dystrophy, dystrophinopathies,[15k,l] or γ-sarcoglycanopathy.[15e] In inflammatory myopathies, apoptotic nuclei are detected in inflammatory cells but not within the muscle fibers.[15k,l]

Miscellaneous nuclear structures and nuclear abnormalities. In addition to the nucleolus, different types of nuclear structures have been identified in the normal interphase mammalian nucleus, first by ultrastructural[15m,n] and subsequently by immunocytochemical[16,17] criteria. These include interchromatin and perichromatin granules, perichromatin fibrils, coiled bodies (Fig. 31-14F), fibrillar bodies showing ring-like structure (Fig. 31-14C), and dot-like promyelocytic leukemia (PML) bodies. The coiled bodies vary from 1 to 1.3 µm in diameter, and up to five coiled bodies appear in normal nuclei. These structures are enriched in P80-coilin, fibrillarin, small nuclear ribonucleoprotein (snRNP) splicing factors, and RNA polymerase transcription factors; they are thought to be involved in snRNP biogenesis and trafficking. The coiled bodies associate with twin-like structures ("gemini" or "gems") of similar size. The gems are devoid of snRNP, contain high concentrations of the survival motor neuron (SMN) protein, and play an important role in the biogenesis of splicesosomal snRNP. Deletion mutations in the telomeric copy of *SMN* cause spinal muscular atrophy, and the affected patients have a reduced number of gems in their nuclei.[16,17] The PML bodies are enriched in the promyelocytic leukemia protooncoprotein. Some 10 to 30 PML bodies are present per nucleus; these bodies are 0.2 to 1 µm in size and have a doughnut-like shape consisting of a dense fibrillary ring surrounding a central core.[18] They likely function as negative growth regulators and are targeted by DNA viruses that accumulate within the PML bodies and then disrupt them.

Structures resembling PML bodies have been observed in *dermatomyositis and polymyositis*.[2] Another nuclear inclusion occasionally detected in these diseases is rod-shaped, is 0.3 to 2 µm long and 0.2 µm wide, and contains closely packed is thin filaments. Other nuclear alterations—such as condensation and margination of chromatin, increase in perichromatin or interchromatin granules, clusters of dense granules, osmiophilic spots (Fig. 31-14F), and fragmented, hypertrophic, or multiple nucleoli—have also been observed in inflammatory myopathies.

Filamentous inclusions are a characteristic feature of *oculopharyngeal dystrophy* and inclusion body myositis. In oculopharyngeal dystrophy, the inclusions are composed of 2- to 3-µm unbranched rectilinear filaments that interlace randomly or form palisades. The inclusions incorporate the expanded and probably misfolded polyadenylate binding protein as well as ubiquitin and proteasomal components. These inclusions are further described and illustrated in Chap. 40.

In *inclusion body myositis* there is progressive replacement of some nuclei by interlacing bundles of 13- to 18-nm-wide tubulofilaments (Fig. 31-14A). These inclusions are further discussed in Chap. 50. Collections of irregularly coiling 14- to 50-nm-wide tubules and cisternae were observed by us in a single case of inclusion body myositis (Fig. 31-14D).

Intranuclear nemaline rods that have the characteristic periodicity of cytoplasmic nemaline rods can occur in *nemaline myopathy* (Fig. 31-14E).

In *X-linked Emery-Dreifuss dystrophy* caused by mutations in emerin, ultrastructural studies have revealed condensation of chromatin, discharge of chromatin into the cytoplasm, and curious intranuclear canaliculi.[18a] Another study reports decreased peripheral chromatin and thickening of the nuclear lamina.[18b] In *autosomal dominant Emery-Dreifuss dystrophy* caused by mutations in lamin A/C, condensation of chromatin and detachment of heterochromatin from the nuclear envelope were noted[18d,e] (see also Chap. 35).

ALTERATIONS OF THE T TUBULES

The T-tubular system (or T system) represents an inward extension of the muscle fiber plasma membrane. In addition to its role in transverse impulse conduction, this system also plays an important role in muscle pathology. The tubules can become dilated with electrolyte movements,[19,20] in hypertonic external media,[21] and in muscle stimulated to fatigue.[21a] Light microscopy affords no insight into the reactions of this orangelle.

Normal T tubules range from about 20 to 40 nm in diameter (Fig. 31-1B), but dilations up to 200 nm, possibly related to fixative hypertonicity, can occur near the surface of normal fibers (Fig. 31-15A). Normal T tubules may anastomose or may run parallel to the long axis of the muscle fiber (Fig. 31-15B). The reactions of the T tubules include *displacement* from the normal position in degenerating fiber regions; *focal dilation, proliferation, and labyrinthine network formation* in degenerating and regenerating fibers; *generation of membranes for autophagic vacuoles* of all sizes; *delivery of lysosomal enzymes to autophagic vacuoles;* and *generation of membrane for the elongation and/or repair of the muscle fiber plasma membrane.* In some instances—e.g., in regenerating fiber regions or in

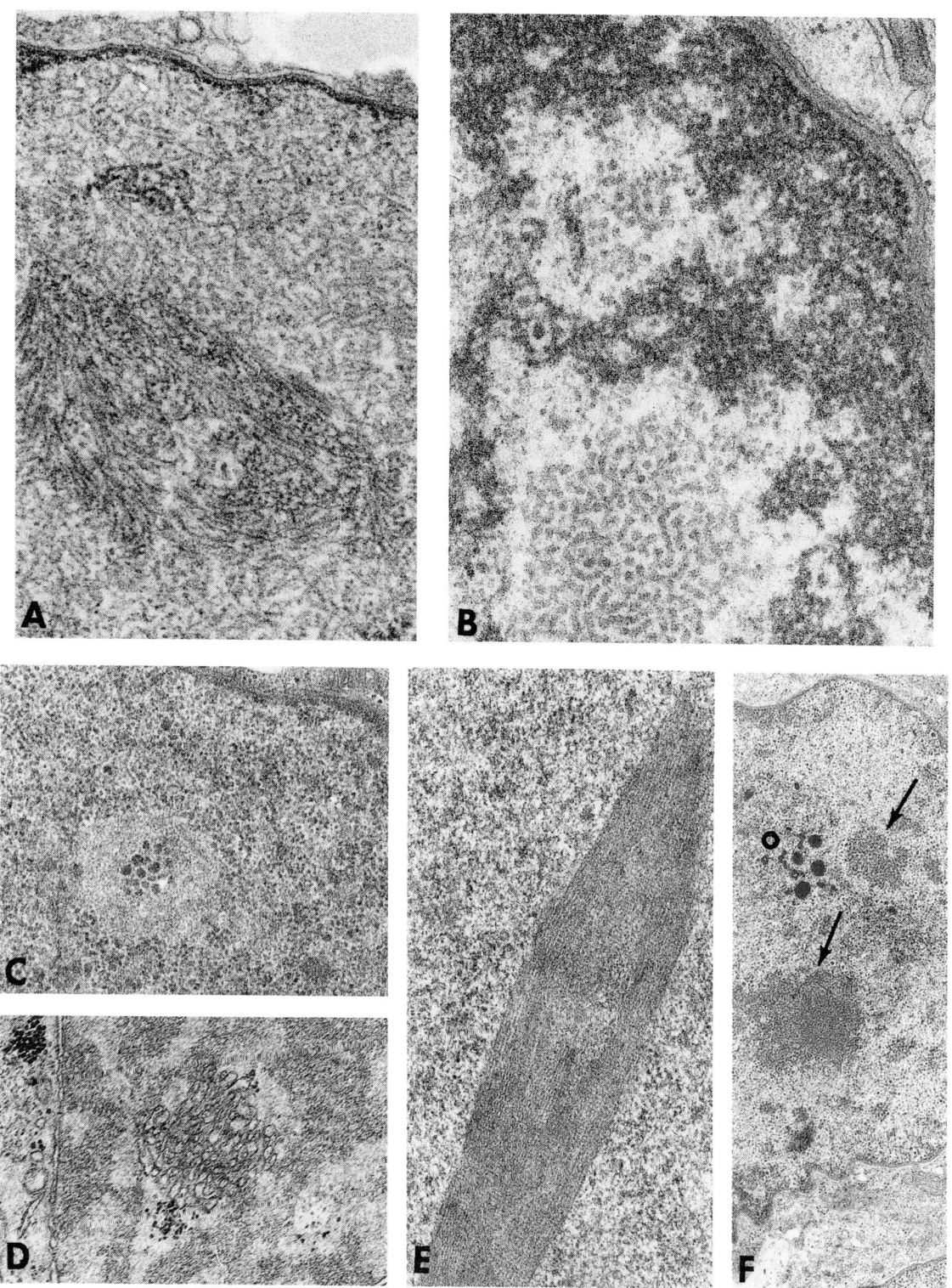

FIGURE 31-14. Miscellaneous nuclear inclusions. *A.* Filamentous nuclear inclusions in inclusion body myositis. *B.* Tubular inclusions in a granulomatous myopathy. *C.* Simple nuclear bodies. *D.* Coiling intranuclear tubules of varying diameter in inclusion body myositis. *E.* An intranuclear nemaline rod in late-onset nemaline myopathy. *F.* Osmiophilic spots (o) and coiled bodies (arrows) in dermatomyositis. *A,* ×37,000; *B,* ×55,000; *C,* ×39,300; *D,* ×29,900; *E,* ×39,300; *F,* ×15,000.

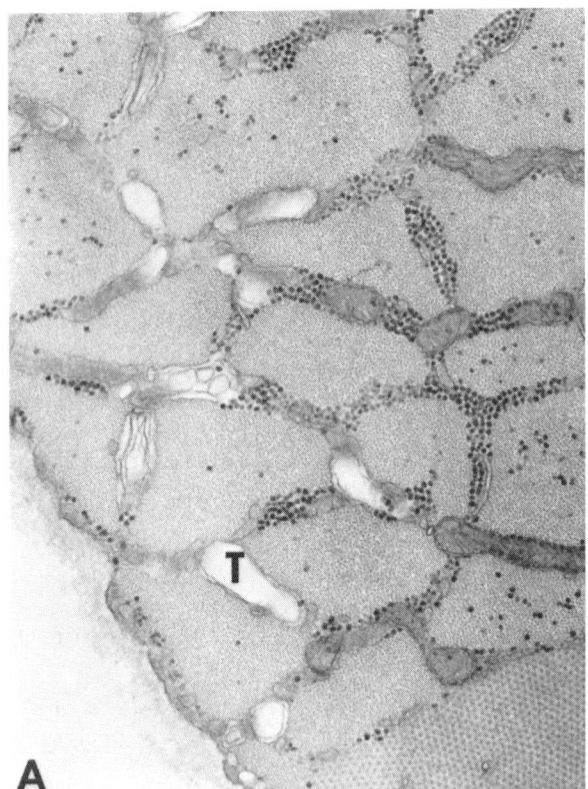 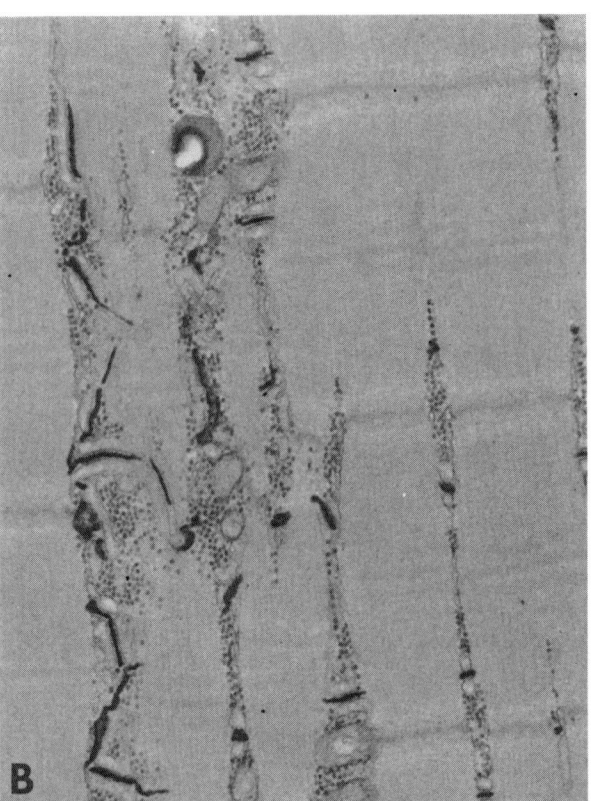

FIGURE 31-15. *A.* Focally dilated T tubules (T) in normal human muscle. *B.* Obliquely or longitudinally oriented triads consisting of T tubules and junctional SR in normal rat gastrocnemius. In *B*, electron-dense material in T tubules is due to osmium-potassium ferrocyanide fixation. *A*, ×34,100; *B*, ×25,100.

periodic paralysis,[7,22,23] sarcotubular myopathy,[24] or chloroquine myopathy[25]—T-tubule and SR reactions occur in various combinations.

Displacement. This occurs commonly in degenerating fiber regions and especially in areas of focal myofibrillar degeneration (Fig. 31-16). The dislocated T tubules are usually associated with dislocated junctional SR components (Fig. 31-16).

Focal dilatation. Focal dilatations more extensive than fixation artifacts can occur in any myopathy (Figs. 31-17*D*, 31-18, 31-35*C*, 31-79, 31-80*A*, 31-98*C*) and are especially prominent in periodic paralysis. When both T-system and SR components react pathologically, dilated T and SR components may be difficult to distinguish from one another. In these instances, T tubules, T-tubule-derived structures, and spaces communicating with them can be identified with horseradish peroxidase or other electron-dense markers that can enter the T tubules from the extracellular fluid (Figs. 31-18*A*, 31-19, 31-30*E*, 31-91*E* and *F*),[7,22–25] whereas the SR components can be recognized by their reactivity for a Mg-dependent ATPase (Figs. 31-18*B*, 31-25*D*, 31-30*B* to *D*).[7,23–25]

Proliferation. T-system proliferation, first noted in denervated rat muscle,[26] was subsequently described in a variety of pathologic states (reviewed in Ref. 12). Further studies of myopathies in which autophagic mechanisms are prominent, such as acid maltase deficiency,[6,26,27] chloroquine myopathy,[25] and periodic paralysis,[22] established that the proliferating T system plays an important role in autophagic mechanisms.

Proliferating T tubules produce complicated labyrinthine networks. The smallest of these arise as evaginations from normal or dilated T tubules (Fig. 31-17*A*). The three-dimensional organization of the networks is still unclear, but when the networks are loaded with peroxidase from the extracellular fluid, an orderly array of convoluted tubules that are continuous with normal T tubules can be observed (Fig. 31-19*C*).

T-system networks occur in otherwise normal fiber regions (Fig. 31-17*B*, *C*, and *D*), in sarcoplasmic masses (Fig. 31-80*B* and *C*), in fiber regions containing aggregates of mitochondria and glycogen (Fig. 31-98*C*), or in hyaline bodies (Fig. 31-62*C*). The functional significance of the networks at these sites is unclear. The networks are also common in

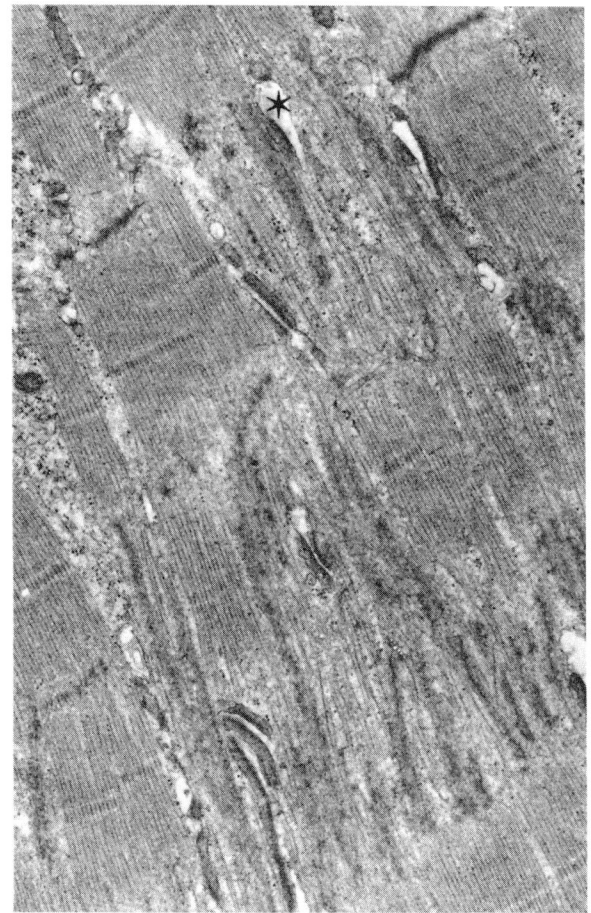

FIGURE 31-16. Horizontally oriented triads in an area of focal myofibrillar degeneration. In some triads the T tubules are dilated (asterisk). Polymyositis, ×18,200.

regenerating fiber regions (Figs. 31-11, 31-20, 31-89A and B), where they are often positioned near dilated SR vesicles (Figs. 31-20, 31-89A and B) and prominent Golgi complexes (Figs. 31-20, 31-89A). T-system networks consistently appear adjacent to and fuse with autophagic vacuoles (Figs. 31-34, 31-92B, 31-94, 31-101A); they also occur near sites where new plasma membrane is formed (Figs. 31-107B, 31-115A).

Generation of membranes for autophagic vacuoles.

Sequestration of cytoplasmic organelles or regions into autophagic vacuoles is initiated by T tubules and networks. Small adjacent vacuoles coalesce to form larger ones, and T tubules and networks coalesce with autophagic vacuoles of all sizes. Thus it is clear that the T system initiates the formation of, and serves as a membrane source for, autophagic vacuoles (Figs. 31-19, 31-21, 31-22, 31-34, 31-86E and F, 31-92B, 31-94, 31-101A).[7] Peroxidase-loading experiments indicate that the extracellular marker enters not only the T tubules and networks that limit the autophagic vacuoles but also the lumina of the vacuoles (Fig. 31-19D).[7,22,25] Thus the T system may also serve as a conduit through which degraded vacuolar contents can exit from the fiber and extracellular fluid can enter autophagic vacuoles. Autophagic mechanisms are further discussed under "Focal Cytoplasmic Degradation and Autophagic Mechanisms," later in this chapter.

Delivery of lysosomal enzymes to autophagic vacuoles.

Vesicles derived from proliferating T-system networks, and the networks themselves, react for acid phosphatase, and the reactive vesicles and networks fuse with autophagic vacuoles (Fig. 31-22).[7,26,27] Thus the T system can deliver lysosomal enzymes to the vacuoles. Acid phosphatase reactivity in muscle also appears in Golgi components,[25] and it is well established that in different types of cells lysosomal enzymes flow from the rough endoplasmic reticulum to the Golgi system.[28-30] Packages of these enzymes eventually appear in the *trans*-most Golgi cisternae, from which they detach as coated vesicles to become primary lysosomes.[31] Few coated vesicles can be observed to fuse with autophagic vacuoles in muscle (Fig. 31-22A), and it has not been established that coated vesicles represent the major or direct pathway for the delivery of lysosomal enzymes to autophagic vacuoles. If the Golgi system is the only source of primary lysosomes in muscle, then the T-system-derived vesicles act as intermediate carriers of lysosomal enzymes to the autophagic vacuoles.

Elongation and/or repair of the muscle fiber plasma membrane.

That elongation or repair occurs is suggested by the following observations:

1. T-system networks occasionally abut on infolding plasma membranes during longitudinal fiber splitting. However, this occurs infrequently, and the T system is probably not a significant membrane source during fiber splitting.
2. T-system networks (Fig. 31-115A) or caveolar inpocketings (Fig. 31-112B) abut on the membranous boundaries of nascent satellite cells and may contribute to the extra layer of plasma membrane required for the separation of the satellite cell from the parent fiber.
3. In nonnecrotic muscle fibers invaded by cytotoxic lymphoid cells, fiber regions near the invading cells frequently contain T-system networks, and some networks coalesce with segments of the muscle fiber plasma membrane facing the invading cells (Fig. 31-107B).[5] This may allow elongation of the plasma membrane around the spike-like processes of the invading cells or may repair membrane defects induced by the cytotoxic cells. It is interesting to note, however, that T-system networks are not present near the focal membrane defects of nonnecrotic muscle fibers in Duchenne dystrophy.

Other T-tubule reactions.

Markedly elongated, coiled, and branching T-tubule profiles associated with SR profiles in various stages of dilation are found in periodic paralysis[22] and occasionally in other myopathies. The abnormal membrane assemblies degenerate, forming dense osmiophilic lamellae and irregularly arrayed myeloid structures (Fig. 31-29).

In sarcotubular myopathy, T-tubule profiles abut on, indent, or become invaginated into abnormally dilated and coalescing SR components (Fig. 31-30).[24]

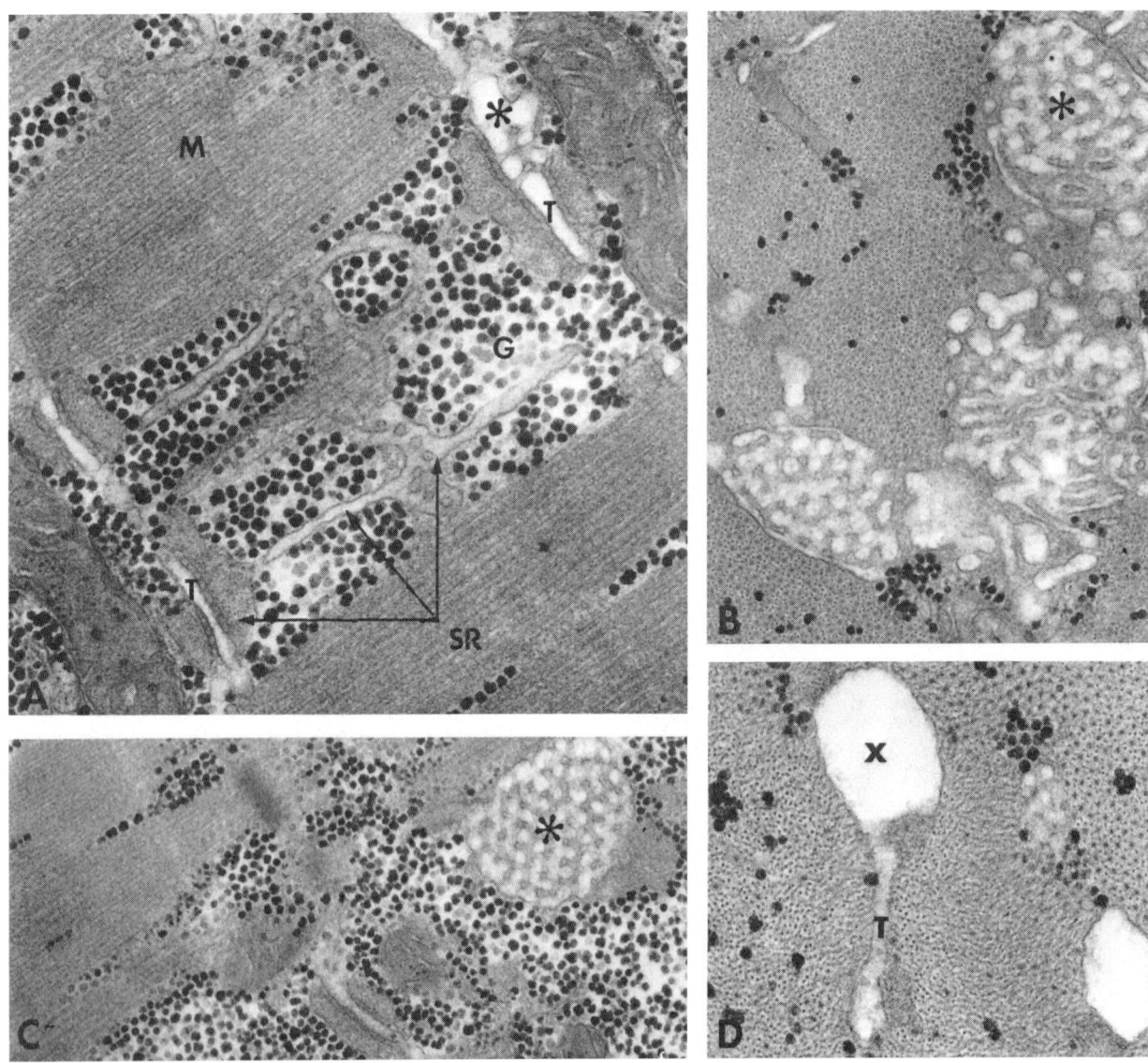

FIGURE 31-17. Proliferating (asterisk) and dilated (x) T tubules. In *A*, note that small T-system network is arising by budding from a T tubule. T, T tubule; SR, sarcoplasmic reticulum; M, M band. Primary hypokalemic periodic paralysis. *A*, ×50,500; *B*, ×42,500; *C*, ×36,400; *D*, ×53,000. *(Reproduced by permission from Engel AG, Mayo Clin Proc 45:774, 1970.)*

Anastomoses between T tubules and SR components have been described in various neuromuscular disorders.[32] The evidence for this rests on the entry of lanthanum in fixed muscle into tubules that course parallel to the long axis of the muscle fiber. However, the evidence is incomplete because (1) T tubules can course horizontally even in normal muscle (Fig. 31-15*B*); (2) in regenerating, degenerating, or denervated fibers T and SR components can become displaced from their normal position and cannot be consistently identified by simple inspection; (3) the anastomoses have not been demonstrated by loading unfixed muscle with peroxidase or another extracellular marker; (4) the putative SR components filling with lanthanum have not been shown to react for an SR marker such as the SR-associated Mg-dependent ATPase.[7,24,25]

ALTERATIONS OF THE SARCOPLASMIC RETICULUM

Since the anatomy of the normal SR is clearly described in Chap. 11, only a few points need mention here. Normal human muscle contains less SR than mouse or rat muscle. Longitudinal sections of human muscle commonly show the junctional SR (Fig. 31-1) but seldom display the tubular and

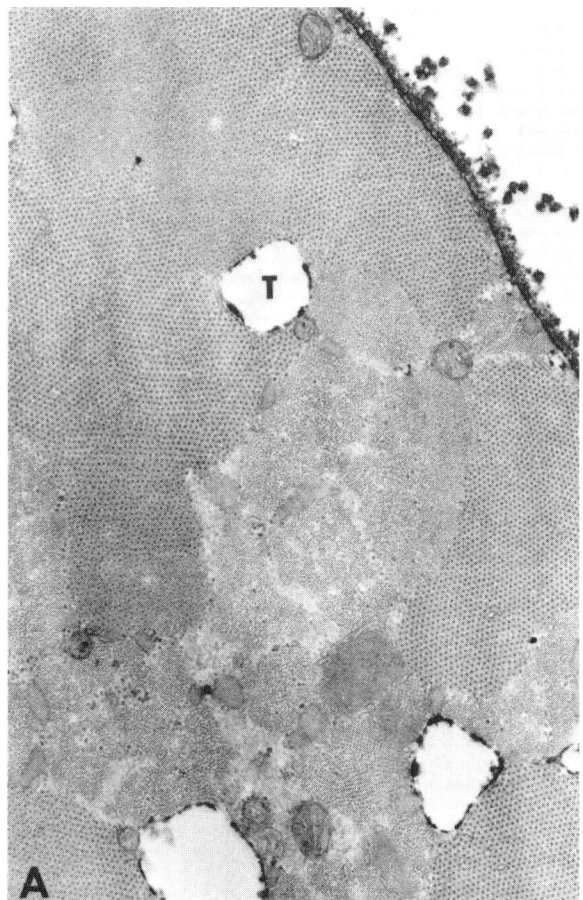
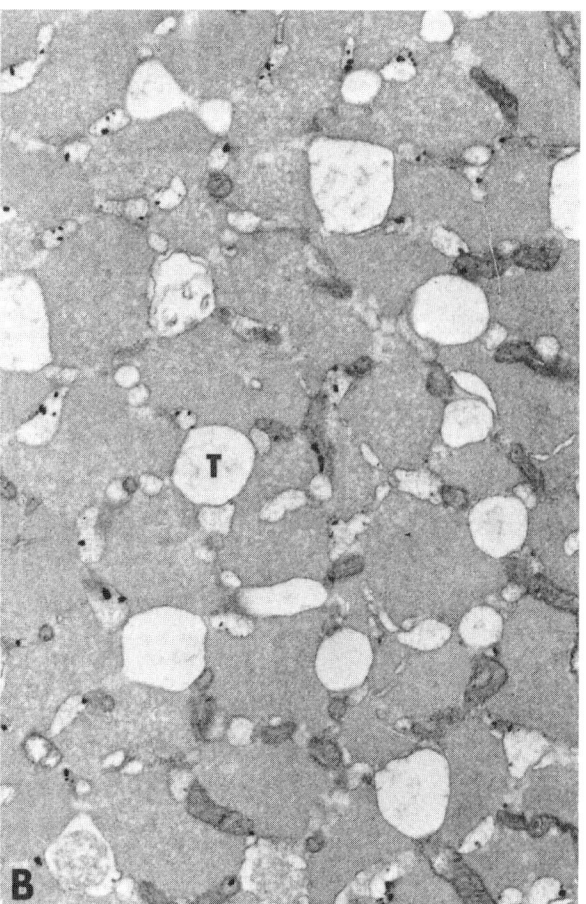

FIGURE 31-18. Focally dilated T tubules in primary hyperkalemic periodic paralysis. Muscle shown in A has been immersed in extracellular fluid containing horseradish peroxidase. The marker is observed over the surface membrane of the fiber and within the dilated T tubules. Muscle shown in B has been reacted for a Mg-dependent, SR-specific ATPase. The electron-dense reaction product appears in small membrane-bound profiles that are distinct from the dilated T tubules. A, ×20,900; B, ×19,200.

fenestrated SR (Fig. 31-17A). In transverse sections of normal muscle it is difficult to distinguish between SR and T tubule transections (Fig. 31-2), except when grazing sections of T tubules also expose the adjacent junctional SR (Fig. 31-15A). In material doubly fixed by glutaraldehyde and osmium the SR has a finely granular content.

The pathologic reactions of the SR include *focal dilation; proliferation* of the entire organelle, the junctional SR, and the tubular SR; *mineralization; storage of homogeneous electron-dense material;* and *degeneration*. As mentioned under "Alterations of the T Tubules," above, both T tubules and SR often react jointly in a given abnormal fiber region.

Focal dilation. Focal dilation of the SR can occur in any myopathy, although it is particularly common in periodic paralysis (Fig. 31-23). The dilated vesicles initially retain the finely granular content of the normal SR. Clusters of SR vesicles together with T-system networks and prominent Golgi systems occur in regenerating fiber regions (Figs. 31-20, 31-89A and B). Dilated SR vesicles are also common in denervated fibers (Fig. 31-81C); in the junctional sarcoplasm of end plates in the slow-channel syndrome, or when acetylcholinesterase is absent or inhibited; under conditions where the electrolyte milieu, and particularly the calcium content, of the junctional sarcoplasm is altered[11,34]; and in delta lesions in Duchenne dystrophy (Fig. 31-9A).

Proliferation. This can involve all SR components or predominantly the junctional or tubular SR.

Proliferation of all SR components occurs in denervated muscle fibers.[33] Many of the membranous profiles are also dislocated from their normal positions, so that T and SR components may be difficult to distinguish (Figs. 31-24A, 31-81A, B, and E).

Proliferation of junctional SR and T tubules produces pentads, heptads, or even longer arrays composed of alternating T and SR profiles (Figs 31-24B, 31-124B and C). Dilated SR vesicles may also occur in the arrays. These formations appear in regenerating, degenerating, and denervated fibers.[34]

Proliferation of junctional SR components but not of T tubules is an infrequent nonspecific finding (Fig. 31-24C).

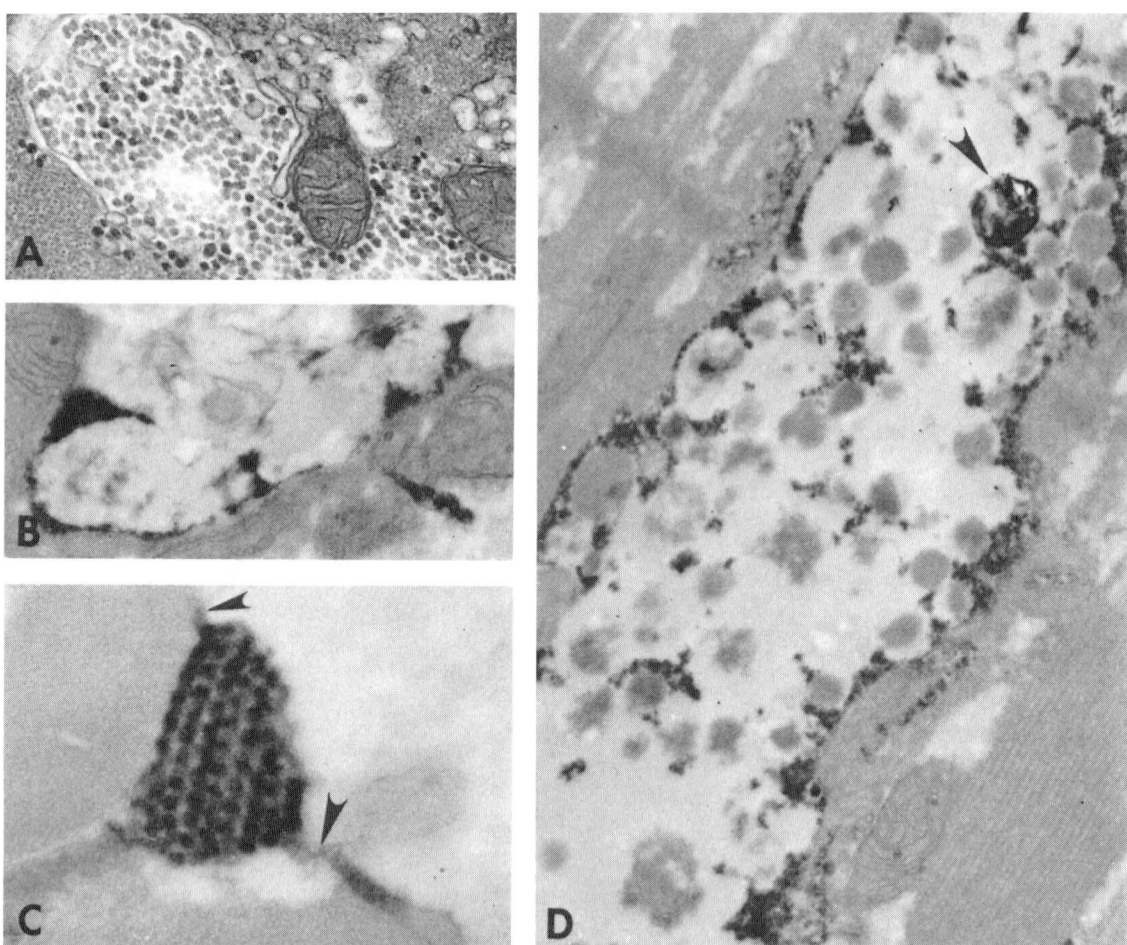

FIGURE 31-19. Sequestration of cytoplasmic organelles by the T system in acid maltase deficiency. In A, T tubule continuous with a small T network sequesters glycogen. B shows an identical configuration to that seen in A, but the T system has been loaded with peroxidase. In C, a peroxidase-filled T-system network continuous with T tubules (arrowheads) embraces the border of an autophagic vacuole. In D, peroxidase-filled tubules surround and limit an autophagic vacuole that has heterogenous contents. T tubules also open into the vacuole, and some peroxidase has entered into the lumen of the vacuole. The circular dense deposit (arrowhead) may indicate endogenous peroxidase activity. A and B, ×43,200; C, ×54,300; D, ×32,000. [A is reproduced by permission from Engel AG, Macdonald RD, Excerpta Medica ICS 199:71–89, 1970; B, C, and D are reproduced by permission from Engel AG, in Pearson CM (ed): The Striated Muscle, Baltimore: Williams & Wilkins, 1973, pp.301–341.]

Proliferation of the tubular SR produces tubular aggregates (Figs. 31-25, 31-26). These occur in a variety of disorders, such as periodic paralysis; the slow-channel congenital myasthenic syndrome; other congenital myasthenic syndromes[35]; muscle disorders associated with cramps, pain, or stiffness; alcoholic myopathy; after exposure to various drugs; and in anoxic rat fast-twitch muscle (for a review, see Ref. 36 and Chap. 30). Finally, we have also observed such aggregates in the C57B/10 inbred strain of mice. The tubules in the aggregates contain the fine granular material seen in normal SR. In some aggregates the tubules have a double lumen (Fig. 31-25A) or a clear space intervenes between the tubular membrane and the granular material in the lumen (Fig. 31-25C). Some aggregates also contain glycogen or lipofuscin granules (Fig. 31-26) or are composed of a mixture of SR tubules and dilated SR vesicles (Figs. 31-25C and D, 31-26A). The tubules and vesicles in the aggregates react for an SR-associated Mg-dependent ATPase (Fig. 31-25D).

Novel tubular aggregates composed of 30- to 200-nm-wide tubules containing 1 to 21 tubulofilamentous structures 14 to 18 nm in size were observed in a dominantly inherited adult-onset myopathy associated with type 1 fiber predominance. Other abnormalities of the SR, consisting of proliferating junctional cisternae as well as the above-described tubular aggregates, were also present.[36a]

Mineralization. Concentric rings of dense to highly dense material appear in dilated SR vesicles in periodic paralysis. These vesicles usually occur in clusters in developing or mature vacuoles.[22] Transitions from dilated vesicles

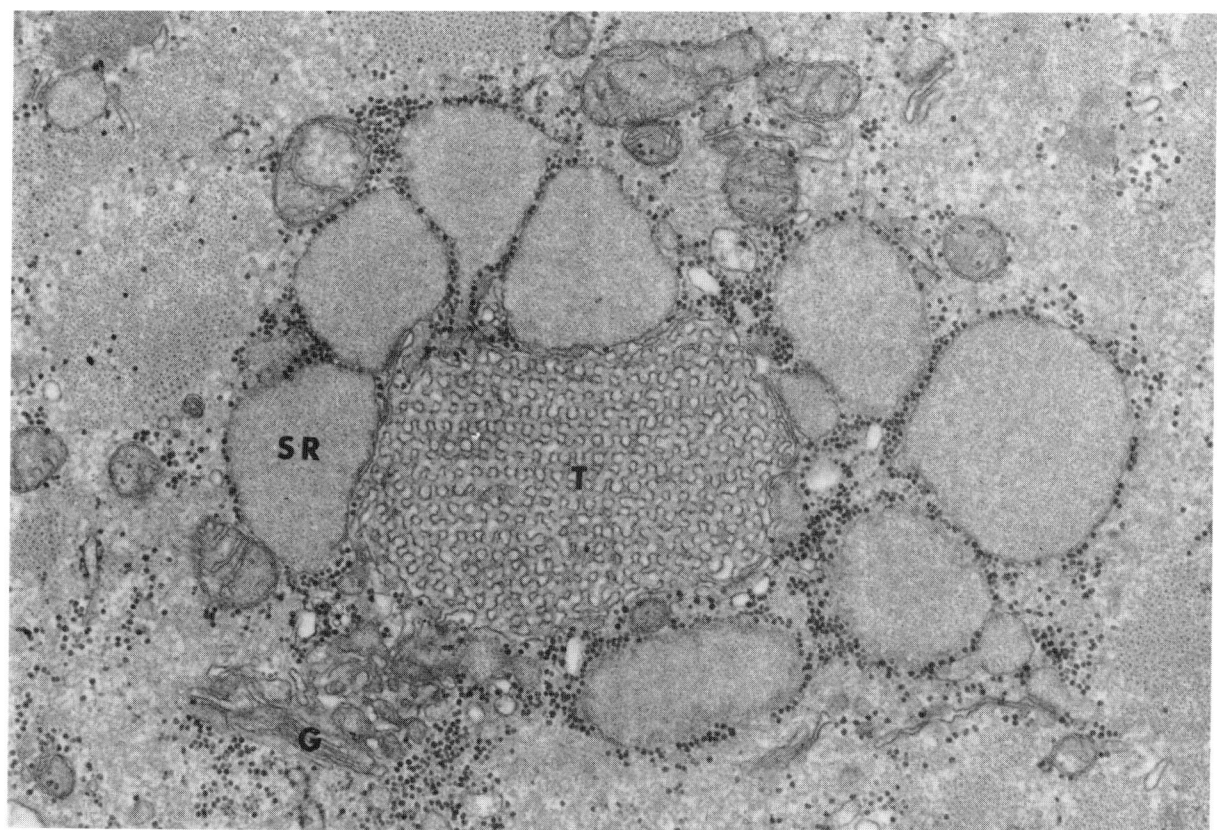

FIGURE 31-20. Large T-system network (T) is surrounded by several dilated SR vesicles (SR) and prominent Golgi apparatus (G). Glycogen granules appear between dilated SR vesicles. Polymyositis, ×30,800.

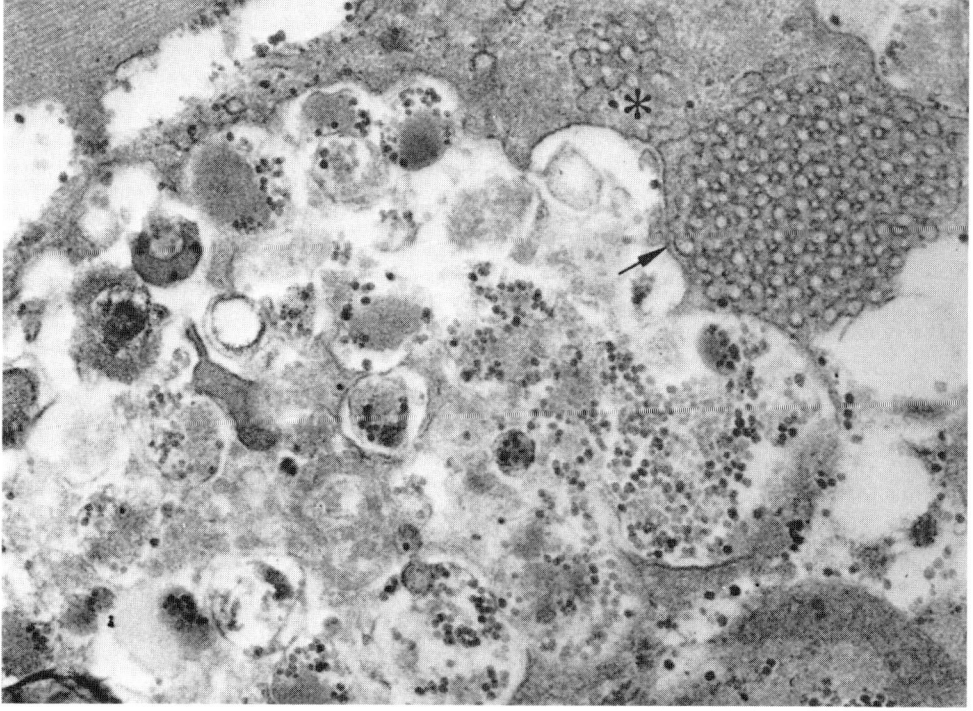

FIGURE 31-21. T-system network merges with the border of an autophagic vacuole. Tubule apposed to border (arrow) results in double limiting membrane. To left of T-system network, tubules and vesicles derived from network (asterisk) are also fusing with vacuole. ×46,000. *(Reproduced by permission from Engel AG, Brain 93:599, 1970.)*

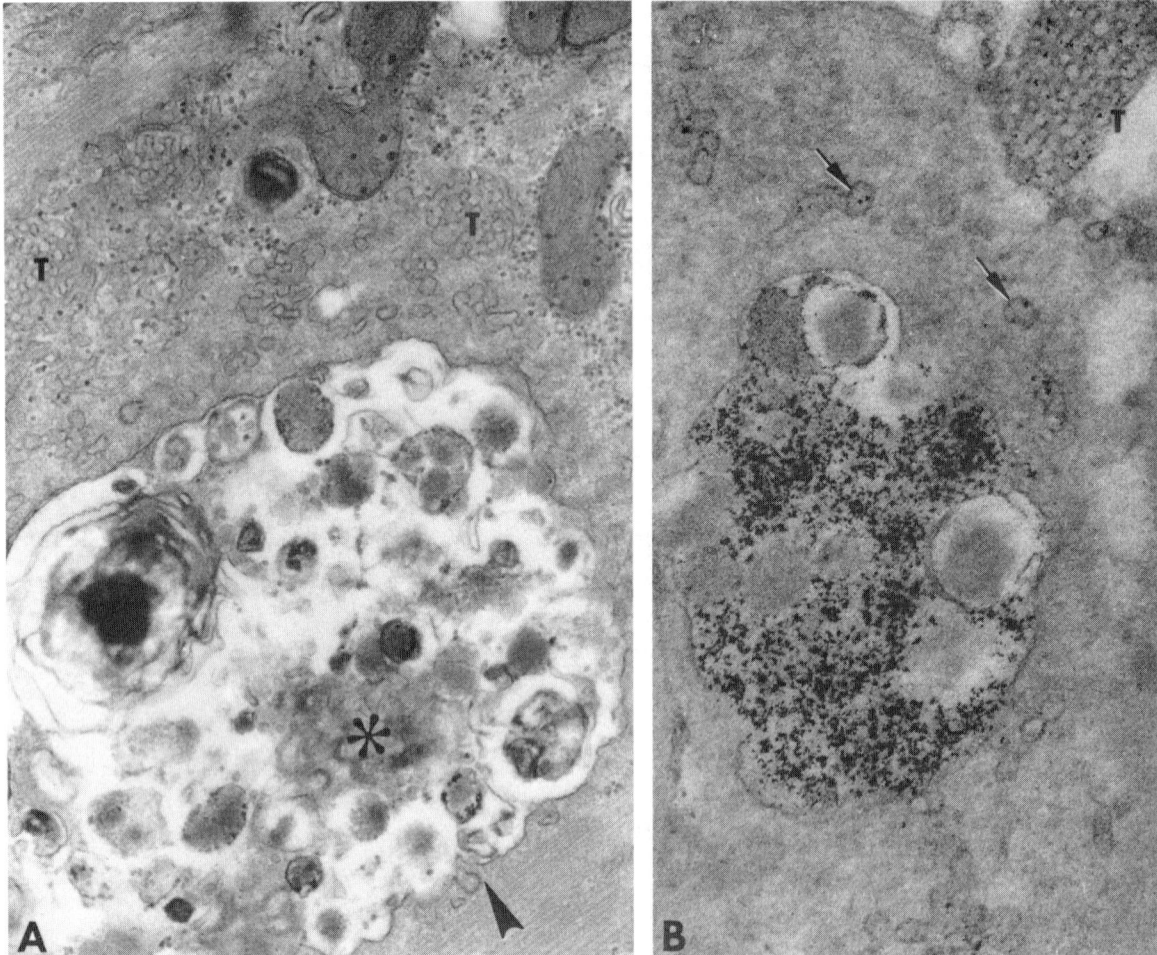

FIGURE 31-22. Autophagic vacuoles surrounded by T-system networks (T) and multiple small vesicles. Some of the vesicles appear to arise by budding from the T-system networks, and others are merging with the vacuolar borders. In *A*, note curvilinear arrangement of degraded material in center of vacuole (asterisk). A single coated vesicle is fusing with the vacuole (arrowhead). *B* has been reacted for acid phosphatase. The reaction product appears within the T network, in vesicles between the T network and the vacuole (arrows), in vesicles coalescing with the vacuole, and in the lumen of the vacuole. *A.* Experimental chloroquine myopathy, ×28,200. *B.* Acid maltase deficiency, ×52,500. *[A is reproduced by permission from Macdonald RD, Engel AG, J Neuropathol Exp Neurol 29:479, 1970; B is reproduced by permission from Engel AG, in Pearson CM (ed): The Striated Muscle. Baltimore: Williams & Wilkins; 1973, pp 301–341.]*

containing amorphous material to others with multiple concentric rings can be seen (Fig. 31-27). The latter resemble the rings of Liesegang that develop when an inorganic salt precipitates in a supersaturated colloidal gel. The deposits probably contain calcium salts, because the SR serves as a calcium sink in muscle and because abnormal calcific deposits that correspond in size and location to those observed in the electron microscope can be demonstrated cytochemically in cryostat sections (Color Plate 13G to I).[22]

Storage of homogeneous electron-dense material in the SR. This is an uncommon ultrastructural reaction. We have encountered it in numerous muscle fibers in a vacuolar myopathy of undetermined etiology (Fig. 31-28D), in some cases of myofibrillar myopathy, in a few muscle fibers in a granulomatous myopathy (Fig. 31-28A, C, and G), in experimental hypokalemic myopathy in rats (Fig. 31-28B, E, and F), in periodic paralysis (Fig. 31-29), and in a patient with chronic progressive and relapsing neuromyopathy.[36b]

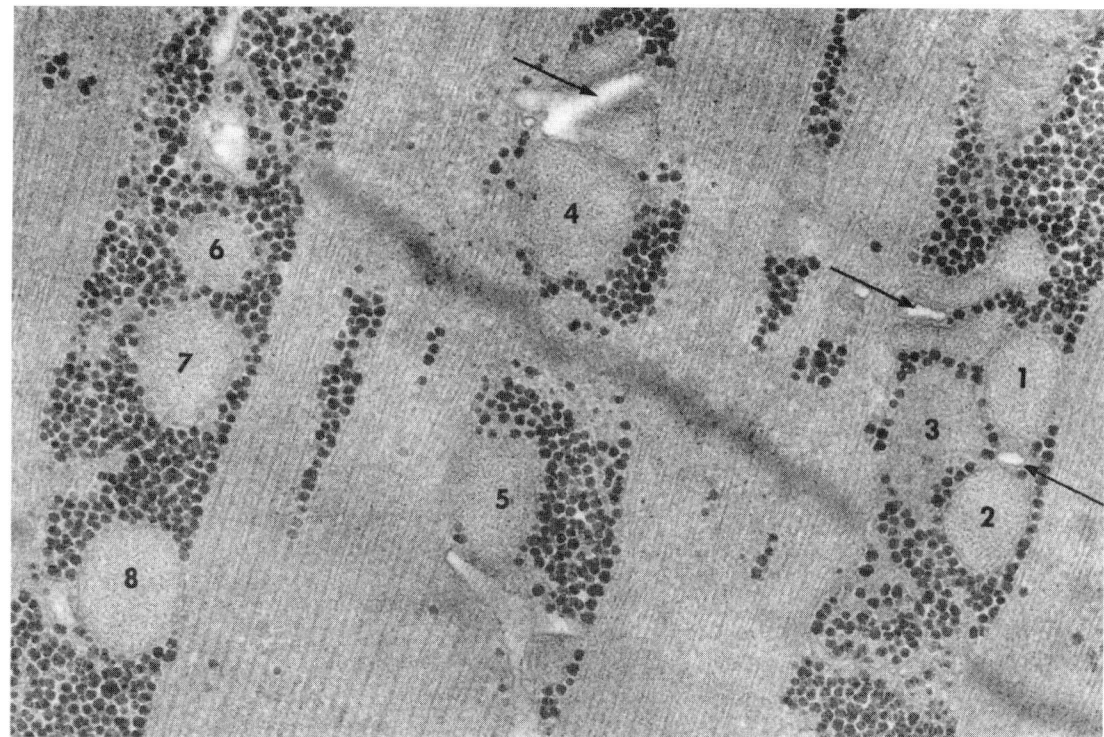

FIGURE 31-23. Eight dilated SR vesicles (numbers) are shown. Glycogen granules surround vesicles. Arrows indicate T tubules in triadic relation with SR vesicles. Primary hypokalemic periodic paralysis, ×45,000. (*Reproduced by permission from Engel AG, Mayo Clin Proc 45:774, 1970.*)

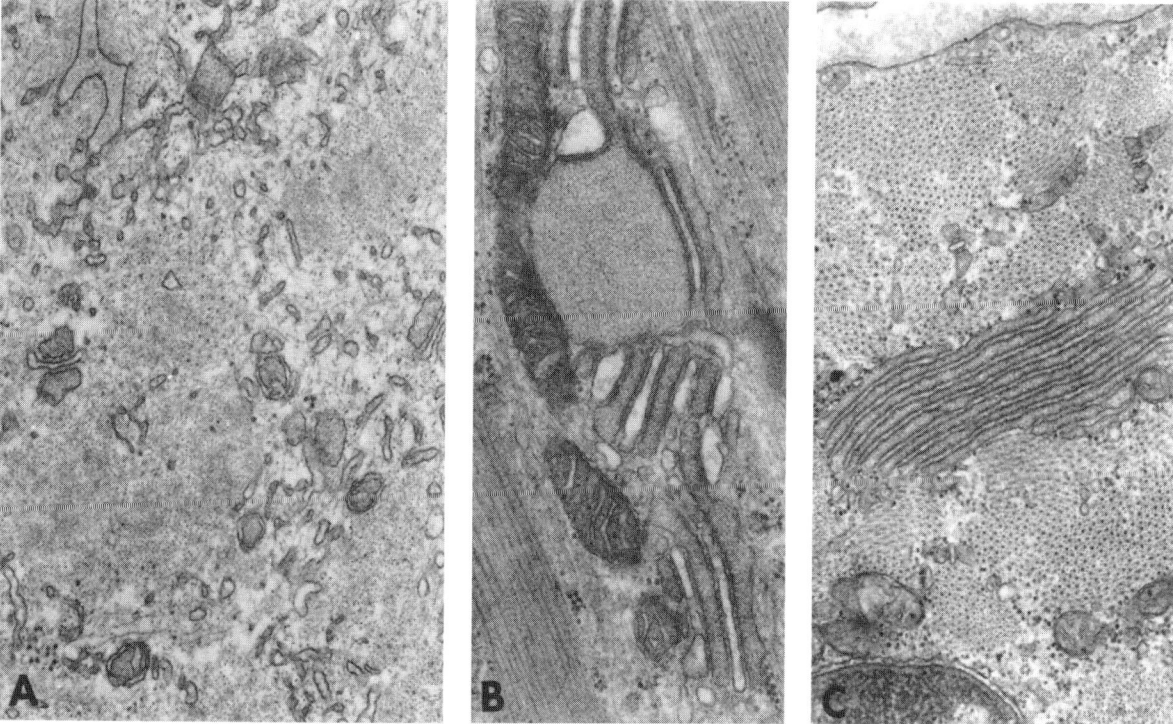

FIGURE 31-24. *A.* Numerous SR profiles, some in triadic relation to T tubules, surround atrophic myofibrils. *B.* Alternating T and SR profiles appear between myofibrils; some SR profiles are dilated. *C.* Parallel tubules with undulating borders and finely granular content suggest proliferation of the junctional SR. *A.* Peripheral neuropathy, ×46,700. *B.* Granulomatous myopathy, ×35,100; *C.* Seventy-day-denervated rat gastrocnemius, ×29,600. (*B is reproduced by permission from Engel AG, Macdonald RD, Excerpta Medica ICS 199:71, 1970; C is reproduced by permission from Engel AG, Stonnington HH, Ann NY Acad Sci 228:68, 1974.*)

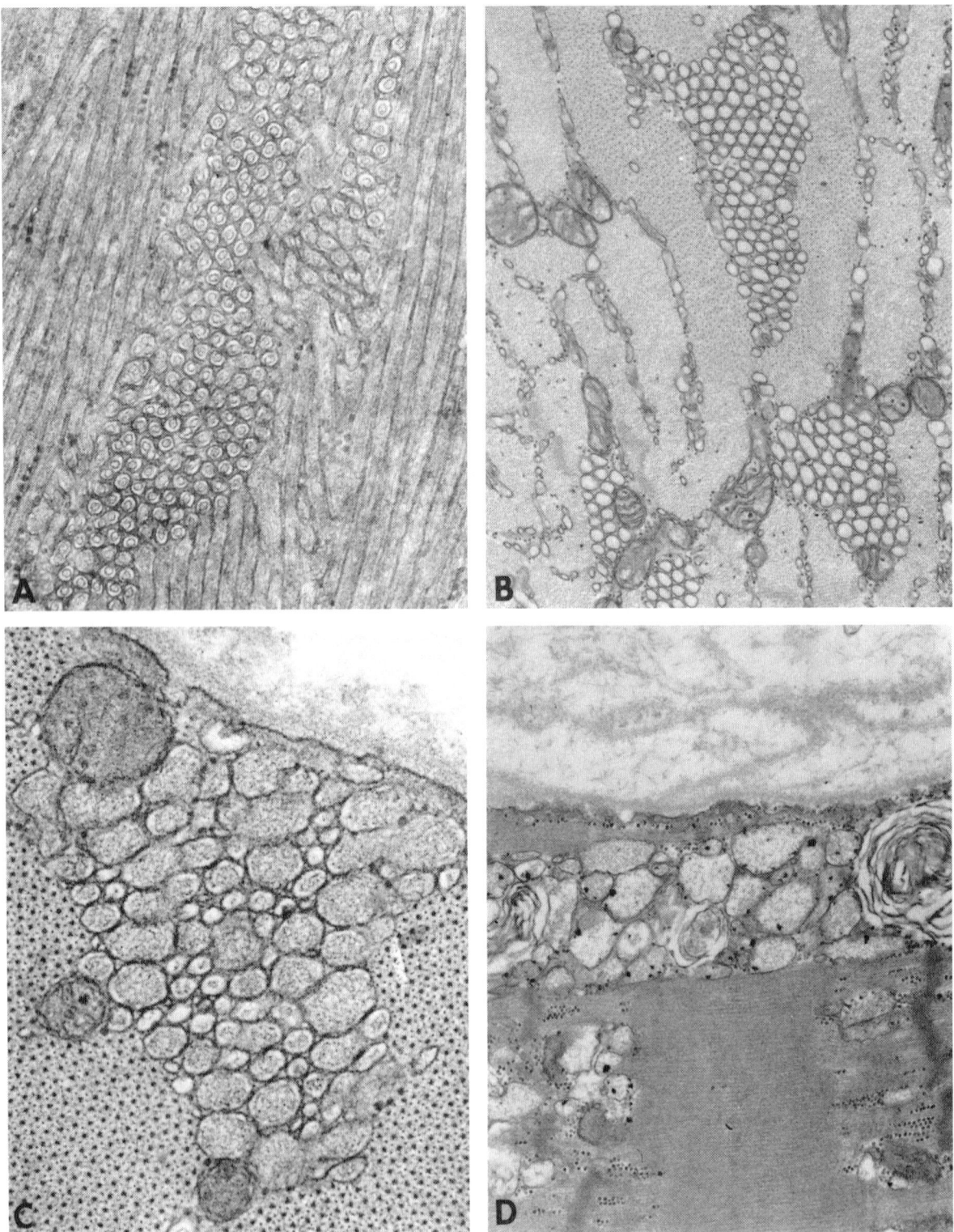

FIGURE 31-25. Aggregates of tubular SR in polymyositis *(A)*, in the C57B/10 mouse *(B)*, and in primary hyperkalemic periodic paralysis *(C* and *D)*. *D* demonstrates reactivity of SR profiles for a Mg-dependent SR-specific ATPase. *A*, ×44,600; *B*, ×25,900; *C*, ×64,400; *D*, ×28,400.

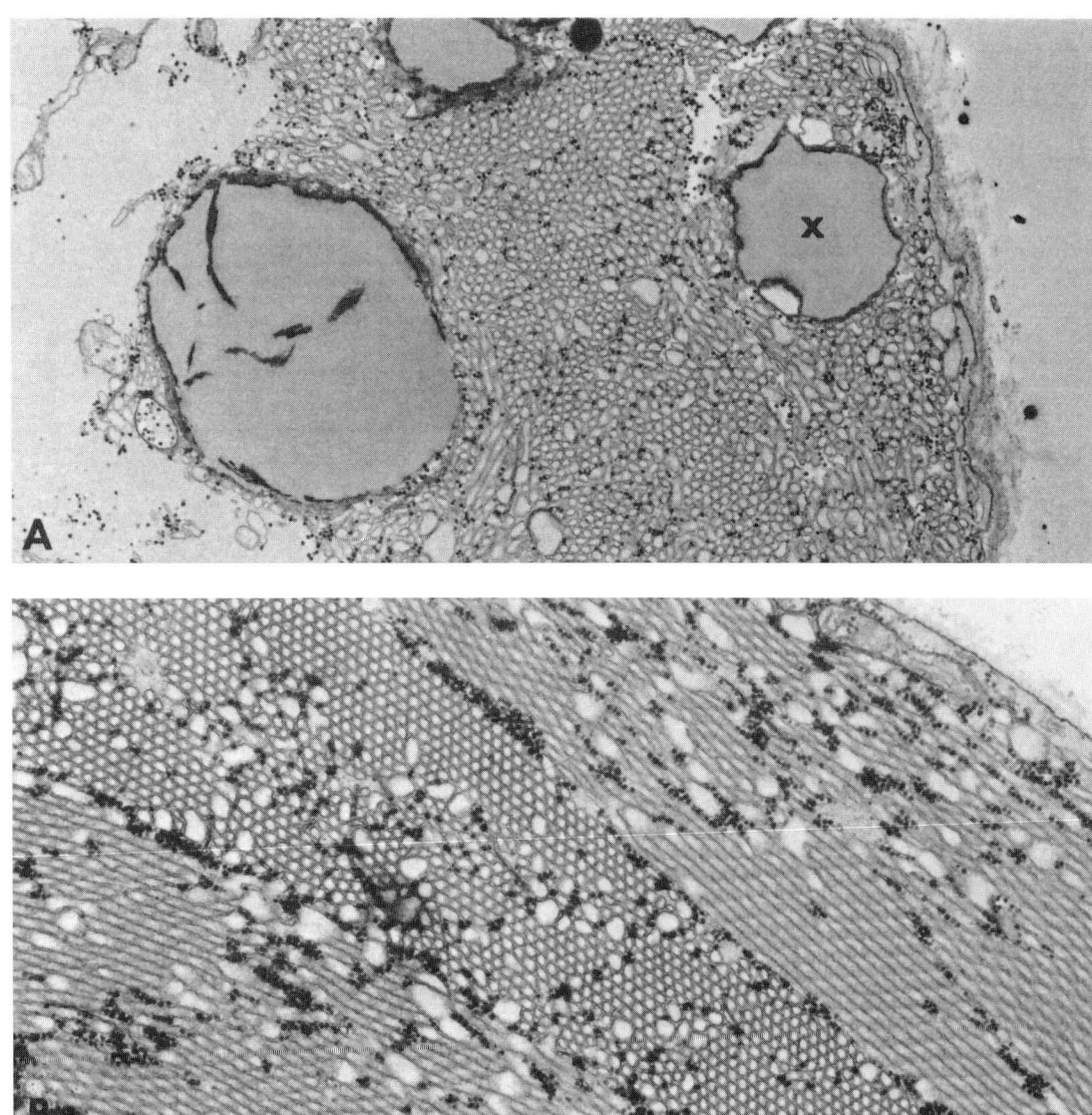

FIGURE 31-26. Aggregates of tubular SR in a myopathy associated with muscle cramps and aching *(A)* and in the slow-channel myasthenic syndrome *(B)*. Lipofuscin (x) and glycogen granules are intermingled with the tubules. *A*, ×20,700, *B*, ×24,000.

Dilated vesicles containing floccular material (Figs. 31-28*A*, 31-29*B*) and autophagic vacuoles are also present in some fibers in which the dense material is accumulating. In periodic paralysis the vesicles containing the dense material appear in fiber regions in which there is also extensive proliferation, dilation, and degeneration of T and SR components (Fig. 31-29).

The abnormal material is optically dense in the phase microscope (Fig. 31-28*G*). In frozen sections it fails to stain for lipid, glycogen, or acid mucins and is nonmetachromatic. In the electron microscope the abnormal material is always limited by a single membrane. It accumulates in circular spaces (Fig. 31-28*A*), in elongated and irregularly lobulated cisternae that extend along the long axis of the fiber (Fig. 31-28*B* and

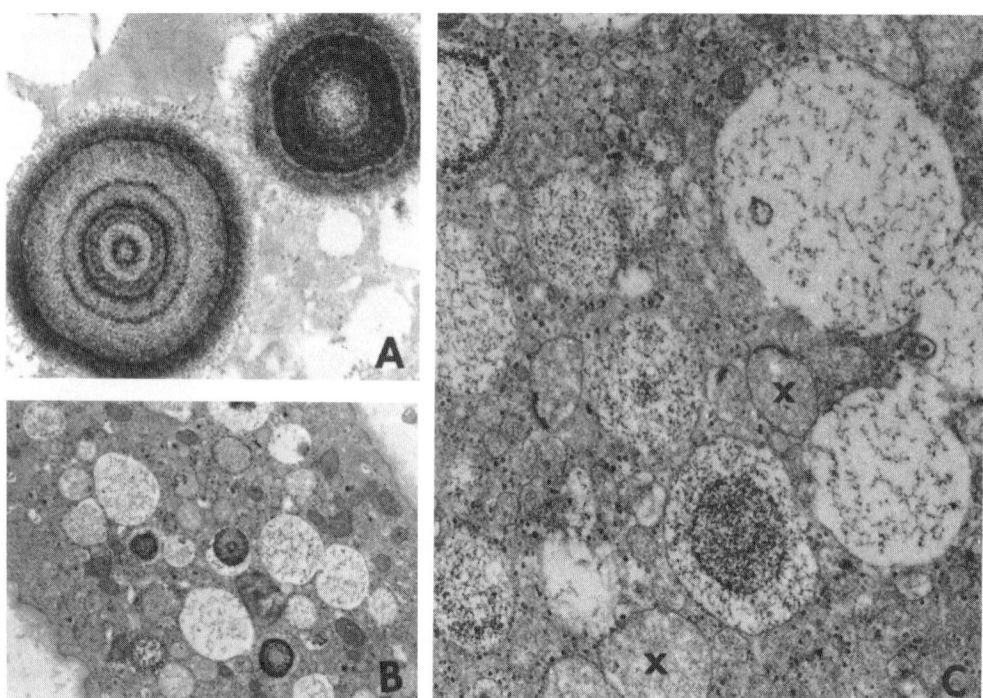

FIGURE 31-27. Dilated and mineralized SR vesicles in primary hypokalemic periodic paralysis. Some vesicles display numerous Liesegang rings. Other vesicles (x) retain amorphous content of normal SR. A few mitochondria and glycogen granules appear between the vesicles in C. A, ×16,700; B, ×8000; C, ×27,600. (*Reproduced by permission from Engel AG, Mayo Clin Proc 45:774, 1970.*)

C), and in tubules that communicate with the larger cisternae (Fig. 31-28C and D). The smallest deposits occur in the SR components of triads, and some of the smallest vesicles containing the abnormal material display the undulating border of the junctional SR (Fig. 31-28E and F).

Degeneration. Degeneration of the SR together with other membranous organelles is common in myopathies in which autophagic mechanisms become excited and is conspicuous in the toxic myopathy induced by lovastatin[36c]; however, it can occur in any other myopathy. Dilation, loss of granular material from the lumen, increased osmiophilia of the limiting membrane, appearance of frayed membranes or myeloid formations in the lumen, and replacement of the entire organelle by a myeloid structure are progressive steps in the degeneration of the SR (Figs. 31-29, 31-30).

Proliferation, dilation, and degeneration of the SR are the predominant pathologic alterations in congenital sarcotubular myopathy (Fig. 31-30).[24]

Membrane glycogen complexes. These have been observed in young mouse or newborn rat muscle, denervated rat muscle, normal rabbit extraocular muscle (Fig. 31-31B),[33,37] and tissues other than muscle.[37] In muscle, the tubules in the complex could be of SR origin, but this has not been definitely established. In random sections of rabbit extraocular muscle, about 5 percent of the complexes abut on the Golgi apparatus.[37]

ALTERATIONS OF THE ENDOPLASMIC RETICULUM

Increases in smooth and rough endoplasmic reticulum profiles appear in regenerating fibers and fiber regions and are considered later in this chapter, under "Muscle Fiber Regeneration."

The formation of concentric cisternae of the rough endoplasmic reticulum is an infrequent reaction in regenerating fiber regions. The sarcoplasmic matrix between the cisternae contains many clusters of ribosomes. The ribosomal particles are readily distinguished from larger and more electron-dense glycogen granules (Fig. 31-31A).

The microtubular inclusions that accumulate in the smooth endoplasmic reticulum are considered under "Miscellaneous Inclusions," below.

ALTERATIONS OF THE GOLGI APPARATUS

In normal mature muscle fibers the Golgi system occurs in the hof region of subsarcolemmal nuclei and in the junctional sarcoplasm near motor end plates.

Prominent Golgi networks appear in regenerating fibers and fiber regions, as mentioned earlier (Figs. 31-11, 31-20, 31-89A and B, 31-121).

In acid maltase deficiency, Golgi cisternae contribute membranes to lysosomal sacs containing only glycogen

Chapter 31. Ultrastructural Changes in Diseased Muscle

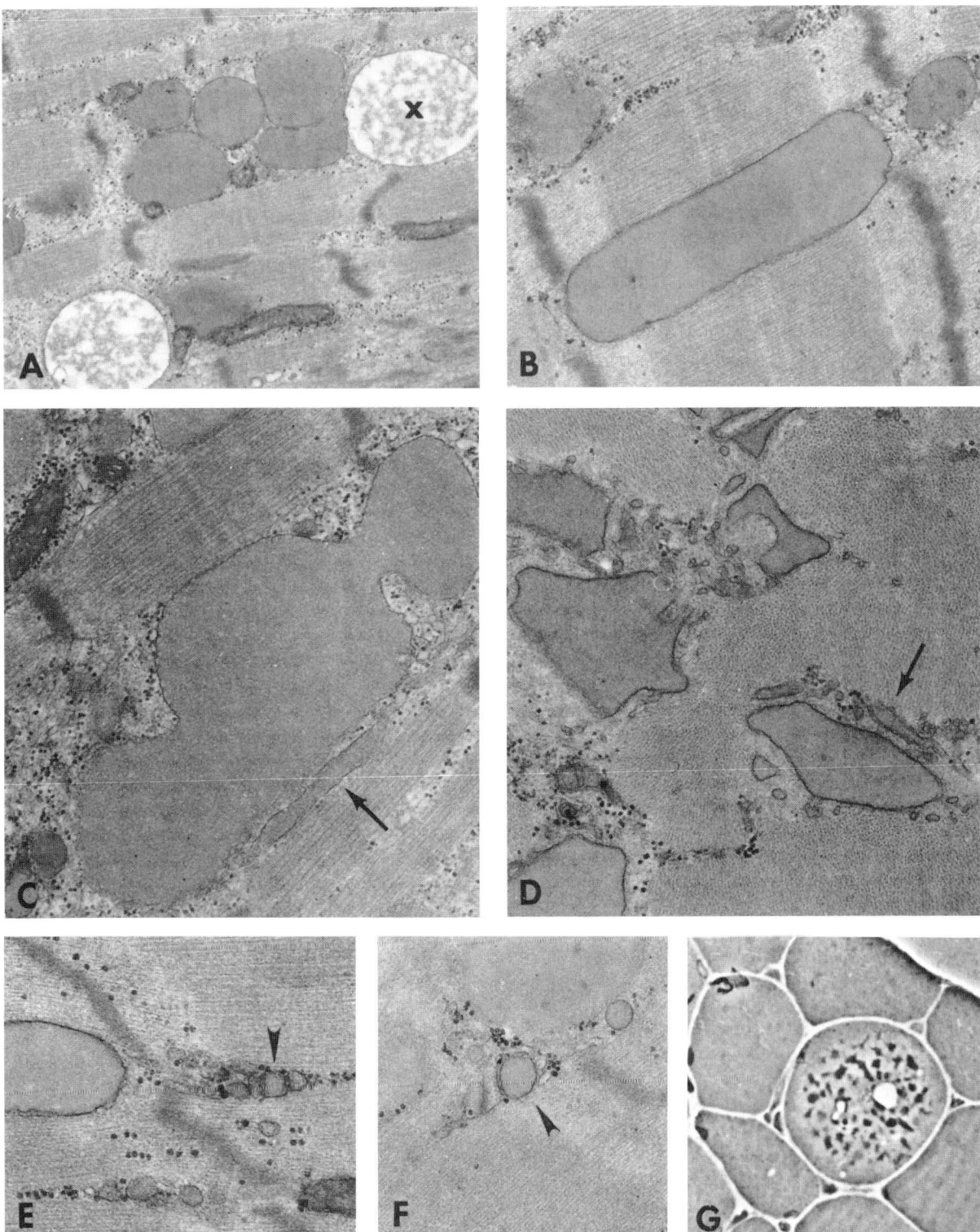

FIGURE 31-28. Accumulation of homogeneous material in dilated SR cisternae in granulomatous myopathy (A, C, and G), in experimental hypokalemic myopathy (B, E, and F), and in a vacuolar myopathy of undetermined etiology (D). Tubular profiles (arrows) containing similar material communicate with the larger cisternae and with normal SR components. In E and F, dilated vesicles with undulating borders and in triadic relation to T tubules (arrowheads) contain similar material. Dilated vesicles with floccular contents (X) also occur in some of the abnormal fiber regions. In semithin resin section (G) the abnormal material is phase optically dense. A, ×20,400; B, ×30,200; C and D, ×32,600; E, ×43,000; F, ×33,400; G, ×380.

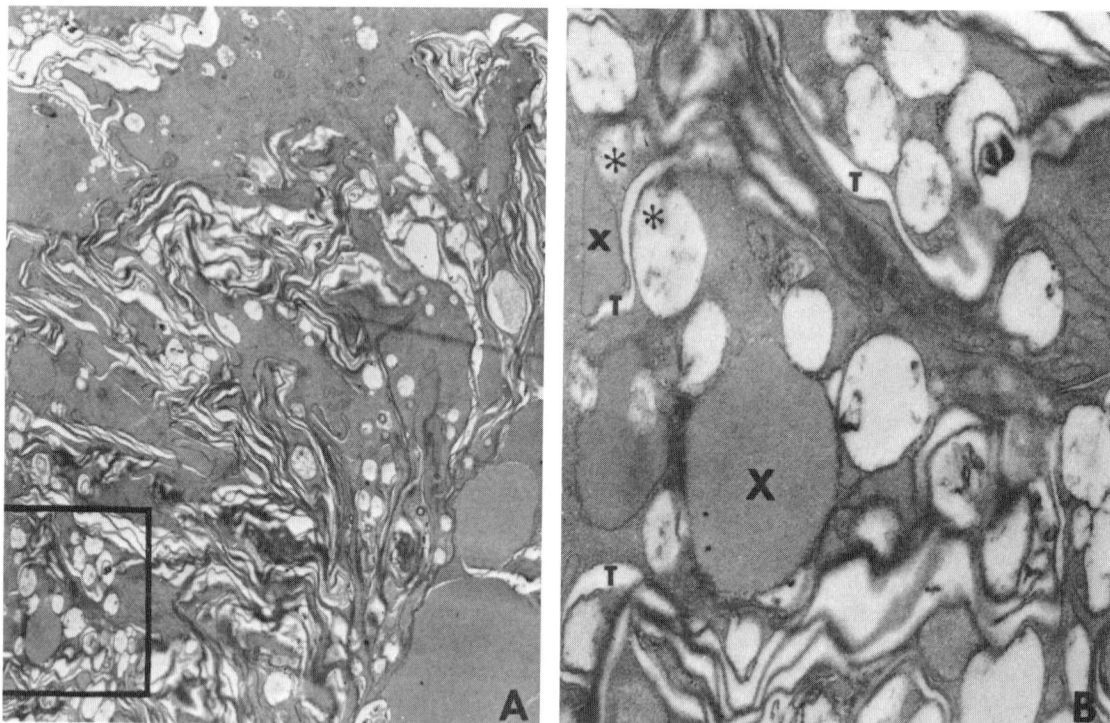

FIGURE 31-29. Abnormal fiber region in primary hypokalemic periodic paralysis. A. Bizarre T tubules (T), irregularly curving osmiophilic lamellae, and dilated vesicles are present. B. Higher magnification of bracketed region in A shows transitions from tubular membranes (T) to irregularly curving lamellae. Two vesicles (asterisks) are in triadic relation to tubules. Large membrane-bound structure (X) contains amorphous material of intermediate density and resembles the abnormal SR cisternae shown in Fig. 31-28. Smaller space of the same type (x) abuts on a T tubule. A, ×5000; B, 22,900. (Reproduced by permission from Engel AG, Mayo Clin Proc 45:774, 1970.)

(Fig. 31-101B) and often appear near such sacs (Fig. 31-102A).[26,27] In other myopathies in which autophagic mechanisms are prominent, Golgi elements appear in fiber regions near the autophagic vacuoles (Fig. 31-92A), presumably to provide packages of lysosomal enzymes for the secondary lysosomes.[31]

ALTERATIONS OF MITOCHONDRIA

In normal human muscle, the average mitochondrial fraction of the muscle fiber volume ranges from 3 to 5 percent.[38] The abundance of mitochondria varies with histochemical fiber type, but human muscle fiber types are difficult to identify in the electron microscope either by simple inspection or by morphometric criteria. Most mitochondrial profiles are adjacent to the I band; those adjacent to the A band are small and sparse (Figs. 31-1 and 31-2). Subsarcolemmal mitochondrial aggregates are less common in normal human muscle than in mouse or rat muscle, but do occur (Fig. 31-35A).

Alterations in the distribution of mitochondria in muscle fibers are best assessed by light microscopic histochemical studies of the organelle's oxidative enzyme activities, as described in Chap. 30. However, decreases or increases in enzyme activity cannot be interpreted as indicating change in the size, number, or structural integrity of the mitochondria. Longitudinal sections of fibers fixed at rest length by fixatives known to preserve mitochondrial enzyme activity (paraformaldehyde or hydroxyadipaldehyde) are essential for demonstration of small areas of decreased activity.[39,40] Except for selected cytochemical observations, such as loss of cytochrome oxidase activity or immunocytochemical evidence for loss of DNA,[40a,b] light and electron microscopic studies provide little insight into altered biochemical properties of mitochondria.

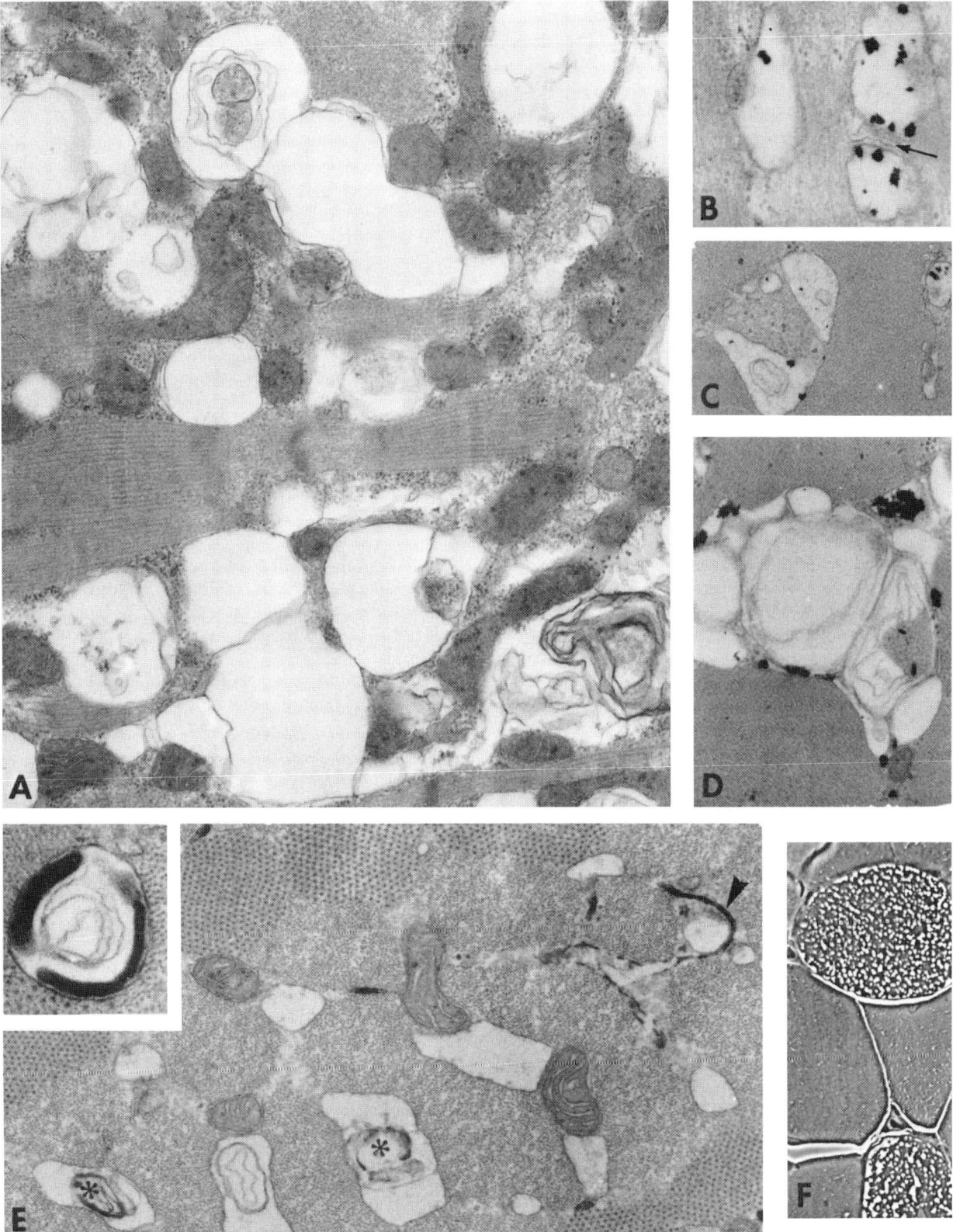

FIGURE 31-30. Sarcotubular myopathy. In *A*, numerous dilated SR vesicles are present, and some of these are degenerating. *B, C,* and *D* show reactivity of the dilated vesicles for a Mg-dependent, SR-specific ATPase. Some of the dilated vesicles are in triadic relation to T tubules (arrow). In *E*, peroxidase-loaded T tubules partially encircle (arrowhead), abut on, or are invaginated into (asterisks) the dilated SR vesicles. Inset shows an invaginated T tubule at a higher magnification. F represents semithin resin section viewed in phase optics. Myriad small vacuoles appear in the affected fibers. *A,* ×24,600; *B,* 51,000; *C* and *D,* ×30,500; *E,* ×35,300; inset to *E,* ×62,500; *F,* ×520. (*Reproduced by permission from Jerusalem F, Engel AG, Gomez MR, Neurology 23:897, 1973.*)

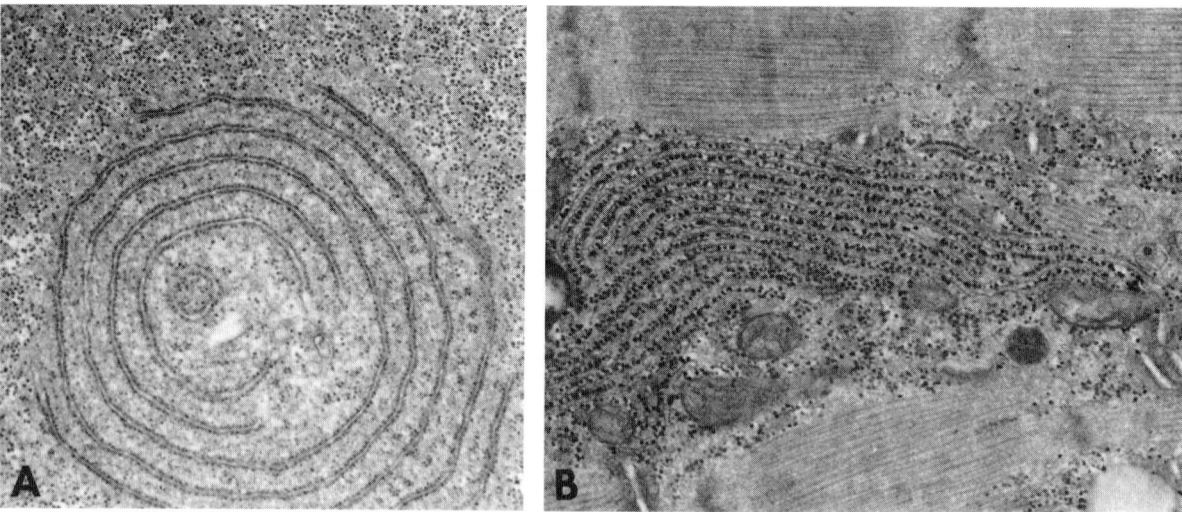

FIGURE 31-31. *A.* Concentrically arrayed rough endoplasmic reticulum profiles in regenerating fiber. *B.* Glycogen membrane complex in 56-day-denervated rat gastrocnemius. *A,* ×20,000; *B,* ×26,800. *(B is reproduced by permission from Engel AG, Stonnington HH, Ann NY Acad Sci 228:68, 1974.)*

The reactions of mitochondria include *fixation artifacts* and *anoxic effects; disappearance; degeneration and inclusion in autophagic vacuoles; increase in size or number; formation of aggregates; abnormal cristae;* and *inclusions* consisting of abnormally large dense granules, circular, moderately dense deposits (possibly phospholipid), and crystalloids.

Fixation artifacts and anoxic effects. Mitochondria may swell and become vacuolated during immersion fixation with glutaraldehyde. These changes are most marked in the deeper regions of the specimen, which the fixative penetrates last. The addition of 1% sodium azide to the fixative, an inhibitor of mitochondrial respiration, reduces mitochondrial swelling during immersion fixation.[41] Marked mitochondrial swelling occurs if fixation is initiated after a period of anoxia or fatigue,[41a] or if cut muscle fibers are fixed,[41b] or if fixation is initiated postmortem (Fig. 31-32), and the mitochondria of the neuromuscular junction are selectively severely affected. Anoxia also induces the formation of plate-like inclusions within mitochondrial cristae (Fig. 31-32); the inclusions consist of a protein and can be dissolved with pepsin.[42]

Swelling and vacuolation of mitochondria also occur after prolonged and fatiguing stimulation of animal muscles.[42a]

Disappearance. Decreases in mitochondria are readily observed and represent the most consistent morphologic feature of core, multicore, and target formations (Figs. 31-72 to 31-77 and Color Plate 7C and D). Focal loss of mitochondria from fiber regions that vary widely in shape and size can occur in any myopathy (Figs. 31-46*A* to *C*, 31-88*B* and *C*, 31-91*A*, *B*, and *D*) and in denervation atrophy,[43] and can be experimentally induced in rats by emetine[40] or glucocorticoid[44] therapy.

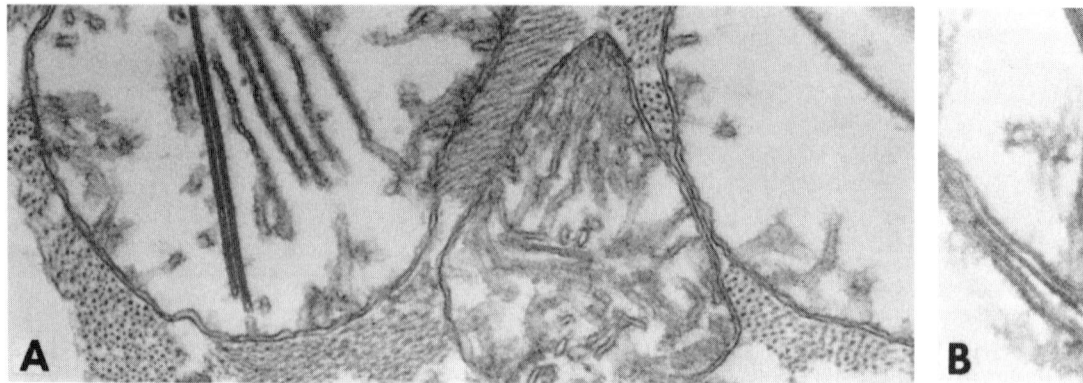

FIGURE 31-32. Anoxic mitochondria in autopsy specimen of human muscle with markedly swollen matrix and plate-like inclusions in their cristae *(A and B).* The intracristal inclusions consist of multiple closely spaced parallel lamellae *(B). A,* ×49,600; *B,* ×125,000.

An association exists between mitochondrial loss from a given fiber region and focal myofibrillar degeneration that begins at the Z disk in that region (Figs. 31-46A to C, 31-72 to 31-77, 31-88B and C, 31-91A, B, and D). The following generalizations can be made[12,43]:

1. Decrease in mitochondrial density can be observed without focal myofibrillar degeneration.
2. When myofibrillar degeneration occurs in the area of mitochondrial loss, the area of myofibrillar degeneration is small or of the same size as but as not larger than the area of mitochondrial decrease.
3. In experimental myopathies in the rat, mitochondrial loss commonly results in myofibrillar degeneration in type 1 fibers but seldom in type 2 fibers.[40,44]
4. Focal myofibrillar degeneration (which begins at the Z disk) can occur in myofibrillar myopathy. In other myopathies this occurs seldom without a concomitant or antecedent decrease in mitochondrial density (Fig. 31-46D).

Thus mitochondrial loss is an important but not unique cause of myofibrillar degeneration. The relationship between mitochondria and myofibrillar integrity is further discussed under "Alterations of the Z Disk," below.

The manner in which mitochondria disappear from muscle fibers is not always clear. When degenerating mitochondrial profiles are observed, as in some of the inflammatory and toxic myopathies (Figs. 31-33, 31-34), the decrease can be attributed to increased destruction of the organelle. In other instances, as in core or target formations, the mitochondrial "loss" could be due to increased destruction (for which there is no evidence), or to decreased biogenesis (i.e., the rate at which mitochondria subdivide to form new mitochondria), or to an abnormal regulation of the distribution of mitochondria in the muscle fiber.

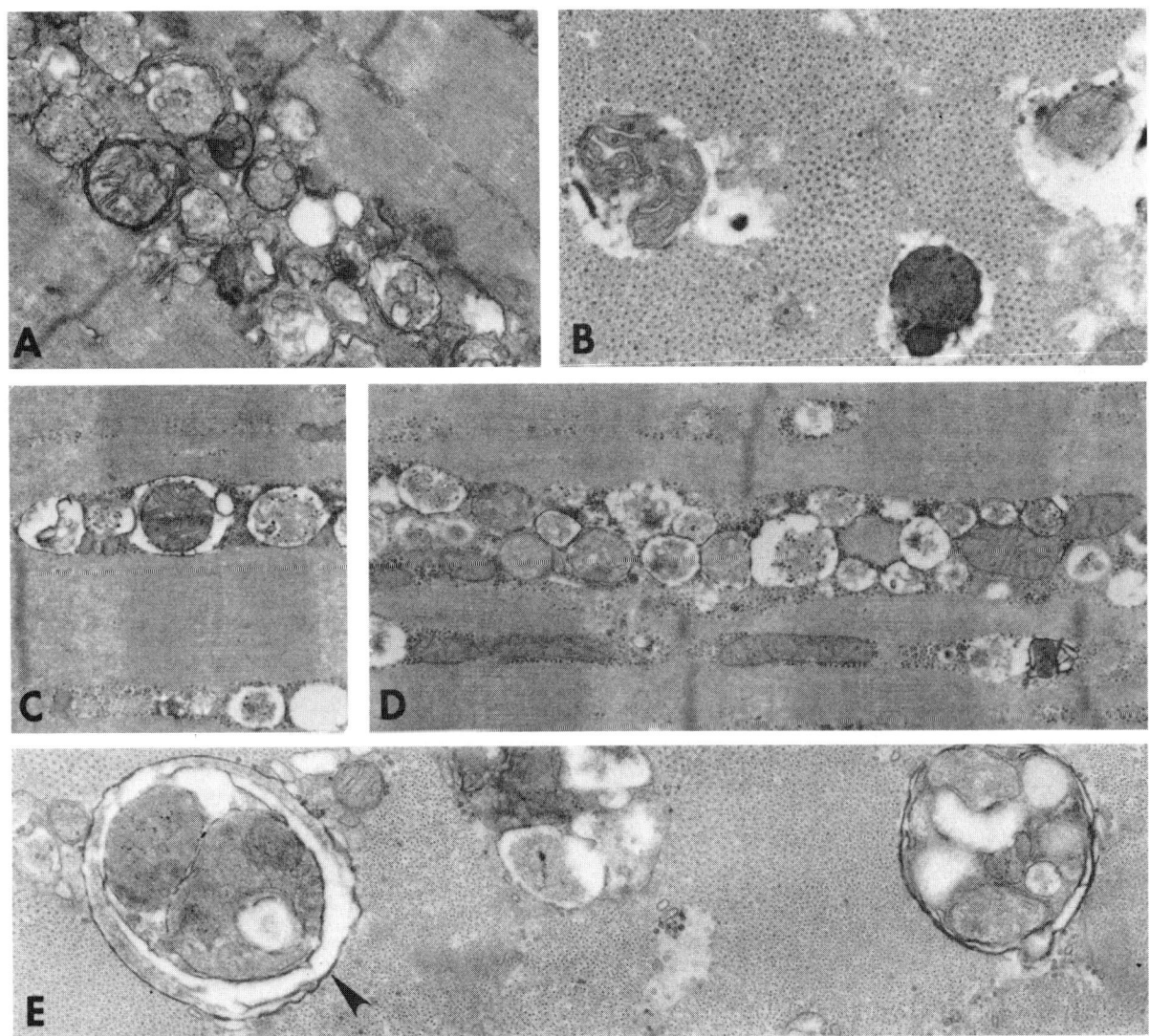

FIGURE 31-33. Degenerating mitochondria in experimental emetine myopathy (A), ocular–limb muscle dystrophy (B), and polymyositis (C, D, and E). Some of the degenerating organelles are enclosed in membrane-bound spaces, and the limiting membranes of some of these spaces are also degenerating (arrowhead in E). A, ×17,000; B, ×39,300; C, ×18,400; D, ×19,400; E, ×30,000.

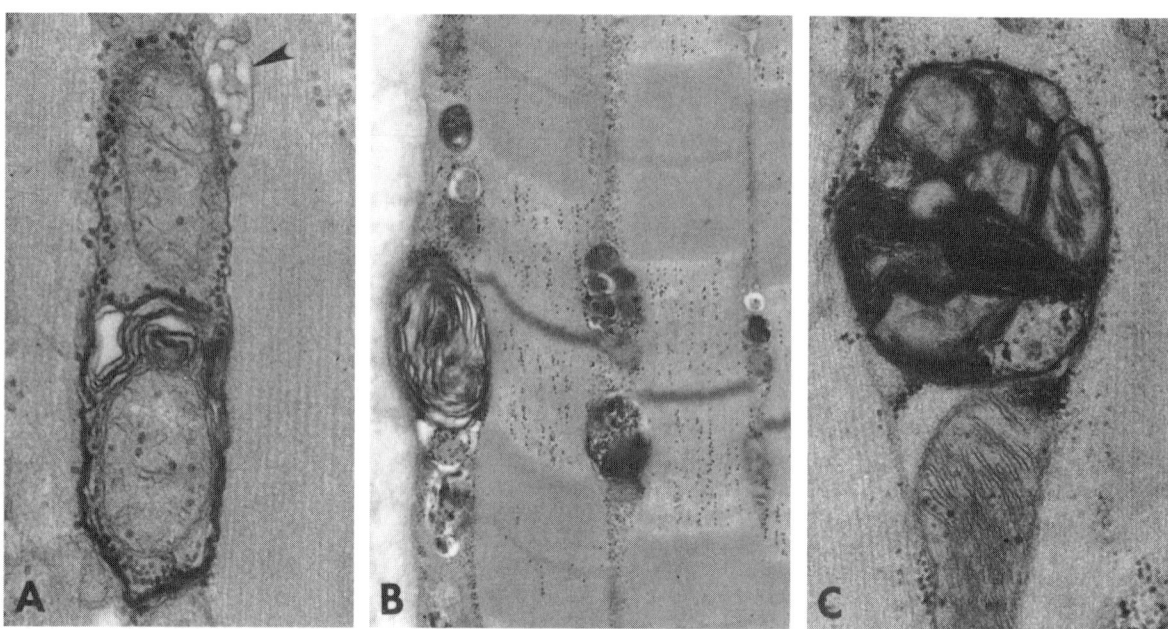

FIGURE 31-34. Degenerating mitochondria in ploymyositis (A), limb-girdle dystrophy (B), and experimental chloroquine myopathy (C). In A, a T-system network (arrowhead) abuts on membrane surrounding degenerating mitochondria. A, ×49,600; B ×20,000; C, ×40,600.

Degeneration and inclusion in autophagic vacuoles. Early signs of mitochondrial degeneration consist of increase in the density, thickness, and splitting of the inner or outer mitochondrial membranes (Figs. 31-33A, 31-34A and C) or distention of the intracristal space by amorphous material (Fig. 31-33B and C). More advanced changes consist of replacement of the cristae and matrix by amorphous or granular material of intermediate density (Fig. 31-33C, D, and E) or by homogeneous dense material (probably phospholipid) (Fig 31-33B), or conversion of the entire organelle to a myeloid structure (Fig. 31-34B). Degenerating mitochondria are often enclosed in small membrane-bound spaces (Figs. 31-33C and E, 31-34A), and T-system networks contribute to the membranes that limit these spaces (Fig. 31-34A). The limiting membranes may also degenerate (Figs. 31-33E, 31-34A), and smaller spaces coalesce, forming larger ones (Figs. 31-91 to 31-93). The membrane-bound spaces containing the degenerating mitochondria react for acid phosphatase and are therefore autophagic vacuoles, or secondary lysosomes.

Increase in size or number and aggregates. Individual transverse or longitudinal sections of a given fiber provide inadequate information on the size and number of mitochondria. For example, an increase in mitochondrial transections can result from elongation or increase in complexity of individual mitochondria; or an apparent increase in the size of the organelle in longitudinal sections, as in recently denervated muscle,[33] can be due to reorientation of the organelle in space. The combined study of longitudinal and transverse sections and morphometric analysis can help in assessing the size, orientation, and density of mitochondria.[33,38]

Large mitochondria and an increase in mitochondrial density occur in human (Fig. 31-35C) and experimental thyrotoxic myopathy[45,46] and in many mitochondrial myopathies (Figs. 31-36 to 31-38).

Mitochondrial aggregates occur in mitochondrial myopathies (Figs. 31-36A, 31-37A, 31-38A and B, and Color Plate 7E and F), in human and experimental corticosteroid-induced myopathy,[44,47] in myxedema myopathy (Figs. 31-35A, 31-98B and C), and in other myopathies. The mitochondria are usually associated with glycogen granules in the aggregates. Small mitochondrial aggregates abut at intervals on the bundles of aberrant myofibrils in lobulated fibers (Fig. 31-51A) and on the annular myofibrils in ring fibers (Fig. 31-50), but mitochondria are sparse or absent between the abnormally coursing myofibrils (Figs. 31-50, 31-51A). The lobulated distribution of oxidative enzyme activity in the lobulated fibers is due to these aggregates.

A paradoxical decrease in mitochondria and focal myofibrillar degeneration accompanies the proliferative changes in mitochondria in thyrotoxic and corticosteroid-induced myopathy.[44,45] In diverse other myopathies focal increases and decreases of mitochondria can be found in the same fibers (Fig. 31-90A and B). In light microscopic histochemical studies these fibers display a mottled distribution of oxidative enzyme activity.

Abnormal cristae. Mitochondria with sparse (Fig. 31-37D), concentrically arrayed (Fig. 31-37A, B, and C), or bizarre cristae and intracristal crystalloid inclusions (Fig. 31-38) can be found in various mitochondrial myopathies and occasionally in other myopathies.

Chapter 31. Ultrastructural Changes in Diseased Muscle

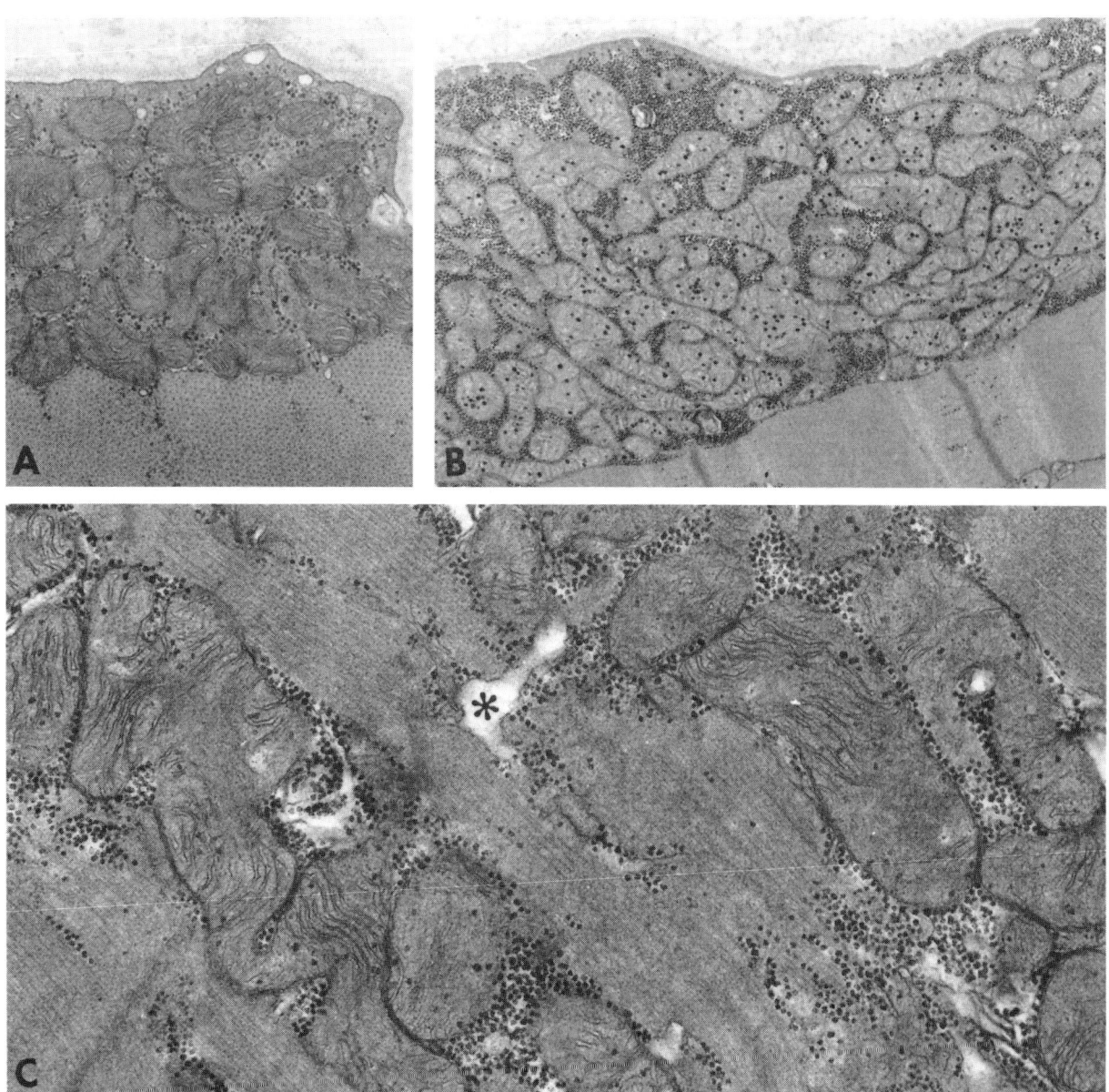

FIGURE 31-35. Mitochondrial aggregates in normal human muscle *(A)*, myxedema myopathy *(B)*, and thyrotoxic myopathy *(C)*. In *B* and *C*, the mitochondria contain an increased number of electrondense granules. Glycogen particles surround the mitochondria. Asterisk in *C* indicates dilated T tubule. In *B* and *C*, the mitochondrial profiles are abnormally large for longitudinally sectioned fibers. *A*, ×20,400; *B*, ×16,500; *C*, ×28,000. *(C is reproduced by permission from Engel AG, Mayo Clin Proc 47:919, 1972.)*

Inclusions. More than one type of inclusion can occur in one mitochondrion. Cytoplasmic material such as glycogen can become invaginated into abnormal, degenerating mitochondria. Plate-like intracristal inclusions appear after anoxia, as mentioned in the paragraph "Fixation Artifacts and Anoxic Effects," above.

Small, electron-dense granules that represent divalent cation-binding sites are present in normal mitochondria (Figs. 31-1, 31-2, 31-35*A*). These granules can increase in number and/or size in mitochondrial and other myopathies, such as acid maltase deficiency or myxedema myopathy (Figs. 31-35*B*, 31-38*D, E,* and *G*, 31-98*B* and *C*).

Less dense and circular inclusions of varying size (probably phospholipid) and crystalloid inclusions appear in a variety of mitochondrial and other myopathies (for reviews see Chap. 58 and Ref. 48).

The crystalloid inclusions typically appear in enlarged, oval, polygonal, or prism-shaped mitochondria that range

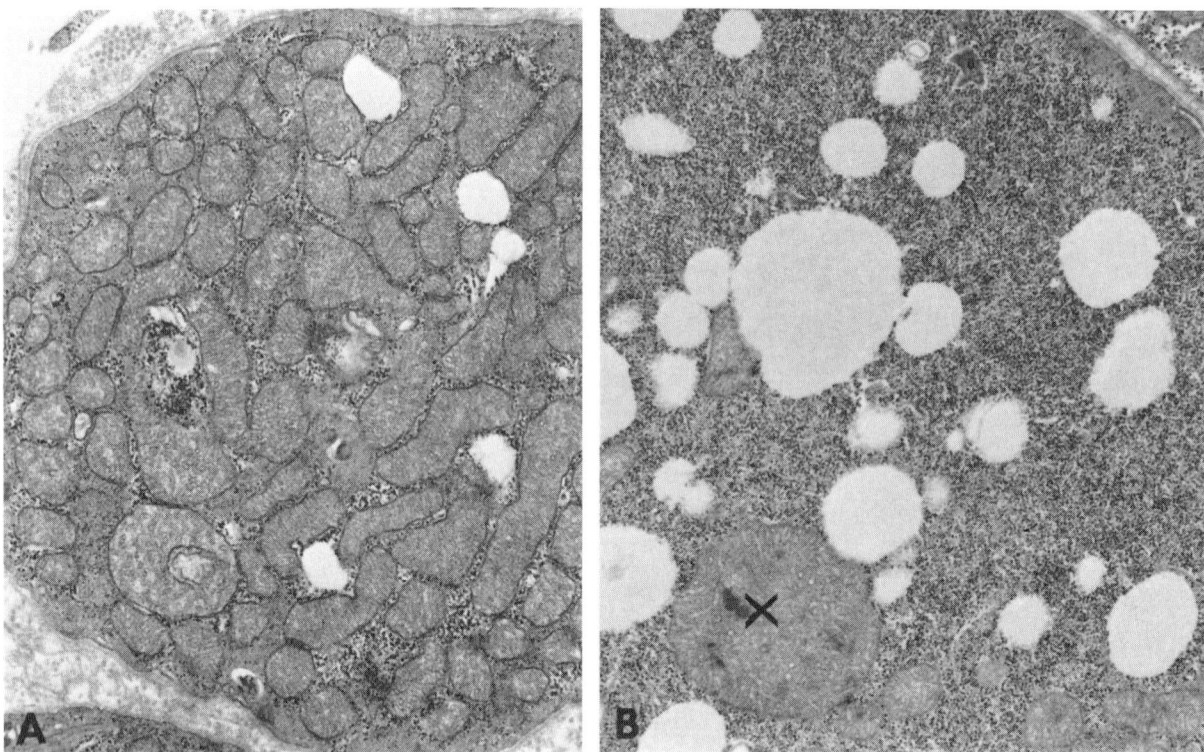

FIGURE 31-36. Transversely sectioned muscle fibers in infantile mitochondrial myopathy. Fiber in A is almost completely filled with mitochondria separated by glycogen granules and a few lipid droplets. Fiber in B contains large amounts of glycogen, lipid droplets of varying size, and one enlarged mitochondrion with prominent dense granules (X). A and B, ×14,000. *(Reproduced by permission from Jerusalem F, Angelini C, Engel AG, Groover RV, Arch Neurol 29:162, 1973.)*

up to 1.5 μm wide and up to 8 μm long (Fig. 31-38). The inclusions are rectangular, and from 1 to more than 40 inclusions can be found in a single mitochondrion. When multiple inclusions are present in one mitochondrion, they tend to form parallel stacks (Fig. 31-38). The inclusions are always in the outer mitochondrial space (i.e., either between the inner and outer mitochondrial membrane or in the intracristal space) (Fig. 31-38E, F, and G). The narrowest inclusions are about 50 nm wide and consist of a fourfold array of 4-nm-thick lines separated by a 6-nm interval from each other and by an 8-nm gap from the investing mitochondrial membranes (Fig. 31-38F). Wider inclusions contain two to more than four sets of fourfold lines (Fig. 31-38B, C, D, and E). In favorable sections the lines are connected by short transverse projections at 9-nm intervals (Fig. 31-38C and F). Examination of ultrathin sections at high tilt angles shows the lines to consist of closely spaced 8-nm particles, and the particles of adjacent lines form a hexagonal pattern. Strands connect the central particles of each hexagon to a similar particle in an adjacent hexagon or to the cristal membrane.[48a]

The crystalloid inclusions are a nonspecific indicator of disturbed mitochondrial energy metabolism. They can be induced by uncoupling agents[49] or temporary ischemia.[49a] Crystalloid inclusions in mitochondria resembling those found in human muscle fibers were observed in rat cardiomyocytes cultured in a creatine-deficient medium. These inclusions were enriched in mitochondrial creatine kinase by immunoelectron microscopy criteria. Creatine kinase is also the major constituent of the crystalloid inclusions in human mitochondrial myopathies.[49b]

ALTERATIONS OF THE Z DISK

The Z disk plays a key role in linking sarcomeres together and in maintaining the structural integrity of myofibrils. Therefore reactions of the Z disk are described here before other myofibrillar reactions are considered.

The normal Z disk ranges from less than 50 to more than 100 nm in width. It is wider in type 1 than type 2 fibers, but its width is not in itself sufficient for typing muscle fibers at the ultrastructural level. However, a significant correlation does exist between Z-disk width and mitochondrial density in human muscle fibers.[38]

In longitudinal sections, thin filaments approaching the Z disk are parallel to each other and spaced at 18 to 20 nm. At the lateral border of the disk, each thin filament gives rise to Z filaments that traverse the disk (Figs. 31-39, 31-40A and C). According to the Z-disk model originally proposed by Knappeis and Carlsen,[50] each thin filament on one side of

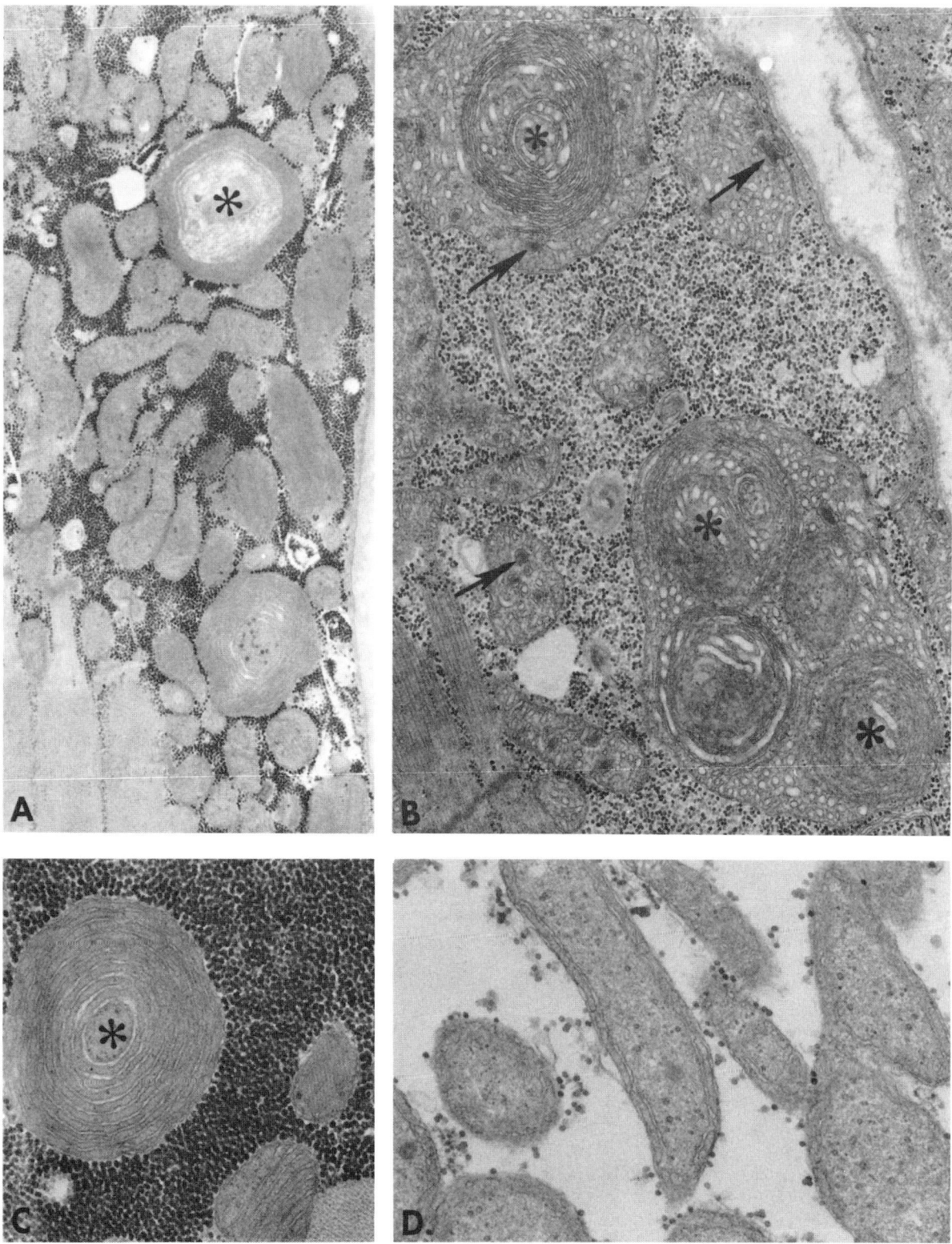

FIGURE 31-37. Abnormal mitochondria containing concentrically arrayed tubular cristae (asterisks in *A, B,* and *C*) or too few cristae and too many dense granules *(D)*. Mitochondria with crystalloid inclusions are also present in *A* and *C*. Arrows in *B* indicate small, dense intracristal deposits. The mitochondria are surrounded by glycogen particles. *A, C,* and *D* are from limb muscles of patients with Kearns-Sayre syndrome; *B* is from an infant with benign reversible cytochrome c oxidase deficiency. *A,* ×16,700; *B,* ×20,700; *C* and *D,* 39,300. *(B is reproduced by permission from Jerusalem F, Angelini C, Engel AG, Groover RV, Arch Neurol 29:162, 1973.)*

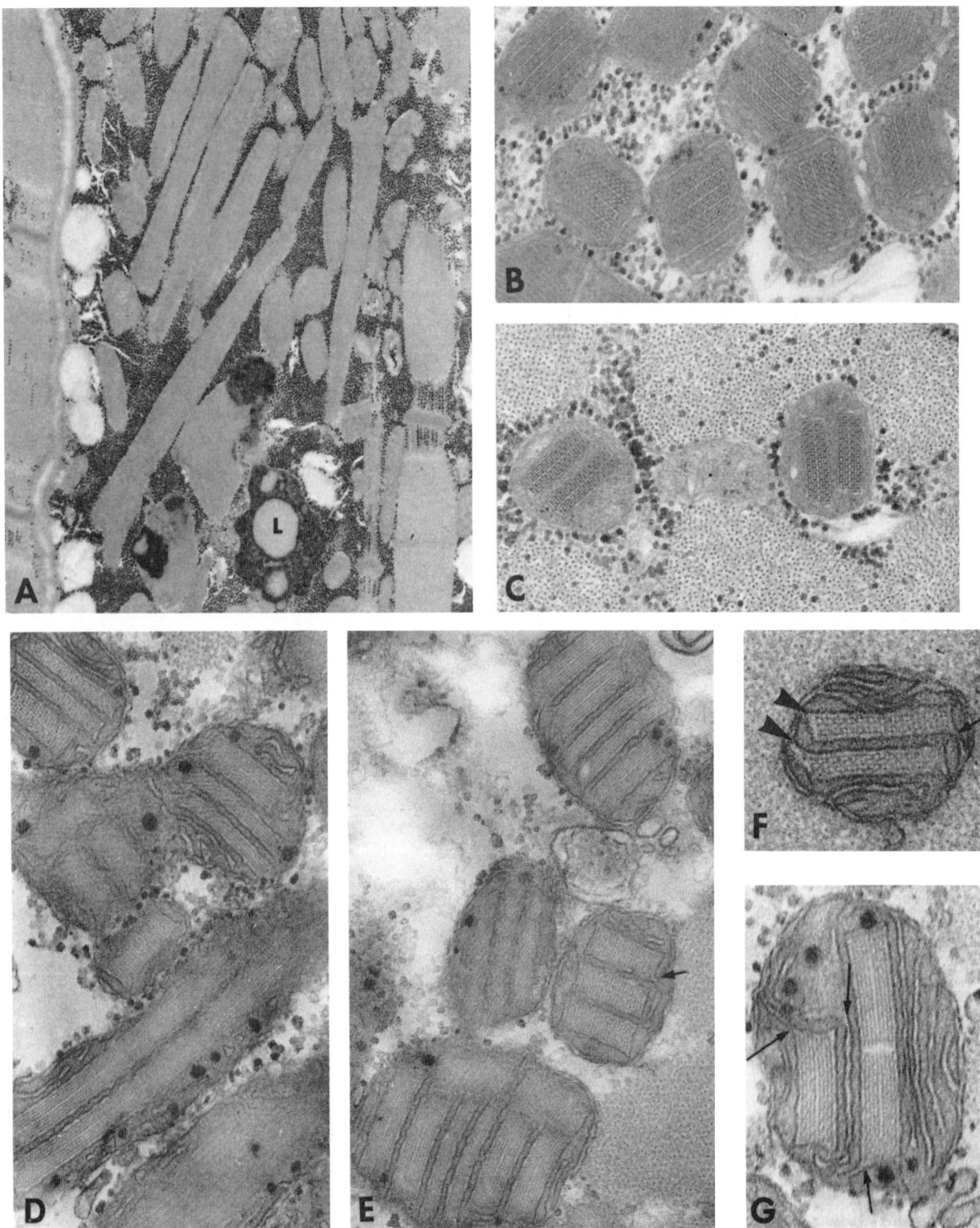

FIGURE 31-38. Mitochondria containing crystalloid inclusions in Kearns-Sayre syndrome (A, B, and C), and in a patient with late-onset acid maltase deficiency (D to G). Many mitochondria are also enlarged (A, D, E, and G), and the mitochondria are surrounded by glycogen particles. The crystalloid inclusions are covered by membrane, which is continuous with cristal membranes (arrows in E, F, and G) or with the inner mitochondrial membrane (arrowheads in F). Various geometric patterns are seen in inclusions. A, ×16,700; B, ×49,600; C, ×39,300; D, ×56,000; E, ×50,300; F, ×91,000; G, ×75,000. (D, E, F, and G are reproduced by permission from Engel AG, Dale AJD: Mayo Clin Proc 43:233, 1968.)

the disk connects with four thin filaments on the other side of the disk by means of four Z filaments. The Z filaments are surrounded by an amorphous and moderately dense material (Figs. 31-39, 31-41, 31-47A) that is better preserved after double fixation with glutaraldehyde and osmium than after osmium fixation alone.[51] An additional set of short linking filaments located 10 to 15 nm from the center of the Z disk occurs between actin filaments of the same polarity.[51a]

Digestion of the Z disks with a calcium-activated protease removes amorphous material and Z filaments from the disk and reveals interdigitating tips of thin filaments of opposite polarity within the disk.[52] This finding implies that Z-disk, width may be determined by the amount of overlap of thin filaments of opposite polarity within the disk. If this is correct, then it also follows that in wider Z disks, more than a single set (i.e., two or more sets) of four Z filaments arises at intervals from the terminal portion of each thin filament. The presence of periodic lines spaced at 14 to 20 nm in wider Z disks is consistent with this notion.

In a transverse section of the glutaraldehyde-and-osmium-fixed Z disk, the thin filaments adjacent to the disk form the corners of 18- to 20-nm squares; within the disk, Z filaments occupy the lateral borders and subdivide the interior of these squares, forming a small square net spaced at 9 nm; and the small squares are not rotated relative to the orientation of the larger squares (Figs. 31-41, 31-47A). After osmium fixation alone, the thin filaments form the corners of 22-nm squares and the Z filaments form a basket-weave lattice spaced at 15 nm that is rotated 45° relative to the larger squares. Nemaline rods, which represent a proliferative anomaly of the Z disk, show the same variation of lattice pattern with fixation as the normal Z disk (Fig. 31-40E and F).[51,53] Macdonald and Engel proposed a simple explanation and model for these observations[51]: Glutaraldehyde fixation preserves the Z filaments in a more acutely curving state than osmium fixation alone. Goldstein and coworkers[53a] suggest that the Z-disk lattice oscillates between the small square net existing in relaxed muscle and the basket-weave pattern when the myofibrils are under tension. When projected on the transverse plane, more acutely curving Z filaments produce a small square net which is unrotated relative to the array of the thin filaments; the less acutely curving Z filaments project the image of a larger basket-weave lattice which appears rotated 45° relative to the thin-filament array (Fig. 31-40). According to this model, Z filaments must traverse the Z disk. Other plausible models of Z-disk structure have also been proposed.[54,55]

The molecular composition of the Z disk and of its proliferative anomaly, the nemaline rod, has been of considerable interest. Chemical extraction of thin filaments disintegrates Z disk and rods, leaving an amorphous or finely filamentous debris behind[56]; cross-sectioned rods always display thin filaments[51]; and partial digestion of the disk and rods with a calcium-activated protease, which does not digest actin, shows that thin filaments interdigitate in the disk and traverse the entire length of the rods.[52] Therefore thin filaments and thin-filament-associated proteins are structural components of Z disks and rods. α-Actinin, a 4- by 50-nm rod-like protein with 74 percent helical content, is a dimer of two 95,000-Da peptide chains.[57] It cross-links actin filaments in vitro, is extracted from the Z disk by low-ionic-strength solutions[57,58] or calcium-dependent proteases,[59,59a] and immunolocalizes at the Z disk and nemaline rods.[60,61]

Actin, α-actinin, nebulin, and titin represent major components of the Z disk.[62,62a] Other Z-disk-associated proteins include telethonin,[62a] myotilin,[63] myozenin (FATZ or calsarcin 2),[64] myopalladin,[65] and Nsp11.[66a] The biologic and clinical significance of these and other Z-disk-related proteins is discussed further in Chaps. 7, 37, 43, and 54.

In mature muscle, 10-nm-wide desmin filaments encircle Z disks[66b] and are linked to each other and to the sarcolemma by the intermediate-filament-associated protein plectin.[66c] This network organizes the myofibrils at the Z-disk level and likely protects them from disruption during

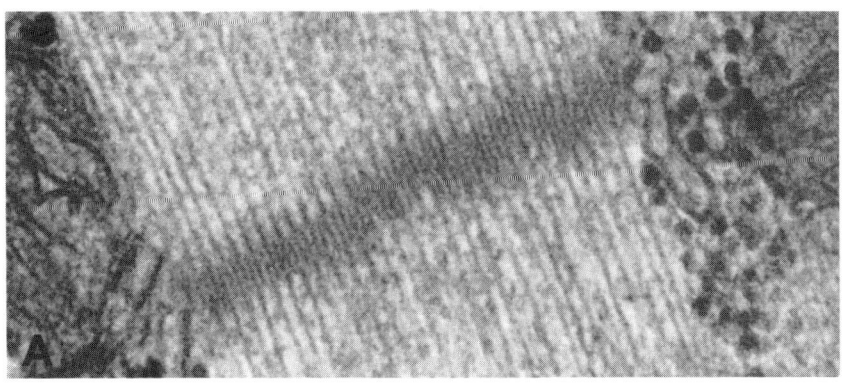 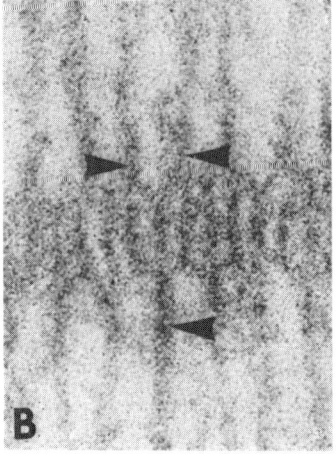

FIGURE 31-39. Longitudinal sections of Z disk in rat gastrocnemius after double fixation with glutaraldehyde and osmium. In A, thin filaments approach and extend into the disk region, where they give rise to thinner Z filaments. Amorphous material surrounds the filaments within the disk. In B, lower arrowhead points to a thin filament that extends into the disk and there gives rise to two arching Z filaments that extend to thin filaments on the opposite side of the disk (upper arrowheads). A, ×124,000; B, ×340,000. (Reproduced by permission from Macdonald RD, Engel AG, J Cell Biol 48:431, 1971.)

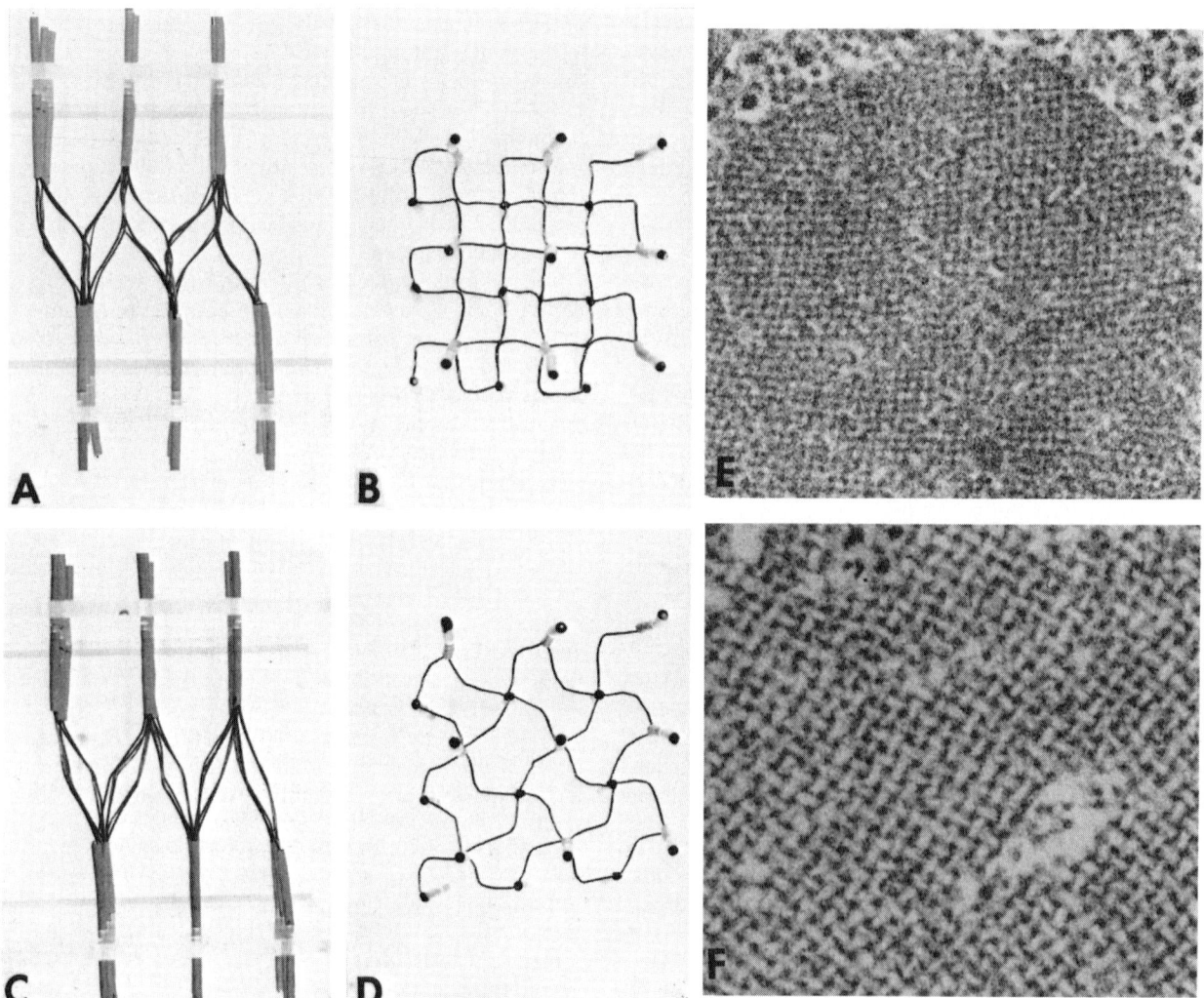

FIGURE 31-40. Wire models of the Z disk in the small square net (A and B) and basket-weave (C and D) conformations in longitudinal (A and C) and transverse (B and D) sections. The small square net conformation is observed after double fixation with glutaraldehyde and osmium; the basket-weave pattern appears after either osmium fixation alone or low-ionic-strength extraction followed by double fixation. The small square net model (A and B) was obtained from the basket-weave model (C and D) by substituting more acutely bending wires for Z filaments than those used in the basket-weave model. E is a transverse section of a nemaline rod after double fixation; F is a transverse section of a nemaline rod after low-ionic-strength extraction followed by double fixation. Compare B with E and D with F. E and F, ×155,000. *(Reproduced by permission from Macdonald RD, Engel AG, J Cell Biol 48:431, 1971.)*

force generation. αB-crystallin, a small heat-shock protein that also localizes to the Z disk, is a molecular chaperone for desmin as well as for tubulin and a variety of soluble enzymes.[66d]

The reactions of the Z disk include *rod formation, cytoplasmic body formation, streaming and disintegration,* and *duplication.*

Nemaline rods. Rod formation is the hallmark of congenital nemaline myopathy, in which it occurs without significant involvement of other organelles (Figs. 31-42B, 31-43A to D, 31-44A, and Color Plate 7A and B). It is also the predominant pathologic alteration in late-onset nemaline myopathy, but here other organelles are also affected and the rod-bearing fibers undergo progressive atrophy (Fig. 31-43E and F). Small rod formations appear consistently in regenerating fibers and fiber regions (Figs. 31-44B, 31-87E, 36-89C, 31-121, 31-122, 31-124C) and occasionally in denervated fibers (Fig. 31-85B). They are also found in tenotomized muscles,[67] in end plate myopathies induced by prostigmine,[68,69] in a variety of other myopathies,[70-75] in some normal adult myotendinous junctions,[76] and in aging or hypertrophied heart muscle.[52]

In some of the myopathies, as in the end plate myopathy induced by prostigmine or tenotomy,[66,67,69] rod formation is a transient event during myofibrillar regeneration; a similar mechanism probably accounts for the small rod formations in polymyositis and dermatomyositis (Figs. 31-87E, 31-89C, 31-121, 31-122), but larger rod structures than those in regen-

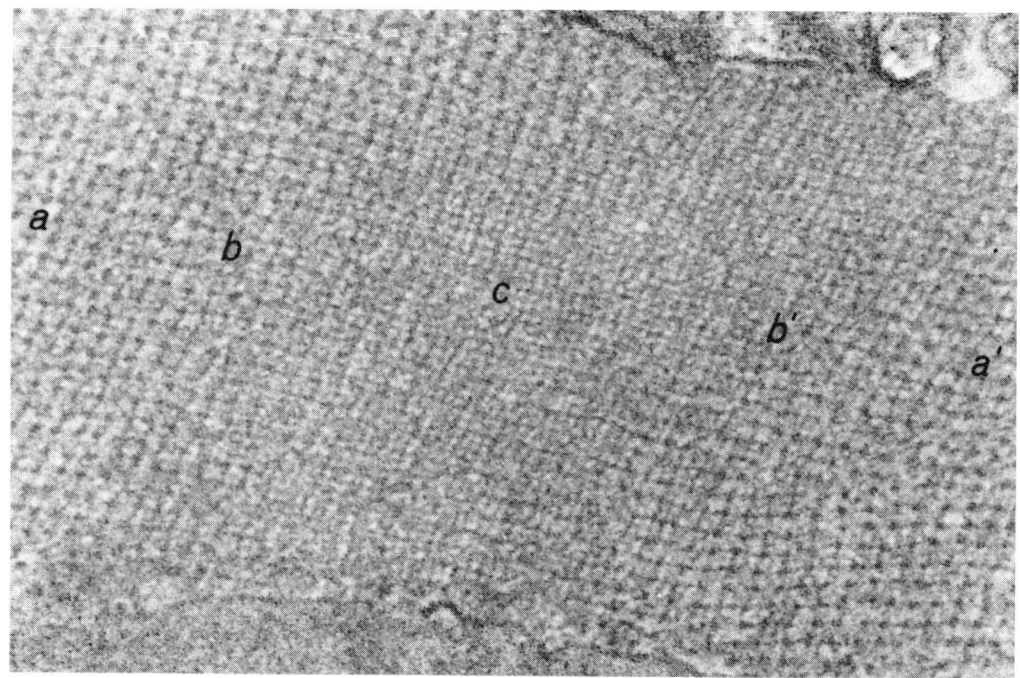

FIGURE 31-41. Transversely sectioned frog sartorius Z disk displays the small square net pattern after double fixation with glutaraldehyde and osmium, ×155,000. *(Reproduced by permission from Macdonald RD, Engel AG, J Cell Biol 48:431–437, 1971.)*

erating fibers have been described in an inactive case of polymyositis,[70] in some mitochondrial myopathies,[72,73] and in cricopharyngeal dysphagia.[74]

The rods have five distinct morphologic features:

1. Origin in the Z disk (Figs. 31-42B, 31-43C, D, and F, 31-44)
2. A 9-nm square net in transverse sections that is identical with the Z disk lattice (Figs. 31-40E, 31-47A and B)
3. Structural continuity with thin filaments (Figs. 31-43B and E, 31-44)
4. Periodic lines at 14- to 20-nm intervals perpendicular to the long axis of the rods (Fig. 31-43B and E).
5. Periodic lines at 8- to 12-nm intervals parallel to the long axis of the rods (Fig. 31-43B and E)

Osmium fixation without glutaraldehyde prefixation converts the small square net rod lattice into a larger basket-weave lattice and reveals that thin filaments traverse the rods (Fig. 31-40F).[51] On digestion with a calcium-activated protease, which removes α-actinin, the rods lose their Z filaments and perpendicular periodicity and display a backbone of thin filaments.[52] Further, three-dimensional reconstruction studies of the rods suggest that within the rods, actin filaments of opposite polarity are connected by linking filaments composed of two α-actinin dimers.[76a] Thus the rods

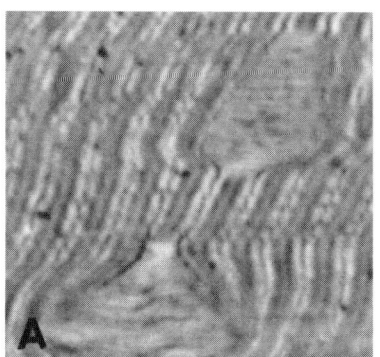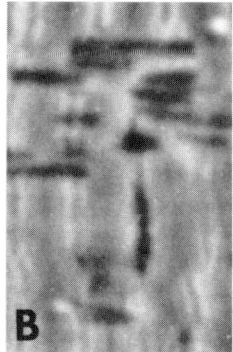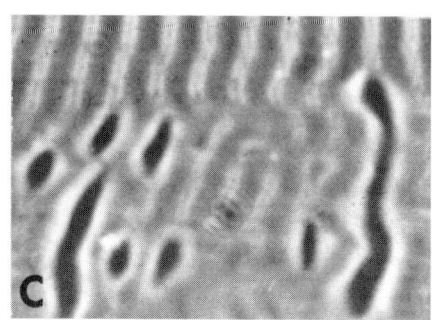

FIGURE 31-42. Phase micrographs of Z-disk streaming and disintegration *(A)*, nemaline rods *(B)*, and cytoplasmic bodies *(C)*. A, ×1700; B, ×3300; C, ×2300. [B is reproduced by permission from Engel AG, Gomez MR, J Neuropathol Exp Neurol 26:601, 1976; C is reproduced by permission from Macdonald RD, Engel AG, Acta Neuropathol (Berl) 14:99, 1969.]

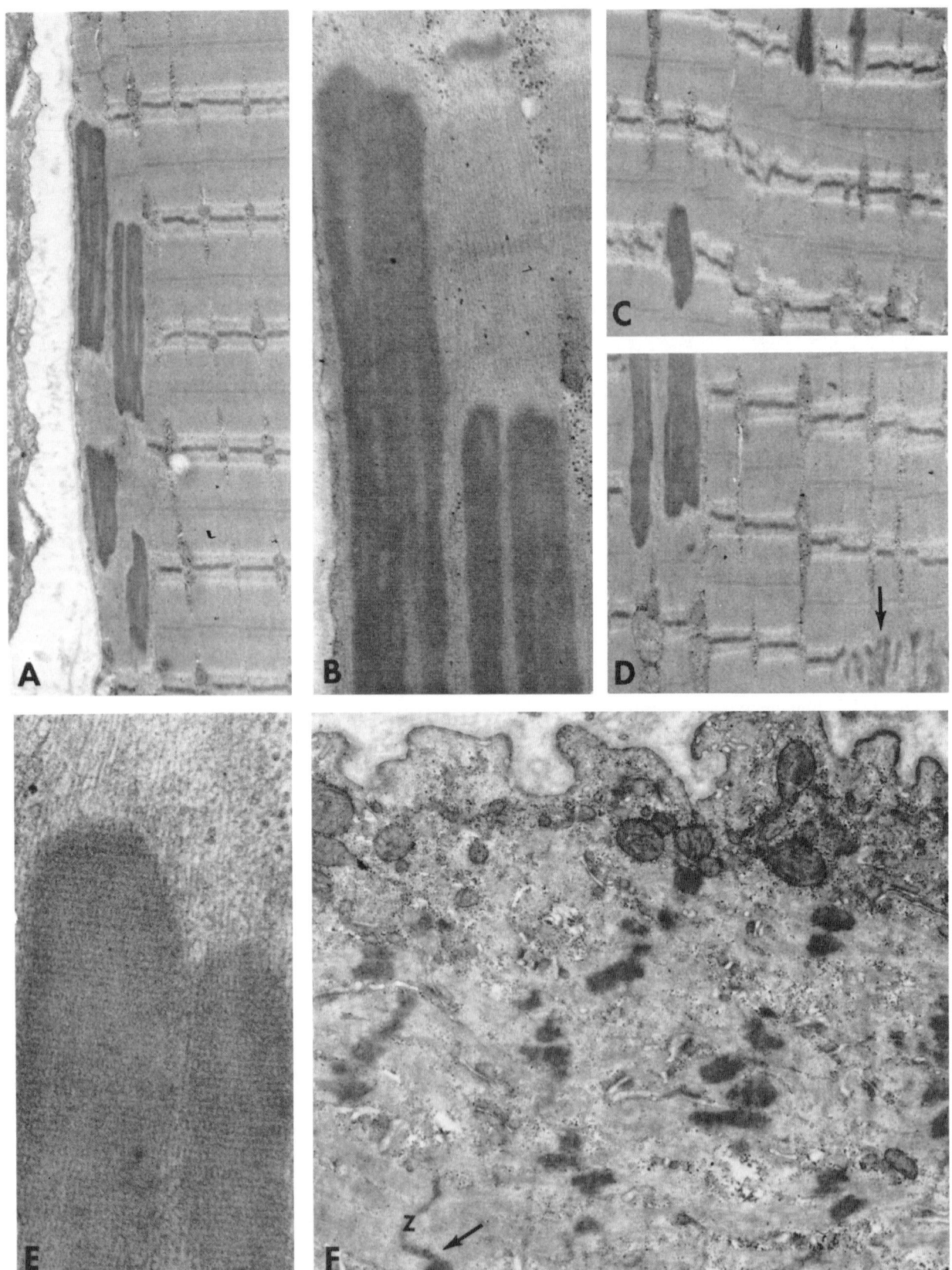

FIGURE 31-43. Nemaline rods in congenital (A through D) and late-onset (E and F) nemaline myopathy. The rods arise in the Z disk (C and D), thin filaments insert into the rods (B and E), and there are periodic lines parallel and perpendicular to the long axis of the rods (E). Arrows in D and F show early rod formations. A, ×9300; B, ×30,000; C and D, ×10,600; E, ×79,700; F, ×14,000. (A through D are reproduced by permission from Engel AG, Gomez MR, J Neuropathol Exp Neurol 26:601, 1967; F is reproduced by permission from Engel AG, Mayo Clin Proc 41:713, 1966.)

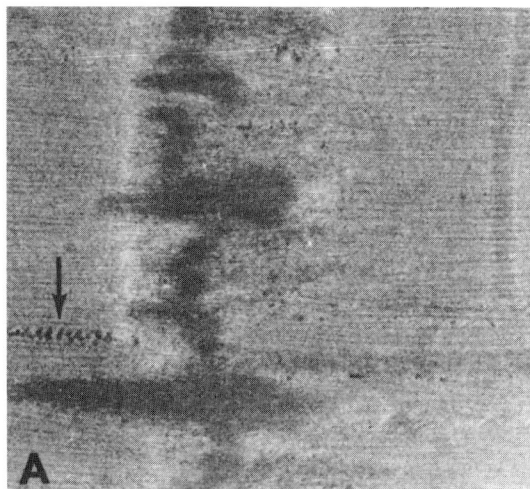 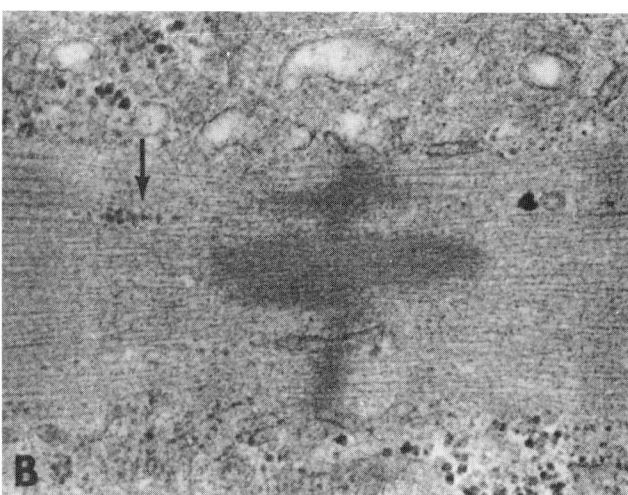

FIGURE 31-44. Small rod bodies in congenital nemaline myopathy *(A)* and in regenerating muscle fiber in polymyositis *(B)*. Arrows indicate helical polyribosomes. *A*, ×39,300; *B*, ×49,600.

represent a proliferative anomaly of the Z disk, and the length of both rods and Z disks may be determined by the amount of overlap of actin filaments of opposite polarity.[52]

Cytoplasmic bodies. Cytoplasmic bodies represent a nonspecific degenerative abnormality of the Z disk. They occur in any myopathy and even in denervated fibers. It has been suggested that these formations constitute the predominant pathologic change in cytoplasmic body myopathy (see Chap. 43). The cytoplasmic body has the following characteristic features[77]: (1) origin in the Z disk; (2) a dense filamentous core: (3) a surrounding lighter halo; (4) randomly oriented thin and finer filaments in the halo; and (5) lack of a square filamentous array regardless of the plane of sectioning (Figs. 31-42*C*, 31-45, 31-47*D*).

Streaming and disintegration of the Z disk. This is the commonest reaction of the Z disk, a common reaction in any myopathy and denervation atrophy,[43] and a reaction that initiates focal myofibrillar degeneration. The light microscopic correlate is a focal loss of cross striations (Fig. 31-42*A*).

As mentioned under "Alterations of Mitochondria," above, Z-disk streaming is frequently associated with mitochondrial decrease and is thus seen in cores (Figs. 31-72, 31-73), multicores (Figs. 31-76, 31-77), target formations (Figs. 31-74, 31-75), "moth-eaten fibers" (Figs. 31-88*B* and *C*, 31-90*A*, *B*, and *D*), or any other lesion associated with decrease in mitochondria (Fig. 31-46*A* to *C*). Less frequently, Z-disk streaming occurs without mitochondrial loss (Fig. 31-46*D*). It also can be seen in normal muscle in which myofibrils bifurcate or display vernier shifts.[78] Foci of Z-band streaming were present in 3.5 ± 4.6 percent (overall mean ± SD) of muscle fibers in 34 healthy adults; and in 0.6 ± 1.1 percent of the fibers the size of at least one lesion exceeded three or more adjacent myofibrils *and* three or more continuous sarcomeres.[79]

In phase optics the affected fiber regions are irregular in outline and vary in size. Small lesions extending over one or two sarcomeres resemble rods, but in the electron microscope rods of that size and Z-disk streaming are clearly different. Some of the affected sarcomeres are stretched so that the lesions become irregularly widened (Fig. 31-42*A*). In the electron microscope, in the initial stage of the change, the Z disk is slightly widened and irregular (Figs. 31-46*A*, 31-73*B*, 31-76). At this stage the Z-disk abnormality cannot be distinguished from the earliest alteration that occurs during rod formation (Figs. 31-43*C*, and 31-44*A*) or cytoplasmic body formation (Fig. 31-45*A*). At a slightly more advanced stage, amorphous material emanating from the Z disk extends into the adjacent I band (Fig. 31-46*A* and *B*) and then into the A band (Fig. 31-46*A* and *D*). The material released from the disk could be a preexisting normal constituent, or some additional normal or abnormal substance could be formed. In large lesions adjacent sarcomeres are affected (Figs. 31-46*C*, 31-74*A*, 31-85*B* and *C*, and 31-90*A*), and SR and T-tubule components may be dislocated (Fig. 31-16) and reduced in number (Figs. 31-88*B* and *C*, 31-74, 31-75, 31-77). In transverse sections amorphous material can be observed between myofilament profiles (Figs. 31-47*C*, 31-75, 31-77), or the filament profiles may be obscured by the dense deposits. In some portions of larger lesions thick-filament profiles are no longer recognizable. Loss of thick filaments from larger lesions is indicated in frozen sections by a loss of reactivity for myofibrillar ATPase.

Streaming and disintegration of the Z disk in areas of mitochondrial decrease is more commonly observed in type 1 than in type 2 muscle fibers in tenotomized animals[67] and in experimental myopathies induced by emetime[40] or corticosteroids.[44] This suggests that Z-disk integrity is more dependent on mitochondria in type 1 than in type 2 fibers.

Further insight into the mechanism of Z-disk breakdown has come from studies of end plate myopathies induced by

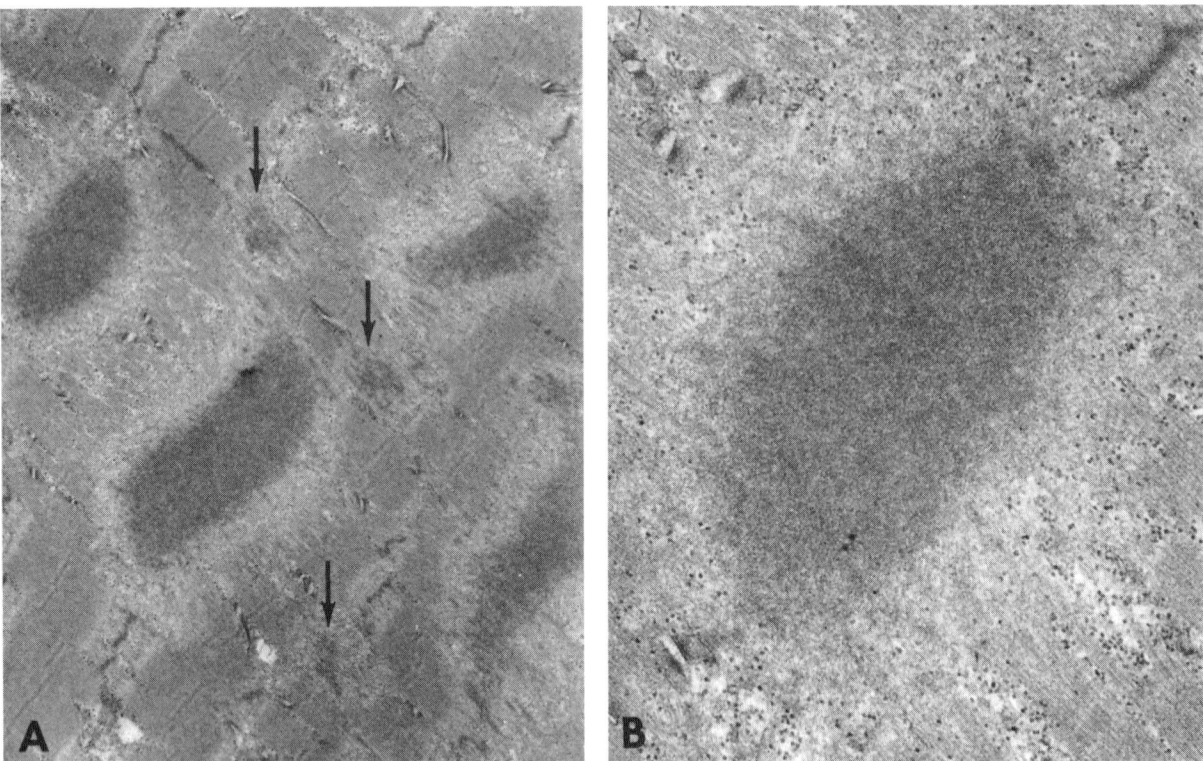

FIGURE 31-45. Cytoplasmic bodies. A. Four cytoplasmic bodies arising in the Z disks extend across several myofibrils. Arrows indicate early Z-disk lesions. B. The dense core of the cytoplasmic body is composed of short, fine, irregularly oriented filaments. These filaments are best seen at the edge of the cytoplasmic body. A, ×11,000; B, ×58,200. [Reproduced by permission from Macdonald RD, Engel AG, Acta Neuropathol (Berl) 14:99, 1969.]

cholinesterase inhibitors[68,69,80] or carbamylcholine[34] and of the slow-channel myasthenic syndrome.[11] In these disorders calcium accumulates in the junctional region because of abnormally frequent or prolonged openings of the acetylcholine receptor (AChR) ion channel.[11,69] The pathologic changes include dilation of the SR, damage to mitochondria, and Z-disk streaming and breakdown. The alterations induced by carbamylcholine in vitro can be prevented by omitting calcium from the extracellular fluid[34]; and leupeptin, a protease inhibitor, partially protects the Z disks from the effects of carbamylcholine.[81] Thus, at least the acutely induced end plate myopathies are calcium-dependent, and Z-disk damage is at least partly mediated by the calcium-activated protease found at the Z disk.

Less is known about the mechanism of Z-disk streaming and disintegration in the many other disorders in which it occurs. Low- and high-calcium-requiring proteases exist in muscle. The former species is half-maximally activated at a calcium concentration of 45 μM,[82] but the normal calcium concentration in the myofilament space in the resting state is less than 1 μM. The calcium concentrations in the adjacent spaces (SR 16 to 20 mM,[83] mitochondria 1 to 2.5 mM,[84] extracellular space 2.5 mM) are three to four orders of magnitude higher than in the myofilament space. The low calcium concentration in the myofilament space is regulated by the plasma membrane, the SR, the mitochondria, and the soluble calcium-binding proteins calmodulin, parvalbumin, and troponin C (reviewed in Ref. 85). Accordingly, a structural or metabolic abnormality involving any of the regulating factors could result in calcium excess in the myofilament space provided that the other regulatory factors could not handle the extra load. One may also speculate that a decrease in mitochondrial density, or a metabolic factor that interferes with the uptake of calcium by this organelle, could result in abnormally high calcium transients in the myofilament space when calcium is released from the SR. If these did occur, they would be more prolonged and more damaging in type 1 than in type 2 fibers because the SR calcium pump is less active in the type 1 fibers. A combined decrease or metabolic lesion in both mitochondria and SR, or a reduced ability of the plasma membrane to extrude calcium by means of its specific ATPase and Na^+-Ca^{2+} exchanger,[85] or structural plasma membrane defects could readily compromise calcium homeostasis and induce focal myofibrillar degeneration beginning at the Z disk. Marked focal calcium increases do occur in delta lesions beneath surface membrane defects in Duchenne dystrophy[1,86] but paradoxically Z-disk streaming is not conspicuous in delta lesions.

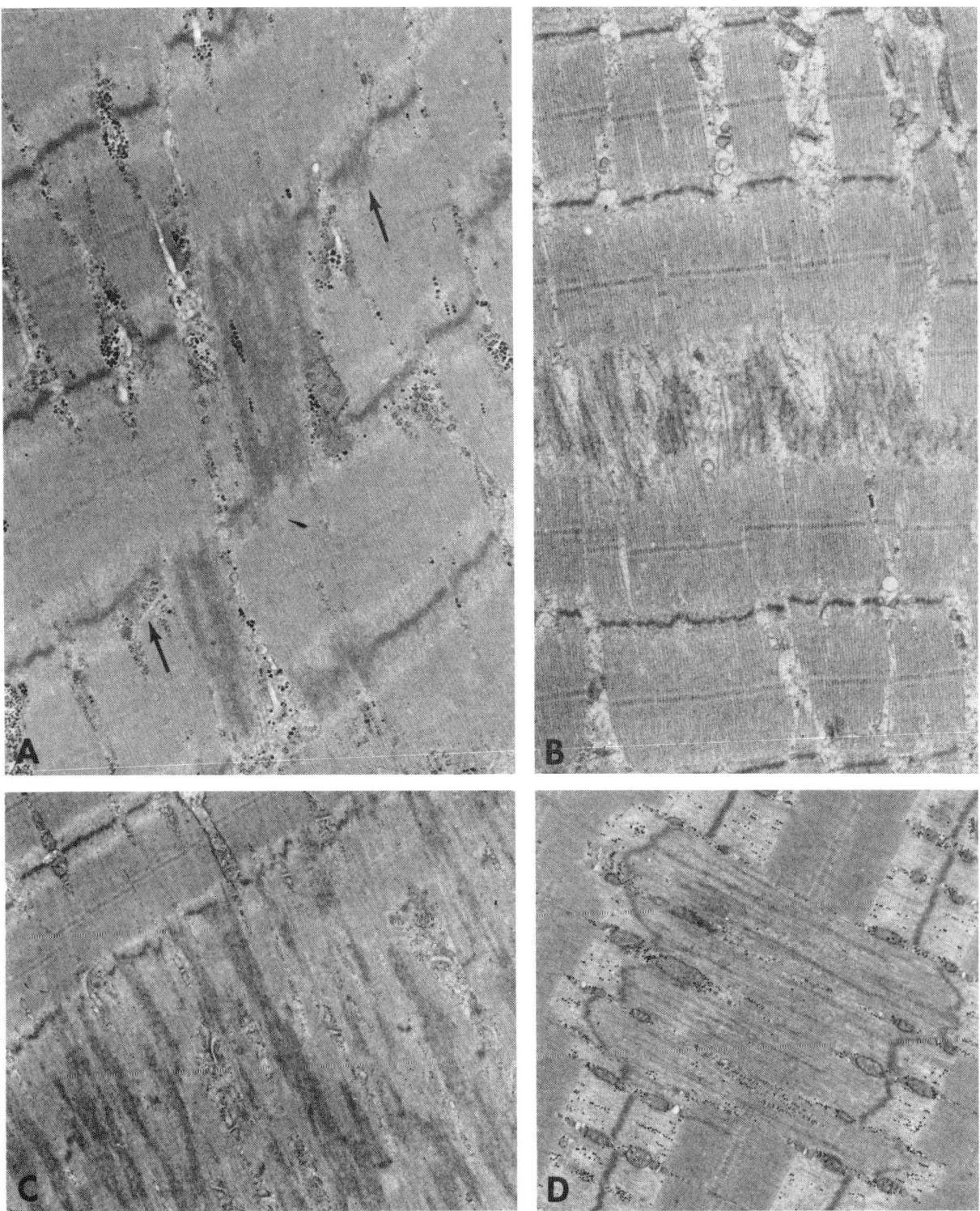

FIGURE 31-46. Z-disk streaming in acid maltase deficiency *(A)*, in myopathy associated with malabsorption syndrome *(B)*, in hyperkalemic periodic paralysis *(C)*, and in a Kearns-Sayre syndrome *(D)*. Arrows in *A* indicate early Z-disk lesions. Mitochondrial density is reduced in the abnormal fiber regions in *A* to *C* but not in *D*. *A*, ×18,000; *B*, ×14,400; *C*, ×10,000; *D*, ×12,300.

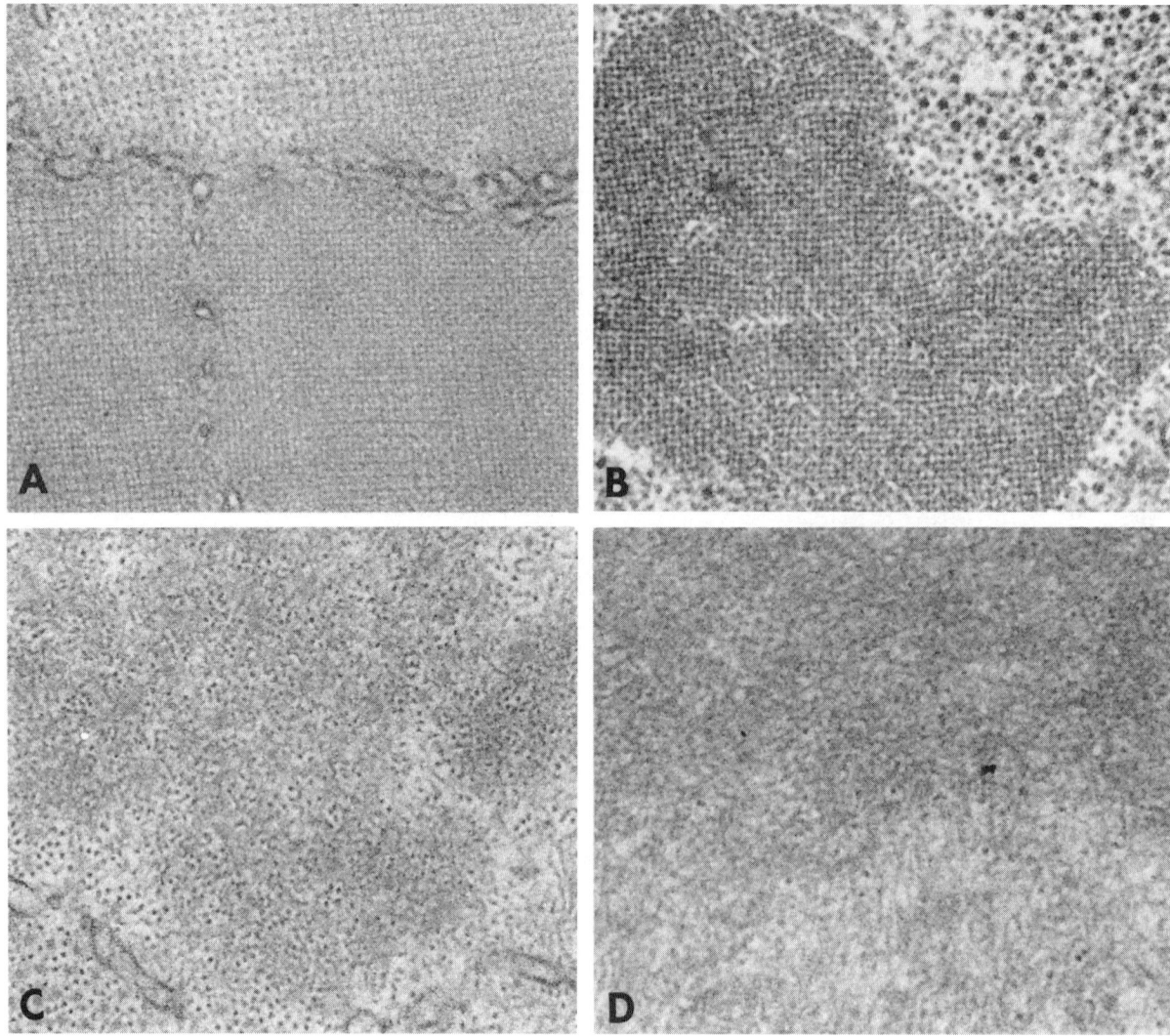

FIGURE 31-47. Transverse sections of normal Z disk (A), nemaline rod (B), Z-disk streaming (C), and cytoplasmic body (D). In B, the section traverses the A band, and the rod is surrounded by a double array of thick and thin filaments. In C, the section traverses the I band, and amorphous material of Z-disk origin surrounds the thin filaments. D shows the core (upper part) and halo (lower part) of the cytoplasmic body. Thin filaments in the halo extend to the core. The core contains an irregular array of shorter and thinner filaments than those in the halo. A to D, ×99,500. [Reproduced by permission from Macdonald RD, Engel AG, Acta Neuropathol (Berl) 14:99, 1969.]

Duplication. Duplication of the Z disk, together with widening of the Z disks and small rod formations, occurs in regenerating fibers and fiber regions (Fig. 31-124)[12] and at normal myotendinous junctions.[76]

OTHER MYOFIBRILLAR ALTERATIONS

Other myofibrillar reactions include *loss of thick filaments, annular myofibrils* (Ringbinden), *aberrant myofibrils, leptomeres,* and *alterations at the myotendinous junction.* Other formations related to myofibrillar components or filamentous structural proteins (e.g., filamentous bodies, concentric laminated bodies, fingerprint bodies, spheroid bodies, hyaline bodies, and granulofilamentous bodies) are discussed under "Miscellaneous Inclusions," at the end of this section.

Loss of thick filaments. Loss of thick filaments and disappearance of reactivity for myofibrillar ATPase occurs eventually in the course of myofibrillar degeneration that begins at the Z disk.

Selective loss of thick filaments associated with widespread muscle fiber atrophy is a prominent feature of the critical illness myopathy (acute quadriplegic myopathy) that affects patients who receive high doses of corticosteroids and, in addition, are also treated by muscle relaxants[86a,b,c] or have multiple medical problems with anoxia, hypercapnia, or acidosis.[87,88] In the affected muscle fibers, there are multiple foci where there is partial or complete loss of thick filaments (Figs. 31-48, 31-49, and Color Plate 15H–I). The affected myofibrils initially remain in register but eventually become disorganized (Figs. 31-48A to C and 31-49A), and the adjacent organelles (SR, T tubules, and mitochondria)

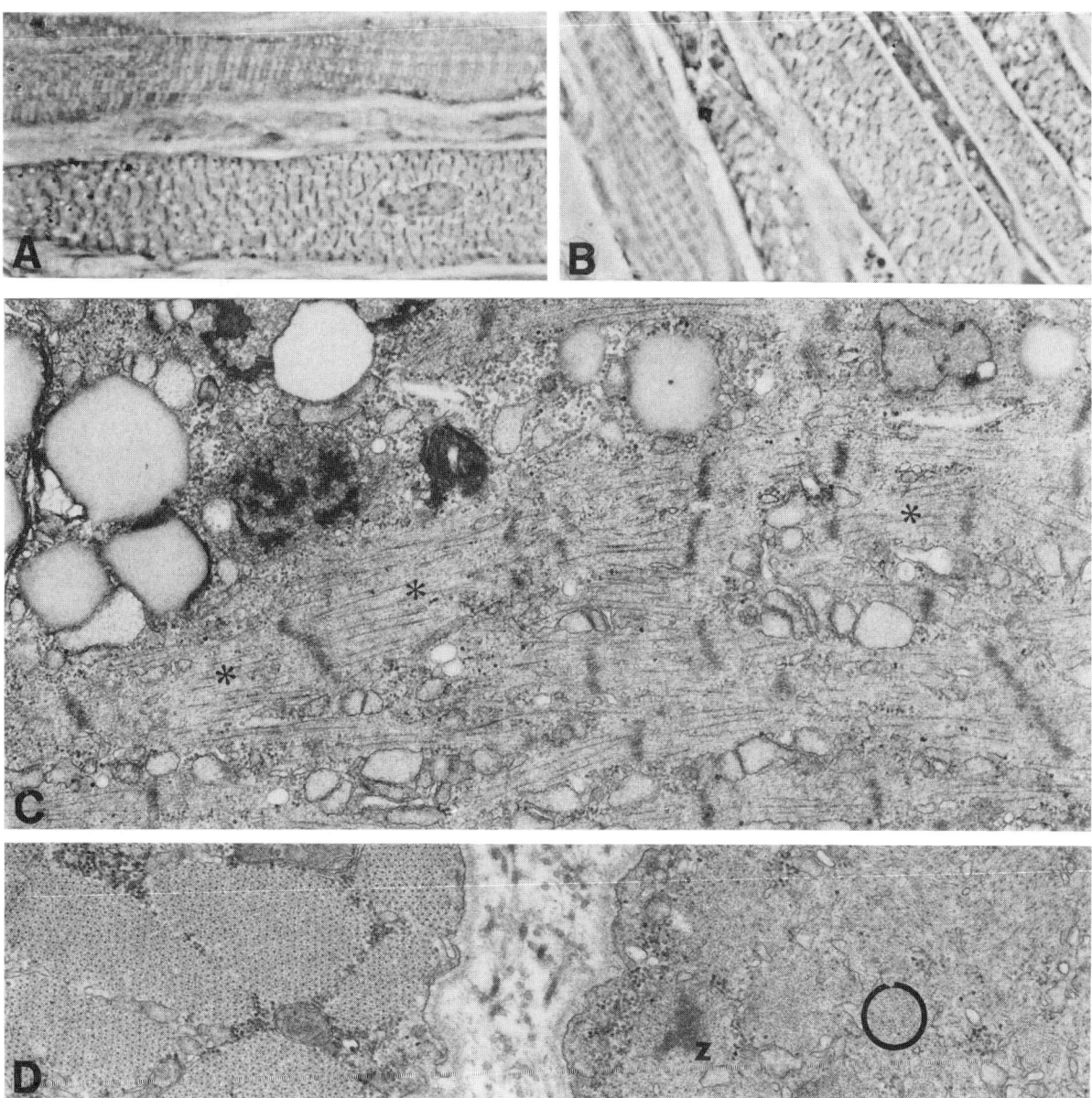

FIGURE 31-48. Thick-filament loss in critical illness myopathy. A and B. Phase micrographs. The parallel alignment of the myofibrils is disrupted, and many sarcomeres are stretched or collapsed in the abnormal fibers. C. There is partial thick-filament depletion in all sarcomeres (asterisks). The myofibrils are disorganized. SR and T-system components are displaced from their normal positions and the SR elements are dilated. Lipid droplets, lipofuscin bodies, and glycogen granules are accumulating in the upper part of the field. D. Transversely sectioned muscle fibers. The fiber on the right contains a reduced number of thick filaments (see circle). The fiber on the left displays the normal double hexagonal array of thick and thin filaments. Z, Z disk. A, ×1040; B, ×1240; C, ×15,500; D, ×25,900.

become displaced from their normal positions (Fig. 31-48C). Some muscle fibers also show dilated SR cisternae and focal accumulations of lipid droplets, lipofuscin bodies, and glycogen granules (Figs. 31-48C and 31-49A). In the most severely affected fibers, there are large regions that contain only thin-filament "brushes" attached to Z disks, few dilated vesicles, and sparse glycogen granules (Fig. 31-49B). Depletion of thick filaments has also been observed in de-

nervated soleus muscles of rats receiving large-dose glucocorticoids.[88a,b] In this model there is also failure of the majority of muscle fibers to generate action potentials.[88c] Detailed studies of action potential generation in human critical illness myopathy have not been carried out to date.

Thick-filament loss was also described in two patients with congenital myopathies.[89,90] In one patient the thick filaments were absent from superficial myofibrils in about 10

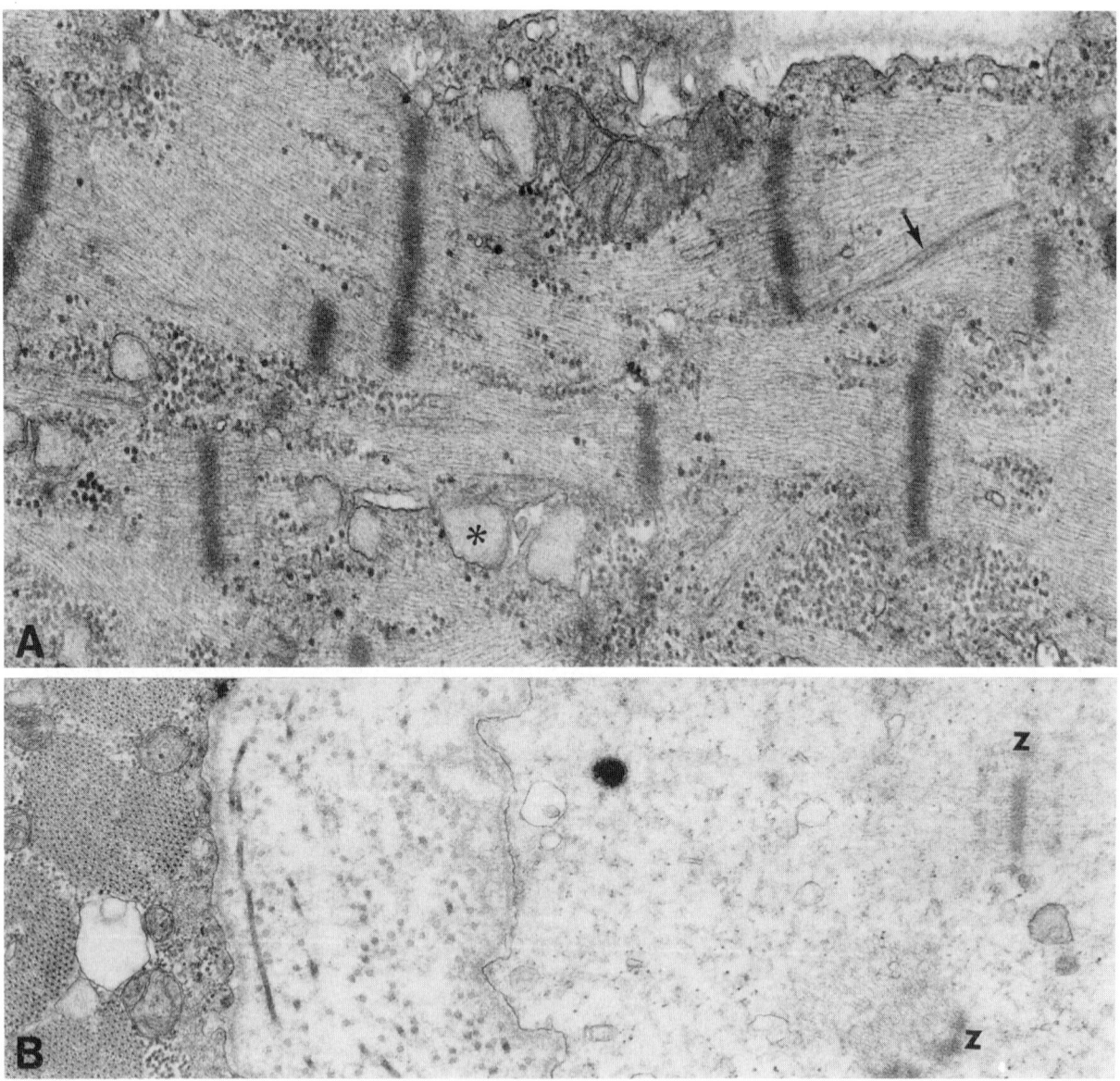

FIGURE 31-49. Thick-filament loss in critical illness myopathy. In *A*, the sarcomeres are spanned by thin filaments; only two thick filaments remain (arrow). The myofibrils have lost their usual alignments, and some of the sarcomeres have collapsed. The lateral cisternae of the SR are dilated (asterisks). In *B*, the fiber imaged at the right only contains thin-filament "brushes" attached to Z disks, few small vesicles, and sparse granules; the fiber at the left contains normal myofibrils. *A*, ×44,000; *B*, ×25,900.

percent of the muscle fibers. In the other patient with congenital myopathy, described under the name of *cap disease*,[90] 70 percent of the muscle fibers contained superficial zones lightly reactive for ATPase and strongly reactive for glycogen, phosphorylase, and oxidative enzymes. In the electron microscope, the abnormal regions contained aberrant myofibrils in which Z disks and thin filaments but no thick filaments were discerned (see also Chap. 54).

Annular myofibrils (Ringbinden). These occur in myotonic dystrophy, limb girdle and other types of dystrophy, occasionally in other myopathies, in denervated or reinnervated muscle fibers, and occasionally in normal muscle. The annular myofibrils course in a plane perpendicular to the long fiber axis encircling the periphery of the fiber. Occasionally some of the peripherally coursing myofibrils turn inward and traverse deeper regions of the fiber or run obliquely to the long fiber axis. Sarcotubular elements and glycogen granules are associated with the annular myofibrils. Mitochondria are sparse between the individual myofibrils constituting the ringlet but form small clusters along the inner or outer border of the entire ringlet (Fig. 31-50).

Aberrant myofibrils. These either are organized into bundles or are disorganized. Organized aberrant myofibrils appear in lobulated fibers. Here bundles of myofibrils course obliquely to the long fiber axis. Many bundles, each com-

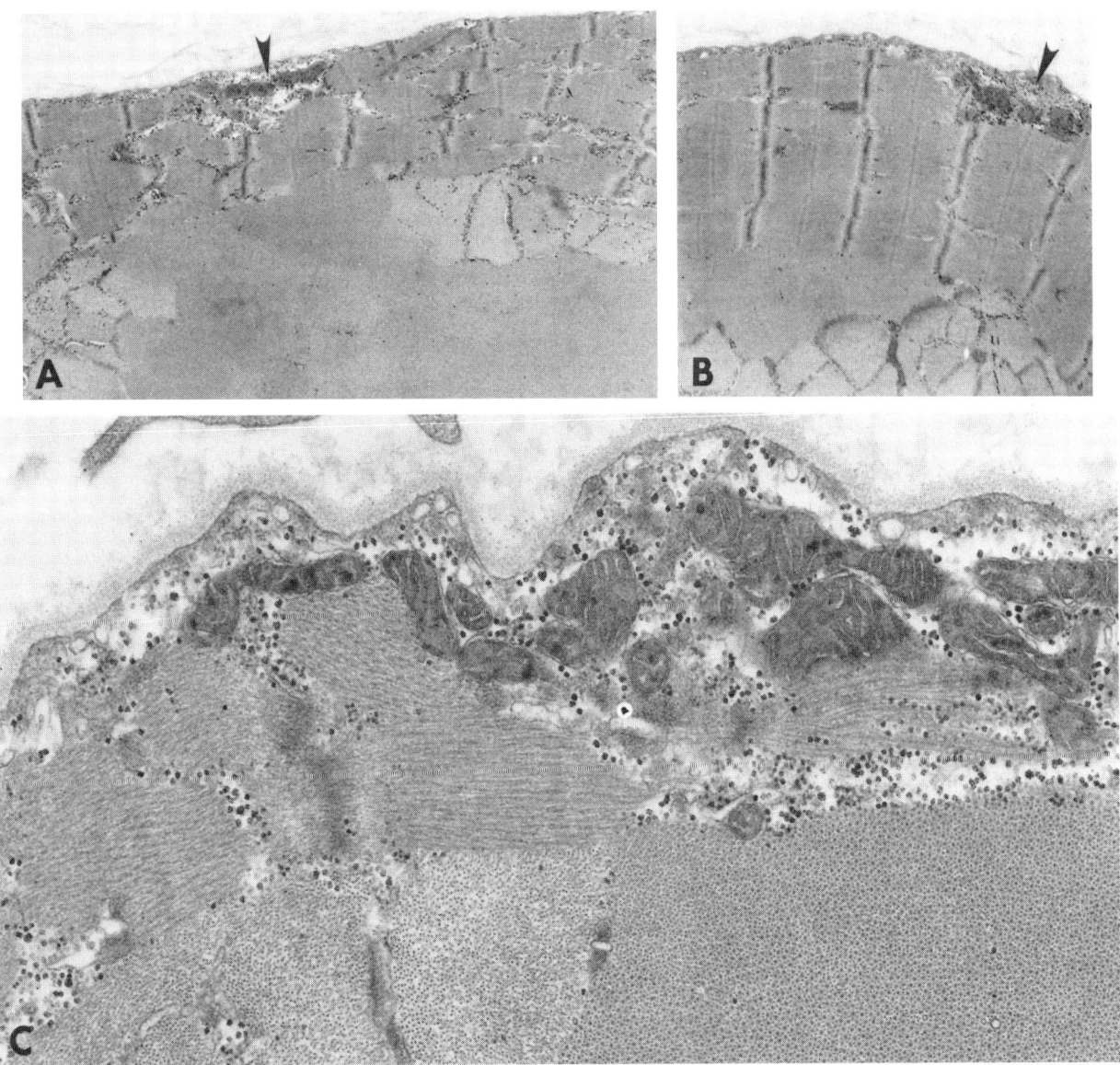

FIGURE 31-50. Annular myofibrils in limb-girdle dystrophy. Arrowheads indicate small clusters of mitochondria along outer border of the ring formation. *A* and *B*, ×11,200; *C*, ×32,000.

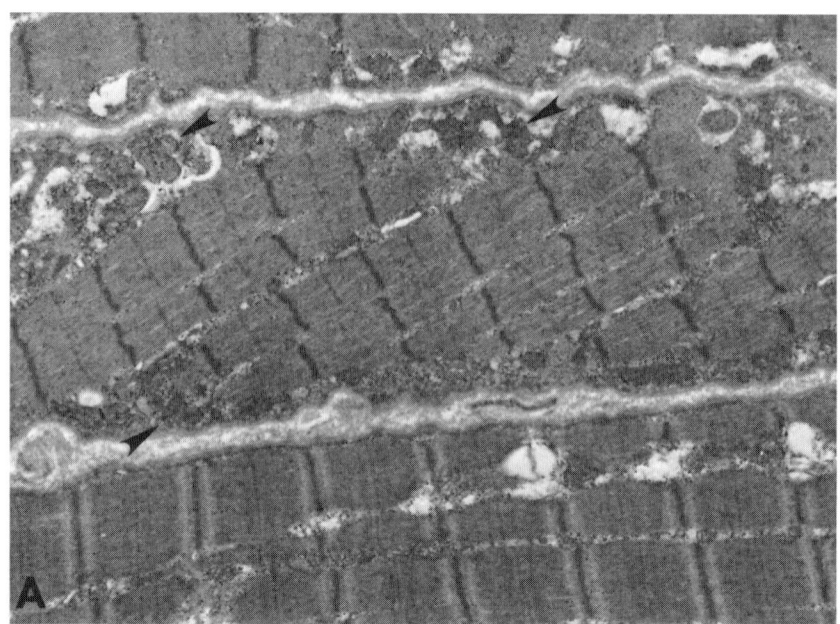

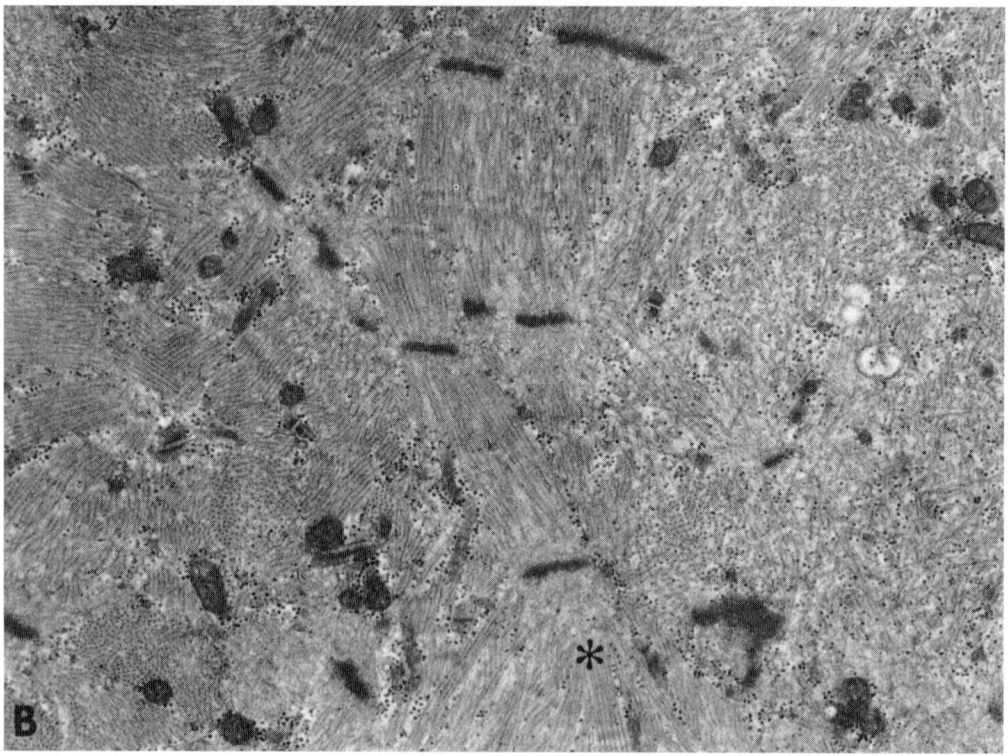

FIGURE 31-51. *A.* Organized aberrant myofibrils in lobulated fiber in fingerprint body myopathy. *B.* Disorganized aberrant myofibrils in inflammatory myopathy. *A*, ×8100; *B*, ×20,400. *(A is reproduced by permission from Engel AG, Angelini C, Gomez M, Mayo Clin Proc 47:377, 1972.)*

prising a variable number of myofibrils, occur in a given fiber, and the obliquely spiraling bundles intertwine like skeins in a rope. Mitochondria are sparse within the bundles (i.e., between individual myofibrils) but form clusters at various sites between the bundles (Fig. 31-51*A*). This results in a lobulated distribution of oxidative enzyme activity in frozen sections. Lobulated fibers typically occur in chronic myopathies and were especially frequent in Bethlem myopathy caused by mutations in collagen VIA.[91,91a]

Disorganized aberrant myofibrils curve irregularly and intertwine randomly; individual myofibrils are seldom parallel to each other; and some myofibrils split into smaller fibrils or sheaves of filaments that also course irregularly (Fig. 31-51B). Disorganized aberrant myofibrils can be observed in any myopathy (Fig. 31-90C), in chronically denervated fibers (Fig. 31-86C), in regenerating fiber regions (Figs. 31-124B and C), and in some areas in sarcoplasmic masses (Figs. 31-79C and 31-80A).

The faulty alignment of the annular and aberrant myofibrils suggests faulty myofibril-cytoskeleton interactions. These interactions are developmentally regulated, and the cytoskeleton itself becomes reorganized as myofibrils appear, increase in girth, associate with other organelles, and fall into register.[66] Thus, either a derangement in the maturational sequence of the cytoskeletal supporting and anchoring elements or failure of the developing myofibrils to associate with the appropriate cytoskeletal components at the appropriate time could result in faulty myofibrillar alignment.

Probable lysis of myofibrils in type 1 fibers. This reaction was described in two siblings with a benign congenital myopathy. Muscle biopsy specimens in both showed type 1 fiber predominance and atrophy, and large, abnormal peripheral zones in type 1 fibers. These zones appeared pale in the modified trichrome stain, lacked oxidative enzyme activity, and reacted intensely for myofibrillar ATPase. Ultrastructurally, the abnormal zones contained fine granular material in which few nuclei and sparse mitochondria and glycogen granules were present.[91b] This disease is morphologically identical with hyaline body myopathy, which is now known to be caused by a dominant mutation in *MYH7* that encodes slow/β-cardiac myosin (MyHC I). Also see below, under "Myosin Storage Myopathy, alias Hyaline Body Myopathy."

Excess of thin filaments. Masses of haphazardly arranged thin filaments replacing normal sarcomeres were observed in a congenital myopathy.[91c] Intranuclear and sarcoplasmic nemaline rods were also detected in some fibers. This disorder is now known to stem from a mutation in actin.[91d]

Leptomere formations. These have been described also as *microladder formations* or *zebra bodies*. They range from a few to several microns long or wide and consist of dense striae linked by fine crisscrossing filaments. The striae are spaced at 0.15- to 0.2-μm intervals, and the filamentous interspace sometimes contains two indistinct lines parallel to the striae. The striae resemble Z disks in density and sometimes appear structurally continuous with Z disks.[92] Digestion with pronase or pepsin removes Z disks and striae, but with 2.5 M urea the striae are more resistant to extraction than the Z disks. The protein composition of the fine connecting filaments has not been investigated.[92] Leptomeres appear in cardiac muscle in both Purkinje and contractile fibers.[92,93] In normal skeletal muscle leptomeres occur near sensory nerve contacts in intrafusal fibers[94] and are particularly prominent at a point just proximal to the intercellular bridge. The leptomeres are usually located near the surface of the fiber, and their axial orientation differs from that of the myofibrils (Fig. 31-52A).[94a] The leptomeres are also present at the myotendinous junction and elsewhere in extrafusal fibers and in developing muscle fibers (reviewed in Refs. 76 and 93).

Leptomeres were also described in a congenital myopathy, in which they occurred together with a variety of other myofibrillar abnormalities.[95] We have encountered only a few of these formations in diverse myopathies. Thus far, the leptomere formations have no known role in either normal or pathologic muscle.

Alterations at the myotendinous junction. At the myotendinous junction the muscle fibers end in finger-like projections. The projections are surrounded by a thick layer of basal lamina and interdigitate with the surrounding connective tissue elements. The cytoplasmic surface of the projections is buttressed by deposits of moderately electron-dense material, and thin filaments of the terminal sarcomeres insert into this material (Fig. 31-52B).[76] In detergent-extracted muscle, fine (2 to 7 nm) connecting filaments extend from the terminal thin filaments through the electron-dense intracellular layer into the extracellular basement membrane. The connecting filaments therefore traverse the plasma membrane and transmit tension from the myofibrils to the basal lamina.[96] Alterations that would be interpreted as abnormal elsewhere in the muscle fiber occur at the normal myotendinous junction. These include leptomere formations, duplication of Z disks, nemaline rods,[76] lipofuscin granules, and internal nuclei (Fig. 31-52B).

MISCELLANEOUS INCLUSIONS

Filamentous bodies. These are oblong or ovoid structures ranging from less than 1 μm to a few microns in length and from about 0.3 to more than 1 μm in width. They are typically subsarcolemmal and either abut on the myofibrils or are surrounded by glycogen. Occasionally mitochondria, Golgi membranes, or lipofuscin granules appear near the formations (Fig. 31-53A). The formations consist of densely packed, parallel 6-nm filaments that resemble thin filaments (Fig. 31-53B) and, in favorable sections, are continuous with thin filaments emanating from I bands of adjacent sarcomeres (Fig. 31-53C). Thus the filamentous body is a proliferative anomaly of the thin filaments. Filamentous bodies occur infrequently and lack pathologic significance or specificity.

Concentric laminated bodies. These occur in a variety of neuromuscular disorders (for reviews see Refs. 97 and 98) and especially in type 2 fibers.[97] The inclusions are about 0.2 to 1 μm wide and 1 to 3 μm long, and randomly oriented inclusions appear in subsarcolemmal aggregates of varying size (Fig. 31-54). Most inclusions surround a cytoplasmic core filled with glycogen particles, and glycogen particles usually surround the inclusions. The walls of the inclusions consist of spiraling 6- to 8-nm filaments separated by 7- to 10-nm intervals. In favorable sections one can note that the filaments are studded with twin subunit densities at 22- to 24-nm intervals (Fig. 31-54B).[98] The twin subunits are separated by a 3-nm gap, and each subunit rests on a 6-nm base and projects 6 to 9 nm away from the filament. Subunits on adjacent filaments are in register and project in the same direction. When the filaments are examined at different tilt angles, superimposition of adjacent filaments and their sub-

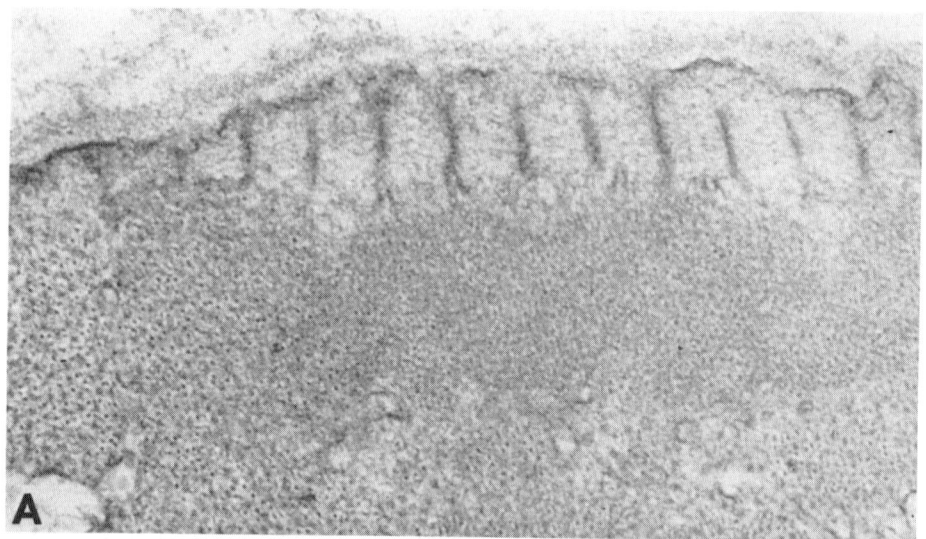
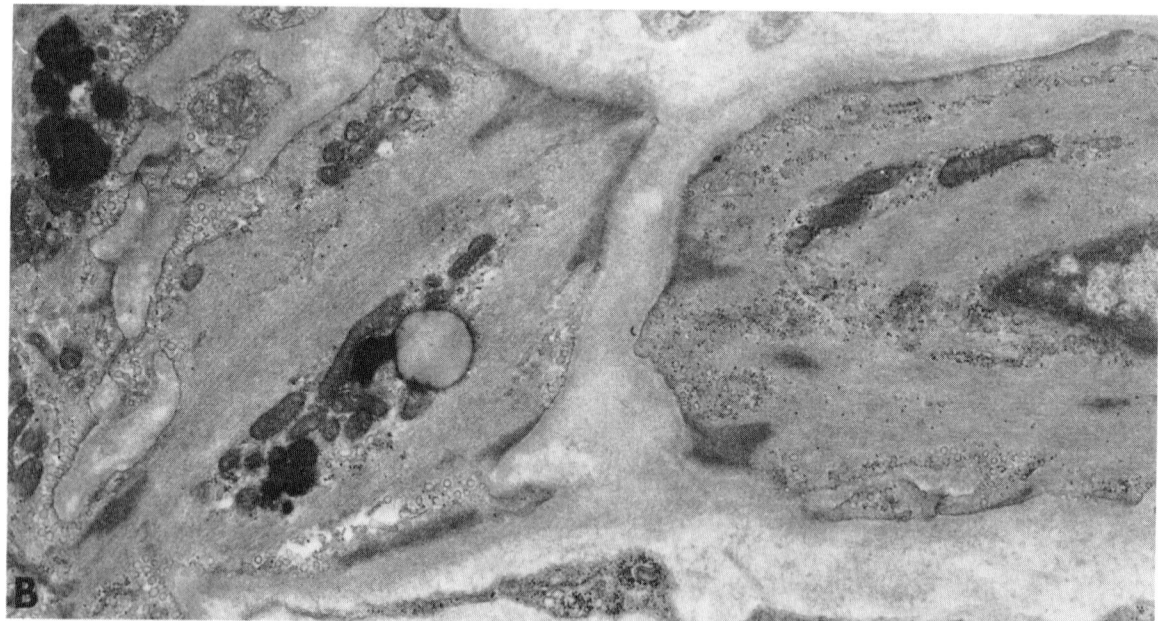

FIGURE 31-52. *A.* Leptomere (microladder) formation in intrafusal muscle fiber, ×65,300. *B.* Myotendinous junction. Note lipofuscin granules, central nucleus, and numerous subsarcolemmal caveolae. The collagen fibrils in the connective tissue are unstained. ×16,400. *[A is reproduced by permission from Banker BQ, Girvin JP, in Banker BQ, Przybylski RJ, Van Der Meulen JP, Victor M (eds): Research in Muscle Development and the Muscle Spindle, Excerpta Medica ICS 240:267, 1972.]*

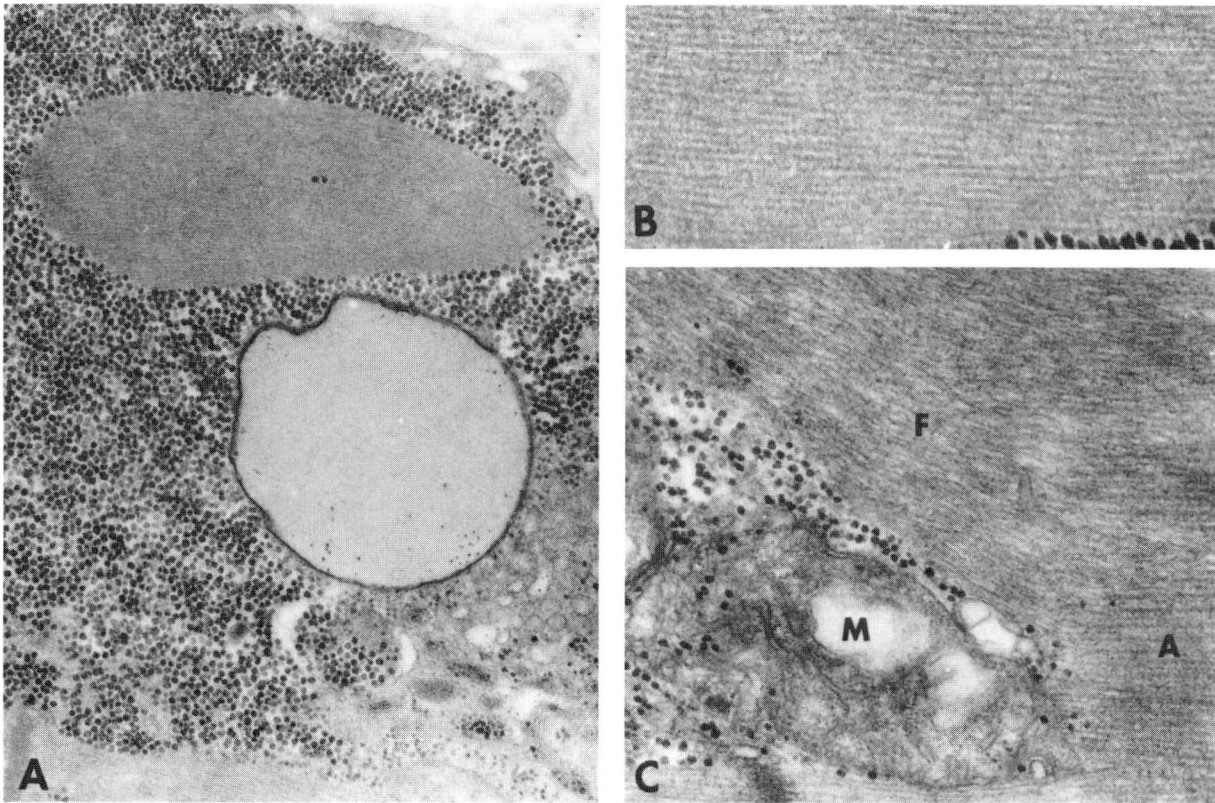

FIGURE 31-53. Filamentous bodies in Kearns-Sayre syndrome. In A, the abnormal formation is surrounded by glycogen particles and is close to a lipofuscin granule. In B, the filaments of the filamentous body are rectilinear and about 6 nm in diameter. In C, the filaments in the filamentous body (F) are continuous with thin filaments in I bands of adjacent sarcomeres. A, A band; M, mitochondrion. A, ×33,200; B, ×106,600; C, ×49,600.

units within the depth of the section produces a pattern of striations that reflects the spacings of the subunits (Fig. 31-55). The concentric laminated bodies had been originally described in the mitochondrial myopathy associated with extrathyroidal hypermetabolism and had been thought to be mitochondrial in origin.[99] Other workers have observed that thin filaments terminate in the inclusions.[97] We have observed that inclusions arise from or are attached to the A bands of myofibrils (Fig. 31-54C). The protein composition of the inclusions is not known.

Fingerprint bodies. These structures show no enzyme activity in frozen sections and resemble myofibrils in their staining properties with the hematoxylin-eosin and trichrome stains. In phase optics they appear as dense, irregularly oval or circular inclusions, usually subsarcolemmal and frequently juxtanuclear, varying from 0.5 to 10 μm in length and from 0.4 to 4 μm in width. In the electron microscope they are composed of convoluted, complex lamellae arranged in fingerprint patterns (Fig. 31-56).[100] The lamellae are spaced 30 to 36 nm apart and consist of sawtooth-like projections, about 6 nm wide and 16 nm high, spaced at intervals of 14 to 16 nm (Figs. 31-56, 31-57). Adjacent projections in a given lamella point in the same direction, but projections of adjacent lamellae point in different directions (Fig. 31-57). Some of the fingerprint bodies abut on myofibrils, and some appear in the midst of whirling filamentous profiles.[100]

The fingerprint bodies are different from the curvilinear fingerprint-like lysosomal profiles observed in chloroquine myopathy[101] and in neural, muscle, and other cells in neuronal ceroid lipofuscinosis (see Chap. 30).

The fingerprint bodies cannot be extracted from glycerinated muscle fibers by a low-ionic-strength solution that extracts material from the M band and Z disks or by solutions that extract either the thick filaments or the thin filaments.[100] These findings suggest that the fingerprint body consists of normal or abnormal cytoskeletal protein(s).

Numerous fingerprint bodies were first observed in type 1 fibers in a patient with congenital myopathy associated with type 1 fiber atrophy and predominance[100]; they were also abundant in other patients with benign congenital myopathies[101a–104] and appear to be specific for type 1 fibers.[104] Fingerprint bodies occur infrequently in other disorders, such as oculopharyngeal dystrophy,[105] myotonic dystrophy, and other myopathies.[106,107]

Inclusions in myofibrillar myopathy. The microscopic features consist of multiple abnormal fiber regions of varying shape and size within which normal myofibrillar markings are replaced by amorphous or granular material or by spherical or irregularly curving hyaline structures (Figs.

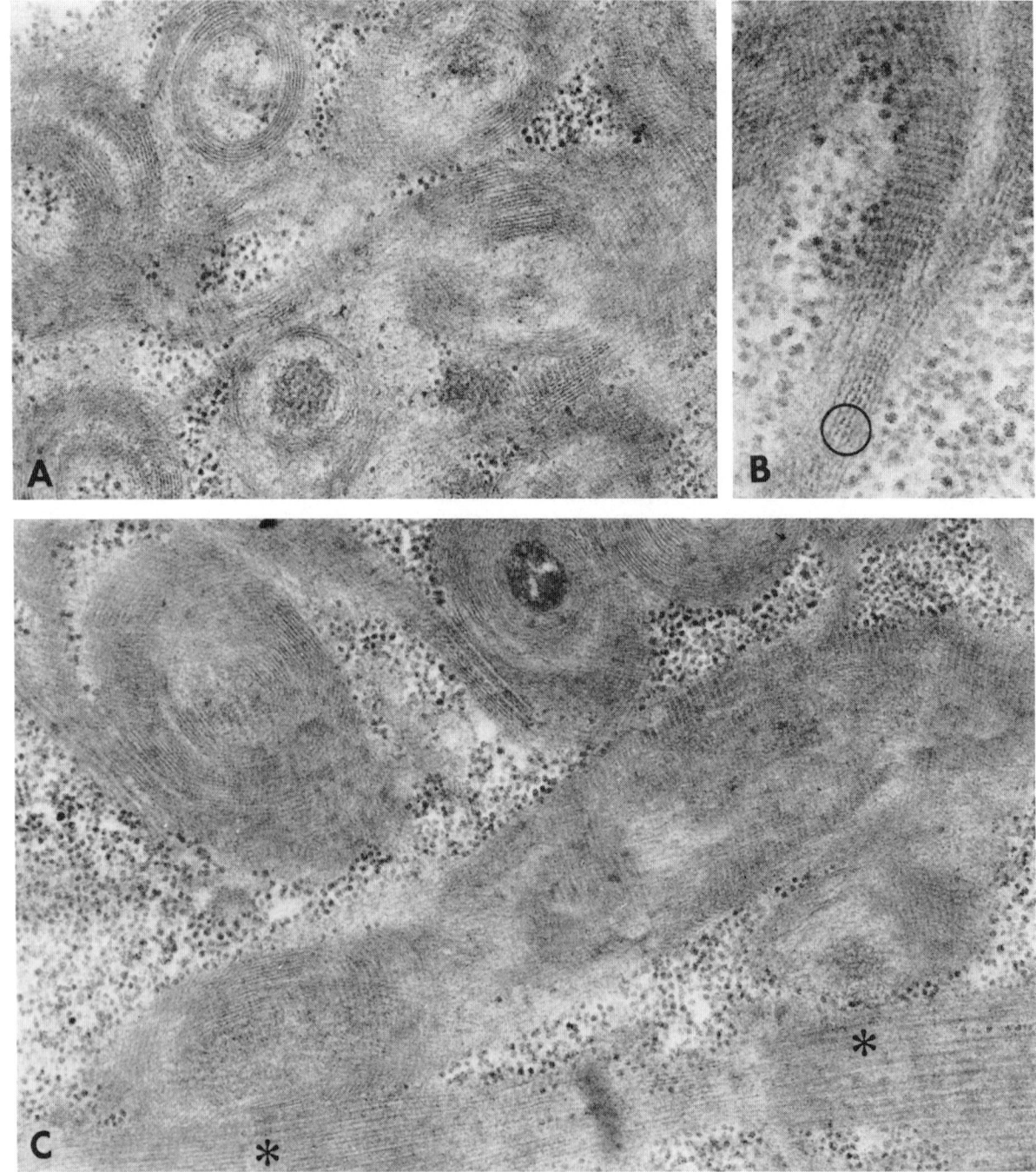

FIGURE 31-54. Concentric laminated bodies in juvenile spinal muscular atrophy. Glycogen granules surround and appear in the center of the abnormal formations. The laminated bodies consist of filaments that display periodic twin subunit densities (circle in B). In C, the concentric laminated bodies abut on and appear to merge with A bands (asterisks). A, ×24,600; B, ×66,500; C, ×44,000.

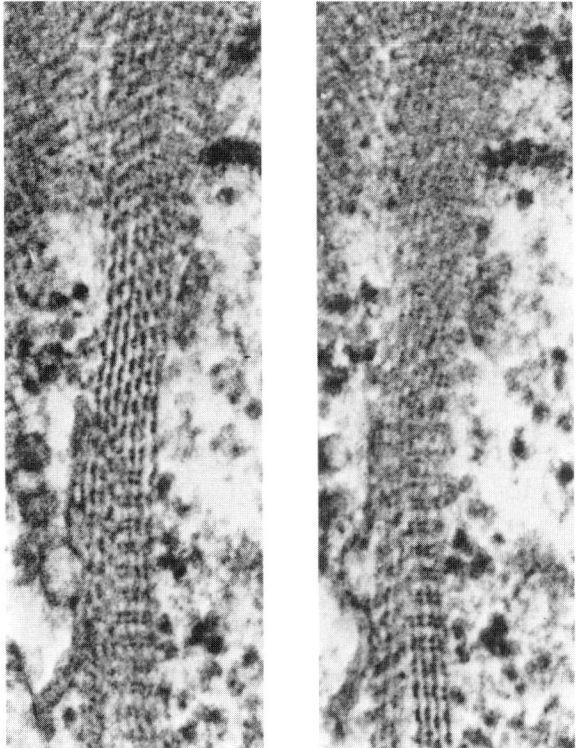

FIGURE 31-55. Stereo-pair electron micrographs of concentric laminated body. The tilt angle difference between the two micrographs is 52°. Comparison of the two figures indicates that the striations in the laminated bodies are due to superimposition of adjacent filaments and their subunits within the depth of the section. ×115,000.

31-58A, E, and 31-59). The majority of the abnormal fiber regions react positively for desmin (Fig. 31-58B and C), myotilin, αB-crystallin, dystrophin, and NCAM, and many abnormal deposits are congophilic (Color Plate 10). Other frequently associated features consist of rimmed vacuoles and signs of denervation atrophy. The disorder presents in children or adults, is sporadic or inherited, and can be associated with peripheral neuropathy and cardiomyopathy.[107a,108,109,109a] The earliest lesions arise from the Z disk (Figs. 31-58D and 31-60C) and are composed of a fine filamentous network (Fig. 31-60C), granulofilamentous material (Fig. 31-60A and B), or circular deposits speckled with material of Z-disk density (Fig. 31-60D). Immunocytochemical and ultrastructural analysis of the hyaline structures reveals that they comprise degraded remnants of myofibrils.[108,109,109a] Recent studies have revealed genetic heterogeneity of myofibrillar myopathy. Some cases are caused by mutations in desmin[110–112] or αB-crystallin[113]; other cases are linked to different chromosomal loci.[113a] The genetic background of the majority of cases remains undeciphered. Chapter 43 presents a detailed discussion of myofibrillar myopathy.

Myosine storage myopathy, alias hyaline body myopathy. The hyaline bodies occur subsarcolemmally in type 1 fibers, stain green with the modified trichrome stain, and lack reactivity for glycogen or oxidative enzymes. They extend up to 50 μm in length or width, retain reactivity for myofibrillar ATPase, and are sometimes surrounded by a halo of increased reactivity for glycogen and oxidative enzymes (Fig. 31-61). Ultrastructurally, the hyaline bodies consist of fine filamentous or granular material (Fig. 31-62). Rare mitochondria, sparse glycogen granules, and occasional T-system networks occur within the hyaline bodies (Fig. 31-62A and C), and some are surrounded by mitochondria and glycogen granules (Fig. 31-62B). Hyaline bodies were observed by us in 10 to 15 percent of the muscle fibers of a patient who had an adult-onset, slowly progressive neuromyopathy, scapuloperoneal distribution of weakness, and electrical but no clinical myotonia. The hyaline bodies were present in hypertrophic but not in atrophic fibers. Essentially identical structures in type 1 fibers were described by Sahgal and Sahgal in a patient with a nonprogressive congenital myopathy in which there was absence of the sternocleidomastoid and middle trapezius muscles and scapuloperoneal distribution of weakness.[114] Masuzugawa and coworkers observed the same structures in a dominantly inherited scapuloperoneal syndrome,[114a] whereas Barohn and coworkers identified them as the predominant pathologic finding in two unrelated patients with nonprogressive congenital muscle weakness.[114b]

Ultrastructurally, the hyaline bodies resemble the abnormal fiber regions in the congenital myopathy attributed to abnormal lysis of myofibrils in type 1 fibers.[91a] The formations attributed to focal lysis of the myofibrils and the hyaline bodies described by Sahgal and Sahgal[114] are the end result of a similar pathologic process. Immunocytochemical studies reveal that the hyaline bodies react strongly for the slow but not for the fast type of myosin heavy chain.[114a] This disorder was recently shown to be a myosin storage myopathy caused by a dominant mutation (R1845W) in MYH7 that encodes the slow/β cardiac myosin heavy chain I expressed in type 1 fibers in skeletal muscle and in cardiac muscle. The mutation is in the rod region of the myosin heavy chain and does not cause cardiomyopathy, indicating that the mutated residue is important for myosin assembly in skeletal but not in cardiac muscle.[114c]

Sarcoplasmic protein crystals. These crystals occur mainly in type 2 muscle fibers. The crystals are nonbirefringent, eosinophilic, stain bright red with the modified trichrome stain, react strongly for tyrosine, and are removed by tryptic digestion. In the electron microscope the crystals appear rhomboid or rectangular in shape, lack orientation, and are less than 5 μm long. They are not membrane-bound and have a compact granular substructure with no discernible periodicity (Fig. 31-63).[115] These crystals were an isolated morphologic finding in about 3 percent of the muscle fibers of an adult who had diffuse aches and muscle fatigue unrelated to exertion.[115] The crystals resemble the cystine crystals detected in fibroblasts in nephropathic cystinosis,[115a] but in this disease cystine crystals do not appear in the muscle fibers, and the patient whose muscle fibers contained the crystals shown in Fig. 31-63 had no signs of nephropathic cystinosis. Recent studies indicate that these crystals in muscle immunostain for tubulin and may thus be a consequence of a defect in tubulin synthesis, processing, or degradation.[115b]

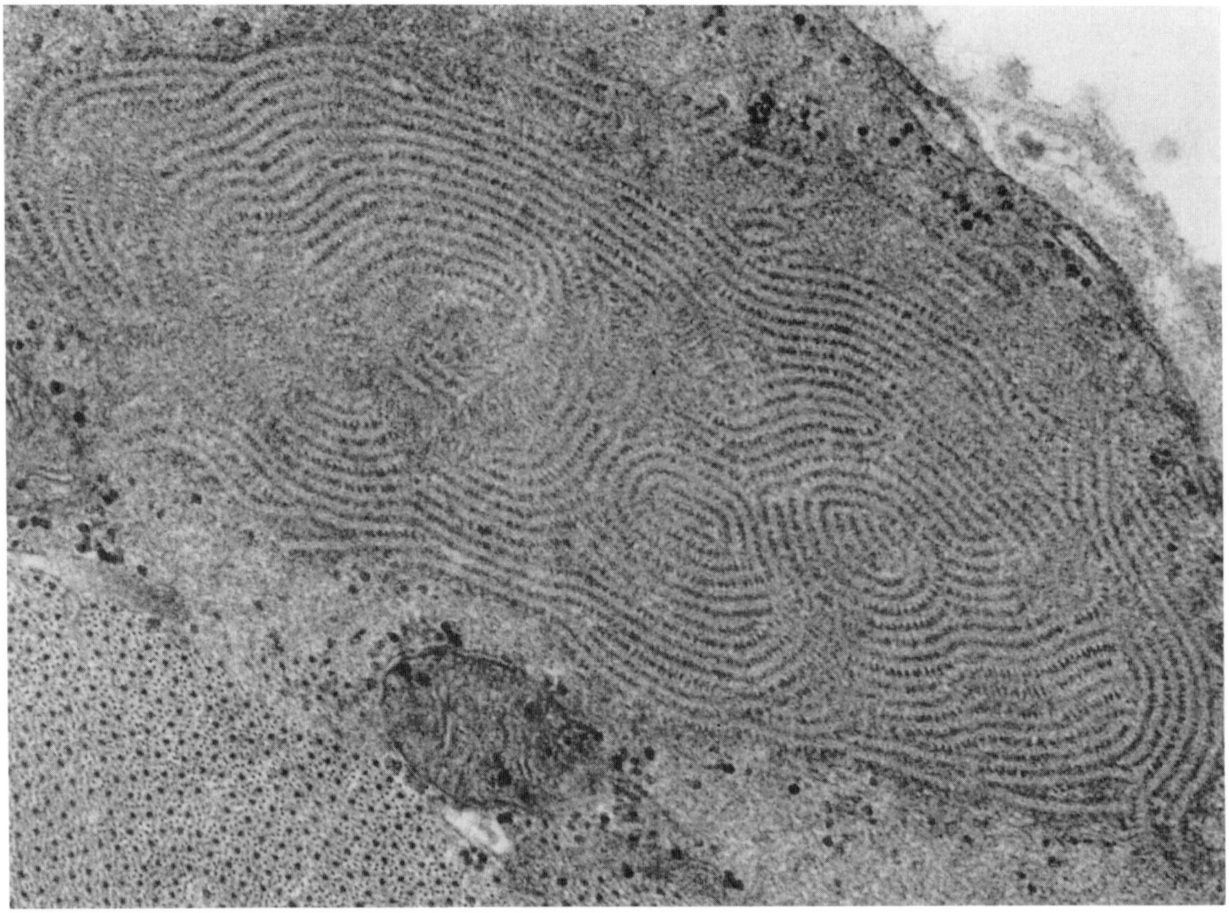

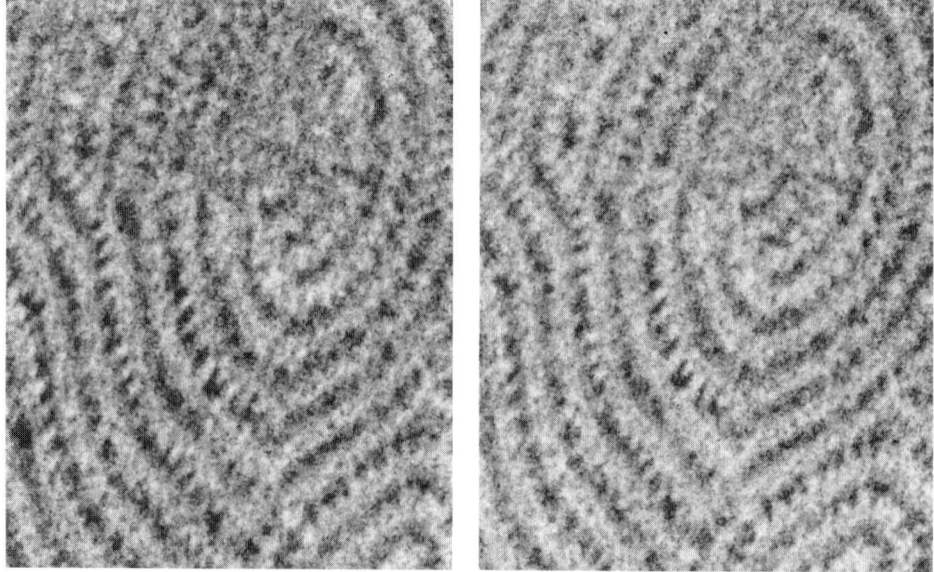

FIGURE 31-56. Fingerprint body in congenital fingerprint body myopathy, ×58,800. *(Reproduced by permission from Engel AG, Angelini C, Gomez M, Mayo Clin Proc 47:377, 1972.)*

FIGURE 31-57. Stereo-pair electron micrographs of fingerprint body. The tilt angle difference between the two micrographs is 12°. ×170,800. *(Reproduced by permission from Engel AG, Angelini C, Gomez M, Mayo Clin Proc 47:377, 1972.)*

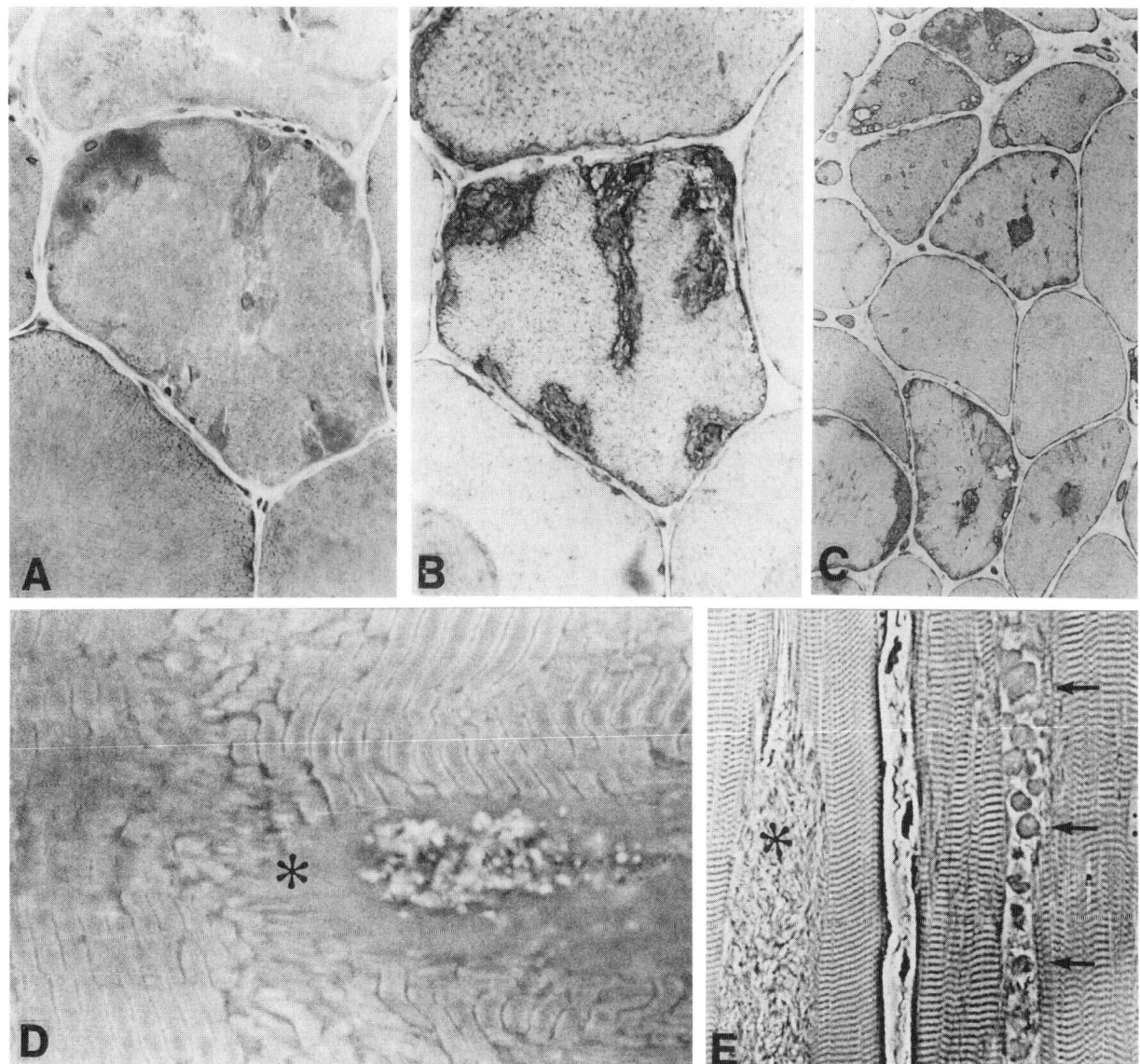

FIGURE 31-58. Myofibrillar myopathy. Cryostat sections stained with trichrome (A) and immunoreacted for desmin (B and C). A trichromatically stained muscle fiber harbors multiple abnormal regions filled with homogeneous material (A); the abnormal deposits are strongly desmin-positive (B). A low-power view reveals desmin-positive regions of varied shape and size in most muscle fibers (C). D and E. Semithin resin sections viewed in phase optics. In D, homogeneous material emanating from Z disks (asterisk) fills a large region in the center of the fiber. Multiple small vacuoles appear in the center of this region. In E, fiber on the left contains a central zone filled with small, irregularly shaped and oriented optically dense structures (asterisk); fiber on the right harbors multiple spheroid bodies (arrows). A and B, ×260; C, ×105; D, ×1800; E, ×450.

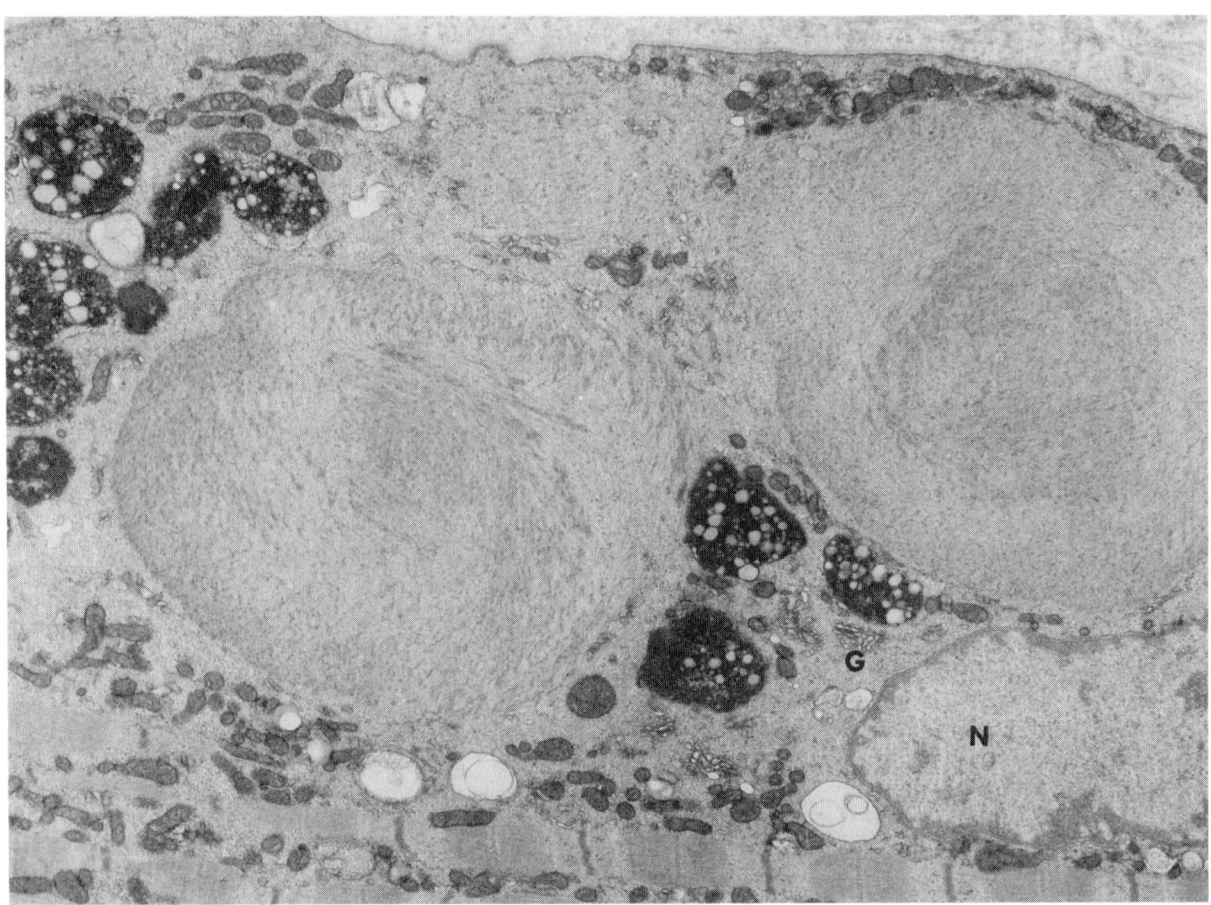

FIGURE 31-59. Two large subsarcolemmal spheroid bodies surrounded by glycogen granules, lipofuscin bodies, and mitochondria. Note streaks and speckles of dense material within the spheroids. G, Golgi system; N, nucleus. ×9300.

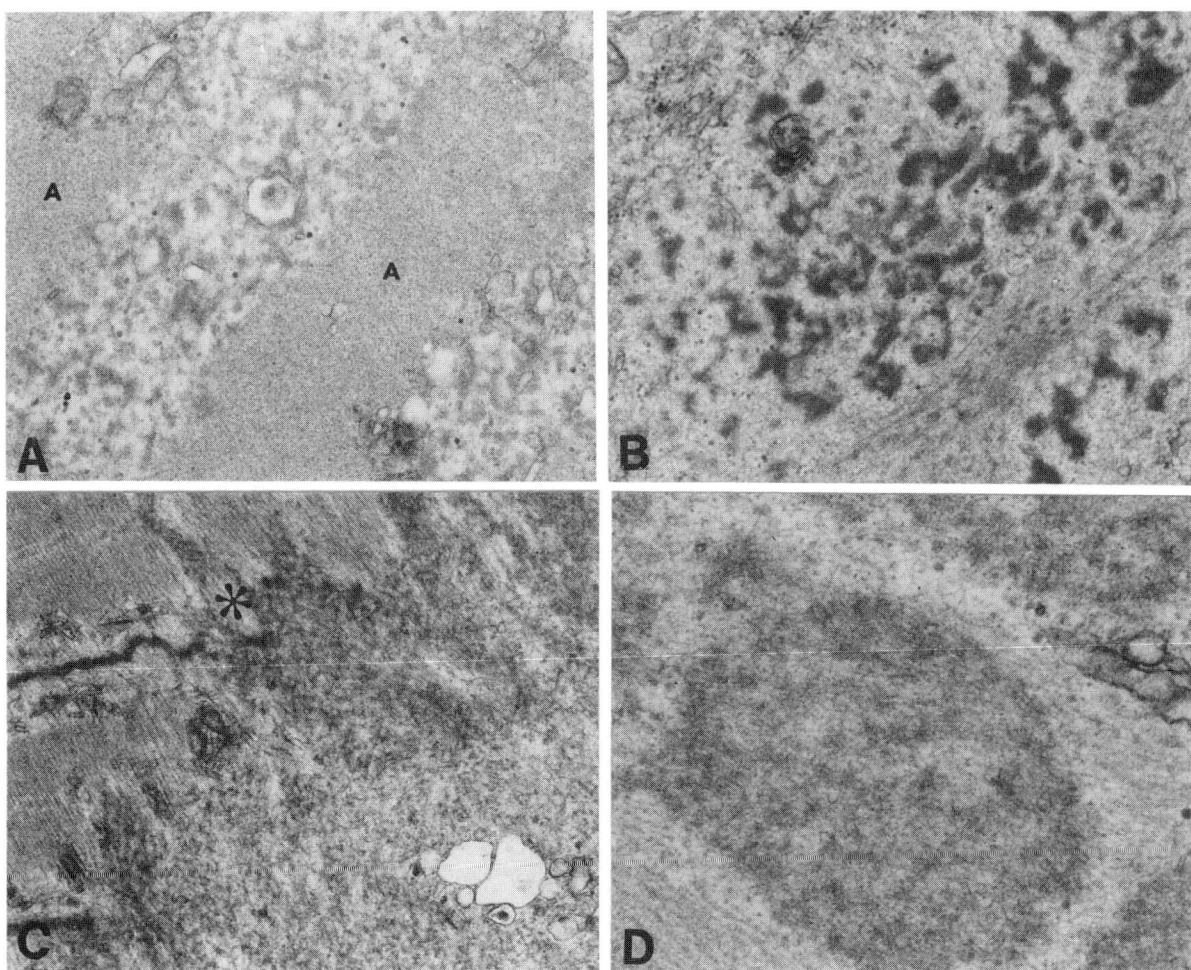

FIGURE 31-60. *A* and *B*. Small, irregularly shaped deposits of the same or higher density than Z disks are accumulating between the myofibrils. *C*. Osmiophilic material emanating from the Z disk (asterisk) is contiguous with a lake of granular and finely filamentous material. This field represents the electron microscopic image of the region marked with an asterisk in Fig. 31-58D. *D*. Circular abnormal deposit speckled with material of Z-disk density intermingled with fine filaments. *A*, ×33,700; *B*, ×25,900; *C*, ×15,500; *D*, ×57,000.

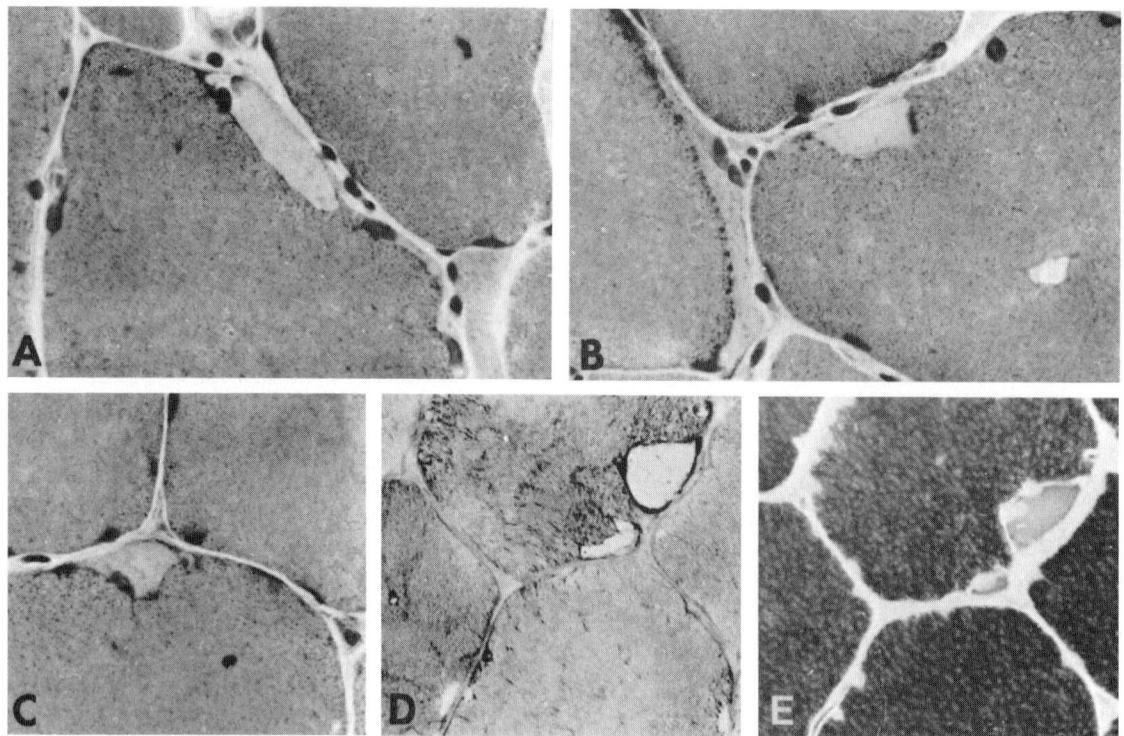

FIGURE 31-61. Cryostat sections of hyaline bodies in patient with hyaline body myopathy. In trichromatically stained sections (A, B, and C), the hyaline bodies are light and show no intermyofibrillar membranous network. In NADH dehydrogenase reacted section (D), increased enzyme activity appears around the inclusions. In the ATPase reaction after preincubation at pH 4.3 (E), the inclusions display weak enzyme activity. A, B, and C, ×430; D and E, ×270.

Cylindrical spirals. These interesting inclusions were first observed in 1979 and have been reported a few times since then.[116–120b] They typically appear in type 2B fibers[119] and tend to form subsarcolemmal clusters that extend parallel to the long fiber axis. The clusters are 5 to 30 μm wide and 10 to 300 μm long, and more than one cluster can occur in a given fiber (Fig. 31-64). In frozen sections the clusters stain bright red[116] or dark purple[117,119] with the modified trichrome stain and may thus mimic nemaline rods, acquire the brown color of monoformazan in the NADH dehydrogenase reaction, do not react for succinic dehydrogenase, and stain lightly in the periodic acid–Schiff (PAS) reaction.[116]

In phase optics the individual inclusions are rod-like, measuring 1 to 2 μm in diameter and up to 10 μm in length, and are positioned with their long axis parallel or oblique to that of the fiber (Fig. 31-64).

In the electron microscope the inclusions consist of spiraling membranous lamellae. Transversely sectioned inclusions display from 6 to 30 lamellae wrapped around a central cytoplasmic core that contains glycogen granules and a few vesicles (Fig. 31-65A). The most peripherally placed lamellae are connected by a mesaxon-like structure to a surrounding membranous envelope, or are structurally continuous with tubules and vesicles of undetermined origin (Fig. 31-65A), or are surrounded by glycogen granules (Fig. 31-65B), or abut on myofibrils. In longitudinally sectioned inclusions the lamellae are arranged in parallel stacks on either side of the central cytoplasmic core; each lamella ends in a club-like expansion, and the outer lamellae are shorter than the inner lamellae (Fig. 31-65B). The origin of the cylindrical spirals has not been determined. They are not continuous with the extracellular space and hence are not of T-system origin.[116] Each half of a longitudinally sectioned cylindrical spiral resembles a stack of Golgi cisternae, but the transversely sectioned inclusions do not resemble Golgi cisternae. In one patient the cylindrical spirals appeared in the midst of tubular aggregates, suggesting that they may have arisen from a component of the SR.[120a]

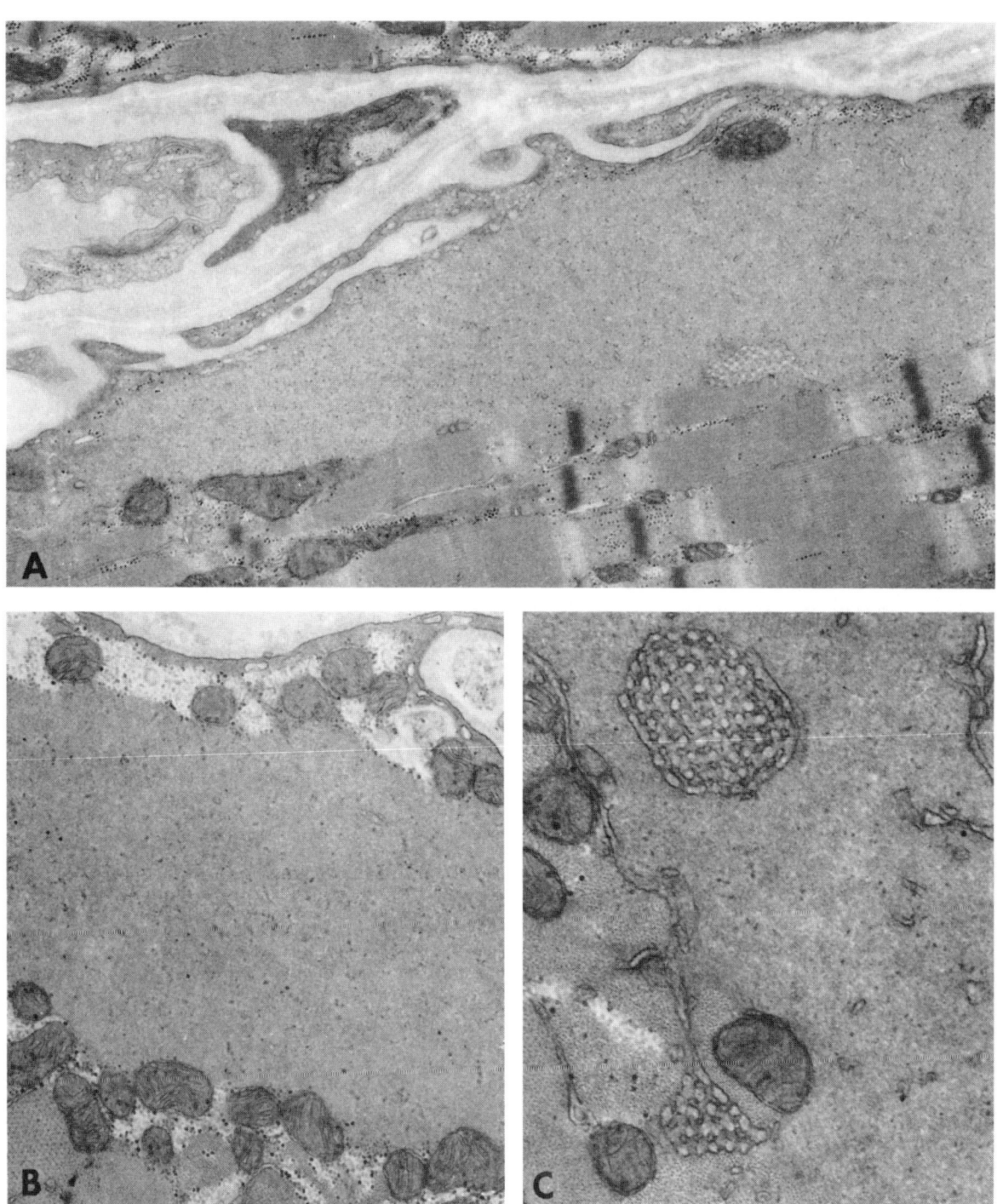

FIGURE 31-62. Hyaline bodies in patient with hyaline body myopathy. The hyaline bodies contain no recognizable myofibrils. Mitochondria and glycogen granules surround and seldom penetrate the abnormal formations *(A* and *B)*. T-system networks and other tubular profiles are found in some of the hyaline bodies *(C)*. A, ×20,000; B, ×31,900; C, ×50,600.

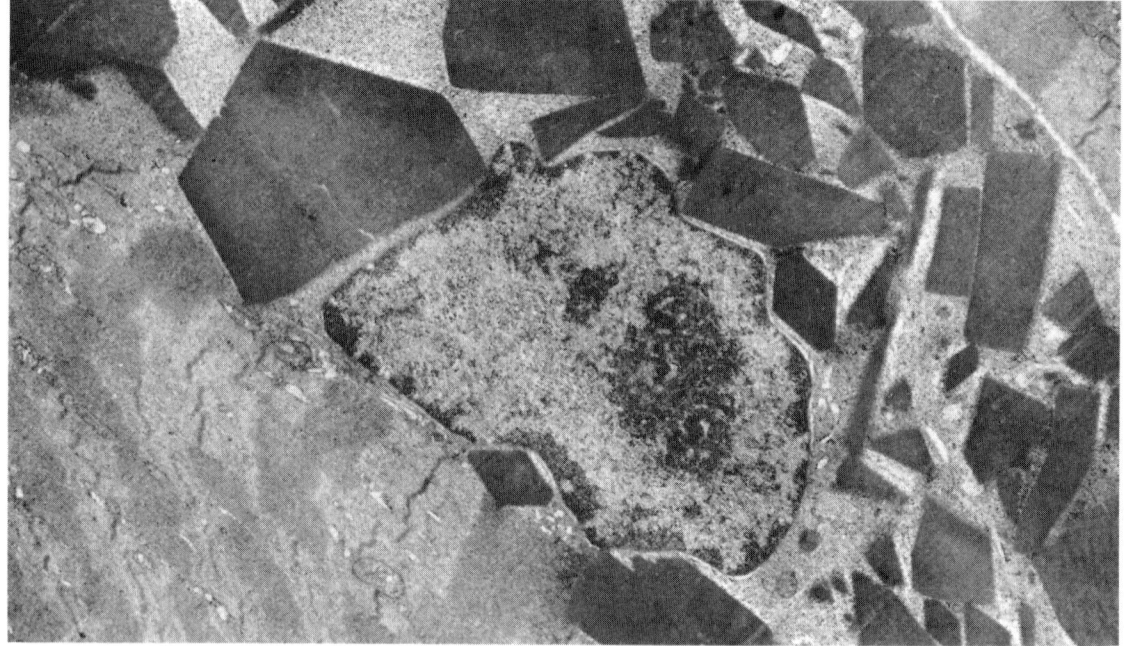

FIGURE 31-63. Sarcoplasmic protein crystals in a patient with diffuse muscle aches and fatigue unrelated to exertion. ×7100. Courtesy of Dr. Abraham Eastwood.

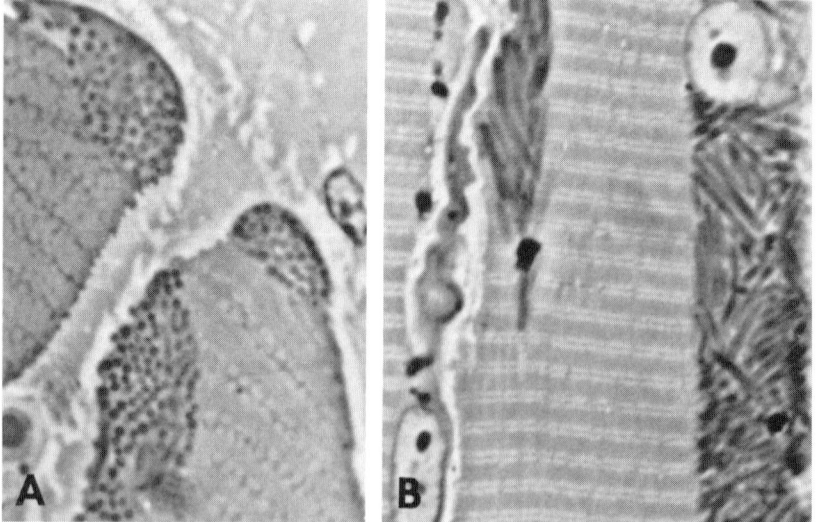

FIGURE 31-64. Cylindrical spirals demonstrated in semithin resin sections stained with para-phenylenediamine. *A* and *B*, ×1500. Courtesy of Dr. Ellen Gibbels. *(Reproduced by permission from Gibbels E, Henke U, Schädlich H-J, et al, Muscle Nerve 6:646–655, 1983.)*

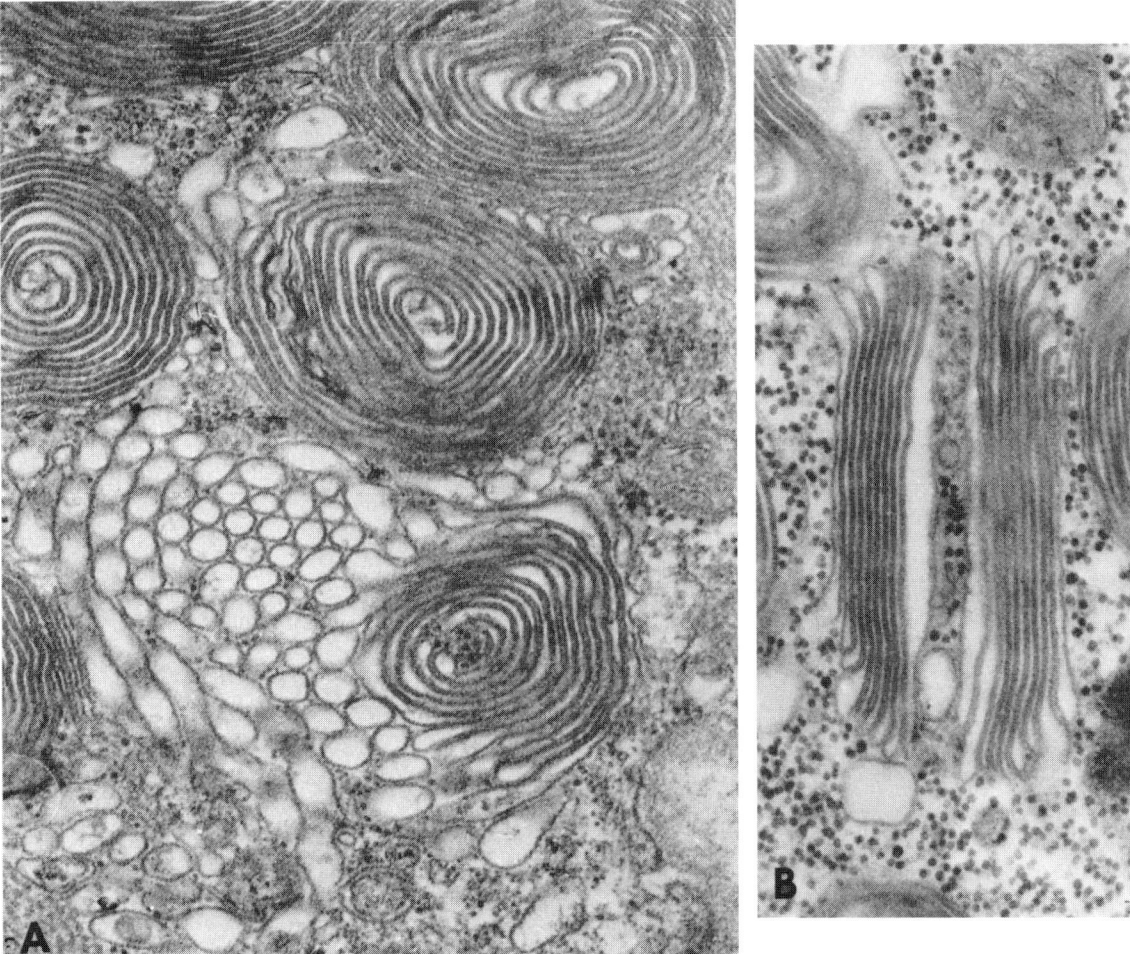

FIGURE 31-65. Cylindrical spirals. In *A*, the cylindrical spirals are in continuity with abundant tubular structures of unknown origin. In *B*, sarcoplasmic material extends into the center of a longitudinally sectioned cylindrical spiral. *A*, ×52,000; *B*, ×60,000. Courtesy of Dr. Ellen Gibbels. *(Reproduced by permission from Gibbels E, Henke U, Schädlich H-J, et al, Muscle Nerve 6:646, 1983.)*

Cylindrical spirals have been observed in a variety of disorders: muscle cramps and malignancy[116]; an unusual form of spinocerebellar degeneration[116]; a dominant disorder associated with myotonia, cramps, and myalgias[117]; a case of myalgia with tubular aggregates[120a]; melorheostosis[118]; polyneuropathy and muscle stiffness[119]; a mitochondrial myopathy[120]; a late-onset autosomal dominant neuromyopathy associated with muscle pain, stiffness, and weakness[120b]; and an asymptomatic patient with a high serum creatine kinase level.[120c]

Lipofuscin. In the light microscope, lipofuscin appears in the form of small yellow-brown subsarcolemmal and perinuclear granules. The granules are autofluorescent and PAS-positive but diastase-fast and react for acid phosphatase (see Chap. 30). In the electron microscope, lipofuscin granules appear oval, oblong, or irregular in shape; vary from a fraction of a micron to several microns in diameter; and have heterogeneous contents (Fig. 31-66). Four components appear in most lipofuscin granules: (1) a finely granular matrix of low electron density; (2) homogeneous droplets of low electron density that resemble lipid droplets but are surrounded by a thin rim of more electron-dense material; (3) 8- to 50-nm globules of moderate to high electron density; and (4) finely granular material of high electron density. The different components are present in varying proportions in different lipofuscin granules (Fig. 31-66) or in different sections of the same granule, and some components may be missing in a given plane of sectioning. Lipofuscin granules are often partly or completely surrounded by a single continuous or discontinuous membrane.

Lipofuscin granules represent residual bodies remaining after lysosomal degradation of normal or abnormal organelles. Only sparse lipofuscin granules are found in normal muscle in young adults (Fig. 31-3*A*). The granules increase in

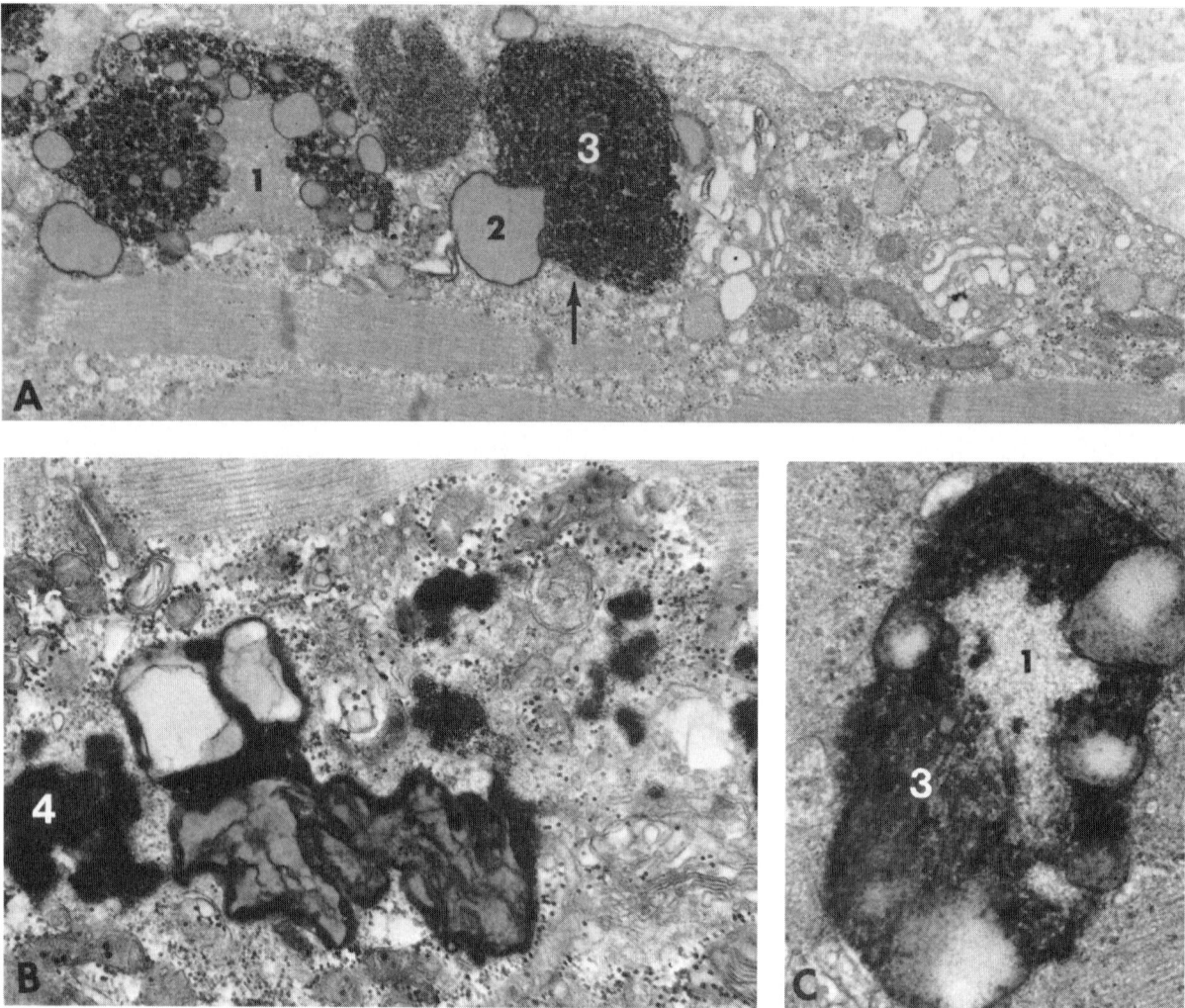

FIGURE 31-66. Lipofuscin granules in inflammatory myopathies. Numbers refer to different types of granule components described in the text. A, ×20,000; B, ×26,000; C, ×65,000.

size and number with age, denervation atrophy (Figs. 31-81D, 31-86D), and various myopathies and are conspicuous in some lysosomal disorders, as in Fabry disease and Batten disease. However, in the latter disorders other and more specific structures (e.g., curvilinear bodies in neuronal lipofuscinosis) also appear in muscle. These inclusions are described in Chap. 30.

Giant lysosomes in human vitamin E deficiency. The giant lysosomes in vitamin E deficiency share with lipofuscin granules the cytochemical features of secondary lysosomes (autofluorescence and reactivity for acid phosphatase and glycolipids) but differ from lipofuscin granules in size, shape, ultrastructural components, and position in the muscle fiber.[121,123–125] The giant lysosomes are consistently oval or oblong in shape, range from 0.7 to 7 μm in length and from 0.5 to 1.5 μm in width, and appear in single files between the myofibrils with their long axis parallel to that of the myofibrils (Fig. 31-67 inset). Ultrastructurally, these bodies are membrane-bound and contain only one type of highly electron-dense and finely granular material (Fig. 31-67A and C). The smallest formations arise from degenerating mitochondria (Fig. 31-67B).[121] The electron-dense content of the giant lysosomes resembles that of peroxisomes, but the giant lysosomes react for acid phosphatase (Fig. 31-67D and E), whereas peroxisomes react for catalase but not for acid phosphatase.[122]

The giant lysosomes in human vitamin E deficiency were first described in a woman with progressive ataxia, peripheral neuropathy, retinal degeneration, hypoparathyroidism, and malabsorption, but serum vitamin E levels were not determined in the patient at the time of the report.[121] Subsequent studies demonstrated identical bodies in human muscle in vitamin E deficiency due to any cause,[123–125] and when the patient in whom these inclusions were first noted was restudied, she also was found to have a markedly decreased level of serum vitamin E (M. R. Gomez and A. G. Engel, unpublished data).

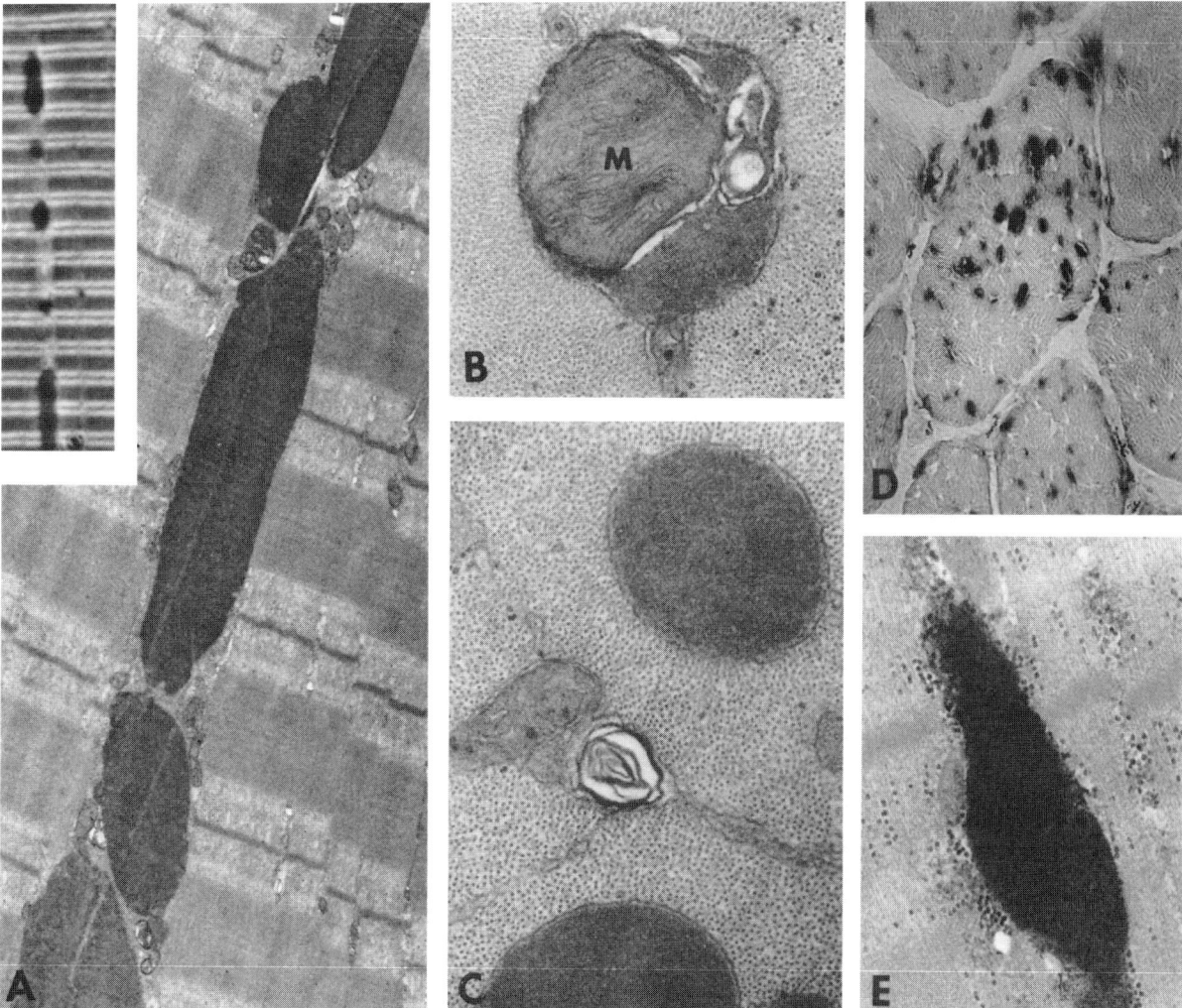

FIGURE 31-67. Giant abnormal lysosomes in human vitamin E deficiency. Inset in A is phase micrograph. The elongated lysosomes are axially oriented in the fibers (A and E), are membrane-bound (C), arise from mitochondria (B), and react for acid phosphatase light microscopically (D) and electron cytochemically (E). Inset for A, ×1350; A, ×10,000; B and C, ×52,300; D, ×400; E, ×34,800. (Reproduced by permission from Gomez MR, Engel AG, Dyck PJ, Neurology 22:849, 1972.)

Microtubular (microreticular) inclusions in the endoplasmic reticulum. These inclusions are composed of 18- to 26-nm undulating, osmiophilic tubules that form networks ranging from 0.4 to more than 4 μm in size (Fig. 31-68). The networks occur within dilated cisternae of the smooth endoplasmic reticulum and originate as invaginations of the endoplasmic reticulum membrane.[126] In human muscle they appear in dermatomyositis[2,127–129] and systemic lupus erythematosus[127] in endothelial cells (Figs. 31-68C and D, 31-131) and less frequently in pericytes, satellite cells (Fig. 31-68A), and myoblasts (Fig. 31-68B). The networks also occur within endothelial cells of blood vessels within skin, kidney, and synovial tissues in patients with various autoimmune disorders, especially systemic lupus erythematosus; in endothelial cells and macrophages in the brain in herpes simplex encephalitis; in human tumor cells; in lymphocytes exposed to 5-bromo-2-deoxyuridine; in hepatocytes of suckling mice treated with mouse α/β interferon,[129a] in cultured human endothelial cells treated with recombinant interferon[129b]; in small intestinal absorptive cells of mice following a high fructose load; and in young cells of the normal cotton plant (for reviews see Refs. 2, 126, and 130 to 132). Abundant microtubular inclusions were detected in endothelial and mononuclear cells in several tissues of 10 patients with the clinical features of AIDS (acquired immunodeficiency syndrome),[133] and leukocyte interferon has been implicated in the formation of the inclusions.[134] The suggestion that these inclusions are viral structures[130] has never been confirmed. However, the inclusions could represent a host cell response to virus(es), to increased levels of serum α interferon, to circulating immune complexes, or to a combination of these factors.[133]

Reducing bodies. These are round to irregularly oval structures from a few microns to about 30 μm in diameter found adjacent to nuclei or between myofibrils. In frozen

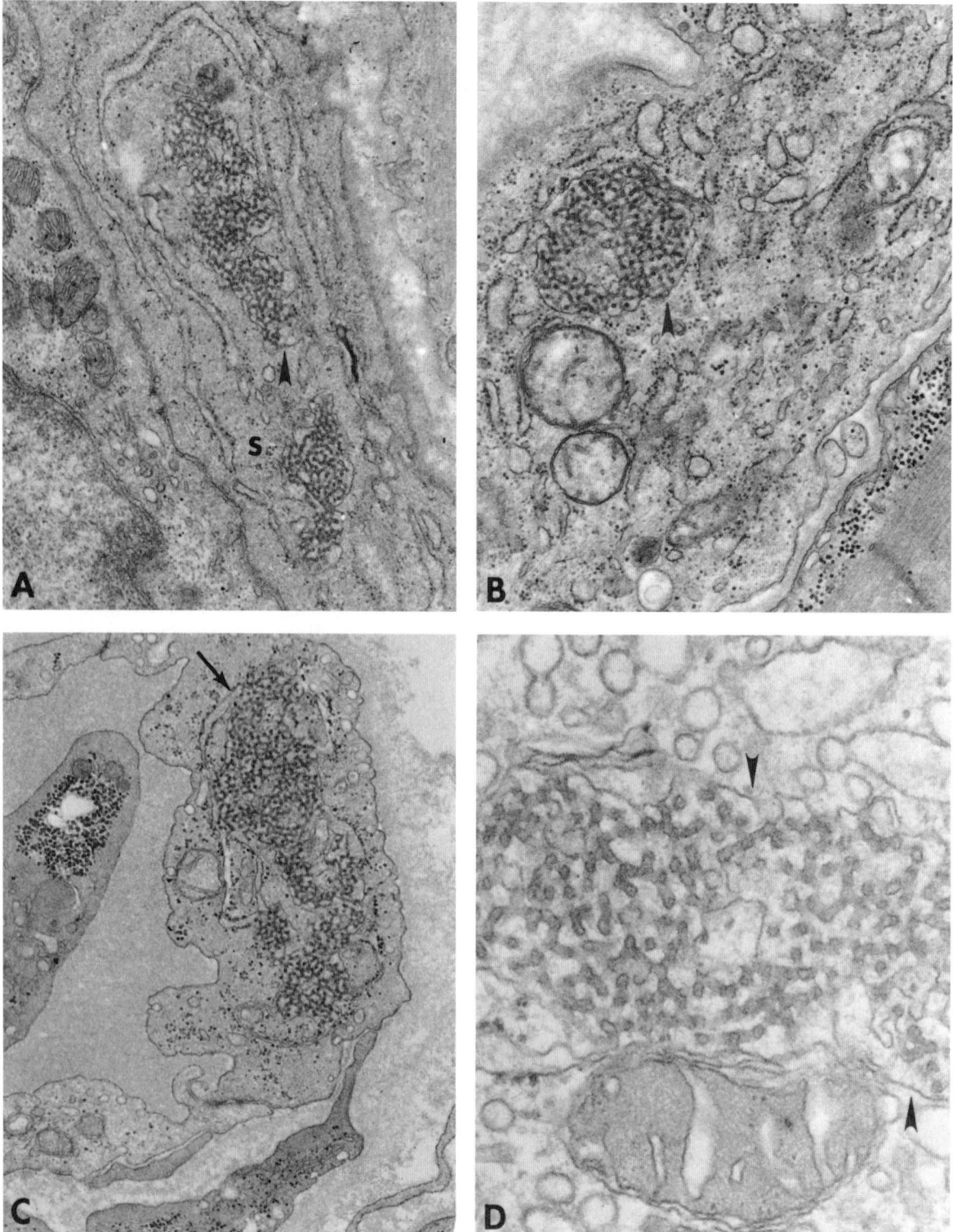

FIGURE 31-68. Microtubular inclusions in dermatomyositis in satellite cell *(A)*, myoblast *(B)*, and capillary endothelium *(C and D)*. Inclusions are surrounded in part by membranes of the endoplasmic reticulum (arrowheads in *A, B,* and *D*) and appear close to rough endoplasmic reticulum profiles (arrow in *C*). A, ×21,800; B, ×26,900; C, ×21,600; D, ×85,700. *(C and D are reproduced by permission from Jerusalem F, Rakusa M, Engel AG, Macdonald RD, J Neurol Sci 23:391, 1974.)*

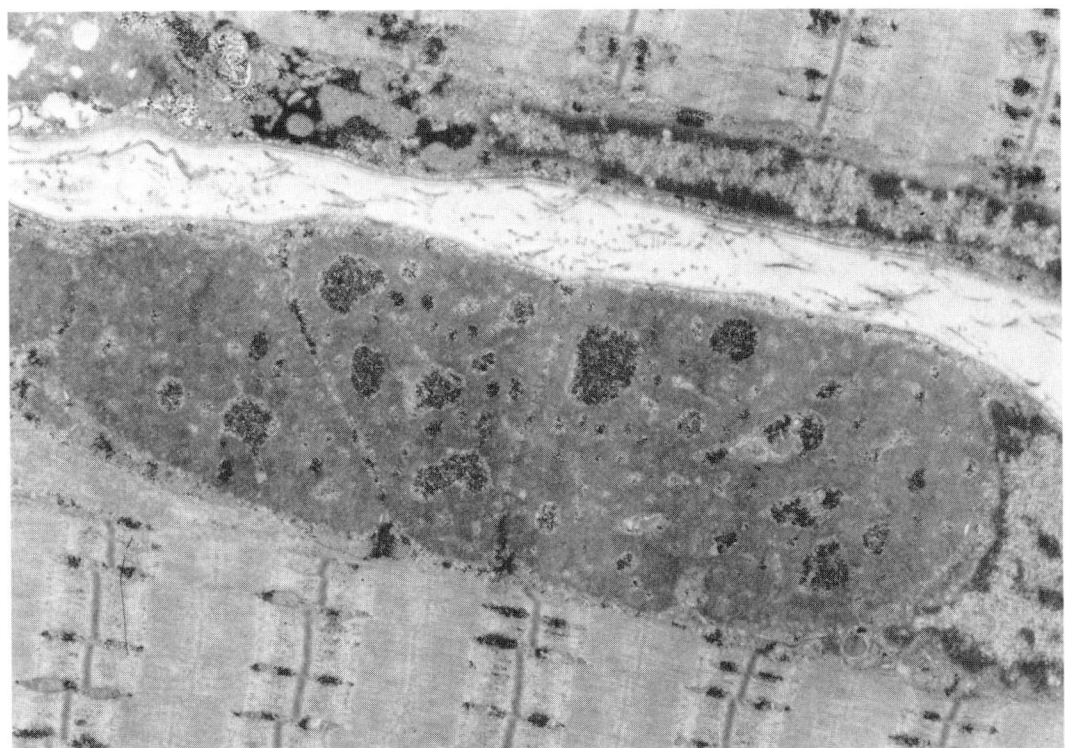

FIGURE 31-69. Reducing body in congenital reducing body myopathy. The subsarcolemmally located inclusions are adjacent to a nucleus and are honeycombed by small spaces containing glycogen. ×12,500. Courtesy of Dr. Hans E. Neville. *[Reproduced by permission from Neville HE, in Vinken PJ, Bruyn GW (eds): Handbook of Clinical Neurology, vol 41, Amsterdam: North-Holland Publishing Company; 1979, pp 63–123.]*

sections they are brightly eosinophilic, stain gray-purple with the modified trichrome stain, and transfer electrons to nitroblue tetrazolium in the presence of menadione. They stain positively for sulfhydryl groups but lack mitochondrial or myofibrillar enzyme activity.[135–137] They also stain positively for pyronine and are autoflourescent.[137a] In the electron microscope the reducing bodies are highly osmiophilic, lack limiting membrane, contain 10- to 15-nm granules or tubules, and may contain small spaces filled with glycogen or other sarcoplasmic material (Fig. 31-69). The origin of the reducing bodies has not been established to date. Their proximity to nuclei in the first report[135] suggested that they contain an abnormal material of nuclear origin, but in other cases the association with nuclei was inconsistent.

Reducing bodies were present in a high proportion of the muscle fibers of two children who had congenital muscle weakness and died in infancy of respiratory failure.[135] Other instances of inclusion body myopathy with fatal outcome owing to respiratory muscle weakness were observed in the past two decades (see Chap. 54). Similar inclusions were observed in less than 1 percent of the muscle fibers in two other children with clinically more benign congenital myopathies.[136,137]

Filamentous inclusions in inclusion body myositis and distal myopathies. These inclusions occur in the nucleus (see "Alterations of the Nucleus," above, and Fig. 31-14A) and in the cytoplasm. The intranuclear inclusions may consist of only a few filaments or may be so large that they completely fill or even distend the nucleus. The ovoid contours of some cytoplasmic inclusions suggest that they arose in preexisting nuclei (Fig. 31-70A and C). Other cytoplasmic inclusions appear in sheaves or bundles of varying size and complexity (Fig. 31-71A and C). The cytoplasmic inclusions characteristically occur adjacent to abnormal fiber regions filled with cytoplasmic degradation products.

In light microscopic studies the cytoplasmic and intranuclear inclusion bodies measure up to 4 by 7 μm, are eosinophilic (Color Plate 7G) and phase optically dense, and lack enzyme activity. Those fiber regions containing cytoplasmic degradation products are imaged as rimmed vacuoles (Chap. 30).

In the electron microscope the filaments are straight (Fig. 31-70B) or curve gently (Fig. 31-71A and C) and range from 10 to 21 nm in diameter. There is a wider distribution in the diameter of cytoplasmic than of intranuclear filaments; in some nuclei the filament diameters are in the 10- to 15-nm

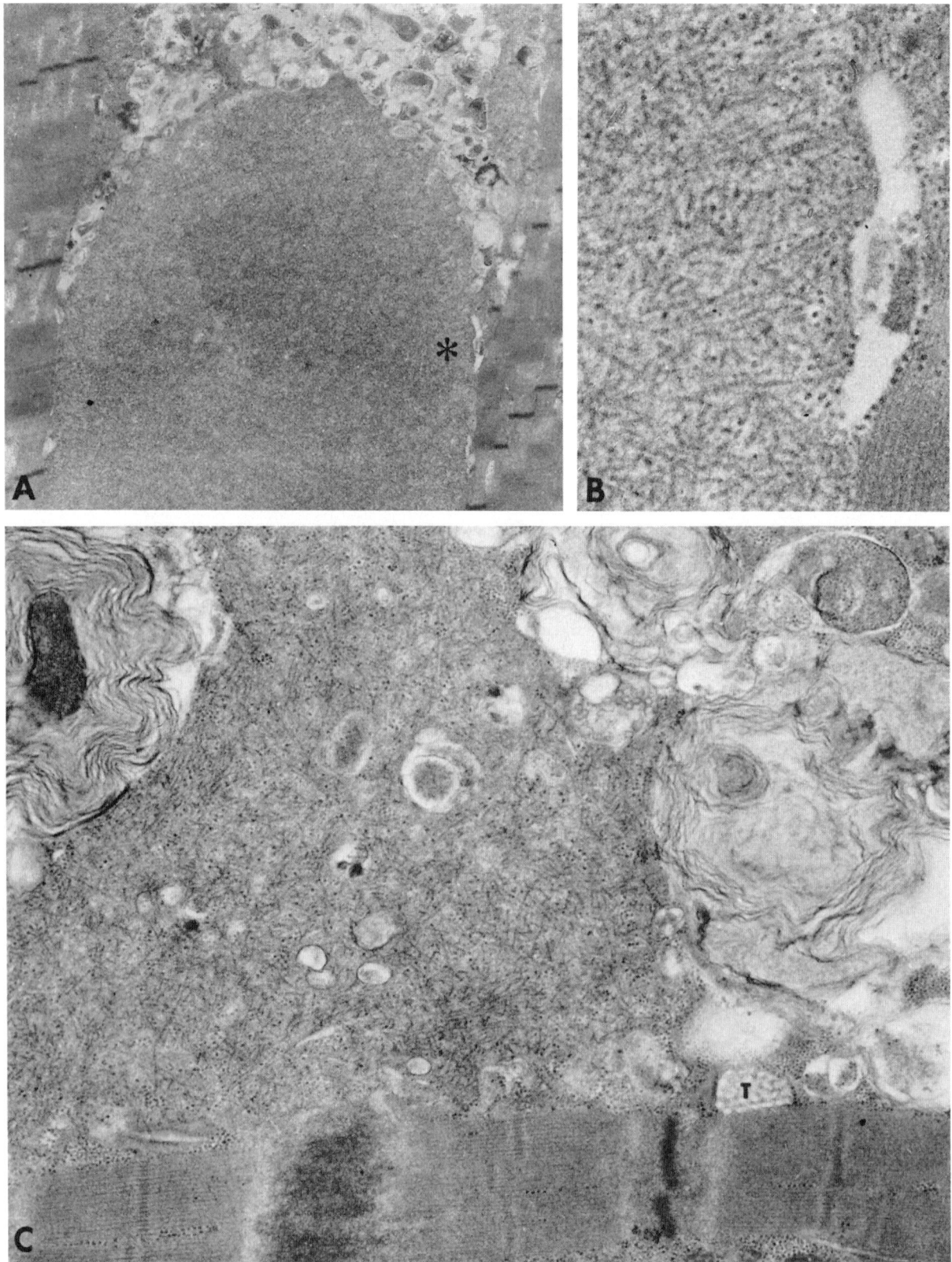

FIGURE 31-70. Filamentous inclusions in inclusion body myositis. In *A*, large inclusion resembles a nucleus in its shape. Region indicated by asterisk is shown at a higher magnification in *B*. In *A* and *C*, the filamentous inclusions abut on myeloid structures and other degraded organelles. T-system network (T) appears near the inclusion in *C*. *A*, ×12,700; *B*, ×76,700; *C*, ×24,500.

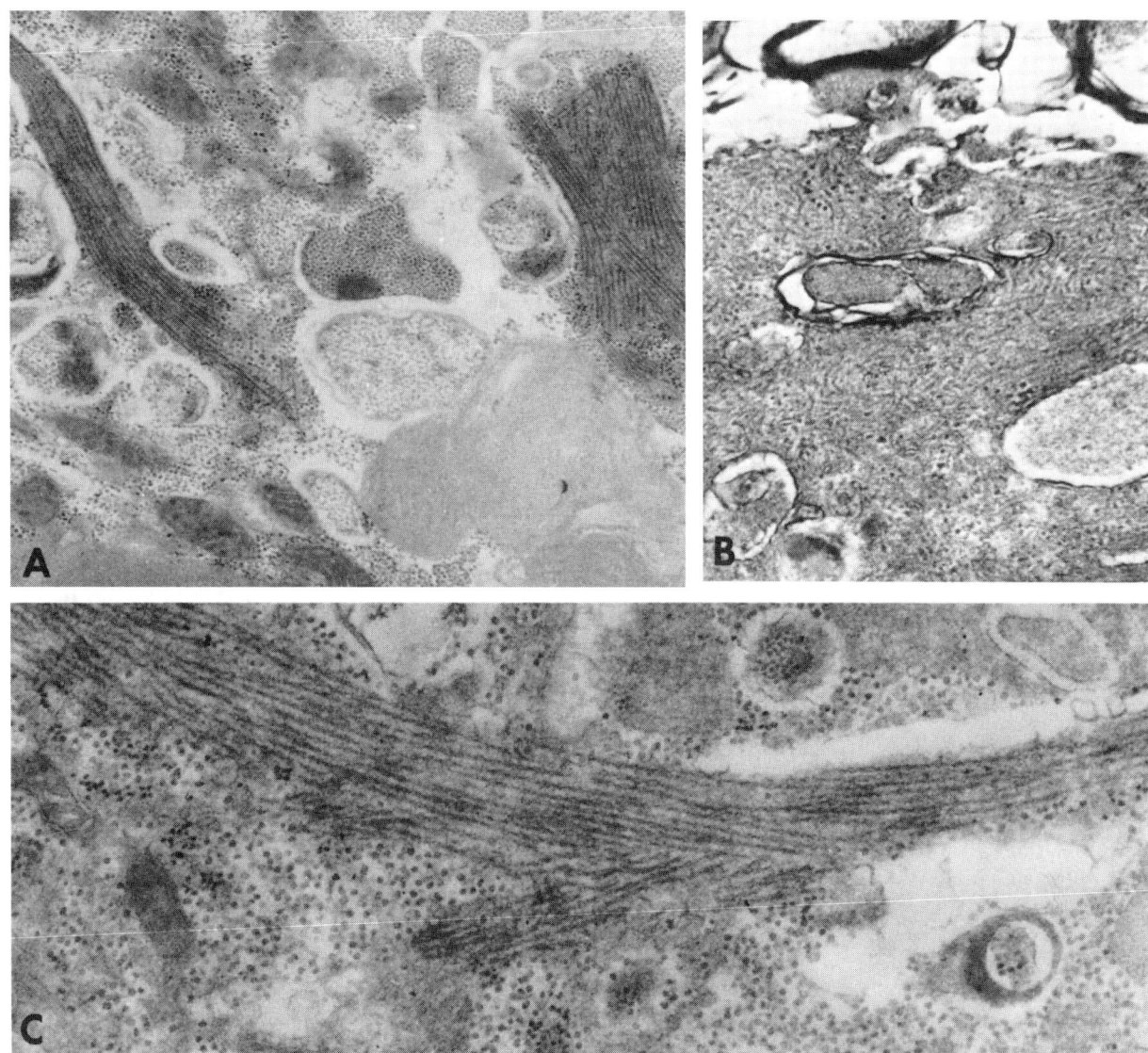

FIGURE 31-71. Filamentous inclusions in inclusion body myositis. In A and C, the filaments are surrounded by glycogen granules, mitochondrial profiles, and small membrane-bound structures containing dense material and glycogen granules. In A and B, the filaments are more elongated and slightly thicker than those imaged in Fig. 31-70. A, ×24,800; B, ×39,000; C, ×44,300.

range, and most cytoplasmic filaments vary from 15 to 21 nm in diameter. However, the measurements are imprecise because the filaments have indistinct or serrated borders. In some preparations the filaments also display a 6-nm lumen.[3,138–144] Some filaments are short and form an interlacing meshwork (Figs. 31-14A, 31-70, 31-71B). Other filaments are elongated, reaching more than 1 μm in length, appear in parallel arrays in bundles, and are thicker and more osmiophilic than the filaments in the interlacing meshworks (Fig. 31-71A and C). In some fiber regions the abnormal filaments appear near myofibrils and resemble thick-filament profiles.[140,142] However, it has not been established that the thick filaments give rise to the abnormal filaments.

The filamentous inclusions had been originally described in chronic polymyositis,[3,138–140] and their presence in some cases of chronic polymyositis had prompted the rubric of *inclusion body myositis*.[140] This term was subsequently applied to a disorder associated with variable inflammation, rimmed vacuoles, filamentous inclusion bodies, small groups of atrophic fibers without type grouping, slow progression of weakness, and refractoriness to immunosuppressant therapy.[141] Because the filaments in muscle bear some resemblance to those observed in cultured cells infected with myxovirus, it has been postulated that the filaments in muscle are possibly incomplete myxovirus virions.[3,138–140] Until recently, attempts to identify or isolate a virus in inclusion body myositis have failed except in one case in which an adenovirus was isolated from muscle (Ref. 144 and Chap. 50). Further, the filaments are not morphologically identical with known viral structures; and similar filamentous inclusions, together with rimmed vacuoles, also occur in familial distal myopathies.[145,146] Although the mumps virus antigen was identified by an immunoperoxidase method in inclusions in nuclei and in rimmed vacuoles,[146a] others have failed to confirm this and in situ hybridization studies show no mumps virus genetic material in muscle in inclusion body myositis.[146b]

The inclusions bind Congo red at pH 10.5 to 11[146c] and immunoreact for β-amyloid protein,[9c] β-amyloid precursor protein,[146d] and ubiquitin.[9b] Immunogold electron microscopy studies identified three distinct components associated with the inclusions: (1) the 15- to 21-nm filaments, which immunoreact for ubiquitin; (2) heretofore overlooked 6- to 10-nm amyloid-like fibrils, which immunoreact for β-amyloid protein; and (3) some dense floccular material, in close proximity to the 15- to 21-nm filaments, which immunoreacts for ubiquitin, β-amyloid protein, and β-amyloid precursor protein[9d] (see also Chap. 50).

It is now apparent that the inclusions are not specific for inclusion body myositis, for they also occur in familial inclusion body myopathies and with mutations in myosin heavy chain IIa and in the *GNE* gene (see Chap. 48). The origin and pathogenetic significance of these inclusions remain elusive.

Spherical particles in hexagonal arrays. These crystalline arrays are composed of 14- to 20-nm particles. The arrays appear between myofibrils, subsarcolemmally, or near nuclei; occupy irregularly contoured zones up to several microns long or wide; and are *not* associated with other pathologic change. They have been reported in muscle in 2 of 40 biopsy specimens in diverse muscle diseases[147]; in six of eight autopsied patients with Reye's syndrome and in six of eight autopsied children and adults who died of diverse diseases[148]; in an autopsied patient with a chronic muscle disease in which coxsackievirus type A9 was also isolated from muscle[149]; and in an autopsied patient with malignant hyperthermia.[150] In another patient who died of Reye's syndrome, numerous crystalline arrays were found in muscle 2 h after death, but no arrays were present in muscle only 1 h before death.[151] The findings of the last report, the much higher incidence of the arrays in autopsy than in biopsy specimens, and the lack of association with other pathologic change suggest that the arrays appear in muscle under unusual conditions, and especially during or after the agonal state. The particles in the arrays resemble β-glycogen granules in size and staining properties, and digestion with diastase results in their removal.[148] However, another study has localized nucleic acids in the particles found at autopsy in a traffic accident victim, and this might indicate that the particles are virions.[152] Further, the picornavirus arrays in mouse muscle in experimental coxsackievirus myositis[153] are strikingly similar to the spherical particle arrays found in human muscle at autopsy. In the experimental viral myositis, however, inflammation, fiber necrosis and phagocytosis, and myriad compound membrane-vesicle complexes are associated with the viral particles.[153] Additional immunocytochemical studies and investigations employing DNA probes for detecting viral material will be required to define the origin and significance of the hexagonally arrayed spherical particles in human muscle.

Ultrastructural Alterations in the Muscle Fiber

CORE, MULTICORE, AND TARGET FORMATIONS

A similar pattern of ultrastructural alterations can be observed in core formations (Figs. 31-72, 31-73), target formations (Figs. 31-74, 31-75), and multicore formations (Figs. 31-76, 31-77). However, the three types of formation can be distinguished by their distribution and three-dimensional profile in the muscle fibers (Chap. 30 and Color Plate 7C and D).

The basic ultrastructural changes in all three formations are a decrease or disappearance of mitochondria from a fiber region, focal myofibrillar degeneration within the confines of the mitochondrial decrease, decreases in sarcotubular elements and glycogen in the abnormal region, and variable alterations in mitochondria at the border of the lesion. Cytochemical features of cores and targets are described in Chap. 30.

The mitochondrial decrease is the most constant feature of the abnormal formations and typically is more extensive than the myofibrillar degeneration (Figs. 31-72, 31-76).[12,39,43] In core formations the zone of mitochondrial decrease is a long cylinder that probably extends through the entire fiber (Color Plate 7C). In target formations this zone is oblong or cigar-shaped, with its long axis parallel to the fiber axis, and the long axis of the lesion seldom exceeds 10 times the diameter of the affected fiber. In most multicore formations the zones of mitochondrial loss range from a few microns to about 30 μm in length and width, and the long axis of the abnormal zones is either parallel or perpendicular to the fiber axis (Color Plate 7D).

In each formation the focal myofibrillar degeneration begins with streaming and disintegration of the Z disk, as described under "Alterations of the Z Disk," above. The myofibrillar alterations tend to be less extensive in core than in target formations (Figs. 31-72 to 31-75). In some central cores (Figs. 31-72B) and multicores (Fig. 31-76) the Z disks show little streaming, and in some central cores the Z disks are wider than in the adjacent fiber regions (Fig. 31-72). However, these differences are not sufficiently consistent to distinguish between the three types of formation ultrastructurally.

The decreases in sarcotubular profiles and glycogen usually occur together with focal myofibrillar degeneration and are less extensive than the area of mitochondrial decrease (Fig. 31-77A and B).

An increase in mitochondrial profiles may or may not be present at the borders of either core (Fig. 31-72) or target (Fig. 31-75B) formations, and swollen and possibly degenerating mitochondria may occur at the borders of target formations (Figs. 31-74B and 31-75A). These alterations are also unreliable for distinguishing between the different types of formation.

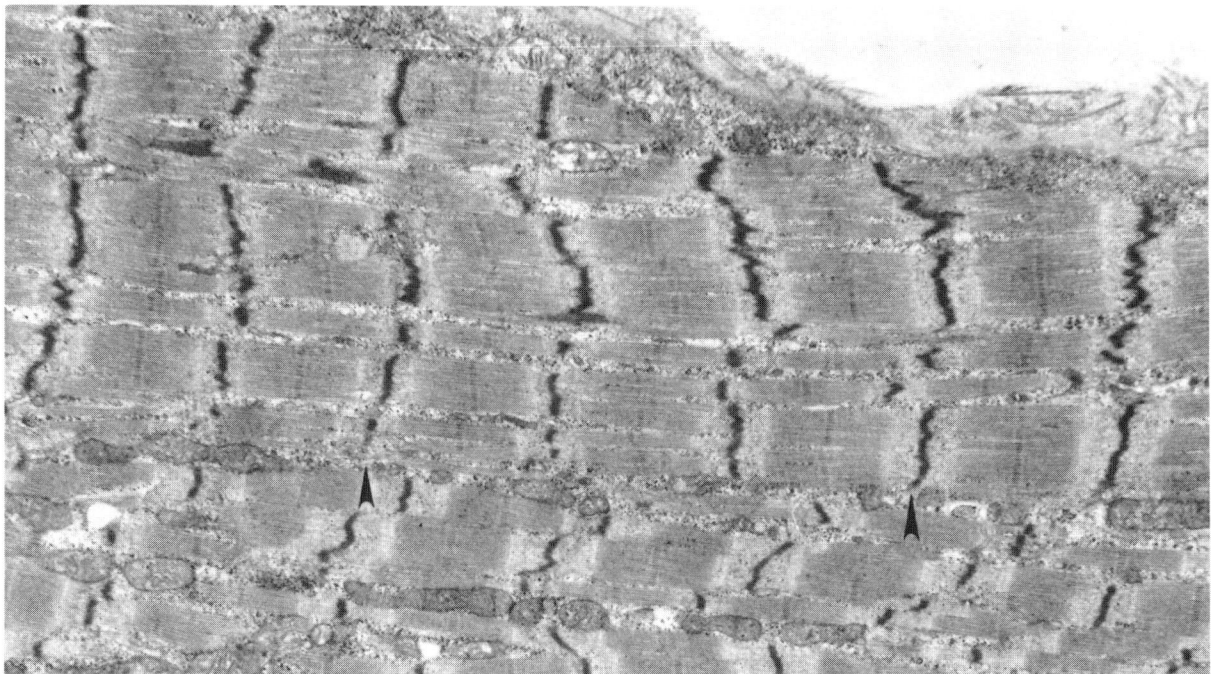

FIGURE 31-72. Peripherally located "central" core in central core disease. The mitochondrial profiles are reduced, and the Z disks are widened and irregular in the core formation. Arrowheads indicate the border of the core. ×13,000.

SARCOPLASMIC MASSES

The abnormal fiber regions vary from a few micrometers in length or width to large areas that encompass nearly the entire muscle fiber (Fig. 31-78). The abnormal masses are superficial or deep in location and extend for variable distances along the long fiber axis. Multiple sarcoplasmic masses can occur in a single fiber (Fig. 31-78). The masses appear blue in the trichrome stain, show a diffuse (instead of granular) reaction product of variable intensity in the NADH dehydrogenase reaction, react for phosphorylase and glycogen (Fig. 31-78A to C), and are faintly reactive or unreactive for myofibrillar ATPase (Chap. 30).

In the electron microscope the sarcoplasmic masses contain scattered mitochondria and glycogen granules, normal or dilated T tubules and T system networks (Figs. 31-79, 31-80), smooth-surfaced tubules, scattered ribosomal particles, rough endoplasmic reticulum profiles (Fig. 31-80B), and myofibrillar elements. The latter consist of poorly organized and randomly oriented thick and thin filaments and fragments of wide Z disks (Figs. 31-79C, 31-80A). The abundance and degree of organization of the myofibrillar elements varies between different sarcoplasmic masses and within a given sarcoplasmic mass.

Sarcoplasmic masses are conspicuous in some cases of myotonic dystrophy but also occur in other dystrophies, in inflammatory or metabolic myopathies, and occasionally in denervated muscle fibers. The presence of ribosomes, rough endoplasmic reticulum profiles, and wide Z disks suggests attempts at regeneration, and the incompletely assembled and organized myofibrils may indicate inadequate interaction between cytoskeletal and myofibrillar elements. Further, it is tempting to speculate that abnormal regeneration within the sarcoplasmic masses may result in the formation of annular or aberrant myofibrils. The sequence of ultrastructural changes that result in the formation of sarcoplasmic masses has not been investigated to date.

DENERVATION ATROPHY

The ultrastructural effects of denervation on the muscle fiber are difficult to evaluate in human muscle, because in most neurogenic disorders both denervated and reinnervated fibers are present in the same specimen. Highly atrophic fibers in such disorders are likely to be denervated, but the less atrophic fibers could be either denervated or reinnervated. Ultrastructural analysis is further complicated by secondary myopathic alterations that can occur in nondenervated fibers during chronic neurogenic atrophy. Denervation effects would be easier to analyze when reinnervation has failed to occur, as in muscles whose nerve supply has been severed or in the acute form of infantile spinal muscular atrophy. However, totally denervated human muscles are seldom biopsied for ultrastructural studies; and in acute spinal muscular atrophy some of the highly atrophic fibers may be noninnervated rather than denervated. On the other hand, denervation atrophy can be sequentially analyzed in completely denervated animal muscles. We therefore first describe the ultrastructural changes in experimentally de-

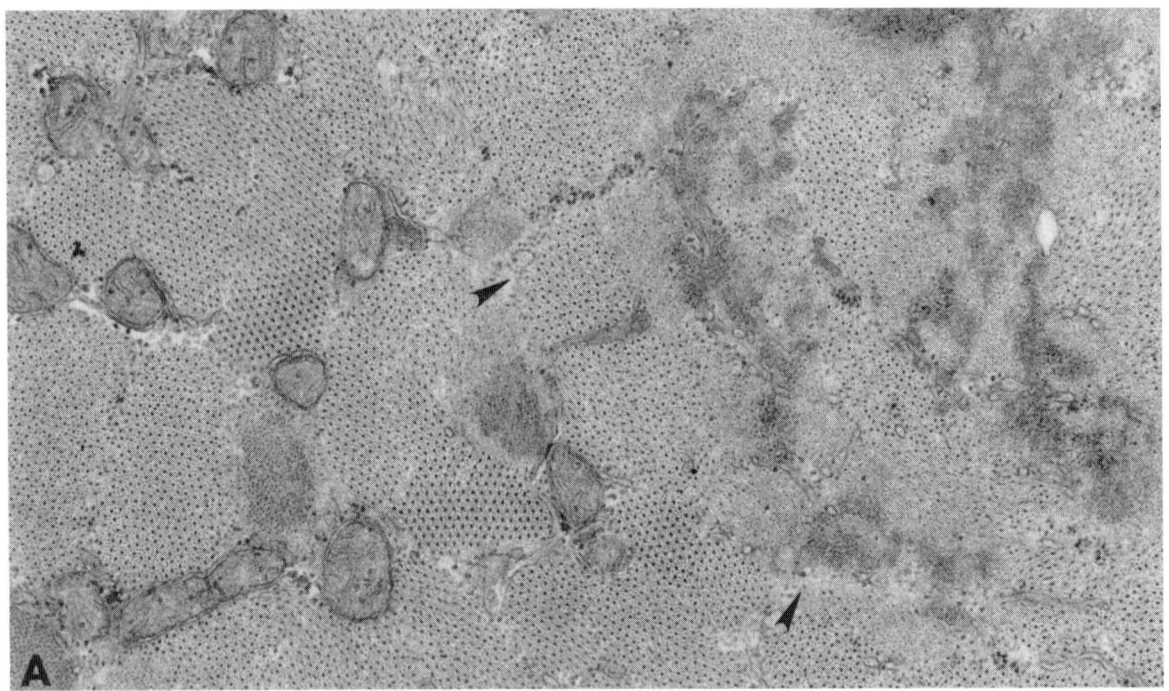
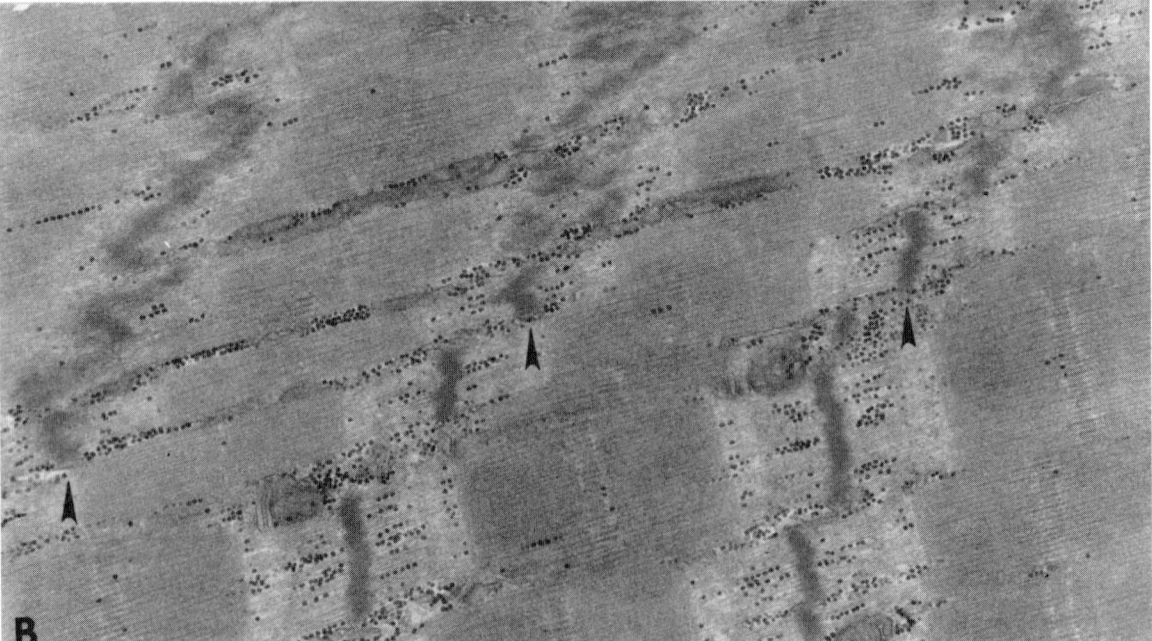

FIGURE 31-73. Longitudinal and transverse sections of central cores in central core disease. The Z disks are irregular (B), and material of Z-disk origin has spread into the adjacent I bands but not into the A bands (A and B). Arrowheads indicate border of the core. A, ×30,200; B, ×24,300.

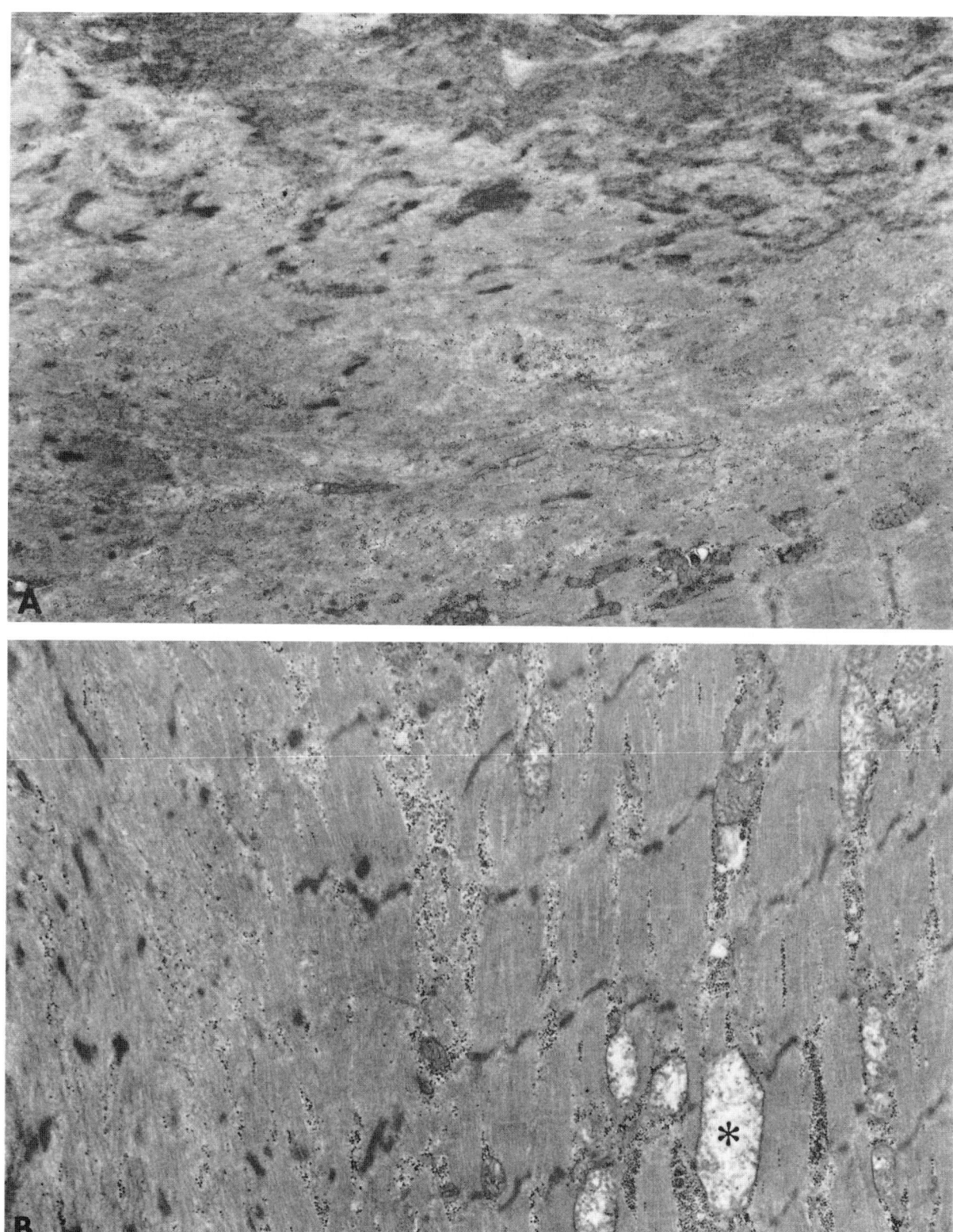

FIGURE 31-74. Longitudinal sections through target formations in chronic neurogenic atrophy. In *A*, extensive streaming and disintegration of Z disks and loss of myofibrillar markings has occurred in the center of the target formation. At the peripheral zone of the target the Z disks are indistinct, and here scattered glycogen granules and dislocated sarcotubular profiles can be observed. In *B*, the fiber region adjacent to the target formation contains enlarged and possibly degenerating mitochondria. *A*, ×9900; *B*, ×13,600.

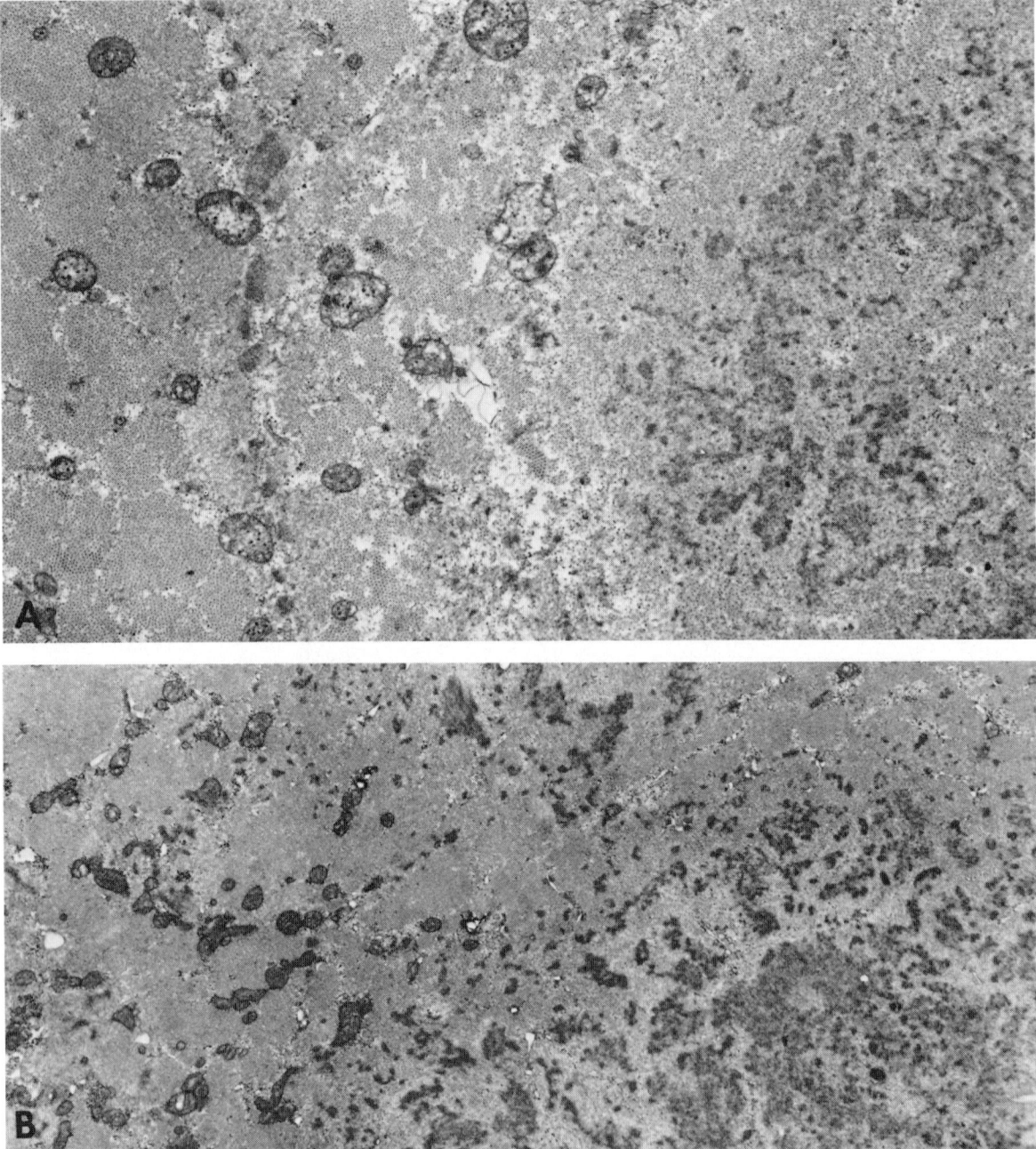

FIGURE 31-75. Transverse sections through target formations in chronic neurogenic atrophy. Extensive myofibrillar degeneration has occurred in the center of the target formation. The peripheral zone of the target formation contains an increased number of mitochondria, some of which are swollen. *A*, ×9000; *B*, ×8400.

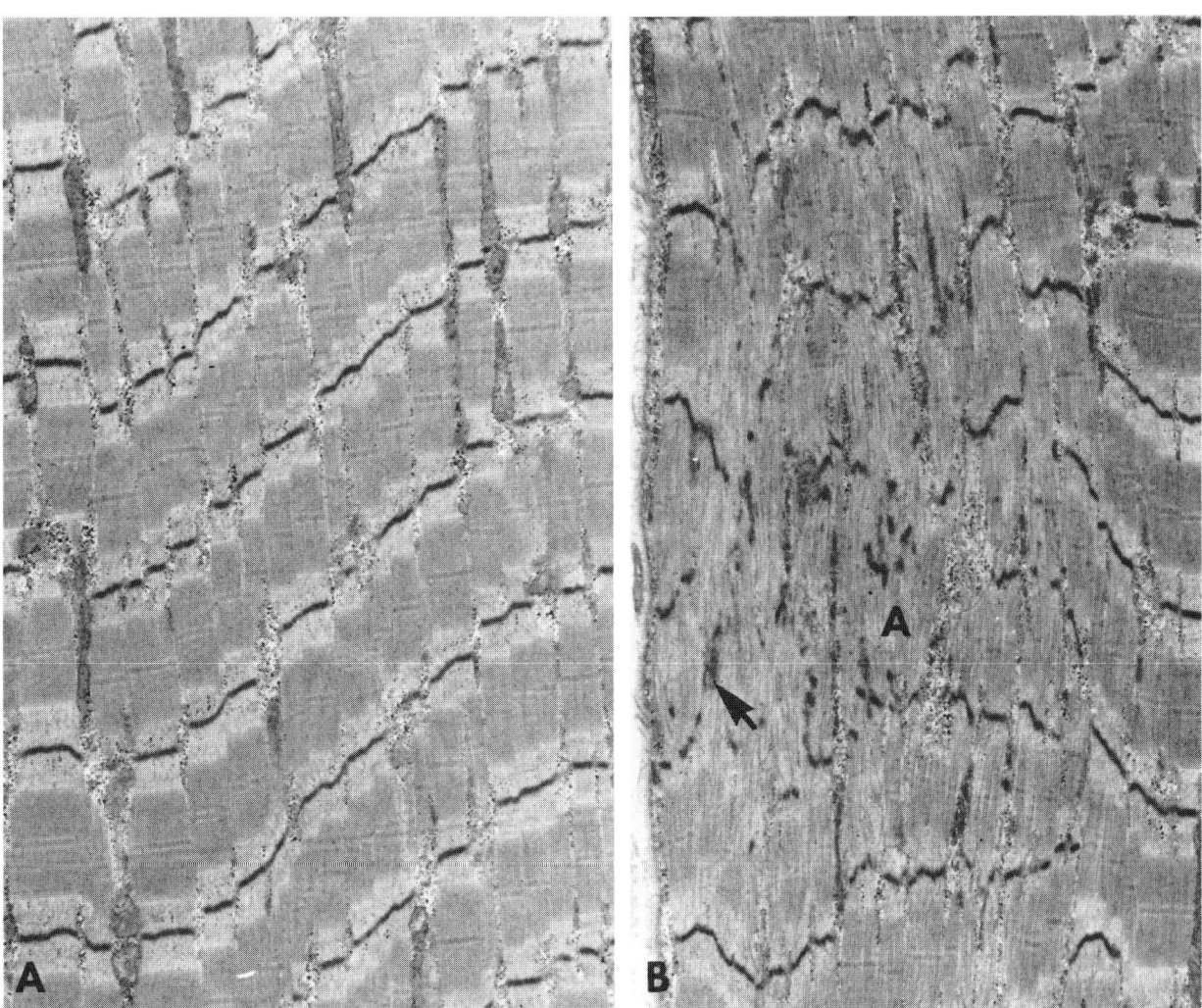

FIGURE 31-76. Multicore disease. In A, the abnormal fiber region lacks mitochondria. In B, the abnormal fiber region lacks mitochondria and shows focal myofibrillar degeneration beginning at the Z disks (arrow). In the center of the lesion the sarcomeres are pulled apart and are out of register. A bands (A) are still recognizable in the lesion. A, ×9500; B, ×9600. *(Reproduced by permission from Engel AG, Gomez MR, Groover RV, Mayo Clin Proc 46:666, 1971.)*

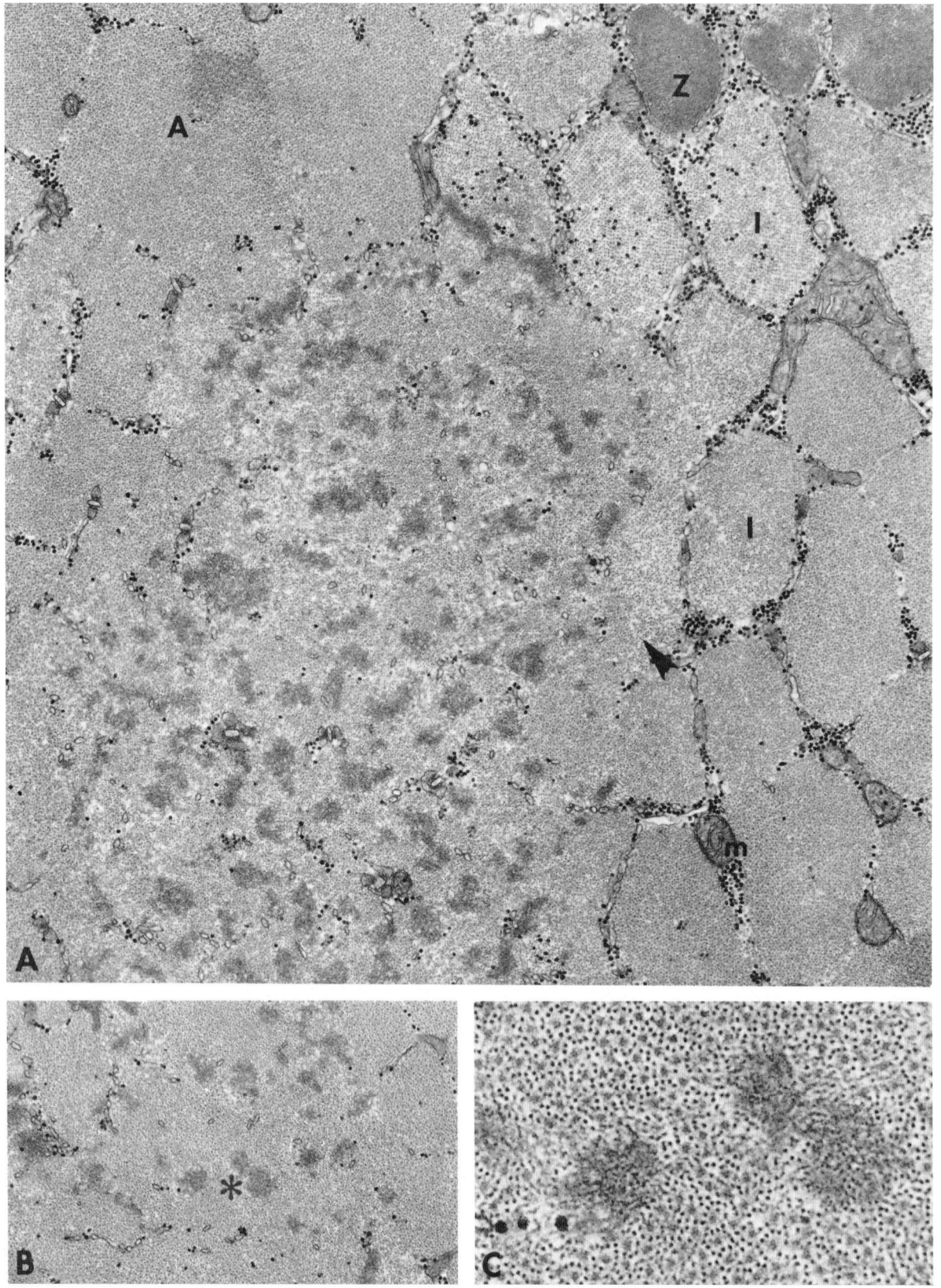

FIGURE 31-77. Multicore disease, transverse sections. A relatively large lesion is shown in A. At upper right, section traverses the Z disk (Z) and I bands (I); rest of section is through A bands (A). Z-disk material has spread into A bands at center and lower left. Disorganized sarcotubular profiles and glycogen granules appear in lower part of abnormal area. Arrowhead points to upper part of lesion, where glycogen granules are sparse. Mitochondria (m) are absent from lesion. B shows part of a multicore formation at the
(continued on bottom of next page)

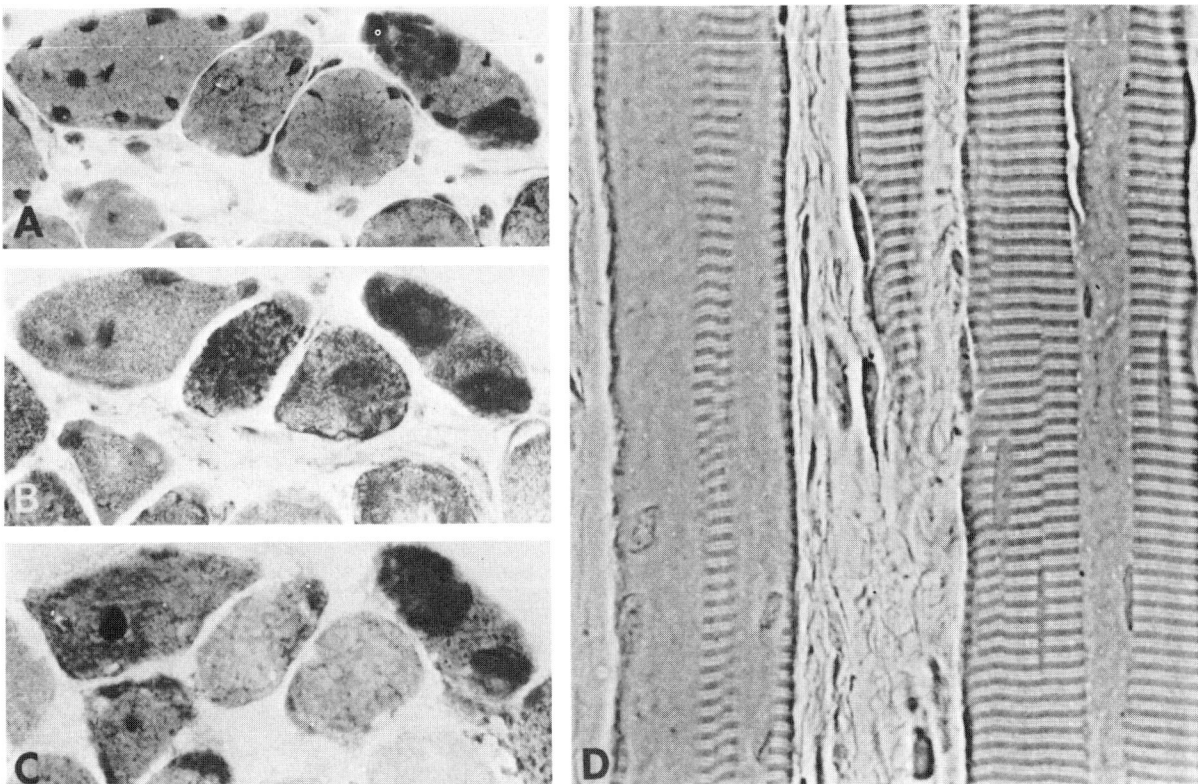

FIGURE 31-78. Sarcoplasmic masses in myotonic dystrophy; cryostat sections *(A to C)* and semithin resin section viewed in phase optics *(D)*. The sarcoplasmic masses stain darkly with the trichrome stain *(A)* and react relatively strongly for NADH dehydrogenase *(B)* and phosphorylase *(C)*. In the resin section, the sarcoplasmic masses contain a few nuclear profiles but no other clearly identifiable structures *(D)*. A, B, and C, ×270; D, ×750.

nervated rat muscle fibers[33] and then those in highly atrophic, denervated human muscle fibers.

Sequential Ultrastructural Changes in Experimentally Denervated Muscle Fibers

Rat soleus and gastrocnemius muscles were studied between 1 and 84 days after sciatic nerve section at midthigh level.[33] Results of a sequential and quantitative analysis were as follows.

Immediately after denervation the muscle fibers began to atrophy. The muscle fiber atrophy is most rapid during the first 2 weeks after denervation and proceeds more slowly thereafter. Myofibrillar atrophy is essentially proportionate to the atrophy in fiber size. Irregular Z disks and streaming

◀ FIGURE 31-77 *(continued)*
level of the A band. C is a higher magnification of the region indicated by the asterisk in B. In B and C, moderately electron-dense amorphous material of Z-disk origin appears in small, irregularly shaped zones. Glycogen granules, sarcotubular profiles, and the double array of thick and thin filaments are preserved. *A,* ×29,600; *B,* ×23,600; *C,* ×83,200. *(Reproduced by permission from Engel AG, Gomez MR, Groover RV, Mayo Clin Proc 46:666–681, 1971.)*

of dense material from the disks are often observed, but massive streaming, as seen in some target or core formations, is not encountered.

During the first week of denervation, while fiber size and contractile elements decrease rapidly, there is both an absolute and a relative increase in sarcotubular profiles (T tubules and SR) (Fig. 31-81*A*). Focal dilations of both the SR and the T system (Fig. 31-81*A*) and T-system networks appear in the fibers and are present even 70 days after denervation (Fig. 31-81*B* and *C*).

After the first week of denervation the sarcotubular profiles decrease in density, but this decrease is less than in the contractile elements, with the net result that the concentration of sarcotubular profiles continues to increase (Fig. 31-81*B* to *E*). As the sarcotubular profiles become relatively more abundant, their spatial arrangement becomes increasingly irregular, and T and SR profiles are frequently difficult to distinguish from each other (Fig. 31-81*B* to *E*).

Mitochondria also increase in density during the first week of denervation. In addition, they become reoriented in the muscle fiber so that their longest and largest profiles appear in longitudinal instead of transverse sections. After the first week of denervation there is a decrease in mitochondrial density. This decrease is more rapid than that in sarcotubular surface density, so that the concentration of

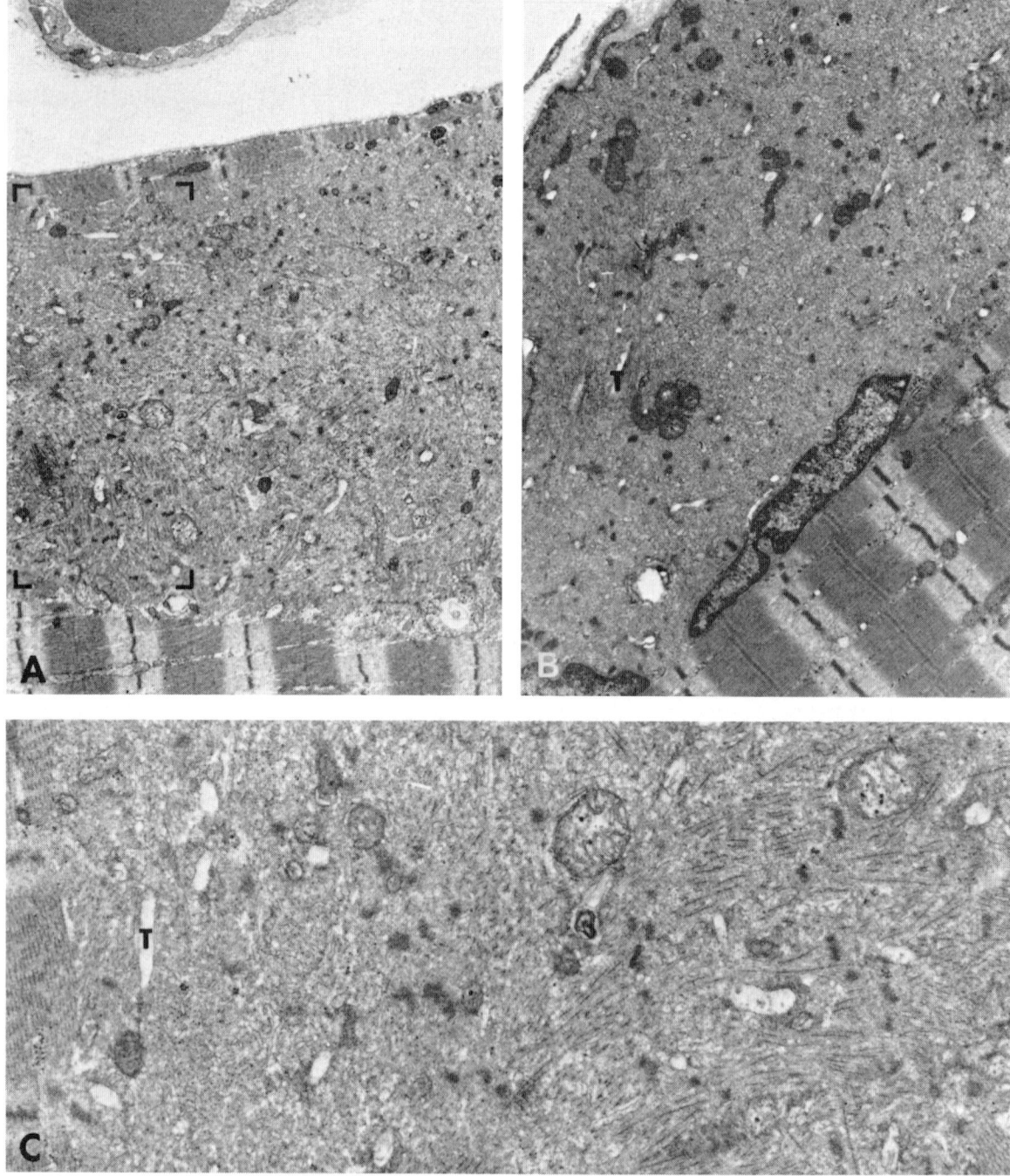

FIGURE 31-79. Subsarcolemmal sarcoplasmic masses in myotonic dystrophy contain irregularly oriented and disorganized myofibrillar components, mitochondria, and dilated tubules, some of T-system origin (T). Bracketed region in A is shown at a higher magnification in C. A, ×6400; B, ×9400; C, ×16,600.

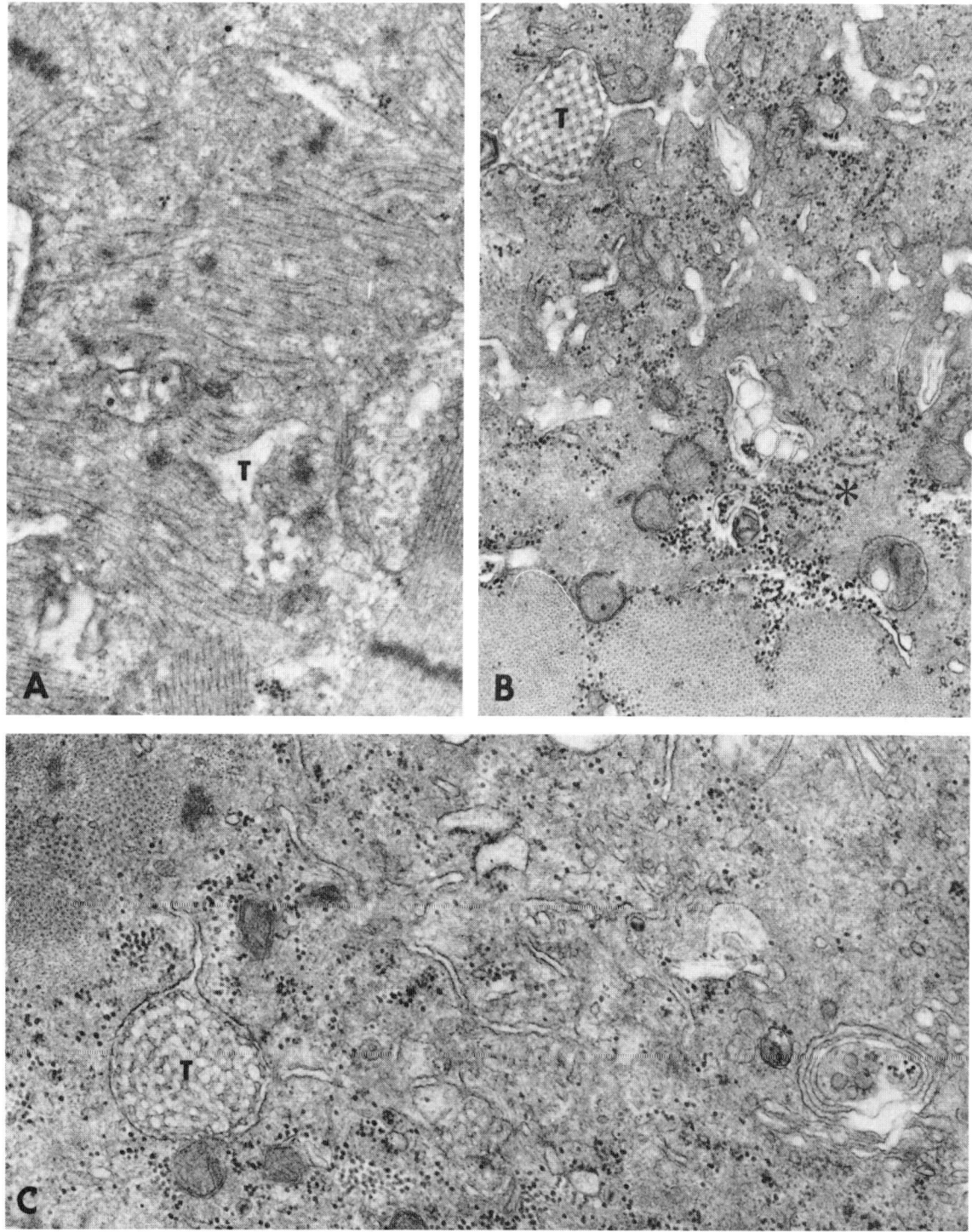

FIGURE 31-80. Sarcoplasmic masses in myotonic dystrophy *(A* and *B)* and in a myopathy of undetermined type *(C)* contain irregularly oriented myofibrillar components *(A)*, T-system networks, dilated T tubules (T), and rough endoplasmic reticulum profiles (asterisk). *A*, ×29,800; *B*, ×28,000; *C*, ×39,300.

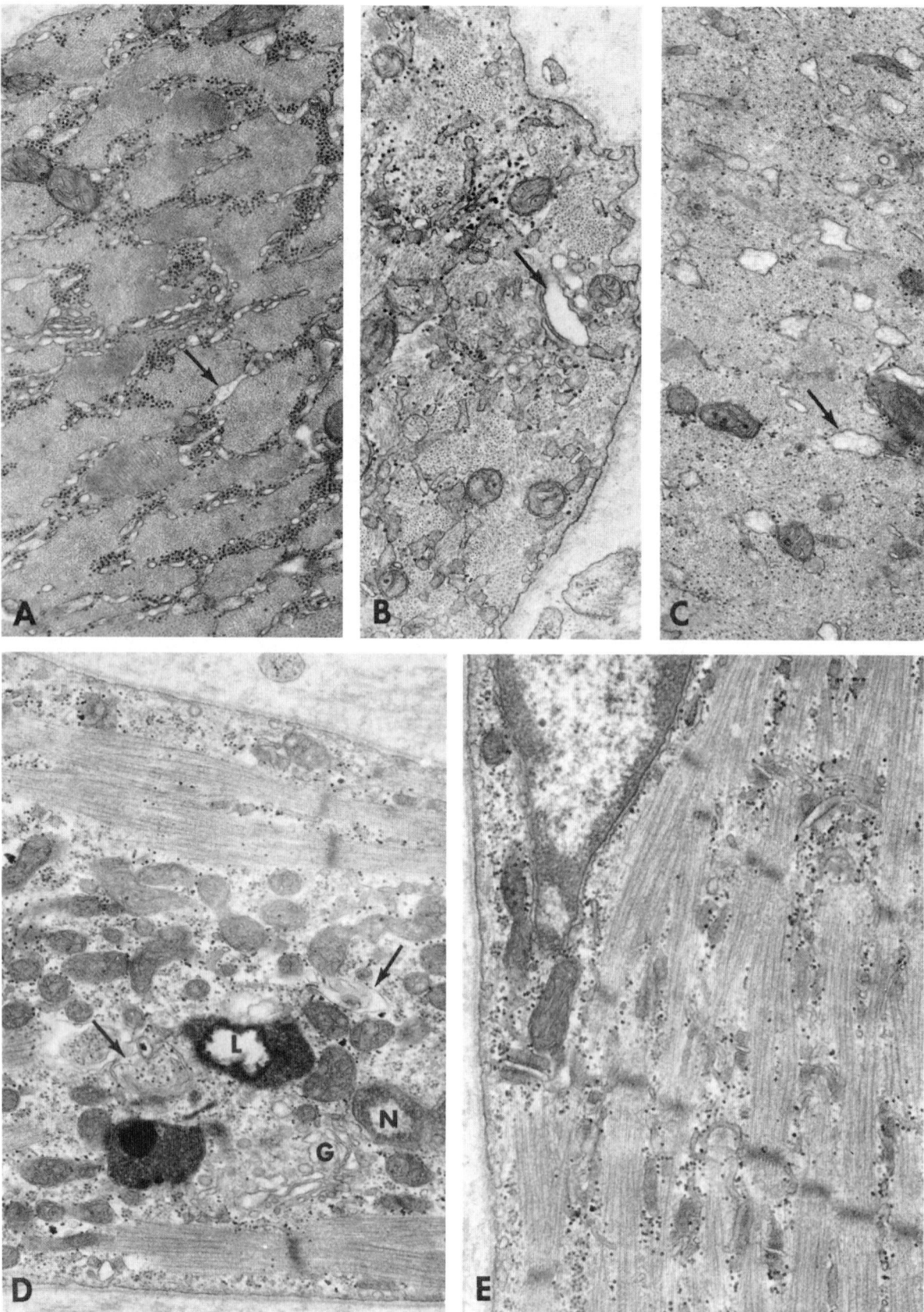

FIGURE 31-81. Denervated rat gastrocnemius (*A, B, D,* and *E*) and soleus (*C*) muscles 6 days (*A*), 70 days (*B* and *C*), and 84 days (*D* and *E*) after denervation. In the transverse sections (*A, B,* and *C*), the mitochondrial profiles have changed from elongated to round configuration. The sarcotubular profiles are prominent, irregularly disposed, and sometimes dilated (arrows). In *D,* prominent Golgi

(continued on bottom of next page)

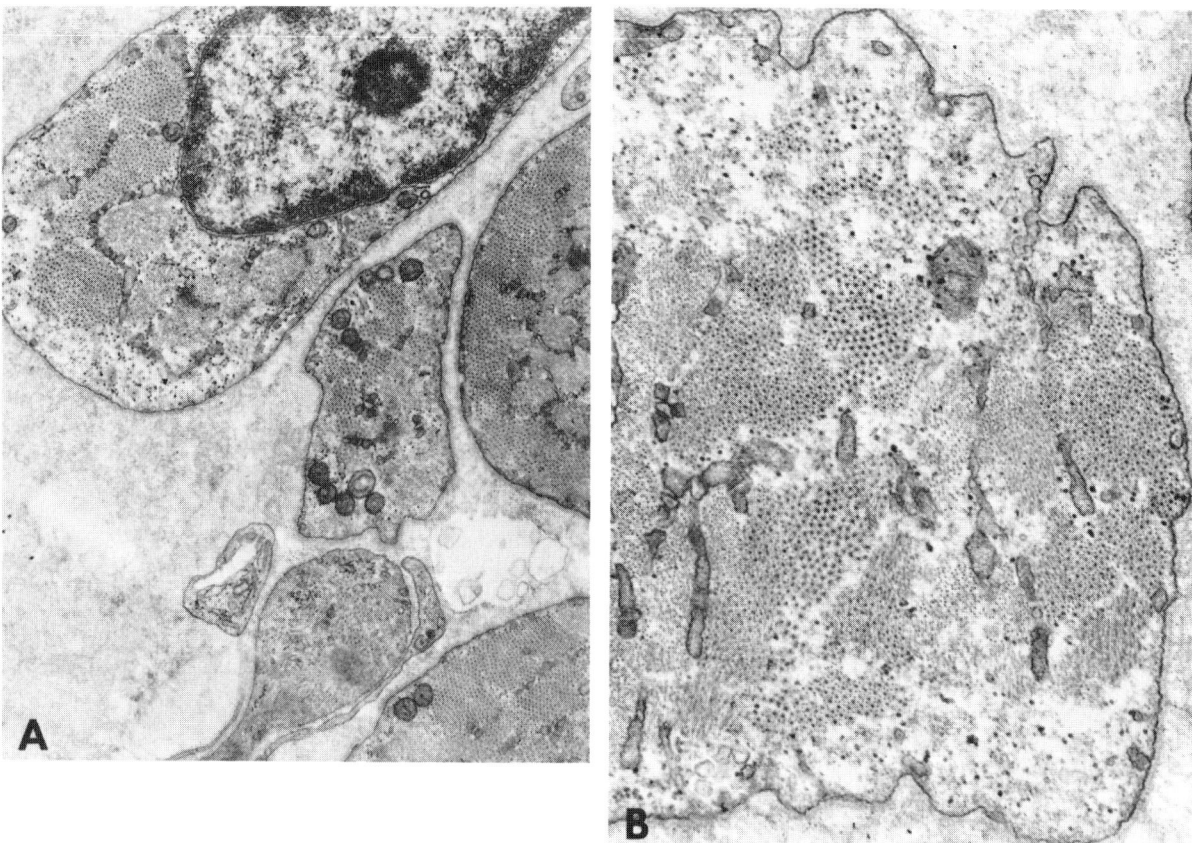

FIGURE 31-82. Seventy-day-denervated rat gastrocnemius muscle fibers. Myofibrillar atrophy is present at the periphery as well as in the interior of the fiber. Some of the mitochondria appear in small clusters. *A*, ×14,800; *B*, ×29,900. (*B is reproduced by permission from Engel AG, Stonnington HH, Ann NY Acad Sci 228:68, 1974.*)

mitochondria returns to normal values after the first month of denervation. However, the relatively uniform distribution of mitochondria in the muscle fiber is altered, and mitochondria tend to aggregate into small clusters (Figs. 31-81*D*, 31-82*A*).

Lipofuscin granules, small autophagic vacuoles, and central nuclei with prominent Golgi networks in their hof region appear with moderate frequency after the first week of denervation (Fig. 31-81*D*). Increased numbers of ribosomal particles, some associated with tubules, are observed soon after denervation under the sarcolemma, near the nucleus, and between myofibrils (Fig. 31-83).

In chronically denervated muscles the difference in the width of Z disks in soleus and gastrocnemius fibers becomes less apparent. Myofibrillar atrophy that began at the periphery of the muscle fibers is now also observed in the fiber interior (Fig. 31-82). Some fibers contain glycogen-membrane arrays (Fig. 31-31*B*) or parallel arrays of the junctional SR (Fig. 31-24*C*). Papillary projections of the muscle fiber surface and redundant loops of basal lamina can be observed around some atrophic fibers.

Increasing times of denervation are accompanied by a progressive decline in the number of nuclei per muscle fiber and an initial rise and a subsequent fall in satellite cell number.[153a] Some 2 to 4 months after denervation, satellite cells show signs of activation. As denervation progresses, activated satellite cells become separated from the parent fiber by basal lamina; some satellites detach or form bridges between adjacent fibers. Long-term denervated muscles also show signs of capillary loss and interstitial fibrosis.[153b]

Highly Atrophic Denervated Human Muscle Fibers

The myofibrils are atrophic or normal in size (Figs. 31-24, 31-84, 31-85). Disorganized myofibrils (Figs. 31-84, 31-85*B* and *C*, 31-86*C*), widened Z disks (Fig. 31-85*C*), or small nemaline rods (Figs. 31-85*B*, 31-86*C*) appear in some atrophic fibers. Numerous and irregularly oriented SR and T-tubule profiles occur between the myofibrils (Figs. 31-24*A*,

◀ FIGURE 31-81 *(continued)*
apparatus (G), lipofuscin granules (L), small autophagic vacuoles (arrows), and a cluster of mitochondria appear in the hof region of the nucleus (N). In *E*, abundant sarcotubular profiles are disposed irregularly between atrophic myofibrils. *A*, ×17,500; *B*, ×31,400; *C*, ×26,900; *D*, ×23,000; *E*, ×27,400. (*Reproduced by permission from Engel AG, Stonnington HH, Ann NY Acad Sci 228:68, 1974.*)

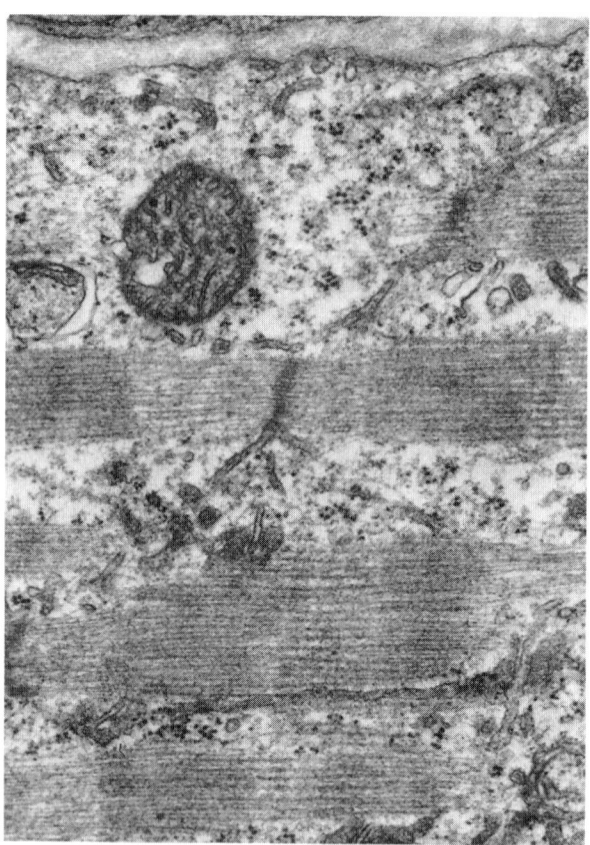

FIGURE 31-83. Numerous ribosomal particles occur under the surface membrane and between myofibrils in 21-day-denervated rat gastrocnemius muscle. ×33,000. (Reproduced by permission from Engel AG, Stonnington HH, Ann NY Acad Sci 228:68, 1974.)

31-85A and C). Dilated SR profiles (Fig. 31-86B) and T-system networks are occasionally observed. Widened subsarcolemmal and intermyofibrillar spaces contain cytoskeletal filaments (Fig. 31-85A and C), glycogen granules (Figs. 31-85C, 31-86B), and scattered mitochondria (Fig. 31-85A and C). Circumscribed fiber regions devoid of myofibrils contain lipofuscin granules, smooth-surfaced tubules, small vesicles, and scattered ribosomes (Fig. 31-86D). Central nuclei occur in some fibers (Fig. 31-86). Papillary projections of the surface membrane (Fig. 31-86A, C, and D) and redundant loops of basal lamina (Fig. 31-86A) occur but are not constant findings. Thus, most features that eventually appear in experimentally denervated muscle fibers are also present in chronically denervated human muscle fibers.

MYOGENIC MUSCLE FIBER ATROPHY

The possible causes of myogenic muscle fiber atrophy include type 2 fiber atrophy; recurrent cycles of cytoplasmic degradation and exocytosis; proliferation of a single organelle, such as nemaline rods, accompanied by disappearance of other fiber components; destruction of segments of nonnecrotic muscle fibers by cytotoxic mononuclear cells; and degeneration or segmental fiber destruction followed by incomplete regeneration or repair. Longitudinal fiber splitting causes an apparent decrease in fiber size in a given plane of sectioning, but the split-off fiber segments remain connected to the parent fiber by anastomoses distal to the plane of sectioning. The light microscopic aspects of these reactions were reviewed in Chap. 30.

An adequate ultrastructural study of type 2 fiber atrophy has not been published to date, and the sequence of events associated with this type of fiber atrophy remains to be elucidated.

The fiber atrophy in late-onset myopathy was considered under "Alterations of the Z Disk," above (Fig. 31-43F). Fiber splitting (Fig. 31-6) and exocytosis (Fig. 31-5A) were discussed under "Alterations of the Surface Membrane," above. The effects of cytotoxic mononuclear cells on nonnecrotic muscle fibers (Figs. 31-103 to 31-107) are reviewed under "Muscle Fiber Invasion and Destruction by T Cells and Macrophages," below. Muscle fiber degeneration or destruction followed by inefficient, incomplete, or abortive regeneration may play an important role in muscle fiber atrophy in dermatomyositis.

The Perifascicular Atrophy of Dermatomyositis

A selective atrophy of muscle fibers occurs at the periphery of the fascicles in dermatomyositis. The reasons for the increased vulnerability of the fibers in this region and for the prominence of this change in dermatomyositis are still not known, but ischemia due to capillary necrosis may be an important contributing factor.[2,154] Several ultrastructural alterations are observed in the atrophic fibers, suggesting different but still related pathogenic mechanisms.

Necrotic fibers (Fig. 31-87B) and regenerating fibers (Fig. 31-87C to E) are present at the periphery of the fascicles in some acute cases of dermatomyositis. Myoblasts, presumably arising from activated satellite cells, can be observed within the necrotic fiber remnants (Fig. 31-87C), where they may fuse to form a new fiber. The embryonal form of fiber regeneration, during which myoblasts derived from activated satellite cells fuse to form myotubes outside the confines of the basal lamina of the necrotic fiber, may also occur. Since the putative factor(s) that caused fiber necrosis (ischemia, circulating immune complexes, antibody-dependent complement-mediated cytotoxicity, or a combination of these) persist as long as the disease is active, one could envision repeated cycles of necrosis involving incompletely differentiated fibers. Alternatively, these factor(s) might cause degeneration of regenerating fibers or might interfere with regeneration without causing further fiber necrosis. The presence of atrophic fibers undergoing vacuolar degeneration (Fig. 31-87A) would be consistent with such mechanisms. Thus, one possible reason for the appearance of atrophic fibers would be ongoing fiber necrosis associated with a failure of the regenerating fibers to fully mature and regain their girth.

There are reasons, however, to suggest that perifascicular atrophy can occur even without antecedent fiber necrosis. If

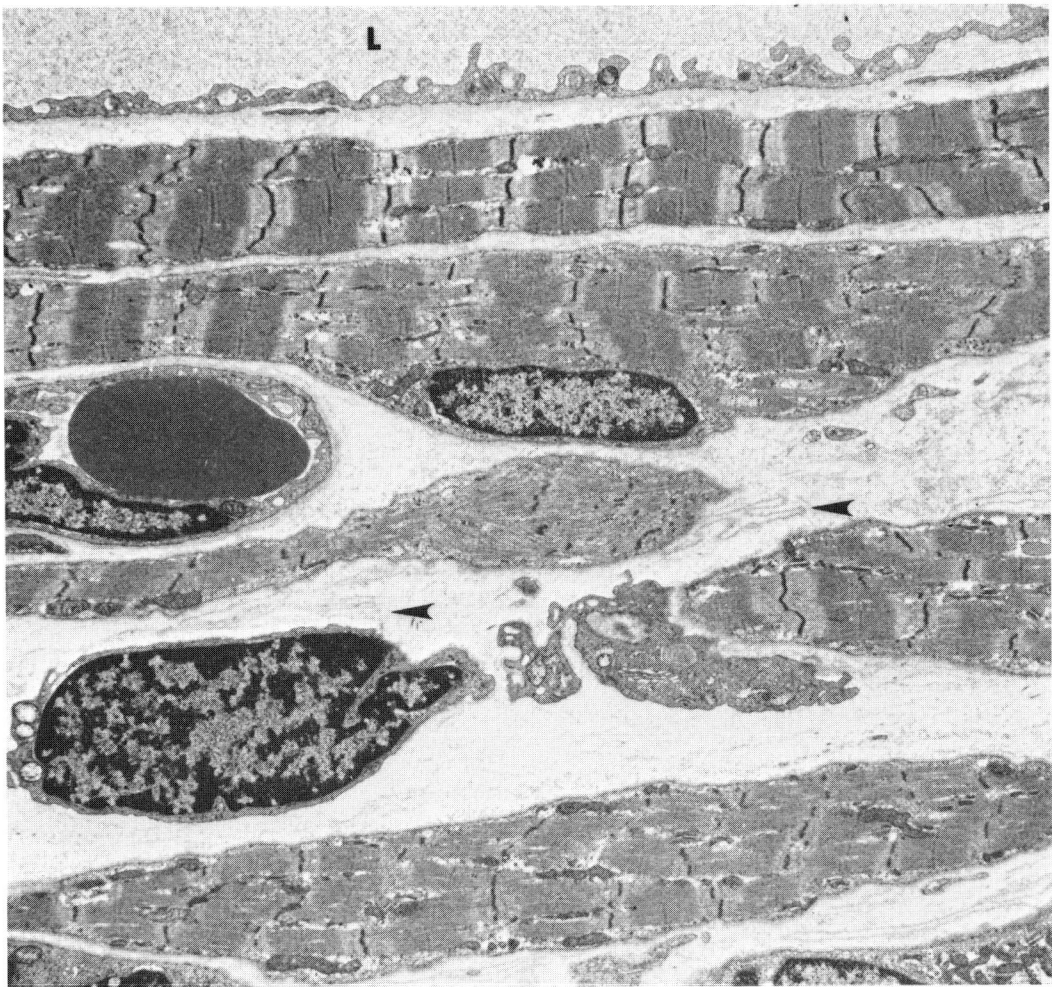

FIGURE 31-84. Highly atrophic muscle fibers in acute infantile spinal muscular atrophy. Arrowheads indicate redundant loops of basal lamina around atrophic fibers. Aberrant myofibrils appear in some of the fibers. L, lymphatic. ×6100.

one defines a necrotic fiber by its staining properties in the trichrome stain and reactivity for the complement membrane attack complex,[155] then the mean incidence of necrotic fibers in children and adults with dermatomyositis is 0.6 and 1.3 percent, respectively.[156] Further, light microscopic histochemical studies frequently reveal nonatrophic "moth eaten fibers" at the periphery of the fascicles (Chap. 30). Ultrastructurally, these fibers show a focal decrease in mitochondria associated with focal myofibrillar degeneration (Fig. 31-88B and C). In other nonatrophic fibers, circumscribed regions from which myofibrils have disappeared (probably because of focal myofibrillar degeneration) are filled with glycogen granules, dislocated sarcotubular components, or debris (Fig. 31-88D). Still other fibers display cytoplasmic bodies, another sign of myofibrillar degeneration, sometimes with clusters of mitochondria around the cytoplasmic body (Fig. 31-88A).

Other atrophic or nonatrophic perifascicular fibers contain regenerating areas adjacent to internal nuclei. The regenerating regions are composed of large Golgi complexes, numerous ribosomal particles, and rough endoplasmic reticulum profiles (Fig. 31-89A); or clusters of dilated SR vesicles intermingled with T-system networks, glycogen granules, and ribosomes (Fig. 31-89B); or primitive, disorganized myofibrils with wide Z disks or small nemaline rods (Fig. 31-89C). These findings suggest that focal muscle fiber degeneration and regeneration can occur without antecedent fiber necrosis and satellite cell activation, and that a decrease in fiber size may also result from inefficient, incomplete, or abortive regeneration within continuously degenerating nonnecrotic fibers.

The highly atrophic perifascicular fibers continue to show signs of injury and repair, such as myofibrillar degeneration (Fig. 31-90A and D), focal increases and decreases of mitochondria (Fig. 31-90A and B), proliferating and degenerating membranous profiles (Fig. 31-90E), and disorganized myofibrils with widened Z disks or small nemaline rods (Fig. 31-90C). Some atrophic fibers also display an increased

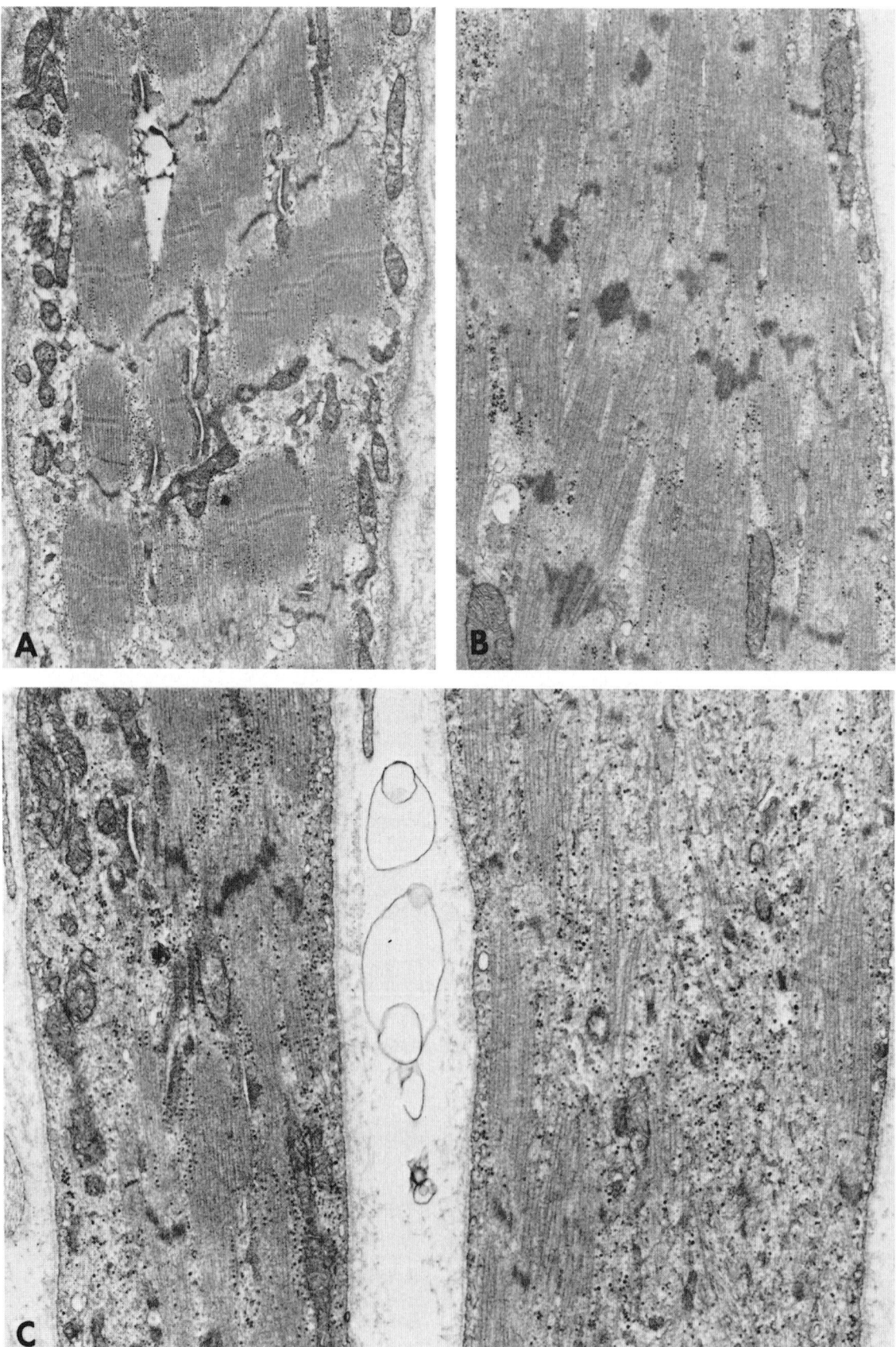

FIGURE 31-85. Atrophic muscle fibers in acute spinal muscular atrophy. Note widened subsarcolemmal and intermyofibrillar spaces containing glycogen granules, scattered mitochondria, and cytoskeletal filaments (A, B, and C), widened Z disks (B and C), and small nemaline rods (B). A, ×12,800; B, ×18,700; C, ×25,600.

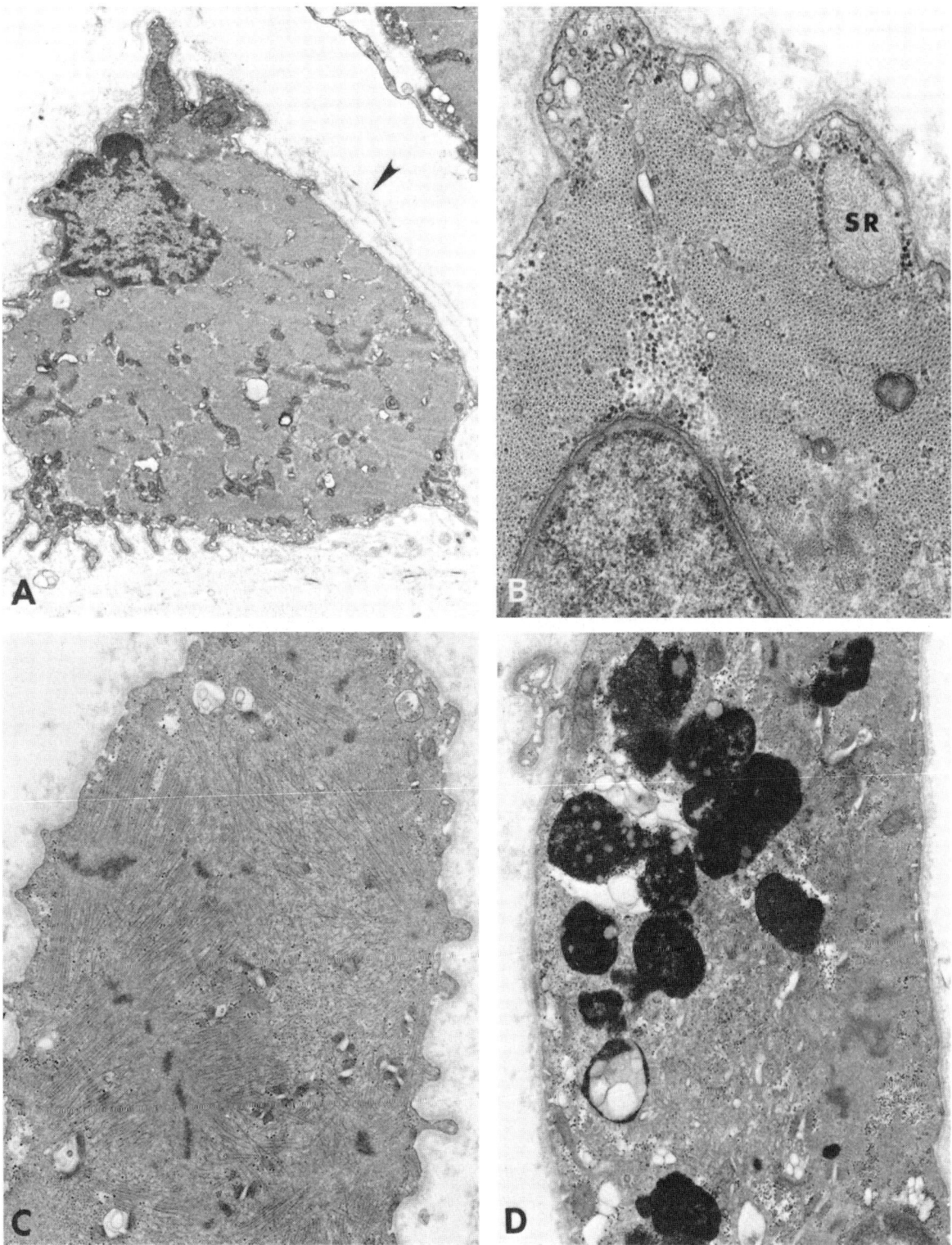

FIGURE 31-86. Highly atrophic denervated muscle fibers in peripheral neuropathy. Some atrophic fibers display papillary projections (A and C) and are surrounded by redundant loops of basal lamina (arrowhead in A). Dilated SR profiles (B), disorganized aberrant myofibrils (C), and fiber regions filled with lipofuscin granules and membranous organelles but devoid of myofibrils (D) can be observed. A, ×7900; B, ×30,500; C, ×15,400; D, ×12,900.

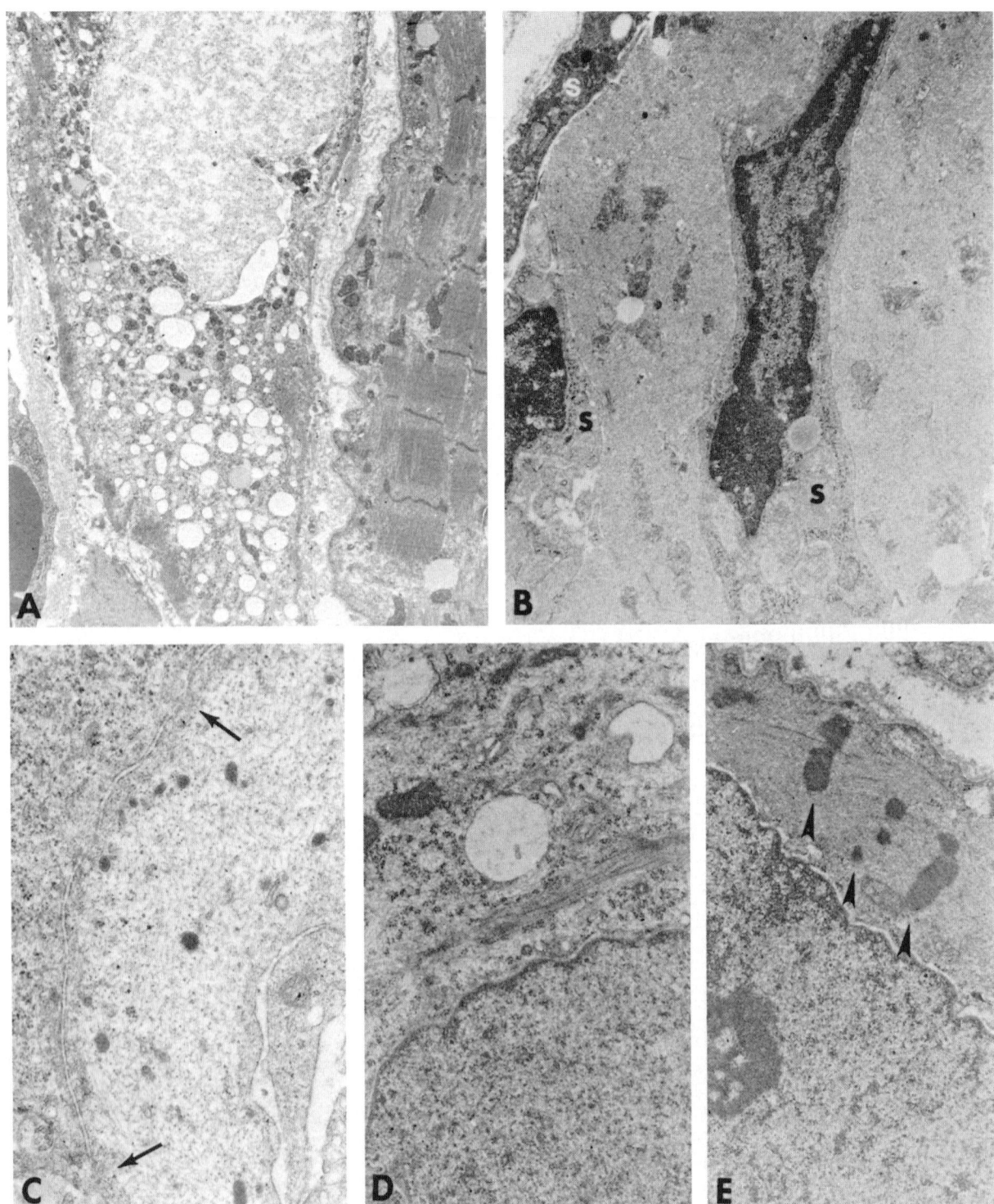

FIGURE 31-87. Degenerating *(A)*, necrotic *(B)*, and regenerating *(C to E)* perifascicular muscle fibers in childhood dermatomyositis. In *A*, myriad dilated vesicles and mitochondria surround a larger abnormal space that may represent a swollen nucleus. In *B*, the necrotic muscle fiber has lost its plasma membrane and contains satellite cells (S). In *C*, adjacent myoblasts are fusing (arrows). In *D*, abundant ribosomes, cytoskeletal filaments, and mitochondria surround the central nucleus. In *E*, early myofibrils display nemaline rods (arrowheads). *A*, ×6100; *B*, ×13,100; *C*, ×22,300; *D* and *E*, ×15,800.

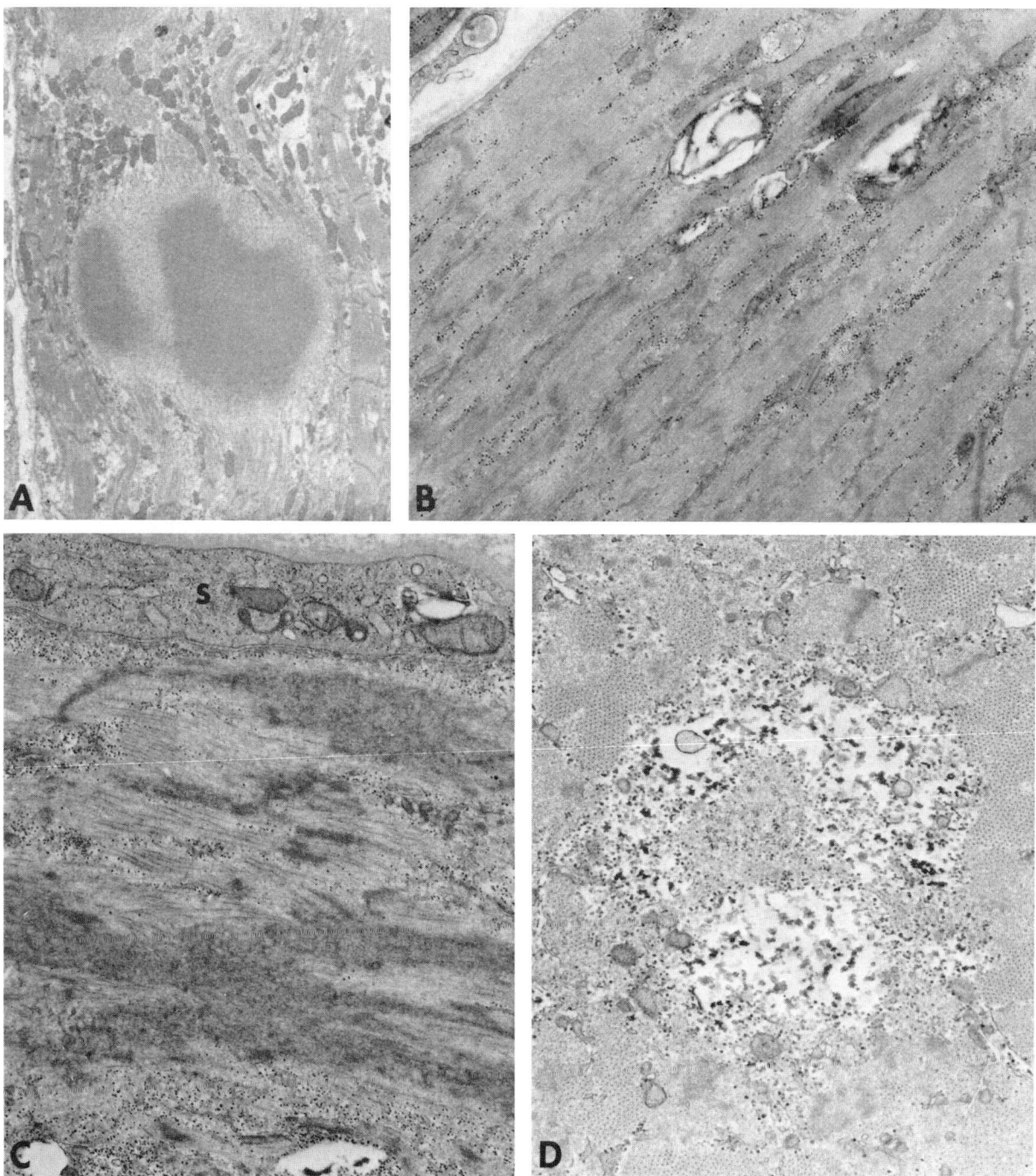

FIGURE 31-88. Abnormal perifascicular muscle fibers in dermatomyositis display a large cytoplasmic body *(A)*, focal mitochondrial loss and myofibrillar degeneration *(B and C)*, and a circumscribed area of myofibrillar destruction filled with glycogen granules *(D)*. A, ×4900; B, ×18,200; C, ×16,800; D, ×20,000.

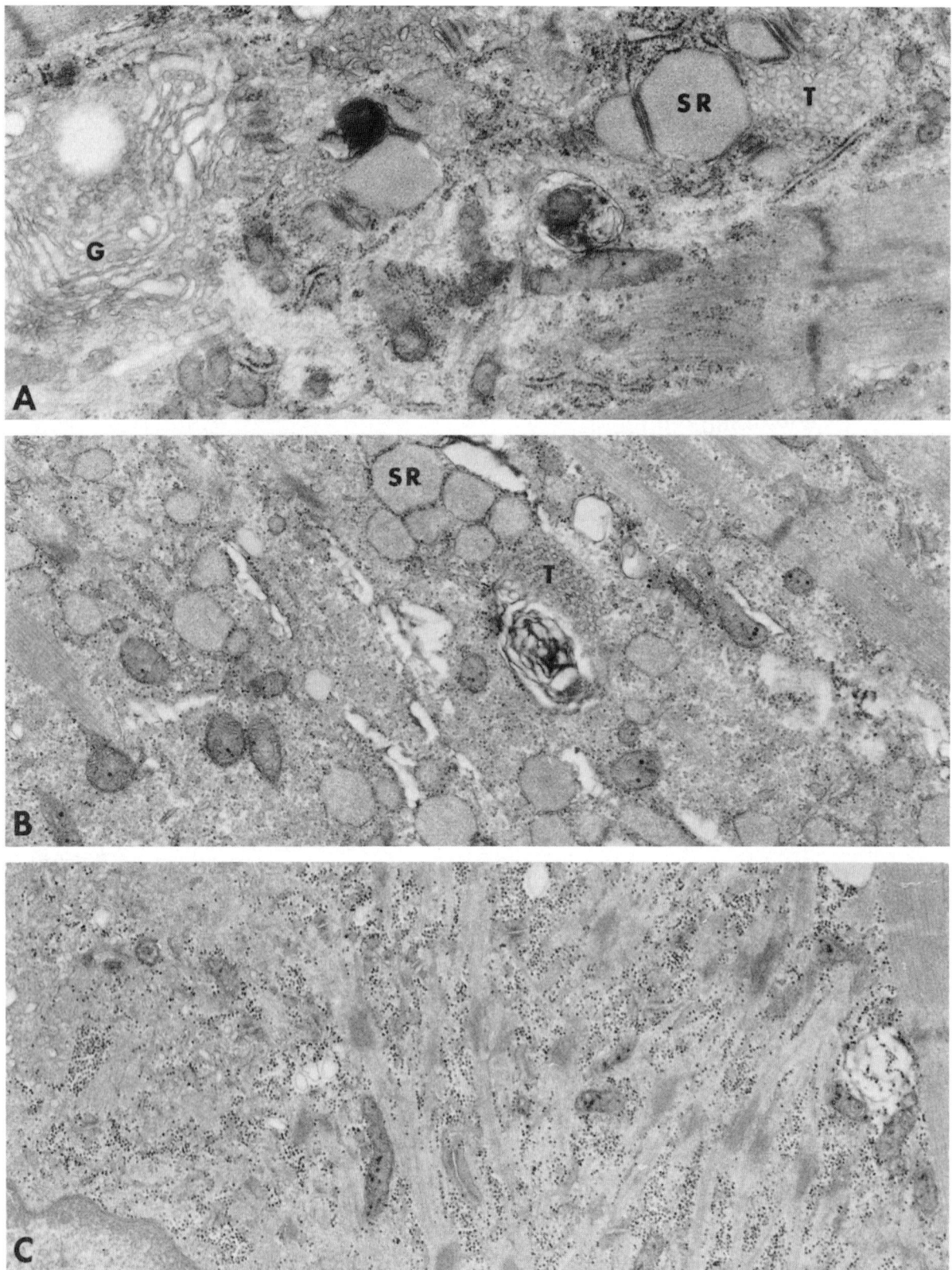

FIGURE 31-89. Regenerating regions in perifascicular muscle fibers in dermatomyositis. Prominent Golgi *(A)*, numerous rough endoplasmic reticulum profiles *(A)*, clusters of dilated SR vesicles *(A* and *B)*, T-system networks (T), and primitive myofibrils with wide Z disks and small nemaline rods *(C)* can be observed. *A* and *B*, ×25,000; *C*, ×19,500.

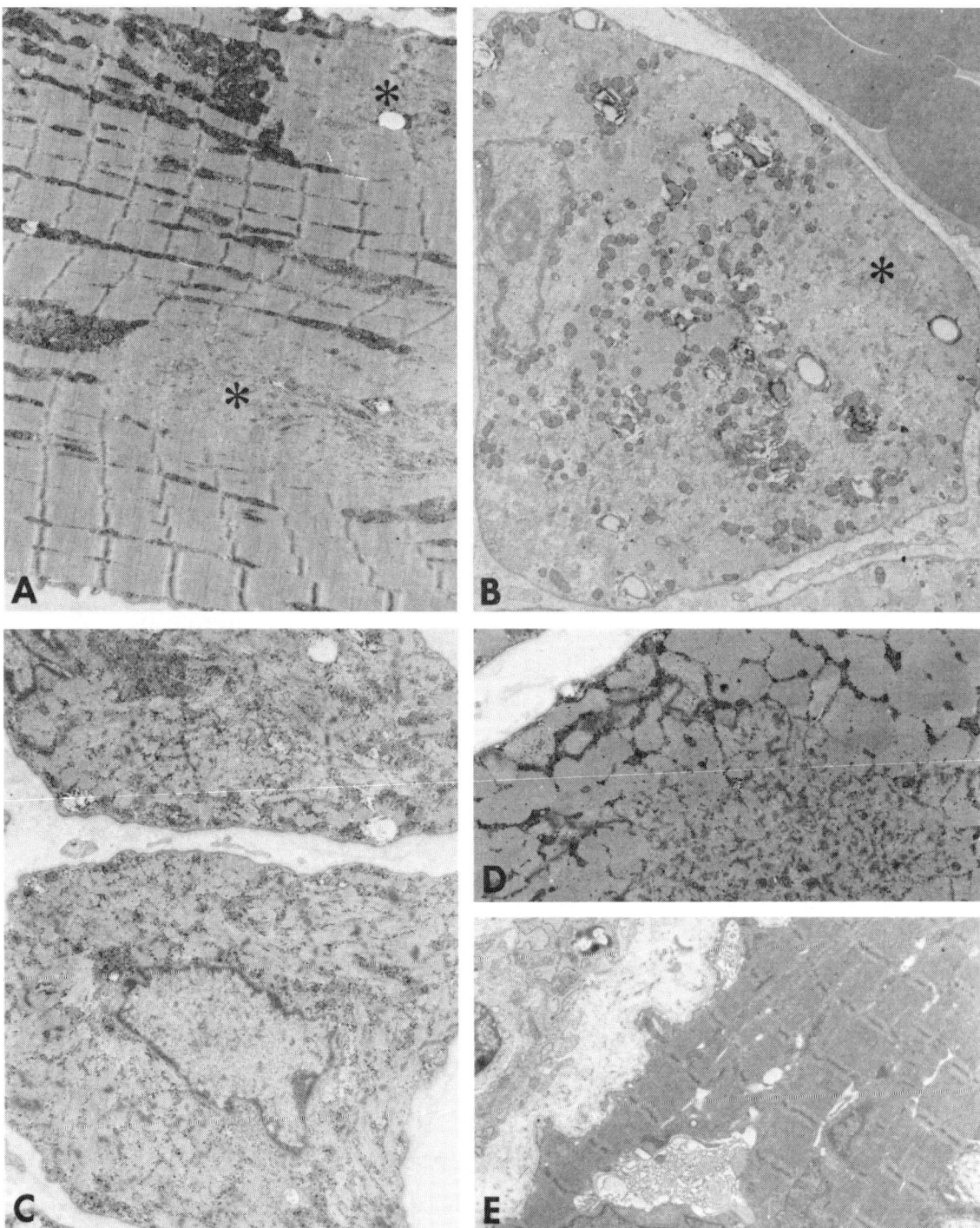

FIGURE 31-90. Highly atrophic perifascicular muscle fibers in dermatomyositis show focal mitochondrial loss associated with myofibrillar degeneration *(A, B, and D)*, clusters of mitochondria *(A and B)*, central nucleus and aberrant myofibrils with nemaline rods *(C)*, and abnormal spaces occupied by proliferating and degenerating membranous organelles *(E)*. A, ×4200; B, ×5600; C and D, ×7000; E, ×4900.

number of small lipid droplets (Fig. 31-90B), central nuclei (Fig. 31-90C), and papillary projections of the surface membrane (Fig. 31-90E).

FOCAL CYTOPLASMIC DEGRADATION AND AUTOPHAGIC MECHANISMS

Focal cytoplasmic degradation can occur within or outside autophagic vacuoles. However, when it begins outside the autophagic vacuoles, the partially degraded organelles can be subsequently entrapped within autophagic vacuoles in which their degradation is completed.

Autophagic Vacuoles

Definition and distribution. An autophagic vacuole is a secondary lysosome. It is limited by membrane, contains cytoplasmic degradation products, and reacts for acid phosphatase (Figs. 31-22, 31-91G). Lysosomal enzymes synthesized in the rough endoplasmic reticulum are further processed by the Golgi apparatus and are released as primary lysosomes from the *trans*-most Golgi cisternae. When lysosomal enzymes are delivered to membrane-bound spaces containing sequestered cytoplasmic material (autophagosomes), these spaces become secondary lysosomes, or autophagic vacuoles.[28]

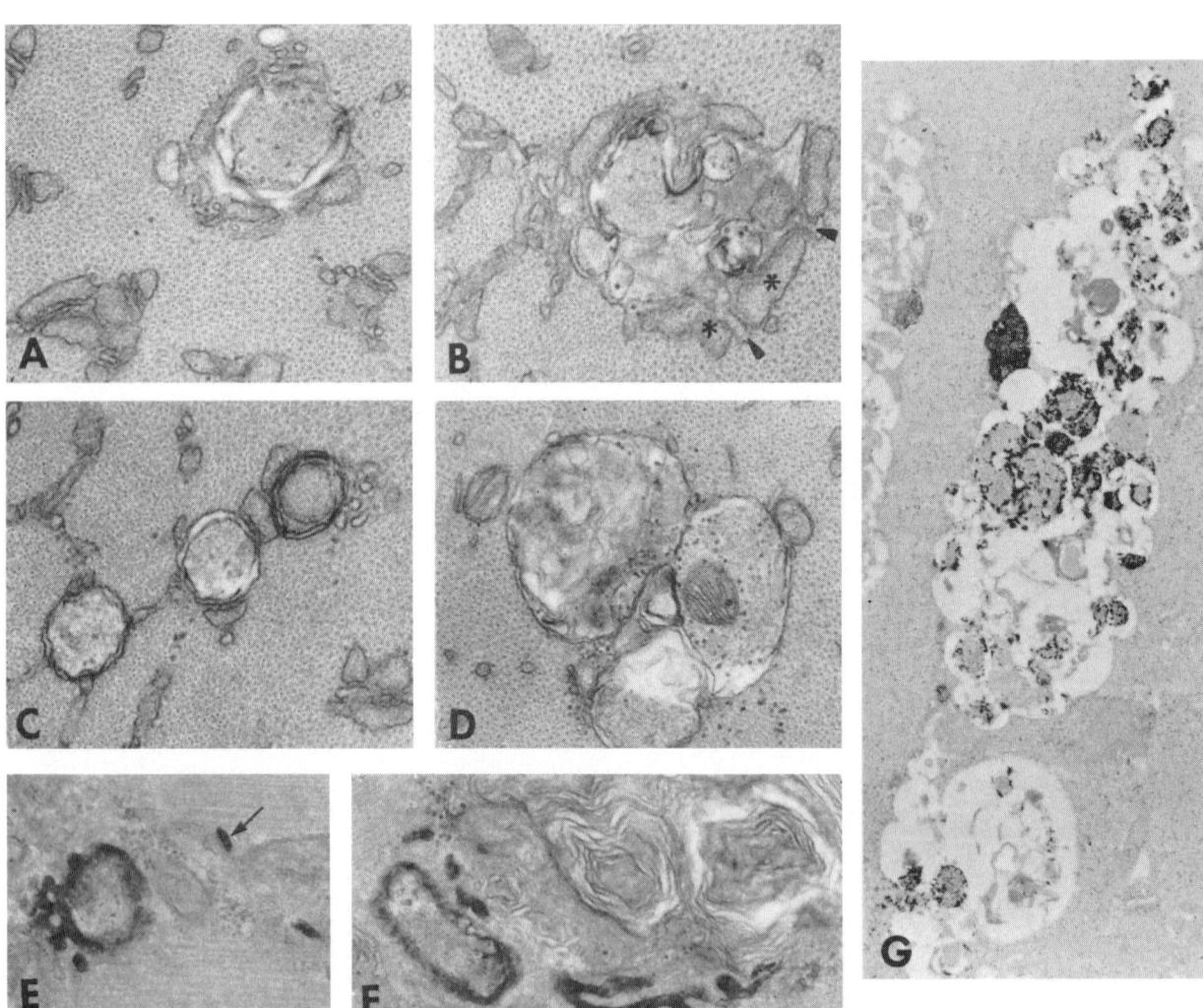

FIGURE 31-91. Autophagic mechanisms in experimental chloroquine myopathy. A to D show the entrapment of organelles into small vacuoles; E and F show that the T tubules provide membranes for the early vacuoles; G demonstrates acid phosphatase activity in a large autophagic vacuole. In A, membranous organelles incompletely surround a small area of cytoplasm. In B, alternating T (arrowheads) and junctional SR (asterisks) profiles and other membranes of undetermined origin surround a small cytoplasmic region. In C, three small abnormal spaces are surrounded by double membrane. The inner limiting membrane is incomplete in places, and the outer limiting membrane is thickened at the upper right. In D, three small spaces limited by frayed double membrane are coalescing to form a larger lobulated space that contains mitochondrion, glycogen granules, and amorphous or degraded cytoplasmic material. In E and F, peroxidase-loaded T tubules partially or completely surround small areas of cytoplasm. In G, the reaction product for acid phosphatase is associated with vacuolar contents. A to D, ×49,000; E and F, ×31,000; G, ×17,500. [A to F are reproduced by permission from Macdonald RD, Engel AG, J Neuropathol Exp Neurol 29:479, 1970; G is reproduced by permission from Engel AG, in Pearson CM (ed): The Striated Muscle. Baltimore: Williams & Wilkins; 1973, pp 301–341.]

Normal skeletal muscle contains only small lysosomal structures, identifiable by the acid phosphatase reaction, in the hof region of nuclei and in the junctional folds and cytoplasm at the neuromuscular junction.[157] Autophagic vacuoles are not found in normal muscle fibers but are prominent in some inflammatory myopathies (Figs. 31-92A and B, 31-93A, 31-94A); in lysosomal storage disorders, especially acid maltase deficiency (Figs. 31-19, 31-21, 31-22B, 31-101, 31-102)[6,7,26]; in LAMP-2 deficiency (Danon disease)[157a]; colchicine myopathy[157b]; in chloroquine myopathy (Figs. 31-22A, 31-91)[7,25]; in various types of periodic paralysis[7,22]; and in human (Fig. 31-92C) and experimental hypokalemic myopathy. They also occur in myofibrillar myopathy (Chap. 43); in oculopharyngeal dystrophy (Chap. 40); in sporadic or familial distal myopathies[145,146,158–161] (Chap. 42); in experimental[162] and human vitamin E deficiency (see "Miscellaneous Inclusions," above); and in experimental vincristine myopathy.[163,164]

Factors promoting autophagic vacuole formation. A number of stimuli promote the formation of autophagic vacuoles. These include deficiency of a lysosomal enzyme (e.g., acid maltase); impaired degradation of lysosomal contents due to an increase in lysosomal pH, as in chloroquine myopathy[165]; or inhibition of phospholipid catabolism, as in vincristine myopathy.[163] In each of these instances the stimulus for lysosomal proliferation is a defect in the digestive power or impaired control of the action of lysosomes. In other disorders, as in periodic paralysis, emetine myopathy (Fig. 31-33A), some of the end plate myopathies, and some of the inflammatory myopathies (Fig. 31-33D) and dystrophies (Fig. 31-33B), an extralysosomal degradation of organelles appears to act as a stimulus for their entrapment into autophagic vacuoles, where their destruction can be completed. Temporary experimental ischemia or cardiac muscle is followed by the appearance of numerous autophagic vacuoles during reoxygenation.[165] The stimuli promoting autophagic vacuole formation in sporadic or familial distal myopathies are not known, but it is somewhat tempting to speculate that at least some of these myopathies could be conditioned by a lysosomal enzyme defect.

The content of autophagic vacuoles. The content of these vacuoles can vary with the disorder in which the vacuoles occur, but similar autophagic vacuoles can be found in different disorders, and different types of autophagic vacuole

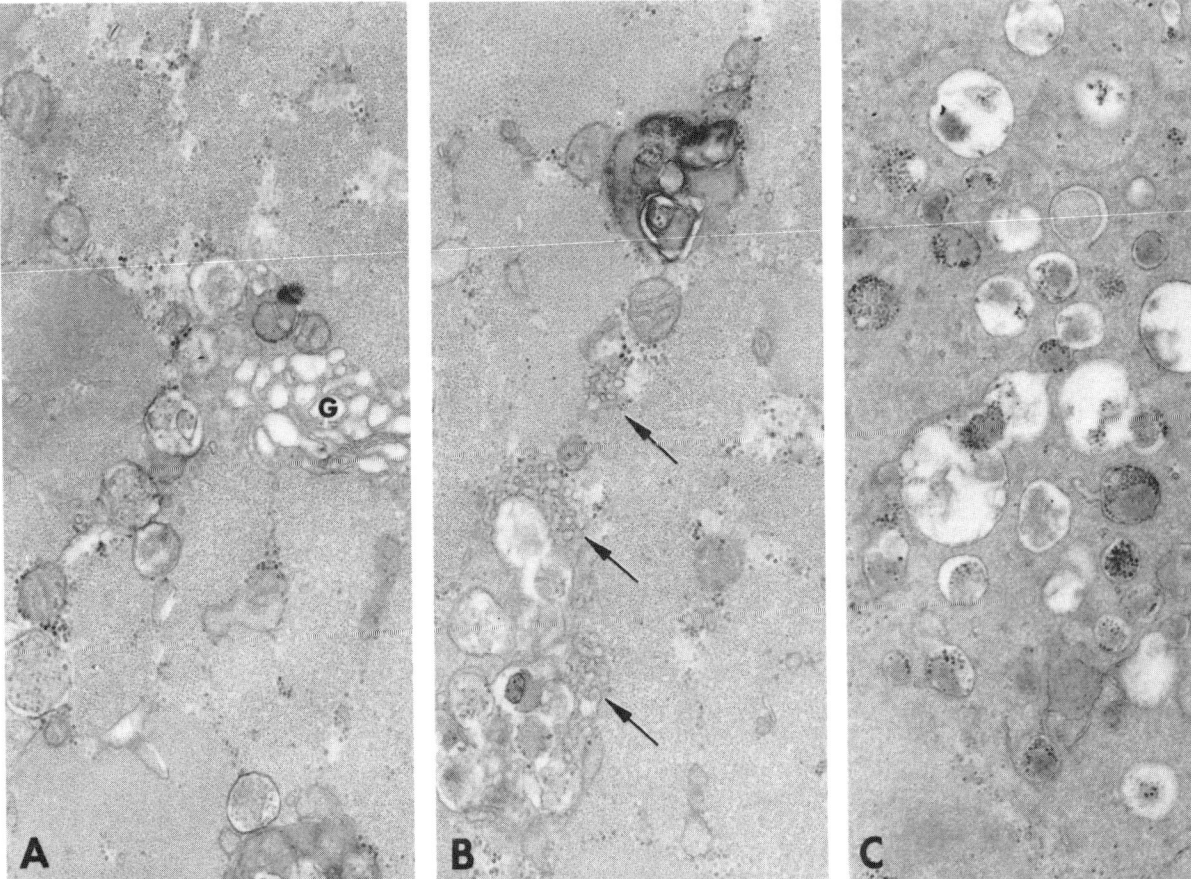

FIGURE 31-92. Autophagic mechanisms in polymyositis (A and B) and hypokalemic myopathy (C). Degenerating organelles are entrapped in small membrane-bound spaces (A, B, and C); T-system networks (arrows) provide membrane for the abnormal spaces (B); and the smaller abnormal spaces coalesce to form larger ones (B and C). G, Golgi network. A and B, ×24,800; C, ×20,000.

may appear in a given disorder. The commonest, or ordinary, autophagic vacuole is one with heterogeneous contents that include small dense bodies studded with glycogen particles, membrane fragments, myeloid structures, and debris (Figs. 31-21, 31-92, 31-93B). This type of vacuole is observed in most disorders in which an autophagic mechanism is excited, such as acid maltase deficiency, chloroquine myopathy, distal myopathies, or hypokalemic myopathy.

A number of vacuolar components are associated with, but not specific for, different disorders. These include the electron-dense curvilinear bodies found in neuronal lipofuscinosis (Chap. 30) and in some vacuoles in chloroquine myopathy (Fig. 31-22A); the spheromembranous bodies in experimental vincristine myopathy[163,164]; and the homogeneous dark material which is the only component of the giant secondary lysosomes in human vitamin E deficiency (Fig. 31-67). Also, glycogen granules are the only component of one type of autophagic vacuole in acid maltase deficiency (Figs. 31-101, 31-102); and mineralized SR vesicles are found in some autophagic vacuoles in periodic paralysis (Fig. 31-27).

The source of membranes for autophagic vacuoles. The T system is the principal membrane source for autophagic vacuoles (see "Alterations of the T Tubules," above, and Figs. 31-19, 31-21, 31-34A, 31-91, 31-92, 31-101A). In addition, the Golgi cisternae also provide membranes for autophagic vacuoles in acid maltase deficiency (Fig. 31-101B).

The development of autophagic vacuoles. The development of these vacuoles has been investigated in detail in experimental chloroquine myopathy[25] (Fig. 31-91), but the general scheme appears to be identical in other myopathies studied to date (Figs. 31-19, 31-34A, 31-92). The initial step is the encirclement of small cytoplasmic areas containing normal or abnormal organelles by a double membrane (Figs. 31-19A, 31-34A, 31-91A and C). The small double-membrane-bound spaces gradually enlarge and fuse to form somewhat larger, lobulated vacuoles with scalloped borders limited mostly by a single but in places still by a double membrane (Figs. 31-91D, 31-92B and C). The latter, in turn, coalesce to form even larger autophagic vacuoles (Figs. 31-21, 31-22A, 31-93B). When the T system is marked by peroxidase, the proliferating tubules that partly or completely encircle small areas of cytoplasm (Fig. 31-91E and F) and the membrane networks and tubular structures that contribute to the walls of larger vacuoles (Figs. 31-19B to D) become filled with peroxidase.

The delivery of lysosomal enzymes to autophagic vacuoles. The electron cytochemical localization of acid phosphatase indicates that the T system also plays a role in the delivery of lysosomal enzymes to the autophagic vacuoles (Fig. 31-22B).[7,26] However, coated vesicles may also participate in lysosomal enzyme transport. This subject also has been discussed under "Alterations of the T Tubules," above.

The fate of autophagic vacuoles. Ordinary autophagic vacuoles containing partially degraded material are able to move about within the muscle fiber or are vectorially translated in the direction of the surface membrane. On reaching the surface membrane, they discharge their contents by exocytosis, as described under "Alterations of the Surface Membrane." Interestingly, autophagic vacuoles that have a more uniform content (such as curvilinear bodies or only glycogen granules) seldom exocytose their contents.

Some autophagic vacuoles that entrap partially degraded or degenerating organelles degrade their contents completely and become filled with an amorphous matrix (Fig. 31-94). At an intermediate stage of development these vacuoles contain partially degraded organelles surrounded by matrix material (Fig. 31-94A), but when mature they contain only matrix material (Fig. 31-94B). This type of vacuole is also lined by membranes of T-system origin, communicates with the T system and via the T system with the extracellular fluid (Fig. 31-94), and can be loaded with peroxidase from the extracellular fluid.[7,22] Vacuoles of this type do not undergo exocytosis, but one can infer that liquefied degradation products can exit from them and from the fiber via the T tubules. These vacuoles represent the mature and most frequently encountered vacuoles in periodic paralysis.[7,22] They also appear in the end plate myopathy associated with the slow-channel myasthenic syndrome[11] and, occasionally, in polymyositis (Fig. 31-94) and myotubular myopathy. Membranes of these vacuoles are reinforced by the cytoskeletal components dystrophin and β-spectrin[165a] (Color Plate 13Q, R, and S).

Cytoplasmic Degradation in Inclusion Body Myositis and in Some Distal Myopathies

Abundant cytoplasmic degradation products accumulate in abnormal muscle fibers in inclusion body myositis (Figs. 31-70, 31-71, 31-95) and in some sporadic or familial distal myopathies.[145,146,158–161] On light microscopic observation, the smaller abnormal fiber regions show a loss of myofibrillar markings and react for acid phosphatase; the larger abnormal regions appear as rimmed vacuoles that either react for acid phosphatase at their periphery and/or center or fail to react for the enzyme.[141,146,160,161] In unfixed cryostat sections, acid phosphatase reactivity is more prominent with naphthol AS-BI phosphate than with sodium β-glycerophosphate as the substrate, but some of the rimmed vacuoles do not react even with the latter substrate.

In the electron microscope the large abnormal fiber regions always contain prominent myeloid structures of varying size and electron density. Small, dense bodies studded with glycogen granules, freely dispersed glycogen granules, small vesicles of unknown origin, and debris are present in variable amounts (Figs. 31-70A and C, 31-71, 31-95). Filamentous inclusions appear within or adjacent to the abnormal regions in inclusion body myositis and in some of the sporadic or familial myopathies (see "Miscellaneous Inclusions," above, and Refs. 145 and 146). A given large abnormal fiber region differs from a single autophagic vacuole in that it is not surrounded by a continuous limiting membrane, but numerous small degraded and membrane-bound structures occur within it (Figs. 31-70A, 31-95). T-system networks abut on some of the large abnormal regions (Fig. 31-70C) but fail to entrap the contents of the entire region and never form membranes around the filamentous inclusions. The above findings suggest that both lysosomal and ubiquitin-dependent proteosomal destruction or organelles occurs in inclusion body myositis and in some of the distal myopathies and that the ability of the affected fibers to

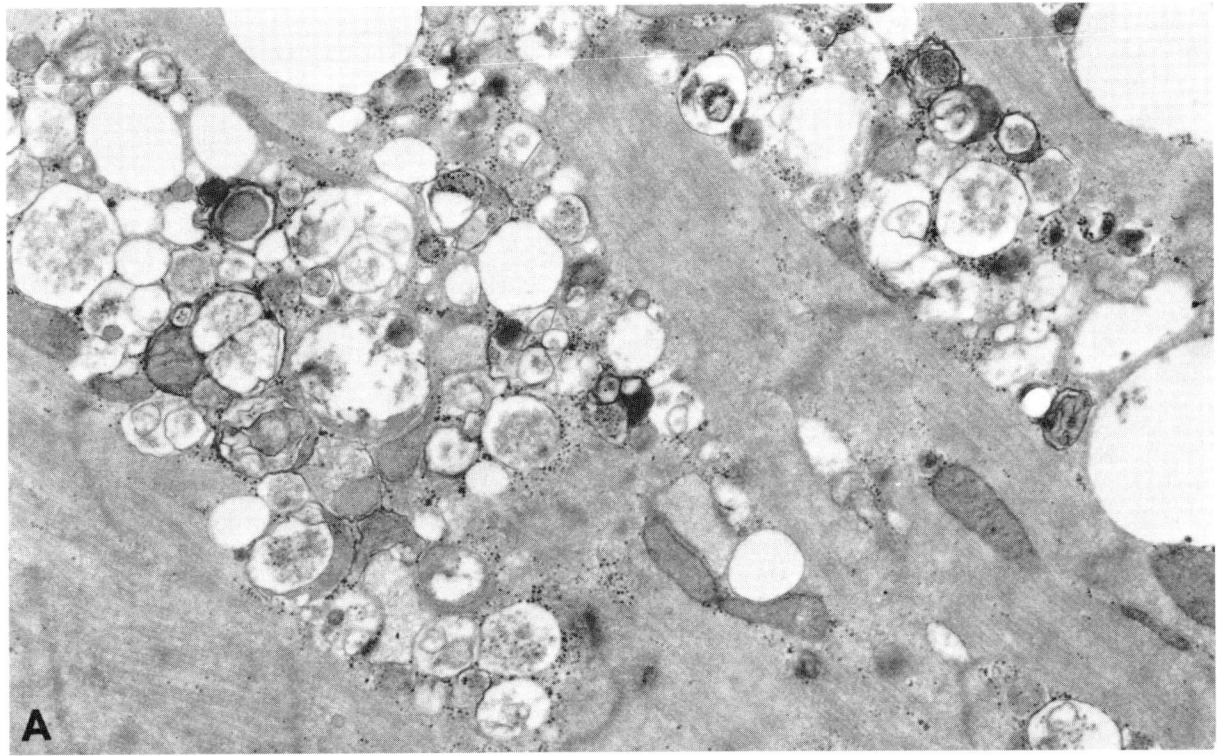
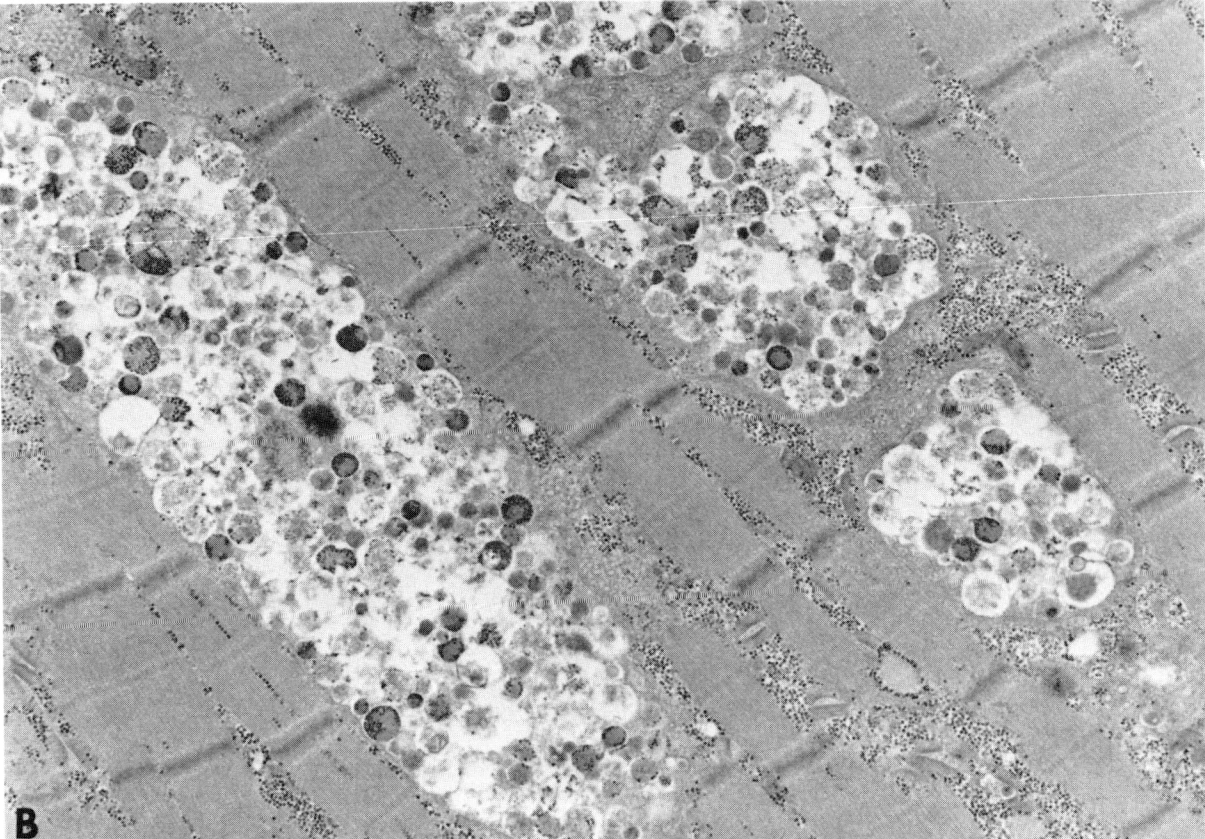

FIGURE 31-93. Autophagic mechanisms in polymyositis *(A)* and acid maltase deficiency *(B)*. In *A*, multiple small adjacent autophagic vacuoles occupy abnormal fiber regions; in *B*, large autophagic vacuoles with lobulated contours arise by coalescence of multiple small adjacent autophagic vacuoles. *A*, ×20,000; *B*, ×16,700.

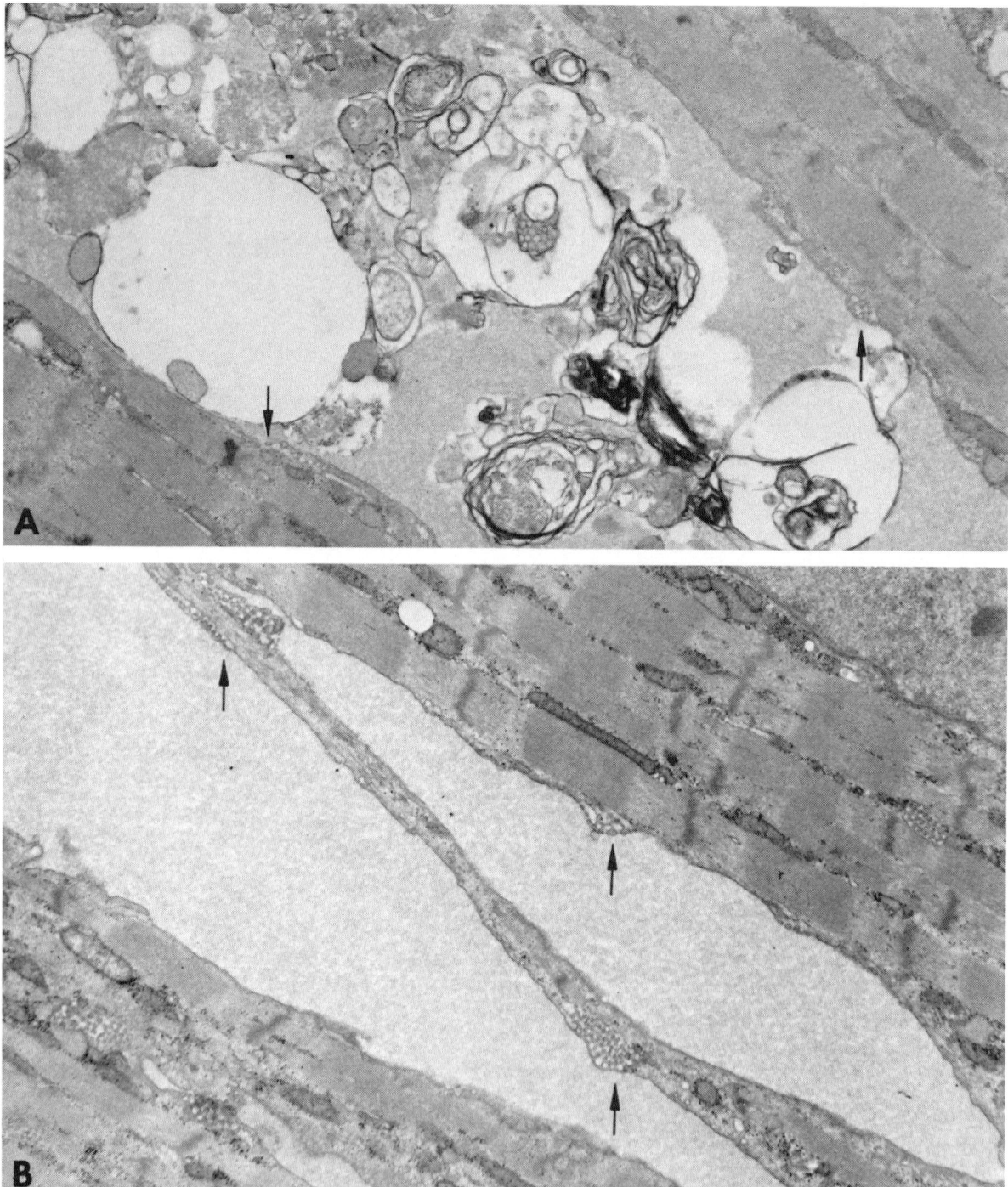

FIGURE 31-94. Autophagic mechanisms in polymyositis. Large vacuoles contain partially degraded organelles, myeloid structures, and debris surrounded by amorphous material (A), or amorphous material only (B). Numerous T-system networks abut on and communicate with the lumen of the vacuole. Vacuoles of this type are commonly observed in periodic paralysis. A and B, ×13,600.

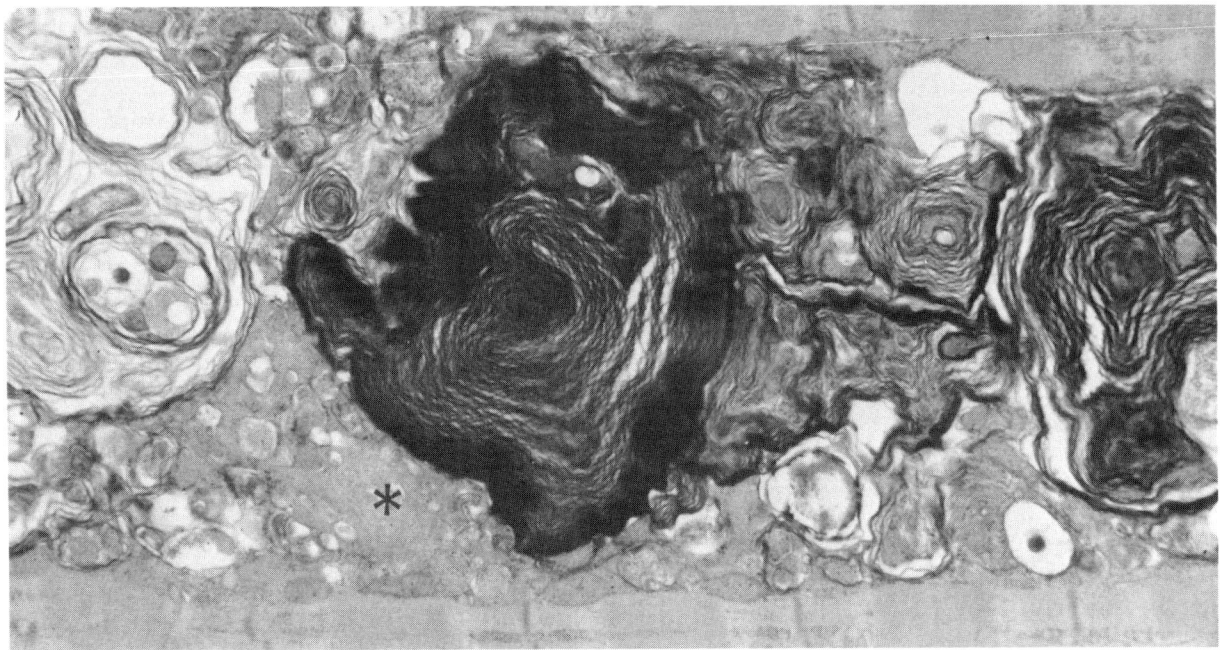

FIGURE 31-95. Large myeloid structures, partially degraded organelles, and filamentous inclusion (asterisk) in inclusion body myositis. Although multiple small abnormal membrane-bound spaces appear in the large abnormal region, the region itself is not surrounded by a single membrane. ×11,000.

sequester, degrade, and eliminate the accumulating degradation products may be compromised. Electron cytochemical localization of acid phosphatase in these disorders would be informative but has not been done to date.

LIPID ACCUMULATION IN MUSCLE FIBERS

Normal human muscle fibers contain a few small (less than 0.5 μm in diameter) neutral fat droplets. The droplets are typically adjacent to the I bands and are more commonly observed in type 1 than in type 2 fibers. They are electron-lucent and non-membrane-bound, but traces of slightly more electron-dense material can appear around or within the droplets. In 10 healthy subjects the percentage of the fiber volume occupied by lipid droplets was less than 0.3 percent.[166] The lipid fraction of the fiber volume may increase with obesity; with primary disturbances of lipid or mitochondrial metabolism (Figs. 31-36, and Color Plate 7J and P); and in scattered fibers in inflammatory (Fig. 31-90B), endocrine, and other myopathies. Lipid droplets together with glycogen granules generally accumulate near mitochondrial aggregates in mitochondrial myopathies (Figs. 31-37A, 31-38A) and in myxedema myopathy (Fig. 31-98C).

In primary carnitine deficiency or in other disorders of lipid metabolism affecting skeletal muscle, the mean lipid fraction of the fiber volume can be as high as 10 percent, and up to 30 percent of the volume of some type 1 fibers consists of lipid droplets.[166,167] The lipid droplets appear in long rows between the myofibrils and under the sarcolemma, and adjacent droplets coalesce to form larger, irregularly lobulated bodies that may exceed 10 μm in diameter (Fig. 31-96 and Color Plate 7P). Mitochondria usually abut on the lipid droplets, and the mitochondrial content of the muscle fibers is also increased.[167] Much less lipid accumulates in muscle fibers in carnitine palmityltransferase deficiency than in carnitine deficiency.[166] Marked neutral lipid excess occurs in muscle fibers and in many other tissues in a disorder associated with congenital ichthyosis,[167a] also known as Chanarin-Dorfman disease. The biochemical basis of this disorder is impaired utilization of endogenously synthesized triglycerides owing to a defect in a lipolytic enzyme encoded by CGI-58 on chromosome 3.[167b]

GLYCOGEN ACCUMULATION IN MUSCLE FIBERS

Normal human muscle fibers contain numerous 20- to 25-nm β-glycogen granules. Most granules are adjacent to the I bands (Figs. 31-1, 31-2); a few appear between the myofilaments within the I bands (Fig. 31-2B), but few or none occur in relation to the A bands (Figs. 31-1, 31-2A). In normal fibers the glycogen granules do not compress the myofibrils. A few normal fibers contain small subsarcolemmal glycogen deposits.

The abundance of glycogen in muscle varies with the nutritional state and physical activity, and type 2 fibers contain more glycogen than type 1 fibers. However, from simple inspection of electron micrographs one cannot classify the fibers by their glycogen content or make reliable inferences about the patient's nutritional state.

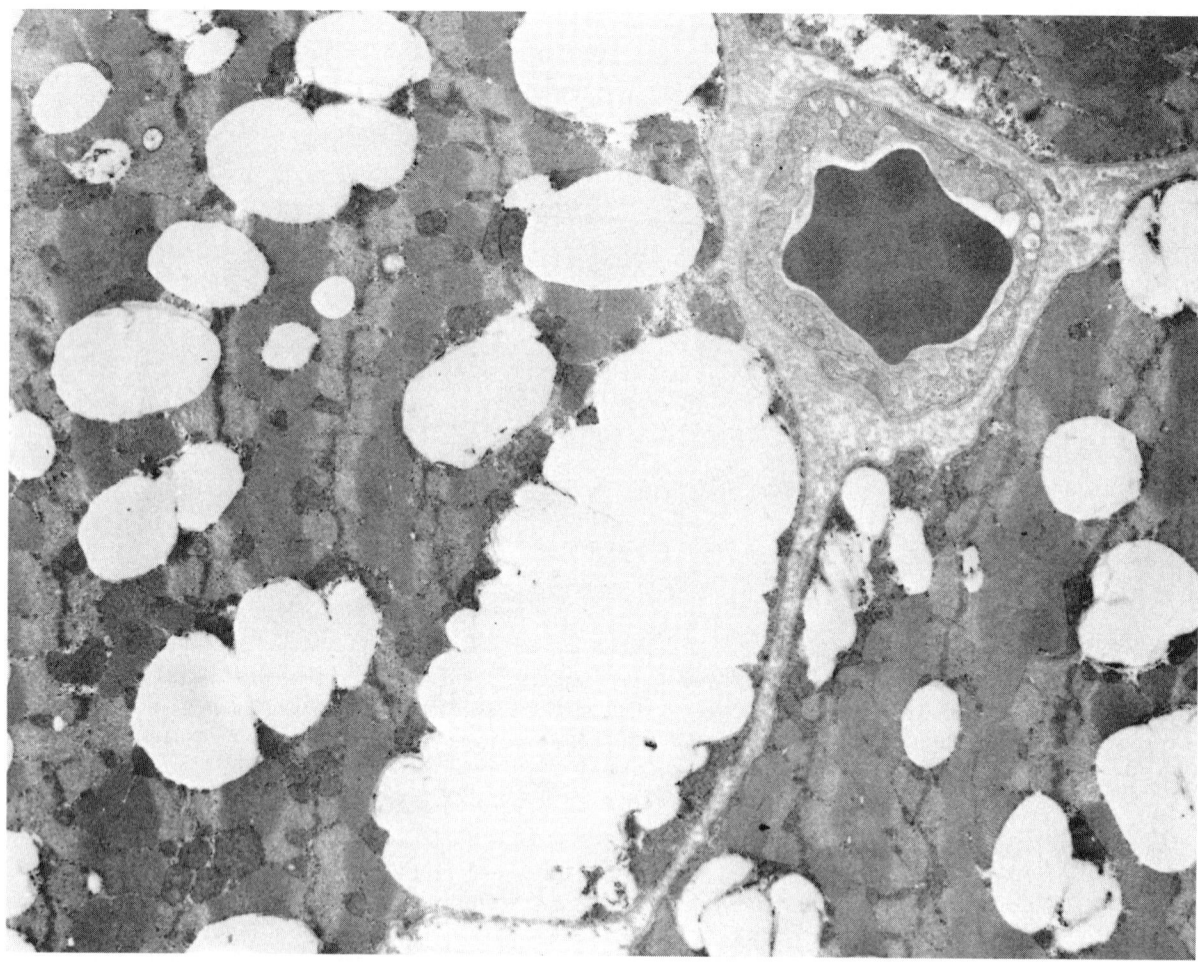

FIGURE 31-96. Lipid storage in muscle carnitine deficiency. Abnormal spaces of varying sizes lack limiting membrane, and some are coalescing. Largest lipid deposit is subsarcolemmal. ×7800. [Reproduced by permission from Engel AG, in Pearson CM (ed): The Striated Muscle. Baltimore: Williams & Wilkins; 1973, pp 301–341.]

Inadequate fixation, or prolonged storage of glutaraldehyde-fixed muscle in buffer before osmium fixation, or prolonged en bloc staining with aqueous uranyl acetate at an acid pH can result in loss of glycogen granules from the fibers, so that the spaces previously occupied by glycogen granules appear empty (Fig. 31-12B). The use of phosphate-buffered glutaraldehyde or treatment of the tissues with potassium ferrocyanide during or after osmication increases the affinity of the glycogen granules for lead electron stains and makes it easier to distinguish them from the slightly smaller and less electron-dense ribosomal particles.

Glycogen Accumulation in Miscellaneous Disorders

Glycogen granules tend to accumulate passively in fiber regions from which all other organelles have disappeared (Figs. 31-85C, 31-86B, 31-88D, 31-97A). They also accumulate around filamentous bodies (Fig. 31-53), concentric laminated bodies (Fig. 31-54), and cylindrical spirals (Fig. 31-64).

Typically, abundant glycogen granules are associated with aggregates of normal or abnormal mitochondria in mitochondrial myopathies (Figs. 31-28A, 31-37). Marked glycogen excess is found in some muscle fibers in benign infantile cytochrome c oxidase deficiency[168,169] (Fig. 31-36 and Color Plate 7L).

In hypothyroid myopathy glycogen accumulates in abnormal fiber regions that also contain mitochondria, lipid droplets, and proliferating, dilated, and degenerating T tubules (Figs. 31-35B, 31-98B and C).[170–173] Entrapment of glycogen granules in lysosome-like structures may also occur in hypothyroid myopathy.[171] Increases in glycogen in relation to mitochondrial aggregates have been observed in corticosteroid-induced myopathy.[174]

Small lakes of glycogen appear in some regenerating fibers (Fig. 31-123) and in the hof regions of central nuclei in centronuclear (myotubular) myopathy (Fig. 31-12B).

Glycogen and Polysaccharide Storage Disorders

Since the ultrastructural features of the glycogen storage disorders are discussed in Chaps. 55 and 56, only a brief summary is presented here.

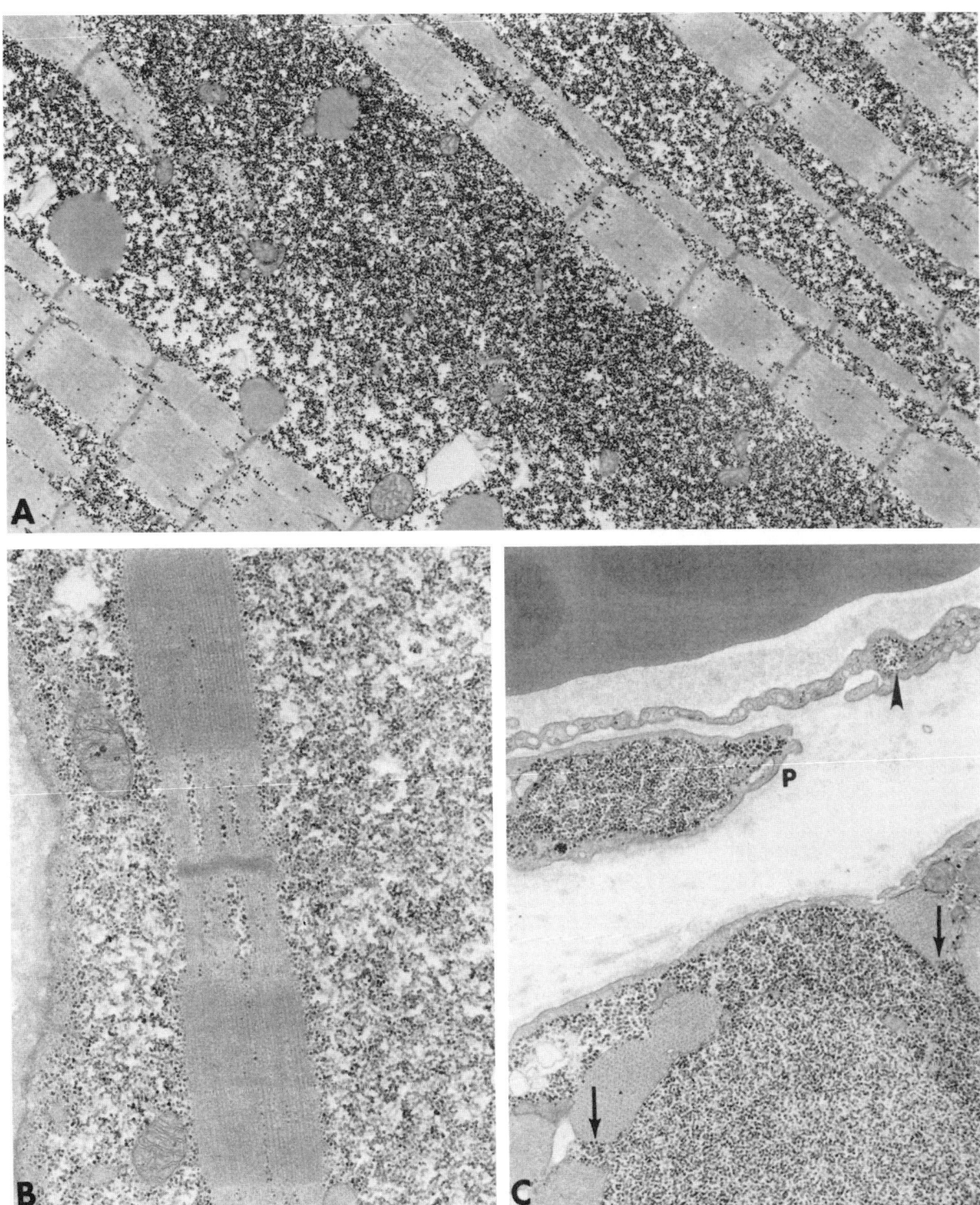

FIGURE 31-97. Glycogen accumulation in a myopathy of undetermined type *(A)* and in acid maltase deficiency *(B* and *C)*. In *A* and *B*, the glycogen accumulations are non-membrane-bound; in *C*, membrane-bound glycogen appears in capillary endothelial cell (arrowhead), pericyte (P), and muscle fiber. Holes in membrane around glycogen deposit (arrows) may allow glycogen granules to enter or escape from lysosomal space. *A*, ×11,900; *B*, ×22,000; *C*, ×20,400.

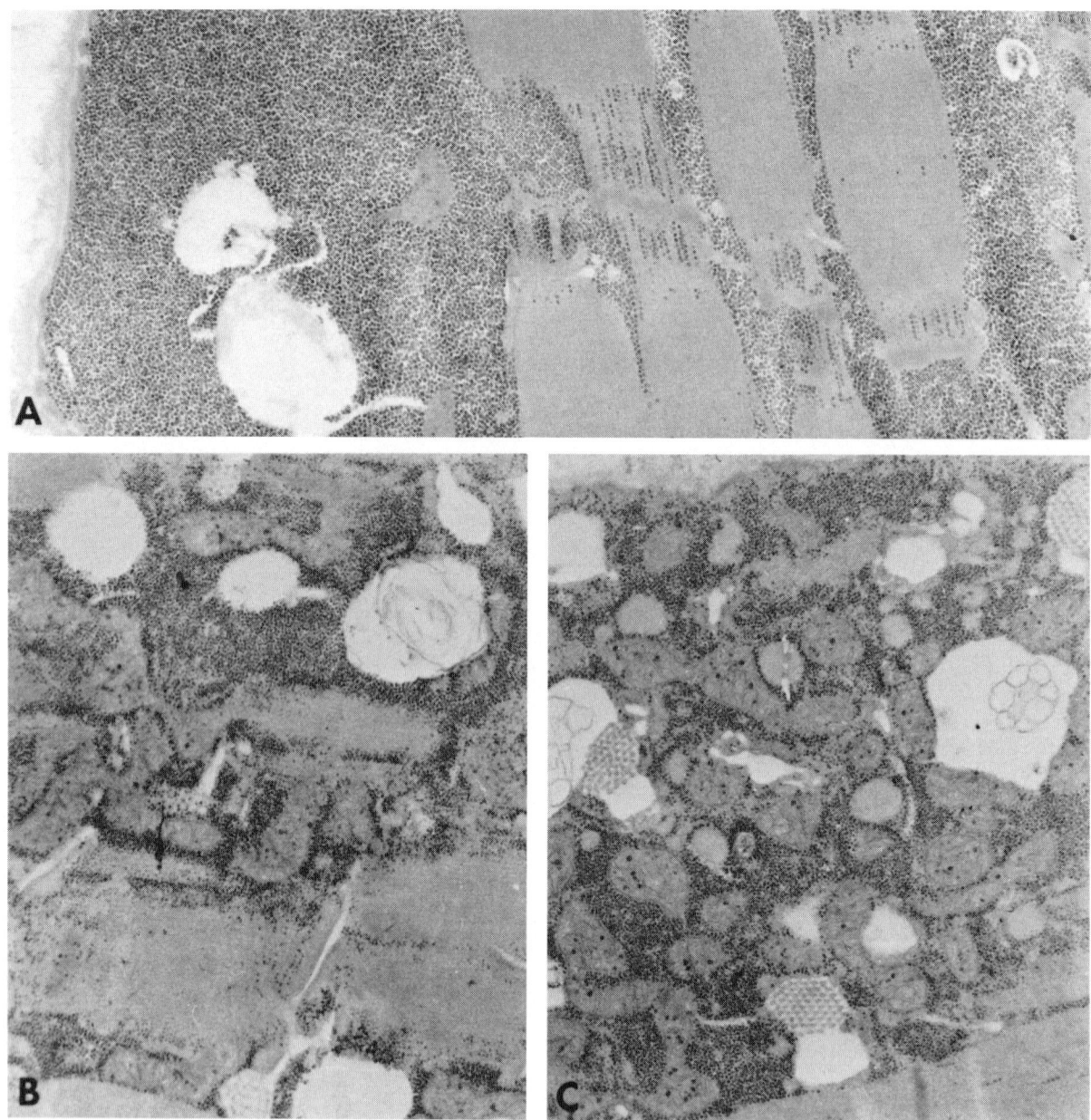

FIGURE 31-98. Intermyofibrillar and subsarcolemmal glycogen accumulation in muscle phosphorylase deficiency (A) and in myxedema myopathy (B and C). A few lipid droplets are associated with glycogen in A. Lipid droplets, T-system networks, dilated T tubules, and clusters of mitochondria are intermingled with glycogen in B and C. A, B, and C, ×20,400.

Defects in the classic glycolytic pathway. The ultrastructural aspects of glycogen storage are similar in deficiencies of debranching enzyme, phosphorylase, phosphofructokinase, phosphoglycerate kinase, and phosphoglycerate mutase. In each of these disorders β-glycogen granules accumulate in subsarcolemmal pockets and in deeper fiber regions, where they displace, replace, and compress the myofibrils and other organelles (Fig. 31-98A).

Additional morphologic features have been noted in debranching enzyme deficiency and phosphofructokinase deficiency. In debranching enzyme deficiency small lysosomal structures appear within large glycogen deposits, but there is

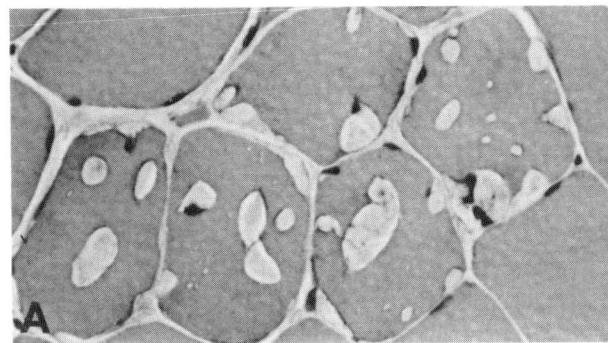 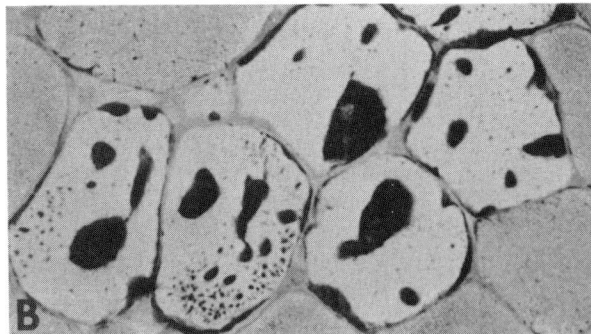

FIGURE 31-99. Neuromyopathy associated with polyglucosan storage; cryostat sections stained with hematoxylin and eosin (A), and with PAS after diastase digestion (B). The vacuoles appear empty in A and are filled with diastase-fast PAS-positive material in B. A and B, ×300.

no significant lysosomal storage of glycogen.[175] In three patients with phosphofructokinase deficiency, amylopectin (glucosan) also accumulated in some muscle fibers.[176,177] Lipofuscin granules and small membrane-bound glycogen deposits were noted near the amylopectin deposits.[176]

Branching enzyme deficiency. β-Glycogen granules and amylopectin accumulate in branching enzyme deficiency.[178-180] Amylopectin is a PAS-positive polysaccharide that differs from normal glycogen in being diastase-fast and in having abnormally long chains and too few branch points. Ultrastructurally, it is composed of short, 6- to 8-nm-wide, randomly oriented, and occasionally branching filaments. The affected muscle fibers contain large, sharply circumscribed vacuoles in which peripherally situated glycogen granules surround the more centrally positioned amylopectin filaments. The vacuoles are not membrane-bound and typically appear in type 1 fibers.

Polyglucosan accumulation in other disorders. In addition to branching enzyme deficiency and some cases of phosphofructokinase deficiency, amylopectin (glucosan) deposits also appear in the nervous system and in muscle in Lafora myoclonus epilepsy (Chap. 30 and Refs. 181 and 182); in neuronal processes and glial cells[183,183a,b]; and in corpora amylacea in the central nervous system with aging. Interestingly, in a subgroup of patients with adult polyglucosan body disease, branching enzyme deficiency was found in leukocytes and peripheral nerves, and mutations in branching enzyme were identified.[183c,d]

Large glucosan deposits in muscle fibers also occur in polyglucosan body disease. This disorder presents in children or adults with skeletal or cardioskeletal myopathy. Glucosan deposits are found in skeletal, cardiac, and smooth muscle; hepatocytes; adrenal medullary cells; epithelium of sweat glands; and glial elements of the nervous system.[183d,e,f]

In a patient with this disorder observed by us, a middle-aged woman who had a slowly progressive myopathy and peripheral neuropathy, many type 1 muscle fibers harbored large polyglucosan deposits that intermingled with glycogen granules (Figs. 31-99, 31-100A, and Color Plate 7M, N, and O). In this patient phosphofructokinase and other glycolytic enzymes were normally active in muscle, and branching enzyme activity (determined by Dr. Barbara Brown) was normal in cultured fibroblasts. Finally, we have encountered large polyglucosan deposits in occasional fibers in soleus muscles of normal rabbits (Fig. 31-100B).

Acid maltase deficiency. There is marked glycogen accumulation in all tissues in infantile acid maltase deficiency (Color Plate 12A to F). Less glycogen accumulates and skeletal muscle is predominantly affected in the childhood cases. The glycogen excess is least marked and only skeletal muscle is clinically affected in the adult cases (Color Plates 7H and 12J to L). Acid mucins as well as glycogen accumulate in muscle in the infants and children but not in the adults (Color Plate 12G to I).[184] In all cases of acid maltase deficiency, glycogen is stored in four types of spaces[6,7,26]: (1) freely dispersed in the cytoplasm, where it displaces, replaces, and compresses preexisting organelles (Figs. 31-97B, 31-101C, and 31-102A); (2) in sacs limited by single or double membranes that contain only glycogen (Figs. 31-101 and 31-102); (3) in ordinary autophagic vacuoles with heterogeneous contents (Figs. 31-21 and 31-93B); and (4) in spaces transitional between the above types (Figs. 31-97C and 31-101C). Both the T system (Figs. 31-19, 31-21, and 31-101A) and Golgi cisternae (Fig. 31-101B) contribute to the vacuolar membranes. The membrane-bound vacuoles react for acid phosphatase and are therefore secondary lysosomes. In some sacs the glycogen granules are decreased in size (Fig. 31-102A), perhaps because they have been partially degraded.

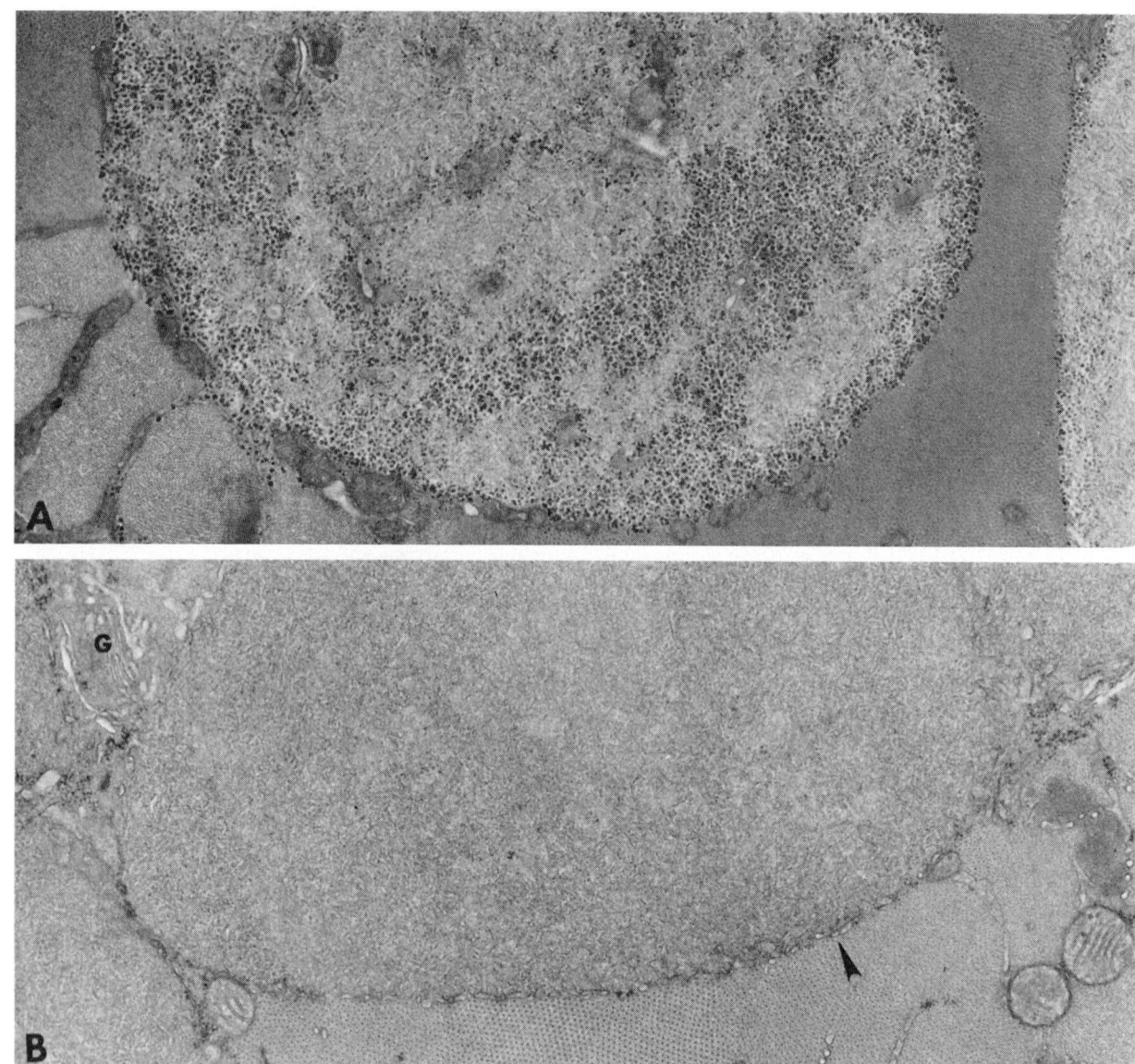

FIGURE 31-100. Polyglucosan deposits composed of 6- to 8-nm-wide short filaments in a patient with polyglucosan neuromyopathy not due to branching enzyme or phosphofructokinase deficiency (A) and in soleus muscle of normal rabbit (B). In A, glycogen granules and sarcotubular components intermingle with the stored material. In B, the glucosan deposit is surrounded by sarcotubular profiles (arrowhead) and is adjacent to a Golgi complex (G). A and B, ×24,800.

MUSCLE FIBER INVASION AND DESTRUCTION BY T CELLS AND MACROPHAGES

Invasion and destruction of nonnecrotic fibers by mononuclear cells occurs relatively frequently in polymyositis and inclusion body myositis (Color Plate 8G to L), infrequently in dermatomyositis and scleroderma, and seldom in genetic myopathies such as Duchenne dystrophy (Chaps. 30, 34, and 49 and Refs. 156 and 185). The mononuclear cells that focally surround and invade the nonnecrotic fibers are either T lymphocytes or macrophages. Among those cells in immediate contact with the surface of the invaded fiber (i.e., the invading cells), about two-thirds are CD8[+], and one-half of these are activated; 20 to 30 percent

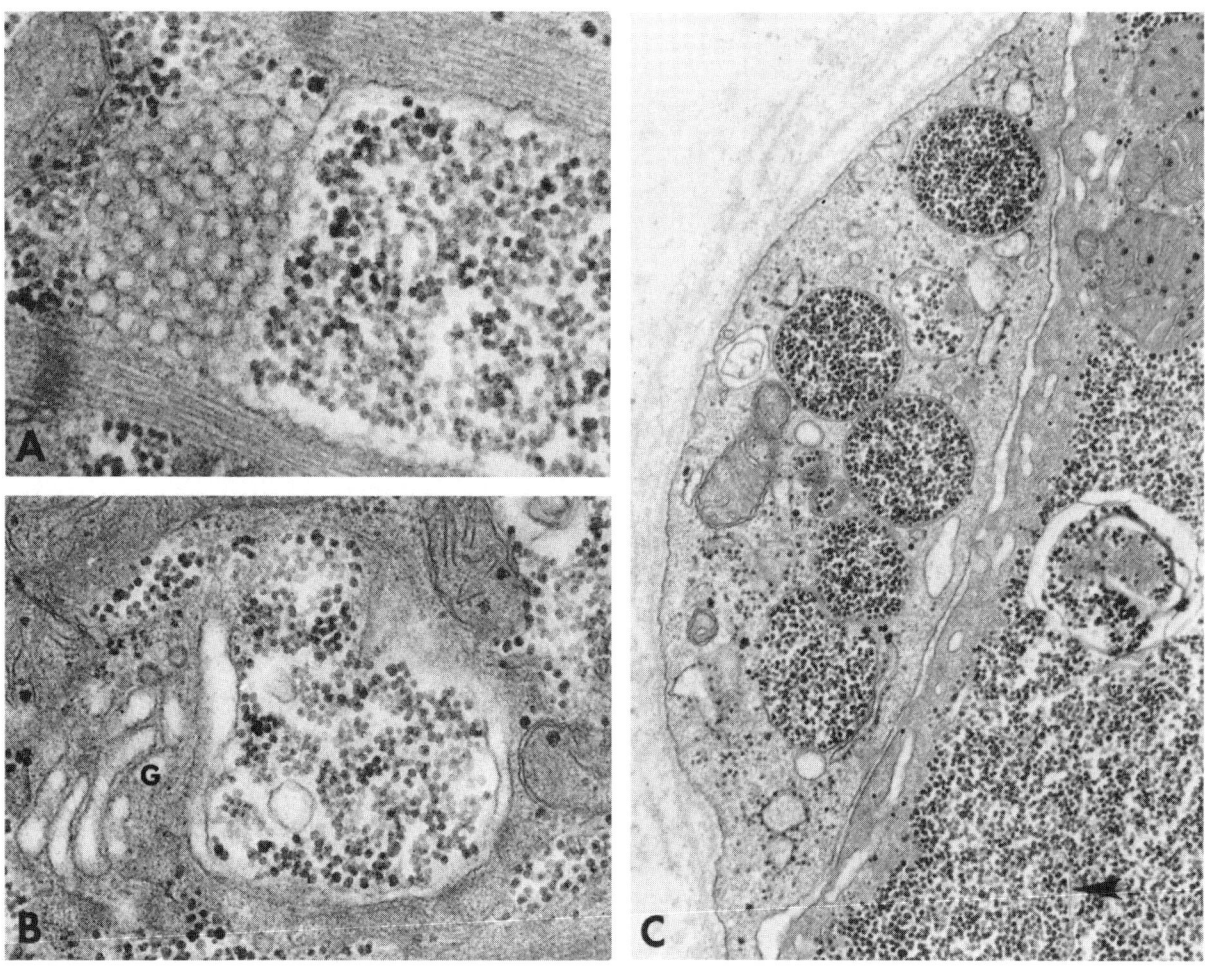

FIGURE 31-101. Lysosomal glycogen sacs in acid maltase deficiency. In A, T-system network merges with membrane around glycogen deposit. In B, glycogen deposit near Golgi complex (G) is incompletely enveloped by double membrane, which appears to have arisen from a Golgi cistern. In C, glycogen sacs appear in satellite cell; parent fiber contains both intra- and extrasaccular glycogen deposits separated by membrane profiles (arrowhead). A, ×59,000; B, ×44,700; C, ×21,000. [A and B are reproduced by permission from Engel AG, Brain 93:599, 1970; C is reproduced by permission from Engel AG, in Pearson CM (ed): The Striated Muscle. Baltimore: Williams & Wilkins; 1973, pp 301–341.]

are macrophages; and less than 10 percent are CD4+ cells (Color Plate 8I to L).[185] These findings are especially significant in view of the known cytotoxic capability of CD8+ cells and because histocompatibility factors permit CD8+ but not CD4+ cells to recognize an antigen on the muscle fiber surface membrane.[186]

Invasion and destruction of nonnecrotic muscle fibers by mononuclear cells can be readily observed in cryostat sections (Chap. 30 and Color Plate 8G to L). That the invaded fibers are not necrotic is indicated by their staining properties with the modified trichrome stain and by their lack of reactivity for the C5b-9 complement membrane attack complex (MAC).[155,185] Cell-mediated fiber destruction is also apparent in semithin resin sections (Fig. 31-103), and immunoelectron microscopic studies demonstrate at a higher level of resolution how different types of mononuclear cells interact with the invaded muscle fiber.[5,5a] Lymphocyte surface markers can be immunolocalized in biopsy specimens with optimal sensitivity and preservation of fine structure by applying monoclonal antibodies to glutaraldehyde-prefixed 20-μm frozen sections in which immunoreactivity of antigens is restored by $NaBH_4$ reduction.[5,5a] After treatment with a biotinylated second antibody and the avidin-biotin-peroxidase complex,[187] the sections are processed for electron microscopy. The following sequence of events is observed[5,5a]:

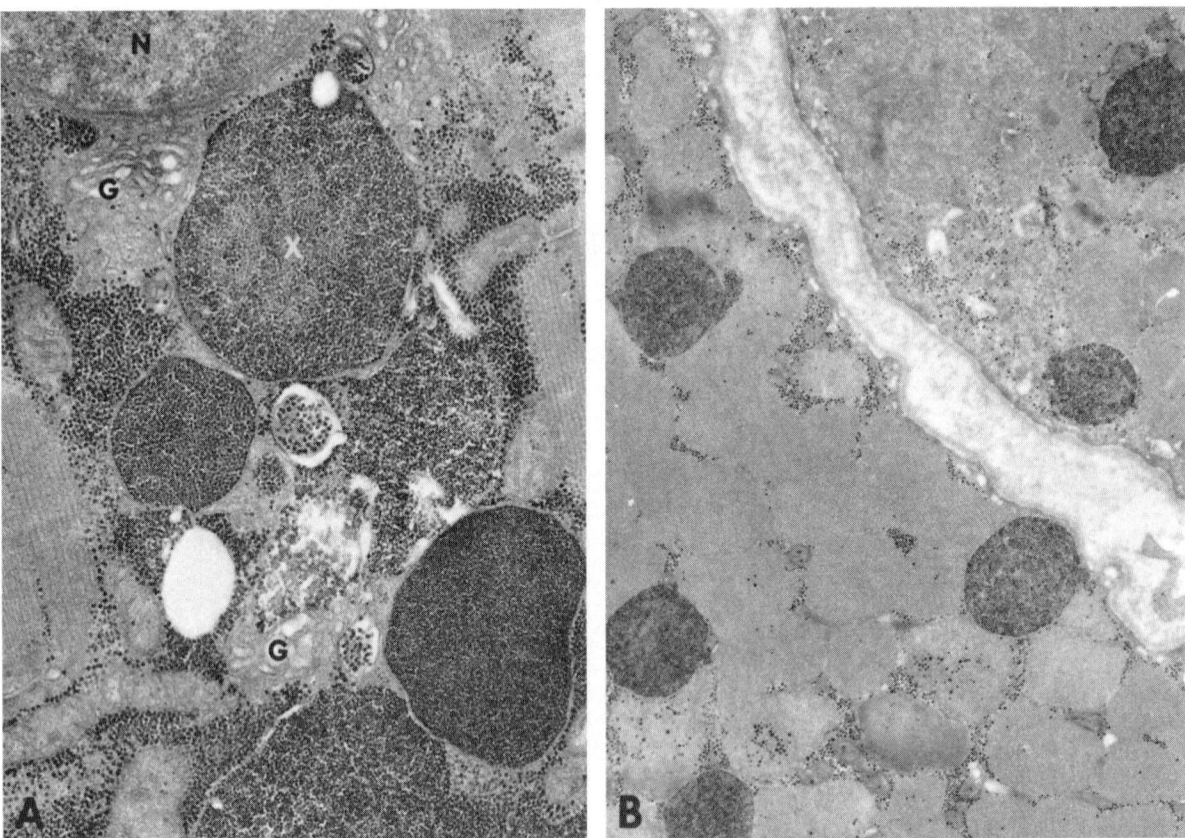

FIGURE 31-102. Lysosomal glycogen sacs in acid maltasedeficiency. In B, multiple small glycogen sacs represent the only abnormality in two adjacent fibers. In A, larger glycogen sacs (X) occur in hof region of nucleus (N), and freely dispersed glycogen appears at lower left. G, Golgi complex. A, ×13,600; B, ×24,400. [A is reproduced by permission from Engel AG, Excerpta Medica ICS 199:236, 1970; B is reproduced by permission from Engel AG, in Pearson CM (ed): The Striated Muscle. Baltimore: Williams & Wilkins; 1973, pp 301–341.]

1. CD8+ cells, alone or accompanied by macrophages, are apposed against the surface membrane of the non-necrotic fiber.
2. CD8+ cells and/or macrophages push spike-like processes into the muscle fiber. The spikes indent but do not perforate the muscle fiber plasma membrane.
3. CD8+ cells, with or without accompanying macrophages, traverse the basal lamina and further deform the muscle fiber plasma membrane (Figs. 31-5B, 31-104, 31-105). Some of the invading cells move into deeper regions of the muscle fiber but remain separated from the fiber interior by the muscle fiber plasma membrane (Figs. 31-104, 31-105, 31-107B). Therefore, the deeply migrating cells must cause an infolding of the muscle fiber plasma membrane, with or without the formation of new plasma membrane. Both the superficial and the deeply located invading cells continue to push spikes into the fiber (Figs. 31-5B, 31-104, 31-105, 31-107C).
4. An increasing number of CD8+ cells and macrophages traverse the basal lamina; these cells focally replace, displace, and compress the fiber (Figs. 31-105, 31-106, and Color Plate 8G to L); and spikes from these cells honeycomb the adjacent fiber regions (Fig. 31-106). The integrity of the muscle fiber surface membrane facing the invading cells is maintained, or the membrane is rapidly repaired.
5. Infrequently, CD57+ killer/natural killer cells also accompany the invading CD8+ cells and macrophages (Color Plate 8L). CD4+ cells usually do not penetrate the fibers.
6. The invading macrophages lack heterophagic vacuoles (Figs. 31-105, 31-107A) and therefore act in a cytotoxic rather than phagocytic capacity.

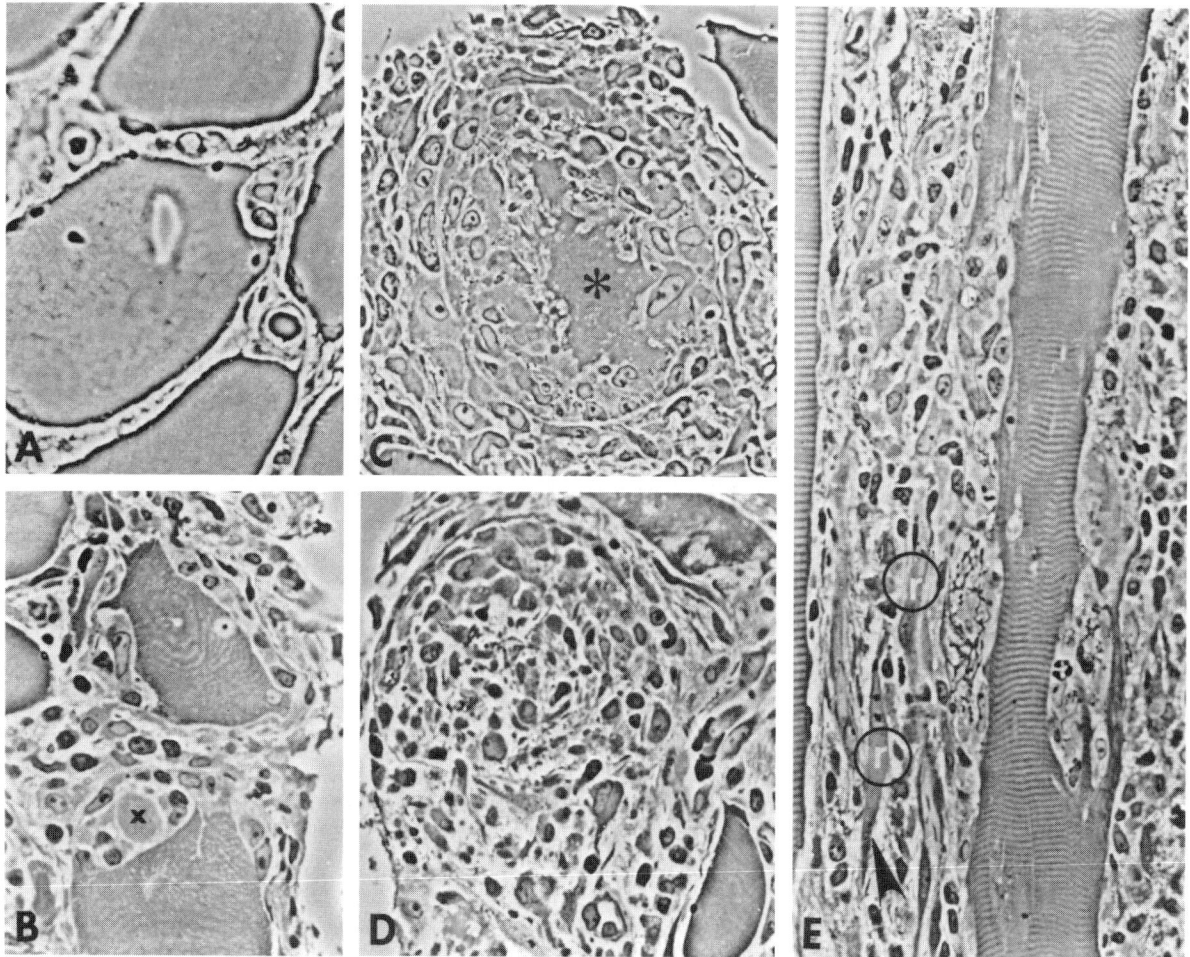

FIGURE 31-103. Polymyositis. Semithin resin sections viewed in phase optics demonstrate focal invasion (A), progressive replacement (B, C, and E), and eventual destruction (D) of nonnecrotic muscle fibers by mononuclear cells. In E, slender regenerating fibers (arrowhead and r) surrounded by inflammatory cells appear adjacent to partially destroyed fiber. x in B indicates fiber fragment nearly completely surrounded by invading cells; asterisk in C is positioned over irregularly lobulated fiber remnant. A, ×720; B and C, ×530; D and E, ×440.

7. The muscle fiber regions immediately underlying the invading cells appear normal (Fig. 31-104), or display proliferating T tubules (Fig. 31-107B), or show a regenerating zone devoid of myofibrils and occupied by smooth and rough endoplasmic reticulum profiles, Golgi networks, and intermediate-size filaments (Fig. 31-107A and C). In other fiber regions close to the invading cells, mitochondrial loss, myofibrillar alterations (Figs. 31-105, 31-106), or small empty spaces filled with debris (Fig. 31-104) can be observed.

8. The invaded muscle fiber becomes markedly reduced in size. The mononuclear cells that had replaced the peripheral zones of the fiber now surround its central remnant (Color Plate 8K). Eventually this, too, is replaced by the invading cells (Fig. 31-103C, D, and E).

The cellular mechanisms by which the invading cells destroy the muscle fiber without phagocytosis or membrane lysis are still unclear. In experimental models of T-cell-mediated cytotoxicity, sensitized T cells adhere to their target

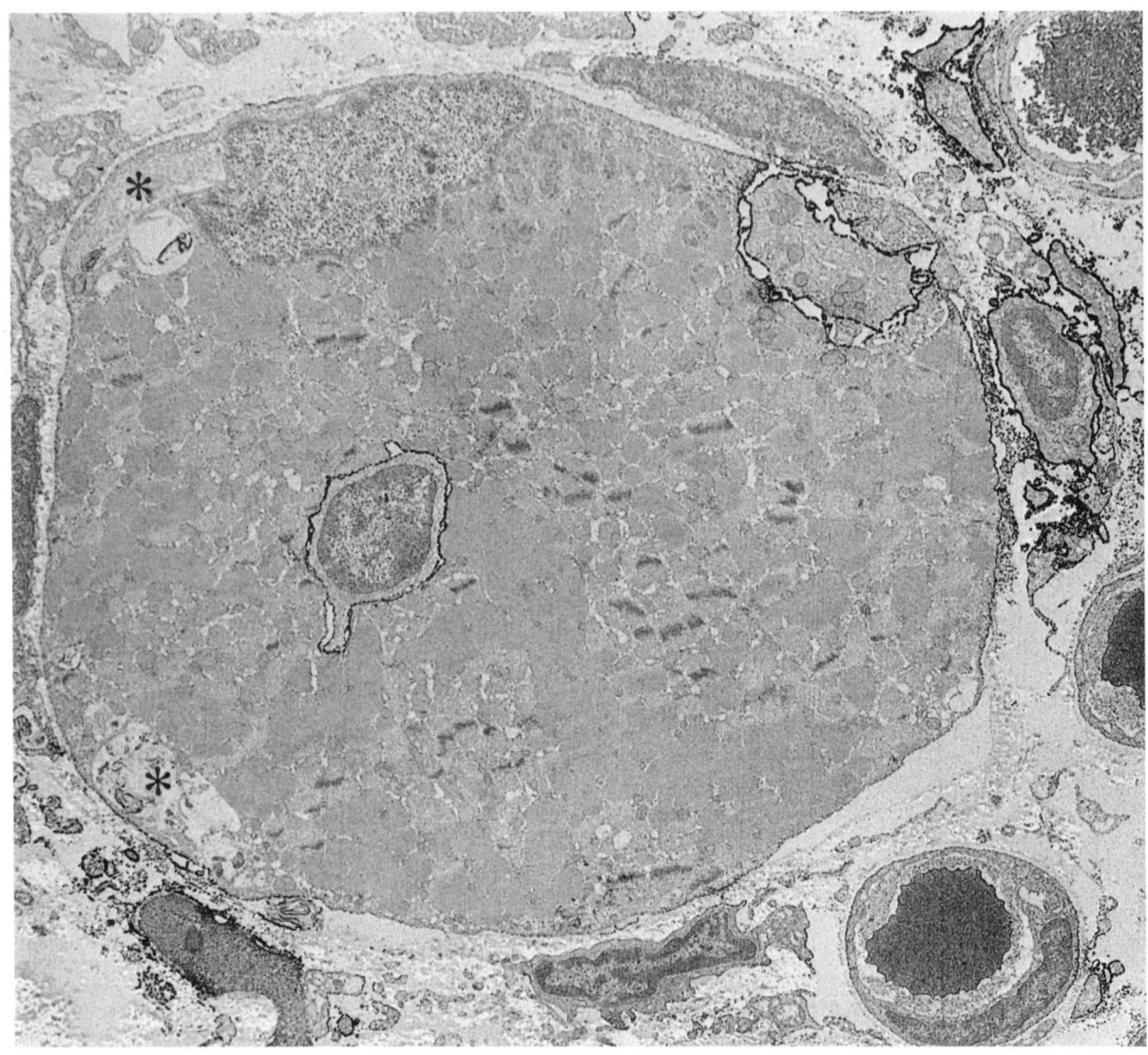

FIGURE 31-104. Nonnecrotic muscle is focally invaded by CD8+ cytotoxic lymphocytes. Invading cell at upper right has penetrated the basal lamina; another invading cell has reached the center of the fiber and sends spike-like projections into the surrounding fiber region. Regions marked by asterisks contain debris. The CD8 antigen is localized with monoclonal CD8 antibody and the immuno-peroxidase technique. Inclusion body myositis. ×6000. *(From Arahata K, Engel AG, Ann Neurol 19:112, 1986. Reproduced by permission.)*

(another lymphocyte or a cultured tumor cell) and send spike-like projections into it. The surface membrane and organelles of the target cell remain intact over a latent period of a few minutes to a few hours, but then the target cell membrane boils violently (*zeiosis*) and the target cell disintegrates.[188–190] During cell-mediated muscle fiber destruction, the initial events resemble those observed in model systems, but the subsequent steps differ in several respects: (1) Zeiosis does not occur; (2) the muscle fiber is physically replaced by the invading cells; (3) the invaded fibers proba-

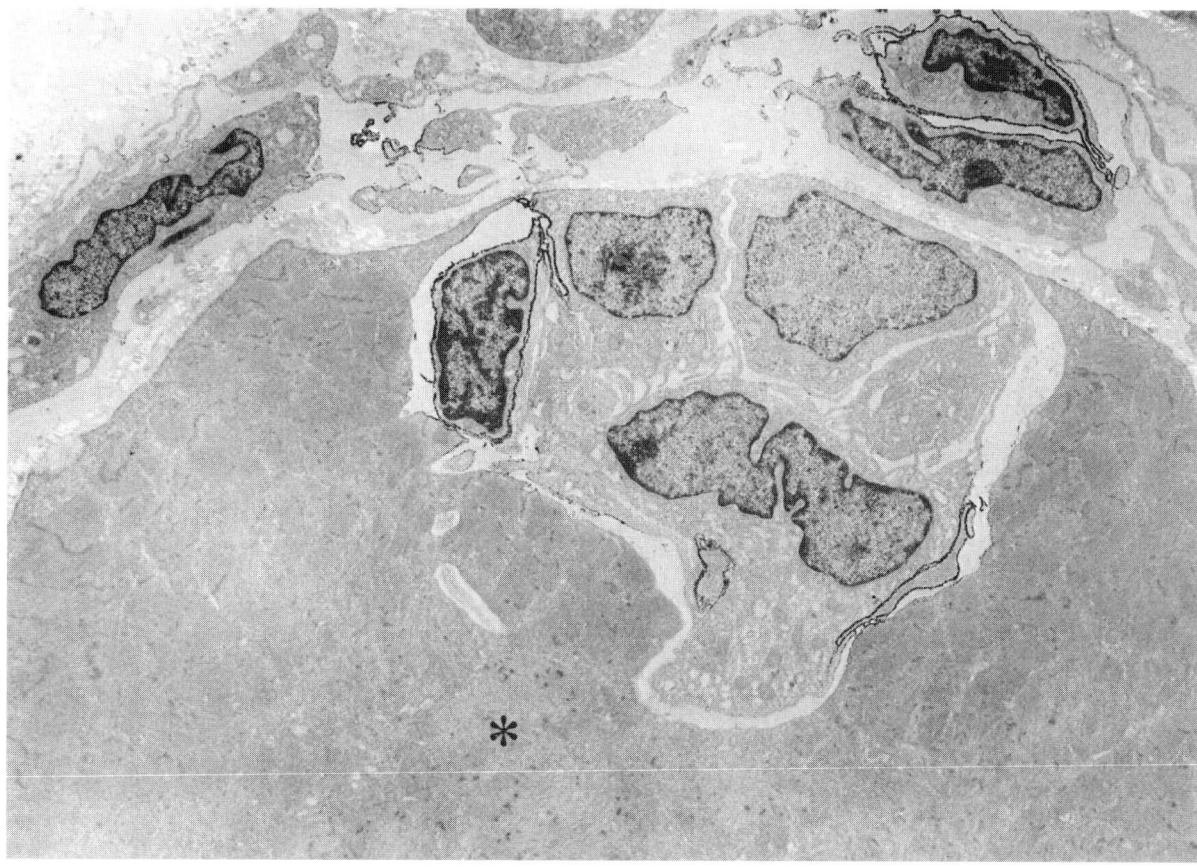

FIGURE 31-105. More advanced focal invasion of nonnecrotic muscle fiber by CD8+ lymphocytes and macrophages. Fiber region close to invading cells contains disorganized aberrant myofibrils with widened Z disks (asterisk). The CD8 antigen is demonstrated with monoclonal CD8 antibody and the immunoperoxidase method. Inclusion body myositis. ×4400

bly survive for more than a few hours, and certainly long enough to show regenerative changes; (4) both T cells and macrophages participate in cell-mediated muscle fiber destruction.

Cytolytic granules that can induce the assembly of tubular macromolecules resembling the membranolytic polymer of complement C9 have been found in both T cells and natural killer cells.[191] These granules, containing the cytotoxic mediator perforin, are located vectorially in the invading CD8+ T cells toward the surface of the invaded nonnecrotic muscle fiber. This is consistent with specific recognition by the T-cell receptor of an antigen on the muscle fiber surface and implies a perforin- and secretion-dependent mechanism of muscle fiber injury.[191a] However, the perforin-induced membrane defects are so small and focal that they cannot be detected electron microscopically in sections of resin-embedded material.

MUSCLE FIBER NECROSIS

Definition and light microscopic features. Muscle fiber necrosis is a stereotyped response in vivo to a variety of pathogenic stimuli and represents the final common pathway in many neuromuscular disorders. It is always associated with a break in the integrity of the muscle fiber surface

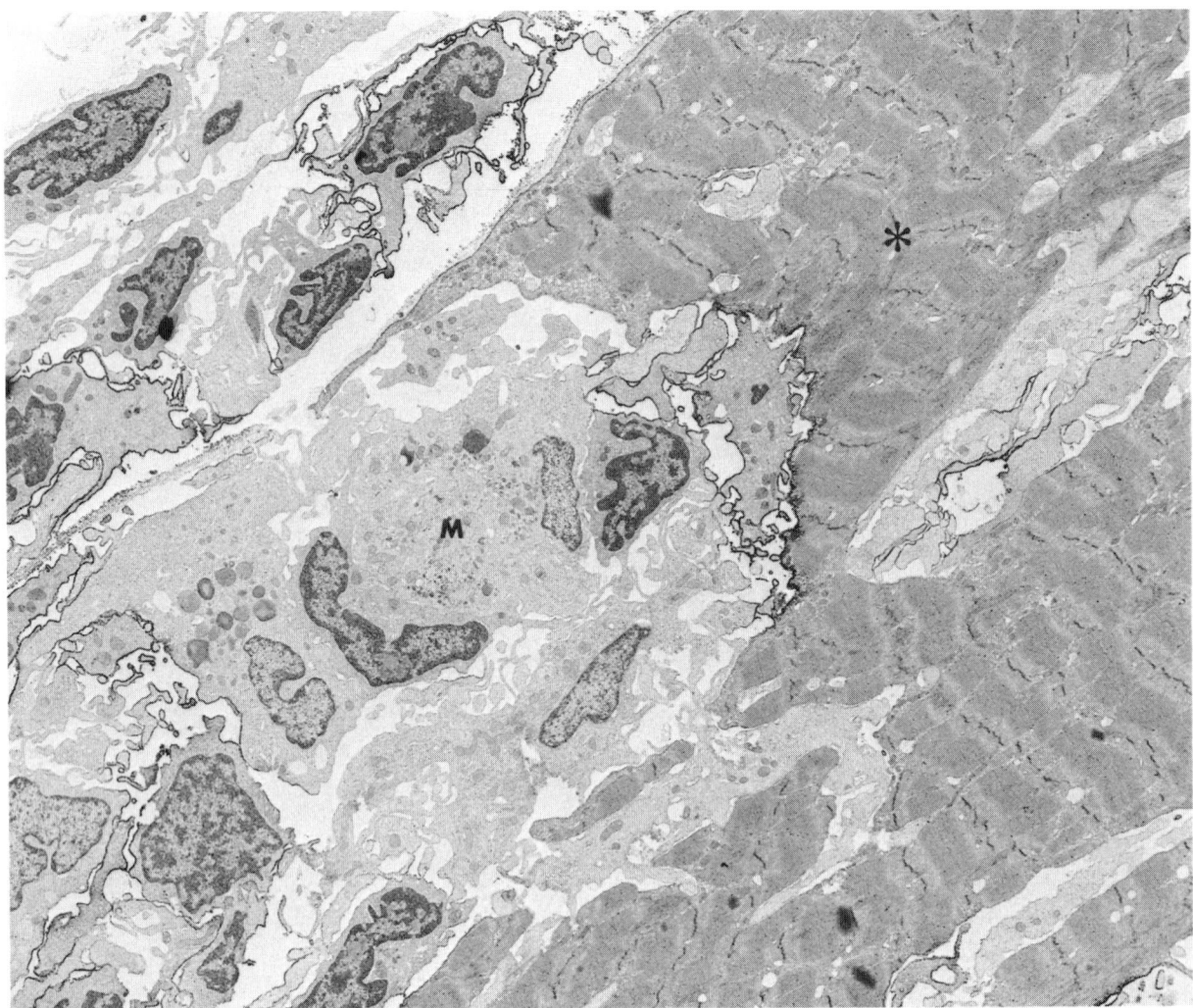

FIGURE 31-106. Extensive invasion of nonnecrotic fiber by CD8+ lymphocytes and macrophages (M). The remaining fiber shows focal myofibrillar degeneration (asterisk) and is honeycombed by spikelike processes of the invading cells. The CD8 antigen is demonstrated with monoclonal CD8 antibody and the immunoperoxidase method. Inclusion body myositis. ×4400. *(From Arahata K, Engel AG, Ann Neurol 19:112, 1986. Reproduced by permission.)*

membrane and results in irreversible injury to all organelles of the entire fiber, a segment of the fiber, or a circumscribed region of the fiber that is subsequently either absorbed or removed by macrophages. In trichrome-stained cryostat sections of unfixed muscle, the necrotic fiber has a green-blue color (normal color, deep blue); shows an absent, attenuated, or clumped intermyofibrillar network; and may or may not be invaded by macrophages (Color Plate 8*A, B, D,* and *E*). A necrotic fiber remnant and regenerating fiber elements can coexist in the confines of the basal lamina that had previously surrounded a single preexisting nonnecrotic fiber. The necrotic fiber or fiber segment invariably reacts for the neoantigenic determinants of complement MAC (Chap. 30, Color Plate 8*C, D, F,* and Ref. 155).

The presence of MAC in necrotic fibers implies that during necrosis (1) circulating complement components enter the fiber; (2) complement activation and MAC assembly occur within the fiber; (3) MAC participates in destruction of fiber organelles; and (4) complement split products formed during complement activation (C5A, C3b, and perhaps Bb) recruit macrophages and stimulate phagocytosis of the necrotic fiber.[155] The entry of circulating complement components into the necrotic fiber also indicates that the integrity of the muscle fiber surface membrane has been breached and is consistent with the observation that necrotic fibers are diffusely overloaded with calcium.[86,192]

Ultrastructural features. In either longitudinal or transverse sections the plasma membrane is invariably absent from all or most of the imaged fiber surface. The basal lamina is characteristically preserved and covers the denuded fiber surface (Figs. 31-108, 31-109, 31-111*B*).

In the earliest stages of necrosis, partially lysed and highly contracted myofibrils are still present in the fiber. These are

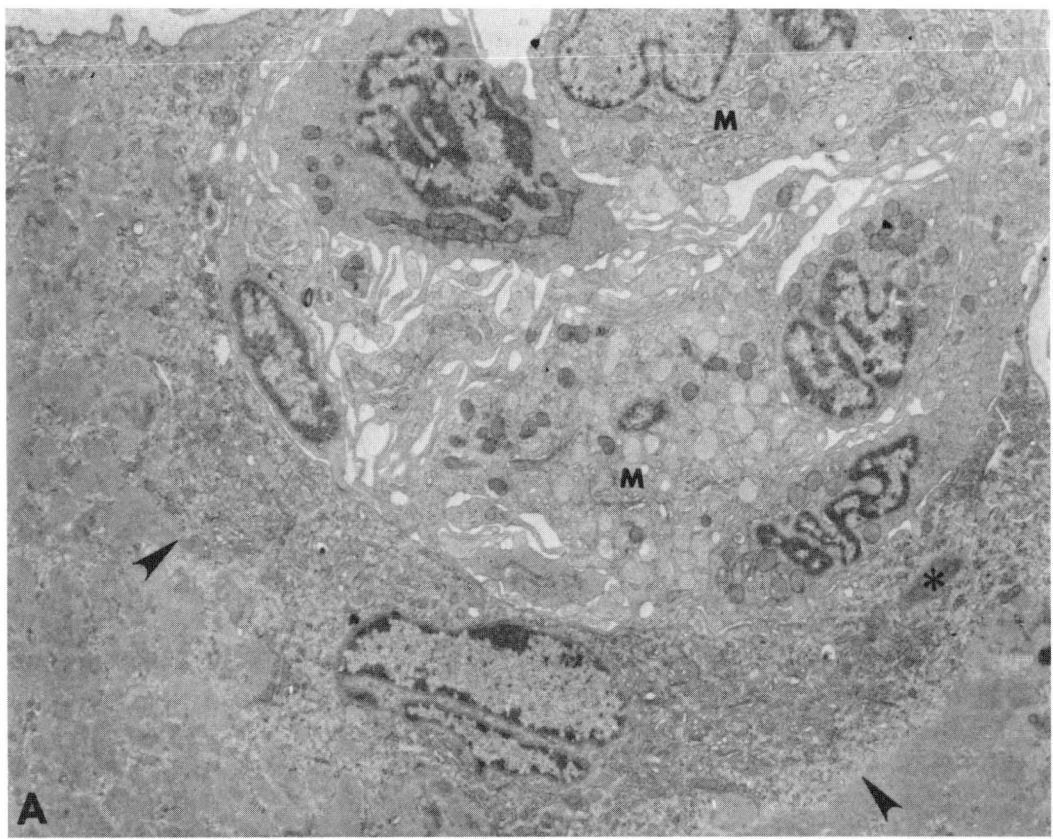

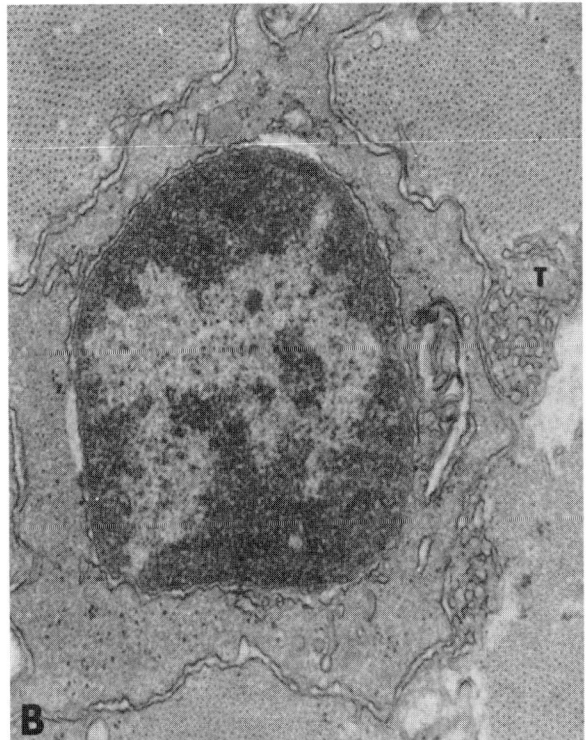
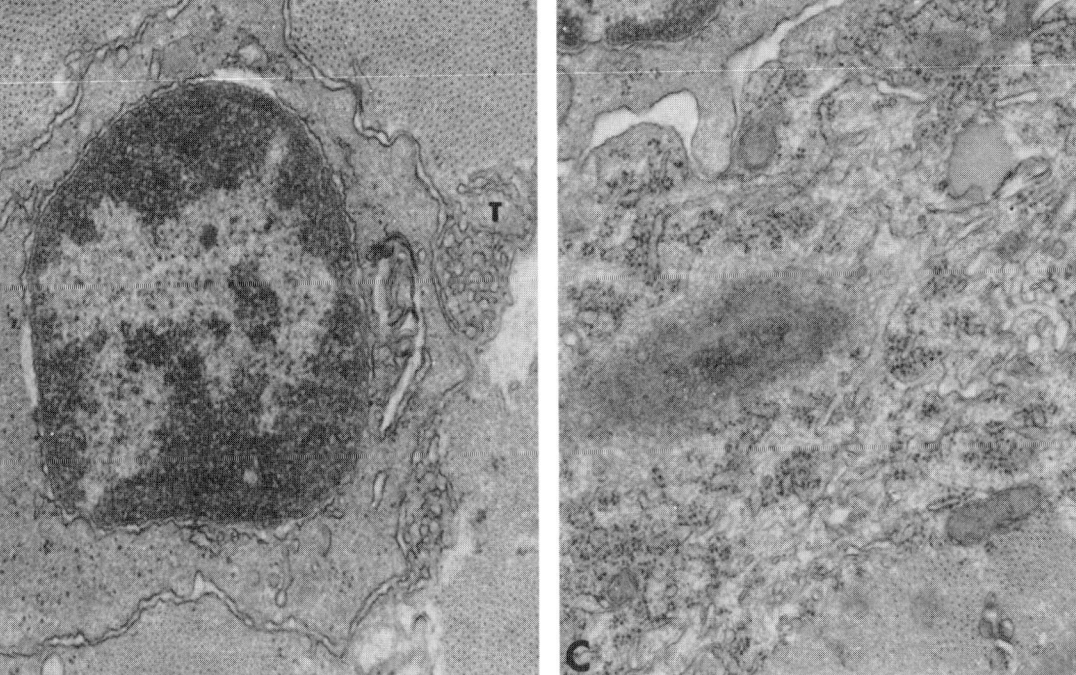

FIGURE 31-107. Regenerative changes in muscle fibers invaded by cytotoxic mononuclear cells. In A, muscle fiber region between arrowheads and invading cells contains numerous ribosomes, smooth and rough endoplasmic reticulum profiles, Golgi complexes, and nuclei. C is higher magnification of region marked by asterisk in A. Spike-like process of invading cell indents but does not disrupt the muscle fiber plasma membrane. B shows deep penetration of a cytotoxic lymphocyte into the muscle fiber. The muscle fiber plasma membrane is intact. T-system network (T) abuts on the muscle fiber plasma membrane where it faces the invading cell. Polymyositis. A, ×6300; B, ×33,300; C, ×25,600. (From Arahata K, Engel AG, Ann Neurol 19:112, 1986. Reproduced by permission.)

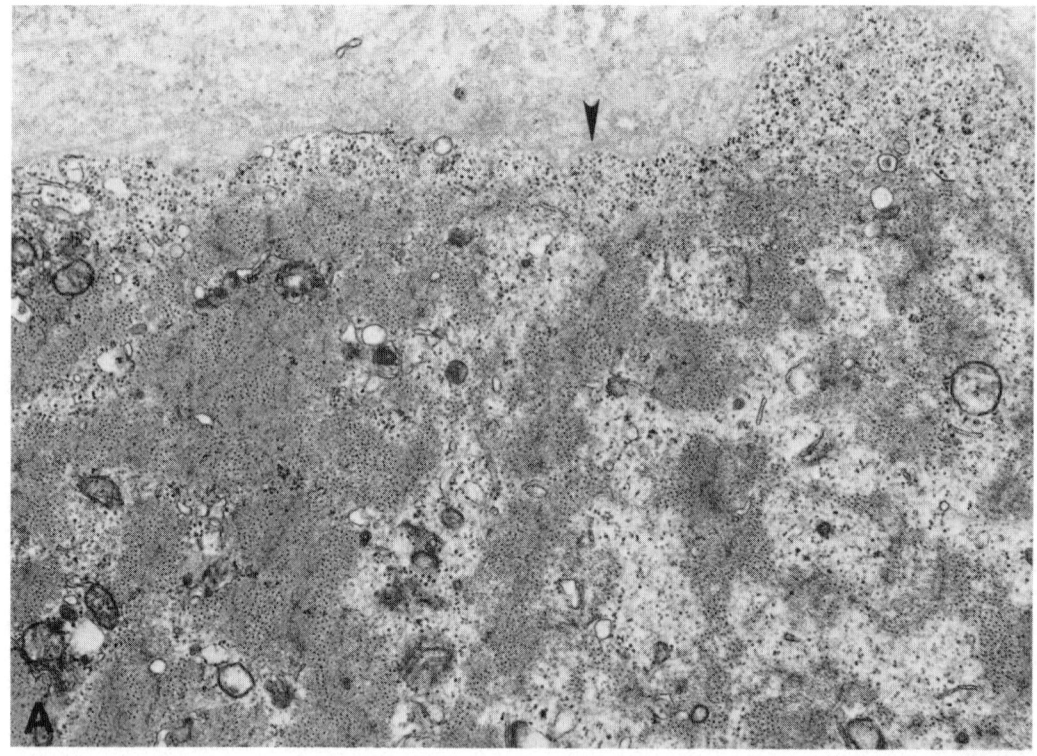
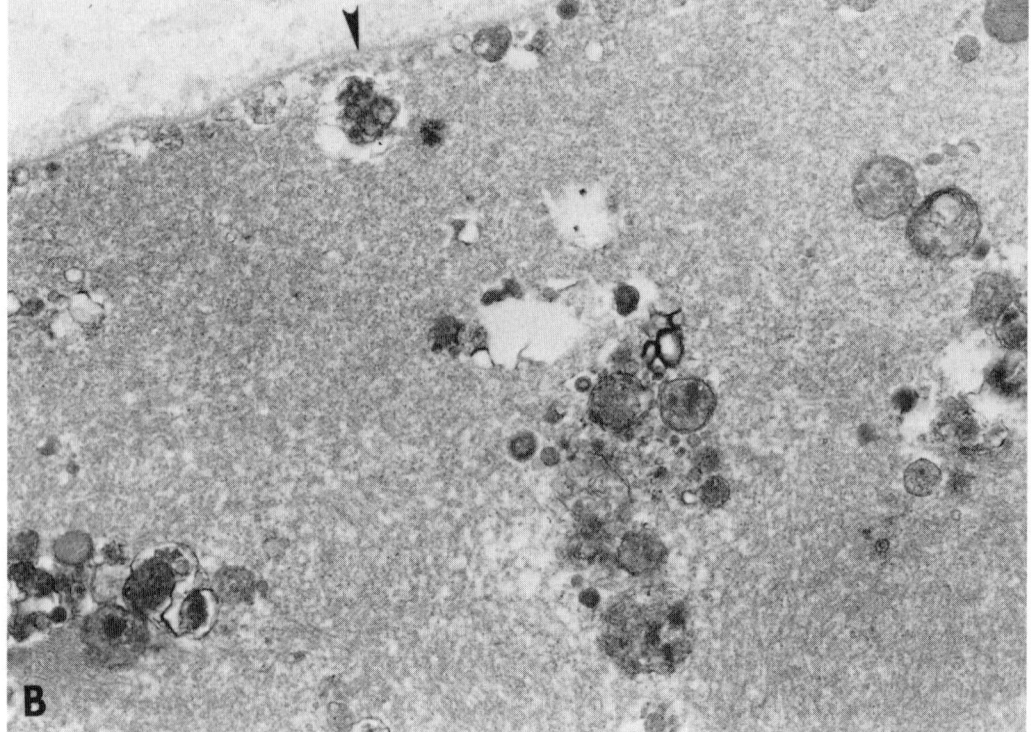

FIGURE 31-108. Necrotic fibers. The plasma membrane is absent from nearly the entire imaged fiber surface in A and from the entire imaged fiber surface in B. The basal lamina (arrowheads) persists. In A, highly contracted and partially lysed myofibrils are still present in the fiber. In B, the fiber contains only granular or filamentous debris and clumps of degenerating organelles. A. Polymyositis, ×16,800. B, Dermatomyositis, ×20,000.

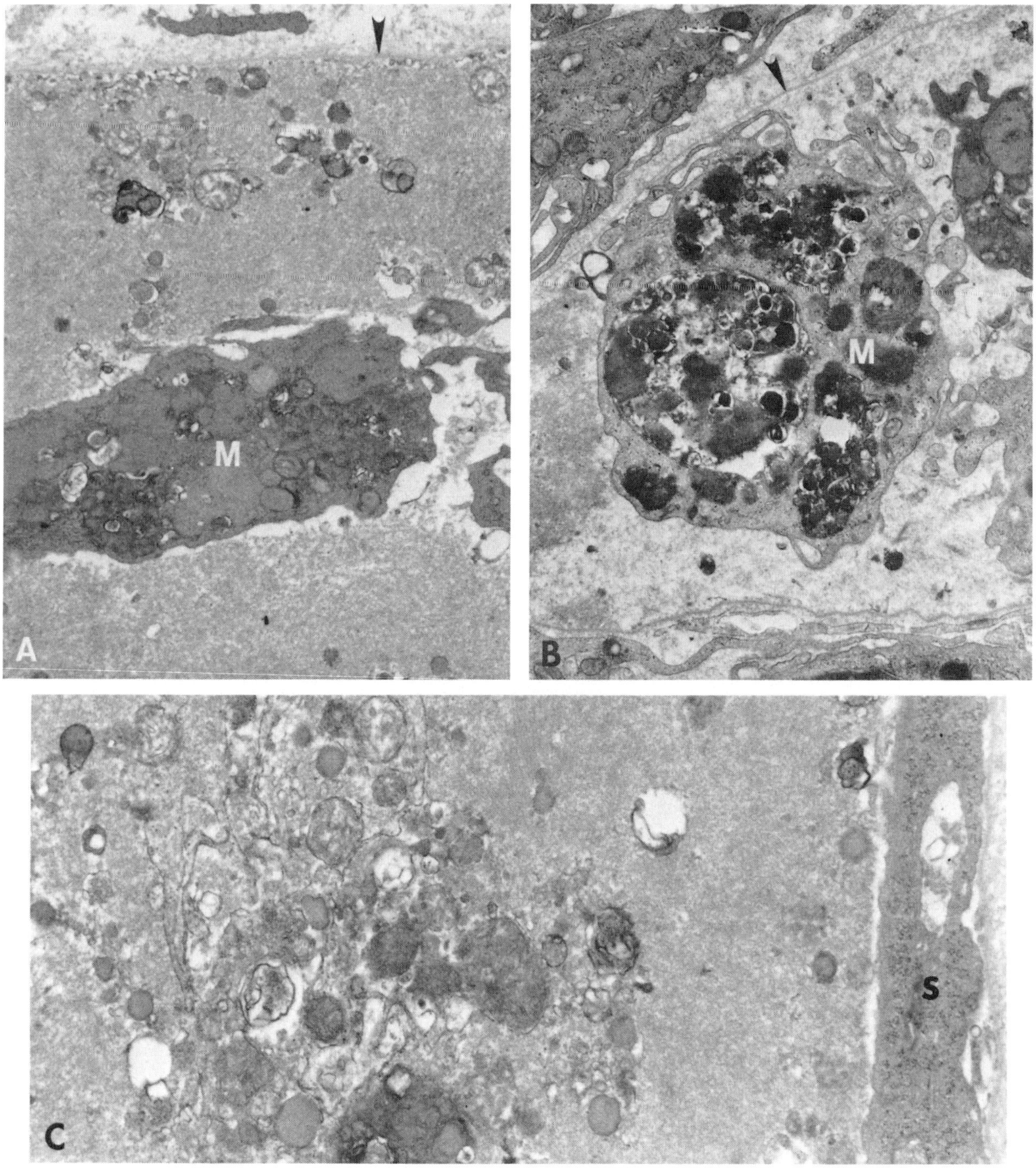

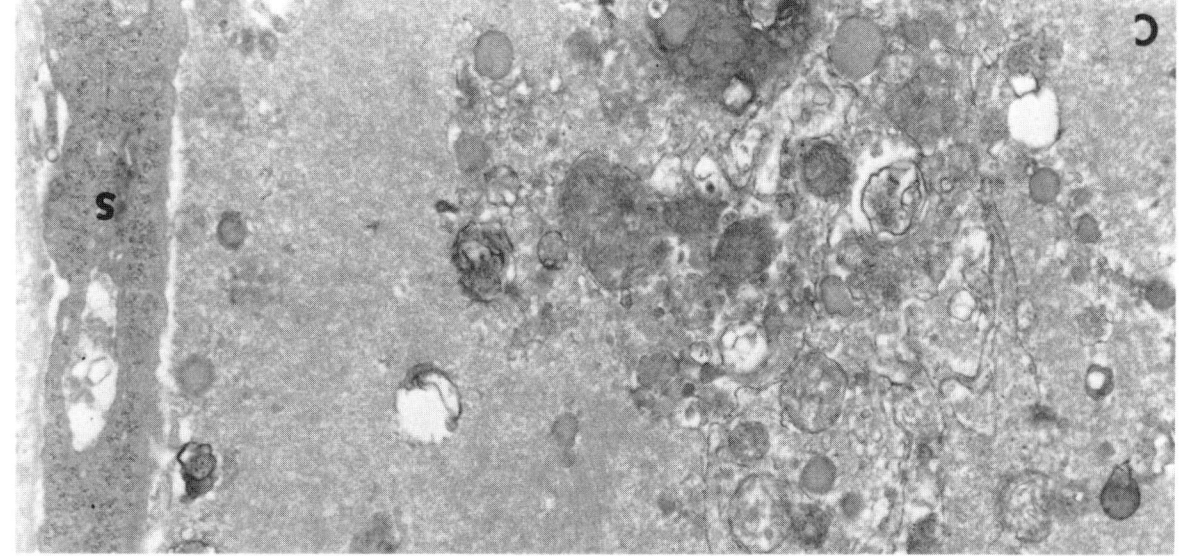

FIGURE 31-109. In A and B, macrophages (M) containing heterophagic vacuoles appear within the necrotic fibers. Arrowheads indicate persistent basal lamina. In C, a satellite cell (or myoblast) can be observed under the basal lamina of the necrotic fiber. A. Dermatomyositis, ×13,400. B. Muscular dystrophy, ×10,100. C. Dermatomyositis, ×20,000.

separated by irregular spaces that contain sparse glycogen granules, normal or abnormal mitochondria, and scattered sarcotubular elements (Fig. 31-108A). The contracted state of the myofibrils is due to the ingress of extracellular calcium (Chap. 13), and their lysis can be attributed to calcium-activated sarcoplasmic proteases (Chap. 23).

At a more advanced stage of necrosis, the fiber contains granular or filamentous debris and clumps of degenerating membranous organelles. Myofibrillar and sarcotubular components are no longer recognizable (Fig. 31-108B). However, in some cases of polymyositis, in ε-aminocaproic acid–induced myopathy, and in experimental myositis of guinea pigs, the A bands resist lysis and are removed only when macrophages invade the fiber.[193]

Macrophages commonly invade necrotic fibers and ingest remaining fiber components into heterophagic vacuoles (Figs. 31-109A and B, 31-110, 31-111B and C). Activated satellite cells can also appear in superficial regions (Fig. 31-109C)

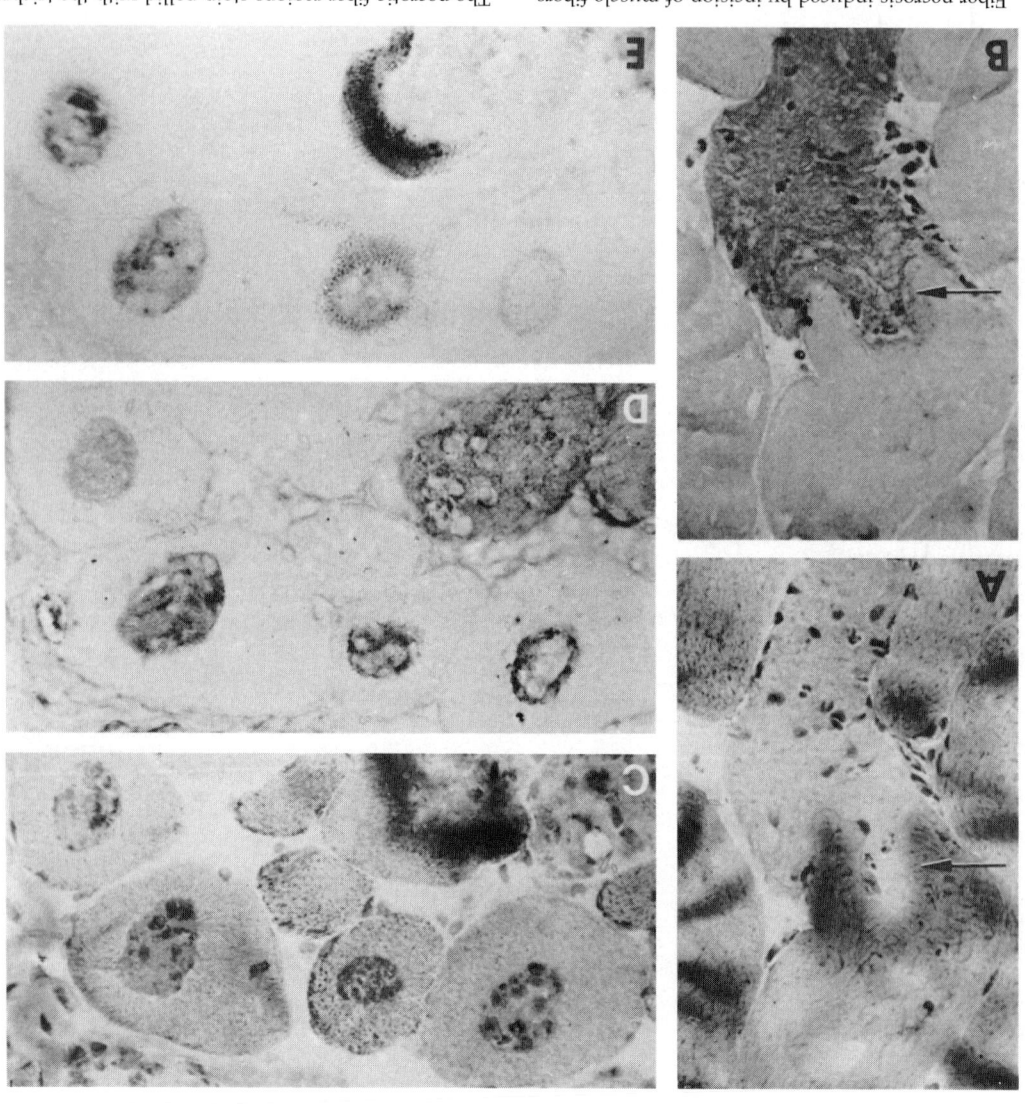

FIGURE 31-110. Fiber necrosis induced by incision of muscle fibers 14 h before biopsy. The biopsy was taken 3 mm from where the muscle fibers were transected. Cryostat sections stained with trichrome (A and C), reacted for complement component C9 (B and D), and stained for calcium with the glyoxal bis-(2-hydroxyanil) reagent (E). A and B, and also C, D, and E, are nonconsecutive serial sections. The necrotic fiber regions stain pallid with the trichrome stain (A), are invaded by macrophages (A and C), react for complement component C9 (B and D), and are overloaded with calcium (E). The necrotic zones have cone-shaped tips (arrows in A and B); transverse sections through these tips show central fiber necrosis. ×300.

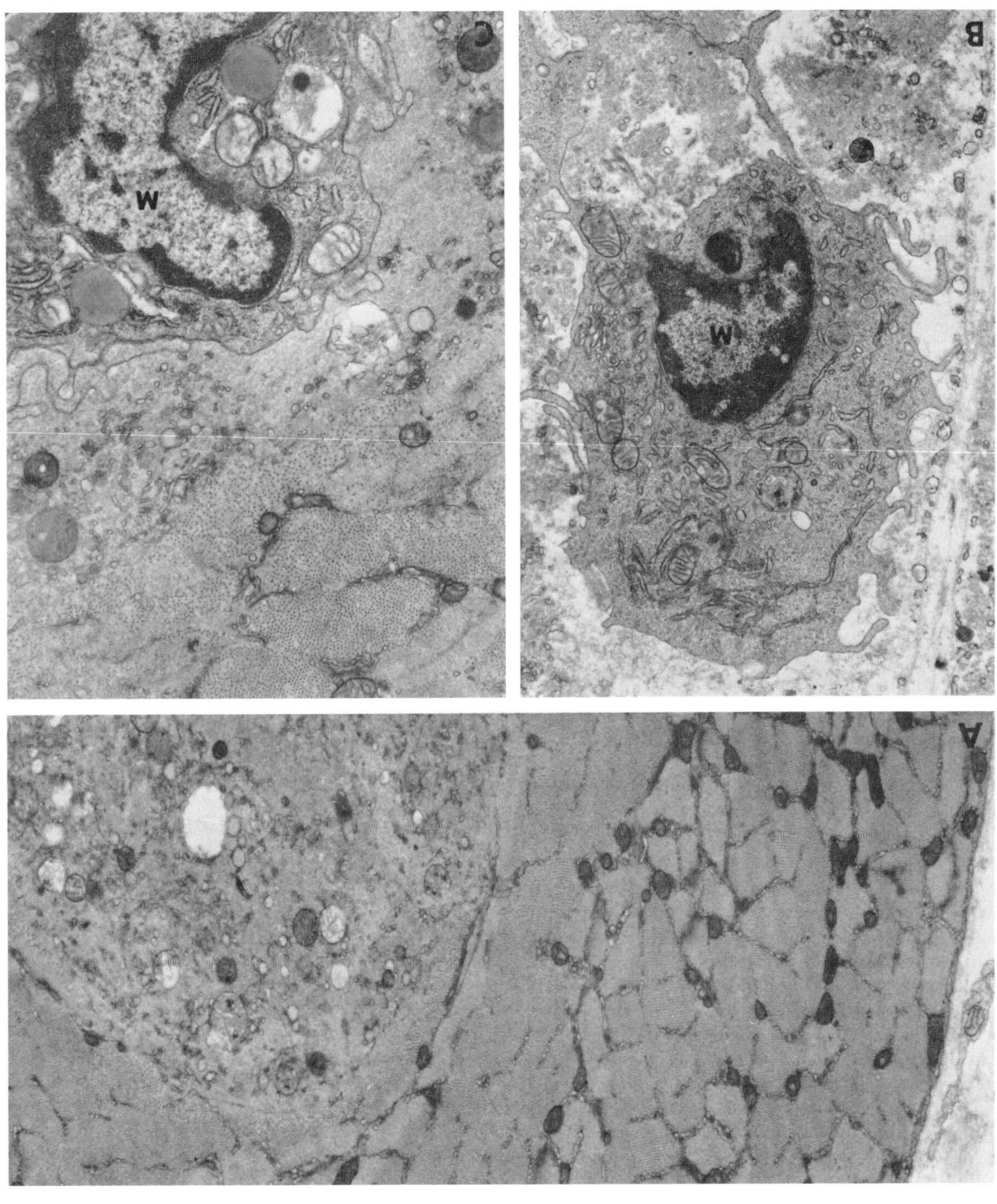

FIGURE 31-111. Electron micrographs of biopsy specimen described in Fig. 31-110. Transverse sections through the tip (A and C) and through the middle (B) of the necrotic zone. The tip of the necrotic zone contains degenerating organelles, debris (A), and macrophages (C) and is surrounded by a normal fiber zone. The plasma membrane overlying this region of the fiber is intact. In the midportion of the necrotic zone, the entire fiber is necrotic and the plasma membrane has disappeared. Macrophages can readily enter the fiber in this region. M, macrophages. A, ×11,900; B, ×12,400; C, ×16,700.

and deeper regions (Fig. 31-87B) of the necrotic fibers, where they may fuse to form a new fiber.

Experimentally induced segmental muscle fiber necrosis is followed within a few hours by demarcation of the injured fiber segment by new sarcoplasmic membrane.[193a,b]

Central fiber necrosis. In some instances the central regions of transversely sectioned fibers appear necrotic and are partly or completely filled with macrophages, yet peripheral parts of these fibers appear normal. An explanation for this is found in longitudinal sections that show that the necrotic central region is a cone-shaped or cylindrical extension of an adjacent zone in which the entire fiber is necrotic. Central fiber necrosis can be readily observed in a simple experimental model that also provides insights into the mechanism of fiber necrosis. The midportion of rat gastrocnemius is incised perpendicularly to the direction of the fibers with a razor blade, and the overlying subcutaneous tissues and skin are then closed. The incision initiates fiber necrosis, which spreads in either direction from the incision. Fourteen hours after injury, the necrotic changes extend for a distance of about 3 mm from the site of injury. The advancing front of the necrotic zone is cone-shaped, and the tip of the cone is in the center of the immediately adjacent nonnecrotic fiber region (Fig. 31-110). Transverse sections through the advancing tip demonstrate central fiber necrosis (Figs. 31-110C to E, 31-111A and C). The necrotic zone is overloaded with calcium (Fig. 31-110E), reacts for complement component C9 (Fig. 31-110B and D), and is invaded by macrophages (Figs. 31-110A and C, 31-111B and C). Electron microscopic studies show that the plasma membrane disintegrates beyond the site of the original incision and is absent from those fiber regions that are completely necrotic (Fig. 31-111B). This, in turn, implies that alteration of the intracellular ionic milieu and/or complement or protease activation initiates a vicious circle with further destruction of the plasma membrane and lateral spread of the zone of necrosis. The intramuscular injection of the calcium ionophore A23187 also induces plasma membrane lysis and focal necrosis,[194] indicating that massive calcium overloading of the fiber itself can initiate the vicious circle.

SATELLITE CELLS

The fine structure, functional role, and reactions of the satellite cell are discussed in Chap. 3 and are considered only briefly here. Satellite cells are associated with intrafusal and extrafusal fibers in skeletal muscle but are absent from smooth or cardiac muscle.[94,195,196] Each cell consists of a nucleus surrounded by a small amount of cytoplasm and plasma membrane and is wedged under the basal lamina of the parent fiber. The inner surface of the satellite cells is separated from the parent fiber by a 10- to 50-nm gap from which the basal lamina is absent. The cytoplasm of the satellite cell contains ribosomes, polyribosomes, a few rough endoplasmic reticulum profiles, Golgi apparatus, sparse mitochondria, and few or no glycogen granules. The satellite cell nucleus is oval or slightly indented and typically heterochromatic (Figs. 31-112 to 31-114, 31-115B). In normal sub-

jects, satellite cell nuclei constitute about 4 percent of all nuclei within the muscle fiber basal lamina.[197]

Autoradiographic studies with tritiated thymidine indicate that in developing muscle satellite cells associated with muscle fibers undergo mitosis, after which one or more daughter nuclei are incorporated into the parent fiber. Thus, during ontogenesis, satellite cells function as myoblasts.[198] When satellite cells are labeled in uninjured muscles of young rats and the muscles are transplanted, the labeled cells appear as regenerating myoblasts[199] and give rise to myotubes.[200] Finally, labeled satellite cells in cloned tissue cultures and in minced muscle implants also appear as labeled myoblasts that fuse to form labeled nuclei in myotubes.[201] These data support the notion that satellite cells are dormant myoblasts and become activated when the parent fiber is injured. Studies of muscle fiber regeneration in vitro also indicate that satellite cells become myoblasts, whereas myonuclei do not.[196,202–205]

An additional possible source of satellite cells in mature muscle might be muscle fiber nuclei that split away from the parent fiber with a small amount of cytoplasm. That this could be so is suggested by the following ultrastructural findings in diseased muscles in vivo:

1. Partial separation of a small nucleus-bearing cytoplasmic region from the parent fiber can be observed (Fig. 31-112A).
2. Cytoplasmic continuity exists between some satellite cells and their parent fibers (Figs. 31-112B, 31-115A, 31-116A).
3. Proliferating T-system and caveolar networks, which can provide new plasma membrane, occur immediately adjacent to partially separated satellite cells (Figs. 31-112B, 31-115A).
4. Satellite cells also appear in infolded pockets of the plasma membrane in longitudinally splitting fibers (Fig. 31-113), and these cells must have separated from the parent fiber only *after* the plasma membrane had become invaginated into the parent fiber.

One might argue, however, that cytoplasmic continuities between satellite cells and parent fibers indicate fusion rather than separation, and it has been suggested that longitudinal fiber splitting is always due to incomplete lateral fusion of regenerating fibers rather than to infolding of the plasma membrane of mature fibers.[206] Further studies will be required to prove or disprove the possibility that satellite cells can not only fuse with but also split away from differentiated fibers.

FIGURE 31-112. Satellite cells. B to F show typical satellite cells wedged under the basal lamina of the parent fiber. In B, C, and D a papillary projection of the parent fiber partially covers the external surface of the satellite cell. In B there are two cytoplasmic bridges between parent fiber and satellite cell (arrows), and a caveolar network (circle) abuts on one of the bridges. In A there is partial separation of a small nucleus-bearing cytoplasmic region from the parent fiber; arrow indicates developing cleft. A, ×11,000; B, ×13,500; C, ×17,100; D, ×15,500; E, ×17,500; F, ×21,800. (A and B reproduced by permission from Engel AG, Macdonald RD, Excerpta Medica ICS 199:71, 1970.)

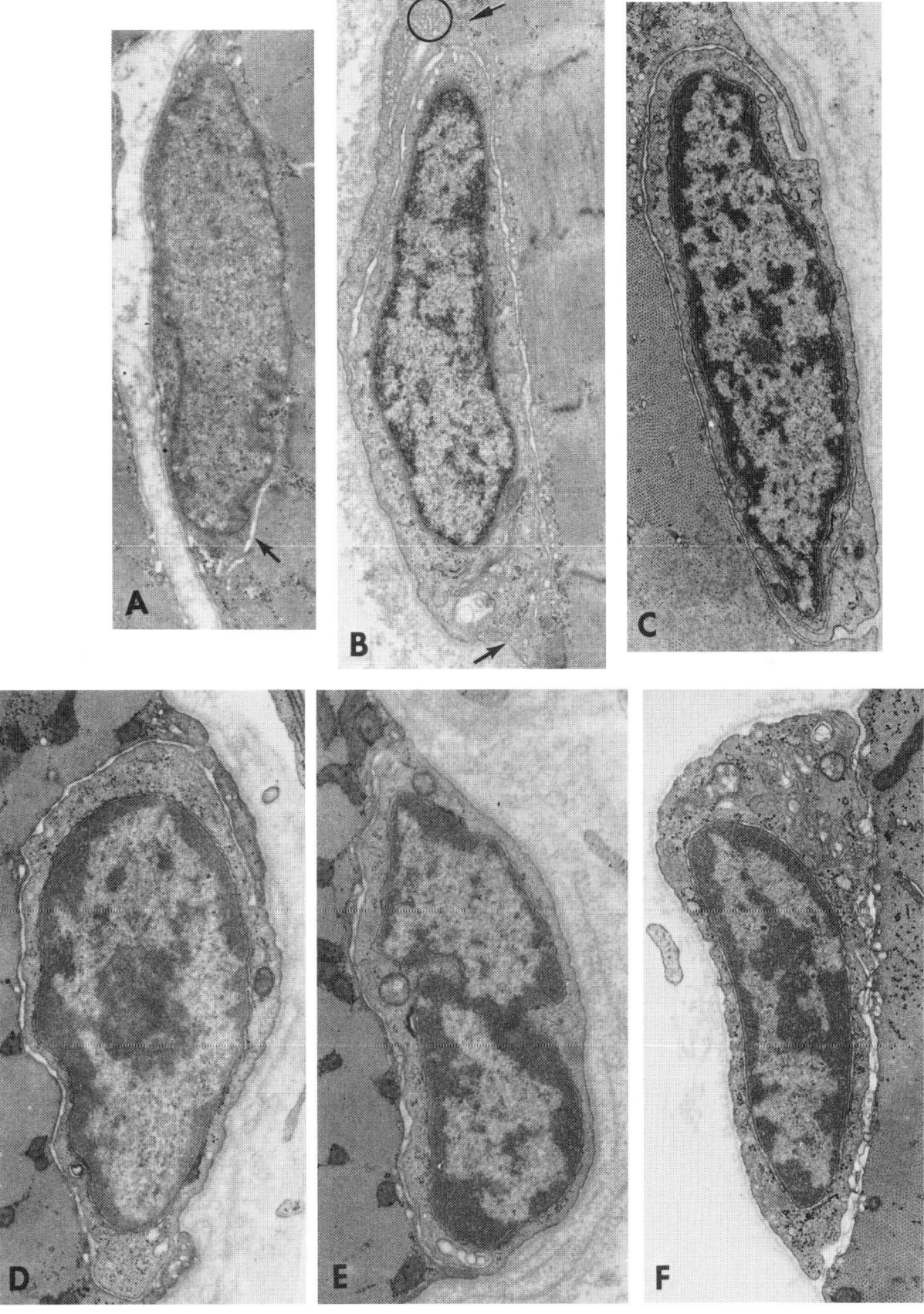

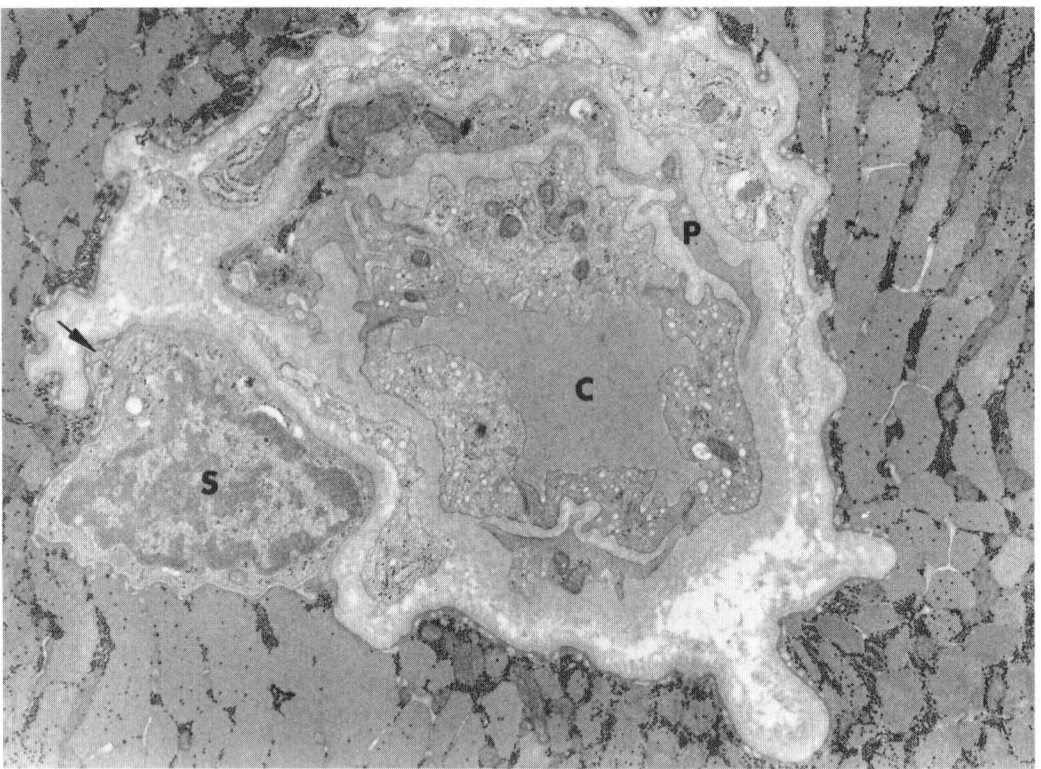

FIGURE 31-113. Satellite cell (S) abuts on infolded pocket of plasma membrane of a longitudinally splitting muscle fiber. Note multiple tubules and caveolae near left upper corner of satellite cell. C, capillary; P, pericyte. ×10,300. (Reproduced by permission from Engel AG, Mayo Clin Proc 45:774–814, 1970.)

Satellite cells are remarkably immune to stimuli that damage the muscle fiber. Infrequently, however, they degenerate (Fig. 31-115B); and in lysosomal storage disorders, such as acid maltase deficiency, they contain abnormal lysosomes (Fig. 31-101C). An increase in the number of satellite cell nuclei relative to the number of fiber nuclei has been observed in Duchenne dystrophy.[207]

Activation of satellite cells occurs not only in response to injury of the underlying muscle fiber but also in response to a single bout of strenuous exercise. Here the proliferative response is attributed to leakage of a mitogenic factor through small membrane disruptions.[207a] Migration of satellite cells occurs extensively during both embryogenesis and regeneration. Experimental studies indicate that transforming growth factor beta (TGF-β), produced by platelets and inflammatory cells, is chemotactic for satellite cells. Crushed muscle releases both mitogenic and chemotactic factors; the chemotactic factors likely comprise both hepatocyte growth factor (HGF) and TGF-β.[207b]

Activated satellite cells have more abundant cytoplasm and more extensive Golgi networks and rough endoplasmic reticulum membranes than resting satellite cells (Fig. 31-114B). The role of the satellite cell in muscle fiber regeneration is again discussed in the next section.

MUSCLE FIBER REGENERATION

Patterns of Muscle Fiber Regeneration

Muscle fiber regeneration can occur in three situations: focally within an injured but nonnecrotic fiber; within the basal lamina cylinder of a fiber that has become necrotic; and adjacent to necrotic or nonnecrotic fibers but not within the basal lamina cylinder of a preexisting fiber.

Focal regeneration in nonnecrotic fibers. This can be observed after focal muscle fiber injury in the end plate myopathy induced by prostigmine,[68,69] in tenotomized muscles,[68] in the hof region of centrally migrated nuclei (Fig. 31-11), in some parts of sarcoplasmic masses (Fig. 31-81B), in some muscle fibers in polymyositis (Fig. 31-20) and dermatomyositis (Fig. 36-89), and in nonnecrotic muscle fibers invaded by cytotoxic mononuclear cells (Fig. 31-107A and C). The regenerating fiber regions contain prominent Golgi networks (Figs. 31-11, 31-20, 31-89A, 31-107A), abundant ribosomes, polyribosomes or rough endoplasmic reticulum (Figs. 31-11, 31-20, 31-80A, 31-89A, 31-107C), a variable admixture of T-system networks and clusters of dilated SR vesicles (Figs. 31-11, 31-20, 31-80, 31-89A and B), and poorly organized myofibrils with widened Z disks or small nema-

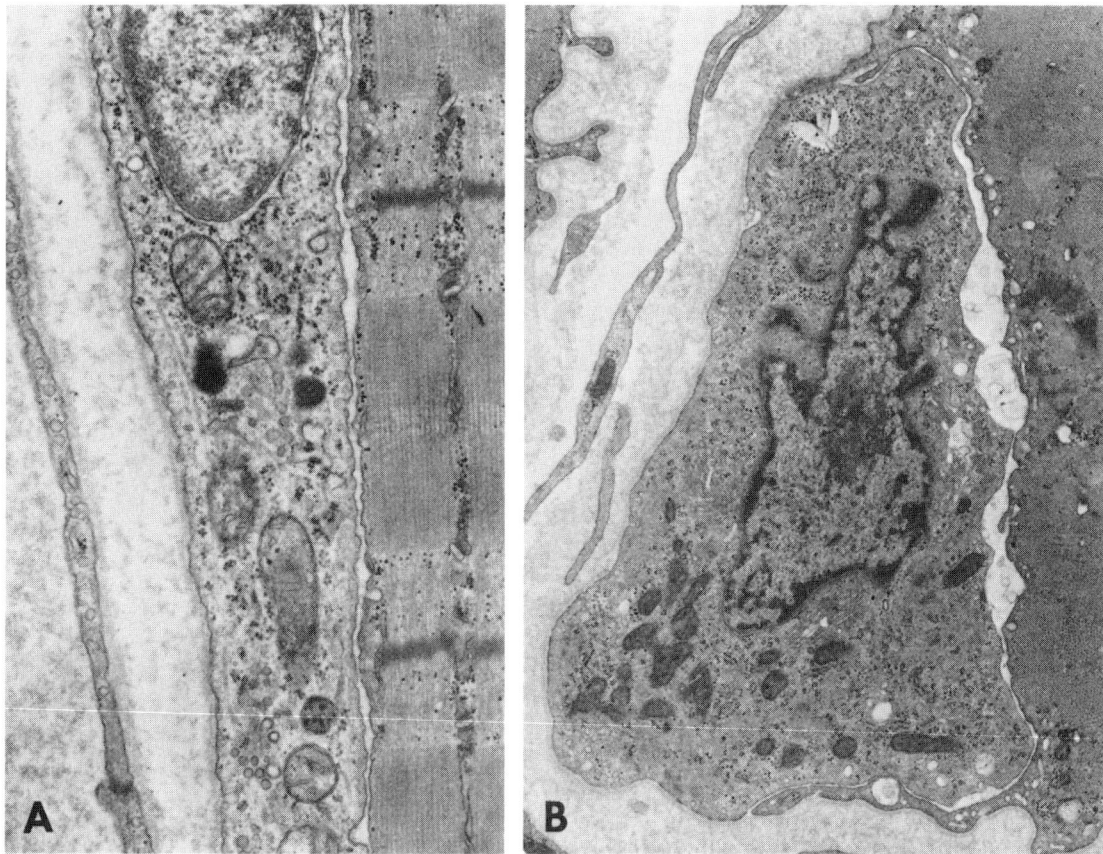

FIGURE 31-114. Satellite cells. A. Part of an elongated satellite cell in experimental emetine myopathy. B. Activated satellite cell in polymyositis. Irregularly widened cleft containing small membrane fragments between the parent fiber and the satellite cell suggests that the satellite cell is becoming detached from the parent fiber. Surface of the parent fiber is studded with caveolae. A, ×21,000; B, ×11,900.

line rods (Fig. 31-89C). The stimuli that induce focal regeneration as well as the pattern and outcome of the regenerative process vary in different disorders. For example, successful regeneration occurs in the experimental end plate myopathy induced by prostigmine or tenotomy, but small nemaline rods may persist in the repaired fiber regions.[68,69] Despite attempts at regeneration, the muscle fibers eventually decrease in size and show aberrant myofibrils in dermatomyositis; some muscle fibers invaded by cytotoxic lymphocytes in inclusion body myositis and polymyositis eventually vanish. Finally, the annular and aberrant myofi-brils in various myopathies suggest unsuccessful focal myofibrillar regeneration.

Regeneration within the basal lamina cylinder of a fiber that has become necrotic. This is the usual form of muscle fiber regeneration, in which a segment of a muscle fiber becomes necrotic but the basal lamina of the fiber is spared (Fig. 31-87B to E). The genome that codes for regeneration resides in the surviving myogenic nuclei, and an extensive body of evidence indicates that the nuclei are those of satellite cells (for reviews see Refs 196, 202, 208, and 209). This is the *discontinuous* form of regeneration, and it recapitulates the events of embryonal myogenesis.

In an alternative scheme of regeneration, referred to as *continuous* regeneration, cytoplasmic buds are thought to grow directly into the destroyed fiber region from the adjacent nonnecrotic fiber stump. This scheme was originally based on light microscopic studies in which the presence or absence of plasma membrane around the cytoplasmic buds and the origin of the nuclei associated with the buds could not be clearly defined. It seems unlikely, however, that viable cytoplasmic material can grow into a destroyed fiber region unless it is surrounded by plasma membrane, and an ultrastructural study that describes regeneration from such buds does not show the tips of the cytoplasmic buds.[210] In another possible scheme, myoblasts that grow into the destroyed fiber region originate from preexisting

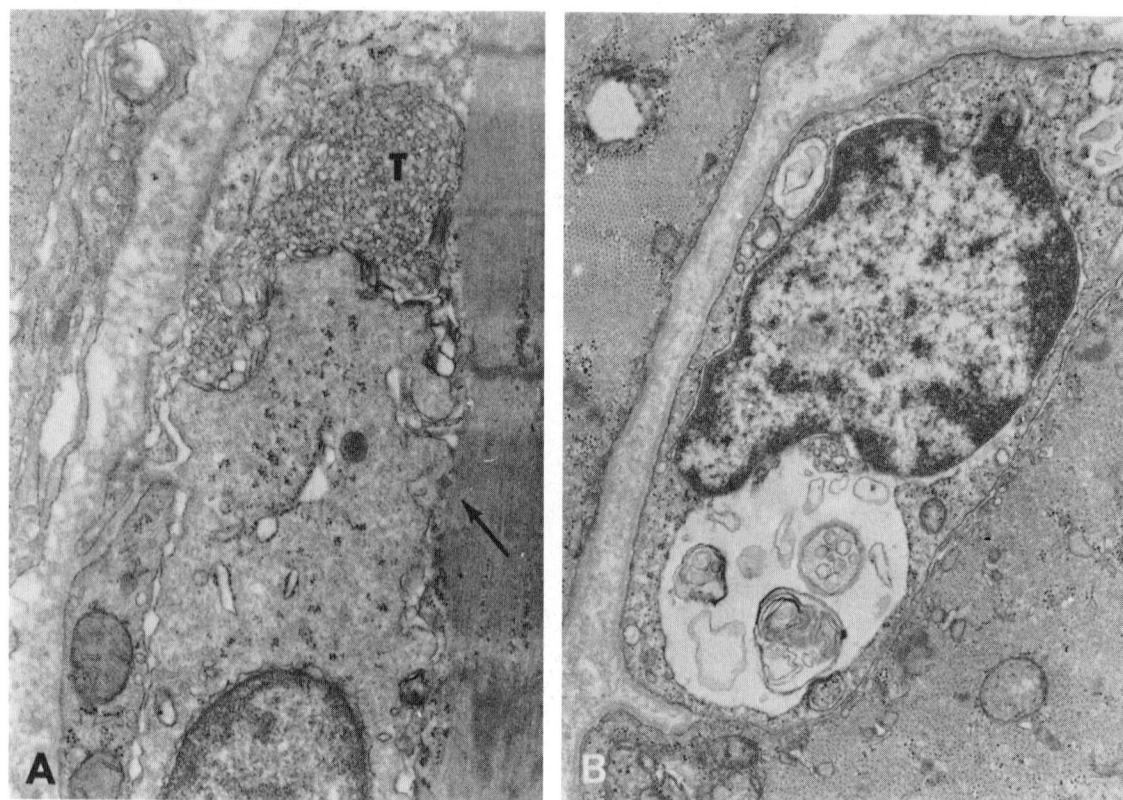

FIGURE 31-115. Satellite cells. *A.* T-system network (T) in the parent fiber abuts on satellite cell near a cytoplasmic bridge between the satellite cell and the parent fiber (arrow). *B.* Degenerating satellite cell. A. Polymyositis, ×17,400. B. Dermatomyositis, ×15,000.

myofiber nuclei that gather plasma membrane and pass through a satellite cell stage, rather than from those satellite cells that survive the local injury.[211] As mentioned under "Satellite Cells," above, differentiated muscle fibers might generate satellite cells by splitting off a small area of cytoplasm containing a nucleus, but it is uncertain that this mechanism can operate effectively in the stump region of injured fibers.

Regardless of the origin of the myogenic cells, the basic events during regeneration of the necrotic fiber segment consist of (1) mitosis of the myogenic cells; (2) fusion of the postmitotic myogenic cells with one another to form myotubes and with myotubes that have already formed; (3) elongation of the myotubes to bridge the necrotic zone; and (4) fusion of the myotubes to fill the entire circumference of the basal lamina cylinder.[196,202]

The stumps of the two surviving fiber segments that face the intervening necrotic segment must be sealed off by plasma membrane while the myogenic cells proliferate and fuse within the zone that has undergone necrosis. Eventually this membrane should vanish as the newly formed myotubes bridge the gap between the two stumps. The source of the membrane that temporarily seals off the nonnecrotic stumps has not been determined. Regenerating, necrotic, and well-differentiated muscle fiber elements within the same basal lamina cylinder can be observed in different myopathies (Fig. 31-117). One may infer that here the sectioning plane traverses the sealed-off portion of the non-necrotic stump, the adjacent regenerating elements, and remnants of the necrotic segment.

Failure of the myotubes to fuse laterally will result in the appearance of parallel slender muscle fibers that resemble longitudinally split fibers.[206] It has been argued that this phenomenon always accounts for longitudinal fiber splitting,[206] but in our experience longitudinal fiber splitting due to infolding of the plasma membrane can occur without antecedent fiber necrosis.[6,25]

Regeneration outside the basal lamina cylinder of a preexisting fiber. If a muscle is transected in vivo or is excised and minced and then either reimplanted or placed in a culture system, or if a single isolated muscle fiber is deliberately injured, proliferating myogenic cells leave the disrupted muscle fiber through tears in the basal lamina and attempt to form myotubes adjacent to the disrupted fiber.[196, 202,203,208,209] The extent to which regeneration succeeds and the morphology of the regenerated fiber depend on the availability of a suitable substrate for the attachment of the myogenic cells, the prevailing physiologic conditions, and whether nerve sprouts are available to innervate the newly formed myotubes.[202,208]

In denervated muscles[212,213] or in muscles undergoing compensatory hypertrophy,[214] satellite cells can migrate even through intact basal lamina into the interstitial space and form new fibers there. Two facts suggest that in human myopathies satellite cells also can migrate into the endomysium and form new fibers there: (1) Myogenic cells molded to nonnecrotic fibers but separated from them by basal lamina can be observed. Such cells may represent activated satellite cells separating from their parent fibers (Figs. 31-68B, 31-116B). (2) Slender endomysial myotubes can be noted that are surrounded by connective tissue on all sides, are not apposed to the stump of another fiber, and are not positioned within the basal lamina cylinder of a preexisting fiber (Figs. 31-116, 31-118 to 31-121). The slender endomysial regenerating fibers in some of the inflammatory myopathies (Figs. 31-116, 31-118, 31-119B, 31-120, 31-121) and some of the small regenerating fibers in Duchenne dystrophy (31-119A) may possibly arise by this mechanism. Finally, activated satellite cells leaving normal muscle fibers have been observed when rat muscle is injured by the local injection of the snake venom taipoxin.[214a]

Organelle Development in Regenerating Muscle Fibers

Since the development of muscle fiber organelles is considered in Chaps. 1, 2, 7, and 11, only a brief review is presented here. Organelle development in regenerating fibers resembles that in embryonic muscle. Myotubes arising by the fusion of postmitotic myoblasts contain euchromatic nuclei, well-developed Golgi, scattered mitochondria, ribosomes, polyribosomes, abundant rough endoplasmic reticulum, microtubules, and cytoskeletal filaments (Figs. 31-87C, 31-119B). At a slightly later stage, abundant axially oriented cytoskeletal filaments appear and the organelles become axially aligned (Fig. 31-120). Myofibrillar assembly begins with the simultaneous appearance of clusters of axially aligned thick and thin filaments. Z disks develop subsequently and allow the formation of sarcomeres and elongation of the myofibrils (reviewed in Ref. 215). The newly formed myofibrils contain wide Z disks and frequently display small nemaline rods (Figs. 31-44B, 31-121). The axially oriented cytoskeletal filaments provide scaffolding for the nascent myofibrils (Fig. 31-121). During further development the cytoskeletal elements are reorganized and the myofibrils increase in size, number, and length. Eventually the myofibrils fall into register and are linked to one another, to other organelles, and to the sarcolemma by cytoskeletal filaments.[66]

The nuclear envelope is the putative membrane source for the rough endoplasmic reticulum. The SR develops from the latter organelle[215,216] after myofibril formation has begun, and the earliest SR tubules course parallel or obliquely relative to the early myofibrils (Fig. 31-122). The superficial components of the T-tubule system arise from caveolar inpocketings of the plasma membrane[217]; the more deeply positioned tubules arise in the perinuclear regions and penetrate most parts of the myotube before their connections with the plasma membrane are established.[217a] The SR and T components initially associate with each other near the plasma membrane (Fig. 31-123) and later on in deeper regions of the fiber. During subsequent development triads appear, but they are axially oriented at first. The normal disposition of the T tubules and SR relative to one another and to the myofibrils is attained only after myofibrillar development is complete and the sarcomeres are in register.[218–220]

Although the sequence of organelle development is stereotyped in a given myotube, regions of differing maturity can be observed in a given regenerating fiber. This is readily explained by fusion of myotubes of differing maturity with one another and with myoblasts during fiber development.[215]

Myofibril formation is coded for by postmitotic nuclei in myotubes, but myofibril formation has been described in satellite cells fusing to degenerating fibers in human myopathies.[221] However, serial sections demonstrating that the "satellite cells" were not fused to other satellite cells (which would have established that mononuclear myogenic cells rather than myotubes were observed) were not obtained in this study.

Recently regenerated human muscle fibers have central nuclei. Hof regions of these nuclei contain ribosomes, rough endoplasmic reticulum, and prominent Golgi cisternae (Fig. 31-124A). With further maturation, the nuclei become subsarcolemmal and the organelles in the hof region become less conspicuous. By contrast, in rodents, muscle fibers that had regenerated remain centronucleated indefinitely. Some recently regenerated fibers in human myopathies display irregularly oriented aberrant myofibrils, wide or double Z disks, small nemaline rods, proliferating T tubules, and irregularly disposed triads, pentads, and heptads (Fig. 31-124B and C). The abnormal organelle development in these fibers may be due to lack of innervation, to insufficient longitudinal tension on the fiber,[202] or to faulty myofibril-cytoskeleton interactions.[66]

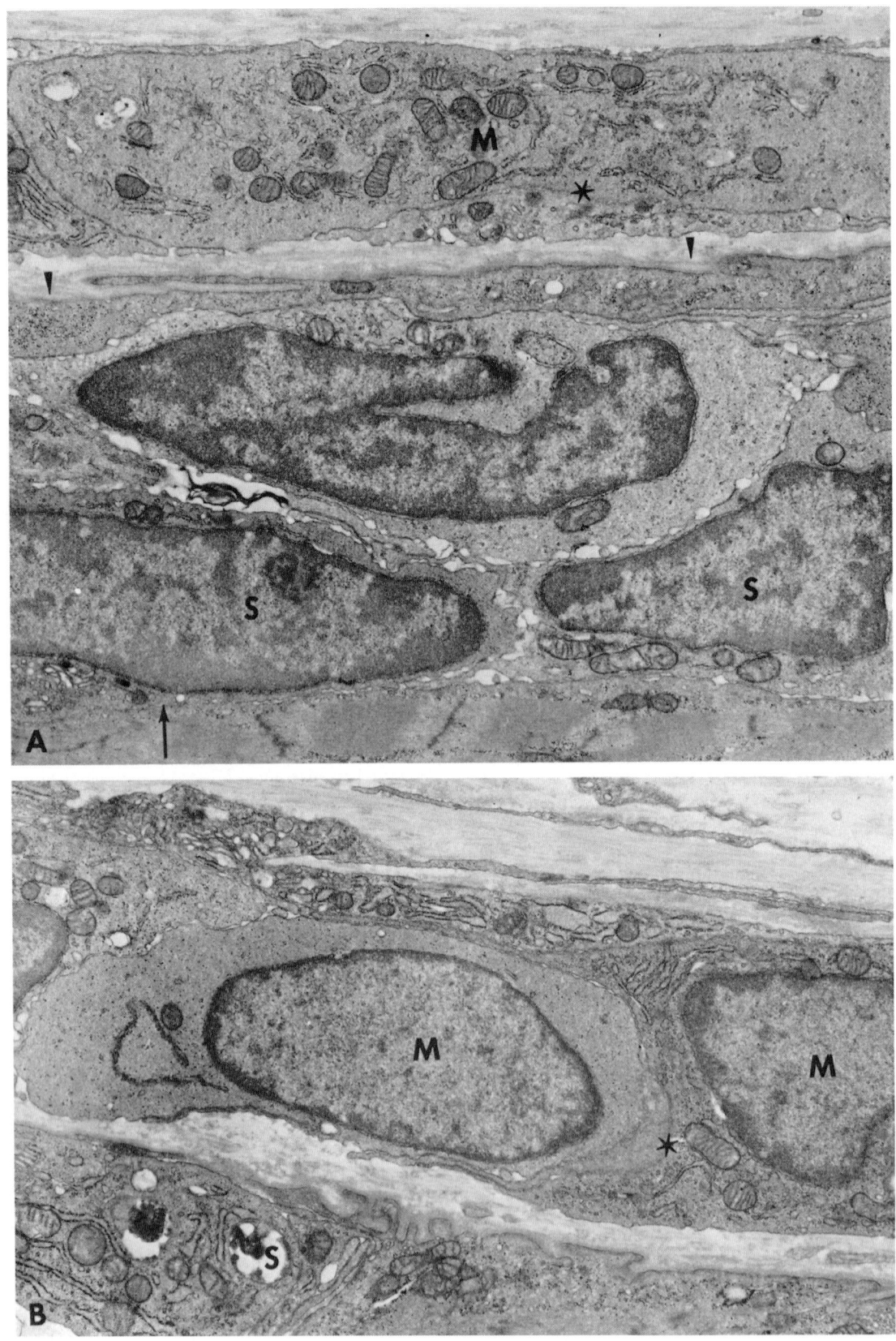

FIGURE 31-116. Satellite cells and muscle fiber regeneration. *A.* In the lower third of the field, a muscle fiber segment is covered by twin satellite cells (S). A cytoplasmic bridge is seen between one of these cells and the parent fiber (arrow). A second layer of satellite cells is positioned above the twin satellite cells and is separated from the interstitial space by basal lamina (arrowheads). At the top, myoblasts (M) in the intrestitial space are coalescing (asterisk) to form an early myotube. This picture can be interpreted in two ways. (1) Satellite cells become detached from the parent fiber, pass into the interstitial

(continued on bottom of next page)

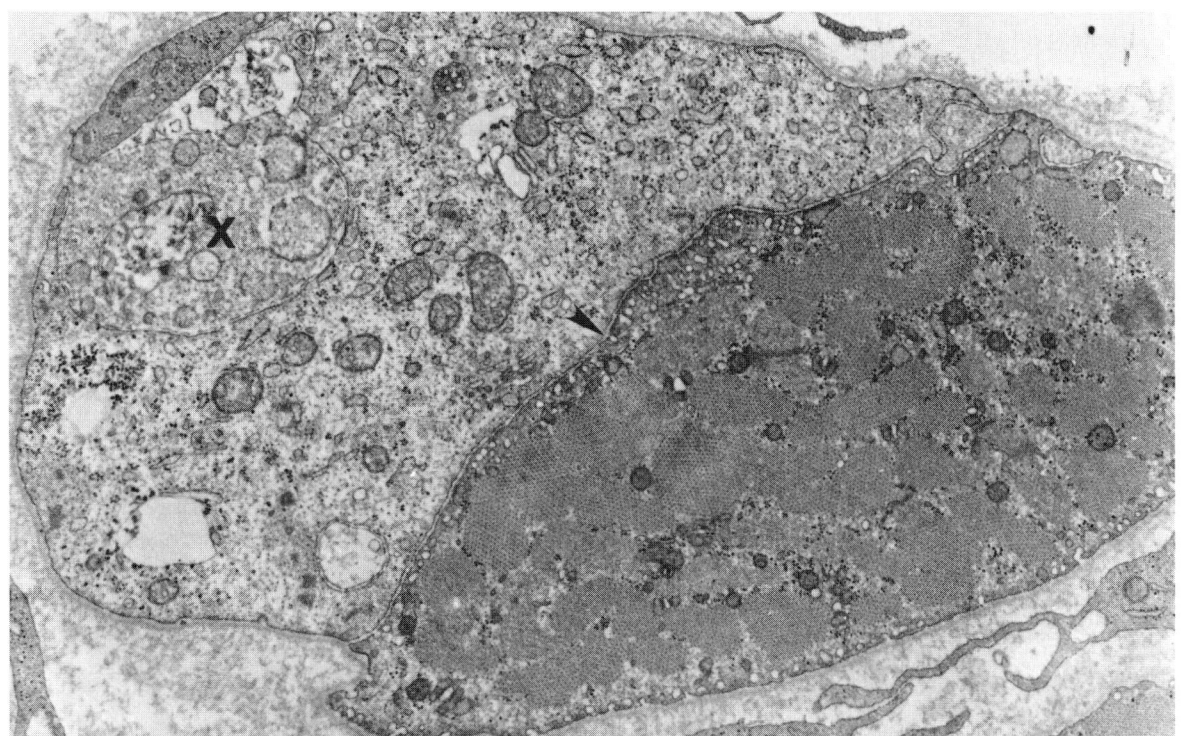

FIGURE 31-117. Necrotic (X), regenerating, and normal fiber elements within the same basal lamina cylinder. Borders of normal fiber segment are studded with caveolae (arrowhead). Dermatomyositis, ×37,700.

Alterations at the Neuromuscular Junction

This section summarizes the principal pathologic reactions of the pre- and postsynaptic regions of the neuromuscular junction (NMJ). Chap. 15 describes the ultrastructure of the normal NMJ, and Chaps. 64, 65, and 66 review the pathologic changes in the NMJ in myasthenia gravis and myasthenic syndromes.

PRESYNAPTIC ALTERATIONS

Degeneration of the nerve terminal. Degenerating nerve terminals are seldom observed in the electron microscope, perhaps because they persist only for a short time before they disappear. Distention of the nerve terminal by neurofilaments is a characteristic feature of acrylamide dying-back neuropathy (Fig. 31-125C),[222] but a few nerve terminals in normal muscle are also engorged by neurofilaments.[223] Myeloid structures appear in the nerve terminal in chloroquine neuromyopathy.[224]

Disappearance of the nerve terminal. Nerve terminals disappear from the NMJ after irreversible injury of the anterior horn cell or its axon and in the course of dying-back neuropathies. In either instance, remnants of the nerve ter-

◀ FIGURE 31-116 (continued)
space, and fuse to form myotubes. (2) Myoblasts exist in the interstitial space, where they either fuse to form myotubes or fuse to adjacent fibers to become satellite cells. In either case, satellite cells must have passed through the basal lamina of the parent fiber to reach the interstitial space. B. Activated satellite cell (s) has features of myoblast. Immediately above it, myoblasts (M) are fusing (asterisk) in the interstitial space to form a primitive myotube. A. Polymyositis, ×10,000. B. Dermatomyositis, ×11,900. (B is reproduced by permission from Engel AG, Macdonald RD, Excerpta Medica ICS 199:71, 1970.)

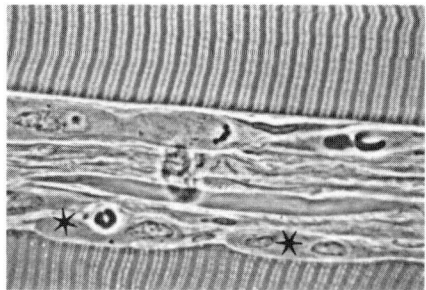

FIGURE 31-118. Slender myotubes (asterisks) positioned immediately adjacent to a nonnecrotic fiber and in the interstitial space. Compare with Fig. 31-116. Semithin resin section viewed in phase optics, ×330. (Reproduced by permission from Engel AG, Macdonald RD, Excerpta Medica ICS 199:71, 1970.)

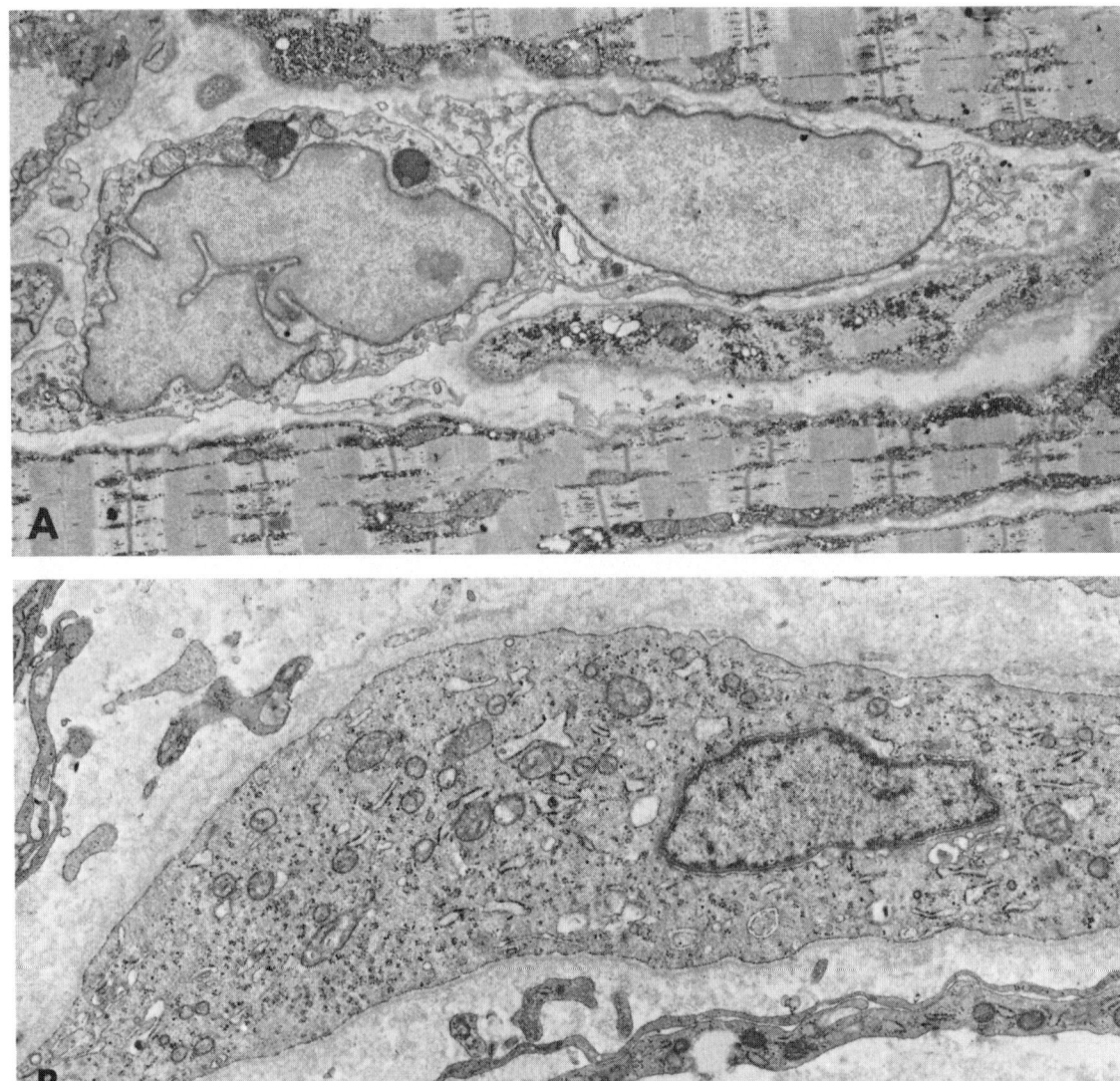

FIGURE 31-119. *A.* Closely adjacent myoblasts in the interstitial space between normal muscle fibers. *B.* Slender endomysial myotube covered by basal lamina. *A.* Duchenne dystrophy, ×10,000. *B.* Polymyositis, ×13,000.

minal are phagocytosed by the Schwann cell (Fig. 31-125*B*). Experimental section of a motor nerve is followed by a latent period during which the nerve terminal appears normal. The duration of this period depends on the distance between the lesion and the NMJ. In the rat diaphragm the nerve terminals remain normal for 8 to 12 h after phrenic nerve section at the cervical level. During the next 8 to 10 h the mitochondria become swollen, the synaptic vesicles conglutinate, osmiophilic material accumulates in the terminal, and the terminal splits into fragments that are phagocytosed by the Schwann cell.[225] After the nerve terminal is destroyed, the empty synaptic gutter is occupied by the Schwann cell for many weeks (Fig. 31-125*A*). If reinnervation fails to occur, the Schwann cell eventually retracts from the synaptic gutter.

Abnormally small nerve terminals. Reliable estimation of nerve terminal size requires morphometric analysis. However, the nerve terminal is likely to be small if it occupies only a small fraction of the synaptic gutter (Fig. 31-126).[223] Random sections through a NMJ whose nerve ter-

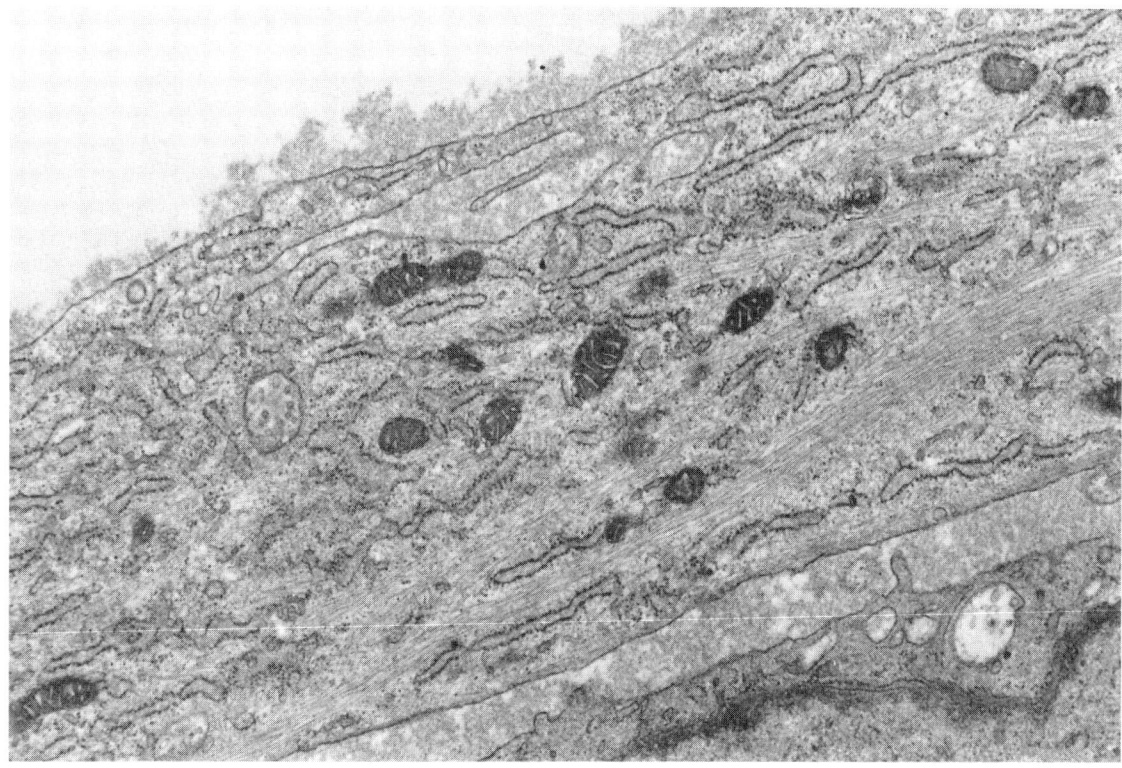

FIGURE 31-120. Early myotube covered by basal lamina on all sides contains axially oriented cytoskeletal filaments, rough endoplasmic reticulum, and mitochondria. Polymyositis, ×20,800.

minals are small may show empty synaptic gutters, and serial sections are required to distinguish this type of NMJ from a chronically denervated NMJ. Small nerve terminals occur at newly formed or recently reinnervated NMJs (Fig. 31-126) and in the congenital myasthenic syndrome associated with NMJ acetylcholinesterase deficiency (Fig. 31-127C).[10]

Sprouting. *Collateral sprouting* of motor axons begins at a node of Ranvier, whereas *ultraterminal sprouting* begins at the NMJ. The ultraterminal sprouts may reach the NMJ on another muscle fiber, may remain on the same muscle fiber and within the existing synaptic gutter of the NMJ from which they originate (intraterminal sprouting), or may remain on the same muscle fiber but migrate beyond the existing synaptic gutter to establish new junctional sites on the fiber (Chap. 15).

Denervation induces both ultraterminal and collateral sprouting, and the sprouts attempt to reach denervated NMJs. Ultraterminal sprouting also occurs after inactivity due to a variety of causes (e.g., botulism, tetrodotoxin blockade, periodic paralysis, hereditary motor end plate disease, and in winter frogs) and is probably stimulated by yet unidentified humoral factor(s) released by inactive muscle. Intraterminal sprouting may be a feature of local synaptic regeneration.

Ultraterminal sprouting resulting in new synaptic contacts on the same muscle fiber occurs in botulism without antecedent postsynaptic damage and in other diseases in which the postsynaptic region is severely damaged. The latter disorders include autoimmune myasthenia gravis (Chap. 64 and Ref. 226), the slow-channel myasthenic syndrome (Chap. 66 and Ref. 11; Fig. 31-127D), and the end plate myopathy induced by chronic prostigmine treatment.[227] Repeated cycles of destruction of the postsynaptic region followed by sprouting and formation of new synaptic contacts result in progressive separation of end plate regions on the surface of the muscle fiber.[11,226]

Depletion of presynaptic membrane active zones.

Depletion of presynaptic membrane active zones occurs in the Lambert-Eaton myasthenic syndrome and is described in Chap. 65.

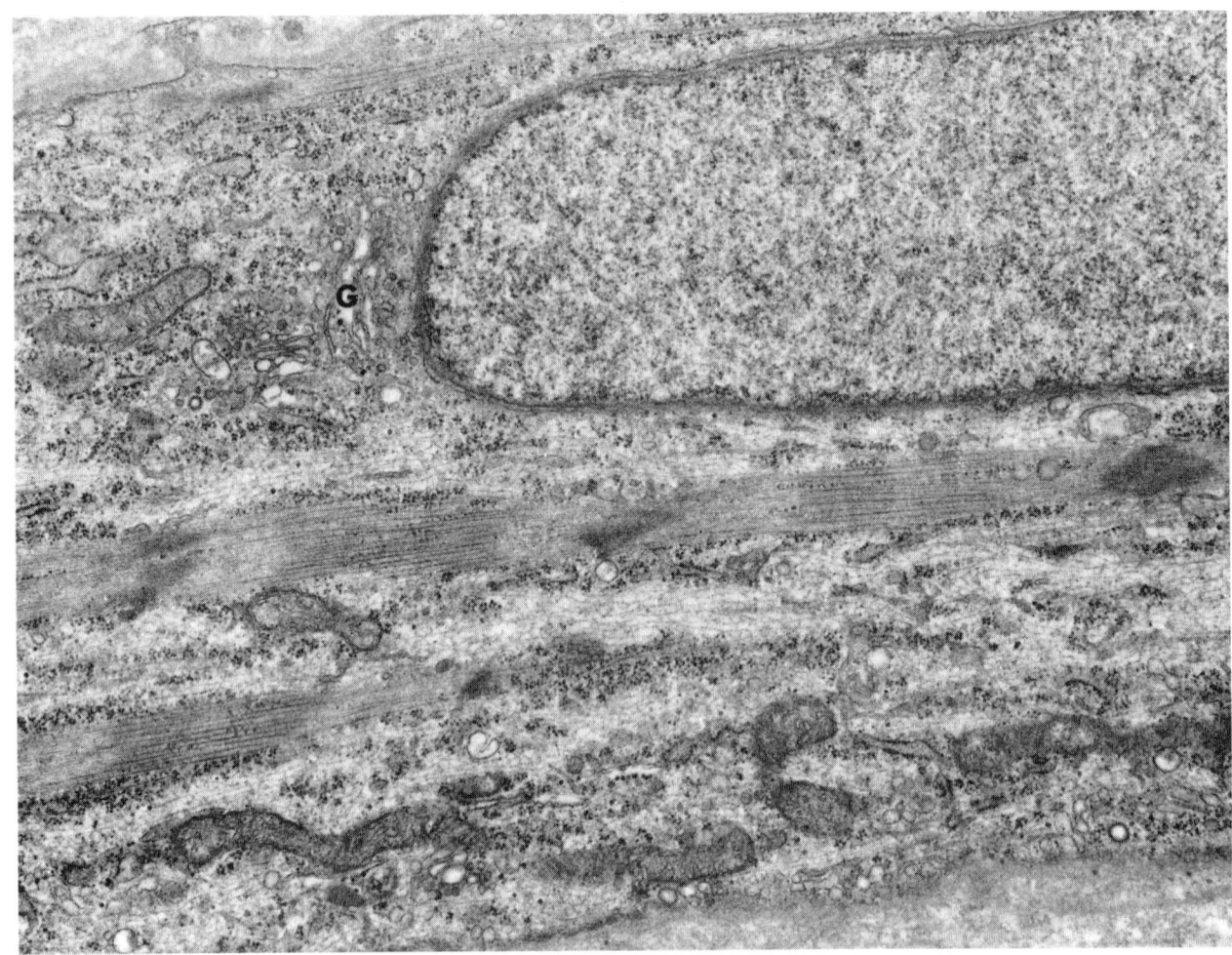

FIGURE 31-121. Myotube covered by basal lamina contains axially oriented cytoskeletal filaments, early myofibrils with small nemaline rods, abundant ribosomes, rough endoplasmic reticulum, and Golgi (G). Uneven distribution of organelles may be due to fusion of myotubes of differing maturity with each other and with myoblasts. Polymyositis, ×20,800.

POSTSYNAPTIC ALTERATIONS

Pathologic alterations in the postsynaptic region can be associated with a net loss of the acetylcholine receptor (AChR) from the NMJ. These alterations include degeneration and destruction of the junctional folds and the formation of immature junctions with few or no junctional folds. Destruction of the junctional folds will also hinder the reinsertion of new AChR into the NMJ. Accelerated internalization of AChR cross-linked by antibody (modulation) may also reduce the AChR of the NMJ if AChR resynthesis and reinsertion cannot keep up with the rate of AChR destruction. Modulation in itself is not known to be associated with a pathologic change in the NMJ, and it has not been clearly established that it can cause clinically significant depletion of the AChR of the NMJ unless there is also concomitant destruction or injury of the junctional folds.[228]

Degeneration of the junctional folds. The common mechanism for destruction of the junctional folds is an altered subsynaptic ionic milieu, especially focal calcium excess.[228] This can be induced by antibody and complement, as in acquired autoimmune myasthenia gravis (Fig. 31-127A; also see Chap. 64)[226]; by too frequent openings of the AChR ion channel, as in those myopathies induced by cholinergic agonists or cholinesterase inhibitors (Fig. 31-127B)[80,229]; and by abnormally prolonged opening episodes

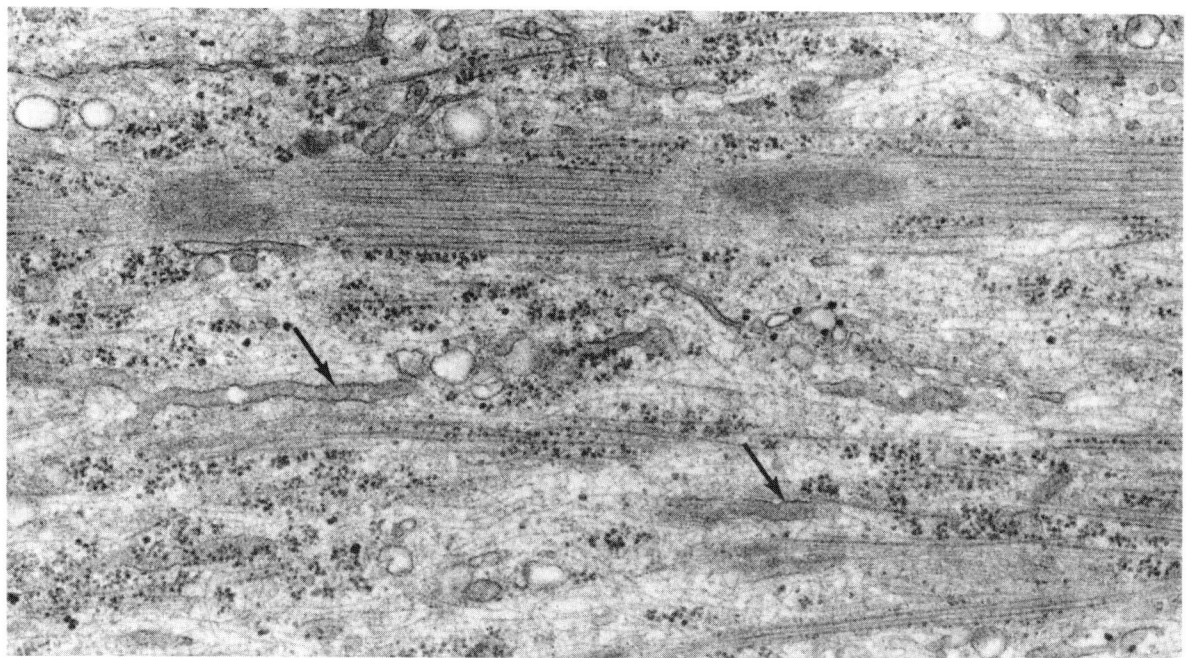

FIGURE 31-122. Myotube with axially oriented early SR tubules (arrows), myofibrils, and cytoskeletal filaments. Polymyositis, ×33,900.

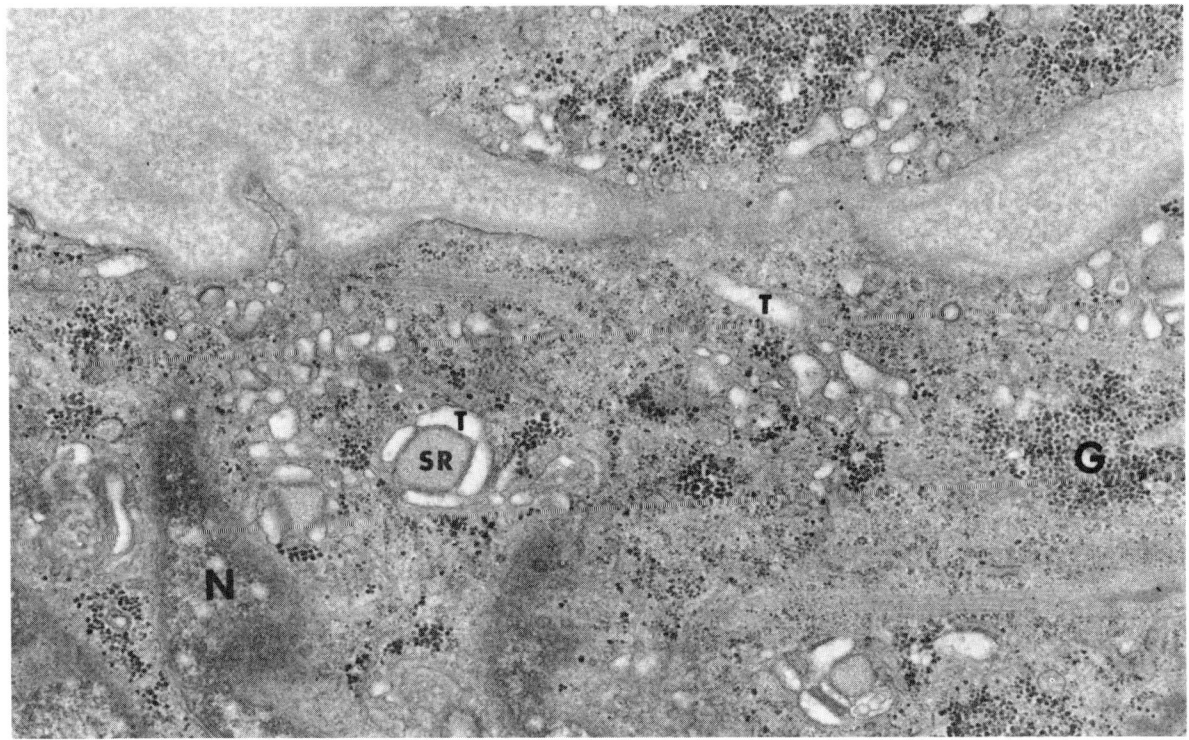

FIGURE 31-123. Myotube containing numerous subsarcolemmal T tubules (T), small lakes of glycogen (G), and early myofibrils. Several T tubules associate with dilated SR (SR) vesicles. N, nucleus. Dermatomyositis, ×20,400.

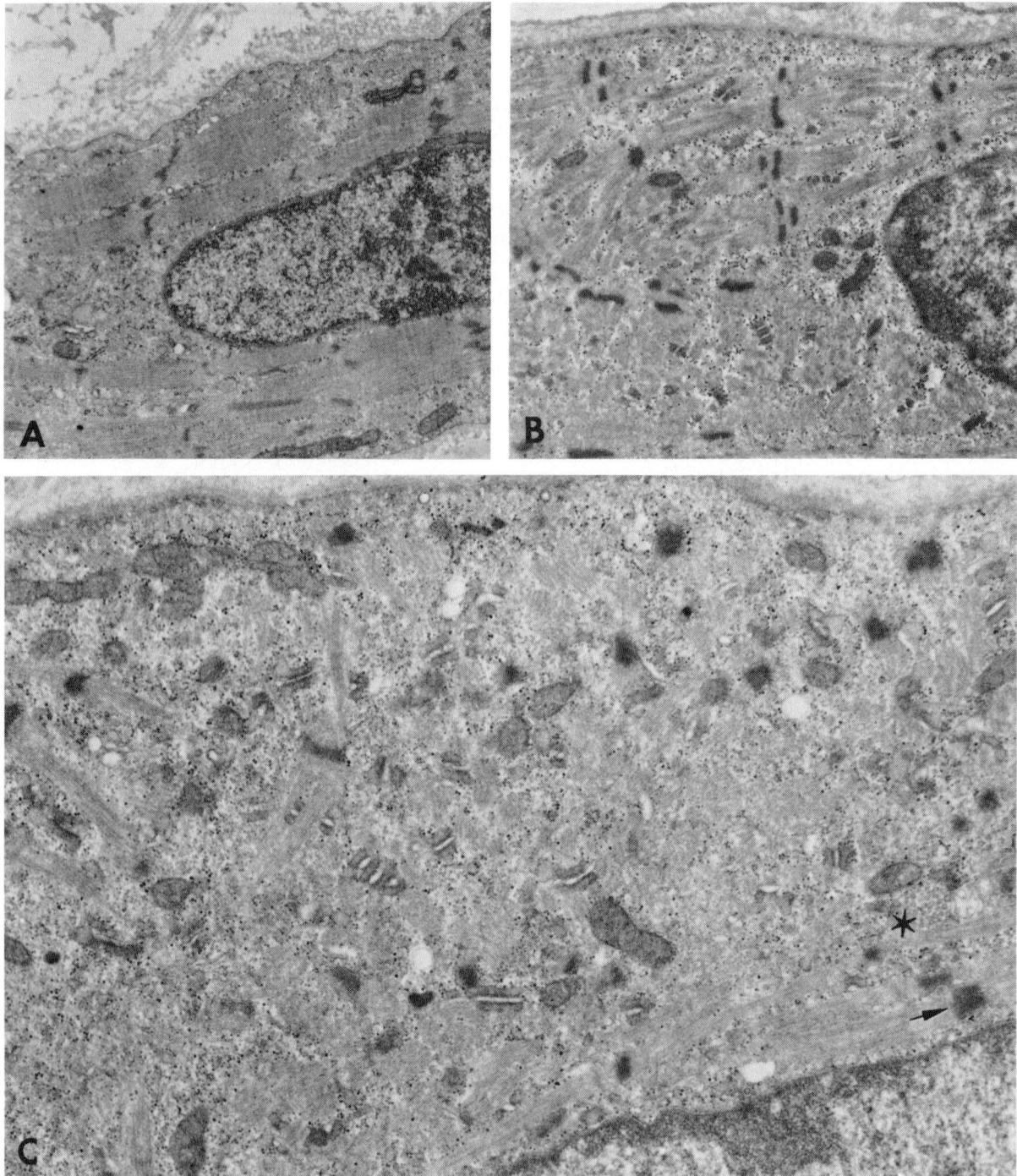

FIGURE 31-124. Differentiated myotubes with central nuclei and with normally aligned (A) and aberrant (B and C) myofibrils. Note wide Z disks (A, B, and C); double Z disks (B); small nemaline rods (arrow in C); irregularly disposed triads, pentads, and heptads (B and C); and T-system network (asterisk in C). A. Granulomatous myopathy, ×11,200. B. Limb-girdle dystrophy, ×6100. C. Limb-girdle dystrophy, ×15,800.

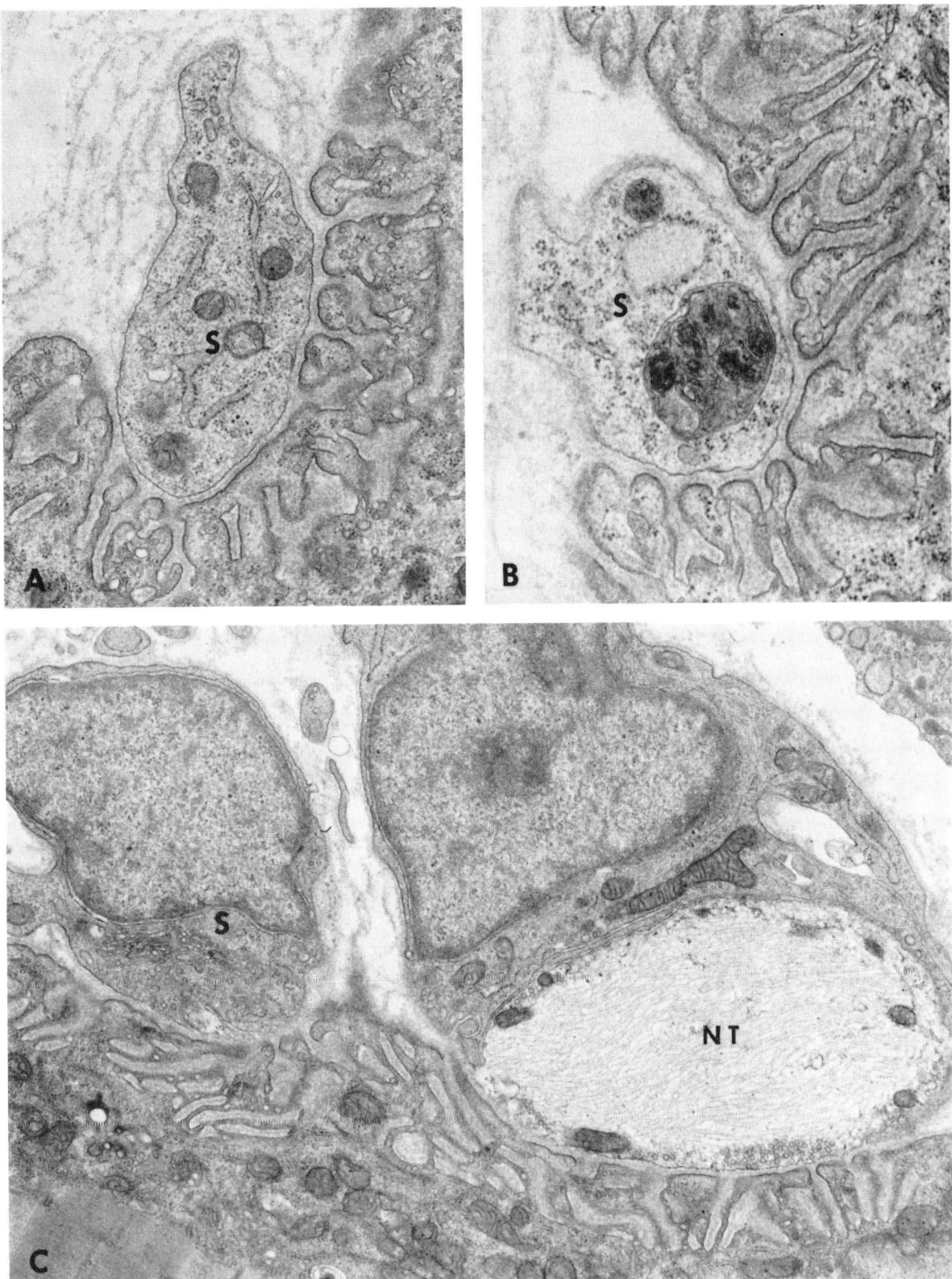

FIGURE 31-125. Experimental acrylamide neuropathy. Schwann cells (S) replace nerve terminals at end plate regions imaged in *A* and *B* and at the left of *C*. In *B*, Schwann cell contains degraded remnants of nerve terminal in a heterophagic vacuole. At the right of *C*, the nerve terminal (NT) is engorged by neurofilaments and contains few synaptic vesicles. *A*, ×23,700; *B*, ×28,000; *C*, ×15,300. (Reproduced by permission from Tsujihata M, Engel AG, Lambert EH, Neurology 24:849, 1974.)

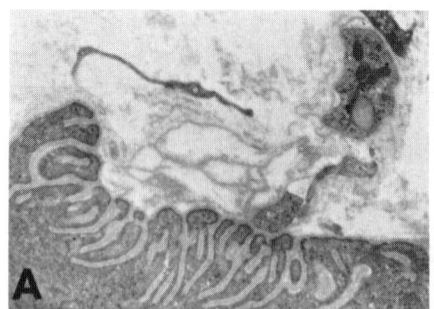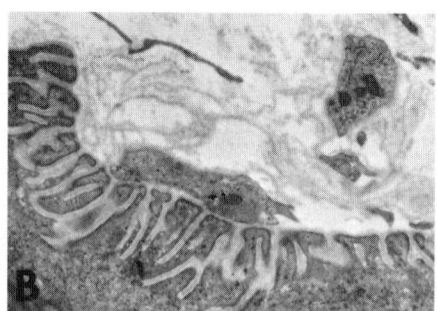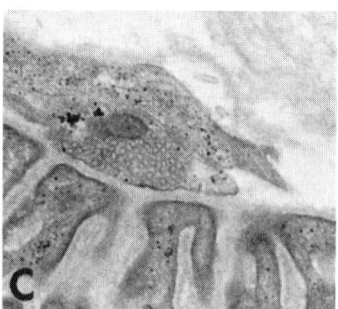

FIGURE 31-126. Sections through different planes of an end plate region in amyotrophic lateral sclerosis. Postsynaptic region is denuded of its nerve terminal in A, but a small nerve terminal appears in B. This is shown at a higher magnification in C. A and B, ×1600; C, ×15,800. (*Reproduced by permission from Engel AG, Jerusalem F, Tsujihata M, Gomez MR, Excerpta Medica ICS 360:132, 1975.*)

of the AChR ion channel, as in the slow-channel myasthenic syndrome (Fig. 31-128D).[11]

In autoimmune myasthenia gravis, activation of the lytic phase of the complement reaction sequence (Color Plate 14B and C) results in the formation of transmembrane ion channels. This is likely to cause an uncontrolled influx of extracellular ions, focal calcium excess,[230] protease activation, and destruction of cytoskeletal elements within the junctional folds. The subsequent shedding of injured segments of the folds bearing AChR, IgG, and complement (for illustrations, see Chap. 64) may be the outcome of disturbed membrane dynamics and impaired cytoskeletal support. The postsynaptic membrane reseals itself over the folds, which are now shorter and contain less AChR than the preexisting folds. Repeated cycles of these events result in a simplified postsynaptic region in which widened synaptic clefts contain material shed from the junctional folds (Fig. 31-127A). The nerve terminals abandon severely injured postsynaptic regions and seek new sites of contact with the muscle fiber.

The junctional folds are also injured in experimental myopathies induced by cholinergic agonists or anticholinesterase drugs (Fig. 31-127B) and in the slow-channel myasthenic syndrome (Fig. 31-127D). The changes in the folds are similar to those found in myasthenia gravis, but IgG and complement are not present on the folds. Focal degeneration of the junctional folds also occurs in Duchenne dystrophy,[231] in the *mdx* mouse,[231a] and occasionally in other dystrophies.[69] This, too, may be caused by calcium excess for in Duchenne dystrophy and in the *mdx* mouse the abnormal fragility of the dystrophin-deficient junctional plasma membrane can result in focal plasma membrane defects and an uncontrolled ingress of calcium from the extracellular fluid.

Phagocytosis of the junctional folds. This occurs in acute and passively transferred experimental autoimmune myasthenia gravis[232,233] but seldom if ever in human myasthenia gravis.[233a] In the experimental disease, opsonization of the junctional folds by IgG and complement precedes the phagocytic removal of the folds; and some muscle fibers undergo focal necrosis centered on the NMJ. The focal fiber necrosis here is probably due to complement-mediated lysis of a large segment of the postsynaptic membrane that allows a massive influx of extracellular fluid into the fiber near the NMJ. The exact reason for the selective susceptibility of the junctional folds to phagocytosis in acute and passively transferred experimental autoimmune myasthenia gravis has not been established.

Labyrinthine membranous networks in the junctional folds. These arise from caveolar inpocketings of the plasma membrane and resemble T-system networks. They are frequently observed in congenital NMJ acetylcholinesterase deficiency (Fig. 31-127C)[10] and in the slow-channel myasthenic syndrome.[11] The networks may protect AChR from excessive exposure to acetylcholine or may represent an attempt to generate new postsynaptic membrane.

Simple postsynaptic regions. These are observed after extensive destruction of the junctional folds and at newly formed NMJs. Simple postsynaptic regions also occur on normal intrafusal and on some normal extraocular muscle fibers (Chap. 6). When the simplification is caused by destruction of the folds, the primary and remaining secondary synaptic clefts are irregularly widened and contain degenerated remnants and basal lamina envelopes of preexisting folds (Fig. 31-127A, B, and D).

New NMJs formed by ultraterminal nerve sprouts (Fig. 31-128A) resemble developing NMJs in newborn animals (Fig. 31-128B). These junctions contain few or no secondary synaptic clefts and show no signs of antecedent destruction of the junctional folds. At simple, newly formed junctions the sites for AChR as well as sodium channel insertion are

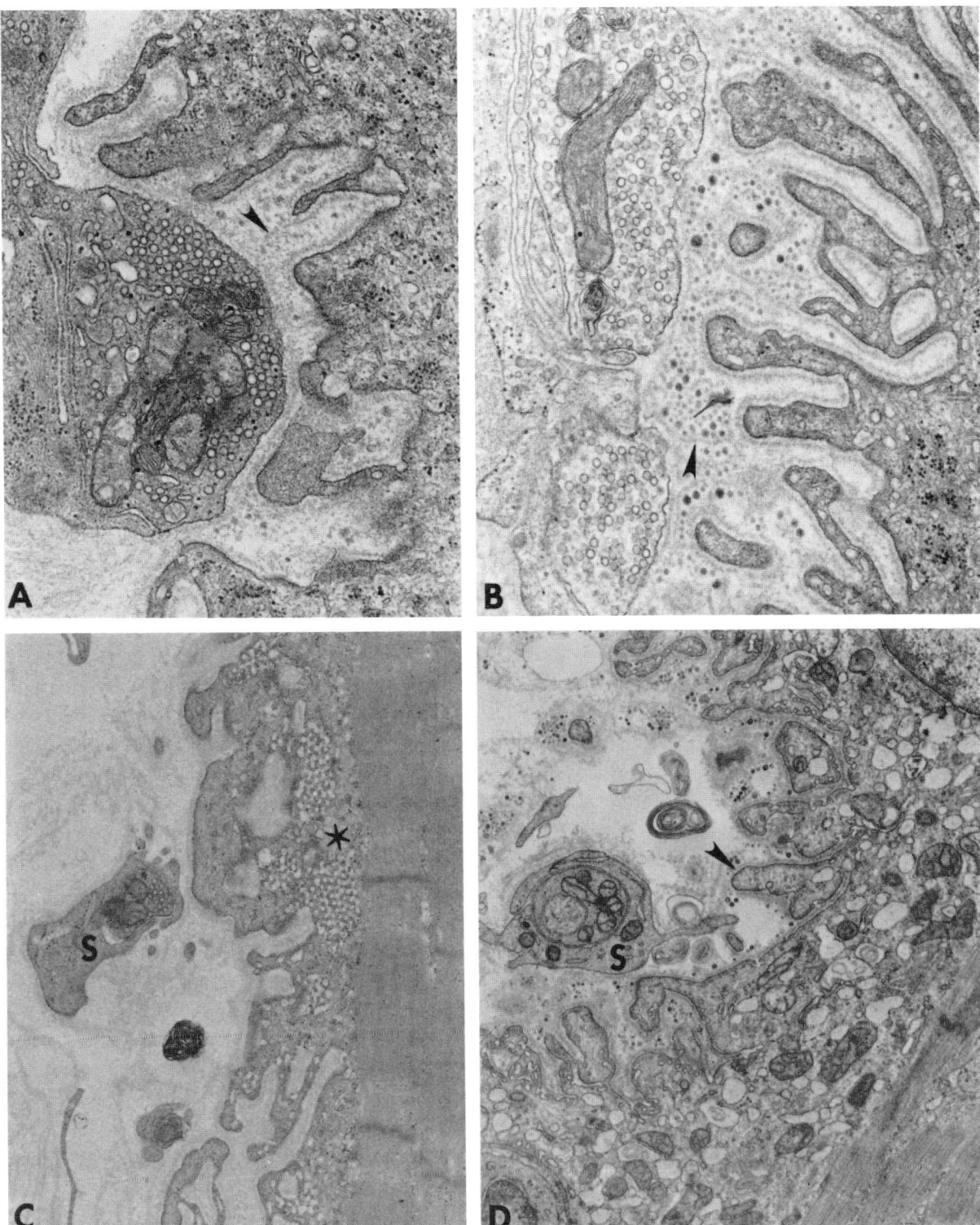

FIGURE 31-127. Motor end plate abnormalities in autoimmune myasthenia gravis (A), experimental prostigmine-induced end plate myopathy (B), congenital end plate acetylcholinesterase deficiency (C), and slow-channel myasthenic syndrome (D). Note degenerating junctional folds in A, B, and D. Basal lamina envelopes (arrowheads) and small globules mark sites from which junctional folds have disappeared. In C and D, small nerve terminals completely surrounded by Schwann cell (S) are nerve sprouts approaching or receding from postsynaptic region. In C, the junctional folds are honeycombed by caveolar or T-system networks (asterisk). A, ×31,900, B, ×25,400, C and D, ×13,500. (A is reproduced by permission from Engel AG, Tsujihata M, Lindstrom J, et al, Ann NY Acad Sci 274:60, 1976; B is reproduced by permission from Engel AG, Lambert EH, Santa T, Neurology 23:1273, 1973; D is reproduced by permission from Engel AG, Lambert EH, Mulder DM, et al, Ann NY Acad Sci 377:614, 1981.)

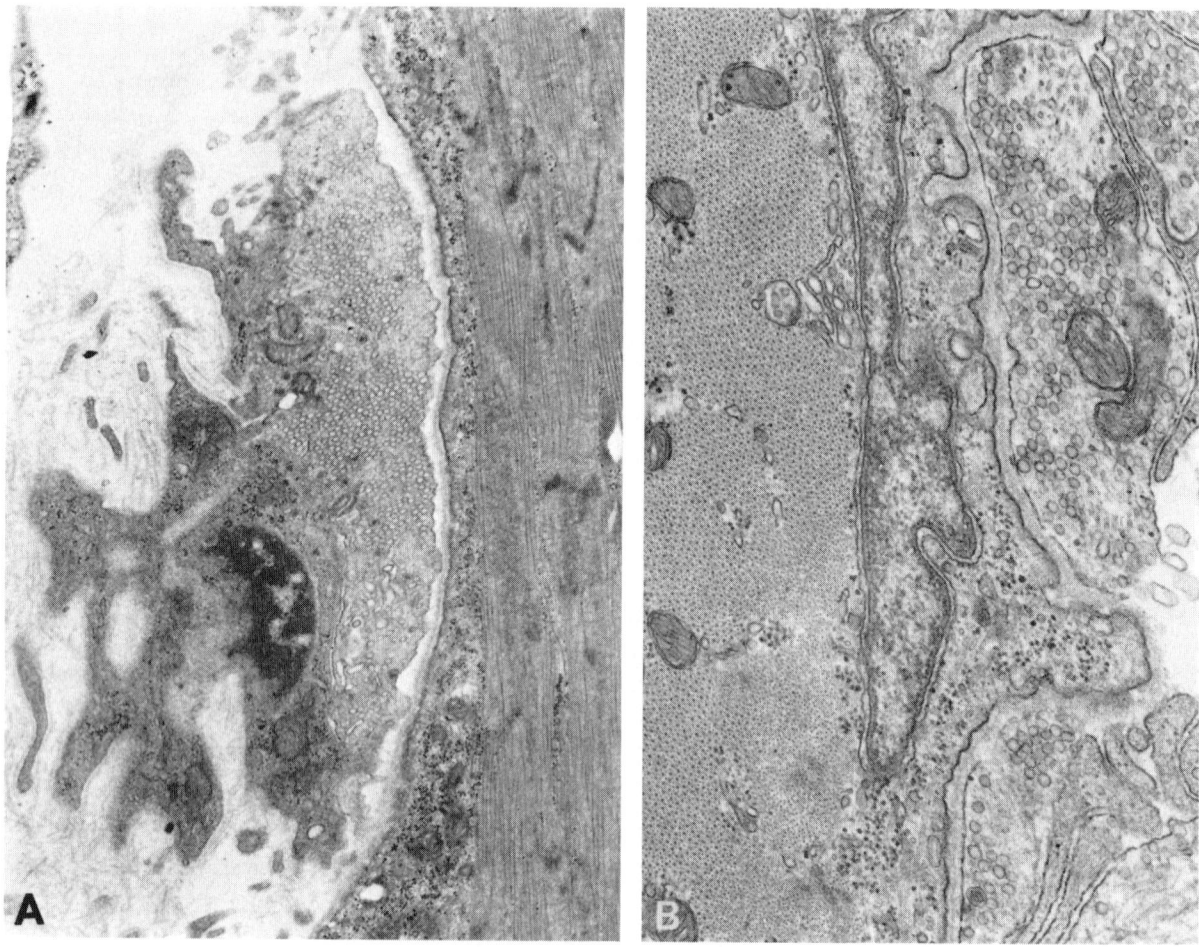

FIGURE 31-128. Simple postsynaptic regions associated with an ultraterminal nerve sprout in human botulism (A) and in gastrocnemius muscle of a newborn rat (B). A, ×11,200; B, ×30,800.

limited by the lack of junctional folds, and this reduces the safety margin of synaptic transmission.

Alterations in junctional sarcoplasm. An increase in the amount of junctional sarcoplasm can be observed at many NMJs in acquired autoimmune myasthenia gravis.[234] The increased junctional sarcoplasm at these junctions is consistent with the notion that here accelerated destruction or synthesis (or both) of AChR is taking place.

A spectrum of pathologic alterations can be observed in the junctional sarcoplasm and nearby fiber regions in the end plate myopathies induced by cholinesterase inhibitors,[68,69,80] cholinergic agonists,[34] and the slow-channel myasthenic syndrome.[11] These include dilation (Fig. 31-127D), proliferation and degeneration of SR vesicles, degeneration and disappearance of mitochondria, focal myofibrillar degeneration, proliferating T-system and Golgi elements, nuclear degeneration and apoptosis (Fig. 31-13C and D), and the entrapment and degradation of degenerating organelles in vacuoles. Dilation of SR vesicles, mitochondrial alterations, and Z-disk streaming are rapidly induced in the experimental end plate myopathies. These changes are calcium-mediated[34,69] and at least partially protease-mediated.[81] The additional pathologic changes that appear in the slow-channel myasthenic syndrome may depend on more chronic alterations of the local electrolyte milieu (Chap. 66).

Alterations of the Muscle Microvasculature

The ultrastructure of normal intramuscular blood vessels is described in Chap. 22. This section summarizes the more

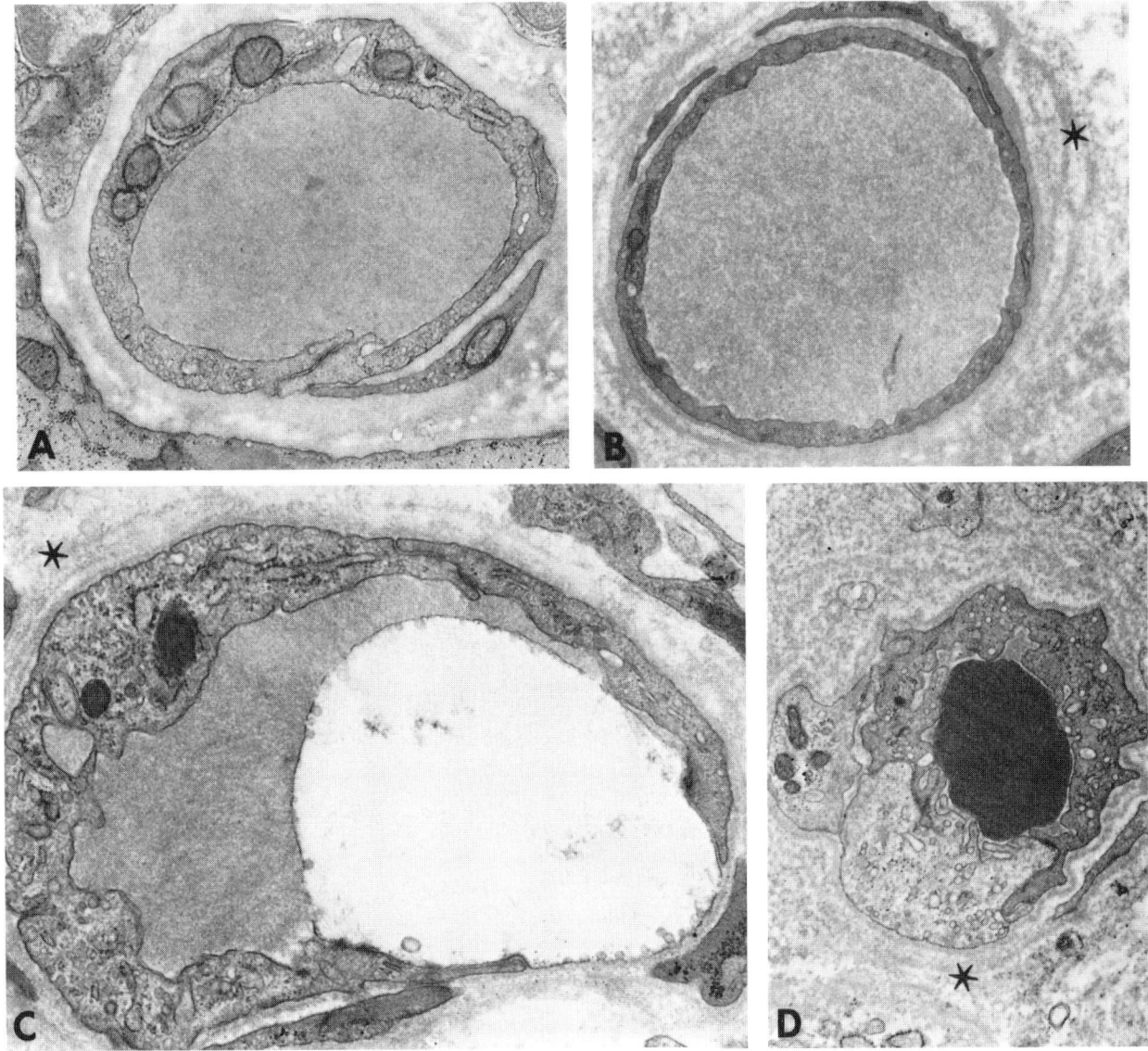

FIGURE 31-129. Muscle capillaries in normal subject *(A)* and in Duchenne dystrophy *(B)* and dermatomyositis *(C and D)*. Note replication of basal lamina (asterisks) in *B, C,* and *D* and pale and swollen endothelial cells in *C* and *D.* *A,* ×12,700; *B,* ×12,200; *C,* ×21,900; *D,* ×15,800. *(A, B, and D are reproduced by permission from Jerusalem F, Engel AG, Gomez MR, Brain 97:115–122, 1974; C is reproduced by permission from Jerusalem F, Rakusa M, Engel AG, Macdonald RD, J Neurol Sci 23:391, 1974.)*

common pathologic reactions of the small intramuscular blood vessels.

Replication of the basal lamina. This is a nonspecific alteration involving small blood vessels. It can be observed in more than half the capillaries in dermatomyositis (Figs. 31-129D, 31-130A), scleroderma, systemic lupus erythematosus, and Duchenne dystrophy (Fig. 31-129B) and significantly less often in other dystrophies and in neurogenic atrophies.[235] Replication and thickening of the muscle capillary basal lamina occur after experimentally induced capillary necrosis and in diabetes mellitus (reviewed in Ref. 235). Thus, replication of the capillary basal lamina may indicate antecedent capillary destruction followed by regeneration or remodeling of the capillary bed in response to varying tissue requirements for capillaries.

Thickening of the basal lamina and pipestem vessels. Thickening of the capillary basal lamina can occur (1) in diabetes mellitus, (2) in partially denervated muscle, (3) in the eosinophilia-myalgia syndrome related to L-tryptophan ingestion,[235a] (4) in a necrotizing myopathy associated with microvascular deposition of the complement MAC,[235b] or (5) as an isolated finding. Marked thickening of the basal lamina confers a pipestem appearance on the capillaries.[235b] Partially denervated human gastrocnemius muscle displays this alteration more frequently than other denervated muscles, perhaps because of increased hydrostatic pressure. Ultrastructurally, the pipestem vessels are embedded in amorphous material laced with concentrically arrayed collagen fibrils (Fig. 31-130).[235b] Compact globules of the same material, sometimes containing cellular debris or extravasated erythrocytes, represent sites from which capillaries had disappeared (asterisks in Fig. 31-130A and C). These deposits correspond to "hyaline globules" found in the endomysium in trichrome-stained frozen sections.[235b]

Decrease in capillary density. A decrease in muscle capillaries has been found in scleroderma, systemic lupus erythematosus,[236] and dermatomyositis[128,236a] but not in inclusion body myositis,[4] polymyositis,[237] or Duchenne dystrophy.[236]

Increase in capillary size. Morphometric studies indicate that the average capillary area is increased in Duchenne dystrophy,[235] dermatomyositis, scleroderma, and systemic

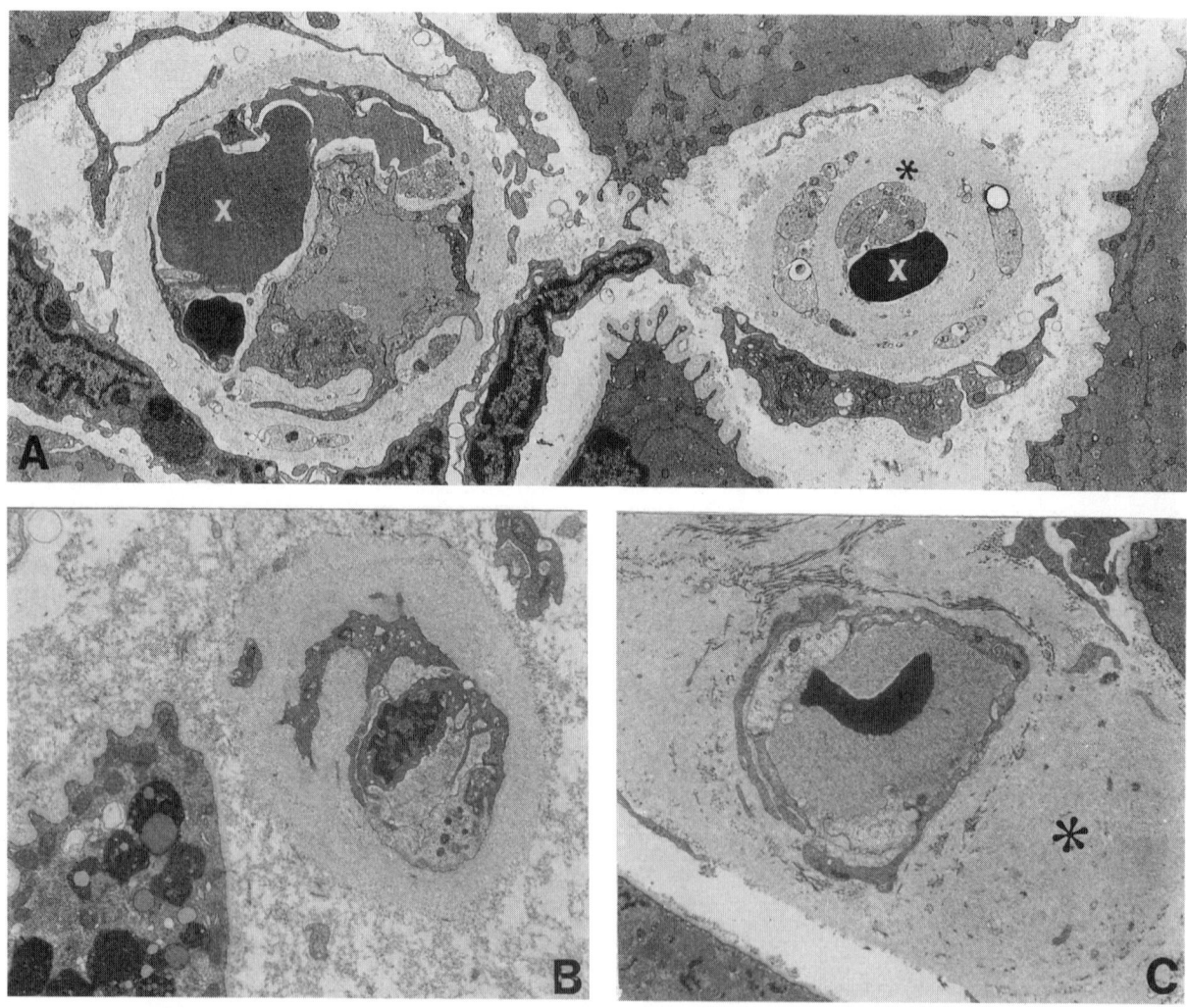

FIGURE 31-130. Pipestem vessels. *A.* At the left, a patent capillary abuts on extravasated erythrocytes (X) flanked by pericytes. All are surrounded by a heavy coat of amorphous material. At the right, an erythrocyte (X) and capillary remnants are embedded in a globule of amorphous material (asterisk). *B.* Capillary and pericyte are surrounded by a heavy coat of amorphous material. *C.* A capillary displaying two swollen endothelial cells is embedded in a thick coat of amorphous material interlaced with collagen fibrils. The asterisk adjacent to it indicates a globular collection of the same material. *A,* ×5700; *B,* ×6500; *C,* ×5700. *(Reproduced by permission from Emslie-Smith AM, Engel AG, Neurology 4:936, 1991.)*

lupus erythematosus.[127] In Duchenne dystrophy the dimensions of endothelial cells and pericytes are increased in proportion to the overall increase in the capillary area. The density of pinocytotic vesicles in the endothelial cells is slightly but significantly reduced, but the other capillary organelles are normal.[235] In dermatomyositis, polymyositis, scleroderma, and systemic lupus erythematosus there is hypertrophy of the endothelial cells and pericytes (Figs. 31-131A, 31-132A). This is accompanied by an increase in the density of mitochondrial and rough endoplasmic reticulum profiles and a decrease in the density of pinocytotic vesicles in the endothelial cells. In dermatomyositis and scleroderma the average number of tight junctions per capillary transection is increased from the normal value or 1.6 to 2.6, indicating that an extra endothelial cell has become incorporated into the enlarged capillary wall.[127] The abundant rough endoplasmic reticulum in the hypertrophied endothelial cells (Figs. 31-131A, 31-132A) suggests that these cells are regenerating.

Pale, swollen endothelial cells. These occur in 20 percent of the capillaries in dermatomyositis (Fig. 31-129C and D) and in a smaller proportion of the capillaries in other inflammatory muscle diseases and in Duchenne dystrophy.[127,235] The significance of this alteration is uncertain. However, some, at least, of the pale endothelial cells may be regenerating (Fig. 31-129D).

Microtubular inclusions in endothelial cells. These occur in endothelial cells and less frequently in pericytes, satellite cells, and myoblasts in dermatomyositis and systemic lupus erythematosus. The morphology of these inclusions (Figs. 31-68 and 31-132B) and their possible significance were discussed under "Miscellaneous Inclusions," earlier in this chapter. Their presence in hypertrophied (Fig. 31-132A) and in degenerating (Fig. 31-131B) endothelial cells links them to disease activity, but it is not known whether they instigate other pathologic alterations or are a concomitant morphologic reaction.

Degeneration and necrosis of endothelial cells. Concentrically arrayed layers of basal lamina surrounding small empty areas in the interstitial space represent the

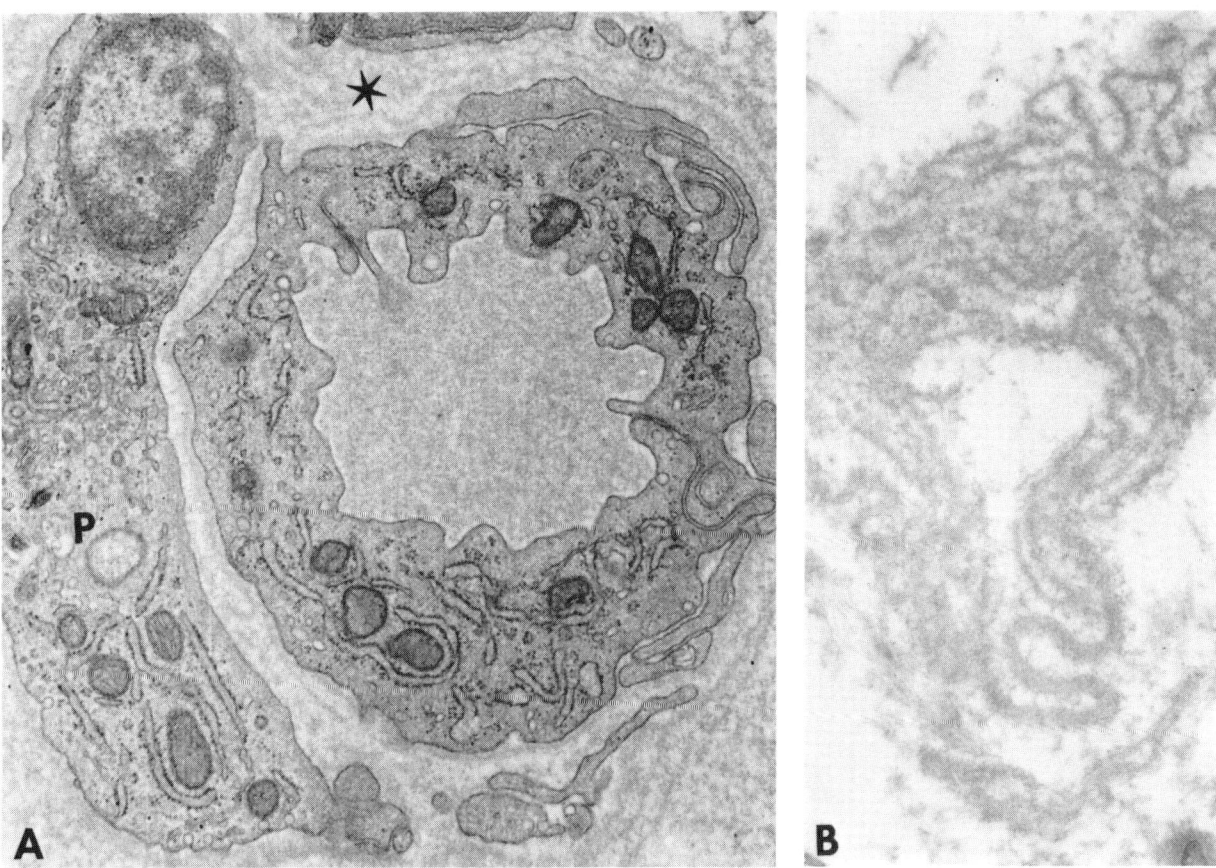

FIGURE 31-131. *A.* Hypertrophied capillary and pericyte (P). Endothelial cells contain abundant rough endoplasmic reticulum and sparse pinocytotic vesicles. Asterisk marks replicated basal lamina. *B.* Collapsed basal lamina residues surround space from which capillary has disappeared. *A.* Dermatomyositis, ×19,400; *B.* Scleroderma, ×16,600. (*Reproduced by permission from Jerusalem F, Rakusa M, Engel AG, Macdonald RD, J Neurol Sci 23:391, 1974.*)

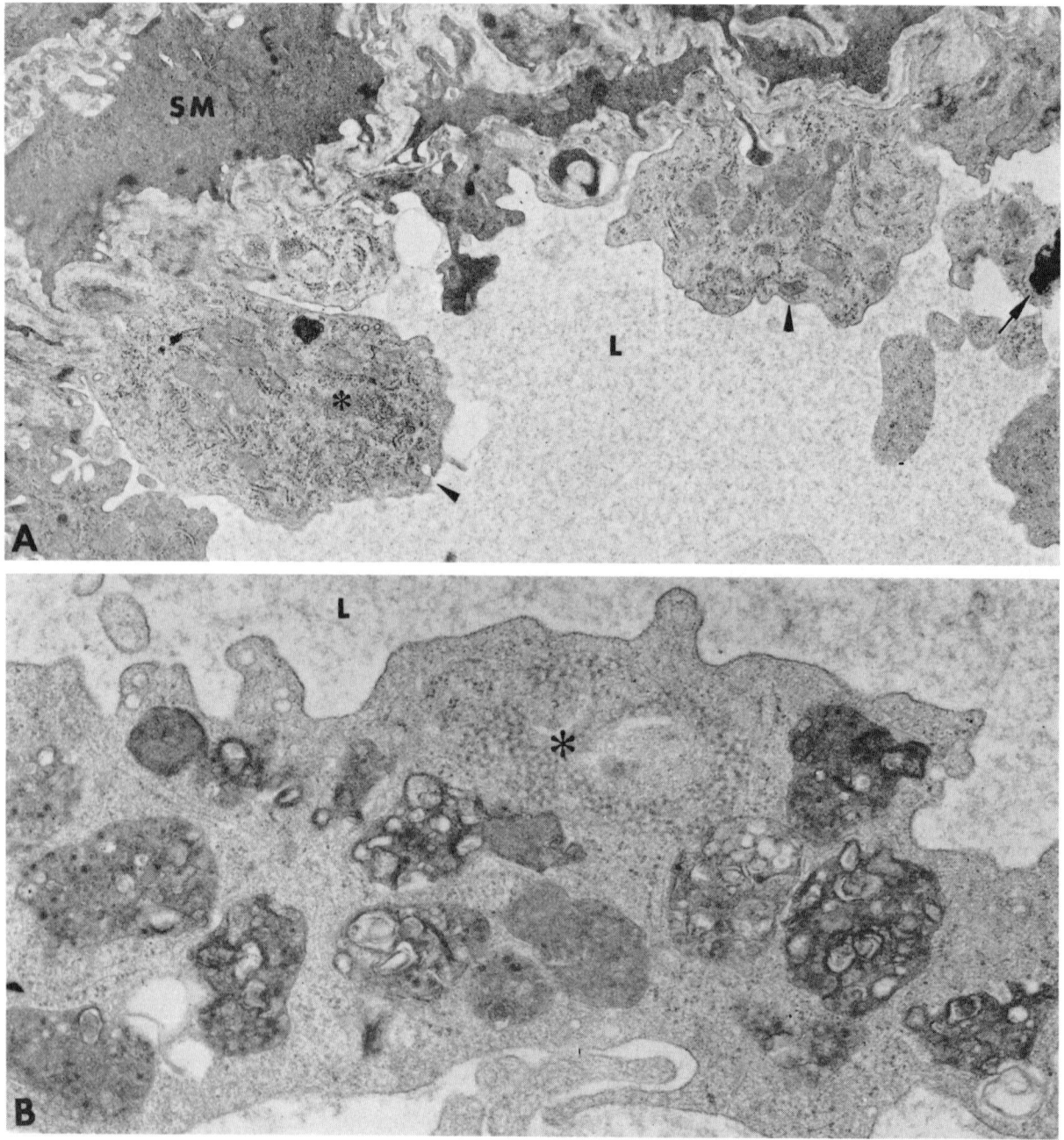

FIGURE 31-132. Abnormal small blood vessels in dermatomyositis. In *A*, lumen of arteriole is lined by enlarged regenerating endothelial cells (arrowheads) and degenerating endothelial cells (arrow). Microtubular inclusion (asterisk) appears in one regenerating cell. In *B*, endothelial cell contains numerous autophagic vacuoles and a microtubular inclusion (asterisk). L, lumen; SM, smooth muscle. *A*, ×11,600; *B*, ×34,000.

"tombstones" of capillaries that have undergone necrosis (Fig. 31-131B). These formations appear in inflammatory myopathies[127] and occasionally in denervated muscle, and are more abundant in dermatomyositis and in the eosinophilia myalgia syndrome than in the other disorders.[237a–c] Capillary necrosis in dermatomyositis is initiated or propagated by complement (Color Plate 9B). The sequential changes that lead to capillary necrosis in different disorders have not been described in detail, but the degenerating endothelial cells in dermatomyositis have been well characterized (Fig. 31-132).[2,128] These contain abundant small autophagic vacuoles filled with cytoplasmic degradation products, with or without the additional presence of microtubular inclusions (Fig. 31-132B). In some capillaries and small blood vessels, regenerating and degenerating endothelial cells appear side by side (Fig. 31-132A).

Amyloid infiltration. Amyloid infiltration of skeletal muscle, and especially of the tongue, can occur in systemic amyloidosis.[238] In this condition the abnormal deposits are filamentous, and each amyloid filament is made up of a series of thin lamellae in which the polypeptide chains are arranged perpendicularly to the axis of the filament.[239]

The clinically affected muscles either atrophy, partly at least because of concomitant amyloid neuropathy, or hypertrophy. Infrequently, systemic amyloidosis presents as a hypertrophic myopathy.[240,241]

The histochemical aspects of amyloid infiltration of muscle are described in Chap. 30 and Color Plate 9F to N. In semithin resin sections the amyloid deposits appear as homogeneous material between and around the mural elements of small vessels and immediately adjacent to the muscle fiber surface membrane (Fig. 31-133). The lumen of the infiltrated blood vessels is not compromised.

In the electron microscope, the amyloid filaments are short, rectilinear, nonbranching, and about 10 nm in diameter (Figs. 31-134 and 31-135). In some deposits the amyloid filaments are intermingled with amorphous material that may represent unpolymerized immunoglobulin light chains. In small arterioles and venules the amyloid filaments accumulate externally to the contraluminal surface of the endothelial cells, disrupt the internal elastica, separate and compress the smooth muscle fibers of the media, and may extend for a variable distance into the adventitia and the surrounding interstitial region (Fig. 31-134). Amyloid filaments also accumulate around capillary endothelial cells; here they surround but spare the adjacent pericytes and fibroblasts, spread for a variable distance into the nearby interstitial space, and may merge with those deposits that surround muscle fibers. The deposits around the muscle fibers vary from a fraction of a micron to several microns in thickness and are often covered by a fibroblast process (Fig. 31-135C and D). Superficial regions of muscle fibers surrounded by amyloid may be devoid of myofibrils; these regions contain abundant rough endoplasmic reticulum profiles, Golgi cisternae, mitochondria, and a few myeloid structures (Fig. 31-135C). Concentric muscle fiber splitting also occurs in amyloid myopathy (see under "Alterations of the Surface Membrane" and Figs. 31-7 and 31-8).

The presence of amyloid deposits in inclusion body myositis was discussed earlier in this chapter under "Miscellaneous Inclusions."

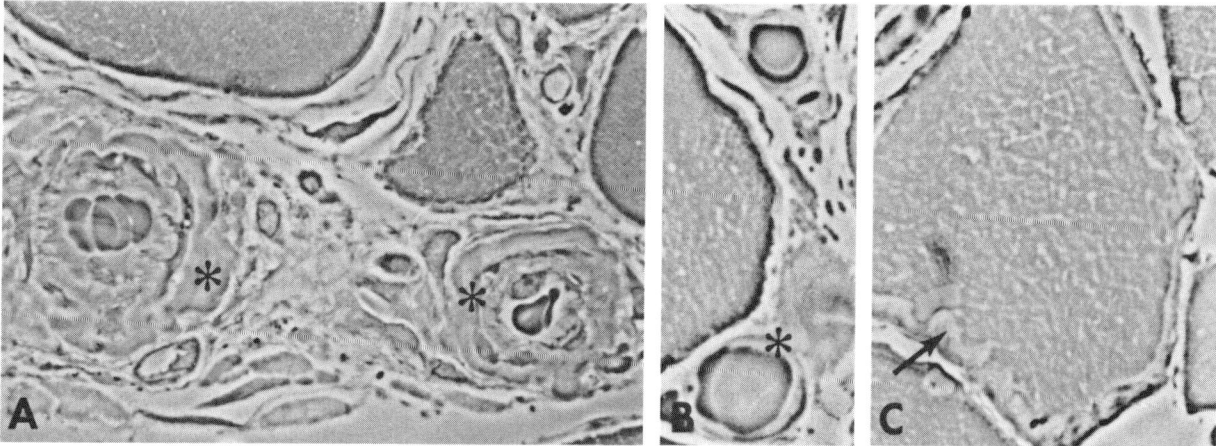

FIGURE 31-133. Amyloid myopathy; semithin resin section viewed in phase optics. Amyloid accumulates between mural elements of small blood vessels (asterisks in A) and around capillaries (asterisk in B) and muscle fibers (arrow in C). A, ×950; B, ×1400; C, ×1200.

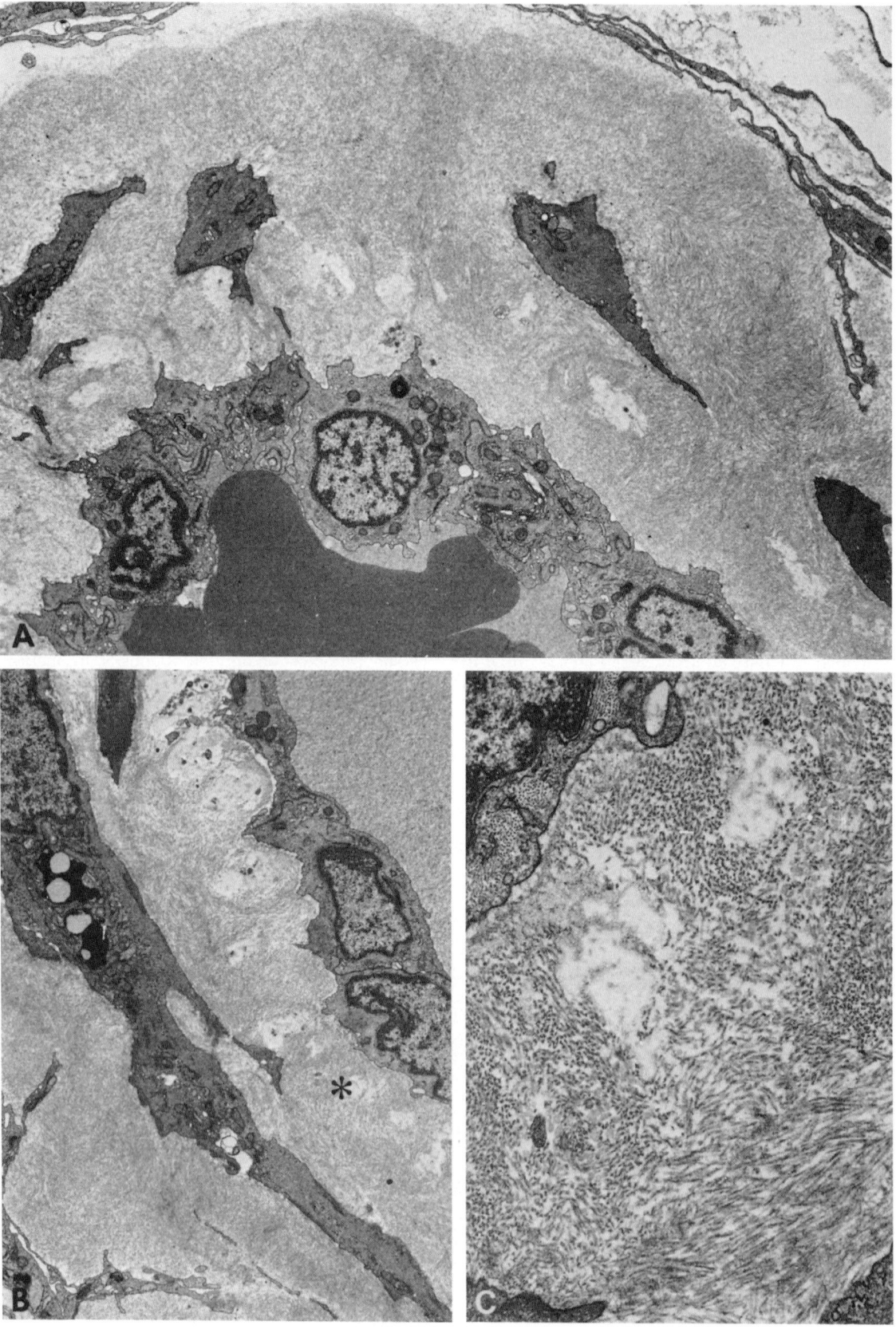

FIGURE 31-134. Amyloid myopathy. *A* and *B*. Amyloid fibrils accumulate between the intima and adventitia of small blood vessels. The smooth muscle fibers and internal elastica are disrupted in *A*. *C* is a higher magnification of region marked by asterisk in *B*. The amyloid filaments are rectilinear, course in bundles, and do not branch. *A*, ×8000; *B*, ×6700; *C*, ×29,400.

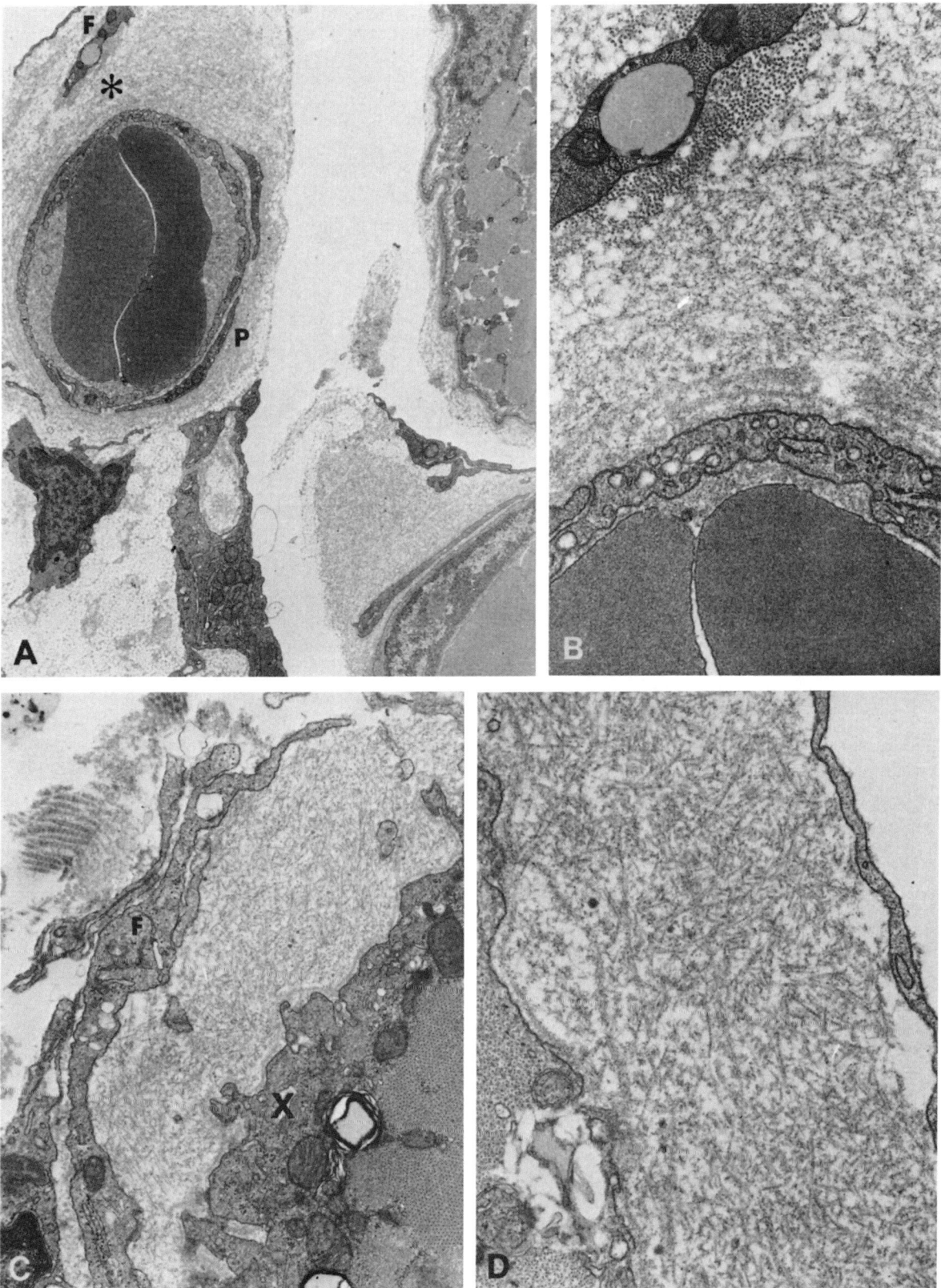

FIGURE 31-135. Amyloid myopathy. Amyloid deposits around capillaries *(A and B)* and muscle fibers *(C and D)*. B is a higher magnification of region marked by asterisk in *A*. In *C*, the superficial region of the muscle fiber surrounded by amyloid shows loss of myofibrils and regenerative activity (X). P, pericyte; F, fibroblast process. *A*, ×7300; *B*, ×35,400; *C*, ×16,700; *D*, ×38,600.

List of Abbreviations

AChR	acetylcholine receptor	PML	promyelocytic leukemia
AIDS	acquired immunodeficiency syndrome	SMN	survival motor neuron
ATPase	adenosine triphosphatase	snRNP	small nuclear ribonucleoprotein
HGF	hepatocyte growth factor	SR	sarcoplasmic reticulum
MAC	membrane attack complex	T tubule	transverse tubule
NMJ	neuromuscular junction	TGF-β	transforming growth factor beta

References

1. Mokri B, Engel AG: Duchenne dystrophy: Electron microscopic findings pointing to basic or early abnormality in the plasma membrane of the muscle fiber. *Neurology* 25:1111, 1975.
1a. Selcen D, Stilling G, Engel AG: The earliest pathologic alterations in dysferlinopathy. *Neurology* 56:1472–1481, 2001.
2. Banker BQ: Dermatomyositis of childhood. Ultrastructural alterations of muscle and intramuscular blood vessels. *J Neuropathol Exp Neurol* 34:46, 1975.
3. Chou S-M: Myxovirus-like structures and accompanying nuclear changes in chronic polymyositis. *Arch Pathol* 86:649, 1968.
4. Carpenter S, Karpati G, Heller I, et al: Inclusion body myositis: A distinct variety of idiopathic inflamatory myopathy. *Neurology* 28:8, 1978.
5. Arahata K, Engel AG: Immunoelectron microscopic analysis of cell mediated muscle fiber injury in polymyositis and inclusion body myositis. *J Neuropathol Exp Neurol* 44:361, 1985.
5a. Arahata K, Engel AG: Monoclonal antibody analysis of mononuclear cells in myopathies: III. Immunoelectron microscopic aspects of cell mediated muscle fiber injury. *Ann Neurol* 19:112, 1986.
6. Engel AG, Dale AJD: Autophagic glycogenosis of late onset with mitochondrial abnormalities: Light and electron microscopic observations. *Mayo Clin Proc* 43:233, 1968.
7. Engel AG: Vacuolar myopathies: Multiple etiologies and sequential structural studies, in Pearson CM (ed): *The Striated Muscle*. Baltimore: Williams & Wilkins; 1973, pp 301–341.
8. Engel AG, Lindstrom J, Lambert EH, Lennon VA: Ultrastructural localization of the acetylcholine receptor in myasthenia gravis and in its experimental autoimmune model. *Neurology* 27:307, 1977.
9. Engel AG, Lambert EH, Howard FM: Immune complexes (IgG and C3) at the motor end-plate in myasthenia gravis: Ultrastructural and light microscopic localization and electrophysiologic correlations. *Mayo Clin Proc* 52:267, 1977.
9a. Pellissier JF, Pouget J, Charpin C, et al: Myopathy associated with desmin type intermediate filaments: An immunoelectron microscopic study. *J Neurol Sci* 89:49, 1989.
9b. Askanas V, Serdaroglu P, Engel WK, et al: Immunolocalization of ubiquitin in muscle biopsies of patients with inclusion body myositis and oculopharyngeal muscular dystrophy. *Neurosci Lett* 130:73, 1991.
9c. Askanas V, Engel WK, Alvarez RB: Light and electron microscopic localization of beta-amyloid protein in muscle biopsies of patients with inclusion-body myositis. *Am J Pathol* 141:31, 1992.
9d. Askanas V, Alvarez RB, Engel WK: β-Amyloid precursor epitopes in muscle fibers of inclusion body myositis. *Ann Neurol* 34:551, 1993.
10. Engel AG, Lambert EH, Gomez MR: A new myasthenic syndrome with end-plate acetylcholinesterase deficiency, small nerve terminals, and reduced acetylcholine release. *Ann Neurol* 1:315, 1977.
11. Engel AG, Lambert EH, Mulder DM, et al: A newly recognized congenital myasthenic syndrome attributed to a prolonged open time of the acetylcholine induced ion channel. *Ann Neurol* 11:553, 1982.
12. Engel AG, Macdonald RD: Ultrastructural reactions in muscle disease and their light microscopic correlates. *Excerpta Medica ICS* 199:71, 1970.
12a. Schmalbruch H: Muscle fiber splitting and regeneration in diseased human muscle. *Neuropathol Appl Neurobiol* 2:3, 1976.
13a. Bormioli SP, Schiaffino S: Myomuscular junctions in re-innervated rat skeletal muscle. *J Anat* 124:359, 1977.
13b. Bulfield G, Siller WG, Wight PAL, Moore KJ: X chromosome-linked muscular dystrophy (mdx) in the mouse. *Proc Natl Acad Sci USA* 81:1189, 1984.
13c. Fadic R, Waclawik AJ, Lewandoski PJ, et al: Muscle pathology and clinical features of the sarcolemmopathies. *Pediatr Neurol* 16:79–82, 1997.
13d. Li M, Dickson DW, Spiro AJ: Sarcolemmal defect and subsarcolemmal lesion in a patient with γ-sarcoglycan deficiency. *Neurology* 50:807–809, 1998.
13e. Hack AA, Ly CT, Jiang F, et al: Gamma-sarcoglycan deficiency leads to muscle membrane defects and apoptosis independent of dystrophin. *J Cell Biol* 142:1279–1287, 1998.
13f. Straub V, Duclos F, Venzke DP, et al: Molecular pathogenesis of muscle degeneration in the delta-sarcoglycan-deficient hamster. *Am J Pathol* 153:1623–1630, 1998.
13g. Richard I, Roudaut C, Marchand S, et al: Loss of calpain 3 proteolytic activity leads to muscular dystrophy and to apoptosis-associated IkappaBalpha/nuclear factor kappaB pathway perturbation in mice. *J Cell Biol* 151:1583–1590, 2000.
13h. Straub V, Rafael J, Chamberlain JS, et al: Animal models for muscular dystrophy show different patterns of sarcolemmal disruption. *J Cell Biol* 139:375–385, 1997.
14. Carpenter S, Karpati G: Duchenne muscular dystrophy: Plasma membrane loss initiates muscle cell necrosis unless it is repaired. *Brain* 102:147, 1979.
14a. Minetti C, Bado M, Morreale G, et al: Disruption of muscle basal lamina in congenital muscular dystrophy with merosin deficiency. *Neurology* 46:1354–1358, 1996.
14b. Osari S, Kobayashi O, Yamashita Y, et al: Basement-membrane abnormality in merosin-negative congenital muscular dystrophy. *Acta Neuropathol* 91:332–336, 1996.
14c. Arahata K, Hayashi YK, Koga R, et al: Laminin in animal models for muscular dystrophy. *Proc Jpn Acad* 69, Ser B:259–264, 1993.
14d. Miyagoe Y, Hanaoka K, Nonaka I, et al: Laminin α2 chain null-mutant mice by targeted disruption of the *Lama2* gene: A new model of merosin (laminin 2)-deficient congenital muscular dystrophy. *FEBS Lett* 415:33–39, 1997.
14e. Vajsar J, Ackerley C, Chitayat D, et al: Basal lamina abnormality in the skeletal muscle of Walker-Warburg syndrome. *Pediatr Neurol* 22:139–143, 2000.
14f. Ishii H, Hayashi YK, Nonaka I, et al: Electron microscopic examination of basal lamina in Fukuyama congenital muscular dystrophy. *Neuromuscul Disord* 7:191–197, 1997.
14g. Ishikawa H, Sugie K, Murayama K, et al: Ullrich's disease: Collagen VI deficiency: EM suggests new basis for muscular weakness. *Neurology* 59:920–923, 2002.
14h. Torres LFB, Duchen LW: The mutant *mdx*: Inherited myopathy in the mouse. Morphological studies of nerve, muscles and end-plates. *Brain* 110:269, 1987.
15. Banker BQ: A phase and electron microscopic study of dystrophic muscle: I. The pathological changes in the two-week-old Bar Harbor 129 dystrophic mouse. *J Neuropathol Exp Neurol* 26:259, 1967.
15a. Kerr JFR, Gobé GC, Winterford CM, et al: Anatomical methods in cell death. *Methods Cell Biol* 46:1–27, 1995.
15b. Mirabella M, Di Giovanni S, Silvestri G, et al: Apoptosis in mitochondrial encephalomyopathies with mitochondrial DNA mutations: A potential pathogenic mechanism. *Brain* 123:93–104, 2000.
15c. Monici MC, Toscano A, Girlanda P, et al: Apoptosis in metabolic myopathies. *Neuroreport* 9:2431–2435, 1998.
15d. Chae J, Minami N, Jin Y, et al: Calpain 3 gene mutations: Genetic and clinico-pathologic findings in limb-girdle muscular dystrophy. *Neuromuscul Disord* 11:547–555, 2001.
15e. Goebel HH, Anderson JR, Hübner C, et al: Congenital myopathy with excess of thin myofilaments. *Neuromuscul Disord* 7:160–168, 1997.
15f. Ikezoe K, Yan C, Momoi T, et al: A novel congenital myopathy with apoptotic changes. *Ann Neurol* 47:531–536, 2000.
15g. Sasaki K, Suga K, Tsugawa S, et al: Muscle pathology in Marinesco-Sjögren syndrome: A unique ultrastructural feature. *Brain Dev* 18:64–67, 1996.
15h. Tews DS, Goebel HH: DNA fragmentation and BCL-2 expression in infantile spinal muscular atrophy. *Neuromuscul Disord* 6:265–273, 1996.
15i. Yamada H, Nakagawa M, Higuchi I, et al: Detection of DNA fragmentation of myonuclei in myotonic dystrophy by double staining with anti-emerin antibody and by nick end-labeling. *J Neurol Sci* 173:97–102, 2000.

15j. Sandri M, El Meslemani AH, Biol D, et al: Caspase 3 expression correlates with skeletal muscle apoptosis in Duchenne and fascioscapulohumeral muscular dystrophy. A potential target for pharmacologic treatment? *J Neuropathol Exp Neurol* 60:302–312, 2001.
15k. Migheli A, Mongini T, Doriguzzi C, et al: Muscle apoptosis in humans occurs in normal and denervated muscle, but not in myotonic dystrophy, dystrophinopathies or inflammatory muscle disease. *Neurogenetics* 1:81–87, 1997.
15l. Olivé M, Martinez-Matos J, Montero J, et al: Apoptosis is not the mechanism of cell death of muscle fibers in human muscular dystrophies and inflammatory myopathies. *Muscle Nerve* 20:1328–1330, 1997.
15m. Monneron A, Bernhard W: Fine structural organization of the interphase nucleus in some mammalian cells. *J Ultrastruct Res* 27:266–288, 1969.
15n. Brasch K, Ochs RL: Nuclear bodies (NBs): A newly "rediscovered" organelle. *Exp Cell Res* 202:211–223, 1992.
16. Schul W, de Jong L, van Driel R: Nuclear neighbors: The spatial and functional organization of genes and nuclear domains. *J Cell Biochem* 70:159–171, 1998.
17. Matera AG: Of coiled bodies, gems and salmons. *J Cell Biochem* 70:181–192, 1998.
18. Hodges M, Tissot C, Howe K, et al: Structure, organization, and dynamics of promyelocytic leukemia protein nuclear bodies. *Am J Hum Genet* 63:297–304, 1998.
18a. Fidzianska A, Toniolo D, Hausmanowa-Petrusevicz I: Ultrastructural abnormality of sarcolemmal nuclei in Emery-Dreifuss muscular dystrophy. *J Neurol Sci* 159:88–93, 1998.
18b. Ognibene A, Sabatelli M, Petrini S, et al: Nuclear changes in a case of X-linked Emery-Dreifuss muscular dystrophy. *Muscle Nerve* 22:864–869, 1999.
18c. Sabatelli P, Lattanzi G, Ognibene A, et al: Nuclear alterations in autosomal-dominant Emery-Dreifuss muscular dystrophy. *Muscle Nerve* 24:826–829, 2001.
18d. Sewry CA, Brown SC, Mercuri E, et al: Skeletal muscle pathology in autosomal dominant Emery-Dreifuss muscular dystrophy with lamin A/C mutations. *Neuropathol Appl Neurobiol* 27:281–290, 2001.
18e. Sabatelli P, Lattanzi G, Ognibene A, et al: Nuclear alterations in autosomal-dominant Emery-Dreifuss muscular dystrophy. *Muscle Nerve* 24:826–829, 2001.
19. Freygang WG, Goldstein DA, Hellam DC, Peachey LD: The relation between the late after potential and the size of the transverse tubular system of frog muscle. *J Gen Physiol* 48:235, 1964.
20. Emberson JW, Muir AR: Changes in the ultrastructure of rat myocardium induced by hyperkalemia. *J Anat* 104:411, 1969.
21. Howarth JW: The behavior of frog muscle in hypertonic solutions. *J Physiol (Lond)* 144:167, 1958.
21a. Gonzales-Serratos H, Somlyo AV, McClellan G, et al: Composition of vacuoles and sarcoplasmic reticulum in fatigued muscle: Electron probe analysis. *Proc Natl Acad Sci* 75:1329, 1978.
22. Engel AG: Evolution and content of vacuoles in primary hypokalemic periodic paralysis. *Mayo Clin Proc* 45:774, 1970.
23. Santa T, Engel AG: Histochemical, electron microscopic and electron histochemical studies of vacuoles and tubular structures in periodic paralysis. *Clin Neurol (Tokyo)* 14:792, 1974.
24. Jerusalem F, Engel AG, Gomez MR: Sarcotubular myopathy: A newly recognized, benign, congenital, familial muscle disease. *Neurology* 23:897, 1973.
25. Macdonald RD, Engel AG: Experimental chloroquine myopathy. *J Neuropathol Exp Neurol* 29:479, 1970.
26. Engel AG: Acid maltase deficiency in adults: Studies in four cases of a syndrome which may mimic muscular dystrophy or other myopathies. *Brain* 93:599, 1970.
27. Engel AG: Acid maltase deficiency in adult life. Morphologic and biochemical data in 3 cases of a syndrome simulating other myopathies. *Excerpta Medica ICS* 199:236, 1970.
28. Marzella L, Glaumann H: Biogenesis, translocation, and function of lysosomal enzymes. *Int Rev Exp Pathol* 25:239, 1983.
29. Sabatini DD, Kreibich G, Morimoto T, Adesnik M: Mechanisms for the incorporation of proteins in membranes and organelles. *J Cell Biol* 92:1, 1982.
30. Arstila AU, Trump BF: Studies on cellular autophagocytosis: The formation of autophagic vacuoles in the liver after glucagon administration. *Am J Pathol* 53:687–733, 1968.
31. Alberts B, Johnson A, Lewis J, et al (eds): *Molecular Biology of the Cell,* 4th ed. New York: Garland; 2003.
32. Chou SM, Miike T: Ultrastructural abnormalities and perifascicular atrophy in childhood dermatomyositis: With special reference to transverse tubular systems sarcoplasmic reticulum junctions. *Arch Pathol Lab Med* 105:76, 1981.
33. Engel AG, Stonnington HH: Morphological effects of denervation of muscle: A quantitative ultrastructural study. *Ann NY Acad Sci* 228:68, 1974.
34. Leonard JP, Salpeter MM: Agonist-induced myopathy at the neuromuscular junction is mediated by calcium. *J Cell Biol* 82:811, 1979.
35. Dobkin BH, Verity MA: Familial neuromuscular disease with type 1 fiber hypoplasia, tubular aggregates, cardiomyopathy and myasthenic features. *Neurology* 28:1135, 1978.
36. Schiaffino S, Severin E, Cantini M, Sartore S: Tubular aggregates induced by anoxia in isolated rat skeletal muscle. *Lab Invest* 37:223, 1977.
36a. Schroeder JM, Vielhaber S, Brunn A, et al: Dominantly inherited myopathy with novel tubular aggregates containing 1–21 tubulofilamentous structures. *Acta Neuropathol* 102:27–35, 2001.
36b. Lach B, Christie S, Preston D: Chronic progressive and relapsing neuromyopathy with massive dilations of endoplasmic reticulum in muscle fibers. *Acta Neuropathol* 80:611, 1990.
36c. Waclawik AJ, Lindal S, Engel AG: Experimental Lovastatin myopathy. *J Neuropathol Exp Neurol* 52:542, 1993.
37. Davidowitz J, Philips G, Breinin GM: Membrane-glycogen complexes in rabbit extraocular muscle. *J Ultrastruct Res* 82:64, 1983.
38. Jerusalem F, Engel AG, Peterson HA: Human muscle fiber fine structure: Morphometric data on controls. *Neurology* 25:127, 1975.
39. Engel AG, Gomez MR, Groover RV: Multicore disease: A recently recognized congenital myopathy associated with multifocal degeneration of fibers. *Mayo Clin Proc* 46:666, 1971.
40. Duane DD, Engel AG: Emetine myopathy. *Neurology* 20:733–739, 1970.
40a. Andreetta F, Tritschler H-J, Schon EA, et al: Localization of DNA in normal and pathological muscle using immunological probes: A new approach to the study of mitochondrial myopathies. *J Neurol Sci* 105:88, 1991.
40b. Tritschler H-J, Andreetta F, Moraes CT, et al: Mitochondrial myopathy of childhood associated with depletion of mitochondrial DNA. *Neurology* 42:209,1992.
41. Minassian H, Huang S-N: Effect of sodium azide on the ultrastructural preservation of tissues. *J Microsc* 117:243, 1979.
41a. Lännergren J, Westerblad H, Flock B: Transient appearance of vacuoles in fatigued *Xenopus* muscle fibers. *Acta Physiol Scand* 140:437, 1990.
41b. Lotz BP, Engel AG: Are hypercontracted muscle fibers artifacts and do they cause rupture of the plasma membrane? *Neurology* 37:1466, 1987.
42. Hanzlikova V, Schiaffino S: Mitochondrial changes in ischemic skeletal muscle. *J Ultrastruct Res* 60:121, 1977.
42a. Transient appearance of vacuoles in fatigued muscle fibers. *Acta Physiol Scand* 140:437–445, 1990.
43. Engel AG: Pathological reaction of the Z disk. *Excerpta Medica ICS* 147:398, 1967.
44. Tice LW, Engel AG: The effects of glucocorticoids on red and white muscles in the rat. *Am J Pathol* 50:311, 1967.
45. Engel AG: Neuromuscular manifestations of Graves' disease. *Mayo Clin Proc* 47:919, 1972.
46. Gustafsson R, Tata JR, Lindberg O, et al: The relationship between the structure and activity of rat skeletal muscle mitochondria after thyroidectomy and thyroid hormone treatment. *J Cell Biol* 26:555, 1965.
47. Engel AG: Electron microscopic observations in thyrotoxic and corticosteroid induced myopathies. *Mayo Clin Proc* 41:785, 1966.
48. Kamienieckka Z, Schmalbruch H: Neuromuscular disorders with abnormal muscle mitochondria. *Int Rev Cytol* 65:321, 1980.
48a. Mokherjee TM, Dixon BR, Blumbergs PC, et al: The fine structure of the intramitochondrial crystalloids in mitochondrial myopathy. *J Submicrosc Cytol* 18:595, 1986.
49. Melmed C, Karpati G, Carpenter S: Experimental mitochondrial myopathy produced by in vivo uncoupling of oxidative phosphorylation. *J Neurol Sci* 26:305, 1975.
49a. Sjöström M, Neglén P, Fridén J, Eklöf B: Human skeletal muscle metabolism and morphology after temporary incomplete ischemia. *Eur J Clin Invest* 12:69, 1982.
49b. Stadhouders AM, Jap PHK, Winkler H-P, et al: Mitochondrial creatine kinase: A major constituent of pathological inclusions in mitochondrial myopathies. *Proc Natl Acad Sci USA* 91:5089–5093, 1994.
50. Knappeis GG, Carlsen F: The ultrastructure of the Z disk in skeletal muscle. *J Cell Biol* 13:323, 1962.
51. Macdonald RD, Engel AG: Observations on organization of Z-disk components and on rod-bodies of Z-disk origin. *J Cell Biol* 48:431, 1971.
51a. Luther PK: Three-dimensional reconstruction of a simple Z-band in fish muscle. *J Cell Biol* 113:1043, 1991.
52. Yamaguchi M, Robson RM, Stromer MH: Evidence for actin involvement in cardiac Z-lines and Z-line analogues. *J Cell Biol* 96:435, 1983.
53. Luther PK: Symmetry of a vertebrate muscle basketweave Z-band. *J Struct Biol* 115:275–282, 1995.
53a. Goldstein MA, Schroeter JP, Sass RL: Two structural states of the vertebrate Z band. *Electron Microsc Rev* 3:227, 1990.
54. Schroeter JP, Breatudiere JP, Sass RL, et al: Three-dimensional structure of the Z band in a normal mammalian skeletal muscle. *J Cell Biol* 133:571–583, 1996.
55. Franzini-Armstrong C: The structure of a simple Z line. *J Cell Biol* 58:630, 1973.

56. Engel AG, Gomez MR: Nemaline (Z disk) myopathy: Observations on the origin, structure, and solubility properties of the nemaline structures. *J Neuropathol Exp Neurol* 26:601, 1967.
57. Suzuki A, Goll DE, Singh I, et al: Some properties of purified skeletal muscle α-actinin. *J Biol Chem* 251:6860, 1976.
58. Etlinger JD, Fischman DA: M and Z band components and the assembly of myofibrils. *Cold Spring Harbor Symp Quant Biol* 37:511, 1972.
59. Dayton WR, Goll DE, Stromer MH, et al: Some properties of a Ca^{++}-activated protease that may be involved in myofibrillar protein turnover, in Reich E, Rifkin DB, Shaw E (eds): *Proteases and Biological Control*, vol 2. New York: Cold Spring Harbor Laboratory; 1975, pp 551–577.
60. Schollmeyer JE, Stromer MH, Goll DE: Alpha-actinin and tropomyosin localization in normal and diseased muscle. *Biophys J* 12:280a, 1972.
61. Jockusch BM, Veldman H, Griffiths G, et al: Immunofluorescence microscopy of a myopathy. α-Actinin is a major constituent of nemaline rods. *Exp Cell Res* 127:409, 1980.
62. Tang J, Taylor DW, Taylor KA: The three-dimensional structure of alpha-actinin obtained by cryoelectron microscopy suggests a model for Ca^{2+}-dependent actin binding. *J Mol Biol* 310:845–858, 2001.
62a. Faulkner G, Lafranchi G, Valle G: Telethonin and other new proteins of the Z-disc of skeletal muscle. *Life* 51:275–282, 2001.
63. Hauser MA, Horrigan SK, Salmikangas P, et al: *Myotilin* is mutated in limb girdle muscular dystrophy 1A. *Hum Mol Genet* 9:2141–2147, 2000.
64. Takada F, Vander Woude DL, Tong HQ, et al: Myozenin: An α-actinin- and γ-filamin-binding protein of skeletal muscle Z lines. *Proc Natl Acad Sci USA* 98:1595–1600, 2001.
65. Bang M-L, Mudry RE, McElhinny AS, et al: Myopalladin, a novel 145-kilodalton sarcomeric protein with multiple roles in Z-disk and I-band protein assemblies. *J Cell Biol* 153:413–427, 2001.
66. Zhou Q, Chu PH, Huang C, et al: Ablation of Cypher, a PDZ-LIM domain Z-line protein, causes a severe form of congenital myopathies. *J Cell Biol* 155:605–612, 2001.
66a. Geisler JG, Palmer RJ, Stubbs LJ, et al: Nspl1, a new Z-band-associated protein. *J Muscle Res Cell Motil* 20:661–668, 1999.
66b. Lazarides E, Granger BL, Gard DL: Desmin- and vimentin-containing filaments and their role in the assembly of the Z-disk in muscle cells. *Cold Spring Harbor Symp Quant Biol* 46:351–378, 1993.
66c. Hijikata T, Murakami T, Imamura M, et al: Plectin is a linker of intermediate filaments to Z-discs in skeletal muscle fibers. *J Cell Sci* 112:867–876, 1999.
66d. Derham BK, Harding JJ: Alpha-crystallin as a molecular chaperone. *Prog Retin Eye Res* 18:463–509, 1999.
67. Shafiq SA, Gorycki MA, Asiedu SA, Milhorat AT: Tenotomy: Effect on the fine structure of the soleus muscle of the rat. *Arch Neurol* 20:625, 1969.
68. Osame M, Kawabuchi M, Igata A, Sugita H: Changes at the neuromuscular junctions in the affected muscles of neostigmine-treated rats, tenotomized rats and a patient with nemaline myopathy. *Acta Histochem Cytochem* 10:70, 1977.
69. Kawabuchi M: Neostigmine myopathy is a calcium ion-mediated myopathy initially affecting the motor end-plate. *J Neuropathol Exp Neurol* 41:298, 1982.
70. Cape CA, Johnston WW, Pitner SE: Nemaline structure in polymyositis. *Neurology* 20:494, 1970.
71. Danon MJ, Giometti CS, Manaligod JR, et al: Adult-onset nemaline rods in a patient treated for suspected dermatomyositis. *Arch Neurol* 38:761, 1981.
72. Fukunaga H, Osame M, Igata A: A case of nemaline myopathy with ophthalmoplegia and mitochondrial abnormalities. *J Neurol Sci* 46:169, 1980.
73. Kornfeld M: Mixed nemaline-mitochondrial "myopathy." *Acta Neuropathol (Berl)* 51:185, 1980.
74. Hanna W, Henderson RD: Nemaline rods in cricopharyngeal dysphagia. *Am J Clin Pathol* 74:186, 1980.
75. Mukuno K: Electron microscopic studies on the human extraocular muscles under pathologic conditions. *Jpn J Ophthalmol* 13:35, 1969.
76. Mair WGP, Tomé FMS: The ultrastructure of the adult and developing human myotendinous junction. *Acta Neuropathol (Berl)* 21:239, 1972.
76a. Morris EP, Nneji G, Squire JM: The three-dimensional structure of the nemaline rod Z-band. *J Cell Biol* 111:2961, 1990.
77. Macdonald RD, Engel AG: The cytoplasmic body: Another structural anomaly of the Z disk. *Acta Neuropathol (Berl)* 14:99, 1969.
78. Schmalbruch H: Noniusperioden und Längenwachstum der quergestreiften Muskelfaser. *Z Mikrosk Anat Forsch* 79:493, 1968.
79. Meltzer HY, Kuncl RW, Click J, Yang V: Incidence of Z band streaming and myofibrillar disruptions in skeletal muscle from healthy young people. *Neurology* 26:853, 1976.
80. Salpeter MM, Kasprzak H, Feng H, Fertuck H: End plates after esterase inactivation in vivo: Correlation between esterase concentration, functional response and fine structure. *J Neurocytol* 8:95, 1979.
81. Leonard JP, Salpeter MM: Calcium-mediated myopathy at neuromuscular junctions of normal and dystrophic muscle. *Exp Neurol* 76:121, 1982.
82. Dayton WR, Schollmeyer JV, Lepley RA, Cortés LR: A calcium-activated protease possibly involved in myofibrillar protein turnover: Isolation of a low-calcium-requiring form of the protease. *Biochim Biophys Acta* 659:48, 1981.
83. Endo M: Calcium release from the sarcoplasmic reticulum. *Physiol Rev* 57:71, 1977.
84. Mezon BJ, Wrogemann K, Blanchaer MC: Differing populations of mitochondria isolated from the skeletal muscle of normal and dystrophic hamsters. *Can J Biochem* 52:1024, 1974.
85. Carafoli E: The regulation of intracellular calcium. *Adv Exp Med Biol* 151:461, 1982.
86. Bodensteiner J, Engel A: Intracellular calcium accumulation in Duchenne dystrophy and other myopathies: A study of 567,000 muscle fibers in 114 biopsies. *Neurology* 28:439, 1978.
86a. Waclawick A, Sufit RL, Beinlich BR, et al: Acute myopathy with selective degeneration of myosin filaments following status asthmaticus treated with methylprednisolone and vercuronium. *Neuromuscul Disord* 2:19, 1992.
86b. Hirano M, Ott BR, Raps EC, et al: Acute quadriplegic myopathy: A complication of treatment with steroids, nondepolarizing blocking agents, or both. *Neurology* 42:2082, 1992.
86c. Danon MJ, Carpenter S: Myopathy with thick filament (myosin) loss following prolonged paralysis with vecuronium during steroid treatment. *Muscle Nerve* 14:1131, 1991.
87. Carpenter S, Karpati G, Rothman S, Watters G: The childhood type of dermatomyositis. *Neurology* 26:952, 1976.
88. Sher JH, Shafiq SA, Schutta HS: Acute myopathy with selective lysis of myosin filaments. *Neurology* 29:100, 1979.
88a. Rouleau G, Karpati G, Carpenter S, et al: Glucocorticoid excess induces preferential depletion of myosin in denervated skeletal muscle fibers. *Muscle Nerve* 10:428, 1987.
88b. Massa R, Carpenter S, Karpati G: Preferential loss of myosin heavy-chain rod portion in denervated soleus muscle of rats receiving large-dose glucocorticoids. *Neurology* 40(suppl 1):121, 1990.
88c. Rich MM, Pinter MJ, Kraner SD, et al: Loss of electrical excitability in an animal model of acute quadriplegic myopathy. *Ann Neurol* 43:154–155, 1988.
89. Yarom R, Shapira Y: Myosin degeneration in a congenital myopathy. *Arch Neurol* 34:114, 1977.
90. Fidzianska A, Badurska B, Ryniewicz B, Dembek I: "Cap disease": New congenital myopathy. *Neurology* 31:1113, 1981.
91. Bethlem J, Van Wijngaarden GK: Benign myopathy, with autosomal dominant inheritance. *Brain* 99:91, 1976.
91a. Jobsis GJ, Keizers H, Vreijling JP, et al: Type VI collagen mutations in Bethlem myopathy, an autosomal dominant myopathy with contractures. *Nat Genet* 14:113–115, 1996.
91b. Cancilla PA, Kalyanaraman K, Verity MA, et al: Familial myopathy with probable lysis of myofibrils in type I fibers. *Neurology* 21:579, 1971.
91c. Goebel HH, Anderson JR, Hübner C, et al: Congenital myopathy with excess of thin myofilaments. *Neuromuscul Disord* 7:160–168, 1997.
91d. Nowak KJ, Wattanasirichaigoon D, Goebel HH, et al: Mutations in skeletal muscle α-actin gene in patients with actin myopathy and nemaline myopathy. *Nat Genet* 23:208–212, 1999.
92. Bogusch G: Enzymatic digestion and urea extraction on leptomeric structures and normomeric myofibrils in heart muscle cells. *J Ultrastruct Res* 55:245, 1976.
93. Bogusch G: Electron microscopic investigations on leptomeric fibrils and leptomeric complexes in hen and pigeon heart. *J Mol Cell Cardiol* 7:733, 1975.
94. Katz B: The terminations of the afferent nerve fibre in the muscle spindle of the frog. *Philos Trans R Soc Lond [Biol]* 243:221, 1961.
94a. Banker BQ, Girvin JP: The ultrastructural features of the normal and deafferented mammalian muscle spindle, in Banker BQ, Przybylski RJ, Van Der Meulen JP, Victor M (eds): *Research in Muscle Development and the Muscle Spindle*. Amsterdam: Excerpta Medica; 1972, pp 267–298.
95. Lake BD, Wilson J: Zebra body myopathy. Clinical, histochemical and ultrastructural studies. *J Neurol Sci* 24:437, 1975.
96. Trotter JA, Corbett K, Avner BP: Structure and function of the murine muscle-tendon junction. *Anat Rec* 201:293, 1981.
97. Payne CM, Curless RG: Concentric laminated bodies. Ultrastructural demonstration of muscle fiber type specificity. *J Neurol Sci* 29:311, 1976.
98. Gambarelli D, Hassoun J, Pellissier JF, et al: Concentric laminated bodies in muscle pathology. *Pathol Eur* 9:289, 1974.
99. Luft T, Ikkos D, Palmieri G, et al: A case of severe hypermetabolism of nonthyroid origin with a defect in the maintenance of mitochondrial respiratory control: A correlated clinical, biochemical and morphological study. *J Clin Invest* 41:1776, 1962.
100. Engel AG, Angelini C, Gomez M: Fingerprint body myopathy. A newly recognized congenital disease. *Mayo Clin Proc* 47:377, 1972.
101. Neville HE, Maunder-Sewry CA, McDougall J, et al: Chloroquine-induced cytosomes with curvilinear profiles in muscle. *Muscle Nerve* 2:376, 1979.

101a. Fardeau M, Tomé FMS, Derambure S: Familial fingerprint body myopathy. *Arch Neurol* 33:724, 1976.
102. Gordon AS, Rewcastle NB, Humphrey JG, et al: Chronic benign congenital myopathy: Fingerprint body type. *Can J Neurol Sci* 1:106, 1974.
103. Jadro-Santel D, Grcević N, Dogan S, et al: Centronuclear myopathy with type 1 fibre hypotrophy and "fingerprint" inclusions associated with Marfan's syndrome. *J Neurol Sci* 45:43, 1980.
104. Payne CM, Curless RG: Fingerprint inclusions. Ultrastructural demonstration of muscle fiber type specificity. *J Neurol Sci* 31:379, 1977.
105. Julien J, Vital CL, Vallat JM, et al: Oculopharyngeal muscular dystrophy: A case with abnormal mitochondrial and "fingerprint" inclusions. *J Neurol Sci* 21:165, 1974.
106. Tomé FMS, Fardeau M: "Fingerprint inclusions" in muscle fibres in dystrophia myotonica. *Acta Neuropathol (Berl)* 24:62, 1973.
107. Sengel A, Stoebner P: Une inclusion musculaire atypique rare: Les "corps en empreintes digitales" ou "fingerprint bodies." *Acta Neuropathol (Berl)* 27:61, 1974.
107a. Pellissier JF, Pouget J, Charpin C, et al: Myopathy associated with desmin type intermediate filaments: An immunoelectron microscopic study. *J Neurol Sci* 89:49, 1989.
108. Nakano S, Engel AG, Waclawik AJ, et al: Myofibrillar myopathy with abnormal foci of desmin positivity. I. Light and electron microscopy analysis. *J Neuropathol Exp Neurol* 55:549–562, 1996.
109. De Bleecker JL, Engel AG, Ertl BB: Myofibrillar myopathy with abnormal foci of desmin positivity. II. Immunocytochemical analysis reveals accumulation of multiple other proteins. *J Neuropathol Exp Neurol* 55:563–577, 1996.
109a. Selcen D, Ohno K, Engel AG: Myofibrillar myopathy. Clinical, morphological, and genetic studies in 63 patients. *Brain* 127:439–451, 2004.
110. Goldfarb LG, Park KY, Cervenáková L, et al: Missense mutations in desmin associated with familial cardiac and skeletal myopathy. *Nat Genet* 19:402–403, 1998.
111. Dalakas MC, Park KY, Semino-Mora C, et al: Desmin myopathy, a skeletal myopathy with cardiomyopathy caused by mutations in the desmin gene. *N Engl J Med* 342:770–780, 2000.
112. Munoz-Mármol AN, Strasser G, Isamat M, et al: A dysfunctional desmin mutation in a patient with severe generalized myopathy. *Proc Natl Acad Sci USA* 95:11312–11317, 1998.
113. Vicart P, Caron A, Guicheney P, et al: A missense mutation in the αB-crystallin chaperone gene causes a desmin-related myopathy. *Nat Genet* 20:92–95, 1998.
113a. Engel AG: Myofibrillar myopathy. *Ann Neurol* 46:681–683, 1999.
114. Sahgal V, Sahgal S: A new congenital myopathy. A morphological, cytochemical and histochemical study. *Acta Neuropathol (Berl)* 37:225, 1977.
114a. Masuzugawa S, Kuzuhara S, Narita Y, et al: Autosomal dominant hyaline body myopathy presenting as scapuloperoneal syndrome: Clinical features and muscle pathology. *Neurology* 48:253–257, 1997.
114b. Barohn RJ, Brumback RA, Mendell JR: Hyaline body myopathy. *Neuromuscul Disord* 4(3):257–262, 1994.
114c. Tajsharghi H, Thornell L-E, Lindberg C, et al: Myosin storage myopathy associated with a heterozygous missense mutation in *MYH7*. *Ann Neurol* 54:494–500, 2003.
115. Hays AP, Braun CW, Eastwood: Crystalline inclusion myopathy. A new disorder. *Abstracts of Free Communications*. Fifth International Congress of Neuromuscular Diseases, Marseilles, France, September 1982.
115a. Gahl WA, Dalakas M, Charnas L, et al: Myopathy and cystine storage in muscle in a patient with nephropathic cystinosis. *N Engl J Med* 319:1461, 1988.
115b. Vu TH, Hays AP, Tanji K, et al: Myopathy with tubulin-reactive crystalline inclusions. *Neurology* 57:149–152, 2001.
116. Carpenter S, Karpati G, Robitaille Y, Melmed C: Cylindrical spirals in human skeletal muscle. *Muscle Nerve* 2:282, 1979.
117. Bové KE, Iannaccone ST, Hilton PK, Samaha F: Cylindrical spirals in a familial neuromuscular disorder. *Ann Neurol* 7:550, 1980.
118. McDougall J, Wiles CM, Edwards RHT: Spiral membrane cylinders in the skeletal muscle of a patient with melorheostosis. *Neuropathol Appl Neurobiol* 6:69, 1980.
119. Gibbels E, Henke U, Schädlich H-J, et al: Cylindrical spirals in skeletal muscle: A further observation with clinical, morphological, and biochemical analysis. *Muscle Nerve* 6:646, 1983.
120. Sahashi K, Mizuno Y, Ibi T, Sobue G: A case of a mitochondrial myopathy with cylindrical spirals. *Clin Neurol (Tokyo)* 22:244, 1982.
120a. Danon MJ, Carpenter S, Harati Y: Muscle pain associated with tubular aggregates and structures resembling cylindrical spirals. *Muscle Nerve* 12:265, 1989.
120b. Taratuto AL, Matteucci M, Barreirro C, et al: Autosomal dominant neuromuscular disease with cylindrical spirals. *Neuromuscul Disord* 1:433–441, 1991.
120c. Rapuzzi S, Prelle A, Moggio M, et al: High serum creatine kinase levels associated with cylindrical spirals at muscle biopsy. *Acta Neuropathol* 90:660–664, 1995.
121. Gomez MR, Engel AG, Dyck PJ: Progressive ataxia, retinal degeneration, neuromyopathy, and mental subnormality in a patient with true hypoparathyroidism, dwarfism, malabsorption, and cholelithiasis. *Neurology* 22:849, 1972.
122. Goldfischer S, Reddy JK: Peroxisomes (microbodies) in cell pathology. *Int Rev Exp Pathol* 26:45, 1984.
123. Burck U, Goebel HH, Kuhlendahl HD, et al: Neuromyopathy and vitamin E deficiency in man. *Neuropaediatrie* 12:267, 1981.
124. Neville HE, Ringel SP, Guggenheim MA, et al: Ultrastructural and histochemical abnormalities of skeletal muscle in patients with chronic vitamin E deficiency. *Neurology* 33:483, 1983.
125. Werlin SL, Harb JM, Swick HJ, Blank E: Neuromuscular dysfunction and ultrastructural pathology in children with chronic cholestasis and vitamin E deficiency. *Ann Neurol* 13:291, 1982.
126. Baringer JR, Swoveland P: Tubular aggregates in endoplasmic reticulum: Evidence against their viral nature. *J Ultrastruct Res* 41:270, 1972.
127. Jerusalem F, Rakusa M, Engel AG, Macdonald RD: Morphometric analysis of skeletal muscle capillary ultrastructure in inflammatory myopathies. *J Neurol Sci* 23:391, 1974.
128. Carpenter S, Karpati G, Rothman S, Watters G: The childhood type of dermatomyositis. *Neurology* 26:952, 1976.
129. Oshima Y, Becker LE, Armstrong DL: An electron microscopic study of childhood dermatomyositis. *Acta Neuropathol* 47:189, 1979.
129a. Moss J, Woodrow DF, Gresser I: Cytochemistry of the tubular aggregates found in hepatocytes of interferon-treated suckling mice. *Histochem J* 17:33, 1985.
129b. Feldman D, Goldstein AL, Cox DC, et al: Cultured human endothelial cells treated with recombinant leukocyte A interferon: Tubuloreticular inclusion formation, antiproliferative effect, and 2-5 oligoadenylate synthetase induction. *Lab Invest* 58:584, 1988.
130. Györkey F, Siukovics JG, Miu KW, Györkey PH: A morphologic study on the occurrence and distribution of structures resembling viral nucleocapsids in collagen diseases. *Am J Med* 53:148, 1972.
131. Grimley PM, Barry DW, Schaff Z: Induction of tubular structures in the endoplasmic reticulum of human lymphoid cells by treatment with 5-bromo-2-deoxyuridine. *J Natl Cancer Inst* 51:1751, 1973.
132. Grimley PM, Schaff Z: Significance of tubuloreticular inclusions in the pathobiology of human diseases, in Ioachim HL (ed): *Pathobiology Annual*. New York: Appleton-Century-Crofts; 1976, pp 221–257.
133. Kostianovsky M, Kang YH, Grimley PM: Disseminated tubuloreticular inclusions in acquired immunodeficiency syndrome (AIDS). *Ultrastruct Pathol* 4:331–336, 1983.
134. Carrette S, Klippel JH, Preble OT, et al: Association of human leukocyte interferon and lymphocyte tubuloreticular inclusions in systemic lupus erythematosus (SLE). *Arthritis Rheum* 25:557, 1982.
135. Brooke MB, Neville HE: Reducing body myopathy. *Neurology* 22:829, 1972.
136. Tomé FMS, Fardeau M: Congenital myopathy with "reducing bodies" in muscle fibres. *Acta Neuropathol (Berl)* 31:207, 1975.
137. Oh SJ, Meyers GJ, Wilson ER, Alexander CB: A benign form of reducing body myopathy. *Muscle Nerve* 6:278, 1983.
137a. Carpenter S, Karpati G, Holland P: New observations in reducing body myopathy. *Neurology* 35:818–827, 1985.
138. Sato T, Walker DL, Peters HA, et al: Chronic polymyositis and myxovirus-like inclusions: Electron microscopic and viral studies. *Arch Neurol* 24:409, 1971.
139. Jerusalem F, Baumgartner G, Wyler R: Virus-Ehnliche einschlüsse bei chronischen neuro-muskulären Prozessen: Elektronenmikroskopische Biopsiebefunde von 2 Fällen. *Arch Psychiatr Nervenkr* 215:148, 1972.
140. Yunis EJ, Samaha FJ: Inclusion body myositis. *Lab Invest* 25:240, 1971.
141. Carpenter S, Karpati G, Heller I, Eisen A: Inclusion body myositis: A distinct variety of idiopathic inflammatory myopathy. *Neurology* 28:8, 1978.
142. Tomé FMS, Fardeau M, Lebon P, Chevallay M: Inclusion body myositis. *Acta Neuropathol (Berl)* 7(suppl):287, 1981.
143. Julien J, Vital CL, Vallat JM, et al: Inclusion body myositis. Clinical, biological and ultrastructural study. *J Neurol Sci* 55:15, 1982.
144. Mikol J, Felten-Papaiconomou A, Ferchal F, et al: Inclusion body myositis: Clinicopathological studies and isolation of an adenovirus type 2 from muscle biopsy specimen. *Ann Neurol* 11:576, 1982.
145. Matsubara S, Tanabe H: Hereditary distal myopathy with filamentous inclusions. *Acta Neurol Scand* 65:363, 1982.
146. Fukuhara N, Kumamoto T, Tsubaki T: Rimmed vacuoles. *Acta Neuropathol (Berl)* 51:229, 1980.
146a. Chou SM, Mizuno Y: Mumps virus antigen in inclusion body myositis (IBM). *Neurology* 35(suppl):204, 1985.
146b. Nishino H, Engel AG, Rima BK: Inclusion body myositis—The mumps virus hypothesis. *Neurology* 25:260, 1989.
146c. Mendell JR, Sahenk Z, Paul L: Amyloid filaments in inclusion body myositis: Novel findings provide insight into nature of filaments. *Arch Neurol* 48:1229, 1991.
146d. Villanova M, Kawai M, Lübke U, et al: Rimmed vacuoles of inclusion body myositis and oculopharyngeal dystrophy contain amyloid precursor protein and lysosomal markers. *Brain Res* 603:343, 1993.

147. Schmalbruch H: Kristalloide in menschlichen Skelettmuskelfasern. Z Naturwissenschaften 19:519, 1967.
148. Collins DN, Gilbert EF: Glycogen complexes in muscle in Reye's syndrome simulating virus-like particles. Lab Invest 36:91, 1977.
149. Tang TT, Sedmak GV, Siegesmund KA, McCreadie SR: Chronic myopathy associated with coxsackievirus type A9: A combined electron microscopical and viral isolation study. N Engl J Med 292:608, 1975.
150. Schiller HH: Chronic viral myopathy and malignant hyperthermia. N Engl J Med 292:1409, 1975.
151. Hanson PA, Urizar RE: Reye's syndrome—Virus or artifact in muscle? N Engl J Med 293:505, 1975.
152. Fukuhara N: Electron microscopical demonstration of nucleic acids in virus-like particles in the skeletal muscle of a traffic accident victim. Acta Neuropathol (Berl) 47:55, 1979.
153. Sato T, Chou S-M: Effect of denervation on Coxsackie A virus myositis in mice: An electronmicroscopic study. Neurology 28:1232, 1978.
153a. Viguie CA, Lu D-X, Huang S-K, et al: Quantitative study of the effects of long-term denervation of the extensor digitorum longus muscle of the rat. Anat Rec 248:346–354, 1997.
153b. Lu D-X, Huang S-K, Carlson BM: Electron microscopic study of long-term denervated rat skeletal muscle. Anat Rec 248:355–365, 1997.
154. Carpenter S, Karpati G, Rothman S, Watters G: The childhood type of dermatomyositis. Neurology 26:952, 1976.
155. Engel AG, Biesecker G: Complement activation in muscle fiber necrosis: Demonstration of the membrane attack complex of complement in necrotic fibers. Ann Neurol 12:289, 1982.
156. Arahata K, Engel AG: Monoclonal antibody analysis of mononuclear cells in myopathies: I. Quantitation of subsets according to diagnosis and sites of accumulation and demonstration and counts of muscle fibers invaded by T cells. Ann Neurol 16:193, 1984.
157. Fumagalli G, Engel AG, Lindstrom J: Ultrastructural aspects of acetylcholine receptor turnover at the normal end-plate and in autoimmune myasthenia gravis. J Neuropathol Exp Neurol 41:567, 1982.
157a. Nishino I, Fu J, Tanji K, et al: LAMP-2 deficiency causes X-linked vacuolar cardiomyopathy and myopathy (Danon disease). Nature 406: 906–910, 2000.
157b. Fernandez C, Figarella-Branger D, Alla P, et al: Colchicine myopathy: A vacuolar myopathy with selective type I muscle fiber involvement. An immunohistochemical and electron microscopic study of two cases. Acta Neuropathol 103:100–106, 2002.
158. Markesbery WR, Griggs RC, Herr B: Distal myopathy: Electron microscopic and histochemical studies. Neurology 27:727, 1977.
159. Vaccario ML, Scoppetta C, Bracaglia R, Uncini A: Sporadic distal myopathy. J Neurol 224:291, 1981.
160. Nonaka I, Sunohara N, Ishiura S, Satoyoshi E: Familial distal myopathy with rimmed vacuole and lamellar (myeloid) body formation. J Neurol Sci 51:141–155, 1981.
161. Kumamoto T, Fukuhara N, Nagashima M, et al: Distal myopathy: Histochemical and ultrastructural studies. Arch Neurol 39:367, 1982.
162. Howes EL, Price HM, Blumberg JM: The effects of a diet producing lipochrome pigment (ceroid) on the ultrastructure of skeletal muscle in the rat. Am J Pathol 45:599, 1964.
163. Clarke JTR, Karpati G, Carpenter S, Wolfe LS: The effect of vincristine on skeletal muscle in the rat: A correlative histochemical, ultrastructural and chemical study. J Neuropathol Exp Neurol 31:247, 1972.
164. Anderson PJ, Song SK, Slotwiner P: The fine structure of spheromembranous degeneration of skeletal muscle induced by vincristine. J Neuropathol Exp Neurol 26:15, 1967.
165. Wattiaux R, Wattiaux-De Coninck S: Effects of ischemia on lysosomes. Int Rev Exp Pathol 26:85, 1984.
165a. DeBleecker JL, Engel AG, Winkelmann JC: Localization of dystrophin and β-spectrin in vacuolar myopathies. Am J Pathol 143:1200–1208, 1993.
166. Engel AG, Santa T, Stonnington HH, et al: Morphometric study of skeletal muscle ultrastructure. Muscle Nerve 2:229, 1979.
167. Engel AG, Banker BQ, Eiben RM: Carnitine deficiency: Clinical, morphological and biochemical observations in a fatal case. J Neurol Neurosurg Psychiatry 40:313, 1977.
167a. Chanarin I, Patel A, Slavin G, et al: Neutral-lipid storage disease: A new disorder of lipid metabolism. Br Med J 1:553, 1975.
167b. Lefevre C, Jobard F, Caux F, et al: Mutations in CGI-58, the gene encoding a new protein of the esterase/lipase/thioesterase family. Am J Hum Genet 69:1002, 2001.
168. Jerusalem F, Angelini C, Engel AG, Groover RV: Mitochondria-lipid-glycogen (MLG) disease of muscle. Arch Neurol 29:162, 1973.
169. DiMauro S, Nicholson JF, Hays AP, et al: Benign infantile mitochondrial myopathy due to reversible cytochrome c oxidase deficiency. Ann Neurol 14:226, 1983.
170. Khaleeli AA, Gohil K, McPhail G, et al: Muscle morphology and metabolism in hypothyroid myopathy: Effects of treatment. J Clin Pathol 36:519, 1983.
171. McKeran RO, Slavin G, Ward P, et al: Hypothyroid myopathy: A clinical and pathological study. J Pathol 132:35, 1980.
172. Godet-Guillain J, Fardeau M: Hypothyroid myopathy. Histological and ultrastructural study of an atrophic form. Excerpta Medica ICS 199:512, 1970.
173. Norris FH, Panner BJ: Hypothyroid myopathy. Clinical, electromyographical, and ultrastructural observations. Arch Neurol 14:574, 1966.
174. Engel AG: Electron microscopic observations in thyrotoxic and corticosteroid induced myopathies. Mayo Clin Proc 41:785, 1966.
175. DiMauro S, Hartwig GB, Hays A, et al: Debrancher deficiency; Neuromuscular disorder in 5 adults. Ann Neurol 5:422, 1979.
176. Agamanolis DP, Askari AD, DiMauro S, et al: Muscle phosphofructokinase deficiency: Two cases with unusual polysaccharide accumulation and immunologically active enzyme protein. Muscle Nerve 3:456, 1980.
177. Hays AP, Hallett M, Delfs J, et al: Muscle phosphofructokinase deficiency: Abnormal polysaccharide in a case of late-onset myopathy. Neurology 31:1077, 1981.
178. Schochet SS, McCormick WF, Koransky J: Light and electron microscopy of skeletal muscle in type IV glycogenosis. Acta Neuropathol (Berl)19:137, 1971.
179. Ishihara T, Uchino F, Adachi H, et al: Type IV glycogenosis—A study of two cases. Acta Pathol Jpn 25:613, 1975.
180. Ferguson IT, Mahon M, Cumming WJK: An adult case of Andersen's disease—Type IV glycogenosis. A clinical, histochemical, ultrastructural and biochemical study. J Neurol Sci 60:337, 1983.
181. Coleman DL, Gambetti P, DiMauro S, Blume RE: Muscle in Lafora disease. Arch Neurol 31:396, 1974.
182. Neville HE, Brooke MH, Austin JH, Denver MD: Studies in myoclonus epilepsy (Lafora body form). Arch Neurol 30:466, 1974.
183. Robitaille Y, Carpenter S, Karpati G, DiMauro S: A distinct form of adult polyglucosan body disease with massive involvement of central and peripheral neuronal processes and astrocytes: A report of four cases and a review of the occurrence of polyglucosan bodies in other conditions such as Lafora's disease and normal ageing. Brain 103:315, 1980.
183a. Gray F, Gherardi R, Marshall A, et al: Adult polyglucosan body disease (APBD). J Neuropathol Exp Neurol 47:459, 1988.
183b. Cafferty MS, Lovelace RE, Hays AP, et al: Polyglucosan body disease. Muscle Nerve 14:102, 1991.
183c. Bruno C, Servidei S, Shanske S, et al: Glycogen branching enzyme deficiency in adult polyglucosan body disease. Ann Neurol 33:88, 1993.
183d. Greene GM, Weldon DC, Ferrans VJ, et al: Juvenile polysaccharidosis with cardioskeletal myopathy. Arch Pathol Lab Med 111:977, 1987.
183e. Thompson AJ, Swash M, Cox EL, et al: Polysaccharide storage myopathy. Muscle Nerve 11:349, 1988.
183f. Moses SW, Parvari R: The variable presentations of glycogen storage disease type IV: A review of clinical, enzymatic and molecular studies. Curr Mol Med 2:177–188, 2002.
184. Engel AG, Gomez MR, Seybold ME, Lambert EH: The spectrum and diagnosis of acid maltase deficiency. Neurology 23:95, 1973.
185. Engel AG, Arahata K: Monoclonal antibody analysis of mononuclear cells in myopathies: II. Phenotypes of autoinvasive cells in polymyositis and inclusion body myositis. Ann Neurol 16:209, 1984.
186. Janeway CA, Travers P, Walport M, Capra JD (eds): Immunobiology. The Immune System in Health and Disease, 4th ed. London: Current Biology Publications; 2003.
187. Hsu S-M, Raine L, Fanger H: Use of avidin-biotin-peroxidase complex (ABC) in immunoperoxidase techniques: A comparison between ABC and unlabeled antibody (PAP) procedures. J Histochem Cytochem 29:577, 1981.
188. Sanderson CJ: The mechanism of lymphocyte-mediated cytotoxicity. Biol Rev 56:153, 1981.
189. Sanderson CJ: Morphological aspects of lymphocyte mediated cytotoxicity. Adv Exp Med Biol 146:3, 1982.
190. Sanderson CJ: The mechanism of T cell mediated cytotoxicity. V. Morphological studies by electron microscopy. Proc R Soc Lond [Biol] 198:315. 1977.
191. Podack ER, Konigsberg PJ: Cytolytic T cell granules: Isolation, structural, biochemical and functional characterization. J Exp Med 160:695, 1984.
191a. Goebels N, Michaelis D, Engelhardt M, et al: Differential expression of perforin muscle-infiltrating T cells in polymyositis and dermatomyositis. J Clin Invest 97:2905–2910, 1996.
192. Oberc MA, Engel WK: Ultrastructural localization of calcium in normal and abnormal skeletal muscle. Lab Invest 36:566, 1977.
193. Cullen MJ, Fulthorpe JJ: Phagocytosis of the A band following Z line, and I band loss. Its significance in skeletal muscle breakdown. J Pathol 138:129, 1982.
193a. Carpenter S, Karpati G: Segmental necrosis and its demarcation in experimental micropuncture injury in skeletal muscle fibers. J Neuropathol Exp Neurol 48:154, 1989.
193b. Papadimitriou JM, Robertson TA, Mitchell CA, et al: The process of new plasmalemma formation in focally injured muscle fibers. J Struct Biol 103:124, 1990.
194. Pestronk A, Parhad IM, Drachman DB, Price DL: Membrane myopathy: Morphological similarities to Duchenne muscular dystrophy. Muscle Nerve 5:209, 1982.
195. Mauro A: Satellite cell of skeletal muscle fibers. J Biophys Biochem Cytol 9:493, 1961.
196. Campion DR: The muscle satellite cell: A review. Int Rev Cytol 87:225, 1984.
197. Schmalbruch H, Hellhammer U: The number of satellite cells in normal human muscle. Anat Rec 185:279, 1976.

198. Moss FP, Leblond CP: Satellite cells as the source of nuclei in muscles of growing rats. *Anat Rec* 179:421, 1971.
199. Snow MH: Myogenic cell formation in regenerating rat skeletal muscle injured by mincing: II. An autoradiographic study. *Anat Rec* 188:201, 1977.
200. Snow MH: An autoradiographic study of satellite cell differentiation into regenerating myotubes following transplantation of muscles in young rats. *Cell Tissue Res* 186:535, 1978.
201. Lipton BH, Schultz E: Developmental fate of skeletal muscle satellite cells. *Science* 205:1292, 1979.
202. Allbrook D: Skeletal muscle regeneration. *Muscle Nerve* 4:234, 1981.
203. Bischoll R: Tissue culture studies on the origin of myogenic cells during muscle regeneration in the rat, in Mauro A (ed): *Muscle Regeneration*. New York: Raven Press; 1979, pp 13–29.
204. Königsberg IR: Regeneration of single muscle fibers in culture and in vivo, in Mauro A (ed): *Muscle Regeneration*. New York: Raven Press; 1979, pp 41–56.
205. Hsu L, Trupin GL, Roisen FJ: The role of satellite cells and myonuclei during myogenesis in vitro, in Mauro A (ed): *Muscle Regeneration*. New York: Raven Press; 1979, pp 115–120.
206. Schmalbruch H: Manifestations of regeneration in myopathic muscles, in Mauro A (ed): *Muscle Regeneration*. New York: Raven Press; 1979, pp 121–129.
207. Wakayama Y, Schotland DL, Bonilla E, Orecchio E: Quantitative ultrastructural study of muscle satellite cells in Duchenne dystrophy. *Neurology* 29:401, 1979.
207a. Jacobs SCJM, Wokke JHJ, Bar PR, et al: Satellite cell activation after muscle damage in young and adult rats. *Anat Rec* 242:329–336, 1995.
207b. Bischoff R: Chemotaxis of skeletal muscle satellite cells. *Dev Dyn* 208:505–515, 1997.
208. Carlson BM: The regeneration of skeletal muscle—A review. *Am J Anat* 137:119, 1973.
209. Snow MH: Myogenic cell formation in regenerating rat skeletal muscle injured by mincing: I. A fine structural study. *Anat Rec* 188:181, 1977.
210. Shafiq SA, Gorycki MA: Regeneration in skeletal muscle of mouse: Some electron microscope observations. *J Pathol Bacteriol* 90:123, 1965.
211. Reznik M: Origin of myoblasts during muscle regeneration: Electron microscopic observations. *Lab Invest* 20:353, 1969.
212. Shultz E: Changes in the satellite cells of growing muscle following denervation. *Anat Rec* 190:299, 1978.
213. McGeachie J, Allbrook DB: Cell proliferation in skeletal muscle following denervation or tenotomy. *Cell Tissue Res* 193:259, 1978.
214. Salleo A, Anastasi G, Spada G, et al: New muscle fiber formation during compensatory hypertrophy. *Med Sci Sports Exerc* 12:268, 1980.
214a. Maltin CA, Harris JB, Cullen MJ: Regeneration of skeletal muscle following the injection of the snake-venom toxin, taipoxin. *Cell Tissue Res* 232:565, 1983.
215. Fischman DA: Development of striated muscle, in Bourne G (ed): *The Structure and Function of Muscle*. New York: Academic Press; 1973, pp 75–148.
216. Ezerman EB, Ishikawa H: Differentiation of the sarcoplasmic reticulum and T system in developing chick skeletal muscle in vitro. *J Cell Biol* 35:405, 1967.
217. Ishikawa H: Formation of elaborate networks of T-system tubules in cultured skeletal muscle with special reference to the T-system formation. *J Cell Biol* 38:51, 1968.
217a. Flucher BE, Terasaki M, Chin H, et al: Biogenesis of transverse tubules in skeletal muscle *in vitro*. *Dev Biol* 145:77, 1991.
218. Walker SM, Schrodt GR: Triads in skeletal muscle fibers of 19-day fetal rats. *J Cell Biol* 37:564, 1968.
219. Edge MB: Development of apposed sarcoplasmic reticulum at the T system and sarcolemma and the change in orientation of triads in rat skeletal muscle. *Dev Biol* 23:634, 1970.
220. Schiaffino S, Margreth A: Coordinated development of the sarcoplasmic reticulum and T system during postnatal differentiation of rat skeletal muscle. *J Cell Biol* 41:855, 1969.
221. Chou SM, Nonaka I: Satellite cells and muscle regeneration in diseased human skeletal muscles. *J Neurol Sci* 34:131, 1977.
222. Tsujihata M, Engel AG, Lambert EH: Motor endplate fine structure in acrylamide dying-back neuropathy: A sequential morphometric study. *Neurology* 24:849, 1974.
223. Engel AG, Jerusalem F, Tsujihata M, Gomez MR: The neuromuscular junction in myopathies: A quantitative ultrastructural study. *Excerpta Medica ICS* 360:132, 1975.
224. Fardeau M: Normal ultrastructural aspect of human motor end-plate and its pathologic modifications, in Pearson CM, Mostofi FK (eds): *The Striated Muscle*. Baltimore: Williams & Wilkins; 1973, pp 342–363.
225. Miledi R, Slater CR: On the degeneration of rat neuromuscular junctions after nerve section. *J Physiol (Lond)* 207:507, 1970.
226. Sahashi K, Engel AG, Lambert EH, Howard FM: Ultrastructural localization of the terminal and lytic ninth complement component (C9) at the motor endplate in myasthenia gravis. *J Neuropathol Exp Neurol* 39:160, 1980.
227. Engel AG, Santa T: Motor endplate fine structure. Quantitative analysis in disorders of neuromuscular transmission, in Desmedt JE (ed): *New Developments in Electromyography and Clinical Neurophysiology*, vol 1. Basel: Karger; 1973, pp 41–54.
228. Engel AG, Fumagalli G: Mechanisms of acetylcholine receptor loss from the neuromuscular junction, in *Receptors, Antibodies and Disease*. Ciba Foundation Symposium 90. London: Pitman; 1982, pp 197–224.
229. Engel AG, Lambert EH, Santa T: Study of long-term anticholinesterase therapy: Effects on neuromuscular transmission and on motor end-plate fine structure. *Neurology* 23:1273, 1973.
230. Campbell AK, Daw RA, Luzio JP: Rapid increase in intracellular free Ca^{2+} induced by antibody plus complement. *FEBS Lett* 107:55, 1979.
231. Jerusalem F, Engel AG, Gomez MR: Duchenne dystrophy. II. Morphometric study of motor end-plate fine structure. *Brain* 97:123, 1974.
231a. Nagel A, Lehmann-Horn F, Engel AG: Neuromuscular transmission in the *mdx* mouse. *Muscle Nerve* 13:742, 1990.
232. Engel AG, Tsujihata M, Lambert EH, et al: Experimental autoimmune myasthenia gravis: A sequential and quantitative study of the neuromuscular junction ultrastructure and electrophysiologic correlations. *J Neuropathol Exp Neurol* 35:569, 1976.
233. Engel AG, Sakakibara H, Sahashi K, et al: Passively transferred experimental autoimmune myasthenia gravis: Sequential and quantitative study of the motor end-plate fine structure and ultrastructural localization of immune complexes (IgG and C3), and of the acetylcholine receptor. *Neurology* 29:179, 1979.
233a. Nakano S, Engel AG: Myasthenia gravis: Quantitative immunocytochemical analysis of inflammatory cells and detection of complement membrane attack complex at the end-plate in 30 patients. *Neurology* 43:1167, 1993.
234. Engel AG, Sahashi K, Fumagalli G: The immunopathology of acquired myasthenia gravis. *Ann NY Acad Sci* 377:158, 1981.
235. Jerusalem F, Engel AG, Gomez MR: Duchenne dystrophy: I. Morphometric study of the muscle microvasculature. *Brain* 97:115, 1974.
235a. Martin RW, Duffy J, Engel AG, et al: The clinical spectrum of the eosinophilia-myalgia syndrome associated with L-tryptophan ingestion: Clinical features in 20 patients and aspects of pathophysiology. *Ann Intern Med* 113:124, 1990.
235b. Emslie-Smith AM, Engel AG: Necrotizing myopathy with pipestem capillaries, microvascular deposition of the complement membrane attack complex (MAC), and minimal cellular infiltration. *Neurology* 41:936, 1991.
236. Norton WL, Hurd ER, Lewis DC, Ziff M: Evidence of vascular injury in scleroderma and systemic lupus erythematosus: Quantitative study of the microvascular bed. *J Lab Clin Med* 71:919, 1968.
237. Jerusalem F, Simona F, Fontana A: Myopathologische und immunologische Befunde zur Diagnose und Pathogenese der Polymyositis und Dermatomyositis. *Nervenarzt* 51:255, 1980.
237a. Kissel JT, Mendell JR, Rammohan KW: Microvascular deposition of complement membrane attack complex in dermatomyositis. *N Engl J Med* 314:331, 1986.
237b. Emslie-Smith AM, Engel AG: Microvascular changes in early and advanced dermatomyositis. A quantitative study. *Ann Neurol* 27:343, 1990.
237c. Nakano S, Emslie-Smith A, Engel AG: Ultrastructural and cytochemical aspects of the angiopathy associated with the eosinophilia-myalgia syndrome (EMS). *Neurology* 41(suppl 1):394, 1991.
238. Kyle RA, Greipp PR: Amyloidosis (AL): Clinical and laboratory features in 229 cases. *Mayo Clin Proc* 58:665, 1983.
239. Glenner GG, Ignaczak TF, Page DL: The inherited systemic amyloidoses and localized amyloid deposits, in Stanbury JB, Wyngaarden JB, Fredrickson DS (eds): *The Metabolic Basis of Inherited Disease*, 4th ed. New York: McGraw-Hill; 1978, pp 1308–1339.
240. Whitaker JN, Hashimoto K, Quinones M: Skeletal muscle pseudohypertrophy in primary amyloidosis. *Neurology* 27:47, 1977.
241. Ringel SP, Claman HN: Amyloid-associated muscle pseudohypertrophy. *Arch Neurol* 39:413, 1982.

Chapter 32
Immune Mechanisms in Muscle Diseases

REINHARD HOHLFELD

Introduction
The Innate Immune Response
   THE COMPLEMENT SYSTEM
   PATTERN-RECOGNITION RECEPTORS
   NATURAL KILLER (NK) CELLS
Adaptive (Specific) Immunity
   B AND T LYMPHOCYTES
   ANTIGEN RECOGNITION BY B CELLS AND ANTIBODIES
   ANTIGEN RECOGNITION BY T CELLS
   COOPERATION BETWEEN B AND T CELLS
   ROLE OF THE THYMUS
   ANTIGEN-PRESENTING CELLS
   ANTIBODY- AND CELL-MEDIATED CYTOTOXICITY
Principles of Cellular Communication
   ADHESION AND MIGRATION OF IMMUNE CELLS
   CYTOKINES AND CHEMOKINES
   THE IMMUNOLOGIC SYNAPSE
Mechanisms of Autoimmunity
Novel Targets for Therapeutic Modulation
   TRIMOLECULAR COMPLEX
   COSTIMULATORY MOLECULES
   ADHESION- AND MIGRATION-RELATED MOLECULES
   CYTOKINES AND CHEMOKINES AS THERAPEUTIC TARGETS
Immunologic Properties of Cultured Myoblasts
   EXPRESSION OF CLASSIC AND NONCLASSIC MHC (HLA) MOLECULES
   EXPRESSION OF ADHESION AND COSTIMULATORY MOLECULES
   SECRETION OF CYTOKINES AND CHEMOKINES
   FUNCTIONAL INTERACTION WITH T CELLS

Introduction

Immunologic mechanisms are crucially involved in the pathogenesis of autoimmune, dysimmune, and inflammatory muscle diseases, including myasthenia gravis, polymyositis and dermatomyositis syndromes, inclusion body myositis, and infectious myopathies. Further, immunologic reactions may occur in response to degenerative changes in some of the hereditary myopathies. Notable examples include Duchenne muscular dystrophy,[1] facioscapulohumeral muscular dystrophy,[2] and some dysferlinopathies.[3] Muscle inflammation may also occur as a local or generalized response to toxic agents—as, for example, in macrophagic myofasciitis.[4,5]

This chapter provides a general overview of current immunologic concepts as they are relevant to an understanding of the immunopathogenesis of inflammatory muscle disorders. Disease-specific immune mechanisms are discussed in the chapters on individual diseases. For additional reading on general immunology, the reader is referred to the major textbooks on this subject [e.g., Janeway CA, Travers P, Walport M, Shlomchik M: *Immunobiology: The Immune System in Health and Disease.* New York: Garland, 2001; Paul WE (ed): *Fundamental Immunology.* Philadelphia: Lippincott Raven, 1999]. Additional sources of useful information are the review journals *Trends in Immunology* and *Nature Reviews Immunology* and the review series *Annual Reviews of Immunology.*

A better understanding of the mechanisms of autoimmunity and immunoregulation should eventually lead to improved therapy of autoimmune disorders. Unlike the presently available nonselective and often toxic immunosuppressive agents, novel agents that aim at selective manipulation of autoimmune processes are currently being developed. These novel strategies are discussed in a separate section of this chapter. Conventional immunosuppressive treatment of specific disorders is discussed in chapters on individual diseases.

The last section emphasizes the important concept that muscle is not just a passive target of various immune reactions.[6] On the contrary, muscle cells (myoblasts) can themselves express and transmit a large array of immunologic signals, including various cytokines, chemokines, adhesion molecules, and costimulatory molecules. This enables them to participate actively in immune reactions—for example, as antigen-presenting cells.[6]

The Innate Immune Response

The immune system can be divided into innate (antigen-nonspecific) and adaptive (antigen-specific) responses. The adaptive response, which centers around antigen-specific B and T cells, is discussed in the next section. The innate immune response uses a variety of effector mechanisms to clear or contain an infection until the pathogen can be recognized by the adaptive immune system. These effector mechanisms are regulated by receptors that can distinguish between noninfected self and infectious nonself ligands. In this section, three components of the innate immune response are considered: the complement system, pattern recognition receptors, and natural killer (NK)* cells (for a more detailed review of the innate immune system, see Ref. 7).

THE COMPLEMENT SYSTEM

The complement system includes at least 20 plasma glycoproteins. These are activated in a cascade sequence, with different amplification stages (Fig. 32-1). The classic pathway is triggered directly by pathogen or indirectly by antibody binding to the pathogen surface. The alternative pathway is stimulated by polysaccharides from yeasts and gram-negative bacteria. The more recently identified mannan-binding lectin pathway feeds into the classic sequence by activating it independently of the C1rs complex and is stimulated by mannose-

---

*A list of abbreviations used in this chapter is given at the end of the chapter.

containing proteins and carbohydrates on microbes, including viruses and yeasts. All three pathways converge with the activation of the central C3 convertase enzyme, which cleaves C3 to produce the active complement component C3b (Fig. 32-1). This leads to a final common pathway, with assembly of C5-C9 forming a transmembrane pore (membrane attack complex) in the cell surface membrane and subsequent death by osmotic lysis. Normal host cells bear the complement receptor type 1 and decay accelerating factor, which inhibit C3 convertase and prevent progression of complement activation. In addition to lysis, complement has opsonic functions (C3b), vasoactive functions (C3a and C5a), and chemotactic activity (C5a). Complement also has a role in the specific immune response. Its activation and deposition in immune complexes targets these to complement-receptor–bearing antigen-presenting cells, such as B lymphocytes, macrophages, and dendritic cells.

PATTERN-RECOGNITION RECEPTORS

In contrast to the antigen-specific receptors of B and T lymphocytes, which are somatically rearranged, the receptors of the innate immune system are encoded in the germline. They are expressed on many cells of the innate immune system, especially macrophages, dendritic cells, and B cells. These receptors recognize a few highly conserved structures present in large groups of microorganisms and are therefore called pattern-recognition receptors. An example of such pattern-recognition receptors is the recently identified receptors of the toll family, the so-called toll-like receptors (TLRs).[7] These are homologs of a *Drosophila* transmembrane protein called toll, which is involved in the immune response of insects. The first identified human toll-like receptor (TLR-4) is involved in the recognition of lipopolysaccharide and activates the NF-κB signaling pathway, inducing the expres-

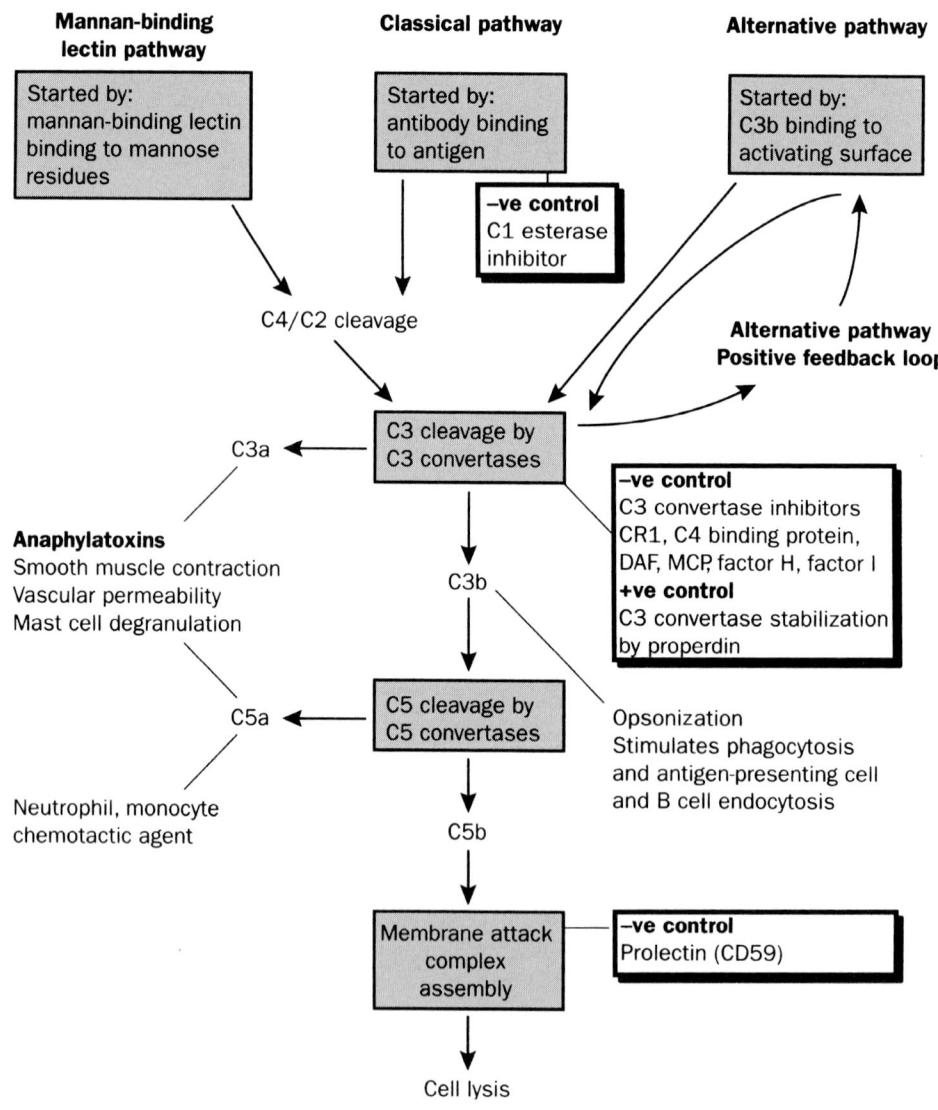

FIGURE 32-1. The complement system. *(Adapted from Allen JE, Maizels RM: Th1-Th2: Reliable paradigm or dangerous dogma? Immunol Today 18:387–392, 1997. With permission.)*

sion of a variety of cytokines and costimulatory molecules crucial to the adaptive immune response. At least 10 mammalian TLRs likely involved in recognition of the major microbial patterns that trigger innate immune responses have been identified. For example, bacterial unmethylated CpG dinucleotides seem to be recognized by TLR9,[8] and heat-shock proteins can stimulate macrophages via TLR2 and TLR4. Thus, TLRs can be viewed as eyes of the innate immune cells turned outward to identify conserved molecular patterns of pathogens and danger signals originating from stressed or injured cells.[8]

NATURAL KILLER (NK) CELLS

NK cells have the morphology of lymphocytes but do not express somatically rearranged antigen-specific receptors. They recognize abnormal cells in two ways. First, they bind antibody-coated targets via Fc receptors, leading to antibody-dependent cellular cytotoxicity (see "Antibody- and Cell-Mediated Cytotoxicity," below). Second, they have various surface receptors that recognize molecular flags on target cells, indicating that the target cell is potentially dangerous and must be eliminated. NK activity is stimulated by cytokines, such as interferons and macrophage-derived cytokines like interleukin- (IL-) 12.

NK cells are functionally identified by their ability to kill certain lymphoid tumor cell lines in vitro without prior immunization or activation. Their mechanism of killing is identical to that used by cytotoxic T cells (CTLs) in the adaptive immune response (see "Antibody- and Cell-Mediated Cytotoxicity," below). However, in contrast to CTL, NK-cell killing is triggered not by variable antigen-specific receptors but by invariant receptors. These NK-cell receptors may be stimulatory or inhibitory.[9] They recognize various ligands on the surface of potential target cells, and their response is controlled by integrated signals from various receptors, recognizing the presence or absence of ligands on target cells. For example, loss of MHC class I antigens on target cells, because of either tumor transformation or viral infection, lowers the threshold of NK activation because of reduced signaling from inhibitory receptors. This event, together with an upregulation of ligands for activating receptors, favors NK-cell activation. In this way, NK cells are probably controlled by the array of ligands for activating receptors and the amount of MHC class I present on antigen-presenting cells as well as the activation state of the NK cells, which is influenced by local cytokines and chemokines.[9]

Adaptive (Specific) Immunity

B AND T LYMPHOCYTES

B and T lymphocytes express specific receptors for antigen recognition. In the case of B cells, the antigen receptor is a heterodimer of immunoglobulin light and heavy chains. In the case of T cells, the antigen receptor is a heterodimer of one α and one β chain (the $\alpha\beta$ T-cell receptor) or one γ and one δ chain (the $\gamma\delta$ T-cell receptor).

The immune repertoire of B and T cells comprises an enormous number of different antigen specificities, each of which is represented by a different cell clone. This diversity is created by somatic gene rearrangements of the genes encoding the antigen receptors of B and T cells (Fig. 32-2).[10–12] Each B- or T-cell clone selects one gene segment from each of several pools of germline segments and combines these segments into the functional genes coding for the protein chains of B-cell receptors (immunoglobulin light and heavy chains) or T-cell receptors (α and β or γ and δ chains). Part of the diversity of the rearranged immunoglobulin and T-cell receptor genes results from random combinatorial joining of the different gene segments. Additional diversity results from the deletion or insertion of nucleotides at the junctional borders between the different rearranged gene segments (Fig. 32-2).

B cells manufacture antibody and have the capacity to present antigens to T cells.[13] In response to antigen contact and modulation from other cells, B cells undergo clonal expansion and differentiation into antibody-synthesizing plasma cells. T cells function as regulatory cells or effector cells. Two major subsets of T cells are defined by expression of the CD4 and CD8 differentiation antigens. The majority of CD4+ T cells act as antigen-specific helper (Th2) or proinflammatory (Th1) cells. The two cell types can be distinguished by their pattern of cytokine secretion: Th1 cells produce IL-2 and interferon-γ, whereas Th2 cells produce IL-4, IL-5, IL-10, and related "Th2-type" cytokines (Fig. 32-3).[14] CD8+ T cells act as antigen-specific killer cells. A small minority of T cells, the $\gamma\delta$ T cells, are predominantly CD3+CD4-CD8-. Most $\gamma\delta$ T cells have cytotoxic potential in vitro, but their in vivo functions are largely unknown.[15]

ANTIGEN RECOGNITION BY B CELLS AND ANTIBODIES

Newly generated B cells initially express IgM and soon thereafter also express IgD (Fig. 32-4).[16] During an immune response, B cells switch the isotype of the immunoglobulins they express. This isotype switch, which is thought to occur in germinal centers of lymph nodes and spleen, leads to the appearance of memory B cells that express IgG, IgA, or IgE. The memory B cells have mutated variable regions of their Ig molecules. Somatic hypermutation of genes coding for the variable chains of antigen receptors occurs only in B cells, not in T cells. This process adds to the great potential diversity already available through large numbers, combinations, and junctional diversity of germline variable regions.

In germinal centers of lymph nodes and spleen, antigen is retained for prolonged periods of time on the surface of follicular dendritic cells (Fig. 32-4).[17] Continuous encounter with antigen selects B cells with high-affinity receptors among the pool of antigen-specific B cells that have mutated Ig variable chains. Antibody-secreting plasma cells resulting from these clones will also be of high affinity. A prototypic soluble (secreted) immunoglobulin monomer (IgG) is composed of two heavy (55-kDa) chains and two light (25-kDa) chains (Fig. 32-2). The four polypeptide chains are held

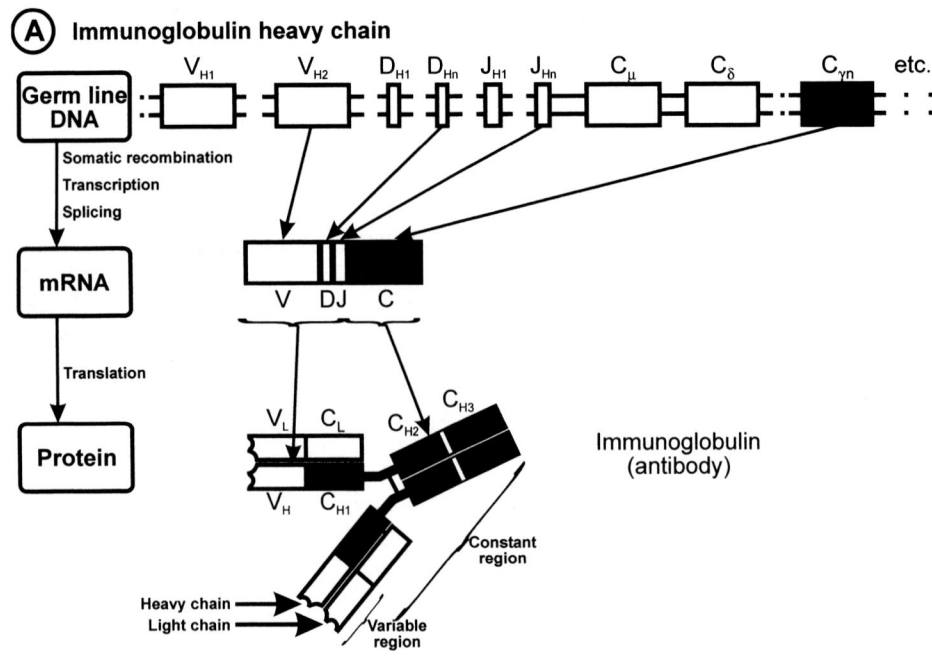

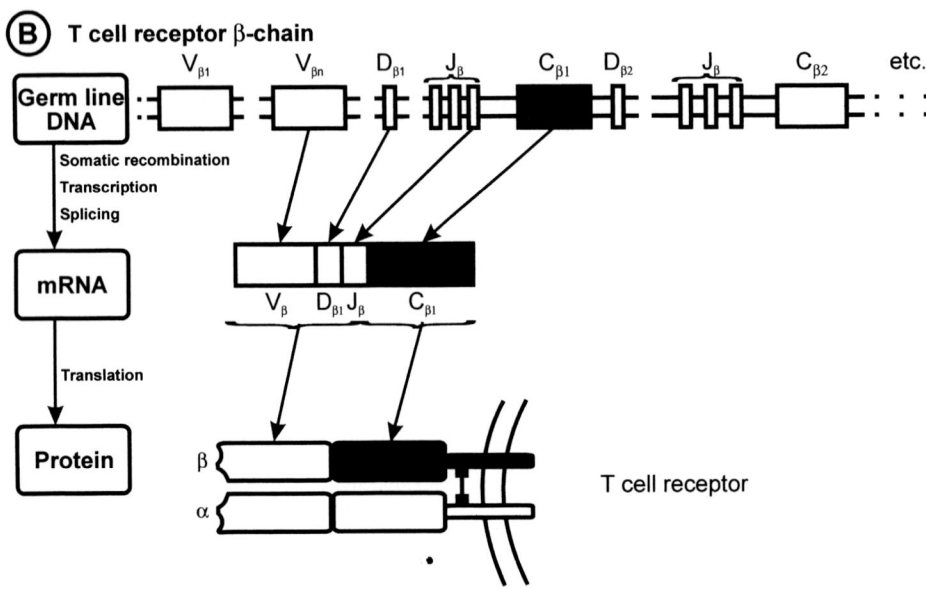

FIGURE 32-2. Somatic rearrangement of immunoglobulin and T-cell receptor genes. The germline DNA is somatically rearranged before it is transcribed into mRNA. This process, which is unique to the immune system, creates the enormously diverse im-mune repertoire of antigen receptors of B cells (*A*) and T cells (*B*). (*From Hohlfeld R: Biotechnological agents for the immunotherapy of multiple sclerosis. Principles, problems and perspectives. Brain 120: 865–916, 1997. With permission.*)

together by noncovalent interactions and stabilized by disulfide bonds, forming the shape of a Y. The arm segments of the Y (called Fab) contain the light chains, part of the heavy chain (Fd), and the ligand-binding activity. The stem of the Y (called Fc) is a dimer of the carboxy-terminal halves of the heavy chains that determines all the metabolic and effector properties of an immunoglobulin. These effector functions include neutralization of toxins, complement activation, opsonization of bacteria for phagocytosis, and sensitization of tumor and infected cells for antibody-dependent cytotoxic attack by NK cells.

Each B cell expresses only one functionally rearranged heavy-chain gene and one light-chain; thus, in a given antibody molecule, the heavy and light chains are identical. There are five heavy-chain isotypes (γ, α, μ, δ, ε) and two light-chain isotypes (κ, λ). Some of the isotypes split further

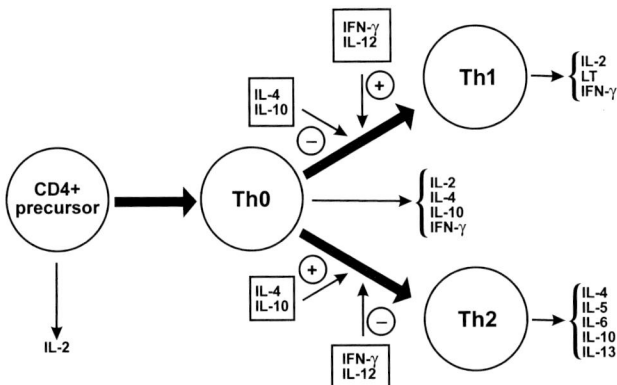

FIGURE 32-3. Differentiation of Th1 and Th2 cells. CD4+ precursor cells mature into Th0 cells. Under the positive or negative influence of various cytokines, Th0 cells differentiate into Th1 or Th2 cells. Fat arrows indicate differentiation pathways; thin arrows indicate positive or negative regulatory influences or cytokine secretion. IFN = interferon. (*From Hohlfeld R: Biotechnological agents for the immunotherapy of multiple sclerosis. Principles, problems and perspectives. Brain 120:865–916, 1997. With permission.*)

into subtypes. For example, human γ splits into γ-1, -2, -3, and -4. The variable amino-terminal domains of both heavy and light chains have three hypervariable clusters, the complementarity-determining regions (CDRs). The CDRs cooperate to form the antigen-binding sites. X-ray crystallographic studies have revealed at least two types of binding sites: a deep cleft that snugly surrounds small ligands such as peptides and other low-molecular-weight organic molecules and a broad face that is complementary to an equally broad epitope on large protein antigens. Antibodies and ligands are not rigid but rather dynamic entities that undergo conformational adjustments, which may be required for proper binding.

In general, B cells need no specific antigen-presenting cell to evoke a response. However, in germinal centers, follicular dendritic cells, which bear Fc and complement receptors, trap and retain antigens in the form of immune complexes and transfer antigen to B cells.[17] These "follicular dendritic cells" need to be distinguished and are distinct from the "dendritic cells" (see "Antigen-Presenting Cells," below) in that they do not belong to the leukocyte family, are not derived from bone marrow precursors, are not phagocytic, and do not express MHC class II proteins. Macrophages can also present antigens to B cells, but in this instance B cells see an altered, processed form of the antigen. Most antibodies and B cells, however, recognize antigens in their native conformation provided that a native protein was used as the immunogen. Fig. 32-4 summarizes B lymphocyte development from stem cell to plasma cell.

ANTIGEN RECOGNITION BY T CELLS

T cells recognize antigen in a processed form on the surface of antigen-presenting cells (APCs), and the uptake and processing of antigen by APCs is a crucial initial step in the cascade of antigen-induced immune reactions.[18] The prototypes of APCs are macrophages and dendritic cells (see "Antigen-Presenting Cells," below). Antigen processing may take two principal pathways, often referred to as the MHC class I ("endogenous") and MHC class II ("endocytic") pathways (Figs. 32-5 and 32-6). The endogenous pathway leads to the presentation of endogenously synthesized antigens in the molecular context of HLA class I molecules. HLA class I–associated antigens are recognized by CD8+ T cells. The endogenously synthesized peptides may be derived either from self proteins or from foreign (e.g., viral) proteins.

The endocytic pathway leads to the presentation of antigens in the molecular context of HLA class II (Fig. 32-6). HLA class II–associated antigens are recognized by CD4+ T cells. In comparison to HLA class I, HLA class II molecules have a relatively restricted tissue distribution. They are constitutively expressed mainly on B cells, macrophages, and dendritic cells. Thus, the capacity to stimulate CD4+ T cells is normally confined to B cells and professional APCs. Many of the antigens presented in this pathway derive from surface molecules of APCs.

Soluble proteins can be internalized via fluid-phase or receptor-mediated endocytosis after binding to surface immunoglobulin (expressed only on B cells) or after antigen-antibody complexes bind to different types of immunoglobulin Fc domain receptors (Fc receptors are expressed on many cells, including monocytes, macrophages, and B cells). The receptor-mediated endocytotic mechanisms serve to concentrate specific antigens, so that their peptide fragments can be presented more efficiently to CD4+ T cells.[13] In the case of antigen-antibody complexes, the antibody can influence the degradation and processing of the bound antigen.

COOPERATION BETWEEN B AND T CELLS

There is a "reciprocal dialogue" between B and T cells. Activation of antigen-specific T cells depends on interactions between T cells and APCs, which can themselves be B cells.[13] Once active, the T cells promote B-cell activation by releasing T-cell–derived cytokines—such as IL-2, IL-4, and IL-5—and by direct intercellular contact.

Perhaps the most important example of the reciprocal interaction between B and T cells is the immunoglobulin class (isotype) switching that occurs in B cells when they are "helped" by antigen-specific T cells. In this collaboration, the B cell uses IgM molecules on its surface to capture the antigen and presents the processed antigen to the T cell. Contact between the collaborating lymphocytes is enhanced by complementary pairs of adhesion molecules. Some of these molecules, such as CD4 and HLA class II molecules, are constitutively expressed on the surface of T and B cells, respectively. Others, by contrast, are induced. For example, contact between B and T cells induces the T cell to express a ligand for the B-cell surface molecule CD40. In turn, CD40 interacts with the newly expressed CD40 ligand on the T cell, and this leads to the expression of another B-cell surface molecule, B7. The partners of B7 on the surface of the T cell are CD28 and CTLA-4. These cooperative interactions between the T and B cells induce the secretion of cytokines, such as IL-2 and IL-4. Isotype switching requires two signals. The first is delivered

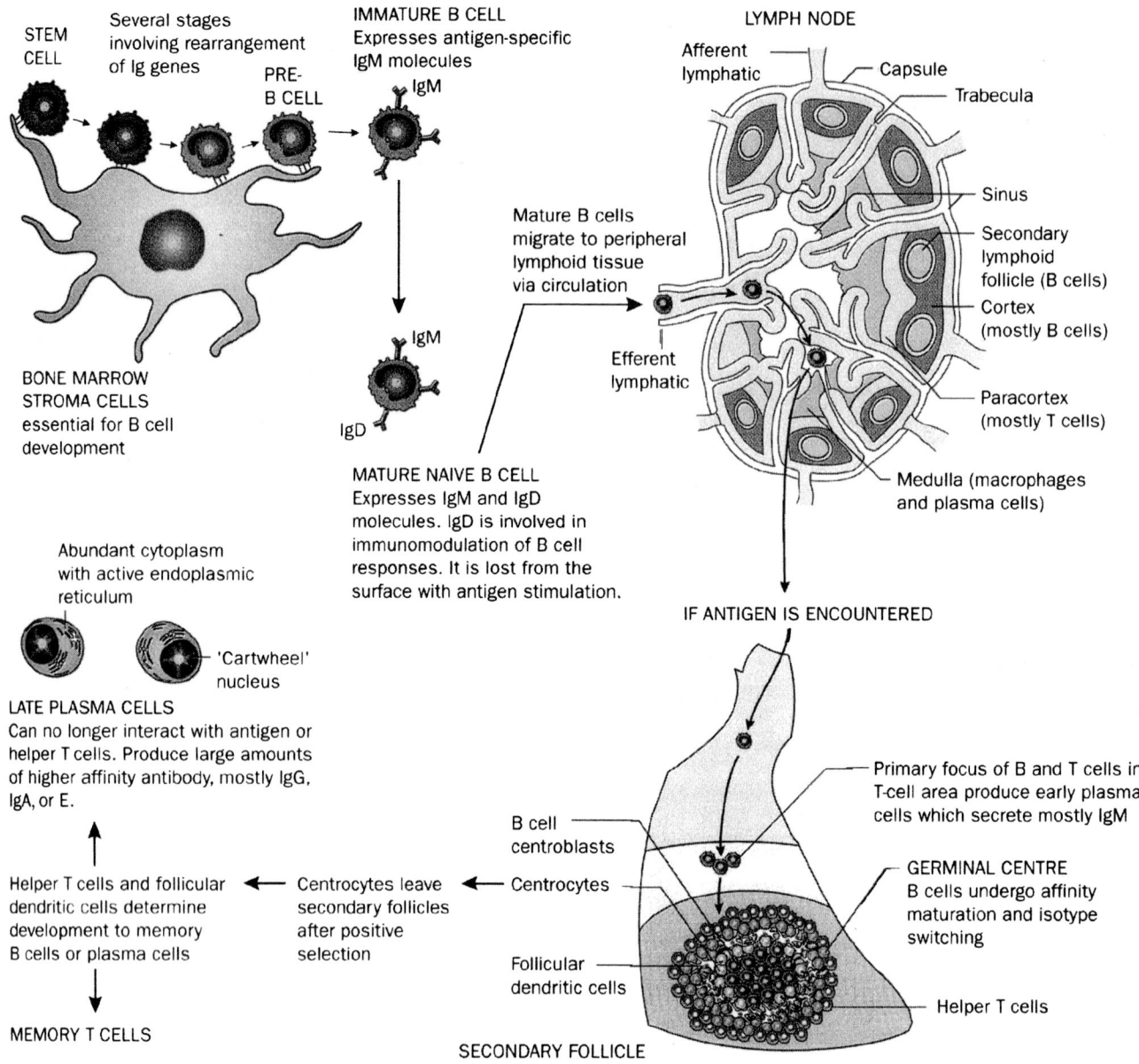

FIGURE 32-4. The pathway of B lymphocyte development from stem cell to plasma cell. (*Modified from Parkin J, Cohen B: An overview of the immune system. Lancet 357:1777–1789, 2001. With permission.*)

by an interleukin and the second by the binding of CD40 to its ligand on the T cell.

B cells recognizing a specific antigen by their antigen-specific surface immunoglobulin internalize the antigen by receptor-mediated endocytosis and present its peptide fragments to T cells with high efficiency.[13] The specific surface Ig plays two roles in this process. First, it efficiently internalizes antigen and directs it to relevant internal compartments of the B cell. Second, signal transduction events triggered by antigen binding enhance expression of both adhesion and HLA class II molecules on the B-cell surface. These, and possibly other events, promote the general ability of the antigen-recognizing B cell to present the antigen to a specific helper T cell.

After receptor-mediated endocytosis of the antigen, the immunoglobulin may sterically influence the rate at which different parts of the antigen are processed in the B cell. Thus, different B cells bearing different surface immunoglobulin would process the antigen differently, in contrast to nonspecific APCs, which process the antigen in a uniform manner. By this mechanism, B-cell specificity could lead to selective antigen presentation to helper T cells and therefore to selective T-cell help for certain specific epitopes. Thus, helper T cells and B cells can reciprocally influence each other's specificity. These basic mechanisms are crucial for understanding of antibody-dependent autoimmune reactions, as they occur, for example, in myasthenia gravis (see Chap. 64).

ROLE OF THE THYMUS

A major function of the thymus gland is to generate immunocompetent mature T cells. Immature T-cell progenitors enter the gland, then proliferate rapidly, interact sequentially with various components of the thymic stroma, and eventually leave the gland as immunocompetent T cells (Fig. 32-7). The education of the T cells in the gland results in diversification of the T-cell antigen receptor, and this confers subset-specific functions on clones of T cells.

The primitive, bone marrow–derived progenitor cells entering the thymus initially settle in the cortex of the gland (Fig. 32-7). The differentiating and maturing T-cell progenitors then move through different thymic compartments, eventually reaching the medulla. The T cells arriving here are predominantly immunocompetent virgin T cells.

The thymus is composed of cells of diverse origin. The microenvironments of the gland are determined by the local stromal cells, and the composition and character of stromal cells is controlled by the local T cells. For example, thymuses of severe combined immunodeficiency (SCID) mice or those of mice treated with cyclosporine lack a differentiated medulla, but the medulla regenerates when these animals are reconstituted with intact T cells.[19] Conversely, the composition of stromal cells determines how the local microenvironment functions in T-cell differentiation. Particular sets of cell adhesion molecules fit and hold T cells in various stages of development at various loci for a sufficient time to allow a given differentiation step to go to completion. The induction of the consecutive steps of differentiation likely depends on membrane signals and on soluble mediators.

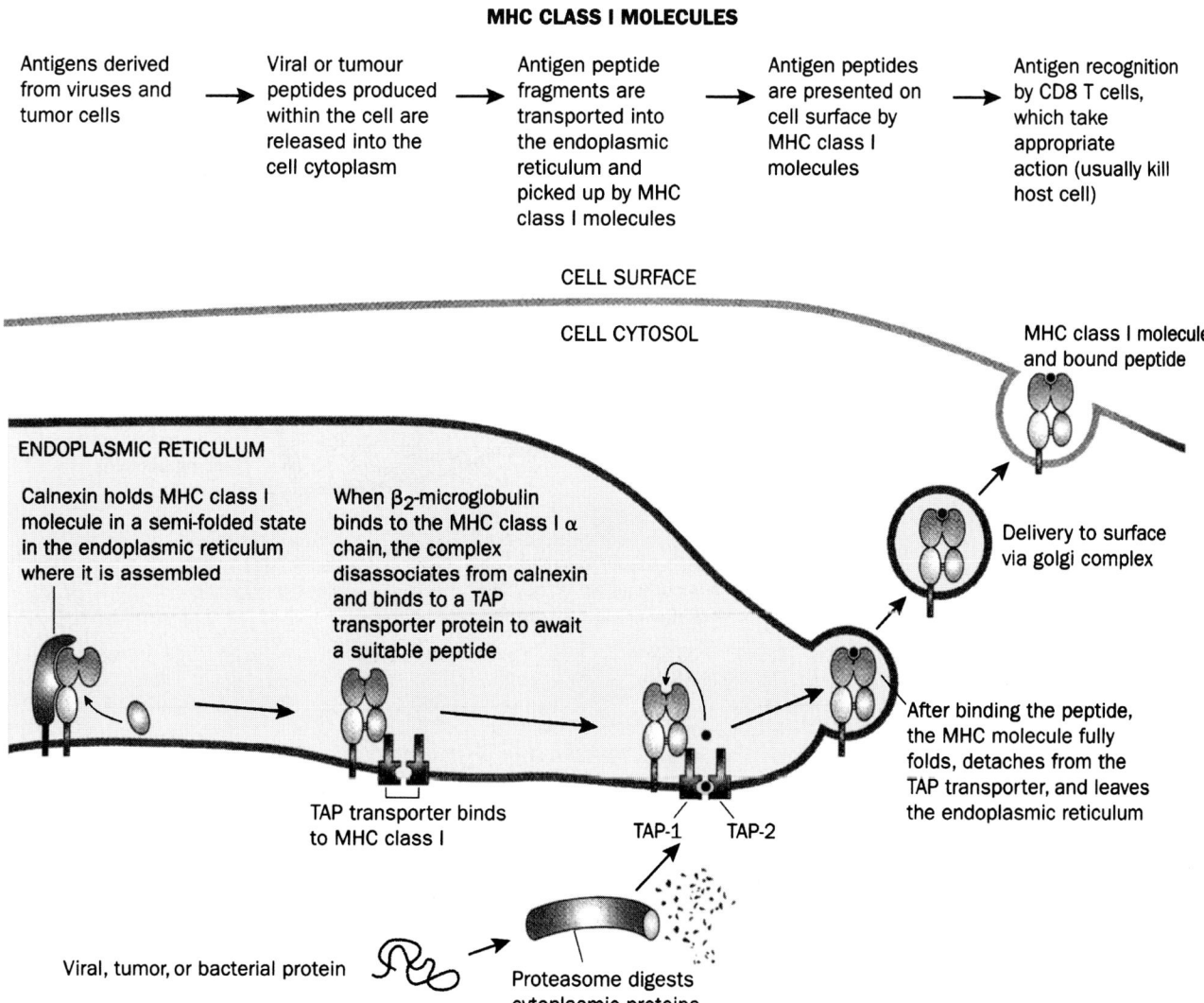

FIGURE 32-5. The pathway of endogenous antigen delivery to class I MHC molecules. Endogenously synthesized proteins are processed in the cytoplasm. The resulting peptides bind to a "transporter associated with antigen processing" (TAP). TAP is responsible for the ATP-dependent transport of peptides from the cytoplasm into the lumen of the endoplasmic reticulum (ER). In the ER, the peptide binds to a nascent MHC class I molecule. Peptide binding alters and stabilizes the conformation of the MHC class I molecule. (Modified from Parkin J, Cohen B: An overview of the immune system. Lancet 357:1777–1789, 2001. With permission.)

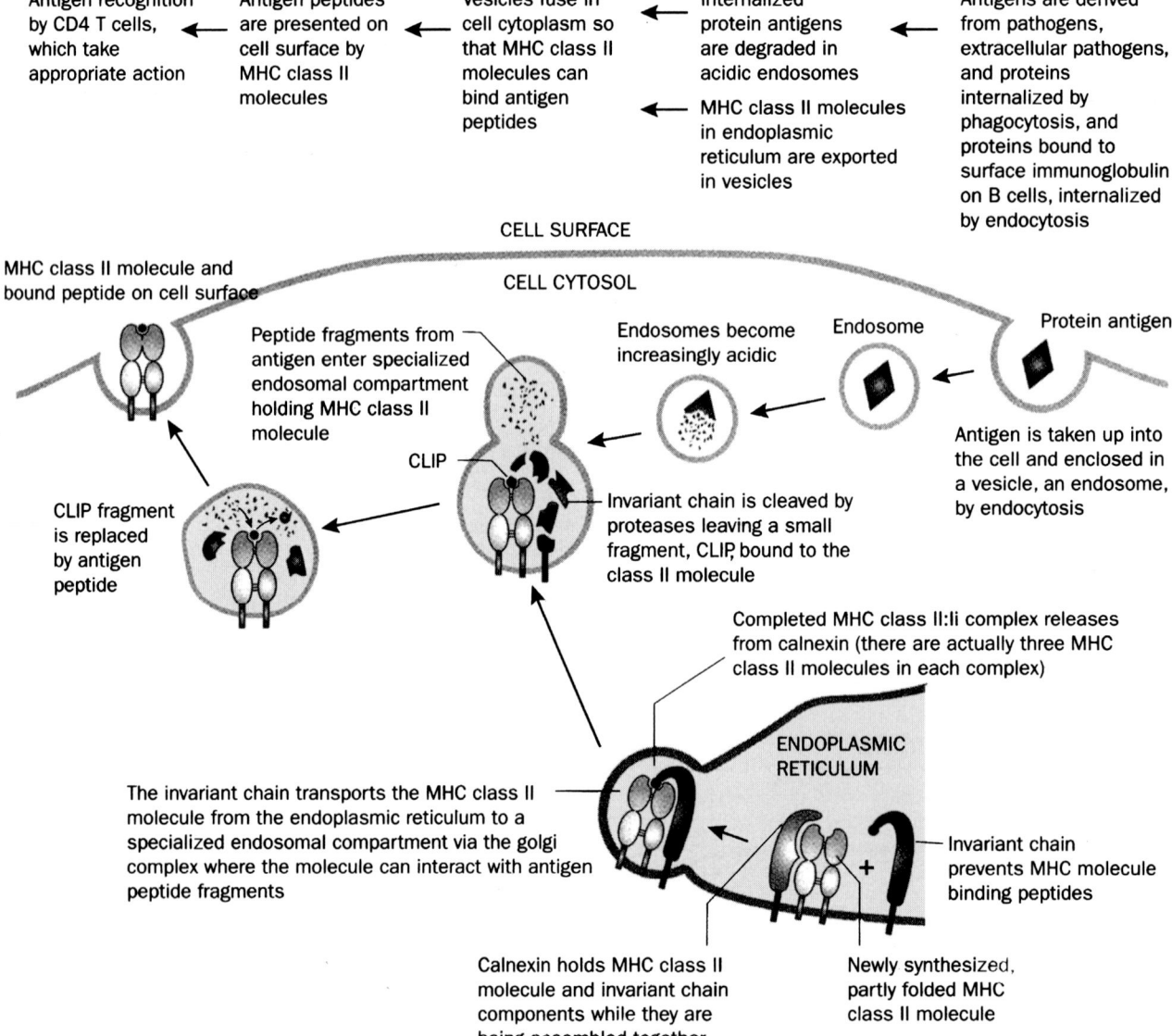

FIGURE 32-6. The pathway of exogenous antigen delivery to class II MHC molecules. MHC class II molecules assemble in the endoplasmic reticulum (ER) as a complex with the invariant chain (Ii). The MHC class II–Ii complex moves to specialized endosomal compartments. A small fragment of Ii, called CLIP, remains bound to the MHC class II molecule until it is replaced by an antigenic peptide. The bound peptide is further trimmed, and the peptide–MHC class II complex is expressed on the cell surface. (*Modified from Parkin J, Cohen B: An overview of the immune system. Lancet 357:1777–1789, 2001. With permission.*)

The factors that characterize each thymic microenvironment are still unidentified. Clearly, epithelial cells must act in concert with bone marrow–derived stromal cells, such as thymic interdigitating cells and macrophages. Consistent with diverse microenvironments in the gland, monoclonal antibody studies indicate regional diversity among thymic epithelial cells.[20]

The huge subcapsular cortical epithelial cells interact with differentiating thymic T cells in an unusual manner. T cells first bind to the surface of these large cells, which then engulf as many as 50 T cells. Some of the engulfed T cells persist and proliferate in membrane-bound vacuoles within the epithelial "nurse" cells.[21] A comparable number of T cells undergo apoptotic, programmed cell death, indicated by fragmentation of their nuclei. It is still not known whether the thymic nurse cells play a role in the positive selection of proliferating thymocytes or participate in negative selection, eliminating the undesirable cells by apoptosis, or both. It is clear, however, that the architectural integrity of the thymus is crucial for the normal development and organization of the immune system. For example, disruption of the structure of the gland by infection or by graft-vs.-host attack can profoundly disturb T-cell production, causing reduced resistance to microbial pathogens or an autoimmune disease.

The development and differentiation of thymic T-cell subsets can be monitored by changes in surface markers and in the expression of the T-cell receptor (TCR) genes. Productive of rearrangement of the TCR genes is an initial and key event in T-cell differentiation, and the progressive changes in TCR expression are closely linked to the induction and surface expression of the CD4 and CD8 markers on the differentiating cells.

Progenitor T cells arriving from the bone marrow lack rearranged TCRs and express neither the CD4 nor the CD8 marker (Fig. 32-7). At this stage, the structural genes of the TCR are still located in germline formations at separate chromosomal loci. Components of the TCR β-chain gene rearrange first, and the gene products appear on the cell membrane together with a primitive surrogate α chain. This is the signal for several differentiation steps. The first of these steps is induction of CD4 and CD8 expression; this is followed by rearrangement of the TCR α genes and the appearance of CD4/CD8 double-positive thymocytes expressing the TCR. These cells are now ready to undergo further maturational steps that eventually produce an intact, functional T-cell repertoire composed of CD4 or CD8 single-positive lymphocytes (Fig. 32-7).[22]

Generation of the mature T-cell repertoire involves intensive interactions between the TCR of the developing T cells

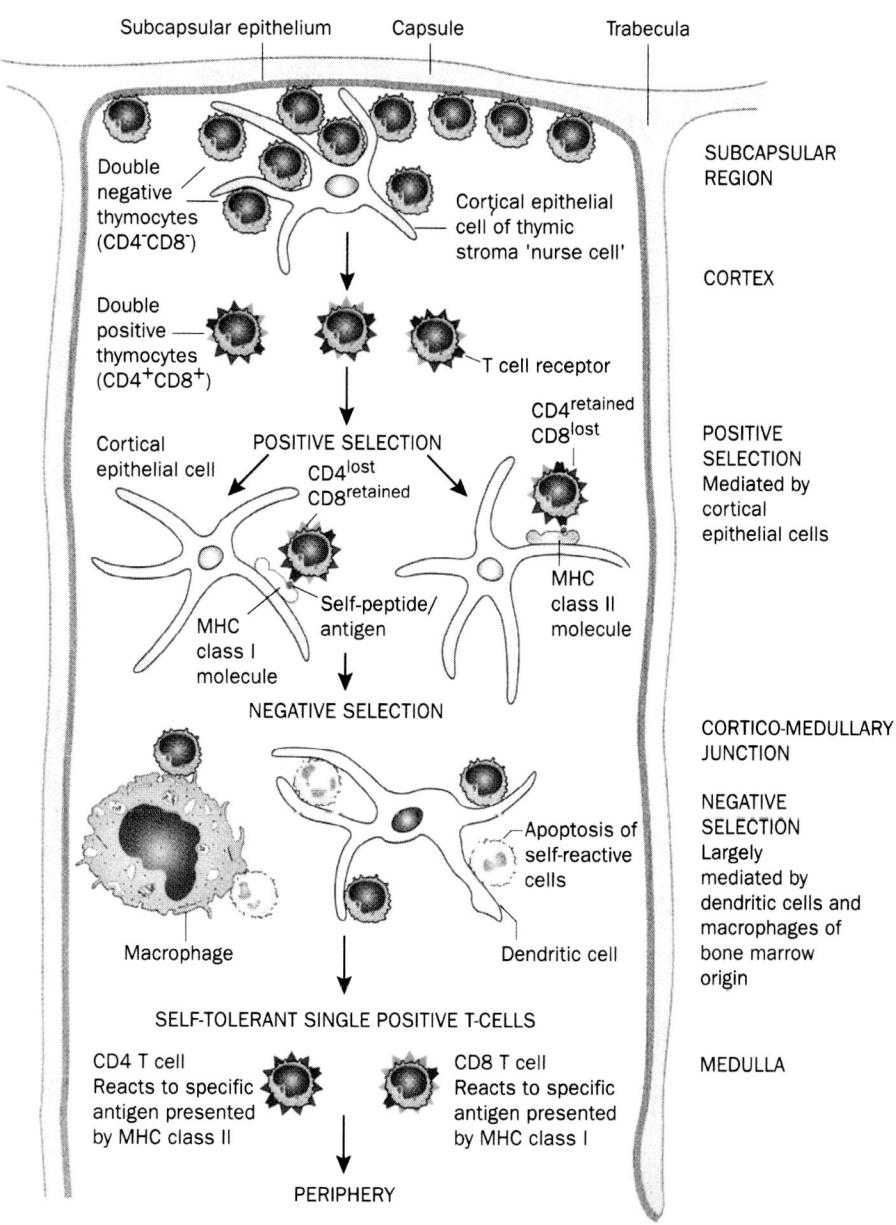

FIGURE 32-7. T-cell development in the thymus. Thymocytes enter the thymus in the subcapsular region. Cells bearing a T-cell receptor that recognizes self-MHC are positively selected in the cortex and pass into the corticomedullary junction. Here, T cells that react with self-antigens are deleted by apoptosis (negative selection). The cells that exit are self-tolerant but able to recognize foreign antigen when presented with self-MHC. (*Modified from Parkin J, Cohen B: An overview of the immune system. Lancet 357:1777–1789, 2001. With permission.*)

and the self-peptides expressed in the context of MHC molecules on the surface of thymic stroma cells. Two separate global rounds of T-cell selection take place. First, there is *positive* selection: All thymocytes are pushed into proliferation and express TCRs that bind to self-peptide/MHC complexes available within the thymus gland. During this phase of the self-recognition process, thymocytes that bind with low affinity to a readily available self-peptide/MHC complex, or with higher affinity to a rare self-peptide/MHC complex, are positively selected; high-avidity binding to a self-peptide is not a selective advantage.[23]

Next, there is a round of *negative* selection: Now all T-cell clones that bind with high affinity to highly concentrated self-antigen/MHC complexes are eliminated. Obviously, this is to prevent the generation of autoreactive T-cells that would attack the body's own tissues upon activation in the peripheral immune system.[24]

To summarize, T-cell differentiation in the thymus is an extremely complex process. It requires the sequential expression of genes by the differentiating cells as well as positive selection for T cells recognizing MHC and then negative selection of T cells directed against self-antigens. These events ultimately result in a T-cell population that efficiently reacts against foreign antigens but tolerates self-antigens. During the differentiation, the T cells traverse different, specialized stromal microenvironments and then enter the circulation. It also follows that a defect in the structure of any thymic compartment (or a disturbed thymic microenvironment) could cause, or be a consequence of, an immunologic aberration. This simple fact is particularly important for understanding the pathogenesis of myasthenia gravis (see Chap. 64).

ANTIGEN-PRESENTING CELLS

In contrast to B cells that can recognize soluble antigens via their immunoglobulin receptors, T cells can recognize only antigens presented on the surface of APCs. The most important APCs are the dendritic cells, whose only known function is to process and present antigens.[25,26] An important property of dendritic cells is that they can activate "naive" T cells—that is, T cells that have not previously been confronted with antigen. Together with macrophages and B cells, dendritic cells are known as "professional APCs." Under appropriate conditions, other cell types can also present antigens to T cells. Usually these "facultative APCs" need to be stimulated in some way to acquire antigen-presenting properties. A notable example of facultative APCs is myoblasts (see "Functional Interaction with T Cells," below). When stimulated with cytokines like interferon-γ, they upregulate MHC class I and II molecules on their surface and become capable of antigen presentation.

Dendritic cells arise from myeloid progenitor cells in the bone marrow. They migrate to peripheral tissues, where they display an immature phenotype—that is, they express low levels of MHC molecules and lack costimulatory B7 molecules. At this immature stage, they are not capable of antigen presentation. However, they are very active in taking up antigens. (Typical examples of immature dendritic cells are Langerhans cells in the skin.) After they have taken up antigens, they migrate via the lymphatics to the local lymphoid tissues, where they convert into mature dendritic cells, which have a totally different phenotype. The mature dendritic cells are no longer able to ingest antigens but express very high and stable levels of MHC molecules, adhesion molecules, and costimulatory molecules. These newly acquired properties enable them to stimulate naive T cells.

Dendritic cells are crucial not only for the defense against foreign pathogens and cancer cells but also for the induction and maintenance of self-tolerance. Some dendritic cells take up ubiquitous self-antigens, but in the absence of infection, they lack the appropriate costimulatory molecules to fully activate autoreactive T cells. On the contrary, they can render T cells tolerant or anergic. This mechanism contributes to the phenomenon of "peripheral tolerance." In addition, subsets of dendritic cells can influence the differentiation of T cells into Th1 and Th2 cells.[27]

ANTIBODY- AND CELL-MEDIATED CYTOTOXICITY

The destruction of antibody-coated target cells by NK cells is called antibody-dependent cell-mediated cytotoxicity (ADCC). This type of cytotoxic reaction is triggered when Fc receptors on the surface of NK cells interact with antibody bound to the target cell. NK cells express Fc-γ receptor III (CD16), which recognizes antibodies of IgG1 and IgG3 subclasses. The actual killing mechanism employed by NK cells is identical to that of cytotoxic T cells (CTLs), involving the release of cytotoxic granules containing perforin and granzymes (see below).

CTLs can kill by several different mechanisms.[28,29] A main pathway of cytotoxicity is mediated by the secretion of the pore-forming protein perforin by the cytotoxic T cell. An alternative, nonsecretory pathway relies on the interaction of the Fas ligand that is upregulated during T-cell activation with the apoptosis-inducing Fas receptor on the target cell. The perforin-dependent killing mechanism has central importance in polymyositis (see below and Chap. 49).

The central killing mechanism of CTLs involves the calcium-dependent release of lytic granules upon recognition of antigen on a target cell. The granules contain at least two distinct classes of cytotoxic proteins, perforin and granzymes. Perforin polymerizes to form transmembrane pores in the target-cell membrane. The pores allow the entry of cytotoxic mediators such as granzymes. The term *granzymes* refers to a group of at least three different serine proteases which seem to be able to induce apoptosis in any type of target cell.

In addition to the perforin-mediated killing mechanism, cytotoxic T cells can kill by a nonsecretory, ligand-mediated mechanism.[28,29] This second killing mechanism requires the interaction between Fas (expressed on the target cell) and Fas ligand (expressed on the T cell) (Fig. 32-8). Ligation of Fas (CD95) recruits adaptor molecules (such as procaspase-8 and -10) to the receptor. By being brought into proximity with one another, these procaspases cleave their nearest neighbors to form active, mature caspases.[30] The active caspases efficiently cleave procaspase-3 and other executioner caspases, and apoptosis proceeds (Fig. 32-8).

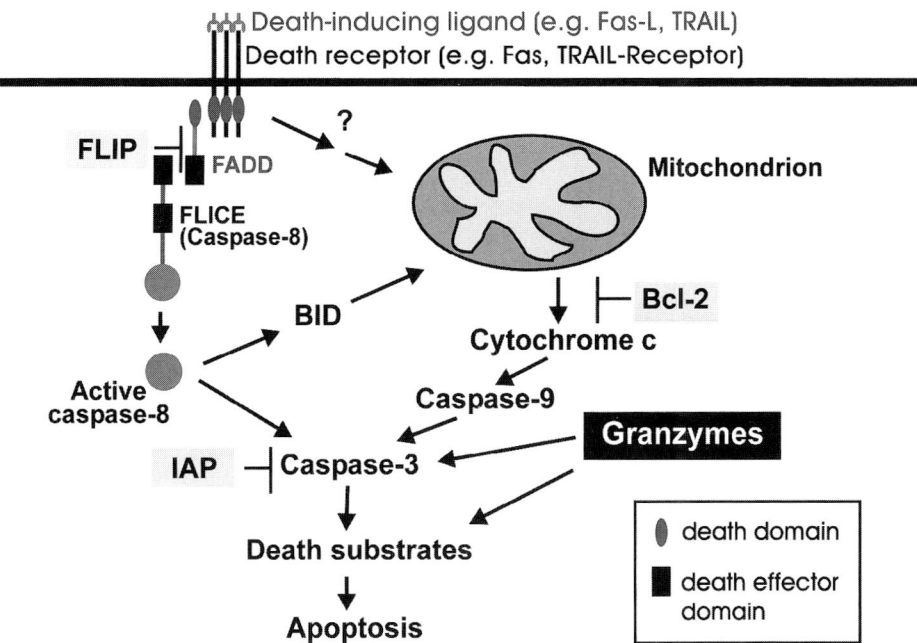

FIGURE 32-8. Scheme of the signaling pathways that induce cell death (apoptosis). Apoptosis can occur via extrinsic and intrinsic pathways. Both pathways converge into proteolytic cleavage events mediated by "effector" caspases, such as caspase 3. Caspase 3 is activated by "initiator" caspases, such as caspases 8 and 9, and inhibited by inhibitor of apoptosis protein (IAP). The extrinsic pathway can be mediated by ligand-dependent signals [e.g., Fas-ligand; TNF-related apoptosis-inducing ligand (TRAIL), or secretion (as by granzyme)]. Ligand binding to "death receptor" complexes leads to the recruitment of procaspase-8 via the adaptor molecule [Fas-associated death domain (FADD)]. This pathway is modulated by several factors, including FLIP (FLICE inhibitory protein; FLICE is an alternative designation for caspase-8).

Intrinsic death signals are communicated through the mitochondrial release of cytochrome c. This pathway is highly dependent on the stoichiometry of anti- versus proapoptotic Bcl-2 family members. Controversy surrounds the degree to which cross talk occurs between the extrinsic and intrinsic pathways in vivo. At a molecular level, this appears to occur via the proteolysis of BID, which normally serves an antiapoptotic role within the intrinsic pathway until it is truncated by caspase-8 (derived from the extrinsic pathway). (BID is not an abbreviation but a conventional designation for one of approximately 20 members of the Bcl-2 protein family).

Cytotoxic T cells (CTL) kill by extrinsic signals, mediated either by the binding of Fas-ligand (expressed on the CTL) to Fas (expressed on the target cell), or by secretion-dependent pathways. Secretion-dependent killing depends on proteolytic enzymes called granzymes, which are secreted by the CTL. The granzymes enter the target cell, where they act on caspase-3 and other components of the apoptotic pathway.

Principles of Cellular Communication

ADHESION AND MIGRATION OF IMMUNE CELLS

Adhesion molecules are cell-surface proteins that participate in leukocyte circulation, homing to tissues and inflammatory sites, and transendothelial migration. Interaction of these molecules with their specific ligands mediates adherence of leukocytes to other cells, the vascular endothelium, and the extracellular matrix (reviewed in Ref. 31). In particular, adhesion molecules participate in essentially all cellular interactions between immune cells. The classes of "adhesion molecules" and "costimulatory molecules" (see below) overlap, because many of these molecules mediate not only adhesion but also transmission of costimulatory signals.

Adhesion molecules are classified into several groups, including selectins, integrins, and members of the immunoglobulin superfamily (Table 32-1).[31] *Selectins* are expressed on leukocytes, platelets, and endothelial cells. Their common structural component is an N-terminal lectin-binding domain. Accordingly, selectins bind to glycosylated and sialylated ligands with a rapid association and dissociation constant. Selectins mediate leukocyte "rolling" along the endothelial cell wall and are involved in the initial localization of leukocytes to inflammatory sites (Fig. 32-9). There, the slowed, rolling leukocytes are exposed to chemoattractants and cytokines, leading to leukocyte activation, upregulation of additional adhesion molecules, adherence to the endothelial lining, and eventually diapedesis and chemotaxis (Fig. 32-9). The most prominent *chemoattractants* that bind to specific receptors with seven transmembrane domains and transmit intracellular signals through G proteins include various chemokines, activated complement component C5 (C5a), platelet-activating factor (PAF), leukotriene B4 (LTB4), and formyl peptides.

Integrins are heterodimeric adhesion molecules composed of noncovalently bound α and β subunits. Different combinations of subunits form functionally different receptors.

Table 32-1 ADHESION MOLECULES

Adhesion Molecule	Tissue Distribution	Ligand
Immunoglobulin superfamily		
ICAM-1	Endothelial cells, monocytes, T and B cells, dendritic cells, keratinocytes, chondrocytes, epithelial cells	LFA-1
ICAM-2	Endothelial cells, monocytes, dendritic cells, subpopulations of lymphocytes	LFA-1
ICAM-3	Lymphocytes	LFA-1, Mac 1
VCAM-1	Endothelial cells, kidney epithelium, macrophages, dendritic cells, myoblasts, bone marrow fibroblasts	VLA-4
PECAM-1	Platelets, T cells, endothelial cells, monocytes, granulocytes	?
MAdCAM-1	Endothelial venules in mucosal lymph nodes	$\alpha 4\beta 7$ integrin and L-selectin
Selectin family		
E-selectin/ELAM-1	Endothelial cells	?
L-selectin	Lymphocytes, neutrophils, monocytes	CD34
P-selectin	Megakaryocytes, platelets, and endothelial cells	?
Integrin family		
VLA subfamily		
VLA-1 to VLA-4	Endothelial cells, resting T cells, monocytes, platelets and epithelial cells	Various molecules including laminin, fibronectin, collagen, and VCAM1
VLA-5 (fibronectin receptor)	Endothelial cells, monocytes and platelets	Laminin
VLA-6 (laminin receptor)	Endothelial cells, monocytes and platelets	Laminin
$\beta 1\alpha 7$	Endothelial cells, ?	Laminin
$\beta 1\alpha 8$	Endothelial cells, ?	?
$\beta 1\alpha$	Platelets and megakaryocytes	Fibronectin
$\beta 2$	Widely distributed	Collagen, laminin, vitronectin
Leucam subfamily		
LFA-1	Leucocytes	ICAMs-1 to 3
Mac-1	Endothelial cells, ?	ICAM-1, fibrinogen, C3bi
Cytoadhesin subfamily		
Vitronectin receptor	Platelets and megakaryocytes	Vitronectin, fibrinogen, laminin, fibronectin, von Willebrand factor, thrombospondin
$\beta 4\alpha 6$	Endothelial cells, thymocytes and platelets	Laminin
$\beta 5\alpha$	Platelets and megakaryocytes, ?	Vitronectin, fibronectin
$\beta 6\alpha$	Platelets and megakaryocytes, ?	Fibronectin
$\beta 7\alpha 4$/LPAM-1	Endothelial cells, thymocytes, monocytes	Fibronectin, VCAM-1
$\beta 8\alpha$	Platelets and megakaryocytes, ?	?

SOURCE: From Parkin J, Cohen B: An overview of the immune system. *Lancet* 357:1777–1789, 2001.[83] Reproduced by permission.
ABBREVIATIONS: ICAM = intercellular adhesion molecules; VCMA = vascular cell adhesion molecule; MAdCAM-1 = mucosal addressin; E-selectin or ELAM = endothelial leukocyte adhesion molecule; LPAM = lymphocyte Peyer's patch adhesion molecule; PECAM = platelet/endothelial cell adhesion molecule; VLA = very late antigen.

Integrins bind to a variety of extracellular matrix proteins (e.g., fibronectin, vitronectin, laminin, collagen) and to receptors of the immunoglobulin superfamily. Two prototypical integrin adhesion molecules are the leukocyte function antigen (LFA)-1 and the very late antigen (VLA)-4. LFA-1 is expressed on most circulating leukocytes, binds to intercellular adhesion molecules (ICAM)-1 and -2, and acts as a cell adhesion and costimulatory molecule in T-cell activation. VLA-4, also found on activated leukocytes, adheres to fibronectin and vascular cell adhesion molecule (VCAM)-1, an adhesion receptor of the immunoglobulin family expressed on vascular endothelial cells. An important feature of integrins is that they exist in different conformational states. An activated cell can transmit a signal from its cytoplasm, which modifies the conformation of the extracellular domains of integrins on the cell surface, increasing the affinity of the integrins for their ligands ("inside-out signaling").

CYTOKINES AND CHEMOKINES

Cytokines are soluble peptides that mediate intercellular communication. They act by binding to high-affinity receptors expressed on target cells and by inducing biochemical signals within those cells. Cytokines are released not only by cells of the immune system but also by many other cell types. Many effects of cytokines are redundant; that is, different cytokines can induce similar or identical effects. Furthermore, most cytokines have a multitude of different biological effects; that is, they are "pleiotropic" (Tables 32-2 and 32-3).

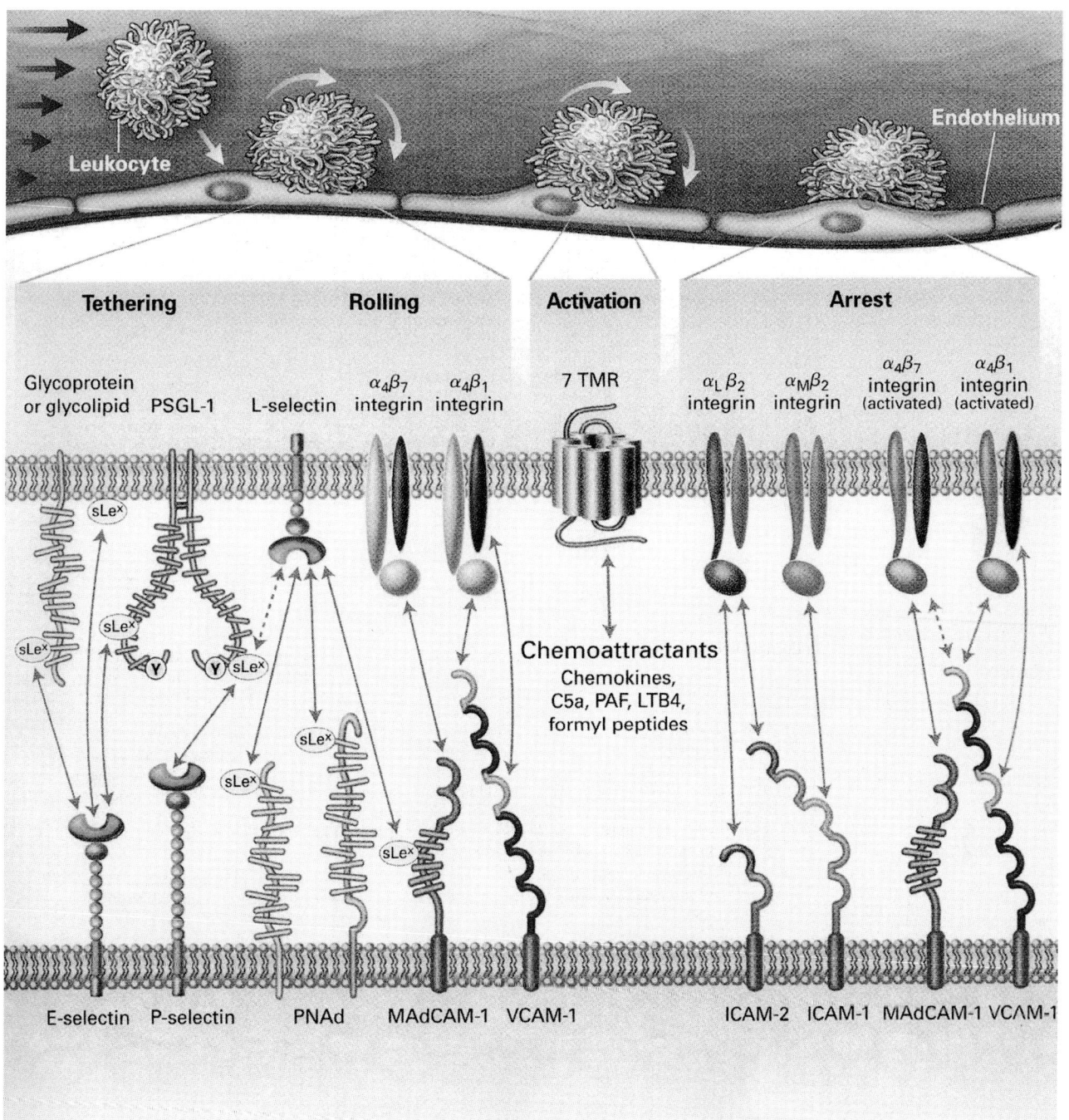

FIGURE 32-9. Molecules of the adhesion cascade. Leukocytes in the bloodstream become tethered to endothelial cells and roll slowly downstream. The most efficient tethering molecules are L-selectin and P-selectin. Rolling leukocytes respond to chemoattractants on endothelial cells because they express specific receptors with seven transmembrane domains (7 TMR), which transmit intracellular signals through G proteins. The activating signal induces activation of different integrins, which bind to members of the endothelial immunoglobulin superfamily. *Abbreviations:* C5a, activated complement component 5; ICAM-1 (2), intercellular adhesion molecule 1 (2); LTB4, leukotriene B4; MAdCAM-1, mucosal addressin-cell adhesion molecule type 1; PAF, platelet-activating factor; PNAd, peripheral-node addressin; sLe^x, sulfated sialyl-Lewis^x; PSGL-1, P-selectin glycoprotein ligand 1; VCAM-1, vascular-cell adhesion molecule 1; Y, N-terminal motif containing three tyrosines. (*Modified from von Andrian UH, Mackay CR: T-cell function and migration. Two sides of the same coin. N Engl J Med 343:1020–1034, 2000. With permission. See also Table 32-1.*)

Table 32-2 CYTOKINES AND THEIR RECEPTORS

Family	Cytokine (alternative names)	Size (no. of amino acids) and form	Receptors ("c" Denotes common subunit)	Producer Cells	Actions	Effect of Cytokine or Receptor Knockout (where known)
Hematopoietins (four-helix bundles)						
	Epo (erythropoietin)	165, monomer	EpoR	Kidney cells, hepatocytes	Stimulates erythroid progenitors	Epo or EpoR: embryonic lethal
	IL-2 (T-cell growth factor)	133, monomer	CD25(α), CD122 (β), CD132 (γc)	T cells	T-cell proliferation	IL-2: deregulated T-cell proliferation, colitis IL-2Rα: incomplete T-cell development; IL-2Rβ: increased T-cell autoimmunity; IL-2γ: severe combined immunodeficiency
	IL-3 (multicolony CSF)	133, monomer	CD123, βc	T cells, thymic epithelial cells	Synergistic action in early hematopoiesis	IL-3: impaired eosinophil development; bone marrow unresponsive to IL-5, GM-CSF
	IL-4 (BCGF-1, BSF-1)	129, monomer	CD124, CD132 (γc)	T cells, mast cells	B-cell activation, IgE switch suppresses Th1 cells	IL-4: decreased IgE synthesis
	IL-5 (BCGF-2)	115, homodimer	CD125, βc	T cells, mast cells	Eosinophil growth, differentiation	IL-5: decreased IgE, IgG1 synthesis (in mice); decreased levels of IL-9, IL-10 and eosinophils
	IL-6 (IFN-β_2 BSF-2 BCDF)	184, monomer	CD126, CD130	T cells, macrophages, endothelial cells	T- and B-cell growth and differentiation, acute phase protein production fever	IL-6: decreased acute phase reaction, reduced IgA production
	IL-7	152, monomer	CD127, CD132 (γc)	Non-T cells	Growth of pre-B cells and Pre-T cells	IL-7: early thymic and lymphocyte expansion severely impaired
	IL-9	125, monomer	IL-9R, CD132 (γc)	T cells	Mast-cell enhancing activity, stimulates Th2	
	IL-11	178, monomer	IL-11R, CD130	Stromal fibroblasts	Synergistic action with IL-3 and IL-4 in hematopoiesis	
	IL-13 (P600)	132, monomer	IL-13R, CD132 (γc) (may also include CD24)	T cells	B-cell growth and differentiation, inhibits macrophage inflammatory and cytokine production and Th1 cells	IL-13: defective regulation of isotype-specific responses
	G-CSF	?, monomer	G-CSFR	Fibroblasts and monocytes	Stimulates neutrophil development and differentiation	Defective myelopoiesis, neutropenia
	IL-15 (T-cell growth factor)	114, monomer	IL-15R, CD122 (1L-Rβ) CD132 (γC)	Many non T-cells	IL-2-like, stimulates growth of intestinal epithelium, T cells and NK cells	
	GM-CSF (granulocyte-macrophage colony stimulating factor)	127, monomer	CD116, βc	Macrophages, T cells	Stimulates growth and differentiation of myelomonocytic lineage cells, particularly dendritic cells	GM-CSF, GM-CSFR: pulmonary alveolar proteinosis

Name	Size (aa), form	Receptors	Actions	Effect of knockout or (deficiency)
OSM (OM/oncostatin M)	196, monomer	OSMR cr LIFR, CD130	T cells, macrophages	Stimulates Kaposi's sarcoma cells, inhibits melanoma growth	
LIF (leukemia inhibitory factor)	179, monomer	LIFR, CD130	Bone marrow stroma, fibroblasts	Maintains embryonic stem cells, like IL-6, IL-11, OSM	LIFR: die at or soon after birth; decreased hematopoietic stem cells
Interferons					
IFN-γ	143, homodimer	CD119, IFNGR2	T cells, NK cells	Macrophage activation, increased expression of MHC molecules and antigen processing components, Ig class switching, suppresses Th2	IFNγ, IFNγR: decreased resistance to bacterial infection, especially mycobacteria and certain viruses, impaired Th1 responses
IFN-α	166, monomer	CD118, IFNAR2	Leukocytes	Antiviral, increased MHC class I expression	IFN-α: impaired antiviral defences
IFN-β	166, monomer	CD118, IFNAR2	Fibroblasts	Antiviral, increased MHC class 1 expression	
Immunoglobulin superfamily					
B7.1 (CD80)	262, dimer	CD28, CTLA-4	Antigen-presenting cells	Costimulation of T-cell responses	CD28: decreased T-cell responses
B7.2 (B70, CD86)		CD28, CTLA-4	Antigen-presenting cells	Costimulation of T-cell responses	B7.2: decreased co-stimulator response to alloantigen. CTLA-4: massive lymphoproliferation, early death
TNF family					
TNF-α (cachectin)	157, trimers	p55, p75, CD120a, CD120b	Macrophages, NK cells, T cells	Local inflammation, endothelial activation	TNF-αR: resistance to septic shock, susceptibility to *Listeria* STNF-αR: periodic febrile attacks
TNF-β (lymphotoxin LT, LT-α)	171, trimers	p55, p75, CD120a, CD120b	T cells, B cells	Killing, endothelial activation	TNF-β: absent lymph nodes, decreased antibody, increased IgM
LT-β	Transmembrane, trimerizes with TNF-β, (LT-α)	LTβ3 or HVEM	T cells, B cells	Lymph node development	Defective development of peripheral lymph nodes, Peyer's patches and spleen
CD40 ligand (CD40L)	Trimers	CD40	T cells, mast cells	B-cell activation, class switching	CD40L: poor antibody response, no class switching, diminished T-cell priming (hyper-IgM syndrome)
Fas ligand (FasL)	Trimers	CD95 (Fas)	T cells, stroma?	Apoptosis, Ca²⁺ independent cytotoxicity	Fas, FasL: mutant forms lead to lymphproliferation and autoimmunity
CD27 ligand (CD27L)	Trimers (?)	CD27	T cells	Stimulates T-cell proliferation	
CD30 ligand (CD30L)	Trimers (?)	CD30	T cells	Stimulates T- and B-cell proliferation	CD30: increased thymic size, alloreactivity
4-1BBL	Trimer (?)	4-1BB	T cells	Co-stimulates T and B cells	
Trail	281, aa trimers	DCR4, DR5, DCR1, DCR2, DCR6, and OPG	T cells, monocytes	Apoptosis of activated T cells and tumor cells	
OPG-L (Rank-L)	316, aa trimers	RANK/OPG	Osteoblasts, T cells	Stimulates osteoclasts and bone resorption	OPG-L: osteopetrotic, runted, toothless; OPG: osteoporosis

(Continued)

Table 32-2 (Continued). CYTOKINES AND THEIR RECEPTORS

Family	Cytokine (alternative names)	Size (no. of amino acids) and Form	Receptors (c Denotes common subunit)	Producer Cells	Actions	Effect of Cytokine or Receptor Knockout (where known)
Unassigned	TGF-β	112, homo- and heterotrimers	TGF-βR	Chondrocytes, monocytes, T cells	Inhibits cell growth, anti-inflammatory, induces IgA secretion	TGF-β: lethal inflammation
	IL-1α	159, monomer	CD121a (IL-1RI) and CD-121b (IL-1RII)	Macrophages, epithelial cells	Fever, T-cell activation, macrophage activation	IL-1RI: decreased IL-6 production
	IL-1β	153, monomer	CD121a (IL-1RI) and CD121b (IL-1RII)	Macrophages, epithelial cells	Fever, T-cell activation, macrophage activation	IL-1β: impaired acute phase response
	IL-1 RA	?, monomer	CD121a	Monocytes, macrophages, neutrophils, hepatocytes	Binds to but does not trigger IL-1 receptor, acts as a natural antagonist of IL-1 function	IL-1RA: reduced body mass, increased sensitivity to endotoxins (septic shock)
	IL-10 (cytokine synthesis inhibitor F)	160, homodimer	IL-10Rα, CRF2-4 (IL-10Rβ)	T cells, macrophages, EBV-transformed B cells	Potent suppressant of macrophage functions	IL-10 or CRF2-4: reduced growth, anemia, chronic enterocolitis
	IL-12 (NK-cell stimulatory factor)	197 and 306, heterodimer	IL-12Rβ1 IL-12Rβ2	B cells, macrophages	Activates NK cells, induces CD4 T-cell differentiation to Th1-like cells	IL-12: impaired in IFN-γ production and Th1 responses
	MIF	115, monomer		T cells, pituitary cells	Inhibits macrophage migration, stimulates macrophage activation, induces steroid resistance	MIF: resistance to septic shock
	IL-16	130, homotetramer		CD4 T cells, mast cells, eosinophils	Chemoattractant for CD4 T cells, monocytes, and eosinophils; antiapoptotic for IL-2 stimulated T cells	
	IL-17 (mCTLA-8)	150, monomer		CD-4 memory cells	Induce cytokine production by epithelia, endothelia, and fibroblasts	
	IL-18 (IGIF, IFN-γ inducing factor)	157, monomer	Il-1Rrp(IL-1R related protein)	Activated macrophages and Kupffer cells	Induces IFN-γ production by T cells and NK cells, favors Th1 induction and later Th2 responses	Defective NK activity and Th1 responses.

SOURCE: From Janeway CA: *Immunobiology: The Immune System in Health and Disease.* New York: Garland, 2001.[84] Reproduced by permission.

Table 32-3 PROPERTIES OF SELECTED CHEMOKINES

Class	Chemokine	Produced by	Receptors	Cells Attracted	Major Effects
CXC	IL-8	Monocytes, macrophages, fibroblasts, keratinocytes, endothelial cells	CXCR1, CXCR2	Neutrophils, naive T cells	Mobilizes, activates, and degranulates neutrophils, angiogenesis
	PBP, β-TG, NAP-2	Platelets	CXCR2	Neutrophils	Activates neutrophils, clot resorption, angiogenesis
	GROα, β, γ	Monocytes, fibroblasts, endothelium	CXCR2	Neutrophils, naive T cells, fibroblasts	Activates neutrophils, fibroplasia, angiogenesis
	IP-10	Keratinocytes, monocytes, T cells, fibroblasts, endothelium	CXCR3	Resting T cells, NK cells, monocytes	Immunostimulant, antiangiogenic, promotes Th1 immunity
	SDF-1	Stromal cells	CXCR4	Naive T cells, progenitor (CD34+) B cells	B-cell development, lymphocyte homing, competes with HIV-1
	BLC	Stromal cells	CXCR5	B cells	Lymphocyte homing
CC	MIP-1α	Monocytes, T cells, mast cells, fibroblasts	CCR1, 3, 5	Monocytes, NK and T cells, basophils, dendritic cells	Competes with HIV-1, antiviral defense, promotes Th1 immunity
	MIP-1β	Monocytes, macrophages, neutrophils, endothelium	CCR1, 3, 5	Monocytes, NK and T cells, dendritic cells	Competes with HIV-1
	MCP-1	Monocytes, macrophages, fibroblasts, keratinocytes	CCR2B	Monocytes, NK and T cells, basophils, dendritic cells	Activates macrophages, basophil histamine release, promotes Th2 immunity
	RANTES	T cells, endothelium, platelets	CCR1, 3, 5	Monocytes, NK and T cells, basophils, eosinophils, dendritic cells	Degranulates basophils, activates T cells, chronic inflammation
	Eotaxin	Endothelium, monocytes, epithelium, T cells	CCR3	Eosinophils, monocytes, T cells	Role in allergy
	DC-CK	Dendritic cells	?	Naive T cells	Role in activating naive T cells
C	Lymphotactin	CD8 > CD4 T cells	?	Thymocytes, dendritic cells, NK cells	Lympocyte trafficking and development
CXXXC (CX$_3$C)	Fractalkine	Monocytes, endothelium, microglial cells	CX$_3$CR1	Monocytes, T cells	Leukocyte-endothelial adhesion, brain inflammation

SOURCE: From Janeway CA: *Immunobiology: The Immune System in Health and Disease.* New York: Garland, 2001.[84] Reproduced by permission.

The receptors for cytokines can be grouped into families. Signaling by these receptors depends on their association with a family of protein tyrosine kinases termed Janus kinases (Jaks), which couple ligand binding to tyrosine phosphorylation of intracellular signaling proteins recruited to the receptor complex. Among these are the signal transducers and activators of transcription (STATs), a family of transcription factors that contribute to the diversity of cytokine responses.[32] The functional redundancy of cytokines can partly be explained by different members of a subfamily sharing a common signal-transducing receptor component.

The ligand cytokines can also be grouped into families on the basis of their structure, genetic organization, and cellular source.[33] Cytokine families include the hematopoietins, interferons, immunoglobulin superfamily members (Table 32-2), and chemokines[33] (Table 32-3). It appears that cytokines and their receptors have diversified together during evolution. In higher animals, the "cytokine network" has reached such an enormous complexity that it is impossible to conceptualize it in a simple scheme. The complexity of the cytokine network is further increased by the fact that the functional network involves not only soluble cytokines but also soluble cytokine receptors in addition to membrane-associated receptors and, in some cases, membrane-associated cytokines ("tethered ligands"). A soluble form of receptor exists for many if not most cytokines and is usually generated by proteolytic cleavage of the receptor protein or by alternative splicing of its messenger RNA.[34]

The principles of immune regulation via the cytokine network can be illustrated with the paradigm of T helper 1 (Th1) and T helper 2 (Th2) cells.[14] Th1 cells act as "inflammatory" T cells, which induce and directly participate in inflammatory ("delayed type-hypersensitivity") reactions and contribute to tissue injury. In contrast, Th2 cells stimulate antibody production by B cells and enhance eosinophil functions. For example, in myasthenia gravis, Th2 cells are thought to play a pivotal role by stimulating autoreactive B cells to produce the pathogenic anti-AChR autoantibodies. Th1 and Th2 cells each produce a characteristic and distinct spectrum of cytokines.[14] Th1 cells secrete IL-2, interferon-γ, and lymphotoxin, whereas Th2 cells produce IL-4, IL-5, IL-6, IL-9, IL-10, and IL-13. Several other cytokines are secreted by both Th1 and Th2 cells, including IL-3, TNF-α, granulocyte-macrophage colony-stimulating factor (GM-CSF) and members of the chemokine families (see below). T cells that produce both Th1 and Th2 cytokines are sometimes referred to as "Th0" cells. Individual T-cell clones may show rather complex patterns of cytokine production, but it appears that the majority can be broadly categorized as either Th1, Th2, or Th0. Differences between cells in cytokine expression may represent distinct stable phenotypes, transient developmental stages, or transient responses to stimulation conditions.[35]

The characteristic cytokine products of Th1 and Th2 cells are mutually inhibitory for the differentiation and effector functions of the reciprocal phenotype. For example, interferon-γ selectively inhibits the proliferation of Th2 cells, and IL-10 inhibits cytokine synthesis by Th1 cells. It is likely that in vivo, cytokine-induced changes in the overall pattern of cytokine secretion are brought about by changes at both the population and single-cell levels. Any disturbance in the delicate balance between Th1 and Th2 cells may favor pathologic autoimmune reactions, mediated either by autoaggressive inflammatory T cells (which would be stimulated by Th1 cytokines) or by pathogenic B cells and autoantibodies (which would be stimulated by Th2 cytokines). It should be noted, however, that this appealingly simple scheme is an oversimplification, and that many exceptions occur where Th1 or Th2 cytokines have unexpected or even paradoxical effects.[36]

Another example for a complex cytokine cascade is the IL-1 system. IL-1 is a major proinflammatory cytokine produced by monocytes and macrophages.[37] Two types of IL-1 (IL-1α and IL-1β) have been described, which display similar activities. The production and action of IL-1 are regulated by multiple control pathways, some of which are unique to this cytokine.[37] In addition to the two agonists, the IL-1 system consists of a specific activation system (IL-1 converting enzyme, or ICE), a receptor antagonist (IL-1ra) produced in different isoforms, and two (type I and II) high-affinity receptors. The biological activity of IL-1 is counterbalanced by three types of inhibitors, namely (1) the naturally occurring IL-1 receptor antagonist, which competitively binds IL-1 receptor without inducing signal transduction; (2) soluble IL-1 receptors, which bind IL-1 and diminish the free concentration of the soluble cytokine, thus hampering its binding to the cell surface receptor; and (3) the membrane-associated "decoy" (type II) receptor, a nonsignaling molecule whose function is to prevent the ligand from interacting with the signal-transducing (type I) receptor on the same cell. Recombinant IL-1 receptor antagonist and soluble IL-1 receptor constructs might be useful for therapeutic modulation of the immune system[38] (see "Novel Targets for Therapeutic Modulation," below, for a more detailed discussion of immunomodulatory strategies).

Chemokines are a subgroup of cytokines with chemoattractant properties. Chemokines direct the migration of leukocytes toward sites of inflammation.[39,40] The receptors of chemokines are single-chain transmembrane molecules coupled to G proteins. Some chemokine receptors are promiscuous in ligand binding.

The chemokines are divided into several closely related polypeptide families, which display and are named after conserved cysteine amino acid residues. The CXC chemokine family has the first two amino-terminal cysteines separated by one nonconserved residue; the CC chemokine family has the first two amino-terminal cysteines in juxtaposition; the C chemokine (lymphotactin) has one lone amino-terminal cysteine; and the CXXXC chemokine (fractalkine) has two cysteines separated by three indifferent amino acids (Table 32-3). The CC chemokines include RANTES, macrophage inflammatory protein (MIP)-1α, MIP-1β, monocyte chemoattractant protein (MCP)-1, MCP-2, and MCP-3. The CXC chemokines include IL-8, interferon-γ–inducible protein-10 (IP-10), and other members. The CXC chemokines can be divided further by the presence or absence of an amino acid triplet (glutamic acid-leucine-arginine, or ELR) preceding the first of these invariant cysteines. All the chemokines that attract neutrophils have this motif, whereas most of the other CXC chemokines lack it. Most CC chemokines attract monocytes and T cells. Some CXC chemokines also attract T cells (Table 32-3). Furthermore, the CC chemokines MIP-1α and -1β, RANTES, and MCP-1 can provide costimulatory signals to T cells.[41]

THE IMMUNOLOGIC SYNAPSE

The activation of antigen-specific immune cells, that is, B-lymphocytes and T-lymphocytes, is an intricate, still incompletely understood process. In many respects the contact and signaling between an APC and a T cell resembles the contact and signaling between neurons and has therefore been aptly termed the *immunologic synapse* (Fig. 32-10).

The center of the synapse is formed by the "trimolecular complex" (TMC). It consists of the antigenic peptide, which is typically 10 to 20 amino acids long and bound to a major histocompatibility complex (MHC or HLA) molecule on the surface of the APC, and the clonotypic antigen-specific receptor of the T cell. Signaling is mediated by the invariant proteins of the CD3 complex associated with the T-cell receptor (TCR). The efficiency of TCR triggering depends on the capacity of a peptide/MHC ligand to stimulate the TCR long enough for the necessary phosphorylation steps of the cytoplasmic signaling cascade to be completed. This leads to recruitment and activation of zeta-associated protein-70 (ZAP-70) and transmission of the signal to downstream adaptors.[42] The coreceptors CD4 and CD8, which bind to relatively invariant sites on MHC class II and class I molecules, respectively, serve to "boost" recognition of the ligand by the TCR.

Before signaling via the TCR can occur, the T cell has to come into close physical contact with the APC. This adhesion process depends on interactions between various adhesion molecules expressed on the surface of the T cell (e.g., integrins such as LFA-1 and VLA-4, and nonintegrin molecules such as CD2) and their counterreceptors on the APC (ICAM-1, ICAM-2, VCAM, CD58) (Table 32-1 and Fig. 32-10). T cells initially bind APCs through low-affinity, integrin-mediated adhesion interactions. Subsequent signaling through the TCR induces a conformational change in the integrins, which causes them to bind with higher affinity to their partner molecules on the antigen-presenting cell. The activated integrins then help to stabilize the association between the antigen-specific T cell and the APC.

The kinetics of synapse formation has been studied in living cells.[43] Initially, peptide/MHC complexes are located in an outer ring of the nascent synapse. Within minutes, these complexes are transported into the center of the synapse. In the mature synapse, the integrin-related adhesion molecules form an outer ring around the centrally located TCRs (not shown in Fig. 32-10; reviewed in Ref. 43). Interestingly, agrin has recently been shown to have an important role in formation of the immunologic synapse. Lymphocytes express the Z$^-$ isoform of agrin. In activated lymphocytes, agrin colocalizes with clustered T-cell receptors and seems to be impor-

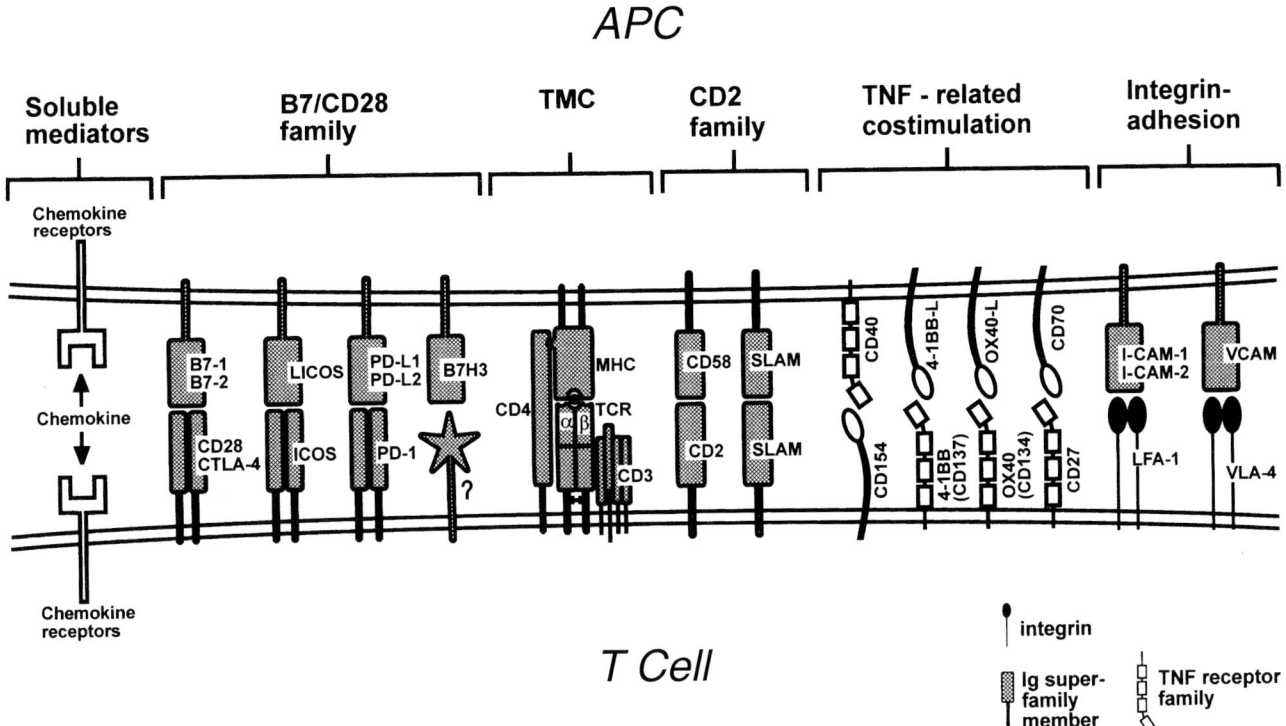

FIGURE 32-10. Schematic view of the "immunologic synapse." The figure shows some of the molecular interactions that occur at the interface between an antigen-presenting cell (APC) (top) and a CD4+ T cell (bottom). The interacting molecules are grouped into soluble mediators; costimulatory molecules of the B7/CD28, CD2, and TNF/TNF-R families; adhesion molecules of the integrin family; and the trimolecular complex (TMC). See text for details. *Abbreviations:* CD, cluster of differentiation nomenclature; CTLA-4, cytotoxic T lymphocyte antigen 4; ICAM, intercellular adhesion molecule; ICOS, inducible costimulator; LFA, leukocyte function–associated antigen; LICOS, ligand of the inducible costimulator; MHC, major histocompatibility complex; SLAM, signaling lymphocyte activation molecule; TCR, T-cell receptor for antigen; TMC, trimolecular complex; TNF, tumor necrosis factor; VCAM, vascular-cell adhesion molecule; VLA, very late antigen.

tant in the reorganization of membrane lipid microdomains and setting the threshold for T-cell signaling. Thus it appears that agrin induces the aggregation of signaling proteins and the creation of signaling domains in both the immune and nervous systems through a common lipid raft pathway.[44]

It has been known for a long time that T cells require two types of signal for activation: Signal 1 is provided through the TCR, and a second, costimulatory signal (signal 2) is provided through one or several "costimulatory molecules." For example, the CD28 molecule on T cells binds to B7-1 or B7-2 on APCs, thereby providing signal 2 for initiation of "naive" T-cell responses. Despite convincing evidence that CD28 provides a critical costimulus, not all T-cell-mediated responses are CD28-dependent. Indeed, many other molecules have been identified which have an accessory or costimulatory function in T-cell activation.[45] CD28 plays a predominant role in providing costimulatory signals to naive CD4+ T cells. Other costimulatory receptors of the CD28 family, CD2 family, TNF receptor family, and integrin family also play a role in T-cell activation. It should be noted, however, that not all "costimulatory molecules" can provide a classic signal 2 in the same way as CD28.

The CD28 family includes the cytotoxic T-lymphocyte antigen 4 (CTLA-4) and the newly identified inducible costimulator (ICOS). In contrast to CD28, CTLA-4 is primarily a negative regulator of T-cell activation. ICOS is expressed only on activated T cells. It seems to facilitate the cooperation between helper T cells and B cells, as it occurs in germinal centers. Signaling lymphocyte activation molecule (SLAM), or CDw150, is a member of the CD2 subfamily of the immunoglobulin superfamily found on activated T and B cells. In contrast to CD2, which can act on resting T cells, SLAM appears to act only on memory cells and upregulates interferon-γ production. In addition to members of the CD28 and CD2 families, several members of the TNF receptor family are involved in T-cell activation. These molecules include CD40, 4-1BB, OX 40 (CD134), and CD27 and their respective ligands CD40-L (CD154), 4-1BBL, OX40L, and CD70.

The immunologic synapse is a highly dynamic structure that integrates various costimulatory signals (which occur in many different combinations) and translates them into a (graded) T-cell response. It is important to keep in mind that T cells can "respond" in many different ways—e.g., by cytotoxicity, proliferation, cytokine secretion, or differentiation into various subsets of helper cells, cytotoxic cells, or memory cells. Each of these different types of response has a different threshold of activation, which is triggered by different combinations of costimulatory signals.

Mechanisms of Autoimmunity

Because the antigen-specific receptors of B cells and T cells are generated by random somatic rearrangements of antigen receptor genes (Fig. 32-2), it is inevitable that some B- and T-cell clones carry receptors that recognize self-antigens. Some of these autoreactive lymphocytes are destroyed (deleted) early during development. Others are not deleted but are inactivated by various mechanisms, inducing a state of self-tolerance in which the immune system responds only to foreign antigens and not to self-antigens. Loss of this acquired property results in autoimmune disorders.[46]

The cells mainly responsible for immunoregulation and maintenance of immune tolerance are the T lymphocytes. Self-tolerance is induced and maintained by several different mechanisms. Many potentially autoaggressive T cells die in the thymus (clonal deletion). Other autoreactive T cells are not deleted but receive different types of inactivating signals leading to clonal anergy[47] or clonal suppression. Still others do not need to be deleted or inactivated, because they never have a chance to "see" their autoantigen (clonal ignorance).[46]

Loss of tolerance may result from activation of autoreactive T cells that are normally exposed to self-antigen(s) but do not react to them because they are anergic or otherwise inactivated. For example, T-cell anergy might be reversed by "antigenic mimicry." Peptide sequences of bacterial or viral antigens may be identical or similar to sequences of self-antigens to which the T cells are anergic. During infection, these foreign sequences may be presented in such a way that the state of anergy is reversed and a secondary autoimmune reaction is triggered. Furthermore, anergic or inactivated autoreactive T cells could be stimulated by microbial "superantigens." Superantigens bind HLA class II molecules and stimulate powerful proliferative responses of large numbers of T cells sharing particular TCR V-β sequences. During bacterial or viral infection, superantigens might stimulate anergic or inactivated autoreactive T cells expressing the appropriate TCR V-β chains. This could lead to reversal of anergy and, consequently, to autoimmune disease. Finally, in addition to antigenic mimicry and superantigen stimulation, self-tolerance may be broken by purely nonspecific mechanisms: During infections many proinflammatory mediators and cytokines are released locally and systemically. These factors can stimulate autoreactive T cells nonspecifically, leading to a loss of immune tolerance and subsequent development of autoimmune disease.[46]

Another mechanism for loss of tolerance is the loss or weakening of the suppressive mechanisms that normally help to keep the autoreactive T cells in check. One such mechanism seems to be mediated by "suppressor cells." Cellular suppressor mechanisms were not well understood until recently. But now there is evidence that a distinct population of CD4+CD25+ regulatory cells is crucial for maintaining self-tolerance.[48,49] These suppressor cells, which are generated in the thymus, exert their suppressive function by direct cell-to-cell contact with other T cells, but the precise mechanisms of their function and dysfunction have yet to be defined.

In the case of ignorant T cells, loss of tolerance presumably involves a change in the level or site of expression of the target antigen. Potential autoantigens may be sequestered at sites where they are not reached by circulating T cells, or they may not be expressed under normal conditions. Expression of "neoautoantigens" might be induced, for example, by viruses, either by activation of normally silent genes or by changes in cellular protein metabolism. Further, certain cells may not express self-peptides on their surface because they do not express HLA molecules. Upregulation of HLA molecules can have many causes, including infection, injury, malignant transformation, or degeneration of cells. In all these cases, some of the upregulated HLA molecules would be expected to be associated with self-peptides that could stimulate previously anergic or ignorant autoreactive T cells.

The relationship between (viral) infection and autoimmune disease has been elucidated in a transgenic mouse model expressing a T-cell-receptor transgene specific for a self-peptide of the cornea.[50] Herpes stromal keratitis (HSK) is a T-cell-dependent autoimmune response that destroys corneal tissue after infection with a murine herpesvirus. The disorder seems to be provoked by antigenic mimicry: Infection with the murine herpesvirus stimulates a population of T cells that cross-react with a self-peptide of the cornea.[50] Experiments with T cells from T-cell-receptor transgenic mice indicate that (1) direct activation of T cells by the molecular mimic peptide is required to induce disease in normal nonprimed animals containing limiting numbers of autoreactive T cells and (2) innate (antigen-nonspecific) immune mechanisms are sufficient to trigger disease in animals that contain expanded numbers of autoantigen-specific T cells.[50] These results open the possibility that subclinical infection by a virus that expresses a mimic epitope can "prime" the host for an autoimmune response upon infection of the target organ by an unrelated virus, thus complicating the search for viral mimics in established autoimmune diseases.

Novel Targets for Therapeutic Modulation

TRIMOLECULAR COMPLEX

The ultimate target for selective (antigen-specific) immunotherapies is the trimolecular complex of T-cell receptor, antigenic peptide, and MHC molecule.[51] In principle, each component of the TMC can be targeted. The MHC molecule could be blocked by anti-MHC antibodies or "blocking peptides"; the TCR can be targeted with anti-TCR antibodies or by vaccination with whole T cells or TCR-derived peptides; and the antigen (or antigenic peptide) can be chemically modified or applied in such a way that the autoreactive T cells are inhibited or modified rather than stimulated (e.g., by administering "altered peptide ligands").

MHC blocking agents are not very selective. At the other extreme, anti-TCR strategies may be too selective; in most cases, autoimmune reactions are mediated by a diversity of T cells, not by a single T-cell clone.[51] Therefore, antigen-based strategies are perhaps the most practical and promising of the TMC-directed approaches. Altered peptide ligands are peptides that have been modified from an autoantigenic peptide in such a way that the original MHC binding moieties are retained, whereas one or several of the TCR-binding amino acids have been changed. Altered peptide ligands (APLs) can bind to TCR without triggering the full program of T-cell activation. For example, an APL may partially activate a helper T cell to produce IL-4 and help B cells, but fail to induce proliferation. (As mentioned above, the antigen-induced stimulation of T cells is a graded response rather than an "all-or-nothing" phenomenon.)

In principle, stimulation of T cells by APLs can have several different consequences that may be useful for immunotherapy. Most desirable for therapeutic purposes would be a long-lasting change of the properties of autoreactive T cells. For example, some APLs induce a form of "anergy" in T cells (anergic T cells are unable to respond to stimulatory ligand). A less attractive, presumably only transient effect of APLs is simple competition with the unaltered ligand for TCR binding ("TCR antagonism").

APL therapy is facing the same problems as other peptide-mediated therapies, especially problems relating to peptide delivery and bioavailability. On the one hand, if APL therapy affected only T cells capable of reacting with the APLs, then this strategy would likely fail in human disease. On the other, if the encouraging data suggesting a more widespread effect of APL treatment on bystander T cells ("bystander suppression") can be corroborated, then this treatment could hold substantial promise (reviewed in Ref. 52). But even then, the autoimmune reaction could find a way to evade the effects of APL therapy—for example, by epitope spreading.

COSTIMULATORY MOLECULES

Another attractive target for immunotherapy is the *costimulatory signals* generated at the immunologic synapse (Fig. 32-10). Interfering with these costimulatory signals may result in T-cell "anergy" (antigen-specific nonresponsiveness). In this connection, the B7/CD28/CTLA-4 family of costimulatory molecules is of particular importance. CD28 and CTLA-4 appear to have opposing effects on T cells. CD28 lowers the threshold for effective TCR activation. In contrast, CTLA-4 may increase the threshold for T-cell activation, and thereby prevent undesired activation of autoimmune responses.[53] Examples of experimental therapies targeting these costimulatory molecules include anti-B7 monoclonal antibody, anti-CTLA-4 antibody, soluble CTLA-4 constructs, and anti-CD28 monoclonal antibodies. For example, a recent phase I clinical trial demonstrated that blockade of T-lymphocyte costimulation with soluble CTLA-4-Ig fusion protein is very effective in psoriasis.[54]

The great complexity and diversity of these costimulatory molecules and pathways may be an obstacle to successful therapy in vivo.[53] For example, CTLA-4 blockade can enhance or inhibit the clonal expansion of different T cells that respond to the same antigen, depending on both the T-cell activation state and the strength of the T-cell receptor signal delivered during T-cell stimulation.[55] Furthermore, therapeutic CTLA-4 blockade may result in the preferential activation of a Th2 T-cell response (if strong stimulating signals are present) or may result in the expansion of both Th1 and Th2 populations (if the stimulating signals are weak).[55] These observations emphasize that the antigen and stimulation conditions critically influence the results of therapeutic manipulation of the CD28/CTLA-4 costimulatory pathways.

It is noteworthy that some of the classic "costimulatory molecules" are expressed not only on immune cells but also on other cell types, where they may have different functions. This is highlighted by the unexpected adverse effects of a monoclonal antibody against the CD40 ligand (CD154). Therapy with this antibody induced severe thromboembolic complications in monkeys who had received a kidney allograft.[56] This complication is likely to be related to the presence of CD40-L (CD154) on platelets and endothelial cells.

ADHESION- AND MIGRATION-RELATED MOLECULES

Adhesion molecules and chemokine receptors are promising targets for new anti-inflammatory therapies. "Small molecules" are probably the drugs of choice for manipulating adhesion and migration processes. There are already several potent small molecule antagonists of chemokine receptors. In addition, numerous monoclonal antibodies, recombinant soluble adhesion molecules, and receptor-blocking mutant chemokines are being evaluated as treatments for asthma, inflammatory bowel disease, arthritis, and psoriasis. In multiple sclerosis, short-term treatment with a monoclonal antibody against α-4 integrin (VLA-4) resulted in a significant reduction of the number of new active lesions on MRI.[57] Further studies are under way to determine the long-term effectiveness of this treatment. It should be noted that anti-adhesion therapies are relatively nonselective. Effective anti-adhesion agents are likely to affect leukocyte migration in general and could thus have undesired effects in situations requiring a strong inflammatory reaction. Furthermore, because many adhesion molecules are widely expressed in many tissues, therapeutic manipulation of adhesion molecules could adversely affect important "nonimmunologic" tissue reactions such as wound repair, hemostasis, and fertility.

CYTOKINES AND CHEMOKINES AS THERAPEUTIC TARGETS

Cytokine-based immunotherapies follow one of three basic strategies. The first strategy is to administer or induce "downregulatory" cytokines. It should be kept in mind, however, that cytokines with exclusively downregulatory (or conversely exclusively proinflammatory) properties do not exist. The second strategy is to administer inhibitors of proinflammatory cytokines. The third, overlapping strategy is to induce a global and lasting shift in the balance of the cytokine network in favor of beneficial cytokines (the so-called *immune deviation* approach). One consequence of the complexity of the cytokine network is that it is virtually impossible to predict the overall effect that a given cytokine or cytokine inhibitor may have in vivo. Although it is obviously essential to test the safety and efficacy of cytokine-based therapies in animal models, totally unexpected effects may occur in human clinical trials.

A growing subclass of cytokines that is receiving increasing attention is the chemokines (Table 32-3). Chemokines are secreted as polypeptides that bind to specific surface receptors, which transmit signals through G proteins.[31] To date, more than 50 chemokines and 18 chemokine receptors have been identified.[31] Like adhesion molecules, chemokine receptors can be upregulated or downregulated, allowing leukocytes to coordinate their migratory routes with their immunologic function. Some chemokines trigger intravascular adhesion, whereas others direct the migration of leukocytes into the extravascular space. Not surprisingly, chemokines and their receptors are considered promising targets for immunotherapy.[58]

Immunologic Properties of Cultured Myoblasts

Numerous studies have shown that cultured myoblasts can express a surprising variety of immunologically important molecules, including MHC molecules and costimulatory molecules. Furthermore, myoblasts can secrete various cytokines and chemokines (reviewed in Ref. 59). For these reasons, myoblasts should be considered as active participants rather than passive targets of immune reactions.[6] This concept has central importance for all immune reactions that can occur in muscle—e.g., in inflammatory myopathies and also after intramuscular vaccination, therapeutic myoblast transfer, and gene therapy.[60,61]

Human myoblasts (myogenic stem cells) can be isolated and purified from muscle biopsy specimens and expanded in culture.[62–64] In contrast to fibroblasts, myoblasts express the cytoskeletal protein desmin and the neural cell adhesion molecule N-CAM (CD56/Leu 19/NKH-1).[6] Highly purified myoblast preparations can be obtained by immunostaining with a myoblast-specific antibody and isolation with a fluorescence-activated cell sorter (FACS) or an immunomagnetic bead procedure (Fig. 32-11).[63,64]

EXPRESSION OF CLASSIC AND NONCLASSIC MHC (HLA) MOLECULES

Myoblasts constitutively express the classical HLA class I antigens HLA-A, -B, and -C. Interferon-γ, a cytokine secreted by T cells and NK cells, induces myoblasts to express the HLA class II antigen HLA-DR.[64–66] HLA-DP and HLA-DQ are also inducible by interferon-γ, but the kinetics of induction and the levels of expression vary with the different HLA class II molecules[64] (Table 32-4). The expression of the different HLA class II molecules seems to be developmentally regulated in that more differentiated myotubes can be induced to express HLA-DR but not DQ and DP on their surfaces.[67] In vivo, neither MHC class I nor MHC class II antigens are detectable on normal mature muscle fibers, but MHC class I antigens[68,69] (and questionably also MHC class II antigens[70,71]) are upregulated in various inflammatory myopathies. In mice, intramuscular injection of oligonucleotides containing unmethylated CpG motifs induces synthesis of chemokines [monocyte chemoattractant protein-1 (MCP-1)] by muscle fibers, which attracts inflammatory cells secreting IFN-γ.[72] This cytokine induces expression of MHC class II and other molecules involved in antigen presentation on the surface of muscle cells. These results are relevant to intramuscular vaccination with "naked DNA" vaccines.[72]

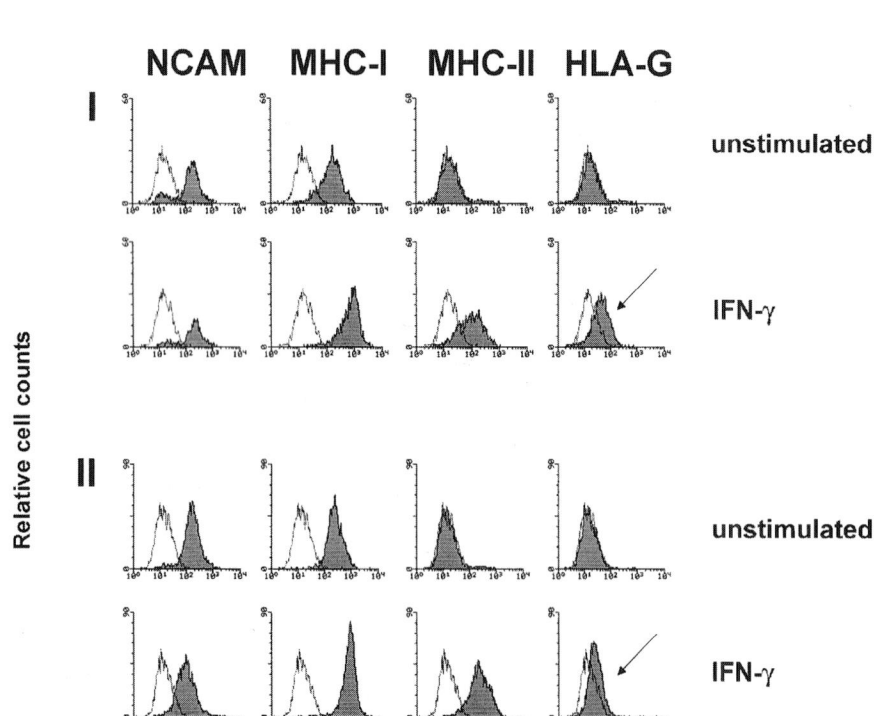

FIGURE 32-11. FACS analysis of HLA-G surface expression on cultured human myoblasts. Purified unstimulated NCAM+ myoblasts express MHC class I but are negative for MHC class II and HLA-G. Weak surface expression of HLA-G is detectable after 48 h of induction with interferon (IFN)-γ (arrows), as shown for myoblast cultures from two different donors (labeled I and II). Histograms show staining with the designated antibodies (dark curves) underlaid with isotype controls (white curves). (From Wiendl H, Behrens L, Maier S, et al: Muscle fibers in inflammatory myopathies and cultured myoblasts express the nonclassical major histocompatibility antigen HLA-G. Ann Neurol 48:679–684, 2000. With permission.)

Table 32-4. IMMUNOLOGICALLY RELEVANT SURFACE MOLECULES EXPRESSED ON HUMAN MYOBLASTS[a]

Surface Antigen	Constitutive Expression	IFN-γ-Stimulated Expression
Differentiation marker		
NCAM-1 (CD56)	+	+
HLA molecules		
Classic HLA class I	(+)	+
HLA-DR	—	+
HLA-DP	—	+
HLA-DQ	—	(+)
HLA-G	—	+
Adhesion molecules		
ICAM-1 (CD54)	—	+
LFA-3 (CD58)	(+)	(+)
Costimulatory molecules		
B7.1 (CD80)	—	—
B7.2 (CD86)	—	—
LiCOS	(+)	(+)
B7-H1	—	+
CD40	+	+

[a]Data from Refs. 64, 65, 67, 73, 73a, 75a, 75b, 85. With permission.

In addition to the classical MHC class I and II molecules, myoblasts can be induced to express the nonclassic MHC class I molecule HLA-G[73, 73a] (Fig. 32-11; Table 32-4). HLA-G expression was first observed in cytotrophoblasts of the human placenta. The function of HLA-G is not yet known. Like the classic HLA class I molecules, HLA-G binds antigenic peptides and CD8. It should therefore be capable of presenting antigenic peptides to T cells in a way similar to the classic HLA class I molecules. For example, in polymyositis, some of the autoaggressive T cells may recognize their antigen in the molecular context of HLA-G. In muscle infections, HLA-G might present bacterial or viral peptides to cytotoxic T cells. After vaccination or intramuscular injection of vectors for gene therapy,[60] HLA-G may present peptides of the immunizing antigen or vector-encoded peptides. After therapeutic transfer of myoblasts, HLA-G may be involved in allograft rejection. Furthermore, HLA-G interacts with different receptors expressed on various types of lymphocytes, monocytes, and dendritic cells. It is thought that the recognition of HLA-G induces immunoregulatory functions in these cells,[73a] raising the possibility that HLA-G plays a role as a tissue-protective molecule in inflammatory responses not just in muscle but also in other peripheral tissues.

EXPRESSION OF ADHESION AND COSTIMULATORY MOLECULES

Human myoblasts constitutively express a low level of lymphocyte function-associated (LFA-) molecule 3 (LFA-3, CD58) (Table 32-4). Interferon-γ stimulates myoblasts to express ICAM-1.[64–66] TNF-α, a cytokine secreted by macrophages, T cells, and NK cells, induces myoblasts to express the intercellular adhesion molecule-1 (ICAM-1, CD54).[64] Thus, many molecules of the "immunologic synapse" are indeed inducible on myoblasts. These results suggest that myoblasts have sufficient immunologic "potential" to qualify them to act as facultative antigen-presenting cells. For example, they might (re)stimulate memory and effector T cells in muscle. It is not clear, however, to what extent they can stimulate naive (unprimed) T cells. Myoblasts do not express the classical costimulatory molecules B7.1 (CD80) and B7.2 (CD86),[74] but they do express CD40, another important costimulatory molecule.[74,75] Furthermore, a subpopulation of myoblasts expresses BB-1, a B7-related molecule that has not been molecularly defined.[74] In addition, myoblasts can express the B7-related inducible costimulatory molecule LiCOS[75a] and the B7-related molecule B7-H1.[75b] The presence of these costimulatory molecules further emphazises the important immunologic role of myoblasts.

SECRETION OF CYTOKINES AND CHEMOKINES

Human myoblasts can express various cytokines and chemokines, either constitutively or after stimulation.[76–78] For example, myoblasts secrete IL-6 under basal conditions[79] and in response to several proinflammatory agents, including IL-1β, TNF-α, and lipopolysaccharide (LPS).[76] Furthermore, myoblasts express IL-1α constitutively, whereas IL-1β and TNF-α were detected only after stimulation with proinflammatory cytokines.[77] TNF-α was expressed after stimulation with TNF-α, indicating the presence of an autocrine loop.[77] The chemokines IL-8 and RANTES were expressed constitutively, whereas MCP-1 was expressed after stimulation with TNF-α and interferon-γ.[77]

FUNCTIONAL INTERACTION WITH T CELLS

Cultured myotubes and myoblasts express HLA class I molecules. This qualifies them as potential targets of CD8+ CTL. Lysis of myotubes by CTL was shown in different experimental situations. On the one hand, myotubes were lysed by allogeneic CD8+ CTL lines raised against the allogeneic HLA antigens expressed by the myotubes.[80] Autologous control myotubes were not lysed. Lysis involved the recognition of allogeneic class I HLA antigens, since it was completely blocked by a monoclonal antibody against a monomorphic determinant of HLA class I.[80] Furthermore, myotubes were lysed by autologous polyclonal CD8+ T-cell lines directly expanded from muscle of patients with different inflammatory myopathies.[81] The results obtained in this model system clearly establish that cultured myotubes are fully susceptible to HLA class I–restricted lysis by CD8+ CTL. The autoreactive myocytotoxicity is consistent with the hypothesis that some of the CTL isolated from muscle recognize the same antigen on myotubes in vitro that they recognize on muscle fibers in vivo (see discussion of polymyositis in Chap. 48).

Antigen presentation to CD4+ T cells depends on the constitutive or induced expression of HLA class II on the presenting cell. Myoblasts can be induced to express HLA class II by γ-interferon.[65] Highly purified human myoblasts were tested for their ability to present various protein antigens to autologous CD4+ T-cell lines specific for tuberculin, tetanus toxoid, or myelin basic protein.[64] Noninduced myoblasts or myoblasts treated with TNF-α alone could not present any of these antigens to T cells. However, interferon-γ–treated myoblasts induced antigen-specific T-cell proliferation and were killed by the T cells only in the presence of the relevant antigen.[64] Antigen-specific lysis was reduced to background level by adding the anti-HLA-DR monoclonal antibody L-243. These results suggest that HLA class II–positive human myoblasts can act as facultative local antigen-presenting cells in muscle by providing the signals necessary to trigger both antigen-specific lysis and T-cell proliferation. In addition to presentation of exogenous antigens processed in the classic MHC class II–restricted pathway, human myoblasts seem to be capable of presenting endogenous antigen to MHC class II–restricted CD4+ T cells.[82]

In conclusion, myoblasts can participate as facultative APCs in both MHC class I–dependent and MHC class II–dependent immune reactions. They secrete a surprising number of soluble factors, including important cytokines and chemokines, and they can be stimulated to express several costimulatory molecules. Thus, myoblasts can form a functional immunologic synapse with T cells, at least in vitro. Although some of these molecules are less abundantly expressed in more differentiated myotubes and muscle fibers, it seems likely that even mature muscle fibers can actively participate in various immune reactions.

List of Abbreviations

C5a	activated complement component 5	NK	natural killer
CD	cluster of differentiation nomenclature	PAF	platelet-activating factor
CTLA-4	cytotoxic T-lymphocyte antigen 4	PNAd	peripheral-node addressin
ICAM	intercellular adhesion molecule	PSGL-1	P-selectin glycoprotein ligand 1
ICAM-1 (-2)	intercellular adhesion molecule 1 (2)	SLAM	signaling lymphocyte activation molecule
ICOS	inducible costimulator	sLe^x	sulfated sialyl-Lewis^x
LFA	leukocyte function–associated antigen	TCR	T-cell receptor for antigen
LICOS	ligand of the inducible costimulator	TMC	trimolecular complex
LTB4	leukotriene B4	TNF	tumor necrosis factor
MAdCAM-1	mucosal addressin-cell adhesion molecule type 1	VCAM	vascular-cell adhesion molecule
		VCAM-1	vascular-cell adhesion molecule 1
MHC	major histocompatibility complex	VLA	very late antigen

References

1. Arahata K, Engel AG: Monoclonal antibody analysis of mononuclear cells in myopathies. I. Quantitation of subsets according to diagnosis and sites of accumulation and demonstration and counts of muscle fibers invaded by T cells. *Ann Neurol* 16:193–208, 1984.
2. Munsat TL, Piper D, Cancilla P, Mednick J: Inflammatory myopathy with facioscapulohumeral distribution. *Neurology* 22:335–347, 1972.
3. McNally EM, Ly CT, Rosenmann H, et al: Splicing mutation in dysferlin produces limb-girdle muscular dystrophy with inflammation. *Am J Med Genet* 91:305–312, 2000.
4. Cherin P, Gherardi RK: Macrophagic myofasciitis. *Curr Rheumatol Rep* 2:196–200, 2000.
5. Gherardi RK, Coquet M, Cherin P, et al: Macrophagic myofasciitis lesions assess long-term persistence of vaccine-derived aluminium hydroxide in muscle. *Brain* 124:1821–1831, 2001.
6. Hohlfeld R, Engel AG: The immunobiology of muscle. *Immunol Today* 15:269–274, 1994.
7. Medzhitov R, Janeway CA: Innate immunity. *N Engl J Med* 343:338–344, 2000.
8. Wagner H: Toll meets bacterial CpG DNA. *Immunity* 14:499–502, 2001.
9. Lanier LL: On guard—activating NK cell receptors. *Nat Immunol* 2:23–27, 2001.
10. Thompson CB: New insights into V(D)J recombination and its role in the evolution of the immune system. *Immunity* 3:531–539, 1995.
11. Wagner SD, Neuberger MS: Somatic hypermutation of immunoglobulin genes. *Annu Rev Immunol* 14:441–457, 1996.
12. Matis LA: The molecular basis of T-cell specificity. *Annu Rev Immunol* 8:65–82, 1990.
13. Lanzavecchia A: Receptor-mediated antigen uptake and its effects on antigen presentation to class II–restricted T lymphocytes. *Annu Rev Immunol* 8:773–794, 1990.
14. Romagnani S: Lymphokine production by human T cells in disease states. *Annu Rev Immunol* 12:227–257, 1994.
15. Born W, Cady C, Jones-Carson J, et al: Immunoregulatory functions of gamma delta T cells. *Adv Immunol* 71:77–144, 1999.
16. Hardy RR, Hayakawa K: B cell development pathways. *Annu Rev Immunol* 19:595–621, 2001.
17. MacLennan ICM: Germinal centers. *Annu Rev Immunol* 12:117–139, 1994.
18. Germain RN: MHC-dependent antigen processing and peptide presentation: Providing ligands for T lymphocyte activation. *Cell* 76:287–299, 1994.
19. Surh CD, Ernst B, Sprent J: Growth of epithelial cells in the thymic medulla is under the control of mature T cells. *J Exp Med* 176:611–616, 1992.
20. Van Ewijk W, Shores EW, Singer A: Crosstalk in the mouse thymus. *Immunol Today* 15:214–217, 1994.
21. Wekerle H, Ketelsen U-P: Thymic nurse cells—Ia-bearing epithelium involved in T-lymphocyte differentiation? *Nature* 283:402–404, 1980.
22. Robey E, Fowlkes BJ: Selective events in T cell development. *Annu Rev Immunol* 12:675–705, 1994.
23. von Boehmer H: Positive selection of lymphocytes. *Cell* 76:219–228, 1993.
24. Allen PM: Peptides in positive and negative selection: A delicate balance. *Cell* 76:593–596, 1994.
25. Lanzavecchia A, Sallusto F: The instructive role of dendritic cells on T cell responses: Lineages, plasticity and kinetics. *Curr Opin Immunol* 13:291–298, 2001.
26. Liu YJ, Kanzler H, Soumelis V, Gilliet M: Dendritic cell lineage, plasticity and cross-regulation. *Nat Immunol* 2:585–589, 2001.
27. Moser M, Murphy KM: Dendritic cell regulation of TH1-TH2 development. *Nat Immunol* 1:199–205, 2000.
28. Kägi D, Ledermann B, Bürki K, et al: Molecular mechanisms of lymphocyte-mediated cytotoxicity and their role in immunological protection and pathogenesis in vivo. *Annu Rev Immunol* 14:207–232, 1996.
29. Liu C-C, Young LHY, Young JDE: Lymphocyte-mediated cytolysis and disease. *N Engl J Med* 335:1651–1659, 1996.
30. Green DR: Apoptotic pathways: Paper wraps stone blunts scissors. *Cell* 102:1–4, 2000.
31. von Andrian UH, Mackay CR: T cell function and migration. Two sides of the same coin. *N Engl J Med* 343:1020–1034, 2000.
32. Ihle JN: STATs: Signal transducers and activators of transcription. *Cell* 84:331–334, 1996.
33. Paul WE, Seder RA: Lymphocyte responses and cytokines. *Cell* 76:241–251, 1994.
34. Heaney ML, Golde DW: Soluble cytokine receptors. *Blood* 87:847–857, 1996.
35. Coffman RL, Reiner SL: Instruction, selection, or tampering with the odds? *Science* 284:1283, 1285, 1999.
36. Allen JE, Maizels RM: Th1-Th2: Reliable paradigm or dangerous dogma? *Immunol Today* 18:387–392, 1997.

37. Dinarello CA: Biologic basis for interleukin-1 in disease. *Blood* 87: 2095–2147, 1996.
38. Dinarello CA: The role of interleukin-1 receptor antagonist in blocking inflammation mediated interleukin-1. *N Engl J Med* 343:732–734, 2000.
39. Zlotnik A, Yoshie O: Chemokines: A new classification system and their role in immunity. *Immunity* 12:121–127, 2000.
40. Mackay CR: Chemokines: Immunology's high impact factors. *Nat Immunol* 2:95–101, 2001.
41. Taub DD, Turcovski-Corrales SM, Key ML, et al: Chemokines and T lymphocyte activation: I. β Chemokines costimulate human T lymphocyte activation in vitro. *J Immunol* 156:2095–2103, 1996.
42. Lanzavecchia A, Sallusto F: From synapses to immunological memory: The role of sustained T cell stimulation. *Curr Opin Immunol* 12:92–98, 2000.
43. Dustin ML, Cooper JA: The immunological synapse and the actin cytoskeleton: Molecular hardware for T cell signaling. *Nat Immunol* 1:23–29, 2000.
44. Khan AA, Bose C, Yam LS, et al: Physiological regulation of the immunological synapse by agrin. *Science* 292:1681–1686, 2001.
45. Watts TH, DeBenedette MA: T cell costimulatory molecules other than CD28. *Curr Opin Immunol* 11:286–293, 1999.
46. Kamradt T, Mitchison NA: Tolerance and autoimmunity. *N Engl J Med* 344:655–664, 2001.
47. Wells AD, Walsh MC, Bluestone JA, Turka LA: Signaling through CD28 and CTLA-4 controls two distinct forms of T cell anergy. *J Clin Invest* 108:895–904, 2001.
48. Shevach EM: Certified professionals: CD4(+)CD25(+) suppressor T cells. *J Exp Med* 193:F41–F46, 2001.
49. Shevach EM, McHugh RS, Thornton AM, et al: Control of autoimmunity by regulatory T cells. *Adv Exp Med Biol* 490:21–32, 2001.
50. Panoutsakopoulou V, Sanchirico ME, Huster KM, et al: Analysis of the relationship between viral infection and autoimmune disease. *Immunity* 15:137–147, 2001.
51. Hohlfeld R: Biotechnological agents for the immunotherapy of multiple sclerosis. Principles, problems and perspectives. *Brain* 120:865–916, 1997.
52. Steinman L: A few autoreactive cells in an autoimmune infiltrate control a vast population of nonspecific cells: A tale of smart bombs and the infantry. *Proc Natl Acad Sci USA* 93:2253–2256, 1996.
53. Anderson DE, Sharpe AH, Hafler DA: The B7-CD28/CTLA-4 co-stimulatory pathways in autoimmune disease of the central nervous system. *Curr Opin Immunol* 11:677–683, 2000.
54. Abrams JR, Kelley SL, Hayes E, et al: Blockade of T lymphocyte costimulation with cytotoxic T lymphocyte-associated antigen 4-immunoglobulin (CTLA4Ig) reverses the cellular pathology of psoriatic plaques, including the activation of keratinocytes, dendritic cells, and endothelial cells. *J Exp Med* 192:681–693, 2000.
55. Anderson DE, Bieganowska KD, Bar-Or A, et al: Paradoxical inhibition of T cell function in response to CTLA-4 blockade: Heterogeneity within the human T cell population. *Nat Med* 6: 211, 2000.
56. Kawai T, Andrews D, Colvin RB, et al: Thromboembolic complications after treatment with monoclonal antibody against CD40 ligand. *Nat Med* 6:114, 2000.
57. Miller DH, Khan OA, Sheremata WA, et al: A controlled trial of natalizumab for relapsing multiple sclerosis. *N Eng J Med* 348:15–23, 2003.
58. Ransohoff RM: Mechanisms of inflammation in MS tissue: Adhesion molecules and chemokines. *J Neuroimmunol* 98:57–68, 1999.
59. Hohlfeld R, Engel AG, Goebels N, Behrens L: Cellular immune mechanisms in inflammatory myopathies. *Curr Opin Rheumatol* 9:520–526, 1997.
60. Prud'homme GJ, Lawson BR, Chang Y, Theofilopoulos AN: Immunotherapeutic gene transfer into muscle. *Trends Immunol* 22:149–155, 2001.
61. Blau HM, Springer ML: Muscle-mediated gene therapy. *N Engl J Med* 333:1554–1556, 1995.
62. Blau HM, Webster C: Isolation and characterization of human muscle cells. *Proc Natl Acad Sci USA* 78:5623–5627, 1981.
63. Webster C, Pavlath GK, Parks DR, et al: Isolation of human myoblasts with the fluorescence-activated cell sorter. *Exp Cell Res* 174:252–265, 1988.
64. Goebels N, Michaelis D, Wekerle H, Hohlfeld R: Human myoblasts as antigen presenting cells. *J Immunol* 149:661–667, 1992.
65. Hohlfeld R, Engel AG: Induction of HLA-DR expression on human myoblasts with interferon-gamma. *Am J Pathol* 136:503–508, 1990.
66. Mantegazza R, Hughes SM, Mitchell D, et al: Modulation of MHC class II antigen expression in human myoblasts after treatment with IFN-γ. *Neurology* 41:1128–1132, 1991.
67. Michaelis D, Goebels N, Hohlfeld R: Constitutive and cytokine-induced expression of human leukocyte antigens and cell adhesion molecules by human myotubes. *Am J Pathol* 143:1142–1149, 1993.
68. Karpati G, Pouliot Y, Carpenter S: Expression of immunoreactive major histocompatibility complex products in human skeletal muscles. *Ann Neurol* 23:64–72, 1988.
69. Emslie-Smith AM, Arahata K, Engel AG: Major histocompatibility complex class I antigen expression, immunolocalization of interferon subtypes, and T cell-mediated cytotoxicity in myopathies. *Hum Pathol* 20:224–231, 1989.
70. Bartoccioni E, Gallucci S, Scuderi F, et al: MHC class I, MHC class II and intercellular adhesion molecule-1 (ICAM-1) expression in inflammatory myopathies. *Clin Exp Immunol* 95:166–172, 1994.
71. Inukai A, Kuru S, Liang Y, et al: Expression of HLA-DR and its enhancing molecules in muscle fibers in polymyositis. *Muscle Nerve* 23:385–392, 2000.
72. Stan AC, Casares S, Brumeanu TD, et al: CpG motifs of DNA vaccines induce the expression of chemokines and MHC class II molecules on myocytes. *Eur J Immunol* 31:301–310, 2001.
73. Wiendl H, Behrens L, Maier S, et al: Muscle fibers in inflammatory myopathies and cultured myoblasts express the nonclassical major histocompatibility antigen HLA-G. *Ann Neurol* 48:679–684, 2000.
73a. Wiendl H, Mitsdoerffer M, Hofmeister V, et al: The non-classical MHC molecule HLA-G protects human muscle cells from immune-mediated lysis: Implications for myoblast transplantation and gene therapy. *Brain* 126:176–185, 2003.
74. Behrens L, Kerschensteiner M, Misgeld T, et al: Human muscle cells express a functional costimulatory molecule distinct from B7.1 (CD80) and B7.2 (CD86) in vitro and in inflammatory lesions. *J Immunol* 161:5943–5951, 1998.
75. Sugiura T, Kawaguchi Y, Harigai M, et al: Increased CD40 expression on muscle cells of polymyositis and dermatomyositis: Role of CD40-CD40 ligand interaction in IL-6, IL-8, IL-15, and monocyte chemoattractant protein-1 production. *J Immunol* 164:6593–6600, 2000.
75a. Wiendl H, Mitsdoerffer M, Schneider D, et al: Muscle fibers and cultured muscle cells express the B7.½-related inducible co-stimulatory molecule, ICOSL: Implications for the pathogenesis of inflammatory myopathies. *Brain* 126:1026–1035, 2003.
75b. Wiendl H, Mitsdoerffer M, Schneider D, et al: Human muscle cells express a B7-related molecule, B7-H1, with strong negative immune regulatory potential: A novel mechanism of counterbalancing the immune attack in idiopathic inflammatory myopathies. *FASEB J* 17:1892–1894, 2003.
76. Gallucci S, Provenzano C, Mazzarelli P, et al: Myoblasts produce IL-6 in response to inflammatory stimuli. *Int Immunol* 10:267–273, 1998.
77. De Rossi M, Bernasconi P, Baggi F, et al: Cytokines and chemokines are both expressed by human myoblasts: Possible relevance for the immune pathogenesis of muscle inflammation. *Int Immunol* 12:1329–1335, 2000.
78. Nagaraju K, Raben N, Merritt G, et al: A variety of cytokines and immunologically relevant surface molecules are expressed by normal human skeletal muscle cells under proinflammatory stimuli. *Clin Exp Immunol* 113:407–414, 1998.
79. Bartoccioni E, Michaelis D, Hohlfeld R: Constitutive and cytokine-induced production of interleukin-6 by human myoblasts. *Immunol Lett* 42:135–138, 1994.
80. Hohlfeld R, Engel AG: Lysis of myotubes by alloreactive cytotoxic T cells and natural killer cells. Relevance to myoblast transplantation. *J Clin Invest* 86:370–374, 1990.
81. Hohlfeld R, Engel AG: Coculture with autologous myotubes of cytotoxic T cells isolated from muscle in inflammatory myopathies. *Ann Neurol* 29:498–507, 1991.
82. Curnow J, Corlett L, Willcox N, Vincent A: Presentation by myoblasts of an epitope from endogenous acetylcholine receptor indicates a potential role in the spreading of the immune response. *J Neuroimmunol* 115:127–134, 2001.
83. Parkin J, Cohen B: An overview of the immune system. *Lancet* 357:1777–1789, 2001.
84. Janeway CA: *Immunobiology: The Immune System in Health and Disease.* New York: Garland, 2001.
85. Behrens L, Kerschensteiner M, Misgeld T, et al: Human muscle cells express a functional costimulatory molecule distinct from B7.1 (CD80) and B7.2 (CD86) in vitro and in inflammatory lesions. *J Immunol* 161:5943–5951, 1998.
86. von Andrian UH, Mackay CR: T-cell function and migration. Two sides of the same coin. *N Engl J Med* 343:1020–1034, 2000.

Chapter 33

The Tools of Molecular Genetics and Their Application to the Study of Muscle Diseases

ERIC A. SCHON

Fundamentals of Molecular Biology
   THE STRUCTURE OF NUCLEIC ACIDS AND CHROMOSOMES
   GENES AND GENE STRUCTURE
   RNA STRUCTURE: TRANSCRIPTION AND TRANSLATION
   REGULATION OF GENE EXPRESSION
   TYPES OF DNA MUTATIONS AND THEIR CONSEQUENCES
   MITOCHONDRIAL GENETICS

The Tools of Molecular Biology
   ENZYMOLOGY OF DNA AND RNA
   CLONING GENES
   ANALYZING CLONED GENES
   USING CLONED GENES

The Molecular Biology of Muscle
   MUSCLE-SPECIFIC GENE REGULATION
   MUSCLE-SPECIFIC GENES

Molecular Genetics in the Study of Muscle Disease
   FORWARD GENETICS
   REVERSE GENETICS
   MITOCHONDRIAL MYOPATHIES

Future Prospects

Almost any paper that describes the molecular genetics of an inherited disease is written with the implicit assumption that the reader is conversant with the language of molecular biology. In this chapter, we first review relevant concepts and nomenclature to make this language easier to understand and then discuss how the techniques of molecular biology have been applied to the study of muscle gene regulation and inherited muscle diseases.

Fundamentals of Molecular Biology

The past two decades saw an unprecedented growth of knowledge of molecular biology. For details not covered in this chapter, the reader is referred to standard texts on molecular biology.

THE STRUCTURE OF NUCLEIC ACIDS AND CHROMOSOMES

The "central dogma" of molecular biology states that "DNA encodes RNA and RNA encodes protein." Deoxyribonucleic acid (DNA),* the stable genetic material that is the major component of the chromosomes that pass from one generation to the next, is the template for the synthesis of ribonucleic acid (RNA), using DNA as the template. The subset of RNAs called messenger RNAs are further templates for the synthesis of all the proteins required for the cell's function.

Both DNA and RNA are polymerized chains of one fundamental unit, the nucleotide (Fig. 33-1A). The nucleotide monomer consists of three elements: (1) a five-membered *pentose sugar*, which is the backbone of the polymer, (2) a *phosphate* group attached to the pentose at the 5' carbon, and (3) a cyclic *base* attached to the pentose at the 1' carbon. The "prime" notation of the sugar carbons is used to differentiate them from the carbons and nitrogens of the bases ("unprimed" notation).

RNA is called *ribonucleic acid* because the sugar is *ribose*, a pentose with hydroxyl groups at the 1', 2', 3', and 5' positions on the ring (Fig. 33-1B). However, in DNA, the OH group at the 2' position is missing (it is replaced by a hydrogen atom); the pentose in DNA is thus *deoxyribose*, and the biopolymer is therefore called *deoxyribonucleic acid*. In both DNA and RNA, polymerization of the *nucleic acid* chain (it is acidic because of the ionizable phosphate groups) takes place through an esterification reaction between the phosphate group on the 5' carbon of one nucleotide and the hydroxyl group at the 3' carbon of the adjacent nucleotide. These *phosphodiester bonds* link the nucleotides to form the linear polymer (Fig. 33-1C). Because the phosphodiester bond between any two nucleotides involves a 5'-3' link, the overall linear polymer has a directionality or *polarity*, which is conventionally written as the $5' \rightarrow 3'$ *orientation*.

There are five kinds of bases (Fig. 33-1D): cytosine (C), thymine (T), and uracil (U) are cyclic 6-membered *pyrimidines* (containing 4 carbons and 2 nitrogens), while adenine (A) and guanine (G) are bicyclic 9-membered *purines* (5 carbons and 4 nitrogens). These bases are attached to the pentose of the nucleotide at the nitrogen located at the #1 position of the pyrimidine (N-1) or the #9 of the purine (N-9).

The bases of the nucleotides of DNA are A, G, C, and T; those of RNA are A, G, C, and U. Thus, in RNA, uracil replaces the thymine found in DNA. The *base-pairing rule* of Watson and Crick states that, because of favorable hydrogen bonding between specific purines and pyrimidines, the purine adenine can base-pair with the pyrimidines thymine or uracil, and the purine guanine can base-pair with the pyrimidine cytosine (Fig. 33-2A). G-C has three hydrogen bonds, and is about 50 percent stronger than A-T or A-U, which have two. The G-C, A-T, and A-U base pairs are called *complementary*, and are the most stable and thermodynamically favored.

Two individual strands of nucleic acid with complementary bases can form a series of hydrogen bonded bases that allow the two strands to *anneal* together to form a *duplex* (Fig. 33-2A). The two strands can anneal, or *hybridize*, only if the strand running $5' \rightarrow 3'$ bonds to the complementary strand running $3' \rightarrow 5'$; in other words, the duplex consists of two *antiparallel* strands. Two complementary, antiparallel strands of DNA normally wind around each other in a right-handed

---

*A list of abbreviations used in this chapter is given at the end of the chapter.

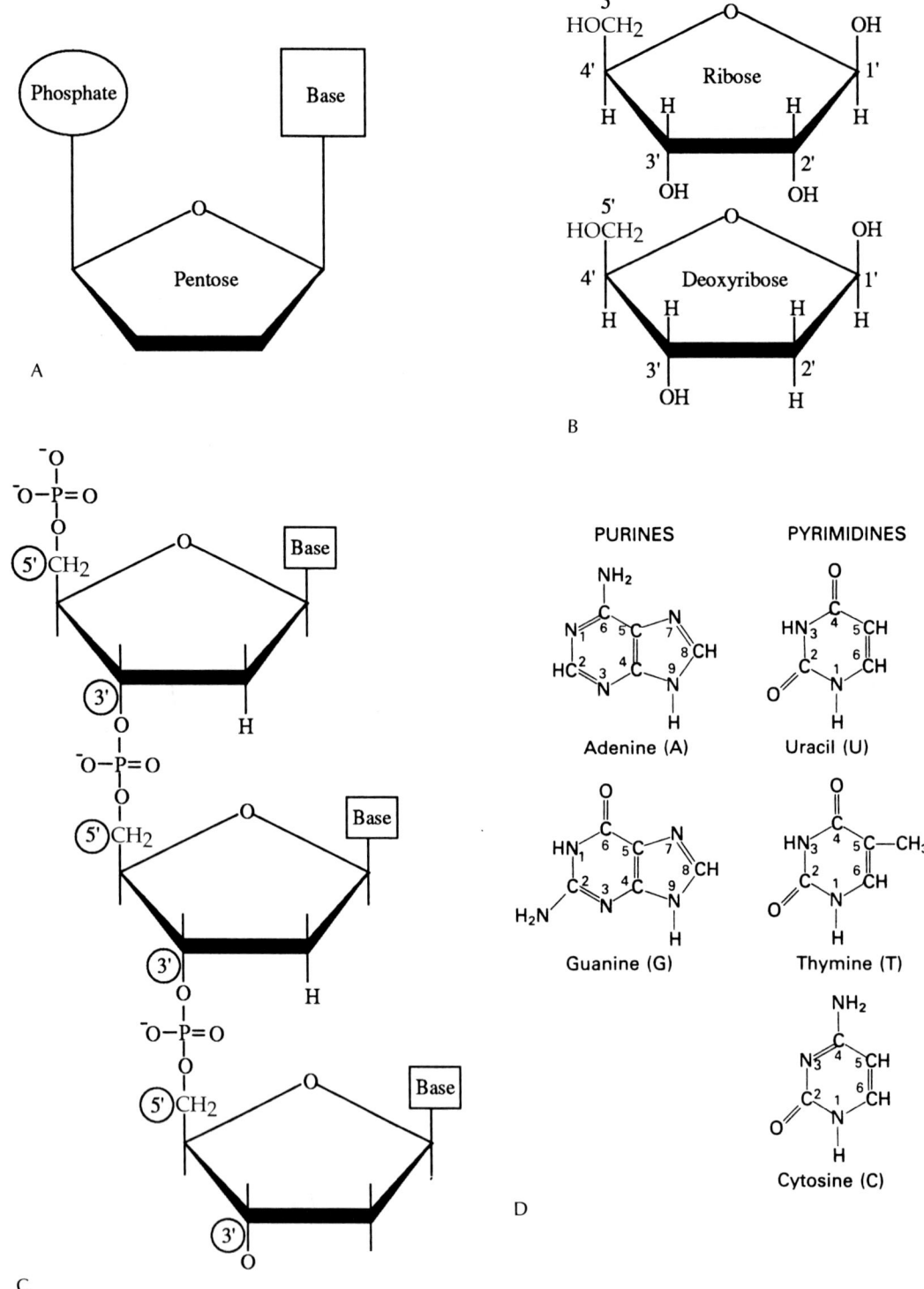

FIGURE 33-1. Structure of nucleic acids. *A.* The three elements comprising a nucleotide: a base and a phosphate group attached to a pentose sugar. *B.* Ribose and deoxyribose. *C.* Polymerization of nucleotides into a polynucleotide. *D.* Structures of the bases. (*Adapted from Darnell J, Lodish H, Baltimore D: Molecular Cell Biology. New York: Scientific American/WH Freeman, 1986. Copyright © 1986 by Scientific American Books, Inc. Reprinted with permission of W.H. Freeman and Company.*)

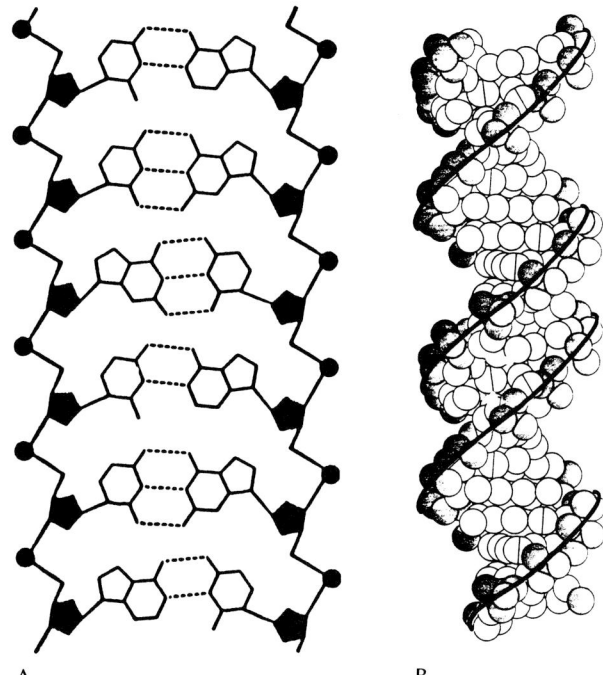

FIGURE 33-2. The structure of DNA. *A.* Duplex DNA; note the hydrogen bonding between purine-pyrimidine pairs (dotted lines). (*Adapted from Watson JD, Tooze J, Kurtz DT (eds): Recombinant DNA: A Short Course. New York: Scientific American/WH Freeman, 1983. Copyright © 1983 by Scientific American Books, Inc. Reprinted with permission of W.H. Freeman and Company.*) *B.* Space-filling model of the αhelix. (*Adapted from Darnell J, Lodish H, Baltimore D: Molecular Cell Biology. New York: Scientific American/WH Freeman, 1986. Copyright © 1986 by Scientific American Books, Inc. Reprinted with permission of W.H. Freeman and Company.*)

the diploid complement of DNA in a single cell were stretched out, it would be nearly 2 m long! Because there is so much DNA in the eukaryotic genome, the DNA must be packaged in a way that allows it to be contained physically within the confines of the nucleus. The solution to this problem was the development of chromosomes. A *chromosome* may be defined as a discrete, large-scale unit of the genome, consisting of genomic DNA plus its associated proteins (called *chromatin*), which is visible as a subcellular entity, usually during some phases of cell division. Chromosomes enable the genome to be broken down into more manageable pieces (46 such pieces in the diploid human genome), while the chromosomal proteins allow the DNA to be "wound up" into a compact structure that occupies an astonishingly small volume relative to the amount of DNA being packaged.

The packaging of chromatin into a chromosome (Fig. 33-4) is accomplished by a set of hierarchical foldings of the chromatin, starting with the *nucleosome*, 200 bp of DNA wrapped around a core of basic *histone* proteins. This "beads-on-a-string" chromatin structure (the *10-nm fiber*) is itself coiled into a solenoid shape (the *30-nm fiber*), which is folded fur-

spiral—the well-known α *helix* (Fig. 33-2*B*). The sugarphosphate "backbone" lies on the outside of the helix, with the bases facing inwards, perpendicular to the central helical axis. There are about 10 base pairs (*bp*) in each helical turn, with a "rise" of 0.34 nm between bases (i.e., 3.4 nm/helical turn).

The two complementary strands are *isomorphic structures*: If the sequence of bases on one strand is known, the base-pairing rules can be used to infer directly the antiparallel sequence of the other strand. This is the basis of the heritable nature of double-stranded (*ds*) DNA, as each strand can be used as a template to make a new, complementary strand, using the enzyme *DNA polymerase*, in a process called *DNA replication*.

DNA replication is a *semiconservative* process (Fig. 33-3): Each new daughter duplex consists of one old parental strand and one newly synthesized strand. The original strand is preserved, no matter how many times it serves as template for the synthesis of a new strand, although obviously, after many rounds of replication, the original "parental" strand is present in vanishingly small amounts as each new "daughter" strand becomes a template for subsequent rounds of replication.

The amount of DNA in a human cell is enormous: 3×10^9 bp in the haploid genomes of sperm and ova and double that in the diploid genomes of somatic cells. Put another way, if

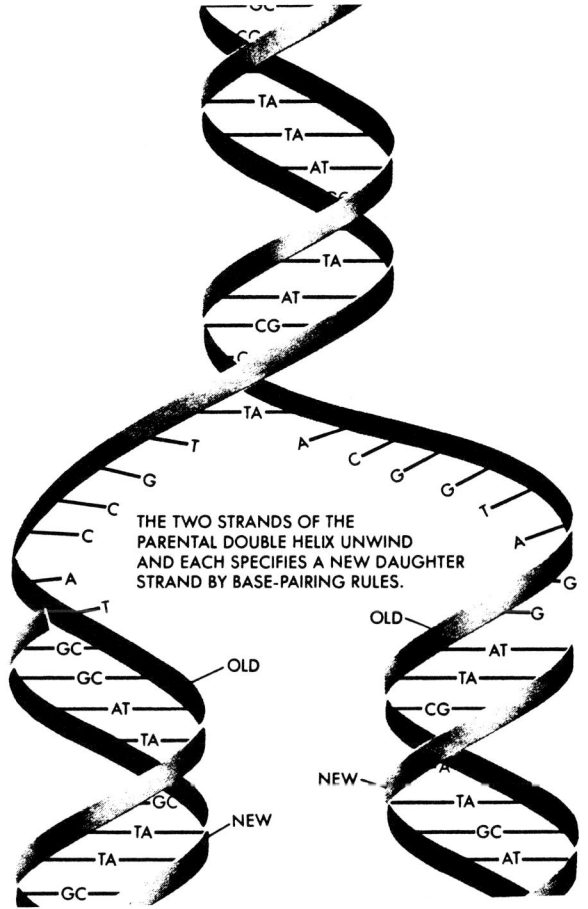

FIGURE 33-3. DNA replication. New daughter double helices are produced via semiconservative replication of parental DNA. (*From Watson JD, Tooze J, Kurtz DT (eds): Recombinant DNA: A Short Course. New York: Scientific American/WH Freeman, 1983. With permission. Copyright © 1983 by Scientific American Books, Inc. Reprinted with permission of W.H. Freeman and Company.*)

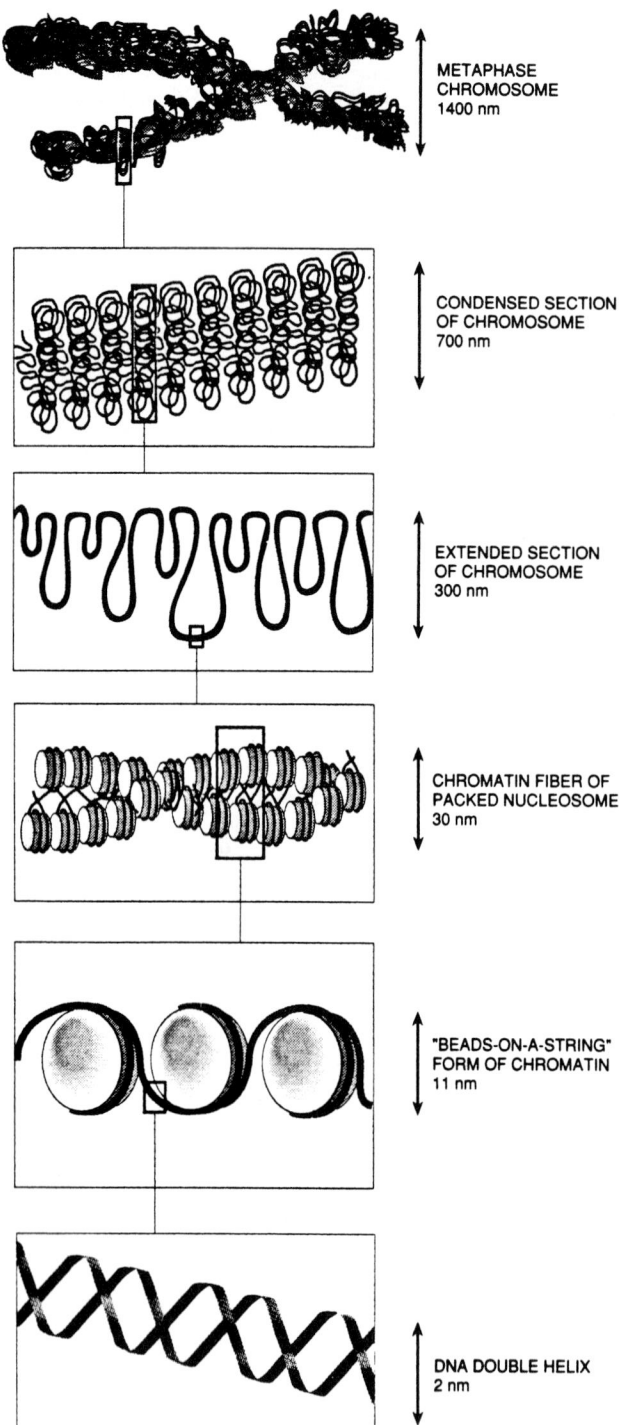

FIGURE 33-4. Hierarchy of chromatin organization. Panels from bottom to top: 2-nm naked DNA; the structure of a nucleosome—140 bp of DNA wrapped around a core octamer of histones—comprising the 10-nm fiber; the 30-nm fiber as a solenoid of cylindrically folded nucleosomes; the 300-nm extended section of the chromosome; the 700-nm condensed section of one of the two sister chromatids; and the 1400-nm metaphase chromosome consisting of two sister chromatids attached at the centromere. (*From Gelehrter TD, Collins FS (eds): Principles of Medical Genetics. Baltimore: Williams & Wilkins, 1990. With permission. Copyright © 1990 by Williams & Wilkins.*)

ther into a *300-nm extended large-loop structure*, and then into a *700-nm condensed section* of the chromosome; the latter constitutes one of the two *sister chromatids* comprising the *replicated chromosome*. Only four levels of chromatin folding are required to package anywhere from 100 to 300 million bp of DNA in a single metaphase chromosome; while the packaging diameter increases by a factor of 350, the amount of DNA packaged increases by a factor of 1 million. A typical chromosome only 5 μm long contains enough DNA in each chromatid to extend 5 cm in length.

The chromosome itself has a macroscopic structure, which is most easily observed just prior to cell division, when the replicated sister chromatids are joined at the *centromere* with their arms extending outwards to the four *telomeres*. When stained with appropriate dyes, the condensed sections of each chromosome display unique banding patterns (e.g., G bands when Giemsa stain is used) due to local variations in AT- or GC-richness. A single G band contains around 10 million bp of DNA.

GENES AND GENE STRUCTURE

A *genome* may be defined as the total heritable informational content of an organism as contained in its DNA. In most human cells, which contain DNA not only in the nucleus but also in mitochondria (see below), there are actually two genomes present. One can therefore consider the nuclear and mitochondrial genomes as separate entities, or consider the entire human genome as comprising all forms of DNA in the cell.

The genome may be represented by a *map*, either linear or circular, with genes placed at appropriate intervals along its length. The earliest maps were *genetic maps*, in which the genes were ordered on the basis of *recombination frequency* (see below). However, the genome may also be drawn as a *physical map*, with known landmarks [e.g., genes, restriction endonuclease recognition sites (see below), or other features of the DNA] located at discrete intervals. The ultimate physical map is the DNA sequence itself.

The definition of a *gene* keeps undergoing revision as more is learned about genomic organization. The definition we will use is that *a gene is an integral unit of "usable" genetic information*. Most genes encode structural proteins, but some genes encode RNA [for example, the ribosomal RNAs (*rRNAs*) and transfer RNAs (*tRNAs*) that are used in protein translation]. It is now estimated that there are approximately 20,000 to 30,000 genes in the human genome, accounting for a mere 5 percent of the total genomic DNA; the remaining 95 percent serves no obvious role.

The organization of a gene is relatively simple (Fig. 33-5*A*). There is a coding region of DNA (whether for a polypeptide, a tRNA, or a rRNA) flanked at the 5' and 3' ends by regulatory regions of DNA (the direction or polarity of genes is conventionally represented as reading 5' to 3', from left to right, in the "message sense" of the transcribed RNA, as described below). In prokaryotic protein-coding genes, a single contiguous piece of DNA encodes a single polypeptide. However most eukaryotic protein-coding genes are segmented, with coding regions, or *exons*, separated by non-

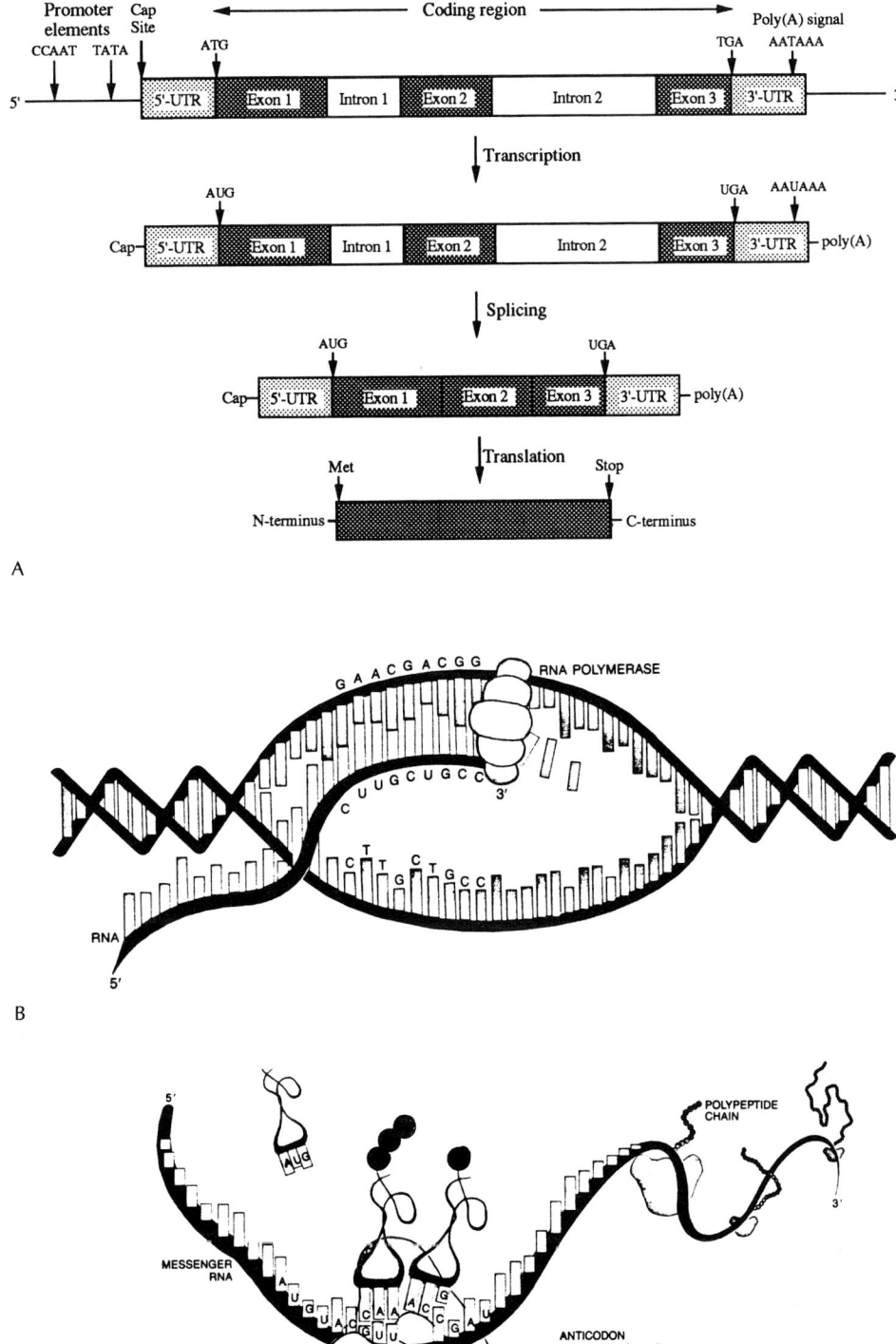

FIGURE 33-5. Transcription and translation. *A.* Structure of a eukaryotic gene; transcription of the gene to form the primary transcript; splicing of the primary transcript to form mature mRNA; and translation of the mature mRNA into a polypeptide. *B.* Schematic of transcription by RNA polymerase. Note that the coding strand of DNA has a sequence complementary to the message sense of the RNA. *C.* Translation of mRNA on a ribosome, using tRNAs to incorporate specific amino acids into the growing polypeptide chain. [*B* and *C* from Micklos DA, Freyer FA (eds): *DNA Science: A First Course in Recombinant DNA Technology.* Cold Spring Harbor, NY: Cold Spring Harbor Laboratory Press, 1990. Copyright © 1990 by Carolina Biological Supply Company.]

coding *intervening sequences*, or *introns*. The RNA *transcribed* from a split gene has the same exon/intron organization (i.e., the *precursor* RNA). In the processing of the precursor RNA, the introns are *spliced out* and the mature RNA transcript is exported from the nucleus into the cytoplasm to be *translated* into protein. Most of the excised intron sequence appears to be "junk" DNA; however, small regions of each intron contain signals that are required for correct splicing. Some eukaryotic genes do not have introns (e.g., rRNA genes).

Besides structural genes, eukaryotic genomes contain *pseudogenes*. These are regions of DNA that "look" like genes but are not genes in our definition because they are mutated, nonfunctional versions of an ancestral functional gene (i.e., they do not encode for a functional gene product). Both functional genes and their evolutionarily related inactive pseudogenes coexist in the genome, often (but not necessarily) at the same chromosomal locus. There are two types of pseudogenes: (1) those derived by *gene duplication* of a functional gene, followed by subsequent inactivation by mutation of one of the duplicated copies, and (2) those derived by *retroposition*, in which the processed RNA of a functional gene is *reverse transcribed* from RNA back into DNA and is inserted at a new chromosomal location lacking the appropriate DNA control signals for proper gene function, thereby rendering the gene inactive. Many "single-copy" functional genes are actually members of *gene families*, including functional genes that encode proteins of related function as well as pseudogenes.

Besides low-copy-number genes and gene families, the genome also contains families of medium- and high-copy-number elements, which are all repeated sequences of various types. These include (1) about 10 families of *satellite DNA*, each consisting of multiple (around 1 million) tandem repeats of a short (7- to 10-bp) repeating unit, located near the centromeres of chromosomes; (2) at least 14 families of *MERs*, or medium reiteration-frequency elements, ranging in size from 150 to 500 bp and present at a frequency of 200 to 10,000 copies[1]; (3) *LINEs*, or large interspersed repeated elements, which are multiple sequences 1000 to 7000 bp long scattered throughout the genome (e.g., the human *Kpn family*, with about 50,000 members); and (4) *SINEs*, or small interspersed repeated elements, which are also multiple sequences 100 to 300 bp long, dispersed randomly throughout the genome (e.g., the family of human *Alu sequences*, with more than 500,000 members[2]). Alu elements are primate-specific and are often used as markers of human DNA in recombinant DNA experiments.

RNA STRUCTURE: TRANSCRIPTION AND TRANSLATION

Transcription is the synthesis of RNA using one of the two DNA strands as the template, using the enzyme *RNA polymerase* to read, or transcribe, the DNA into RNA. Although the term applies to all RNAs, we will focus on transcription of eukaryotic *messenger RNAs*, or *mRNAs*, which encode proteins.

Transcription of an mRNA begins with the binding of RNA polymerase II upstream of the coding region of the gene (Fig. 33-5A and B) (RNA polymerases I and III transcribe other classes of RNAs, including rRNAs, tRNAs, and some repetitive elements). The polymerase advances in the 5' → 3' direction (i.e., by convention, this is usually denoted as the *top strand* of the DNA duplex, which is in the *message-sense* orientation) by reading the *bottom, antimessage strand* (also called the *coding strand*) of the DNA. At some point beyond the end of the coding region, the polymerase disengages from the DNA, thus terminating transcription.

A *transcription unit* is defined as the distance between sites of initiation and termination of a single RNA transcript (Fig. 33-5A). It contains signals that specify the beginning and the end of transcription, called the *promoter* and the *terminator*, respectively. The protein-coding region itself has "start" and "stop" signals for protein synthesis, or *translation*, that flank the part of the RNA encoding the polypeptide itself. The transcription unit, longer than the coding region, is flanked at both the 5' and 3' ends of the message by regions of *5'- and 3'-untranslated sequence* that are specified by the promoter and terminator in the DNA.

In eukaryotes, the message transcribed in the nucleus is actually a *precursor RNA*, because it includes both exons and introns, and also requires further modifications prior to export of the mature message from the nucleus to the cytoplasm, where translation takes place. Two important modifications are attachment of a *cap* structure (an unusual guanine nucleotide) to the 5' end of the transcript (nucleotide #1 of the primary transcript is often called the *cap site*) and the addition of a long stretch of polyadenylic acid (between 50 and 200 A's) to the 3' end of the transcript, about 10 to 30 nt downstream of the sequence AAUAAA (called the *polyadenylation signal*).

During the RNA maturation process, the introns are removed and the exons are ligated to each other, in a process called *splicing*. There are specific sequences at the 5' and 3' ends of the introns that are required for splicing: The dinucleotide GT is almost invariably found at the 5' end of each intron, while the dinucleotide AG, preceded by a polypyrimidine stretch, is found at the 3' end. The intron splicing machinery, called the *spliceosome*, is a complex *ribonucleoprotein* particle (i.e., it contains both proteins and RNA) that recognizes both the 5' and 3' splice signals, as well as a short sequence about 20 to 50 nt preceding the 3' splice site. This latter site is a signal for *lariat* formation: The G at the 5' end of the intron is ligated in a unique 2' to 5' phosphodiester bond to an A within the "lariat site," forming an authentic lariat-shaped structure. Following formation of the lariat (which is discarded and degraded), the flanking exons, still bound to the spliceosome, are brought together and ligated to each other.

In messages with more than 2 exons, *alternative splicing* may occur, often in a tissue-specific manner.[3,4] In this situation, an upstream exon may be ligated, not to its immediately following exon, but to an exon further downstream (Fig. 33-6). For example, rat troponin T contains 18 exons and 17 introns, but in fast skeletal muscle exon 3 is often ligated to exon 9, skipping exons 5 to 8.

Translation (Fig. 33-5C) takes place on ribosomes, which are giant ribonucleoprotein particles consisting of *ribosomal RNAs* (the two main ones are called *18S* and *28S rRNA*) and a few dozen *ribosomal proteins*. The ribosome straddles the mRNA and advances down the message from 5' to 3', reading the

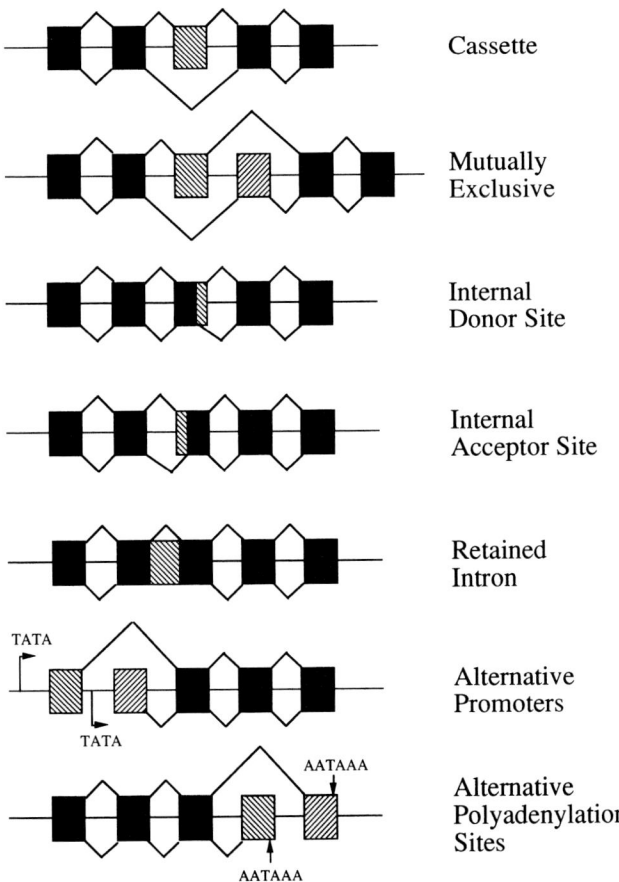

FIGURE 33-6. Patterns of alternative splicing. Exons (black boxes) and alternatively spliced sequences (shaded boxes) are spliced by different pathways (compare upper and lower connecting lines in each pattern). (Adapted from Breitbart RE, Andreadis A, Nadal-Ginard B: Alternative splicing: A ubiquitous mechanism for the generation of multiple protein isoforms from single genes. Annu Rev Biochem 56:467–495, 1987. With permission from the Annual Review of Biochemistry. Copyright © 1987 by Annual Reviews, Inc.)

RNA sequence of the coding region in groups of 3 nucleotides, called *triplets* or *codons* [each codon specifies a single amino acid, as determined by the *genetic code* (Fig. 33-7)], and incorporating the appropriate amino acid using one of the 20 amino acid–specific *transfer RNAs*, or *tRNAs*. Almost all polypeptides start with the triplet AUG, the codon that specifies the amino acid methionine. This AUG is the "start" signal for translation, and thus methionine is found at the *amino terminus* of most proteins (in many proteins, however, the *initiator Met* is removed in a posttranslational processing event). Translation terminates at the *carboxy terminus* of the protein when the cell's translation system encounters one of the three *stop codons*, UAA, UAG, or UGA. In between the initiator Met codon and the stop codon is the coding region itself, which is read by the translation system in RNA codons specifying one of the 20 amino acids, as defined by the genetic code. As there are 64 possible triplets of 4 bases (i.e., 4^3) but only 20 amino acids, the genetic code is *degenerate*, because most amino acids are specified by more than one codon; 3 of the 64—the stop codons—specify no amino acid at all.

REGULATION OF GENE EXPRESSION

The investigation of the nature of the signals in the DNA that specify the position and mode of expression of the transcription units is only partly understood and is one of the most intensively studied areas in all of biology. Not surprisingly, the regulation of transcription is turning out to be quite complex.[5] Specifically, small DNA sequences controlling or modulating transcription of mRNAs in mammalian cells by RNA polymerase II can be located at many places, both upstream and downstream of the transcription start site. These sites are targets for the binding of proteins, acting either singly or in combination, that can act as positive or negative regulators: *Positive* regulatory proteins bind to a control sequence to assist in transcription initiation, while *negative* ones usually bind to a site and repress transcription until they are removed from the binding site by other factors. Some of these control sites are located quite close to the transcription start site (within a few hundred bp), which is called the *promoter* region.

Two main control elements in the promoter region specify the accuracy and efficiency of transcription initiation (Fig. 33-8). One is called the *TATA box*, which is an AT-rich region (typical sequence TATAA) located about 30 nt prior to the cap site (i.e., nt -30), and which is the place on the DNA where the RNA polymerase binds in order to initiate transcription at the cap site (i.e., nt +1). The other element is called the *CCAAT box*, so called because the nucleotides CCAAT

	U	C	A	G	
U	UUU - Phe UUC - Phe UUA - Phe UUG - Phe	UCU - Ser UCC - Ser UCA - Ser UCG - Ser	UAU - Tyr UAC - Tyr UAA - Stop UAG - Stop	UGU - Cys UGC - Cys **UGA - Stop** UGG - Trp	U C A G
C	CUU - Leu CUC - Leu CUA - Leu CUG - Leu	CCU - Pro CCC - Pro CCA - Pro CCG - Pro	CAU - His CAC - His CAA - Gln CAG - Gln	CGU - Arg CGC - Arg CGA - Arg CGG - Arg	U C A G
A	AUU - Ile AUC - Ile **AUA - Ile** AUG - Met	ACU - Thr ACC - Thr ACA - Thr ACG - Thr	AAU - Asn AAC - Asn AAA - Lys AAG - Lys	AGU - Ser AGC - Ser **AGA - Arg** **AGG - Arg**	U C A G
G	GUU - Val GUC - Val GUA - Val GUG - Val	GCU - Ala GCC - Ala GCA - Ala GCG - Ala	GAU - Asp GAC - Asp GAA - Glu GAG - Glu	GGU - Gly GGC - Gly GGA - Gly GGG - Gly	U C A G

FIGURE 33-7. The genetic code. Note that except for codons specifying methionine and tryptophan, the code is degenerate—more than one codon can specify the same amino acid. The genetic code for human mitochondrial DNA differs from the universal code at the four codons shown in bold (in mtDNA, AUA = Met; UGA = Trp; AGA = Stop; AGG = Stop).

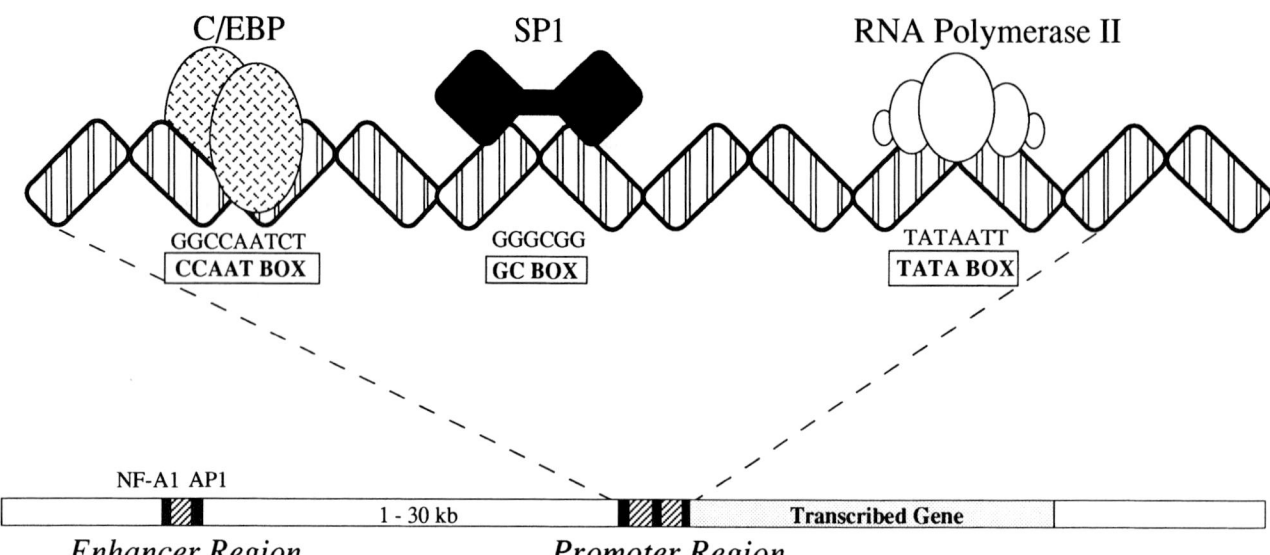

FIGURE 33-8. Promoters and enhancers. Examples of DNA-binding proteins and their target DNA sequences in the promoter region immediately upstream of a gene, relative to more distantly located enhancer elements (e.g., binding sites for nuclear factors NF-A1 and AP1). (Adapted from Micklos DA, Freyer FA (eds): DNA Science: A First Course in Recombinant DNA Technology. Cold Spring Harbor, NY: Cold Spring Harbor Laboratory Press, 1990. Copyright © 1990 by Carolina Biological Supply Company.)

are often part of the element's structure. It is located around nt position -80, and seems to regulate the efficiency of initiation. The TATA and CCAAT boxes are found upstream of many, but by no means all, genes. While CCAAT and TATA are generic promoter elements, other elements are specific to a gene type. For example, muscle-specific genes and genes induced by stress ("heat-shock" genes), growth factors, hormones, and environmental agents such as heavy metals all contain additional specialized elements in the 5'-flanking region.

As opposed to TATA, CCAAT, and some gene-specific promoter elements, other control elements lie very far away [up to 30 kilobases (kb)] from the cap site, both 5' and 3' to the gene, and can function independently of their orientation. These elements are called *enhancers*. Enhancers appear to be distal target sequences for DNA-binding proteins that operate in concert with other soluble factors and binding proteins to control the assembly of RNA polymerase in the proximal promoter region.

It has been found that the DNA-binding domains of identified transcription factors share a number of motifs, many with colorful names.[6] One such motif is called the *leucine zipper*.[7] This is a polypeptide motif in which the amino acid (aa) leucine is found repeated at 7-aa intervals along α-helical regions of various proteins; the 7-aa spacing aligns the leucines (usually 4 within a 28-aa stretch) along one face of the helix (Fig. 33-9A). When the protein dimerizes in antiparallel fashion, the two monomer faces align with the leucines interdigitated: hence the name zipper. The zipper domain promotes dimerization, thus facilitating DNA binding, which is located in an adjacent basic–amino acid DNA-binding domain. Thus, a leucine zipper protein dimer is like a pair of tongs: The zipper dimer forms the "handles," and the two basic DNA-binding domains form the "teeth" that grab the DNA. The leucine zipper was first found in a protein binding the CCAAT box, and was therefore called C/EBP (CCAAT/enhancer-binding protein). Since then, many DNA-binding proteins have been found to contain zipper domains, including the protooncogenes *fos, jun,* and *myc*.

A second motif is the *zinc finger*, in which a Zn^{2+} ion is coordinately bound tetrahedrally to two pairs of specific amino acids (cysteine or histidine) within the polypeptide, with a

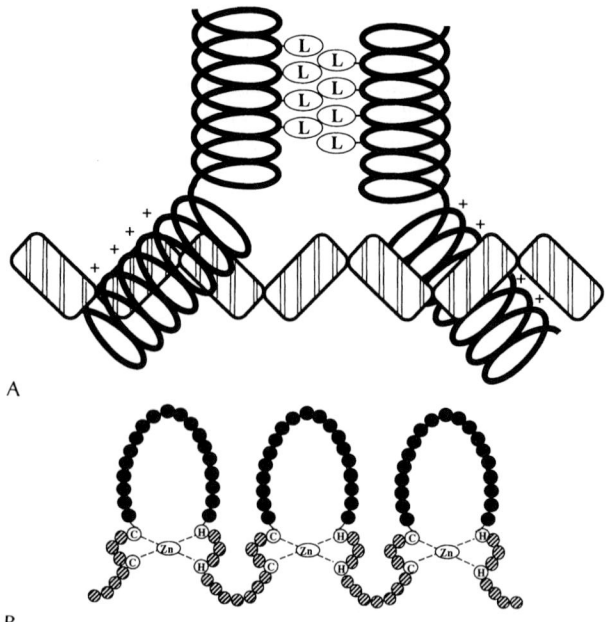

FIGURE 33-9. Transcription factor–binding motifs. A. The leucine zipper. The leucines (L's in ovals) are spaced at 7–amino acid intervals and associate as interdigitated dimers; the positively charged helical region may bind the negatively charged DNA. B. The zinc finger. Pairs of cysteine (C) and/or histidine (H) residues bind a zinc ion in a tetravalent coordinate complex, looping out intervening amino acids as the "fingers." (Both adapted from Lewin B: Genes IV. Cambridge, MA: Cell Press, 1990. With permission. Copyright © 1990 by Cell Press.)

peptide "finger" looped out between the pairs (Fig. 33-9B). Two examples of zinc finger proteins are the transcription factor Sp1, which binds to a GC-rich control element,[8] and the glucocorticoid receptor steroid-responsive element.[9]

A third motif is called the *homeodomain*, encoded by a DNA sequence called the *homeobox*, which is a sequence conserved across many species encoding a 60–amino acid polypeptide found to be important in cell- and tissue-specific pattern development during embryogenesis.[10,11] The homeodomain motif is related to the *helix-loop-helix* proteins, so named because the polypeptide contains a pair of α-helix peptides flanking a looped-out region of amino acids. The helix-loop-helix, or HLH, motif has been found in *MyoD*, the first identified member of a group of muscle-specific regulatory proteins.[12] Homeodomain motifs have been found in Pit-1, a pituitary-specific factor[13]; in the octamer-binding factors of immunoglobulin control regions,[14] such as Oct-1 and Oct-2; and in the Unc-86 regulatory protein in nematodes.[15] Besides the homeodomain, these proteins contain another consensus region (the POU box); the entire motif has been designated the *POU domain* (so named after Pit, Oct, and Unc).[16] Other known DNA-binding proteins, such as the *serum response factor*,[17] which is associated with binding to the *serum response element*, a muscle-specific gene regulatory sequence, belong to a different group of transcription factors containing the so-called MADS box.[18]

How do these DNA-binding proteins operate? In brief, these factors, either singly or in combination, bind to regions that regulate the transcription of specific genes, presumably by determining whether RNA polymerase can bind productively to initiate transcription of a specific gene. Interestingly, these regulatory mechanisms can operate both *in cis* (i.e., the binding protein acts on the segment of DNA containing the gene being regulated) or *in trans* (i.e., the binding protein acts "at a distance" and binds to a region of DNA located far from the gene it regulates, and in fact, may act at a locus on a totally different chromosome).

A well-studied example of *cis*-acting regulation is the "locus control region" (LCR) that regulates the developmental expression of the six globin genes located at the human β-globin locus on chromosome 11 (Fig. 33-10A).[19] An LCR is a segment of DNA that is able to enhance expression of a linked gene(s); in the case of the β-globin locus, the LCR elements are located between 6 and 22 kb upstream of the embryonic ε-globin gene, the first gene in the series. One model for *cis*-activation is a "looping" model, in which proteins bound to the LCR are brought into proximity of a downstream gene by looping of the upstream DNA so that proteins bound at the LCR are brought into contact with proteins located at the promoter, thereby activating transcription (Fig. 33-10B). Other models, such as those in which the LCR-bound proteins "track" along the DNA until they find the promoter region, have also been proposed. More than 30 LCR-like elements have been identified, including an LCR regulating expression of the human β-myosin heavy-chain gene in muscle.[20]

Regulation *in trans* is exemplified by the "Swi/Snf" nucleosome remodeling complexes.[21] Although the terms Swi and Snf derive from yeast sucrose fermentation mutants, the Swi/Snf family is highly conserved in evolution, and is present in humans.[22,23] In essence, Swi/Snf is a multisubunit complex (at least eight polypeptides) that can bind to chromatin and reposition nucleosomes, thus presumably allowing the transcription to proceed (or to be repressed) at specific genes, including at least one muscle-specific gene, *MYOD*.[24] Such activation/repression may occur via binding directly to the transcriptional machinery (e.g., to RNA polymerase II or to TATA-binding protein), or via binding to an activator protein located near the gene promoter.

Thus, the cell can regulate transcription by controlling whether transcription factors are, or are not, available to bind DNA and initiate transcription in a tissue- or temporal-specific manner. However, many transcription factors are promiscuous, in the sense that they can bind to dozens, or

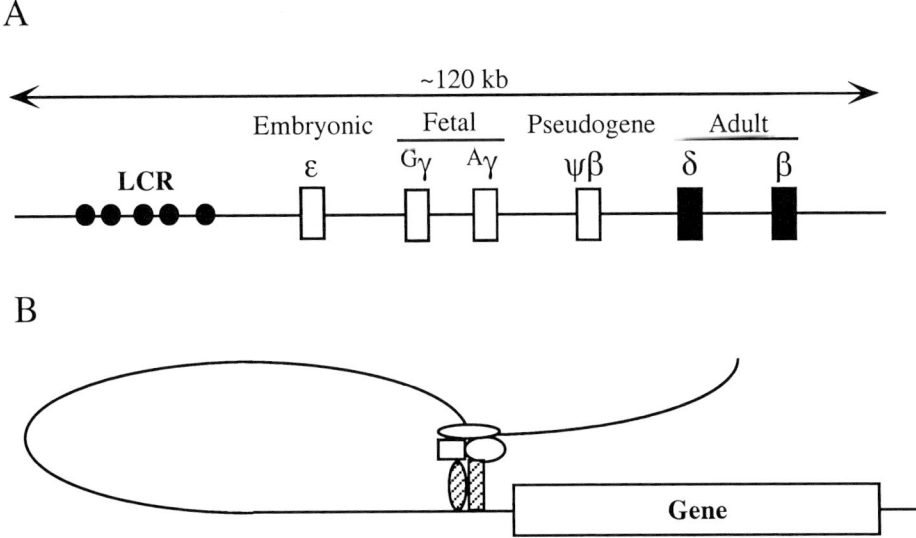

FIGURE 33-10. *Cis*-acting gene regulation. *A*. The locus control region (LCR) in the human β-globin locus. Map distances are not to scale. *B*. The "looping" model for *cis*-activation at the LCR.

even hundreds, of gene promoters, and yet there are circumstances where such a factor will initiate transcription of only a subset of these genes. The fact that some genes are turned "on" while many others are "off" thus begs the question as to how the cell can distinguish between "transcription-competent" and "transcription-incompetent" regions of the chromosome. In general, transcriptional competence is determined epigenetically, that is, via effects on gene expression arising from "transient" modifications of the genome that are not inherited unalterably. The main modification controlling transcription is (reversible) DNA methylation in so-called CpG islands (i.e., methylation of a cytosine to ^{CH_3}C specifically when present in the dinucleotide CG) located in the upstream regions of genes.[25] Other epigenetic phenomena, many of which are set down in the germline, are reprogramming of the genome during development, mainly via genomewide changes in DNA methylation patterns,[26] covalent modification of histone proteins,[27] X-chromosome inactivation,[28] and genomic imprinting, in which only one of the two parentally inherited genes is expressed, while the other is "silenced."[29] Gene expression can even be regulated post-transcriptionally, through "gene silencing" of transcribed mRNAs via *RNA interference* (RNAi), in which a small (~22-nt) piece of *antisense* RNA binds to the mRNA and initiates a cascade of events resulting in degradation of the message.[30]

TYPES OF DNA MUTATIONS AND THEIR CONSEQUENCES

While almost all the DNA in a person is similar to that in other individuals (especially in the gene regions), it has been estimated that there is a 1-bp difference between any two individuals as frequently as once per 250 to 500 bp. Of course, most (but not all) of these differences are in the non-gene portions of the genome, and have no apparent effect on the phenotype. Such differences, in which different versions of a DNA sequence exist at a particular locus, are called *DNA polymorphisms*. DNA polymorphisms may take many forms. They may be single-base substitutions (an AT pair replacing a GC pair, for example); they may be single or multiple base-pair *insertions* or *deletions* of DNA; they may be *tandem repeats* of a short sequence element, varying among individuals in the number of repeats; or they may be *duplications, inversions*, or other *rearrangements* of DNA regions, caused by various types of *recombination events*.

These types of alterations in DNA can have consequences that affect the phenotype, some of which are fortunate, but which more often are deleterious. These changes are generally called *mutations*, although the term has been applied to all changes in DNA, irrespective of consequence. Hereditary diseases may result from mutations at any level of DNA organization, ranging from single base-pair errors to alterations in whole chromosomes.

Point mutations are single-nucleotide changes in the genome (Fig. 33-11). A point mutation in which one purine is replaced by another purine (e.g., A → G), or a pyrimidine by a pyrimidine (e.g., C → T), is called a *transition*; a replacement of a purine by a pyrimidine or vice versa (e.g., G → T) is called a *transversion*. If the change is in a coding region, the mutation could still be innocuous, because the change might

be "silent" [e.g., a G → A change that converts one glutamate codon (GAG) into another (GAA)]. On the other hand, a deleterious mutation may arise if the change alters the amino acid incorporated into a polypeptide chain [e.g., a G → A change can convert the codon for glutamate (GAG) into one for lysine (AAG)], resulting in a *missense mutation*, which may alter the function of the protein. Alternatively, the mutation may convert a triplet into a stop codon (e.g., a G → T change converting GAG to TAG), resulting in a *nonsense mutation* that causes premature termination of translation and almost always producing a truncated protein with either aberrant function or no function.

While most pathogenic point mutations fall into the two classes of missense and nonsense alterations, there is a remarkable variety of other types of changes that a single base alteration can engender. Point mutations can prevent transcription initiation (e.g., if the mutation is in CCAAT, TATA, or another promoter or enhancer element) or can have effects on the initiation, amount, stability, and/or processing of mRNAs. They can prevent efficient translation [e.g., mutation of the *ribosome-binding site* located in the 5' untranslated region (5'-UTR) of the message]. They can cause errors in RNA splicing if they change the sequences located at the 5' and 3' ends of introns required for correct ligation of the flanking exons, thus causing the excision of exons or the interposition of "meaningless" intron sequences into a mature message, while mutations within exons that create canonical splice sites can cause "premature" splicing starting at the "cryptic" splice site within the exon rather than at the authentic site at the end of the exon. They can prevent transcription termination (if in a downstream termination element) or polyadenylation (e.g., mutation of the polyadenylation signal from AAUAAA to AAUGAA), thereby altering the amount of mRNA produced. An unusual example of an error in the 3'-untranslated region (3'-UTR) was a mutation located in the region downstream of the polyadenylation signal associated with cleavage of the primary transcript for the prothrombin gene: The mutation caused a gain of function by *upregulating* the amount of cleaved mRNA, thereby causing thrombocytopenia.[31]

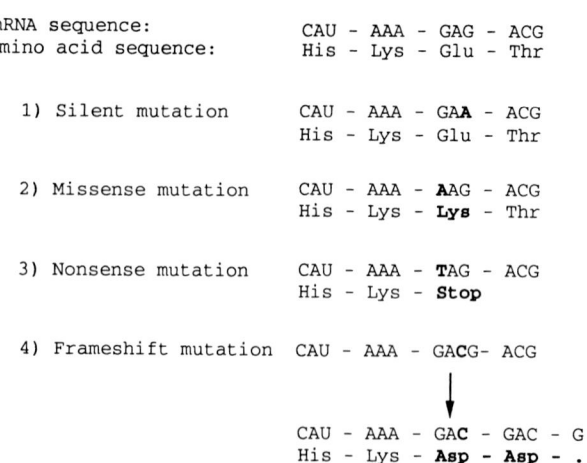

FIGURE 33-11. Point and frameshift mutations in DNA. The wild-type DNA and deduced amino acid sequence (top lines) can be altered by the indicated single-base mutations (bold).

Amazingly, eukaryotic cells have the ability to recognize and degrade mRNAs that contain premature stop codons generated, for example, by nonsense mutations. This process, termed nonsense-mediated mRNA decay (NMD), normally operates as a surveillance mechanism to eliminate those erroneous messages containing inappropriate in-frame stop codons that are inadvertently transcribed from *normal* genes.[32,33] NMD operates posttranscriptionally, with the surveillance mechanism taking place in the nucleus prior to mRNA export. Given the existence of NMD, one might guess that authentic pathogenic stop-codon mutations would be less severe than expected. In fact, NMD does seem to modify the severity of such mutations, with the expression of the disorder related to whether or not the mutation resides in an upstream exon (higher frequency of NMD) or a downstream exon (lower frequency). The graded severity of disease due to different mutations in β-globin (causing β-thalassemia) and in fibrillin 1 (causing Marfan syndrome) has been attributed to NMD.[32]

Equally remarkable, missense mutations and even silent site mutations can also sometimes have deleterious effects on mRNA stability and translation.[34] If the mutation (in the DNA) falls within a region of an exon that contains a so-called exonic splicing enhancer (ESE) or exonic splicing silencer (ESS)—small 6- to 8-nt sequence motifs that bind splicing factors and are required for efficient splicing of the exon in which they reside[35,36]—then exon skipping, alternative splice site choice, or intron inclusion in the precursor or the processed mRNA may result.[37]

Mutations in a coding region in which an extra 1 or 2 bp are inserted or deleted often cause *frameshift mutations* because they throw the triplet reading frame out of register, so that either a new protein with a totally different amino acid sequence (downstream of the point of the mutation, of course) is produced, or a previously out-of-frame stop codon is now brought into frame, causing premature termination and a truncated protein (Fig. 33-11). Small insertions and deletions in noncoding regions can have the same bad effects as those described above with point mutations.

A special case of insertion/deletion mutations is that where the reading frame is maintained, i.e., where the insertion or deletion is a multiple of 3 bp. In the last decade, a large number of "trinucleotide repeat diseases" have been described, in which the coding region contains an insertion of a few dozen repeats of a simple trinucleotide sequence, for example CAG, which specifies the amino acid glutamine (see below).

Mutations caused by large-scale DNA rearrangements are also quite common. These would include the insertion or deletion of large blocks of sequence (up to several kilobases long), substitution of one segment of DNA by another, *tandem duplication* of blocks of sequence, repetitive duplication of sequences (i.e., *amplification*), and *inversions* of sequences (so that the "top" strand is now on the "bottom" and vice versa, causing a region of the coding strand to be "nonsense" DNA). Again, the severity of the mutation will depend on its precise location. The best-known large-scale mutations causing muscle disease are those in the dystrophin gene leading to Duchenne and Becker muscular dystrophy, while facioscapulohumeral muscular dystrophy is due most commonly to expansions of a 3.3-kb segment of DNA on chromosome 4 called D4Z4.[38]

MITOCHONDRIAL GENETICS

Eukaryotic cells contain mitochondria, which are bacterium-sized organelles in which many important cellular functions take place, including the citric acid cycle, lipid metabolism, the respiratory chain, and oxidative phosphorylation.[39] The mitochondrion is the only cellular organelle, besides the nucleus, that contains its own DNA (mtDNA). Mitochondria have their own modes of replication and transcription, as well as their own translational machinery. They also have a genetic code different from the nuclear "universal" code (Fig. 33-7). However, the mitochondrial genome contains few genes, and almost all of the proteins required for mitochondrial function are encoded by nuclear gene products, which are synthesized in the cytoplasm and are then imported into the organelle (see Chap. 58).

Human mtDNA is a 16,569-bp circle of double-stranded DNA.[40] It encodes 13 mRNAs specifying 13 structural polypeptides, plus 2 rRNAs and 22 tRNAs used in the protein translation of the 13 mRNAs (see Chap. 58). The 13 structural genes specify subunits of four of the five complexes making up the respiratory chain/oxidative phosphorylation system, all of which are located in the mitochondrial inner membrane. These include seven subunits of NADH–coenzyme Q oxidoreductase (complex I), one subunit of coenzyme Q–cytochrome *c* oxidoreductase (complex III), three subunits of cytochrome *c* oxidase (complex IV), and two subunits of ATP synthase (complex V). These complexes also contain subunits encoded by nuclear genes, which are imported from the cytoplasm and are coassembled with the mtDNA-encoded subunits. One complex, succinate–coenzyme Q oxidoreductase (complex II), contains no mtDNA-encoded subunits and is encoded entirely by nuclear genes. Most of the nuclear-encoded respiratory chain subunit genes have been cloned; dissection of their promoter regions has revealed that many contain promoter and enhancer elements specific for these genes—the "OXBOX" in the 5′-flanking region of the ADP/ATP translocator gene[41] and the DNA-binding regions for two "nuclear respiratory factors" called NRF-1 and NRF-2.[42]

The replication of mtDNA is unique. The two mtDNA strands (called the *heavy* and *light* strands) are replicated asymmetrically, using two origins of replication—one on each strand, called O_H and O_L—placed at separate locations on the circle, for synthesis of each daughter strand.[43] Mitochondrial transcription is also unusual. The transcription units are *polycistronic*: They are large precursor RNAs, derived from transcription of both the heavy and light strands, containing multiple tRNAs and mRNAs. In a series of posttranscriptional processing events, the tRNAs, which are located between most of the individual protein-coding segments of the precursor message, are excised from the precursor, thereby also releasing the intervening mRNAs. These mRNAs, which contain no introns, are then polyadenylated prior to translation.[44,45]

Mitochondria are inherited exclusively from the mother,[46] Thus, human mtDNA, and, by extension, any genetic defect in the mitochondrial genome, is *maternally inherited*. The mitochondria of most somatic cells contain multiple genomes—about five genomes per organelle[47]—and there are hundreds or thousands of mitochondria per cell, depending on the oxidative requirements of each cell or tissue. Unfertilized eggs[48–50] and platelets[51] apparently contain only one mtDNA per organelle. Usually all the mtDNAs in a person are identical, that is, the population is *homoplasmic*. In some cases, however, including a number of cases in which mtDNA mutations cause disease, two or more populations of mtDNAs (e.g., normal and mutated genomes) can coexist in the same person, a situation known as *heteroplasmy*. There are even cases where some mitochondria are totally devoid of mtDNA, but nevertheless are still viable and can still divide (although, of course, they would be incapable of oxidative phosphorylation).

The Tools of Molecular Biology

Much of the material reviewed in this section can be found in greater detail in specialized texts on techniques in molecular biology and recombinant DNA. The laboratory "bible" in the field is by Sambrook and Russell[52] (historically called "Maniatis," after the original author), although other texts are also excellent.[53,54]

ENZYMOLOGY OF DNA AND RNA

The breakthroughs in our ability to study and manipulate genes are a direct result of the knowledge developed in the last 40 years on the basic biology of prokaryotes and on the metabolism of nucleic acids. Much of the enzymology associated with these two areas has been used to create the fundamental tools of the molecular biologist. With these tools, one can now synthesize, cut, ligate, rearrange, transform, sequence, and otherwise manipulate DNA and RNA so that they can be studied or used for other purposes.

By far the most useful and versatile of these tools are the *restriction endonucleases*, enzymes isolated from prokaryotes that cleave double-stranded DNA at specific DNA sequences. Restriction endonucleases (also called *restriction enzymes*) isolated from different species of bacteria usually have different cleavage *sequence specificities*. As a general rule, most restriction sites are 4-, 6-, or 8-bp *palindromic* sequences; that is, they have the same sequence when read on both the top and bottom strands (e.g., the enzyme *Bam*HI, isolated from *Bacillus amyloliquefaciens* H, cuts within the 6-bp palindrome GGATCC, while *Pvu*II, isolated from *Proteus vulgaris*, cuts within CAGCTG). All else being equal, a "4-cutter," such as *Alu*I (cleavage site AGCT) will cut a genome in many small pieces, because a specific 4-bp sequence is present on average once every 256 bp ($1/4^4$). At the other extreme, an "8-cutter" like *Not*I (recognition sequence GCGGCCGC) should cleave DNA only once every 64,000 bp ($1/4^8$). In fact, *Not*I cuts human DNA even less frequently—about once per million bp—because mammalian DNA is unusually sparse in the dinucleotide CG; *Not*I is thus a very useful enzyme for long-range physical mapping of human DNA.

The position of the *cleavage site* relative to the recognition sequence varies among restriction enzymes (Fig. 33-12). Some cut "dead-center" within the palindrome (e.g., *Sma*I cuts at CCC|GGG (where the line denotes the cleavage position), leaving *blunt-ended* DNA ends. Others cut asymmetrically within the recognition sequence, leaving 5' *overhangs* (e.g., *Eco*RI cuts at G|AATTC) or 3' *overhangs* (e.g., *Pst*I cuts at CTGCA|G). Still others (usually those with nonpalindromic recognition sequences) have their cleavage sites located outside the boundaries of the recognition sequence (e.g., *Mnl*I cuts at GGATCNNNNNNN|, where N is any of the four bases), while yet others cut within the recognition sequence, but in a "degenerate" manner (e.g., *Hin*fI cuts at G|ANTC). Sometimes different species of bacteria produce restriction endonucleases with the same sequence specificity; often, these *isoschizomers* differ in their cleavage positions (e.g., *Hha*I cuts at CGC|G, while *Hin*PI cuts at C|GCG).

There are now hundreds of identified restriction enzymes and sequence specificities, providing powerful tools for many kinds of manipulations, as shown below. Why do bacteria synthesize these enzymes? Simply put, restriction endonucleases are the prokaryotic version of the immune system: Any "foreign" piece of DNA that enters the cell (for example, on a *bacteriophage*, which is a bacterial virus) will be cleaved rapidly by the host's restriction system into smaller harmless DNA fragments. The host bacterium protects its own chromosomal DNA from cleavage by its own restriction enzyme (similar to self-tolerance) by methylating a specific nucleotide—usually adenine or cytosine—located within all the recognition sequences on its own DNA (e.g., the enzyme *Eco*RI *methylase* converts GAATTC to GA^{CH_3}ATTC, which is resistant to cleavage by *Eco*RI). Since the restriction enzyme

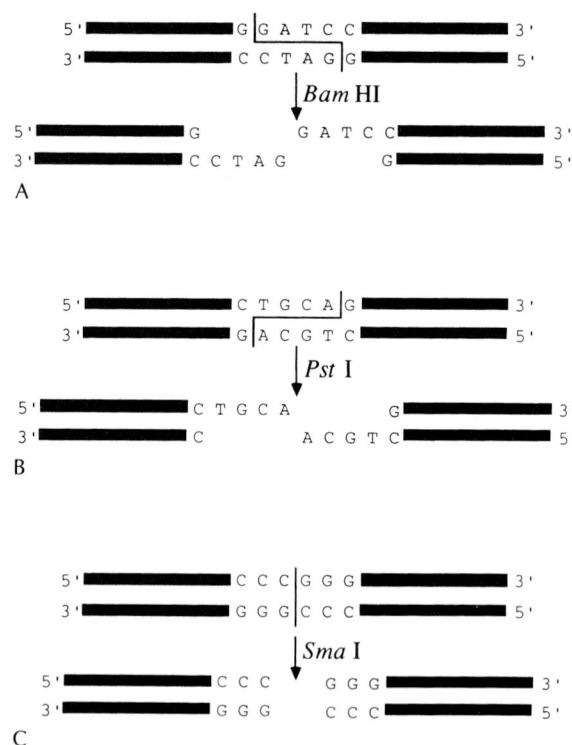

FIGURE 33-12. Restriction endonucleases. *A*. Cleavage of double-stranded DNA to leave a 5' overhang (e.g., *Bam*HI). *B*. Cleavage to leave a 3' overhang (e.g., *Pst*I). *C*. Cleavage to leave a blunt end (e.g., *Sma*I). Note the palindromic nature of the recognition sites.

can cut only within "naked," unmethylated recognition sequences, the methylated chromosome (but not invading, unmethylated, viral DNA) is protected. Because bacteria containing this combined *restriction-modification* system will prevent various genetic engineering manipulations from being carried out, many laboratory bacterial strains are often mutated in these functions.

There is a wide range of DNA and RNA modifying enzymes that, in conjunction with the restriction enzymes, enable one to change or manipulate the structure of nucleic acids in specific ways. *Polymerases* advance along a strand of nucleic acid and synthesize the complementary strand. They come in three types: *DNA-dependent DNA polymerases* (e.g., *Escherichia coli* DNA polymerase I, phage T4 DNA polymerase, mammalian DNA polymerase α; mitochondrial DNA polymerase γ) replicate DNA; *DNA-dependent RNA polymerases* (e.g., phage T7 RNA polymerase, mammalian RNA polymerases I, II, and III) transcribe DNA into RNA; and *RNA-dependent DNA polymerases* (e.g., avian myeloblastosis virus *reverse transcriptase*) reverse-transcribe RNA back into DNA. Two DNA polymerases deserve special mention: (1) *Klenow fragment*, which is a portion of *E. coli* DNA polymerase I lacking the 5' → 3' exonuclease activity, is useful for filling in nucleotides (often radioactively labeled) and for synthesizing intact complementary DNA strands in vitro, and (2) *Taq polymerase*, derived from the thermophilic bacterium *Thermus aquaticus*, which can replicate DNA at high temperatures, making it particularly useful in the polymerase chain reaction (see below).

Nucleases cut at phosphodiester bonds in nucleic acid chains: *Exonucleases* operate only at the edges of DNA or RNA and "nibble" inwards, releasing free mononucleotides, while *endonucleases* cut at phosphodiester bonds anywhere within a DNA or RNA chain to release oligonucleotide fragments (and ultimately free nucleotides); some nucleases have both activities. Nucleases may be specific for DNA (e.g., DNase I) or for RNA (e.g., RNase A, RNase T1, exonuclease VII); they may prefer single-stranded substrates (e.g., S1 nuclease, mung bean nuclease) or double-stranded ones (e.g., DNase I, exonuclease III, Bal-31 nuclease), or cut both indiscriminately. The ribonuclease RNase H has the interesting property of degrading RNA only when the RNA is part of a DNA-RNA duplex.

Other enzymes catalyze the modification of nucleic acids. *Phosphatases* remove 5'-terminal phosphate groups from DNA and RNA, leaving 5'-OH. *Kinases* do the opposite: They add a phosphate group to the 5'-OH on dephosphorylated DNA. *Ligases* covalently bind two DNA or RNA strands in an esterification reaction between the phosphate group at the 5' end of one strand with the hydroxyl at the 3' end of another strand, thereby forming a phosphodiester bond. *Terminal deoxynucleotidyl transferase* adds nucleotides to the ends of DNA, a useful property if one wants to add a polynucleotide *tail* to a DNA fragment; *polynucleotide phosphorylase* adds ribonucleotides to the end of RNA. *Poly(A) polymerase* can add a poly(A) tail to the 3' end of an RNA synthesized in vitro, while *guanylyltransferase* (also called *capping enzyme*) can add the 5'-terminal cap structure; *tobacco acid pyrophosphatase* will remove these caps.

Still other enzymes modify the shape of DNA: These are the *topoisomerases*. Some can introduce superhelical turns into a double-stranded DNA circle (e.g., topoisomerase II, also called DNA gyrase), similar to twisting a rubber band many times, while others (e.g., topoisomerase I) can remove turns from a supercoiled circle and convert it into a "relaxed" circle. Other proteins, such as T4 gene 32 helix destabilizing protein and *E. coli* single-stranded binding protein, bind DNA after it is unwound.

CLONING GENES

Genes are now routinely isolated, or *cloned*, based on the principles and using the tools described in the preceding sections. Most genes are cloned from libraries of recombinant DNA molecules. Below, we describe how libraries are constructed, what the contents of a DNA library are, and how individual clones may be identified. In addition, we describe how, once identified, a clone can be used as a tool to investigate how the DNA sequences contained in that clone are organized in the genome and how one can study the expression of specific genes in tissues.

Libraries. A library may be defined as a place in which reference materials, usually books, are kept for use. Ordinarily, these reference materials are easily accessible because they are catalogued and cross-referenced. In molecular biology, a *library* is a collection of recombinant DNA molecules—the books—that can serve as a source of specific clones. However, the term *library* in this case is not completely analogous, because there is no "Dewey decimal system"—the clones are not catalogued and can be extracted from the library only after a search through the library's entire contents.

The recombinants used in making a library are specific. They are composed of gene sequences that can self-propagate in bacteria (called the *vector*), plus a segment of DNA from another species of interest (the *insert*); both sources of DNA replicate as a single covalent segment of DNA (the *recombinant*). To carry the analogy of the library further, the recombinant is like a book. It has a cover to help protect it and carry it around (the vector), and it is filled with the pages that a reader will be interested in reading (the insert).

Vectors and inserts. The self-replicating vector DNA is derived from a *phage* (a bacterial virus) or a *plasmid* (an autonomous piece of self-replicating, extrachromosomal DNA found in many bacteria). The most commonly used vectors are bacteriophage lambda (λ) and variants of the circular plasmid pBR322 (the lowercase "p" is a common prefix to signify that we are talking about a plasmid) and the circular bacteriophage M13. The size of λ is about 48 kb pairs; pBR322 is 4.5 kb, and M13 is 7.3 kb. All of these vectors can be propagated in the bacterium *Escherichia coli*, which is referred to as the *host*. For technical reasons, λ vectors can accommodate inserts up to only about 20 kb long, while it is difficult to insert fragments greater than about 10 kb into M13 or into plasmids. However, another type of vector has been created by genetic engineering, called a *cosmid*, which combines the best features of both phages and plasmids; in a cosmid, inserts up to 40 to 50 kb can be accommodated.

The recombinants are made by using restriction enzymes. Both the insert and vector DNA are cut with restriction

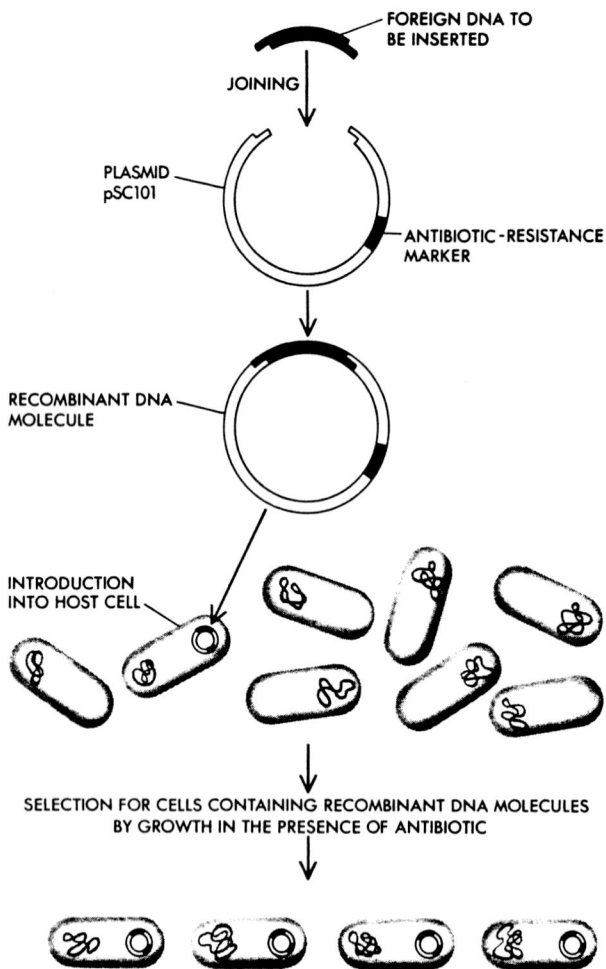

FIGURE 33-13. Creating recombinant DNA molecules. Insertion of a foreign sequence into a plasmid vector using drug selection to select for successful recombinants. (From Watson JD, Tooze J, Kurtz DT (eds): Recombinant DNA: A Short Course. New York: Scientific American/WH Freeman, 1983. Copyright © 1983 by Scientific American Books, Inc. Reprinted with permission of W.H. Freeman and Company.)

Recombinant phage or cosmid DNA can be infected into E. coli by a method called *in vitro packaging*. In this case, the naked DNA is mixed with separate protein components of the phage that are required for packaging of the DNA into its outer protein "coat," or *capsid*. Under appropriate conditions in vitro, the DNA and the *packaging extract* will self-assemble and become an infectious particle that can infect at very high efficiency—perhaps 1 in 20. Practically speaking, plasmid transfection yields about 10^5 *clones* per μg of recombinant DNA, while phage infection yields about $10^7/\mu g$. Each clone is a segment of DNA that has been amplified as a recombinant molecule in bacteria.

Once the DNA transfection or infection has been accomplished, the individual recombinant DNA molecules can be isolated as a single clone from the *library*, which is the total of all the viable plasmid or phage recombinants. Bacteria harboring plasmid recombinants form *colonies* on agar plates; each colony contains several thousand cells, each with one or more identical copies of the recombinant DNA, all of which were derived from transfection of a single cell by a single recombinant plasmid. Since λ phages are bacterial viruses that are lethal to their hosts, E. coli harboring phage λ recombinants do not form colonies but rather *plaques* (clear, circular areas of dead bacteria *lysed* by phage, as visualized against a background "lawn" of uninfected bacteria). Like colonies, however, each plaque represents one *infective center* derived from infection of a single cell with a single recombinant phage (Fig. 33-14). In both cases, an individual colony or plaque can now be picked and grown in bulk to yield 10^9 to 10^{12} identical recombinants per milliliter; up to 200 μg of recombinant DNA can be

enzymes that have compatible restriction sites; the insert and vector are then *ligated* together using DNA ligase (Fig. 33-13). Those recombinants that are viable can be selected by *transforming* (in the case of plasmids) or *infecting* (in the case of phage) them into the host. In transformation, pure, or "naked," DNA is taken up by E. coli bacteria that have been pretreated with calcium; about 1 molecule in 100,000 finds its way into the cell and replicates.

The most useful hosts are those that permit recombinants but not nonrecombinants to grow. Conditions are selected under which the recombinant and host can grow together but the host alone cannot grow. Typically, the plasmid contains a gene for *antibiotic resistance* (usually ampicillin, tetracycline, or kanamycin) to which the host is sensitive; only recombinant-containing hosts will grow when plated on the appropriate antibiotic-containing growth medium. In the case of phages, the phage may carry a lethal mutation that can be *suppressed* only by a host designed for this purpose; this prevents the recombinant from spreading to a natural, nonengineered host.

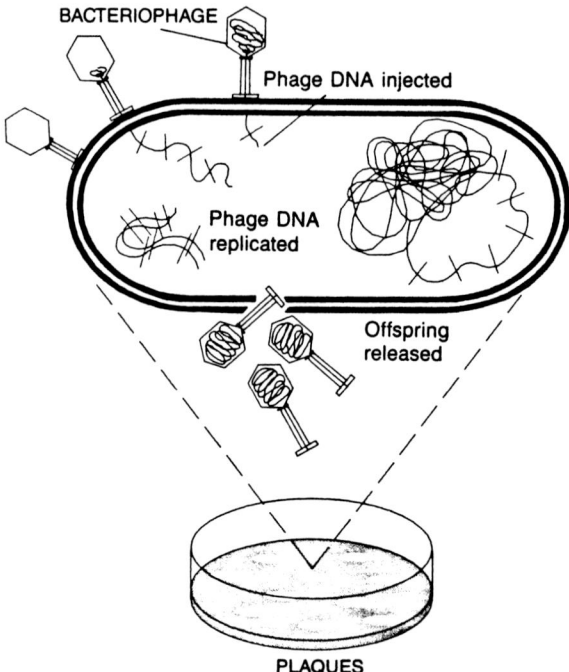

FIGURE 33-14. Phage infection of a bacterium and plaque formation on a lawn of uninfected bacteria. (From Micklos DA, Freyer FA (eds): DNA Science: A First Course in Recombinant DNA Technology. Cold Spring Harbor, NY: Cold Spring Harbor Laboratory Press, 1990. Copyright © 1990 by Carolina Biological Supply Company.)

purified in a day or two from such preparations. The process of obtaining replicas of the DNA from a single cell or organism is what we mean by *cloning*; if the DNA of interest happens to be a gene, we would say that "we have cloned a gene."

Genomic libraries. The complete genome of an organism can be represented in a *genomic library*. The most useful phage vectors for genomic libraries are *replacement vectors*, in which a segment of the wild-type phage has been removed and is now replaced by a similarly sized insert of foreign DNA of interest (Fig. 33-15A). For example, the λ phage called Charon 30 is 46.5 kb long and contains recognition sites for the restriction enzymes *Bam*HI, *Eco*RI, *Hin*dIII, *Sal*I, and *Xho*I. Cleavage of Charon 30 with *Bam*HI releases a *left arm* 22.3 kb long, a *right arm* 9.2 kb long, and two copies of an internal 7.5-kb *stuffer fragment*. The vector is designed so that the 15 kb of eliminated stuffer can be replaced with foreign DNA while still maintaining the viability of the phage. Only molecules of a certain size can be packaged viably in the phage capsid; thus, there is both a "lower" and an "upper" *packaging limit* for the amount of foreign DNA that can be incorporated into the vector. In the case of Charon 30, the limit ranges from 6.9 to 16.6 kb.

The replacement or insert DNA is obtained from the species to be cloned and is cleaved with a restriction enzyme with a recognition site compatible with the cloning sites in the vector. Because of the packaging limits of the vector, complete digestion of genomic DNA with a restriction enzyme such as *Bam*HI would not give a complete library because some *Bam*HI fragments would not fit in the vector. This is because digestion of genomic DNA with *Bam*HI (a "6-cutter" that cuts at 5'-G|GATCC-3') yields a Poisson distribution of sizes centered around 4096 bp, and many fragments would be either too large or too small to fit within the Charon 30 packaging limits. The most common way to circumvent this problem is to do a *partial digestion* using a more frequently recognized but compatible sequence. For example, digestion of genomic DNA with the "4-cutter" *Mbo*I (which cleaves at 5'-|GATC-3') results in fragments that are, on the average only 256 bp long but which have overhanging "*sticky ends*"—GATC—that are identical (and complementary) to the 5' overhangs generated by cleavage with *Bam*HI (see Fig. 33-12). Therefore, the genomic DNA is digested with "suboptimal" amounts of *Mbo*I, so that not every *Mbo*I site is cleaved, and a distribution of partially digested *Mbo*I fragments is obtained with an average length of about 15 kb. Each such fragment, which can now be ligated into the *Bam*HI site of Charon 30, will contain about 60 *Mbo*I sites (i.e., 15,000/250). However, cleavage at the *Mbo*I sites is random, so that a sequence of interest may be found in different, *overlapping* clones. Because the haploid human genome contains about 3×10^9 bp, a human genomic library in phage would require a minimum of 200,000 independent clones (i.e., $3 \times 10^9 / 1.5 \times 10^4$) to cover the entire genome, assuming no missing regions and no overlap of clones.

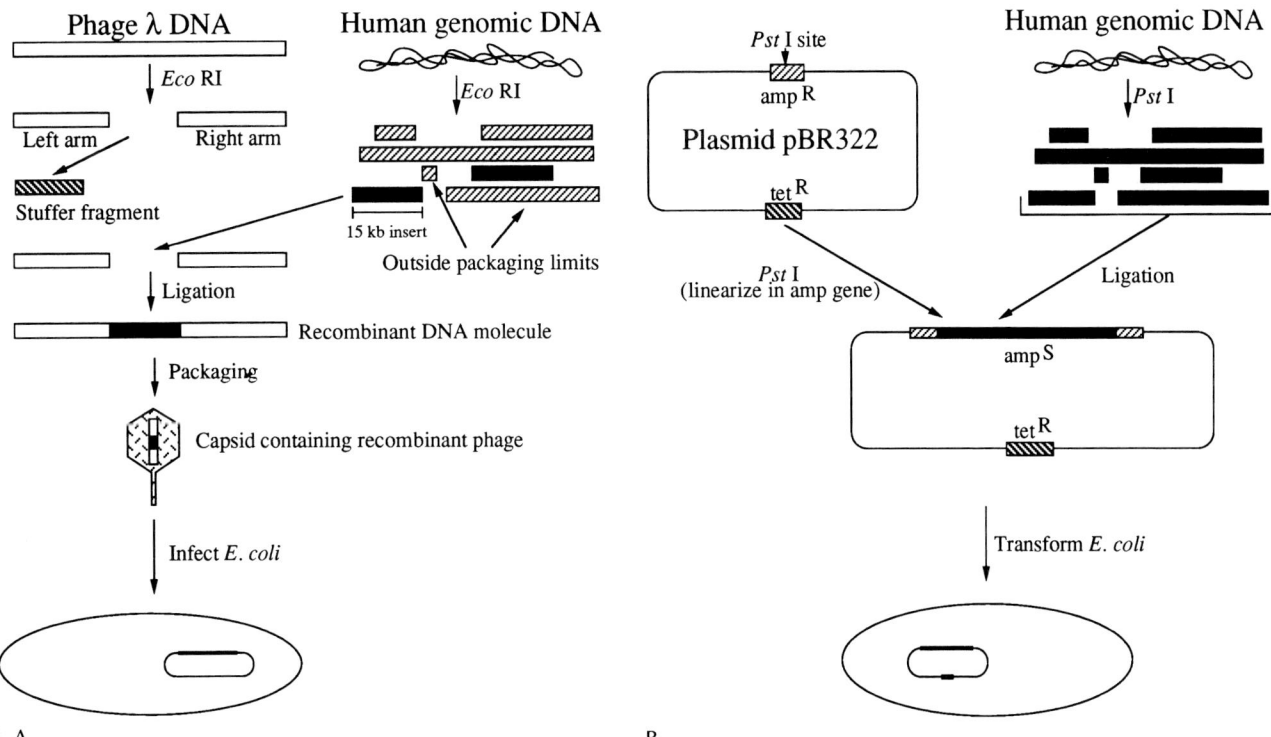

FIGURE 33-15. Making phage and plasmid genomic recombinant libraries. *A.* Making a genomic library in phage λ. (*Adapted from Watson JD, Hopkins NH, Roberts JW, et al: Molecular Biology of the Gene. Menlo Park, CA: Benjamin Cummings, 1987. With permission. Copyright © 1987 by The Benjamin/Cummings Publishing Company, Inc.*) *B.* Making a genomic library in plasmid pBR322. Note that insertion of the foreign DNA into the ampicillin-resistance gene disrupts it and renders the host bacterium ampicillin-sensitive (but still tetracycline-resistant, as are the ampicillin-resistant bacteria harboring nonrecombinants).

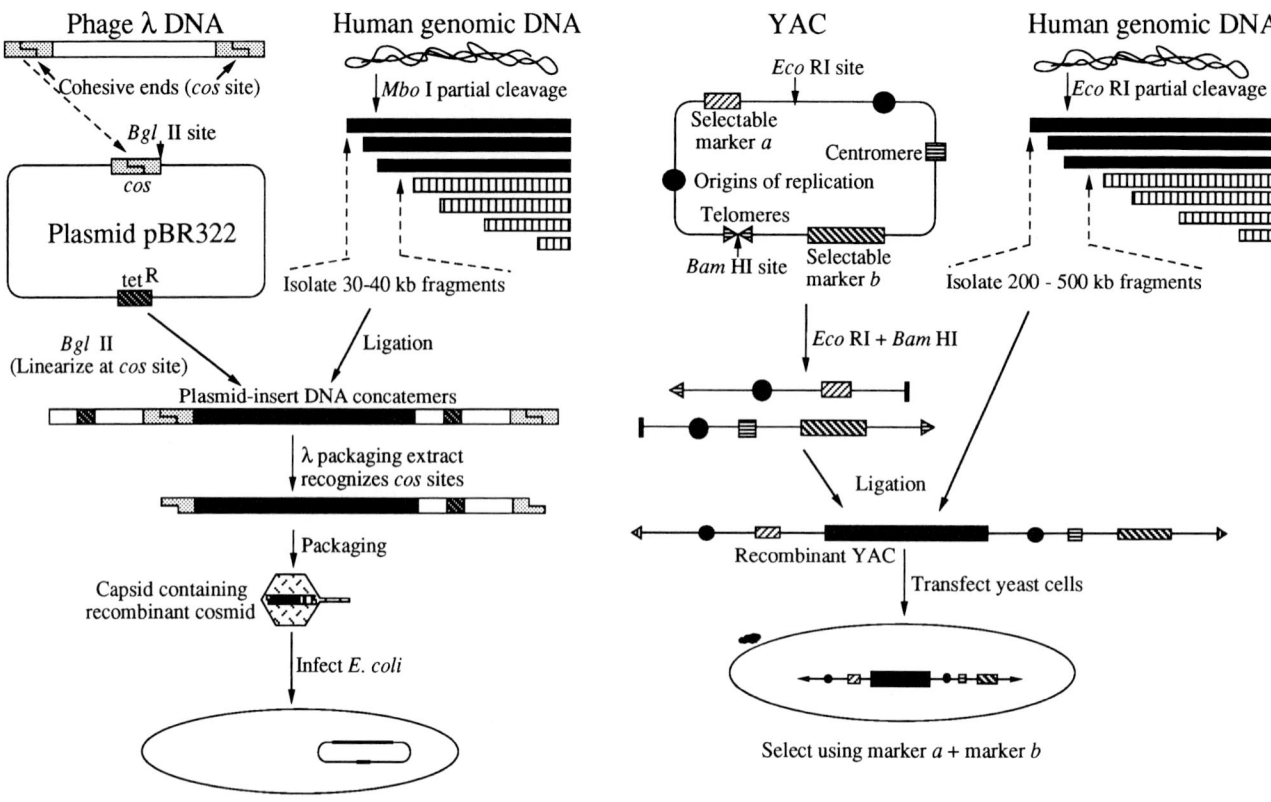

Figure 33-16. Making cosmid and YAC genomic recombinant libraries. *A.* Making a cosmid library, which combines the ability to incorporate large inserts into a phage at high efficiency with the ease of manipulation of a plasmid. Although the initial infection of the bacteria is phage-mediated, there is no cell lysis or plaque formation; the recombinant grows as a plasmid in a bacterial colony. (*Adapted from Watson JD, Tooze J, Kurtz DT (eds): Recombinant DNA: A Short Course. New York: Scientific American/WH Freeman, 1983. Copyright © 1983 by Scientific American Books, Inc. Reprinted with permission of W.H. Freeman and Company.*) *B.* Making a yeast artificial chromosome (YAC) library. Note that the YAC vector plasmid has two origins of replication, two telomeres, two different selectable markers, but only one centromere. Upon linearization with *Eco*RI+*Bam*HI followed by ligation with foreign DNA, a complete yeast artificial chromosome is generated, which can be identified by selecting for yeast cells positive for both selectable markers. (*Adapted from Micklos DA, Freyer FA (eds): DNA Science: A First Course in Recombinant DNA Technology. Cold Spring Harbor, NY: Cold Spring Harbor Laboratory Press, 1990. Carolina Biological Supply Company, 1990. Copyright © 1990 by Carolina Biological Supply Company.*)

Plasmids or cosmids can also be used to make genomic libraries. Plasmids are easier to work with than phage, but they do not accept large inserts easily, and the recombinants are more difficult to screen than are phage. However, under some circumstances, especially when a "minilibrary" is desired, plasmid cloning is practical (Fig. 33-15B).

Cosmid vectors enjoy the theoretical advantages of both plasmid and phage systems (Fig. 33-16A). Cosmids are plasmids that contain a unique cloning site, antibiotic-resistance genes, an origin of replication, and special λ phage sequences, called *cos* sites (hence the word *cosmid*). Because of the *cos* site, the recombinant can be packaged in vitro in phage capsids, and the recombinant DNA can therefore be introduced into *E. coli* by the high-efficiency method of phage infection. Once inside the cell, however, the cosmid acts like a plasmid, and the antibiotic-resistant hosts grow as colonies, not plaques. Since the cosmid vectors are small (4 to 7 kb) and packaging of λ requires 40- to 50-kb molecules, more than 40 kb of foreign DNA can be inserted into these vectors. Thus, relative to phage libraries, only one-third as many recombinants must be screened to find a desired gene sequence.

An even more efficient genomic cloning system is based on the development of *yeast artificial chromosomes,* or *YACs* (Fig. 33-16B). A YAC is a genetically engineered "minichromosome" that can replicate independently when introduced into yeast cells. It contains yeast centromeric and telomeric sequences plus special marker genes that can be used to select for growth of the YAC. Inside this minichromosome, one can insert truly gigantic segments of foreign DNA, ranging in size from 100 to 500 kb. One could thus theoretically create a human genomic YAC library in yeast cells in which the entire human genome was represented by only 6000 YAC clones ($3 \times 10^9 / 5 \times 10^5$), 10-fold fewer than the number of clones required for a cosmid library and 50-fold fewer than for a phage library.

cDNA libraries. Genomic libraries are most useful for isolating regions of the genome. However, biological questions of temporal-, developmental-, or tissue-specific expression are best answered by construction and analysis of *complementary DNA*, or *cDNA*, *libraries*, which are representations of the populations of expressed messenger RNAs within specific cell types. Whereas eukaryotic protein-coding genes have an exon-intron organization, the mature mRNAs are the products of splicing in which only the exons are retained. Thus, a cDNA clone represents only the exons; in a genomic clone of the same gene, these exons would be spread over a much larger span of DNA, with intron-encoding DNA in between.

Experimentally, RNA is much more difficult to deal with than DNA. First, most RNAs are short-lived, with a half-life that is often measured in minutes. Second, RNA is easily degraded by ribonucleases, both inside the cell and in the laboratory. Special care must be taken to work quickly and as free of RNases as possible. Third, there may be a problem in representation. DNA sequences of interest may be present in very low abundance in the genome, but in some tissues the corresponding RNA may account for 1 to 2 percent to even 50 percent of the total RNA in a particular cell type; conversely, some RNAs, especially those with a potential regulatory role or those encoding long-lived proteins, may be present at levels of only 0.001 percent, and may be very difficult to isolate even from a well-made cDNA library. Fourth, an mRNA that is extremely large (greater than 5 kb) will be difficult to represent in one *full-length* cDNA clone.

To make a cDNA library, one takes advantage of the structure of mRNA (Fig. 33-17A). Although mRNAs are heterogeneous in size, they all contain a long stretch of *poly(A)* at their 3' ends. Thus, the first step is to anneal *oligo d(T)* to the poly(A) stretches. The oligo d(T) serves as a *primer* for the action of *reverse transcriptase* to make a *complementary* strand of DNA—*cDNA*—reading in the antimessage sense (on the "bottom" strand). After the reverse transcriptase reaction,

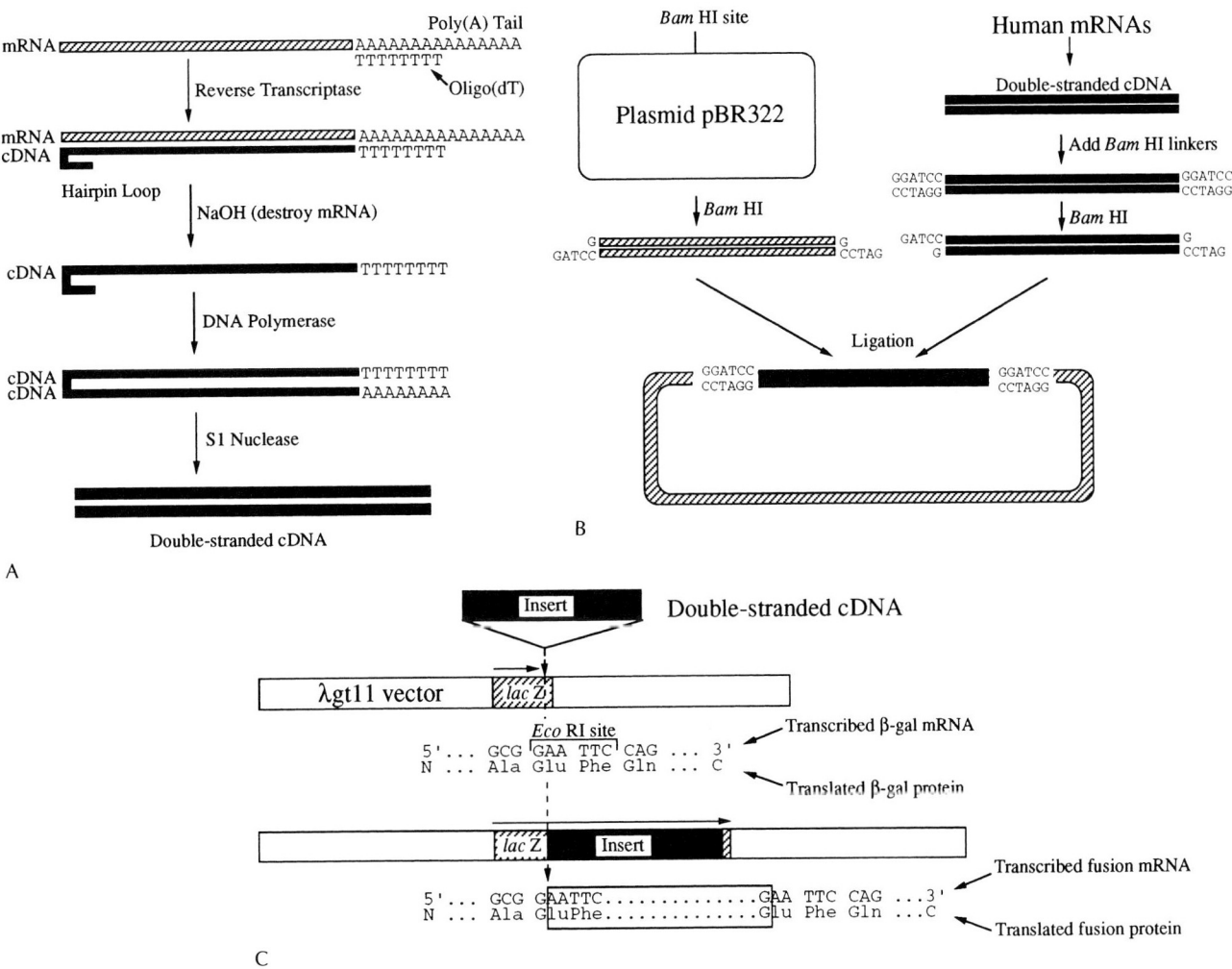

FIGURE 33-17. Making cDNA libraries. *A*. Making double-stranded cDNA from mRNA. *B*. Creating a cDNA library in a plasmid vector using *Bam*HI linkers. (*A and B adapted from Watson JD, Tooze J, Kurtz DT (eds): Recombinant DNA: A Short Course. New York: Scientific American/WH Freeman, 1983. Copyright © 1983 by Scientific American Books, Inc. Reprinted with permission of W.H. Freeman and Company.*) *C*. Creating a cDNA library in the phage λgt11 expression vector. Insertion of foreign DNA into the unique *Eco*RI site disrupts the β-galactosidase (*lacZ*) gene. Upon induction of *lacZ* with the sugar analog IPTG, a *lacZ*-insert fusion protein is translated from the *lacZ*-insert fusion mRNA. The insert portion of the fusion protein can be detected by an antibody specific for the encoded polypeptide.

the RNA is degraded or displaced, and a second ("top") strand of cDNA is synthesized in its place, in the message sense, using *DNA polymerase*. This *double-stranded cDNA* can now be inserted into a suitable vector. With plasmid pBR322, *G-C tailing* is popular. A string of about 20 dC residues is added to both 3' ends of the insert DNA, and pBR322 linearized by *Pst*I digestion is tailed with about 20 dG residues; both reactions are catalyzed using *terminal deoxynucleotidyl transferase*. The dC and dG tails are complementary to each other, so they will self-anneal and, under appropriate conditions, will produce a closed circular recombinant plasmid. These molecules are then used to transform *E. coli*. Inserted cDNAs can be released from the vector sequences by digestion with *Pst*I.

A second method of preparing DNA for insertion into the vector is through the use of *linkers* (Fig. 33-17B). Linkers are small (8- to 12-bp) oligonucleotides that contain one or two restriction sites. The choice of linker depends on the vector cloning site but is usually *Bam*HI or *Eco*RI. The linker is ligated onto the ends of the double-stranded cDNA and then cut with the appropriate restriction enzyme to produce a linkered cDNA with "sticky ends" suitable for ligation into a similarly cut vector (if an *Eco*RI linker is used, all potential *Eco*RI sites *inside* the cDNA are protected from cleavage by pretreatment with *Eco*RI *methylase*). There are phage cDNA vectors, such as λgt10, with a single *Eco*RI cloning site, into which *Eco*RI-linkered cDNA can be ligated. λgt10 has been engineered to accept inserts up to 5.1 kb long.

Some cDNA vectors have been designed so that the peptide encoded by the cDNA insert is produced by the growing *E. coli* host. These are *expression vectors* (Fig. 33-17C), and the cDNA-encoded peptide can be detected by antibodies. Expression vectors contain (1) a promoter for *E. coli* RNA polymerase, (2) the 5' untranslated region for a bacterial gene [often β-galactosidase (see below)], and (3) a translational initiation region located upstream of the cDNA cloning restriction site. If the cDNA is ligated in the correct translational reading frame with the vector sequences (i.e., it is *in frame* with the upstream bacterial gene sequence), a *fusion polypeptide* is produced, which can be detected by the antibody.

Probes. In order to isolate a clone of interest (whether genomic or cDNA), one must have some way of sorting through the library. This is done by using a *probe*. Probes come in many types but fall into two main categories. One is a *hybridization probe* complementary to the sequence of interest. The other uses some type of assay of *structure or function*, such as the *antibody*.

If one knows the amino acid sequence for a protein of interest, one can use a *DNA synthesizer* to synthesize an *oligonucleotide DNA probe* corresponding to a subregion of the protein, using the genetic code as a way to deduce the protein's mRNA sequence. Because the genetic code is degenerate (more than one RNA triplet may encode the same amino acid), "backtranslation" of an amino acid sequence to its mRNA sequence will necessarily involve some ambiguity. This can be overcome, however, by use of more than one nucleotide in the "wobble" position or by incorporation in the wobble position of an "unnatural" nucleotide analogue, such as *inosine*, which will hybridize to any of the four "natural" bases (A, G, C, or T). In order to use it as a probe, the oligonucleotide must be labeled. Ordinarily, this is done by *end-labeling* of the 5' end of the oligonucleotide with ^{32}P-ATP in the presence of the enzyme *T4 polynucleotide kinase* (Fig. 33-18A).

Another kind of DNA probe is cDNA. For example, globin mRNA accounts for more than 50 percent of all polyadenylated mRNA in reticulocytes. cDNA made from reticulocyte poly(A)$^+$ mRNA can be used to screen a reticulocyte cDNA library. A large percentage of clones obtained using this probe should therefore contain globin cDNA inserts, which can be identified by comparison of the amino acid sequence deduced from the cDNA to the known amino acid sequences of globin.

The easiest type of DNA probe to use is a cloned probe already obtained by someone else, perhaps for the same gene but from another species ("clone by phone"). Care must be taken to ensure that a *heterologous* probe is not so evolutionarily diverged from the target sequence that nucleotide mismatch between sequences will preclude hybridization.

cDNA probes are radiolabeled by two main methods. One is *nick translation* (Fig. 33-18B), in which ^{32}P-radiolabeled dNTPs are incorporated into DNA through the action of *E. coli DNA polymerase I* in the presence of tiny amounts of *DNase I*, an endonuclease that introduces nicks into the cDNA (the nicks are required starting points for pol I action). The second, newer method is *random-primer* labeling (Fig. 33-18C). A random set of hexanucleotides, containing all possi-

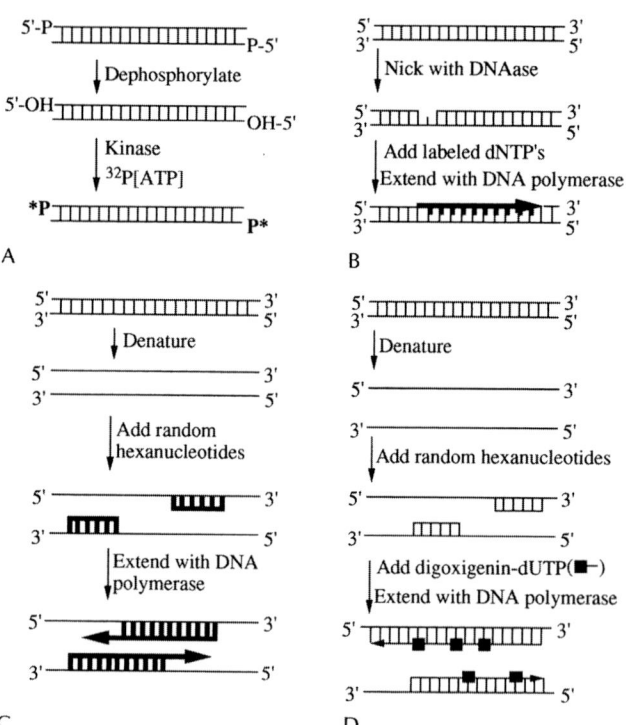

FIGURE 33-18. Labeling DNA. *A.* End-labeling DNA. The asterisk denotes a ^{32}P-labeled deoxynucleotide. *B.* Nick translation with ^{32}P-labeled deoxynucleotides (bold arrows). *C.* Random-primer labeling with "cold" random hexanucleotide primers that are extended by DNA polymerase in the presence of ^{32}P-labeled deoxynucleotides (bold arrows). *D.* "Cold" labeling using nonradioactive digoxigenin-labeled dUTP (black boxes) instead of dUTP in a random-primer labeling reaction.

ble combinations of bases at each of the six positions in the oligonucleotide, is annealed to the cDNA, which has been *denatured* (made single-stranded) by boiling. These hexamers anneal at random to many locations on the cDNA, and become *primers,* which are extended with ^{32}P-dNTPs in the presence of DNA polymerase. Both nick-translation and random-primer labeling produce long (50- to 500-nt) stretches of labeled DNA.

One can also make nonradioactively labeled probes. These "cold" probes have high sensitivity plus the added advantages of safety and storability. Many are based on "sandwich" methodology, in which a specially designed molecule incorporated into the nucleic acid probe is detected by a second molecule, called a *reporter group,* that reacts specifically to it (Fig. 33-18D). For example, digoxigenin (a steroid molecule) bound to deoxyuridine triphosphate can be incorporated into in vitro–synthesized DNA. One can detect this digoxigenin-labeled DNA probe by enzyme-linked immunoassay: An antidigoxigenin antibody conjugated with the enzyme alkaline phosphatase will produce an enzyme-catalyzed color upon reaction with a suitable phosphatase–sensitive substrate and reporter dye (blue in the case of 5-bromo-4-chloro-3-indolyl phosphate plus nitroblue tetrazolium). A similar methodology can be used with biotin-labeled probes, which use alkaline phosphatase–conjugated streptavidin as the reporter. There are even chemiluminescent probe systems, in which the reporter is light. For example, the enzyme horseradish peroxidase is covalently linked to a DNA probe and is detected by a peroxidase-catalyzed oxidation of luminol, a compound that emits light in the presence of a chemiluminescent enhancer.

These second-antibody techniques can also be used to detect a primary antibody specific to a gene product of interest. This is particularly useful in screening for synthesis of fusion proteins in an expression library.

Screening libraries. Once we have both a library and a probe, we are ready to screen the library for our sequence of interest. If we have a DNA hybridization probe, the screening is done on either colonies or plaques.

In *Gruenstein-Hogness screening* (Fig. 33-19A), a plasmid or cosmid library is plated out on agar plates, and the colonies are allowed to grow up overnight. The number of colonies one would plate depends on the expected frequency of the target gene, but ordinarily it would be around 100,000 colonies for cDNA in plasmids and 300,000 colonies for genomic DNA in cosmids; about 30,000 colonies can be plated on one large agar plate. The colonies are then transferred to nitrocellulose or nylon filters by "lifting," usually in triplicate; one filter serves as the "master" to regrow all the colonies, and the other two are used for the screening. The colonies on the replica filters are *lysed* in alkaline buffer and the filters are then "baked" to bind the released DNA to the filter paper covalently. The filters are then treated with a solution containing the radiolabeled probe at a suitable *stringency of hybridization*—a combination of temperature and salt concentration that maximizes hybridization of the probe to the sequence of interest while at the same time minimizing both background hybridization and hybridization to unrelated and unwanted sequences ("garbage clones"). After hybridization for 12 to 18 h, the probe is washed off the filter and the filters are exposed to x-ray film for 1 to 2 days. Positive colonies are those that display a strong hybridization signal above background on both replica filters. These positives are then retrieved off the master plate and another round or two of screening is done to confirm the initial result and obtain a single, pure colony.

In *Benton-Davis* screening (Fig. 33-19B), essentially the same procedure is followed, except that phage plaques, not bacterial colonies, are analyzed. Plaque hybridization is quicker and easier than colony hybridization and gives a lower background. The phage library is plated on a lawn of uninfected *E. coli,* using about 100,000 *plaque-forming units* (pfu) for cDNA libraries and 1 million pfu for genomic libraries. Phage can be plated at 50,000 pfu per large plate. After 4 to 6 h of growth, the clear lysed regions—the plaques—are observable against the translucent lawn and are lifted in duplicate onto filters. No master lift is required; the plate with the leftover plaques serves as the master. The filters are treated as above and plaque-pure clones are obtained after two to three rounds of screening.

Screening of cDNA protein-expression libraries is identical to colony or plaque hybridizations up to the point of the filter lifts. In both cases, once the colonies or plaques are grown, they must then be *induced* to produce the fusion protein that will be detected by the antibody (Fig. 33-19C). The most popular way of doing this is to use a vector containing the *E. coli* gene for β-galactosidase, a sugar-catabolism enzyme, with the cDNA cloning site inside the β-gal gene (see Fig. 33-17C). The β-gal gene (also called *lacZ,* because it is part of the bacterial lactose operon) can be "turned on" using the inducer *IPTG* (isopropylthio-β-D-galactoside). In the case of the most commonly used phage expression vector, λgt11, once the plaques appear on the plates, they are overlaid with a filter saturated with IPTG and placed back in the incubator to induce β-gal mRNA and protein synthesis. Any cDNA inserted within the β-gal cloning site will also be transcribed and, if in frame, translated. The filter is now lifted and treated first with the primary antibody to the protein of interest and then with a second antibody containing a reporter group, such as horseradish peroxidase. When a peroxide-sensitive developing agent, such as diaminobenzidine plus imidazole, is added, any plaque containing the primary/secondary antibody complex will show a small colored "doughnut" of purple stain in the periphery of the plaque. The plaque can then be picked and rescreened to plaque purity in two to three successive rounds of antibody screening. Most cDNA libraries, including λgt11, do not specify the frame orientation of the insert relative to that of the β-gal gene (i.e., there are three possible reading frames and two possible orientations of insertion of the cDNA into the vector). Therefore only one plaque in six will contain the correct orientation and reading frame for a particular fusion protein. For this reason, if one screens 90,000 pfu of a λgt11 library, only 15,000 "real" plaques will be examined.

Plus-minus screening. Some tissue-specific and developmental questions can be addressed by comparing the contents of two different cDNA libraries. Clones common to both libraries can be recognized, but, more importantly, clones represented in one library but not another can also be identified. The simplest way to do this is to use probes against

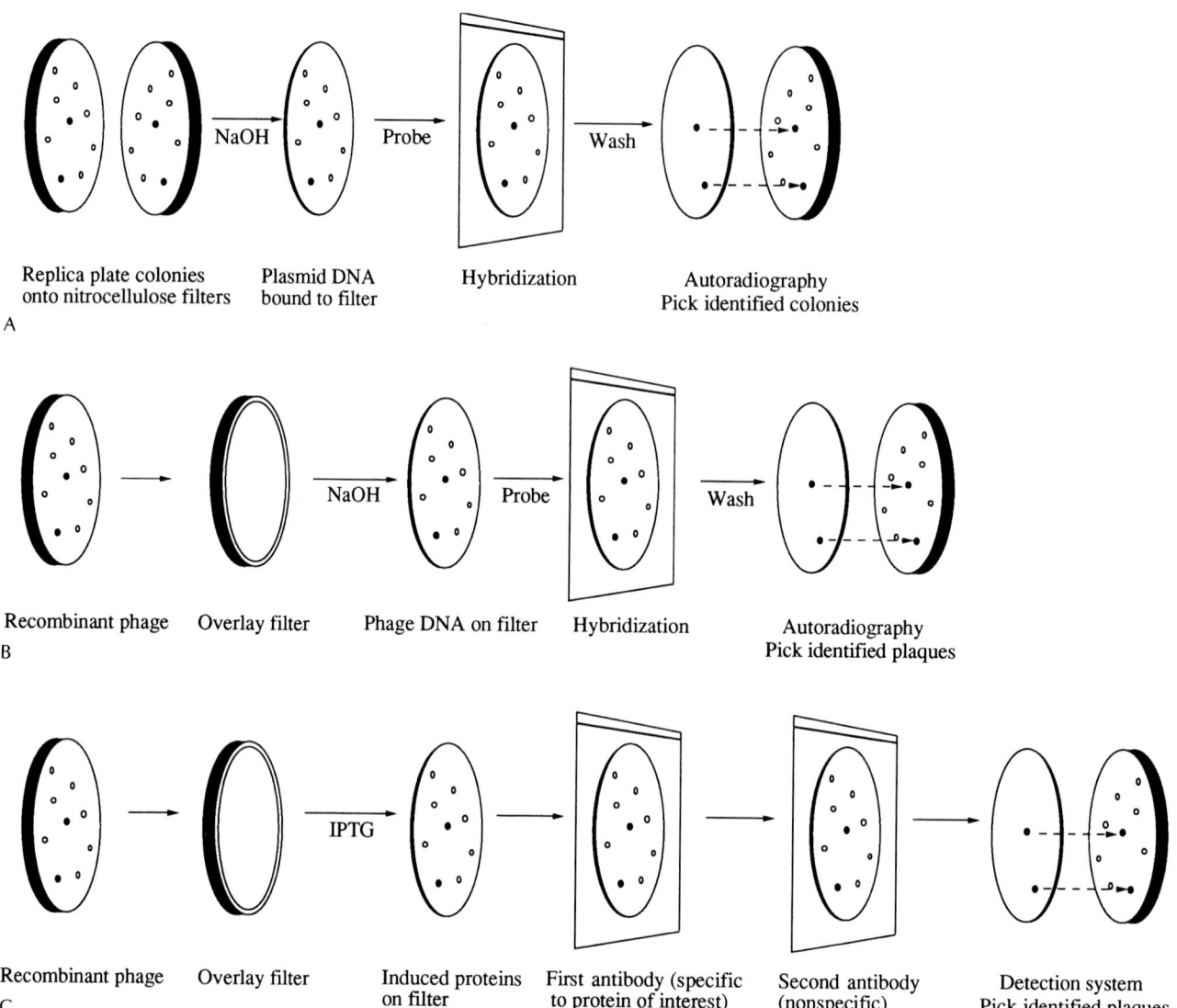

FIGURE 33-19. Screening libraries. A. Gruenstein-Hogness screening of recombinant plasmids or cosmids in bacterial colonies. (Adapted from Watson JD, Tooze J, Kurtz DT (eds): Recombinant DNA: A Short Course. New York: Scientific American/WH Freeman, 1983. Copyright © 1983 by Scientific American Books, Inc. Reprinted with permission of W.H. Freeman and Company.) B. Benton-Davis screening of recombi- nant phages. (Adapted from Micklos DA, Freyer FA (eds): DNA Science: A First Course in Recombinant DNA Technology. Cold Spring Harbor, NY: Cold Spring Harbor Laboratory Press, 1990. Copyright © 1990 by Carolina Biological Supply Company.) C. Antibody screening of recombinant phage expression libraries.

mRNA isolated from two sources; cDNA may be represented in one cell type but not another. For example, if a muscle-specific mRNA is sought, one might select probes that hybridize with muscle but not fibroblast mRNA (see "Northern Blotting," below). Probes of this type would eliminate the "housekeeping" genes that are expressed in all cells.

An alternative approach is to enrich the *single-stranded* cDNA population from one source for the specific messages that are found only in that source or that are quantitatively more abundant. Three such approaches are *subtractive hybridization, differential display,* and *representational difference analysis*. There are also powerful genetic methods, using strange-sounding vectors (e.g., *phagemids* and *lafmids*), to generate subtracted libraries by combined genetic and biochemical means.

The Human Genome Project. The greatest advance in identifying human genes is the success of the Human Genome Project. Using many of the tools described above—the creation of artificial chromosome libraries of human DNA in yeast (YAC) and bacterial artificial chromosome (BAC) vectors in order to manipulate easily relatively large pieces of DNA, subcloning of segments from YACs and BACs into cosmid and plasmid vectors, and DNA sequencing of PCR-amplified fragments (see below)—the entire human genome, 3 billion bp in size, has been sequenced almost in its entirety.[55,56] It is estimated that the human genome contains about 20,000 to 30,000 genes, which is a surprisingly low number, considering that *E. coli* has about 4000 genes, yeast about 6000 genes, and the worm *Caenorhabditis elegans* about 20,000 genes. However, because of the phenomena of alternative splicing and of posttranscriptional and posttranslational modifications, the number of distinct polypeptides that are synthesized in cells is likely to be at least on the order of 100,000 and possibly two or even three times that number. In other words, a relatively small number of genes, almost all of which are composed of a string of intron-punctuated exons (and which are, in essence, small protein-coding modules), can give rise to an incredible diversity of proteins, many of which are expressed in a tissue- or temporal-specific manner.

Much, but not all, of the genomic sequence has been annotated; that is, the locations on the DNA of identifiable landmarks—exons, introns, coding regions, 5'- and 3'-untranslated regions, regulatory elements, and the like—have been mapped to their exact positions in the genome. In parallel, a nearly entire set of mRNAs has also been identified, in various degrees of annotation. Most of the mRNA data are available as *expressed sequence tags*, or *ESTs*. These are essentially short cDNAs, about 500 bp in size, derived from the 3' ends of poly(A)-containing mRNAs amplified by RT-PCR (see below). Similar sets of data are also available for yeast (*Saccharomyces cerevisiae*), worm (*Caenorhabditis elegans*), fly (*Drosophila melanogaster*), plant (*Arabidopsis thaliana*), and numerous prokaryotic organisms, including *E. coli*.

These genomes can be accessed on the Internet; the main site in the United States is the Genbank database curated by the National Center for Biotechnology Information at the National Library of Medicine of the National Institutes of Health (http://www.ncbi.nlm.nih.gov/). Genomic and EST sequences that have been mapped to specific regions of the 23 human chromosomes can be found at http://genome.ucsc.edu/, located at the University of California, Santa Clara.

Using the resources developed by the Human Genome Project, one can often now identify a gene of interest without having to resort to any "wet-bench" experiments at all! If one has even a snippet of protein or DNA sequence information on a gene of interest, even in a distantly related organism, it is often possible to identify a related sequence in the human genome, using a variety of rapid protein and DNA search algorithms (see, for example, the BLAST home page at http://www.ncbi.nlm.nih.gov/BLAST/). Identifying genes in this manner—called *cybercloning* or *cloning in silico*—has become so efficient that our ability to identify new genes has far outstripped our ability to analyze their functions.

ANALYZING CLONED GENES

Extraction of DNA. Once a pure colony or plaque is obtained, it can be grown in quantity and the DNA extracted for further examination. DNA from colonies is usually extracted by *alkaline lysis*. The colony is grown; the bacteria are then pelleted and lysed in alkali plus SDS (sodium dodecyl sulfate, a detergent). The bacterial chromosomal DNA, along with the SDS, is precipitated by the addition of potassium acetate, but the tiny plasmids remain in the supernatant. The plasmids are cleaned up by extractions with phenol and chloroform and then precipitated with ethanol. After drying, the precipitated pellet is taken up in buffer and is ready for use.

DNA from phage is obtained by infecting bacteria with the plaque-pure phage, pelleting the bacterial debris, precipitating the phage (which remain in the supernatant) with NaCl and polyethylene glycol (PEG), and then breaking open the phage capsids with formamide to release the DNA. For large phage preparations, the PEG-pelleted phage are banded on a cesium chloride gradient prior to the formamide step. Cleanup of the DNA is as above.

Gels. Almost all analyses of nucleic acids begin or end with an analysis on an electrophoretic gel. These gels are used to visualize, size, and quantitate DNA and RNA fragments, and although specific methodologies vary, they all work on the same principle. Nucleic acids are negatively charged, and when embedded in a suitable semisolid support and placed in an electric field, they will migrate toward the positively charged electrode (i.e., from the cathode to the anode). All else being equal, the speed of migration will depend almost exclusively on the size of the DNA or RNA fragment. Thus, if one electrophoreses a mixture of DNA fragments, the smallest ones migrate the fastest and the largest fragments the slowest, thus enabling one to separate fragments by size.

Two electrophoretic solid supports are most commonly used: agarose and polyacrylamide. Agarose gels can separate double-stranded DNA fragments ranging in size from 500 to 50,000 bp. Polyacrylamide gels are used to separate smaller DNA fragments 50- to 1000-bp long. Because RNA and single-stranded DNA have regions of self-complementarity, electrophoresis of these molecules is usually performed in *denaturing* gels, such as agarose gels containing formaldehyde or methyl mercuric hydroxide, or polyacrylamide gels containing formamide or urea.

The separated fragments can be visualized by staining the gel with *ethidium bromide*, a positively charged dye that binds to double-stranded nucleic acids by intercalating within the base pairs and that fluoresces in the visible region upon excitation with ultraviolet light.

While useful for analyzing and preparing relatively small fragments of DNA, these types of gels are useless for distinguishing larger fragments in the million-bp [megabase pair (mb)] range. A variant of agarose electrophoresis called *pulsed-field gel electrophoresis* (PFGE) has been developed that will do just that.[57] In PFGE, the electric field is not continuous but varies with time: Every few seconds during the gel run the field is inverted, causing the DNA fragments (sometimes chromosome-sized pieces) to reorient themselves in the gel. Under the proper conditions of field strength, pulsing time, gel geometry, and gel pore size, these gigantic pieces of DNA will slowly move through the gels like undulating pieces of spaghetti, and different-sized fragments in the megabase-size range can be resolved. PFGE has become invaluable in large-scale mapping projects. Many variants on PFGE have now been developed, but they all use this same dynamic principle.

DNA subcloning. Sometimes it is useful to excise the cloned insert from its vector and to *subclone* it into another vector. This is done by cutting the insert out of the vector (e.g., a λ phage) with a restriction enzyme, ligating it with another (usually a circular plasmid that has been linearized by digestion with the same restriction enzyme and has only one restriction site in the circle), and transforming the recombinant into host bacteria by the calcium-shock method. Many of the popular vectors (e.g., pUC19) have *polylinkers*, containing a 50- to 100-bp stretch of synthetic DNA designed to contain up to a dozen unique restriction sites. This allows one to subclone inserts into the vector easily. A second feature of many of these vectors is the ability to identify visually those plasmids that have incorporated the insert within the polylinker. One example of this is *blue-white screening*. The polylinker is placed inside a *lacZ* (β-galactosidase) gene that has been engineered into the vector. Upon induction with IPTG in the presence of X-gal (5-bromo-4-chloro-3-indolyl-β-D-galactopyranoside), a chromogenic substrate for β-gal, the full-length *lacZ* mRNA is transcribed and the translated β-gal protein cleaves the X-gal, producing a bacterial colony with a blue color. However, plasmids with inserts subcloned into the polylinker within the *lacZ* gene prevent production of the β-gal protein, and the colonies remain white.

While most subcloning is done in plasmids of double-stranded DNA, sometimes it is useful to subclone into a vector that can produce single-stranded DNA. The most popular vectors of this type are modified versions of bacteriophage M13 (e.g., M13mp19), which, like pUC19, contain a *lacZ* polylinker suitable for subcloning with blue-white screening.

Restriction mapping. One way of obtaining a *physical map* of a piece of DNA (the linear ordering of specific landmarks on the DNA) is by *restriction mapping*, which is the ascertainment of the location of restriction endonuclease sites on a segment of DNA. This is done by cutting the DNA with one or more restriction enzymes, either singly or in pairs (*double digests*), running the digested fragments on a gel to size them, and then using logic to deduce the location of the various restriction sites with respect to some known starting point.

RFLPs. It has been estimated that the DNA from any two individuals differs in the DNA sequence at a frequency between 1 per 250 and 1 per 500 bp. If, by chance, the base pair at which the DNA of two individuals differs happens to be in a restriction endonuclease recognition sequence, one can then distinguish between the two individuals merely by examining that region of DNA for the absence or presence of the site, as revealed by a difference in the migration of the appropriate restriction fragment on a gel. A difference at a *locus* (position on the chromosome) in the size of a DNA restriction fragment among two or more individuals is called a *restriction fragment length polymorphism* (RFLP) (Fig. 33-20). RFLPs are powerful tools in the analysis of disease genes in pedigrees and are discussed in greater detail below.

Southern blotting. *Southern blotting* is a method used to identify specific DNA fragments through the use of a DNA probe that will identify only the sequence(s) of interest, by virtue of the complementarity of the DNA sequence of the probe to that of the "target." One use of Southern blotting (named after Ed Southern, the inventor of the method) is to identify cloned sequences (Fig. 33-21A): Purified phage or plasmid DNA is digested with one or more restriction

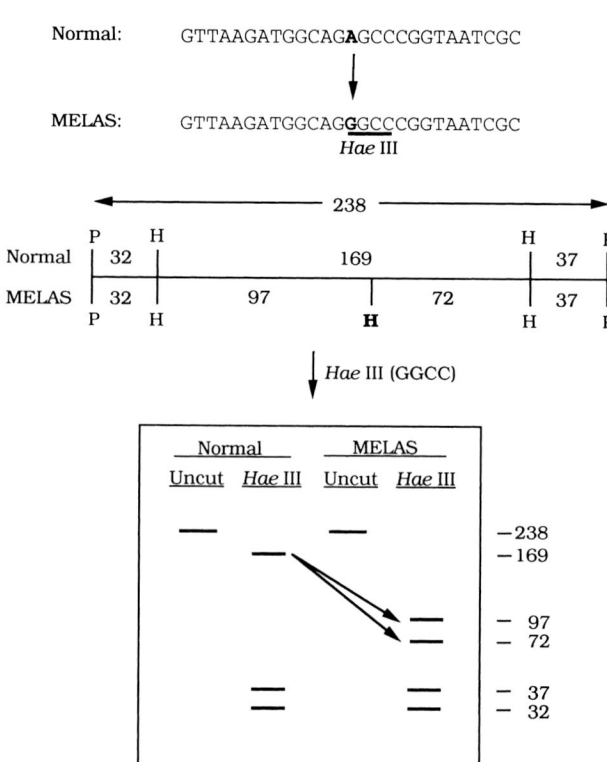

FIGURE 33-20. Restriction fragment length polymorphisms. Schematic of the use of RFLP analysis to detect a point mutation associated with mitochondrial encephalomyopathy, lactic acidosis, and stroke-like episodes (MELAS). An A⇑G transition in the mitochondrial genome at mtDNA position 3243 creates a *Hae*III polymorphism. PCR of mtDNA with primers (P) generates a 238-bp fragment. Cleavage of normal DNA with *Hae*III (H) yields three fragments that are 169, 37, and 32 bp long. The extra *Hae*III site in MELAS mtDNA (**H**) cleaves the 169-bp fragment into two smaller fragments of 97 and 72 bp (arrows on schematic of an electrophoretic gel).

enzymes that release the insert from the vector (say, *Eco*RI), and the products of the digestion reaction are electrophoresed through an agarose slab gel. The bands, which separate by size, may be visualized by staining them with ethidium bromide. The separated bands are then denatured in the gel with alkali to make them single stranded. After neutralization of the excess alkali, the single-stranded DNA is transferred to a nitrocellulose or nylon filter by vacuum, by capillary action, or by electrotransfer (this is the *blotting* step). The filter is then "baked" to bind the DNA to the filter and incubated overnight with a radioactively labeled single-stranded probe (in order for the probe sequences to "find" and hybridize to the complementary "target" sequences bound to the filter). The filter is then washed to remove unbound probe and overlaid with x-ray film for autoradiography, as was done in the library screening. This time, however, only those restriction fragments carrying sequences complementary to the probe will "light up."

A second major use of Southern blotting is in *genomic hybridization* to identify probe-hybridizable regions of the genome (Fig. 33-21B). This is done by isolating genomic DNA (usually from lymphocytes, but it can be from any tissue) and

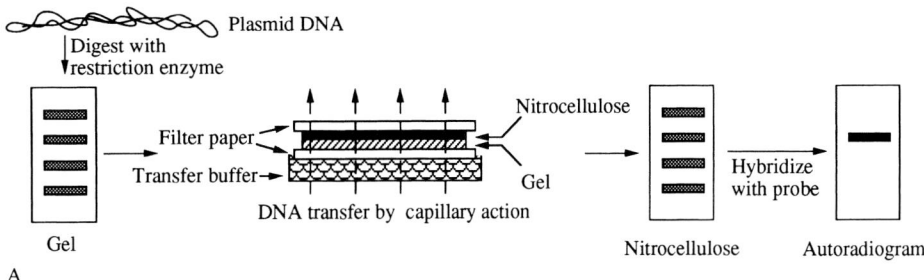
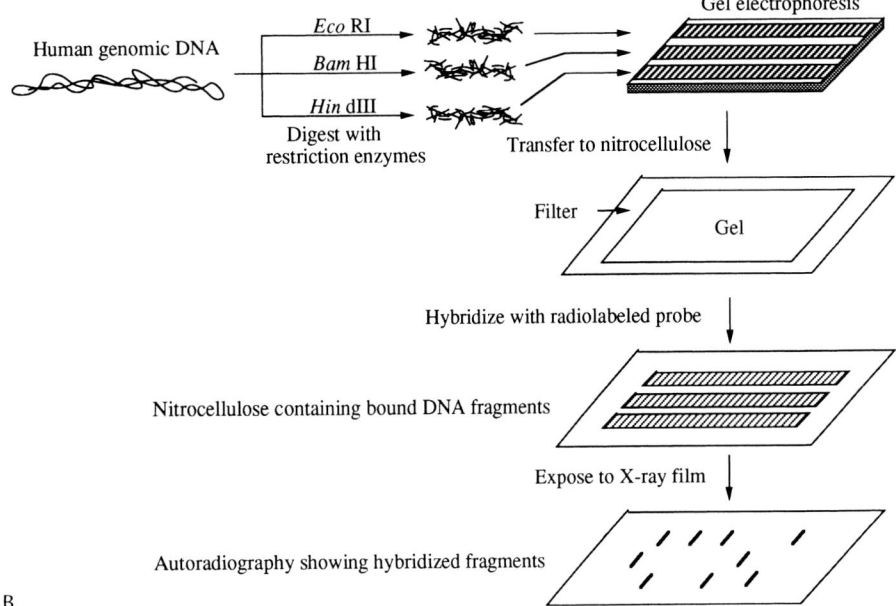

FIGURE 33-21. Filter hybridization. A. Southern blotting of a cloned DNA sequence in a plasmid. (*Adapted from Darnell J, Lodish H, Baltimore D: Molecular Cell Biology. New York: Scientific American/WH Freeman, 1986. Copyright © 1986 by Scientific American Books, Inc. Reprinted with permission of W.H. Freeman and Company.*) B. Southern blotting of genomic DNA. (*Adapted from Watson JD, Hopkins NH, Roberts JW, et al: Molecular Biology of the Gene. Menlo Park, CA: Benjamin Cummings, 1987. With permission. Copyright © 1987 by The Benjamin/Cummings Publishing Company, Inc.*)

then performing the Southern analysis exactly as described above. In the case of Southerns of cloned DNA, the signal comes up on the x-ray in a matter of hours because of the large quantity of target DNA present on the filter. In genomic Southerns, however, gene sequences are often present in only one or a few copies per haploid genome. Thus, the probe has to have a very high specific activity (around 1×10^9 cpm/μg) and the filter usually has to be exposed for at least 1 or 2 days and sometimes for a week. The results of a genomic hybridization can yield information on the genomic organization of a gene, copy number, gene rearrangements, insertions, or deletions; it is also useful in following experiments in which genes are introduced into cells or tissues (e.g., transgenic mice). Clinically, genomic Southern hybridization is indispensable for RFLP and pedigree analysis (see below).

Northern blotting. Instead of using a probe to study DNA organization, one can also use a probe to examine RNA expression in cells or tissues. This is done in a manner analogous to Southern blotting called *Northern blotting*. Total RNA is isolated from cells by homogenizing them in a buffer containing a strong denaturing agent, such as guanidinium isothiocyanate, to denature cellular proteins, including endogenous RNases. After treatment with DNase, the RNA is pelleted, resuspended, phenol-extracted, and reprecipitated.

About 500 to 1000 μg of total RNA can be isolated from about 1 g of tissue, but only 1 percent of it is mRNA. Most of the rest of the RNA is composed of two species of ribosomal RNA, called 18S (about 1850 nt long) and 28S (about 5000 nt long) rRNA (the 18S and 28S rRNAs are often used as internal size markers on Northern blots). The mRNA fraction, which is the only fraction that is polyadenylated, can be isolated by passing the total RNA through an *oligo d(T) column*. The unbound, poly(A)$^-$ fraction is usually discarded, and the poly(A)$^+$ fraction is eluted off in low salt.

The RNA is electrophoresed through a *denaturing* agarose gel to eliminate aberrant migration of individual RNA species (RNA, which is single-stranded, has significant secondary structure due to self-complementarities). After electrophoresis, the gel is stained, transferred, and probed in a manner analogous to the Southern procedure. The resulting autoradiograph displays one or more bands equivalent in size to full-length RNAs expressed in the tissue of interest. The intensity of the band reflects the *steady-state* level of RNA in the tissue; since RNA is constantly being made and degraded, a "standard" Northern provides no information on RNA turnover or half-life.

Dot blots. Instead of performing a Southern or Northern analysis on nucleic acids that have been separated by size on electrophoretic gels, one can simply spot some DNA or RNA on a filter and probe this *dot blot* directly. Dot blots have the advantage of speed; they are useful for quantitating the amount of hybridizing target present in the dot and for rapid screening protocols. They suffer from the disadvantage that no information on target fragment size or on levels of nonspecific background hybridization are obtained.

Polymerase chain reaction. The *polymerase chain reaction* (PCR) is a way of amplifying and cloning a specific DNA sequence without the use of vectors or libraries.[58] The only requirement of PCR is that one must know something about the sequence being amplified.

In PCR (Fig. 33-22), two short (15- to 30-bp) *oligonucleotide primers* are synthesized, with sequences corresponding to the endpoints of the desired *target* sequence (usually a gene segment 500 to 1000 bp long). One primer is complementary to the "top" DNA strand on the "right" edge, while the second primer is complementary to the "bottom" strand on the "left" edge. After heating total genomic DNA to denature the duplex into single-stranded DNA, the DNA is cooled in the presence of a vast molar excess of both primers; each primer (which has a unique and specific DNA sequence) will rapidly anneal and hybridize to a single specific target region, the left or right side of the target. Upon the addition of DNA polymerase, each oligonucleotide will then serve as a primer for the synthesis of a complementary "daughter" strand beginning at the primer and extending in the $5' \rightarrow 3'$ direction. Thus, each "parental" duplex strand is replicated to create two new "daughter" duplexes, but only in the region flanked by the two primers. The daughter DNA is then reheated, reannealed with primers, and reextended with more polymerase to "replicate" the two strands into four "granddaughter" duplexes and, after another cycle, into eight "great-granddaughter" duplexes. After 20 rounds of such annealing-extension-denaturation, a single molecule can theoretically be amplified by a factor of 2^{20}, or a millionfold. With the development of thermostable DNA polymerases that can survive temperatures up to 95°C (e.g., *Taq DNA polymerase* from the thermophile *Thermus aquaticus*, found in the hot springs at Yellowstone Park), the entire PCR procedure can be made self-contained, and each cycle can be performed in about 5 to 10 min; the total amplification can be performed in only a few hours. What used to take months by standard methods of library construction and screening can now be done in an afternoon!

The implications for biotechnology, prenatal diagnosis, and genetic analyses of all types, including anthropology and forensics, are staggering, as specific pieces of DNA can now be amplified starting with as little as a single cell as the source of the template DNA. To give just one example, one can now amplify tiny amounts of mRNA by using *reverse-transcription PCR* (RT-PCR). Using primers specific for a particular mRNA, one can first copy mRNA into cDNA using reverse transcriptase (similar to what is done in making cDNA for a library) and then amplify the cDNA by standard PCR. RT-PCR is a powerful tool for analyzing tiny amounts of RNA, even from single cells.

DNA sequencing. Once a pure clone has been isolated, one can obtain the DNA sequence of the insert. The DNA

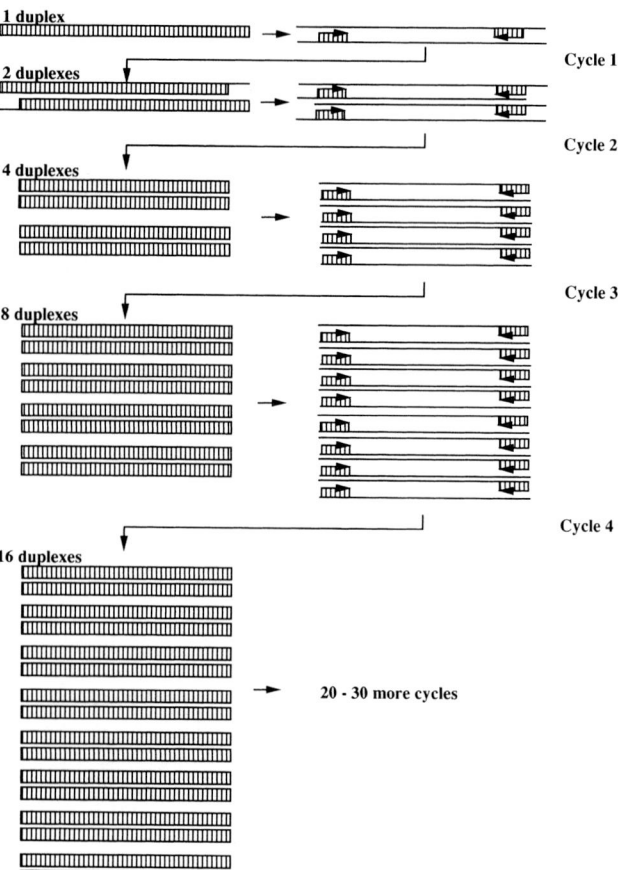

FIGURE 33-22. Polymerase chain reaction. Each PCR cycle consists of three steps: (1) denaturation of duplex DNA into single strands; (2) annealing of sequence-specific "left" and "right" primers (boxes with arrows) to exposed single strands; and (3) extension of each hybridized primer into a "full-length" DNA strand, using the complementary DNA strand as template for DNA synthesis by DNA polymerase. Note the exponential increase in amplified duplexes, as each synthesized duplex becomes the template for synthesis of two daughter duplexes in the next PCR cycle. The PCR-extended daughter strands in cycle 1 are longer than the subsequent PCR-amplified strands in the subsequent cycles due to synthesis using the initial template DNA; duplexes synthesized from preexisting PCR-generated duplexes (the vast majority, i.e., $2^n - 1$ duplexes after n cycles) are of discrete length, equal to the distance between the left and right primers.

sequence is the ultimate physical map, since it is used to order spatially the nucleotides in a fragment of DNA. With cDNA clones, the DNA sequence of the coding region should be an open reading frame from which the encoded polypeptide sequence can be deduced. In fact, it is now easier to deduce an amino acid sequence from a cloned cDNA than to isolate and sequence the protein itself.

The sequence is obtained by one of two methods: the *Maxam-Gilbert chemical cleavage method* or the *Sanger dideoxy enzymatic method*. Although the techniques differ, they embody similar principles. In both procedures, the DNA is marked at one end—for example, by end-labeling with a radioactive nucleotide at the 5'-terminal nucleotide. The

DNA is then divided into four aliquots, and each is subjected to a procedure that results in DNA strands that terminate randomly along the chain in a base-specific manner (i.e., chains terminate at A's in the A-specific tube, at G's in the G-specific tube, and so on). The reaction is done in such a way as to ensure that most DNA molecules are "hit" only once or a few times. Each of the four reaction products is then electrophoresed through a *denaturing polyacrylamide gel* in four adjacent lanes, which separates the DNA strands by size, and the resulting separation pattern is visualized on x-ray film by autoradiography. Only those DNA strands extending from the labeled 5' end to the point of base-specific termination are visualized. In the G-specific lane, therefore, one sees a pattern of labeled bands running up the gel, with each band representing a subpopulation of molecules beginning at the labeled 5' end and ending at one of the G's in the sequence. Each band in the G lane differs in size from the band below it by a distance corresponding to the number of bases from one G to the next G in the sequence. The same holds true for the A-, T-, and C-specific lanes. Thus, by "reading" all four lane patterns at once as the bands ascend the gel, the ordered sequence of all four DNA letters can be deduced.

In Maxam-Gilbert sequencing (Fig. 33-23A), the DNA to be sequenced is a purified fragment marked at one end by radiolabeling and the four reactions are base-specific *chemical* cleavages. In Sanger sequencing, which is an *enzymatic* method (Fig. 33-23B), the DNA to be sequenced remains inserted in the host vector, but it must be in a single-stranded form (hence the utility of single-stranded M13 vectors). The beginning of the DNA region to be sequenced is marked by a small piece of single-stranded *primer* DNA that hybridizes to a known point flanking the insert (e.g., just outside the polylinker region in single-stranded M13 or denatured double-stranded pUC vectors). The four reactions are actually four syntheses of complementary DNA, using the sequencing primer as the start of polymerization. DNA polymerase or Klenow enzyme is used to incorporate radioactive nucleotides into a growing complementary chain, using the single-stranded insert of unknown DNA sequence (located just beyond the primer) as a template. In each reaction, a small amount of a base-specific *nucleotide analogue*, called a *2',3'-dideoxynucleotide* (i.e., ddG, ddA, ddT, or ddC), is added; because polymerase extension in the 5' → 3' direction requires ligation of the hydroxyl group at the 3' position of one nucleotide to the phosphate group at the 5' position of the following nucleotide, incorporation of a dideoxynucleotide lacking a 3'-OH terminates the polymerization reaction at that point. With four ddNTP-specific reactions, four populations of ddNTP-terminated reactions are obtained. These can be read on the sequencing gel just like the Maxam-Gilbert reactions.

Sequencing technology has now become automated. Using the dideoxy technique with fluorescently labeled DNA primers (four colors, one for each base) combined with laser scanning of the separated fragments as they emerge from a small packed column that replaces the polyacrylamide gel, machines can separate, read, and store thousands of base pairs of sequence per day. An example of a printout from an automated sequencing gel is shown in Fig. 33-24.

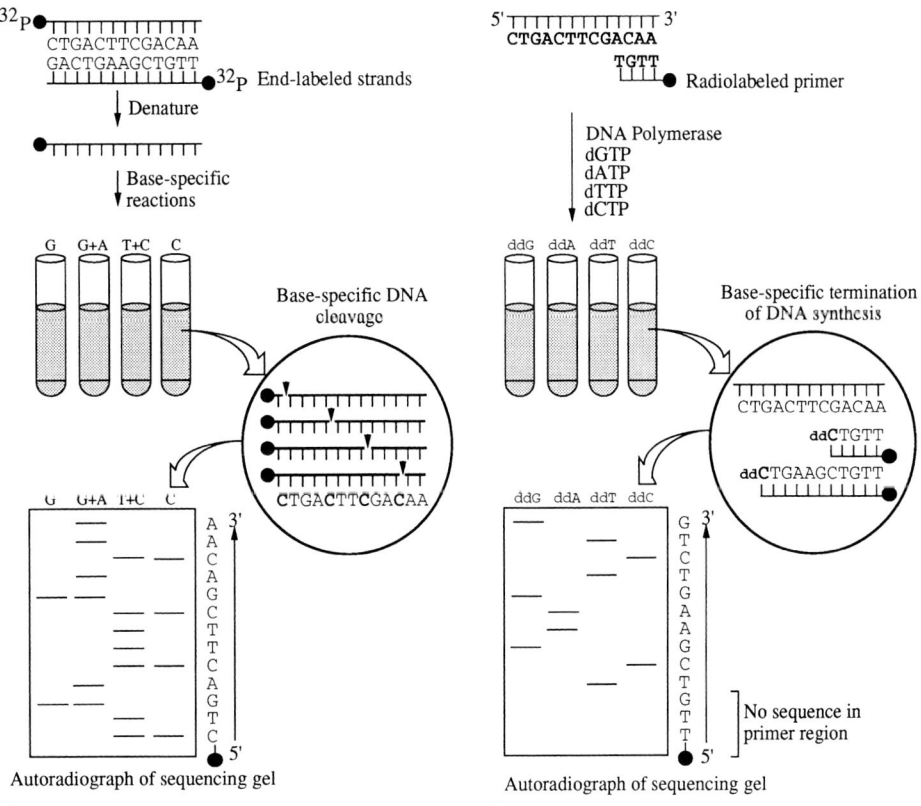

FIGURE 33-23. DNA sequencing. A. Maxam-Gilbert chemical method. B. Sanger dideoxy enzymatic method. (Both adapted from Watson JD, Hopkins NH, Roberts JW, et al: Molecular Biology of the Gene. Menlo Park, CA: Benjamin Cummings, 1987. With permission. Copyright © 1987 by The Benjamin/Cummings Publishing Company, Inc.)

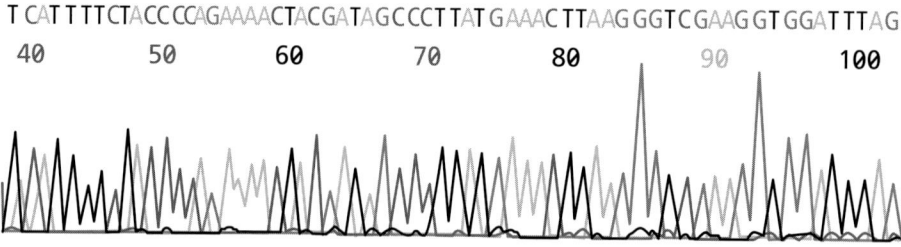

FIGURE 33-24. Automated sequence analysis. The base-specific Sanger sequencing reactions are performed with four different fluorescently labeled primers (e.g., red, black, green, blue), added together, passed through a capillary column, and detected colorimetrically. Rather than visualizing bands on a gel (as in Fig. 33-23), the output (shown in black and white here but actually in color) looks like a chromatogram.

The advent of gene chip technology (see below) has introduced a third method of DNA sequencing, called *sequencing by hybridization*.[59] In this method (Fig. 33-25), a gene of interest, say 1000 bp in length, is depicted as a series of 20-nt oligonucleotides, each designed to represent a 20-nt segment of the gene. Each 20-mer is offset in sequence by one base from its predecessor oligonucleotide in the array in such a way that an overlapping set of 20-mers traverses the DNA in a "sliding window" that represents the entire gene sequence. Importantly, each 20-mer is designed as a quadruplicate set of four related oligonucleotides: In three of the four oligonucleotides, the bases match the target DNA sequence at 19 of the 20 positions, whereas in the fourth oligonucleotide all 20 bases match perfectly (i.e., the set of four 20-mers are perfect matches except for an A, G, C, or T at one "internal" mismatch position). Thus, if a 1000-nt single-stranded DNA or cDNA fluorescent probe corresponding to the sequence represented on the array is hybridized to the chip, all 4000 cells in the array (i.e., all 1000 "tetrads") will light up, but in each tetrad of cells, one of the four will hybridize significantly better than will the other three, due to the perfect match at all 20 bases in that cell. Since the tetrads are arrayed as a sliding window that traverses the sequence, each intensely hybridizing cell in each tetrad represents the one letter out of four that creates the perfect match in that tetrad; in other words, the order of lit-up cells in the set of overlapping tetrads represents the DNA sequence. This method of sequencing not only is rapid but can easily identify mutations in a test sequence (say a myosin gene suspected of being mutated in a patient with a cardiomyopathy) compared to the wild-type reference sequence represented on the chip.

Multiplex analysis of gene expression. The availability of the complete sequence of a genome means that, for the first time, we know essentially the entire set of mRNAs encoded by that genome. In principle, therefore, one ought to be able to ask if the expression of these mRNAs is altered under various conditions (e.g., normal vs. reduced nutrients in the medium or in normal vs. tumor tissue). The analysis

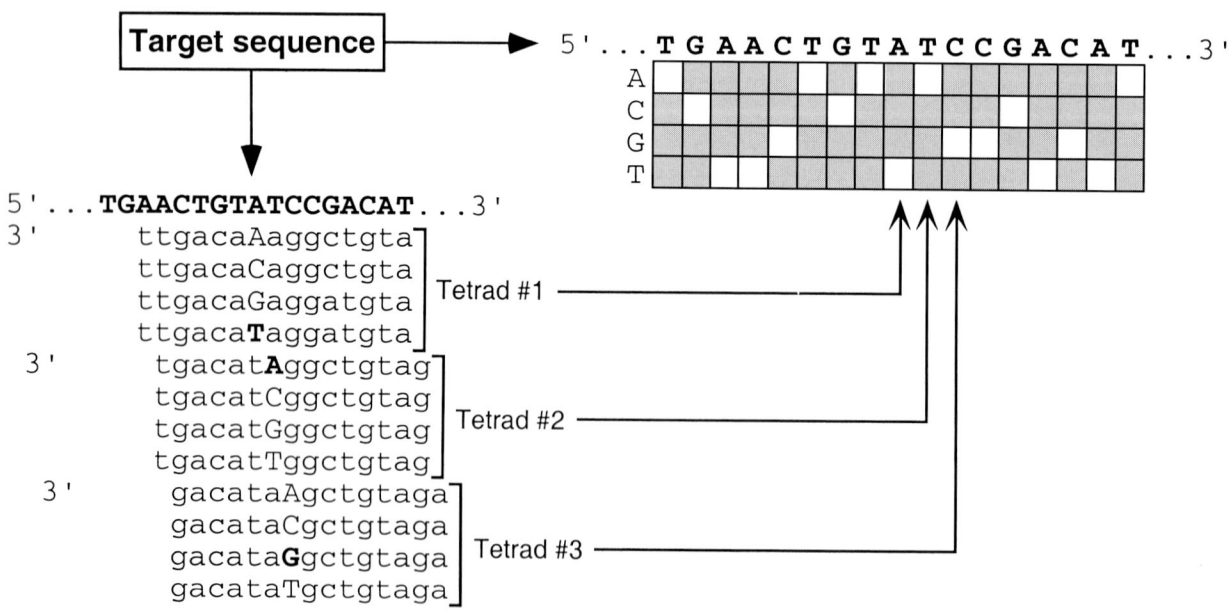

FIGURE 33-25. Sequencing by hybridization. A set of arrayed oligonucleotide "tetrads" representing the sequence of interest is "built up" on a chip (see Fig. 33-26) and "queried" with the target probe. Upper-case letters denote the position of the single internal mismatch in each tetrad; the bold letter denotes the perfect match. See text for details. (*Adapted from Chee M, Yang R, Hubbell E, et al: Accessing genetic information with high-density DNA arrays. Science 274:610–614, 1996. With permission.*)

of the expression of hundreds or even thousands of genes could not possibly be addressed using standard techniques: From a practical standpoint, Northern blot analysis can examine only a handful of mRNAs at a time, and the various subtractive hybridization methods described above are time-consuming and require much laboratory expertise.

Fortunately, a new set of technologies has been developed to deal with this problem. The greatest breakthrough has been in the development of *DNA microarrays*, also known as *gene chips*. Using a microlithography technique similar to that used in designing silicon computer chips, short oligonucleotides (20 to 60 nt in length), each having a defined and unique sequence, can be "built up" on a solid substrate and arrayed on a grid (Fig. 33-26A and B).[60] The grid can be tiny—about the size of a postage stamp—and yet contain up to 64,000 "cells," each with an oligonucleotide repre-

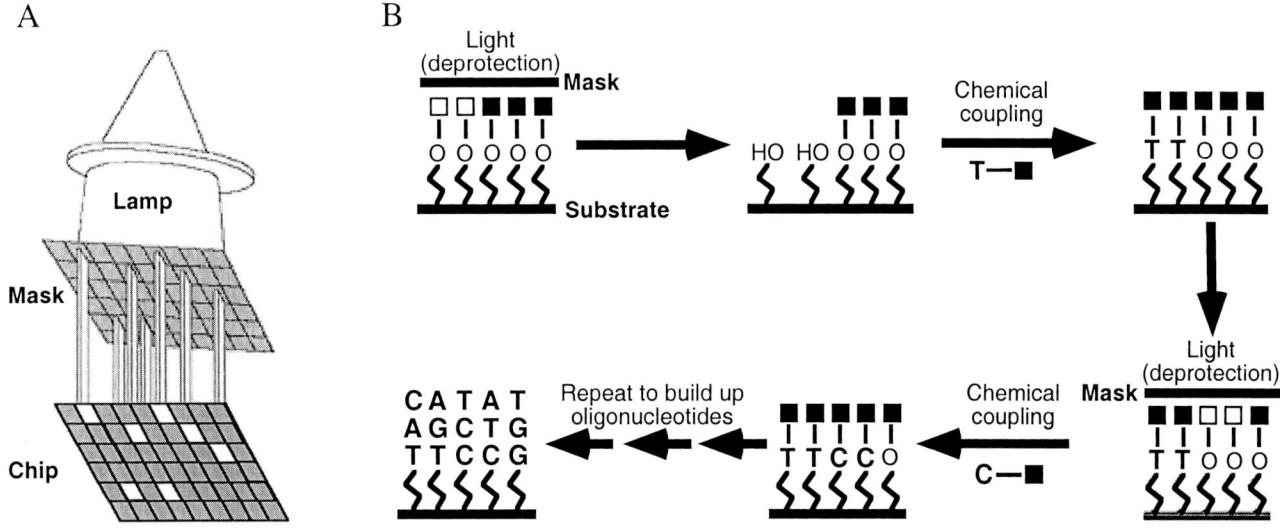

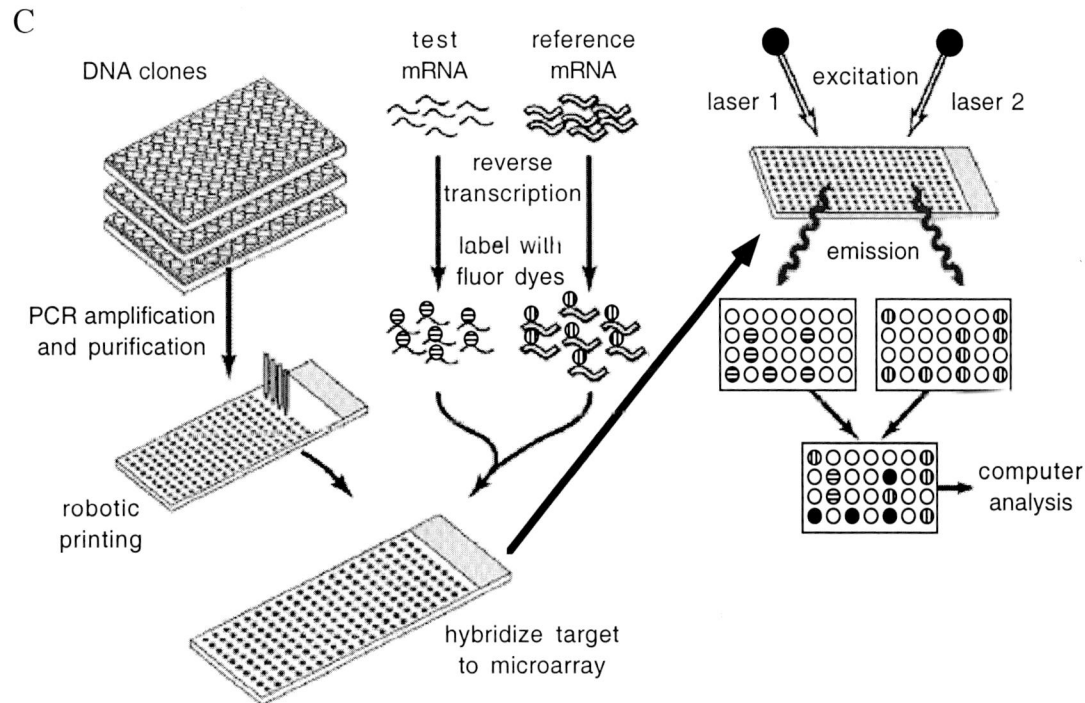

FIGURE 33-26. Microarray technology. *A.* Making a gene chip by microlithography. *B.* The array is "built up" by a series of light-catalyzed protection and deprotection steps. *C.* Expression profiling using PCR-amplified cDNA clones "printed" on a slide. (*Adapted from Lipshutz RJ, Fodor SP, Gingeras TR, et al: High density synthetic oligonucleotide arrays. Nat Genet 21:20–24, 1999. With permission.*)

senting one specific gene or mRNA. The chip can then be queried by hybridizing fluorescently labeled cDNAs derived from mRNAs from two sources (e.g., red cDNA probes from source A and green from source B) and comparing the colored signals derived from each source. Thus, in one experiment, one can determine not only which genes are upregulated (i.e., red signal predominates), which are downregulated (i.e., green signal predominates), and which are unchanged (both red and green signals are equal in intensity, yielding a yellow signal), but also by how much.[61] In a modification of this method, instead of representing each mRNA by a short oligonucleotide, the entire full-length cDNA can be "spotted" on a glass slide (Fig. 33-26C). As with the gene chip, hundreds and in some cases thousands of cDNAs can be arrayed on a microscope slide and analyzed in a similar manner.[62,63]

Besides analyzing differences in expression between two cell types, the same approach can be used to deduce how perturbations in cell function affect gene pathways (e.g., glycolysis, or cell-cycle signaling). Thus, microarray analysis can help us develop "functional maps" in which each gene is a node in an n-dimensional network, with genes "pointing" toward or away from other genes, depending on whether they are upstream or downstream of those gene products in various pathways.[64-66]

A different approach for multiplex analysis of transcription is called *serial analysis of gene expression* (SAGE).[67] In SAGE, each mRNA in a tissue is converted to a cDNA containing a short, unique identifer tag (similar to a bar code) appended to its 3' end. After all the cDNAs have been synthesized, the identifiers are cut away from their cognate cDNAs (which are no longer required in the analysis) and are ligated together into a long string. By sequencing the string of tags (this is the "serial analysis"), one can deduce both the identities and the relative amounts of all the mRNAs initially present in the sample. The advantage of SAGE over microarrays is that SAGE makes no a priori judgments as to the composition of the mRNA pool, because *every* mRNA present in the tissue can theoretically be detected and quantified (in contrast, microarrays can detect only those mRNAs represented on the chip in the first place). The main drawback is that hundreds or thousands of tags need to be sequenced in order to get a statistically relevant answer.

Functional genomics. By analogy to the multiplex analysis of mRNA expression using microarrays, a new field has arisen focused on the study of the proteins expressed from these mRNAs and their interactions with other proteins. The large-scale analysis of proteins, called *proteomics*, includes the analysis and "microsequencing" of proteins separated by high-pressure liquid chromatography or on two-dimensional protein gels, often in conjunction with mass spectrometry; differential display of proteins from two different sources on two-dimensional gels; and the determination of protein-protein interactions.[68-70] In a similar vein, the field of *structural genomics* has begun high-throughput approaches to characterize the three-dimensional crystal strucure of individual proteins as well as developing an inventory of basic protein folds and structures that are used to build those proteins.[71]

Computer-based sequence analysis. With the advent of sequencing machines and arrays, DNA sequence technology has now reached a point where millions of base pairs of DNA sequence are being generated each year. The necessity to store, catalogue, and extract useful information from DNA and protein sequences, and to analyze the massive amounts of data that can be generated in microarray experiments, has created a whole new field: *computational biology*, or *bioinformatics*. There are a number of databases that house these sequences. In the United States, Genbank is the largest such database, holding, as of early 2003, about 28 billion bases of DNA from 22 million sequences derived from all species, of which about 30 percent are human sequences. The European Molecular Biology Laboratory (EMBL) houses a similar database in Europe, as does the DNA Data Bank in Japan (DDBJ). There are also databases for protein sequences and for protein crystal structures.

These databases can be searched for similarity of a newly generated sequence with those already in the database and for detecting biologically relevant features (e.g., coding regions, promoter elements, DNA-binding motifs, secondary structure patterns, and the like). There are a number of commercially available software programs for computer sequence analysis; most present their output numerically and, when appropriate, graphically. Increasingly, the computer is being used for performing "dry" experiments, in which the huge size of the database is taken advantage of in order to reveal features in DNA and protein sequences that would be difficult to deduce experimentally, but that, a posteriori, can be subjected to experimental test.

USING CLONED GENES

Once a gene or other DNA sequence has been cloned, it can be used to study genetic function, both in vivo and in vitro. Along with the techniques already discussed above, such as mapping, sequencing, and blotting, there are a number of other extremely useful methodologies that extend the range of our understanding.

In vitro transcription. Some plasmid vectors contain promoter elements that can be recognized by specific prokaryotic RNA polymerases, located immediately upstream of the polylinker region containing a cloned DNA insert. Upon addition of RNA polymerase, the insert is transcribed into RNA in an in vitro *transcription* reaction. If radioactive ribonucleotides, such as ^{35}S-labeled UTP (uridine triphosphate), are added, one can make a labeled "riboprobe" that can be used for a number of subsequent manipulations, including in situ hybridization.

In vitro translation. One can take a cloned gene, transcribe it in vitro, and add it to a "cocktail" of cellular factors, such as *rabbit reticulocyte lysate* or *wheat germ extract*, and the system will translate the transcribed message into protein. Usually this in vitro *translation* reaction is performed in the presence of ^{35}S-labeled methionine, so that the resulting polypeptide can be visualized on a gel. One can also used a cloned cDNA bound to a piece of filter paper to "pick out" a single mRNA from a mixture of total cellular mRNA (i.e., *hybrid selection*) and use this mRNA (after elution from the filter) for in vitro translation. One can even do the reverse, called *hybridize-arrest in vitro translation*, to confirm the identity of a cloned cDNA: A target mRNA can be immobilized by hybridizing it to a cloned cDNA, and the remaining pool of mRNAs can be analyzed by in vitro translation to see if they do *not* synthesize the expected polypeptide.

In situ hybridization. Southern and Northern hybridizations are essentially in vitro analyses of isolated DNA or RNA fragments immobilized on filter paper; they give only indirect information on the location or amounts of specific sequences in the tissue from which they were extracted. In situ *hybridization* (ISH) is a powerful and elegant technology that makes it possible to perform Northerns and Southerns in vivo.

In situ techniques are fundamentally identical to the filter-based methods. Tissue sections (e.g., sections from a muscle biopsy) are mounted on a slide and overlaid with a hybridization solution containing radioactive DNA or RNA probes. After incubation, the probe is washed off and the section exposed to x-ray film to give a macroscopic view of the hybridization pattern. For a microscopic view, the slides are dipped in photographic emulsion to expose individual silver grains. In combination with the classic morphologic methods of cytochemistry and immunocytochemistry, genetic analysis by in situ hybridization is rendered even more powerful as an analytic tool. With the advent of commercially available in situ hybridization "kits," this technology can sometimes be used for diagnostic purposes.

In situ PCR. In situ PCR is conceptually identical to in situ hybridization in that the topographic location of specific RNA transcripts (or, on occasion, DNA) can be identified in tissue segments. Rather than using a DNA probe to identify the transcript of interest, RT-PCR is performed on the tissue section to amplify the transcript of interest. The PCR product can be visualized by using radioactive or fluorescent primers, but often the PCR product is visualized by in situ hybridization using an ISH probe specific for the predicted RT-PCR product. Since the RT-PCR product is highly abundant, the ISH probe can detect it relatively easily compared to detection of the mRNA that was the PCR template. This method is particularly useful for low-abundance messages.

Site-directed mutagenesis. With the advent of PCR and oligonucleotide synthesis, it is now a relatively simple matter to introduce a known point mutation, insertion, or deletion into a piece of cloned DNA by using an oligonucleotide synthesized to contain a known "mismatch" as one of the PCR primers. The resulting mutated DNA, which often mimics a mutation in a human disease gene, can then be studied in vitro.

Conformational analysis. It is now possible to search for and distinguish a mutant (or polymorphic) allele of a segment of DNA that differs at only a single base pair from its normal counterpart. One way is to use *conformational analysis*, in which the normal and mutant DNAs migrate differently on gels based on topologic differences in DNA structure arising from the difference in sequence. In *single-strand conformation polymorphism analysis* (SSCP), the normal and mutant DNAs are first denatured at low concentration and then allowed to reanneal intramolecularly into a thermodynamically stable secondary structure.[72] The two types of molecule usually migrate at different rates through a nonde-

naturing polyacrylamide gel due to their slightly different shapes, resulting in an apparent length polymorphism on the gel. In *denaturing gradient gel electrophoresis* (DGGE), the normal and mutant double-stranded DNAs are electrophoresed through a gel containing a gradient of a DNA denaturant, such as formamide or temperature. At some position in the gel (determined by the formamide concentration or by the temperature at that position), the duplex DNA denatures into single-stranded DNA, and its rate of migration slows down. Even a single base-pair difference in the mutant sequence will cause it to migrate a different distance in the gradient gel prior to denaturing, thereby making it possible to distinguish the two alleles. A third type of conformational analysis is actually a variant of Southern blotting. This method uses two *allele-specific oligonucleotides* (ASOs) that differ in sequence by only one nucleotide, as hybridization probes of cloned or genomic DNA. Under specific conditions, only one or the other but not both probes will hybridize, thus distinguishing the alleles.

Heteroduplex analysis. The presence of polymorphic alleles can be monitored by *heteroduplex analysis*. Two populations of duplex DNA that differ at an allele are denatured and allowed to reanneal, so that a subpopulation of reannealed duplexes forms, containing the sequence of one allele on the top strand and the other allele on the bottom. This *heteroduplex* can be analyzed by DGGE or by using nucleases, such as S1 or mung bean nuclease, that digest heteroduplex DNA at mismatches. If in vitro–transcribed riboprobes are used to synthesize one of the two strands, single strand–specific RNases can also be used to detect the mismatches.

Another way to monitor alleles is to look for an RFLP due to the mutated base. If the mutation creates a new restriction site, the region can be amplified by PCR and cut by the relevant restriction enzyme. The mutant allele will be cut, while the normal one will not be (or vice versa). If the mutation does not create an RFLP, a PCR primer can be used that is so designed as to *introduce* an RFLP into one allele but not the other by site-directed mutagenesis.

Primer extension and nuclease protection. The transcription start site of an mRNA can be deduced by annealing a radiolabeled oligonucleotide complementary to a region of the mRNA near the 5' end and synthesizing cDNA using reverse transcriptase. The enzyme will fall off the mRNA at the cap site, generating a labeled, *primer-extended* fragment that can be sized on a gel. Alternatively, a piece of cloned genomic DNA can be labeled and, with the antimessage sense hybridized to total DNA, treated with S1 nuclease (or RNase if a riboprobe was used). Only the region of the probe protected by the mRNA will survive nuclease treatment, and this fragment can be sized on a gel. *S1-protection analysis* is highly useful in analyzing mutations that cause alterations in mRNA length.

Gel retardation. If a region of regulatory DNA has been cloned, it may well interact with a DNA-binding protein. One way to search for this interaction is to use a *gel-retardation* assay. The cloned fragment is mixed with a cellular fraction containing potential DNA-binding proteins or with a purified candidate DNA-binding protein. If the DNA binds to the protein specifically, it will migrate on a nondenaturing gel more slowly than will the cloned "naked" DNA alone: Its mobility will be retarded. The gel-retardation assay can then be used as a bioassay in the subsequent purification of the protein.

DNA footprinting. If the protein binds a fragment of DNA at a specific site (similar to a restriction enzyme binding at a restriction site), it will protect the DNA from attack by various chemical agents (e.g., dimethyl sulfate) or enzymes (e.g., DNases). A radiolabeled fragment protected in this way can be visualized and sized on a polyacrylamide gel. The size of the protected fragment is directly related to the region on the DNA covered by the DNA-binding protein, called the protein's *footprint* on the DNA. The specific location of the footprint on the DNA can be deduced by electrophoresing the footprinted DNA next to the sequence of the same DNA fragment loaded in four adjacent lanes on the gel; the protected region will have the sequence of the corresponding comigrating DNA sequence.

Linkage analysis. Cloned pieces of DNA can be localized to specific regions of the chromosome by Southern blotting or by in situ hybridization techniques. Once localized, they can then be used as probes in *linkage analysis*, the most powerful method currently available to isolate disease-causing genes that have no known gene product.

Linkage analysis is based on the principle that the farther apart two DNA sequences are on a chromosome, the more likely it is that they will be transmitted separately to daughter germline cells during meiosis owing to a *recombination event* between sister chromatids that *unlinks* them (Fig. 33-27). Conversely, the closer the interval between two sequences (called *linkage markers*), the less likely it is that recombination will unlink them and the more likely that they will be transmitted (and inherited) together. These distances are expressed in *centimorgans* (cM): One cM equals 1 percent of recombination—that is, the distance between markers is such that, for every 100 meiotic events analyzed, 1 recombination event unlinking the markers will be observed. Since recombination events occur during meiosis, they can be observed by examining the linkage markers in related individuals within the same pedigree.

If one of the two DNA markers is a piece of DNA whose sequence and chromosomal position is known and the second DNA marker is a gene of interest whose function and chromosomal position are initially unknown [e.g., the gene causing spinal muscular atrophy (SMA)], then the sequence marker can be used to see whether it is linked to the disease phenotype expressed by the gene of interest (in this case SMA) as the disease gene "passes" through a pedigree. As with any two markers, the closer the known marker is to the disease gene allele, the more likely it is that the two will be inherited together without recombination. There is one feature that the known DNA marker must exhibit: It must be *polymorphic*—that is, there must be at least two *alleles* (versions of the gene or DNA sequence at the same position on two different chromosomes) of the marker that differ in some detectable way (for example, they may vary at a single nucleotide within a restriction enzyme recognition sequence and thus be distinguishable as an RFLP). If one allele of the DNA marker is tightly linked to the disease gene, all indi-

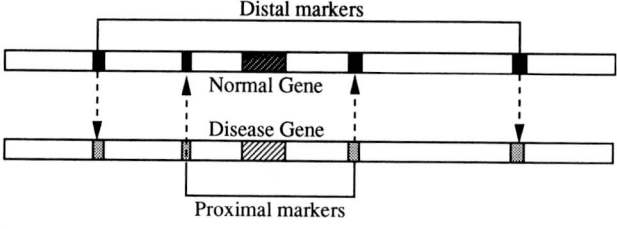

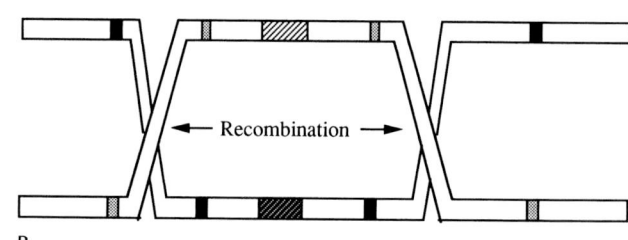

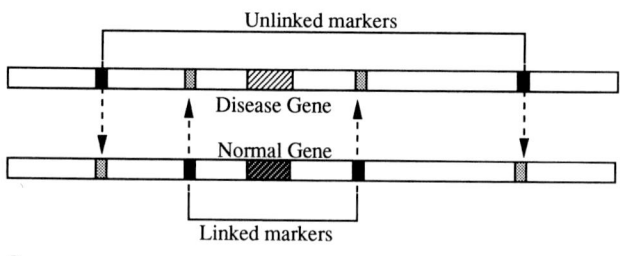

FIGURE 33-27. Recombination of markers near alleles of a disease gene during meiosis. *A*. Pairing of sister chromatids during first meiotic division. *B*. Recombination during crossing over of chromatids. Markers proximal (linked) to the disease gene of interest remain with original chromatid, while distal (unlinked) markers become separated. *C*. Resolution and segregation of chromatids following crossing over. Note how the proximal markers on each chromatid "stayed" with each respective gene allele even though a recombination event occurred to separate the more distantly located markers. *From Micklos DA, Freyer FA (eds): DNA Science: A First Course in Recombinant DNA Technology. Cold Spring Harbor, NY: Cold Spring Harbor Laboratory Press, 1990. Copyright © 1990 by Carolina Biological Supply Company.*

viduals carrying the disease should also carry the identical marker allele linked to it at a nearby chromosomal position (*linkage disequilibrium*). On the other hand, those pedigree members who do not carry the disease gene should more frequently carry the other allele(s) of the marker.

If, in fact, analysis of a pedigree shows that one allele of a marker *segregates* with the disease in a statistically significant way, while all other alleles do not, then the chromosomal position of the marker defines the neighborhood (say, within 1 cM) in which the unknown disease gene resides. The logarithm of the probability that the two sequences (in our case the DNA marker at the known chromosomal location and the SMA gene at an unknown chromosomal location) are near each other, or *linked*, is called the "log of the odds" score, or *lod score*. Thus, in order to get linkage to a disease gene, one must find a large pedigree in which affected and unaffected members can be analyzed and then find a DNA marker that, when tested on the DNA of pedigree members, generates a large lod score, usually 3.0 (i.e., 1000:1 odds that the marker and the disease are linked) or higher. The problem is that to get within 1 cM of a disease gene at a lod of 3, one might have to test hundreds or even thousands of DNA markers. This tedious work has been successful in SMA: Markers located on chromosome 5 defined a small region where the disease gene must lie, and that gene, called *SMN*, was cloned.

Length polymorphisms that do not rely on RFLPs are even more useful in linkage analysis. One example of this type of analysis takes advantage of *variable-number tandem repeats* (VNTRs). As its name implies, a VNTR is a series of tandemly repeated identical sequences that are flanked by unique sequences at one or a few locations in the genome. The number of repeats may vary among individuals or even differ between the two allelic chromosomal loci within an individual. Thus, using suitable VNTR probes on Southern blots, one can track a VNTR length polymorphism pattern through a pedigree. An extreme example of a repeated sequence length polymorphism is the *dinucleotide-repeat* polymorphism. A sequence of dinucleotides (e.g., CA) may be repeated a number of times [e.g., $(CA)_{10}$] within a region of unique, single-copy DNA. Instead of $(CA)_{10}$, other alleles may contain $(CA)_9$ or $(CA)_{11}$ flanked by the unique DNA. A PCR fragment of this piece of unique DNA containing these highly polymorphic CA repeats could then serve as useful markers, because each allele will differ from the other alleles by an integral multiple of two nucleotides, which can be observed easily on polyacrylamide gels. Other repeated elements, such as the so-called *minisatellite repeats*, are also highly variable in length and location[73] and can be used for producing essentially unique DNA profiles of an individual (a "fingerprint") that are useful not only in linkage analysis but in other areas as well, including anthropology and forensics.

Length polymorphisms are now being superseded by *single-nucleotide polymorphisms*, or SNPs (pronounced "snips"). As the name implies, SNPs are differences at a single base pair (often neutral changes) in a candidate region of the genome (and often in the candidate gene itself) in which the nucleotide that is inherited in affected members of a pedigree differs from that in the analogous sequence in the unaffected members. Since there are hundreds of thousands of SNP variants in the normal human genome, the use of SNPs as linkage markers will make the search for culprit genes both rapid and efficient.

Protein-protein interactions. Since many proteins function as members of multiprotein complexes, it is often important to determine if a polypeptide encoded by a cloned gene does or does not interact with other proteins. A number of techniques have been developed to identify and ultimately purify such interacting partners, but two in particular stand out. The first is the *pull-down assay*, in which the polypeptide of interest (the "bait") is expressed as a "fusion protein" derived from the coding region of the polypeptide's cDNA ligated in-frame to sequences encoding an "affinity tag" that can be used to mark and separate interacting proteins within a milieu of noninteracting proteins. A common affinity tag is glutathione-S-transferase (GST), which can be used to immobilize the expressed fusion protein on glutathione-coupled beads in an affinity column.[74] The expressed GST-protein fusion gene (the GST tag is typically positioned upstream of the polypeptide's N terminus but can be located anywhere as long as it does not impede function) is mixed with labeled proteins (e.g., a cell lysate containing ^{35}S-Met-labeled proteins) together with glutathione-coupled Sepharose beads. After incubation to allow for protein-protein interactions to take place, the beads are centrifuged in order to "pull down" the interacting proteins. The putatively interacting proteins in the pellet are resolved on an SDS-polyacrylamide gel and identified by fluorography to detect the ^{35}S-Met label. Column chromatography approaches employing the same scheme can be used to isolate the interacting protein in sufficient quantities for identification via amino acid sequencing.

As opposed to the biochemical approach embodied in the GST pull-down assay, the *yeast two-hybrid system* employs a genetic approach to accomplish the same task.[75] In brief, the "bait" protein is fused to a DNA-binding domain in such a way that the expressed fusion protein binds to a promoter activation region located upstream of a reporter gene, such as β-galactosidase (similar to the blue-white screening described above). This construct is transfected into yeast containing a library of cDNAs encoding potential interacting partners. Importantly, each member of the cDNA library is also engineered to be expressed as a fusion protein, except that now the fusion tag is the β-gal-activation domain. Transcription of the β-galactosidase gene requires the interaction of the β-gal DNA-binding domain (now fused to the bait protein) with the β-gal-activation domain (now fused to the potential "prey" cDNAs). Thus, β-galactosidase can be synthesized only if the two domains are in sufficiently close proximity to activate transcription, and the only way the DNA-binding and β-gal-activation domains can interact is if the bait binds to a prey protein. Upon interaction, β-galactosidase is produced and, in the presence of the substrate X-gal, the yeast colony turns from white to blue. There are now numerous variations on both approaches, but the principle remains the same.[52]

Expression of cloned genes in cells. Instead of transcribing and translating a cDNA in vitro, a more efficient technique to produce a polypeptide is to insert the plasmid harboring the cDNA into a bacterium and have the cell produce the protein in vivo. This is the basis of the genetic engineering techniques drug companies now use to produce—actually overproduce—commercially valuable rare biologicals from recombinant DNA (e.g., insulin, tissue plasminogen activator, erythropoetin, interferon, restriction enzymes). In the laboratory, expression of a cloned gene in bacteria is useful for synthesizing enough pure protein to inject into mice or rabbits to produce a specific antibody against the polypeptide of interest.

While technically more difficult, it is also possible to express a cloned gene in eukaryotic cells (e.g., mammalian or insect cells). This is usually done when the polypeptide of interest has important posttranslational modifications, such as glycosylation, that bacteria do not incorporate into the translation product.

One method of studying a gene's expression in mammalian cells is to disrupt its function and study the phenotypic consequences of the disruption. One way of doing this is to transfect cells with a plasmid construct that is capable of synthesizing large amounts of *antisense RNA*, that is, RNA complementary in sequence to a normally transcribed message.[76] The antisense RNA hybridizes to the normal message-sense mRNA and thus either induces RNA interference (see above) or prevents the normal message from being spliced or translated. The net effect is to sequester the normal mRNA and prevent translation of the gene product.

A second, even more powerful method of disruption is to disable the normal gene by homologous recombination. In one such method, a genomic sequence is constructed in a vector containing selectable drug markers and is transfected into mammalian cells. The drug selection scheme will allow only those cells to grow in which the exogenous gene has recombined with and disrupted the endogenous chromosomal gene.

Expression of cloned genes in animals. One of the greatest advances in the use of cloned genes has been the direct insertion of a gene into the germline of an animal, usually a mouse, in order to study its effects in vivo. The generation of *transgenic mice* has been a technical tour de force, and the information obtained in these experiments has been invaluable in the study of all aspects of gene regulation. The basic strategy is to microinject a piece of foreign genomic DNA (often human) containing the gene of interest plus its flanking regulatory regions into the pronucleus of a fertilized mouse embryo. The embryo is then implanted into a pregant foster mother mouse and allowed to develop normally in utero. When successful, the foreign *transgene* will be integrated into the mouse's chromosomes, and the transgenic mice will have a distinct phenotype as well as the transgenic genotype. Because the foreign gene is integrated randomly in the mouse genome, the analogous mouse endogenous gene is unaffected.

Rather than express an introduced extra copy of a gene, one can ablate the endogenous mouse gene by inserting a "null" version of the mouse gene (e.g., removal of exons or mutatgenesis to ensure truncation of the polypeptide) via homologous recombination (Fig. 33-28A), so that the endogenous gene is replaced with the truncated transgene at the same locus.[77,78] The insertion of such a *knockout* gene is done in mouse *embryonic stem cells*—totipotent cells that can be grown and manipulated in tissue culture and then injected into mouse blastocysts.[79] Mice born following injection of ES cells are chimeric for the transgene, but some animals will harbor the knockout allele in the germline. Mating of such heterozygous mice will result in some progeny homozygous for the knockout construct. Knockout animals are useful in determining the function of a gene on a whole-animal basis, but there are more than a few cases where the phenotype of the knockout mouse was either diferent from that predicted or unexpectedly benign.

The technique of homologous recombination can also be used to make *knock-in* mice (Fig. 33-28B), in which a mutated version of the endogenous mouse gene encoding, for example, the mouse analogue of a pathogenic point mutation in a human gene is inserted at the endogenous mouse locus. Such animals are typically used as animal models of human genetic disorders in order to study the natural history and course of the disorder and pathogenesis of the disease and as a test bed to assess treatment strategies.

The Molecular Biology of Muscle

The molecular revolution, using the concepts and tools described above, has begun to pay off for those interested in the study of the contraction, function, gene regulation, and diseases of muscle. In the last few years, a large number of human muscle-specific genes have been cloned, and the pace of gene isolation shows no sign of letting up. Moreover, a series of breakthroughs has now shed light on one of the most fundamental questions in biology: the control of cellular differentiation. In particular, genes have now been cloned that have the remarkable property of being intimately involved in the control of muscle differentiation—that is, they are true regulatory genes. The elucidation of their mode of function is described in much greater detail in Chap. 1 and is outlined here only briefly.

MUSCLE-SPECIFIC GENE REGULATION

The fact that muscle-specific genes exist begs the question of how the cell identifies such genes and then transcribes them and no others at the right time in development and in the right tissue. This problem, which is one of the most fundamental in cell biology, became amenable to analysis at the molecular genetic level in 1987, when Harold Weintraub and colleagues isolated a gene controlling myogenic differentiation, called *MYOD*, that is expressed only in skeletal muscle.[80] When introduced experimentally into nonmuscle cells, such as fibroblasts, *MYOD* activates muscle-specific gene expression, thereby converting fibroblasts into myoblasts. Significantly, *MYOD* is not expressed in cardiac or smooth muscle, even though those cells express many genes that are also expressed in skeletal muscle. It has been found that the MyoD polypeptide, which is the product of the *MYOD* gene, is a DNA-binding helix-loop-helix (HLH) protein that apparently activates myogenesis by binding as a dimer to DNA elements in the control regions of muscle-specific genes.[81,82] Because of these properties, *MYOD* has been called a "master regulatory gene."[83] The basic/HLH domains found in MyoD are found in other DNA-binding proteins (referred to collectively as the *myc* homology family), and it is probably significant that oncogenes such as *c-myc*, *c-fos*, and *c-mos* can also promote myogenesis.

Myogenic-determination proteins like MyoD bind to muscle-specific regulatory sequences, foremost among them the "E-box" and "CArG" motifs.[84-87] Both of these elements are small DNA sequences located near the 5' ends of muscle-specific genes that share an overall palindromic motif. The E-box is a hexamer beginning with CA and ending with TG; the internal two nucleotides are variable (i.e., CANNTG). Similarly, the CArG (C – AT-rich – G) motif is a decamer, beginning with CC and ending with GG, with six adenine or thymine nucleotides in between [i.e., $CC(A/T)_6GG$]. Two "named" elements, the *serum response*

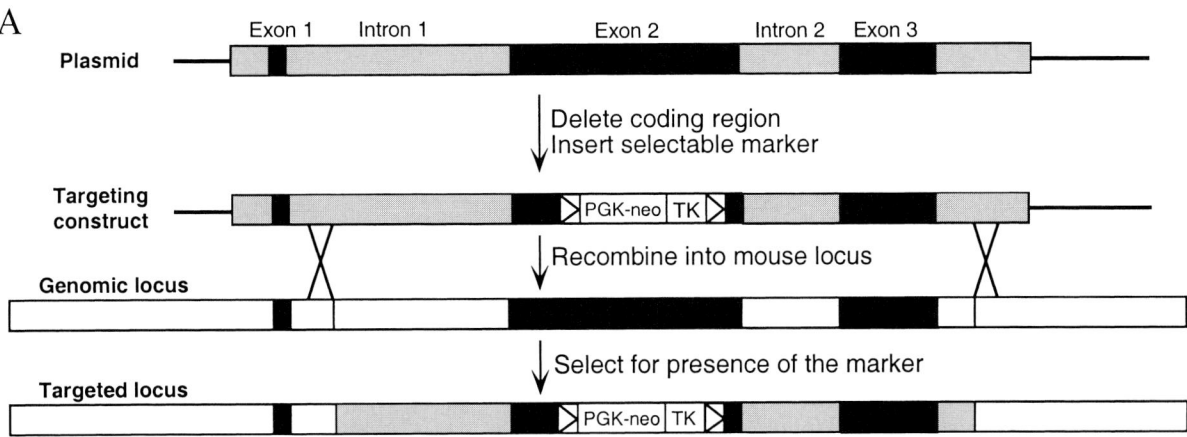

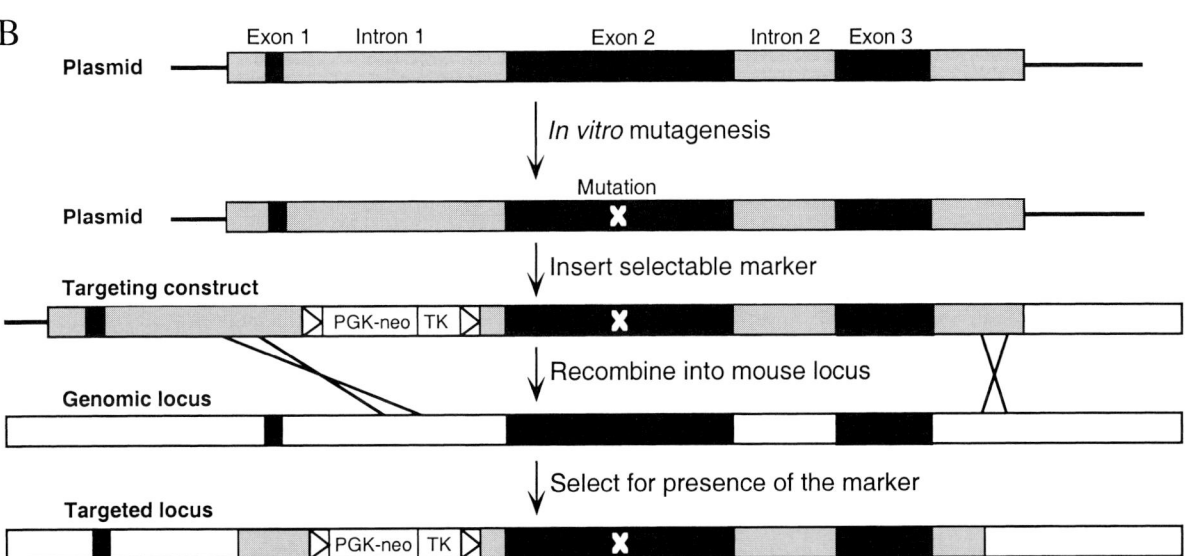

FIGURE 33-28. Transgenic mouse technology. *A.* Strategy to knock out a gene. *B.* Strategy to knock in a gene. PGK-neo (neomycin resistance gene driven by the phosphoglycerate kinase promoter) and TK (thymidine kinase) denote typical selectable markers.

element[84] and the *muscle regulatory element*,[88] are actually CArG boxes. Other consensus muscle-regulatory elements have also been identified. One is called *muscle CAT* or *M-CAT*,[89] due to the similarity of its sequence—CATTCCT—to the CCAAT box. Since the discovery of the E-box, numerous other regulatory elements have been identified in a number of muscle-specific genes, such as SURE (slow troponin I upstream regulatory element) and FIRE (fast troponin I intronic regulatory element).[90]

Following the discovery of *MYOD*, a related set of mammalian muscle-specific regulatory genes, all with basic amino acid and HLH DNA-binding motifs, were identified.[91] These include *myogenin*,[81] *myf-5*,[92] and *myf-6* (also called *MRF-4* and *herculin*),[92–94] and a single-stranded DNA-binding protein called *MF3* (for muscle factor 3),[95] which can bind to the MCAT, CArG, and E-box motifs.

It is important to note that these muscle-specific enhancer elements and DNA-binding proteins are *necessary but not sufficient* for myogenesis. To cite just two examples, motifs like the E-box are also present in the enhancers of nonmuscle genes and, as alluded to above, the expression of MyoD protein does not automatically initiate myogenesis. It has become clear that *MYOD* itself is regulated (for example, by a gene called *ID*, for inhibitor of differentiation[96,97]) and that other gene products are required for the controlled regulation of myogenesis. This is why Weintraub called *MYOD* a "nodal point" for specification of the muscle cell lineage.[83]

Other types of myogenic-regulatory genes, some of which have no sequence similarity to the *MYOD* family, have also been identified.[82] Many *positive regulators* are transcriptional activators themselves—for example, the *serum response factor*, or SRF.[98] Others are muscle-specific transcription factors, such as MEF2C and the muscle LIM protein (MLP), both of which bind to myogenic bHLH proteins to activate transcription,[99,100] and nuclear hormone receptors, such as the thyroid hormone and retinoic acid receptors, both of which appear to interact directly with MEF2.[101] During embryonic development, homeodomain-containing proteins, such as PAX3 and SIX1, interact to regulate myogenesis.[102] The ability of proteins such as MyoD to initiate the myogenic program can also be regulated postively and directly via phosphorylation by kinases of specific amino acid residues on the transcription factor itself. While most kinases are ubiquitously expressed, two, CDK9[103] and the *stress-activated protein kinase* p38,[104] are particularly noteworthy. A more indirect mechanism of positive regulation of myogenesis is *coactivation* of transcription, via, for example, remodeling of chromatin domains containing muscle-specific genes. Two such proteins, PCAF and p300, acetylate histone proteins and sequence-specific transcription factors, thereby allowing for the access of other transcription factors to the DNA.[105–107]

Many *negative regulators* of muscle-specific transcription also operate via protein-protein interaction, except that in this case, the binding of the regulatory protein *prevents* the initiation of transcription. A well-studied negative regulator is the Id family of HLH proteins, which prevent MyoD and Myf5 from forming heterodimers with other HLH proteins, such as E2A, thereby preventing DNA binding.[96] Other negative regulators—with exotic names like Twist,[108] Mist1,[109] I-mf,[110] MyoR,[111] Notch,[112] and ZEB[113]—behave in a fundamentally similar way. Just as PCAF can stimulate transcription via acetylation, the corepressor N-CoR can silence transcription by *deacetylating* target proteins.[114]

Finally, a new group of muscle regulatory genes is exemplified by two proteins that have recently been identified to be regulators of muscle atrophy. Both proteins, called MURF1 (for muscle-specific ring finger 1)[115] and MAFBX [for muscle atrophy F-box protein (also called atrogin-1)[115,116] are ubiquitin protein ligases. Ubiquitin is, as the name implies, a ubiquitously expressed gene; it encodes a polypeptide required for the turnover of cellular proteins. Covalent attachment of ubiquitin to a target polypeptide initiates a "ubiquitin pathway" for the degradation of that protein. MURF1 and MAFBX are muscle-specific gene products that stimulate turnover (and ultimately loss) of muscle-specific proteins via this pathway.

MUSCLE-SPECIFIC GENES

Cloned genes specifying proteins expressed only in muscle fall into two main groups: muscle-specific genes encoding proteins associated primarily with muscle function, and non-muscle-specific genes encoding proteins having muscle-specific isoforms. While many such genes have been cloned from many organisms, the focus here is on cloned human genes. A list of gene products expressed predominantly or even exclusively in muscle is shown in Table 33-1. While not exhaustive, it illustrates the fact that besides genes that are obviously associated with muscle function, many that are not are nevertheless expressed in a muscle-specific fashion.

Genes encoding proteins specific for muscle function. This group includes four types of genes. The first comprises genes specifying components of the muscle cytoskeleton, such as desmin and dystrophin. The second includes the protein components of the contractile apparatus, such as actin, myosin, nebulin, titin, and tropomyosin. The third includes genes specifying proteins required for muscle function distinct from those involved in the mechanical contractile apparatus itself, such as the acetylcholine receptor,[117,118] histidine-rich calcium-binding protein, myoglobin,[119] phospholamban,[120] and the calcium-channel of the sarcoplasmic reticulum (also called the ryanodine receptor). Finally, the developmental program for muscle differentiation requires the expression of numerous genes (some described above), many of which are muscle-specific. Detailed descriptions of the function of many of these gene products may be found in the appropriate chapters in Part 1.

One of the interesting things about these genes, and especially those associated with the contractile apparatus, is that many of them exist in tissue- and developmental-specific isoforms. In some cases, each isoform is specified by a different gene (e.g., aortic- and enteric-type smooth muscle actins); but in a surprising number of cases (e.g., the skeletal muscle myosins, tropomyosins, and troponins), the different isoforms are translated from alternatively spliced mRNAs derived from a precursor RNA transcribed from a single gene.[3,121] For example, the two isoforms of myosin alkali light chain found in fast skeletal muscle (i.e., MLC1 and MLC3) are derived from a single gene with 9 exons. Seven exons (exons 1, 4, 5, 6, 7, 8, and 9) are spliced to form the mRNA encoding MLC1, while a different set of 7 exons (exons 2, 3, 5, 6, 7, 8, and 9) form the mRNA for MLC3. Similarly, the smooth muscle myosin heavy-chain gene specifies at least four isoforms.[122] An even more extreme example is found in α-tropomyosin, which also has 9 exons. In this case, 6 mRNAs are made (2 skeletal muscle isoforms, 1 smooth muscle isoform, and 3 nonmuscle isoforms) using 6 splicing patterns: exons 1, 3, 4, 5, 7, and 8 are found in all 6 mRNAs, but different "combinations" of exons 2, 6, and 9 are found in each isoform. Similarly, a single rat troponinT gene with 18 exons is alternatively spliced to produce at least 10 different mRNAs; only 9 of the 18 exons are present in all 10 transcripts.

Genes encoding non–muscle-specific proteins having muscle-specific isoforms. This group of genes includes a number of *housekeeping* genes, that is, genes whose protein products are required in all cell types (e.g., in amino acid metabolism, the citric acid cycle, nucleic acid metabolism, respiratory chain function, oxidative phosphorylation, and the like). Because these proteins are present ubiquitously, it was surprising to find that many of them exist as isoforms in different cell types, with the most common pattern being that of a pair of isoforms, one found only in muscle and the other found in all other tissues (sometimes including muscle). These observations at the protein level have been confirmed at the genetic level, with the cloning of an ever-increasing number of muscle-specific isoform genes (Table 33-1).

While the isoforms of many muscle contractile proteins are produced by alternative splicing, many "housekeeping" protein isoforms are products of separate genes (e.g., phosphoglycerate mutase[123,124]); of course, alternatively spliced isoforms of housekeeping genes also exist (e.g., NCAM[125]).

Chapter 33. The Tools of Molecular Genetics and Their Application to the Study of Muscle Diseases

Table 33-1. SOME GENE PRODUCTS EXPRESSED PREDOMINANTLY OR EXCLUSIVELY IN MUSCLE

GENE PRODUCT	SYMBOL
General metabolism	
Acylphosphatase 2, muscle-specific isoform	ACYP2
Adenosine monophosphate deaminase 1, isoform M, sk m	AMPD1
Adenine nucleotide translocator 1 (mitochondrial), sk m, h	SLC25A4
Apo B mRNA editing catalytic polypeptide-like 2, sk m, h	APOBEC2
ATP receptor, smooth muscle	P2X1
ATPase subunit alpha (mitochondrial), h isoform	ATP5A1
ATPase subunit gamma (mitochondrial), h isoform	ATP5C1
Calpain 3, large subunit, sk m-specific	CAPN3
Carbonic anhydrase III	CA3
Carboxypeptidase-like protein ACLP, aortic smooth muscle	[ACLP]
Carnitine palmitoyltransferase I (mitochondrial), muscle type	CPT1B
Creatine kinase, muscle isoform	CKMM
Creatine kinase (mitochondrial), muscle isoform	CKMT2
Cytochrome c oxidase subunit VIa-H (mitochondrial), sk m, h	COX6A2
Cytochrome c oxidase subunit VIIa-H (mitochondrial), sk m, h	COX7A1
DNAse 1-like protein, sk m, h	DNASE1L1
Enolase, muscle-specific (MSE)	ENO3
Fatty-acid-binding protein (FABP), h	FABP3
Fructose-1,6-bisphosphatase, isozyme 2, sk m	FBP2
Glutathione S-transferase GSTA4-4, sk m isoform	GSTA4
Glycogen debranching enzyme, 3 muscle-specific isoforms	GDE
Glycogen phosphorylase, muscle-specific	PYGM
Glycogen synthase, sk m	GYS1
Glycogenin, skeletal muscle-specific isoform	GYG
GPI-linked NAD(P)(+)-arginine ADP-ribosyltransferase, sk m	ART1
Heat shock protein, 27 kD protein 2, sk m, h	HSPB2
Hexokinase II (muscle isoform) (mitochondrial)	HK2
Iinositol phosphatase, 43-kDa isoform, sk m and kidney	[SKIP]
Inositol 1,4,5-triphosphate receptor, type 2, sk m, h	TIPR2
Lactate dehydrogenase, skeletal muscle type	LDHA
Lactate dehydrogenase, heart type	LDHB
Lysosomal-associated membrane protein 2, isoform B, sk m, h	LAMP2
Myoadenylate deaminase	AMPD1
Myoglobin	MB
Nucleolar protein 3 (ARC, NOP), sk m, h	NOL3
Rribosomal protein L3-like protein, sk m	RPL3L
Ribosomal protein MRP-L5 (mitochondrial), h-specific isoform	[MRP-L5V1]
Phosphodiesterase, cAMP-specific, isoform PDE7A2	PDE7A1
Phosphodiesterase, cGMP-specific, alt spl isoforms	PDE5A
Phosphofructokinase, muscle isoform	PFKM
Phosphoglucomutase 1 (alt spl)	PGM1
Phosphoglycerate mutase, muscle isoform (also in blood)	PGAMM
Phosphorylase B kinase, alpha subunit, muscle isoform	PHKA1
Phosphorylase B kinase, gamma subunit, muscle isoform	PHKG1
Protein phosphatase 1 gamma catalytic subunit	PPP1CC
Protein phosphatase type 1, glycogen-binding reg subunit, sk m	PPP1R3
Pyruvate kinase, muscle type (M1), sk m, h, b	PKM2
Succinyl CoA synthetase (mitochondrial), h	SUCLG1
Ubiquitin-conjugating enzyme, sk m	UBE2G1
Ubiquitin specific protease 28, alt spl forms in sk m, h	USP28
Uncoupling protein, isoform 3 (mitochondrial), sk m, h	UCP3
Muscle differentiation, regulation, and signalling	
Acetylcholine receptor-associated protein, 43 kDa	RAPSN
ADAM12 metalloprotease-disintegrin (2 isoforms) (meltrin alpha)	ADAM12
Adenylyl cyclase type V, cardiac	ADCY5
Agrin	[AGRN]
Apoptosis receptor with CARD (mainly in myogenic cells)	ARC
Calsequestrin (calmitine) (mitochondrial), sk m isoform	CASQ1
Calcipressin 1, sk m, h, brain	DSCR1
Calsequestrin, sk m, h	CASQ2
Contraction regulatory protein	ID2B
Delta-like protein 3 (mouse kyphoscoliosis protein), sk m	DLL3
14-3-3 protein tau (activates MEF2D)	YWHAQ
Growth factor receptor-bound protein 10, sk m	GRB10
Histidine-rich calcium binding protein, sarcomeric	HRC
Histone deacetylase 4, sk m, h	HDAC4
Histone deacetylase 5, sk m, h	HDAC5
Homeobox protein sine oculis 1, sk m	SIX1
Homeobox protein sine oculis 2, sk m	SIX2
Insulin receptor binding protein (Grb-IR/hGrb10), sk m	GRB10
Insulin receptor substrate-1	IRS1
Interferon gamma-responsive transcript IRT-1, sm m	AIF1
Keratinocyte transcription factor protein, gamma isoform	KET
LIM protein (mouse Enigma homolog protein), sk m. h	LIM
LIM-protein 1 (SLIM1, SLIMMER isoforms), sk m, h	FHL1
LIM- protein 2 (mitochondrial), sk m	FHL2
LIM- protein 3 (mitochondrial), sk m	FHL3
MafG, sk m, h, brain	MAFG
Minibrain protein kinase homolog (MNBHb/DYRK1), sk m, h, alt spl	MNBH
Mitogen-activated protein kinase 6 (ERK3), p97 isoform	MAPK6
Mitogen-activated protein kinase 12 (ERK6), sk m	MAPK12
Mitogen-activated protein kinase kinase 6, sk m-specific isoform	MKK6
Muscle atrophy ubiquitin ligase F-box protein (atrogin-1), sk m, h	[MAFBX]
Muscle atrophy ubiquitin ligase RING finger 1 (MURF1), sk m, h	RNF28
Muscle specific ring finger protein 2 (MURF-2)	RNF29
Muscle specific ring finger protein 3 (MURF-3)	RNF30
Muscle LIM protein, sk m, h	MLP
Muscle TFII-I repeat domain-containing protein 1	WBSCR11
Myocyte enhancer factor 2A (alt spl isoforms)	MEF2A
Myocyte enhancer factor 2B (alt spl isoforms)	MEF2B
Myocyte enhancer factor 2C (alt spl isoforms), sk m-specific	MEF2C
Myocyte enhancer factor 2D (alt spl isoforms)	MEF2D
Myogenic factor 3 (Myf-3)	MYOD1
Myogenic determination transcription factor Myf-4 (myogenin)	MYOG
Myogenic factor 5 (Myf5)	MYF5
Myogenic factor 6 (herculin)	MYF6
Myogenic factor LIM3 (CSRP3)	CSRP3
Myogenic repressor (musculin), embryonic sk m	MSC
Myostatin (growth/differentiation factor 8 [GDF-8]), sk m	MSTN
Myotonin protein kinase (alt spl isoforms), sk m, h	DMPK
Nuclear receptor ROR-gamma, sk m	RORC
Orphan nuclear receptor, fetal m (but adult liver, brain, thyroid)	NAK1
PDZ and LIM domain protein 1 (elfin), sk m, h	PDLIM1
Phospholamban	PLN
Protein tyrosine phosphatase type IVA, member 3, ak m isoforms	PTP4A3
Ras-related protein RAB-11B	YPT3
Serine/threonine protein kinase 1, muscle-specific	MSSK1
Sex comb on midleg homolog 1 isoform 1 (SCMH1)	SCMH1
SEX protein (plexin-4), sk m	SEX
Skeletal muscle abundant protein (nuclear receptor coactivator?)	SMAP
Ski protooncogene, alt spliced isoform Snol, sk m	[SNO1]
Smooth muscle activation-specific gene 64	SMAG-64
Steroid receptor coactivator-1, sk m, h	[SRC-1]
Transcription factor SOX-4 (heart, testis, brain)	[SOX4]
Transcription factor SOX-10 (h, sm m, brain)	[SOX10]
Tyrosine kinase receptor, muscle specific (MUSK)	MUSK
Cytoskeleton	
Alpha-actinin, isoform 2, sk m, h	ACTN2
Alpha-actinin, isoform 3, sk m, h	ACTN3
Alpha-actinin-2 associated LIM protein	ALP
Alpha-sarcoglycan (adhalin-35, dystroglycan 2) (alt spl forms)	SGCA
Alpha-syntrophin	SNT A1
Ankyrin 1, muscle-specific isoform	ANK1
Ankyrin 2 (stretch-responsive ankyrin-repeat protein), sk m	ANKRD2
Beta1 integrin cytoplasmic domain binding protein	MIBP
Beta-sarcoglycan	SGCB
Beta1-syntrophin	SNT B1
Beta2-syntrophin	SNT B2
Cadherin-15, muscle-specific	CDH15
Caveolin-3, sk m	CAV3
Clathrin heavy chain, muscle-specific isoform	CLTCL1
Cofilin 2, sk m	CFL2
Delta-sarcoglycan	SGCD
Desmin (class-III intermediate filament), sk m	DES
Desmuslin (dystrobrevin-interacting protein), sk m, h	[DMN]
Dysferlin, sk m	DYSF
Dystrobrevin-alpha (sk m, brain; isoforms 7 & 8 in heart)	DTNA
Dystroglycan (dystrophin-associated glycoprotein) (sk m)	DAG1
Dystrophin (sk m, brain)	DMD
Emerin	EMD
Filamin-2, sk m-specific isoform (gamma-filamin, FLNC, ABPL)	FLN2
Fukutin	FCMD
Gap junction alpha-1 protein (connexin-43), cardiac	GJA1
Genethonin 1 skeletal muscle internal membrane proteins	None
Genethonin 2 skeletal muscle internal membrane proteins	None
Genethonin 3 skeletal muscle internal membrane proteins	None
Integrin alpha-7, sk m	ITGA7
Lamin A/C, alt spl	LMNA
Melusin (beta1 integrin cytoplasmic domain interactor), sk m, h	ITGB1BP2
Neural cell adhesion molecule (N-CAM), sk m-specific isoform	NCAM1
Protein 4.1-G (in skeletal protein 4.1 (EPB41) gene family)	EPB41L2
Sarcosin (Kelch-related protein 1; KRP1), sk m	SARCOSIN
Sarcospan (isoform 1 only in heart, sk m)	SSPN
Smoothelin (alt spl isoforms), sm m	SMTN
Smooth muscle protein SM22alpha, 22 kDa	SM22
Spectrin, beta isoform (alt spl)	SPTR
Supervillin, isoform 2, sk m	SVIL
Tenascin-X (cardiac, sm m, sk m)	TNXB
Tubulin alpha-8 chain, sk m, heart, testis	TUBA8
Utrophin	UTRN
Meta-vinculin muscle-specific variant of vinculin	VCL
Zonula occludens 2, sm m	[ZO2]
Contractile proteins	
Alpha-actin, sk m	ACTA1
Alpha-actin, aortic sm m	ACTA2
Ankyrin protein 2 (stretch responsive muscle), sk m	ANKRD2
Caldesmon, smooth muscle isoform (H-CAD) (alt spl isoforms)	CALD1
Calponin H1, sm m	CNN1
Calponin H2 (neutral calponin), sm m, h	CNN2
Mitofilin, heart motor protein (HMP) (mitochondrial)	IMMT
Myomesin 1 (190-kDa titin-associated protein), sk m	MYOM1
Myomesin 2 (165-kDa titin-associated protein), sk m	MYOM2

KEY: alt spl, alternative splicing; h, heart; sk m, skeletal muscle; sm m, smooth muscle. Gene symbols in brackets are unofficial.

Table 33-1 (Continued). SOME GENE PRODUCTS EXPRESSED PREDOMINANTLY OR EXCLUSIVELY IN MUSCLE

GENE PRODUCT	SYMBOL	GENE PRODUCT	SYMBOL
Contractile proteins (cont.)		Troponin T, slow skeletal muscle (alt spl isoforms)	TNNT1
Myosin alkali light chain, sm m isoform (MLC 1sm) (alt spl)	MYL6	Troponin T2, cardiac (alt spl isoforms)	TNNT2
Myosin binding protein C, cardiac type	MYBPC3	Troponin T, fast skeletal muscle isoform beta	TNNT3
Myosin binding protein C, fast type	MYBPC2	Telethonin (titin cap protein)	TCAP
Myosin binding protein C, slow type	MYBPC1	Titin (connectin), heart and skeletal muscle isoforms	TTN
Myosin binding protein H	MYBPH	Triadin	TRDN
Myosin heavy chain IIx/d, sk m, adult 1	MYH1	Z-band PDZ-motif protein (ZASP), sk m, h alt spl isoforms	ZASP
Myosin heavy chain IIa, sk m, adult 2	MYH2		
Myosin heavy chain, fast skeletal muscle, embryonic	MYH3	**Channels and transporters**	
Myosin heavy chain IIb, sk m, fetal	MYH4	Acetylcholine receptor, beta chain, mature sk m (CHRNB1)	ACHRB
Myosin heavy chain, cardiac muscle alpha isoform	MYH6	Acetylcholine receptor, epsilon chain, mature sk m	ACHRE
Myosin heavy chain, cardiac muscle beta isoform	MYH7	Acetylcholine receptor, gamma chain, immature sk m	ACHRG
Myosin heavy chain, sk m, perinatal	MYH8	Calcium ATPase, plasma membrane (alt spl forms)	HPMCA2
Myosin heavy chain, smooth muscle (alt spl isoforms SM1/SM2)	MYH11	Calcium ATPase, plasma membrane (alt spl forms), isoform K	ATP2B1
Myosin heavy chain, extraocular muscle	MYH13	Calcium ATPase, plasma membrane (alt spl forms)	ATP2B4
Myosin heavy chain, smooth muscle isoform SMemb	[SMEMB]	Calcium ATPase 1 (adult/neonatal alt spl forms) (SERCA1)	ATP2A1
Myosin light chain 1, embryonic skeletal muscle isoform	MLC1	Calcium ATPase 2 (sk m isoform SERCA2A by alt spl)	ATP2A2
Myosin light chain 1, skeletal muscle isoforms	MYL1	Calcium-activated potassium channel alpha subunit, sm m	KCNMA1
Myosin light chain 1, slow twitch muscle B/ventricular isoform	MYL3	Calcium-activated potassium channel beta subunit, sm m	KCNMB1
Myosin light chain 1, embryonic muscle/atrial isoform	MYL4	Calcium-activated potassium channel MaxiK alpha subunit, sm m	MAXIK
Myosin light chain 1, slow twitch muscle A isoform	MLC1SA	Calcium-activated potassium channel MaxiK beta subunit, sm m	KCNMB1
Myosin light chain 2	None	Calcium channel alpha 1c subunit, L-type voltage-gated	CACNA1C
Myosin light chain 2, cardiac isoform	MYL2	Calcium channel alpha 1s subunit, L-type voltage-gated	CACNA1S
Myosin light chain kinase, smooth-muscle isoform	MYLK	Calcium channel beta-1M subunit, L-type voltage-gated	CACNB1
Myosin light chain kinase (BA243J16.3), sk m	MYLK2	Calcium channel gamma-1 subunit, L-type voltage-gated	CACNG1
Myosin light chain phosphatase, regulatory subunit (MYPT2)	PPP1R12B	Calcium release channel, sk m	RYR1
Myosin regulatory light chain, h isoform (HUMMLC2At)	[MYL2A]	Calcium release channel 2, cardiac	RYR2
Myosin regulatory light chain 2, smooth muscle isoform	MYRL2	Chloride channel, muscle-specific	CLCN1
Myosin regulatory light chain 5, fetal sk m (also retina)	MYL5	Glucose transporter 4, insulin responsive (GLUT4), sk m, h, fat	SLC2A4
Myosin X	MYO10	Potassium channel H-EAG, in sk m myoblasts at onset of fusion	EAG
Myotilin (Z-disc protein)	TTID	Potassium channel, inwardly rectifying, heart	KCNJ2
Myozenin (filamin-, actinin-, telethonin-binding protein), sk m	MYOZ	Potassium channel, inwardly rectifying, Kir2.2, sk m, brain	KCNJ12
Nebulette (actin-binding Z-disc protein)	NEBL	Potassium channel modulatory protein 2 (KCHIP2), h (alt spl forms)	KCNIP2
Nebulin	NEB	Purinoreceptor 6, sk m	P2RXL1
Calsarcin (sarcomeric calcineurin-binding protein), sk m, h	C4ORF5	Sodium/potassium exchanger (alt spliced isoforms)	SLC8A1
Reticulon-2 (NSP-like protein 1), sk m isoform	RTN2	Voltage-gated potassium channel (HK1), heart	KCNA4
Stretch responsive muscle protein, sk m	SMPX	Voltage-gated potassium channel (HK2), heart	KCNA5
Tropomyosin, alpha chain, sk m	TPM3	Voltage-gated potassium channel HERG, h	KCNH2
Tropomyosin, alpha chain, sk m, sm m	TPM1	Voltage-gated potassium channel beta subunit, h (alt spl forms)	KCNAB1
Tropomyosin, beta chain, sk m	TPM2	Voltage-gated potassium channel, IsK slow voltage (MinK), heart	KCNE1
Troponin C, slow skeletal muscle, cardiac	TNNC1	Voltage-gated sodium channel alpha subunit type V, heart	SCN5A
Troponin C, fast skeletal muscle	TNNC2	Voltage-gated sodium channel alpha subunit, heart and uterus	SCN6A
Troponin I, slow twitch isoform	TNNI1	Voltage-gated sodium channel alpha subunit, skeletal muscle	SCN4A
Troponin I, fast twitch isoform	TNNI2	Voltage-gated sodium channel type I, beta-1 subunit	SCN1B
Troponin I, cardiac isoform	TNNI3		

KEY: alt spl, alternative splicing; h, heart; sk m, skeletal muscle; sm m, smooth muscle. Gene symbols in brackets are unofficial.

In some gene systems these are called the M (for muscle) and B (for brain, but in reality found in all tissue types) isoforms. As a general rule, for any one gene family, the B-isoform gene seems to be the evolutionarily more ancient gene from which the M-isoform gene later evolved, usually by gene duplication. This may explain why B-type genes are usually present in the human genome in multiple copies (i.e., functional genes plus many pseudogenes), while the M-type genes are more often present in few copies (i.e., fewer pseudogenes) or even in a single copy (i.e., no pseudogenes). Another observation is that the 3'-untranslated regions of a number of M-isoform mRNAs (e.g., creatine kinase,[126,127] phosphoglycerate mutase,[123,128,129] and cytochrome *c* oxidase subunits VIa[130] and VIIa[131]) are much shorter than the analogous regions in the B-isoform mRNAs. While this may be related to requirements for message stability, it is also possible that this region of the gene, either as DNA or as RNA, is involved in muscle-specific gene regulation.

Molecular Genetics in the Study of Muscle Disease

As a result of the human genome project, about 30,000 human genes have been identified, including many which, when mutated, cause inherited disease. Among these, molecular genetic techniques have been used to identify mutations in specific genes that cause more than 100 specific neuromuscular disorders (Table 33-2). While identifying pathogenic genes that seems almost mundane, this was far from true in the mid '80s, when hunting for disease-causing genes began in earnest. Perhaps the most spectacular and conceptually important of those advances was the cloning of the dystrophin gene, which, when mutated, causes Duchenne and Becker muscular dystrophy.[132] That event ushered in a new era in the study of the hereditary diseases of muscle and foreshadowed our ability to dissect the molecular basis of many myopathies. This effort is already providing new insights into the study of normal muscle function and gene regulation and will certainly lead to new and effective treatments for these debilitating and often fatal disorders.

There are a number of chapters in Part 3, covering the entire range of muscle disease, in which the respective authors describe the role of molecular biology in finding the etiology, pathogenesis, and in a few cases treatment of muscle diseases. For this reason, the disorders described below are not discussed in any great detail. Rather, they are presented as exemplars of the different kinds of molecular genetic approaches that have been taken to study various types of neuromuscular diseases.

FORWARD GENETICS

Forward genetics is the term applied to the isolation of a gene whose gene product is already known, based on the knowl-

Table 33-2. GENES MUTATED IN NEUROMUSCULAR DISEASES

DISEASE	INH	MUTATED GENE PRODUCT	SYMBOL	LOCUS
Muscular dystrophies				
Congenital muscular dystrophy	AR	Laminin, alpha2 chain (merosin)	LAMA2	6q22.33
Congenital muscular dystrophy	AR	Integrin, alpha7 form	ITGA7	12q13.2
Congenital muscular dystrophy (Fukuyama)	AR	Fukutin	FCMD	9q31.3
Duchenne/Becker muscular dystrophy	XR	Dystrophin (DYS)	DMD	Xp21.1
Emery-Dreifuss muscular dystrophy	XR	Emerin	EMD	Xq28
Emery-Dreifuss muscular dystrophy	AD	Lamin A/C	LMNA	1q23.1
Epidermolysis bullosa/late-onset musc. dystr.	AR	Plectin (hemidesmosomal protein)	PLEC1	8q24
Hereditary inclusion body myositis	AR	UDP epimerase/kinase	GNE	9p13.2
Limb-girdle muscular dystrophy, type 1A	AD	Myotilin	TTID	5q31.2
Limb-girdle muscular dystrophy, type 1C	AD	Caveolin-3	CAV3	3p25.3
Limb-girdle muscular dystrophy, type 2A	AR	Calpain 3, large subunit	CAPN3	15q15.1
Limb-girdle muscular dystrophy, type 2B	AR	Dysferlin (also Miyoshi myopathy)	DYSF	2p13.2
Limb-girdle muscular dystrophy, type 2C	AR	Gamma-sarcoglycan	SGCG	13q12.13
Limb-girdle muscular dystrophy, type 2D	AR	Alpha-sarcoglycan	SGCA	17q21.33
Limb-girdle muscular dystrophy, type 2E	AR	Beta-sarcoglycan	SGCB	4q12
Limb-girdle muscular dystrophy, type 2F	AR	Delta-sarcoglycan	SGCD	5q33.3
Limb-girdle muscular dystrophy, type 2G	AR	Telethonin (titin cap protein)	TCAP	17q21.1
Limb-girdle muscular dystrophy (Bethlem)	AD	Collagen type VI, alpha1 subunit	COL6A1	21q22.3
Limb-girdle muscular dystrophy (Ullrich)	AD	Collagen type VI, alpha2 subunit	COL6A2	21q22.3
Limb-girdle muscular dystrophy (Bethlem)	AD	Collagen type VI, alpha3 subunit	COL6A3	2q37.3
Myotonic muscular dystrophy, type 1 (DM1)	AD	Myotonin-protein kinase	DMPK	19q13.31
Oculopharyngeal muscular dystrophy	AD	Poly(A) binding protein 2 (PABPN1)	PABP2	14q11.2
Rigid spine muscular dystrophy	AR	Selenoprotein N	SEPN1	1p36.11
Channelopathies and conduction disorders, including congenital myasthenic syndromes				
Brody disease	AR	Sarcoplasmic reticulum Ca-ATPase (SERCA1)	ATP2A1	16p12.1
Central core disease	AD	Calcium release channel (ryanodine receptor)	RYR1	19q31.1
Familial polymorphic ventricular tachycardia (VPFT)	AD	Cardiac muscle-type ryanodine receptor	RYR2	1q42.3
Stress-induced polymorphicventricular tachycardia (VTSIP)	?	Cardiac muscle-type ryanodine receptor	RYR2	1q42.3
Episodic ataxia/myokymia	AD	Voltage gated K-channel	KCNA1	12p
Fast channel syndrome	AR	Acetylcholine receptor, epsilon subunit	CHRNE	17p13
Hyperkalemic periodic paralysis	AD	Sodium channel, alpha subunit	SCN4A	17q23
Hypokalemic periodic paralysis; malignant hyperthermia	AD	Ca channel alpha-1S subunit (dihydropyridine receptor)	CACNA1S	1q32.1
Malignant hyperthermia	AD	Calcium release channel (ryanodine receptor)	RYR1	19q13.1
Long QT syndrome	AD	Voltage-gated potassium channel (HERG)	KCNH2	7q35-q36
Long QT syndrome	AD	Voltage-gated potassium channel protein KQT-like 1 (KVLQT1)	KCNQ1	11p15.5
Long QT syndrome	AR	Voltage-gated potassium channel protein KQT-like 1 (KVLQT1)	KCNQ1	11p15.5
Long QT syndrome	AD	IsK slow voltage-gated potassium channel protein (MinK)	KCNE1	21q22
Long QT syndrome	AR	IsK slow voltage-gated potassium channel protein (MinK)	KCNE1	21q22
Long QT syndrome	AR	Minimum potassium ion channel-related peptide 1 (MIRP1)	KCNE2	21q22.1
Long QT syndrome	AD	Cardiac sodium channel, alpha subunit	SCN5A	3p21
Myotonia (Thomsen)	AD	Muscle chloride channel (CLC1)	CLCN1	7q34
Myotonia (Becker)	AR	Muscle chloride channel (CLC1)	CLCN1	7q34
Paramyotonia congenita	AD	Sodium channel, alpha subunit	SCN4A	17q23
Slow channel congenital myasthenic syndrome	AD	Acetylcholine receptor, alpha subunit	CHRNA1	2q31.1
Slow channel congenital myasthenic syndrome	AD	Acetylcholine receptor, beta subunit	CHRNB1	17p13.1
Slow channel congenital myasthenic syndrome	AD	Acetylcholine receptor, epsilon subunit	CHRNE	17p13.1
Spinocerebellar ataxia	AD	Voltage-dependent Ca channel alpha-1A subunit	CACNA1A	19p13.2
Ventricular tachycardia	AD?	Potassium channel modulatory protein 2 (KCHIP2)	KCNIP2	10q24.32
Congenital myopathies				
Congenital myasthenic syndrome	AR	Collagen Q	COLQ	3p25.1
Desmin-related myopathy	AD	Desmin	DES	2q35
Desmin-related myopathy	AD	Alpha B-crystallin	CRYAB	11q23.1
Dilated cardiomyopathy !a	AD	Lamin A/C	LMNA	1q23.1
Familial hypertrophic cardiomyopathy	AD	Cardiac myosin heavy chain, alpha subunit	MYH6	14q11.2
Familial hypertrophic cardiomyopathy	AD	Cardiac myosin heavy chain, beta subunit	MYH7	14q11.2
Familial hypertrophic cardiomyopathy	AD	Cardiac troponin T	TNNT2	1q32.1
Familial hypertrophic cardiomyopathy	AD	Cardiac myosin binding protein	MYBPC3	11p11.2

KEY: Inh, mode of inheritance; AD, autosomal dominant; AR, autosomal recessive; XD, X-linked dominant; XR, X-linked recessive; ?, mode of inheritance unclear.

(Continued)

edge of the properties of the polypeptide encoded by that gene. It is the "easiest" type of cloning possible, as the knowledge of the gene product provides the basis for designing a probe to isolate the gene. Usually that probe is either an oligonucleotide based on the polypeptide's known amino acid sequence (for use in screening cDNA or genomic libraries) or an antibody against that polypeptide (for use in screening expression libraries).

Many of the metabolic disorders affecting muscle are due to deficiencies of housekeeping enzymes or of muscle-specific isoforms of these enzymes (see Table 33-2). These include myopathies due to deficiencies in enzymes involved in glycolysis (e.g., phosphoglycerate mutase, phosphofructokinase), glycogenolysis (phosphorylase, phosphorylase kinase), the respiratory chain (e.g., cytochrome *c* oxidase), and fatty acid metabolism (e.g., carnitine palmitoyltransferase). In most if not all of these cases, much was known about the biochemical, kinetic, and immunologic properties of the enzyme as well as the amino acid sequences of the purified constituent polypeptide(s). This information was used to isolate cDNA and genomic clones specifying these polypeptides using the methods described above. Once isolated, these clones were used as probes to clone the analogous defective gene sequences from patients with inherited enzyme defects (usually recessive diseases). Comparison of the DNA sequences between the wild-type and mutated

Table 33-2 (Continued). GENES MUTATED IN NEUROMUSCULAR DISEASES

DISEASE	INH	MUTATED GENE PRODUCT	SYMBOL	LOCUS
Congenital myopathies *(cont.)*				
Familial hypertrophic cardiomyopathy	AD	Alpha tropomyosin	TPM1	15q22.2
Familial hypertrophic cardiomyopathy	AD	Myosin regulatory light chain	MYL2	12q24.11
Familial hypertrophic cardiomyopathy	AD	Essential myosin light chain	MYL3	3p21.31
Familial hypertrophic cardiomyopathy	AD	Cardian troponin I	TNNI3	19q13.42
Familial hypertrophic cardiomyopathy	AD	Cardiac alpha actin	ACTC	15q14
Myotubular myopathy	XR	Myotubularin	MTM1	Xq28
Nemaline myopathy	AD	Alpha-tropomyosin	TPM3	1q23.1
Nemaline myopathy	AD	Alpha actin, skeletal muscle	ACTA1	1q42.13
Nemaline myopathy	AR	Alpha actin, skeletal muscle	ACTA1	1q42.13
Nemaline myopathy	AR	Nebulin	NEB	2q23.3
Neuropathies and motor neuron disorders				
Adrenoleukodystrophy	XR	Adrenoleukodystrophy protein (ALDP)	ABCD1	Xq28
Amyloidosis Type IV (Iowa)	AD	Apolipoprotein A1	APOA1	11q23.3
Amyloidosis Type V (Finnish)	AD	Gelsolin	GSN	9q34.11
Barth syndrome	XR	Taffazin	TAZ	Xq28
Charcot-Marie-Tooth neuropathy, Type IA	AD	Peripheral myelin protein P22	PMP22	17p11.2
Charcot-Marie-Tooth neuropathy, Type IB	AD	Peripheral myelin protein P0	MPZ	1q23.3
Charcot-Marie-Tooth neuropathy, Type IIA	AD	Kinesin motor protein 1B, isoform beta	KIF1B	1p36.22
Charcot-Marie-Tooth neuropathy, Type IIE	AD	Neurofilament, light chain	NEFL	8p21.2
Charcot-Marie-Tooth neuropathy, Type IV	AD	Early growth response protein 2	ERG2	10q21.3
Charcot-Marie-Tooth neuropathy, Type IVA	AD	Ganglioside-induced differentiation-associated protein	GDAP1	8q21.11
Charcot-Marie-Tooth neuropathy, Type IVB	AR	Myotubularin-relayed protein 2	MTMR2	11q21
Charcot-Marie-Tooth neuropathy, Type IVD	AR	N-myc downstream-regulated gene-1	NDRG1	8q24.22
Charcot-Marie-Tooth neuropathy, Type IVE	AR	Transcription factor SOX-10	SOX10	22q13.1
Charcot-Marie-Tooth neuropathy, Type IVF	AR	Periaxin (L and S alternatively spliced forms)	PRX	19q13.13
Charcot-Marie-Tooth neuropathy, Type X1	XD	Connexin-32 (CX32)	GJB1	Xq13.2
Familial amyloid neuropathy	AD	Transthyretin	TTR	18q12.1
Familial amyotrophic lateral sclerosis	AD	Cu, Zn superoxide dismutase	SOD1	21q22.11
Familial amyotrophic lateral sclerosis	AR	Cu, Zn superoxide dismutase	SOD1	21q22.11
Familial dysautonomia	AR	IkappaB-kinase complex-associated protein	IKBKAP	9q32
Friedrich ataxia	AR	Frataxin	FRDA	9q13
Friedrich ataxia with vitamin E deficiency	AR	Alpha tocopherol transfer protein	TTPA	8q12.3
Hereditary motor neuropathy w pressure palsies	AD	Peripheral myelin protein P22	PMP22	17p11.2
Hereditary spastic paraplegia	AD	Spastin	SPG4	2p22.3
Hereditary spastic paraplegia	AR	Paraplegin	SPG7	16q24.3
Hereditary spastic paraplegia	XR	Neural cell adhesion molecule L1	LICAM	Xq28
Hereditary spastic paraplegia	XR	Myelin proteolipid protein	PLP1	Xq22.2
Spastic ataxia (Charlevoix-Saguenay)	AR	Sacsin	SACS	13q12.2
Spinal and bulbar muscular atrophy (Kennedy)	XR	Androgen receptor	AR	Xq13.1
Spinal muscular atrophy (Werdning-Hoffmann)	AR	Survival motor neuron protein	SMN	5q13.2
Spinal muscular atrophy (Kugelberg-Welander)	AR	Survival motor neuron protein	SMN	5q13.2
Spinocerebellar ataxia	AD	Ataxin-1	SCA1	6p22.3
Spinocerebellar ataxia	AD	Ataxin-2	SCA2	12q24.12
Spinocerebellar ataxia with macular dystrophy	AD	Ataxin-7	SCA7	3p14.1
Spinocerebellar ataxia (Machado-Joseph)	AD	Ataxin-3 (josephin)	MJD	14q32.12
Spinocerebellar ataxia	AD	Protein phosphatase regulatory subunit B	PPP2R2B	5q32
Metabolic muscle diseases				
Carnitine deficiency	AR	Carnitine transporter (OCTN2)	SLC22A5	5q31.1
Carnitine palmitoyltransferase II deficiency	AR	Carnitine palmitoyltransferase II	CPT2	15q25.2
Exercise-induced myopathy	AR	Myoadenylate deaminase	AMPD1	1p13.2
Glycogenosis, type II (Pompe)	AR	Alpha glucosidase (acid maltase)	GAA	17q25.3
Glycogenosis, type V (McArdle)	AR	Phosphorylase, muscle type	PYGM	11q13.1
Glycogenosis, type VII (Tarui)	AR	Phosphofructokinase, muscle type	PFKM	12q13.11
Glycogenosis, type IX	XR	Phosphoglycerate kinase	PGK1	Xq21.1
Glycogenosis, type X	AR	Phosphoglycerate mutase, muscle type	PGAM2	7p13
Glycogenosis, type XI	AR	Lactate dehydrogenase, muscle type	LDHA	11p15.1
Glycogenosis, X-linked	AR	Phosphorylase kinase, alpha-1 subunit	PHKA1	Xq13.2
Lysosomal glycogen storage disease (Danon)	XR	Lysosomal-associated membrane protein 2	LAMP2	Xq24

KEY: Inh, mode of inheritance; AD, autosomal dominant; AR, autosomal recessive; XD, X-linked dominant; XR, X-linked recessive; ?, mode of inheritance unclear.

versions of the gene, coupled with analysis of the genotypes in affected vs. unaffected pedigree members, enabled researchers to pinpoint the exact nature of the genetic lesion.

Phosphofructokinase deficiency. A nice example of the power of forward genetics was the elucidation of Tarui disease, or muscle-specific phosphofructokinase deficiency (see Chap. 55). The normal cDNA specifying PFK-M was cloned by Tarui's group in 1987.[133] In 1990, they cloned PFK-M cDNAs from a muscle cDNA library of a patient with the disease and showed that there was a 75-nucleotide in-frame deletion of coding sequence in the mRNA that removed 25 amino acids from the PFK-M polypeptide.[134] Using PCR, they then amplified the genomic DNA of the patient, using PCR primers flanking the region of the deletion found in the mRNA (as cDNA). DNA sequencing of the genomic PCR product (which was *not* deleted and had a length *identical* to that of the wild-type gene) showed a single base-pair difference between patient and control DNA: There was a mutation from G → T in the patient's gene at the 5' splice site of exon 13. Instead of the sequence CAG | **G**TATGG (where the line denotes the exon/intron boundary), the patient's DNA had CAG | **T**TATGG. As a result, a "cryptic" 5' splice site located 75 bp upstream of the normally used splice site was used as the 5' splice site instead (sequence ACT | GTGAGG, inside exon 13). This aberrant splice ligated only the portion of exon 13 proximal to the new splice site to exon 14 and deleted the distal 75 nt of exon 13, resulting in the deleted processed mRNA.

Phosphoglycerate mutase deficiency. A second example of this approach is the elucidation of the molecular defect responsible for muscle phosphoglycerate mutase (PGAM-M) deficiency (see Chap. 55). PGAM-M deficiency is a rare autosomal recessive disorder characterized by cramps, muscle necrosis, and myoglobinuria following strenuous exercise. The cDNA encoding PGAM-M was cloned in 1987,[123] and the genomic clone was isolated soon thereafter.[128,129] Using PCR, the exons of the PGAM-M gene were amplified from three patients. All three had an identical G → A transition mutation in exon I at deduced amino acid position 78, which converted a codon encoding Trp (T**G**G) into a stop codon (T**A**G). This base change also created a new *Alu*I restriction site at this position in the PGAM-M gene; *Alu*I digestion of PCR-amplified DNA from the patients and carrier relatives (parents and siblings) showed that the patients were homozygotes and the carriers heterozygotes for the G → A mutation.[135] Another patient with PGAM-M deficiency from an ethnic background different from the first three patients had a different mutation, also in exon I; it was a C → T transition in codon 90, which converted Arg (**C**GG) to Trp (**T**GG).

REVERSE GENETICS

Reverse genetics is the term applied to the isolation of a gene whose gene product is unknown and for which no direct probes are available. The main strategy for isolating genes in this category is based on ascertaining whether the inheritance of a suspected chromosomal region containing the defective gene in a pedigree of affected and unaffected family members correlates with the disease phenotype. The key tactic in finding such a region is linkage analysis, which was described briefly above. Once a chromosomal region is identified through linkage analysis, other, more precise methods must be used to "walk" from the nearest linked marker to the defective gene itself.

Reverse genetic techniques are most often required for dominant diseases, where heterozygotes express the phenotype, as in myotonic muscular dystrophy and hyperkalemic periodic paralysis. However, recessive genes have also been located in this fashion, initially in the cases of Duchenne/Becker muscular dystrophy, Kennedy disease, and malignant hyperthermia. Since the advent of the human genome project, the strategy of reverse genetics has been applied with increasing frequency to recessive disorders, to the point where almost every new culprit gene, whether dominant or recessive, is now being found by "reverse" methodologies.

Dystrophies: Duchenne/Becker muscular dystrophy. The isolation in 1986 of the dystrophin gene, which is mutated in Duchenne/Becker muscular dystrophy, was a landmark event and is described in Chap. 34. DD and BD were both known to be X-linked disorders, and "classic" linkage analysis using markers on the X chromosome had localized the DD region to the short, or "p," arm of the chromosome. One breakthrough in cloning the gene, however, came from two related events. First, Uta Francke and her colleagues discovered a boy (named B.B.) with DD who had a huge deletion of a region of Xp.[136] The deleted region was so large that it was observable microscopically in the karyotype analysis, and, in fact, this patient had not only DD but also retinitis pigmentosa, mental retardation, McLeod syndrome, and chronic granulomatous disease, all presumably due to loss of a number of genes at this locus. Second, Louis Kunkel and colleagues used a novel subtraction hybridization approach to isolate regions in normal DNA that were missing in patient B.B.[137] These pieces of DNA turned out to be segments of the DD locus[132,138] encoding the giant muscle protein now called dystrophin.[139] Using dystrophin cDNA and genomic DNA as probes, it was found that many DD/BD mutations are large-scale deletions in the dystrophin gene.

Channelopathies. A relatively large number of muscle diseases are caused by mutations in ion channels. The earliest example of such a disease was malignant hyperthermia (MH), an autosomal recessive neuromuscular disorder involving calcium release and susceptibility to anesthetics (see Chap. 59). As with DD and BD, linkage analysis was used to localize the MH susceptibility locus. In this case, the glucose phosphate isomerase (GPI) gene was used as a candidate gene for linkage analysis because it had been known that an almost identical genetic disorder in pigs was linked to the porcine GPI locus. In humans, the *GPI* gene maps to 19q12-13.2 and, in fact, MH was found to map to this region of chromosome 19 by linkage analysis.[140] Because the gene encoding the ryanodine receptor[141] (RYR; also called the Ca^{2+}-release channel of the sarcoplasmic reticulum) had been mapped to 19q13.1, it became a candidate gene for the gene responsible for MH.[142] It has now been shown that mutations in the RYR gene probably cause both porcine and human MH. For example, a C → T transition at nucleotide position 1843 in the porcine RYR gene [converting Arg (**C**GC) to Cys (**T**GC) at amino acid position 615] correlates with porcine MH,[143,144] and the corresponding C→T base substitution at position 1840 in the human RYR gene (also converting Arg → Cys) is responsible for at least one form of human MH.[145] Malignant hyperthermia has now been found to be caused by mutations in another ion channel, the α-1S subunit of the muscle calcium channel (*CACNA1S*), also called the dihydropyridine receptor.

Similarly, the molecular basis of an autosomal dominant disease, hyperkalemic periodic paralysis (*HYPP*), was elucidated using a combination of linkage analysis and cloning of a candidate gene. HYPP is characterized by episodic skeletal muscle weakness and paralysis resulting from depolarization of the muscle cell membrane (see Chap. 46). Linkage analysis had localized the mutated gene to the long arm of chromosome 17[146] in a region containing the α-subunit of the adult muscle sodium channel (*SCN4A*). Sequence analysis showed an A → G transition, resulting in a Met → Val substitution (**A**TG → **G**TG) in the last membrane-spanning domain of the polypeptide.[147] Remarkably, it was found that paramyotonia congenita (PMC), a dominant disorder featuring cold-induced myotonia (see Chap. 46), is allelic to HYPP and is due to mutations in a different region of the sodium channel α-subunit gene. Two such mutations, resulting in Gly → Val and Thr → Met substitutions, were localized to a loop region of the protein that connects two of the membrane-spanning domains.[148]

The identification of mutations in *RYR* and *SCN4A* led to a new classification of muscle disease, the *channelopathies*, in which mutations in ion channel proteins (e.g., sodium, potassium, calcium) cause clinically distinct phenotypes.[149,150] More than 20 muscle disorders (and, of course, nonmuscle disorders too, such as epilepsy[151]) have been associated with mutations in ion channels, including various subtypes of long-QT syndrome, which affects cardiac pacemaking by interfering with potassium gradients.[152]

Trinucleotide repeat disorders. In the last 10 years, a completely new class of genetic disorder has been defined: the *trinucleotide repeat disorders*. These diseases are characterized by generation-to-generation changes in the composition of a gene via expansion or contraction of a simple-sequence repeat element.[153,154] The expansion (and sometimes contraction) of the repeat is typically due to a slipped-mispairing event during DNA replication in meiosis (i.e., the repeat size changes in the germline but is fundamentally stable in somatic cells). Because many of the repeat expansions are in the coding regions of genes, the repeats are typically three bases in length, such that the reading frame of the translated mRNA is maintained. The number of these coding-region repeats tends to be relatively small, with approximately 20 repeats in the normal version of the gene, compared to between 50 and 100 repeats in the mutated, pathogenic, gene. Diseases in this class ("moderate" expansions) include spinobulbar muscular atrophy, or Kennedy disease (expansion in the androgen receptor gene), Huntington disease (huntingtin gene), dentatorubropallidoluysian atrophy (atrophin gene), Machado-Joseph disease (josephin gene), and spinocerebellar ataxias (genes for ataxin 1, 2, 3, and 7, and the α1A calcium channel). The repeat is typically CAG, which encodes the amino acid glutamine. In a number of cases, the expanded number of repeats in these *polyglutamine disorders* affects the solubility of the protein (e.g., the affected protein is deposited as inclusions within the cell).[155]

Often, however, the trinucleotide expansion is located outside the coding region, for example, in the 5'-UTR,[156] in the 3'-UTR,[157] and in introns.[158] In these cases, there is almost no limit to the size to which the repeat expansion can grow, and there are examples of pathogenic expansions into the hundreds of repeats and in some instances into the thousands. Diseases in this class ("massive" expansions) include fragile X syndrome (expansion in the 5'-UTR of the *FMR1* and *FMR2* genes),[156] Friedreich ataxia (intron of the frataxin gene),[156] and at least two muscle diseases, progressive myoclonic epilepsy (5'-UTR of the cystatin B gene)[159] and myotonic muscular dystrophy (3'-UTR of the *DMPK* gene[156,160–162] and intron 1 of the *ZFN9* gene[163]).

The mechanisms underlying the pathology in these disorders are unclear. While the CTG repeats in myotonic muscular dystrophy (DM), an autosomal dominant disorder that is the most common dystrophy affecting adults (see Chap. 35), are located in the 3'-UTR of a gene on chromosome 19 called *DMPK* (dystrophia myotonica protein kinase), there is no evidence that the DMPK polypeptide itself is involved in the pathogenesis of the disease. One leading hypothesis is that the poly-CUG stretch in the DMPK 3-UTR affects other genes *in trans*, especially those with poly-CUG in their transcripts, perhaps via affects on an RNA-binding protein called CUGBP.[164] Indirect support of this idea comes from the finding that repeat expansions (a CCTG *tetranucleotide*) located in an intron of *ZNF9*, a second gene causing DM located on chromosome 3, encodes a nucleic acid-binding protein.[163]

Conundrums. The power of molecular biology to uncover the genetic basis of muscle disease has also led to "culprit" genes which, on the surface, ought not to be pathogenic. Two cases in point are Charcot-Marie-Tooth disease type 1A (CMT1A) and facioscapulohumeral muscular dystrophy (FSHD). In both cases, the problem apparently resides not in the gene itself but in its copy number. CMT1A is clearly due to a large-scale tandem (megabase-sized) duplication of DNA on chromosome 17p11.2 containing the gene specifying peripheral myelin protein P22 (*PMP22*). The duplication arose via an unequal crossing-over recombination event between two of three long direct repeats in the region. Importantly, there is no obvious mutation in the *PMP22* gene itself; rather, the mere presence of the duplicated segment is sufficient to cause the disease, but it is unclear whether this is merely a gene dosage effect. Interestingly, the reciprocal recombination product of the unequal crossing-over event, namely deletion of the *PMP22* gene on one allele, causes a completely different disorder called hereditary neuropathy with liability to pressure palsies (HNPP).[165]

The second example of a disease associated with an ostensibly normal segment of DNA, FSHD, is an autosomal dominant disorder (see Chap. 36). The affected locus, on chromosome 4q35, contains tandem repeats of a 3.3-kb segment of DNA, with the number of repeats correlating inversely with the severity of the disorder.[38,166] No specific FSHD gene has been identified. In a sense, this appears to be a trinucleotide repeat disorder "writ large."

MITOCHONDRIAL MYOPATHIES

The advances in deducing the molecular bases of the mendelian-inherited muscle diseases have been paralleled by a veritable explosion of knowledge concerning the molecular bases of mitochondrial diseases resulting from defects in mitochondrial DNA (mtDNA). With a few notable exceptions, the mitochondrial diseases all result in myopathies or encephalomyopathies and fall into three main classes: point mutations, deletions, and quantitative errors. In addition to mutations in mtDNA, mitochondrial disorders can also be inherited as classic mendelian traits for the simple reason that the vast majority of mitochondrial proteins are actually specified by nuclear DNA. For a complete overview of these disorders, see Chap. 58.

Future Prospects

The role of molecular biology, molecular genetics, and recombinant DNA technology in the isolation of genes involved in muscle biogenesis and regulation, in the study of muscle in both normal and diseased states, and in the characterization of mutated genes responsible for muscle disorders has been nothing short of revolutionary. What now lies ahead?

The sequencing of the genomes of other organisms shows no signs of abating. From a muscle perspective, genomic information from numerous vertebrates (e.g., human, mouse, pufferfish) and invertebrates (e.g., fruitfly, worm, sea urchin), as well as from seemingly "muscle-unrelated" organisms such as prokaryotes and plants, will begin to provide insight into the ontogeny, development, and physiology of muscle in hitherto unforeseen ways.

Only now are we starting to analyze the interactions among multiple expressed genes in a coherent way. The way is being blazed by the yeast community, which is creating "gene expression maps" in which master regulatory genes lie at n-dimensional nodes that are the recipients of inputs from other genes and/or are the sources of signals to other genes and nodes.[66] It is clear that the days of "single-gene expression analysis" in complex higher eukaryotes are numbered. The outcome of the "industrialization" of gene analysis will initially be chaotic, due to an almost uncontrollable amount of information, but with the help of bioinformatics, that confusion will soon give way to clarity. Presumably, this gain in knowlege will not only provide insight into basic muscle biology but also have clinical benefits, especially in the area of gene therapy.

One major theme of the last decade has been the realization of the fundamental role that *apoptosis*, or programmed cell death, plays in regulating the overall integrity of organisms. Apoptotic pathways, along with related phenomena such as the ubiquitination pathways discussed earlier, will affect our understanding of the programming of muscle development and our definition of pathogenetic mechanisms in muscle disease.

The redefinition or recategorization of muscle diseases based on genetics has allowed us to think about muscle disorders in new ways. While many muscle diseases described in this book are distinct phenotypes, some nevertheless display symptoms that overlap with other phenotypes. Often, the overlap had been such that it was impossible to classify two or more diseases as distinct entities or as variations of an underlying single disorder. The deduction of the genetic basis of these disorders has changed our perspective, most clearly in the cases of the channelopathies and the dystrophinopathies.

The cloning of animals, while currently considered almost a novelty, will continue, and in spite of the enormous ethical ramifications of performing such experiments, "therapeutic cloning" for the purpose of generating mammalian (including human) pluripotent stem cells will likely have far-reaching effects on our ability to understand and treat intractable muscle diseases.

In spite of all these advances, there are a number of areas in the field of the molecular biology of muscle that are true stumbling blocks to further advances in the field. Two disparate examples will suffice. First, there is still no good technique to target a gene or a gene product specifically to muscle. It is paradoxical that muscle, which comprises the greatest proportion of the body's mass, should also be one of the least accessible parts. Combined with the almost total inaccessibility of the brain, this means that targeting genes involved in neuromuscular diseases will be stymied until this problem can be solved. Second, while transfecting DNA into bacterial cells or into the nuclei of mammalian cells has become commonplace, there is still no system to transform mammalian mitochondria with exogenous DNA. Progress in understanding and treating mitochondrial myopathies cannot occur until this obstacle is overcome.

List of Abbreviations

aa	amino acid	LHON	Leber hereditary optic neuropathy
ASO	allele-specific oligonucleotide	mb	megabase
BAC	bacterial artificial chromosome	MELAS	mitochondrial encephalomyopathy, lactic acidosis, and stroke-like episodes
BD	Becker muscular dystrophy	MH	malignant hyperthermia
bp	base pair	mtDNA	mitochondrial DNA
cDNA	complementary DNA	NMD	nonsense-mediated mRNA decay
cM	centimorgan	PCR	polymerase chain reaction
CMT1A	Charcot-Marie-Tooth disease type 1A	PEG	polyethylene glycol
DD	Duchenne muscular dystrophy	PFGE	pulsed-field gel electrophoresis
DDBJ	DNA Data Bank in Japan	PFK	phosphofructokinase
DM	myotonic muscular dystrophy	pfu	plaque-forming units
DMPK	dystrophia myotonica protein kinase	PGAM	phosphoglycerate mutase
DNA	deoxyribonucleic acid	PMC	paramyotonia congenita
EMBL	European Molecular Biology Laboratory	RFLP	restriction fragment length polymorphism
ESE	exonic splicing enhancer	RNA	ribonucleic acid
ESS	exonic splicing silencer	rRNA	ribosomal RNA
EST	expressed sequence tag	RT-PCR	reverse-transcription PCR
FSHD	facioscapulohumeral muscular dystrophy	RYR	ryanodine receptor
GPI	glucose phosphate isomerase	SAGE	serial analysis of gene expression
GST	glutathione-S-transferase	SDS	sodium dodecyl sulfate
HLH	helix-loop-helix	SMA	spinal muscular atrophy
HNPP	hereditary neuropathy with liability to pressure palsies	SNP	single-nucleotide polymorphism
HYPP	hyperkalemic periodic paralysis	SSCP	single-strand conformation polymorphism
IPTG	isopropylthio-β-D-galactoside	tRNA	transfer RNA
ISH	in situ hybridization	UTR	untranslated region
kb	kilobase	VNTR	variable-number tandem repeat
lacZ	β-galactosidase	YAC	yeast artificial chromosome
LCR	locus control region		

References

1. Kaplan DJ, Jurka J, Solus JF, et al: Medium reiteration frequency repetitive sequences in the human genome. *Nucleic Acids Res* 19:4731–4738, 1991.
2. Deininger PL, Batzer MA: Alu repeats and human disease. *Mol Genet Metab* 67:183–193, 1999.
3. Breitbart RE, Andreadis A, Nadal-Ginard B: Alternative splicing: A ubiquitous mechanism for the generation of multiple protein isoforms from single genes. *Annu Rev Biochem* 56:467–495, 1987.
4. Grabowski PJ, Black DL: Alternative RNA splicing in the nervous system. *Prog Neurobiol* 65:289–308, 2001.
5. Lemon B, Tjian R: Orchestrated response: A symphony of transcription factors for gene control. *Genes Dev* 14:2551–2569, 2000.
6. Beyersmann D: Regulation of mammalian gene expression. *EXS* 89:11–28, 2000.
7. Landschulz WH, Johnson PF, McKnight SL: The leucine zipper: A hypothetical structure common to a new class of DNA binding proteins. *Science* 240:1759–1764, 1988.
8. Lania L, Majello B, De Luca P: Transcriptional regulation by the Sp family proteins. *Int J Biochem Cell Biol* 29:1313–1323, 1997.
9. Karin M, Chang L: AP-1-glucocorticoid receptor crosstalk taken to a higher level. *J Endocrinol* 169:447–451, 2001.
10. Levine M, Hoey T: Homeobox proteins as sequence-specific transcription factors. *Cell* 55:537–540, 1988.
11. Relaix F, Buckingham M: From insect eye to vertebrate muscle: Redeployment of a regulatory network. *Genes Dev* 13:3171–3178, 1999.
12. Yun K, Wold B: Skeletal muscle determination and differentiation: Story of a core regulatory network and its context. *Curr Opin Cell Biol* 8:877–889, 1996.
13. Ingraham HA, Chen RP, Mangalam HJ, et al: A tissue-specific transcription factor containing a homeodomain specifies a pituitary phenotype. *Cell* 55:519–529, 1988.
14. Wirth T, Staudt L, Baltimore D: An octamer oligonucleotide upstream of a TATA motif is sufficient for lymphoid-specific promoter activity. *Nature* 329:174–178, 1987.
15. Finney M, Ruvkun G, Horvitz HR: The C. elegans cell lineage and differentiation gene unc-86 encodes a protein with a homeodomain and extended similarity to transcription factors. *Cell* 55:757–769, 1988.
16. Phillips K, Luisi B: The virtuoso of versatility: POU proteins that flex to fit. *J Mol Biol* 302:1023–1039, 2000.
17. Chang PS, Li L, McAnally J, et al: Muscle specificity encoded by specific serum response factor-binding sites. *J Biol Chem* 276:17206–17212, 2001.
18. Shore P, Sharrocks AD: The MADS-box family of transcription factors. *Eur J Biochem* 229:1–13, 1995.
19. Li Q, Harju S, Peterson KR: Locus control regions: Coming of age at a decade plus. *Trends Genet* 15:403–408, 1999.
20. Knotts S, Rindt H, Robbins J: Position independent expression and developmental regulation is directed by the beta myosin heavy chain gene's 5' upstream region in transgenic mice. *Nucleic Acids Res* 23:3301–3309, 1995.
21. Sudarsanam P, Winston F: The Swi/Snf family nucleosome-remodeling complexes and transcriptional control. *Trends Genet* 16:345–351, 2000.
22. Muchardt C, Yaniv M: The mammalian SWI/SNF complex and the control of cell growth. *Semin Cell Dev Biol* 10:189–195, 1999.
23. Phelan ML, Sif S, Narlikar GJ, et al: Reconstitution of a core chromatin remodeling complex from SWI/SNF subunits. *Mol Cell* 3:247–253, 1999.
24. de la Serna IL, Carlson KA, Imbalzano AN: Mammalian SWI/SNF complexes promote *MyoD*-mediated muscle differentiation. *Nature Genet* 27:187–190, 2001.
25. Jones PA, Takai D: The role of DNA methylation in mammalian epigenetics. *Science* 293:1068–1070, 2001.
26. Reik W, Dean W, Walter J: Epigenetic reprogramming in mammalian development. *Science* 293:1089–1093, 2001.
27. Jenuwein T, Allis CD: Translating the histone code. *Science* 293:1074–1080, 2001.
28. Park Y, Kuroda MI: Epigenetic aspects of X-chromosome dosage compensation. *Science* 293:1083–1085, 2001.
29. Ferguson-Smith AC, Surani MA: Imprinting and the epigenetic asymmetry between parental genomes. *Science* 293:1086–1089, 2001.
30. Matzke M, Matzke AJ, Kooter JM: RNA: Guiding gene silencing. *Science* 293:1080–1083, 2001.
31. Gehring NH, Frede U, Neu-Yilik G, et al: Increased efficiency of mRNA 3' end formation: A new genetic mechanism contributing to hereditary thrombophilia. *Nature Genet* 28:389–392, 2001.
32. Frischmeyer PA, Dietz HC: Nonsense-mediated mRNA decay in health and disease. *Hum Mol Genet* 8:1893–1900, 1999.
33. Hentze MW, Kulozik AE: A perfect message: RNA surveillance and nonsense-mediated decay. *Cell* 96:307–310, 1999.
34. Maquat LE: The power of point mutations. *Nat Genet* 27:5–6, 2001.
35. Blencowe BJ: Exonic splicing enhancers: Mechanism of action, diversity and role in human genetic diseases. *Trends Biochem Sci* 25:106–110, 2000.
36. Caudevilla C, Codony C, Serra D, et al: Localization of an exonic splicing enhancer responsible for mammalian natural trans-splicing. *Nucleic Acids Res* 29:3108–3115, 2001.
37. Valentine CR: The association of nonsense codons with exon skipping. *Mutat Res* 411:87–117, 1998.
38. Zhang Y, Forner J, Fournet S, et al: Improved characterization of FSHD mutations. *Ann Genet* 44:105–110, 2001.
39. Scheffler IE: *Mitochondria*. New York: Wiley-Liss, 1999.
40. Anderson S, Bankier AT, Barrell BG, et al: Sequence and organization of the human mitochondrial genome. *Nature* 290:457–465, 1981.
41. Li K, Hodge JA, Wallace DC: OXBOX, a positive transcriptional element of the heart-skeletal muscle ADP/ATP translocator gene. *J Biol Chem* 265:20585–20588, 1990.
42. Scarpulla RC: Nuclear control of respiratory chain expression in mammalian cells. *J Bioenerg Biomembr* 29:109–119, 1997.
43. Clayton DA: Replication of animal mitochondrial DNA. *Cell* 28:693–705, 1982.
44. Clayton DA: Transcription of the mammalian mitochondrial genome. *Annu Rev Biochem* 53:573–594, 1984.
45. Ojala D, Montoya J, Attardi G: tRNA punctuation model of RNA processing in human mitochondria. *Nature* 290:470–474, 1981.
46. Giles RE, Blanc H, Cann HM, et al: Maternal inheritance of human mitochondrial DNA. *Proc Natl Acad Sci USA* 77:6715–6719, 1980.
47. Satoh M, Kuroiwa T: Organization of multiple nucleoids and DNA molecules in mitochondria of a human cell. *Exp Cell Res* 196:137–140, 1991.
48. Michaels GS, Hauswirth WW, Laipis PJ: Mitochondrial DNA copy number in bovine oocytes and somatic cells. *Dev Biol* 94:246–251, 1982.
49. Piko L, Matsumoto L: Number of mitochondria and some properties of mitochondrial DNA in the mouse egg. *Dev Biol* 49:1–10, 1976.
50. Piko L, Taylor KD: Amounts of mitochondrial DNA and abundance of some mitochondrial gene transcripts in early mouse embryos. *Dev Biol* 123:364–374, 1987.
51. Shuster RC, Rubenstein AJ, Wallace DC: Mitochondrial DNA in anucleate human blood cells. *Biochem Biophys Res Commun* 155:1360–1365, 1988.
52. Sambrook J, Russell DW: *Molecular Cloning: A Laboratory Manual*, 3d ed. Cold Spring Harbor, NY: Cold Spring Harbor Press, 2001.
53. Davis LG, Kuehl M, Battey FJ: *Basic Methods in Molecular Biology*, 2d ed. New York: Elsevier, 1994.
54. Micklos DA, Freyer GA: *DNA Science: A First Course in Recombinant DNA Technology*. Cold Spring Harbor, NY: Cold Spring Harbor Laboratory Press, 1990.
55. Venter JC, Adams MD, Myers EW, et al: The sequence of the human genome. *Science* 291:1304–1351, 2001.
56. Lander ES, Linton LM, Birren B, et al: Initial sequencing and analysis of the human genome. *Nature* 409:860–921, 2001.
57. Schwartz DC, Cantor CR: Separation of yeast chromosome-sized DNAs by pulsed field gradient gel electrophoresis. *Cell* 37:67–75, 1984.
58. Saiki RK, Gelfand DH, Stoffel S, et al: Primer-directed enzymatic amplification of DNA with a thermostable DNA polymerase. *Science* 239:487–491, 1988.
59. Chee M, Yang R, Hubbell E, et al: Accessing genetic information with high-density DNA arrays. *Science* 274:610–614, 1996.
60. Lipshutz RJ, Fodor SP, Gingeras TR, et al: High density synthetic oligonucleotide arrays. *Nat Genet* 21:20–24, 1999.
61. Lockhart DJ, Winzeler EA: Genomics, gene expression and DNA arrays. *Nature* 405:827–836, 2000.
62. Duggan DJ, Bittner M, Chen Y, et al: Expression profiling using cDNA microarrays. *Nat Genet* 21:10–14, 1999.
63. Stanton LW: Methods to profile gene expression. *Trends Cardiovasc Med* 11:49–54, 2001.
64. Eisenberg D, Marcotte EM, Xenarios I, et al: Protein function in the post-genomic era. *Nature* 405:823–826, 2000.
65. Xenarios I, Fernandez E, Salwinski L, et al: DIP: The database of interacting proteins: 2001 update. *Nucleic Acids Res* 29:239–241, 2001.
66. Tong AH, Evangelista M, Parsons AB, et al: Systematic genetic analysis with ordered arrays of yeast deletion mutants. *Science* 294:2364–2368, 2001.
67. Polyak K, Riggins GJ: Gene discovery using the serial analysis of gene expression technique: Implications for cancer research. *J Clin Oncol* 19:2948–2958, 2001.
68. Pandey A, Mann M: Proteomics to study genes and genomes. *Nature* 405:837–846, 2000.
69. Mann M, Hendrickson RC, Pandey A: Analysis of proteins and proteomes by mass spectrometry. *Annu Rev Biochem* 70:437–473, 2001.
70. Tong AH, Drees B, Nardelli G, et al: A combined experimental and computational strategy to define protein interaction networks for peptide recognition modules. *Science* 295: 321–324, 2002.
71. Mittl PR, Grutter MG: Structural genomics: Opportunities and challenges. *Curr Opin Chem Biol* 5:402–408, 2001.
72. Orita M, Suzuki Y, Sekiya T, et al: Rapid and sensitive detection of point mutations and DNA polymorphisms using the polymerase chain reaction. *Genomics* 5:874–879, 1989.
73. Jeffreys AJ, MacLeod A, Tamaki K, et al: Minisatellite repeat coding as a digital approach to DNA typing. *Nature* 354:204–209, 1991.
74. Kaelin WG Jr., Pallas DC, DeCaprio JA, et al: Identification of cellular proteins that can interact specifically with the T/E1A-binding region of the retinoblastoma gene product. *Cell* 64:521–532, 1991.

75. Fields S, Song O: A novel genetic system to detect protein-protein interactions. *Nature* 340:245–246, 1989.
76. Jen KY, Gewirtz AM: Suppression of gene expression by targeted disruption of messenger RNA: Available options and current strategies. *Stem Cells* 18:307–319, 2000.
77. Mansour SL, Thomas KR, Capecchi MR: Disruption of the proto-oncogene int-2 in mouse embryo-derived stem cells: A general strategy for targeting mutations to non-selectable genes. *Nature* 336:348–352, 1988.
78. Bronson SK, Smithies O: Altering mice by homologous recombination using embryonic stem cells. *J Biol Chem* 269:27155–27158, 1994.
79. Mills AA, Bradley A: From mouse to man: Generating megabase chromosome rearrangements. *Trends Genet* 17:331–339, 2001.
80. Davis RL, Weintraub H, Lassar AB: Expression of a single transfected cDNA converts fibroblasts to myoblasts. *Cell* 51:987–1000, 1987.
81. Wright WE, Sassoon DA, Lin VK: Myogenin, a factor regulating myogenesis, has a domain homologous to MyoD. *Cell* 56:607–617, 1989.
82. Puri PL, Sartorelli V: Regulation of muscle regulatory factors by DNA-binding, interacting proteins, and post-transcriptional modifications. *J Cell Physiol* 185:155–173, 2000.
83. Weintraub H, Davis R, Tapscott S, et al: The myoD gene family: Nodal point during specification of the muscle cell lineage. *Science* 251:761–766, 1991.
84. Buskin JN, Hauschka SD: Identification of a myocyte nuclear factor that binds to the muscle-specific enhancer of the mouse muscle creatine kinase gene. *Mol Cell Biol* 9:2627–2640, 1989.
85. Church GM, Ephrussi A, Gilbert W, et al: Cell-type-specific contacts to immunoglobulin enhancers in nuclei. *Nature* 313:798–801, 1985.
86. Minty A, Kedes L: Upstream regions of the human cardiac actin gene that modulate its transcription in muscle cells: Presence of an evolutionarily conserved repeated motif. *Mol Cell Biol* 6:2125–2136, 1986.
87. Phan-Dinh-Tuy F, Tuil D, Schweighoffer F, et al: The 'CC.Ar.GG' box. A protein-binding site common to transcription-regulatory regions of the cardiac actin, c-fos and interleukin-2 receptor genes. *Eur J Biochem* 173:507–515, 1988.
88. Walsh K: Cross-binding of factors to functionally different promoter elements in c-fos and skeletal actin genes. *Mol Cell Biol* 9:2191–2201, 1989.
89. Mar JH, Ordahl CP: A conserved CATTCCT motif is required for skeletal muscle-specific activity of the cardiac troponin T gene promoter. *Proc Natl Acad Sci USA* 85:6404–6408, 1988.
90. Calvo S, Vullhorst D, Venepally P, et al: Molecular dissection of DNA sequences and factors involved in slow muscle-specific transcription. *Mol Cell Biol* 21:8490–8503, 2001.
91. Braun T, Arnold HH: The four human muscle regulatory helix-loop-helix proteins Myf3-Myf6 exhibit similar hetero-dimerization and DNA binding properties. *Nucleic Acids Res* 19:5645–5651, 1991.
92. Braun T, Buschhausen-Denker G, Bober E, et al: A novel human muscle factor related to but distinct from MyoD1 induces myogenic conversion in 10T1/2 fibroblasts. *EMBO J* 8:701–709, 1989.
93. Miner JH, Wold B: Herculin, a fourth member of the *MyoD* family of myogenic regulatory genes. *Proc Natl Acad Sci USA* 87:1089–1093, 1990.
94. Rhodes SJ, Konieczny SF: Identification of MRF4: A new member of the muscle regulatory factor gene family. *Genes Dev* 3:2050–2061, 1989.
95. Santoro IM, Yi TM, Walsh K: Identification of single-stranded-DNA-binding proteins that interact with muscle gene elements. *Mol Cell Biol* 11:1944–1953, 1991.
96. Benezra R, Davis RL, Lockshon D, et al: The protein Id: A negative regulator of helix-loop-helix DNA binding proteins. *Cell* 61:49–59, 1990.
97. Benezra R: Role of Id proteins in embryonic and tumor angiogenesis. *Trends Cardiovasc Med* 11:237–241, 2001.
98. Treisman R: The serum response element. *Trends Biochem Sci* 17:423–426, 1992.
99. Kong Y, Flick MJ, Kudla AJ, et al: Muscle LIM protein promotes myogenesis by enhancing the activity of MyoD. *Mol Cell Biol* 17:4750–4760, 1997.
100. Molkentin JD, Olson EN: Combinatorial control of muscle development by basic helix-loop-helix and MADS-box transcription factors. *Proc Natl Acad Sci USA* 93:9366–9373, 1996.
101. Lee Y, Nadal-Ginard B, Mahdavi V, et al: Myocyte-specific enhancer factor 2 and thyroid hormone receptor associate and synergistically activate the alpha-cardiac myosin heavy-chain gene. *Mol Cell Biol* 17:2745–2755, 1997.
102. Heanue TA, Reshef R, Davis RJ, et al: Synergistic regulation of vertebrate muscle development by Dach2, Eya2, and Six1, homologs of genes required for *Drosophila* eye formation. *Genes Dev* 13:3231–3243, 1999.
103. MacLachlan TK, Giordano A: TRAF2 expression in differentiated muscle. *J Cell Biochem* 71:461–466, 1998.
104. Ono K, Han J: The p38 signal transduction pathway: Activation and function. *Cell Signal* 12:1–13, 2000.
105. Eckner R, Ewen ME, Newsome D, et al: Molecular cloning and functional analysis of the adenovirus E1A-associated 300-kD protein (p300) reveals a protein with properties of a transcriptional adaptor. *Genes Dev* 8:869–884, 1994.
106. Struhl K: Histone acetylation and transcriptional regulatory mechanisms. *Genes Dev* 12:599–606, 1998.
107. Giordano A, Avantaggiati ML: p300 and CBP: Partners for life and death. *J Cell Physiol* 181:218–230, 1999.
108. Spicer DB, Rhee J, Cheung WL, et al: Inhibition of myogenic bHLH and MEF2 transcription factors by the bHLH protein Twist. *Science* 272:1476–1480, 1996.
109. Lemercier C, To RQ, Carrasco RA, et al: The basic helix-loop-helix transcription factor Mist1 functions as a transcriptional repressor of MyoD. *EMBO J* 17:1412–1422, 1998.
110. Chen CM, Kraut N, Groudine M, et al: I-mf, a novel myogenic repressor, interacts with members of the MyoD family. *Cell* 86:731–741, 1996.
111. Lu J, Webb R, Richardson JA, et al: MyoR: A muscle-restricted basic helix-loop-helix transcription factor that antagonizes the actions of MyoD. *Proc Natl Acad Sci USA* 96:552–557, 1999.
112. Wilson-Rawls J, Molkentin JD, Black BL, et al: Activated notch inhibits myogenic activity of the MADS-Box transcription factor myocyte enhancer factor 2C. *Mol Cell Biol* 19:2853–2862, 1999.
113. Postigo AA, Dean DC: ZEB represses transcription through interaction with the corepressor CtBP. *Proc Natl Acad Sci USA* 96:6683–6688, 1999.
114. Bailey P, Downes M, Lau P, et al: The nuclear receptor corepressor N-CoR regulates differentiation: N-CoR directly interacts with MyoD. *Mol Endocrinol* 13:1155–1168, 1999.
115. Bodine SC, Latres E, Baumhueter S, et al: Identification of ubiquitin ligases required for skeletal muscle atrophy. *Science* 294:1704–1708, 2001.
116. Gomes MD, Lecker SH, Jagoe RT, et al: Atrogin-1, a muscle-specific F-box protein highly expressed during muscle atrophy. *Proc Natl Acad Sci USA* 98:14440–14445, 2001.
117. Beeson D, Morris A, Vincent A, et al: The human muscle nicotinic acetylcholine receptor alpha-subunit exists as two isoforms: A novel exon. *EMBO J* 9:2101–2106, 1990.
118. Talib S, Leiby K, Wright K, et al: Cloning and expression in *Escherichia coli* of a synthetic gene encoding the extracellular domain of the human muscle acetylcholine receptor α-subunit. *Gene* 98:289–293, 1991.
119. Weller P, Jeffreys AJ, Wilson V, et al: Organization of the human myoglobin gene. *EMBO J* 3:439–446, 1984.
120. Fujii J, Zarain-Herzberg A, Willard HF, et al: Structure of the rabbit phospholamban gene, cloning of the human cDNA, and assignment of the gene to human chromosome 6. *J Biol Chem* 266:11669–11675, 1991.
121. Buckingham ME: The control of muscle gene expression: A review of molecular studies on the production and processing of primary transcripts. *Br Med Bull* 45:608–629, 1989.
122. Babu GJ, Warshaw DM, Periasamy M: Smooth muscle myosin heavy chain isoforms and their role in muscle physiology. *Microsc Res Tech* 50:532–540, 2000.
123. Shanske S, Sakoda S, Hermodson MA, et al: Isolation of a cDNA encoding the muscle-specific subunit of human phosphoglycerate mutase. *J Biol Chem* 262:14612–14617, 1987.
124. Sakoda S, Shanske S, DiMauro S, et al: Isolation of a cDNA encoding the B isozyme of human phosphoglycerate mutase (PGAM) and characterization of the PGAM gene family. *J Biol Chem* 263:16899–16905, 1988.
125. Hamshere M, Dickson G, Eperon I: The muscle specific domain of mouse N-CAM: Structure and alternative splicing patterns. *Nucleic Acids Res* 19:4709–4716, 1991.
126. Trask RV, Strauss AW, Billadello JJ: Developmental regulation and tissue-specific expression of the human muscle creatine kinase gene. *J Biol Chem* 263:17142–17149, 1988.
127. Nigro JM, Schweinfest CW, Rajkovic A, et al: cDNA cloning and mapping of the human creatine kinase M gene to 19q13. *Am J Hum Genet* 40:115–125, 1987.
128. Tsujino S, Sakoda S, Mizuno R, et al: Structure of the gene encoding the muscle-specific subunit of human phosphoglycerate mutase. *J Biol Chem* 264:15334–15337, 1989.
129. Castella-Escola J, Ojcius DM, LeBoulch P, et al: Isolation and characterization of the gene encoding the muscle-specific isozyme of human phosphoglycerate mutase. *Gene* 91:225–232, 1990.
130. Fabrizi GM, Sadlock J, Hirano M, et al: Differential expression of genes specifying two isoforms of subunit VIa of human cytochrome *c* oxidase. *Gene* 119:307–312, 1992.
131. Arnaudo E, Hirano M, Seelan RS, et al: Tissue-specific expression and chromosome assignment of genes specifying two isoforms of subunit VIIa of human cytochrome *c* oxidase. *Gene* 119:299–305, 1992.
132. Monaco AP, Neve RL, Colletti-Feener C, et al: Isolation of candidate cDNAs for portions of the Duchenne muscular dystrophy gene. *Nature* 323:646–650, 1986.
133. Nakajima H, Noguchi T, Yamasaki T, et al: Cloning of human muscle phosphofructokinase cDNA. *FEBS Lett* 223:113–116, 1987.
134. Nakajima H, Kono N, Yamasaki T, et al: Genetic defect in muscle phosphofructokinase deficiency. Abnormal splicing of the muscle phosphofructokinase gene due to a point mutation at the 5'-splice site. *J Biol Chem* 265:9392–9395, 1990.
135. Tsujino S, Shanske S, Sakoda S, et al: The molecular genetic basis of muscle phosphoglycerate mutase (PGAM) deficiency. *Am J Hum Genet* 52:472–477, 1993.
136. Francke U, Ochs HD, de Martinville B, et al: Minor Xp21 chromosome deletion in a male associated with expression of Duchenne muscular dystrophy, chronic granulomatous disease, retinitis pigmentosa, and McLeod syndrome. *Am J Hum Genet* 37:250–267, 1985.

137. Kunkel LM, Monaco AP, Middlesworth W, et al: Specific cloning of DNA fragments absent from the DNA of a male patient with an X chromosome deletion. *Proc Natl Acad Sci USA* 82:4778–4782, 1985.
138. Koenig M, Hoffman EP, Bertelson CJ, et al: Complete cloning of the Duchenne muscular dystrophy (DMD) cDNA and preliminary genomic organization of the DMD gene in normal and affected individuals. *Cell* 50:509–517, 1987.
139. Hoffman EP, Brown RH Jr, Kunkel LM: Dystrophin: The protein product of the Duchenne muscular dystrophy locus. *Cell* 51:919–928, 1987.
140. McCarthy TV, Healy JM, Heffron JJ, et al: Localization of the malignant hyperthermia susceptibility locus to human chromosome 19q12-13.2. *Nature* 343:562–564, 1990.
141. Zorzato F, Fujii J, Otsu K, et al: Molecular cloning of cDNA encoding human and rabbit forms of the Ca^{2+} release channel (ryanodine receptor) of skeletal muscle sarcoplasmic reticulum. *J Biol Chem* 265:2244–2256, 1990.
142. MacLennan DH, Duff C, Zorzato F, et al: Ryanodine receptor gene is a candidate for predisposition to malignant hyperthermia. *Nature* 343:559–561, 1990.
143. Fujii J, Otsu K, Zorzato F, et al: Identification of a mutation in porcine ryanodine receptor associated with malignant hyperthermia. *Science* 253:448–451, 1991.
144. Otsu K, Khanna VK, Archibald AL, et al: Cosegregation of porcine malignant hyperthermia and a probable causal mutation in the skeletal muscle ryanodine receptor gene in backcross families. *Genomics* 11:744–750, 1991.
145. Gillard EF, Otsu K, Fujii J, et al: A substitution of cysteine for arginine 614 in the ryanodine receptor is potentially causative of human malignant hyperthermia. *Genomics* 11:751–755, 1991.
146. Fontaine B, Khurana TS, Hoffman EP, et al: Hyperkalemic periodic paralysis and the adult muscle sodium channel α-subunit gene. *Science* 250:1000–1002, 1990.
147. Rojas CV, Wang JZ, Schwartz LS, et al: A Met-to-Val mutation in the skeletal muscle Na+ channel α-subunit in hyperkalaemic periodic paralysis. *Nature* 354:387–389, 1991.
148. McClatchey AI, Van den Bergh P, Pericak-Vance MA, et al: Temperature-sensitive mutations in the III-IV cytoplasmic loop region of the skeletal muscle sodium channel gene in paramyotonia congenita. *Cell* 68:769–774, 1992.
149. Felix R: Channelopathies: Ion channel defects linked to heritable clinical disorders. *J Med Genet* 37:729–740, 2000.
150. Ptacek LJ: Channelopathies: Ion channel disorders of muscle as a paradigm for paroxysmal disorders of the nervous system. *Neuromuscul Disord* 7:250–255, 1997.
151. Lerche H, Jurkat-Rott K, Lehmann-Horn F: Ion channels and epilepsy. *Am J Med Genet* 106:146–159, 2001.
152. Keating MT, Sanguinetti MC: Molecular and cellular mechanisms of cardiac arrhythmias. *Cell* 104:569–580, 2001.
153. Bowater RP, Wells RD: The intrinsically unstable life of DNA triplet repeats associated with human hereditary disorders. *Prog Nucleic Acid Res Mol Biol* 66:159–202, 2001.
154. Evert BO, Wullner U, Klockgether T: Cell death in polyglutamine diseases. *Cell Tissue Res* 301:189–204, 2000.
155. Ross CA, Wood JD, Schilling G, et al: Polyglutamine pathogenesis. *Philos Trans R Soc Lond B Biol Sci* 354:1005–1011, 1999.
156. Inoue SB, Siomi MC, Siomi H: Molecular mechanisms of fragile X syndrome. *J Med Invest* 47:101–107, 2000.
157. Ueda H, Ohno S, Kobayashi T: Myotonic dystrophy and myotonic dystrophy protein kinase. *Prog Histochem Cytochem* 35:187–251, 2000.
158. Palau F: Friedreich's ataxia and frataxin: Molecular genetics, evolution and pathogenesis (Review). *Int J Mol Med* 7:581–589, 2001.
159. Lalioti MD, Mirotsou M, Buresi C, et al: Identification of mutations in cystatin B, the gene responsible for the Unverricht-Lundborg type of progressive myoclonus epilepsy (EPM1). *Am J Hum Genet* 60:342–351, 1997.
160. Brook JD, McCurrach ME, Harley HG, et al: Molecular basis of myotonic dystrophy: Expansion of a trinucleotide (CTG) repeat at the 3' end of a transcript encoding a protein kinase family member. *Cell* 68:799–808, 1992.
161. Buxton J, Shelbourne P, Davies J, et al: Detection of an unstable fragment of DNA specific to individuals with myotonic dystrophy. *Nature* 355:547–548, 1992.
162. Harley HG, Brook JD, Rundle SA, et al: Expansion of an unstable DNA region and phenotypic variation in myotonic dystrophy. *Nature* 355:545–546, 1992.
163. Liquori CL, Ricker K, Moseley ML, et al: Myotonic dystrophy type 2 caused by a CCTG expansion in intron 1 of ZNF9. *Science* 293:864–867, 2001.
164. Timchenko NA, Cai ZJ, Welm AL, et al: RNA CUG repeats sequester CUGBP1 and alter protein levels and activity of CUGBP1. *J Biol Chem* 276:7820–7826, 2001.
165. Chance PF: Molecular basis of hereditary neuropathies. *Phys Med Rehabil Clin North Am* 12:277–291, 2001.
166. Kissel JT: Facioscapulohumeral dystrophy. *Semin Neurol* 19:35–43, 1999.

INDEX

Note: Page numbers followed by f indicate figures; those followed by t indicate tables.

A band, 130f, 131
Acetazolamide
  for hypokalemic periodic paralysis, 1288
  for sodium channel myotonias, 1278
Acetazolamide-responsive myotonia, 1268
Acetylcholine
  quantal release of
    events after, 1801–1802
    morphologic correlates of, 343, 344f
  uptake by small, clear synaptic vesicles, 336
Acetylcholine receptor(s), 397–416
  activation of, 384
    saturating disk model for, 387
  binding site of, 405–406
  bursting kinetics of, 385–386, 386f
  cation channel and its gate and, 406
  channel blockers and, 386
  deficiency of, end plate, without mutation in AChR or rapsyn, 1839
  degradation of, 355, 358, 358f
  desensitization of, 388–389
  destruction of, 412, 413f
  evolution of, 400–401
  excess, 388, 388f
  fetal, maternal antibodies inhibiting, arthrogryposis multiplex congenita caused by, 1759
  historical perspective on, 397–398
  in inclusion body myositis, 1378
  kinetics of, 1818
  low-expressor mutations with no or minor kinetic abnormality, 1831f–1833f, 1831–1832
  as members of gene superfamily, 398
  muscle
    antibody-mediated autoimmune response to, in myasthenia gravis, 413–414
    antigenic structure of, 414–415
    function of, 406–407, 407f
    subtypes of, 398–399, 399f
    in myasthenia gravis, 413–414
      therapy and, 415–416
  of neuromuscular junction, metabolic stability of, 362
  neuronal
    diseases associated with, 409–410
    function of, 407–411
    subtypes of, 399f, 399–400
  neurotransmitter release and, 383–387
  permeability of channel and, 383–384
  of postsynaptic region, 347, 349–351, 351f–355f
    structure-function correlates of, 350–351
  properties at human end plate, 387
  recording from single channels, 384–385, 385f, 386f
  regulation of distribution and kinetic properties of, 362–363
  regulation of expression of, 412
  size and shape of, 401, 404f, 404–405, 405f
  structure of, 1817–1818, 1818t
  subtypes of, 398–400, 399f
  subunit sequences of, 401, 402f, 403f
  synthesis of, 355, 358, 358f, 411–412, 412f
Acetylcholine receptor antibodies
  in myasthenia gravis
    pathogenic effects of, 1767, 1768f, 1769–1772
    properties of, 1766–1767
  tests for, in myasthenia gravis, 1773–1774
Acetylcholinesterase, 423–438
  asymmetrical, of synaptic basal-z-lamina, 346
  in blood, forms of, 436–437
  cellular distribution of, 433–437
  end plate, congenital deficiency of, 1811–1817
    clinical features of, 1811, 1811f
    diagnosis of, 1817
    electrophysiologic features of, 1812, 1812f
    molecular studies of, 1814–1815, 1816f, 1817
    morphologic features of, 1812, 1813f–1815f
    pathogenesis of, 1812
    therapy for, 1817
  expression at neuromuscular junction, 363
  function of, 429–433
    enzymatic mechanisms of, 429–431
    methods for detection, localization, and quantitation and, 432–433, 433f
    at neuromuscular junction, modeling, 431–432
  gene encoding
    structure of, 427–428
    transcriptional control of, 428–429
  immune reaction against, myasthenia gravis versus, 1776
  inhibitors of, 429–430
  muscle, forms of, 433–436
  neuronal, forms of, 436
  physical properties of, 426
  structure of, 424–429
    associated noncatalytic subunits and, 426–427
    classification of forms and, 424–426, 425f
    mRNA expression and localization and, 428
    primary, 427
    three-dimensional subunit of catalytic subunit and, 424, 424f
  synthesis of, 437–438
  turnover of, 438
Acid lipase deficiency, 574t, 586
Acid maltase deficiency, 574t, 730, 737f, 1559–1580
  acid maltases and, 1559–1561
  adult, 1563f, 1563–1565, 1564f, 1852
  cellular injury in, 1570
  childhood, 1562f, 1562–1563

I-1

Acid maltase deficiency *(Cont.)*
  definition of, 1559
  diagnosis of, 1572–1574, 1573t
  differential diagnosis of, 1573–1574
  electromyography in, 1565
  electron microscopy in, 1566–1569, 1567f–1569f
  experimental models for, 1577–1578
  genetic variability in, 1574, 1574t–1577t, 1576–1577
  historical background of, 1559, 1560f
  infantile, 1562, 1562f
  light microscopy in, 1565f, 1565–1566, 1566f
  molecular aspects of, 1571–1572
  neutral maltases and, 1561, 1570–1571
  pathogenesis of, 1569–1571
  residual enzyme hypothesis of, 1570
  serum enzymes in, 1565
  therapy for, 1578–1580
  ultrastructural features of, 845, 847f, 848f
  variability of, 1570–1571
Acidophilic hyalinization, 697
Acromegaly
  electrodiagnostic studies in, 642
  myopathy associated with, 1729–1730
  neuropathy with, 1916
Actin, 132t
  dystrophin binding to, 459–461
  filamentous, in myofibrillar myopathies, 1190
  polymerization of, to form thin filaments, 147–150, 148f, 149f
  of thin filaments, 156, 156f
α-Actin, 132t
β-Actinin, 132t
  of thin filaments, 156
  of Z line, 158
α-Actinin, of Z line, 158
Actin-myosin complex, 174
Action potentials
  compound, *in vitro*, 1905, 1905f
  of skeletal muscle, 213–225
    characteristics of, 213–214, 214f
    conduction velocity of, 224
    currents conducted during, 214
    patch-clamp technique and, 225f, 225–228
    spread of electrical activity and, 224–225
    T-tubules and, 224–225
    voltage-gated ion channels essential for, 214–224, 215f
Activator deficiency, 572t, 577–579, 580f, 1872–1873
Activity
  increased, microcirculatory remodeling and, 522–524, 523f
  protein metabolism and, 554–556
Actomyosin
  energy transduction by, 188. *See also* Lever-arm hypothesis; Sliding filament theory
  kinetics of, 168–170, 170f
Actomyosin-ATPase system, magnesium-activated, features enabling regulation of, 282–283
Acute inflammatory demyelinating and axonal polyradiculoneuropathy, 1910–1911
Acylcarnitine translocase
  deficiency of, 1610, 1642
  mitochondrial β-oxidation and, 1593–1594
Acyl-CoA dehydrogenase
  deficiency of
    medium-chain, 1606–1607
    multiple, 1607–1609, 1609f
    short-chain, 1610
    very long chain, 1603–1604
  mitochondrial β-oxidation and, 1594
Acyl-CoA synthases, mitochondrial β-oxidation and, 1592
Adaptive immunity. *See* Immunity, adaptive (specific)
Adductor muscle, molluscan, thick filament regulation in, 299f, 299–300, 300t
Adenine nucleotide translocase, 1642
Adeno-associated virus infection, 1395–1396
Adenosine triphosphate
  ATP-ubiquitin-proteasome proteolytic pathway and, 543–546, 544t, 545f
  cross-bridge cycle and. *See* Cross-bridge cycle
Adhesion molecules, 899–900, 900t, 901f, 1349–1350
  expression of, 911
  in inclusion body myopathy, 1372
  neural cell, in myofibrillar myopathies, 1190
  as therapeutic target, 909
Adrenal dysfunction
  electrodiagnostic studies in, 642
  insufficiency
    myopathy associated with, 1721–1722
    periodic paralysis secondary to hyperkalemia in, 1279
  myopathy associated with, 1715–1722
    adrenal insufficiency and, 1721–1722
    adrenocorticotropic hormone excess and, 1721
    glucocorticoid excess and, 1715–1721
Adrenocorticotropic hormone excess, myopathy associated with, 1721
Adrenoleukodystrophy, X-linked, peripheral neuropathy associated with, 1920
Adrenomyeloneuropathy, 1873
  X-linked, 1920
Adult-onset distal myopathy, 1170t
Aeromonas hydrophila myonecrosis, 1464
African trypanosomiasis, 1423–1425
  clinical manifestations of, 1424
  geographic location and, 1423–1424, 1424f
  laboratory studies in, 1424–1425
  pathology of, 1425
  transmission to humans, 1424
  treatment of, 1425
Afterload, 194
Agammaglobulinemia, echovirus infection and myositis associated with, 1393, 1393f
Agenesis, of muscle spindles, 743
Aging, mitochondrial encephalopathy due to, 1652
Agrin, neuromuscular junction and, 360f, 360–361
Alanine, production and release from muscle, 539f, 539–540, 540f
Albuterol, myositis due to, 1704
Alcohol
  myoglobinuria due to, 1687
  myopathy due to, 1705–1707
    hypokalemic, 1705–1706, 1706f
  neuropathy associated with, 1919
  toxicity of, electrodiagnostic studies in, 643
Aldolase A deficiency, 1551
Allele-specific oligonucleotides, 943
Allergic granulomatosis, myositis in, 1455

Allotypical muscles, fiber types in, 92
ALS2, amyotrophic lateral sclerosis and, 1878, 1878f, 1879f
Alzheimer disease
  neuronal acetylcholine receptors and, 410
  similarities with inclusion body myositis, 1376–1379
Ambenonium chloride, for myasthenia gravis, 1776t, 1776–1777
American trypanosomiasis, 1425–1427
  clinical manifestations of, 1426
  geographic location and, 1425
  laboratory studies in, 1426
  pathology of, 1426, 1427f
  transmission to humans, 1425–1426
  treatment of, 1426–1427
Amiloride, for hypokalemic periodic paralysis, 1289
Amines, urinary, in dystrophinopathies, 979
Amino acid metabolism, 537–541
  alanine production and release and, 539f, 539–540, 540f
  glutamine production and release and, 540t, 540–541
  muscle energy metabolism and, 538–539
  oxidation of branched-chain amino acids and, 537–538
Amiodarone, myopathy due to, 1700
Ammonia, production of, in forearm exercise, monitoring of, 668–669, 669f
Amorphin, of Z line, 158
Amphiphilic myopathy, toxic, 1694t, 1696, 1699–1701
Amyloid
  deposition of, 728–729, 736f
  infiltration of microvasculature by, ultrastructural features of, 879, 879f–881f
Amyloid myopathy, electrodiagnostic studies in, 636
Amyloidosis
  inherited, peripheral neuropathy associated with, 1921
  neuropathy with, 1916–1917
Amyloid β peptide, in inclusion body myositis, 1376–1377
β-Amyloid precursor protein
  in inclusion body myositis, 1377
  in myofibrillar myopathies, 1190
Amylopectinosis, 730, 738f
Amyotonia congenita, 1846

Amyotrophic lateral sclerosis, 1852, 1865–1882
  clinical diagnostic features of, 1866–1869, 1867t, 1868t
    autonomic system involvement, 1869
    bulbar and pseudobulbar palsy, 1868
    dementia, 1869
    extrapyramidal disease, 1868–1869
    lower and upper motor neuron signs in limbs and, 1866–1868
    sensory system impairment, 1869
  differential diagnosis of, 1873–1876
  epidemiology of, 1865–1866
  etiology of, 1876–1880
    autoimmunity and inflammation in, 1880
    endogenous toxins and, 1880
    glutamate toxicity and, 1880
    infectious, 1880
    Kennedy syndrome and, 1878
    Mendelian gene defects in, 1876t, 1876–1878, 1877f
    neurofilament mutations/intermittent filaments in, 1878–1880
  juvenile, 1871–1873
    familial disorders related to, 1872–1873
    possibly heritable variants of, 1872
    recessively inherited, 1872
    sporadic, 1871
  laboratory diagnosis of, 1869–1871
    creating kinase in, 1870–1871
    electrodiagnostic studies in, 1869–1870
    muscle biopsy in, 1870
    mutation analysis of motor neuron disease genes in, 1871
    radiographic imaging in, 1870
    respiratory function tests in, 1871
    spinal fluid examination in, 1870
  pathology of, 1869
  therapy for, 1880–1882
    primary, 1880–1881, 1881t
    symptomatic, 1881–1882
Amyotrophy, monomelic, amyotrophic lateral sclerosis versus, 1873
Amysin, exocytosis and, 338
Anatomic muscles
  coordination of myotome and tendon differentiation and, 33–34, 35f

  limb formation and muscle patterning and, 34, 36–37
  migration of muscle progenitors to anatomic sites, 30–31, 31f
  myocyte fusion and muscle fiber formation and, 32f, 32–33
  myotome formation and, 33, 34f
  specification of, 31–32
Ancylostoma caninum infection, 1439
Andersen disease, 1551–1553
  glycogenosis type 4, 730, 738f
  ultrastructural features of, 845
Andersen syndrome, 1289f, 1289–1290
Anencephaly, with anterior horn dysgenesis, arthrogryposis multiplex congenita and, 1941–1942, 1942f
Anesthesia
  in congenital myopathies, 1521, 1523
  in hypokalemic periodic paralysis, 1289
  for malignant hyperthermia-susceptible patients, 1667
  in myotonia congenita, 1264
  in myotonic dystrophy, 1045
  in nemaline myopathy, 1483
Angiotensin II, protein metabolism in muscle and, 551
Angulated fibers, 710, 713f
Anterior horn dysgenesis
  anencephaly with, arthrogryposis multiplex congenita and, 1941–1942, 1942f
  arrhinencephaly with encephalocele and, arthrogryposis multiplex congenita and, 1941
Antibiotic resistance genes, 929
Antibody-dependent cytotoxicity, 898
  in dermatomyositis, 1351–1352
Antibody epitopes, muscle acetylcholine receptors and, 414–415
Anticholinesterase drugs
  in myasthenia gravis diagnosis, 1772
  for myasthenia gravis therapy, 1776t, 1776–1777
α_1 Antichymotrypsin
  in inclusion body myositis, 1377
  in myofibrillar myopathies, 1190
Anticipation, in myotonic dystrophy, 1059–1061
Antigenic modulation, in myasthenia gravis, by acetylcholine receptor antibody effects, 1769, 1771

Antigen-presenting cells, 893, 895f, 896f, 898, 1351
Antimicrotubular myopathy, toxic, 1695t, 1701–1703
Antinuclear antibodies, in polymyositis/dermatomyositis, 1331
Antipsychotic drugs, myoglobinuria due to, 1685–1686
Antisense RNA, 924
Antisynthetase syndrome, myositis and, 1329
Anti-tumor necrosis factor-α, for polymyositis/dermatomyositis, 1347
Apolipoprotein A-I amyloidosis, peripheral neuropathy associated with, 1921
Apolipoprotein E, in inclusion body myositis, 1377
Apoptosis
  myopathy with, 1516–1517, 1517f
  plasma membrane defects and, 1004
Arachnodactyly, contractural, congenital, arthrogryposis multiplex congenita and, 1952
Arnold-Chiari syndrome, arthrogryposis multiplex congenita and, 1942f, 1942–1944, 1943f
Arrhinencephaly, with encephalocele and anterior horn dysgenesis, arthrogryposis multiplex congenita and, 1941
Arrhythmogenic cardiomyopathy, 1241
Arteries, fine structure of, 515–516
Arterioles, fine structure of, 516, 516f
Arthrogryposes, 616
  distal, 1953t, 1953–1954
Arthrogryposis multiplex congenita, 1931–1955, 1932f, 1957
  caused by maternal antibodies inhibiting fetal acetylcholine receptors, 1759
  connective tissue types, 1952–1954
    congenital contractural arachnodactyly, 1952
    distal, 1953t, 1953–1954
    Marfan syndrome, 1952–1953
  experimental studies of, 1954–1955
  motor end plate types, 1951–1952
    congenital myasthenic syndromes and, 1951–1952
    maternal curare treatment and, 1951
    maternal myasthenia gravis and, 1951
  myopathic types, 1949–1951
    autosomal dominant hereditary inclusion body myopathy, 1950
    central core disease, 1949
    with congenital mitochondrial myopathy, 1951
    congenital muscular dystrophy, 1949–1950
    myotonic muscular dystrophy, 1950
    nemaline myopathy, 1949
    with phosphofructokinase and phosphorylase deficiencies, 1950
    with phosphorylase b-kinase deficiency, 1951
  neurogenic types, 1933–1949
    with anencephaly with dysgenesis of anterior horns, 1941–1942, 1942f
    with Arnold-Chiari malformation, 1942f, 1942–1944, 1943f
    with Bruch syndrome, 1948
    with caudal regression syndrome, 1944f, 1944–1945
    with central nervous system dysgenesis, 1935–1940, 1936f–1940f
    with cerebrohepatorenal syndrome, 1945–1946, 1946f, 1947f
    with craniocarpotarsal syndrome, 1941
    with dysgenesis of anterior horns of spinal cord and motor nuclei of brainstem, 1933–1935, 1934f, 1935f
    with encephalocele and arrhinencephaly, 1941
    with Gaucher disease, 1948
    with Gordon syndrome, 1947
    misoprostol and, 1948
    with muscle fiber-type predominance or disproportion, 1933, 1933f
    with peripheral neuropathy, 1949
    with renal tubular dysfunction, cholestasis, and ichthyosis, 1946–1947
    with Waardenburg syndrome, 1945
    with Werdnig-Hoffman disease, 1948–1949
    spinal muscular atrophy with, 1860f, 1860–1861
  ultrasonography in, 1954
Artificial electron acceptors, for mitochondrial encephalopathy, 1653
Aspartylglucosaminuria, 573t
Assisted ventilation, for dystrophinopathies, 1012
Astrologist's posture, 1148
ATP synthase deficiency, 1641–1642
A/T-rich sties, muscle-specific promoters and, 25
Autoimmune disorders.
  See also specific disorders
  association of myasthenia gravis with, 1760
  Lambert-Eaton myasthenic syndrome association with, 1792
  peripheral nerve hyperexcitability associated with, 1304
  stiff-man syndrome as, 1746
Autoimmunity, 1351
  in amyotrophic lateral sclerosis, 1880
  mechanisms of, 908
Autonomic impairment, in amyotrophic lateral sclerosis, 1869
Autonomic neuropathies, in diabetes mellitus, 1915
Autophagic mechanisms, ultrastructural features of, 836–841
Autophagic vacuoles, 714–715, 836–838
  content of, 837–838
  definition and distribution of, 836f, 836–837, 837f, 839f, 840f
  development of, 838
  factors promoting formation of, 837
  fate of, 838
  liposomal enzyme delivery to, 838
  lysosomal enzyme delivery to, ultrastructural features of, 765
  membrane generation for, ultrastructural features of, 765, 769f, 770f
  mitochondrial inclusion in, ultrastructural features of, 780
  source of membranes for, 838
Axonal atrophy, distal, 1902–1903
Axonal spheroids, 1902
5-Azacytidine, myositis due to, 1704

Azathioprine
  for myasthenia gravis, 1778
  for polymyositis/dermatomyositis, 1345–1346
Azidothymidine (AZT), myopathy associated with, 1406–1413, 1407t, 1408f–1411f, 1696
  experimental induction of AZT toxicity and, 1409, 1411f, 1412f
  management of, 1409, 1413
  mechanism of, 1407, 1409

Bacterial infections, muscle pain associated with, 1741t, 1742t
Bare H zone. *See* Pseudo-H zone
Bartter syndrome, 1292
Basal lamina, 471
  composition of, 474
  defects of, muscular dystrophies caused by, 463
  endoneurial, 471
  satellite cell crossing of, 72
  synaptic, 345f, 345–347, 346f
  ultrastructural features of, 875f, 875–876, 876f
Basement membrane, 471
Base-pairing rule, 915, 917f
Basket nerve endings, 327f, 331
Bassoon, exocytosis and, 338
B cells, 891, 892f
  antigen recognition by, 891–893, 894f
  cooperation between T lymphocytes and, 893–894
  functions of, 1348
Becker muscular dystrophy, 961. *See also* Dystrophinopathies
  cardiac involvement in, 976
  cardiomyopathy in, 1244–1246, 1245f
  carriers of, cardiac involvement in, 976
  central nervous system involvement in, 976
  clinical features of, 974–975
  dystrophin expression in sarcolemma in, 998–999
  dystrophin gene mutation in, 968
  immunoblot studies in, 1000f, 1000–1001
  retinal involvement in, 977
  reverse genetics in, 953
Becker myotonia. *See* Myotonia congenita
Behavioral modification, for sodium channel myotonias, 1278

Behçet disease, myositis in, 1459
Benton-Davis screening, 933, 934f
Beta-receptor blocking agents, myositis due to, 1704
Bethlem myopathy, 1110, 1135–1145
  cardiac involvement in, 1138–1139
  clinical features of, 1136, 1138f, 1138–1139, 1139f, 1140t
  collagen VI in, 1139–1141, 1143f
  definition of, 1135
  diagnosis of, 1111, 1142–1143
  differential diagnosis of, 1143–1144
  etiology of, 1135–1136, 1137t
  histopathology of, 1139, 1141f–1143f
  historical background of, 1135, 1136f, 1137f
  laboratory features of, 1139, 1141f
  management of, 1144
  pathophysiology of, 1141–1142
  pulmonary involvement in, 1139
  unsolved problems in, 1144–1145
Bezafibrate, myopathy due to, 1697
Biopsy. *See* Muscle biopsy
Bleeding, into peripheral nerves, 1898
B leukocytes, in myasthenia gravis, 1765
Blocking, in single-fiber electromyography, 629
Blood, acetylcholinesterase forms in, 436–437
B lymphocytes, 891, 892f
  antigen recognition by, 891–893, 894f
  cooperation between T lymphocytes and, 893–894
  functions of, 1348
Bornholm disease, 1392
Botulism
  myasthenia gravis versus, 1775t, 1775–1776
  neurodiagnostic studies in, 646
Brain
  in Becker muscular dystrophy, 976
  in Duchenne muscular dystrophy, 976
  in Fukuyama congenital muscular dystrophy, 1218
  in mitochondrial encephalomyopathies, 1633
  in muscle-eye-brain disease, 1220, 1220f
  in Walker-Warburg syndrome, 1222, 1222f
Brain dystrophin promoter, 963–964

Brainstem, dysgenesis of motor nuclei of, in arthrogryposis multiplex congenita, 1933–1935, 1934f, 1935f
Brainstem nuclei, dysgenesis of, arthrogryposis multiplex congenita and, 1933, 1938f–1940f, 1938–1940
Branching enzyme deficiency, 1551–1553
  type 4, 730, 738f
  ultrastructural features of, 845
Broad A-band disease, 1518f, 1518–1519
Brown-Vialetto-Van Laere syndrome, 1858, 1858f
Bruch syndrome, arthrogryposis multiplex congenita and, 1948
Bulbar palsy, 1858, 1858f
  in amyotrophic lateral sclerosis, 1868
Bumetanide, myositis due to, 1704

Cachexia, in cancer, protein metabolism and, 557–558
Caffeine, T-tubule activation and inactivation effects of, 260–261, 262f
Calcium
  disorders of metabolism of, myopathy associated with, 1731–1734
    hyperparathyroidism and metabolic bone disease, 1731–1733
    hypoparathyroidism and pseudo-hypoparathyroidism, 1733–1734
  external, effects on T-tubule activation and inactivation, 259–260
  in muscle contraction, 281–303
    calcium-binding proteins and, 284–285, 285t
    calcium transients and, 283f, 283–284
    chromosome locations of genes expressing regulatory proteins of thin filaments and, 301–302, 302t
    I filament regulation and, 285f–290f, 285–295, 292f
    isolated contractile systems and, 281–282
    magnesium-activated actomyosin-adenosine triphosphatase system features enabling its regulation and, 282–283

Calcium *(Cont.)*
  myosin-binding protein C and, 300
  parvalbumins and, 300–301
  phosphorylation of regulatory proteins of thin filament and, 295–296
  thick filament regulation and, 296–300
  whole intact cells and, 281
  neurotransmitter release and, 376–378, 377f
  protein metabolism and, 555–556
  release into cytosol, 312–313
Calcium-binding proteins, 284–285, 285t
Calcium channels
  abnormal activity of, plasma membrane defects and, 1003–1004
  properties of, 377
  voltage-gated, 221–222
    kinetics and potential dependency of, 221, 222f
    modifying subunits of, 221–222
    as target antigens in Lambert-Eaton myasthenic syndrome, 1793, 1796f, 1797t
Calcium pumps, 307–310, 308f
  proteins modulating, 310–312
Calcium release channel(s). *See* Ryanodine receptors
Calcium release channel genes, malignant hyperthermia and central core disease and, 1668, 1668f
Calcium release units, 233–234
  assembly of, 58–60
    blocking and maturation of units and, 58f, 59f, 59–60
    targeting of components to junctional domains and, 58–59
  composition and structure of, 246, 247f, 248, 248f
  shapes of, 239, 241f–243f
  structural relationships between components of, 248–253, 249f, 250f
Calcium transients, 283f, 283–284
  depolarization-induced, 263–264, 264f
Calmodulin, ryanodine receptor modulation by, 316
Calmodulin-dependent protein kinase, 317

Calpain(s), 542–543
  calpain 3 in limb-girdle muscular dystrophy and, 1081t
Calpain 3, in limb-girdle muscular dystrophy, 1087–1088
Calpainopathy, 1089–1091
  clinical features of, 1089, 1090f
  diagnosis of, 1091, 1091f, 1111, 1112
  epidemiology of, 1089
  genetics of, 1089–1091
  treatment of, 1091
Calreticulin, 318
Calsarcin 2, 132t
Calsequestrin, 317–318, 318f
Cancer. *See* Malignancies
Candidal myositis, 1465
Canine dystrophinopathy, 1002
Cap disease, 1517–1518
Capillaries
  find structure of, 516–518, 517f
  morphometry of, 515, 515t
  perfusion and, 519
  ultrastructural features of, 876–877, 877f, 878f
Capping proteins, of thin filaments, 156, 156f
Capsids, 929
CapZ, 132t
  of thin filaments, 156
  of Z line, 158
Carbimazole, myositis due to, 1704
Carbonic anhydrase inhibitors
  for hypokalemic periodic paralysis, 1288–1289
  for sodium channel myotonias, 1278
Carcinoma, neuropathies associated with, 1917
Carcinomatous neuropathy, 1913
Cardiac muscle
  ryanodine receptor mutations in, diseases resulting from, 314–315
  titin in, 147
  transcription enhancers and control elements and, 27–28
Cardiac therapy, for Emery-Dreifuss muscular dystrophy, 1034
Cardiomyopathy, 1239–1254
  alcoholic, 1707
  arrhythmogenic, 1241
  classification, etiology, and pathogenesis of, 1232t, 1233f, 1241–1242, 1243t
  clinical picture of, 1240f, 1240–1241, 1241f, 1241t

  in complex III deficiency, 1650
  dilated, 1240, 1241f
    X-linked, 1246–1247
  in distal dystrophies, 1251
  dystrophinopathic, 1242–1247
    in Becker muscular dystrophy, 1244–1246, 1245f
    of carriers, 1247
    dilated, X-linked, 1246–1247
    in Duchenne muscular dystrophy, 1243–1244
  emerin defects causing, 1249–1250
  in Emery-Dreifuss muscular dystrophy, 1028–1029
  in facioscapulohumeral muscular dystrophy, 1251
  in fukutin-negative muscular dystrophy, 1251
  future prospects for, 1254
  historical background of, 1239–1240
  hypertrophic, 1240, 1241f
    familial, sarcomere in, 161
    myosin mutations in, 181–182
  lamin defects causing, 1250
  in merosin-negative muscular dystrophy, 1251
  in myofibrillar myopathies, 1251
  in myotonic dystrophies, 1250–1251
  preclinical, 1241, 1241f, 1241t
  restrictive, 1241
  in sarcoglycanopathies, 1247–1249
  spinal muscular atrophy with, 1861
  therapy for, 1251–1253
    for arrhythmogenic cardiomyopathies, 1252
    during aspecific intermediate stage, 1252
    for dilated cardiomyopathies, 1252–1253, 1253t
    during end stage, 1253
    for heterotrophic cardiomyopathies, 1252
    during preclinical stage, 1251t, 1251–1252
  unsolved problems with, 1253–1254
  X-linked, due to dystrophinopathy, 977–978
L-Carnitine, for lipid metabolism disorders, 1614
Carnitine deficiency, primary, 1600–1601
Carnitine palmitoyltransferases
  deficiency of, 1601–1603
  mitochondrial β-oxidation and, 1592–1593

Carnitine translocase
   deficiency of, 1610, 1642
   mitochondrial β-oxidation and, 1593–1594
Caspaces, protein metabolism and, 546
CAST, exocytosis and, 338
Catecholamines, protein metabolism in muscle and, 551
Cation-chloride cotransporters, 212
Caudal regression syndrome, arthrogryposis multiplex congenita and, 1944f, 1944–1945
Caveolae, 234, 235f
Caveolin-3
   binding to β-dystroglycan and dysferlin, 459
   in dystrophinopathies, 999
      limb-girdle muscular dystrophy, 1080t, 1085–1086
   n-NO synthase binding to, 459
   signaling by, 466
Caveolin-1, in inclusion body myositis, 1378
Caveolinopathy, 1104–1105, 1106f, 1180
CD30, soluble, in polymyositis/dermatomyositis, 1330–1331
Cell adhesion molecules, 899–900, 900t, 901f, 1349–1350
   expression of, 911
   in inclusion body myopathy, 1372
   neural cell, in myofibrillar myopathies, 1190
   as therapeutic target, 909
Cell division cycle kinase 2, in myofibrillar myopathies, 1190
Cell-mediated cytotoxicity, 898, 899f
   in polymyositis, 1352–1353
Cell membrane, 457–471
   complexes obtained from fractions of, 458f, 458–459
   dystrophin binding to actin filament and β-dystroglycan and, 459–461, 461f
   glycoprotein complex of, 457–458
   in vitro binding of dystrophin–dystrophin-associated protein complex to other proteins and, 459, 459f
Cell therapy, for dystrophinopathies, 1009–1010
Cellular infiltrates, plasma membrane defects and, 1004
Cellulitis, associated with myonecrosis, 1464–1465
Central core(s), 707–708, 708f

Central core disease, 1475–1480
   arthrogryposis multiplex congenita and, 1949
   clinical features of, 1475f, 1475–1476
   differentiation between malignant hyperthermia and central core disease mutants and, 1672f, 1672–1673
   genetic basis for, 1668–1671
      alternative loci and, 1669–1671
      calcium release channel genes and, 1668, 1668f
      guidelines for genetic determination of susceptibility and, 1669
      linkage to *RYR1* and, 1669, 1670t, 1671t
   genetics of, 1479–1480
   investigations in, 1476
   malignant hyperthermia association with, 1668
   muscle pain associated with, 1742t
   pathologic features of, 1476f–1478f, 1476–1479
   physiologic basis for, 1671–1673
   ryanodine receptor mutations in, 314
Central nervous system. *See also* Brain; Spinal cord
   in congenital muscular dystrophy, 1226
   dysgenesis of
      of brainstem nuclei, 1933–1935, 1934f, 1935f, 1938
      cerebrohepatorenal syndrome with, arthrogryposis multiplex congenita and, 1945–1946, 1946f, 1947f
      myelomeningocele with, arthrogryposis multiplex congenita and, 1942f, 1942–1944, 1943f
      with partial deletion of long arm of chromosome 18, 1937
      of spinal cord, 1938f–1940f, 1938–1940
      with trisomy 18, 1935–1936, 1936f–1938f
      with trisomy 21, 1936–1937
   in laminin α2 deficiency, 1211f, 1211–1212
   in myotonic dystrophy, 1044t, 1045–1046
   in nemaline myopathy, 1482–1483
   structural lesions of, amyotrophic lateral sclerosis versus, 1873

Centronuclear myopathy, 1490–1491, 1494–1495
   clinical features of, 1494
   differential diagnosis of, 1495
   genetics of, 1495
   pathologic features of, 1494–1495, 1495f, 1496f
Cerebrohepatorenal syndrome, arthrogryposis multiplex congenita and, 1945–1946, 1946f, 1947f
Ceroid accumulation, muscle fiber contour and, 702–703
Ceroid lipofuscinosis, 574t, 579–581, 581f, 582f, 731–732, 739f
Cervical muscles, testing of, 604t
Cestode infections, myositis caused by, 1430–1437. *See also specific infections*
Chain fibers, 489
Chanarin-Dorfman disease, 1612–1613, 1613f
Channelopathies, 1748, 1748t, 1749t
   reverse genetics in, 953–954
Charcot-Marie-Tooth disease, 1318, 1856, 1856f
   reverse genetics in, 954
Charge movement, depolarization-contraction coupling and, 261–263, 262f
   complexities of charge movement and, 262–263
   voltage sensors in dihydropyridine receptor proteins and, 262
Chemokines, 1350
   in intercellular communication, 900, 905t, 906
   secretion of, 911
   as therapeutic target, 909–910
Chloride channels
   lack of contribution to resting potential, 209
   voltage-dependent, 222–224, 223f, 224f
Chloroquine
   myopathy due to, 1699f, 1699–1700, 1700f
   toxicity of, electrodiagnostic studies in, 643
Cholesterol, in inclusion body myositis, 1378
Cholesterol ester storage disease. *See* Acid lipase deficiency
Choline acetyltransferase deficiency, 1805–1807
   clinical features of, 1806, 1806f

Choline acetyltransferase deficiency (Cont.)
  electrophysiologic features of, 1807
  end plate studies in, 1807, 1807f
  molecular studies in, 1807, 1808f, 1809t
  treatment of, 1807
Chondrodystrophic myotonia, 1292–1294, 1293f, 1748
  electrodiagnostic studies in, 642
  laboratory findings and microscopy in, 1293, 1293f
  differential diagnosis of, 1294
  molecular genetics of, 1293
  pathogenesis of, 1294
Chromatin, 917–918, 918f
Chromatin remodeling complexes, in Emery-Dreifuss muscular dystrophy, 1033, 1034f
Chromosomes, structure of, 915, 916f–918f, 917–918
Chronic inflammatory demyelinating and axonal polyradiculoneuropathy, 1911–1912
Ciguatera poisoning, myopathy due to, 1703
Cimetidine, myositis due to, 1704
Claudication, 1740
Clinical examination, 599–617
  clinical features found in, 614–617
  cranial muscle testing in, 603
  gait inspection in, 602–603
  history taking in, 599–601
  manual muscle testing in, 603, 609, 610f–612f, 610t
  palpation of muscles and nerves in, 609, 612–613
  percussion of muscles in, 613
  reactions and reflexes in, 613–614
  simple inspection at rest in, 500
  weakness and atrophy in, 601–602
Clinical history, 599–601
Clofibrate, myopathy due to, 1697
Cloning, 927–946
  analysis of cloned genes and, 935–942
    computer-based sequence analysis for, 942
    DNA extraction for, 935
    DNA sequencing for, 938–940, 939f, 940f
    DNA subcloning for, 935–942
    dot blots for, 937–938
    functional genomics and, 942
    gels for, 935
    multiplex analysis of gene expression and, 940–942, 941f
    Northern blotting for, 937
    polymerase chain reaction for, 938, 938f
    restriction fragment length polymorphisms for, 936, 936f
    restriction mapping for, 936
    Southern blotting for, 936–937, 937f
  cDNA libraries and, 930–932, 931f
  genomic libraries and, 929f, 929–930, 930f
  Human Genome Project and, 934–935
  libraries and, 927
  plus-minus screening and, 933–934
  probes and, 932f, 932–933
  screening libraries and, 933, 934f
  uses of cloned genes and, 942–946
  vectors and inserts and, 927–929, 928f
Clostridial myonecrosis, 1464
Clubfoot, 1955–1956
Coats disease, 1127
Cocaine, myoglobinuria due to, 1686
Coenurosis, 1434–1435
Coenzyme Q10 deficiency, 1636–1637
  encephalomyopathic presentation of, 1636–1637, 1637t
  ataxic presentation of, 1637
Cofactors, for mitochondrial encephalopathy, 1653
Colchicine, myopathy due to, 1701–1703
Cold, myoglobinuria due to, 1683
Collagen(s), in limb-girdle muscular dystrophy, 1080t
Collagen VI, 457t
  in Bethlem myopathy, 1139–1141, 1143f
Complement
  activation of, plasma membrane defects and, 1003
  in myasthenia gravis, acetylcholine receptor antibody effects on, 1769, 1770f, 1771f
Complementary DNA libraries, 930–932, 941f
Complement system, 889–890, 890f
Complex I deficiency, 1635–1636, 1636t, 1649–1650, 1650t
Complex II deficiency, 1636
Complex III deficiency, 1637–1638, 1650
Complex IV deficiency, 1638–1641, 1650–1651
  encephalomyopathies in, 1639–1641, 1640f
  multiple mitochondrial defects in, 1641
  myopathies in, 1638–1639, 1639f
Complex repetitive discharges, on electromyography, 625
Complex V deficiency, 1641–1642, 1651
Compression injury, of peripheral nerves, 1897–1898
Computational biology, 942
Computed tomography, 655, 656, 656t
Concentric laminated bodies, ultrastructural features of, 797, 799, 800f, 801f
Conduction block, persistent, multifocal motor mononeuropathy with, 1912
Conduction defect, with cardiac involvement, 1029
Conduction velocity, action potential spread and, 224
Conformational analysis, 943
Congenital deformities. *See specific deformities*
Congenital muscular dystrophies, 1203–1232
  arthrogryposis multiplex congenita and, 1949–1950
  classification of, 1205–1207, 1206f, 1206t, 1207t
  with contractural phenotypes, 1226
  α-dystroglycanopathies, 1213–1216
    etiology and pathogenesis of, 1213t, 1213–1215, 1214f–1216f
    muscle pathology in, 1215–1216
  electrodiagnostic studies in, 640
  epidemiology of, 1205
  fukutin-related, cardiomyopathy in, 1251
  Fukuyama, 1206t, 1216–1218
    clinical features of, 1217–1218, 1218f
    gene and protein in, 1217
    molecular pathology of, 1217
  genetic counseling and, 1232
  historical background of, 1203–1205, 1204f
  with integrin deficiency, 1206t, 1230–1231
  with laminin α2 deficiency, 1206t, 1207–1213
    animal models of, 1210

central nervous system in, 1211f, 1211–1212
complete, clinical features of, 1210f, 1210–1211
heart in, 1212
LAMA2 gene and molecular pathology of, 1208–1209
laminin role in striated muscle and, 1207–1208, 1208f
muscle pathology in, 1209f, 1209–1210
partial, 1212
peripheral nerves in, 1212
prenatal diagnosis of, 1212–1213
skin in, 1212
LARGE mutation causing, 1225
muscle-eye-brain disease, 1206t, 1218–1220, 1226
clinical features of, 1219f, 1219–1220, 1220f
gene and protein in, 1219, 1219f
with nervous system involvement, 1226
prenatal diagnosis of, 1232
with prominent contractures, 1230
rare forms of, 1206t, 1231, 1231t
rigid-spine, 1206t, 1226–1227, 1227f, 1228f
therapy for, 1231–1232
type 1B, 1206t, 1225–1226
type 1C, 1206t, 1222–1225
clinical features of, 1223
FKRP mutations causing, 1223f–1225f, 1223–1225
gene and protein in, 1223
Ullrich, 1206t, 1227–1230
clinical features of, 1229f–1230f, 1229t, 1229–1230
collagen genes and etiopathogenesis of, 1228–1229
muscle pathology in, 1230, 1230f
Walker-Warbug syndrome, 1206t, 1220–1222
clinical features of, 1221f, 1221–1222, 1222f
gene and protein in, 1220
phenotypic heterogeneity in, 1221
Congenital myasthenic syndromes, 1803–1839
arthrogryposis multiplex congenita and, 1951–1952
classification of, 1803–1804, 1804t
clinical features of, 1804–1805
electrodiagnostic studies in, 645–646

electromyography in, 1805
intravenous edrophonium test in, 1805
investigation of, 1804, 1804t
myasthenia gravis versus, 1775t
partially characterized, 1839
postsynaptic, 1817–1839
acetylcholine receptor kinetics and, 1818
acetylcholine receptor structure and, 1817–1818, 1818t
fast-channel, 1827f, 1827–1831
low-expressor acetylcholine receptor mutations with no or minor kinetic abnormality and, 1831–1832
with plectin deficiency, 1838–1839
rapsyn deficiency and, 1833–1835, 1834f, 1835f
slow-channel, 1818–1827
sodium channel myasthenia, 1835–1838, 1836f–1838f, 1839t
presynaptic, 1805–1811
choline acetyltransferase deficiency and, 1805–1807, 1807f, 1808f, 1809t
Lambert-Eaton–like syndrome, 1809, 1810f
paucity of synaptic vesicles and reduced quantal release and, 1807, 1809, 1809f, 1810f
serologic tests in, 1805
synaptic basal lamina-associated syndrome. *See* Acetylcholinesterase, end plate, congenital deficiency of
therapy for, response to, 1805
Congophilic deposits, in inclusion body myopathy, 1369, 1371f
Connectin, 133t
Connective tissue
increased, dystrophin deficiency and, 720, 721f
increase in, in polymyositis/dermatomyositis, 1332
Core formations, ultrastructural features of, 816, 817f–822f
Core-rod myopathy, 1489–1490
Cori-Forbes disease. *See* Debrancher deficiency
Cortical dystrophin promoter, 963–964
Corticosteroids
for Duchenne muscular dystrophy, 1008–1009
for myasthenia gravis, 1777–1778

myopathy due to, 1694t, 1698
for polymyositis/dermatomyositis, 1345
for thyroid-associated ophthalmopathy, 1727
Costameres, 55–56, 335–339, 337f, 461–462
Costimulatory molecules, 1350
expression of, 911
as therapeutic target, 909
Coxsackievirus infection, myositis due to, 1392–1394, 1393f
C protein, myosin-binding, muscle contraction and, 300
Cramp-fasciculation syndrome, 1747
amyotrophic lateral sclerosis versus, 1874
Cramps, 600, 1744, 1744t, 1746–1747
benign, 1744, 1746–1747
neurodiagnostic studies in, 646
pathologic, 1744
Cranial muscles, testing of, 603
Craniocarpotarsal syndrome, arthrogryposis multiplex congenita and, 1941
Creatine, urinary, in dystrophinopathies, 978–979
Creatine kinase
of M line, 143
serum, in dystrophinopathies, 978
Creatinine, urinary, in dystrophinopathies, 978–979
Critical illness myopathy, 1719t, 1719–1721
Cross-bridge(s), 187, 188f
sliding filaments and, 134
Cross-bridge cycle, 187–200
caged molecules and, 198–199, 199f
eccentric contractions and, 196, 196f
isometric contractions and, 191, 191f, 192f
energetics of, 193–194
isotonic contractions and, 194f, 194–195
length-tension curves and, 191–193, 193f
mechanical transients and, 197–198, 198f
mechanics in vitro and, 199–200, 200f
stiffness and, 197
structural correlates of, 187, 188f
working contractions and, 195–196
working hypothesis of, 188–190, 189f, 190f

Crush syndrome, myoglobinuria due to, 1683–1684
Cryptococcus neoformans myositis, 1465
αB-Crystallin
  expression in muscle fibers, in inclusion body myositis, 1379, 1379f, 1380f, 1381
  in myofibrillar myopathies, 1190
    functional importance of, 1195, 1197
    mutations in, 1197–1198
αB-Crystallinopathy, 1170t
Cunninghamella bertholletiae myositis, 1465
Curare
  maternal treatment with, arthrogryposis multiplex congenita and, 1951
  neuromuscular transmission safety factor and, 632
Cushing disease. *See* Glucocorticoid excess
Cutaneous larva migrans, 1439
Cutaneous nerve endings, quantitation of, 1905
Cyclophosphamide
  for myasthenia gravis, 1778
  myositis due to, 1704
  for polymyositis/dermatomyositis, 1345, 1346
Cyclosporine
  for myasthenia gravis, 1778
  myositis due to, 1704
  for polymyositis/dermatomyositis, 1346
Cylindrical spirals, ultrastructural features of, 806, 808f, 809, 809f
Cylindrical spirals myopathy, 1508, 1508f
Cysteine string protein, exocytosis and, 338–339
Cysticercosis, 1430–1431, 1432f
Cystinosis, 574t, 584
Cytochrome oxidase deficiency, 739, 740f
Cytokines, 1350
  in inclusion body myositis, 1378
  in intercellular communication, 900, 902t–904t, 905–906
  protein metabolism and, 556–558
  secretion of, 911
  as therapeutic target, 909–910
Cytoplasmic bodies, 703–704, 706f
  ultrastructural features of, 789, 790f

Cytoplasmic body myopathy, 704
Cytoplasmic degradation, ultrastructural features of, 836f, 836–841, 837f, 839f–841f
Cytoskeleton, 443–451
  components of, 457t
  costamere structure and, 445–449, 447f
    myotendinous and neuromuscular junctions and, 448f, 448–449, 449f
  cytoskeletal components of nerve terminal above active zones and, 339, 339f
  dystrophin system of, 455–466
  integrins and, 449–451
    functions of, 450–451
    general properties of, 449
    of skeletal muscle, 449–450
  links to extracellular matrix, 445, 446f
  microtubules and, 451
  myofibrils and, 55f, 55–56
  sarcolemmal network and transverse collecting system of, 443–445, 444f
Cytosol
  calcium release into, 312–313
  calcium removal from, 307–310
Cytotoxicity, antibody-dependent, in dermatomyositis, 1351–1352

Danazol, myositis due to, 1704
Danon disease. *See* Lysosome-associated membrane protein-2 deficiency
Dantrolene
  for Duchenne muscular dystrophy, 1008
  as malignant hyperthermia antidote, 1663, 1666, 1666t
Debrancher deficiency, 1543–1545
  biochemistry of, 1543–1544
  clinical features of, 1543
  genetics of, 1543
  laboratory studies in, 1543
  molecular genetics of, 1544
  pathology of, 1543, 1543f
  therapy for, 1544–1545
  type 3, 730, 738f
Deflazacort, for Duchenne muscular dystrophy, 1008–1009
Dementia. *See also* Alzheimer disease
  in amyotrophic lateral sclerosis, 1869

  familial juvenile amyotrophic lateral sclerosis with, 1872
Demyelinating polyneuropathy, inflammatory, chronic, amyotrophic lateral sclerosis versus, 1874
Demyelination, inflammatory, of peripheral nerves, 1899
Dendritic cells, 898
  functions of, 1351
Denervation
  microcirculatory remodeling and, 525
  muscle spindle alterations and, 740–741
  proteolysis in skeletal muscle and, 569
Denervation atrophy
  dystrophin deficiency and, 724, 726
  muscle fiber diameter and, 696
  protein metabolism and, 555
  ultrastructural features of, 817, 823, 826f–831f, 827–828
Dermatomyositis. *See also* Polymyositis/dermatomyositis
  in adults, 1324–1326
    cardiac involvement in, 1325
    prognosis of, 1326
    pulmonary involvement in, 1325–1326
  childhood, 1322–1324, 1323f–1325f
  electrodiagnostic studies in, 634f, 634–635
  humoral effector mechanisms in, 1351–1352
  morphology of, 1352
  muscle fiber nuclei in, ultrastructural features of, 762
  muscle pain associated with, 1742t
  parvovirus B19 infection and, 1395
  pathologic features of, 1333–1340
  perifascicular atrophy of, ultrastructural features of, 828–829, 832f–835f, 836
Desmin, 132t, 457t
  defects of, myopathies caused by, 464
  in dystrophinopathies, 999
  of intermediate filaments, 160
  in myofibrillar myopathies, 1190
    functional importance of, 1191
    mutations of, 1191, 1198f
  in myofibrillar myopathies, 1195
Desmin intermediate filaments, 462, 462f

Desminopathy, 1170t
Desmuslin, 457t
Diabetes mellitus
    muscle microcirculation in, 528–529
    neuropathy with, 1914–1915
2,4-Dienoyl-CoA reductase deficiency, 1610
Dietary therapy, for hypokalemic periodic paralysis, 1288
Dihydropyridine receptors, 248f, 248–251, 249f
    calcium release channel modulation by, 313f, 313–314
    excitation-contraction coupling in skeletal muscle and. *See* Excitation-contraction coupling, in skeletal muscle
    isoforms of, 251, 251f
    ratio to ryanodine receptors, variations in, 251
    structure of, 266f, 266–268
    voltage sensors in, 262
Diphtheria, neuropathy due to, 1907
Direct muscle stimulation, 633
Distal myopathies, 1169–1182
    adult-onset, 1170t
    definition of, 1169
    differential diagnosis of, 1181t, 1181–1182
    early-onset, 1170t
    historical background of, 1169–1170, 1170t
    Laing, 1179–1180
    late-onset, 1170t, 1172–1176
        laboratory findings in, 1173, 1173f
        molecular genetics of, 1172–1173
        molecular pathogenesis of, 1175–1176, 1186f
        muscle pathology in, 1173f–1175f, 1173–1175
        treatment and management of, 1176
    Miyoshi (dysferlinopathy), 1170t, 1176–1178, 1177f, 1178f
    new Finnish, 1170t
    Nonaka (with rimmed vacuoles), 1170t, 1178–1179, 1179f
    oculopharyngeal, 1170t, 1180
    with pes cavus and areflexia, 1170t
    with respiratory failure, 1170t
    with rimmed vacuoles, 1170t, 1178–1179, 1179f
    tibial, 1170t, 1172, 1172f
    variable-onset, 1170t
    very late onset, 1170t

    with vocal cord and pharyngeal signs, 1170t
    Welander, 1170t, 1170–1171, 1171f
Diuretics, for sodium channel myotonias, 1278
DM1, myotonic dystrophy and, 1058, 1058f
DMPK ZFN9, in limb-girdle muscular dystrophy, 1081t
DMWD, in myotonic dystrophy, 1065
DNA
    deletions of, in inclusion body myopathy, 1370
    extraction of, 935
    instability of, in myotonic dystrophy, 1061–1063, 1063f
    mutations of, 924f, 924–925
    structure of, 915, 916f–918f, 917–918
    subcloning of, 935–936
DNA footprinting, 944
DNA microarrays, 941f, 941–942
DNA polymerases, 917, 927, 932
DNA polymorphisms, 924
DNA sequencing, 938–940, 939f, 940f
DOD1 gene, amyotrophic lateral sclerosis and, 1876t, 1876–1878, 1877f
Dot blots, 937–938
Down syndrome, arthrogryposis multiplex congenita and, 1936–1937
Doxorubicin, myositis due to, 1704
DP proteins, 965
Dracunculiasis, 1439–1441
    clinical manifestations of, 1440
    geographic location and, 1439–1440
    laboratory studies in, 1440
    pathology of, 1440, 1440f
    transmission to humans, 1440
    treatment of, 1440–1441
Dropped head syndrome, electrodiagnostic studies in, 643
DRP2, 964
Drug-induced myoglobinuria, 1684t, 1685–1687
Drug-induced neuropathy, 1919
Duchenne muscular dystrophy, 961, 962. *See also* Dystrophinopathies
    adverse anesthetic reactions in, 972
    cardiac involvement in, 975–976, 1243–1244
    carriers of, 973–974, 975f
        cardiac involvement in, 976
    cardiomyopathy in, 1247
    central nervous system involvement in, 976

    clinical features of, 969–974
        early descriptions of, 969–970, 970f–972f
    clinical heterogeneity in, 972–973, 974f
    dystrophin expression in sarcolemma in, 997–998, 998f
    electron microscopy in, 989–997
        freeze-fracture studies and, 996
        intramuscular nerves and endplates on, 996, 997f
        muscle fiber alterations associated with plasma membrane defects on, 995–996
        muscle microvasculature on, 996–997
        plasma membrane defects in nonnecrotic fibers on, 990, 990f–995f, 993, 995
        satellite cells on, 996
    in females, 973, 974
    hearing loss in, 977
    immunoblot studies in, 999–1000, 1000f
    light microscopic studies in. *See* Dystrophinopathies, light microscopy in
    natural history of, 970–973, 973f
    retinal involvement in, 977
    reverse genetics in, 953
    smooth muscle involvement in, 976
    treatment of, muscle gene regulatory regions in, 28–29
Duty ratio, of myosin, 170
Dynactin, amyotrophic lateral sclerosis and, 1878
Dysferlin, 457t
    caveolin-3 binding to, 459
    in limb-girdle muscular dystrophy, 1080t, 1086
Dysferlinopathy, 1091–1095
    clinical features of, 1091–1093, 1092f
    diagnosis of, 1093, 1094f, 1095f, 1111
    distal, 1170t, 1176–1178, 1177f, 1178f
    genetics of, 1093
    treatment of, 1095
Dyskalemic periodic paralysis, with arrhythmia and dysmorphia, 1289f, 1289–1290
Dystrophinopathies, 961–1012. *See also* Becker muscular dystrophy; Duchenne muscular dystrophy
    animal models of, 1001–1002
        canine, 1002
        feline, 1002
        murine, 1001

Dystrophinopathies (Cont.)
  biochemical abnormalities in body fluids in, 978–979
    serum, 978
    urinary, 978–979
  cardiac involvement in, 975–976
  carrier detection for, 1007–1008
  central nervous system involvement in, 976
  diagnosis of, 1005–1007
    algorithms for, 1006
    genomic, 1005, 1005f
    immunoblotting and immunostaining in, 1006
    mRNA analysis in, 1005–1006
    prenatal, 1008
  differential diagnosis of, 1006–1007
  dystrophin and. See Dystrophin(s)
  electrodiagnostic studies in, 639, 979
  electron microscopy in, 989–997
  gonadal mosaicism in, 1007–1008
  hearing loss in, 977
  historical perspective on, 962
  immunoblot studies in, 999–1001
  immunocytochemical studies of cryostat sections in, 997–999
    caveolin-3 and, 999
    dystrophin-associated proteins and, 999
    plectin and, 999
    sarcolemmal dystrophin expression and, 997–999, 998f
    titin and desmin and, 999
    vinculin and, 999
  light microscopy in, 980–989
    calcium-loaded nonnecrotic fibers on, 988
    central nuclei on, 986
    distribution of histochemical fiber types on, 984–985
    fiber size on, 985–986, 986f, 987f
    grouping of necrotic and regenerating fibers on, 982, 984
    hypercontracted fibers on, 986, 988
    inflammatory cells on, 988–989, 989f
    necrotic fibers on, 980–981, 981f–984f
    regenerating fibers on, 981–982, 985f, 986f
  management of, 1011–1012
    family and, 1011
    physical and orthopedic therapy in, 1011
    ventilatory support in, 1012
  morphologic studies in, 980–957
    electron microscopic, 989–997
    historical background of, 980
    light microscopic, 980–989
  mosaicisms in, 968–969
  pathogenesis of, 1002–1005
    sarcolemmal structural weakness in, 1002–1003
    secondary consequences of membrane defects in, 1003–1005
  prevention of, 1007–1008
  retinal involvement in, 977
  smooth muscle involvement in, 976
  therapy for, 1008–1011
    cell therapy for, 1009–1010
    conventional therapeutic agents for, 1008–1009
    gene therapy for, 1009, 1010–1011
  X-linked dilated cardiomyopathy due to, 977–978
Dystrobrevin, 456–457, 457t, 964
  binding to syntrophins, 459, 459f
  defects of, muscular dystrophies caused by, 464
  dystrophin binding to, 459, 459f
  in limb-girdle muscular dystrophy, 1079
Dystroglycan(s), 455–456, 457t
  caveolin-3 binding to, 459
  glycosylation defects of, in limb-girdle muscular dystrophy, 1083–1084
  in limb-girdle muscular dystrophy, 1083
Dystroglycan complex, 455–456
  defects of, muscular dystrophies caused by, 463
α-Dystroglycanopathies, 1213–1216
  etiology and pathogenesis of, 1213t, 1213–1215, 1214f–1216f
  muscle pathology in, 1215–1216
Dystrophin(s), 455–466, 457t, 961
  binding of
    to actin, 459–461
    to dystrobrevin, 459, 459f
    to β-dystroglycan, 459–461
    to sarcoglycan complexes, 458, 458f
    to syntrophins, 459, 459f
  complexes obtained from muscle cell membrane functions and, 458–459
  costameric distribution of, 965
  defects of, muscular dystrophies caused by, 463
  deficiency of, 717–729, 720f
    amyloid deposition and, 728–729, 736f
    compensation for, 28–30
    connective tissue increase and, 720, 721f
    denervation atrophy and, 724, 726
    histochemical diagnosis of dystrophies with monoclonal antibodies and, 719, 720t
    infarction and, 720–722, 722f–725f, 724
    inflammation and, 726–728, 728f–735f
    muscle fiber loss and, 720
    myogenic atrophy and, 726, 727f
    perifascicular atrophy and, 724, 726f
  domains of, 964–965
  expression in sarcolemma, 997–999, 998f
  glycoprotein complex and, 457–458
  interactions within dystrophin-based fixation bolt and, 461
  in limb-girdle muscular dystrophy, 1080t
  mitigation of mdx phenotype by, 463–464
  in myofibrillar myopathies, 1190
  phosphorylation of, 465
  short, 964
  structure of, 455–457, 456f, 457t
  transverse fixation system and intermediate filaments, costameres, and fixation bolts of, 461–462, 462f
  proteins responsible for muscular dystrophies in, 462–464
  in vitro binding of dystrophin-associated proteins to other proteins, 459
Dystrophin-associated proteins, 965
  in dystrophinopathies, 999
  in limb-girdle muscular dystrophy, 1079
  in vitro binding to other proteins, 459, 459f
Dystrophin--dystrophin-associated protein complex
  developmental expression of, 464–465

as signaling system, 465–466
structure of, 457
subcomplexes of, 458, 458f
Dystrophin gene, 962f, 962–963, 963f
  mutations of, 966–967
    deletion-induced exon skipping and, 966–967, 967f
    frameshift rule and, 966
    germline and somatic, 968–969
    in mice, 1001
    mutant-gene transcripts and, 966
    patterns of, 966
    protein products of, 967–968
    splice-site, 966–967
Dystrophin promoters, 963–964
  cortical, 963–964
  lymphoid cell, 964
  muscle, 963
  Purkinje cell, 964
Dystrophin protein family, 964

Early-onset distal myopathy, 1170t
Eccentric contraction, 196, 196f
Echinococcosis. See Hydatidosis
Echovirus infection, myositis associated with, 1393, 1393f
Edema, of peripheral nerves, 1898–1899
Elasticity, modulus of, 197
Electrodiagnostic studies, 619–648. *See also* Electromyography; Nerve conduction studies; Repetitive stimulation testing; *specific conditions*
  in congenital myopathies, 640, 641t
  in critical illness myopathy, 643–644
  direct muscle stimulation for, 633
  in disorders of altered cell membrane excitability, 636–639
  in infiltrative myopathies, 636
  in inflammatory myopathies, 633–636
  in metabolic muscle disorders, 640–643, 641t
  motor-unit number estimates and, 633
  in muscle spasms and related phenomena, 646–647
  in muscular dystrophies, 639–640
  nerve accommodation testing as, 633
  in neural diseases, 647–648
  in neuromuscular transmission disorders, 644–646
  in neuromyopathies, 648, 648t

Electromyography, 620–630. *See also* Electrodiagnostic studies; *specific conditions*
  macroelectrode, 629–630
  needle, 620–628
    abnormal motor unit potentials on, 626–628, 628f
    abnormal spontaneous activity on, 623f, 623–625, 624t, 626f
    electrodes for, 620, 620f
    normal activity on, 620–623, 621f–623f
  of peripheral nerves, 1904
  single-fiber, 628–629, 629f
  surface recordings using, 630
Electron acceptors, artificial, for mitochondrial encephalopathy, 1653
Electron transferring flavoprotein, mitochondrial β-oxidation and, 1594
Embryogenesis, satellite cell development from myogenic cells during, 68–69
Embryonic origins of skeletal muscles, 3–37
  building muscle anatomy and, 30–37
  mesoderm and skeletal muscle progenitor specification and, 4–18
  molecular control of muscle differentiation and, 18–30
Embryonic stem cells, 946
Emerin
  defects in, cardiomyopathy due to, 1249–1250
  in limb-girdle muscular dystrophy, 1080t
Emerinopathy, presenting as limb-girdle muscular dystrophy, 1109
Emery-Dreifuss cardiomyopathy, 1249–1250
Emery-Dreifuss muscular dystrophy, 1027–1035
  animal models of, 1033
  autosomal dominant, muscle fiber nuclei in, ultrastructural features of, 762
  cell transfection studies of, 1033
  clinical features of, 1027–1030, 1028f
  definition of, 1027
  diagnosis of, 1111, 1112
  genetic alterations in, 1031–1032
  historical background of, 1027

  laboratory investigations in, 1030–1031
  pathophysiology of, 1032–1033
  spinal muscular atrophy versus, 1852
  therapy for, 1033–1035
  X-linked, muscle fiber nuclei in, ultrastructural features of, 762
Emery muscular dystrophy. *See* Emery-Dreifuss muscular dystrophy
Emetine, myopathy due to, 1695t, 1701, 1701f, 1702f
Encephalocele, with arrhinencephaly and anterior horn dysgenesis, arthrogryposis multiplex congenita and, 1941
Encephalomyopathies
  in complex I deficiency, 1649
  in complex IV deficiency, 1650
  in complex V deficiency, 1651
  mitochondrial. *See* Mitochondrial encephalomyopathies
End-brush nerve endings, 327f, 331
Endocrine disorders, in myotonic dystrophy, 1044t, 1046t, 1046–1047, 1047t
Endocrine myopathies, 1713–1734
  with adrenal dysfunction, 1715–1722
    adrenal insufficiency and, 1721–1722
    adrenocorticotropic hormone excess and, 1721
    glucocorticoid excess and, 1715–1721
  with calcium and vitamin D metabolism disorders, 1731–1734
    hyperparathyroidism and metabolic bone disease, 1731–1733
    hypoparathyroidism and pseudohypoparathyroidism, 1733–1734
  cellular actions of hormones and, 1713t, 1713–1715, 1714f, 1714t
    membrane receptors and, 1713–1714
    nuclear receptors and, 1715
  muscle pain associated with, 1742t
  with pituitary dysfunction, 1729–1731
    acromegaly, 1729–1730
    hypopituitarism, 1730–1731
  with thyroid disease, 1722–1729
    endocrine ophthalmopathy, 1726–1727
    hypothyroidism, 1727–1729

Endocrine myopathies (Cont.)
  thyrotoxic myopathy, 1722–1725
  thyrotoxic periodic paralysis, 1725–1726
Endocytosis, synaptic vesicle formation and, 343–344
Endomysial tubes, regeneration within, 78
Endomysium, 471, 471f
Endonucleases, 927
Endoplasmic reticulum
  microtubular inclusions in, ultrastructural features of, 810–811, 812f
  transition to sarcoplasmic reticulum, 57–58
  ultrastructural reactions of, 774, 778f
Endothelial cells, ultrastructural features of, 877, 877f, 878f, 879
Endothelial-leukocyte interactions, microcirculatory remodeling and, 527–528
End plate acetylcholinesterase deficiency, congenital. See Acetylcholinesterase deficiency, congenital, end plate
End plate currents
  decaying phase of, factors determining, 388
  generation of, 387–388
  rising phase of, factors determining, 387
End plate noise, 621
End plate potentials
  facilitation, augmentation, potentiation, and depression of, 378–380, 379t, 380f
  measuring transmitter release with, 374
  measuring with voltage clamp, 374–375, 375f
  miniature, facilitation, augmentation, and potentiation of, 381
  in single-fiber electromyography, 628–629, 629f
End plates, in Duchenne muscular dystrophy, 996, 997f
Energy metabolism, amino acid contribution to, 538–539
Energy utilization, in exercise, 665–667, 666f, 666t, 667f
En grappe nerve endings, 327f, 331
β-Enolase deficiency, 1551
2-Enoyl-CoA hydratase, mitochondrial β-oxidation and, 1594

En plaque nerve endings, 327f, 331
Entrapment neuropathies, in diabetes mellitus, 1915
Enzyme(s). See also specific enzymes
  in limb-girdle muscular dystrophy, 1087–1088
  proteolytic, in inclusion body myositis, 1377
  restriction, 926f, 926–927
Enzyme replacement therapy, for acid maltase deficiency, 1578–1579
Eosinophilia, diffuse fasciitis with, 1446, 1447f, 1448f
Eosinophilia-myalgia syndrome, 1447, 1449–1450, 1704, 1742t, 1743–1744
  electrodiagnostic studies in, 643
Eosinophilic polymyositis, 1445–1446
Epilepsy
  frontal lobe, nocturnal, autosomal dominant, neuronal acetylcholine receptors and, 409
  myoclonic, spinal muscular atrophy with, 1861
Epimysium, 471, 471f
Epinephrine, lipid metabolism and, 1590
Epinephrine test, 632
Epineurium, 471
Epsilon aminocaproic acid myopathy, 1697
Equatorial region, of intrafusal bundle, 489
Erythrocyte sedimentation rate, in polymyositis/dermatomyositis, 1330
Essential light chain, 168
Esterase, end plate current and, 388, 388f
ETF:ubiquinone oxidoreductase, mitochondrial β-oxidation and, 1594
Excitation-contraction coupling, 191
Excitation-contraction coupling, in skeletal muscle, 257–277
  activation and inactivation relations and, 257–261, 258f, 259f
  caffeine effects on, 260–261, 261f
  external calcium effects on, 259–260
  strength-duration relation to attain contraction threshold and, 260, 260f
  depolarization-induced calcium transients and, 263–266, 264f

  dihydropyridine receptors, 268–269, 270f
    alphacentric view and, 269–271, 270f, 271f
    betacentric view and, 275–277, 276f, 277f
    biochemical interactions between dihydropyridine receptors and ryanodine receptors and, 274f, 274–275
  molecular basis of, 266–277
  ryanodine receptors and dihydropyridine receptors and, 270f
    alphacentric view and, 269–271, 270f, 271f
    betacentric view and, 275–277, 276f, 277f
    biochemical interactions of, 274f, 274–275
    peptide fragment application to isolated ryanodine receptors and, 271f, 271–272
    RyR1 domains and, 272f–274f, 272–274
  structure of, 266f, 266–268
  voltage-dependent charge movement and, 261–263, 262f
Exercise
  in congenital myopathies, 1523–1524
  energy utilization in, 665–667, 666f, 666t, 667f
  extreme, myoglobinuria due to, 1681–1682
  glycogen as fuel for, 1536
  lysosomes and, 568–569
  muscle metabolism in, 667–673, 668t
    cycle ergometry assessment of oxidative metabolism and, 673
    magnetic resonance spectroscopy evaluation of, 669–670, 670f, 671f
    monitoring glycogenolysis and ammonia production in forearm exercise and, 668–669, 669f
    monitoring of oxidative metabolism and, 671–673
    near infrared spectroscopy evaluation of, 671–672, 672f
    venous effluent oxygen levels and, 672, 672f
  pathophysiology in muscle energy defects and, 673–677
    in fatty acid oxidation defects, 677
    in glycogenolysis disorders, 675–677

in respiratory chain and related disorders, 673–675
purine nucleotide cycle and, 538–539
skeletal muscle regulation mediated by, 27
Exertional myalgia, 600, 1740–1741, 1741t, 1742t
Exocytosis, 336–339, 337f
proteins modulating, 337–339
SNARE complex and, 336–337
steps in, 338
synaptotagmin I and, 337–338
Exon skipping, antisense-induced, for dystrinopathies, 1010
Exophthalmos, 1726t, 1726–1727
Expression vectors, 931f, 932
Extracellular matrix, 471–484
acetylcholinesterase collagen-tailed form association with, 435–436
basal lamina of. *See* Basal lamina
components of, 473–475
in cultured muscle, 477, 478f
in developing muscle, 476–477, 477f
mechanical strength and, 477, 479
morphology of, 471, 472f–473f, 473
muscle maintenance and, 479
muscle regeneration and, 479–480
myogenesis and, 479
in myotendinous junctions, 476
in neuromuscular junction, 475f, 475–476, 476f
functions of, 480–484
pathology of, 484
Extraocular muscles, 119–126
anatomy of, 119
cellular organization of, 119, 120f
congenital fibrosis of, myasthenia gravis versus, 1775t
development of, 125–126
in diseases, 125
innervation autonomic nervous synapses of, 122, 122f, 123f
layers of, 119–121, 121f, 121t
pathologic reactions of, 125
physiologic aspects of, 122–123
proprioception by, 124f, 124–125
structure-function correlations of, 123–124
testing of, 603
Extrapyramidal disease, in amyotrophic lateral sclerosis, 1868–1869
Eye(s). *See also* Extraocular muscles
in Becker muscular dystrophy, 977

in Duchenne muscular dystrophy, 977
in Fukuyama congenital muscular dystrophy, 1218
in muscle-eye-brain disease, 1220
myasthenia gravis affecting, therapy for, 1780
in myotonic dystrophy, 1044t, 1047, 1047t
in Walker-Warburg syndrome, 1221

Fabry disease, 572t, 576–577, 734–735, 739f
Facial muscles, testing of, 604t
Facioscapulohumeral muscular dystrophy, 1109, 1123–1130, 1318
cardiomyopathy in, 1251
clinical features of, 1123, 1125f–1127f, 1125–1127
differential diagnosis of, 1130
electrodiagnostic studies in, 640
genetics of, 1128–1129
historical background of, 1123, 1124f
laboratory, electrophysiologic, and pathologic features of, 1127–1128
molecular pathogenesis of, 1129–1130
reverse genetics in, 954
therapy of, 1130
Facioscapulohumeral muscular syndrome, 1313
F-actin
atomic model of, 149–150, 150f
cross-bridges and, 187
Familial hypertrophic cardiomyopathy, sarcomere in, 161
Familial partial lipodystrophy, clinical features of, 1029–1030
Family, dystrophinopathy management and, 1011
Family history, 599–600
Farber lipogranulomatosis, 572t
Fasciculation(s), 616–617, 1746–1747
in amyotrophic lateral sclerosis, 1867
benign, amyotrophic lateral sclerosis versus, 1874
in clinical examination, 602
Fasciculation potentials, 625
Fasciitis
diffuse, with eosinophilia, 1446, 1447f, 1448f
toxic, 1695t

Fast-channel congenital myasthenic syndromes, 1827f, 1827–1831
εA411P mutation and, 1831
clinical features of, 1827–1828, 1828f
diagnosis of, 1829
εD175N mutation and, 1830
electrophysiologic studies in, 1828, 1829f
kinetic consequences of fast-channel mutations and, 1829–1831
molecular studies in, 1828–1829
morphologic features of, 1828
mutations in long cytoplasmic domain between TMD3 and TMD4 and, 1830
six-residue duplication STRDQE in ε subunit and, 1830
therapy for, 1829
αV285I mutation and, 1830
αV132L mutation and, 1830
Fast fibers, specification of, 94–96
Fasting
long-term, protein balance in muscle and, 553
short-term, protein balance in muscle and, 552–553
Fatigability, 616
Fatigue, 1750–1751
differential diagnosis of, 1750–1751
epidemiology of, 1750
pathogenesis of, 1750
Fatty acid(s), uptake, synthesis, and transport of, 1588, 1590
Fatty acid oxidation
biochemistry of, 1591–1594
of microsomal ω-oxidation, 1596
of mitochondrial β-oxidation, 1592–1595, 1593f
of peroxisomal β-oxidation, 1595–1596
defects of, 677
disorders of, 1596–1600
clinical manifestations of, 1596–1597
diagnosis of, 1599–1600
pathologic findings in, 1598, 1598f, 1599f
pathophysiology of, 1597–1598
FATZ, 132t
Fazio-Londe disease, 1858, 1872
Feedback, neurotransmitter release and, 383
Feeding difficulties, in congenital myopathies, 1523
Feline dystrophinopathy, 1002

Feline immunodeficiency virus infection, 1406
Fenfibrate, myopathy due to, 1697
Fenn effect, 195
Fiber-type disproportion
 in arthrogryposis multiplex congenita, 1933, 1933f
 congenital, 1502–1503
  clinical features of, 1502
  genetics of, 1503
  pathologic features of, 1502, 1502f
  secondary causes of, 1503, 1593t
Fibric acid derivatives, myopathy due to, 1697
Fibrillation potentials, 623f, 623–625, 624t
Fibroblast growth factors, satellite cell cell cycle modulation in response to, 74
Fibromyalgia, 1739, 1739t, 1741, 1742t, 1743
Filamentous bodies, ultrastructural features of, 797, 799f
Filamentous inclusions
 in inclusion body myopathy, 1373f–1376f, 1373–1376
 ultrastructural features of, 813, 814f, 815f, 815–816
γ-Filamin, 132t
 of Z line, 158
Fingerprint bodies, 710–711, 714f
 ultrastructural features of, 799, 802f
Fingerprint body myopathy, 1503–1505
 clinical features of, 1503
 differential diagnosis of, 1505
 genetics of, 1505
 pathologic features of, 1503–1505, 1504f
Fixation bolts, 462
FK506-binding protein, ryanodine receptor modulation by, 315–316
Flavivirus infection, 1396
Floppy infant syndrome, 1851
Focal adhesions, 55
Force output
 gradation by motor neuron firing rate, 113f, 113–115, 114f
 mechanisms controlling, 111
 of muscle units, 110, 110f
Foreign substances, injection into peripheral nerves, 1898
Forward genetics, 950–953
Frameshift mutations, 925
Freeman-Sheldon syndrome, arthrogryposis multiplex congenita and, 1941

Frontal lobe epilepsy, nocturnal, autosomal dominant, neuronal acetylcholine receptors and, 409
Fucosidosis, 573t, 583–584, 584f
Fukutin, in limb-girdle muscular dystrophy, 1081t
Fukutin-related protein
 deficiency of, 1206t, 1222–1225
  clinical features of, 1223
  FKRP mutations causing, 1223f–1225f, 1223–1225
  gene and protein in, 1223
 in limb-girdle muscular dystrophy, 1081t
Fukutin-related proteinopathy, 1101f, 1101–1102, 1111
Fukuyama congenital muscular dystrophy, 1206t, 1216–1218
 clinical features of, 1217–1218, 1218f
 gene and protein in, 1217
 molecular pathology of, 1217
Functional genomics, 942
Fused tetanus, 191

GAA gene, genomic and cDNA structure of, 1571–1572
G-actin
 atomic structure of, 148–149, 149f
 cross-bridges and, 187
Gait, inspection of, 602–603
Galactosialidosis, 573t, 586
Galactosylceramide lipidosis, 572t, 737
GalNAc transferase, therapeutic uses of, 30
Gangliosidoses
 G_{M1}, 572t, 577, 580f, 733–734
 G_{M2}, 572t, 577–579, 580f
  motor neuron variants of, 1872–1873
Gas gangrene, myositis in, 1464
Gastrostomy, in amyotrophic lateral sclerosis, 1882
Gaucher disease, 572t
 infantile, arthrogryposis multiplex congenita and, 1948
Gel(s), for analysis of cloned genes, 935
Gel retardation, 943–944
Gelsolin, in myofibrillar myopathies, 1190
Gelsolin amyloidosis, peripheral neuropathy associated with, 1921
Gemfibrozil, myopathy due to, 1697
Gene(s), 918, 919f, 920
 cloning of. *See* Cloning

 muscle-specific, 948, 949t–950t, 950
 regulation of, 946–948
Gene chips, 941f, 941–942
Gene expression
 altered, in Emery-Dreifuss muscular dystrophy, 1033
 of cloned genes
  in animals, 946, 947f
  in cells, 945–946
 multiplex analysis of, 940–942, 941f
 regulation of, 921–924, 922f, 923f
Gene families, 920
Gene therapy, 30
 for acid maltase deficiency, 1579–1580
 for dystrophinopathies, 1009, 1010–1011
 for Emery-Dreifuss muscular dystrophy, 1034–1035
 for mitochondrial encephalopathy, 1654
Genetic code, 921, 921f
Genetic counseling. *See specific conditions*
Genetic helix, cross bridges and, 187
Genetic maps, 918
Genomes, 918
Genomic hybridization, 936–937, 937f
Genomic libraries, 929f, 929–930, 930f
Genomics
 functional, 942
 structural, 942
Germanium, myopathy due to, 1696
Giant axonal neuropathy, 1873
Giant cell arteritis, myositis in, 1456, 1458f, 1459, 1459f
Globoid cell leukodystrophy, 572t, 737
Glucocorticoid(s)
 cellular actions of, 1714t
 protein turnover in muscle and, 550–551, 551t
Glucocorticoid excess, 1715–1721
 clinical pattern of, 1715
 epidemiology of, 1715
 myopathy associated with
  critical illness myopathy and, 1719t, 1719–1721
  electromyography in, 1716
  experimental corticosteroid myopathy and, 1716, 1717f
  histology in, 1716, 1716f
  myopathic potential of glucocorticoid preparations and, 1715
  pathogenesis of, 1716–1718, 1718f, 1719f
  treatment of, 1718–1719

Glucose
  lipid metabolism and, 1590
  protein turnover in muscle and, 547–548
Glucosylceramide liposis, 572t
  infantile, arthrogryposis multiplex congenita and, 1948
Glutamate toxicity, amyotrophic lateral sclerosis and, 1880
Glutamine, production and release from muscle, 540t, 540–541
Glycerol kinase deficiency, with dystrinopathy, 977
Glycogen
  accumulation in muscle fibers, ultrastructural features of, 841–845, 843f–848f
  as fuel for exercise, 1536
  metabolism of, disorders of, electrodiagnostic studies in, 641
Glycogenolysis
  disorders of
    anaerobic and aerobic metabolic implications of, 675–676
    myoglobinuria due to, 1680
  in forearm exercise, monitoring of, 668–669, 669f
Glycogenoses
  nonlysosomal, 1535f, 1535–1553
    aldolase A deficiency, 1551
    debrancher deficiency, 1543f, 1543–1545
    β-enolase deficiency, 1551
    glycogen as fuel for exercise and, 1536
    historical background of, 1535–1536
    lactate dehydrogenase deficiency, 1550–1551
    Lafora disease, 1553
    phosphofructokinase deficiency, 1545f, 1545–1549, 1546f, 1547t, 1548f
    phosphoglycerate mutase deficiency, 953, 1549–1550, 1550f
    phosphorylase b kinase deficiency, 1536t, 1536–1537
    phosphorylase deficiency, 1537–1542, 1538t, 1539f, 1540f, 1542f
    triosephosphate isomerase deficiency, 1551
    type IV, 1551–1553
    type II. See Acid maltase deficiency
    type III. See Debrancher deficiency

type IV, 730, 738f
  ultrastructural features of, 845
type IX, 1549
type V. See Phosphorylase deficiency
type VII. See Phosphofructokinase deficiency
type VIII. See Phosphorylase b kinase deficiency
type X, 1549–1550, 1550t
  forward genetics in, 953
type XI, 1550–1551
type XII, 1551
type XIII, 1551
type XIV, 1551
Glycogen storage disorders, 730–731
  peripheral neuropathy associated with, 1921
  ultrastructural features of, 842, 844–845
Glycolysis, disorders of
  myoglobinuria due to, 1680
  ultrastructural features of, 844f, 844–845
Glycoprotein complex, 457–458
GNE, in limb-girdle muscular dystrophy, 1081t
Golgi apparatus, ultrastructural reactions of, 774, 776
Gordon syndrome, arthrogryposis multiplex congenita and, 1947
Gowers' maneuver, 614, 615f
Graft-versus-host disease, 1463–1464
Granulomatosis
  allergic, myositis in, 1455
  Wegener's, myositis in, 1455–1456, 1457f
Granulomatous neuropathy, 1913
Granzymes, 898
Grape-like nerve endings, 327f, 331
Ground substance, 471
Growth factors
  myoblast proliferation and, 19–20
  satellite cell cell cycle modulation in response to, 73–76
Growth hormone
  cellular actions of, 1714t
  protein turnover in muscle and, 548
Gruenstein-Hogness screening, 933, 934f
Guillain-Barré syndrome, myasthenia gravis versus, 1775t

Hansen's disease, myositis in, 1466
Hearing loss, in Duchenne muscular dystrophy, 977

Heart. See also Cardiomyopathy
  in Becker muscular dystrophy, 976
  in Becker muscular dystrophy carriers, 976
  in Bethlem myopathy, 1138–1139
  in Duchenne muscular dystrophy, 975–976
  in Duchenne muscular dystrophy carriers, 976
  in laminin α2 deficiency, 1212
  in mitochondrial encephalomyopathies, 1633
  in myotonic dystrophy, 1044, 1044t
  in nemaline myopathy, 1482
  in polymyositis/dermatomyositis, in adults, 1325
Heart failure, muscle microcirculation in, 529
Heat, myoglobinuria due to, 1682–1683
Heat-shock proteins
  exocytosis and, 339
  in polymyositis, 1355
  rimmed, 570
Helix-loop-helix proteins, 923
Hemopexin, serum, in dystrinopathies, 978
Hepatic disease, neuropathy with, 1916
Hepatic lipid metabolism, 1591
Hepatitic steatosis, lactic acidosis and myopathy with, 1413
Hepatitis C infection, 1394
Hereditary motor and sensory neuropathy, 1922
  axonal varieties of, 1922
  demyelinating varieties of, 1922, 1923f
Hereditary motor neuronopathies, 1856, 1856f
Hereditary sensory and autonomic neuropathies, 1923–1925, 1924t
Herpes zoster infection, neuropathy due to, 1906–1907
Heteroduplex analysis, 943
Heteroplasmy, 1628
  skewed, 1628, 1628t
Hexosaminidase A deficiency, 1852
Histidine-rich calcium-binding protein, 319
Histochemistry, of muscle fibers
  motor unit types and, 108–109, 109f
  muscle fiber diversity recognition by, 88f, 88–90, 89t
  pattern of fiber types and. See Muscle fibers, pattern of fiber types and

Histogenesis, fiber-type diversity related to, 96f–98f, 96–99
Histones, 917
History taking, 599–601
HIV infection. *See* Human immunodeficiency virus infection
HMG-CoA reductase inhibitors, myopathy due to, 1697
Homeobox, 923
Homeodomains, 923
Homeostasis, altered, myoglobinuria due to, 1683
Hormones. *See also* Endocrine disorders; Endocrine myopathies; *specific hormones*
   cellular actions of, 1713t, 1713–1715, 1714f, 1714t
      membrane receptors and, 1713–1714
      nuclear receptors and, 1715
   microcirculatory control by, 522
   microcirculatory remodeling and, 524
Hormone-sensitive lipase, 1590
Human coxsackie-adenovirus receptors, in human muscle tissue, 1390
Human foamy retrovirus infection, 1405
Human Genome Project, 934–935
Human immunodeficiency virus infection
   myositis and, 1396–1404
      clinical and histologic findings in, 1396t, 1396–1398, 1397f–1399f
      immunopathogenesis of, 1403f, 1403–1404
      incidence and natural history of, 1401
      inclusion body, 1398, 1400f
      motor neuron-like disorder and, 1401
      myasthenia gravis and, 1400
      myoglobinuria and, 1399–1400
      pathogenesis of, 1401
      pyomyositis and, 1400–1401
      subclinical neuromuscular involvement in, 1398–1399
      treatment of, 1404
      virological studies in, 1401–1403, 1402f
      wasting syndrome and, 1399, 1400f
   neuropathy and, 1909
Human leukocyte antigen, 1351
   myasthenia gravis associations with, 1760, 1763

Human T-cell lymphotropic virus type I myositis, 1404–1405, 1405f
Hunter disease, 573t, 585, 585f
Hurler disease, 573t, 584–585, 585f
Hurler-Scheie syndrome, 573t, 584–585, 585f
Hutchinson's posture, 1148
Hyaline body myopathy, 1508–1510
   clinical features of, 1509
   genetics of, 1510
   pathologic features of, 1509f, 1509–1510
Hyalinization, of muscle fiber, 697
Hyaluronate, in polymyositis/dermatomyositis, 1330
Hydatidosis, 1432–1434
   clinical manifestations of, 1433
   geographic location and, 1432–1433
   laboratory studies in, 1433–1434
   pathology of, 1434, 1434f
   transmission to humans, 1433
   treatment of, 1434
3-Hydroxyacyl-CoA dehydrogenase
   deficiency of, long-chain, 1604–1605, 1606
   mitochondrial β-oxidation and, 1594–1595
L-3-Hydroxyacyl-CoA dehydrogenase deficiency, short-chain, 1610
Hydroxychloroquine
   myopathy due to, 1699f, 1699–1700, 1700f
   toxicity of, electrodiagnostic studies in, 643
Hyperemia, functional, coordinated control of, 521–522, 522f
Hyperkalemic periodic paralysis, 1268–1269, 1269f, 1270f, 1273
   equine model of, 1280, 1280f
   with multiple sleep-onset periods of rapid eye movement, 1279
   secondary to sustained hyperkalemia, 1279–1280
   X-linked, 1279
Hyperparathyroidism, myopathy associated with, 1731–1733
Hypersensitivity myositis, 1456
Hypertension, muscle microcirculation in, 528
Hyperthermia, malignant. *See* Malignant hyperthermia
Hyperthyroidism
   association of myasthenia gravis with, 1761

   electrodiagnostic studies in, 642
   muscle pain associated with, 1742t
Hypertrophic cardiomyopathy, 1240, 1241f
   familial, sarcomere in, 161
   myosin mutations in, 181–182
Hypertrophy
   in clinical examination, 602
   compensatory
      lysosomal enzymes and, 569
      microcirculatory remodeling and, 524
Hypervitaminosis E, myopathy due to, 1697
Hypoaldosteronism, infantile, recessive, periodic paralysis secondary to hyperkalemia in, 1280
Hypokalemia, drug-induced, myoglobinuria due to, 1686
Hypokalemic myopathy, toxic, 1694t, 1698, 1705–1706, 1706f
Hypokalemic periodic paralysis, familial, 1280–1289, 1281f
   correlations between structural changes, electrolyte shifts, and clinical features in, 1284–1285
   electromyography in, 1282
   microscopy in, 1282, 1283f–1286f, 1284
   molecular diagnosis of, 1286–1287, 1287f
   pathogenesis of, 1288, 1288f
   provocative tests in, 1282, 1283f
   therapy for, 1288–1289
Hypoparathyroidism, myopathy associated with, 1733–1734
Hypopituitarism, myopathy associated with, 1730–1731
Hypothyroidism
   muscle pain associated with, 1742t
   myopathy associated with, 1727–1729
      clinical pattern in, 1727–1728
      electrodiagnostic evaluation in, 1728
      metabolic alterations in, 1728–1729
      structural alterations in, 1728
      treatment of, 1729
   myopathy in, electrodiagnostic studies in, 642
Hypoxia, microcirculatory remodeling and, 524

I band, 130f, 131
I-cell disease, type II, 574t, 581–582, 582f, 583f
Ice tests, in myasthenia gravis diagnosis, 1772
Imaging, 655t, 655–662
  general pathologic features and, 656, 656t, 657f–659f
  in inflammatory myopathy, 657–658, 660, 660f
  in metabolic myopathies and mitochondrial disorders, 660, 661f
  in muscular dystrophy, 657, 659f, 660f
  in neurogenic disorders, 661f, 661–662, 662f
  value of, 662
Immune cells
  adhesion and migration of, 899–900, 900t, 901f
  phenotypes and functions of, 1348–1349
  types of, 1351
Immune complexes, in dermatomyositis, 1351–1352
Immune neuropathy. See Peripheral neuropathy, infectious
Immune response
  afferent limb of
    in myasthenia gravis, 1762–1766
    in polymyositis/dermatomyositis, 1348–1351
  efferent limb of
    in myasthenia gravis, 1766–1772
    in polymyositis/dermatomyositis, 1351–1356
  innate, 889–891
    complement system and, 889–890, 890f
    natural killer cells and, 891
    pattern-recognition receptors and, 890–891
Immune-response genes, in Lambert-Eaton myasthenic syndrome, 1792
Immune system, 889–912
  autoimmune mechanisms and, 908
  cellular communication and, 899–907
    adhesion and migration of immune cells and, 899–900, 900t, 901f
    cytokines and chemokines in, 900, 902t–905t, 905–906

immunologic synapse and, 906–907, 907f
immunologic properties of cultured myoblasts and, 910f, 910–912
  adhesion and costimulatory molecule expression and, 911
  classic and nonclassic MHC molecule expression and, 910–911, 911t
  cytokine and chemokine secretion and, 911
  functional interaction with T cells and, 911–912
Immunity
  adaptive (specific), 891–898
    antibody- and cell-mediated cytotoxicity and, 898, 899f
    antigen-presenting cells and, 898
    antigen recognition by B cells and antibodies and, 891–893, 894f
    antigen recognition by T cells and, 893, 895f, 896f
    B and T lymphocytes and, 891, 892f, 893f
    cooperation between B and T cells and, 893–894
    thymus in, 895–898, 897f
  humoral, in dermatomyositis, 1351–1352
Immunologic synapse, 906–907, 907f
Immunotherapy
  for polymyositis/dermatomyositis, 1357
  therapeutic targets for, 908–910
    adhesion- and migration-related molecules as, 909
    costimulatory molecules as, 909
    cytokines and chemokines as, 909–910
    trimolecular complex as, 908–909
Inactivity, microcirculatory remodeling and, 524
Inclusion bodies, 716–717, 719f
Inclusion body myopathies
  autosomal dominant, with congenital joint contractures, ophthalmoplegia, and rimmed vacuoles, 1950
  hereditary, 1170t, 1178–1179, 1311–1319
    brain white matter disease and, 1313

    clinical features of, 1312t, 1312–1313
    controversies and future prospects for, 1318–1319
    definition of, 1311
    diagnosis and differential diagnosis of, 1317–1318
    electromyography in, 1314
    electron microscopy, 1316, 1316f, 1317f
    epidemiology of, 1314
    genetics of, 1314
    immunohistochemistry in, 1316
    inclusion body myopathy compared with, 1369
    inclusion criteria for, 1311–1312
    muscle biopsy in, 1314–1316, 1315f, 1316f
    nerve conduction studies in, 1314
    pathogenesis of, 1317
  sporadic, 1318
Inclusion body myositis, 717, 719f, 1367–1384
  adhesion molecules in, 1372
  clinical aspects of, 1367–1368
  congophilic deposits in, 1369, 1371f
  αB-crystallin expression in muscle fibers in, 1379, 1379f, 1380f, 1381
  cytoplasmic degradation in, ultrastructural features of, 838, 841, 841f
  demographic features of, 1367
  diagnosis of, 1382–1383
  differential diagnosis of, 1383
  disorders associated with, 1368
  electromyography in, 1368
  filamentous inclusions in, ultrastructural features of, 813, 814f, 815f, 815–816
  hereditary inclusion body myopathies compared with, 1369
  histochemical studies in, 1369, 1370f
  historical background of, 1367
  HLA associations in, 1368
  human immunodeficiency virus, 1398, 1400f
    pathogenesis of, 1401
  imaging studies in, 1368
  inflammatory cell phenotypes in, 1370–1371, 1372f
  laboratory studies in, 1368
  light microscopy in, 1368–1373

Inclusion body myositis (Cont.)
  matrix metalloproteinases in, 1371–1372
  microvasculature in, 1372
  mitochondrial abnormalities and DNA deletions in, 1369–1370
  muscle fiber nuclei in, ultrastructural features of, 762, 763f
  paraffin sections in, 1368–1373, 1369f
  paramyxovirus infection and, 1395
  pathogenesis of, 1381–1382
  peripheral nerves in, 1372–1373
  similarities with Alzheimer disease, 1376–1379
  therapy for, 1383–1384
  ultrastructural studies in, 1373–1376
    filamentous inclusions and, 1373f–1376f, 1373–1376
  virologic studies in, 1381
Industrial exposures, neuropathy caused by, 1919
Infarction, dystrophin deficiency and, 720–722, 722f–725f, 724
Infection(s). See also specific infections
  bacterial, muscle pain associated with, 1741t, 1742t
  myoglobinuria due to, 1687–1688
  parasitic, muscle pain associated with, 1741t, 1742t
  of peripheral nerves, 1899–1900
  viral. See Viral infections; specific viral infections
Infectious diseases
  amyotrophic lateral sclerosis and, 1880
  amyotrophic lateral sclerosis versus, 1874–1875
Infectious neuropathy, 1906–1909
  diphtheritic, 1907
  herpes zoster, 1906–1907
  in HIV infection, 1909
  in leprosy, 1907–1909
  in Lyme disease, 1909
Infiltration, of peripheral nerves, 1899, 1900f, 1901f
Inflammation
  in amyotrophic lateral sclerosis, 1880
  dystrophin deficiency and, 726–728, 728f–735f
  muscle spindle alterations and, 743
  in polymyositis/dermatomyositis, 1332–1333, 1334f
Inflammatory cells
  in dystrinopathies, 988–989, 989f
  phenotypes of, in inclusion body myopathy, 1370–1371, 1372f
Inflammatory demyelinating polyneuropathy, chronic, amyotrophic lateral sclerosis versus, 1874
Inflammatory demyelination, of peripheral nerves, 1899
Inflammatory myopathies
  electrodiagnostic studies in, 633–636
  microcirculatory remodeling and, 525
  muscle imaging in, 657–658, 660, 660f
  muscle pain associated with, 1742t
  toxic, 1695t, 1703–1704
Inflammatory polyganglionopathy, 1913
Influenza virus infection, myositis and, 1394–1395
Infrared optical trap, 199
Inherited neuropathy, 1919–1925
Inherited system atrophies, peripheral neuropathies associated with, 1921
Inner mitochondrial membrane, defects of, 1642–1643
Inserts, in cloning, 927–929, 928f
In situ hybridization, 943
Inspection
  of gait, 602–603
  at rest, 601
Insulin, protein turnover in muscle and, 547–548
Insulin-like growth factors
  for dystrophinopathies, 1011
  protein turnover in muscle and, 548–549
  satellite cell cycle modulation in response to, 74–75
Integrin(s), 449–451, 899–900, 900t
  α7, 457t
  deficiency of, congenital muscular dystrophy with, 1206t, 1230–1231
  functions of, 450–451
  general properties of, 449
  in limb-girdle muscular dystrophy, 1080t
  of skeletal muscle, 449–450
  upregulation of, for dystrophinopathies, 1010–1011
Integrin-cytoskeletal complexes, therapeutic uses of, 30
Intercellular communication, 899–907
  adhesion and migration of immune cells and, 899–900, 900t, 901f
  cytokines and chemokines in, 900, 902t–905t, 905–906
  immunologic synapse and, 906–907, 907f
Interferon alpha, myopathy due to, 1703
Interferon beta-1a, for inclusion body myositis, 1383
Intergenomic signaling, defects of, 1643–1645
Intermediate filament(s)
  in amyotrophic lateral sclerosis, 1878–1879
  desmin, 462, 462f
  developmental changes in, 56f, 56–57
  of skeletal muscle, 160f, 160–161
Intermediate filament network, of transverse connecting system, 444f, 444–445
Intracellular recording, 374, 374f
Intracranial compressive lesions, myasthenia gravis versus, 1775t
Intrafusal muscle fibers, 489, 493–494, 495f
Intramuscular injections, myopathy due to, 1695t, 1707–1708
Intranuclear rods, in nemaline myopathy, 1485, 1486f
Intravenous immunoglobulin
  for inclusion body myositis, 1383
  for myasthenia gravis, 1779
  for polymyositis/dermatomyositis, 1347
  for thyroid-associated ophthalmopathy, 1727
Introns, 920
Ion channels. See also specific ion channels
  action potential of skeletal muscle and. See Action potential, of skeletal muscle
  in myasthenia gravis, acetylcholine receptor antibody effects on, 1767
  resting potential of skeletal muscle and. See Resting potential, of skeletal muscle
  voltage-gated, essential for action potential, 214–224, 215f
  voltage-insensitive, setting resting potential, 204–209, 205f
Ipecac, myopathy due to, 1695t, 1701, 1701f, 1702f
Irradiation, total-body, for polymyositis/dermatomyositis, 1347

Isaacs syndrome. *See* Neuromyotonia
Ischemia
  microcirculatory remodeling and, 525–526, 527f
  muscle pain associated with, 1741t
  neuromuscular transmission safety factor and, 632
  of peripheral nerves, 1899, 1899f
Isoetharine, myositis due to, 1704
Isometric contraction, 191, 191f, 192f
  energetics of, 193–194
Isometric twitches, 191, 191f
Isotonic contraction, 194f, 194–195
  energetics of, 195–196
Iterative discharges, 625, 626f

Jansky-Bielschowsky disease, 574t, 579–581, 581f, 582f, 731–732, 739f
Jiggle, in single-fiber electromyography, 629
Jitter, in single-fiber electromyography, 628, 629f
Joint contractures
  congenital, proximal myopathy with ophthalmoplegia and, 1312–1313
  in congenital myopathies, 1523
Junctin, 316–317
Junctional folds, of postsynaptic region, 347, 348f–350f
Junctophilin, 317

Kearns-Sayre syndrome, 1645–1646
Kennedy syndrome, 1852, 1855t, 1858–1859, 1859f
  amyotrophic lateral sclerosis versus, 1878
3-Ketoacyl-CoA thiolase
  deficiency of, medium-chain, 1610
  mitochondrial β-oxidation and, 1594–1595
Ketoconazole, myositis due to, 1704
Knock-in mice, 946, 947f
Knockout mice, 946
Krabbe disease, 572t, 737
Kuf's disease, 574t, 579–581, 581f, 582f, 731–732, 739f
Kugelberg-Welander disease, 1847t, 1849f, 1849–1850, 1850f

Labetalol, myositis due to, 1704
Labile maintenance heat, 193
Lactate dehydrogenase deficiency, 1550–1551

Lactic acidosis, myopathy and hepatitic steatosis with, 1413
Lafora disease, 735, 1553
LAMA2 gene, in congenital muscular dystrophy, with laminin α2 deficiency, 1208–1209
Lambert-Brody syndrome, 1750
Lambert-Eaton–like syndrome, 1809, 1810f
Lambert-Eaton myasthenic syndrome, 1791–1798
  autoimmune pathogenesis of, 1793–1797
    animal studies of, 1793, 1794f, 1795f
    autonomic disorder and, 1793, 1797
    clinical evidence for, 1793
    synaptotagmin in, 1797
    tumor antigens in, 1797
    voltage-gated calcium channels as target antigens in, 1793, 1796f, 1797t
  autonomic features of, 1792
  diagnosis of, 1797
  disease associations of, 1792
  electrodiagnostic studies in, 645, 1792
  epidemiology of, 1791
  historical background of, 1791
  morphologic studies in, 1792
  pharmacologic studies in, 1792
  prognosis of, 1798
  somatic features of, 1791–1792
  treatment of, 1797–1798
Lambert-Eaton syndrome
  myasthenia gravis versus, 1775t
  neurotransmitter release in, 381
Lamellar body myositis, 1519f, 1519–1520
Lamin(s)
  α2, 457t
  A/C, in limb-girdle muscular dystrophy, 1080t, 1087
  defects in, cardiomyopathy due to, 1250
Lamina densa, 471, 473
Lamina rara, 473, 473f
Laminin(s)
  α2, partial deficiency of, 1109
  binding to dystroglycans, 459, 459f
  in limb-girdle muscular dystrophy, 1080t
  of synaptic basal lamina, 346–347
Laminin receptors, defects of, muscular dystrophies caused by, 463

Laminopathy, 1106–1108
  clinical features of, 1106–1107, 1107f
  diagnosis of, 1108
  genetics of, 1107–1108
  treatment of, 1108
LARGE
  in limb-girdle muscular dystrophy, 1081t
  mutation in, congenital muscular dystrophy caused by, 1225
Larsson-Linderholm syndrome, exercise pathophysiology in, 673–674, 674f
Laryngeal muscles, testing of, 603
Laser tweezers, 199
Latent period, 191
Late-onset distal myopathy, 1170t, 1172–1176
  laboratory findings in, 1173, 1173f
  molecular genetics of, 1172–1173
  molecular pathogenesis of, 1175–1176, 1186f
  muscle pathology in, 1173f–1175f, 1173–1175
  treatment and management of, 1176
Legionnaires' disease
  myoglobinuria due to, 1687
  myositis in, 1465
Lengthening, forced, lysosomal proteolysis and, 569
Length-tension curves, 191–193, 193f
Leprosy
  myositis in, 1466
  neuropathy in, 1907–1909
Leptomere formations, ultrastructural features of, 797, 798f
Leptospirosis, myositis in, 1467
Leucine
  as energy source, 538, 538f
  protein turnover in muscle and, 546–547
Leukapheresis, for polymyositis/dermatomyositis, 1347
Leukodystrophy
  globoid cell, 572t, 737
  metachromatic, 572t, 736–737
Leuprolide acetate, myopathy due to, 1703
Lever-arm hypothesis, 171–174, 173f, 188
  correlation between structural and kinetic states and, 172–174
Levodopa, myopathy due to, 1703
Libraries, 927
  complementary DNA, 930–932, 941f

Libraries (Cont.)
   genomic, 929f, 929–930, 930f
   screening, 933, 934f
Liddle syndrome, 1292
Light-chain domain, in cross-bridge cycle, 187, 188f, 188–190
Limb-girdle muscular dystrophy, 1077–1113, 1318
   autosomal dominant, 1103–1109
     with cardiac involvement, 1029, 1106–1109
     without cardiac involvement, 1104–1106
   autosomal recessive, 1089–1103
     calpainopathy, 1089–1091
     dysferlinopathy, 1091–1095
     fukutin-related proteinopathy, 1101–1102
     sarcoglycanopathies, 1095–1100
     telethoninopathy, 1100
     titinopathy, 1102–1103
     TRIM32-related dystrophy, 1100
   biochemistry and pathophysiology of, 1079, 1080t–1081t, 1082f, 1083–1088
     enzymes and, 1087–1088
     inner nuclear membrane proteins and, 1087
     plasma membrane proteins and, 1079, 1083–1086
     sarcomeric apparatus and, 1086–1087
   current concept of, 1077–1079, 1078t
   diagnostic workup in, 1110–1113
     clinical evaluation in, 1110–1112, 1111t
     muscle LGMD 1C, protein, and genetic studies in, 1112–1113
   disease entities in, 1088
   electrodiagnostic studies in, 639
   other muscular dystrophies presenting with phenotype of, 1109–1110
   spinal muscular atrophy versus, 1852
   type 2I, 1206t, 1222–1225
     clinical features of, 1223
     FKRP mutations causing, 1223f–1225f, 1223–1225
     gene and protein in, 1223
   type 1D, 1108–1109
   type 1E, 1105–1106
   type 1F, 1106
Limb-girdle myasthenia, familial, 1839
Limb morphogenesis, 36f, 36–37

Limb muscles
   progenitors of, 34, 36
   tendons and, patterning of, 37, 37f
Limit dextrinosis, 730, 738f
Linear scleroderma, 1327–1328
Linkage analysis, 944f, 944–945
Linkage disequilibrium, 944
Linked motor unit potentials, 627
Linkers, 931f, 932
Lipid, accumulation in muscle fibers, ultrastructural features of, 841, 842f
Lipid bodies, 716
Lipid-lowering agents, myoglobinuria due to, 1685
Lipid metabolism, 1588, 1590–1591
   fatty acid oxidation and, 1591–1596
     mitochondrial β-oxidation, 1592–1595, 1593f
     peroxisomal ω-oxidation, 1595–1596
     peroxisomal β-oxidation, 1595–1596
   fatty acid uptake, synthesis, and transport and, 1588, 1590
   homeostasis and, 1591
   in liver, 1591
   regulation of, 1590
   in skeletal muscle, 1590–1591
Lipid metabolism disorders, 1587–1614
   carnitine/acylcarnitine translocase deficiency, 1610
   carnitine palmitoyltransferase deficiency, 1601–1603
   Chanarin-Dorfman disease (multisystem triglyceride storage disease), 1612–1613, 1613f
   2,4-dienoyl-CoA reductase deficiency, 1610
   electrodiagnostic studies in, 641–642
   historical background of, 1587–1588, 1589t
   medium-chain acyl-CoA dehydrogenase deficiency, 1606–1607
   medium-chain 3-ketoacyl-CoA thiolase deficiency, 1610
   mitochondrial trifunctional protein deficiency, 1604–1606, 1605f, 1606f
   multiple acyl-CoA dehydrogenase deficiency, 1607–1609, 1609f
   muscle coenzyme Q_{10} deficiency, 1610–1612, 1611f
   myoglobinuria due to, 1680
   primary carnitine deficiency, 1600–1601

   short-chain acyl-CoA dehydrogenase deficiency, 1610
   short-chain L-3-hydroxyacyl-CoA dehydrogenase deficiency, 1610
   treatment of, 1613–1614
   very long chain acyl-CoA dehydrogenase deficiency, 1603–1604
Lipofuscin
   accumulation of, muscle fiber contour and, 702–703
   ultrastructural features of, 809–810, 810f
Lipogranulomatosis, Farber, 572t
Lipoprotein abnormalities, peripheral neuropathy associated with, 1920–1921
Lipoprotein receptors, in inclusion body myositis, 1378
Liposomal enzymes, delivery to autophagic vacuoles, 838
Liver, lipid metabolism in, 1591
Liver disease
   hepatitic steatosis, lactic acidosis and myopathy with, 1413
   hepatitis C, 1394
   neuropathy with, 1916
   LMNA gene, in Emery-Dreifuss muscular dystrophy, 1032
Long-chain 3-hydroxyacyl-CoA dehydrogenase deficiency, 1604–1605, 1606
Lower extremity muscles, testing of, 608t–609t
Lower motor neuron signs, in amyotrophic lateral sclerosis, 1866–1867
Luft disease, 1641–1642
Lungs, 137. See Respiratory entries
Lyme disease
   myositis in, 1467
   Neuropathy in, 1909
Lymphoid cell dystrophin promoter, 964
Lymphoma
   amyotrophic lateral sclerosis and, 1876
   neuropathies associated with, 1917–1918
Lymphoproliferative disease, neuropathies associated with, 1917–1918
Lysosomal enzymes, 565–566, 567t
   delivery to autophagic vacuoles, ultrastructural features of, 765

Man-6-P receptors and, 566–568
processing of, 566
synthesis of, 566
trafficking in skeletal muscle, 570
Lysosomal membrane proteins, 568
Lysosomal storage diseases, 570–592, 1900
acquired, 588, 589f, 590, 590f
clinical diagnosis of, 575
conditions simulating, 590, 590f, 591f, 592
genetics of, 571, 575
inherited, 576–588
laboratory diagnosis of, 575–576
muscle involvement in, 575
pathophysiology of, 570–571, 571t–574t
peripheral neuropathy associated with, 1920
treatment of, 576
Lysosomal storage myopathy, 1699–1701
Lysosome-associated membrane protein-2 deficiency, 574t, 586–587
Lysosome-associated proteins, in inclusion body myositis, 1377
Lysosomes, 565–592
concept of, 565–568, 566f
enzymes of. See Lysosomal enzymes
giant, in vitamin E deficiency, ultrastructural features of, 810, 811f
membrane proteins of, 568
proteolytic process in, 541–542
of skeletal muscle, 568–570

McArdle disease. See Phosphorylase deficiency
McLeod syndrome, 977–978
Macrophages
functions of, 1351
muscle fiber invasion and destruction by, ultrastructural features of, 846–851, 849f–853f
Macrophagic myofasciitis, 1450
Magnesium intoxication, myasthenia gravis versus, 1775t
Magnetic resonance imaging, 655, 656, 656t, 657f, 658f
Magnetic resonance spectroscopy, 655
energy metabolism and, 669–670, 670f, 671f
Maintenance heat, 193
Malaria, 1429–1430
myoglobinuria due to, 1687

Malignancies
amyotrophic lateral sclerosis and, 1876
cachexia associated with, protein metabolism and, 557–558
inherited, peripheral neuropathies associated with, 1921
Lambert-Eaton myasthenic syndrome association with, 1792
neuropathy with, 1917–1919
peripheral neuropathy with metabolic abnormalities and, 1920–1922
polymyositis and dermatomyositis associated with, 1326–1327
stiff-man syndrome and, 1746
Malignant hyperthermia, 1663–1673, 1682
anesthesia for patients susceptible to, 1667
association with central core disease, 1668
clinical presentation of, 1665–1666, 1666t
dantrolene as antidote to, 1663, 1666, 1666t
differentiation between malignant hyperthermia and central core disease mutants and, 1672f, 1672–1673
genetic basis for, 1668–1671
alternative loci and, 1669–1671
calcium release channel genes and, 1668, 1668f
guidelines for genetic determination of susceptibility and, 1669
linkage to RYR1 and, 1669, 1670t, 1671t
historical background of, 1663
incidence of, 1664
mortality associated with, 1664
physiologic basis for, 1671f, 1671–1673, 1672f
susceptibility to, evaluation of, 1667–1668
treatment of, 1666t, 1666–1667
triggering, 1664t, 1664–1665
Mandibular muscles, testing of, 604t
Manganese superoxide dismutase, in polymyositis/dermatomyositis, 1330
O-Mannose beta-1,2-N-acetylglucosaminyltransferase, in limb-girdle muscular dystrophy, 1081t

α-Mannosidosis, 573t, 583
β-Mannosidosis, 573t
O-Mannosyltransferase 1, in limb-girdle muscular dystrophy, 1081t
Marfan syndrome, arthrogryposis multiplex congenita and, 1952–1953
Markesbery-Griggs disease, 1170t, 1172–1176
laboratory findings in, 1173, 1173f
molecular genetics of, 1172–1173
molecular pathogenesis of, 1175–1176, 1186f
muscle pathology in, 1173f–1175f, 1173–1175
treatment and management of, 1176
Matrix metalloproteinases, 1350
in inclusion body myopathy, 1371–1372
Maxam-Gilbert chemical cleavage method, 938–939, 939f
mdx mice, 1001
Mechanical strength, extracellular matrix and, 477, 479
Medium-chain acyl-CoA dehydrogenase deficiency, 1606–1607
Medium-chain 3-ketoacyl-CoA thiolase deficiency, 1610
Membrane systems, 57–61, 232–254. See also Caveolae; Mitochondria; Plasma membrane; Sarcoplasmic reticulum; T tubule(s)
calcium release unit assembly and, 58f, 58–60, 59f
endoplasmic reticulum transition to sarcoplasmic reticulum and, 57–58
T tubule and membrane-to-myofibrillar linkage development and, 60f, 60–61, 61f
Mesenchymal disease, neuropathy with necrotizing vasculitis and, 1913–1914
Mesenchymal dysplasia syndrome, 1940
Mesoderm
formation in vertebrate embryos, 4, 5f
paraxial
formation in vertebrate embryos, 4–5, 6f
segmentation of, 6–8, 7f, 8f
specification of, 5–6

Metabolic bone disease, myopathy associated with, 1731–1733
Metabolic disorders
  amyotrophic lateral sclerosis versus, 1875
  electrodiagnostic studies in, 640–643, 641t
  inherited neuropathy with tumors and, 1920–1922
  myoglobinuria due to, 1681
Metabolic homeostasis, lipid metabolism and, 1591
Metabolic myopathies
  functional evaluation of, 665–677
    energy utilization in exercise and, 665–667, 666f, 666t, 667f
    in muscle energy defects, 673–677
    muscle metabolism in exercise and, 667–673, 668t
    rationale for, 665
  muscle imaging in, 660, 661f
  muscle pain associated with, 1742t
  muscle spasms associated with, 1748–1749
Metabolites, for mitochondrial encephalopathy, 1653
Metachromatic leukodystrophy, 572t, 736–737
Methotrexate
  for inclusion body myositis, 1383
  for polymyositis/dermatomyositis, 1345, 1346
3,4-Methylenedioxymeth-amphetamine, myoglobinuria due to, 1686–1687
Methylprednisone, for myasthenia gravis, 1777
Metolazone, myositis due to, 1704
Mexiletine, for sodium channel myotonias, 1278
Microangiopathy, toxic, 1695t
Microarray transcription analysis, 1350
Microcirculation, 511–529
  in diabetes, 528–529
  fine structure of blood vessels and, 515–518
  in heart failure, 529
  in hypertension, 528
  physiologic control of, 518–522
    capillary perfusion and recruitment and, 519
    conducted responses and cell-cell communication and, 521
    coordinated control of functional hyperemia and, 521–522, 522f
    endothelial, 520–521
    hormonal, 522
    metabolic, 520
    myogenic, 520
    nervous, 519
    site of, 518f, 518–519
  remodeling under pathologic conditions, 525–528
  remodeling under physiologic conditions, 522–524
    compensatory hypertrophy and, 524
    hormones and, 524
    hypoxia and, 524
    increased activity and, 522–524, 523f
    muscle inactivity and, 524
  vascular anatomy and, 511–515
    macroscopic structure and, 511
    microscopic structure and, 511–514, 512f, 513t, 514f
    in muscle spindles, 515, 515t
    nutritive and nonnutritive flow and flow heterogeneity and, 514–515
Microladder formations.
  See Leptomere formations
Microsomal ω-oxidation, 1596
Microsporidiosis, 1427–1429
  clinical features of, 1428
  geographic location and, 1427
  laboratory studies in, 1428
  pathology of, 1428–1429
  transmission to humans, 1428
  treatment of, 1429
Microtubules, 451
  developmental changes in, 56f, 56–57
Microvascular alterations, ultra-structural features of, 874–879
  amyloid infiltration, 879, 879f–881f
  of basal lamina, 875f, 875–876, 876f
  of capillaries, 876–877, 877f, 878f
  of endothelial cells, 877, 877f, 878f, 879
Microvasculature
  in inclusion body myopathy, 1372
  injury of, in dermatomyositis, 1352
  of muscles, in Duchenne muscular dystrophy, 996–997
Microvasculitis, neuropathy with, 1914
Miller-Fisher syndrome, myasthenia gravis versus, 1775t
Miniature end plate potentials, 621
Minisatellite repeats, 945
Misoprostol, arthrogryposis multiplex congenita and, 1948
Missense mutations, 924
Mitochondria
  disorders of
    muscle imaging in, 660
    myoglobinuria due to, 1680–1681
  genetics of, 925–926
  in inclusion body myopathy, 1369–1370
  motility of, defects of, 1643
  positioning of, 242, 245f
  ultrastructural reactions of, 776, 778f–784f, 778–782
Mitochondrial encephalomyopathies, 1623–1655
  acquired defects and, 1651–1652
    age-related, 1652
    iatrogenic, 1651–1652
    toxic, 1651
  biochemical studies in, 1633–1634, 1634f
  brain pathology in, 1633
  clinical heterogeneity of, 1629, 1630t
  epidemiology of, 1654–1655
  genetic counseling for, 1654
  genetics of, 1625–1629, 1626f
    genetic testing and, 1629
    Mendelian, 1625–1626, 1626t
    mitochondrial, 1626–1628, 1627f
    myopathies and, 1628, 1628t
  historical background of, 1623, 1624f, 1625
  laboratory studies in, 1635
  mitochondrial DNA mutations and, 1645–1651
    point mutations in tRNA genes, 1647–1649
    protein-coding gene mutations, 1649–1651, 1650t
    sporadic large-scale rearrangements, 1645–1647, 1646t
  muscle pathology in, 1629–1633, 1631f, 1632f
  nuclear DNA mutations and, 1635–1645
    electron transport chain defects, 1635–1641, 1636t, 1637t, 1639f, 1640f
    inner membrane lipid milieu defects, 1642–1643
    intergenomic signaling defects, 1643–1645, 1644t
    mitochondrial motility defects, 1643

oxidation/phosphorylation
coupling defects, 1641–1642
protein importation disorders, 1642
translocase disorders, 1642
physiologic aspects of, 1634–1635
therapy for, 1652–1654
Mitochondrial encephalomyopathy, lactic acidosis, and stroke-like episodes, 1648–1649
Mitochondrial function, disorders of, electrodiagnostic studies in, 642
Mitochondrial myopathies, 1628, 1628t
congenital, arthrogryposis multiplex congenita and, 1951
myasthenia gravis versus, 1775t
reverse genetics in, 954
toxic, 1696–1697
Mitochondrial β-oxidation, 1592–1595, 1593f
Mitochondrial trifunctional protein, mitochondrial β-oxidation and, 1594–1595
Mitochondrial trifunctional protein deficiency, 1604–1606, 1605f, 1606f
Mitogen, satellite cell cycle modulation in response to, 75f, 75–76
Mitogenic growth factors, cell-cycle regulation of myoblast differentiation and, 18–19, 19f
Mitotic segregation, 1628
Mitoxantrone, myositis due to, 1704
Mitsugumin, 317
Mixed connective tissue disease
myositis and, 1329–1330
pathologic features of, 1343
Miyoshi myopathy, 1170t, 1176–1178, 1177f, 1178f
M line, 130f, 131, 143–145
function of, 145
model of, 144–145
protein components and interactions of, 143–144
structure of, 143, 143f, 144f
MM creatine kinase, 132t
Möbius syndrome, arthrogryposis multiplex congenita and, 1938
Modulus of elasticity, 197
Molecular biology, 915–955.
See also Molecular genetics; specific conditions
DNA mutations and, 924f, 924–925
future prospects for, 954–955
genes and gene structure and, 918, 919f, 920

mitochondrial genetics and, 925–926
of muscle, 946–950
muscle-specific gene regulation and, 946–948
muscle-specific genes and, 948, 949t–950t, 950
nucleic acid and chromosome structure and, 915, 916f–918f, 917–918
regulation of gene expression and, 921–924, 922f, 923f
RNA transcription and translation and, 920–921, 921f
tools of, 926–946
cloning as. See Cloning
enzymology of DNA and RNA as, 926f, 926–927
Molecular genetics, 950–954, 951t–952t.
See also specific conditions
forward, 950–953
future prospects for, 954–955
of mitochondrial myopathies, 954
reverse, 953–954
Monoclonal gammopathies, of undetermined significance, neuropathy associated with, 1918–1919
Monomelic amyotrophy
amyotrophic lateral sclerosis versus, 1873
benign, 1857, 1857f
Mononeuropathy, 1906
inflammatory, 1912
motor, multifocal, with persistent conduction block, 1912
multiple, 1906
inflammatory, 1912
Mononucleated cells
in dermatomyositis, immunophenotype analysis of, 1352
multinucleated muscle fiber formation from, 45–49, 48f–50f
Monoradiculopathy, inflammatory, 1912
Morphea, 1327
Morquio disease, 573t
Morvan fibrillary chorea, 1747
Mosaic fibers, congenital myopathy with interlacing sarcomeres and, 1515–1516, 1516f
Mosaicisms, in dystrophinopathies, 968–969
Motor mononeuropathy, multifocal, with persistent conduction block, 1912

Motor nerves, satellite cell activity and, 79
Motor neuron(s)
fiber type modulation by, 99
firing rate of, motor unit force gradation by, 113f, 113–115, 114f
properties of, interrelations with motor unit properties, 111
Motor neuron diseases, 1865–1882.
See also Amyotrophic lateral sclerosis
neurodiagnostic studies in, 647
segmental, amyotrophic lateral sclerosis versus, 1873
Motor neuron-like disorders, human immunodeficiency virus and, 1401
Motor neuropathies
hereditary, 1872, 1922–1925
multifocal, with conduction block, amyotrophic lateral sclerosis versus, 1874
Motor nuclei, anatomy of, 104–105
Motor unit(s), 104–115, 105f, 115f
in action, 111–115
force gradation by motor neuron firing rate and, 113f, 113–115, 114f
interrelations with motor neurons, 111
mechanisms controlling muscle output and, 111
recruitment control and, 112f, 112–113
anatomy of, 105–106, 106f
force output and innervation ratios of, 110, 110f
in human muscle, 110–111
motor nuclei and, 104–105
muscle architecture and, 105, 106f
physiologic properties of, 106–110, 107f
pools of, 112–113
types of
development of, 109–110
identification of, 107, 107f, 108f
muscle fiber histochemistry and, 108–109, 109t
Motor unit potentials
parasite (linked; satellite), 627
polyphasic, 627
spontaneous
abnormal, 623f, 623–625, 624t, 626–628
normal, 620f, 620–621

Motor unit potentials *(Cont.)*
  voluntary potentials, normal, 621–623, 622f, 623f
M protein, 132t
  of M line, 143–144
mRNA
  acetylcholinesterase, expression and localization of, 428
  dystrophin, 962
mtDNA
  mutations in, mitochondrial encephalopathy due to, 1652
  mutations of, disorders due to, 1645–1651, 1646t, 1650t
mtDNA depletion syndromes, 1644–1645
Mucolipidosis
  type I, 573t
  type II, 574t, 581–582, 582f, 583f
  type III, 574t, 581–582, 582f, 583f
  type IV, 572t, 582–583, 583f
Mucopolysaccharidoses, 732
  type I, 573t, 584–585, 585f
  type II, 573t, 585, 585f
  type III, 573t, 585f, 585–586
  type IVA, 573t
  type IX, 573t
  type VI, 573t, 586
  type VII, 573t
Multicore formations, ultrastructural features of, 816, 817f–822f
Multicores, 708–709, 709f–711f
Multifocal motor mononeuropathy, with persistent conduction block, 1912
Multiminicore disease, 1495–1502
  clinical features of, 1496f, 1496–1497
  differential diagnosis of, 1501–1502
  genetics of, 1501
  investigations in, 1497
  pathologic features of, 1497, 1498f–1500f, 1499, 1501
Multinucleated muscle fibers, formation from mononucleated cells, 45–49, 48f–50f
Multiple acyl-CoA dehydrogenase deficiency, 1607–1609, 1609f
Multiple mononeuropathy, 1906
  inflammatory, 1912
Multiple myeloma, neuropathies associated with, 1918
Multiple sulfatase deficiency, 572t
Multisystem triglyceride storage disease, 1612–1613, 1613f
Munc13, exocytosis and, 338

Munc18, exocytosis and, 338
Murine, dystrophinopathy, 1001
Muscle, congenital absence of, 1957
Muscle action potentials, compound, in nerve conduction studies, 630–631, 631f
Muscle architecture, 105, 106f
Muscle atrophy
  in clinical examination, 601–602
  muscle fiber diameter and, 696
  postpoliomyelitis, 1852
  process of, 558
  progressive, 1846
  protein metabolism and, 554–555
Muscle biopsy, 681–688.
  See also specific conditions
  in Emery-Dreifuss muscular dystrophy, 1030
  histopathologic study of, 691
  muscle selection for, 681
  procedure for, 682f, 682–683
  processing specimens for, 683–688
    biochemical studies for, 688
    cryostat sections for, 683f, 683–685, 684t–686t
    electron microscopy for, 685–688, 687f
    immunoblot analysis for, 688
    molecular genetic studies for, 688
    paraffin sections for, 683
    semithin resin sections for, 685
Muscle coenzyme Q_{10} deficiency, 1610–1612, 1611f
Muscle contraction
  calcium in. *See* Calcium, in muscle contraction
  cross-bridge cycle and. *See* Cross-bridge cycle
  isometric. *See* Isometric contraction
  sliding filaments and, 133–134, 134f
Muscle contractures, 1744
  congenital muscular dystrophy with, 1226, 1230
  electrically silent, 600
  metabolic, 1748–1749
  neurodiagnostic studies in, 647
Muscle dystrophin promoter, 963
Muscle enhancer binding factor 2, muscle-specific promoters and, 24–25
Muscle-eye-brain disease, 1206t, 1218–1220, 1226
  clinical features of, 1219f, 1219–1220, 1220f

  gene and protein in, 1219, 1219f
  prevalent in Italy, 1226
Muscle fiber(s)
  amyloid deposition in, 728–729
  atrophy of, myogenic, ultrastructural features of, 828–829, 832f–835f, 836
  cell-mediated injury of
    animal models of, 1356
    in vitro models of, 1355–1356
  central migration of subsarcolemmal nuclei and, 697, 697f
  central nuclei of, in dystrophinopathies, 986
  contour changes in, 697–717
    angulated fibers and, 710, 713f
    central cores and, 707–708, 708f
    cytoplasmic bodies and, 703–704, 706f
    delta or wedge-shaped lesions and, 698–699, 701f
    within fasciculi, 702
    fingerprint bodies and, 710–711, 714f
    inclusion bodies and, 716–717, 719f
    inclusions in myofibrillar myopathy and, 705
    lipofuscin and ceroid accumulation and, 702–703
    lobulated fibers and, 703, 705f
    moth-eaten fibers and, 703, 706f
    multicores and, 708–709, 709f–711f
    necrosis and, 697, 698f–700f
    ragged red fibers and, 712–714, 715f
    reducing bodies and, 711
    regeneration and, 699, 701, 704f
    ringbinden and, 703, 705f
    rod body formation and, 707, 707f, 708f
    sarcoplasmic masses and, 703, 705f
    splitting or branching and, 699, 702f, 703f
    target fibers and, 710, 712f
    trilaminar configurations and, 711–712
    tubular aggregates and, 712, 714f
    vacuoles and, 714–716, 716f–719f
    Z-band streaming and, 704–705, 706f
  contour of, necrosis and, 697, 698f–700f
  cytoskeleton of. *See* Cytoskeleton

diameter of, in polymyositis/
dermatomyositis, 1332
diameters of, 696
disproportion of types of.
See Fiber-type disproportion
diversity of types of, 87–101
in allotypical muscles, 92
demonstration by contractile
protein isoforms, 91–92
emergence of, muscle histogenesis
related to, 96f–98f, 96–99
fiber type correlation with myosin
heavy-chain isoforms and, 91,
92f
histochemical recognition of, 88f,
88–90, 89t
model for, 92–94, 93f
myosin heavy-chain isoform
recognition of, 90
origins of, 94
physiological property recognition
of, 90–91
stages of muscle specialization
and, 94–101
synaptogenesis and, 100
dystrophin deficiency and.
See Dystrophin(s), deficiency of
enzymatic deficiencies and, 729–740.
See also specific disorders
extrafusal, 489
of extraocular muscles, 120–121,
121t
fast, specification of, 94–96
histochemistry of
analysis of, 691–696
distribution in of types
dystrophinopathies, 984–985
motor unit types and, 108–109,
109f
hypercontracted, in
dystrophinopathies, 986, 988
intrafusal, 489, 493–494, 495f
lobulated, 703, 705f
loss of, dystrophin deficiency and,
720
modulation of types by motor neurons, 99
moth-eaten, 703, 706f
muscle spindle alterations and,
740–743, 741f
necrosis of, 851–852, 856–858
central fiber, 858
contour and, 697, 698f–700f
in dystrophinopathies, 980–981,
981f–984f, 982, 984

ultrastructural features of, 852,
854f–857f, 856, 858
nonnecrotic, calcium-loaded, in
dystrophinopathies, 988
nucleus of, ultrastructural reactions
of, 758–762, 759f–761f, 763f
pattern of fiber types and, 691–694,
692f, 693f, 693t
differentiation into mosaic pattern
and, 692–693
fiber-type predominance and, 693,
694f
normal predominance of fiber
type and, 693
reinnervation and fiber-type
grouping and, 694, 695f
selective fiber-type involvement
and, 694
predominance of types of, in
arthrogryposis multiplex
congenita, 1933, 1933f
size of, in dystrophinopathies,
985–986, 986f, 987f
slow
signal transduction pathways
and expression of, 100–101
specification of, 94–95
typing of, in nemaline myopathy,
1485–1486
ultrastructural reactions of.
See Ultrastructural studies
Muscle gene regulatory regions,
therapeutic applications of,
28–29
Muscle hypertrophy, protein
metabolism and, 554–555
Muscle injury, stimulation of satellite
cell activation and proliferation
by, 78
Muscle length, protein metabolism
and, 555–556
Muscle metabolism, in exercise. See
Exercise, muscle metabolism in
Muscle overuse, satellite cell activation
produced by, 79–80
Muscle pain, 1739–1744
differential diagnosis of,
1741t–1742t, 1743–1744
epidemiology of, 1739, 1739t
in exertional myalgia, 600,
1740–1741, 1741t, 1742t
in fibromyalgia and tension
myalgia, 1741, 1743
pathogenesis of, 1739–1740, 1740f,
1740t

referred, 1741t
at rest, 600
Muscle progenitors
of limb muscles, 34, 36
migration to anatomic sites, 30–31, 31f
specification of
of body muscle progenitors, 8–9,
9f, 10f
developmental signals for, 10–12
of head muscle progenitors, 9–10,
11f
MRF transcription factors for,
12–14, 13f
signaling and transcriptional
networks and, 14f–16f, 14–17
Muscle regeneration. See Regeneration
Muscle regulatory element, 947
Muscle spindles, 489–505, 490f
alterations of, 740–743, 741f
agenesis and, 743
in congenital myopathies, 742
denervation and, 740–741
inflammation and, 743
in myotonic dystrophy, 742–743
regeneration and, 741–742
autonomic innervation of, 499
capsule of, 492
development of, 503–505
organogenesis and innervation
and, 503–504, 504f, 505f
trophic and transcription factors
and, 504–505
distribution of, 492
excess of, 742f, 743
myopathy with, 1520, 1520f
intrafusal fibers of, 493–494
microcirculation in, 515, 515t
motor innervation of, 496–499
β innervation and, 497–498
γ innervation and, 496–497, 497t
pattern of, 498–499, 499f
number of, 491
as receptor, 499–503
functional organization of sensory
terminals and, 502–503
input-output conversion and, 502
input-output properties and,
499–500, 500f, 501f, 502
sensory innervation of, 494–496
number of different axons and,
495–496, 496f
primary endings and, 494, 495f
secondary endings and, 495
types of, 491
vascular supply of, 492–493

Muscle stem cells, for Emery-Dreifuss muscular dystrophy, 1035
Muscle strain, muscle pain associated with, 1741t
Muscle stretch reflexes, testing of, 613–614
Muscle weakness
  in amyotrophic lateral sclerosis, therapy for, 1881
  cold-induced, in paramyotonia congenita, 1267f–1269f, 1267–1268, 1272–1273
  in myotonic dystrophy, 1040, 1040t, 1041f
  proximal, progressive, in hereditary inclusion body myositis, 1313
  transient, in myotonia congenita, evaluation of, 1260–1261, 1261f
Muscular dystrophies. *See also* Dystrophinopathies; *specific types of muscular dystrophy*
  congenital. *See* Congenital muscular dystrophies
  costamere protein defects and, 463–464
  diagnosis of, monoclonal antibodies in, 719, 720t
  distal, electrodiagnostic studies in, 640, 640t
  dystrophin bold defects and, 463–464
  electrodiagnostic studies in, 639–640
  extracellular matrix defects and, 463
  extraocular muscles in, 125
  laminin receptor defects and, 463
  microcirculatory remodeling and, 525
  muscle imaging in, 657, 659f, 660f
  muscle pain associated with, 1742t
  myotonic, arthrogryposis multiplex congenita and, 1950
  oculopharyngeal
    electrodiagnostic studies in, 640
    muscle fiber nuclei in, ultrastructural features of, 762
    myasthenia gravis versus, 1775t
  oropharyngeal. *See* Oropharyngeal muscular dystrophy
  proteins responsible for, in transverse fixation system, 462–464
  spinal muscular atrophies versus, 1852
Mutagenesis, site-directed, 943
Mutations
  of DNA, 924f, 924–925
  of dystrophin genes. *See* Dystrophin gene, mutations of

Myalgia. *See* Muscle pain
Myasthenia
  congenital, with end plate acetylcholinesterase deficiency, 431
  limb-girdle, familial, 1839
Myasthenia gravis, 1755–1781
  acquired, electrodiagnostic studies in, 644–645
  afferent limb of immune response and, 1762–1766
    HLA associations and, 1763
    loss of self-tolerance and, 1762–1763
    penicillamine-induced myasthenia gravis and, 1763
    T- and B-lymphocyte responses and, 1765–1766
    thymus gland and, 1763–1765
  antibody-mediated autoimmune response to muscle acetylcholine receptors in, 413–414
  arthrogryposis multiplex congenita caused by maternal antibodies inhibiting fetal acetylcholine receptors and, 1759
  classification of, 1759–1760
  clinical features of, 1758
  definition of, 1755, 1756f
  diagnosis of, 1772–1774
    antibody tests in, 1773–1774
    anticholinesterase drug effects and tests in, 1772
    electromyography in, 1772–1773
    immunocytochemical studies in, 1774
    provocative tests for, 1772
  differential diagnosis of, 1774–1776, 1775t
  disease associations of, 1760–1761
  drugs with adverse effects on, 1781
  efferent limb of immune response and, 1766–1772
    acetylcholine receptor antibody properties and, 1766–1767
    pathogenic effects of acetylcholine receptor antibodies and, 1767, 1768f, 1769–1772
  end plate region in, 390f, 390–391
  epidemiology of, 1757–1758
  experimental autoimmune, immunosuppressive therapies for, 415–416
  experimental autoimmune myasthenia gravis and, 1761–1762, 1762f–1764f
  extraocular muscles in, 125

  fulminating, therapy for, 1780
  genetic aspects of, 1757–1758
  historical background of, 1755–1757
    autoimmune etiology and, 1757
    early clinical observations and, 1755
    electrophysiologic studies and, 1757
    therapeutic approaches and, 1755, 1757
  human immunodeficiency virus and, 1400
  in infants and children, 1759
  maternal, arthrogryposis multiplex congenita and, 1951
  mild, therapy for, 1780
  muscle-specific kinase autoantibody association of, 1758
  natural course of, 1758–1759
  neonatal, transient, 1759
    electrodiagnostic studies in, 645
    therapy for, 1780
  ocular, therapy for, 1780
  pathogenesis of, 1761–1772
  in pregnancy, therapy for, 1780
  seronegative, therapy for, 1780–1781
  severe, therapy for, 1780
  therapy for, 1776–1781
    anticholinesterase drugs in, 1776t, 1776–1777
    azathioprine in, 1778
    corticosteroids in, 1777–1778
    cyclophosphamide in, 1778
    cyclosporine in, 1778
    experimental approaches for, 1781
    four different grades and types of myasthenia gravis, 1780–1781
    intravenous immunoglobulin in, 1779
    mycophenolate mofetil in, 1778–1779
    plasmapheresis in, 1779
    thymectomy in, 1779–1780
Myasthenic crisis, therapy for, 1780
Myasthenic syndromes. *See* Congenital myasthenic syndromes; Lambert-Eaton syndrome
MyBP-C, 132t
MyBP-H, 132t
Mycobacterium avium-intracellulare myositis, 1465
Mycophenolate mofetil
  for inclusion body myositis, 1384
  for myasthenia gravis, 1778–1779
  for polymyositis/dermatomyositis, 1346

Myeloma
   neuropathies associated with, 1918
   osteosclerotic, neuropathies associated with, 1918
Myelomeningocele, with central nervous system dysgenesis, arthrogryposis multiplex congenita and, 1942f, 1942–1944, 1943f
Myf5 gene, signaling and transcriptional networks for, 14f–16f, 14–17
Myf5 protein, myoblast proliferation and differentiation and, 20
Myoadenylate deaminase deficiency, 740, 741f
Myoblasts, 701. *See also* Satellite cells
   cultured, immunologic properties of, 910f, 910–912
      adhesion and costimulatory molecule expression and, 911
      classic and nonclassic MHC molecule expression and, 910–911, 911t
      cytokine and chemokine secretion and, 911
      functional interaction with T cells and, 911–912
   differentiation of, 18–20
   transfer of, for dystrinopathies, 1009
Myoclonic epilepsy
   with ragged red fibers, 1647–1648
   spinal muscular atrophy with, 1861
Myocytes
   differentiation of, 20–27
      control elements for muscle-specific promoters and enhancers and, 22–26
      muscle-specific promoters and enhancers and, 21–22, 22f
      myoblast specific transcriptional control elements and, 26
      transcriptional control of contractile protein genes and, 20–21
      transgenic analysis of skeletal muscle control elements and, 26–27
   fusion of, 32f, 32–33
MyoD gene, signaling and transcriptional networks for, 14f–16f, 14–17
MyoD protein, myoblast proliferation and differentiation and, 20
Myoedema, 613, 614f

Myofascial pain syndrome, 1739
Myofasciitis, macrophagic, 1450
Myofibril(s), 187
   aberrant, ultrastructural features of, 795–797, 796f
   annular, 703, 705
      ultrastructural features of, 795, 795f
   assembly of, 49–50, 51f–54f, 52–55
   cytoskeleton and, 55f, 55–56
   lysis in type 1 fibers, ultrastructural features of, 797
   membrane linkage to, 60, 61f
   ultrastructural reactions of, 795–797, 796f
Myofibrillar myopathies, 1187–1200
   cardiomyopathy in, 1251
   clinical features of, 1187–1188
   αB-crystallinopathy subset of, 1188
   desminopathy subset of, 1188
   diagnosis of, 1200
   disease mechanisms in, 1199t, 1199–1200
   frozen sections in, 1188, 1189f, 1190
   historical background of, 1187
   immunocytochemical features of, 1190
   inclusions in, 705
   molecular genetics of, 1191, 1195–1199, 1198f
   myotilinopathy subset of, 1188
   with sarcoplasmic bodies, 1170t
   therapy, 1200
   ultrastructural features of, 799, 801, 803f–807f, 1191, 1192f–1198f
Myofibrillar proteins, renewal within muscle cells, 57
Myofibrillogenesis, 49–56
Myofibrils, aberrant, 795–797, 796f
Myogenesis
   extracellular matrix and, 479
   regulators of
      global, 17–18
      in invertebrate embryos, 17–18
      MyoD-related, 18
   of skeletal muscles, 3–37
      building muscle anatomy and, 30–37
      mesoderm and skeletal muscle progenitor specification and, 4–18
      molecular control of muscle differentiation and, 18–30
Myogenic atrophy
   dystrophin deficiency and, 726, 727f

   ultrastructural features of, 828–829, 832f–835f, 836
Myogenic cells
   determination of, 94
   satellite cell development from, 68–69
   satellite cell differences from, 70, 70f
Myogenic regulatory factors
   muscle progenitor specification and, 12–14, 13f
   muscle-specific promoters and, 23–24
Myoglobin, 1677–1678
   function of, 1678
   in polymyositis/dermatomyositis, 1330
   structure of, 1677
Myoglobinemia, serum, in dystrophinopathies, 978
Myoglobinuria, 1678–1689
   acquired causes of, 1681–1688
      altered homeostasis as, 1683
      crush syndrome as, 1683–1684
      drugs and myotoxins as, 1684t, 1684–1687
      extreme exercise as, 1681–1682
      infectious, 1687–1688
      temperature extremes as, 1682–1683
   clinical syndrome of, 1678
   complications of, 1688–1689
   definition of, 1678
   human immunodeficiency virus and, 1399–1400
   inherited causes of, 1680–1681
   laboratory evaluation of, 1678–1679
   myositis with, 1413
   pathophysiology of, 1679t, 1679–1680
   toxic, 1693, 1694t
   treatment of, 1688–1689
Myokymia, 617
   focal, 1303
   neurodiagnostic studies in, 646
Myokymic discharges, 625, 626f
Myomesin, 132t
   of M line, 143–144
Myonecrosis
   Aeromonas hydrophila, 1464
   cellulitis associated with, 1464–1465
   clostridial, 1464
   peptostreptococcal, 1465
   streptococcal, 1464–1465
   Vibrio vulnificus, 1464

Myonuclei, replacement of, from satellite cells, 76
Myopalladin, 132t
　of Z line, 158
Myopathies
　amyloid, electrodiagnostic studies in, 636
　amyotrophic lateral sclerosis versus, 1874
　AZT-associated, 1406–1413, 1407t, 1408f–1411f
　　experimental induction of AZT toxicity and, 1409, 1411f, 1412f
　　management of, 1409, 1413
　　mechanism of, 1407, 1409
　brain white matter disease and, 1313
　centronuclear, 1490–1491, 1494–1495
　　clinical features of, 1494
　　differential diagnosis of, 1495
　　genetics of, 1495
　　pathologic features of, 1494–1495, 1495f, 1496f
　in complex I deficiency, 1649–1650, 1650t
　in complex III deficiency, 1650
　in complex IV deficiency, 1650–1651
　congenital, 1473–1524, 1524, 1524t, 1525t
　　with apoptotic changes, 1516–1517, 1517f
　　broad A-band disease, 1518f, 1518–1519
　　cap disease, 1517–1518
　　central core disease, 1475f–1478f, 1475–1480
　　centronuclear, 1486f, 1494–1495, 1495f
　　core-rod, 1489–1490
　　cylindrical spirals, 1508, 1508f
　　definitions and basic concepts of, 1473–1475, 1474t
　　electrodiagnostic studies in, 640, 641t
　　fiber-type disproportion, 1502f, 1502–1503, 1503t
　　fingerprint body, 1503–1505, 1504f
　　with hexagonally cross-linked tubular arrays, 1514f, 1514–1515
　　hyaline body (myosin storage), 1508–1510, 1509f
　　lamellar body, 1519f, 1519–1520
　　monitoring of, 1521, 1521t–1522t
　　with mosaic fibers and interlacing sarcomeres, 1515–1516, 1516f
　　multiminicore disease, 1495–1502, 1496f, 1498f–1500f
　　muscle pain associated with, 1742t
　　muscle spindle alterations and, 742
　　with muscle spindle excess, 1520, 1520f
　　myotubular/centronuclear, 1490–1491
　　nemaline. See Nemaline myopathy
　　poorly defined, 1515
　　prenatal diagnosis of, 1520–1521
　　prevention of, 1520–1521
　　reducing body, 1512, 1513f
　　risk management and, 1521, 1523
　　sarcotubular, 1510–1512, 1511f
　　treatment of, 1523–1524
　　trilaminar, 1519
　　with tubular aggregates, 1505–1507, 1506f, 1507f
　　X-linked, myotubular, 1491f, 1491–1494, 1492f
　　zebra body, 1515, 1515f
　critical illness, electrodiagnostic studies in, 643–644
　cytoplasmic body, 704
　desmin intermediate filament defects causing, 464
　distal, 1313, 1318
　　childhood-onset, 1313
　　cytoplasmic degradation in, ultrastructural features of, 838, 841, 841f
　　filamentous inclusions in, ultrastructural features of, 813, 814f, 815f, 815–816
　endocrine. See Endocrine myopathies
　end plate, acetylcholinesterase blockade and, 430, 431f
　feline immunodeficiency virus, 1406
　focal, electrodiagnostic studies in, 643
　human foamy retrovirus, 1405
　inflammatory
　　electrodiagnostic studies in, 633–636
　　microcirculatory remodeling and, 525
　　muscle imaging in, 657–658, 660, 660f
　　muscle pain associated with, 1742t
　　toxic, 1695t, 1703–1704
　lactic acidosis and hepatitic steatosis with, 1413
　lysosomal storage, 1699–1701
　metabolic. See Metabolic myopathies
　mitochondrial, 1628, 1628t
　　congenital, arthrogryposis multiplex congenita and, 1951
　　myasthenia gravis versus, 1775t
　　reverse genetics in, 954
　　toxic, 1696–1697
　myofibrillar. See Myofibrillar myopathies
　necrotizing, acute, 1704–1705, 1705f, 1706f
　nemaline. See Nemaline myopathy
　neuromyopathies
　　with bulbar weakness, in hereditary inclusion body myositis, 1313
　　neurodiagnostic studies in, 648, 648t
　nonmetabolic, myoglobinuria due to, 1681
　nutritional deficiencies causing, 1708–1709
　oculopharyngodistal, 1313
　proximal, with ophthalmoplegia and congenital contractures, 1312–1313
　quadriceps-sparing, 1312
　rod body, 707, 707f, 708f
　sarcoid, 1452–1454, 1453f, 1454f
　　electrodiagnostic studies in, 636
　simian immunodeficiency virus, 1405–1406
　simian retrovirus type I, 1405, 1406f
　toxic. See Toxic myopathies
　traumatic, electrodiagnostic studies in, 643
　with tubular aggregates, muscle pain associated with, 1742t
　vacuolar, 714, 715–716
Myophosphorylase deficiency, type 5, 730–731, 738f
Myopodin, 132t
　of Z line, 158
Myoseptal innervation, 331
Myosin, 132t, 167–183
　actin-myosin complex and, 174
　activation oncogene, myosin head organization and, 137–138
　duty ratio of, 170
　historical overview of, 167–168, 168f, 169f
　in hypertrophic cardiomyopathy, 181–182
　kinetic diversity of, 181
　kinetics of, 168–170, 170f

lever-arm hypothesis and, 171–174, 173f
molecular structure of, 135–137, 136f
polymerization of, to form thick filaments, 134–135, 135f, 136f
proteins binding to, 140–143, 141f
  function of, 142–143
  structure and interactions with myosin, 142, 142f
structure and function of, 167–174
structure of, 188f
superfamily of, 174–176, 176f–177f
in vitro expression and assays of function of, 182f, 182–183
Myosin-binding protein C, muscle contraction and, 300
Myosin heads
  molecular arrangement of, 137f–139f, 137–138
  structure of, 136–137
  x-ray, 170–171, 171f, 172f
Myosin heavy chain, in limb-girdle muscular dystrophy, 1081t
Myosin heavy-chain isoforms, 176–177
  correlation of muscle fiber types with, 91, 91f
  muscle fiber diversity recognition by, 90
Myosin light chain(s)
  phosphorylation of, 297–298, 298f
  thick filament regulation and, 296–297, 297f
Myosin light-chain isoforms, 178f, 178–179
  regulatory, phosphorylation of, 179–181, 180f
Myosin storage myopathy, 1508–1510
  clinical features of, 1509
  genetics of, 1510
  pathologic features of, 1509f, 1509–1510
Myositis
  adeno-associated virus protection against, 1395–1396
  African trypanosomiasis and, 1423–1425
  in allergic granulomatosis, 1455
  American trypanosomiasis and, 1425–1427
  in Behçet disease, 1459
  candidal, 1465
  cellulitis associated with myonecrosis and, 1464–1465
  cestode infections causing, 1430–1437. See also specific infections

chronic, electrodiagnostic studies in, 635, 635f
coenurosis and, 1434–1435
coxsackievirus-related, 1392–1394
  in humans, 1392–1393, 1393f
  murine, 1393–1394
Cryptococcus neoformans, 1465
Cunninghamella bertholletiae, 1465
cutaneous larva migrans and, 1439
cysticercosis and, 1430–1431
in diffuse fasciitis with eosinophilia, 1446, 1447f, 1448f
dracunculiasis and, 1439–1441
in eosinophilia-myalgia syndrome, 1447, 1449–1450
eosinophilic polymyositis, 1445–1446
focal, 1451
  muscle pain associated with, 1741t
  proliferative, 1450–1451
in giant cell arteritis, 1456, 1458f, 1459, 1459f
in graft-versus-host disease, 1463–1464
human immunodeficiency virus and. See Human immunodeficiency virus infection, myositis and
human T-cell lymphotropic virus type I, 1404–1405, 1405f
hydatidosis and, 1432–1434
hypersensitivity, 1456
inclusion body, 717, 719f
  electrodiagnostic studies in, 635
influenza virus infection and, 1394–1395
in macrophagic myofasciitis, 1450
malaria and, 1429–1430
microsporidiosis and, 1427–1429
Mycobacterium avium-intracellulare, 1465
nematode infections causing, 1437–1441. See also specific infections
nodular, localized, 1451
orbital, idiopathic, 1461–1462
in polyarteritis nodosa, 1454–1455, 1455f
in polymyalgia rheumatica, 1460
protozoan infections causing, 1419–1430. See also specific infections
in pseudothrombophlebitis syndrome, 1462–1463, 1463f

pyomyositis, 1460–1461, 1461f
rhabdomyolysis and myoglobinuria with, 1413
in rheumatic fever, 1459–1460
Ross River virus infection and, 1396
sarcocystosis and, 1421–1422
sparganosis and, 1435–1437
in toxic oil syndrome, 1449–1450
toxoplasmosis and, 1419–1421
trichinellosis and, 1437–1438
in vasculitis, 1454–1459
  in allergic granulomatosis, 1455
  in Behçet disease, 1459
  in giant cell arteritis, 1456, 1458f, 1459, 1459f
  hypersensitivity, 1456
  in polyarteritis nodosa, 1454–1455, 1455f
  in Wegener's granulomatosis, 1455–1456, 1457f
visceral larva migrans and, 1438–1439
in Wegener's granulomatosis, 1455–1456, 1457f
Myositis ossificans, localized, 1451
Myositis ossificans progressiva, 1451–1452
Myositis-specific antibodies, in polymyositis/dermatomyositis, 1331
Myosonography, 655, 656, 656t, 659f
Myostatin, blockade of, for dystrinopathies, 1011
Myotendinous junctions, 448f, 448–449, 449f
  extracellular matrix in, 476
  ultrastructural reactions of, 797, 798f
Myotilin, 132t
  in limb-girdle muscular dystrophy, 1081t, 1086–1087
  in myofibrillar myopathies, 1190
  functional importance of, 1198
  mutations in, 1198–1199
  of Z line, 158
Myotilinopathy, 1104
Myotome
  differentiation of, coordination with tendon differentiation, 33–34, 35f
  formation of, 33, 34f
Myotonia, 1748, 1748t, 1749t
  acetazolamide-responsive, 1268
  chondrodystrophic. See Chondrodystrophic myotonia
  in clinical examination, 617

Myotonia (Cont.)
  in myotonic dystrophy, 1040, 1042, 1042f, 1043t
  paradoxical, 1267f–1269f, 1267–1268, 1272–1273
  percussion, 613, 613f
  potassium-aggravated, 1266f, 1266–1267, 1267f, 1272
  sodium channel. See Sodium channel myotonias
Myotonia congenita, 1257–1265
  anesthesia in, 1264
  animal models of, 1265, 1265f, 1266f
  blood chemistry in, 1261
  clinical features of, 1258f, 1258–1260, 1259f
  differential diagnosis of, 1264–1265
  electrodiagnostic studies in, 637–638, 638f, 1260, 1260f, 1261f
  microscopy in, 1261f, 1261–1262
  molecular diagnosis of, 1262f, 1262–1263
  pathogenesis of, 1263, 1263f
  therapy for, 1264
  transient weakness in, evaluation of, 1260–1261, 1261f
Myotonia fluctuans, 1266, 1266f
Myotonia permanens, 1267, 1267f
Myotonic discharges, 625
  on electromyography, 625
Myotonic dystrophies, 1039t, 1039–1070, 1109–1110
  anesthesia in, 1045
  cardiac involvement in, 1044, 1044t
  cardiomyopathy in, 1250–1251
  central nervous system alterations in, 1044t, 1045–1046
  childhood-onset, 1050
  congenital, 1047, 1047t, 1048f, 1049t–1051t, 1049–1050
  diagnostic studies in, 1054–1055
  electrodiagnostic studies in, 636–637, 1053, 1053f
  endocrine problems in, 1044t, 1046t, 1046–1047, 1047t
  genetic basis of, 1055f, 1055–1057
    DM2 mutation and, 1057
    myotonic dystrophy mutation and, 1055–1057, 1056f
    population origins and, 1057
  genetic counseling and, 1068
  management and therapy of, 1067–1070
  molecular analysis of muscle in, 1051–1053
  molecular genetics of, 1058–1063
    anticipation and, 1059–1061
    DM1 CTG repeat and, 1058, 1058f
    expanded alleles in DM1 families and, 1058
    genetic counseling and, 1068
    germline instability and anticipation and, 1059–1061
    model systems and molecular mechanisms of DNA instability and, 1061–1063, 1063f
    somatic mosaicism and, 1058–1059, 1059f, 1060f
  molecular pathogenesis of, 1064–1067
  muscle pathology in, 1051, 1052f
  muscle spindle alterations and, 742–743
  muscle weakness in, 1040, 1040t, 1041f
  myotonia in, 1040, 1042, 1042f, 1043f
  ocular abnormalities in, 1044t, 1047, 1047t
  proximal (type 2), 1042–1043, 1043t, 1109–1110, 1852
    expanded CTG repeat and, 1063–1064
    molecular pathogenesis of, 1066–1067
    molecular pathogenicity in, 1066–1067
  respiratory involvement in, 1044t, 1044–1045
  skeletal muscle cell pathophysiology in, 1053–1054, 1054f
  smooth muscle involvement in, 1044t, 1045, 1045t
Myotonic dystrophy, proximal (type 2), electrodiagnostic studies in, 637
Myotonic dystrophy protein kinase, 1064
Myotonic muscular dystrophy, arthrogryposis multiplex congenita and, 1950
Myotonic myopathy, proximal, electrodiagnostic studies in, 637
Myotubes, fusion of, 45, 46f, 47f
Myotubular myopathy, 1490–1491
  x-linked, 1491–1494
    clinical features of, 1491f, 1491–1492
    differential diagnosis of, 1495
    genetics of, 1493–1494
    investigations in, 1492
    pathologic features of, 1492f, 1492–1493
Myozenin, 132t
  of Z line, 158
Myxedema, neuropathy with, 1916

Nalidixic acid, myositis due to, 1704
Narcotics, myoglobinuria due to, 1687
Natural killer cells, 891
Near infrared spectroscopy, oxidative metabolism and, 671–672, 672f
Near-rigor structure, 172
Nebulin, 132t
  in limb-girdle dystrophy, 1081t
  of thin filaments, 155, 155f
Necrosis
  of muscle fibers, 851–852, 856–858
    central fiber, 858
    contour and, 697, 698f–700f
    in dystrophinopathies, 980–981, 981f–984f, 982, 984
    ultrastructural features of, 852, 854f–857f, 856, 858
  in myoglobinuria, 1688
  in polymyositis/dermatomyositis, 1332, 1333f
  Sindbis virus infection and, 1396
Necrotizing myopathies
  acute, 1704–1705, 1705f, 1706f
  toxic, 1693, 1694t, 1697–1698
Necrotizing vasculitis, neuropathy with mesenchymal disease and, 1913–1914
Nemaline myopathy, 1480–1489
  anesthesia in, 1483
  arthrogryposis multiplex congenita and, 1949
  atypical features of, 1483
  cardiac involvement in, 1482
  central nervous system involvement in, 1482–1483
  classification of, 1480–1481, 1482f
  differential diagnosis of, 1487, 1487t
  fiber typing in, 1485–1486
  genetics of, 1487–1489, 1488f–1490f
  immunocytochemistry in, 1486f, 1486–1487
  intranuclear rods in, 1485, 1486f
  investigations in, 1483
  muscle fiber nuclei in, ultrastructural features of, 762, 763f
  muscle involvement in, 1481–1482, 1483f
  muscle pain associated with, 1742t

nemaline bodies in, 1483, 1484f, 1485, 1485f
obstetric issues in, 1483
orthopedic manifestations in, 1482
pathologic studies in, 1487
respiratory involvement in, 1482
Nemaline rods, ultrastructural features of, 786–787, 787f–789f
Nematode infections, myositis caused by, 1437–1441. *See also specific infections*
Neoplasms. *See also* Malignancies
muscle pain associated with, 1741t
neoplastic infiltration of peripheral nerves and, 1900
Neopterin, in polymyositis/dermatomyositis, 1330
Neostigmine bromide, for myasthenia gravis, 1776t, 1776–1777
Nerve(s), intramuscular, in Duchenne muscular dystrophy, 996, 997f
Nerve accommodation testing, 633
Nerve conduction studies, 630–631, 631f. *See also* Electrodiagnostic studies; *specific conditions*
of peripheral nerves, 1904
Nerve endings
cutaneous, quantitation of, 1905
types of, 331
Nerve sprouting, synaptic plasticity and, 364
Nestin, 132t
of intermediate filaments, 160
Neural cell adhesion molecule, in myofibrillar myopathies, 1190
Neural disorders, neurodiagnostic studies in, 647–648, 648t
Neural integrators, 123
Neural tissue, acetylcholinesterase forms in. *See* Acetylcholinesterase, neural
Neurasthenia, myasthenia gravis versus, 1775t
Neuroaxonal dystrophy, infantile, 737, 739
Neurofilament mutations, in amyotrophic lateral sclerosis, 1878–1879
Neurogenic disorders, muscle imaging in, 661f, 661–662, 662f
Neuroleptic malignant syndrome, 1682–1683
Neuromuscular diseases, lysosomal proteolysis and, 569

Neuromuscular junction, 325–364, 448, 480–484
acetylcholinesterase role at, modeling of, 431–432
alterations of
postsynaptic, ultrastructural features of, 868, 872, 874, 874f
presynaptic, ultrastructural features of, 865–867, 871f–873f
ultrastructural features of, 865–874
components of, 1801
definition of, 325, 326f
early light microscopic studies of, 325, 327, 327f–329f
early ultrastructural features of, 327–328
extracellular matrix in, 475f, 475–476, 476f
neuromuscular transmission and, 480
organization of, acetylcholinesterase forms related to, 434–435
patterns of motor innervation and, 330–331
focal, distributed, and myoseptal, 330–331
nerve ending types and, 331
postsynaptic differentiation and, 483–484
postsynaptic region of, 347–358
acetylcholine receptor and, 347, 349–351, 351f–355f
cytoskeletal components of, 351–354, 356f
junctional folds of, 347, 348f–350f
junctional sarcoplasm of, 354–355, 357f, 358
presynaptic differentiation and, 482–483, 483f
presynaptic region of, 331, 332f, 334–344
active zone and, 339–341, 341f–342f
cytochemical components of nerve terminal above active zones and, 339, 339f
endocytotic events and formation of new synaptic vesicles and, 343–344
exocytosis and, 336–339, 337f
morphologic correlates of quantal transmitter release and, 343
nerve terminal and, 331, 333f, 334f, 334–336

voltage-gated calcium channels and, 341–343
reinnervation and, 480, 481f, 482, 482f
remodeling of, 364
structure-function correlations and, 328–330, 330f
synaptic adhesion and, 480
synaptic basal lamina of, 345f, 345–347, 346f
synaptic plasticity and, 363–364
nerve sprouting and, 364
remodeling of neuromuscular junction and, 364
withdrawal of polyaxonal innervation and, 363–364
synaptic space of, 344–345
synaptogenesis and, 359–363
general principles of, 359
structural development of neuromuscular junction and, 359
structure-function correlates and, 359–360
trophic interactions and, 360–363
Neuromuscular preparation, 374, 374f
Neuromuscular transmission, 373–391, 480, 1801–1803
disturbances of, electrodiagnostic studies in, 644–646
electrophysiologic measurements of, 373–375, 374f, 375f
events after release of acetylcholine quantum and, 1801–1802
mechanism of, 373
neuromuscular junction components and, 1801
postsynaptic, 383–389
acetylcholine receptor and, 383–387
desensitization and, 388–389
end plate current generation and, 387–388
presynaptic, 375–383
nonquantal transmitter release and, 382–383
quantal transmitter release and, 375f, 375–378
release proteins and feedback systems and, 383
short-term synaptic plasticity and, 378–382
transmitter release overview and, 375
safety factor in, 389–391, 632

Neuromuscular transmission *(Cont.)*
  safety margin of, 1802
  saturating disk model of, 1803
  transmitter release by repetitive nerve stimulation and, 1802–1803
  transmitter release by single nerve impulse and, 1802
Neuromyopathies
  with bulbar weakness, in hereditary inclusion body myositis, 1313
  neurodiagnostic studies in, 648, 648t
Neuromyotonia, 1301–1308, 1747–1748
  acquired, pathogenesis of, 1304–1306
    autoimmune, 1304–1306
    nonimmune, 1306
  clinical features of, 1301–1302, 1302t, 1747–1748
  clinicopathologic classification of, 1301, 1302t
  course and prognosis of, 1302
  diagnosis and differential diagnosis of, 1306–1307, 1307t
  epidemiology of, 1302–1303
  focal, 1303
  future prospects for, 1307–1308
  hereditary, pathogenesis of, 1306
  morphology, 1302
  neurodiagnostic studies in, 646
  neurophysiology of, 1301f, 1301–1302
  serum and cerebrospinal fluid in, 1304, 1304f
  therapy for, 1307
Neuromyotonic discharges, 625, 626f, 1747
Neuron(s)
  agenesis and maldevelopment of, 1900–1901
  degeneration of, 1901–1902
Neuronal ceroid lipofuscinosis, 574t, 579–581, 581f, 582f, 731–732, 739f
Neuropathy
  carcinomatous, 1913
  granulomatous, 1913
Neurotonic discharges, 625, 626f
Neurotransmitter release, 375.
  See also specific neurotransmitters
  calcium and, 376–378, 377f
  measuring with end plate potential amplitude, 374
  nonquantal, 382–383
  quantal, 375f, 375–378.
    See Quantal release
  reduced, 1809, 1811

by repetitive nerve stimulation, 1802–1803
by single nerve impulse, 1802
Neutral maltases, 1561
New Finnish distal myopathy, 1170t
Nicotine use, neuronal acetylcholine receptors and, 410–411
Niemann-Pick disease, 572t, 732
Nitric oxide synthase
  binding to caveolin-3, 459
  plasma membrane defects and, 1004
  signaling by, 466
  syntrophin binding to, 459
Nonaka myopathy, 1170t, 1178–1179, 1179f
Nonsense mutations, 924
Normokalemic periodic paralysis, 1279
Northern blotting, 937
Nuclear-bag fibers, 489
Nuclear-chain fibers, 489
Nuclear envelope, Emery-Dreifuss muscular dystrophy and, 1032–1033
Nuclear muscle-specific genes, mutations in, 1628
Nuclease(s), 927
Nuclease protection, 943
Nucleic acids, structure of, 915, 916f
Nucleosomes, 917
Nutritional deficiencies, myopathy due to, 1708–1709
Nutritional deficiency, of undetermined significance, 1919
Nutritional status, protein turnover in muscle and, 550–551, 551t

Obstetric complications, in congenital myopathies, 1523
Oculomotor neuropathy, in diabetes mellitus, 1915
Oculopharyngeal distal myopathy, 1170t
Oculopharyngeal muscular dystrophy
  electrodiagnostic studies in, 640
  muscle fiber nuclei in, ultrastructural features of, 762
  myasthenia gravis versus, 1775t
Oculopharyngodistal myopathy, 1313
Ophthalmopathy, thyroid-associated, 1726t, 1726–1727
Ophthalmoplegia, proximal myopathy with congenital contractures and, 1312–1313

Organophosphates
  intoxication by, myasthenia gravis versus, 1774–1775, 1775t
  myopathy due to, 1698
Oropharyngeal muscular dystrophy, 1147–1160, 1318
  clinical features of, 1148–1149, 1149f, 1149t
  definition of, 1147
  diagnosis of, 1157–1158
  differential diagnosis of, 1158–1159
  genetic counseling and, 1158
  histopathology of, 1149–1151, 1150f–1153f, 1153–1154, 1154t
  historical background of, 1147–1148, 1148f
  laboratory findings in, 1149
  molecular genetics of, 1154–1156, 1155f, 1155t
  pathogenesis of, 1156–1157, 1157f
  therapy for, 1159
  unsolved problems in, 1159–1160
Orthomyxovirus infection, myositis and, 1394–1395
Orthopedic disorders, in nemaline myopathy, 1482
Orthopedic surgery, for Emery-Dreifuss muscular dystrophy, 1033–1034
Orthopedic therapy, for dystrinopathies, 1011
Osteomalacia, 1732
Osteosclerotic myeloma, neuropathies associated with, 1918
Oxandrolone
  for Duchenne muscular dystrophy, 1008–1009
  for inclusion body myositis, 1383
Oxidation/phosphorylation coupling, defects of, 1641–1642
  complex V deficiency, 1641
  Luft disease, 1641–1642
Oxidative stress
  indicators of, in inclusion body myositis, 1378
  plasma membrane defects and, 1004
Oxygen radical scavengers, for mitochondrial encephalopathy, 1654

Pacemaker switching, 500
Paget's disease, with limb-girdle muscular dystrophy, 1110
Pain. *See* Muscle pain
Painful legs and moving toes, 1748
Palatal muscles, testing of, 603

Palpation, of muscles and nerves, 609, 612–613
Paramyotonia congenita, 1267f–1269f, 1267–1268, 1272–1273
Paramyxovirus infection, myositis and, 1395
Paranemin, 132t
  of intermediate filaments, 160
Paraneoplastic syndromes, Lambert-Eaton myasthenic syndrome association with, 1792
Parasite motor unit potentials, 627
Parasitic infections, muscle pain associated with, 1741t, 1742t
Parathyroid disorders, electrodiagnostic studies in, 642
Parathyroid hormone
  cellular actions of, 1714t
  myopathy and, 1732–1733
Paraxial mesoderm
  formation in vertebrate embryos, 4–5, 6f
  muscle progenitor specification and body muscle, 8–9, 9f, 10f
    developmental signals for, 10–12
    head muscle, 9–10, 11f
    MRF transcription factors for, 12–14, 13f
    signaling and transcriptional networks and, 14f–16f, 14–17
  segmentation of, 6–8, 7f, 8f
  specification of, 5–6
Parkinson disease
  muscle pain associated with, 1742t
  neuronal acetylcholine receptors and, 409
Parvalbumins, muscle contraction and, 300–301
Parvovirus B19 infection, 1395
Patch-clamp technique, 225f, 225–228
Pearson syndrome, 1647
Penicillamine
  myasthenia gravis induced by, 1763
  myopathy due to, 1703
Peptostreptococcal myonecrosis, 1465
Percussion, of muscles, 613
Perhexiline, myopathy due to, 1700–1701
Perifascicular atrophy, dermatomyositis and, 724, 726f
Perimyositis, toxic, 1695t
Perimysium, 45, 471, 471f
Perineal muscles, testing of, 609t
Perineurial cells, pathology of of, 1900
Perineurium, 471

Periodic paralysis
  dyskalemic, with arrhythmia and dysmorphia, 1289f, 1289–1290
  electrodiagnostic studies in, 638–639
  hyperkalemic, 1268–1269, 1269f, 1270f, 1273
    equine model of, 1280, 1280f
    with multiple sleep-onset periods of rapid eye movement, 1279
    secondary to sustained hyperkalemia, 1279–1280
    X-linked, 1279
  hypokalemic, 1291–1292
    acquired, 1291–1292
    in familial potassium deficiency syndromes, 1292
  myasthenia gravis versus, 1775t
  normokalemic, 1279
  thyrotoxic, 1290–1291, 1725–1726
Peripheral nerves
  generalized hyperexcitability of. See Neuromyotonia
  in inclusion body myopathy, 1372–1373
  in laminin α2 deficiency, 1212
Peripheral nervous system, 1889–1925
  anatomy of, 1889–1890, 1890f
  in congenital muscular dystrophy, 1226
  evaluation of, 1903t, 1903–1905
  interstitial pathologic alterations of, 1895, 1897–1900
    bleeding, 1898
    compression, 1897–1898
    edema, 1898–1899
    infection, 1899–1900
    infiltration, 1899, 1900f, 1901f
    inflammatory demyelination, 1899
    injection of foreign substances, 1898
    ischemia, 1899, 1899f
    neoplastic, 1900
    stretch, 1897
    transection, 1895, 1897, 1897f, 1898f
  microenvironment of nerves and, 1894–1895
  microscopic anatomy, metabolism, and function of, 1890–1892, 1891f–1896f, 1894
  parenchymatous pathology of, 1900–1903
    of neurons, 1900–1903
    of Schwann and perineurial cells, 1900

  pathologic alterations of, 1895, 1897–1905
Peripheral neuropathies, 1906–1925
  arthrogryposis multiplex congenita and, 1949
  definition of, 1889
  immune, 1909–1912
    with acromegaly, 1916
    acute inflammatory demyelinating and axonal polyradiculoneuropathy, 1910–1911
    with alcoholism, 1919
    with amyloidosis, 1916–1917
    carcinomatous, 1913
    chronic inflammatory demyelinating and axonal polyradiculoneuropathy, 1911–1912
    with diabetes mellitus, 1914–1915
    drug-induced, 1919
    granulomatous, 1913
    with hepatic disease, 1916
    industrial exposures and, 1919
    inflammatory monoradiculopathy, mononeuropathy, or multiple mononeuropathy, 1912
    inflammatory polyganglionopathy, 1913
    with malignancy, 1917–1918
    with mesenchymal disease and necrotizing vasculitis, 1913–1914
    with microvasculitis, 1914
    with monoclonal gammopathies of undetermined significance, 1918–1919
    multifocal motor mononeuropathy with persistent conduction block, 1912
    with myxedema, 1916
    with nutritional deficiency, 1919
    sensory, 1912–1913
    in serum sickness, 1909–1910
    with uremia, 1915–1916
  infectious, 1906–1909
    diphtheritic, 1907
    herpes zoster, 1906 1907
    in HIV infection, 1909
    in leprosy, 1907–1909
    in Lyme disease, 1909
  inherited, 1919–1925
    hereditary motor and sensory neuropathy, 1922, 1923f
    hereditary sensory and autonomic neuropathy, 1923–1925, 1924t

Peripheral neuropathies (Cont.)
  with metabolic abnormalities and tumors, 1920–1922
    molecular genetic classification of, 1921–1922
  mononeuropathy, 1906
  multiple mononeuropathy, 1906
  radiculoplexus, 1906, 1907f, 1908f
  signs of, 1904
  symptoms of, 1904
Peroxisomal disorders, peripheral neuropathies associated with, 1920–1921
Peroxisomal β-oxidation, 1595–1596
Perturbation analysis, 197
Phages, 928
Pharyngeal muscles, testing of, 603
Phenytoin, myopathy due to, 1703
Phorphorylase b-kinase deficiency, arthrogryposis multiplex congenita and, 1951
Phosphatases, 927
Phosphodiester bonds, 915, 916f
Phosphofructokinase deficiency, 1545–1549
  animal models of, 1548–1549
  arthrogryposis multiplex congenita with, 1950
  biochemistry of, 1546
  clinical features of, 1545
  forward genetics in, 952–953
  laboratory studies in, genetics of, 1545
  molecular genetics of, 1547t, 1547–1548, 1548f
  muscle biopsy in, 1545f, 1545–1546, 1546f
  pathophysiology of, 1546–1547
  therapy for, 1548
  type 7, 731
Phosphoglycerate kinase deficiency, 1549
Phosphoglycerate mutase deficiency, 1549–1550, 1550f
  forward genetics in, 953
Phospholamban, calcium pump modulation by, 310–311, 311f
Phosphorylase b-kinase deficiency, 1536t, 1536–1537
Phosphorylase deficiency, 1537–1542
  animal models of, 1541–1542
  arthrogryposis multiplex congenita with, 1950
  biochemical findings in, 1539, 1540f, 1541

  clinical features of, 1537–1538, 1538t
  genetics of, 1538–1539
  laboratory studies in, 1538, 1538t
  molecular genetics of, 1541, 1542f
  muscle biopsy in, 1539, 1539f, 1540f
  myophosphorylase, type 5, 730–731, 738f
  pathophysiology of, 1541
  therapy for, 1542
Phosphorylation systems, in inclusion body myositis, 1377
Physical therapy, for dystrophinopathies, 1011
Physical trauma, myoglobinuria due to, 1683–1684
Physiologic properties, muscle fiber diversity recognition by, 90–91
Phytanic acid storage disease, peripheral neuropathy associated with, 1920
Pierre Robin syndrome, arthrogryposis multiplex congenita and, 1938
Pituitary dysfunction, myopathy associated with, 1729–1731
  acromegaly, 1729–1730
  hypopituitarism, 1730–1731
Plasmalemma. See Plasma membrane
Plasma membrane, 471
  composition of, 243
  defects of
    muscle fiber alterations associated with, in Duchenne muscular dystrophy, 995–996
    in nonnecrotic muscle fibers, in Duchenne muscular dystrophy, 990, 990f–995f, 993, 995
    secondary consequences of, 1003–1005
  of muscle fiber, elongation and repair of, ultrastructural features of, 765
  protection from mechanical stress, 445, 446f
  proteins of, in limb-girdle muscular dystrophy, 1079, 1083–1085
  structure of, 244, 246
  ultrastructural reactions of, 749, 752–758, 753f–758f
  ultrastructural studies of, in Duchenne muscular dystrophy, 996
Plasmapheresis
  for myasthenia gravis, 1779
  for polymyositis/dermatomyositis, 1347

Plasmids, 928
Plasticity, synaptic. See Synaptic plasticity
Plateau potentials, 111
Platelet-derived growth factor, satellite cell cell cycle modulation in response to, 75
Plate-like nerve endings, 327f, 331
Plectin, 132t, 457t
  defects of, muscular dystrophies caused by, 464
  deficiency of, postsynaptic congenital myasthenic syndromes with, 1838–1839
  in dystrophinopathies, 999
  of intermediate filaments, 161
  in myofibrillar myopathies, 1190
Pleurodynia, epidemic, 1392
Plus-minus screening, 933–934
Point mutations, 924, 924f
Polar regions, of intrafusal bundle, 489
Poliovirus infection, amyotrophic lateral sclerosis versus, 1875
Poliovirus receptors, in human muscle tissue, 1390, 1390f, 1391f
Poly-A binding protein, in limb-girdle muscular dystrophy, 1081t
Polyadenylation signals, 920
Polyarteritis nodosa, myositis in, 1454–1455, 1455f
Polyaxonal innervation, withdrawal of, synaptic plasticity and, 363–364
Polyganglionopathy, inflammatory, 1913
Polyglucosan, accumulation of, ultrastructural features of, 845, 845f, 846f
Polyglutamine disorders, reverse genetics in, 954
Polymerase(s), 927
Polymerase chain reaction, 938, 938f
  in situ, 943
Polymyalgia rheumatica, 1460, 1742t, 1743
Polymyositis. See also Polymyositis/dermatomyositis
  in adults, 1324–1326
    cardiac involvement in, 1325
    prognosis of, 1326
    pulmonary involvement in, 1325–1326
  cellular effector mechanisms in, 1352–1353
  electrodiagnostic studies in, 634f, 634–635

eosinophilic, 1445–1446
  inflammatory lesion in, characteristic features of, 1353–1354
  mediated by γ/δ cells and heat shock protein expression in muscle fibers, 1355
  muscle fiber nuclei in, ultrastructural features of, 762
  muscle pain associated with, 1742t
  pathologic features of, 1340, 1341f–1343f
Polymyositis/dermatomyositis, 1321–1358. *See also* Dermatomyositis; Polymyositis
  in adults, 1324–1326
    cardiac involvement in, 1325
    prognosis of, 1326
    pulmonary involvement in, 1325–1326
  antibody tests in, 1331
  with associated malignancy, 1326–1327
  definition of, 1321
  electromyography in, 1331–1332
  epidemiology of, 1322
  genetics of, 1322
  imaging studies in, 1332
  in overlap syndromes, 1327–1330
  pathogenesis of, 1348–1357
    afferent limb of immune response in, 1348–1351
    efferent limb of immune response in, 1351–1356
    viral infections in, 1356–1357
  pathologic features of, 1332–1344
    in dermatomyositis, 1333–1340
    in mixed connective tissue disease, 1343
    muscle alterations, 1332–1333
    in polymyositis, 1340, 1341f–1343f
    in rheumatoid arthritis, 1341, 1343, 1344f
    in scleroderma, 1340
    in Sjögren's syndrome, 1343–1344
    in systemic lupus erythematosus, 1340–1341
  serum components in, 1330–1331
  therapy for, 1344–1348
    new immunotherapies, 1357
Polyneuropathy, sensory, diabetic, 1914–1915
Polyphasic motor unit potentials, 627
Polyradiculoneuropathy
  chronic inflammatory demyelinating and axonal, 1911–1912

demyelinating and axonal
  acute inflammatory, 1910–1911
  chronic inflammatory, 1911–1912
Polysaccharide storage disorders, ultrastructural features of, 842, 844–845
Polyunsaturated fatty acid oxidation, enzymes of, mitochondrial β-oxidation and, 1595
Pompe disease. *See* Acid maltase deficiency
Pontocerebellar hypoplasia, spinal muscular atrophy with, 1859–1860, 1860f
Postactivation exhaustion, 632, 632f
Postpoliomyelitis muscular atrophy, 1852
Postpolio syndrome, inclusion body myositis-like myopathy in, 1381
Potassium, for hypokalemic periodic paralysis, 1288
Potassium channels
  calcium-activated, open at high intracellular calcium, 208f, 208–209
  inotopic P2X receptors and, 209
  inwardly rectifying
    open at energy depletion, 205, 207–208
    open at negative potentials, 204–205, 206t–207t
  transient receptor potential channels, 209
  voltage-gated, 220–221
    fast-inactivating, 220
    maintaining resting potential, 209
    slowly activating and inactivating, 220–221
    slowly inactivating, 220
Potassium-chloride cotransporters, 212
Prednisone
  for Duchenne muscular dystrophy, 1008–1009
  for inclusion body myositis, 1383
  for myasthenia gravis, 1777–1778
Pregnancy, myasthenia gravis in, therapy for, 1780
Premyofibrils, 52, 53f, 54–55
Pre-power stroke state, 173
Presynaptic membrane
  active zone of, 339–341, 341f–342f
  cytoskeletal components of nerve terminal above, 339, 339f
  voltage-gated calcium channels and, 341–343

Primer extension, 943
Prion protein
  in inclusion body myositis, 1378
  in myofibrillar myopathies, 1190
Probes, 932f, 932–933
Procainamide, myopathy due to, 1703
Progressive external ophthalmoplegia
  autosomal dominant, 1643–1644, 1644t
  autosomal recessive, 1644
  sporadic, with ragged red fibers, 1646–1647
Progressive muscular atrophy, 1846
Proliferative focal myositis, 1450–1451
Promoters, in RNA transcription, 920
Proprioception, by extraocular muscles, 124f, 124–125
Propylthiouracil, myopathy due to, 1703
Proteases, calcium-dependent. *See* Calpain(s)
Proteasomes, ATP-ubiquitin-proteasome proteolytic pathway and, 543–546, 544t, 545f
Protein C, myosin-binding, muscle contraction and, 300
Protein-calorie malnutrition, myopathy due to, 1708
Protein deficiency, protein balance in muscle and, 553–554
Protein importation, defects of, 1642
Protein kinase
  calmodulin-dependent, 317
  myotonic dystrophy, 1064
Protein metabolism in muscle, 535–537, 541–558
  methods for studying, 535–537
  pathways for, 535, 541–546
    ATP-ubiquitin-proteasome, 543–546, 544t, 545f
    calcium-dependent proteases and, 542–543
    lysosomal process and, 541–542
  physiologic significance of, 535
  regulation of, 546–552
    by angiotensin II, 551
    by catecholamines, 551
    by cytokines, 556–558
    by glucocorticoids, 550–551, 551t
    by growth hormone and insulin–like growth factors, 548–549
    by insulin and glucose, 547–548
    by leucine, 546–547
    muscle activity and, 554–556

Protein metabolism in muscle *(Cont.)*
    by nutrients, 550
        nutritional factors in, 552–554
        by testosterone, 551–552
        by thyroid hormones, 549
Proteinopathy, fukutin-related, 1101f, 1101–1102, 1111
Protein synthesis, impaired, myopathy due to, 1695t, 1701, 1701f, 1702f
Proteolysis
    plasma membrane defects and, 1003
    in skeletal muscle, 569
Proteolytic enzymes, in inclusion body myositis, 1377
Proteomics, 942
Protozoan infections, myositis caused by, 1419–1430. *See also specific infections*
Proximal myotonic dystrophy, 1042–1043, 1043t, 1109–1110, 1852
    expanded CCTG repeat and, 1063–1064
    molecular pathogenesis of, 1066–1067
    molecular pathogenicity in, 1066–1067
Proximal myotonic myopathy, electrodiagnostic studies in, 637
Prune belly syndrome, arthrogryposis multiplex congenita and, 1938f–1940f, 1938–1940
Pseudobulbar palsy, in amyotrophic lateral sclerosis, 1868
Pseudo-Hurler polydystrophy, 574t, 581–582, 582f, 583f
Pseudohypoaldosteronism, periodic paralysis secondary to hyperkalemia in, 1280
Pseudohypoparathyroidism, myopathy associated with, 1733–1734
Pseudo-H zone, 130f, 131
    cross-bridges and, 187
Pseudothrombophlebitis syndrome, 1462–1463, 1463f
Pull-down assay, 945
Pulsed-field gel electrophoresis, 935
Purine(s), 915
Purine nucleotide cycle, exercise and, 538–539
Purkinje cell Dystrophin promoter, 964
Pyknodysostosis, 574t
Pyomyositis, 1460–1461, 1461f
    human immunodeficiency virus and, 1400–1401

Pyridostigmine bromide, for myasthenia gravis, 1776t, 1776–1777
Pyrimidines, 915

Quadriceps-sparing myopathy, 1312
Quantal release
    of acetylcholine
        events after, 1801–1802
        morphologic correlates of, 343, 344f
        reduced, 1809, 1811
            paucity of synaptic vesicles and, 1807, 1809, 1809f, 1810f
Quantitative autonomic tests, 1905
Quantitative sensation tests, 1904–1905
Quinolinic acid, in polymyositis/dermatomyositis, 1330

Rab3a, exocytosis and, 338
Rabies virus receptors, in human muscle tissue, 1390–1391
Rabphilin-3A, exocytosis and, 338
Radiculoplexus neuropathies, in diabetes mellitus, 1915
Radiculoplexus neuropathy, 1906, 1907f, 1908f
Ragged red fibers, 712–714, 715f
Rapsyn
    deficiency of, 1833–1835, 1834f, 1835f
    in inclusion body myositis, 1378
Rate coding, 111
Recombination frequency, 918
Recruitment, 623
    control of, 112f, 112–113
    reduction in, 627
Reducing bodies, 711
    ultrastructural features of, 811, 813, 813f
Reducing body myopathy, 1512, 1513f
Reflexes, testing of, 613–614
Refsum disease, peripheral neuropathy associated with, 1920
Regeneration, 76f, 76–80
    in dystrophinopathies, 981–982, 984, 985f, 986f
    in empty endomysial tubes, 78
    extracellular matrix and, 479–480
    facilitation by removal of necrotic debris, 77f, 77–78
    impaired potential for, plasma membrane defects and, 1004
    injury type and, 76–77
    microcirculatory remodeling and, 525

    motor nerve influence on satellite cells and, 79
    muscle fiber contour and, 699, 701, 704f
    of muscle fibers
        organelle development in, 863, 869f, 870f
        patterns of, 860–863, 864f–868f
    muscle spindle alterations and, 741–742
    myonuclei replacement in, 76
    satellite cell activation by muscle overuse and, 79–80
    stem cells other than satellite cells in, 79
    stimulation of satellite cell activation and proliferation by injury and, 78
    ultrastructural features of, 860–863, 864f–870f
Renal failure
    in myoglobinuria, 1688–1689
    secondary hyperparathyroidism and, myopathies with, 1732
Renal tubular acidosis, distal, hypokalemic periodic paralysis in, 1292
Renal tubular dysfunction, with arthrogryposis multiplex congenita, cholestasis, and ichthyosis, 1946–1947
Reperfusion injury, microcirculatory remodeling and, 526–527
Repetitive stimulation testing, 631f, 631–633, 632f. *See also* Electrodiagnostic studies
Residual-calcium hypothesis, of synaptic plasticity, 382
Residual-factor hypothesis, of synaptic plasticity, 382
Respiratory care, for congenital myopathies, 1523
Respiratory distress, spinal muscular atrophy with, 1859, 1859f
Respiratory failure, distal myopathy with, 1170t
Respiratory system
    in Bethlem myopathy, 1139
    in myotonic dystrophy, 1044t, 1044–1045
    in nemaline myopathy, 1482
    in polymyositis/dermatomyositis, in adults, 1325–1326
Resting potentials, of skeletal muscle, 203–213

active ion transport through sodium-potassium pump and, 209–212
bistability of, 212–213
cation-chloride cotransporters and, 212
lack of contribution of calcium channels to, 209
sodium-calcium exchangers and, 212
voltage-gated potassium channels maintaining, 209
voltage-sensitive cation channels setting, 204–209, 205f
Restless legs syndrome, 1741t, 1743, 1743t
Restriction endonucleases, 926
Restriction enzymes, 926f, 926–927
Restriction fragment length polymorphisms, 936, 936f
Restriction mapping, 936
Reticular fibrils, 471
Reticular lamina, 471
Retina
  in Becker muscular dystrophy, 977
  in Duchenne muscular dystrophy, 977
Retroviral infections, 1396–1406
  feline immunodeficiency virus, 1406
  human foamy retrovirus, 1405
  human immunodeficiency virus, 1396–1404
  human T-cell lymphotropic virus type I, 1404–1405, 1405f
  inclusion body myositis and, 1381
  simian immunodeficiency virus, 1405–1406
  simian retrovirus type I, 1405
Retrovirus receptors, in human muscle tissue, 1390
Reverse genetics, 953–954
Reverse transcriptase, 931
Reye syndrome, 1413
Rhabdomyolysis, myositis with, 1413
Rheumatic fever, 1459–1460
Rheumatoid arthritis
  myositis and, 1329
    pathologic features of, 1341, 1343, 1344f
Riboflavin, for lipid metabolism disorders, 1614
Ribosome(s), 920–921
Ribosome-binding site, 924
Rifampin, myositis due to, 1704
Rigid-spine congenital muscular dystrophy, 1206t, 1226–1227, 1227f, 1228f

Riley-Day syndrome, 1924
RIM, exocytosis and, 338
Rimmed vacuoles, 715
Ringbinden, 703, 705f
  ultrastructural features of, 795, 795f
Rippling muscle disease, 613, 1749–1750
RNA
  sequestration of, in inclusion body myositis, 1378
  structure of, 915, 916f
  toxic, in myotonic dystrophy, 1065–1066, 1066f
  transcription and translation of, 920–921, 921f
RNA splicing, regulation of muscle protein expression by, 28
Rod body myopathy, 707, 707f, 708f
Ross River virus infection, 1396
RSHL1, in myotonic dystrophy, 1065
Ryanodine receptors, 248f, 248–251, 249f
  calcium release into cytosol and, 312f, 312–313
  dihydropyridine receptor ratio to, variations in, 251
  excitation-contraction coupling in skeletal muscle and. *See* Excitation-contraction coupling, in skeletal muscle
  isoforms of, 251, 251f
  mutations in, diseases resulting from, 314–315
  structure of, 266f, 266–268
  RYR1, malignant hyperthermia and central core disease and, 1669, 1670t, 1671t

Salivary excess, in amyotrophic lateral sclerosis, therapy for, 1881–1882
Salla disease, 574t
Sandhoff disease, 572t, 577–579, 580f
  motor neuron variants of, 1872–1873
Sanfilippo disease, 573t, 585f, 585–586
Sanger dideoxy enzymatic method, 938–939, 939f
Sarcalumenin, 318–319
Sarcocystosis, 1421–1422, 1423f
Sarcoglycan(s), 456, 457t
Sarcoglycan, in limb-girdle muscular dystrophy, 1080t, 1084–1085
Sarcoglycan complex, 456
  defects of, muscular dystrophies caused by, 464
  signaling by, 465

Sarcoglycan complexes, binding to, 458f, 458–459
Sarcoglycanopathies, 1095–1100
  cardiomyopathy in, 1247–1249
  clinical features of, 1096f, 1096–1097
  diagnosis of, 1098–1099, 1099f, 1111, 1112–1113
  epidemiology of, 1096
  genetics of, 1097–1098
  treatment of, 1100
Sarcoid myopathy, 1452–1454, 1453f, 1454f
  electrodiagnostic studies in, 636
Sarcolemma, 443, 471, 473f
  dystrophin expression in, 997–999, 998f
  folding of, 445
  nuclei of, central migration of, 697, 697f
  structural weakness of, in dystrophinopathies, 1002–1003
Sarcolipin, calcium pump modulation by, 311–312, 312f
Sarcomeres
  diseases of, 161
  interlacing, congenital myopathy with mosaic fibers and, 1515–1516, 1516f
  molecular structure of, 129–161
    intermediate filaments and, 160f, 160–161
    M line and, 143–145
    structure and function of striated muscle and, 129–134
    thick filament and, 134–143, 135f
    thin filament and, 147–157
    titin filaments and, 145–147
    Z line and, 157–160
Sarcoplasm, junctional, 347f, 354–355, 358
Sarcoplasmic masses, 703, 705f
  ultrastructural features of, 817, 823f–825f
Sarcoplasmic protein crystals, ultrastructural features of, 801, 808f
Sarcoplasmic reticulum, 232–233, 233f, 234f
  calcium release units of. *See* Calcium release units
  endoplasmic reticulum transition to, 57–58
  free
    composition of, 244
    shapes of, 239, 240f
    structure of, 237f, 246, 246f

Sarcoplasmic reticulum *(Cont.)*
  junctional, 252f, 252–253, 253f
  morphometry of, 253–254
  structure-function correlations of, 254
  ultrastructural reactions of, 766–774, 771f–777f
  unusual aggregates of, 240, 242, 244f
Sarcospan, 456, 457t
  defects of, muscular dystrophies caused by, 464
  in limb-girdle muscular dystrophy, 1085
Sarcotubular myopathy, 1510–1512
  clinical features of, 1510
  genetics of, 1510, 1512
  pathologic features of, 1510, 1511f
Sarcotubular system, proteins of, 307–319
  calcium release into cytosol and, 312–313
  calcium removal from cytosol and, 307–310
  calmodulin-dependent protein kinase, 317
  junctin, 316–317
  junctophilin, 317
  luminal, 317–319
  mitsugumin, 317
  modulating calcium pumps, 310–312
  modulating calcium release channels, 313–316
  triadin, 316
Satellite cells, 66–71. *See also* Myoblasts
  cell cycle modulation of, in response to growth factors, 73–76
  as committed stem cells, 70–71, 71f
  in culture, 72–73, 73f, 74f
  definition of, 66
  development from myogenic cells, 68–69
  difference between myogenic cells and, 70, 70f
  distribution and frequency of, 67–68
  in Duchenne muscular dystrophy, 996
  markers of, 66–67, 68f, 69f
  migration and crossing of basal lamina by, 72
  in regeneration. *See* Regeneration
  specialization of, 69–70
  structure of, 66, 67f, 68f
  ultrastructural features of, 858, 859f–862f, 860
Satellite motor unit potentials, 627

Saturating disk model of neuromuscular transmission, 1803
Scapuloperoneal spinal muscular atrophy, 1855t, 1857–1858
Scapuloperoneal syndrome, 1130–1131, 1318
Scheie syndrome, 573t, 584–585, 585f
Schindler disease, 572t
Schizophrenia, neuronal acetylcholine receptors and, 410
Schwann cells
  agenesis or maldevelopment of, 1900
  intoxication of, 1900
Schwannomas, 1900
Schwartz-Jampel syndrome, 1292–1294, 1293f, 1748
  electrodiagnostic studies in, 642
  laboratory findings and microscopy in, 1293, 1293f
  differential diagnosis of, 1294
  molecular genetics of, 1293
  pathogenesis of, 1294
Scleroderma
  linear, 1327–1328
  pathologic features of, 1340
Scleroderma-myositis, 1327–1328
Scoliosis, in congenital myopathies, 1523
Screening, plus-minus, 933–934
Screening libraries, 933, 934f
Selectins, 899, 900t, 901f
Selenium deficiency, myopathy due to, 1709
Selenoprotein
  in limb-girdle muscular dystrophy, 1081t
  in myofibrillar myopathies, mutations in, 1199
Selenoprotein N, deficiency of, 1206t, 1226–1227
Self-tolerance, loss of, myasthenia gravis and, 1762–1763
Senna, myopathy due to, 1696–1697
Sensory impairment, in amyotrophic lateral sclerosis, 1869
Sensory neuropathy, 1912–1913
  hereditary, 1922–1925
SEPN1, in limb-girdle muscular dystrophy, 1081t
Sepsis, protein metabolism and, 556–557
Sequencing by hybridization, 940, 940f
Serial analysis of gene expression, 942
Serine proteases, in inclusion body myositis, 1377
Serotonin syndrome, 1683

Serum response element, 923
Serum response factor, 923
Serum response factor (SRF), muscle-specific promoters and, 24
Serum sickness, neuropathy in, 1909–1910
SGT chaperone complex, exocytosis and, 339
Short-chain acyl-CoA dehydrogenase deficiency, 1610
Short-chain L-3-hydroxyacyl-CoA dehydrogenase deficiency, 1610
Shortening heat, 196
Shoulder rotators
  lateral, testing of, 604t–605t
  medial, testing of, 605t
Sialic acid storage disease, 574t, 584
Sialidosis, 573t
Signaling, paraxial mesoderm specification and, 5–6
Signal transduction, in Emery-Dreifuss muscular dystrophy, 1033
Signal transduction pathways, slow fiber phenotype expression and, 100–101
Simian immunodeficiency virus infection, 1405–1406
Simian retrovirus type I myositis, 1405, 1406f
Simvastatin, myositis due to, 1704
Sindbis virus infection, 1396
Single-nucleotide polymorphisms, 945
Single stranded DNA-binding protein, in inclusion body myositis, 1378
Sister chromatids, 918
SIX5, in myotonic dystrophy, 1064–1065
Six4/MEF3/TREX control elements, muscle-specific promoters and, 26
Size principle, 112
Sjögren's syndrome
  myositis and, 1328
  pathologic features of, 1343–1344
Skelemin, 132t
  of intermediate filaments, 161
  of M line, 144
Skeletal anomalies, in clinical examination, 616
Skeletal muscle
  action potential of. *See* Action potential, of skeletal muscle
  excitation-contraction coupling in. *See* Excitation-contraction coupling, in skeletal muscle

exercise-mediated regulation of, 27
fast and slow muscle enhancers and
    control elements and, 27
integrins of, 449–450
lipid metabolism in, 1590–1591
lysosomes of, 568–570
lysosome trafficking in, 570
muscle cell assembly and, 45–62, 46f
    developmental changes in
        microtubules and intermediate
        filaments and, 56f, 56–57
    membrane system assembly and
        organization and, 57–61
    mononucleated cell fusion to form
        multinucleated muscle fibers,
        45–49, 48f–50f
    myofibrillar protein renewal in
        muscle cells and, 57
    myofibrillogenesis and, 49–56
    in myotonic dystrophy,
        pathophysiology of, 1053–1054,
        1054f
passive electrical properties of
    membrane and, 213
proteolysis in, 569
resting potential of. See Resting
    potential(s), of skeletal muscle
ryanodine receptor mutations in,
    diseases resulting from, 314,
    315f
sodium channel of, structure and
    function of, 1273, 1274f
somatic mtDNA mutations in, 1628,
    1628t
transcription enhancers and control
    elements and, 27–28
viral infection of, in vitro, 1391–1392,
    1392f
Skeletal muscles, embryonic origins of,
    3–37
    building muscle anatomy and,
        30–37
    mesoderm and skeletal muscle
        progenitor specification and,
        4–18
    molecular control of muscle
        differentiation and, 18–30
Skeletofusimotor system, 489
Skin, in laminin α2 deficiency, 1212
Slack test, 195
Sliding-filament model of muscle
    contraction, 133–134, 134f
Sliding filament theory, 188
Slow-channel congenital myasthenic
    syndromes, 1818–1827

clinical features of, 1819, 1819f, 1820f
diagnosis of, 1821, 1825
electrophysiologic features of,
    1820–1821, 1824f, 1825f
mechanistic consequences of
    slow-channel mutations and,
    1825–1827
molecular genetic studies in, 1821
morphologic features of, 1819–1820,
    1820f–1824f
pathologic mechanisms in, 1821
therapy for, 1825, 1826f
Slow fibers
    signal transduction pathways and
        expression of, 100–101
    specification of, 94–95
Sly disease, 573t
Smooth muscle
    in myotonic dystrophy, 1044t, 1045,
        1045t
    vertebrate, thick filament regulation
        in, 298–299
Smooth muscles, in Duchenne muscular
    dystrophy, 976
Snake venoms, myopathy due to, 1698
SNARE complex, 336–337, 337f
Sodium-calcium exchangers, 212
Sodium channel, voltage-gated,
    215–220
    activation and deactivation of, 216,
        217f
    blockers and modifiers of, 219–220
    fast inactivation of, 217–218
    pore-determining part of, 216
    recovery from inactivation of, 218
    selectivity filter of, 216
    single-channel conductance and
        channel density and, 218, 219f
    slow and ultraslow inactivation of,
        218
    steady-state activation and
        inactivation of, 218
    β subunits of, 218–219
    voltage-sensing part of, 215–216,
        216f
Sodium channel myasthenia,
    1835–1838
    clinical features of, 1835, 1836f
    electrophysiologic studies in, 1836,
        1838f
    expression studies in HEK cells in,
        1836–1837, 1838f
    molecular genetic analysis in, 1836,
        1838f
    morphologic studies in, 1836, 1837f

    nerve stimulation studies in, 1836,
        1837f
    relation to other sodium channel
        disorders, 1837–1838, 1839t
    therapy for, 1838
Sodium channel myotonias, 1266–1280
    anesthesia in, 1278–1279
    animal models of, 1280
    blood chemistry and electro-
        cardiogram in, 1270
    differential diagnosis of, 1279–1280
    electromyography in, 1269–1270,
        1270f–1272f
    hyperkalemic periodic paralysis,
        1268–1269, 1269f, 1270f, 1273
    microscopy in, 1272–1273
    molecular genetics and pathogenesis
        of, 1273–1277, 1275t,
        1276f–1278f, 1276t, 1277t
    paramyotonia congenita,
        1267f–1269f, 1267–1268,
        1272–1273
    potassium-aggravated, 1266f,
        1266–1267, 1267f 1272
    provocative tests in, 1271–1272
    sodium channel structure in, 1273,
        1274f
    therapy for, 1277–1278
Sodium-potassium-chloride
    cotransporter, 212
Sodium-potassium pump, active ion
    transport through, 209–212
    ATPase subunits and, 210, 210f
    pump electrical contribution to
        resting potential and, 209–210
    pump mechanism and its effect on
        ion gradients and, 209, 210f
    regulation of sodium pump and,
        212
Somatic mosaicism, in myotonic
    dystrophy, 1058–1059, 1059f,
    1060f
Somites, formation of, 6–8, 7f, 8f
Southern blotting, 936–937, 937f
Sparganosis, 1435–1437, 1436f
Spasms, 1744, 1744t
    of central nervous system origin,
        1745–1746, 1746t
    of muscle origin, 1748–1750
    neurodiagnostic studies in, 646–647
    of peripheral nerve origin,
        1746–1748
Spastic paraplegias, hereditary, 1873
Specific immunity. See Immunity,
    adaptive (specific)

Speech augmentation, in amyotrophic lateral sclerosis, 1882
Spherical bodies, in hexagonal arrays, ultrastructural features of, 816
Sphingomyelin-cholesterol lipidosis, 572t, 732
Spielmeyer-Haltia disease, 574t, 579–581, 581f, 582f, 731–732, 739f
Spinal cord
  agenesis of, lumbosacral, arthrogryposis multiplex congenita and, 1944f, 1944–1945
  dysgenesis of anterior horns of, in arthrogryposis multiplex congenita, 1933–1935, 1934f, 1935f
Spinal muscular atrophies, 1845–1861
  basic concepts of, 1845
  definition of, 1845
  diagnostic criteria for, 1847
  epidemiology of, 1845
  future prospects for, 1861
  historical background of, 1846t, 1846–1847
  nonproximal, 1855t, 1855–1859
    bulbar palsy, 1858, 1858f
    distal, 1855t, 1855–1857, 1856f
    scapuloperoneal, 1855, 1857–1858
    segmental, 1855t, 1857, 1857f
    spinobulbar neuronopathy, 1855t, 1858–1859, 1859f
  proximal, 1847–1855
    animal models of, 1854
    clinical picture in, 1847t, 1847–1850, 1848f–1851f, 1848t
    CNS pathology in, 1851
    differential diagnosis of, 1851–1852
    electrophysiological studies in, 1851
    inheritance of, 1853
    laboratory features of, 1851
    management of, 1854–1855
    molecular biology of, 1853f, 1853–1854
    molecular genetic screening in, 1850, 1852t
    muscle pathology in, 1851, 1852f
    nerve pathology in, 1851
  unsolved problems with, 1861
  variants of, 1859–1861
    with arthrogryposis multiplex, 1860f, 1860–1861
    with cardiomyopathy, 1861
    distal, with vocal cord paralysis, 1861
    with myoclonic epilepsy, 1861
    with pontocerebellar hypoplasia, 1859–1860, 1860f
    with respiratory distress, 1859, 1859f
Spinal muscular atrophy, arthrogryposis multiplex congenita and, 1948–1949
Spinobulbar neuronopathy, 1852, 1855t, 1858–1859, 1859f
  X-linked, amyotrophic lateral sclerosis versus, 1878
Spinocerebellar ataxias, peripheral neuropathies associated with, 1925, 1925t
Spironolactone, for hypokalemic periodic paralysis, 1289
Spliceosomes, 920
STA gene, in Emery-Dreifuss muscular dystrophy, 1031–1032
Steatosis, hepatic, lactic acidosis and myopathy with, 1413
Stem cells, 71–76
  in regeneration, 79
  satellite cells. See Satellite cells
Stem cell therapy, for dystrophinopathies, 1009–1010
Stiff-man syndrome, 1745–1746, 1746t
Stiffness, 197, 600–601
STOP codon skipping strategies, 30
Streptococcal myonecrosis, 1464–1465
Stretch injury, of peripheral nerves, 1897
Striated muscle. See also Skeletal muscle
  laminins in, 1207–1208, 1208f
  muscle fibers of, structure of, 121–133, 129, 130f, 131f
  sarcomeres of. See Sarcomeres
  thick filament regulation in, 298
Structural genomics, 942
Strychnine poisoning, 1745
Succinylcholine, myoglobinuria due to, 1686
Superfast myosin heavy chain, 176
Sural nerve biopsy, 1905
Surface membrane. See Plasma membrane
SV2, exocytosis and, 338
Symptoms, in clinical examination, 600–601
Synapses, immunologic, 906–907, 907f
Synaptic basal lamina-associated syndrome. See Acetylcholinesterase, end plate, congenital deficiency of
Synaptic plasticity, 363–364
  short-term, 378–382
    under conditions of low quantal content, 380–381, 381f
    facilitation, augmentation, potentiation, and depression of, 378–379, 379t, 380f
    in Lambert-Eaton syndrome, 381
    mechanism of depression and, 382
    mechanisms of, 381–382
    MEPP frequency facilitation, augmentation, and potentiation and, 381
    properties of depression and, 382
Synaptic vesicles
  clear, small, 335–336
  coated, 334, 335f
  dense-core, 335
  formation of, endocytotic events and, 343–344
  giant, 334
  neurotransmitter release and, 378
  paucity of, reduced quantal release and, 1807, 1809, 1809f, 1810f
Synaptogenesis, 359–363
  fiber-type diversity and, 100
  general principles of, 359
  structural development of neuromuscular junction and, 359
  structure-function correlates and, 359–360
Synaptophysin, exocytosis and, 338
Synaptotagmin, antibodies to, in Lambert-Eaton myasthenic syndrome, 1797
Synaptotagmin I, exocytosis and, 337–338
Syncoilin, 133t, 457t
  of intermediate filaments, 161
Synemin, 133t
  of intermediate filaments, 160
Syntrophin(s), 457t
Syntrophin, in limb-girdle muscular dystrophy, 1079
Syntrophins, 456
  binding to n-NO synthase, 459
  dystrobrevin binding to, 459, 459f
  dystrophin binding to, 459, 459f
  signaling by, 465–466
α-Synuclein, in inclusion body myositis, 1378
Syphilis, myositis in, 1467–1468
Systemic lupus erythematosus
  myositis and, 1328–1329
  pathologic features of, 1340–1341

Tacrolimus, for polymyositis/
	dermatomyositis, 1346
Taenia solium infection, 1430–1431,
	1432f
Tandem duplication, 925
Tandem repeats, 924
Target fibers, 710, 712f
Target formations, ultrastructural
	features of, 816, 817f–822f
Tarui disease. *See* Phosphofructokinase
	deficiency
Tarui's disease, 731
tau protein, in inclusion body myositis,
	1377
Tay-Sachs disease, 572t, 577–579, 580f
	motor neuron variants of, 1872–1873
T cell(s). *See* T lymphocytes
T-cell epitopes, muscle acetylcholine
	receptors and, 415
TEF1 factors, muscle-specific promoters
	and, 25–26
Telethonin, 133t
	in limb-girdle muscular dystrophy,
		1081t, 1086
Telethoninopathy, 1100
	diagnosis of, 1111
	distal onset in, 1170t, 1180
Temperature extremes, myoglobinuria
	due to, 1682–1683
Temporal arteritis, myositis in, 1456,
	1458f, 1459, 1459f
Tendons
	contractures of, 616
	differentiation of, coordination with
		myotome differentiation, 33–34,
		35f
	limb muscles and, patterning of, 37,
		37f
Tension myalgia, 1739, 1741, 1741t,
	1743
Terminal deoxynucleotidyl transferase,
	932
Terminators, in RNA transcription, 920
Testosterone, protein metabolism in
	muscle and, 551–552
Tetanus, 1745
	fused, 191
	unfused, 191
Tetany, 600, 1733–1734, 1734f
	neurodiagnostic studies in, 646
	symptomatic, 1747
Thick filaments
	loss of, ultrastructural features of,
		792–793, 793f, 794f, 795
	regulation of, 296–300

in molluscan adductor muscle,
		299f, 299–300, 300t
	myosin light chains in, 296–297,
		297f
	in striated muscle, 298
	in vertebrate smooth muscle,
		298–299
of skeletal muscle, 130f, 131,
		134–143, 135f
	backbone structure in, 129–140,
		139f
	molecular arrangement of myosin
		heads and, 137–138, 137f–139f
	myosin-binding proteins in,
		140–143, 141f
	myosin molecule structure and,
		135–137, 136f
	polymerization of myosin to form,
		134–135, 135f, 136f
ultrastructural reactions of, 792–793,
	793f, 794f, 795
Thin filaments
	chromosome locations of genes
		expressing regulatory proteins
		of, 301–302, 302t
	mutations of regulatory proteins
		and, 301–302
	excess of, ultrastructural features of,
		797
	phosphorylation of regulatory
		proteins of, 295–296
	regulation of, 285f–290f, 285–295,
		292f
		tropomyosin in, 286–287
		troponin C in, 288–290, 289t
		troponin complex in, 287–288
		troponin I in, 290–293, 292f, 391t
		troponin T in, 293t, 293–295, 294f
	of skeletal muscle, 130f, 131,
		147–157
		actin polymerization to form,
			147–150, 148f, 149f
		capping proteins and, 156, 156f
		molecular model of, 152–154, 153f
		nebulin and, 155, 155f
		regulatory proteins of, 150–152
		"soluble" enzyme binding to,
			156–157
		structural changes on activation,
			153–154, 154f, 155f
		structure of, 188f
		ultrastructural reactions of, 797
Thomsen disease. *See* Myotonia
	congenita
Threshold effect, 1628

Thrombophlebitis, muscle pain
	associated with, 1741t
Thymectomy, for myasthenia gravis,
	1779–1780
Thymus gland
	immune function of, 895–898, 897f
	myasthenia gravis and, 1763–1765
Thyroid-associated ophthalmopathy,
	1726t, 1726–1727
Thyroid disease
	electrodiagnostic studies in, 642
	myopathy associated with,
		1722–1729
		endocrine ophthalmopathy,
			1726–1727
		hypothyroidism, 1727–1729
		thyrotoxic myopathy, 1722–1725
		thyrotoxic periodic paralysis,
			1725–1726
Thyroid hormones
	cellular actions of, 1714t
	protein turnover in muscle and, 549
Thyrotoxic myopathy, 1722–1725
	clinical presentation of, 1722
	electrodiagnostic evaluation of, 1723
	epidemiology of, 1722
	histology in, 1723
	metabolic alterations related to
		thyrotoxicosis and, 1723–1724
	physiologic alterations associated
		with thyrotoxicosis and,
		1724–1725
	treatment of, 1725
Thyrotoxic periodic paralysis,
	1290–1291, 1725–1726
Tibial distal myopathy, 1170t, 1172,
	1172f
Titin, 133t
	in cardiac muscle, 147
	in dystrophinopathies, 999
	length-tension curves and, 192
	in limb-girdle muscular dystrophy,
		1081t, 1087
Titin filaments, 145–147
	functions of
		mechanical, 146–147, 147f
		in myofibrillogenesis, 146
	molecular structure, interactions, and
		organization of, 145–146, 146f
Titinopathy, 1102–1103
T lymphocytes, 891, 892f, 893f
	cooperation between B lymphocytes
		and, 893–894
	cultured myocyte interaction with,
		911–912

T lymphocytes *(Cont.)*
  functions of, 1348–1349
  muscle fiber invasion and destruction by, ultrastructural features of, 846–851, 849f–853f
  in myasthenia gravis, 1765–1766
  thymus production of, 895–898, 897f895
Togavirus infection, 1396
Tolerance, 1350–1351
Toll-like receptors, 890–891
Tolosa-Hunt syndrome, 1461–1462
Tomosyn, exocytosis and, 338
Tongue muscles, testing of, 603
Topoisomerases, 927
Torticollis, congenital, 1956f, 1956–1957
Total-body irradiation, for polymyositis/dermatomyositis, 1347
Tourette syndrome, neuronal acetylcholine receptors and, 410
Toxic myopathies, 1693–1708
  amphiphilic, 1694t, 1696, 1699–1701
  antimicrotubular, 1695t, 1701–1703
  corticosteroid, 1694t, 1698
  electrodiagnostic studies in, 642–643
  hypokalemic, 1694t, 1698, 1705–1706, 1706f
  inflammatory, 1695t, 1703–1704
  intramuscular injections causing, 1695t, 1707–1708
  mitochondrial, 1696–1697
  muscle pain associated with, 1742t
  myoglobinuria, 1693, 1694t
  necrotizing, 1693, 1694t, 1697–1698
Toxic oil syndrome, 1449–1450, 1703–1704
Toxins
  exogenous, amyotrophic lateral sclerosis and, 1875–1876, 1880
  myoglobinuria due to, 1685
Toxocariasis, 1438–1439
Toxoplasmosis, 1419–1421
  clinical manifestations of, 1420
  geographic location and, 1419
  laboratory studies in, 1420
  pathology of, 1420–1421, 1421f
  transmission to humans, 1419–1420
  treatment of Toxoplasmosis, pathology of, 1421
Trail nerve endings, 327f, 331
Transcription
  of RNA, 920, 921f
  synapse-specific, regulation of, 361, 362f
  in vitro, 942

Transcription factors, paraxial mesoderm specification and, 5–6
Transection, of peripheral nerves, 1895, 1897, 1897f, 1898f
Transforming growth factor β, satellite cell cell cycle modulation in response to, 75
Transgenic mice, 946, 947f
Transitions, 924
Transition stroke state, 173
Translation
  of RNA, 920–921, 921f
  in vitro, 942–943
Translocases, defects of, 1642
Transverse connecting system, 443–445
  intermediate filament network and, 444f, 444–445
  links between cytoskeleton and extracellular matrix and, 445, 446f
Transverse fixation system
  intermediate filaments, costameres, and fixation bolts and, 461–462, 462f
  proteins responsible for muscular dystrophies in, 462–464
Transversions, 924
Triadin, 316
Triad junctions, protein components of, 267–268, 268f
Triamterene, for hypokalemic periodic paralysis, 1289
Trichinellosis, 1437–1438, 1438f
Triglyceride storage disease, multisystem, 1612–1613, 1613f
Trilaminar configurations, 711–712
Trilaminar myopathy, 1519
Trimolecular complex, as therapeutic target, 908–909
TRIM 32, in limb-girdle muscular dystrophy, 1081t
TRIM 32-related dystrophy, 1100
Trinucleotide repeat disorders, reverse genetics in, 954
Triosephosphate isomerase deficiency, 1551
Trisomy 18, arthrogryposis multiplex congenita and, 1935–1936, 1936f–1938f
Trisomy 21, arthrogryposis multiplex congenita and, 1936–1937
tRNA, 921
tRNA genes, point mutations in, 1647–1649

Tropomodulin, 133t
  of thin filaments, 156
Tropomyosin, 133t
  correlation of muscle fiber types with, 91–92
  in limb-girdle muscular dystrophy, 1081t
  phosphorylation of, 295
  thin filament regulation and, 286–287
  of thin filaments, 150–151, 151f
Troponin(s), 133t
  C
    interaction with troponin T, 295
    thin filament regulation and, 288–290, 289t
    of thin filaments, 152, 152f
  correlation of muscle fiber types with, 91–92
  I
    interaction with troponin T, 295
    phosphorylation of, 295–296, 296f
    thin filament regulation and, 290–293, 292f, 391t
    of thin filaments, 151–152
    in limb-girdle muscular dystrophy, 1081t
  T
    interaction with troponin C, 295
    interaction with troponin I, 295
    phosphorylation of, 296
    thin filament regulation and, 293t, 293–295, 294f
    of thin filaments, 152, 153f
  of thin filaments, 151–152
Troponin complex, thin filament regulation and, 287–288
Trunk muscles, testing of, 607t
Trypanosomiasis. *See* African trypanosomiasis; American trypanosomiasis
T tubule(s), 232–233
  action potential spread and, 224–225
  contractile responses to depolarization of, 257–261, 258f, 259f
  development of, 60f, 60–61
  free, composition of, 244
  junctional and free, 235–236, 238f, 239
  morphometry of, 253–254
  networks of, dispositions of, 235, 237f
  openings of, 235, 236f
  structure-function correlations of, 254
  ultrastructural reactions of, 762, 764f–770f, 764–766
  unusual aggregates of, 240, 242, 244f

T-tubule helicoids, 239
Tuberculosis, myositis in, 1465–1466
Tubocurarine, neuromuscular transmission sensitivity to, 390f, 390–391
Tubular aggregates, 712, 714f
  myopathy with, 1505–1507
    clinical features of, 1505–1506
    hexagonally cross-linked aggregates and, 1514f, 1514–1515
    pathologic features of, 1506f, 1506–1507, 1507f
Tularemia, myoglobinuria due to, 1687
Tumor antigens, in Lambert-Eaton myasthenic syndrome, 1797
Twitches, 191, 191f

Ubiquitin
  ATP-ubiquitin-proteasome proteolytic pathway and, 543–546, 544t, 545f
  in inclusion body myositis, 1377
  in myofibrillar myopathies, 1190
  structurally abnormal, in inclusion body myositis, 1378
Ubiquitination, defect in, in limb-girdle muscular dystrophy, 1088
Ullrich congenital muscular dystrophy, 1206t, 1227–1230
  clinical features of, 1229f–1230f, 1229t, 1229–1230
  collagen genes and etiopathogenesis of, 1228–1229
  muscle pathology in, 1230, 1230f
Ultrastructural studies, 749–879. *See also specific conditions*
  microvascular alterations and, 874–879
    amyloid infiltration, 879, 879f–881f
    of basal lamina, 875f, 875–876, 876f
    of capillaries, 876–877, 877f, 878f
    of endothelial cells, 877, 877f, 878f, 879
  muscle fiber alterations and, 816–863
    core, multicore, and target formations, 816, 817f–822f
    denervation atrophy, 817, 823, 826f–831f, 827–828
    focal cytoplasmic degradation and autophagic mechanisms, 836f, 836–841, 837f, 839f–841f
    glycogen accumulation, 841–845, 843f–848f
    lipid accumulation in muscle fibers, 841, 842f
    muscle fiber invasion and destruction by T cells and macrophages, 846–851, 849f–853f
    myogenic muscle fiber atrophy, 828–829, 832f–835f, 832–836
    necrosis, 851–852, 854f–857f, 856–858
    regeneration and, 860–863, 864f–870f
    sarcoplasmic masses, 817, 823f–825f
    satellite cells, 858, 859f–862f, 860
  muscle fiber organelle and component changes and, 749, 752–816
    concentric laminated bodies, 797, 799, 800f, 801f
    cylindrical spirals, 806, 808f, 809, 809f
    of endoplasmic reticulum, 774, 778f
    filamentous bodies, 797, 799f
    filamentous inclusions, 813, 814f, 815f, 815–816
    fingerprint bodies, 799, 802f
    giant lysosomes in vitamin E deficiency, 810, 811f
    of Golgi apparatus, 774, 776
    Leptomere formations, 797, 798f
    lipofuscin and, 809–810, 810f
    microtubular inclusions in endoplasmic reticulum, 810–811, 812f
    of mitochondria, 776, 778f–784f, 778–782
    in myofibrillar myopathy, 799, 801, 803f–807f
    of myofibrils, 795–797, 796f
    at myotendinous junction, 797, 798f
    of nucleus, 758–762, 759f–761f, 763f
    reducing bodies, 811, 813, 813f
    sarcoplasmic protein crystals, 801, 808f
    of sarcoplasmic reticulum, 766–774, 771f–777f
    spherical bodies in hexagonal arrays, 816
    of surface membrane, 749, 752–758, 753f–758f
    of thick filaments, 792–793, 793f, 794f, 795
    of thin filaments, 797
    of T tubules, 762, 764f–770f, 764–766
    of Z disk, 782, 785f–792f, 785–792
  neuromuscular junction alterations and, 865–874
    postsynaptic, 868, 872, 874, 874f
    presynaptic, 865–867, 871f–873f
  patterns of changes in muscle disease, 749, 750f–752f
Unfused tetanus, 191
Upper extremity muscles, testing of, 604t
Upper motor neuron signs, in amyotrophic lateral sclerosis, 1868
Uremia, neuropathy with, 1915–1916
Urethral obstruction malformation complex, 1940
Utrophin, 457t, 964, 965
  therapeutic uses of, 29–30
  upregulation of, for dystrinopathies, 1010
Utrophin-deficient mice, 1001
Utrophin-dystrophin double-deficient mice, 1001

Vacuolar myopathies, X-linked. *See* X-linked vacuolar myopathies
Vacuolar myopathy, 714, 715–716
Vacuoles, 714–716, 716f–719f
  autophagic. *See* Autophagic vacuoles
  rimmed, 715
    lysosomal proteolysis and, 570
Variable-number tandem repeats, 945
Variable-onset distal myopathy, 1170t
Vasculitis, 1454–1459
  in allergic granulomatosis, 1455
  in Behçet disease, 1459
  in giant cell arteritis, 1456, 1458f, 1459, 1459f
  hypersensitivity, 1456
  in polyarteritis nodosa, 1454–1455, 1455f
  systemic, muscle pain associated with, 1742t
  in Wegener's granulomatosis, 1455–1456, 1457f
Vectors
  in cloning, 927–929, 928f
  expression, 931f, 932
Venous effluent oxygen levels, oxidative metabolism and, 672, 672f

Ventilatory support, in amyotrophic lateral sclerosis, 1882
Venules, fine structure of, 516
Very late onset distal myopathy, 1170t
Very long chain acyl-CoA dehydrogenase deficiency, 1603–1604
Vialetto-Van Laere motor neuron disease, Madras variant of, 1872
Vibrio vulnificus myonecrosis, 1464
Vimentin, 132t
 of intermediate filaments, 160
Vincristine, myopathy due to, 1703
Vinculin, in dystrophinopathies, 999
Viral infections, 1389–1413.
 See also specific viral infections
 implicated in muscle diseases in humans and experimental animals, 1392
 inclusion body myositis and, 1381
 muscle pain associated with, 1741t, 1742t
 myoglobinuria due to, 1688
 polymyositis/dermatomyositis and, 1356–1357
 of skeletal muscle, *in vitro*, 1391–1392, 1392f
 viral tropism barriers and viral receptors in human muscle tissue and, 1389–1391, 1390t
Visceral larva migrans, 1438–1439
Vitamin A derivatives, myopathy due to, 1697–1698
Vitamin D
 cellular actions of, 1714t
 deficiency of, myopathy due to, 1709
 metabolism of, disorders of, myopathy associated with, 1731–1734
  hyperparathyroidism and metabolic bone disease, 1731–1733
  hypoparathyroidism and pseudohypoparathyroidism, 1733–1734
 myopathy and, 1732–1733
Vitamin E
 deficiency of
  giant lysosomes in, ultrastructural features of, 810, 811f
  myopathy due to, 1708–1709
 myopathy due to, 1697

Vocal cord paralysis, spinal muscular atrophy with, 1861
Voltage-gated sodium channel antibodies, neuromyotonia and, 1303, 1304, 1304f, 1305, 1306

Waardenburg syndrome, arthrogryposis multiplex congenita and, 1945
Walker-Warbug syndrome, 1206t, 1220–1222
 clinical features of, 1221f, 1221–1222, 1222f
 gene and protein in, 1220
 phenotypic heterogeneity in, 1221
Wasting syndrome, human immunodeficiency virus, 1399, 1400f
Weakness, in clinical examination, 601–602, 614, 615f, 616
Wegener's granulomatosis, myositis in, 1455–1456, 1457f
Welander distal myopathy, 1170t, 1170–1171, 1171f
Werdnig-Hoffman disease, 1846, 1847t, 1847–1848, 1848f
 arrested, 1847t, 1848–1849, 1849f
 arthrogryposis multiplex congenita and, 1948–1949
West Nile virus infection, 1396
Whipple disease, myositis in, 1466–1467
Whistling face syndrome, arthrogryposis multiplex congenita and, 1941
Wolman disease. *See* Acid lipase deficiency
Wrist extensors, testing of, 605t–606t
Wrist flexors, testing of, 606t–607t

X-linked adrenoleukodystrophy, peripheral neuropathy associated with, 1920
X-linked adrenomyeloneuropathy, 1920
X-linked dilated cardiomyopathy, 1246–1247
X-linked hyperkalemic periodic paralysis, 1279
X-linked myotubular myopathy, 1491–1494
 clinical features of, 1491f, 1491–1492
 differential diagnosis of, 1495
 genetics of, 1493–1494
 investigations in, 1492
 pathologic features of, 1492f, 1492–1493
X-linked progressive muscular dystrophy, spinal muscular atrophy versus, 1852
X-linked vacuolar myopathies, 1163–1168
 with cardiomyopathy and mental retardation, 1166–1168
  animal model of, 1167
  clinical features of, 1167
  genetics of, 1167
  historical background of, 1166–1167
  laboratory findings in, 1167
  muscle pathology in, 1167
  pathogenesis of, 1167–1168
 with excessive autophagy, 1163–1166
  clinical features of, 1163, 1164f
  genetics of, 1163–1164
  historical background of, 1163
  laboratory findings in, 1163
  muscle pathology in, 1164–1166, 1165f, 1166f, 1166t

Yeast artificial chromosomes, 930, 930f
Yeast two-hybrid system, 945
Young's modulus, 197

ZASP/Cypher, 133t
Z-band streaming, 704–705, 706f
Z disk, ultrastructural reactions of, 782, 785f–792f, 785–792
Zebra bodies. *See* Leptomere formations
Zebra body myopathy, 1515, 1515f
Zellweger syndrome, arthrogryposis multiplex congenita and, 1945–1946, 1946f, 1947f
Zidovudine, myopathy associated with, 1406–1413, 1407t, 1408f–1411f, 1696
 experimental induction of AZT toxicity and, 1409, 1411f, 1412f
 management of, 1409, 1413
 mechanism of, 1407, 1409
Zinc finger, 922–923
Z line, 130f, 131, 157–160
 composition of, 158
 model of, 158–160, 159f
 structure of, 157f, 157–158